Imaging in Cardiovascular Disease

Imaging in Cardiovascular Disease

Editors

Gerald M. Pohost, M.D.
*Mary Gertrude Waters Professor of
    Cardiovascular Medicine
Faculty Cardiologist
Department of Medicine
University of Alabama at Birmingham
Birmingham, Alabama*

Robert A. O'Rourke, M.D.
*Charles Conrad and Anna Sahm
    Brown Distinguished Professor of
    Medicine
Department of Medicine
Division of Cardiology
University of Texas Health Science
    Center at San Antonio
San Antonio, Texas*

Daniel S. Berman, M.D.
*Professor of Medicine
University of California–Los Angeles
    School of Medicine
Director, Nuclear Cardiology
Department of Imaging/Nuclear Medicine
Cedars-Sinai Medical Center
Los Angeles, California*

Pravin M. Shah, M.D., F.A.C.C.
*Professor of Medicine
Loma Linda University School of Medicine
Loma Linda, California
Medical Director
Noninvasive Cardiac Imaging and
    Academic Programs
Hoag Memorial Hospital Presbyterian
Newport Beach, California*

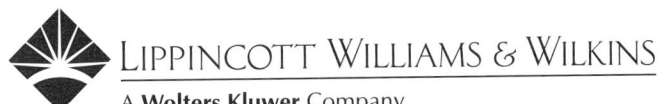
LIPPINCOTT WILLIAMS & WILKINS
A **Wolters Kluwer** Company
Philadelphia · Baltimore · New York · London
Buenos Aires · Hong Kong · Sydney · Tokyo

Acquisitions Editor: Ruth W. Weinberg
Developmental Editor: Ellen DiFrancesco
Production Editor: Deirdre Marino
Manufacturing Manager: Kevin Watt
Cover Designer: Christine Jenny
Compositor: Maryland Composition Company, Inc.
Printer: Edwards Brothers

© **2000 by LIPPINCOTT WILLIAMS & WILKINS**
530 Walnut Street
Philadelphia, PA 19106 USA
LWW.com

Printed in the USA

Library of Congress Cataloging-in-Publication Data

Imaging in cardiovascular disease / Gerald M. Pohost . . . [et al.].
    p.   ; cm.
    Includes bibliographical references and index.
    ISBN 0-397-51591-X
    1. Cardiovascular system—Imaging. 2. Heart—Imaging. 3. Cardiovascular system—
Diseases—Diagnosis. 4. Heart—Diseases—Diagnosis. I. Pohost, Gerald M.
    [DNLM: 1. Cardiovascular Diseases—diagnosis. 2. Diagnostic Imaging. WG 141 I31 2000]
RC683.5.I42 I43 2000
616.1′0754—dc21
                                     00-023282

10 9 8 7 6 5 4 3 2 1

To the memory of Ryan Robert O'Rourke,
who died too young at age 20.

Contents

Section I.   Technology of Cardiovascular Imaging
Section Editors: D. S. Berman, P. M. Shah, and G. M. Pohost

Subsection A.   Ultrasound-based Methods

Subsection B.   Radionuclide-based Methods/Nuclear Cardiology

**Section III.   The Implication of Health Care Delivery System on
Imaging Applications**
Section Editor: G. M. Pohost

Contributing Authors

Abass Alavi, M.D.
Professor
Department of Radiology
University of Pennsylvania School of Medicine
Chief, Nuclear Medicine
Department of Radiology
Hospital of the University of Pennsylvania
3400 Spruce Street
Philadelphia, Pennsylvania 19104

Muayed Al-Zaibag, M.D.
Associate Professor
Department of Cardiology
Loma Linda University Medical Center
11234 Anderson Street
Loma Linda, California 92354
Chairman, Department of Cardiac Sciences
King Fahad National Guard Hospital
Riyadh, Saudi Arabia

James A. Arrighi, M.D.
Assistant Professor
Section of Cardiovascular Medicine
Yale University
333 Cedar Street
New Haven, Connecticut 06520
Chief, Section of Nuclear Medicine
Veterans Administration Healthcare System
950 Campbell Avenue
West Haven, Connecticut 06516

Shaul Atar, M.D.
Cardiology Research Fellow
Cardiology Division
Cedars-Sinai Medical Center
8700 Beverly Boulevard
Los Angeles, California 90048

Stephen L. Bacharach, Ph.D.
Head, Imaging Sciences Group
Imaging Science Program
National Institutes of Health
9000 Rockville Pike
Bethesda, Maryland 20892

Robert S. Balaban, Ph.D.
Chief, Laboratory of Cardiac Energetics
National Institutes of Health
10 Center Drive
Bethesda, Maryland 20892

Edmund R. Becker, Ph.D.
Professor
Department of Health Policy and Management
Rollins School of Public Health at Emory University
1518 Clifton Road Northeast
Atlanta, Georgia 30322

Frank M. Bengel, M.D.
Nuklearmedizinische Klinik
Technical University of Munich
Ismaninger Strasse 22
D-81675 Munich, Germany

Daniel S. Berman, M.D.
Professor of Medicine
University of California–Los Angeles School of Medicine
805 Hilgard Avenue
Los Angeles, California 90025
Director, Nuclear Cardiology
Department of Imaging/Nuclear Medicine
Cedars-Sinai Medical Center
8700 Beverly Boulevard
Los Angeles, California 90048

Robert W. W. Biederman, M.D.
Chief, Cardiology Fellows
Department of Cardiovascular Disease
Center for Nuclear Magnetic Resonance Research and Development
Associate in Cardiology
Department of Medicine
University of Alabama at Birmingham
1808 7th Avenue South
Birmingham, Alabama 35223

Robert O. Bonow, M.D.
Professor of Medicine
Chief, Division of Cardiology
Northwestern University Medical School
Chief, Division of Cardiology
Northwestern Memorial Hospital
251 East Huron Street
Chicago, Illinois 60611

Elias H. Botvinick, M.D.
Professor of Medicine
Division of Cardiology
University of California–San Francisco Medical
Center
San Francisco, California 94143

Jens Bremerich, M.D.
Department of Radiology
University of Basel
Petersgraben 4
CH-4031 Basel, Switzerland

Blase A. Carabello, M.D., F.A.C.C.
Professor
Department of Medicine
Baylor College of Medicine
One Baylor Plaza
Chief, Medical Service
Department of Medicine
Veterans Administration Medical Center
2002 Holcombe Boulevard
Houston, Texas 77030

Joseph R. Carver, M.D.
Senior Medical Director
AETNA U.S. Health Care
980 Jolly Road
Blue Bell, Pennsylvania 19422

Constance E. Cephus, R.N., M.S.N., N.N.P.
Nurse Practitioner
Pediatric Cardiology
Loma Linda University Medical Center and
Children's Hospital
11234 Anderson Street
Loma Linda, California 92354

P. Anthony N. Chandraratna, M.D.
Professor of Medicine
University of California–Irvine
101 The City Drive
Orange, California 92868
Chief of Cardiology
Cardiology Section
Long Beach Veterans Administration Medical
Center
5901 East 7th Street
Long Beach, California 90822

George P. Chatzimavroudis, Ph.D.
Assistant Professor
Department of Chemical Engineering
Cleveland State University
1960 East 24th Street
Cleveland, Ohio 44115
Adjunct Assistant Professor
Departments of Radiology and Biomedical
Engineering
The Cleveland Clinic Foundation
9500 Euclid Avenue
Cleveland, Ohio 44195

César E. Coello, M.D.
Clinical Instructor
Department of Medicine
University of Vermont
111 Colchester Avenue
Burlington, Vermont 05401

Steven D. Culler, Ph.D.
Associate Professor
Department of Health Policy and Management
Rollins School of Public Health at Emory University
1518 Clifton Road Northeast
Atlanta, Georgia 30322

Jucyléa M. Cwajg, M.D.
Staff Physician
Department of Cardiology
Echocardiography Laboratory
Hospital Barra d'Or
Avenida Ayrton Senna 2541
Rio de Janeiro 22793-000, Brazil

Michael W. Dae, M.D.
Professor of Radiology and Medicine
Department of Radiology
University of California–San Francisco
San Francisco, California 94143

Peter G. Danias, M.D., Ph.D.
Instructor
Department of Medicine
Harvard Medical School
Director, Nuclear Cardiology
Cardiovascular Division
Department of Medicine
Beth Israel Deaconess Medical Center
330 Brookline Avenue
Boston, Massachusetts 02115

Vasken Dilsizian, M.D.
Adjunct Professor of Medicine and Radiology
Georgetown University School of Medicine
3800 Reservoir Road Northwest
Washington, District of Columbia 20007
Director of Nuclear Cardiology
Department of Cardiology and Nuclear Medicine
National Institutes of Health
9000 Rockville Pike
Bethesda, Maryland 20892

Mark Doyle, Ph.D.
Associate Professor
Department of Medicine
University of Alabama at Birmingham
1808 7th Avenue South
Birmingham, Alabama 35294

Eric A. Dubois, M.D.
Department of Cardiology
Academic Medical Center
University of Amsterdam
Meibergdreef 9
1105 AZ Amsterdam, The Netherlands

Alex Durairaj, M.D.
Chief Fellow
Division of Cardiology
Keck School of Medicine
Southern California Medical Center
1355 San Pablo Street
Chief Fellow
Division of Cardiology
Los Angeles County and University of Southern
*   California*
1200 North State Street
Los Angeles, California 90033

Robert R. Edelman, M.D.
Professor
Department of Radiology
Harvard Medical School
Director, Magnetic Resonance Imaging
Department of Radiology
Beth Israel Deaconess Medical Center
330 Brookline Avenue
Boston, Massachusetts 02115

Michael D. Ezekowitz, M.D., Ph.D., F.A.C.C.
Professor of Medicine
Department of Cardiology
Director, Clinical Trials Office
Yale University
47 College Street
New Haven, Connecticut 06510

Brian A. Foley, M.D.
Assistant Professor
Department of Medicine
Division of Cardiology
University of Alabama at Birmingham
1900 University Boulevard
Birmingham, Alabama 35294

John D. Friedman, M.D.
Department of Cardiology/Nuclear Medicine
Cedars-Sinai Medical Center
8700 Beverly Boulevard
Los Angeles, California 90048

Anthon R. Fuisz, M.D.
Assistant Professor
Division of Cardiology
Department of Medicine
Director, Clinical Cardiovascular Nuclear Magnetic
*   Resonance Imaging*
University of Alabama at Birmingham
1808 7th Avenue South
Birmingham, Alabama 35294

Hasan Garan, M.D.
Professor
Department of Medicine
University of Texas Medical School at Houston
Director, Cardiac Electrophysiology
University of Texas Health Science Center at
*   Houston*
Hermann Hospital
6431 Fannin
Houston, Texas 77030

Guido Germano, Ph.D., M.B.A.
Associate Professor
Department of Radiological Sciences
University of California–Los Angeles School of
*   Medicine*
405 Hilgard Avenue
Los Angeles, California 90024
Director, AIM Program and Nuclear Medicine
*   Physics*
Department of Medicine
Cedars-Sinai Medical Center
8700 Beverly Boulevard
Los Angeles, California 90048

Linda D. Gillam, M.D., F.A.C.C.
Associate Professor of Medicine
Department of Medicine
University of Connecticut
263 Farmington Avenue
Farmington, Connecticut 06032
Director of Echocardiography
Department of Cardiology
Hartford Hospital
80 Seymour Street
Hartford, Connecticut 06102

Steven A. Goldstein, M.D.
Director, Noninvasive Cardiology Laboratory
Department of Cardiology
Washington Hospital Center
110 Irving Street Northwest
Washington, District of Columbia 20010

Camilo R. Gomez, M.D.
Professor
Department of Neurology
Director, Comprehensive Stroke Center
University of Alabama at Birmingham
1202 Jefferson Tower
Birmingham, Alabama 35294

Charles B. Higgins, M.D.
Professor
Department of Radiology
University of California–San Francisco Medical
  School
505 Parnassus Avenue
San Francisco, California 94143

Brian D. Hoit, M.D.
Professor
Department of Medicine
Case Western Reserve University
Co-director, Echocardiography
Department of Cardiology
University Hospitals of Cleveland
11100 Euclid Avenue
Cleveland, Ohio 44106

Eileen Judkins, M.D.
Research Associate
School of Medicine
Loma Linda University
11234 Anderson Street
Loma Linda, California 92354

Roberto Kalil-Filho, M.D.
Associate Professor of Cardiology
Heart Institute
Capoto Viscente 361
CEP-05409-010 São Paulo, Brazil

Anita M. Kelsey, M.D.
Assistant Clinical Professor
Department of Internal Medicine
University of Connecticut
263 Farmington Avenue
Farmington, Connecticut 06032
Assistant Director of Echocardiography
Department of Cardiology
Hartford Hospital
80 Seymour Street
Hartford, Connecticut 06102

Ban-An Khaw, Ph.D.
Director
George D. Behrakis Professor
Department of Pharmaceutical Sciences
Bouvé College of Health Sciences/Northeastern University
360 Huntington Avenue
Boston, Massachusetts 02115
Associate Biochemist/Radiochemist
Department of Cardiac/Nuclear Medicine
Massachusetts General Hospital
Fruit Street
Boston, Massachusetts 02114

Philip J. Kilner, M.D., Ph.D.
Senior Research Fellow
Cardiovascular Magnetic Resonance Unit
Royal Brompton Hospital
Sydney Street
London, England SW3 6NP

M. Eduardo Kortright, Ph.D.
Assistant Professor
Department of Computer Science
University of New Orleans
Lakefront Campus
New Orleans, Louisiana 70148

Christopher M. Kramer, M.D.
Associate Professor
Director, Cardiac Magnetic Resonance Imaging
Departments of Medicine and Radiology
University of Virginia
Charlottesville, Virginia 22908

Howard C. Lewin, M.D.
Assistant Professor
Department of Medicine
University of California–Los Angeles School of
  Medicine
Los Angeles, California 90024
Staff Physician
Department of Imaging/Cardiology
Cedars-Sinai Medical Center
8700 Beverly Boulevard
Los Angeles, California 90048

Martin M. LeWinter, M.D.
Professor
Department of Medicine
University of Vermont
Director, Cardiology Unit
Fletcher Allen Health Care
111 Colchester Avenue
Burlington, Vermont 05401

Lieng H. Ling, M.B.B.S., M.R.C.P.
Senior Lecturer
Department of Medicine
National University of Singapore
10 Kent Ridge Crescent
Singapore 119260
Consultant
Cardiac Department
National University Hospital
5 Lower Kent Ridge Road
Singapore 119074

Michael J. Longo, M.D.
Virginia Mason Medical Center
1100 9th Avenue
Seattle, Washington 98111

Warren J. Manning, M.D.
Associate Professor
Departments of Medicine and Radiology
Harvard Medical School
Boston, Massachusetts 02114
Co-director, Cardiac Magnetic Resonance Center
Associate Director, Noninvasive Cardiac Imaging
Beth Israel Deaconess Medical Center
330 Brookline Avenue
Boston, Massachusetts 02115

James G. Miller, Ph.D.
Albert Gordon Hill Professor of Physics
Department of Physics
Washington University
One Brookings Drive
St. Louis, Missouri 63130

Radd H. Mohiaddin, M.D., Ph.D., F.E.S.C., F.R.C.R.
Cardiovascular Magnetic Resonance Unit
Royal Brompton Hospital
Sydney Street
London, England SW3 6NP

Navin C. Nanda, M.D.
Professor
Department of Medicine
Director, Heart Station
Echocardiography Laboratories
University of Alabama at Birmingham
619 South 19th Street
Birmingham, Alabama 35249

H. Joachim Nesser, M.D.
Director, Department of Medicine
Division of Cardiology
KH d. Elisabethinen Hospital
Fadingerstrasse 1
A-4010 Linz, Austria

Jae K. Oh, M.D.
Professor
Department of Internal Medicine
Mayo Medical School
Consultant
Department of Cardiovascular Diseases
Mayo Clinic
200 1st Street Southwest
Rochester, Minnesota 55905

Mohammed A. Oraby
Research Fellow
Department of Medicine/Cardiology
University of Texas Health Science Center at San Antonio
7703 Floyd Curl Drive
Research Fellow
Department of Medicine/Cardiology
University Hospital
4502 Medical Drive
San Antonio, Texas 78229

Robert A. O'Rourke, M.D.
Charles Conrad and Anna Sahm Brown Distinguished Professor of Medicine
Department of Medicine
Division of Cardiology
University of Texas Health Science Center at San Antonio
7703 Floyd Curl Drive
San Antonio, Texas 78284

Anne P. Osher, D.V.M., R.D.C.S.
Pediatric Echosonographer
Pediatric Echograph Laboratory
Loma Linda Children's Hospital
Loma Linda, California 92354

Ramdas G. Pai, M.D., F.R.C.P.(E), F.A.C.C.
Director of Echocardiography
Department of Cardiology
Jerry L. Pettis Veterans Hospital
11201 Benton Street
Loma Linda, California 92357

Igor F. Palacios, M.D.
Associate Professor
Department of Medicine
Harvard Medical School
Director, Cardiac Catheterization Laboratory
Director, Interventional Cardiology
Department of Medicine
Massachusetts General Hospital
55 Fruit Street
Boston, Massachusetts 02114

Natesa G. Pandian, M.D., F.A.C.C.
Associate Professor of Medicine and Radiology
Tufts University School of Medicine
Director, Cardiovascular Imaging and
*   Hemodynamic Laboratory*
Tufts-New England Medical Center
750 Washington Street
Boston, Massachusetts 02111

Dudley J. Pennell, M.D., F.R.C.P., F.A.C.C.,
**   F.E.S.C.**
Senior Lecturer
National Heart and Lung Institute
Imperial College
Exhibition Road
London, England SW7 2AZ
Honorary Consultant
Director, Cardiovascular Magnetic Resonance Unit
Royal Brompton Hospital
Sydney Street
London, England SW3 6NP

Julio E. Pérez, M.D.
Professor of Cardiology
Department of Medicine
Washington University
660 South Euclid
Director of Echocardiography
Barnes-Jewish Hospital
St. Louis, Missouri 63110

Gerald M. Pohost, M.D.
Mary Gertrude Waters Professor of Cardiovascular
*   Medicine*
Faculty Cardiologist
Department of Medicine
University of Alabama at Birmingham
1808 7th Avenue South
Birmingham, Alabama 35294

Steven C. Port, M.D., F.A.C.C.
Clinical Professor
Department of Medicine
University of Wisconsin
600 Highland
Madison, Wisconsin 53792
Cardiologist
Department of Medicine
St. Luke's Medical Center
2900 West Oklahoma Avenue
Milwaukee, Wisconsin 53215

Thomas R. Porter, M.D.
Associate Professor
Department of Internal Medicine
Section of Cardiology
University of Nebraska Medical Center
981165 Nebraska Medical Center
Director, Diagnostic Cardiac Ultrasound and Noninvasive
*   Diagnostics*
Department of Internal Medicine
Section of Cardiology
Nebraska Health System/University Hospital
989510 Nebraska Medical Center
Omaha, Nebraska 68198

Gautham P. Reddy, M.D., M.P.H.
Assistant Professor
Department of Radiology
University of California–San Francisco
505 Parnassus Avenue
San Francisco, California 94143

Paulo A. Ribeiro, M.D., Ph.D.
Director, Cardiology Fellowship
Associate Professor of Medicine
Department of Cardiology
Loma Linda University Hospital
11234 Anderson Street
Loma Linda, California 92354

John A. Rumberger, Ph.D., M.D.
HeartCare, Inc.
Gahanna, Ohio 43230

Ernesto E. Salcedo, M.D.
Head, Echocardiography Laboratory
Department of Cardiology
St. Vincent's Medical Center
1801 Barrs Street
Jacksonville, Florida 32204

Colleen Sanders, M.D.
Associate Professor
Department of Radiology
University of Alabama at Birmingham
Chief, Cardiopulmonary Radiology
Department of Radiology
University of Alabama Hospitals
619 South 19th Street
Birmingham, Alabama 35249

Axel Schmermund, M.D.
Assistant Professor of Medicine
Department of Cardiology
University Clinic Essen
Hufelandstrasse 55
45122 Essen, Germany

Markus Schwaiger, M.D.
Klinikum rechts der Isar
Technical University of Munich
Ismaninger Strasse 22
D-81675 Munich, Germany

Maria G. Sciammarella, M.D.
Cardiologist
Division of Cardiology and Nuclear Medicine
University of California–San Francisco
San Francisco, California 94143

Ralph Shabetai, M.D.
Professor of Medicine Emeritus
Attending Physician
Department of Medicine
University of California–San Diego
Veterans Administration Health Care System
La Jolla, California 92161

Pravin M. Shah, M.D., F.A.C.C.
Professor of Medicine
Loma Linda University School of Medicine
Loma Linda, California 92350
Medical Director
Noninvasive Cardiac Imaging and Academic
  Programs
Hoag Memorial Hospital Presbyterian
One Hoag Drive
Newport Beach, California 92663

Leslee J. Shaw, M.D.
Associate Professor
Department of Medicine, Health Policy and
  Management
Emory University
1518 Clifton Road Northeast
Atlanta, Georgia 30322

Girish S. Shirali, M.B.B.S.
Assistant Professor
Department of Pediatrics
Medical University of South Carolina
Director, Echocardiography
Medical University of South Carolina Children's
  Hospital
165 Ashley Avenue
Charleston, South Carolina 29425

Robert J. Siegel, M.D., F.A.C.C.
Professor
Department of Medicine
University of California–Los Angeles School of
  Medicine
10833 Le Conte Avenue
Los Angeles, California 90095
Director, Cardiac Noninvasive Laboratory
Department of Cardiology
Cedars-Sinai Medical Center
8700 Beverly Boulevard
Los Angeles, California 90048

Vincent L. Sorrell, M.D., F.A.C.C.
Assistant Professor of Medicine
Section of Cardiology
East Carolina University Brody School of Medicine
Medical Director
Graphics and Exercise Physiology Laboratories
PCMH-TA 378 Moye Boulevard
Greenville, North Carolina 27858

Benigno Soto, M.D.
Professor
Department of Radiology
University of Alabama at Birmingham Medical Center
619 19th Street South
Birmingham, Alabama 35233

Peter C. Spittell, M.D.
Assistant Professor of Medicine
Mayo Medical School
Consultant
Department of Internal Medicine
Division of Cardiovascular Diseases
Mayo Medical Center
200 First Street Southwest
Rochester, Minnesota 55905

Mark P. Starling, M.D.
Professor of Medicine
Division of Cardiology
Veterans Administration Medical Center
2215 Fuller Road
Ann Arbor, Michigan 48105

Marcus F. Stoddard, M.D.
Associate Professor
Department of Medicine
University of Louisville
530 South Jackson Street
Director, Noninvasive Cardiology
Department of Medicine
Division of Cardiology
University Hospital
550 South Jackson Street
Louisville, Kentucky 40292

Eiji Tadamura, M.D., Ph.D.
Assistant Professor
Department of Nuclear Medicine and Diagnostic
  Imaging
Kyoto University Graduate School of Medicine
Chief, Department of Nuclear Medicine
Kyoto University Hospital
54 Shogoinkawahara
Sakyo, Kyoto 606-8507, Japan

A. Jamil Tajik, M.D., F.A.A.C.
Thomas J. Watson, Jr., Professor of Medicine and
*   Pediatrics*
Chair, Division of Cardiovascular Diseases
Mayo Clinic
200 First Street Southwest
Consultant
Division of Cardiovascular Diseases
Rochester Methodist and Saint Mary's Hospitals
Rochester, Minnesota 55905

Nagara Tamaki, M.D., Ph.D.
Professor
Department of Radiology
Hokkaido University School of Medicine
Chairman, Department of Nuclear Medicine
Hokkaido University Hospital
N-15 W-7 Kita-ku
Sapporo 060-8638, Japan

John J. Tzeng, M.D.
Clinical Assistant Professor
Department of Medicine
Division of Cardiology
University of Southern California School of
*   Medicine*
1355 San Pablo Street
Los Angeles, California 90033

Mario S. Verani, M.D.
Professor
Department of Medicine/Cardiology
Baylor College of Medicine
6550 Fannin
Director, Department of Nuclear
*   Cardiology*
The Methodist Hospital
6565 Fannin
Houston, Texas 77030

Szilard Voros, M.D.
Instructor
Chief Medical Resident
Department of Medicine
University of Alabama at Birmingham
1808 7th Avenue South
Birmingham, Alabama 35233

Edward W. Webster, Ph.D.
Professor of Radiology (Physics)
Department of Radiology
Harvard University
25 Shattuck Street
Boston, Massachusetts 02115
Chief, Radiological Sciences
Department of Radiology
Massachusetts General Hospital
32 Fruit Street
Boston, Massachusetts 02114

Robert G. Weiss, M.D.
Associate Professor
Department of Medicine
Johns Hopkins University School of Medicine
Adult Cardiologist
Johns Hopkins Hospital
600 North Wolfe Street
Baltimore, Maryland 21287

Patrick W. Wilkerson, M.S.M.E.
Graduate Student
Department of Mechanical/Bioengineering
Georgia Institute of Technology
315 Ferst Drive
Atlanta, Georgia 30332

Daniel F. Worsley, M.D., F.R.C.P.C.
Assistant Professor of Radiology
University of British Columbia
Division of Nuclear Medicine
Vancouver General Hospital
899 West 12th Avenue
Vancouver, British Columbia V5Z 1M9
Canada

Jiefen Yao, M.D.
Research Fellow
Instructor of Medicine
Cardiology Division
Department of Medicine
New England Medical Center
Tufts University School of Medicine
750 Washington Street
Boston, Massachusetts 02111

Ajit P. Yoganathan, Ph.D.
Regents' Professor/Associate Chair
Department of Biomedical Engineering
Georgia Tech/Emory University
315 Ferst Drive
Atlanta, Georgia 30332

Miguel Zabalgoitia, M.D.
Associate Professor
Department of Medicine
Director, Department of Echocardiography
University of Texas Health Science Center at San
  Antonio
7703 Floyd Curl Drive
San Antonio, Texas 78229

Michael J. Zellweger, M.D.
Cardiology Fellow
Department of Cardiology
University Hospital Basel
Petersgraben 4
CH-4031 Basel, Switzerland

Marco A. Zenteno, M.D.
Professor
Department of Radiology
Director, Neuroimaging Service
Instituto Nacional de Neurologia y Neurocirugia
Periferico Sur 3697-Torre Angeles
DF CP 10700 Mexico City, Mexico

Sibylle I. Ziegler, Ph.D.
Nuklearmedizinische Klinik
Technical University of Munich
Ismaninger Strasse 22
D-81675 Munich, Germany

Foreword

The editors of this book have provided a comprehensive and up-to-date review of the methods used for cardiovascular imaging. There are 66 chapters that provide thorough reviews of each of the cardiovascular imaging techniques presently available. Included in this book are reviews of ultrasound-based methods; myocardial perfusion techniques; radionuclide methods for evaluating ventricular function and metabolism; x-ray methods for studying the heart, chest, and coronary arteries, including computed tomography and electron-beam computed tomography; and magnetic resonance-based methods, including discussions of magnetic resonance imaging to evaluate cardiac structure and function, myocardial perfusion, angiography of the great vessels and the coronary arteries, and magnetic resonance spectroscopy. Future directions for development of each of these imaging techniques are also discussed by experts working in each of these areas. Analytical approaches to cost-effectiveness and outcomes measurements in cardiovascular imaging are also provided.

Following the discussion of each of the imaging techniques, there is a separate section on clinical applications. Included in this review is a section on ischemic heart disease and the application of these imaging methods to patients with chronic stable angina, acute coronary syndromes, and following coronary interventional therapies. There is an evaluation of the utility of each of the cardiac imaging methods in the detection of myocardial viability, valvular heart disease, cardiomyopathies and congestive heart failure, and cardiac allograft rejection. A separate section on the evaluation of pericardial diseases is also provided with detailed clinical discussions and the potential application of myocardial imaging techniques to the care of patients with these problems is also provided. Sections on congenital heart disease, pulmonary heart disease, diseases of the aorta and peripheral vessels, imaging techniques and cerebrovascular disease, cardiac arrhythmias, cardiovascular trauma, and intraoperative echocardiography are also provided. Finally, the book concludes with a discussion of present and future implications of healthcare delivery systems on imaging applications.

This is the most thorough and ''real-time'' useful book on cardiovascular imaging available today. Each of the sections is written by experts in the field. The discussions are generally even and balanced as the advantages and potential limitations of each of the methods are described. The potential for clinical application of each of the methods is also presented in a fair manner. The lead editor of the book, Dr. Gerald Pohost, is one of the pioneers in imaging in cardiovascular disease. His career has been devoted to the development of imaging techniques that will be useful in the evaluation of patients with cardiovascular diseases. He began by helping to develop myocardial perfusion techniques, especially the thallium-201 myocardial imaging method. He and his colleagues were among the first to point out the clinical and physiological importance of a reversible perfusion defect and the mechanisms by which it occurs in experimental animal models and patients with coronary heart disease. He contributed to the development of the antimyosin imaging technique for the detection of myocardial infarction. In recent years, his efforts have been primarily devoted to the development of magnetic resonance imaging in the detection of cardiovascular disease, including the delineation of myocardial function, perfusion, and metabolism. Thus, Dr. Pohost is an ideal editor to lead the development of a book of this magnitude and insight. Dr. Daniel Berman is a pioneer and major contributor to nuclear cardiology, including perfusion and functional studies. His contributions to this field have been very important. Drs. Robert O'Rourke and Pravin Shah are major contributors to echocardiography and to clinical cardiology as investigators and teachers. Thus, this team of editors is outstanding and the book they have created reflects their talents and experience.

I recommend this book, *Imaging and Cardiovascular Disease*, to all who are interested in and have the professional need to utilize myocardial and vascular imaging techniques in the care of patients with cardiovascular disease. This book will be a very useful addition to each of our libraries.

James T. Willerson, M.D.

Preface

During the past few decades, there have been remarkable developments in technology, leading to dramatic changes in diagnosis and therapy. Now, the clinician is faced with a complex array of choices for appropriately diagnosing and treating patients. Furthermore, healthcare reform has added to the complexity of choosing the best cost-effective management for each patient. Accordingly, familiarity with new technologies is essential for "best practices." The optimal diagnostic imaging strategy is noninvasive, nontraumatic, highly reliable, and inexpensive.

The new imaging technologies are capable of better diagnostic power by defining and improving the clinical observations of patients with cardiac and vascular disease. Such imaging technologies use diverse physical principles, such as sound (ultrasound), x-rays (fluoroscopy), gamma rays (SPECT imaging), and magnetic fields with superimposed radio waves (MRI). This book comprehensively reviews the physical principles and presents the usefulness of contemporary imaging technologies in a clinically relevant and easily understandable format. The book has been edited and authored by internationally known experts in imaging technologies and their clinical applications. The imaging methods have been discussed in a manner that will be helpful to all physicians and technologists with an interest in the diagnosis of cardiovascular diseases.

The first section of this book describes the physical principles, limitations, and major applications of each of the imaging categories. The second section provides an in-depth clinical description of major disease categories and explores the appropriate applications of each noninvasive method. The third section details the impact of managed care on cardiac imaging modalities in order to understand the current environment and to prepare for the future success of providers and laboratories performing cardiac imaging studies.

The book is a unique and comprehensive volume that appropriately bridges the gap between journal reports, cardiology texts, and other texts on imaging methods. It is *not* the usual series of chapters touting the virtues of each imaging technology. This book should be informative for a wide-ranging audience, including medical educators, students, and practitioners in medicine, surgery, radiology, and nuclear medicine. The book should also be valuable to healthcare administrators and members of pharmaceutical companies.

The text is greatly enhanced by numerous tables and figures that improve the understanding of the technologies and illustrate their applications. The book is appropriately referenced so that the reader can rapidly answer specific questions in cardiovascular imaging. This unique book provides comprehensive information on the sometimes confusing array of diagnostic methods for evaluating the cardiovascular system, and it provides a critical perspective on the appropriate uses of these techniques for the diagnosis of cardiovascular diseases.

Gerald M. Pohost
Robert A. O'Rourke
Daniel S. Berman
Pravin M. Shah

SECTION I

Technology of
Cardiovascular Imaging

CHAPTER 1

Basics of Ultrasound

Ajit P. Yoganathan, George P. Chatzimavroudis,
and Patrick W. Wilkerson

Echocardiography represents what is arguably the most important addition to noninvasive diagnostic cardiology in the second half of the twentieth century. Its most fundamental contribution lies in the replacement of invasive techniques for analyzing structural abnormalities and blood flow hemodynamics. To apply these techniques, one must recognize certain limitations and not become carried away with visually appealing images such as those obtained by color Doppler flow mapping. The far reaching capabilities of two-dimensional and Doppler echocardiography and its associated limitations can only be appropriately applied by first understanding the basic principles of instrument physics.

The purpose of this chapter is to provide a foundation of important points on ultrasound physics and instrumentation to aid in the assimilation of pioneering diagnostic concepts currently being presented in the cardiology literature.

The chapter is divided into three parts. The first part is a brief review of echocardiography as used to image anatomic cardiac structures. These techniques have been used for some time now and alone represent an important ability to diagnose abnormalities related to solid structure morphology of the heart. Furthermore, all velocity measurement techniques must be considered in the context of these anatomic imaging capabilities. The second part is a discussion of Doppler physics and what is known as "conventional" Doppler. The third part addresses color Doppler flow mapping (CDFM) techniques that combine, in a visually appealing, two-dimensional format, anatomic imaging and Doppler blood flow measurements. The approach will be to consider CDFM in "light" of conventional Doppler, since the major

difference between the two is their respective abilities to quantitate blood flow physiology.

ECHOCARDIOGRAPHIC IMAGING OF CARDIAC STRUCTURES

The major role of blood velocity measurement techniques is to assess changes in flow fields resulting from disease. The extent of these changes can then be used to characterize the disease. In most cases, the flow field changes are a result of physical changes in cardiac structure morphology or temporal behavior. Therefore, visualizing these moving structures in real time plays an important role in the interpretation of Doppler velocity measurements, as well as providing convenient visualization of structural abnormalities that are independent of blood flow.

Visualization of cardiac structures is achieved by passing ultrasound into the body and monitoring the returning signal. The nature of the interaction between the ultrasound and the structures allows delineation of their location and morphology.

To produce waves in the ultrasonic range (>20 KHz), a high frequency of vibration from the sound source is required. This is provided in ultrasound instruments by piezo-electric crystals. Such crystals alter their shape under the application of an electric voltage, and the change is, for all practical purposes, immediate. Therefore, to produce sound with a frequency of 3 MHz, the applied voltage simply must be varied at such a frequency.

As the ultrasound passes into the body, it is attenuated due to both distance and absorption. The ultrasound wave front spreads radially as it moves away from the transducer, and the energy originally imparted at the transducer is dissipated over this increased area. Due to the radial spread of the wave front, the intensity decreases proportional to the square of the distance from the transducer.

By making a geometric assumption, such as the radial spread of the wave front above, one could calculate ultra-

A. P. Yoganathan: Department of Biomedical Engineering, Georgia Tech/Emory University, Atlanta, Georgia 30332.

G. P. Chatzimavroudis: Department of Chemical Engineering, Cleveland State University, Cleveland, Ohio 44115; Departments of Radiology and Biomedical Engineering, The Cleveland Clinic Foundation, Cleveland, Ohio 44195.

P. W. Wilkerson: Department of Mechanical/Bioengineering, Georgia Institute of Technology, Atlanta, Georgia 30332.

sound intensity at any point based on that information and the original energy of the issuing wavefront at the level of the transducer. However, such a calculation would overestimate the actual intensity, because energy is lost to the molecules of the medium as the sound passes through. That is, as the vibrations are transferred through the molecules, some energy is dissipated as heat, as the molecules interact with one another. This attenuation, due to absorption, is analogous to viscous effects in fluid flow.

A measure of the ability of a medium to conduct ultrasound is the impedance of the medium. The impedance is defined as the ratio of the acoustic pressure to particle speed. Acoustic pressure is the variation in local pressure, with respect to resting conditions, required to produce a compression in response to an acoustic perturbation. The particle speed is the speed of a vibrating particle at a point through which the sound is being transferred.

One-dimensional M-mode Echocardiography

The cardiologist was first able to visualize cardiac structures in the 1950s, with the development of M-mode echocardiography. By passing a line of ultrasound through the heart, a plot of solid structure position against time can be displayed. Figure 1 shows an M-mode image of mitral valve motion in diastole. The images are obtained as the ultrasound beam moves through the interface of two media with different acoustic impedance. Some of the ultrasound is reflected back to the transducer to produce the image. The ultrasound beam typically samples the positions of the individual target structures approximately 1,000 times per second, allowing excellent resolution of spatial position along the line of the

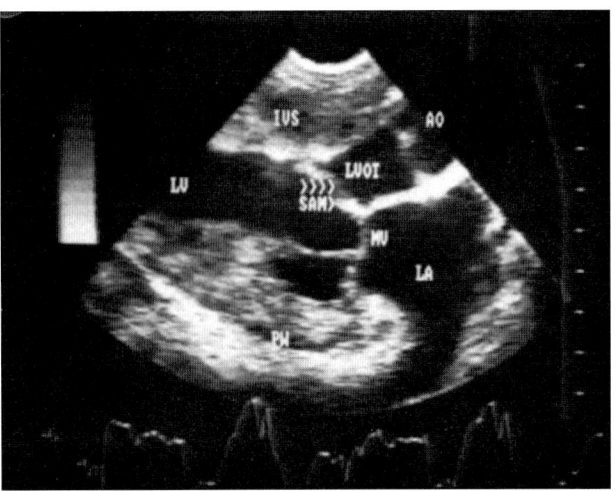

FIG. 2. Two-dimensional echo of patient with hypertrophic cardiomyopathy. The two-dimensional echo allows full visualization of the left ventricle (*LV*) in real time. This long-axis frame clearly shows the enlarged interventricular septum (*IVS*) from which hypertrophic cardiomyopathy gets its name. Also observed during this systolic moment is systolic anterior motion (*SAM*) of the mitral valve (*MV*). The point of coaptation of the tip of the posterior leaflet is not at the tip of the anterior leaflet, but instead displaced toward its (the anterior leaflet's) base. The residual portion of the anterior leaflet has then moved up into the outflow tract and actually contacted the septum. Papillary muscle and chordae tendineae structures are also seen in this frame. *AO*, aorta; *LVOT*, left ventricular outflow tract; *LA*, left atrium; *PW*, posterior wall.

ultrasound beam. The fact that the one-dimensional image is plotted against time provides an excellent assessment of temporal behavior.

Two-dimensional B-mode Echocardiography

A significant extension was made to M-mode echocardiography with the development of two-dimensional B-mode echocardiography. Using a phased-array or mechanical transducer, the "M-mode line" can be swept across a 30- to 60-degree sector at a frequency of about 30 frames per second. With the sweeping frequency being high relative to the frequency of cardiac events, ratio of about 30:1, two dimensional images of the cardiac structures are obtained which are, for all practical purposes, in real time. Figure 2 shows a B-mode frame of a patient with hypertrophic cardiomyopathy. The structural abnormality of systolic anterior motion of the mitral valve can be clearly detected, and, by viewing frame-to-frame images, its time course can be delineated.

Higher frequency transducers produce better spatially resolved images, since more sound is absorbed by the tissue media. The depth available for penetration, however, is lower for higher frequencies. A compromise must therefore be made considering both depth and resolution requirements.

Limitations in spatial resolution of these techniques pro-

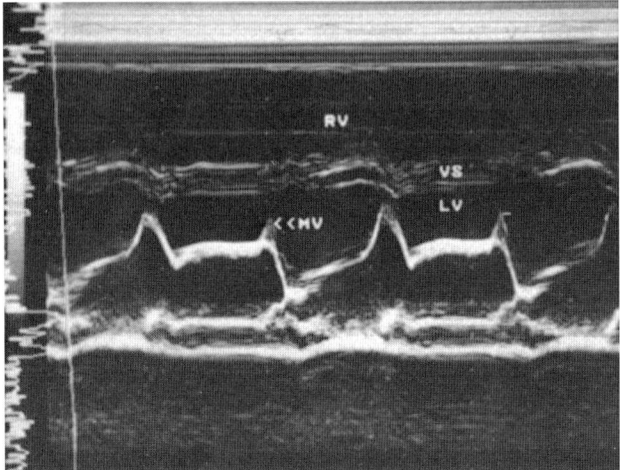

FIG. 1. M-mode of mitral valve—normal subject. Shown above is the M-mode trace of the anterior mitral leaflet in a subject with an undiseased mitral valve (*MV*). Full movement of the leaflet into the left ventricle (*LV*) is observed during diastole, with stable positioning just below the level of the annulus during systole. *RV*, right ventricle; *VS*, ventricular septum.

hibit accurate quantification of stenotic valve areas, and certainly do not allow measurement of regurgitant lesion diameters. In both cases, the resultant hemodynamics must be considered in combination with the structural abnormality. In such cases, Doppler velocity measurements are combined with echocardiography.

Care must also be taken to avoid misinterpretation of reverberations that may cause artifacts to appear on the two-dimensional image. When the ultrasound passes into a medium with a dramatic density difference, such as bone structures or heart valve prostheses, little sound is absorbed and the resultant image on the screen is not spatially accurate. Structures may actually appear in a chamber known to have no structures, such as the ventricle. Therefore, special cases, such as patients with artificial heart valves, must be carefully interpreted.

CONVENTIONAL DOPPLER

Conventional Doppler ultrasound techniques allow noninvasive measurement of blood velocities. By sampling the frequency shift of an ultrasound beam scattered by a moving blood cell, the Doppler unit can calculate the velocity of the cell, which is proportional to the frequency shift. This basic concept is covered extensively in the literature (1) and details will therefore not be reiterated here. Basically, the velocity of blood cells, passing parallel through the ultrasound beam, is given by

$$V_d = (cf_d)/(2f_o) \qquad [1]$$

where

c = the velocity of sound in the medium (about 1560 m/s in blood)
f_o = transmitted frequency
f_d = Doppler frequency shift

If the particles are passing at an angle to the ultrasound beam, only the component of velocity parallel to the beam will be obtained. The relationship between the actual velocity, V_a and the Doppler measured velocity, V_d, is therefore

$$V_a = V_d/\cos\theta$$

In modifying Eq. 1 to correct for angle, we are left with

$$V_a = (cf_d)/(2f_o\cos\theta) = V_d/\cos\theta \qquad [2]$$

This equation represents the fundamental calculation for all the velocity measurement modalities to be discussed. By continuously emitting the signal, pulsing the signal, or using multiple crystals to obtain a two-dimensional grid of discrete sample volumes, we obtain all of the modalities to be discussed. They each have their own advantages and limitations, and these are all related to the processing of information from Eq. 2.

For details on the theory of ultrasound scattering in blood, the reader is referred to Angelson (1) and a review of that is provided in Hatle and Angelson (2). In the next section,

the various Doppler modalities obtained by different applications of Eq. 2 will be discussed.

Continuous-wave Conventional Doppler

To avoid becoming overindulgent in engineering vernacular, the different modes of Doppler ultrasound will be introduced by considering the clinical motivation for each technique, although, in true chronology, the technique may not have resulted from such a straightforward need.

Clinical Motivation

Doppler ultrasound has been most useful in the assessment of valvular heart disease. Pathologically affected valves, such as in the cases of valvular stenosis or insufficiency, result in characteristically altered blood velocity patterns. These altered velocity patterns lend themselves beautifully to assessment by Doppler, since velocities are precisely the quantities obtained.

In valvular stenosis, an obstruction to blood flow is provided by a valve that does not open to its full extent. Such an obstruction results in an elevated pressure gradient across the valve, thereby placing additional pumping requirements on the heart that can result in hypertrophy. Since the systemic pressure is essentially independent of valvular disorders, the elevated pressure is reflected mainly in the proximal chamber (such as the left ventricle in aortic stenosis) and can lead to regurgitation in associated valves (such as the mitral valve). Therefore, it is the pressure gradient across the valve which best characterizes the severity of the lesion. Traditionally, this gradient was measured invasively by catheterization techniques. However, since conservation of energy requirements state that the pressure drop (or loss of potential energy) is accompanied by an increase in velocity (or kinetic energy), elevated velocities can be used to calculate decreased pressures. The physiologic impact of the stenosis is most accurately assessed by the maximum pressure drop, or the maximum velocity. Since this maximum velocity may occur at the level of the leaflets or distal to them—if a significant vena contracta exists (3)—a technique, with which maximum velocity could be obtained regardless of its location along the entire path of blood, would be most effective in obtaining this clinically relevant quantity.

Continuous-wave Doppler fits such specifications perfectly. In this technique, ultrasound is continuously emitted and received by the transducer. Frequency shifts are converted to velocities based on Eq. 2 and displayed in spectral form. Because of the continuous emission/reception of signal, the locations of velocity measurement cannot be defined due to lack of spatial resolution. Therefore, for a given continuous-wave spectrum, velocities throughout the range of the ultrasound beam are displayed. Due to the nature of the data, by reading the peak signal displayed at a given temporal location on the spectrum, one automatically obtains the maximum velocity, regardless of where it occurs along the ultra-

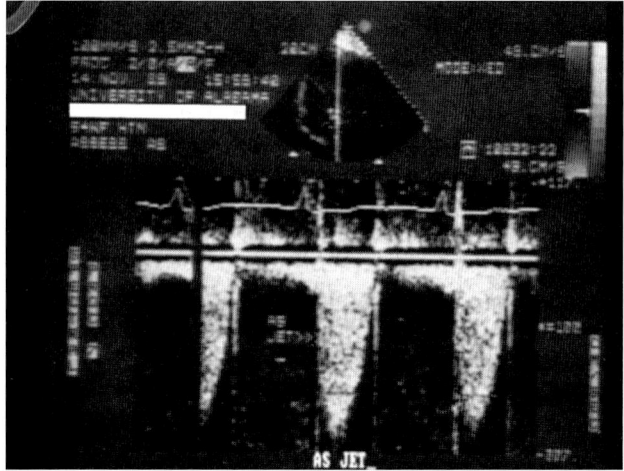

FIG. 3. Continuous-wave spectrum of patient with aortic stenosis (*AS*). This patient with aortic stenosis has a peak aortic ejection velocity of 2 m/s, and this value is quickly and easily obtained by continuous-wave Doppler. The velocity can then be converted into a pressure gradient of 16 mm Hg via the simplified Bernoulli equation to provide an estimate of the severity of the stenosis. Traditionally, such a pressure gradient would have been measured painstakingly by catheterization.

sound beam. Clinically, then, if the continuous-wave beam is passed down the ascending aorta and through the barrel of the stenotic aortic valve, for example, the maximum systolic velocity is immediately obtained and can be converted to the characterizing maximum pressure gradient by an appropriate expression relating the two forms of energy (i.e., kinetic to potential energy by the Bernoulli equation). Figure 3 shows a continuous-wave spectrum of a patient with aortic stenosis.

Limitation

Because of the continuous nature of ultrasound emission in this modality, there is no maximum velocity limit. The only limitation to such a modality is the lack of range resolution, which actually is an advantage for the assessment of valvular stenosis. Techniques, using continuous-wave Doppler developed to replace catheterization in the assessment of stenosis, have been quite successful over the past decade (1).

Pulsed-wave Conventional Doppler

Clinical Motivation

The relationship used to convert Doppler velocities to stenotic pressure gradients is generally the simplified Bernoulli equation:

$$\Delta P = 4V^2 \qquad [3]$$

where

ΔP = pressure drop (mm Hg)
V = continuous-wave maximal velocity (m/s)

To derive such a simplified equation, three deletions were made from the complete Bernoulli (energy balance) equation. The first two, acceleration and viscous effects, have been demonstrated to be valid omissions both *in vitro* and *in vivo* for the obstructive geometries generally presented in valvular stenosis (3). The third, neglecting the proximal velocities, is not always clinically valid. If such an assumption is not made, the Bernoulli equation appears as

$$\Delta P = 4(V_2^2 - V_1^2) \qquad [4]$$

where

V_2 = the maximal distal velocity appearing in Eq. 3
V_1 = a proximal velocity; the distance from this velocity to V_2 is the distance over which the pressure drop occurs.

Since the distal velocity V_2 in a stenotic jet usually significantly exceeds any proximal velocity (and this is especially true for the squares of the values), the proximal velocity is neglected to enable ease of application in the form of Eq. 3 with continuous-wave Doppler. However, in some cases, such as combined valvular insufficiency and stenosis for the same valve, or systolic anterior motion of the mitral valve in hypertrophic cardiomyopathy, or even septal hypertrophy alone, blood cell velocities are already elevated beyond normal at a location proximal to the stenotic valve. In the case of valvular insufficiency, velocities proximal to the valve are also often elevated. These situations can be identified with two-dimensional echocardiography and in such cases, measurement of the proximal velocity is necessary to correct, in effect, Eq. 3 (i.e., to evaluate Eq. 4). Continuous-wave Doppler does not provide the range resolution necessary to obtain such velocities.

In the case of valvular insufficiency, few truly quantitative techniques are clinically available, although promising ones have been successfully tested *in vitro* and in animal models (4). These techniques uniformly demonstrate not only the importance of orifice (lesion level) velocities, but the combined importance of the form of decay of jet velocities, i.e., the magnitude of distal jet velocities at known locations.

Pulsed-wave Doppler provides accurate measurement of velocities at precise locations subject to few limitations. As opposed to continuous-wave Doppler, the transducer emits a burst of ultrasound at speed c, waits a time interval, t, then samples the returning frequency signal. Like continuous-wave measurements, Eq. 2 is used to convert the shifted frequency into velocity. However, by considering the pulsing frequency, it is necessary that the returning signal must have returned from a sample volume a distance d away, where

$$d = ct/2 \qquad [5]$$

The size of the sample volume is determined by the transducer and pulsing interval (interval being the length of a pulse). A longer interval would result in a longer axial dimension of the sample volume. Note that as the length of the pulse approaches infinity, the axial length of the sample volume goes to infinity (subject to the strength of the beam) and we have continuous-wave Doppler. The lateral dimension of the sample volume is determined by the focusing configuration of the transducer. At greater distal positions, the beam becomes gradually defocused, producing a larger sample volume in the lateral dimension.

Limitations

As compared to continuous-wave Doppler, pulsed-wave has the advantage of range resolution. The origin of the velocity signal is precisely known (sample volume dimensions are generally small compared to heart chamber dimensions). Pulsed-wave Doppler, however, has two significant disadvantages that must be considered.

Pulsed-wave Doppler has a limit to the upper velocity that can be measured. This upper velocity corresponds to the Nyquist limit for frequency shift. This is expressed symbolically using the nomenclature of Hatle and Angelson as

$$f_d = f_s/2 \qquad [6]$$

where

f_d = the Nyquist limit Doppler frequency shift to be inserted into Eq. 2

f_s = the sampling frequency or pulse repetition frequency

Velocities exceeding the Nyquist limit will alias and be displayed as negative, starting at the lower limit of the negative velocity scale. The velocities determined by the Nyquist limit can be quite low when considering some physiologic flows (regurgitant jets, for example), and it is difficult to unwrap the aliased signal. To increase the maximum velocity limit, the baseline may be shifted to devote the entire scale to positive or negative velocities, depending on the situation at hand. Another way to increase the maximum velocity limit is to increase the pulse repetition frequency, f_s, as indicated by Eq. 6. This adjustment to high pulse repetition frequency (PRF), however, results in a second disadvantage of pulsed-wave Doppler.

In addition to upper threshold limits of velocity measurement, pulsed-wave Doppler is also subject to range ambiguity. A consideration of Eq. 5 reveals that it is possible—given a pulsing frequency—for the returning signal to have come not only from a sample volume at a distance of $ct/2$, but also from any integer multiple of this quantity. Using high PRF to increase the velocity limit increases the number of sample volumes per unit distance. By lowering the pulse repetition frequency, f_s, "extra" ambiguous sample volumes would form far away from the point of interest, preferably in a solid structure or in a low velocity region (such as proximal to a jet orifice), where contributions to the resultant spectrum would be negligible and nonconfusing (not misleading).

In light of these considerations, a decision must be made in practice as to the trade-off between these two factors. Increasing pulse repetition frequency allows higher velocity measurements, but increases the chance of range ambiguity. Decreasing pulse repetition frequency results in the opposite, so the nature of the clinical situation at hand must be examined constantly when making this decision. In general, the normal upper limit of pulsed-wave Doppler measurements is around 2 m/s. Using high PRF, velocities of around 4 to 5 m/s can be obtained.

In summary, conventional Doppler allows for accurate noninvasive quantification of blood flow velocities. Continuous-wave Doppler provides measurement of maximal blood velocity along a line of ultrasound, with essentially no upper bound. Pulsed-wave Doppler allows selection of the position of velocity measurement, but is subject to an upper limit on velocity measurement. Increasing this limit, by amplifying the pulse repetition frequency, increases the possibility of range ambiguity and so the trade-off between these two factors must be considered for each clinical situation.

COLOR DOPPLER FLOW MAPPING

Clinical Motivation

The advantage of conventional Doppler modalities (continuous-wave and pulsed-wave) lies in their quantitative accuracy. Contemporary instruments provide quite precise measurements. The only serious problem with these techniques would lie in the accuracy of transducer placement. Using two-dimensional echocardiography, the clinician has a good idea of the location of cardiac structures, but must translate this blindly to the invisible path of the ultrasound beam. This problem is further complicated by the general lack of understanding of blood flow physiology by many clinicians.

The development of color Doppler flow mapping (CDFM) in the mid-1980s extended the application of Eq. 2 to a new dimension. With CDFM, color-coded velocity patterns can be superimposed on two-dimensional echocardiographic images. In simplified form, an explanation of the mechanism of CDFM follows below.

CDFM transducers have many crystals (64 to 128) arranged along the face of the transducer. The configuration of these phased-array transducers allows many sample volumes (typically 64) to be arranged along a single line extending perpendicular to the face of the transducer and parallel to oncoming flows. This line is then swept back and forth across a 15-degree to 90-degree sector at a high frequency (7 to 30 frames per second). With this frequency being quite high compared to characteristic cardiac cycle frequencies (of the order of 1 Hz), temporally varying velocities are available throughout the two-dimensional sector in what essentially appears as real time. These velocities are then color-coded, usually with red for flow toward the transducer and blue for flow away from the transducer. Within a direction, increasing intensity corresponds to higher velocity in that direction. Therefore, a CDFM image consists of moving white or gray cardiac anatomic structures (echocardiographic images) on a black background, with superimposed color-coded blood flow—all imaged in quasi-real time.

For reasons to be discussed below, CDFM provides only semiquantitative velocity information in its present state. It does, however, provide extremely useful information to aid conventional Doppler measurements, for example demonstrating the direction of jet flow, so that conventional measurements can be corrected for angle or transducer position modified.

Attempts are currently being made to extend the CDFM technique, especially spatial measurements of jet images, to quantitative methods. Therefore, the consistency of the spatial color image is of great importance. Unfortunately, these images can vary depending on technical factors for a constant flow situation. After a discussion of the limitations of CDFM, the effect of various instrument settings on the resultant image will be discussed.

Due to the increased amount of data processing requirements with respect to conventional Doppler, the two-dimensional modality utilizes an autocorrelation technique in place of direct spectral analysis. Other than this, however, probably the most important fact to remember about CDFM is that it is simply another extension of pulsed-wave Doppler using Eq. 2. All we are seeing is velocity values, not flow itself. That is, CDFM is not analogous to angiography, and ignorance of that fact seems to have misled many investigators in attempts at quantification. Color appears above a certain velocity threshold (as determined by machine settings). Once the blood cells slow beyond that threshold, they disappear from the image. Blood cells either below this limit originally or off angle to the ultrasound beam (producing a Doppler velocity below the color threshold), never show up at all.

Because of the two-dimensional spatial visualization requirements of CDFM, the presence of range ambiguity would destroy the usefulness of the technique. Therefore, pulse repetition frequencies are necessarily set very low, and Nyquist velocities are then also very low by Eq. 6. With these low Nyquist velocities, aliasing frequently occurs for physiologic flows, especially in high velocity situations such as mitral regurgitation or aortic stenosis. The concept of aliasing in color flow, as can be intuitively extended from the conventional Doppler discussion, results in a ''wraparound'' of color to that corresponding to the opposite flow direction. Such multiple aliasing has restricted color image quantification to a simple measurement of the color boundary. Quantitative distinction of velocities within the jet is virtually impossible for high velocity flows.

M-mode Color Doppler Flow Mapping

To obtain better color and temporal resolution with the sacrifice of the lateral dimension, one-dimensional M-mode color flow mapping can be used. The concept is perfectly analogous to the relationship between B-mode and M-mode echocardiography, that is, color along a line of ultrasound is plotted against time. Such techniques have not found much use to date. However, techniques for quantification of regurgitant lesions, which depend on the location of Nyquist transition, may benefit from an application of the more temporally resolved color M-mode after spatial location on the color flow map.

Three-dimensional Echocardiography

While two-dimensional (2-D) echocardiography is a routinely applied imaging method in cardiology, standard 2-D techniques have severe limitations with respect to volume and functional quantification, especially in patients with distorted ventricles, in which standard geometric assumptions are invalid. The limitations of 2-D echocardiography have provided the motivation for the development of three-dimensional (3-D) reconstruction techniques, which eliminate the need for geometric assumptions in the quantitative analysis for evaluation of cardiac chamber size and shape, ventricular function, and complex structural defects.

Three-dimensional echocardiography involves the acquisition and processing of all three spatial dimensions, as a variation of time, providing a complete visualization and analysis of moving cardiac structures. The recent significant progress in 3-D echocardiography is a result of advances in computational hardware and mathematical tools that allow complete 3-D analysis and animation (5). The development of rendering and segmentation techniques have been extremely useful in this regard. Two types of rendering techniques are mainly used: surface and volume rendering. Surface rendering involves wrapping a sheet over a 3-D wire cage, which represents lines connecting points in physical space derived from 2-D images. A major advantage of surface rendering is the ability to obtain quantitative information for stroke volume, endocardial surface area, and wall motion (endocardium has been segmented). Volume rendering is a different process without segmentation known a priori. Regular pixels are placed in a 3-D grid of voxels. The whole set of data is filled and the resulting 3-D image provides invaluable visualization and morphological analysis (the major advantage over surface rendering) of structures and diseases, such as congenital heart defects, valve anomalies, and vegetations. However, because the data are not segmented (as in surface rendering), no quantitative information is directly available (5).

The critical step in 3-D echocardiography is image acquisition, because: (i) geometrical distortions must be avoided; (ii) the images must be acquired rapidly to avoid patient motion; and (iii) the mechanism that localizes the transducer must not interfere with the regular examination. The four major acquisition techniques are tilt, axial, rotational and toroidal scanning.

Initial transesophageal scanning techniques used axial or

parallel acquisition. Current protocols mainly use rotational scanning, in which a cone of data is acquired by rotating the multiplane probe from 0 degrees to 180 degrees (5). The parallel scan is useful for imaging of structures like the aorta, because no rearrangement of the data is needed. Nevertheless, rotational scanning may be preferable, because it can be performed from a single-transducer esophageal location, without any additional discomfort for the patient.

In transthoracic acquisition, it is more difficult to control the location of the probe. Various solutions have been used, some older, such as mechanical localizers and mechanical 3-D probes, and some newer, such as remote acoustic or magnetic localizers. Mechanical localizers involve the simplest way to manipulate the transducer. A mechanical arm is used to mount the transducer. This arm permits the transducer to move in any orientation and angle. With mechanical 3-D probes, the entire system can be hand-held, allowing the translation or rotation of the transducer by a computer-controlled motor. Remote localization includes the use of either acoustic or magnetic localizers to measure the transducer's position and angle in space. The operator manually moves the transducer without constraints, while the localizer monitors its movement. The most common approach is the acoustic localizer that uses sound-emitting devices mounted on the transducer and small microphones to detect sound. The transducer can be localized in space by knowing the speed of sound in air, the locations of the microphones, and the time of flight of the sound pulse. An alternative is to use a magnetic positioning device to localize the transducer. This device produces a spatially varying magnetic field and has a small magnetic sensor mounted on the transducer.

Harmonic Imaging

Contrast echocardiography began more than 25 years ago with the injection of air bubbles as a means of delineating the cavities of the ventricles and great vessels. Nevertheless, it is only recently that contrast echocardiography has become a clinical reality, because of the availability of intravenously injected agents, which can pass through the lungs and cause opacification of the left ventricular cavity (6). These microbubble-type contrast agents can significantly enhance Doppler signals, because of the difference in the acoustic properties between gas and blood. The degree of contrast enhancement depends on the ultrasonic characteristics of the microbubbles, their density, and the properties of the surrounding medium (7).

A new method that aims to solve the problems of small vessel flow detection by suppressing the signal from the solid tissue and provide signal from only the moving blood is harmonic imaging. Application of an ultrasonic field causes the microbubbles (that undergo resonant oscillation) to develop a nonlinear motion. The nonlinearity of the microbubbles is higher than that of tissues. As a result, the backscattered ultrasound from the medium containing these microbubbles contains frequency components at the funda-

mental frequency as well as harmonics, just as the resonant strings of a musical instrument. The first of these harmonics, which is called the second harmonic frequency, is the strongest of all harmonics and is higher for the contrast agent than for the tissue. Therefore, ideally, there should be no confusion from tissue motion artifact or large vessel blood flow. This property of the microbubbles has been exploited to create a new contrast-based imaging modality called harmonic imaging.

Harmonic imaging uses the nonlinear properties of microbubble-based contrast agents by transmitting at the fundamental frequency, but receiving at the second harmonic frequency. Processing backscattered signals to enhance the second harmonic frequency over the fundamental frequency should produce images that enhance the bubble-containing blood pool compared with the surrounding cardiac structures (8). Therefore, the signal-to-noise ratio for backscattered signals from microbubble contrast agents should be higher than that from non-bubble scatterers. In other words, harmonic imaging creates contrast by decreasing the signal intensity of the tissue rather than increasing the intensity of the contrast material. By studying the second harmonic component of the backscattered echo, which is greater in magnitude for the contrast agent than for the tissue, problems involving tissue artifact and inadequate blood signal with respect to tissue signal intensity are overcome. Since harmonic imaging has the ability to suppress the tissue backscattered signal, the simultaneous application of Doppler can quantify blood flow more reliably, since no significant signal from tissue is detected (6). Whereas the spectrum from conventional Doppler shows a large solid tissue clutter component, this is not a problem in harmonic imaging, because the signal from the tissue is rejected without the loss of information about the flow. This, in combination with the improvement in vessel visualization that harmonic imaging provides, highlights the potential of this technique for the detection of slow moving blood flow through small vessels in the presence of tissue structures.

In vivo studies (7) have shown that harmonic imaging significantly improved left ventricular cavity opacification compared with fundamental imaging. Harmonic Doppler quantified the coronary blood flow velocities at rest and after vasodilation, allowing the noninvasive evaluation of coronary vasodilator reserve. It was also shown that the duration of contrast enhancement was significantly longer in harmonic than in conventional ultrasound imaging. In addition, harmonic images seem to be less susceptible to artifacts such as acoustic shadowing.

In practice, the application of harmonic imaging currently involves some uncertainties due to technical limitations of the existing scanners. The transducers used in harmonic imaging are wideband and may emit energy, not only at the fundamental, but also at the second harmonic frequency. Also, tissue becomes more nonlinear at higher pressures, and some tissue-generated second harmonic components may be contained in the detected echo. In addition, since the energy of the harmonic echo depends on the viscosity of the medium, the type of contrast agent and the scanning parameters used can affect image quality and diagnostic capability.

In conclusion, harmonic imaging has potential in clinical echocardiography. By enhancing the ability of B-mode scanners to distinguish microbubbles within vascular space from tissue, it has the ability to better distinguish blood cavities from wall tissue and to detect blood flow in small vessels surrounded by moving tissue (capillaries, coronary arteries). Further progress in echocardiography technology, together with incorporation of three-dimensional reconstruction techniques in harmonic image acquisition, will strengthen this potential (7).

Tissue Doppler Echocardiography

Two-dimensional echocardiography is commonly used for noninvasive assessment of ventricular wall motion. However, quantitative assessment requires off-line computer analysis of two-dimensional echocardiograms, except when automated border detection is used. If the Doppler signals from the cardiac wall can be analyzed by the Doppler auto-correlation technique, ventricular wall motion can be imaged in a color-coded fashion. However, analysis of the Doppler signals, associated with cardiac wall motion, is technically difficult, because the wall motion velocity is too slow to be captured by conventional color Doppler. To overcome these difficulties, tissue Doppler echocardiography (TDE) imaging was developed. TDE is a Doppler echocardiographic imaging technique, which analyzes the wall motion velocity by autocorrelation techniques to generate two-dimensional color images of wall motion. The recently developed TDE allows the acquisition of wall motion velocities on-line during an ultrasound examination (9,10).

Doppler ultrasound has traditionally been used for measurement of blood flow velocities rather than cardiac wall motion. Between blood flow and wall motion, there are two major differences in the acoustic characteristics of the Doppler signals. First, wall motion velocity is much lower than blood flow velocity and second, Doppler signal intensity of wall motion is much greater than that of Doppler signals coming mainly from red blood cells. Hence, in blood flow the moving red blood cells reflect low amplitude Doppler signals at a relatively high velocity, while moving tissue (such as the myocardium) typically reflects at a low velocity, but with very high amplitude Doppler signals.

The acoustic characteristics therefore present an opportunity to visualize the tissue motion by rearranging the Doppler filter to improve the low velocity sensitivity of the color Doppler system used to measure blood flow. Further, by selecting the amplitude of the Doppler signal input to the velocity-measuring unit, elimination of the blood flow signals can be accomplished, thus measuring only the Doppler signals from wall motion. In a conventional Doppler system, a high pass filter is incorporated to eliminate low velocity signals and the gain settings are increased to amplify the signals reflected by moving blood. Hence, to display tissue velocities in TDE, alterations are made to the Doppler signal, processing. First, the Doppler signals derived from cardiac tissue motion are input directly into the auto-correlator, bypassing the high pass filter. In addition, a lower gain amplification is used to eliminate the weaker intensity blood flow signals (9–11).

The tissue Doppler velocities may be displayed either in spectral pulsed or in color-encoded M-mode or two-dimensional mode. The technical principles and limitations of any of these modalities are similar to those encountered with standard Doppler flow systems, with spectral pulsed-wave Doppler providing the highest temporal and velocity range resolution and two-dimensional color providing high spatial but low temporal and velocity range resolution (9). Tissue Doppler echocardiography can be used clinically to measure myocardial tissue motion, though validation of the technique has not been completely verified due to the limited number of studies that have been completed. Further analysis of the technique, including strengths and weaknesses, will continue, so that full realization of the advantages of this technique can be explored.

Instrument Settings

Several instrument parameter settings play an important role in the resultant spatial image of a flow (such as a jet) obtained by CDFM. The ''jet'' will be taken as the example of choice throughout the following discussion.

Gain

Gain may be thought of as the sensitivity of the machine. For a constant jet flow, varied gain can essentially produce three types of images. A gain setting that is too high will cause noise (random color) to appear outside the boundary of the jet—actually throughout the color sector. The jet boundary is difficult to distinguish with such a setting. If the gain is reduced to the point where the noise just disappears, the maximum jet area will be obtained. Continuing to decrease gain will result in a smaller jet for the same flow. The unfortunate fact is that the gain level required to produce the optimum jet varies depending on physical factors, such as hematocrit and the presence of low frequency signals, as well as interaction with other machine settings.

Pulse Repetition Frequency

Increasing pulse repetition frequency increases the Nyquist velocity limit, allowing more extensive display of legitimate colors before aliasing. This directly affects prototype quantitation techniques, which involve image processing and in which aliased velocity interpretation is questionable. In most contemporary CDFM units, the depth available for imaging decreases with increasing pulse repetition frequency in order to eliminate the possibility of range ambiguity.

Wall Filter Settings

Low frequency signals from moving cardiac structures can cause interference with velocity signals and results in unwanted noise. Increasing wall filter settings eliminates these low frequency signals and produces a smoother jet. That is, transition from color to color, moving laterally across a jet, seems to be better defined. It must be remembered, though, that increasing this filter also eliminates actual low velocities that might be present (on the periphery of a jet, for example).

Carrier Frequency

Higher frequency transducers provide clearer images than low frequency ones. But increasing carrier frequency limits the depth of penetration. For example, 5 MHz transducers are often used on infants, but do not provide adequate depth for imaging of adults.

Frame Rate

All of the previously discussed instrument settings have conventional Doppler analogs. The mechanism by which a two-dimensional image is obtained in CDFM introduces another important technical factor, unique to the two-dimensional modality. The single line of sample volumes produced by the multiple crystal array must be swept throughout the color imaging sector (generally, a 15-degree to 90-degree slice). The frequency of sweeping, or frame rate, directly affects the appearance of the jet on the map. A slower frame rate produces a smoother, more accurately colored jet, since more time is allowed for data processing. Faster frame rates produce a jet with a granular type appearance. Although the image obtained with a slow frame rate is more desirable in terms of local spatial accuracy, the fact that frame rates can be as low as 7 frames per second—not much faster than a typical cardiac cycle frequency of 1.12 Hz (resting) or 2.5 Hz (exercise)—may cause the problem of nonsimultaneous physiologic events appearing to be simultaneous on the color map. For example, as the scanning lines sweep from a posterior to an anterior position in a parasternal long-axis view, we might observe simultaneously opened mitral and aortic valves, with corresponding flows.

Limitations

In addition to drawbacks imparted by variability in currently nonstandardized machine settings, two additional limitations exist.

Lateral Resolution Effects

As in the case of conventional Doppler, the ultrasound beam defocuses as it moves away from the focal point of the transducer. This results in larger sample volumes in the far field. Velocity signals are obtained from such a volume and assigned a single color within that volume. Therefore, the detail with which color can be added is less than in the near field. This can cause artifacts with respect to spatial resolution. For example, the flow in a constant diameter vessel may appear wider in the far field than in the near field due to defocusing.

Variance Algorithm

Most state-of-the-art color Doppler instruments have a variance calculation algorithm that can supposedly be used to indicate turbulent or disturbed flow. Variance is calculated from the velocity signals by standard statistical definition and is usually displayed as green on the color flow map if it is above a certain threshold. There are problems with this technique, though, since nonrandom spatial or temporal velocity variation within a sample volume can trigger the variance algorithm in the absence of actual flow turbulence.

SUMMARY

This chapter has described the capabilities of state-of-the-art Doppler echocardiography. The current importance of these techniques in diagnostic cardiology cannot be overstated. The major contribution lies in the replacement of invasive catheter techniques. The two modalities of conventional and color Doppler each have their own limitations, but can complement each other to produce extremely rich information on patient cardiac physiology and pathology.

The two types of conventional Doppler (continuous and pulsed-wave) provide highly quantitative measurements of blood flow velocities in the heart, which can be directly related to the severity of disease from engineering hydrodynamic principles. Color Doppler flow mapping allows visualization of blood flow and cardiac structure movement, providing valuable information on the nature of altered pathologic flow patterns and aiding in accurate transducer placement for conventional Doppler measurements. The most recent developments of echocardiographic techniques (3-D echocardiography, harmonic imaging, and tissue Doppler echocardiography) have furthered the possible uses of echocardiographic imaging. Further development of these techniques, as well as further development of the more widely used techniques, promise even more quantitative applications in the future.

REFERENCES

1. Angelson B. A theoretical study of the scattering of ultrasound from blood, *IEEE Trans Biomed Eng BME* 1980;27:61.
2. Hatle L, Angelson B. *Doppler ultrasound in cardiology: physical principles and clinical applications.* Philadelphia: Lea & Febiger, 1985.
3. Yoganathan AP, Cape EG, Sung HW, Williams FP, Jimoh A. Review of hydrodynamic principles for the cardiologist: applications to the

study of blood flow and jets by imaging techniques. *J Am Coll Cardiol* 1988;12:1344.

4. Cape EG, Skoufis EG, Weyman AE, Yoganathan AP, Levine RA. A new method for noninvasive quantification of valvular regurgitation based on conservation of momentum: *in vitro* validation. *Circulation* 1989;79:1343.

5. Salgo IS. Three-dimensional echocardiography. *J Cardiothorac Vasc Anesth* 1997;11(4):506–516.

6. Burns PN. Harmonic imaging with ultrasound contrast agents. *Clin Radiol* 1996;51[Suppl 1]:50–55.

7. Mulvagh SL, Foley DA, Aeschbacher BC, Klarich KK, Seward JB. Second harmonic imaging of an intravenously administered echocardiographic contrast agent—visualization of coronary arteries and mea-surement of coronary blood flow. *J Am Coll Cardiol* 1996;27(5): 1519–1525.

8. Schwarz KQ, Chen X, Steinmetz S, Phillips D. Harmonic imaging with Levovist. *J Am Soc Echocardiogr* 1997;10(1):1–10.

9. Garcia MJ, Thomas JD, Klein AL. New Doppler echocardiographic applications for the study of diastolic function. *J Am Coll Cardiol* 1998; 32(4):865–875.

10. Miyatake K, Yamagishi M, Tanaka N, et al. New method for evaluating left ventricular wall motion by color-coded tissue Doppler imaging: *in vitro* and *in vivo* studies. *J Am Coll Cardiol* 1995;25:717–724.

11. Sutherland GR, Stewart MJ, Groundstroem KWE, et al. Color Doppler myocardial imaging: a new technique for the assessment of myocardial function. *J Am Soc Echocardiogr* 1994;7:441–458.

CHAPTER 2

Principles of Echocardiographic Approaches

M-mode, Two-dimensional and Spectral Doppler, and Color Flow Imaging

John J. Tzeng and P. Anthony N. Chandraratna

PRINCIPLES OF ECHOCARDIOGRAPHY

Echocardiography utilizes sonic frequency of 1 to 10 million cycles/second, or 1 to 10 megahertz (MHz) to examine the heart and record the reflected sonic waves (1). The transducer used in echocardiography has a piezoelectric element that vibrates very rapidly and produces ultrasound when activated by an electrical current (2). Ultrasonic waves will travel in a straight line if the medium through which the sound travels is homogeneous. However, different acoustic properties are produced if the ultrasound strikes an interface between two media of different acoustic impedance. The quantity of ultrasonic energy reflected is then proportional to the differences of acoustical impedances of the object and its surrounding media. Acoustic shadowing is the condition in which ultrasonic energy does not transverse the object and no images are obtained behind the object if the interface is a very strong reflector of sound. Ultrasonic instrumentation provides adjustment of depth compensation and thereby corrects for the usually gradual loss of ultrasonic energy

(attenuation) as the beam traverses tissues. The resolution of ultrasound varies directly with the frequency and inversely with the wavelength. High frequency (short wavelength) ultrasound can distinguish objects that are less than 1 mm apart, while ultrasound with lower frequencies and longer wavelengths have poorer resolution. The penetration of ultrasound is inversely proportional to the frequency of the signal. A high-frequency (3.5 to 10 mHz) ultrasonic beam is unable to penetrate a thick chest wall and is used for children with a relatively thin chest wall. Lower frequency (2 to 3.5 mHz) ultrasonic transducers are commonly used in adult echocardiography with resolution ability of separating objects that are 1 to 2 mm apart.

M-mode Echocardiography

Background

The M-mode presentation (''M'' refers to motion) permits recording of the rate of motion and the amplitude of moving objects with sampling rate of 1,000 pulses/sec, i.e., the repetition rate of the transducer. With timing as the second dimension on M-mode tracings, this display is not truly one-dimensional on the M-mode. The ultrasonic transducer is conventionally placed along the left sternal border of the chest and the ultrasonic beam is directed toward the part of the heart to be examined. The electrocardiogram is displayed

J. J. Tzeng: Department of Medicine, Division of Cardiology, University of Southern California School of Medicine, Los Angeles, California 90033.

P. A. N. Chandraratna: University of California–Irvine, Orange, California 92868; Cardiology Section, Long Beach Veterans Administration Medical Center, Long Beach, California 90822.

TABLE 1. *Normal M-mode values*

M-mode	Normal values
Fractional shortening	28–40%
E-point septal separation	≤6 mm
Left atrium	19–40 mm
Aorta	22–37 mm
Aortic cusp excursion	1.5–2.5 cm
Left ventricle internal Diameter-end diastole	35–57 mm
Left ventricle internal Diameter-end systole	22–40 mm
Interventricular septum	6–11 mm
Posterior wall	6–11 mm
Left ventricular mass	93 ± 22 g/m^2 (men)
—	76 ± 18 g/m^2 (women)

on the oscilloscope together with the echocardiogram and there is a sweep from left to right with the transducer displayed at the top of the oscilloscopic image. The ultrasound beam can pass through a portion of the right ventricle, the interventricular septum, left ventricular cavity, and posterior wall of the left ventricle. Cardiac walls and valves produce strong echoes, while the blood-filled cavities are relatively echo free. The principal advantages of the M-mode study are the high temporal resolution inherent in sampling cardiac motion at about 1,000 times per second and its ability to demonstrate subtle motion of cardiac structures. An M-mode study can reveal a normal mitral valve with detailed motion of the anterior and posterior mitral leaflets, which are less clearly appreciated on a real-time two-dimensional echocardiography. Another advantage of M-mode echocardiography is that it permits accurate measurement of cardiac chambers and wall thickness (Table 1). Several M-mode measurements are used in clinical practice, such as chamber dimensions of left ventricle, left atrium, and aortic root. Left ventricular mass can be derived from the measurement of interventricular septum and posterior wall thickness (3). One can also use an empirical formula to calculate left ventricular volumes and provide an estimation of ejection fraction. Fractional shortening of the left ventricle can be obtained by measuring the diastolic and systolic dimensions of the left ventricle. The other applications of such measurements are to determine the presence of left ventricular hypertrophy and to detect thinning of LV walls in myocardial infarcts (4).

Assessment of Left Ventricular Function by M-mode Echocardiography

M-mode may be used to provide an estimate of the overall left ventricular size and the performance of the left ventricle (LV) in many patients. The M-mode technique may be used to record a dimension of the left ventricle between the left side of the interventricular septum and the endocardial surface of the posterior left ventricular wall in end diastole and end systole. Such measurements of a single dimension can then be used to roughly estimate ventricular volume, with some errors in such calculations with the assumption of a three-dimensional object (5).

Fractional shortening can be formulated as: $[(LVIDd - LVIDs)/LVIDd] \times 100\%)$, where $LVIDd$ is the left ventricular internal diameter at end diastole, and $LVIDs$ is the left ventricular internal diameter at end systole; i.e., the difference between the end-diastolic and end-systolic dimension provides information about left ventricular systolic function. The quotient of fractional shortening and ejection time is derived from the mean fractional or circumferential shortening (6). Normal fractional shortening ranges from 28% to 40% (Table 1). Limitations of the fractional shortening measurement include the following: (i) global left ventricular function is estimated based on the assumption that the ventricle is contracting uniformly, which may not always be the case, (ii) these measurements only assess the basal portion of the chamber and must be interpreted with caution in patients with segmental wall motion abnormalities due to coronary artery disease (7), (iii) abnormal septal movement in left bundle-branch block, (iv) off-axis measurement with a poor echocardiographic window, and (v) a dilated right ventricle may produce paradoxical septal motion.

E-point septal separation (*EPSS*), another M-mode echocardiographic technique for assessing ventricular performance, is a measure of the distance between the E point of the mitral valve and the left side of the interventricular septum (8). Since the opening of the mitral valve is largely related to the volume of blood passing through that mitral orifice, the amplitude of the E point is decreased if the mitral valve flow or left ventricular stroke volume diminishes. The upper normal limit of mitral EPSS is approximately 6 mm (Table 1). EPSS is inversely correlated with the left ventricular ejection fraction. EPSS increases in LV dysfunction because of LV dilatation and decreased opening of the mitral valve. However, when thickened and calcified mitral leaflets with limited excursion are present, e.g., mitral stenosis, an increase in EPSS may be seen even in the presence of normal left ventricular function. Patients with severe aortic regurgitation usually have reduced mitral valve excursion in the presence of normal mitral leaflets. Thus, EPSS should not be used as a measure of left ventricular function in patients with mitral stenosis and aortic regurgitation.

Assessment of Diastolic Function by M-mode Echocardiography

M-mode recordings of the mitral valves can provide information about LV dysfunction and anatomic abnormalities. Premature closure of the mitral valve (i.e., prior to the onset of the R wave on the electrocardiogram) is seen in severe acute aortic regurgitation, and it is the result of a marked rise of LV diastolic pressure that exceeds the left atrial pressure (9). Absence of the smooth and continuous A and C points with an extra ''B bump'' immediately prior to ventricular contraction signifies an elevated left ventricular end-diastolic pressure of more than 20 mm Hg (10). M-mode echocardiography has also been used to evaluate left ventricular diastolic function with recording of the rate of relaxation of the left ventricle by digitizing the borders of the left ventricular cavity and comparing the rapidity with which the left ventricular dimension increases in early diastole.

Measurement of Left Ventricular Mass by M-mode Echocardiography

Left ventricular mass (LVM) is related to wall thickness and chamber volume of the left ventricle. The calculation of the LVM is based on the assumption that the interventricular septum is a part of the left ventricle and that the left ventricle is uniformly surrounded with walls of even thickness. Left ventricular mass can be estimated from a Penn convention. The formula: $LVM = 1.04 \times [(LVID + PW + IVS)^3 - (LVID)^3] - 13.6$; where $LVID$ is the left ventricular internal diameter at end diastole, PW is the posterior wall thickness, IVS is the interventricular septum thickness. The normal LVM is 93 ± 22 g/m^2 for men and 76 ± 18 g/m^2 for women in healthy people. One major limitation of the M-mode technique in the measurement of left ventricular wall thickness is the variation in thickness from point to point.

M-mode Echocardiography of Cardiac Valves

Mitral Valve

M-mode echocardiography provides a sensitive assessment of the motion and thickness of the mitral valve leaflets. With the transducer placed along the left sternal border in approximately the third or fourth intercostal space, the ultrasonic beam can be swept in a sector from the base to the apex of the heart in the parasternal long-axis view. Figure 1A shows the M-mode recording of a normal mitral valve. The motion of the anterior mitral leaflet has an M-shaped configuration and the posterior mitral leaflet has a W-shaped configuration. The D point occurs at the onset of diastole when leaflets separate to the maximal diastolic excursion of E point. With the decrease of diastolic inflow, the mitral leaflets move toward each other and reach middiastolic F point at the end of the rapid filling period. The A point occurs at the phase of peak leaflet separation following atrial contraction. With the onset of ventricular systole, the B point, there is a rapid closure of the valve (Fig. 1B). The C point occurs at the time of leaflet coaptation.

The M-mode echocardiogram in patients with calcific *mitral stenosis* shows the following abnormalities: (i) the motion of the mitral valve is considerably altered from the normal pattern with inadequate separation of the anterior and posterior leaflets of the valve during diastole and paradoxical anterior motion of the posterior leaflet, (ii) the normal M-shaped configuration during diastole is no longer present, (iii) the number of echoes originating from the valve is increased when it is thickened or fibrotic or calcified, (iv) the absence of valve closure in middiastole, (v) the disappearance of the reopening of the valve with atrial contraction in late diastole, (vi) the absence of the A wave, (vii) decreased or flattened diastolic (E–F) slope (11) (Fig. 1C).

Echo findings of normal mitral valve motion may be altered in *aortic regurgitation*. The excursion of anterior mitral leaflet is impeded by the aortic regurgitant jet and reveals reduced amplitude of motion and diastolic fluttering of the anterior leaflet (Fig. 1D). Premature closure of the mitral valve (prior to onset of QRS on an electrocardiogram) occurs in acute aortic regurgitation. The M-mode echocardiographic patterns of *mitral valve prolapse* include: (i) "U" or hammock-shaped mitral leaflets due to pansystolic posterior movement and (ii) prominent posterior displacement of leaflets in mid-systole with displacement 3 mm or more posterior to the C through D segments (Fig. 1E). The common M-mode echocardiographic findings of *ruptured chordae tendineae* are (i) chaotic diastolic flutter of the mitral valve, (ii) systolic fluttering of the mitral valve, and (iii) paradoxical anterior motion of the posterior leaflet in early diastole. In hypertrophic obstructive cardiomyopathy (HOCM), a prominent systolic anterior motion (SAM) of the anterior mitral leaflet is observed on M-mode echocardiography (Fig. 1F).

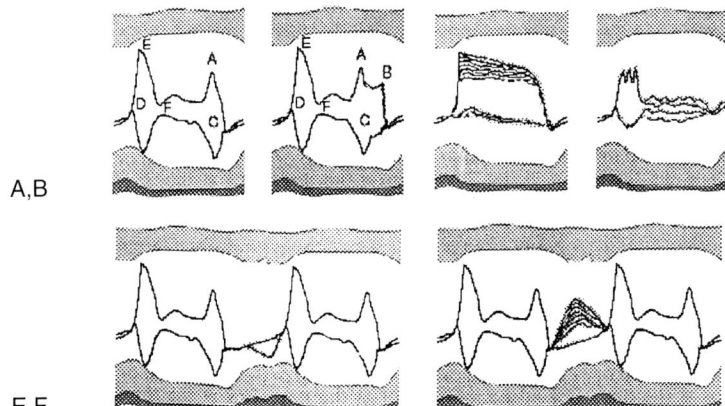

A,B

C,D

E,F

FIG. 1. M-mode configurations of mitral valve. **A:** Normal mitral leaflets. **B:** High left ventricular end-diastolic pressure with "B" bump. **C:** Mitral stenosis. **D:** Fluttering of mitral leaflet in severe aortic regurgitation. **E:** Mitral valve prolapse. **F:** Systolic anterior motion (SAM) of mitral leaflets in hypertrophic obstructive cardiomyopathy. A, atrial contraction; C, mitral closure; D, end systole; E, mitral valve opening.

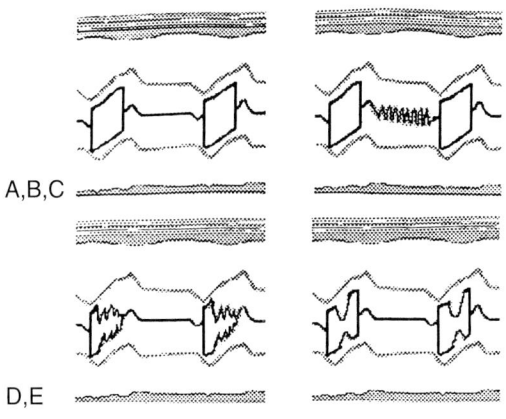

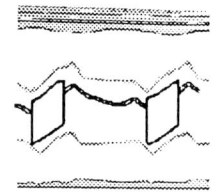

FIG. 2. M-mode configurations of aortic valve. **A:** Normal aortic valve. **B:** Flail aortic valve. **C:** Bicuspid aortic valve. **D:** Discrete subaortic stenosis. **E:** Hypertrophic obstructive cardiomyopathy.

Aortic Valve

M-mode echocardiogram of aortic valve can be obtained by tilting the transducer superiorly and medially with the ultrasound beam traversing the root of the aorta, the leaflets of the aortic valve, and the body of the left atrium in the parasternal long-axis view. The typical "box-like" appearance of the aortic valve in systole is noted (Fig. 2**A**). The right coronary cusp of the aortic valve is located anteriorly and the noncoronary cusp posteriorly. The coapted aortic leaflets appear as a linear image in the middle of the aortic root during diastole. With the onset of left ventricular contraction, the two aortic leaflets separate rapidly, parallel to the anterior and posterior aortic wall with a rectangular configuration during the systole. Systolic flutter of aortic leaflets is a normal echocardiographic finding, while diastolic flutter may indicate the presence of flail leaflet (Fig. 2**B**). The normal cusp motion of the aortic valve depends on the flow and volume through the valve. The normal cusp excursion ranges from 1.5 to 2.5 cm as measured in the widest opening of rectangle-shaped valve on M-mode. Eccentric cuspid closure is observed in patients with bicuspid aortic valve with distorted rectangle-configuration on the M-mode echocardiogram (Fig. 2**C**).

Obstruction of the left ventricular outflow tract may alter the motion of aortic valve. Discrete subaortic stenosis is characterized by normal valve opening followed by rapid partial closure of the valve and systolic fluttering (12) (Fig. 2**D**). In hypertrophic obstructive cardiomyopathy, the aortic leaflets open initially, followed by midsystolic closure due to decreased forward cardiac output, and then reopening in late systole (Fig. 2**E**). The presence of midsystolic closure in HOCM signifies a resting left ventricular outflow (LVOT) gradient. Gradual closure of the aortic valve throughout systole is observed in patients with poor left ventricular stroke volume or severe mitral regurgitation. The aortic valve may open earlier before ventricular systole in patients with severe aortic regurgitation and markedly elevated left ventricular diastolic pressure.

Tricuspid Valve

The M-mode echocardiogram of the tricuspid valve is recorded by directing the transducer medially from the aortic valve to obtain a right ventricular inflow view. The motion pattern of the tricuspid valve is similar to the M-mode of mitral leaflets with anterior and posterior tricuspid leaflet motion (Fig. 1**A**). The letter designation of tricuspid leaflet motion is similar to that used for mitral motion. The tricuspid leaflets usually close 40 msec later than the mitral leaflets. The M-mode pattern of tricuspid stenosis is similar to that of mitral stenosis with flattened E-F slope, inadequate separation of tricuspid leaflet during diastole, and disappearance of the reopening of the valve with atrial contraction in late diastole with disappearance of normal M-shaped configuration. Tricuspid valve prolapse is characterized by thickening of the valve and posterior displacement of tricuspid leaflets in mid-systole posterior to the C–D segment. Endocarditis with vegetation in the tricuspid valve is a common finding in intravenous drug abusers and is revealed as distortion of M-shaped configuration, dense echogenic masses, and evidence of flail leaflet.

Pulmonary Valve

The M-mode echocardiogram of the pulmonary valve can be obtained by tilting the transducer superiorly and laterally from the aortic valve in the parasternal short-axis at the right ventricular outflow view. However, the M-mode motion of the pulmonary valve is more difficult to record than other valves due to the technical limitation in passing the cursor perpendicular to the valve plane. Moreover, the image is obscured by overinflated lungs and by the expanding lung of inspiration. The posterior pulmonary leaflet is more commonly recorded than the anterior leaflet. The valve moves posteriorly to open during systole and anteriorly to close during diastole. The motion of pulmonary valve has been designated as follows: "a" point denotes atrial contraction, "b" point the onset of right ventricular contraction, "c"

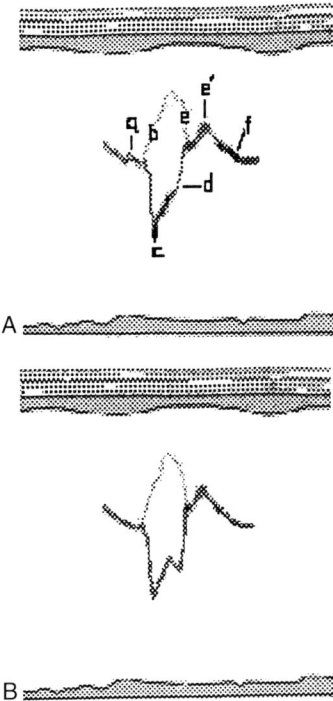

FIG. 3. M-mode configurations of pulmonary valve. **A:** Normal pulmonary valve. a, atrial contraction; b, onset of RV contraction; c, maximal opening; d, end of ejection; e, rapid closure. **B:** Pulmonary valve in the presence of pulmonary hypertension.

point the maximal opening position, ''d'' point designates the end of ejection, ''e'' rapid closure, ''e''' for transmitted aortic motion, and ''f'' point for posterior movement during diastole (Fig. 3**A**). An increase in pulmonary artery pressure may produce the following changes of pulmonary valve motion: (i) elimination of atrial systolic motion and the absence of the pulmonary valve ''a'' wave; this ''a'' wave may reappear if right ventricular failure occurs with pulmonary hypertension and (ii) midsystolic closure of the pulmonary valve (13) (Fig. 3**B**).

M-mode Echocardiography of Pericardial Effusion

Pericardial effusion produces characteristic changes on the M-mode echocardiogram. M-mode echocardiography may detect as little as 20 mL of pericardial fluid (14). The hallmarks of pericardial effusion are an echo-free space anterior or posterior to the heart, absence of motion of the pericardium, and a reduction of the space at the junction of the left ventricle and left atrium due to insertion of the pulmonary vein (15). However, the echo-free space may extend beyond the posterior wall of the left atrium into the oblique pericardial sinus when there is a large amount of pericardial effusion. M-mode echocardiography may also reveal collapse of right ventricular wall in the early diastole in patients with cardiac tamponade. The volume of pericardial effusion can be roughly estimated using M-mode echocardiography and is classified as mild, moderate, and large effusions. With

a large pericardial effusion, a large echo-free space may be imaged posteriorly and anteriorly. However, such estimation may be erroneous when there is a loculated pericardial effusion. Serial echocardiographic studies of pericardial effusion are useful in assessing the clinical course of patients who received pericardiocentesis or pericardial window.

Two-dimensional Echocardiography

Image Orientation

Two-dimensional echocardiography images a sector so that a pie-shaped slice of the heart is obtained. An infinite number of slices of the heart can theoretically be obtained using echocardiography. Multiple ultrasonic elements are fired in sequence using phased array principles (16). The American Society of Echocardiography has standardized and simplified two-dimensional examinations into three orthogonal planes that include long-axis, short-axis, and four-chamber views of the heart.

The *long-axis plane* is the imaging plane that transects the heart perpendicular to the dorsal and ventral surfaces of the body and parallel to the long axis of the heart. The long-axis view can be obtained with the transducer in the apical position, or the parasternal position (left sternal border). The right ventricle, right atrium, and tricuspid valve can all be recorded from a parasternal long-axis position.

The *short-axis plane* is perpendicular to the dorsal and ventral surfaces of the body. A short-axis view can be obtained with the transducer in the parasternal position or in the subcostal (subxiphoid) position. It cuts across the heart so that the left ventricle resembles a circle and the right ventricle curves around the left ventricle. The short-axis views are usually obtained at the levels of the apex, the papillary muscles, the mitral valve, and the base of the heart.

The *four-chamber plane* transects the heart approximately parallel to the dorsal and ventral surfaces of the body. The four-chamber view can be obtained with the transducer over the cardiac apex or with the transducer in the subcostal position. This view permits the examination of all four cardiac chambers simultaneously.

The *subcostal transducer* location produces examinations roughly in the four-chamber and short-axis planes. The subcostal four-chamber view is particularly helpful in examining the interatrial and interventricular septa. The transducer can be rotated 90 degrees to provide a subcostal short-axis examination of the heart. By directing the transducer in a slightly modified short-axis examination, one can obtain an excellent view of the right side of the heart. The subcostal location also permits an opportunity to direct the ultrasonic beam through the inferior vena cava and hepatic veins (16). This examination provides information concerning right-sided hemodynamics and is helpful in assessing the central venous pressure. An increase in pressure dilates the veins and eliminates the normal respiratory variation in the size of the inferior vena cava.

A two-dimensional *suprasternal view* can be obtained by

placing the transducer in the suprasternal notch either parallel or perpendicular to the arch of the aorta. The parallel suprasternal view reveals the aorta, pulmonary artery and left atrium. The perpendicular suprasternal view shows a circular aorta and the horizontal cut of right and left pulmonary arteries.

Two-dimensional Echocardiography of Left Ventricular Function

It is a common practice for the physician interpreting echocardiograms to merely estimate left ventricular function on the basis of visual inspection, which is obviously qualitative and is highly subjective (17). Hence, the assessment of left ventricular volume and ejection fraction is advantageous. Two-dimensional echocardiography also provides an opportunity to automate the quantitation of left ventricular function by using a technique whereby the endocardial border is automatically detected and the cross-sectional area of the left ventricle is instantly measured (18). This technique can be used to obtain volumes as well as area changes.

Left Ventricular Volume and Mass Measured by Two-dimensional Echocardiography

Two-dimensional echocardiography can be used to measure LV volume and LV mass (LVM). The LV muscle volume (Vm) is equal to the total LV volume contained within the epicardial surface (Vt) minus the total chamber volume contained within the endocardial surface (Vc), i.e., $Vm = Vt - Vc$. Then, the Vm can be converted to LVM by multiplying the specific gravity of myocardium of 1.05, i.e., $LVM = Vm \times 1.05$.

Two-dimensional Echocardiography of Cardiac Valves

Two-dimensional echocardiography provides an opportunity to visualize spatial images of the valve, the annulus, the chordae tendineae, and the papillary muscles; to measure the flow-restricting orifice of the stenotic valve directly; and to assess fibrosis and pliability of the valve apparatus, especially with subvalvular adhesions; it also allows measurement of valvular orifice area.

Mitral Valve

The mitral valve can be examined by using the parasternal long-axis of the left ventricle, parasternal short-axis of left ventricle at the mitral valve level, and the apical four-chamber views of the two-dimensional echocardiography. The parasternal long-axis view depicts both anterior and posterior leaflets from their insertion points of mitral annulus to their free tips (Fig. 4A). It also images the mitral annulus, which may be unusually bright in the presence of mitral annular calcification (MAC). The parasternal short-axis of the LV at the mitral valve level allows direct visualization of the mitral orifice and is used for assessing the mitral valve area by planimetry and for detecting the location and extent

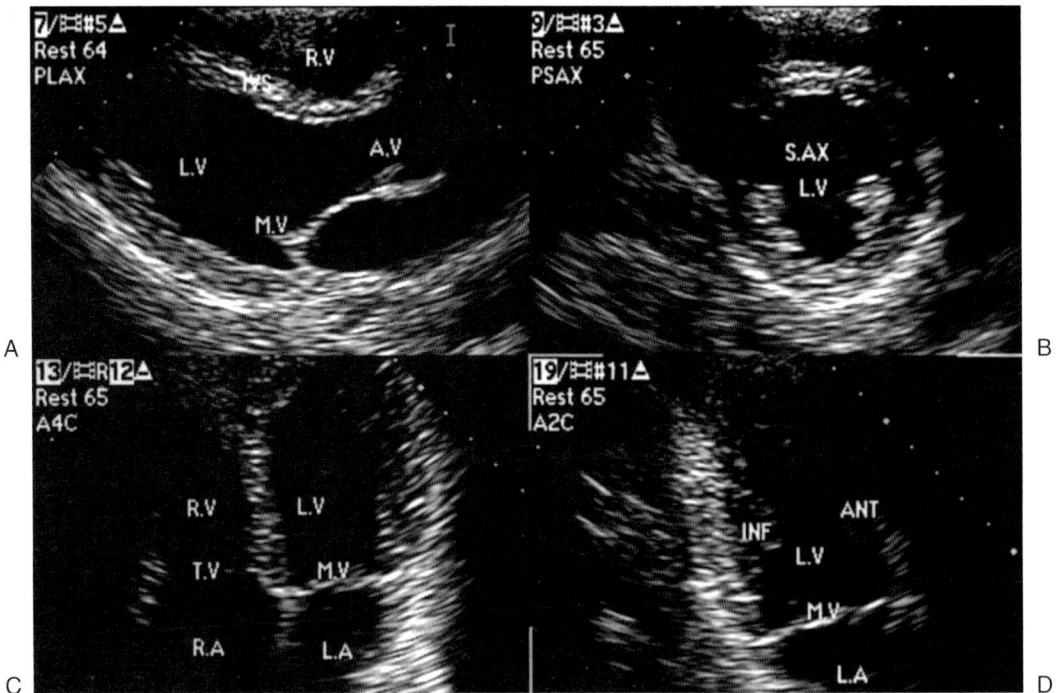

FIG. 4. Two-dimensional echocardiogram. **A:** Parasternal long-axis view. **B:** Parasternal short-axis view at mitral valve level. **C:** Apical four-chamber view. **D:** Apical two-chamber view. *LV*, left ventricle; *RV*, right ventricle; *MV*, mitral valve; *AV*, aortic valve; *TV*, tricuspid valve; *ANT*, anterior wall; *INF*, inferior wall.

of local valvular lesions (Fig. 4**B**). The apical four-chamber view depicts the leaflets and allows visualization of leaflet motion in relation to blood flow (Fig. 4**C**). The apical two-chamber view depicts the mitral leaflets and allows visualization of wall motion of the anterior and inferior walls of left ventricle (Fig. 4**D**).

Aortic Valve

The aortic valve is primarily examined by using parasternal long-axis and short-axis views at the aortic valve level. The transducer transects the aortic valve in the anterior-posterior direction in the parasternal long-axis view (Fig. 4**A**). A linear image of the valve is recorded during diastole when the cusps coapt. During systole, the right coronary leaflet is located anteriorly and the noncoronary leaflet is posterior. In the parasternal short-axis view, the three cusps are recorded during diastole and the open leaflets can be visualized during systole. The two-dimensional echo findings of bicuspid aortic valve are leaflet redundancy, eccentric valve closure, two cusps and two commissure pattern, doming of the valve in systole, and reverse doming in diastole. The findings of aortic stenosis are thickening, doming, calcification, and restricted motion of aortic cusps.

Tricuspid Valve

The tricuspid valve is primarily examined by using parasternal long-axis of the right ventricular inflow tract, the parasternal short-axis of the right ventricular inflow tract at the tricuspid level, and apical four-chamber view. In the parasternal long-axis view, the motion of the anterior and posterior tricuspid leaflets, the annulus, chordae tendineae, and papillary muscles can be imaged. The parasternal short-axis view allows direct visualization and spatial configuration of tricuspid leaflets and annulus. In the apical four-chamber view, the anterior tricuspid leaflet is located laterally and the septal leaflet medially (Fig. 4**C**). The tricuspid valve is inserted closer to the cardiac apex than the mitral valve. It allows visualization of the right-sided atrioventricular ring, the relative location of septal leaflet to the mitral leaflet, and the insertion of septal leaflet into the interventricular septum.

Two-dimensional echocardiography is able to provide spatial morphology of *vegetations on cardiac valves* affected by endocarditis.

Two-dimensional Echocardiography of Pericardial Effusion

Two-dimensional echocardiography is superior to M-mode echocardiography in that the distribution of fluid can be better assessed and loculation of pericardial fluid can be detected. This makes the two-dimensional echocardiography the standard procedure for identifying loculated and circumferential pericardial effusions (15). Two-dimensional echo-

cardiography of a patient with a large pericardial effusion can be detected in the parasternal long-axis view and apical four-chamber view. The pericardial effusion can be differentiated from pleural effusion by the relationship to the position of the descending aorta. Pericardial fluid is located anterior to the descending aorta, whereas pleural fluid accumulates posterior to the aorta. The amount of pericardial fluid can be estimated by the size of echo-free space surrounding the heart.

Cardiac tamponade is associated with the following abnormalities: (i) swinging of the heart in the pericardial sac, (ii) phasic respiratory variations in the left and right ventricular dimensions, (iii) diastolic collapse of the right ventricular anterior free wall (19) in the parasternal short- and long-axis and four-chamber views, (iv) collapse of right atrial free wall in the four-chamber view, which is more sensitive but less specific than right ventricle (RV) collapse, and (v) less frequently collapse of left atrium and left ventricle. Two-dimensional echocardiography can be used for guidance of pericardiocentesis. Using two-dimensional echocardiography along with bubble contrast technique to visualize a pericardiocentesis needle and verify the location of the tip of the needle within the pericardial sac can facilitate pericardiocentesis (15). The echo transducer is usually placed at the apex while pericardiocentesis is performed via the subcostal approach. The two-dimensional echocardiography is continuously recorded during the procedure and is useful in identifying the appearance of microbubbles in the pericardial sac or in a cardiac chamber if perforation has occurred. Serial echocardiographic studies are useful in following the clinical course of pericardial effusion and the disappearance or reaccumulation of fluid following pericardicentesis or institution of a pericardial window.

Two-dimensional Echocardiography of Cardiac Masses

Two-dimensional echocardiography may reveal the tumors in the ventricles as well as in the atria including myomas, rhabdomyomas, and fibromas (20). Two-dimensional echocardiography findings include mobile tumors moving from above the mitral valve into the left ventricle during diastole and pedunculated right ventricular masses prolapsing into the pulmonary artery simulating pulmonic stenosis. Several types of valvular neoplasms can also be detected by two-dimensional echocardiography including: (i) primary myxoma of the mitral valve (21), (ii) cardiac papillary fibroelastomas of the valve leaflets, (iii) rhabdomyosarcoma involving the mitral valve.

The following findings may mimic a cardiac mass: (i) mobile echoes produced by Chiari network within the right atrium (22), (ii) benign lipomatous hypertrophy of the interatrial septum, (iii) moderator bands seen in the right ventricle and left ventricular bands or false tendons straddling the left ventricular chamber frequently can be imaged (23), and (iv) catheters such as Swan-Ganz catheter, pacemaker wires, or defibrillator catheters.

Spectral Doppler and Color Flow Echocardiography

According to the Doppler principle, if an ultrasound beam encounters a moving object (e.g., red cells), it undergoes a change in frequency such that the frequency shift is proportional to the velocity of the object (24). The Doppler shift reveals the difference between the reflected and transmitted frequencies. Blood flow velocity is calculated with the equation: $Fd = Fr - Ft = 2\ Ft \times (V \times \cos\theta/C)$, where Fd denotes Doppler frequency, C is the velocity of sound tissue, the angle (θ) is between the direction of the moving target and the path of the ultrasound beam and the velocity (V) of the moving target. The transmitted frequency (Ft) equals the reflected frequency (Fr) if the ultrasonic beam is reflected by a stationary subject, however, the Fr is greater than the Ft if the object is moving toward the transducer, and the Fr is less than the Ft if the object is moving away from the transducer.

Pulsed-wave Ultrasound

Pulsed-wave (PW) ultrasound can be utilized to obtain the Doppler information with only one transducer. PW Doppler is site-specific, i.e., it allows measurement of blood velocity at a particular region. Pulsed-wave Doppler is most useful in localizing the site of flow disturbance and for measurements of flow velocity, pulmonary venous and hepatic vein velocity profiles, and diastolic filling profiles. However, flow velocity recording of pulsed Doppler is limited by the pulse repetition frequency (PRF) of the system. A phenomenon known as aliasing (25) occurs when the blood velocity exceeds the Nyquist limit and the signal gets wrapped around so that the peak velocity cannot be determined. High pulse repetition frequency Doppler is an alternative means of recording high velocities of flow.

Continuous-wave Ultrasound

The continuous-wave (CW) Doppler utilizes two transducers, one continuously transmits ultrasonic energy that travels to the target of interrogation and the other continuously receives the reflected ultrasonic signals. The Doppler frequency shift is derived by subtracting the frequencies of the reflected from the transmitted bursts of ultrasound. CW Doppler is able to record very high velocities within the cardiovascular system. CW has been used to measure high-velocity flow in valvular stenosis or aortic regurgitation and mitral regurgitation. The advantage of CW Doppler is its ability to measure high velocities without aliasing. The major limitation of CW Doppler is its inability to define the site of a high velocity jet. In contrast, the pulsed-wave Doppler has the ability to locate the site of high frequency jet; however, because of aliasing, the pressure velocity cannot

TABLE 2. *Pulsed-wave vs. continuous-wave ultrasound*

	Pulsed wave	Continuous wave
Velocity detection	Low-velocity jet	High-velocity jet
Ability to detect site of jet	Yes	No
Limited by aliasing	Yes	No

be determined (Table 2). Thus PW and CW Doppler provide complementary information and should be used in concert during diagnostic studies.

Doppler Color Flow Imaging

Color flow imaging is a computer-enhanced pulsed-wave Doppler that provides the information of blood flow direction and velocities with similar Nyquist limit like PW Doppler. It is created by multiple Doppler gates that are spatially corrected formats superimposed on an M-mode or two-dimensional echocardiogram that display the movement of the blood flow (26). The direction of the blood flow is displayed in color with red depicting blood flow toward the transducer and blue depicting blood flow away from the transducer. As color flow imaging is a pulsed Doppler technique, it exhibits the phenomenon of aliasing, which is manifested as a change in color, e.g., red to blue. Aliasing effect occurs with high velocities and is reflected by a reversal of color pattern.

The major advantage of color flow imaging is to measure and localize the position and direction of the abnormal flow including valvular regurgitation, stenotic lesions, or intracardiac shunts. The flow is best detected when it is parallel to the ultrasonic beam and the velocity reflects the angle between moving jet and the ultrasound beam. Mitral regurgitation can be demonstrated by means of color flow Doppler on a two-dimensional view with the area of yellow and green indicating the turbulent flow of regurgitation (Fig. 5; see also Color Plate 1 following page 294). The severity of regurgitation can be semiquantitated by measuring the ratio of the area of the maximum regurgitant jet to the area of the left atrium. However, this method is limited by various factors influencing the size of the flow jet, such as different gain settings of echocardiography machine, various frequencies of transducers, and variations in different cardiac cycles, and various chamber views.

Doppler Evaluation of Blood Flow and Pressure Gradients

Doppler echocardiography is now the major ultrasonic technique used to obtain hemodynamic information. It does so by measuring the velocity of intracardiac blood flow, thus deriving the quantitative data of blood flow and intracardiac pressures—provided that there is no regurgitant flow. The Doppler technique for measuring blood flow can be utilized to measure cardiac output or stroke volume (27). Cardiac output can be obtained by measuring the blood flow in the

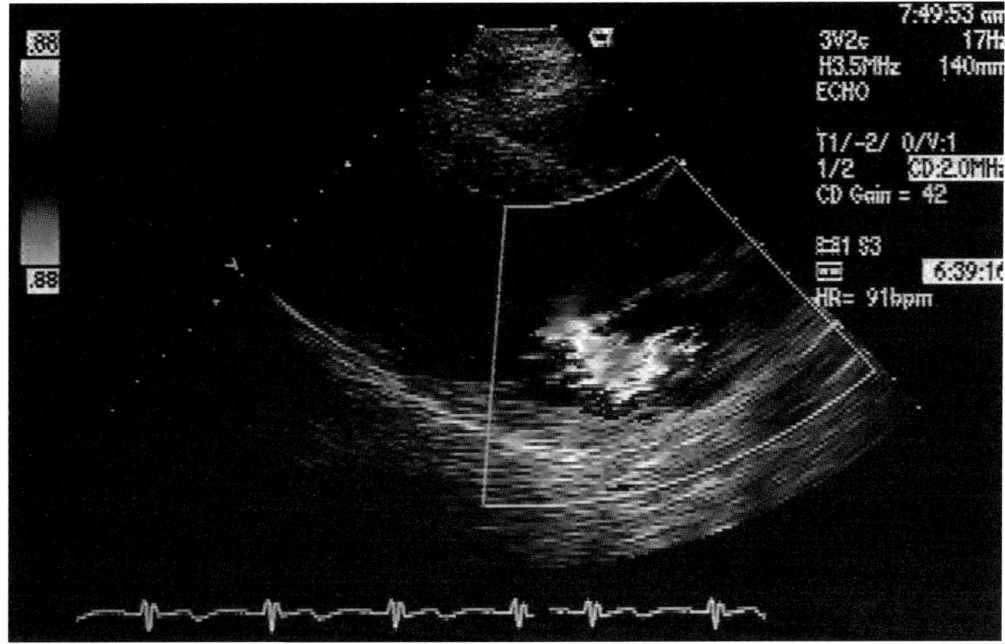

FIG. 5. Color flow Doppler of mitral regurgitation. (See also Color Plate 1 following page 294.)

ascending aorta by calculating the velocity time integral of the aortic flow velocity signal and cross-sectional area of the ascending aorta. Cardiac output (*CO*) can be derived from the equation: $CO = TVI \times CSA \times HR$, where TVI = time velocity integral, CSA = cross-sectional area, and HR = heart rate. The cross-sectional area of the vessel can be obtained directly with two-dimensional echocardiography or indirectly by measuring the diameter on M-mode echocardiography to derive the area.

Pulmonary blood flow can also be measured by multiplying the Doppler pulmonary artery velocity time integral and the cross-sectional area of the pulmonary artery. The blood flow through the mitral and tricuspid valves can also be calculated in a similar way. The effectiveness of Doppler echocardiography for measuring flow has been validated (28). The other applications of blood flow measurement are to quantitate the shunt ratio and regurgitant fraction. The pulmonary to systemic flow ratios (*Qp/Qs*) can be obtained by measuring the time velocity integrals and cross-sectional areas of pulmonary artery and aortic flows (29). Calculating the aortic flow and mitral valve flow can be derived from the regurgitant fraction of mitral regurgitation (30).

Calculation of Pressure Gradients

The pattern of the Doppler flow velocities can be utilized to provide hemodynamic information. By utilizing a modified Bernoulli equation, the Doppler echocardiography can calculate the pressure gradient across a stenotic part of the blood flow in the cardiovascular system (31). The Bernoulli equation establishes the pressure difference across a stenosis

of the vessel or between two chambers. The pressure gradient can be calculated by condensing the Bernoulli equation to a formula of $DP = 4 \times V^2$, i.e., the difference in pressure (*DP*) equals 4 times the square of the velocity (*V*) across the stenotic lesion. The accuracy and validity of this formula have been verified (32).

Doppler echocardiography can be used to assess the difference in pressure across a stenotic valve as well as a regurgitant valve. The difference in pressure across the tricuspid regurgitation between the right ventricle and the right atrium in systole can be obtained by measuring the peak velocity of the regurgitant jet (33). The pulmonary artery systolic pressure can then be derived from adding the estimated right atrial pressure to the pressure differential between the right ventricle and right atrium if there is no obstruction to right ventricular outflow. The right ventricular systolic pressure can also be derived by subtracting the pressure gradient between the left and right ventricles from a known left ventricular systolic pressure, if the velocity of blood flow across a ventricular septal defect is calculated (34).

REFERENCES

1. Carlsen EN. Ultrasound physics for the physician: a brief review. *J Clin Ultrasound* 1975;3:69.
2. Wells PNT. *Ultrasonics in clinical diagnosis*, 2nd ed. New York: Churchill Livingstone, 1977.
3. Devereux RB, Alonso DR, Lutas EM, et al. Echocardiographic assessment of left ventricular hypertrophy: comparison to necropsy findings. *Am J Cardiol* 1986;57:450.
4. Goldberg SJ. Analysis and interpretation of thickening and thinning phases of left ventricular wall dynamics. *Ultrasound Med. Biol* 1984; 10:797.
5. Teichholz LE, Kreulen T, Herman MV, et al. Problems in echocardio-

graphic volume determinations: echocardiographic-angiographic correlations in the presence or absence of asynergy. *Am J Cardiol* 1976;
37:7.

6. Quinones MA, Gaasch WH, Alexander JK. Echocardiographic assessment of left ventricular function: With special reference to normalized
velocities. *Circulation* 1974;50:42.

7. Feigenbaum H. Echocardiographic examination of the left ventricle.
Circulation 1975;51:1.

8. Ahmadpour H, Shah AH, Allen JW, et al. Mitral E point septal separation: A reliable index of left ventricular performance in coronary artery
disease. *Am Heart J* 1983;106:21.

9. Botvinick EH, Schiller NB, Wickramasekaran R, et al. Echocardiographic demonstration of early mitral valve closure in severe aortic
insufficiency. Its clinical implications. *Circulation* 51:836.

10. Konecke LL, Feigenbaum H, Chang S. Abnormal mitral valve motion
in patients with elevated left ventricular diastolic pressures. *Circulation*
1973;47:989.

11. Duchak JM, Jr, Chang S, Feigenbaum H. The posterior mitral valve
echo and the echocardiographic diagnosis of mitral stenosis. *Am J Cardiol* 1972;29:628.

12. Sabbah HN, Stein PD. Mechanism of early systolic closure of the aortic
valve in discrete membranous subaortic stenosis. *Circulation* 1982;65:
399.

13. Weyman AE, Dillon JC, Feigenbaum H, et al. Echocardiographic patterns of pulmonary valve motion with pulmonary hypertension. *Circulation* 1974;50:905.

14. Horowitz MS, Schultz CS, Stinson EB. Sensitivity and specificity of
echocardiographic diagnosis of pericardial effusion. *Circulation* 1974;
50:239.

15. Chandraratna PAN. Echocardiiography and Doppler ultrasound in the
evaluation of pericardial disease. *Circulation* 1991;84:1–303.

16. Moreno FLL, Hagan AD, Holman JR, et al. Evaluation of size and
dynamics of the inferior vena cava as an index of right-sided cardiac
function. *Am J Cardiol* 1984;53:579.

17. Wong M, Bruce S, Joseph D, et al. Estimating left ventricular ejection
fraction from two-dimensional echocardiograms: Visual and computer-
processed interpretations. *Echocardiography* 1991;8:1.

18. Waggoner AD, Miller JG, Perez JE. Two-dimensional echocardiographic automatic boundary detection for evaluation of left ventricular
function in unselected adult patients. *J Am Soc Echocardiogr* 1994;7:
459.

19. Armstrong WF, Schilt,BF, Helper DJ, et al. Diastolic collapse of the
right ventricle with cardiac tamponade: an echocardiographic study.
Circulation 1982;65:1491.

20. Meller J, Teichholz LE, Pichard AO, et al. Left ventricular myxoma.
Echocardiographic diagnosis and review of the literature. *Am J Med*
1977;63:816.

21. Grosse P, Herpin D, Roudaut R, et al. Myxoma of the mitral valve
diagnosed by echocardiography. *Am Heart J* 1986;111:803.

22. Cloez JL, Neimann JL, Chivoret G, et al. Echocardiographic rediscov-
ery of an anatomical structure: The Chiari network. Apropos of 16
cases. *Arch Mal Coeur* 1983;76:1284.

23. Casta A, Wolf WJ. Left ventricular bands (false tendons): Echocardiographic and angiocardiographic delineation in children. *Am Heart J*
1986;111:321.

24. Burns PN. The physical principles of Doppler and spectral analysis. *J
Clin Ultrasound* 1987;15:567.

25. Bom K, deBoo J, Rijsterborgh H. On the aliasing problem in pulsed
Doppler cardiac studies. *J Clin Ultrasound* 1984;12:559.

26. Stevenson JG. Appearance and recognition of basic concepts in color
flow imaging. *Echocardiography* 1989;6:451.

27. Nishimura RA, Callahan MJ, Schaff HV, et al. Non-invasive measurement of cardiac output by continuous-wave Doppler echocardiography:
Initial experience and review of the literature. *Mayo Clin Proc* 1984;
59:484.

28. Lloyd TR, Shirazi F. Nongeometric Doppler stroke volume determination is limited by aortic size. *Am J Cardiol* 1990;66:883.

29. Jenni R, Ritter M, Vieli A, et al. Determination of the ratio of pulmonary
blood flow to systemic blood flow by derivation of amplitude weighted
mean velocity from continuous wave Doppler spectra. *Br Heart J* 1989;
61:167.

30. Goldberg SJ, Allen HD. Quantitative assessment by Doppler echocardiography of pulmonary or aortic regurgitation. *Am J Cardiol* 1985;56:
131.

31. Hatle L, Angelsen B. *Doppler ultrasound in cardiology: physical principles and clinical applications*, 2nd ed. Philadelphia: Lea & Febiger,
1984.

32. Stamm RB, Martin RP. Quantification of pressure gradients across
stenotic valves by Doppler ultrasound. *J Am Coll Cardiol* 1983;2:707.

33. Yock PG, Popp RL. Non-invasive estimation of right ventricular systolic pressure by Doppler ultrasound in patients with tricuspid regurgitation. *Circulation* 1984;70:657.

34. Silbert DR, Brunson SC, Schiff R, Diamant S. Determination of right
ventricular pressure in the presence of a ventricular septal defect using
continuous wave Doppler ultrasound. *J Am Coll Cardiol* 1986;8:379.

CHAPTER 3

Transthoracic Echocardiography

Assessment of Left Ventricular Function

Ramdas G. Pai and Pravin M. Shah

Following its introduction in Europe, use of echocardiography was pioneered in the United States by Joyner and Reid nearly forty years ago. An initial application of M-mode echo was in detection of mitral stenosis. Feigenbaum reported its use in diagnosis of pericardial effusion in 1965. Gramiak, Shah, and colleagues described systolic anterior motion in hypertrophic obstructive cardiomyopathy, diagnosis of mitral valve prolapse, definition of normal aortic valve and pulmonary valve and the use of contrast echocardiography. Additional applications included diagnosis of left atrial myxoma, left ventricular function, cardiac output, and diagnosis of congenital heart disease. Two-dimensional echocardiography was developed in mid-1970s, followed by pulsed- and continuous-wave Doppler; and, subsequently, by color flow imaging. The current echocardiographic approaches consist of two-dimensional echo imaging, cursor derived M-mode echo, and appropriate Doppler techniques to examine intracardiac blood flow.

CROSS-SECTIONAL IMAGES AND ANATOMIC CORRELATIONS

Two-dimensional echocardiography is a cross-sectional imaging technique providing visualization of different components of cardiac structures in cross sections obtained by placing a transducer at specified locations on the chest wall. Theoretically, one could have an infinite number of planes, by varied placements and angulations of transducer over the acoustic precordial window. The American Society of Echocardiography developed standards for obtaining and describing imaging planes, and this approach succeeds in providing standard anatomic references and improved communication.

There are at least seven routinely used echocardiographic cross sections in evaluation of the adult patient.

1. Long-axis cross sections
2. Short-axis view
3. Right ventricular inflow view
4. Four-chamber view
5. Five-chamber view
6. Two-chamber view
7. Subcostal view

Long-axis Cross Sections

These long-axis cross sections (Fig. 1) may be obtained from the parasternal approach or from the apical window. The anatomic structures and landmarks are nearly the same, although apex of the left ventricle is better visualized from the apical window.

This cross section demonstrates ascending aorta, aortic root and aortic valve (generally right and noncoronary cusps), and the left atrium posteriorly. The mitral valve morphology consists of two leaflets and the papillary muscles are generally not visualized. The left ventricular (LV) wall

R. G. Pai: Department of Cardiology, Jerry L. Pettis Veterans Hospital, Loma Linda, California 92357.
P. M. Shah: Loma Linda University School of Medicine, Loma Linda, California 92350; Noninvasive Cardiac Imaging and Academic Programs, Hoag Memorial Hospital Presbyterian, Newport Beach, California 92663.

segments are the anterior ventricular septum in its basal, mid-, and apical segments and the inferolateral wall segments at basal, mid-, and apical levels. The posteromedial papillary muscle along with postero-inferior walls may be imaged by medial angulation of the transducer.

Short-axis Views

These are short-axis cross sections obtained at basal, mitral valve level and at papillary muscle levels. The basal short axis examines the right ventricular infundibulum, the pulmonic valve and the pulmonary artery branches, the aortic root with valve cusps and the origin of major coronary arteries, the left atrium, the interatrial septum, the right atrium, and the tricuspid valve. The short axis at mitral valve level visualizes the mitral valve orifice and the circumferential basal segments of the left ventricle. At the papillary muscle level, the mid-segments of the left ventricle are visualized. At times, short-axis sections of the apex are visualized in younger adults.

Right Ventricular Inflow View

This cross section visualizes the right ventricle, the right atrium, and the tricuspid valve and is generally obtained from parasternal transducer position.

Four-chamber View

All four chambers of the heart can be visualized through a number of positions, the apical and the subcostal transducer locations. The two ventricles, two atria, and both atrioventricular valves are noted, with the tricuspid valve having a slightly more apical (or caudal) attachment as compared to the mitral. The interventricular septum image consists of posterior septum at the base and anterior septum at mid- and apical segments. The lateral wall image comprises posterolateral wall at the base, and lateral segments at mid- and apical portions.

Five-chamber View

An anterior angulation from the four-chamber view brings out left ventricular outflow tract, aortic valve and root, in addition to the four chambers described above. In this view, the basal septum is anterior septum and basal lateral segment the true lateral wall.

Two-chamber View

This view can be obtained from the apex with transducer rotated so that only the left ventricle and the left atrium, along with the mitral valve, are imaged. In this view, the basal, mid- and apical segments of anterior and inferior walls are seen.

Subcostal Views

The four-chamber view with visualization of right ventricular free wall, right atrium, interatrial septum, and inferior vena cava are emphasized. The transducer may be rotated to produce a short-axis view showing right ventricular inflow and outflow. The short-axis cross sections of aorta and left ventricle may also be imaged.

A "ROUTINE" PROTOCOL FOR EXAMINATION IN AN ADULT PATIENT

A comprehensive transthoracic echo evaluation should include a routine format so as to diagnose clinically unsuspected pathologies in addition to answering a clinical question. The approach should be modified to image unusual pathologies.

Parasternal Long-axis View

1. Visualize the ascending aorta 2 to 5 cm downstream from the aortic valve.
2. Image the LV, LA, mitral and aortic valves. Maximize LV cavity dimensions.
3. Color flow image of aortic and mitral valves.

Right Ventricular Inflow View

1. Image the RV, RA, and the tricuspid valve.
2. Color flow image of the tricuspid valve.
3. Continuous-wave Doppler of tricuspid regurgitation, if proper alignment is obtained.

Short-axis Views

1. Image the basal views to include aortic root and RV outflow and pulmonary artery.
2. Color flow image of pulmonic valve and pulmonary artery, aortic valve and tricuspid valve, left atrium and interatrial septum.
3. Image at mitral valve.
4. Obtain color flow image of the mitral orifice.
5. Image at papillary muscle level.

Apical Views

1. Obtain four-chamber cross section.
2. Rotate through two-chamber and apical long-axis cross sections.
3. Obtain color flow image through all the cross sections.
4. Obtain pulsed-wave Doppler tracing of the open mitral valve.
5. Obtain pulsed-wave Doppler of pulmonary veins.
6. Obtain pulsed-wave Doppler of LV outflow tract.
7. Obtain continuous-wave Doppler—lesion specific (tricuspid regurgitation/mitral regurgitation/mitral stenosis/aortic regurgitation/aortic stenosis).

Subcostal Views

1. Image four-chamber view.
2. Obtain color flow image to assess interatrial septum and tricuspid regurgitation.
3. Obtain short-axis view.
4. Obtain IVC at held inspiration.
5. Image abdominal aorta.

Suprasternal View

1. Image aortic arch.
2. Complete a lesion-specific Doppler examination.

SEGMENTAL CORONARY PERFUSION

Echocardiography is extremely versatile in assessment of regional myocardial function employing the various cross-sectional images. This provides a basis for its application in coronary artery disease, largely characterized by segmental dysfunction relating to a diseased coronary artery branch. The pattern of coronary arterial tree and perfusion of seg-

ments subserved by a given artery and its branches is variable. However, a general pattern of coronary flow distribution can be recognized. Figures 1 through 6 provide a framework for commonly observed coronary artery flow distribution in various segments visualized using the standard cross sections as described above (see also Color Plates 2–7 following page 294. The coronary perfusion territories show considerable variations among patients; however, a general pattern of distribution is generally predictable.

ECHOCARDIOGRAPHIC ASSESSMENT OF LEFT VENTRICULAR SYSTOLIC FUNCTION

Assessment of left ventricular (LV) systolic function is important in clinical cardiology. It is commonly expressed in terms of its ejection fraction (EF), which is the fraction of the LV end-diastolic volume that is emptied during systole. The EF can be obtained by contrast or radionuclide left ventriculography, by echocardiography, or by magnetic resonance imaging. Echocardiography has the advantage of being a portable technique that is noninvasive and relatively

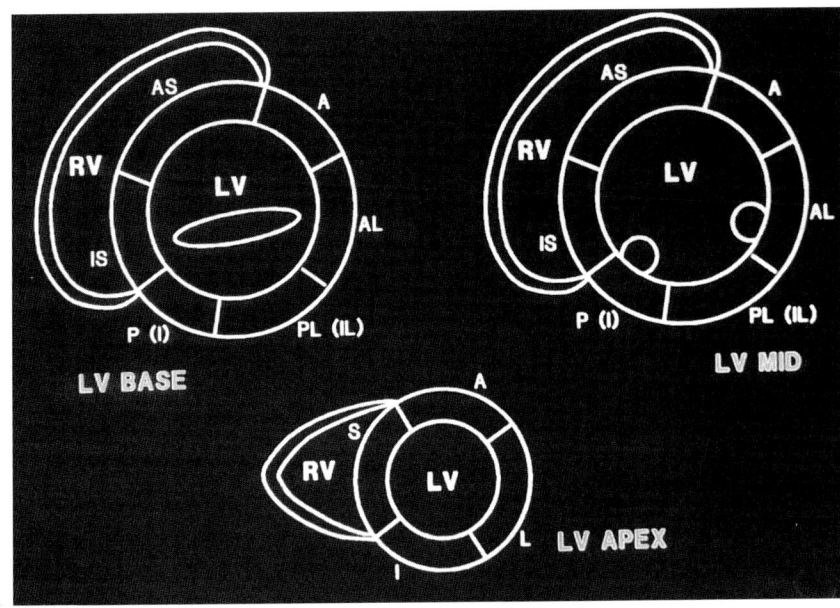

A

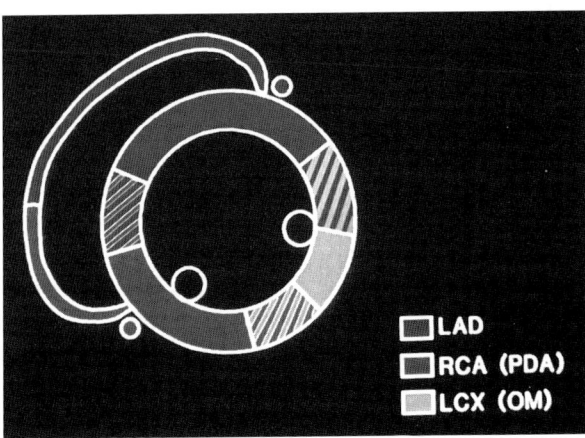

B

FIG. 1. A: Short-axis cross sections with wall segments at basal, mid- and apical levels. **B:** The segments at papillary muscle level and expected coronary distribution. The cross-hatched areas in this and subsequent five figures represent overlapping perfusion territories. *A*, anterior; *AL*, arterolateral; *AS*, anterior septum; *I*, inferior; *IL*, inferolateral; *IS*, inferior septum; *LAD*, left anterior descending artery; *LCX*, left circumflex; *LV*, left ventricle; *OM*, obtuse marginal; *P*, posterior; *PDA*, posterior descending artery; *PL*, posterolateral; *RCA*, right coronary artery; *RV*, right ventricle. (See also Color Plate 2 following page 294.)

METHOD	GEOMETRIC ASSUMPTION	FORMULA

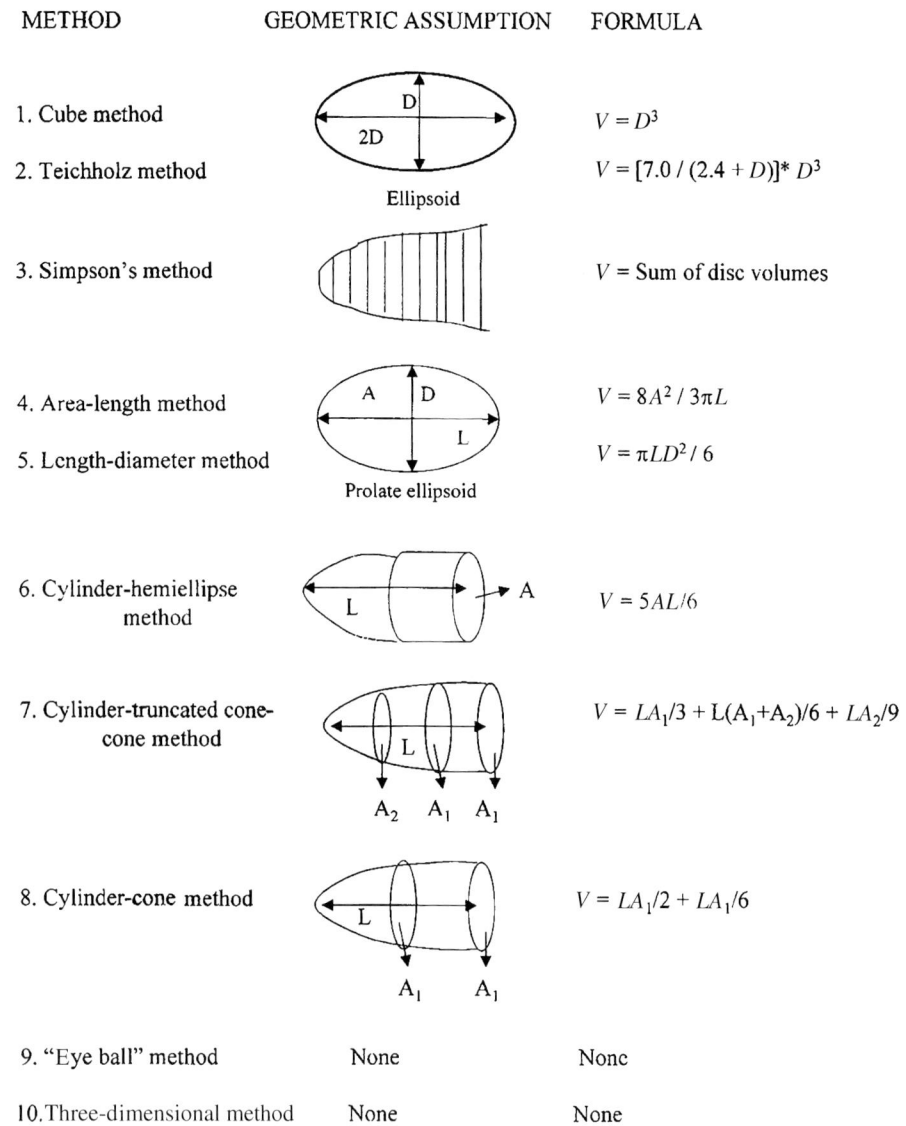

1. Cube method — Ellipsoid — $V = D^3$

2. Teichholz method — $V = [7.0 / (2.4 + D)]* D^3$

3. Simpson's method — $V = $ Sum of disc volumes

4. Area-length method — Prolate ellipsoid — $V = 8A^2 / 3\pi L$

5. Length-diameter method — $V = \pi L D^2 / 6$

6. Cylinder-hemiellipse method — $V = 5AL/6$

7. Cylinder-truncated cone-cone method — $V = LA_1/3 + L(A_1+A_2)/6 + LA_2/9$

8. Cylinder-cone method — $V = LA_1/2 + LA_1/6$

9. "Eye ball" method — None — None

10. Three-dimensional method — None — None

FIG. 7. Figure illustrating the various geometric models used in the calculation of left ventricular volumes and the associated mathematical formulas.

The mode methods (cube and Teichholz methods) try to give the volume, which is a three-dimensional physical quantity, from a single dimension. These equations tend to be inaccurate in the presence of segmental abnormalities of LV contraction.

Simpson's Method

This method divides the LV into stack discs and summates the disc volumes to arrive at the volume. This can be done using the single (four-chamber) or biplane (four- and two-chamber) images of the LV. The three-dimensional method does not make any geometric assumptions.

Area-length Method

This method assumes a prolate ellipsoid LV geometry as shown in Figure 1.

Length-diameter Methods

This again assumes prolate ellipsoid geometry.

Cylinder-hemiellipse Method

As the name suggests, LV is assumed to be composite of a cylinder and a hemiellipse with equal lengths.

Cylinder-truncated Cone-cone Method

LV is a composite of a cylinder, a truncated cone, and a cone of equal lengths.

Cylinder–cone Method

LV is viewed as a composite of a cylinder and a cone.

to arrive at an EF. The accuracy is dependent on operator experience.

Quantitative Three-dimensional Methods

Dynamic three-dimensional LV volume may be computed from a variety of methods (Fig. 8). The three-dimensional data can be obtained either by reconstruction from multiple two-dimensional planes along with precise spatial and temporal registration of the images or in a three-dimensional format using the volumetric scanner developed.

Left Ventricular Fractional Shortening

Fractional shortening (FS) is derived from the LV minor axis M-mode and is obtained as (*LV end-diastolic diameter–LV end-systolic diameter*)/*LV end-diastolic diameter* (Fig. 9). The normal value is 0.26 to 0.40. Like the EF, it is also load dependent.

Left Ventricular Circumferential Fiber Shortening

Left ventricular circumferential fiber shortening (V_{cf}) is a measure of the rate of shortening of LV circumferential fibers and is given by the formula *FS/LVET* where *LVET* is

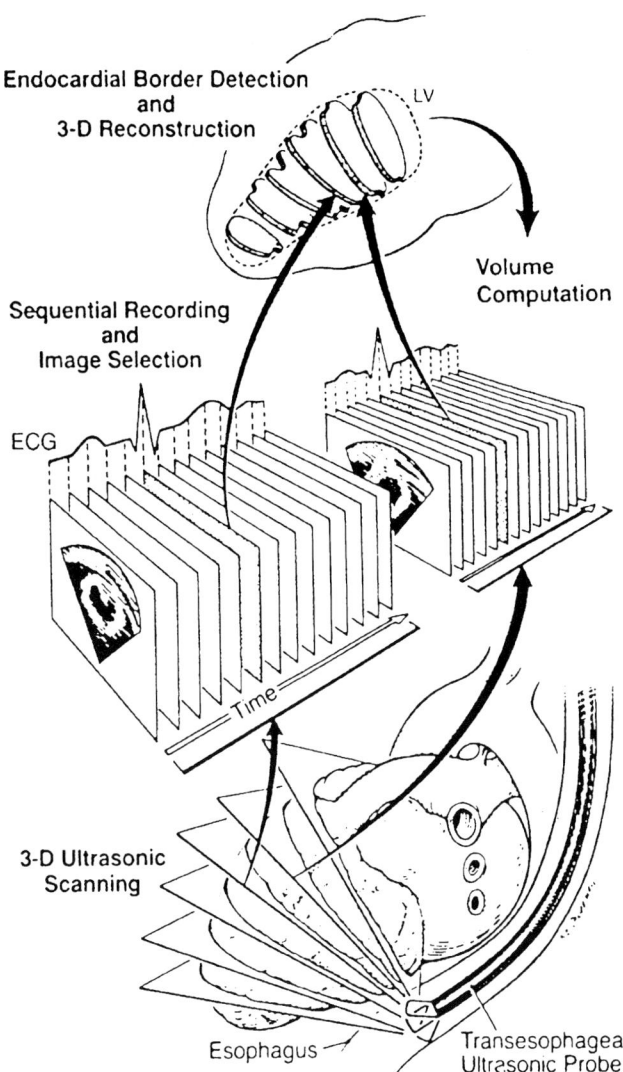

FIG. 8. Principles of three-dimensional computation of left ventricular volume. The dynamic three-dimensional data cube is constructed from a series of two-dimensional images with precise temporal registration in the cardiac cycle and spatial registration. Respiratory gating is necessary to eliminate spatial misregistration. From this data cube, LV volume can be computed using Simpson's method by summating the true volumes of individual discs. This method is independent of any geometric assumptions and should be accurate irrespective of LV shape distortions. The volumetric scanner captures the three-dimensional data online and obviates the need for reconstruction from two-dimensional images. (From ref. 11, with permission.)

Qualitative Three-dimensional or the ''Eye Ball'' Method

Visual estimation of EF from multiple tomographic planes by an experienced echocardiographer agrees very well with that obtained by radionuclide ventriculography. The interpreter constructs a three-dimensional image of the LV in his own mind from the multiple tomographic planes

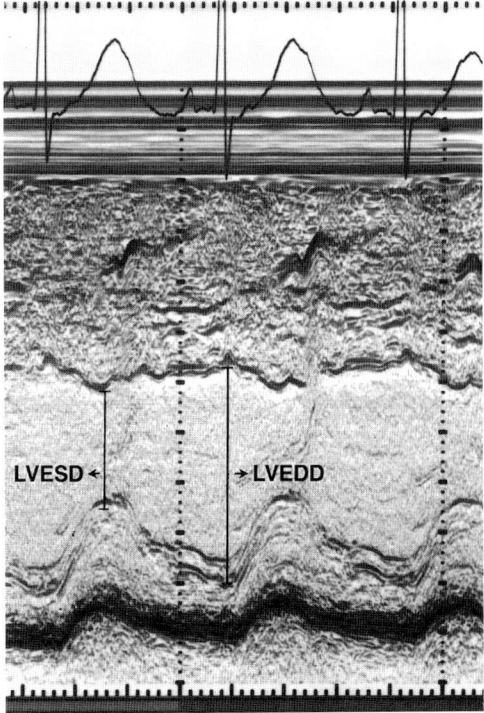

$$FS = \frac{LVEDD - LVESD}{LVEDD} = \frac{4.4 - 2.4}{4.4} = 0.45$$

FIG. 9. Calculation of LV fractional shortening (FS). From the LV M-mode, this calculation is obtained as the LV minor axis shortening as a fraction of its end-diastolic diameter (LVEDD). *LVESD,* LV end-systolic diameter. Normal FS is 0.25 to 0.40.

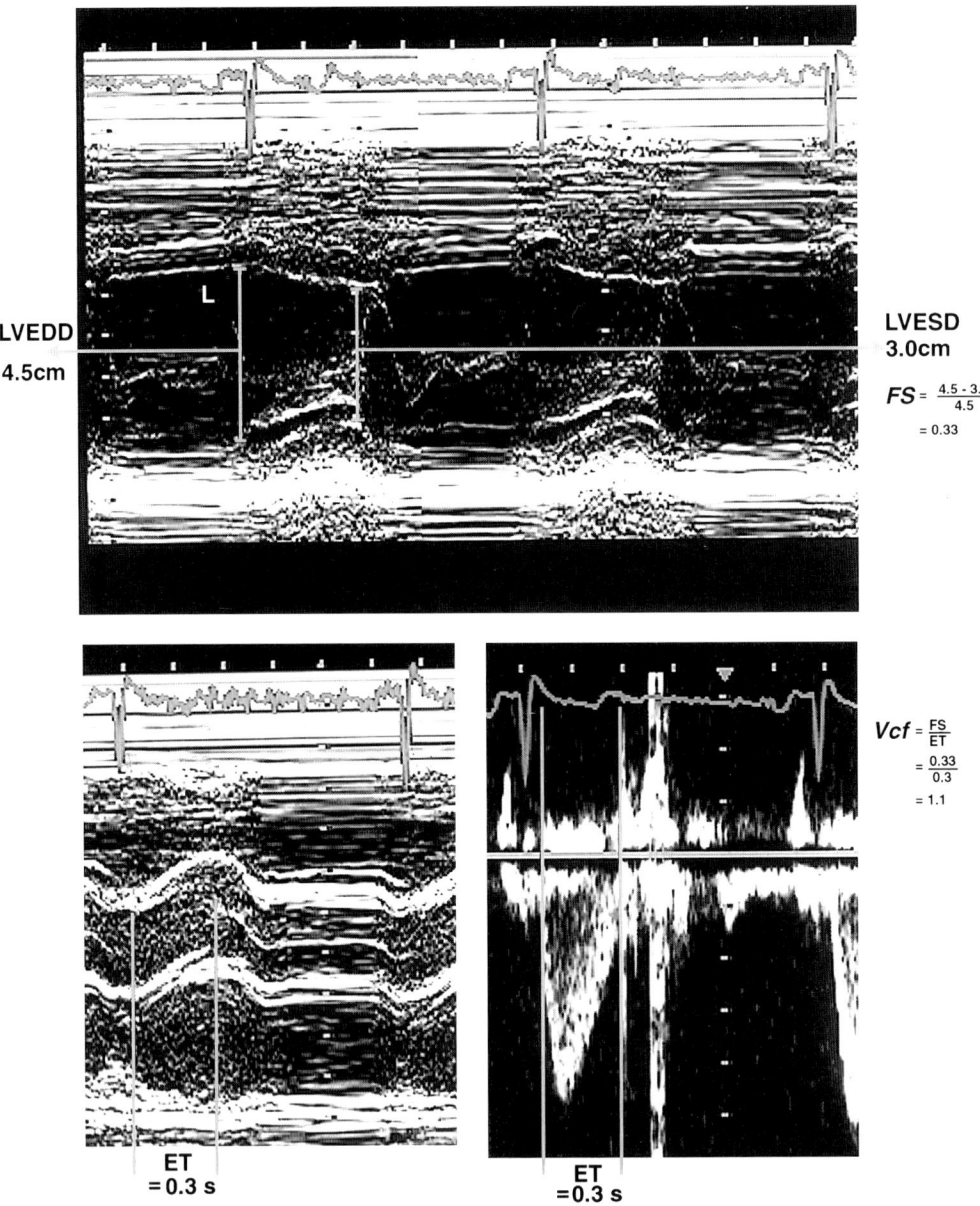

FIG. 10. Calculation of velocity of circumferential fiber shortening (V_{cf}): This is the ratio of FS and the LV ejection time (ET). ET may be obtained as the duration of aortic valve opening on the aortic M-mode or as the duration of LV ejection from the aortic Doppler. Normal V_{cf} is 0.9 to 1.1 circumferences per second.

the LV ejection time measured in seconds (Fig. 10). LVET may be obtained from the duration of opening of the aortic valve by its M-mode examination or from the duration of LV ejection by the Doppler examination of the aortic flow. Normal V_{cf} is about 0.9 to 1.1 circumferences per second.

Left Ventricular Area Change during the Cardiac Cycle Using Automatic Endocardial Border Detection Techniques

This is an approach based on backscatter technology and is available for endocardial border detection and tracking continuously. Using these techniques, one can continuously

record the LV area in a given view or volume with geometric assumption. EF and the first derivative volume over time (dV/dt) can be computed from this (Fig. 11). The accuracy of this method depends on accurate gain setting and true definition of the area of interest.

Left Ventricular Volume, Ejection Fraction, Fractional Shortening, or V_{cf} corrected for Left Ventricular End-systolic Pressure or Wall Stress

The LV end-systolic volume, EF, FS or V_{cf} are affected by the afterload reflected by the LV end-systolic pressure or more accurately by the LV end-systolic wall stress

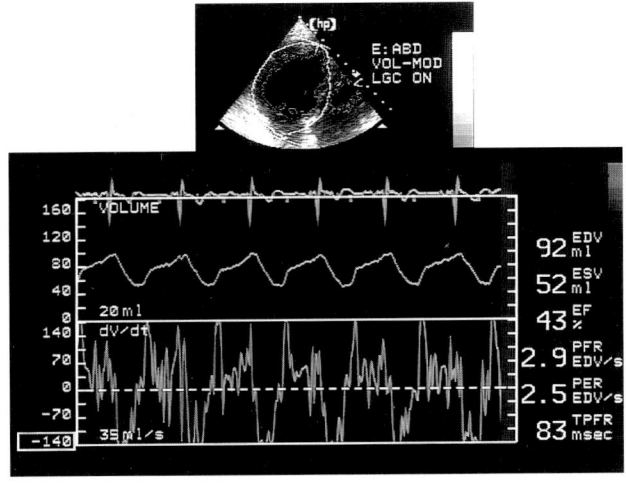

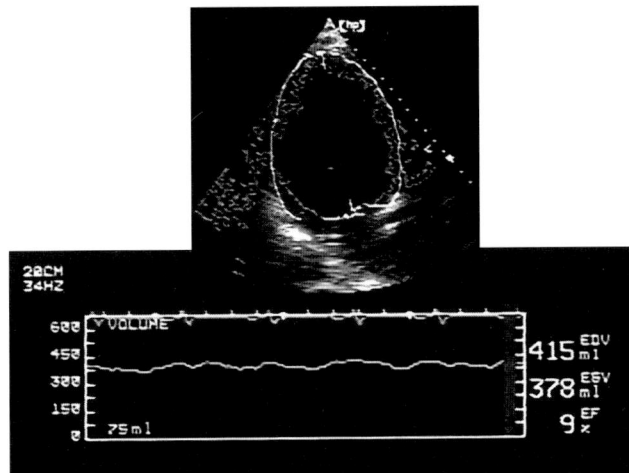

FIG. 11. LV volume changes during the cardiac cycle using automatic border detection in two different patients. The endocardial border can also be tracked with other techniques in an automated fashion. This technique gives single-plane LV volume using any of the formulas and also the instantaneous and peak LV filling and ejection rates. **A:** LV volume is continuously plotted as a function of time and, in this example, the EF is 43%. The tracing in the bottom shows the LV filling and ejection rates on the time axis (*dV/dt*). **B:** In this patient, the LV is grossly dilated and has an EF of 9%.

(ESWS). An increased afterload would increase the LV end-systolic volume but reduce its EF, FS, and V_{cf}. A drop in afterload would have the opposite effect and this needs to be kept in mind when LV loading is markedly altered. Nomograms for various levels of afterload are available in the literature.

For computation of LV ESWS, the cuff blood pressure and the carotid wave forms are recorded. The systolic and diastolic pressures are assigned to the peak and the nadir of the carotid wave form assigning pressure to the *Y*-axis. The resulting wave form has been shown to correlate well with the central aortic pressure with the incisura representing the endsystolic pressure. The LV ESWS is calculated as follows:

$$ESWS = [(1.35) \cdot P_{es} \cdot D_{es}]/[4h_{es}(1 + h_{es}/D_{es})]$$

where P_{es} is the aortic end-systolic pressure, D_{es} is the LV end-systolic diameter, and h_{es} is the mean LV systolic wall thickness. In this equation, 1.35 is the factor used to convert pressure in mm Hg to g/cm^2, and $(1 + h_{es}/D_{es})$ is the geometric correction factor.

LV Volume, EF, FS, or V_{cf} Response to Induced Changes in LV End-systolic Pressure or Wall Stress (LV Contractility)

For example, with an induced increase in ESWS, FS falls minimally in a normal ventricle and the FS / ESWS slope could be used as a measure of myocardial contractility (Fig. 12). Nomograms with 95% confidence intervals for the relationship between FS and LV ESWS have been published. From this, one can roughly evaluate the appropriateness of the FS for patients' ESWS without methoxamine challenge. If the V_{cf} is used instead of FS, the equation for the regression line is as follows:

$$V_{cf} = -0.0045 \cdot ESWS + 1.36$$

In a similar way, the relationship between rate corrected V_{cf} or FS and ESWS can be obtained.

Preejection Indices Including Left Ventricular dP/dt

The LV preejection period and the isovolumic contraction period are prolonged with LV dysfunction, but not used routinely in clinical practice. However, with better understanding of the applications of Doppler, it has been possible to reconstruct LV systolic pressure in subjects with mitral regurgitation using the simplified Bernoulli equation, from

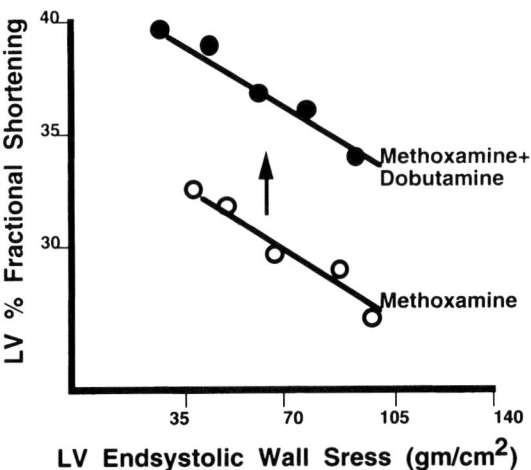

FIG. 12. Assessment of LV contractile function for a given level of inotropy and its contractile reserve. The LV fractional shortening is inversely related to its end-systolic wall stress, which can be increased with methoxamine infusion. Upward shift of this relationship with dobutamine infusion suggests the presence of contractile reserve. Fractional shortening may be substituted by V_{cf} or EF.

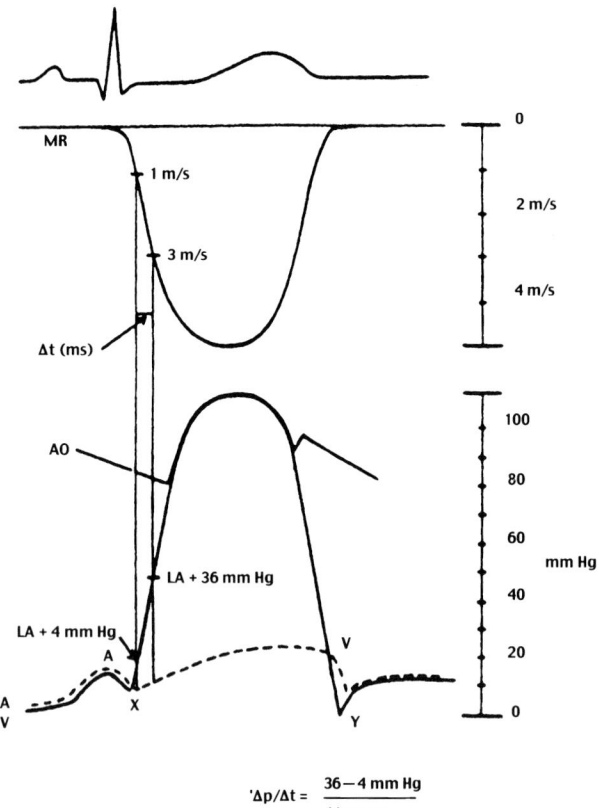

$$'\Delta p/\Delta t = \frac{36-4 \text{ mm Hg}}{\Delta t \text{ msec}}$$

FIG. 13. Calculation of the rate of LV pressure rise from the mitral regurgitation signal: The time (Δ t) taken for the mitral regurgitation (MR) velocity to rise from 1 to 3 m/sec is measured. Assuming constant left atrial (LA) pressure, this corresponds to a rise in LV/LA pressure gradient is from 4 to 36 mm Hg using simplified Bernoulli equation. Assuming that there is relatively little change in the LA pressure during this period, this would amount to a net rise in the LV pressure of 32 mm Hg. Hence, 32/Δ t gives the average rate of rise in LV pressure during early systole, which is referred to as *LV dP/dt*.

Though not instantaneous, it correlates very well with instantaneous *LV dP/dt*. *LV dP/dt* is a good indicator of myocardial contractile function, but is also dependent on preload, heart rate, and the sequence of LV contraction. It is increased by increases in heart rate and preload and is reduced in the presence of left bundle-branch block or LV pacing. (From ref. 12, with permission.)

which left ventricular $\Delta P/\Delta$ t can be obtained (Fig. 13). A simple assessment of the rate of rise of LV systolic pressure in the preejection period can be obtained by measuring the time (Δ t) taken for the mitral regurgitation velocity to rise from 1 to 3 m/s, which corresponds to a rise in LV pressure of 32 mm Hg assuming that the left atrial pressure does not rise significantly during this period (2). The LV $\Delta P/\Delta t$ would approximately be 32 / Δt. It is an isovolumic index and is unaffected by LV afterload, but is likely to be affected by preload, contractility, heart rate, sympathetic tone, and the sequence of LV activation as left bundle branch block. This measurement of LV performance is not truly isovolumic in

the presence of mitral regurgitation but does measure muscle function in the preejection phase of systole. The $\Delta P/\Delta t$ in a normal subject exceeds 1200 mm Hg/s/s and a value of less than 1000 correlates with depressed function.

Left Ventricular Long-axis Shortening

During systole, LV shortens in both its short and long axis reducing the size of its cavity. Downward systolic excursion of the mitral annulus during systole is a measure of its long axis shortening and the mean excursion of the medial and lateral parts of the anulus correlates well with radionuclide LV ejection fraction (Fig. 14). Normal excursion of the mitral anulus averages about 13 to 18 mm and can be measured by an M-mode from the LV apex passing through the annulus.

Myocardial Velocities Using Doppler Tissue Imaging

Doppler tissue imaging allows recording of mitral annular velocities during systole and diastole as shown in Figure 15. Mitral annular descent velocity correlates with EF determined by radionuclide ventriculography. In one study, the 6-site mean mitral annular descent velocity correlated with radionuclide ejection fraction (r = 0.86, ejection fraction in % = 8.2 × Mitral Annular Descent Velocity + 3). The average mitral annular velocity of >5.4 cm/s was 88% sensitive and 97% specific for an ejection fraction of >50%.

ECHOCARDIOGRAPHIC ASSESSMENT OF LEFT VENTRICULAR DIASTOLIC FUNCTION

Comprehensive evaluation of LV diastolic function would ideally consist of assessment of its early diastolic relaxation, the late diastolic stiffness, the filling pressures and the LV diastolic pressure profile (3). This can only be obtained by using high fidelity LV pressure recordings and simultaneous assessment of volumes. Abnormal LV diastolic function is also associated with abnormal LV filling patterns, changes in diastolic flow wave propagation inside the LV and abnormalities in myocardial velocities. Table 1 lists some of these echo-Doppler recordings, which are helpful in the evaluation of LV diastole.

Clues from Two-dimensional Echocardiography

Abnormal LV diastolic function may be suspected from the two-dimensional echocardiogram because of the presence of LV hypertrophy, the sparkling appearance of the myocardium, or isolated left atrial (LA) enlargement in the absence of LV systolic dysfunction or mitral valve disease. Left atrial enlargement in such a case indicates that the left atrium was presumably subjected to high diastolic pressure secondary to LV diastolic dysfunction (4–8).

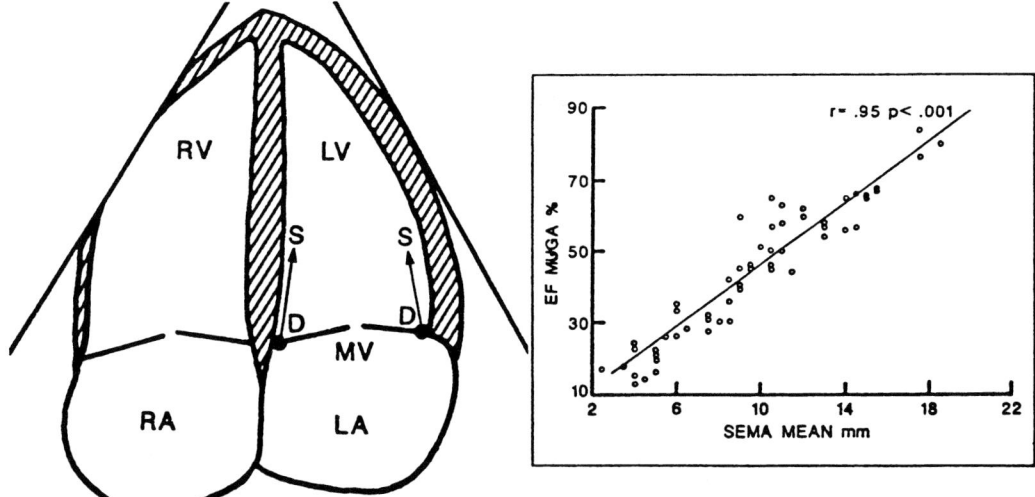

FIG. 14. Relationship between LV long-axis shortening and LV ejection fraction (EF). **Left:** The panel shows the measurement of LV long-axis shortening in terms of mitral annular descent during systole from *D* to *S*. The mean systolic excursion of the medial and lateral portions of the mitral annulus (SEMA mean) correlated well with LV EF by multigated analysis (EF MUGA). *LA*, left atrium; *LV*, left ventricle; *MV*, mitral valve; *RA*, right atrium; *RV*, right ventricle. (From ref. 13, with permission.)

Examination of Mitral and Pulmonary Venous Flow Velocity Profiles

Using the pulsed-wave Doppler technique, mitral and pulmonary flows are recorded from the apical four-chamber view. The sample volume is placed at the tips of the open mitral leaflets to record the transmitral diastolic flow velocities. The normal profile consists of an early rapid filling wave (E wave) and a less prominent flow wave associated with atrial contraction (A wave). The mechanism of genesis of these flow waves is related to the transmitral pressure-flow relationship. The E /A velocity ratio is generally greater than 1, and the deceleration time of the E wave varies from 160 to 240 ms (Fig. 12). The isovolumic relaxation time (IVRT) is measured from the closure of the aortic valve to the opening of the mitral valve, either with dual simultaneous M-modes or from aortic closure to mitral opening click with continuous-wave Doppler or from the end of LV ejection to onset of transmitral flow with a pulsed-wave Doppler sample placed in between the LV outflow and the mitral valve. Normal range for IVRT is 70 and 100 ms. The right upper pulmonary vein (PV) can be interrogated from the apical cross section in the majority of patients and the flow velocity profile can be recorded with sample volume placed about a centimeter inside the vein. The pulmonary venous flow pro-

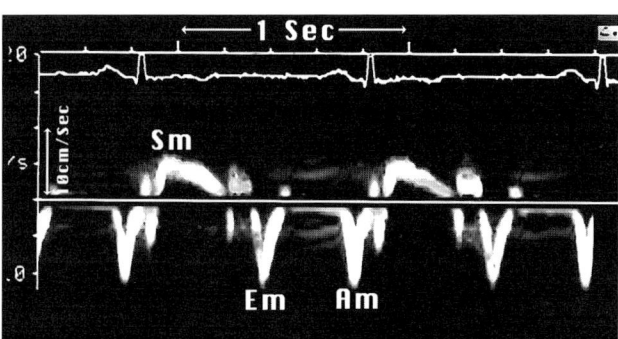

FIG. 15. Mitral annular velocities obtained by Doppler tissue imaging. Velocities recorded from the apical view include apically directed systolic velocity (S_m wave), atrially directed early myocardial lengthening velocity (E_m wave), and atrially directed late myocardial lengthening velocity (A_m wave). There were less prominent biphasic velocities during the isovolumic contraction and relaxation phases as well.

TABLE 1. *Echocardiographic assessment of left ventricle diastolic function*

1. Clues on two-dimensional echocardiography:
   LV hypertrophy
   Echo-reflective myocardium
   Left atrial enlargement in the absence of mitral valve disease
2. Mitral and pulmonary vein flow by Doppler:
   Isovolumic relaxation time
   E/A velocity ratio
   E-wave deceleration time
   E/A integral ratio
   S/D ratio
   Amplitude of AR wave
3. Pulmonary vein AR-wave duration minus mitral A-wave duration
4. Mitral aortic regurgitation velocity
   Peak negative *dP/dt*
   τ
5. Mitral E-wave transmission inside the LV
6. Mitral A-wave transmission inside the LV
7. Myocardial velocities using Doppler tissue imaging

AR, atrial reversal; *E/A*, early/atrial filling; *LV*, left ventricle; *S/D*, systolic/diastolic flow.

file consists of a predominant forward systolic wave (S wave). Occasionally, the S wave may be notched with two peaks, S1 and S2; the former is attributed to atrial relaxation and the latter to mitral annular descent. The forward diastolic flow (D wave) is generally less prominent except in young individuals. A reverse or retrograde flow wave (AR wave)

into the PV occurs during atrial contraction. The amplitude of the AR velocity wave is generally about 20 to 25 cm/s and its duration is less than that of the transmitral flow A wave. Table 2 lists the normal values of mitral and pulmonary vein flow derivatives in the adults.

Ventricular hypertrophy, myocardial ischemia, and early

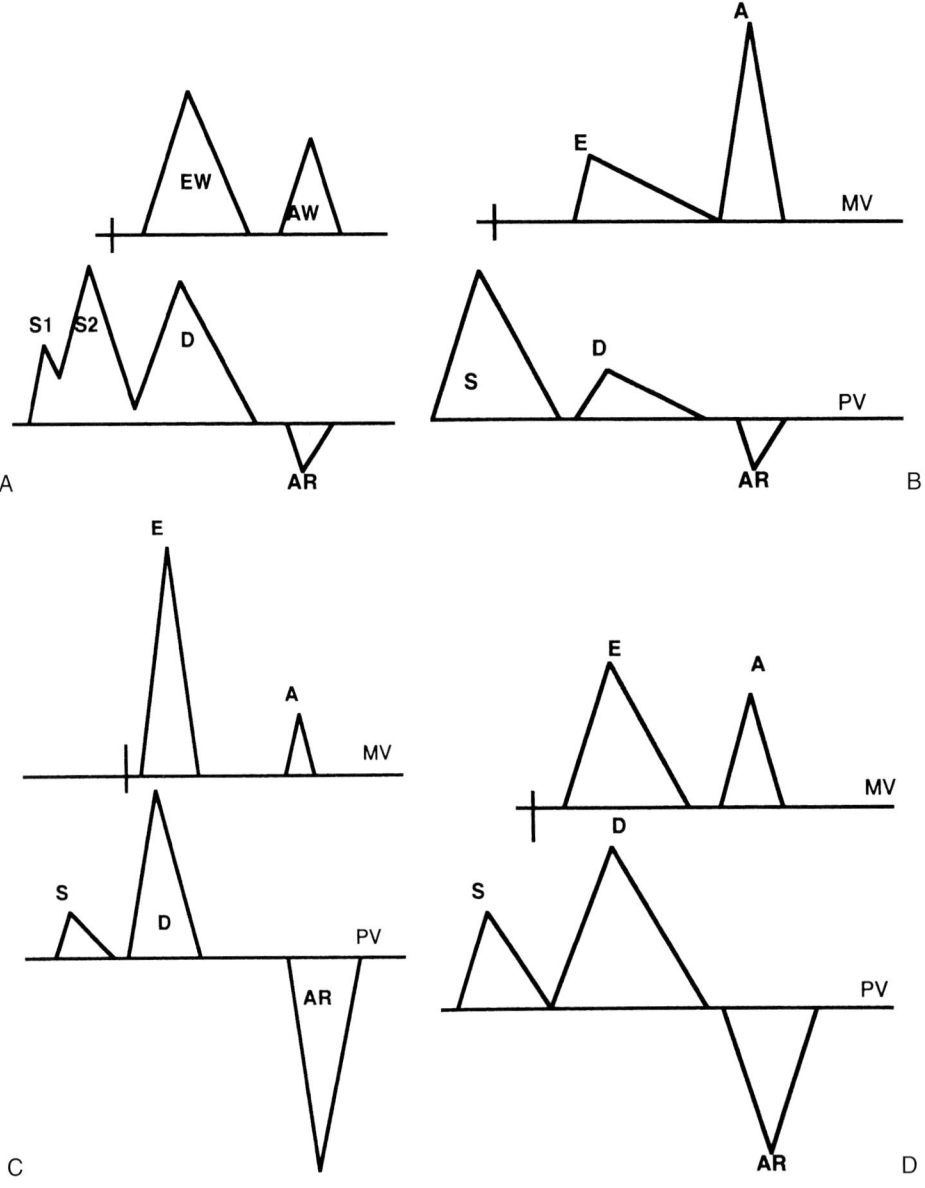

FIG. 16. Transmitral (**upper panel**) and pulmonary venous (**lower panel**) flow with different hemodynamic situations. **A:** Normal: isovolumic relaxation time (IVRT) between 70 and 100 msec, E/A velocity ratio generally >1, but lower in older individuals, E-wave deceleration time between 160 and 240 msec, S/D velocity and integral ratio >1 and AR wave velocity <25 cm/sec and duration less than that of the A wave. **B:** Pattern of abnormal relaxation with prolonged IVRT, reduced E/A velocity ratio, slow E-wave deceleration, and, when LV end-diastolic pressure is elevated, slightly increased AR wave velocity. **C:** High left-atrial pressure gives rise to short IVRT, E/A ratio >2, E-wave deceleration time <160 msec, and a small S wave and a large D wave on pulmonary vein tracing. The amplitude of the AR wave is exaggerated if left atrial systolic function is maintained. **D:** "Pseudonormal" mitral flow pattern with normal-looking mitral flow (here bordering on high left-atrial pressure pattern), but differentiation from normal is made by the amplitude of the AR wave, which is increased at 50 cm/sec in this example, and increased duration of the AR wave. (Adapted from ref. 14, with permission.)

TABLE 2. *Range of normal values of mitral and pulmonary vein flow derivatives in adults*

E-wave velocity amplitude	<100 cm/s
A-wave velocity amplitude	<100 cm/s
E/A velocity ratio	1–1.5
E/A integral ratio	2–3
E-deceleration time	60–240 ms
LV isovolumic relaxation time	70–100 ms
Pulmonary vein S/D velocity ratio	>1
Pulmonary vein AR-wave amplitude	<25 cm/s
AR wave minus A-wave duration	<0

AR, atrial reversal; *E/A*, early/atrial filling; *LV*, left ventricle; *S/D*, systolic/diastolic flow.

phases of myocardial disorders are often associated with slowed ventricular relaxation. This results in a decrease in the rate of ventricular pressure decline so that it takes longer for the mitral valve to open after the aortic valve closure, giving rise to prolongation of IVRT (Figs. 16, 17). Also, following atrio-ventricular pressure crossover, the pressure gradient between the atrium and the ventricle is small resulting in reduced rate of early filling. The early filling wave, E wave, is reduced in amplitude and its deceleration is prolonged. The atrial contraction is stronger as a result of increased residual atrial volume, resulting in a prominent A wave. The salient features of impaired early ventricular relaxation are prolonged IVRT (>100 ms), reduced E amplitude, increased A-wave amplitude, E/A velocity ratio less than 1, and prolonged E-wave deceleration time (>240

msec). The pulmonary venous flow may show a small D wave secondary to reduced early LV diastolic filling and occasionally a prominent AR wave when the LV enddiastolic pressure is elevated. This pattern of abnormal of ventricular relaxation is probably the commonest finding likely to be present as an early manifestation of LV diastolic dysfunction.

Advanced heart failure is associated with an increase in the mean left atrial (LA) pressure and a concomitant increase in the height of the v wave. This results in earlier mitral valve opening and a shorter IVRT. With other factors such as early ventricular relaxation being unchanged, the higher pressure during atrioventricular pressure crossover results in a steeper decline of atrial pressure (i.e., *v* to *y* descent) and higher instantaneous peak early diastolic pressure gradient across the mitral valve. This results in a more prominent early diastolic flow velocity peak (augmented E amplitude) and a more rapid deceleration rate as the augmented early filling rate increases ventricular diastolic pressure abolishing or attenuating the atrioventricular pressure difference. The subsequent atrial contraction is weaker from reduced atrial muscle contractility due to chronic dilation and increased atrial afterload. This pattern of short IVRT, prominent E wave, a more rapid deceleration rate with shortened deceleration time (<160 msec), decreased amplitude of A wave and increased E/A ratio is characteristic of high LV filling pressures (Fig. 16). This pattern has also been termed a "restrictive pattern" when seen in advanced cases of restrictive

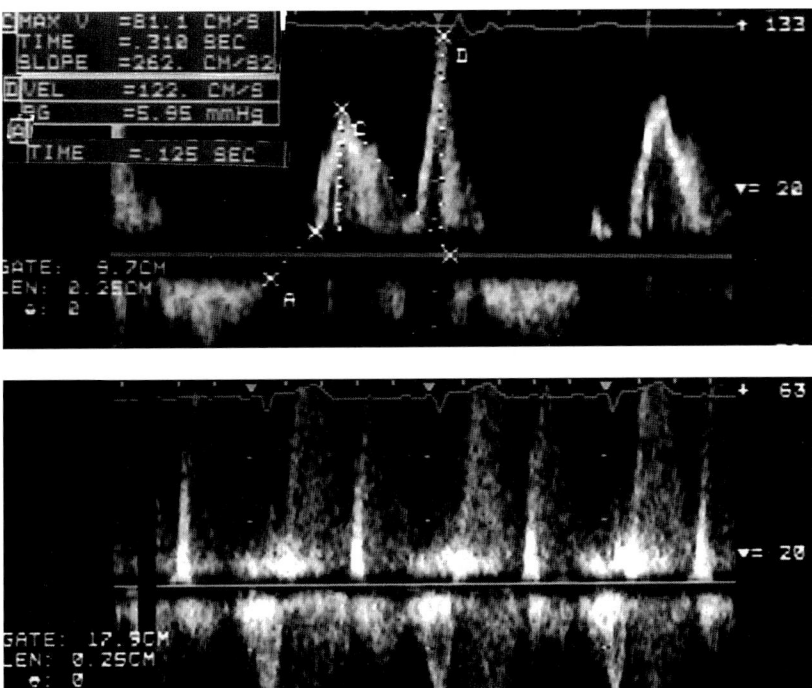

FIG. 17. A patient with abnormal LV relaxation. Note the prolonged LV isovolumic relaxation time of 125 ms, E/A velocity ratio <1, and the E-wave deceleration time of 310 ms. The pulmonary vein AR wave amplitude and duration are increased at 40 cm/s and 175 ms, respectively.

cardiomyopathy, but it is, in fact, representative of elevated left atrial pressure and is seen in most conditions causing left ventricular failure. The high LA pressure also results in a smaller S wave due to high LA systolic pressure and decreased anular descent and an augmented D wave in the PV flow profile (8). In the presence of normal atrial function, an increase in AR-wave amplitude is observed as a result of resistance to late diastolic LV filling. The LV end-diastolic pressure (in mm Hg) is roughly half the AR-wave amplitude in cm/s. It has also been shown that an increase in LV end-diastolic pressure results in abbreviation of the A wave and prolongation of AR-wave durations.

As patients with early diastolic dysfunction and prolonged early relaxation progress to develop increasing atrial filling pressures, the transmitral flow pattern will initially appear to "pseudonormalize," i.e., the E wave increases in amplitude and deceleration time is decreased to normal. This normal appearance of the transmitral flow is a result of combined effects of abnormal relaxation and moderately elevated LA pressure. A distinguishing feature is that the AR wave in the pulmonary vein is generally augmented both in its amplitude and duration secondary to raised LV end-diastolic pressure (Figs. 16,18). The other features that may help to differentiate pseudonormal from the normal pattern include a slower mitral E-wave propagation, reduced early mitral annular ascent velocity, and the response of the mitral flow to preload reduction as with venous cuff occlusion, nitroglycerine administration, or Valsalva maneuver. The pseudonormal pattern would change to the pattern of abnormal relaxation with prolonged E-deceleration time (Table 3).

The Doppler mitral inflow waveform and the E/A velocity ratio are also influenced by a complex interaction of loading conditions, heart rate, and P-R interval as well as relaxation abnormalities, and myocardial stiffness as summarized in

TABLE 3. *Features of pseudonormal as compared to normal mitral flow pattern*

1. Increased pulmonary vein AR-wave duration compared to that of the mitral E wave
2. Slowed E-wave transmission inside the LV
3. Reduced mitral annular E_m wave velocity
4. Abnormal relaxation pattern with preload reduction

AR, atrial reversal; *LV*, left ventricle.

Table 4. The E/A velocity ratio is reduced not only with abnormal relaxation, but with reduced preload (LA pressure), tachycardia, increased P-R interval, increased blood pressure and LV end-systolic volume or with reduced LV recoil. The atrial contribution depends upon its mechanical function and its afterload in terms of LV pre–A-wave diastolic pressure. It is also reduced immediately after electrical cardioversion for atrial fibrillation and the atrial mechanical performance improves gradually over days or weeks. It has been shown that the pattern of abnormal relaxation can normalize with the administration of verapamil; this normalization is not due to improvement in relaxation, but comes about through elevation of left atrial pressure secondary to worsening LV systolic function.

The effects of aging on Doppler indices of diastolic function can be summarized as follows: advancing age is normally associated with a reduction in the E-wave amplitude, with augmentation of the A wave, reduction in E/A velocity ratio, and prolongation of IVRT; an augmented A wave is associated with an audible fourth heart sound. On the other end of the age spectrum, children and younger adults manifest increased early filling with short E-wave deceleration time, which is associated with the physiological third heart sound. An increased E/A velocity ratio is physiological in children.

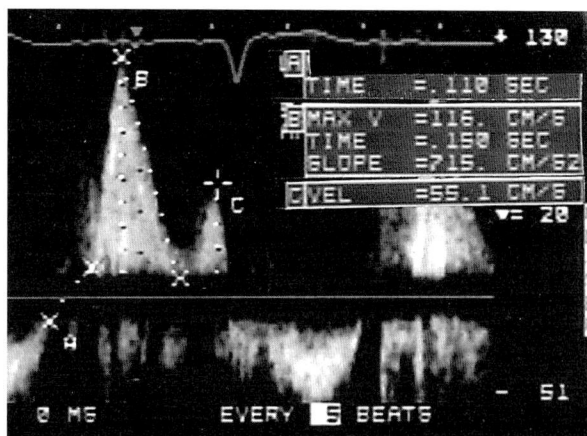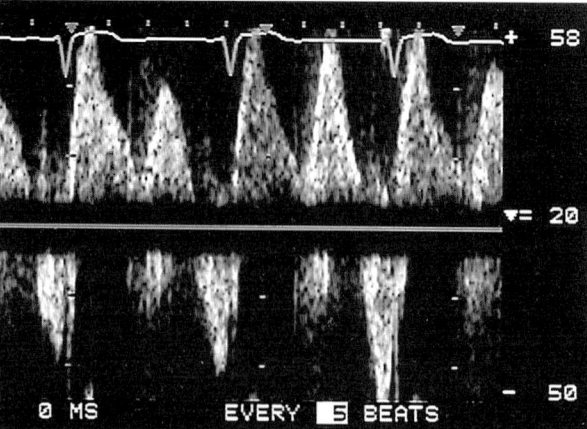

FIG. 18. An example of increased left atrial pressure with good atrial function. **Left panel:** Mitral flow showing IVRT of 110 msec, E-wave velocity of 116 cm/s, E-wave deceleration time of 150 msec, A-wave velocity of 55 cm/s, and the E/A velocity ratio of 2.1. **Right panel:** S-wave amplitude of 60 cm/s, D-wave amplitude of 45 cm/s, and AR-wave amplitude of 60 cm/s. The A-wave duration is 110 msec and that of the AR wave is 220 msec. This patient had a mean pulmonary artery wedge pressure of 24 mm Hg and LV end-diastolic pressure of 39 mm Hg.

TABLE 4. *Factors that affect the E/A velocity ratio*

1. LV relaxation	5. Heart rate
2. LV stiffness	6. P-R interval
3. LV elastic recoil	7. LV afterload
4. LA pressure (or LV preload)	

E/A, early/atrial filling; *LA*, left atrial; *LV*, left ventricle.

AR Duration Minus A-wave Duration (Δdur)

It has been shown by that the relative duration of the pulmonary vein AR wave and mitral A wave (Δdur) is related to LV end-diastolic pressure and LV pre–A-wave pressure (7). There was a positive correlation between this Doppler measure and the LV end-diastolic pressure ($r = 0.68$, $p < 0.001$) and LV A-wave pressure ($r = 0.70$, $p < 0.001$) as shown in Figure 19. The pulmonary vein AR-wave duration exceeding that of the mitral A-wave predicted LV end-diastolic pressure of greater than 15 mm Hg with a sensitivity of 85% and a specificity of 79%.

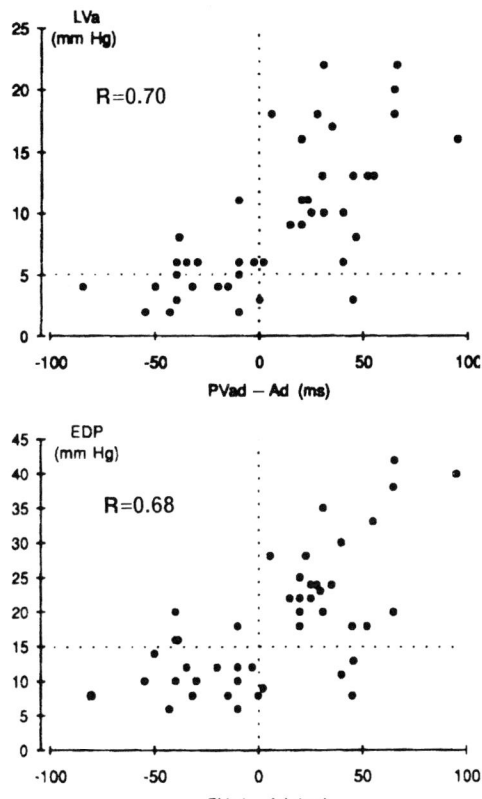

FIG. 19. Relationship between differences in the durations of pulmonary vein 'AR' wave (PVad) and transmitral 'A' wave (Ad), i.e., PVad minus Ad in milliseconds and the left ventricular (LV) end-diastolic pressure (EDP), and the amount of LV pressure rise associated with the A wave (LVa). P Vad longer than Ad identified subjects with an LVEDP >15 mm Hg with a high degree of sensitivity and specificity. (From ref. 7, with permission.)

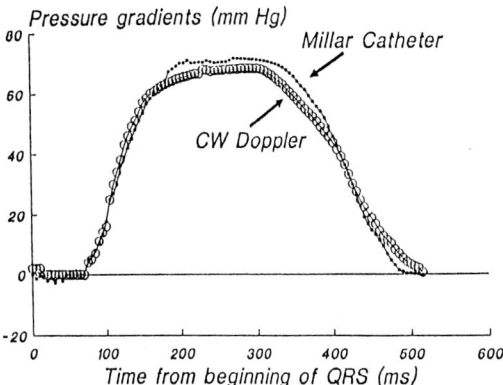

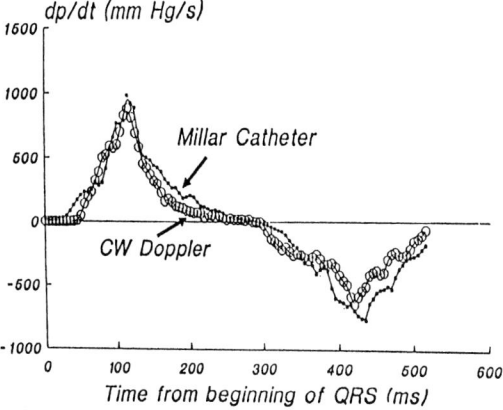

FIG. 20. *LV dP/dt* and τ from the mitral regurgitation signal. Applying simplified Bernoulli principle to the mitral regurgitation (MR) velocity profile (**top panel**), the LV–LA pressure gradient may be obtained. The LV pressure tracing is reconstructed from this by adding measured or estimated left atrial pressure. This LV pressure correlates closely with that measured by high fidelity LV pressure using Millar catheters. From this derived LV pressure profile, one can obtain positive and negative *dP/dt* (**bottom panel**) and τ. (From ref. 2, with permission.)

Determination of Negative dP/dt and τ from the Mitral and Aortic Regurgitation Velocity Profiles

In patients with mitral regurgitation (MR), it is possible to calculate rate of LV pressure rise during systole from the MR velocity signal. The MR velocity profile by continuous wave Doppler reflects the LV–LA pressure gradient during isovolumic contraction, ejection, and isovolumic relaxation periods. From the MR velocity signal, one can obtain the LV–LA pressure gradient throughout systole using the simplified Bernoulli equation. As shown in Figure 20, this can be transformed into LV pressure profile by adding a known LA pressure or an arbitrarily selected LA pressure. Chen et al. (2) have shown that from this reconstructed LV pressure, one can derive the peak negative *dP/dt* and τ, which correlate well with those obtained by high fidelity pressure recording. However, its accuracy in various clinical settings remains to be established. An average rate of fall in LV pressure during isovolumic relaxation can also be obtained as the

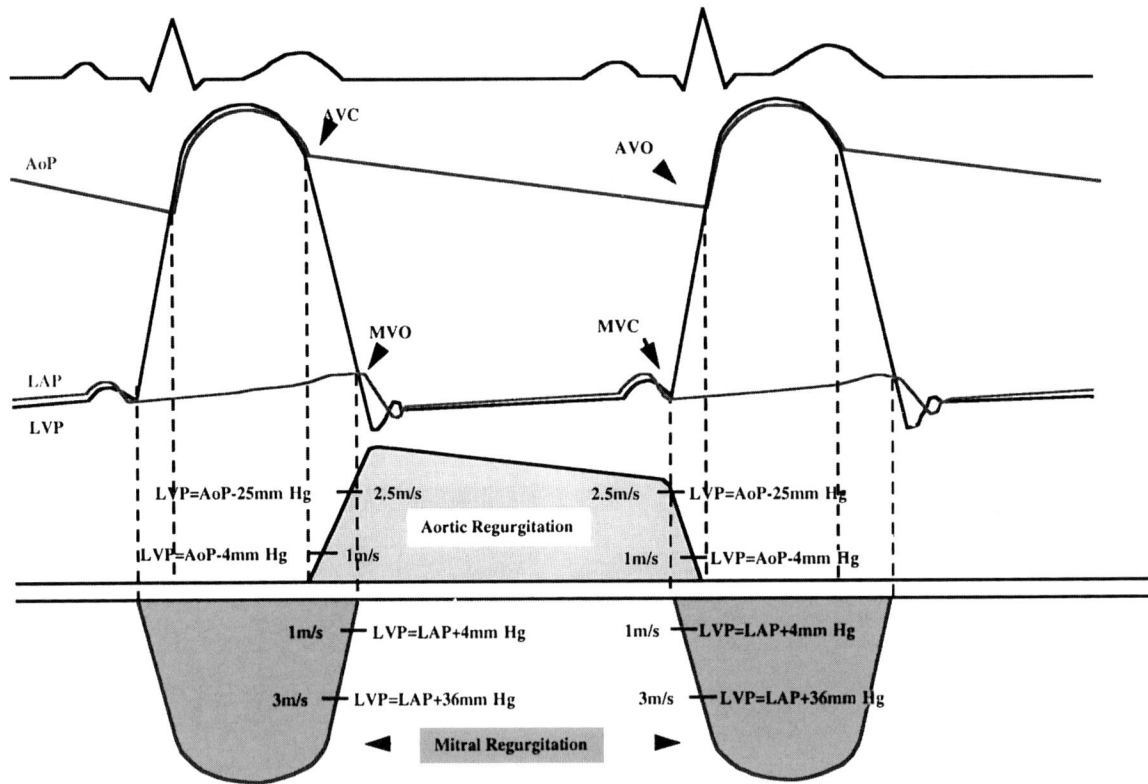

FIG. 21. Schematic illustrating derivation of *LV ΔP/Δ t* from the aortic regurgitation (AR) signal. The negative *LV ΔP/Δ t* from the AR signal was obtained by dividing the time taken for the AR velocity to rise from 1 to 2.5 m/s into 21 mm Hg, which is the amount of LV pressure drop between these two points on the AR signal, assuming the applicability of simplified Bernoulli equation to this situation and the absence of significant changes in the aortic pressures during this time. Using these assumptions, 1 m/s mark on the AR signal corresponds to aortic pressure minus 4 mm Hg and 2.5 m/s to aortic pressure minus 25 mm Hg. In a similar fashion, the LV positive *ΔP/Δ t* was obtained from the fast decelerating portion of the AR signal by dividing the time taken for the AR velocity to drop from 2.5 to 1 m/s into 21 mm Hg. The details of the derivation of left ventricular (LV) *ΔP/Δ t* from the mitral regurgitation signal is described in the text. *AoP*, aortic pressure; *AVC*, aortic valve closure; *AVO*, aortic valve opening; *LAP*, left atrial pressure; *LVP*, left ventricular pressure; *MVC*, mitral valve closure; *MVO*, mitral valve opening. (From ref. 15, with permission.)

ratio of 32 mm Hg to the time taken for the MR velocity to fall from 3 to 1 m/s.

In a similar fashion, the aortic regurgitation (AR) velocity profile reflects the pressure gradient between the aorta and LV during LV isovolumic relaxation period, its filling, and the isovolumic contraction period. As shown in Figure 21, this allows insights into rates of LV pressure fall and rise during the LV isovolumic relaxation and contraction periods, respectively.

Insights from Mitral E-wave Transmission inside the Left Venticle

The propagation of the mitral E wave inside the LV is slowed in those with abnormal relaxation. This leads to an increase in its transit time both to the LV apex and the LV outflow tract, and this can be measured using either a color M-mode of the LV inflow or using the pulsed-wave Doppler flow sampling at the mitral valve and the LV outflow tract. Stugaard et al. (16) measured the transit time of the peak of the early filling wave from the mitral valve to the LV apex using digitized color M-mode from the LV apex. They related this time interval to τ with which there was a strong positive correlation suggesting that the E-wave propagation as judged by computerized analysis of color M-mode is slow in patients with impaired LV relaxation (Figs. 22 and 23). As pseudonormal mitral flow pattern is a combination of abnormal relaxation and elevated left atrial pressure, this can be differentiated from the normal pattern by the presence of abnormally slow E-wave propagation (Fig. 24).

Mitral A-wave Transmission from LV Inflow to Outflow Tract

A series of recent studies in our laboratory have shown that the rate of transmission of the transmitral A wave from

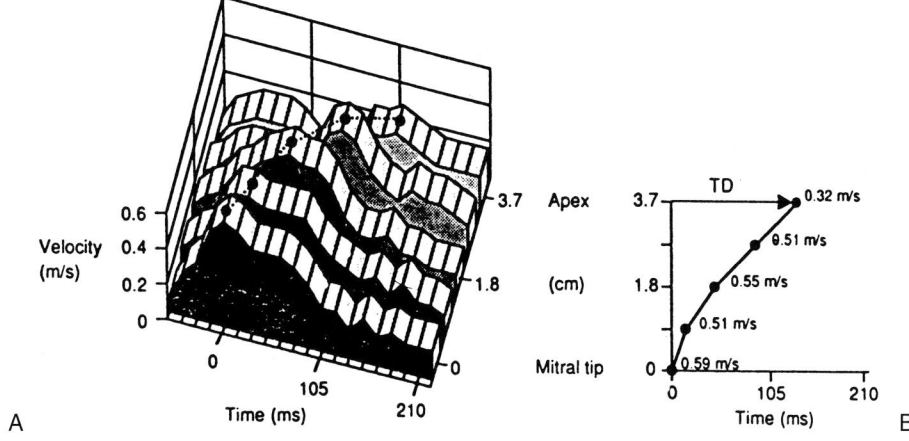

A

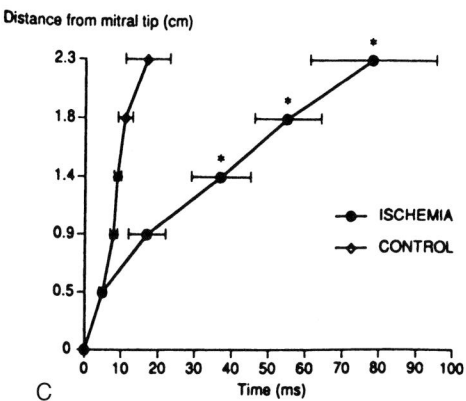

C

FIG. 22. Calculation of the time difference between occurrence of peak velocity in the apical region and at the mitral tip. **A:** Histogram presentation of color M-mode velocities at every 0.92 cm from the mitral valve to the apex. **B:** Computer analysis of the color M-mode recording showing the timing of peak velocity at the different depths from mitral tip toward apex. **C:** Graph showing time difference (TD) of peak filling velocity at the different depths from mitral tip toward apex in animals during control and induction myocardial ischemia. Note that with ischemia, TD is prolonged, and this was associated with an increase in τ, which is a measure of LV relaxation. (From ref. 16, with permission.)

the mitral valve to the LV outflow tract (recorded as AR wave) inside the LV is related to indices of LV late diastolic stiffness as shown in Figure 25. The peak-to-peak A-wave transit time (A–AR interval) of less than 45 ms is associated with increased LV stiffness (9). This phenomenon is similar to pressure and flow wave propagation in the arterial system where the rate of propagation of these wave fronts bears a strong positive relationship to arterial wall stiffness. We have also shown that the duration of the AR wave may be reduced compared to that of the mitral A wave in patients

with elevated LV end-diastolic and A-wave pressures. The A minus AR wave duration of 30 ms predicted an LV end-diastolic pressure of greater than 18 mm Hg with a high degree of accuracy.

Myocardial Velocities Using Doppler Tissue Imaging

Abnormal relaxation would conceivably reduce the rate of myocardial lengthening in early diastole and the E_m wave velocity has been found to be markedly reduced in patients

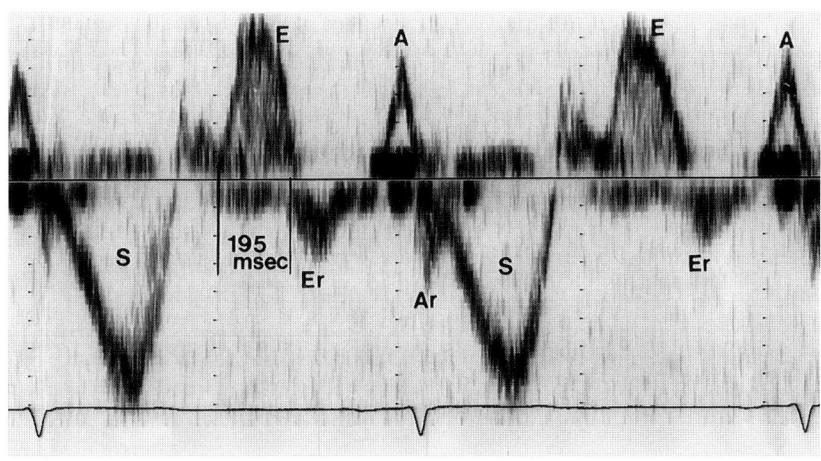

FIG. 23. Mitral E- and A-wave transit time to the LV outflow tract determined by the pulsed-wave Doppler technique. The mitral E-wave transit time (E–Er interval) is measured from the onset of the E wave to the onset of the Er wave in the LV outflow tract referenced to the R wave of the ECG. In a similar fashion, the A-wave transit time, the A–Ar interval, is measured between the onsets of A and Ar waves. The E–Er interval is lengthened with abnormal relaxation, and the A–Ar interval is shortened with elevated LV late diastolic stiffness. (From ref. 17, with permission.)

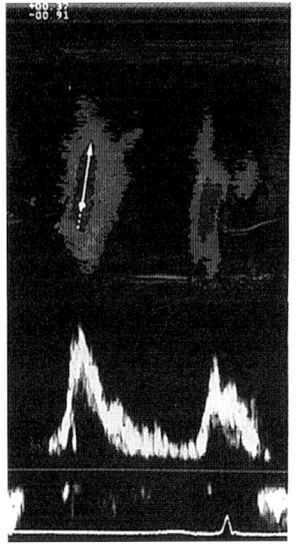
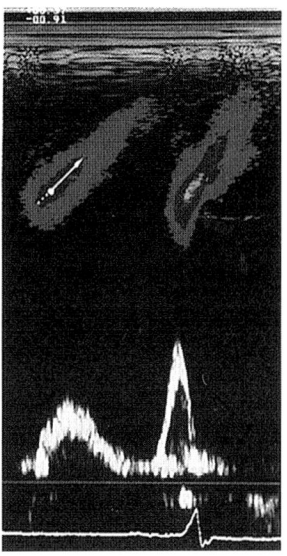
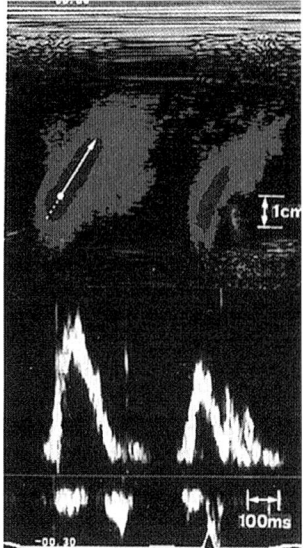

A–C

FIG. 24. Use of color M-mode to differentiate normal from pseudonormal mitral flow patterns. As can be seen from this illustration, the mitral E-wave propagation is slowed in those with a pseudonormal mitral flow pattern (**C**), indicating the presence of underlying abnormal LV relaxation. (From ref. 18, with permission.)

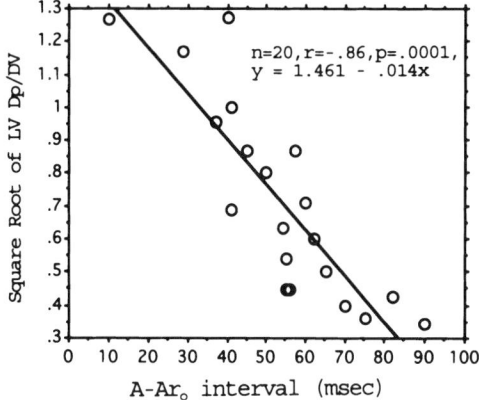

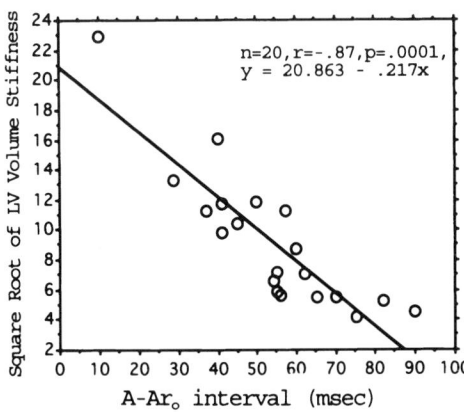

FIG. 25. Graphs showing significant negative correlation between A–Ar$_o$ interval (i.e., onset to onset mitral A-wave transit time) and the square root of *LV Dp/DV* and volume stiffness. A–Ar$_o$ interval had better correlation with measure of LV late diastolic stiffness compared to A–Ar$_p$ (peak-to-peak A-wave transit time) interval. (From ref. 9, with permission.)

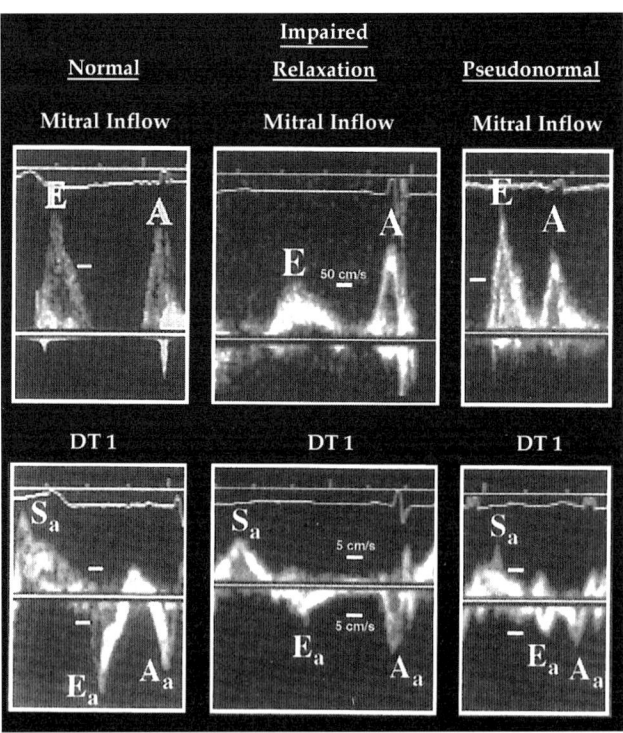

FIG. 26. Application of mitral annular DTI to differentiate normal from pseudonormal mitral filling pattern. Note the markedly reduced Ea (i.e., E$_m$) velocity in patients with pseudonormal and abnormal relaxation patterns. Also note that the E/Ea ratio is markedly increased in patients with a pseudonormal pattern. (From ref. 10, with permission.)

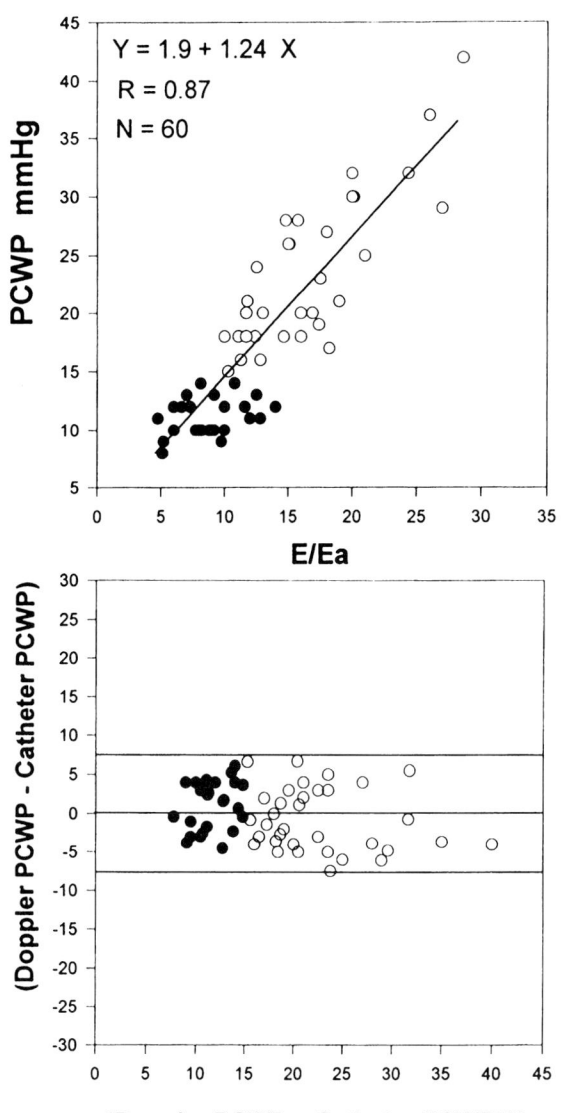

FIG. 27. Figure showing the relationship between E/Ea velocity ratio and pulmonary capillary wedge pressure (PCWP). Note that the PCWP is about 25% greater than the numerical value of this ratio. (From ref.10, with permission.)

with abnormal relaxation. Its amplitude bears a modest negative correlation to τ and has been used to differentiate normal from pseudonormal mitral flow patterns as shown in Figure 26. The E/E_m velocity ratio corrects the mitral E-wave velocity for the rate of LV relaxation and correlates very strongly

with the pulmonary capillary wedge pressure. The numerical value of the ratio roughly corresponds to the pulmonary capillary wedge pressure as shown in Figure 27.

GLOBAL INDEX OF MYOCARDIAL PERFORMANCE

Tei et al. have correlated a new index combining systolic and diastolic parameters (ICT and IRT/ET) with prognosis and outcome in varieties of myocardial disorders, including dilated and restrictive cardiomyopathies.

REFERENCES

1. Pai RG, Shah PM. Noninvasive assessment of cardiac hemodynamics and ventricular function. *Curr Probl Cardiol* 1995;20:681–772.
2. Chen C, Rodriguez L, Guerrero L, et al. Noninvasive estimation of instantaneous first derivative of left ventricular pressure using continuous wave Doppler echocardiography. *Circulation* 1991;83:2101–2110.
3. Shah PM, Pai RG. Diastolic heart failure. *Curr Probl Cardiol* 1992; 17:783–845.
4. Appleton CP, Hathe LK, Popp RL. Relation of transmitral flow velocity pattern to left ventricular diastolic function: new insights from a combined hemodynamic and Doppler cardiographic study. *J Am Coll Cardiol* 1988;12:426–440.
5. Klein AL, Tajik AJ. Doppler assessment of pulmonary venous flow in healthy subjects and in patients with heart disease. *J Am Soc Echocardiogr* 1991;4:379–392.
6. Choong CY, Herrmann HC, Weyman AE, et al. Preload dependence of Doppler-derived indexes of left ventricular diastolic function in humans. *J Am Coll Cardiol* 1987;10:800–808.
7. Rossvoll O, Hatle LK. Pulmonary venous flow velocities recorded by transthoracic Doppler ultrasound: relation to left ventricular diastolic pressures. *J Am Coll Cardiol* 1993;21:1687–1696.
8. Pozzoli M, Capomolla S, Pinna G, et al. Doppler echocardiography reliability predicts pulmonary artery wedge pressure in patients with chronic heart failure with and without mitral regurgitation. *J Am Coll Cardiol* 1996;27:883–893.
9. Pai RG, Suzuki M, Heywood JT, et al. The mitral 'A' wave velocity wave transit time to the outflow tract as a measure of left ventricular diastolic stiffness. *Circulation* 1994;89:553–557.
10. Nagueh SF, Middleton KJ, Kopelen HA, et al. Doppler tissue imaging: a noninvasive technique for evaluation of left ventricular relaxation and estimation of filling pressures. *J Am Coll Cardiol* 1997;30:1527–1533.
11. Martin, et al. 3-D LV volume computation. *Anesthesiology* 1989;70: 470–476.
12. Pai RG. *Circulation* 1990;82:514–520.
13. Pai RG. *Am J Cardiol* 1990;67:222–224.
14. Pai RG, Shah PM. *ACC Curr J Rev* 1994;3:30–33.
15. Pai RG, Stoletniy LN. *J Am Soc Echocardiogr* 1998;11:631–637.
16. Stugaard, et al. *Circulation* 1993;88:2705–2713.
17. Pai RG, Stoletniy LN. *J Am Soc Echocardiogr* 1997;10:532–539.
18. Takatsuji H, et al. *J Am Coll Cardiol* 1996;27:365–371.

CHAPTER 4

Transesophageal Echocardiography

Steven A. Goldstein

Remarkable advances have occurred in cardiovascular ultrasound over the past three decades, allowing it to become a cornerstone of modern cardiac diagnostic imaging. There has been a rapid evolution from M-mode echo (early 1970s) to two-dimensional echo (late 1970s) to conventional Doppler (early 1980s) to color Doppler (mid-1980s) and finally to transesophageal echocardiography (late 1980s). The last decade has seen the maturation of transesophageal echo (TEE). TEE overcomes many of the limitations of precordial echocardiography. High resolution images can be obtained because of the proximity of the esophagus to the heart and because high frequency transducers can be used. Improvements in instrument design, including biplane and multiplane probes, and the increasing recognition of its clinical applications have contributed to the enthusiastic acceptance of this technique as a complement to transthoracic echocardiography (TTE).

This chapter will briefly discuss the historical background and technical aspects of transesophageal echocardiography. It will focus on the clinical applications and diagnostic value of TEE compared to TTE, emphasizing the role of TEE in clinical decision-making and cost-effective patient care.

HISTORICAL PERSPECTIVE

In 1976, Frazin and associates first employed a single crystal M-mode transducer to perform TEE in patients with poor precordial images (1). This primitive device failed to gain widespread use because the thin coaxial cable limited its steerability and because of the limitations inherent in M-mode imaging. It represented, however, a landmark in diagnostic ultrasound. One year later, a transesophageal two-dimensional echo probe was introduced by Hisanaga et al.

(2). Their mechanical sector scanner was limited by its cumbersome probe and a limited field of view. In the early 1980s, smaller transducers and electronic phased-array technology connected to more flexible endoscopes from Germany and Japan prompted a significant increase in the interest in TEE.

In the United States, TEE probes were initially used by anesthesiologists for intraoperative monitoring of regional myocardial function in high-risk surgical patients and for the recognition of intracardiac air during neurosurgical procedures. Widespread use was limited as a result of the perception by cardiologists that patient discomfort from esophageal intubation outweighed the benefits of improved imaging. In Europe, on the other hand, investigators pioneered the use of TEE for the diagnosis of a variety of cardiac abnormalities in outpatients.

By the mid-1980s, further improvements in transducer technology and the recognition of broader clinical applications by investigators in Europe and Japan led to a renewed interest in TEE in the United States. Since 1987, the addition of color flow and continuous wave Doppler and the development of biplane, multiplane, and pediatric transducers have lead to a worldwide explosion in the use of TEE. Currently, in the year 2000, TEE is considered to be an extension of the complete TTE examination and no state-of-the-art echocardiography laboratory is without TEE capability.

TECHNIQUE AND ANATOMICAL VIEWS

Technique

Transesophageal echocardiography combines cardiac ultrasound and upper gastrointestinal endoscopy. The TEE probe consists of a modified flexible endoscope containing a miniature phased-array ultrasound transducer interfaced to a standard echocardiographic machine. Current transesophageal transducers are capable of M-mode and two-dimensional imaging and pulsed, continuous-wave and color flow

S. A. Goldstein: Noninvasive Cardiology Laboratory, Department of Cardiology, Washington Hospital Center, Washington, District of Columbia 20010.

Doppler. Controls at the proximal end of the scope allow anteroposterior and lateral flexion of the transducer at the distal end to optimize image quality and orientation. Single-plane probes are no longer recommended. Biplane probes have two perpendicular scanning probes, transverse (horizontal) and longitudinal (vertical), to permit imaging of two separate cross sections of the heart, although not simultaneously. Multiplane probes consist of a single imaging sector that can be rotated around the long-axis of the ultrasound beam, typically in a 180-degree arc, producing a continuum of tomographic imaging.

Transesophageal echocardiography can be performed in outpatients or inpatients, in the echocardiographic laboratory, the operating room, the intensive care unit, and cardiac catheterization laboratory. The technical and procedural aspects of TEE have been reviewed in great detail (3,4) and will only be briefly discussed here.

Although the procedure may be performed on fully conscious patients, it is most often performed using conscious sedation with intravenous agents such as meperidine (Demerol), diazepam (Valium), midazolam (Versed), or fentanyl (Sublimaze). Prior to the TEE exam, the goals, risks, and the nature of the procedure should be discussed in detail with the patient and informed consent obtained. A brief medical history should be obtained to exclude contraindications to esophageal intubation, such as a history of esophageal disease, mediastinal radiation, or recent gastrointestinal surgery (Table 1). A drug and allergy history should also be obtained.

Dentures and oral prostheses are removed prior to the examination. Blood pressure, heart rate, and respirations should be routinely monitored; pulse oximetry is optional but is recommended for patients receiving intravenous sedation. Topical oral pharyngeal anesthesia is administered using either aerosol sprays or liquid gargles. There are no established recommendations for infective endocarditis prophylaxis with antibiotics. Recent studies have indicated that bacteremia is rarely associated with TEE, and some laboratories do not utilize prophylaxis against endocarditis prior to TEE. Others, however, recommend endocarditis prophylaxis in select patients, such as those with prosthetic heart valves, poor dentition, or previous infective endocarditis. With the patient in the left lateral decubitus position to minimize the likelihood of aspiration, the lubricated transesophageal

TABLE 1. *TEE: relative contraindications*

1. Preexisting esophageal pathology
   Obstruction (cancer, stricture)
   Esophageal diverticulum
   Esophageal varices
   Recent esophageal surgery
2. Active UGI bleeding
3. Perforated viscus (known or suspected)
4. Severe cervical arthritis
5. Profound oropharyngeal distortion
6. Unwilling or uncooperative patient

TEE, transesophageal echocardiography; *UGI*, upper gastrointestinal.

transducer is introduced through the mouth and into the esophagus using standard techniques of probe insertion. Because of the relatively large size of the multiplane transducer tip, digital guidance of the probe during esophageal intubation and for depression of the tongue is recommended. The neck should be slightly flexed to facilitate entrance into the esophagus rather than the trachea. Only mild resistance to the advancing probe should be encountered, and force should never be applied. Particular care should be taken in elderly patients, who may have prominent cervical vertebral prominences, and in smaller adults. A bite guard avoids accidental biting and damage to the endoscope.

The average duration of a comprehensive study is 15 to 20 minutes. During the study, oral secretions are removed by suctioning, as needed.

Despite its semi-invasive nature, TEE has an excellent safety record. Major complications (such as perforation of the hypopharynx or esophagus and bleeding) are exceedingly rare. Pathological studies in animals have documented no substantial mucosal or thermal esophageal injuries after prolonged TEE imaging (up to 8.5 hours) and manipulation of the probe. Nevertheless, in order to assure patient safety and maximum image quality, TEE should be performed only by specially trained physicians. Guidelines for appropriate training have been recommended by the American Society of Echocardiography.

Anatomic Imaging Views

Optimal information from TEE can only be obtained by an operator with a thorough understanding of cardiac anatomy. The esophagus lies in the midline of the body, posterior to the left atrium and anterior to the descending thoracic aorta. This location permits excellent imaging of all four chambers of the heart, the inferior and superior vena cavae, the proximal portions of the aorta and pulmonary arteries, the descending thoracic aorta, and the pulmonary veins.

Because the heart is not a symmetrical structure, and because the vertical and horizontal planes of the heart are neither parallel nor perpendicular to the esophagus, a routine TEE exam should include images from a number of scan planes. Therefore, the transducer is placed in the stomach (transgastric views), in the lower esophagus, midesophagus, and upper (or basal) esophagus. In each of these sites a variety of views can be obtained by maneuvering the probe itself (anteflexion and retroflexion, lateral and medial flexion, clockwise and counterclockwise rotation) as well as by switching between horizontal and longitudinal planes (with a biplane probe) or electronically steering the echo beam between 0 degrees and 180 degrees with a multiplane probe. Color and spectral Doppler are used when appropriate. The probe can then be rotated 180 degrees and the entire descending thoracic aorta and most of the aortic arch can be imaged as the probe is withdrawn from the stomach back to the upper esophagus. In most patients, the aortic arch is imaged last because patient discomfort is often experienced when the transducer is manipulated in the upper esophagus. A systematic approach should be used in performing TEE to ensure that all relevant information is obtained. The imaging sequence depends upon the clinical situation, the time available for the study, and the preference of the operator. In an emergency, TEE is goal-directed and a comprehensive evaluation may be precluded.

The TEE study is recorded on videotape. In addition, the audio channel should be recorded (and/or the videotape annotated) to allow comments concerning the image orientation and probe location. This is particularly helpful for subsequent review in comparison with other TEE exams in the same patient.

A detailed description of the various scan planes, anatomic correlations, and image orientation is provided by Pandian et al. (5).

CLINICAL APPLICATIONS

The clinical applications for TEE are numerous and still expanding (6). TEE has already become the definitive noninvasive imaging modality for a broad range of cardiovascular disorders, including the identification of complications of infective endocarditis, thromboembolism of cardiac and aortic origin, prosthetic mitral valve dysfunction, certain disorders of the aorta (such as aortic dissection and atherosclerosis), intracardiac masses, and certain congenital abnormalities. TEE is invaluable for assessing the suitability for and adequacy of a number of surgical procedures, such as mitral valve repair. It has also proved useful as a means of intraoperative monitoring. It is being used increasingly in critically ill patients and to evaluate patients who are being mechanically ventilated or those who are otherwise difficult to image with TTE. In the catheterization laboratory, TEE has been valuable to assist a variety of procedures (such as transseptal puncture, balloon valvuloplasty, and catheter-ablation).

It should be emphasized that most cardiac abnormalities can be reliably evaluated with transthoracic echo, and that TEE, being a semiinvasive procedure, should not be used routinely or indiscriminately. More specifically, TEE should

TABLE 2. *Major clinical applications for TEE*

1. Infective endocarditis
2. Cardiac source of embolism
3. Native valve disease
4. Prosthetic valve disease
5. Thoracic aortic pathology
6. Intracardiac masses
7. Coronary arteries
8. Congenital heart disease
9. Critically ill patients
10. Intraoperative applications
11. Guidance of interventional procedures
12. Stress echo using TEE

TEE, transesophageal echocardiography.

not be performed if the management or outcome of patients would not be expected to be affected by the information gained. Recommendations for the role of transesophageal echocardiography are included in the recent ACC/AHA Guidelines for the Clinical Application of Echocardiography (7). Following is a discussion of some of the commonly accepted clinical applications of TEE (Table 2).

INFECTIVE ENDOCARDITIS

Infective endocarditis continues to be a serious illness with high morbidity and mortality. Early diagnosis is crucial. Prior to echocardiography the diagnosis of infective endocarditis was based on stringent clinical criteria. Although physicians continue to rely on clinical features and characteristic bacteriologic findings for the diagnosis of infective endocarditis, the echocardiographic demonstration of vegetations is assuming increasing importance. Investigators from Duke University have recently proposed new criteria for the diagnosis of infective endocarditis that incorporate echocardiographic findings (8). In fact, the diagnosis of endocarditis may be based solely on echocardiographic findings when blood cultures are negative.

The hallmark lesions of infective endocarditis are vegetations. Pathologically, a vegetation is an amorphus mass of fibrin and platelets containing large colonies of microorganisms and variable numbers of inflammatory cells. Size does not correlate well with microorganisms, with the exception of fungal vegetations, which are typically large. New vegetations are usually soft and friable. The ''healing'' process consists of sterilization, fibrosis, organization, endothelialization, and calcification. Although this sometimes translates echocardiographically into a more echo-dense and bright vegetation, the distinction between a *new* versus *old* vegetation is not reliable. Vegetations usually begin where the endocardium has been damaged by a jet of abnormal flow, such as one resulting from a regurgitant valve. They usually form in locations on which the jet impinges, such as the atrial aspect of the mitral valve (Fig. 1), the ventricular aspect of the aortic valve, and on the right ventricular aspect of a ventricular septal defect. Although vegetations almost always occur on the valves, they can occasionally occur on unusual sites where the endocardium has been disrupted by abnormal flow.

Transthoracic echocardiography has proven to be useful for the diagnosis of infective endocarditis, but suboptimal images in up to 20 to 30% of patients, limited image resolution, and reduced ability to detect perivalvular abscesses in both native and prosthetic valve endocarditis have been major obstacles. TEE, on the other hand, consistently yields high quality images and superior resolution permitting detection of even small vegetations. A number of investigators have documented improved diagnostic accuracy of TEE compared to TTE (Table 3).

TEE has been shown to be superior to TTE for detection of paravalvular abscess, an extremely important complica-

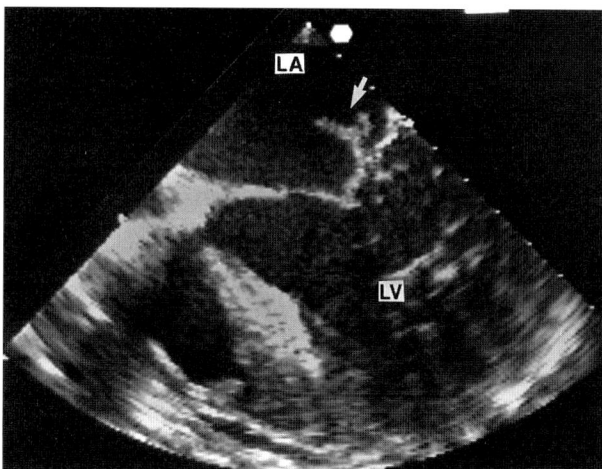

FIG. 1. A four-chamber view illustrating an irregular, "stringy" vegetation (*arrow*) on the left atrial side of the mitral valve. *LA*, left atrium; *LV*, left ventricle.

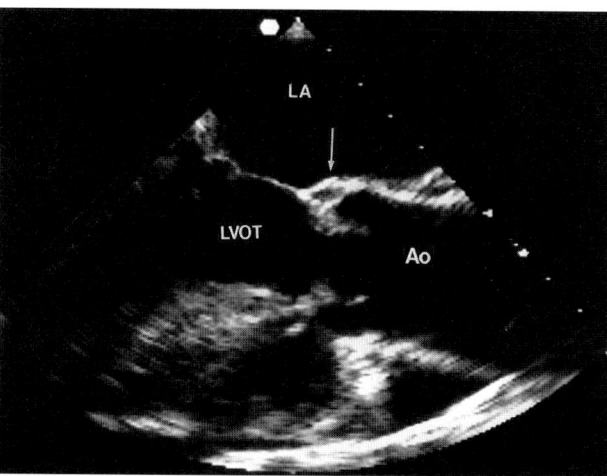

FIG. 2. Longitudinal view of the ascending aorta (*Ao*), aortic root, and left ventricular outflow tract (*LVOT*) illustrating a small posterior perivalvular abscess (*arrow*) which was confirmed at surgery. *LA*, left atrium.

tion of infective endocarditis. Paravalvular abscesses are present in 5 to 30% of patients with infective endocarditis and have important therapeutic and prognostic significance. They typically appear as a relatively echo-free space in the paravalvular region. However, they may also appear as an echo-dense thickening of the wall of the aortic root or ventricular septum. The spectrum of paravalvular destruction varies from simple localized abscesses to large subannular aneurysms with or without perforation into cardiac chambers, extension in the pericardial space, or total disruption of the ventricular-aortic continuity and the mitral-aortic trigone. TEE allows prompt recognition of these conditions before widespread tissue destruction can occur. Karalis et al. found "subaortic" complications (e.g., periaortic abscesses, destruction of the mitral-aortic annular fibrosa [MAIVF], aneurysms of the MAIVF, and aneurysms of both the mitral and aortic leaflets) to be particularly common in patients with aortic valve endocarditis (19).Therefore, many echocardiographers recommend performing TEE early in the course

of all patients with aortic valve endocarditis to detect these complications. Figure 2 shows a small abscess of the aortic annulus.

Indications for TEE in patients with known or suspected endocarditis are currently controversial. Some echocardiographic experts have recommended TEE for all such patients. Others, partly influenced by a desire to contain medical costs, advocate TEE for select patients. Reasonable indications for TEE are listed in Table 4. They are also briefly discussed in the ACC/AHA Guidelines for the Clinical Applications for Echocardiography (7). TEE is probably not required when the clinical picture is clear, for example, when TTE reveals a small focal vegetation and the patient is responding to treatment appropriately. Furthermore, it is not required when there is a low index of suspicion for endocarditis (such as "fever workup" in the absence of new regurgitant murmur, predisposing cardiac abnormalities, or clinical features of endocarditis); and certainly not for all patients with bacteremia.

Even with the high-resolution images provided by TEE, the conclusive identification of vegetation is not always possible. There are situations in which the echocardiographic

TABLE 3. *Diagnosis of infective endocarditis: TTE and TEE*

Author	Year	n	Sensitivity TTE (%)	Sensitivity TEE (%)
Erbel et al. (9)	1988	96	44	82
Daniel et al. (10)	1988	76	60	94
Chan et al. (11)	1989	29	55	90
Mugge et al. (12)	1989	80	58	90
Taams et al. (13)	1990	33	33	100
Shively et al. (14)	1991	62	44	94
Pedersen et al. (15)	1991	24	50	100
Birmingham et al. (16)	1992	29	34	93
Shapiro et al. (17)	1994	64	60	87
Lowry et al. (18)	1994	93	36	93

n, number of patients; *TEE*, transesophageal echocardiography; *TTE*, transthoracic echocardiography.

TABLE 4. *Infective endocarditis: indications for TEE*

1. Strong clinical suspicion for endocarditis and negative or nondiagnostic TTE
2. Persistent bacteremia (abscess suspected)
3. Suspected prosthetic valve endocarditis
4. Hemodynamic instability
5. Clinical embolic event
6. Immediately prior to surgery for infective endocarditis
7. Staph aortic valve endocarditis
8. TTE reveals vegetation, but size, mobility, extent unclear

TEE, transesophageal echocardiography; *TTE*, transthoracic echocardiography.

findings can be particularly confusing and even misleading. For example, vegetation due to infective endocarditis must be distinguished from other masses; ruptured chordae tendineae; myxomatous degeneration and thickening of mitral leaflets; focal, nonspecific thickening or calcium deposits on valves; retained mitral leaflets and chordae after mitral valve replacement; Lambl's excrescences; sutures, pledgets, and other prosthetic material for prosthetic valves; thrombi; and small tumors. In some instances, these conditions can be distinguished by their echocardiographic characteristics; but, always in these situations, echocardiographic findings need to be carefully correlated and integrated with other clinical and microbiologic features.

Although false positive TEE examinations for suspected endocarditis are uncommon, they do occur, perhaps even more commonly than with TTE, because, as the ability of this imaging technology to resolve smaller and smaller structures increases, so does the number of nonvegetative abnormal masses detected. In a small percentage of patients, false negative results may be present, even with TEE. False negative studies usually result from valves that were structurally deformed prior to the endocarditis or from acoustic shadowing by calcified valves or prosthetic devices. Although a negative TEE does not rule out the presence of infective endocarditis completely, the probability of the disease is very low when it is normal. Furthermore, a negative TEE is associated with a good prognosis and a high likelihood that another source of fever will be found (20).

In spite of these limitations, TEE is playing an expanding role in the evaluation of patients with infective endocarditis. Its use substantially improves the ability to diagnose infective endocarditis, enhances the ability to detect its complications, and often facilitates the decision to undertake early surgery. The effect of improved and earlier detection of vegetations by TEE on morbidity and mortality remains to be determined.

CARDIAC SOURCES OF EMBOLISM

Stroke is a major cause of death and disability, and it is estimated that 15 to 20% of strokes are cardioembolic in origin. Identification of those with a cardiac source is a challenging problem (21). However, these features have not proved to be consistent and reliable indicators of embolism from the heart. In other patients, a cardiac source is considered after exclusion of other causes following a thorough neurologic workup, including negative cerebral arteriography. Transesophageal echocardiography has proven to be useful for detecting potential cardiac sources of emboli in such patients. As a result, an increasing number of patients are being referred for this indication. In fact, evaluation for "cardiac source of embolus" is the most common reason for referral for TEE in most laboratories.

Both transthoracic and transesophageal echo play an important role in evaluating these patients. Transthoracic echo has been used for more than 20 years to evaluate patients

TABLE 5. *Studies comparing transthoracic echo with TEE in patients with stroke/transient ischemic attack*

Study	Patients (n)	Potential source of embolism	
		by TTE (%)	by TEE (%)
Pop et al. (22)	72	10	24
Hofmann et al. (23)	153	36	58
Pearson et al. (24)	79	15	57
Cujec et al. (25)	63	14	41
DeRook et al. (26)	66	14	57
Lee et al. (27)	50	0	52

n, number of patients; *TEE*, transesophageal echocardiography; *TTE*, transthoracic echocardiography.

with a possible cardiac source of embolus. However, in unselected series of patients with strokes, TTE has been of limited value, particularly in patients with no clinical evidence of heart disease. In studies that have compared TEE with TTE in groups of patients with cerebral and peripheral embolism, TEE has clearly shown superiority for the identification of potential sources of embolus, such as left atrial appendage or left atrial thrombi, vegetations on native and prosthetic valves, atrial septal aneurysms, and patent foramen ovale (Table 5). The major sources of emboli that can accurately be detected with TEE will be briefly discussed.

Left Atrial/Left Atrial Appendage Thrombi

Transthoracic echocardiography has limited sensitivity for detecting atrial thrombi, in large part due to the posterior location of the left atrium and its limited ability to image the atrial appendage. In contrast, TEE provides detailed imaging of both the left atrium and the left atrial appendage. The latter site is particularly important since it is the most common location for thrombi. The superiority of TEE over TTE for detecting left atrial thrombi is well documented (28). However, the exact sensitivity and specificity are unknown because of the lack of a suitable "gold standard." Several small series, however, suggest that the accuracy is quite high. The echocardiographer must carefully discriminate thrombi from left atrial pectinate muscles, as well as be familiar with the multilobed appearance of the normal left atrial appendage. Although no randomized, prospective studies have been published, biplane and multiplane TEE are generally felt to be superior to single-plane probes for the assessment of left atrial thrombi.

Atrial thrombi are almost always associated with predisposing conditions such as mitral stenosis, prosthetic mitral valves, atrial fibrillation, and severe left ventricular dysfunction. Although TEE is an excellent tool for identifying atrial thrombi, the patients presenting with an embolic stroke and these coexisting conditions are generally treated with chronic warfarin without regard for the TEE findings. Nevertheless, in patients with mitral stenosis, identification of atrial thrombi is particularly important when mitral balloon valvuloplasty is being considered. The presence of a clot in the body of the left atrium or near the "mouth" of the left atrial appendage is a contraindication to this procedure. The significance of small, nonmobile thrombi near the apex of the left atrial appendage is not clear at this time.

TEE is gaining increasing attention as a means of excluding the presence of a left atrial thrombus prior to chemical or electrical cardioversion of atrial fibrillation (29,30). The role of TEE prior to cardioversion for atrial fibrillation is currently being investigated. It is important to note that recent data have shown that a negative TEE for atrial thrombi does *not* preclude the possibility of embolic events if patients are not adequately anticoagulated. This may be due to the phenomenon of "atrial stunning" after cardioversion. Thus, anticoagulation is mandatory at the time of cardioversion and for approximately one month afterward. Whether a management strategy incorporating TEE and including anticoagulation is cost effective and offers lower risk and greater convenience compared with conventional strategy of anticoagulation prior to and after cardioversion, is the subject of ongoing investigation.

Impaired left ventricular function and left atrial enlargement are strongly associated with increased risk of thromboembolism. Despite the superiority of TEE for detecting atrial thrombi, a similar role of TEE for risk stratification in patients with chronic atrial fibrillation and the implications for clinical management of these patients has not been established.

Left Ventricular Thrombi

Although the superiority of TEE for detecting atrial thrombi is clear, this is not the case with ventricular thrombi, probably because the latter are usually apical in location. There are technical difficulties in visualizing the left ventricular apex from the esophagus because of limited resolution at the increased depth of this anterior portion of the heart and because of foreshortening of the left ventricle. With the use of small footprint, high frequency, short focus transducers, transthoracic echo can identify or exclude left ventricular thrombi and distinguish them from trabeculations and false tendons in most patients. Nevertheless, TEE is a reasonable alternative in patients with poor apical windows or in whom TTE data is equivocal. If TEE is used, then both transesophageal and deep transgastric views should be used.

Prosthetic Valve Thrombi

Thrombus formation and subsequent embolization, especially in the setting of suboptimal anticoagulation, may occur in patients with either mechanical or bioprosthetic prostheses in either the mitral or aortic position (Fig. 3). Such thrombi are best detected by TEE; however, the importance of their identification for clinical management is less certain, because patients with prosthetic valves who present with evidence of systemic embolization are generally assumed to have prosthetic valve thrombi (in the absence of infective

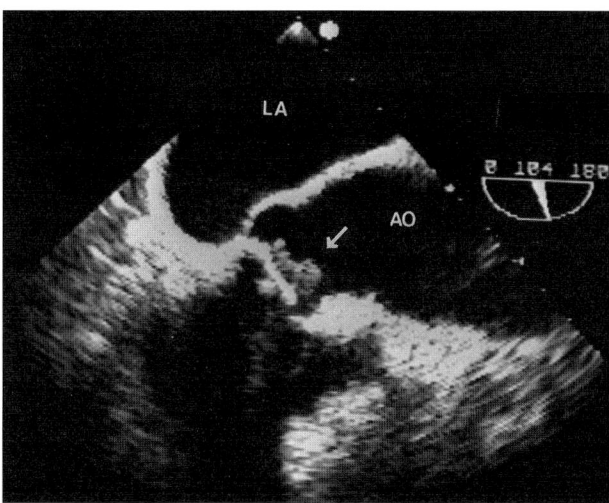

FIG. 3. Longitudinal view (104 degrees) of the ascending aorta (*AO*) illustrating a thrombus (*arrow*) on the aortic side of a prosthetic valve. *LA*, left atrium.

endocarditis) as the etiology and therefore warrant anticoagulation.

Valve "strands" have been detected on both native and prosthetic valves by transesophageal, but not by transthoracic echocardiography (31). These small, mobile, filamentous strands are seen more commonly on prosthetic than native valves and more commonly on mechanical prosthesis than bioprostheses. Moreover, they are identified more commonly on mitral valves than aortic valves. The histology of these "strands" is unclear but they could represent either fibrin, thrombi, or tiny torn chordae. Whether strands on native valves and those on prosthetic valves represent the same morphologic entity is not clear. However, the greater prevalence of such strands on prosthetic valves suggest that strands are related to thrombosis. Several authors have suggested that these strands represent a potential source of embolization (31). Whether strands or fragments of strands embolize or whether they are merely markers for an embolic potential is not known. Definitive therapy for patients with strands who have had an embolic event without another identifiable source of embolism, is undetermined. Prospective TEE follow-up studies are needed to assess the efficacy of anticoagulant and/or antiplatlet therapy in eradicating these strands and in reducing the incidents of embolic events.

Vegetations

The superiority of TEE over TTE for detecting vegetations and confirming the diagnosis of infective endocarditis was discussed in the previous section. Echocardiography also provides important prognostic information related to the risk of systemic embolism. Embolism is more common in patients with TTE- or TEE-detected vegetations than those without. Several investigators have found that patients with vegetations larger than 10 mm, particularly those that are mobile, have a higher incidence of embolic events.

Intracardiac Tumors

Intracardiac tumors, although rare, do have the potential for systemic embolism. In fact, the initial clinical presentation may be thromboembolism, either due to embolization of detached tumor fragments or embolism of overlying thrombotic material from the tumor surface. Atrial myxomas, the most common primary cardiac tumors, characteristically develop in the left atrium attached to the atrial septum. Myxomas occur with decreasing frequency in the right atrium, ventricles, multiple intracardiac sites, or as an isolated tumor attached to the mitral valve. While TTE and TEE have a similar ability to detect myxomas and other tumors, TEE provides useful additional information concerning the exact size, site of attachment, morphology, mobility, and acoustic characteristics (32). Other less common tumors such as sarcomas, papillary fibroelastomas, and fibromas can also be accurately evaluated by TEE.

Thoracic Aortic Atherosclerosis

Until the advent of TEE, the aorta was an underrecognized source of systemic embolism. Several studies have reported an increased frequency of embolic events in patients with atherosclerotic plaques in the thoracic aorta detected by TEE. Embolic events are most frequent in patients with "complex" plaques, defined as those greater than 5 mm thick and those containing protruding (as in Fig. 4) or mobile components. Occasionally, mobile projections from atherosclerotic plaques move freely within the blood stream. TEE is the only imaging technique capable of imaging these small projections.

TEE has provided significant insight into the importance of aortic atherosclerotic material as a source of systemic emboli, yet the management of patients with embolic events and protruding atheromas is still uncertain. Anticoagulation with coumadin and antiplatelet agents have been considered. The safety of coumadin has been questioned by some as it may theoretically remove the thrombin coating (or "cap") from an ulcerated atheroma facilitating microembolization. However, this complication is probably more theoretic than real. Moreover, there is evidence from case reports that the mobile components are, in fact, thrombi and not plaque material. There are also reports of thrombolysis and even surgical debridement in very select patients with clinically severe and recurrent embolism and documented large aortic atherothrombotic masses. Long-term trials comparing the various treatment strategies are still needed. Preliminary data from the SPAF III TEE substudy (33) suggests a possible clinical role for warfarin, but this needs to be more clearly established.

Patent Foramen Ovale

A patent foramen ovale results from lack of complete fusion of the septum primum and septum secundum, setting the stage for right-to-left flow when right atrial pressure exceeds left atrial pressure. Patent foramen ovale (PFO) is detected in up to 30% of patients at necropsy. Similarly, Schneider et al. identified PFO in 26% of a select group of patients having both TEE and autopsy confirmation (34). A PFO can be detected by color flow imaging of the atrial septum. However, contrast echocardiography has been shown to be more sensitive and should be routinely performed. Maneuvers that increase right atrial pressure such as the Valsalva maneuver or "burst coughing" enhance the detection of right-to-left shunting via a PFO. Using TEE as the "gold standard," several prospective studies have

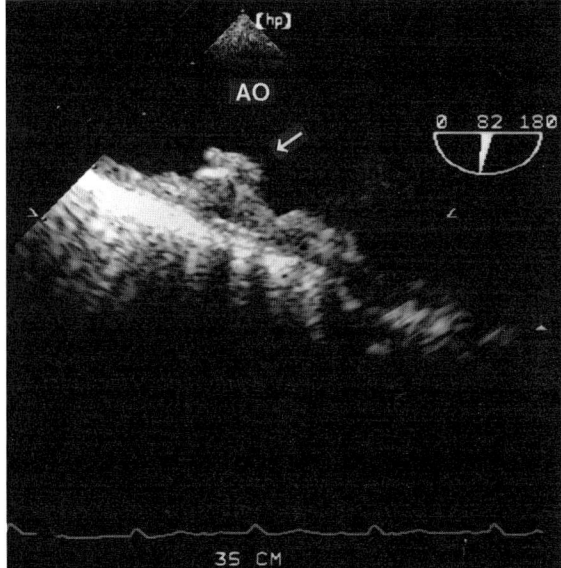 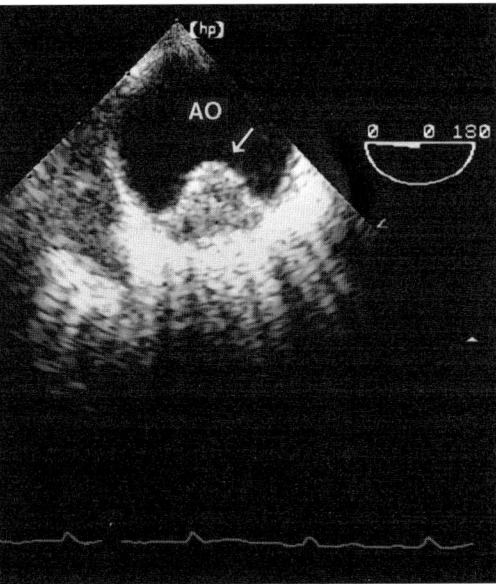

FIG. 4. Two orthogonal views of the descending thoracic aorta illustrating a "lumpy," irregular protruding atherosclerotic plaque (*arrows*). **Left:** longitudinal view; **right:** transverse view.

demonstrated that TEE with contrast is superior to TTE with contrast for the diagnosis of PFO.

Paradoxical embolism of venous thrombi across a PFO can produce a stroke. In a landmark study, Lechat and co-workers emphasized an association of PFO with stroke in young (less than 45 years) adult patients (35). Their findings have been supported by subsequent investigators, who have demonstrated a significantly higher prevalence of PFO in patients with cryptogenic stroke compared to patients with stroke of known cause, regardless of age. Nevertheless, the extent to which paradoxical embolization by way of PFO contributes to the incidence of embolic disease remains speculative. Thus far, only an association between PFO and stroke has been documented. Important questions remain unanswered. Some investigators have suggested that the size of the opening of the PFO as determined by TEE and the degree of right to left contrast shunting (small versus large number of contrast targets) may increase the thromboembolic potential.

If a PFO is the only abnormality detected by TEE in a patient with cryptogenic stroke, a search for lower extremity venous thrombosis or pulmonary embolism appears to be indicated to provide support for a diagnosis of paradoxical embolism. Stollberger et al. made an effort to establish the prevalence of occult venous thrombi by performing lower extremity venographic studies in 42 of 49 stroke patients with patent foramen ovale (36). Venous thrombosis was documented in 24 (57%) even though only a quarter of these were suspected on clinical grounds. Although no control group was used, this study suggests an important association between a potential thromboembolic source and a patent foramen ovale.

Although TEE has improved the ability to detect patent foramen ovale, the clinical implications of this finding remain to be determined in large, prospective trials. Management options, including warfarin, antiplatelet agents, surgical closure, and percutaneous closure, are unclear at the present time.

Atrial Septal Aneurysm

An atrial septal aneurysm (ASA) is a redundant atrial septum, usually located in the fossa ovale region, which bulges 1.5 cm or more beyond the plane of the atrial septum at some point during the cardiac cycle, as in Figure 5. Atrial septal aneurysms may involve only the fossa ovale region, or the entire atrial septum. Atrial septal aneurysms are identified in approximately 1% of all TTEs and up to 3% of all TEEs.

The prevalence of atrial septal aneurysm appears to be higher in patients with unexplained cerebral ischemic events, suggesting an association. Two potential mechanisms have been postulated. One may be paradoxical embolization through an accompanying patent foramen ovale, present in up to 75% of atrial septal aneurysms. Second, the atrial septal aneurysm may provide a nidus for thrombus formation either

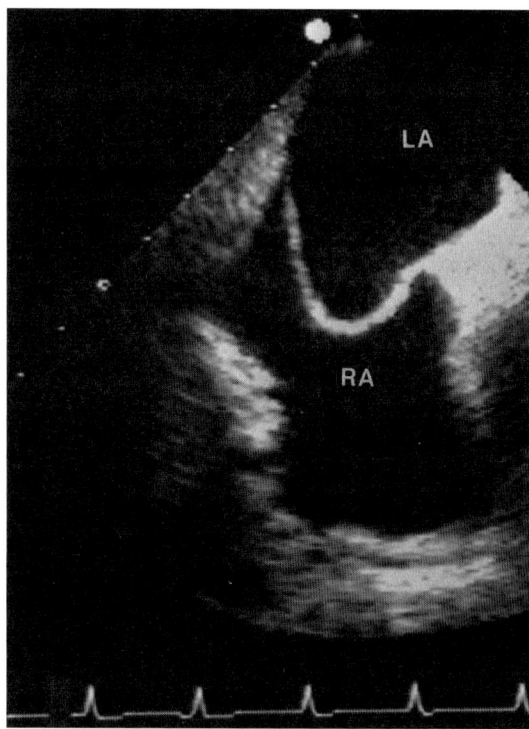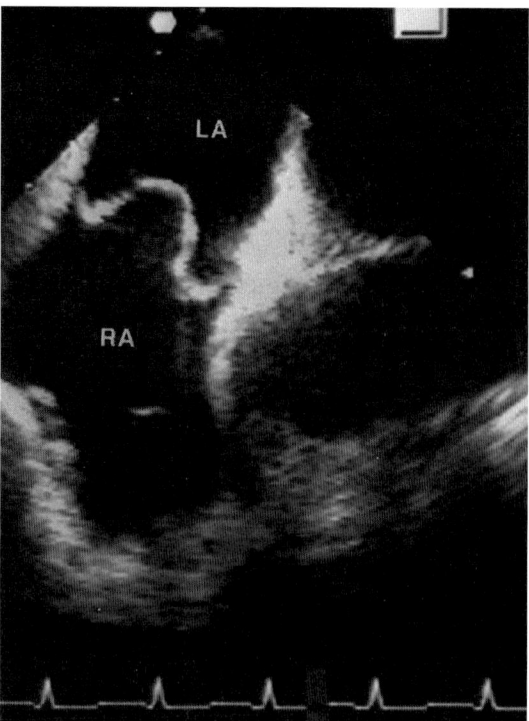

FIG. 5. Two portions of the cardiac cycle illustrating an atrial septal aneurysm which oscillates back-and-forth between the right atrium (*RA*) as shown in the **left panel** and the left atrium (*LA*) as shown in the **right panel**.

within the aneurysm itself, or as tiny fibrin-thrombus tags attached to its roughened or wrinkled surface. Several studies have suggested that the frequency of atrial septal aneurysm is higher in stroke patients than in those examined for other reasons, or in the general population. However, the frequency of ASA in the general population was not defined in these studies.

Although there may be an association between atrial septal aneurysm and cardioembolic stroke, the overall frequency of ASA in stroke populations is very low. Nevertheless, because ASA may constitute a risk factor for cardioembolism in a small subgroup of stroke patients, some authors have suggested that patients with atrial septal aneurysm and unexplained embolic disease should be anticoagulated. However, prospective controlled trials on the treatment of these patients with anticoagulation or surgery require further study. Further studies in larger numbers of patients over a longer period of follow-up and using age-matched controls will be necessary to determine the strength of the association between atrial septal aneurysm and embolic events.

Spontaneous Echo Contrast

Spontaneous echo contrast (SEC) is a phenomenon of amorphus, smoke-like swirling, light gray haze that often spontaneously appears and disappears during imaging. This dynamic swirling appearance resembles and, hence, is often referred to as ''smoke.'' Although the exact mechanism is unknown, it appears that low flow states and low shear rates play a pivotal role in the pathogenesis of SEC. Additional factors may predispose to SEC, such as hypercoagulability or hyperviscosity, but these have not been proven.

SEC is seen most commonly in the presence of conditions associated with low blood flow velocity, such as left atrial enlargement with or without mitral valve disease, atrial fibrillation, left atrial thrombus, left ventricular enlargement and dysfunction (with or without aneurysm formation), and aortic dissection. SEC disappears when flow velocity is normalized, such as after the alleviation of mitral valve stenosis, resection of left ventricular aneurysm, or repair of an aortic dissection.

Although SEC may be detected occasionally with standard transthoracic echocardiography, numerous studies have shown that it is detected with a much greater frequency with transesophageal echo. Indeed, SEC has been reported in up to 19% of patients undergoing TEE, but this high incidence probably reflects patient selection bias.

There appears to be an association between left atrial SEC and left atrial thrombi. In addition, several studies have identified SEC as an independent predictor of embolic events, suggesting that patients with SEC have a high risk for thromboembolism even if atrial thrombi are not detected. Leung and colleagues (37), in a prospective study of 149 patients with nonvalvular atrial fibrillation and no prior thromboembolism, found an embolic rate of 9.5% per year in patients with SEC, which was significantly greater than the rate of 2.2% per year found in patients without SEC. Furthermore, in patients with SEC, the embolic rate was 7% per year in those receiving oral anticoagulants compared with 14% per year in those not receiving them. Thus, it appears that anticoagulation may reduce the occurrence of embolic events in patients with SEC, even though it does not dissipate the SEC. The current consensus is that, absent any contraindication, anticoagulation should be used in all patients with both SEC and atrial fibrillation. There is no convincing evidence that antiplatelet drugs benefit such patients. Moreover, neither warfarin nor antiplatelet agents reduce SEC. Further data are still required with respect to patient management and anticoagulation issues in patients with SEC.

Mitral Annular Calcification

Mitral annular calcification (MAC) is a common TTE finding among elderly patients referred for evaluation of cardiac source of embolus. There is a linear relationship between the incidence of stroke and the severity of mitral annular calcification. Because the diagnosis of MAC is easily made by TTE, TEE is not needed in most patients. Moreover, there are no definitive data on the management of these patients. The empiric use of warfarin in all patients with stroke and mitral annular calcification does not appear to be warranted at the present time.

Mitral Valve Prolapse

Mitral valve prolapse (MVP) is found in approximately 1 to 5% of the general population. Mitral valve prolapse is usually detected by TTE. Although MVP can also be detected using TEE, diagnostic criteria for MVP remain to be determined. Subgroups of patients with mitral valve prolapse have severe myxomatous degeneration, manifest by ''redundant'' or thickened leaflets. Although these patients have a higher likelihood of developing endocarditis, progressive mitral regurgitation, and ruptured chordae tendineae, an increased risk for stroke has not been established (38). Therefore, the finding of MVP on a TEE does not establish a causal or relationship.

Summary

In summary, the role of TEE for evaluating patients with suspected cardiac source of embolus is still evolving. Although the superiority of TEE over TTE in detecting potential cardiac sources of embolism is undisputed, proving causality is most often speculative. Some TEE-detected entities are strongly associated, whereas others, such as patent foramen ovale and atrial septal aneurysm, are less so (Table 6). The impact of TEE on the management of these patients remains undefined for the vast majority of TEE detected findings; therefore, the routine use of TEE for the evaluation and management of these patients is questionable and current recommendations are still being refined. It is logical to con-

TABLE 6. *Sources of systemic embolism detectable by TEE*

High risk of association
 1. Left atrial/left atrial appendage thrombus
 2. Left ventricular apical thrombus
 3. Valvular vegetations
 4. Prosthetic valve thrombus
 5. Intracardiac tumors
 6. Protruding and/or mobile aortic atherosclerotic "debris"
Uncertain risk of association
 1. Patent foramen ovale
 2. Atrial septal aneurysm
 3. Spontaneous echo contrast
 4. Valve "strands"
Low risk of association
 1. Mitral valve prolapse
 2. Mitral annulus calcification

TEE, transesophageal echocardiography.

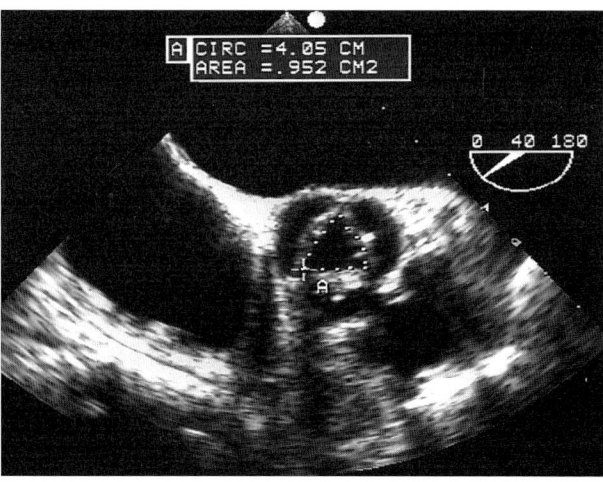

FIG. 6. Cross-sectional view (40 degrees) of a stenotic aortic valve illustrating a planimetered valve area of 0.95 cm^2.

sider performing TEE when it is anticipated that the results may alter management. In patients for whom anticoagulation is indicated regardless of the TEE findings (e.g., atrial fibrillation), TEE is seldom necessary. Several multicenter randomized trials are currently underway to evaluate the efficacy of TEE in patients with cryptogenic stroke or transient ischemic attack. The results of these trials are needed before the role and cost effectiveness of TEE for this purpose are determined.

NATIVE VALVE DISEASE

Transthoracic echo provides all the necessary information for evaluating the vast majority of patients with native valve disease. Patients rarely need to undergo TEE solely for the estimation of the degree of valvular stenosis or regurgitation. Nevertheless, the superior image quality of TEE can provide a more detailed assessment of the valve morphology in individual patients for specific indications.

Valve Stenosis

With meticulous attention to technique, multiplane TEE allows planimetery of the aortic valve area during systole (Fig. 6). Maximal leaflet tip separation can be determined from the longitudinal plane of the left ventricular outflow tract and proximal ascending aorta. The transducer is then rotated 90 degrees until the aortic root appears circular (to avoid an oblique cross-section) and all cusps are included in the image. There is excellent correlation between the TEE results and the cardiac catheterization. Inaccurate results may result from increased reflectances from heavily calcified valves, distorted borders, apical displacement of the aortic valve during systole, and failure to define the smallest orifice of the stenotic valve. Determination of aortic gradients by Doppler TEE is technically difficult and less reliable than by TTE, because it is difficult to align the beam parallel to the stenotic aortic jet.

By contrast, continuous wave Doppler evaluation of the mitral stenotic valve using TEE is feasible and both gradients and valve area correlate closely with TTE measurements (39). Nevertheless, the role of TEE in mitral stenosis is generally limited to patients with technically difficult TTE or the need to assess the presence of left atrial thrombus prior to balloon valvotomy. During balloon mitral valvotomy TEE can be helpful in guiding transseptal puncture, in assessing the extent of post dilatation mitral regurgitation, in detecting procedure related complications, and in detecting the presence of interatrial shunting as a result of transseptal puncture.

Valve Regurgitation

Comprehensive TTE, including precordial, suprasternal, and abdominal windows is generally adequate for the semi-quantitation of aortic regurgitation. TEE usually adds little except when TTE images are suboptimal. TEE is, however, superior for imaging the aortic valve leaflets and aortic root. Therefore, the mechanism of aortic regurgitation (such as dilated aortic root, aortic valve endocarditis, and proximal aortic dissection) is more accurately assessed with TEE than with TTE.

Transesophageal echocardiography plays a much greater role in assessing the severity of mitral regurgitation. Although TTE provides a satisfactory assessment of the severity of MR in most patients, its accuracy may be limited by the presence of eccentric jets (especially in patients with flail leaflets), or the presence of heavy calcification of the mitral valve or annulus that may "block" the ultrasound signal reaching the left atrium (producing underestimation of the severity of regurgitation). Moreover, imaging may be suboptimal in critically ill patients (who are often difficult to image with TTE), and those with tachycardia. In the latter, the frame rate may limit the appreciation of the regurgitant jet size. In addition to its ability to enhance appreciation of the regurgitant jet, TEE provides excellent imaging of the pulmonary veins and allows detection of retrograde regurgitant flow in the pulmonary veins, an indication of severe MR.

TEE is also playing an increasing role in evaluating the structure and function of the mitral apparatus in patients with mitral regurgitation because of the growing enthusiasm for surgical repair of the mitral valve. TEE can help to determine: (i) which patients are candidates for repair, (ii) which type of repair is required, and (iii) whether the repair is adequate.

PROSTHETIC VALVE DISEASE

Although prosthetic valves have greatly improved the prognosis and quality of life of many patients, all are imperfect, and patients with them should not be considered free from heart disease. Echocardiography has played a major role in the detection of complications and abnormal prosthetic function. Listed in Table 7 are complications of prosthetic valves; such structural complications can lead to either prosthetic valve obstruction or regurgitation.

Stenosis

In the vast majority of individuals, transthoracic Doppler examination is still the cornerstone for the assessment of obstruction of a prosthetic valve. Accurate Doppler estimation of valvular pressure gradients requires alignment of the ultrasound beam parallel to the direction of blood flow. This is more easily performed from the transthoracic approach, which allows multiple windows for Doppler interrogation. Although seldom necessary, evaluation of obstruction of mitral and tricuspid prostheses is also possible using TEE with continuous wave Doppler. Elevated mean diastolic gradient, increased antegrade flow velocity, prolonged pressure half-time, and decreased effective orifice area suggest obstruction. In addition, restriction of leaflet or poppet motion is usually better demonstrated by TEE than by TTE (40). On the other hand, transesophageal echo is unreliable for detecting prosthetic aortic valve stenosis, because it is difficult to align the TEE continuous wave cursor parallel to flow through the aortic prosthesis. Occasionally, this can be accomplished using the transgastric view, but the signals are often attenuated because the prosthetic valve is in the far-field of the transducer.

TABLE 7. *Complications of prosthetic valves*

1. Thrombosis
2. Thromboembolism
3. Fibrous tissue ingrowth
4. Infection
5. Dehiscence
6. Degeneration (bioprostheses)
7. Structural deterioration (mechanical prostheses)
8. Prosthetic and periprosthetic regurgitation
9. Obstruction

Regurgitation

Whereas the transthoracic approach is usually sufficient for the evaluation of prosthetic valve obstruction, TTE has significant limitations in evaluating prosthetic valve regurgitation, especially with mitral prostheses. In both parasternal and apical TTE windows, the metallic sewing ring, stents, discs, and poppets of prosthetic valves markedly attenuate ultrasound penetration beyond the prosthesis. This phenomenon known as "flow masking," plus strong reverberations, limit the assessment of flow in the left atrium, masking a central or paravalvular leak, or leading to underestimation of the degree of mitral regurgitation. TEE clearly represents a major advance and overcomes these limitations because the transducer lies immediately behind the left atrium and therefore, provides a clear view of that chamber without interference from the prostheses itself (Fig. 7). Several studies have documented the superiority of TEE over TTE for detecting and quantifying prosthetic mitral valve regurgitation (41). In fact, the assessment of a mitral prosthesis and the quantitation of mitral regurgitation are among the most frequent patterns, indications of TEE. In addition, pulmonary venous flow patterns, detectable by TEE in almost all patients, provides supplemental information for quantitating mitral regurgitation.

Nearly all types of normally functioning mitral prosthetic valves have minor leaks by TEE (around a central strut, through leaflet hinge points, between the sewing ring and disc occluders). The typical patterns of this normal transvalvular prosthetic regurgitation have been well-described and should be recognized by all echocardiographers. Each prosthetic valve type generates its own specific pattern of "physiologic leak." TEE is superior to TTE in differentiating these "physiologic leaks" from pathologic regurgitation.

On the other hand, the transthoracic approach is nearly always sufficient for evaluating prosthetic aortic valve regurgitation, particularly when the appearance of the regurgitant jet by color Doppler is integrated with information from pressure half-time of the regurgitant jet and with the degree of retrograde diastolic flow in the descending thoracic aorta. TEE is less accurate for evaluating prosthetic aortic than mitral regurgitation. Attenuation of the ultrasound beam as it traverses the aortic prosthesis results in "flow masking" of the left ventricular outflow tract and incomplete visualization of bioprosthetic leaflets and mechanical discs. TEE is usually reserved for technically difficult cases, to better define the mechanism of regurgitation, and to assess the aortic root for associated pathology.

Prosthetic Valve Endocarditis

Prosthetic valve endocarditis (PVE) is an infrequent but serious complication of valve replacement occurring in approximately 2 to 4% of cases. Early diagnosis is of the utmost importance as surgical treatment may be lifesaving. Although echocardiography has been the noninvasive tech-

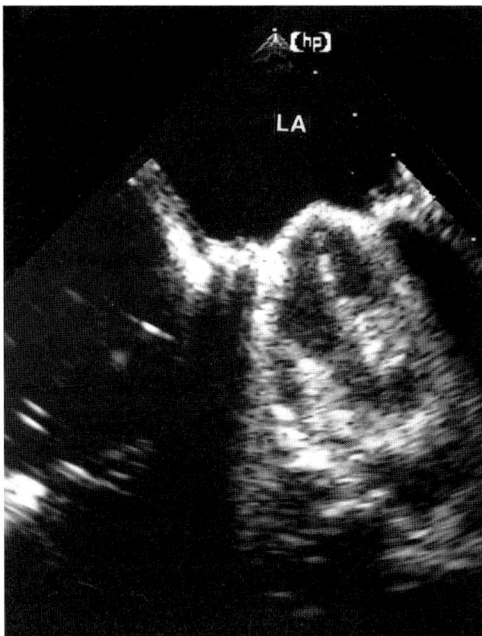 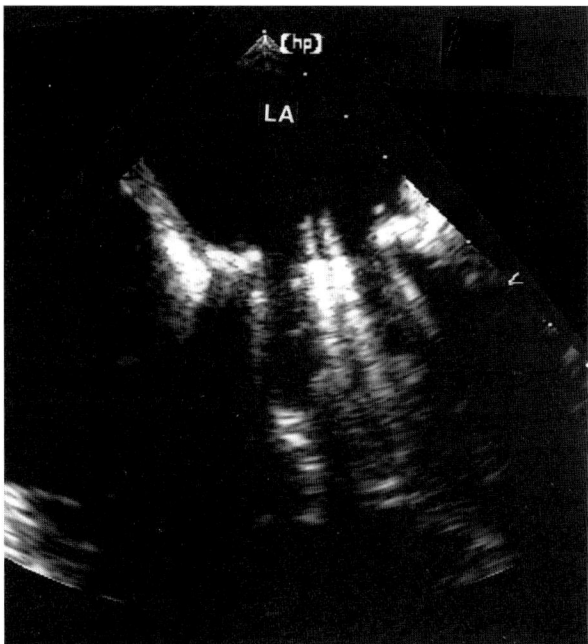

FIG. 7. A four-chamber view (0 degrees) illustrates the high-quality images obtained by TEE of a St. Jude mitral prosthesis. In the **left panel** (systole) the two leaflets form an obtuse angle in the closed position. In the **right panel** (diastole) the two leaflets are aligned nearly parallel in the open position. *LA*, left atrium.

nique of choice for more than 20 years, transthoracic echo has limited ability in the visualization of vegetations and in the detection of paravalvular abscess. These limitations have been overcome to a great extent by TEE and numerous studies have reported the superiority of TEE compared to TTE for these indications.

The ability of TEE to evaluate the atrial surface of mitral prosthesis is of particular importance because thrombi or vegetations are usually attached to the atrial side, an area often inaccessible to TTE in patients with prosthetic valves. The high quality and high resolution images provided by TEE is a "two-edged sword." Very tiny mobile structures above the sewing ring of mitral prosthetic valve are often identified. These so-called "strands" can be extremely difficult to differentiate from vegetations. In addition, microcavitations are frequently imaged immediately after opening and closing of mitral prosthesis. These should not be confused with small masses, such as vegetations or thrombi.

In summary, TEE has become an invaluable complement to a comprehensive transthoracic echocardiogram and Doppler study of patients with prosthetic valves because it provides more detailed structural information. TEE is usually superior to TTE for detecting and quantitating mitral prosthetic regurgitation and marginally superior for evaluating aortic prosthetic regurgitation. In addition, TEE is superior to TTE for detecting masses such as thrombi and vegetations, periprosthetic abscesses, and sewing ring dehiscence. Abnormal gradients across prosthetic valves are generally adequately estimated by TTE; and therefore, standard TEE should always be part of a complete study of prosthetic

valves. Indications for TEE evaluation of prosthetic valves are listed in Table 8.

Thoracic Aortic Pathology

Examination of the thoracic aorta is one of the most important applications of TEE. The proximity of the esophagus to the aorta and the high resolution of TEE transducers make TEE ideally suited for imaging the thoracic aorta. The entire thoracic aorta, with the possible exception of the distal portion of the ascending aorta where the trachea and left mainstem bronchus intervene, can be clearly imaged in almost all patients. With the addition of biplane and multiplane probes, visualization of this previously labeled "blind spot" has improved. Therefore, TEE is playing an increasingly important role in the evaluation of aortic diseases, including

TABLE 8. *Indications for TEE evaluation of prosthetic valves*

1. Inadequate imaging using TTE
2. Suspected embolic event
3. Suspected endocarditis
4. Discordance between clinical and TTE findings
5. To determine etiology of obstruction (e.g., thrombosis, parvus)
6. To assess severity of regurgitation, especially across mitral prosthesis

TEE, transesophageal echocardiography; *TTE*, transthoracic echocardiography.

TABLE 9. *Advantages and disadvantages of TEE for evaluation of aortic dissection*

Advantages
  1. Excellent sensitivity and specificity
  2. Rapid, portable
  3. Safely performed on critically ill patients, even those on ventilators
  4. Can detect, quantify, and define mechanism of aortic insufficiency
  5. Can detect involvement of coronary orifices
  6. Can detect pericardial effusion
  7. Can assess left ventricular function
  8. Can detect intramural hematoma
Disadvantages
  1. Can miss localized dissection of upper ascending aorta
  2. May not define branch vessel involvement
  3. Semiinvasive with a small potential for morbidity
  4. Reverberation artifacts (can be differentiated from flaps in vast majority)

TEE, transesophageal echocardiography.

aortic dissection, aortic aneurysm, aortic atherosclerosis, and aortic trauma.

Aortic Dissection

Rapid and accurate diagnosis of aortic dissection is critical to effective patient management. Four important diagnostic methods are available: aortography, computed tomography (CT), magnetic resonance imaging (MRI), and transesophageal echocardiography. Numerous publications have touted the merits of each of these. In truth, each diagnostic test has strengths and weaknesses. Because of its speed, accuracy, and affordability, TEE has become the first-line diagnostic imaging modality in many centers. However, the choice of diagnostic test should depend not only on the proven accuracy of a given technique, but also the technique available at a given institution and the experience and confidence of the physician performing and interpreting the test. The advantages and disadvantages of TEE for evaluating aortic dissection are listed in Table 9.

It is critically important to establish the diagnosis of aortic dissection with a high level of sensitivity and specificity. TEE has been demonstrated to be highly accurate, and, in

fact, superior to CT scan and aortography. MRI, although as accurate as TEE, is limited by availability, cost, and patient tolerance. Furthermore, in critically ill patients, TEE can be performed more rapidly, can avoid the risks of radioopaque contrast dye and avoid the hazards of transporting patients from heavily monitored critical care areas to radiology suites. Data from a European cooperative study demonstrated TEE to be superior to both aortography and standard CT scan (42). Published results from this multicenter study of 164 consecutive patients with suspected aortic dissection (82 had proven dissection) revealed the sensitivity/specificity of TEE, CT scan, and aortography were 99%/98%, 83%/100%, and 88%/94%, respectively. This large study leaves little doubt as to the accuracy of TEE for the diagnosis of acute dissection. Seventeen patients in that study underwent operation without any other investigative procedure, and the diagnosis of dissection was confirmed in all 17 patients. Subsequent studies have confirmed the accuracy of TEE (Table 10). However, there have been a few reports of failure to recognize type II dissection presumably due to the limited imaging of the distal ascending aorta by TEE. Knowledge of the pitfalls and limitations of the diagnosis of aortic dissection, including the recognition of reverberation and mirror image artifact (48), is important in avoiding incorrect results.

The use of color flow Doppler with TEE helps to identify entry and reentry sites. True and false lumens can almost always be distinguished. TEE is not only useful for detecting and quantitating aortic insufficiency, but can also assist the preoperative planning of the surgical procedure by determining the mechanism of aortic insufficiency. In addition, echocardiography is the procedure of choice for detecting any pericardial effusion that may result from the dissection. Left ventricular function and other significant valvular disease can also be readily assessed.

When the diagnosis of aortic dissection is established by TEE (as in Fig. 8) and all questions necessary to proceed with surgery are answered, no further diagnostic test is required (49). If, however, the diagnosis of aortic dissection is not definitive, then MRI or CT scan is recommended. Aortography is rarely needed except when major side branch involvement is suspected or if information about coronary artery anatomy is necessary. It should also be mentioned

TABLE 10. *Detection of aortic dissection: accuracy of TEE*

Author	Year	n	With diss'n	Sensitivity (%)	Specificity (%)
Erbel et al. (42)	1989	164	82	99	98
Hashimoto et al. (43)	1989	22	22	100	N/A
Adachi et al. (44)	1991	45	45	98	N/A
Ballal et al. (45)	1992	61	34	97	N/A
Simon et al. (46)	1992	32	28	100	100
Nienaber et al. (47)	1993	110	44	98	77
Totals		445	276	98.5	94

n, number of suspected aortic dissections; *TEE*, transesophageal echocardiography; *with diss'n*, number of confirmed dissections.

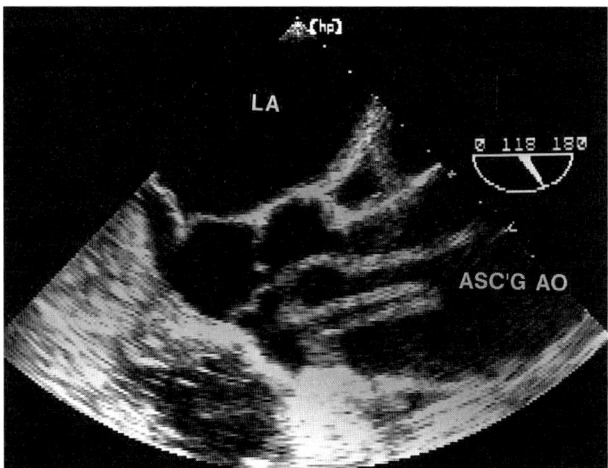

FIG. 8. Longitudinal view (118 degrees) of the ascending aorta (*ASC'G AO*), which contains a convoluted, folded aortic dissection flap. *LA,* left atrium.

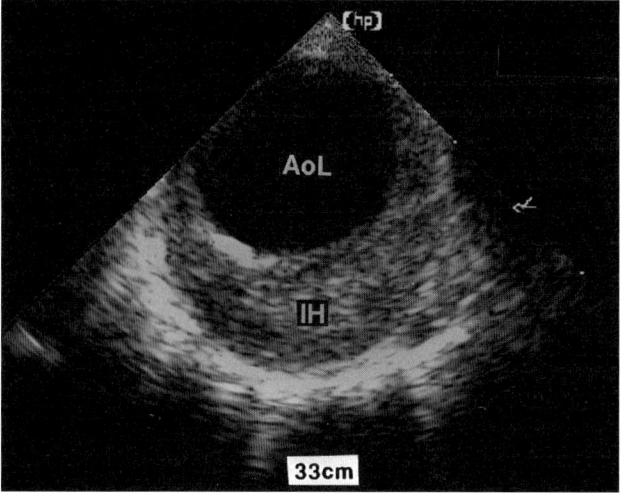

FIG. 9. A cross-sectional view of the proximal descending thoracic aorta, 33 cm from the incisors, which illustrates an intramural hematoma (*IH*), imaged as a crescent-shaped thickening of the aortic wall. *AoL,* aortic lumen.

that a newer and improved type of CT-scan (spiral or helical CT-scan) may become a third alternative (to TEE and MRI) for the initial evaluation of patients with suspected aortic dissection. Spiral CT significantly reduces scan time, reduces respiration and motion artifact, and allows more images during peak levels of contrast enhancement. This technique is capable of three-dimensional imaging, and appears to have a sensitivity and specificity comparable to that of TEE and MRI. A study by Sommer et al. compared the accuracy of spiral CT, MRI, and TEE in 49 patients with suspected aortic dissection (50). Of these, 25 were confirmed to have dissection (18 type A; 7 type B). The sensitivity/specificity of spiral CT, MRI, and TEE were 100%/100%, 100%/94%, and 100%/94%, respectively.

The hallmark of aortic dissection is a dissection flap separating true and false lumens. However, recently, investigators have described an "atypical" type of aortic dissection in which there is no detectable dissection flap in any region of the aorta. This "atypical" type of aortic dissection is detectable by CT scan, MRI, and/or TEE as an abnormally thickened aortic wall, often eccentric and crescent-shaped in cross section (Fig. 9). Aortography usually fails to diagnose this important variant, because the lumen of the aorta is typically normal in size and shape. This "atypical" type

of aortic dissection was termed "aortic dissection without intimal rupture" by Yamada et al. (51), but is more commonly known as intramural hematoma or intramural hemorrhage. Intramural hematomas account for approximately 5 to 15% of all aortic dissections (Table 11). These may occur in either the ascending or descending thoracic aorta, but appear to be more common in the latter region (type B). Although not as thoroughly studied as "classic" aortic dissection, intramural hematomas pose identical risks and should be managed similarly.

TEE provides an excellent means for serial follow-up of patients with aortic dissection (57). It is well tolerated and can be performed on an outpatient basis without exposing patients to radiation or contrast agents. Follow-up by TEE can document healing and stability, or can detect changes, progression, and complications. Items to be evaluated include: diameter of the aorta at various levels (with careful attention to progressive dilatation); aneurysm or pseudoaneurysm formation; competence of the aortic valve after surgical reconstruction; prosthetic aortic valve function; and development of aneurysm or aneurysms of the sinuses of Valsalva, especially in patients with Marfan's syndrome.

TABLE 11. *Intramural hematoma ("atypical" aortic dissection)*

Author	n	Intramural method	Hematoma		Type I	Type II	Type III
Williams et al. (52)	33	CT	8	24%	1	0	7
Nienaber et al. (53)	195	TEE, CT, MRI	25	12.8%	12	0	13
Karen et al. (54)	49	TEE	10	20%	4	1	5
Harris et al. (55)	84	TEE	19	23%	5	4	11
Vilacosta et al. (56)	88	TEE	15	17%	5	4	6
Totals	449		77	17%	27	9	42

n, number; *CT*, computed tomography; *MRI*, magnetic resonance imaging; *TEE*, transesophageal echocardiography.

TABLE 12. *Goals of imaging thoracic aortic aneurysms*

1. Confirm diagnosis
2. Measure maximal diameter of the aneurysm
3. Define longitudinal extent of the aneurysm
4. Determine involvement of aortic valve
5. Determine involvement of arch vessel(s)
6. Detect periaortic hematoma or other signs of leakage
7. Differentiate from aortic dissection
8. Detect mural thrombus

Aortic Aneurysm

The role of TEE for detecting and evaluating thoracic aortic aneurysms is currently evolving (82). The major goals of imaging thoracic aortic aneurysms are listed in Table 12. Both CT-scan and aortography, the most firmly established methods for evaluating thoracic aortic aneurysms, have limitations. TEE promises to overcome some of these limitations and appears to be at least as accurate in identifying the size and location of aneurysms. Although several case studies have been reported, there is only one "large" published study using TEE to evaluate thoracic aortic aneurysms. In this study by Taams and colleagues, 15 patients with thoracic aneurysms were diagnosed by TEE, whereas three of these were missed by CT scan (58). TEE provides detailed information about intraluminal structures such as thrombus (Fig. 10) and atherosclerotic plaque. TEE can also detect compression of adjacent structures such as the pulmonary artery and the left atrium. Moreover, color Doppler may be used to detect complications of aneurysms such as fistulae.

Aortic Trauma

Transesophageal echocardiography has also been used to diagnose traumatic injury to the aorta that usually results from motor vehicle accidents. Traumatic pseudoaneurysms and aortic transections account for 15 to 20% of fatalities from high speed accidents (59).

Traumatic lesions typically occur at the region of the greatest shearing force, the isthmus of the aorta (95%). Only a minority are in the ascending aorta. The majority of aortic tears are horizontal and range from small lacerations to circumferential tears. They typically develop from the inside

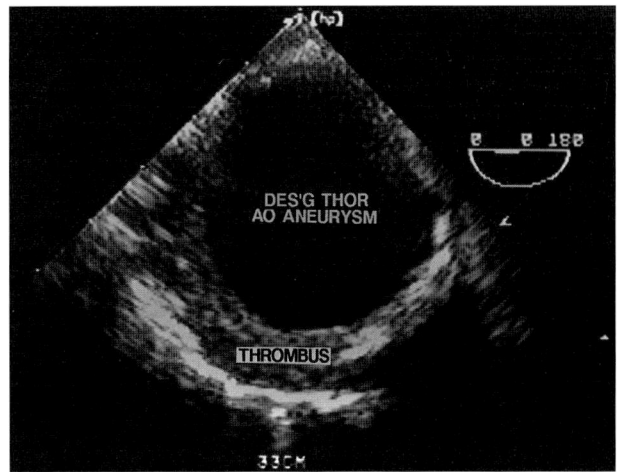

FIG. 10. Cross-sectional view of the proximal descending thoracic aorta (33 cm from incisors) illustrating a 5 cm fusiform aneurysm (*Des'g thor AO aneurysm*) partially lined by *thrombus*.

and progress outward. They may involve the intima only, intima and varying amounts of the media, or the full thickness of the aortic wall. Major dissection is *not* a typical feature of traumatic rupture, probably because there is usually no *medial disease*. The extent of injury ranges from small intimal tears to frank rupture and may include pseudoaneurysms, intramural hematoma, and intramural thrombi. All of these can be detected with transesophageal echocardiography (64). Although aortography remains the "gold standard," recent studies have shown that TEE compares favorably with aortography. Yet as noted in Table 13, results with TEE are inconsistent. This probably reflects the variable experience among individual trauma centers. The main advantage of TEE over aortography is the rapidity with which it can be performed in any area of the hospital and its avoidance of toxic radiographic dyes.

Atherosclerosis

The effectiveness of TEE for the detection, characterization, and embolic potential of atherosclerotic plaques in the thoracic aorta has been previously discussed in the section on cardiac source of embolism.

TABLE 13. *Detection of traumatic injury of the thoracic aorta by TEE*

Author	Year	Suspected rupture	Actual rupture	Sensitivity (%)	Specificity (%)
Shapiro et al. (59)	1991	19	3	67	100
Brooks et al. (60)	1991	21	3	100	—
Kearney et al. (61)	1993	69	7	100	100
Buckmeister et al. (62)	1994	121	14	100	100
Saletta et al. (63)	1994	114	7	62	84
Smith et al. (64)	1994	101	11	100	98
Vignon et al. (65)	1995	32	13	92	100
Minard et al. (66)	1996	34	9	57	91

TEE, transesophageal echocardiography.

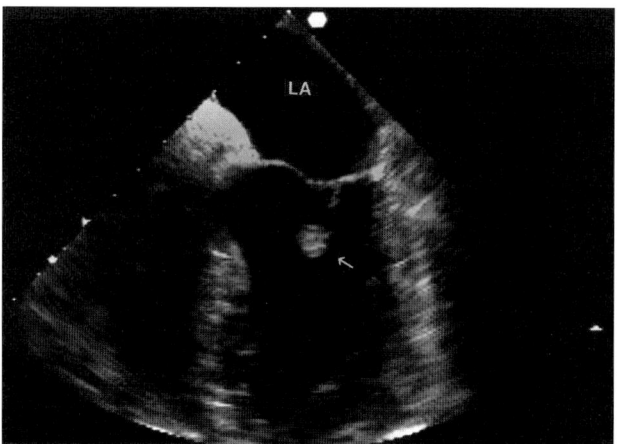

FIG. 11. *Arrow* indicates a small tumor attached to the mitral apparatus. The tumor was surgically removed and pathology confirmed it to be a papillary fibroelastoma. *LA*, left atrium.

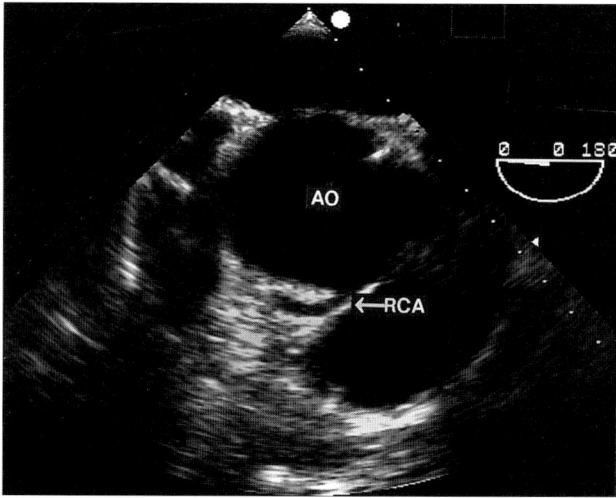

FIG. 12. Cross-sectional view (0 degrees) of the aortic root (*AO*) illustrating the proximal 2 cm of the right coronary artery (*RCA*).

INTRACARDIAC MASSES

Although transthoracic echocardiography is generally excellent for detecting left atrial myxoma, left ventricular thrombi, and other left-sided tumors, TEE is sometimes useful for the further evaluation of these intracardiac masses. TEE can provide additional important information about the site(s) of attachment (Fig. 11), the presence of smaller, secondary lesions, acoustic characteristics, and extension into or impingement upon adjacent structures. These features can be helpful in differentiating malignant from benign masses (32). It is important to emphasize, however, that echocardiography cannot make a histologic diagnosis. Nevertheless, TEE is also often useful in confirming whether or not a mass that is noted by TTE is real or an artifact. Mugge et al. have suggested that masses in or adjacent to the right heart are detected better by TEE than by TTE (67).

The important role of transesophageal echo in identifying left atrial and left atrial appendage thrombi has been discussed earlier (see section on cardiac source of embolus). TEE can also detect pulmonary emboli in the main pulmonary artery and its proximal branches, especially the right pulmonary artery.

CORONARY ARTERIES

Although multiple diagnostic methods are available to visualize the coronary arteries, coronary angiography remains the ''gold standard.'' Noninvasive visualization of the coronary arteries by conventional TTE has been well documented, but the image quality is generally inadequate to permit consistently reliable anatomic details in adult patients. Moreover, TTE imaging of the coronary arteries is time-consuming because the arteries are small and rapidly move in and out of the imaging plane. The superior imaging ability of TEE permits higher resolution and imaging of longer lengths of the coronary arteries than by TTE.

Using TEE, the coronary arteries are imaged just above the level of the aortic valve. The left main and left circumflex coronary arteries are nearly perpendicular to the echo beam and are easily imaged in most patients. The left main coronary artery may almost always be followed to its bifurcation. The left circumflex artery can sometimes be visualized over a distance of 3 to 4 cm. However, the proximal right coronary artery, located further from the TEE echo transducer, is more difficult to image. Nevertheless, it is occasionally visible for several centimeters along its length (Fig. 12). Variable success rates for visualizing the different coronary arteries have been reported (68). The left main coronary artery is visualized in 77 to 100%; the left anterior descending coronary artery (LAD) in 14 to 93%; the left circumflex coronary artery in 33 to 93%; and the right coronary artery in 7 to 82%.

The proximal LAD coronary artery lies almost parallel to the interrogating Doppler beam. This favorable orientation permits adequate pulsed-wave Doppler recordings of coronary blood flow velocity (CBFV) in up to 75% of patients. The normal velocity flow profile is biphasic with a larger diastolic component and a smaller systolic component.

The clinical and pathophysiologic importance of measuring coronary flow reserve is receiving increasing attention. Coronary flow reserve, the difference between baseline (control) and maximal hyperemic flow, is considered to be a better indicator of the functional significance of coronary artery disease than the mere visual anatomic severity of a lesion by coronary angiography. Calculation of coronary flow reserve by TEE Doppler recordings of LAD flow velocity was first described by Iliceto et al. in a select group of patients with and without coronary artery disease (69). Newer contrast agents may improve the feasibility of recording blood flow velocity in the left coronary artery.

Although evaluation of CBFV by TEE is feasible, its clinical value remains to be determined. Certain limitations must be recognized: (i) velocity and not flow is measured (the latter requires accurate measurement of the vessel diameter); (ii) the angle between the Doppler beam and the coronary artery may not be zero degrees, resulting in underestimation of the true velocity; (iii) this method is limited to assessing flow in the LAD artery; and (iv) a clear flow velocity signal during systole is often not present because cardiac motion prevents a stable position of the sample volume within the coronary vessel. Nevertheless, TEE has the advantage of being less invasive and associated with fewer complications than cardiac catheterization. Validation of TEE Doppler methods for the assessment of coronary flow reserve needs to be performed.

Numerous reports have documented the usefulness of TEE in identifying many types of coronary artery anomalies including coronary artery aneurysms, coronary saphenous vein bypass graft aneurysms, coronary arterio-venous fistulae, and abnormal origin of the coronary arteries. TEE can also document the precise drainage site of coronary fistulae in patients in whom angiography has failed to do so.

In summary, TEE is potentially useful for evaluating coronary artery disease in select patients. At present, TEE allows imaging of the proximal coronary arteries, measurement of coronary flow reserve, and identification of coronary artery anomalies.

With technical advances, newer contrast agents, and improvement in operator skills, the role of TEE in evaluating coronary artery disease can be expected to increase.

CONGENITAL HEART DISEASE

Transthoracic echocardiography with Doppler has become an indispensable tool for the evaluation of congenital heart disease and has reduced the need for cardiac catheterization in most pediatric centers. TEE is not required for the majority of these patients. However, children with abnormal heart location, poor precordial ultrasonic windows (e.g., chest wall abnormalities), post-operative patients (especially with previous median sternotomy), children who require detailed imaging of posterior cardiac structures (e.g., pulmonary veins, Fontan circulation), and adults with congenital heart disease may require TEE. Sutherland and Stumper evaluated a group of consecutive patients with congenital heart disease referred for a complete cardiovascular diagnosis (70). Patients were grouped into children between the ages of 0 and 14 years and adolescents over 14 years. Both unoperated and postsurgical patients were included. Transthoracic echo provided a complete, correct morphologic and hemodynamic diagnosis in 93% of infants and children, but in only 57% of adolescents. This difference was felt to reflect the poor acoustic window, lower image resolution, and higher incidence of prior thoracotomy in the adolescent/adult group. Nevertheless, TEE is used extensively in infants, chil-

dren, adolescence, and adults with congenital heart disease. In smaller children and infants, the procedure is usually performed under general anesthesia.

The proximity and orientation of the TEE probe relative to the atrial septum makes TEE a reliable technique for the detection of atrial septal defects (ASDs). Transthoracic echo can detect more than 90% of ostium secundum, nearly 100% of ostium primum, and up to 75% of sinus venosus ASDs. However, the superb imaging of the atrial septum by TEE permits the diagnosis of all three types in almost 100% of patients. In particular, TEE more readily identifies sinus venosus and multiple (fenestrated) atrial septal defects. Furthermore, in patients with ostium primum defects the chordal attachments of both atrioventricular valves can be precisely identified. Moreover, TEE is superior to TTE for measuring the diameter of defects and has become an important tool for appropriate patient selection for transcatheter closure of these defects.

In a study by Shyu et al., TEE provided significantly more diagnostic information than TTE in evaluating 40 patients with patent ductus arteriosus (71). Transesophageal echo can contribute additional valuable information compared to TTE when assessing the morphology and function of either atrioventricular valve and the subvalve apparatus in children with complex congenital heart disease. The mechanism of valve regurgitation, and the site and number of regurgitant jets, can often be defined more accurately. In addition, in patients with either tricuspid or mitral atresia, TEE provides improved differentiation between an imperforate valve and an absent connection. TEE also offers improved insight into the spectrum of lesions producing left ventricular outflow tract obstruction. In 28 adult patients with right ventricular outflow tract lesions (including patients with repaired Fallot's tetralogy and right ventricular outflow tract conduits, pulmonary atresia and unifocalization of pulmonary blood flow, and valvular or subvalvular pulmonic stenosis), Marelli et al. demonstrated the superiority of TTE over TEE for demonstrating anatomic or hemodynamic details of the right ventricular outflow tract.

Transesophageal echocardiography is also an established and reliable intraoperative tool during corrective or palliative repair procedures. Residual shunts, obstructions, and valvular insufficiency can be detected. Among 127 infants and children undergoing operations between one day and 18 years of age, Ritter reported that TEE provided additional information in 56% (72). Transesophageal echo has also proven to be useful in the follow-up of children with surgically corrected congenital heart disease.

TEE has also been used during interventions such as aortic and pulmonic valvotomy, closure of patient ductus arteriosus, Mustard baffle dilatation, and guidance of bedside balloon atrial septostomy in newborns.

Other congenital heart diseases for which TEE plays an important role include Ebstein's anomaly, bicuspid aortic valve, discrete subaortic stenosis, cor triatriatum, supramitral valve stenosing ring, left superior vena cava, coarctation of the aorta, and coronary artery anomalies and fistulas. In summary, the use of TEE in infants and children should be restricted to carefully selected patients. The risks associated with anesthesia or the heavy sedation necessary for the examination should be balanced against the potential benefits.

CRITICALLY ILL PATIENTS

Cardiac emergencies occur anywhere in the hospital including the emergency room, intensive care units, and the operating room. Rapid assessment and diagnosis is often critical for proper management and outcome. Clinical exam, ECG, chest X-ray, and even bedside Swan Ganz catheterization often do not provide all of the necessary information. Cardiac catheterization may be necessary in select patients, but it adds risk and is not available in all centers. Computed tomography and magnetic resonance imaging can be useful, but also have major limitations in emergency situations (time consuming, need to move patient and equipment from the critical care setting, etc). Echocardiography, on the other hand, is rapid, safe, can be performed at the bedside, and provides not only morphologic, but also hemodynamic information. Transthoracic echo (TTE) is still the first line of approach and provides immediate diagnosis in many patients. However, TTE is sometimes limited in critically ill patients and in the intensive care unit setting because of:

1. Suboptimal patient positioning
2. Unresponsive or uncooperative patients
3. Mechanical ventilation
4. Surgical incisions, chest tubes, bandages
5. Respiratory distress
6. Subcutaneous emphysema
7. Intraaortic balloon pump and left ventricular assist devices
8. Tachycardia (limitations with color Doppler)

Transesophageal echo not only overcomes these limitations, but also provides improved resolution compared to TTE. Moreover, TEE can be performed simultaneously with other diagnostic and therapeutic procedures such as laparotomy, fracture repair, and resuscitation. As a consequence, TEE is increasingly being utilized in critically ill patients and in emergency situations. The combination of TTE and TEE has evolved into a powerful diagnostic procedure and is unmatched in terms of versatility and application and in the variety of information that can be obtained. A list of the indications for TEE in critically ill patients is listed in Table 14. The impact of transesophageal echo on the management of these conditions is significant and has been discussed in several studies (73–75). Findings can lead to major changes in medical therapy such as initiation or discontinuation of catecholamines, inotropic drugs, IV fluids, antibiotics, and/ or anticoagulation. The findings can also lead to surgical intervention (e.g., valve replacement or repair, evacuation of pericardial fluid and/or hematoma, and insertion or dis-

TABLE 14. *Indications for TEE in critically ill patients*

1. Unexplained hypotension
2. Hemodynamic instability (low output state)
3. Acute pulmonary edema
4. LV and RV function
5. Complications of acute myocardial infarction
6. Post-op cardiac surgery (acute clinical deterioration)
7. Valvular regurgitation (especially mitral regurgitation)
8. Prosthetic valve dysfunction
9. New neurologic deficit
10. Sepsis, suspected endocarditis
11. Unexplained hypoxemia (suspected shunts)
12. Pulmonary embolism
13. Aortic dissection
14. Trauma
15. Potential heart donor
16. Insertion of/weaning from cardiac support devices
17. Superior vena cava obstruction

LV, left ventricular; *RV*, right ventricular; *TEE*, transesophageal echocardiography.

continuation of ventricular assist devices). The safety of TEE in critically ill patients has been established (73,74).

GUIDANCE OF INTERVENTIONAL PROCEDURES

Although the primary purpose of cardiac ultrasound remains diagnostic, the evolution and technology has permitted the expansion of cardiac ultrasound into what has been termed *interventional echocardiography*. Examples of interventional echocardiography, that is the use of echocardiography to guide invasive techniques, are listed in Table 15.

TEE can provide superb image quality continuously during positioning of catheters and other devices, delineating their relationship to intracardiac structures without interrupting or interfering with catheter manipulation or fluoroscopy (76). In fact, TEE guidance may actually decrease fluoroscopic exposure time. During balloon mitral valvotomy, TEE may guide transseptal puncture (Fig. 13) and balloon positioning, may immediately assess results, and may detect or prevent complications (77). An important lesson learned

TABLE 15. *Role of TEE for guidance of interventional procedures*

1. Intraoperative echocardiography
2. Echo-guided pericardiocentesis
3. Guide endomyocardial biopsy
4. Guide balloon and blade atrial septostomy
5. Guide catheter-based closure of ASD and VSD
6. Transvenous "rescue" of intracardiac foreign bodies
7. Monitor high-risk or complex coronary interventions in the cardiac cath lab
8. Guide catheter ablation of cardiac arrhythmias
9. Guide percutaneous balloon valvotomy
10. Guide surgical or percutaneous transmyocardial laser revascularization

ASD, atrial septal defect; *TEE*, transesophageal echocardiography; *VSD*, ventricular septal defect.

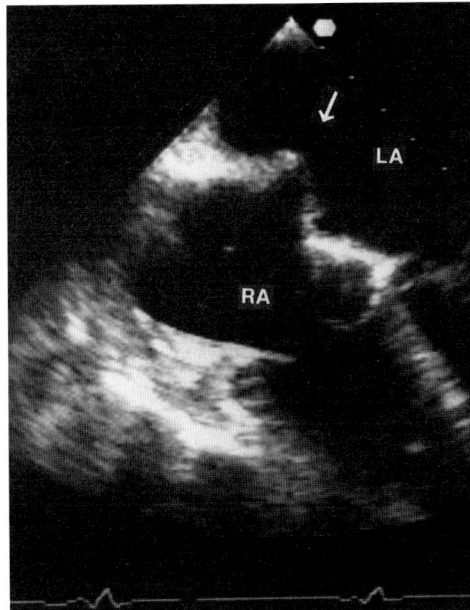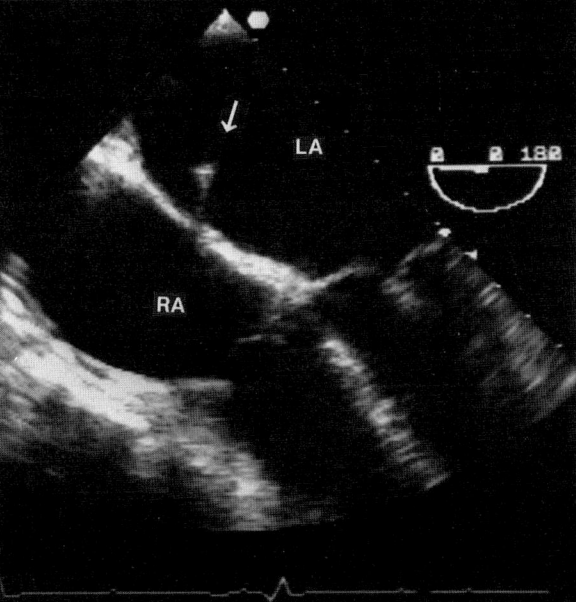

FIG. 13. Transesophageal echo done during balloon mitral valvuloplasty illustrates how echo-imaging can supplement fluoroscopic guidance in the cardiac catheterization laboratory. **Left panel** illustrates "tenting" or bowing (*arrow*) of the atrial septum toward the left atrium (*LA*) due to contact with the advancing transseptal needle. **Right panel** illustrates the tip of the transseptal needle (*arrow*) in the left atrium and return of atrial septum to its normal position. *RA*, right atrium.

from TEE guidance of procedures has been the recognition of the propensity for clot formation on catheters on both sides of the heart (76).

TRANSESOPHAGEAL STRESS ECHOCARDIOGRAPHY

Stress echocardiography is now well established and widely employed as a diagnostic and prognostic test in patients with known or suspected coronary artery disease. The transthoracic approach provides satisfactory image quality in the vast majority of patients. However, a small but significant number of patients have technically inadequate image quality by this approach, even when harmonic imaging is utilized. Recently, several investigators have attempted to overcome this problem utilizing the superior image quality of transesophageal stress testing in conjunction with atrial pacing, dipyridamole, or dobutamine infusion (78,79). These investigators have established the feasibility, accuracy, and safety of this procedure. Moreover, when used in combination with newer myocardial contrast agents, transesophageal stress echocardiography shows promise for the evaluation of myocardial perfusion and blood flow. However, the semi-invasive nature of TEE has limited its widespread use for this purpose. Other disadvantages include limited imaging of the left ventricular apex, patient discomfort, the need for conscious sedation in most patients, and added time and cost.

Therefore, at the present time, the role of transesophageal stress echo appears limited and should be considered as an alternative test only when TTE images are suboptimal and when other stress-imaging modalities, such as stress-Thallium, are not available or additional information about left ventricular function, valvular function, or other cardiac structure is required.

FUTURE ADVANCES

Transesophageal echo has been in widespread use for only a decade. During this time, rapid advances in technology have occurred, and further advances are expected to continue. Small probes have already been developed for pediatric use. Smaller probes also offer new possibilities, including ambulatory monitoring for prolonged imaging. Wide-angle imaging producing "panoramic" views should facilitate comprehension of the heart and surrounding structures. Perhaps even more important is the developing technology of three-dimensional reconstruction. The extensive progress that has been made in this area is expected to reach commercial machines and more widespread use in the near future. Increasing use of digital technology, permitting transfer of images from the operating room or laboratories to remote viewing stations, is expected to grow. Used in conjunction with newer contrast agents, TEE has the potential to assess myocardial perfusion and, therefore, the ability to assess the success of regional myocardial reperfusion postcoronary artery bypass grafting or other forms of coronary revascularization. These, and perhaps other advances, should continue to expand the applications of transesophageal echocardiography.

CONCLUSIONS

Transesophageal echocardiography is a relatively new imaging technology that provides extremely high-resolution images. Nevertheless, transthoracic echocardiography remains the primary echocardiographic imaging technique. TEE is not a substitute for a properly performed and comprehensive conventional echo and Doppler study. Transesophageal echo is currently the echocardiographic procedure of choice for the diagnosis of aortic dissection, intraaortic atheromatous ''debris,'' complications of infective endocarditis, prosthetic valve endocarditis, prosthetic valve dysfunction (especially perivalvular leaks around mitral prostheses), and the intraoperative assessment of mitral and aortic valve repair. In some situations, such as aortic dissection, TEE has eliminated the need for further and often more invasive evaluation, thus reducing cost and improving safety. TEE also plays an important role in evaluating select patients with endocarditis, native valve disease (especially for determining the precise mechanism of valvular regurgitation), congenital heart disease, and intracardiac masses. Its role in evaluating patients with systemic embolism is controversial, but it clearly appears to be useful in select patients.

It should be emphasized that TEE is a semiinvasive procedure associated with a low but identifiable risk, and, therefore, should only be performed by experienced physicians in appropriately selected patients where the findings are expected to alter clinical management.

ACKNOWLEDGMENTS

The author wishes to thank Drs. Joseph Lindsay Jr. and Gary S. Mintz for their helpful review of this manuscript. The author also wishes to thank Pushpa Gulati for her expert assistance in preparing this manuscript.

REFERENCES

1. Frazin L, Talano JV, Stephanides L, et al. Esophageal echocardiography. *Circulation* 1976;54:102–108.
2. Hisanaga K, Hisanaga A, Nagata K, et al. A new transesophageal real-time two-dimensional echocardiographic system using a flexible tube and its clinical applications. *Proc JPN J Med Ultrason* 1977;32:43–44.
3. Seward JB, Khandheria BK, Oh JK, et al. Transesophageal echocardiography: technique, anatomic correlations, implementation, and clinical applications. *Mayo Clin Proc* 1986;63:649–680.
4. Khandheria BK, Seward JB, Tajik AJ. Transesophageal echocardiography (Review). *Mayo Clin Proc* 1994;69:856–863.
5. Pandian NG, Hsu TL, Schwartz SL, et al. Multiplane transesophageal echocardiography. Imaging planes, echocardiographic anatomy, and clinical experience with a prototype phased array Omni plane probe. *Echocardiography* 1992;9:649–666.
6. Daniel WG, Mugge A. Transesophageal echocardiography (Review). *N Engl J Med* 1995;332:1268–1279.
7. Cheitlin MD, Alpert JS, Armstrong WF, et al. ACC/AHA guidelines for the clinical application of echocardiography: a report of the American College of Cardiology/American Heart Association Task Force on Practice Guidelines (Committee on Clinical Application of Echocardiography). *Circulation* 1997;95:1686–1744.
8. Durack DT, Lukes AS, Bright DK. New criteria for diagnosis of infective endocarditis: utilization of specific echocardiographic findings. *Am J Med* 1994;96:200–210.
9. Erbel R, Rohmann S, Drexler M, et al. Improved diagnostic value of echocardiography in patients with infective endocarditis by TEE. A prospective study. *Eur Heart J* 1988;9:43–53.
10. Daniel WG, Schroder E, Mugge A, et al. Transesophageal echocardiography in infective endocarditis. *Am J Cardiac Imaging* 1988;2:78–85.
11. Chan KL, Daniel L, Rakowski H, et al. Transesophageal echocardiography is crucial in the management of endocarditis. *Circulation* 1989; 80(Suppl II):668(abst).
12. Mugge A, Daniel WG, Frank G, et al. Echocardiography in infective endocarditis: reassessment of prognostic implications of vegetation size determined by the transthoracic and the transesophageal approach. *J Am Coll Cardiol* 1989;14:631–638.
13. Taams MA, Gussenhoven EJ, Bos E, et al. Enhanced morphologic diagnosis in infective endocarditis by TEE. *Br Heart J* 1990;63: 109–113.
14. Shively BK, Gurule FT, Roldan CA, et al. Diagnostic value of TEE compared with transthoracic echo in infective endocarditis. *J Am Coll Cardiol* 1991;18:391–397.
15. Pedersen WR, Walker M, Olson JD, et al. Value of transesophageal echocardiography as an adjunct to transthoracic echocardiography in evaluation of native and prosthetic valve endocarditis. *Chest* 1991;100: 351–356.
16. Birmingham GD, Rahko PS, Ballantyne F. Improved detection of infective endocarditis with TEE. *Am Heart J* 1992;123:774–781.
17. Shapiro SM, Bayer AS. Transesophageal and Doppler echocardiography in the diagnosis and management of infective endocarditis. *Chest* 1991;100:1125–1130.
18. Lowry RW, Zoghbi WA, Baker WB, et al. Clinical impact of transesophageal echocardiography in the diagnosis and management of infective endocarditis. *Am J Cardiol* 1994;73:1089–1091.
19. Karalis DG, Bansal RC, Hauck AJ, et al. Transesophageal echocardiographic recognition of subaortic complications in aortic valve endocarditis: clinical and surgical implications. *Circulation* 1992;86:353–362.
20. Sochowski RA, Chan KL. Implications of negative results on a monoplane transesophageal echocardiographic study in patients with suspected infective endocarditis. *J Am Coll Cardiol* 1993;21:216–221.
21. DeRook FA, Comess KA, Albers GW, et al. Transesophageal echocardiography in the evaluation of stroke. *Ann Intern Med* 1992;117: 922–932.
22. Pop G, Sutherland GR, Koudstaal PJ, et al. Transesophageal echocardiography in the detection of intracardiac embolic sources in patients with transient ischemic attacks. *Stroke* 1990;21:560–565.
23. Hofmann T, Kasper W, Meinetz T, et al. Echocardiographic evaluation of patients with clinically suspected arterial emboli. *Lancet* 1990;336: 1421–1424.
24. Pearson AC, Labovitz AJ, Tatineni S, et al. Superiority of transesophageal echocardiography in detecting source of embolism in patients with cerebral ischemia of uncertain etiology. *J Am Coll Cardiol* 1991;17: 66–71.
25. Cujec B, Polasek P, Voll C, et al. Transesophageal echocardiography in the detection of potential cardiac source of embolism in stroke patients. *Stroke* 1991;22:727–733.
26. DeRook FA, Comess KA, Albers GW, et al. Transesophageal echocardiography in the evaluation of stroke. *Ann Intern Med* 1992;117: 922–932.
27. Lee RJ, Bartzokis T, Yeoh TK, et al. Enhanced detection of intracardiac sources of cerebral emboli by transesophageal echocardiography. *Stroke* 1991;22:734–739.
28. Manning WJ, Weintraub RM, Waksmonski CA, et al. Accuracy of transesophageal echocardiography for identifying left atrial thrombi: a prospective, intraoperative study. *Ann Intern Med* 1995;123:817–822.
29. Manning WJ, Silverman DI, Keighley CS, et al. Transesophageal echocardiography facilitated early cardioversion from atrial fibrillation using short-term anticoagulation: final results of prospective 4.5-year study. *J Am Coll Cardiol* 1995;25:1354–1361.
30. Klein AL, Grimm RA, Black IW, et al. Cardioversion guided by transesophageal echocardiography: the ACUTE Pilot Study. A randomized, controlled trial. *Ann Intern Med* 1997;126:200–209.
31. Orsinelli DA, Pearson AC. Detection of prosthetic valve strands by transesophageal echocardiography: clinical significance in patients with suspected cardiac source of embolism. *J Am Coll Cardiol* 1995; 26:1713–1718.
32. Engberding R, Daniel WG, Erbel R, et al. Diagnosis of heart tumours by transesophageal echocardiography: a multicenter study in 154 patients. *Eur Heart J* 1993;14:1223–1228.
33. The Stroke Prevention in Atrial Fibrillation Committee in Echocardiog-

raphy. Transesophageal echocardiographic correlates of thromboembolism in high-risk patients with nonvalvular atrial fibrillation. *Ann Intern Med* 1998;128:639–647.

34. Schneider B, Zienkiewicz T, Jansen V, et al. Diagnosis of patent foramen ovale by transesophageal echocardiography and correlation with autopsy findings. *Am J Cardiol* 1996;77:1202–1209.
35. Lechat PH, Mas JL, Lascault G, et al. Prevalence of patent foramen ovale in patients with stroke. *N Engl J Med* 1988;318:1148–1152.
36. Stollberger C, Slany J, Schuster I, et al. The prevalence of deep venous thrombosis in patients with suspected paradoxical embolism. *Ann Intern Med* 1993;119:461–465.
37. Leung YC, Black JW, Cranney GB, et al. Prognostic implications of left atrial spontaneous echo contrast in nonvalvular atrial fibrillation. *J Am Coll Cardiol* 1994;24:755–762.
38. Marks AR, Choong CY, Sanfilippo AJ, et al. Identification of high-risk and low-risk subgroups of patients with mitral valve prolapse. *N Engl J Med* 1989;320:1031–1036.
39. Stoddard MF, Prince CR, Tuman WL, et al. Angle of incidence does not affect accuracy of mitral stenosis area calculation by pressure half-time: application to transesophageal echocardiography. *Am Heart J* 1994;127:562–572.
40. Daniel WG, Mugge A, Grote J, et al. Comparison of transthoracic and transesophageal echocardiography for detection of abnormalities of prosthetic and bioprosthetic valves in the mitral and aortic positions. *Am J Cardiol* 1993;71:210–215.
41. Khandheria BK, Seward JB, Oh JK, et al. Value and limitations of transesophageal echocardiography in assessment of mitral valve prostheses. *Circulation* 1991;83:1956–1968.
42. Erbel R, Engberding R, Daniel W, et al. Echocardiography in diagnosis of aortic dissection. *Lancet* 1989;1:456–460.
43. Hashimoto S, Kumada T, Osakada G, et al. Assessment of transesophageal Doppler echocardiography in dissecting aortic aneurysm. *J Am Coll Cardiol* 1989;14:1253–1262.
44. Adachi H, Omoto R, Kyo S, et al. Emergency surgical intervention of acute aortic dissection with the rapid diagnosis by transesophageal echocardiography. *Circulation* 1991;84(Suppl III):14–19.
45. Ballal RS, Nanda NC, Gatewood R, et al. Usefulness of transesophageal echocardiography in assessment of aortic dissection. *Circulation* 1991;84:1903–1914.
46. Simon P, Owen AN, Havel M, et al. Transesophageal echocardiography in the emergency surgical management of patients with aortic dissection. *J Thorac Cardiovasc Surg* 1992;103:1113–1118.
47. Nienaber CA, von Kodolitsch Y, Nicolas V, et al. The diagnosis of thoracic aortic dissection by noninvasive imaging procedures. *New Engl J Med* 1993;328:1–9.
48. Appelbe AF, Walker PLG, Yeoh JK, et al. Clinical significance and origin of artifacts in transesophageal echocardiography of the thoracic aorta. *J Am Coll Cardiol* 1993;21:754–760.
49. Goldstein SA, Mintz GS, Lindsay JL. Aorta: comprehensive evaluation by echocardiography and transesophageal echocardiography. *J Am Soc Echocardiogr* 1993;6:634–659
50. Sommer T, Fehske W, Holzknecht N, et al. Aortic dissection: A comparative study of diagnosis with spiral CT, multiplanar transesophageal echocardiography and MR imaging. *Radiology* 1996;199:347–352.
51. Yamada T, Tada S, Harada J. Aortic dissection without internal rupture: diagnosis with MR imaging and CT. *Radiology* 1988;168:347–352.
52. Williams MP, Farrow R. Atypical patterns in the CT diagnosis of aortic dissection. *Clin Radiol* 1994;49:686–689.
53. Nienaber CA, von Kodolitsch Y, Petersen B, et al. Intramural hemorrhage of the thoracic aorta: diagnostic and therapeutic implications. *Circulation* 1995;92:1465–1472.
54. Karen A, Kim CB, Hu BS, et al. Accuracy of biplane and multiplane transesophageal echocardiography in diagnosis of typical acute aortic dissection and intramural hematoma. *J Am Coll Cardiol* 1996;28:627–636.
55. Harris KM, Braverman AC, Gutierrez FR, et al. Transesophageal echocardiographic and clinical features of aortic intramural hematoma. *J Thorac Cardiovasc Surg* 1997;114:619–626.
56. Vilacosta I, Castillo JA, Peral V, et al. Intramural aortic hematoma following intra-aortic balloon counterpulsation. Documentation by transesophageal echocardiography. *Eur Heart J* 1995;16:2015–2016.
57. Masani ND, Banning AP, Jones RA, et al. Follow-up of chronic thoracic aortic dissection: comparison of transesophageal echocardiography and magnetic resonance imaging. *Am Heart J* 1996;131:1156–1163.
58. Taams MA, Gussenhoven WJ, Schippers LA, et al. The value of transesophageal echocardiography for diagnosis of thoracic aortic pathology. *Eur Heart J* 1988;9:1308–1316.
59. Shapiro MJ, Yanofsky SD, Trapp J, et al. Cardiovascular evaluation in blunt chest trauma using transesophageal echocardiography. *J Trauma* 1991;31:835–840.
60. Brooks SW, Young JC, Cmolik B, et al. The use of transesophageal echocardiography in the evaluation of chest trauma. *J Trauma* 1992;32:761–768.
61. Kearney PA, Smith DW, Johnson SB, et al. Use of transesophageal echocardiography in the evaluation of traumatic aortic injury. *J Trauma* 1993;34:696–703.
62. Buckmeister MJ, Kearney PA, Johnson SB, et al. Further experience with transesophageal echocardiography in the evaluation of thoracic aortic injury. *J Trauma* 1994;37:989–995.
63. Saletta S, Lederman E, Kuehler DH, et al. Transesophageal echocardiography as the initial evaluation of the widened mediastinum in trauma patients. *J Trauma* 1994;37:166(abst).
64. Smith MD, Cassidy M, Souther S, et al. Transesophageal echocardiography in the diagnosis of traumatic rupture of the aorta. *New Engl J Med* 1995;332:356–362.
65. Vignon P, Gueret P, Vedrinne JM, et al. Role of transesophageal echocardiography in the diagnosis and management of traumatic aortic disruption. *Circulation* 1995;92:2959–2968.
66. Minard G, Schurr MJ, Croce MA, et al. A prospective analysis of transesophageal echocardiography in the diagnosis of traumatic disruption of the aorta. *J Trauma-Injury Infection and Crit Care* 1996;40:225–230.
67. Mugge A, Daniel WG, Haverich A, et al. Diagnosis of noninfective cardiac mass lesions by two-dimensional echocardiography: comparison of the transthoracic and transesophageal approaches. *Circulation* 1991;83:70–78.
68. Tardif JC, Vannan MA, Taylor K, et al. Delineation of extended lengths of coronary arteries by multiplane transesophageal echocardiography. *J Am Coll Cardiol* 1994;24:909–919.
69. Iliceto S, Marangelli V, Memmola C, Rizzon P. Transesophageal Doppler echocardiography evaluation of coronary blood flow velocity in baseline conditions and during dipyridamole-induced coronary vasodilation. *Circulation* 1991;83:61–69.
70. Sutherland GR, Stumper OFW. Transesophageal echocardiography in congenital heart disease. *Acta Paediatr* 1995;[Suppl] 410:15–22.
71. Shyu K, Lai L, Lin S, et al. Diagnostic accuracy of transesophageal echocardiography for detecting patent ductus arteriosus in adolescents and adults. *Chest* 1995;108:1201–1205.
72. Ritter SB. Transesophageal real-time echocardiography in infants and children with congenital heart disease. *J Am Coll Cardiol* 1991;18:569–580.
73. Pearson AC, Castello R, Labovitz AJ. Safety and utility of transesophageal echocardiography in the critically ill patient. *Am Heart J* 1990;119:1083–1089.
74. Oh JK, Seward JB, Khandheria BK, et al. Transesophageal echocardiography in critically ill patients. *Am J Cardiol* 1990;66:1492–1495.
75. Khoury AF, Afridi J, Quinones MA, et al. Transesophageal echocardiography in critically ill patients: feasibility, safety, and impact on management. *Am Heart J* 1994;127:1363–1371.
76. Goldstein SA, Campbell AN. Mitral stenosis: evaluation and guidance of valvuloplasty by TEE. *Cardiol Clinics* 1993;11:409–425.
77. Tong AD, Rothman A, Shiota T, et al. Interventional cardiac catheterization under transesophageal echocardiographic guidance. *Am Heart J* 1995;129:827–831.
78. Panza JA, Laurienzo JM, Curiel RV, et al. Transesophageal dobutamine stress echocardiography for evaluation of patients with coronary artery disease. *J Am Coll Cardiol* 1994;24:1260–1267.
79. Baer FM, Voth E, Deutsch HJ, et al. Assessment of viable myocardium by dobutamine transesophageal echocardiography and comparison with fluorine—18 fluorodeoxyglucose positron emission tomography. *J Am Coll Cardiol* 1994;24:343–353.

CHAPTER 5

Stress Echocardiography

Linda D. Gillam and Anita M. Kelsey

Stress echocardiography is widely used in the evaluation of patients with known or suspected coronary artery disease. Its use for that purpose is based on the premise that myocardial ischemia induced by a stress-induced mismatch in coronary blood flow and myocardial oxygen demand can be detected by observing changes in wall motion. The normal response to exercise or pharmacologic stress is seen by echocardiography as an increase in both endocardial excursion and myocardial wall thickening. A comparison of stress-to-rest images acquired in multiple views allows the differentiation of resting wall motion abnormalities (infarct or hibernating myocardium) from stress-induced regional wall motion abnormalities (ischemia). Stress echocardiographic techniques for distinguishing hibernating from infarcted myocardium have also been developed.

This chapter discusses the evolution and current practice of exercise and pharmacologic stress echocardiography with an emphasis on clinical techniques and evidence-based applications.

HISTORICAL BACKGROUND

The first reports of wall motion abnormalities detectable during exercise appeared in the early 1970s and used only M-mode echocardiography. In 1979, Wann et al. (1) published the first report of two-dimensional echocardiographic imaging during stress. Later studies took advantage of the technique's ability to visualize all cardiac segments and began to look at stress-induced changes in left ventricular cavity dimensions and regional wall motion. In the early 1980s, stress echocardiography was largely limited to research laboratories because of technical difficulties in image acquisition and the challenge of comparing videotaped rest and stress images. These remained major limitations until

L. D. Gillam: Department of Medicine, University of Connecticut, Farmington, Connecticut 06032; Department of Cardiology, Hartford Hospital, Hartford, Connecticut 06102.
A. M. Kelsey: Department of Internal Medicine, University of Connecticut, Farmington, Connecticut 06032; Department of Cardiology, Hartford Hospital, Hartford, Connecticut 06102.

the mid-to-late 1980s when digital image acquisition and simultaneous rest and stress playback became available. Since then, stress echocardiography has rapidly moved into the clinical mainstream aided by ongoing improvements in echocardiographic image acquisition and digital image manipulation. It is currently possible to obtain diagnostically adequate stress echocardiographic studies in more than 85% of patients evaluated.

The rationale for imaging adjuncts to the ECG and clinical endpoints used in conventional stress testing is illustrated in the ischemic cascade shown in Figure 1. Simply stated, ischemia and regional hypoperfusion elicit regional wall motion abnormalities before either ECG changes or symptoms. It would, therefore, be predicted that stress echocardiography would be a more sensitive method for detecting coronary artery disease than conventional stress testing. This has, indeed, been shown to be the case in clinical studies that have demonstrated increased specificity as well (see section entitled Utility of Stress Echocardiography in the Diagnosis of Coronary Artery Disease).

INDICATIONS

The indications for stress echocardiography parallel those for stress testing in general and overwhelmingly relate to the evaluation of patients with known or suspected coronary artery disease. These include the diagnosis of coronary disease, as well as the detection of viable myocardium, risk stratification, and the evaluation of the outcome of revascularization in patients with known disease. Stress echocardiography is also useful in identifying patients at high risk for cardiac events at the time of noncardiac surgery. The use of exercise stress echocardiography as the *initial* stress modality is indicated in situations where the echocardiogram (ECG) alone is of limited value, such as left bundle-branch block, paced rhythm, nonspecific ST/T wave changes, or use of digoxin. It is also indicated when a prior conventional exercise stress test is thought to be falsely positive or negative.

Pharmacologic stress is indicated whenever a patient can-

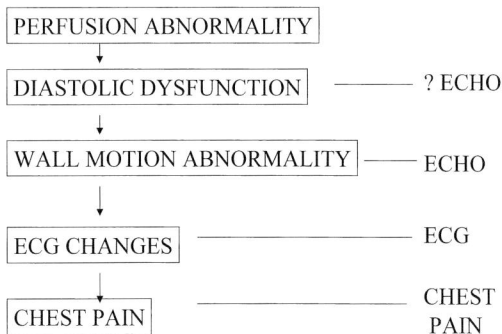

FIG. 1. Demonstration of the cascade of events that occur during myocardial ischemia relative to testing modalities.

not be maximally stressed with exercise. When pharmacologic stress is used, it is imperative that an adjunctive imaging modality be used since the test is unacceptably insensitive if only ECG and clinical endpoints are used.

Stress echocardiography is also useful in nonischemic heart disease, such as valve dysfunction, nonischemic congestive cardiomyopathy, and hypertrophic cardiomyopathy. In these situations, Doppler assessments of hemodynamic parameters, such as gradients and pulmonary artery pressure, complements the technique's imaging capabilities.

METHODS

Stress echocardiography is based on a comparison of baseline and stress images. In clinical practice, the assessment is primarily qualitative or semiquantitative although more quantitative approaches have been used in research applications.

Image Acquisition

Resting transthoracic images are obtained in a minimum of four views: parasternal long-axis view, parasternal short-axis view at the midpapillary muscle level, apical four-chamber and apical two-chamber views (Fig. 2). Additional views, such as the apical long-axis, apical five-chamber, subcostal short-axis, subcostal four-chamber, and parasternal short-axis views at additional levels, may be included to enhance visualization of a particular wall or vascular territory. Comparable views are then acquired during or immediately following stress depending on the form of stress employed (see below). Imaging during stress is desirable since regional wall motion abnormalities may be short-lived. However, with treadmill exercise, this is logistically impossible and peak images obtained within the first 1 to 2 minutes immediately postexercise are generally considered acceptable. Images are stored as digital loops of a single cardiac cycle and displayed side by side with other images from the same view or stage of stress. The display is synchronized with ECG gating. Although the study should also be recorded on videotape, it is not acceptable to rely on sequential videotaped images and one's visual memory of wall motion to interpret the results of the study. However, videotape may be a helpful source of additional beats for analysis if the cycles selected for digital storage prove to be nondiagnostic.

Image Analysis

The recommended approach to wall motion analysis uses the 16 segment model of the left ventricle recommended by the American Society of Echocardiography (2). Stress im-

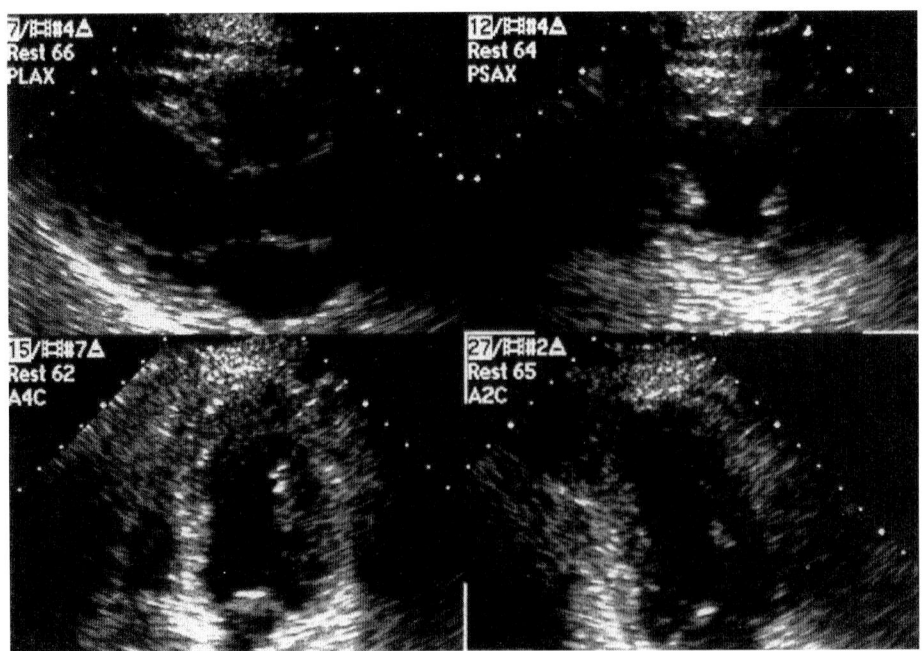

FIG. 2. Standard echocardiographic images acquired digitally during stress echocardiography are presented simultaneously on screen for immediate interpretation.

TABLE 1. *Wall motion score*

	Wall motion
1	Normal
2	Hypokinetic
3	Akinetic
4	Dyskinetic
5	Aneurysmal

ages of each segment are systematically compared to their counterparts at baseline, ensuring that the views are truly comparable. Each segment may then be evaluated using a five-point scoring system as shown in Table 1. A Wall Motion Score Index may be derived by mathematically averaging the individual segment scores for all imaged segments. A normal Wall Motion Score Index would then be 1.0 with higher scores indicating either worsening function within a given segment or dyssynergy that involves more segments. Use of the scoring system provides a standardized method of reporting results and facilitates the comparison of sequential studies in a given patient.

To translate the results of the stress study to the referring physician, the following general approach is used. A normal study is one in which stress induces uniform augmentation of wall motion. Ischemia is identified when a new regional wall motion abnormality is detected, when there is worsening of resting hypokinesis, or when there is regional lack of augmentation of function. Stress that allows continuous imaging (pharmacologic or bicycle), may demonstrate an ischemic biphasic response, in which early augmentation is followed by loss of function. A fixed wall motion abnormality may represent a region of infarction or myocardial hibernation. The approach to differentiating hibernation from infarction is discussed in the section on myocardial viability. There is some controversy concerning the interpretation of akinesis, which progresses to dyskinesis, there being two potential explanations. This phenomenon may represent

either periinfarction ischemia or the passive response of infarcted tissue tethered to normally contracting muscle. Support for the latter hypothesis is presented in the study of Arnese et al. (3). There are some studies that are considered ambiguous since they reveal no stress-induced change in function. This may occur in the setting of global ischemia, nonischemic myopathy, limited exercise, or increased afterload.

Ancillary information that may be helpful in evaluating the ischemic response of patients includes chamber dimensions and an evaluation of the severity of ischemic mitral regurgitation. For example, it has been shown that stress-induced ventricular dilatation is indicative of severe ischemia and triple vessel disease. Theoretically, Doppler indices of diastolic function should be a useful component of stress echocardiography since diastolic dysfunction precedes systolic dysfunction in the ischemic cascade. However, Doppler signals are difficult to interpret at high heart rates due to merging of the mitral E and A waves and signal aliasing. Currently, the assessment of diastolic function during stress remains a research application.

RELATION OF ECHOCARDIOGRAPHIC VIEWS TO CORONARY ARTERY DISTRIBUTION

Figure 3 relates the echocardiographic views used in stress echocardiography to the epicardial coronary distribution. This information has been derived by analyzing the distribution of regional dysfunction following angiographically documented coronary artery occlusion and, more recently, myocardial contrast perfusion studies. As shown, the blood supply to some areas is consistent from subject to subject, while in others, there is more variability. In patients who have undergone coronary artery bypass surgery, these typical distribution patterns may be significantly altered, and it is important to be cognizant of the bypass distribution in interpreting the stress results.

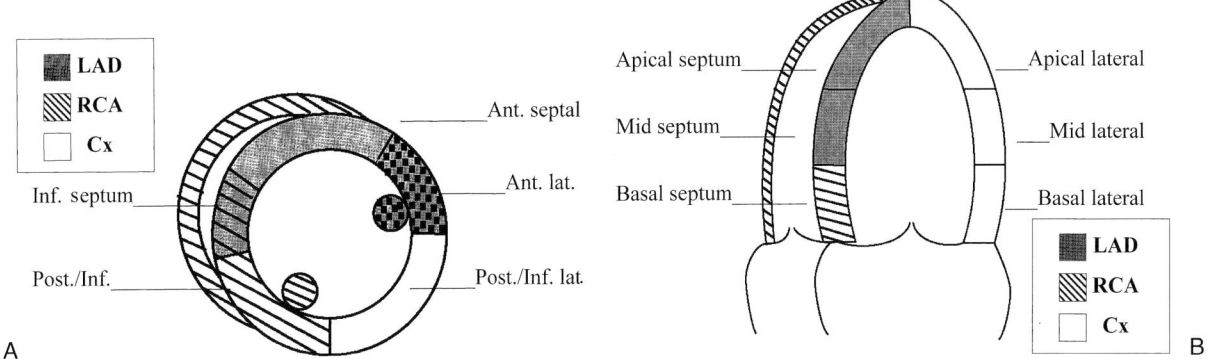

FIG. 3. Shown are five standard views (**A–E**) acquired during stress echocardiographic examination with relative arterial blood supply and standard nomenclature for each wall segment as shown in the key. **A:** parasternal short axis; **B:** apical 4 chamber. *Cx,* circumflex artery; *LAD,* left anterior descending artery; *RCA,* right coronary artery. *(continued)*

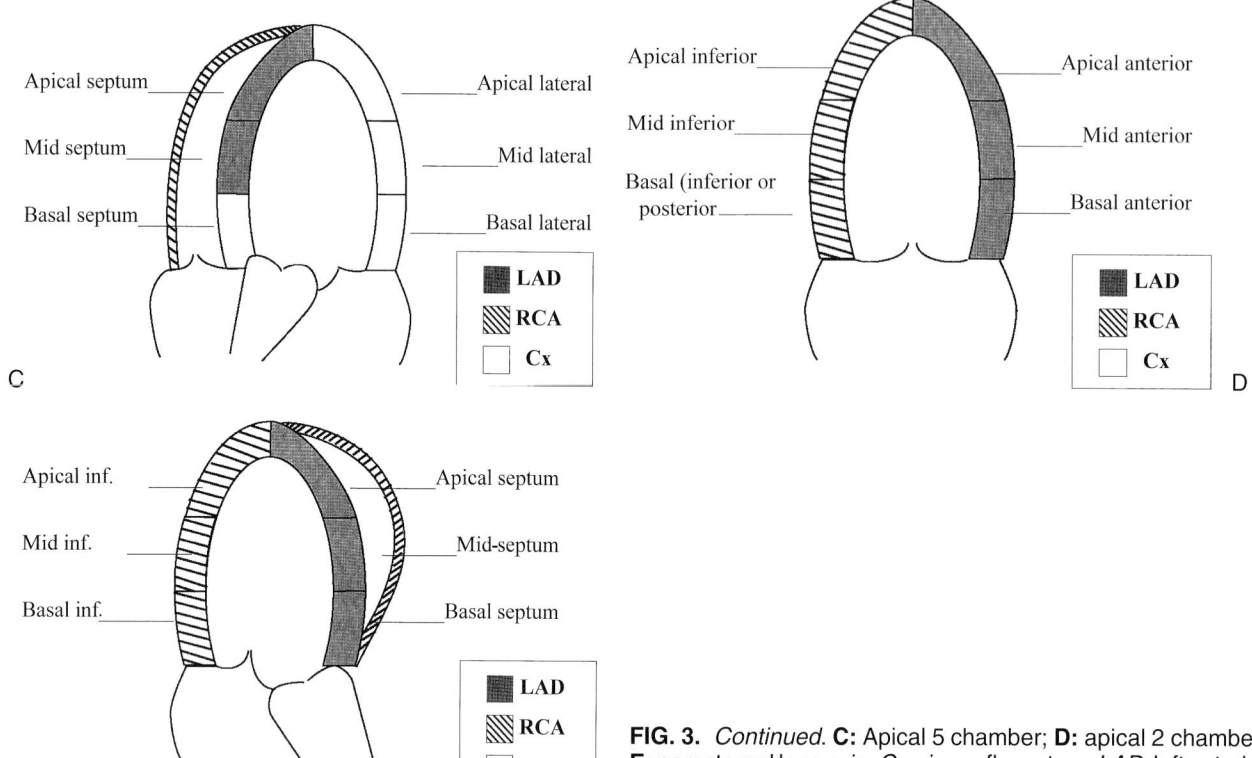

FIG. 3. *Continued.* **C:** Apical 5 chamber; **D:** apical 2 chamber; **E:** parasternal long axis. *Cx*, circumflex artery; *LAD*, left anterior descending artery; *RCA*, right coronary artery.

STRESS TECHNIQUES

Stress echocardiography may be performed with exercise (bicycle or treadmill), pharmacologic stress (inotropes or vasodilators), or miscellaneous stressors including cold pressor, isometric hand grip, mental stress, and pacing. Echocardiographic imaging is typically done transthoracically, although there are rare instances in which a more invasive transesophageal approach may be justified.

Exercise Stress Echocardiography

In most laboratories, exercise is performed using a treadmill. The advantages to treadmill testing include its wide availability and the fact that walking is a universal activity that can be performed by most patients and easily related to one's daily activities. Standard protocols are administered with conventional ECG and blood pressure monitoring. Since wall motion abnormalities may be short-lived, it is imperative that imaging be performed immediately following the cessation of stress (initiated within 20 seconds and completed by 2 minutes). The importance of moving rapidly to the imaging bed as soon as the stress is completed must be emphasized to the patient and, for some, a dry run of this step prior to stress may be helpful. The treadmill must be brought to a stop as rapidly as is safely possible.

Bicycle stress may be performed in either the supine or upright position. While the cost of a bicycle ergometer is comparable to that of a treadmill, laboratories that can afford or accommodate only one piece of stress equipment generally select a treadmill. For many patients, bicycling is not a routine activity and leg fatigue may prematurely terminate the test. Further, cycling is not easily related to the activities of daily living. From a physiologic perspective, treadmill stress tends to elicit higher heart rates but lower systolic and diastolic blood pressures than bicycle stress. Double products are comparable, but the additional venous return associated with supine bicycle stress may result in relatively increased preload and thus increased myocardial oxygen demand.

The major advantage of bicycle over treadmill stress is that it permits echocardiographic imaging during stress (supine bicycle), or both, during and after (supine stress). Peak-stress imaging allows the acquisition of short-lived wall motion abnormalities that would otherwise have resolved by immediate poststress imaging. This increases the sensitivity of the test for ischemia in patients that would otherwise have false negative stress tests (4). Patients in whom imaging during stress may be critical include those with rapidly resolving stress-induced symptoms (as might be seen with long-standing ischemia and collateral arterial distributions) and ECG changes and those with silent ischemia and uninterpretable ECGs. In the latter group, failure to recognize an echocardiographic ischemic endpoint might allow the patient to exercise inappropriately long. These patients may also be candidates for pharmacologic stress. In aggregate, there is no evidence that one exercise modality is superior to another.

Pharmacologic Stress Echocardiography

It is generally accepted that, where possible, maximal exercise stress is superior to pharmacologic stress. However, approximately 30% of candidates for stress testing are unable to exercise adequately and therefore require a pharmacologic alternative.

Pharmacologic echocardiographic stress testing has been performed in conjunction with two classes of stress agents, inotropes (dobutamine and arbutamine) and vasodilators (dipyridamole, adenosine). In North America, inotropic stress with dobutamine is most common; in Europe, dipyridamole is the agent of choice. All forms of pharmacologic stress must be combined with an imaging modality since the use of conventional stress endpoints may result in both false-positive and false-negative results.

Dobutamine

Dobutamine is a synthetic catecholamine, which has beta 1, beta 2, and alpha effects. It increases myocardial oxygen consumption by increasing inotropy, and, to a lesser extent, chronotropy and blood pressure. It is Food and Drug Administration (FDA) approved for use as a short-term inotropic agent. Thus, its use for stress testing is off label. Its onset of action is within 1 to 2 minutes although up to 10 minutes may be required to obtain the peak effect of a given infusion rate. The plasma half-life of the drug is 2 to 3 minutes. It is compatible with most IV solutions and, once mixed, is stable for 24 hours. True hypersensitivity to the drug is extremely rare. One reason for its popularity in North America is its low cost.

The infusion protocol is dependent on the indication. For indications other than the assessment of viability, the standard infusion is 5, 10, 20, 30, and 40 mcg/kg/min typically with increments in dosing every 3 minutes. In some laboratories, the maximum dobutamine dose is 50 mcg/kg/min. If the patient fails to reach the target heart rate (>85% age-predicted maximum) or another endpoint that mandates discontinuation of the infusion, atropine can be added in incremental doses of 0.25 mg up to a total of 1 mg. Isometric hand grip is occasionally used for this purpose but tends to increase heart rate by only a few beats per minute.

Atropine is a parasympatholytic agent, which is used both clinically and in the context of pharmacologic stress to increase heart rate. In most clinical situations, doses of less than 1 mg are not given because of the potential for paradoxical heart-rate slowing. However, high-dose dobutamine infusion eliminates this possible adverse effect, and even small doses will significantly increase heart rate. It has been shown to improve the diagnostic yield of pharmacologic stress echocardiography and is particularly helpful in patients who are beta blocked. The onset of action is within 1 minute. Although it is cleared rapidly from the plasma, it has a physiologic half-life of over 10 minutes. Atropine is contraindicated in the presence of glaucoma, obstructive uropathy and pyloric stenosis.

TABLE 2. *Side effects of dobutamine stress echocardiography*

General	Arrythmias
Chest discomfort (14%)	Atrial fibrillation (0.7%)
Palpitations (12%)	SVT (3–7%)
Tremor (10%)	PVCs (17%)
Headache (9%)	NSVT (3.5–6%)
Dyspnea (6%)	SVT rare
Anxious sensation	Ventricular fibrillation rare
Nausea	

Endpoints for dobutamine stress echocardiography include ischemia, hypertension [systolic blood pressure (SBP) >220 mm Hg, diastolic blood pressure (DBP) >120mm Hg], hypotension (>30 mm Hg fall in SBP), significant arrythmias, or other side effects and achievement of target heart rate (85% maximum predicted). The most desirable ischemic endpoint is regional wall motion abnormality since chest pain or ECG changes in the absence of a regional dysfunction may be considered false-positive.

It may occasionally be necessary to reverse a strongly positive test, particularly if atropine has been given. Nitroglycerin or esmolol 0.5 to 1 mg/kg may be used for this purpose.

Dobutamine stress is generally well tolerated. Test limiting side effects are uncommon (Table 2) and death or nonfatal infarction is extremely rare. It is important to recognize that hypotension occurring during dobutamine stress does not carry the same ominous prognosis that it does in the context of exercise. Indeed, it is not considered to be specific for the presence of coronary disease, and there are several mechanisms that are more common than profound ischemia. These include reduced ventricular filling, peripheral vasodilation, and intraventricular obstruction. The latter has been reported in approximately 20% of patients. Dobutamine is contraindicated in the setting of malignant arrythmias, atrial fibrillation with a poorly controlled ventricular response, and uncontrolled hypertension.

One advantage of dobutamine over exercise stress is that echocardiographic imaging may be virtually continuous. While images from each stage are recorded onto videotape, digital acquisition is generally performed at four stages. Some laboratories record at baseline, low dose (5 or 10 mcg/kg/min), peak dose, and recovery. However, since the recovery images are rarely helpful diagnostically, many laboratories digitize at baseline, low dose, intermediate dose, and high dose and record recovery images exclusively on videotape.

Arbutamine

Arbutamine is a synthetic catecholamine developed exclusively for use as a stress agent. It is the only drug that is approved by the FDA for stress echocardiography. It was perceived that dobutamine is a suboptimal stress agent because its dominant inotropic effects may cause cavity obliter-

TABLE 3. *Side effects of arbutamine*

Side effect	Incidence (%)
Ventricular fibrillation	6.2
Ventricular tachycardia	0.1
Supraventricular tachycardia	3.8
Atrial fibrillation	1.0
Heart block	0.1
Tremor	15
Angina	12
Arrythmias	12
Headache	9
Hypotension	6
Chest pain	4
Dizziness	4
Dyspnea	4
Palpitation	4
Flushing	3
Hot flashes	3
Nausea	3
Paresthesia	2

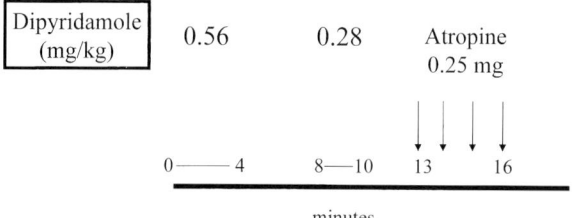

FIG. 4. Infusion protocol for dipyridamole stress echocardiography.

ation and hypotension before the target heart rate is reached. Cavity obliteration may also make it difficult to track endocardial borders. Arbutamine was designed to have balanced inotropic and chronotropic effects. Arbutamine has a rapid onset of action (1 to 2 minutes) and a pharmacodynamic half-life of 16 minutes. Unfortunately, the agent is more expensive than dobutamine and has been made available exclusively for use with a computerized closed-loop feedback system that is based on heart rate. The infusion rate is automatically increased to achieve an 8-bpm slope. The endpoints for arbutamine infusion generally parallel those for dobutamine with the addition of several that are unique to this stressor: a maximum infusion rate of 0.8 mcg/kg/min, a total dose of 10 ug/kg, or heart-rate saturation (plateauing of the heart rate). The agent is generally well tolerated; reported side effects are listed in Table 3.

In multicenter trials, arbutamine has been shown to be an effective stress agent with results that are comparable to those with dobutamine (5). This was confirmed in the one study that directly compared the two agents (6). Since no clear-cut superiority for arbutamine has been established, it is likely that cost considerations will prevail and dobutamine will remain the stress inotrope of choice.

Vasodilators (Dipyridamole and Adenosine)

Dipyridamole

Dipyridamole was developed primarily for use as a coronary vasodilator acting on small resistance arterioles. It increases local adenosine levels by inhibiting reuptake and destruction. Its duration of action is 30 minutes, although in clinical practice, it is frequently reversed with aminophylline. Its use as a stress agent is predicated on the fact that it elicits heterogeneous blood flow in patients with coronary disease and causes a coronary steal from the vascular beds of vessels that are diseased. It has a modest effect on the

rate-pressure product in that it tends to produce a small fall in blood pressure with a reflex rise in cardiac output and heart rate. To generate a positive finding when echocardiographic imaging is used, it must cause absolute ischemia and regional dysfunction rather than simply redistribution of blood flow.

Although dipyridamole has enjoyed widespread use in Europe, the agent is relatively infrequently used for stress echocardiography in North America despite its popularity for use with nuclear perfusion imaging. The reluctance to use the agent has been based on the fact that low doses of dipyridamole (0.56 mg/kg over 4 minutes), such as those used with nuclear imaging, do not reliably generate wall motion abnormalities. Thus, in the early phases of evaluation of the drug with stress echocardiography, the sensitivity was felt to be unacceptably low. More recently, there has been a shift to high-dose protocols (0.84 mg/kg) in which a nondiagnostic low-dose infusion is followed by an additional infusion of 0.28 mg/kg (Fig. 4). If even the high-dose infusion does not produce an ischemic endpoint, it has been reported that the addition of atropine, isometric exercise, or dobutamine may increase test sensitivity without a loss of specificity.

The incidence of side effects with dipyridamole is 1.2% (Table 4). These can generally be quickly reversed with aminophylline 50mg IV. Dipyridamole is contraindicated in the setting of bronchoconstrictive disease, hypotension, second or third degree AV block, and severe congestive heart failure; it may cause a worsening of symptoms in patients with myasthenia gravis who are treated with cholinesterase inhib-

TABLE 4. *Dipyridamole side effects*

Overall incidence (2%)
Hypotension/bradycardia
ST elevation
Ventricular tachycardia
Supraventricular tachycardia
Atrial fibrillation
Atrioventricular block
Bronchospasm
Myocardial infarction
Congestive heart failure
Asystole
Death (1)

(Adapted from ref. 34, with permission.)

itors. Prior to dipyridamole stress, all xanthine-containing medications, such as theophylline, and caffeinated food and beverages must be held for 12 hours since these substances may abolish the desired coronary vasodilatation.

ADENOSINE

Adenosine is an endogenous vasodilator, which exerts an alpha 1 effect on smooth muscle associated with an increase in cyclic guanosine monophosphate (GMP) levels. Since it is the biologic mediator of dipyridamole's effects, it is not surprising that its physiologic profile, side effects, and contraindications are similar to those of dipyridamole. However, in contrast to dipyridamole, it has a very short half-life (less than 10 seconds); this permits a faster testing protocol and a less frequent need for aminophylline. A protocol for adenosine stress is illustrated in Figure 5. As with dipyridamole, the addition of other stressors at peak dose may be helpful.

Choice of Test

A stress echocardiography laboratory should be capable of providing stress using either exercise, an inotrope, or a vasodilator so that the choice of test is based on patient characteristics rather than laboratory preference. If possible, exercise stress should be attempted before resorting to pharmacologic stress due to both the increased sensitivity of exercise testing and the ease of relating exercise to the patient's activities. Inotropic stress is preferred over vasodilator stress in patients with a poor left ventricular ejection fraction, asthma, hypotension, and AV block while vasodilators are preferred in those with hypertension, atrial fibrillation, and ventricular arrhythmias.

Laboratory Setup and Technical Issues

The ability to perform high quality stress echocardiography is dependent on well trained and experienced personnel, good equipment, and an appropriately configured testing area. It should not be assumed that a laboratory that provides good resting transthoracic echocardiography is capable of providing equally good stress services. This fact is recognized by the Intersocietal Commission for the Accreditation of Echocardiography Laboratories, which accredits stress and resting transthoracic services separately.

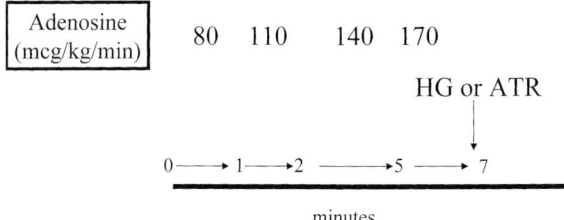

FIG. 5. Infusion protocol for adenosine stress echocardiography.

Personnel

The performance of stress echocardiography requires at least three trained people: a sonographer, an interpreting physician, and an assistant, typically a nurse, to help monitor vital signs, mix and adjust the infusion rate of stress agents, etc. In many laboratories, supervision of the test is performed by another physician or physician extender although there are some advantages to having the same physician perform both supervisory and interpretive functions.

At present, there are no published guidelines for sonographer training in stress echocardiography. However, the sonographer must be an accomplished scanner who is capable of recognizing regional dysfunction and is familiar with digital acquisition techniques. Since the time window for recording images following treadmill stress is extremely short, the sonographer must be adept at rapidly reestablishing the baseline views. This process is facilitated, in some systems, by storing the baseline image settings. Since hyperventilation and increased translation of the heart may contribute to shifting of windows from their baseline position, marking the baseline windows with a skin pencil may not be as helpful as one would hope. It is generally easier to acquire stress images during pharmacologic stress since patient position can be held constant throughout the infusion, respiration less commonly interferes with acquisition, and, if necessary, a stage can often be prolonged.

The American Society of Echocardiography recommendations for physician training and maintenance of skills in stress echocardiography are shown in Table 5. It is expected that physicians who have not had the opportunity to acquire stress echocardiography skills during their fellowship will do so through a combination of visits to an active laboratory and supervision of the performance and interpretation of his or her initial studies by an experienced stress echocardiographer.

It is imperative that all stress echocardiography laboratories regularly compare their results to those of alternate diagnostic procedures, such as coronary angiography.

Equipment

High quality ultrasound equipment is an essential component of stress echocardiography. At a minimum, the machine must have transducers, which can cover a broad range of fundamental frequencies. Harmonic imaging is desirable since it improves endocardial border definition in difficult studies and maximizes the effect of echocardiographic contrast agents. Contrast agents capable of left ventricular opacification are, however, helpful with fundamental imaging alone. It has been suggested that new echocardiographic imaging features, such as Doppler tissue imaging and automatic border tracking, may be useful in patients undergoing stress echocardiography. However, for the time being, these remain research tools.

The performance of stress echocardiography requires the ability to digitize and display baseline and stress images. This capability is now available as a built-in feature of many echocardiographic imaging systems, although stand-alone

TABLE 5. *Summary of recommendations for training in stress echocardiography*

	Fellows-in-training	Postfellowship training	Maintenance of skills
Qualifications for training	• Level 2 training and ability to interpret resting wall motion	• Level 2 training or equivalent • Current active practice of echocardiography	
Conditions for training	• Laboratory performing 40 stress echo studies per month • Supervisor with level 3 training and experience with more than 200 stress echo studies	• Laboratory performing 40 stress echo studies per month • Supervisor with Level 3 training and experience with more than 200 stress echo studies	
Number of cases recommended	• Participation in *performance* of at least 50 exercise echo and/or pharmacologic stress echo studies • *Interpretation* of at least 100 stress echo studies with supervision as above	• Participation in *performance* of at least 50 exercise echo and/or pharmacologic stress echo studies • *Interpretation* of 100 stress echo studies under supervision as above	Interpretation of 15 stress echo studies per month

off-line systems, which are connected to the imaging system during stress, may also be used. Since there is variable degradation of stored images from those seen live, it is important to select a system in which such degradation is minimal. Digital acquisition and storage make it possible to display multiple images on the same screen, most commonly in a quad-screen format. Images may be manipulated so that either all stages for a given view or all views for a given stage are displayed simultaneously. At a minimum, digital stress systems allow the acquisition of four stages using four views (parasternal long-axis, parasternal short-axis, apical four-chamber, and apical two-chamber), but many systems are flexible and permit both additional views and additional stages. A clock, which encodes the delay between the termination of stress and imaging into the digital record, is critical. Videotaping is still an important modality for image storage and typically used for those stages that are not digitized and as a backup should digitized images prove nondiagnostic. It is not acceptable to perform stress echocardiography exclusively by analyzing sequential videotaped segments.

Additional equipment required for stress echocardiography includes a treadmill and/or bicycle, infusion pump, blood pressure monitor, and ECG machine with continuous oscilloscopic display and arrhythmia monitoring capability. Equipment and drugs for cardiopulmonary resuscitation must also be nearby. Imaging beds with cutouts specifically designed to facilitate apical imaging may also be helpful. It should be noted that it is frequently necessary to deviate from the standard precordial electrode placement in order to permit access to the echocardiographic imaging windows. Typically, V2 is moved slightly up and to the right while V4, V5, and V6 are moved down slightly.

Room

The room used for stress echocardiography must be large enough to accommodate all the necessary equipment and the people required for uncomplicated stress testing and to allow the unimpeded influx of any additional equipment and people should cardiopulmonary resuscitation be required. Many rooms that have been designed to permit either resting transthoracic echocardiography or nonimaging stress testing are too small to be used for stress echocardiography. The room must be set up with the bed immediately adjacent to the treadmill to facilitate the rapid initiation of imaging postexercise. Since ECG triggering is a critical element of digital image acquisition, stable ECG monitoring connections must be established. Ideally, the signal from the ECG monitor may be relayed to the echo machine eliminating the need for additional electrodes and wires.

Technical Limitations

The interpretation of stress echocardiograms is recognized as being more difficult for certain patients, including those with left bundle-branch block, left ventricular hypertrophy, atrial fibrillation, and postcardiotomy. Patients with left bundle-branch block are always candidates for imaging stress since their ECGs are uninterpretable. Unfortunately, the assessment of regional wall motion in these subjects is difficult due to the interventricular septal dyssynergy that accompanies the conduction disturbance. Correct interpretation of stress images in these patients relies on a close inspection of wall thickening rather than endocardial excursion. Similar difficulties are encountered following open heart surgery when abnormal translation vectors may complicate the assessment of endocardial excursion. Meticulous assessment of wall thickening is again the key to successful interpretation. Patients with left ventricular hypertrophy have been shown to be more likely than those with normal wall thickness to have false-positive stress echocardiograms when angiographic coronary disease is used as the gold standard. One potential explanation is that such patients are indeed ischemic despite normal epicardial coronaries. Patients with atrial fibrillation, particularly those with a poorly controlled ventricular response or those in whom rate-controlling beta blockade had been withheld prior to stress pose a different problem. First, the irregular cycle lengths introduce load-dependent changes in endocardial excursion. Second, with inotropic pharmacologic stress, there may be an abrupt increase to high heart rates that stress the frame rate capabilities of some echocardiographic imaging systems. These patients are more suitable candidates for vasodilator stress.

The areas that pose the greatest difficulty for stress echocardiographic interpretation are the inferior and lateral walls particularly near the base. The basal segments of these walls are tethered to the mitral annulus as myocardium transitions to the fibrous skeleton of the heart. This is compounded by the fact that endocardial definition in these segments may be suboptimal and short-axis images may be off-axis and somewhat oblique if the only available parasternal window is a low one. The evaluation of more distal segments of the lateral wall may also be difficult because lateral segments are typically the least well imaged. For example, in both the apical four-chamber and parasternal short-axis views, the lateral wall lies parallel to the imaging beam and in the parasternal short-axis view the lateral wall is seen as only a small segment. Harmonic imaging and left ventricular echocardiographic contrast agents appear to be helpful in this regard.

Steps that may help minimize false-positive tests are as follows:

1. Optimize the images by ensuring they are on-axis and that baseline and poststress images display the same segments. When the parasternal window is low and

short-axis images are oblique, consider obtaining additional subcostal short-axis views.
2. Ensure that one's eye is tracking endocardium rather than the midwall. If in doubt, consider using a contrast agent.
3. Take advantage of the imaging redundancy that is available with echocardiography. In a complete study, each wall and vascular territory is seen in more than one view. A true wall motion abnormality will be evident in multiple views.
4. Think in terms of coronary anatomy. A constellation of wall motion abnormalities that make no sense in the context of the usual coronary anatomy is likely to be artifactual or represent nonischemic dysfunction.

The importance of experience in avoiding both false-positive and false-negative studies cannot be overstated.

UTILITY OF STRESS ECHOCARDIOGRAPHY IN THE DIAGNOSIS OF CORONARY ARTERY DISEASE

There is now a large body of literature attesting to the accuracy of stress echocardiography in the diagnosis of coronary artery disease. A detailed discussion of individual studies is beyond the scope of this chapter. However, the results of selected studies are presented in Tables 6 to 10.

Exercise Echocardiography

There are many published studies of the diagnostic sensitivity and specificity of exercise stress echocardiography for angiographically defined coronary disease (Table 6). Since the individual study groups are quite small, it is helpful to

TABLE 6. *Exercise echocardiography sensitivity, specificity, positive and negative predictive value versus ECG alone*

Author	Exercise	N	Sens	Spec	PPV	NPV	Sens	Spec	PPV	NPV	SVD	MVD	LAD	Cx	RCA
Aboul-Enein et al. (35)	TD	101	67	73	78	73	32	75	70	38	36	83	—	—	—
Amanullah & Lindvall (36)	Bike	36	83	50	95	50	61	80	93	31	73	92	—	—	—
Armstrong et al. (37)	TD	123	88	61	97	61	—	—	—	—	81	93	71	13	85
Cohen et al. (38)	Bike	52	78	62	94	62	35	93	93	37	63	90	—	—	—
Dagianti et al. (39)	Bike	100	76	82	73	82	68	80	—	—	70	80	—	—	—
Galanti et al. (40)	Bike	53	93	93	96	93	78	65	—	—	93	92	75	60	58
Hecht et al. (8)	Bike	221	93	86	—	—	52	86	—	—	78	—	95	78	81
Hecht et al. (41)	Bike	71	90	80	—	—	47	83	—	—	77	—	97	83	81
Iliceto et al. (42)	TD	78	82	72	97	72	—	—	—	—	89	90	—	—	—
Kafka et al. (43)	TD	182	85	81	85	81	67	47	62	52	77	96	—	—	—
Limacher et al. (44)	TD	73	86	65	96	65	85	—	—	—	64	—	—	—	—
Marangelli et al. (45)	TD	104	84	86	93	86	—	—	—	—	81	—	—	—	—
Marwick et al. (15)	TD	150	84	63	95	63	88	7	76	14	68	96	—	—	—
Marwick et al. (46)	Bike	86	88	78	91	78	77	43	—	—	82	—	—	—	—
Quinones et al. (47)	TD	292	74	51	96	51	—	—	—	—	58	—	—	—	—
Ryan et al. (48)	TD	64	78	73	100	73	53	100	—	—	76	—	—	—	—
Ryan et al. (16)	Bike	309	91	78	90	81	40	89	—	—	86	95	—	—	—

Cx, circumflex; *ECG*, electrocardiogram; *LAD*, left anterior descending artery; *MVD*, multivessel disease; *N*, number; *NPV*, negative predictive value; *PPV*, positive predictive valve; *RCA*, right coronary artery; *Sens*, sensitivity; *Spec*, specificity; *SVD*, single-vessel disease; *TD*, treadmill.

TABLE 7. *Dobutamine stress echocardiography sensitivity and specificity*

Author	N	Maximum dobutamine dose (mcg/kg/min)	Sensitivity (%)	Specificity (%)	Sensitivity SVD (%)	Sensitivity MVD (%)
Cohen et al. (49)	70	40	86	95	69	94
Previtali et al. (50)	35	40	68	100	50	92
Sawada et al. (51)	55	30	89	85	81	100
Mazeika et al. (52)	50	20	67	93	50	75
Marcovitz & Armstrong (53)	141	30	96	66	95	98
Marwick et al. (54)	97	40	85	82	84	86
Marwick et al. (55)	217	40	72	83	66	77
Hoffmann et al. (56)	64	40	79	81	78	81
Forster et al. (57)	21	40 + atropine	75	89	25	100
Cohen et al. (38)	52		86	87	75	95
Gunalp et al. (58)	27	40	83	89	78	89
Beleslin et al. (59)	136	40	82	77	82	82
Ling et al. (60)	1171	40 + atropine	90	78	—	—
McNeill et al. (61)	80	40 + atropine	70	78	—	—
Pingitore et al. (34)	110	40 + atropine	84	89	—	—
Dagianti et al. (39)	60	40	72	97	60	80

MVD, multivessel disease; *N,* number; *SVD,* single-vessel disease.

summarize the data using preliminary results of a recent metaanalysis (7). This included 57 studies published from 1979 to 1997 in which at least 80% of the patients underwent coronary angiography within 6 months of their exercise echocardiogram. The combined study groups included 5,218 patients. The stress modality was treadmill in 28 series, upright bicycle in 15, supine bicycle in 12, and combined treadmill/bicycle in 2. In the papers reviewed, 92% of patients underwent coronary angiography. The overall sensitivity and specificity of exercise echocardiography for the detection of coronary disease were 84% and 76%, respectively. For comparison, the sensitivity and specificity of the ECG component alone were 56% and 65%, respectively. As might be expected, test sensitivity was higher when more widespread disease was present; sensitivity for single-vessel disease is 75%, double-vessel disease is 88%, and three-vessel disease is 94%. Exercise stress echocardiography is more sensitive for disease in the left anterior descending territory (82%) than either the right coronary artery (72%) or left circumflex artery (56%). The technical limitations of imaging the lateral wall (circumflex territory) have been addressed in a prior section.

The relation between the angiographic severity of disease and test sensitivity has been addressed by Hecht et al. (8). In that study, the sensitivity was greater for critical stenoses (90 to 100% luminal narrowing) than for less severe lesions (50% to 70% luminal narrowing). The relative sensitivities were 91% and 85%, respectively ($P < .05$).

Dobutamine

A selected list of studies evaluating the detection of coronary artery disease with dobutamine stress echocardiography is provided in Table 7. As with exercise stress, the study groups are generally small and the protocols somewhat variable with a trend to higher maximum infusion rates and the use of atropine in more recent studies. Unfortunately, there has as yet been no metaanalysis to help summarize the overall results. While there is a broad range of sensitivities (67% to 97%), the majority are between 70 and 90%. With few exceptions, specificities exceed 80%. As is the case for exercise stress, the sensitivity is lower for single-vessel disease than multiple-vessel disease. The positive predictive values are uniformly high, ranging from 85 to 100%. The negative predictive values tend to be considerably lower, although there is considerable variability (38 to 86%).

TABLE 8. *Sensitivity and specificity of dipyridamole echocardiography for CAD*

Study	N	Max dose (mg/kg)	Overall	Sensitivity (%) SVD	Sensitivity (%) MVD	Overall (%)	Specificity no prior MI (%)	Sensitivity no prior MI (%)
Picano et al. (62)	66	0.56	56	37	85	100	86	N/A
Labovitz et al. (63)	55	0.56	64	N/A	N/A	80	N/A	N/A
Picano et al. (64)	93	0.84	74	50	85	100	82	N/A
Pirelli et al. (24)	75	0.84	71	N/A	N/A	90	75	N/A

CAD, coronary artery disease; *MI,* myocardial infarction; *MVD,* multivessel disease; *N/A,* not available; *SVD,* single-vessel disease.

TABLE 9. *Sensitivity and specificity of adenosine echocardiography*

Author	N	Max Dose (mcg/kg/min)	Overall	Sensitivity (%) SVD	MVD	Overall	Specificity no prior MI (%)	Sensitivity no prior MI (%)
Zoghbi et al. (65)	73	140	85	80	91	92	48	60
Edlund et al. (66)	37	200	89	89	89	—	54	75
Marwick et al. (55)	97	180	58	52	64	87	0	
Amanullah et al. (67)	40	140	74	NA	NA	100	87	62
Tawa et al. (68)	45	170 + HG	91	NA	NA	91	55	*81

* 64%, without HG.
HG, isometric handgrip; *MI*, myocardial infarction; *MVD*, multivessel disease; *N*, number of patients.

Vasodilators

Table 8 provides a limited list of studies evaluating the ability of dipyridamole stress echo to identify patients with coronary disease. As can be seen, the specificity of dipyridamole stress echocardiography has been consistently high. While older low-dose protocols were relatively insensitive, particularly for single-vessel disease, more aggressive high-dose protocols improve sensitivity without a loss of specificity. There are isolated reports using more study-specific protocols in which the addition of atropine, dobutamine, or hand grip to the high-dose protocol may further increase sensitivity. Although not addressed in these tables, the sensitivity of dipyridamole stress is reduced when patients are beta-blocked.

Table 9 provides a summary of data from adenosine stress echocardiographic studies. Consistently good sensitivities and specificities have been reported despite the fact that protocols tend to differ from study to study. As with dipyridamole, higher-dose protocols and the addition of an additional form of stress appear to improve sensitivity.

COMPARISON OF STRESS MODALITIES

There are relatively few studies in which multiple stress modalities are directly compared. Three are listed in Table 10. The findings of these and the indirect comparisons that can be inferred from single modality studies can be summarized as follows: exercise stress echocardiography is more sensitive than either dobutamine or high-dose dipyridamole for the detection of coronary artery disease; exercise stress also appears to be more specific than dobutamine stress but

less specific than dipyridamole; all three modalities have been shown to have diagnostic accuracies that justify their value in the evaluation of patients with known or suspected coronary disease.

EXERCISE TESTING IN SPECIAL GROUPS

Stress Echocardiography in Women

Ischemic heart disease is the most common cause of death in women, and, after decades of relative neglect, heart disease in women is receiving widespread attention from clinicians and scientists and the lay public alike. It has been suggested that stress echocardiography may be particularly valuable in women due to the limitations of conventional stress testing in this group of patients. Before reviewing the relevant stress echocardiographic data, it may, therefore, be helpful to consider the influence of gender on ECG stress testing. Conventional stress testing is considered to be less specific and less sensitive in women than in men. Exercise induced ST-depression appears to be less specific in women in large part due to the lower prevalence of disease in women. It has been reported that both estrogen therapy (9) and the menstrual cycle (10) are a cause of false-positives. In addition, women also have a higher incidence of mitral valve prolapse and Syndrome X that are also associated with false-positive tests (11). Exercise induced ST-depression is also less sensitive in women than men, possibly due to a lower prevalence of severe multivessel disease in women coupled with an inability to exercise to maximum aerobic capacity. However, the American College of Cardiology and the American Heart Association (ACC/AHA) Practice

TABLE 10. *Comparison of stress echocardiographic modalities*

Author	N	Exercise sensitivity (%)	Exercise specificity (%)	Dobutamine sensitivity (%)	Dobutamine specificity (%)	High dose dipyridamole sensitivity (%)	High dose dipyridamole specificity (%)
Belesin (59)	136	88	82	82	77	74	94
Bjornstad (69)	37	84	67	—	—	68	100
Rallidis (70)	62	Positive test = 73% WMSI = 1.73		Positive test = 62% WMSI = 1.57	—	—	—

N, number; *WMSI*, wall motion score index.

TABLE 11. *Stress echocardiographic studies that have exclusively enrolled women*

Author	Stress modality	Number of patients	Sensitivity	Specificity
Sawada et al. (71)	Exercise	57	86	86
Williams et al. (72)	Exercise	70	88	84
Roger et al. (73)	Exercise	100	85	46
Masini et al. (74)	Dipyridamole	83	79	93
Marwick et al. (75)	Exercise	161	81	80

Guidelines for Exercise Testing conclude that these gender differences are not of a magnitude that conventional stress testing in women should be precluded (12).

Table 11 lists the stress echocardiographic studies that enrolled only women. To summarize, stress echocardiography has a high sensitivity and generally high specificity for coronary disease in women. These are higher than those reported for ECG stress alone. The reported sensitivities are similar to those reported in studies that are primarily composed of male patients (13–16), while the specificity and positive predictive value are slightly lower in women. These differences are presumed secondary to the lower prevalence of coronary disease in women than in men. To summarize, while there is no consensus that stress echocardiography should be the initial modality for evaluating women suspected of having coronary disease, it appears to be a cost-effective alternative to angiography when conventional stress testing is considered falsely positive or nondiagnostic.

STRESS ECHOCARDIOGRAPHY FOR RISK STRATIFICATION

Several studies have evaluated the ability of stress echocardiography to identify high-risk patient populations. In a study of patients with chest pain referred for stress echocardiography, Sawada et al. (17) reported that a negative stress echocardiogram carries a favorable prognosis while a positive result predicts a fivefold increase in cardiac events over a mean follow-up of 44 months. In a population of patients with known coronary disease, ischemia during dobutamine infusion was identified as a predictor of cardiac events (18). The prognostic value of dobutamine stress echocardiography has also been evaluated in patients with reduced ejection fraction ($\leq 30\%$). Those with viable ischemic myocardium were at the greatest risk of coronary events in follow up of 16 ± 8 months (19). An ischemic response to dobutamine in that study predicted subsequent events independent of age and ejection fraction with a relative risk ratio of 3.5. These observations have driven efforts to develop reliable methods for identifying viable myocardium (see below). In small studies of early postmyocardial infarction (post-MI), the presence of exercise-induced wall motion abnormalities has been shown to be predictive of future cardiac events in 63 to 80% of patients while the absence of inducible ischemia was predictive of event-free periods (20–22). It should be

noted that post-MI trials of exercise echocardiography preceded the widespread use of acute reperfusion therapy.

STRESS ECHOCARDIOGRAPHY FOLLOWING REVASCULARIZATION

There are several studies in which exercise echocardiography has been used to evaluate patients following myocardial revascularization. Crouse et al. evaluated 125 patients following bypass surgery with treadmill stress. Subsequent coronary angiography provided the gold standard. Stress echocardiography was superior to stress ECG alone for identifying regional coronary insufficiency (>50% luminal reduction); sensitivity 98% versus 41%, specificity 92% versus 67%, positive predictive value of 99% versus 91%, and negative predictive value of 86% versus 12%. Similar results were reported by Kafka et al. in 182 patients undergoing treadmill exercise echocardiography and angiography post-bypass (positive predictive value 85% versus 62% for exercise ECG, negative predictive value 81% versus 52%, respectively. The sensitivity was greater for vascular compromise in multiple regions than in a single region (77% versus 96%). The utility of upright bicycle and dobutamine stress echocardiography in this setting has also been reported (23).

In patients who have undergone angioplasty, stress echocardiography has been shown to be capable of risk stratification. Pirelli et al. (24) used high dose dipyridamole stress echocardiography to evaluate 52 consecutive patients before and after angiographically successful angioplasty. Eight of ten patients with positive postpercutaneous transluminal coronary angioplasty (PTCA) stress echocardiograms had recurrence of angina as compared to only 10 of 42 patients with negative stress studies. Similarly, Dagianti et al. (25) reported that a positive supine bicycle stress echocardiogram performed early after PTCA-predicted clinical restenosis (odds ratio 3.1).

STRESS ECHOCARDIOGRAPHIC METHODS OF ASSESSING MYOCARDIAL VIABILITY

The assessment of myocardial viability is an increasingly important issue in clinical cardiology. Viable noncontractile myocardium is defined as metabolically active dysfunctional tissue that is capable of functional improvement. While it is frequently categorized as stunned or hibernating, some

TABLE 12. *Stress echocardiography in the identification of stunned myocardium*

Author	N	Positive test	STD	SENS	SPEC	PPV	NPV
Pierard et al. (76)	17 AMI	Increase wall thickening	TEE	100	73	67	100
Smart et al. (77)	51 AMI	Improved regional wall motion	TEE	86	90–93	86	90
Watada et al. (78)	21 AMI	Improved regional wall motion	TEE	83	86		

AMI, acute myocardial infarction; N, number; NPV, negative predictive value; PPV, positive predictive value; SENS, sensitivity; SPEC, specificity; STD, stress test modality; TEE, transesophageal echocardiogram.

combination of the two is generally encountered clinically. Stunned myocardium refers to reversible contractile dysfunction seen after reperfusion following a brief coronary occlusion. This situation is encountered clinically in patients with acute myocardial infarction treated successfully with thrombolytics or primary angioplasty. Hibernating myocardium refers to myocardial dysfunction that occurs in the setting of critically reduced resting coronary flow. While the residual perfusion is adequate to support the low energy requiring functions needed to maintain the integrity of the cell membrane, it is inadequate to permit myocardial contraction that has higher energy requirements. Restoration of normal blood flow allows the recovery of contractile function. A clinical model of hibernating myocardium is difficult to identify since ischemic myopathy frequently represents a mixture of hibernating, infarcted, and stunned myocardium. However, it is clinically important to attempt to distinguish infarcted from viable tissue. For example 25 to 40% of patients with heart failure, global LV dysfunction and chronic coronary artery disease will improve with revascularization. Further, patients with viable myocardium do better with surgical versus medical therapy with regard to death and cardiac endpoints. The difficulty lies in identifying patients with viable muscle prior to operation. Both echocardiographic and nuclear cardiology techniques for identifying viable myocardium have been developed. Nuclear methods include positron emission tomography and thallium perfusion imaging. Echocardiographic methods include pharmacologic stress echocardiography, myocardial contrast echocardiography, and tissue characterization. Currently, the latter two are primarily research tools. The gold standard for viability is either postrevascularization improvement in regional wall motion, improved thallium uptake, or an improved overall left ventricular ejection fraction.

The results of animal studies have provided insights into the use of dobutamine stress echocardiography for the identification of viable myocardium. In a porcine model of hibernating myocardium, Chen et al. (26) demonstrated that dobutamine-induced improvement in regional function may be modest, transient, and may occur only at doses lower than 5 mcg/kg/min. In addition, nitroglycerin has been shown to increase the response rate. Therefore, Dobutamine protocols used for viability studies generally use lower doses and longer stages than those used for the diagnosis of coronary artery disease. Infusions typically start at 2.5 mcg/kg/min with increments to 5, 10, 20, 30, and 40 mcg/kg/min. Stages may be prolonged to 5 minutes. Patients should be imaged continuously with digital acquisition when there is a perceived change or at the end of a stage. While the majority of studies have considered improvement in regional wall motion or wall thickening to be a positive test, Afridi et al. (27) reported that a biphasic response (improvement in regional function at low dose followed by deterioration at higher doses) is a better predictor of recovery than monophasic improvement alone. Studies addressing the assessment of myocardial viability with dobutamine stress are listed in Tables 12 and 13. The ability of dobutamine stress echocardiography to identify stunned myocardium has been evaluated in studies of patients with acute myocardial infarction undergoing thrombolysis (Table 12). The use of the technique in patients with hibernating myocardium (Table 13) has been studied in patients with chronic coronary artery disease undergoing revascularization. In both settings, a positive dobutamine stress echocardiogram has been shown to predict recovery of regional function following revascularization. Although the diagnostic accuracy has been shown to be good, the sensitivity and negative predictive values tend to be lower than the specificities and positive predictive val-

TABLE 13. *Stress echocardiography in the assessment of hibernating myocardium*

Author	N	Positive test	STM	SENS	SPEC	PPV	NPV
Barilla et al. (79)	21 MI	Improved regional wall motion	TTE	100	—	—	—
Cigarroa et al. (80)	25 MVD	Increased wall thickening	TTE	82	86	—	—
LaCanna et al. (81)	33 CAD low LVEF	Increased wall thickening and regional wall motion	TTE	87	82	90	77
Afridi et al. (27)	20 prePTCA	Biphasic response	—	74	73	—	—
Perrone-Filardi et al. (82)	18 CAD	Improved regional wall motion	TTE	88	74	73	—
Perrone-Filardi et al. (83)	40 CAD	Improved regional wall motion	TTE	79	83	92	65

CAD, coronary artery disease; LVEF, left ventricular ejection fraction; MI, myocardial infarction; MVD, multivessel disease; N, number; NPV, negative predictive value; PPV, positive predictive value; PTCA, percutaneous transluminal coronary angioplasty; SENS, sensitivity; SPEC, specificity; STM, stress test modality; TTE, transthoracic echocardiography.

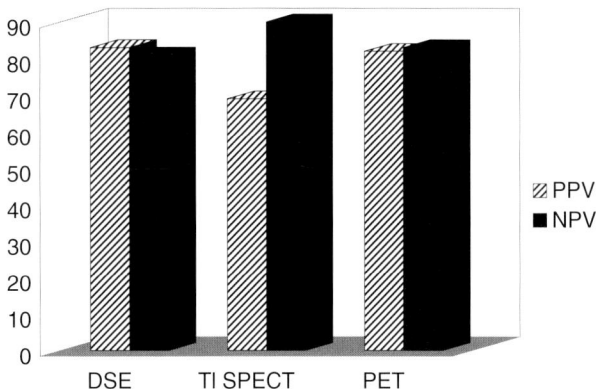

FIG. 6. Comparison of methods for detecting viable myocardium. *PPV*, positive predictive value; *NPV*, negative predictive value. (Adapted from ref. 33, with permission.)

ues. It is therefore worth considering some of the potential explanations for false-negative studies. First, coronary flow reserve may be exhausted to the point that even modest catecholamine stimulation will cause ischemia. Second, the cellular dedifferentiation and dropout of myofibrillar units may result in reduced catecholamine responsiveness. Finally, it is possible that qualitative and semiquantitative echocardiography may be unable to appreciate subtle recruitment of function, particularly if the analysis is based on endocardial excursion rather than wall thickening. Although nuclear methods for assessing myocardial viability are discussed in detail elsewhere in this book, it may be useful to address the relative positive and negative predictive values of the tests (Fig. 6). In general terms, dobutamine stress echocardiography is less sensitive and has a lower negative predictive value than thallium perfusion imaging while its specificity and positive predictive values are relatively higher. Its positive and negative predictive values track closely those of positron emission tomography. These differences are understandable if one considers that thallium positivity may identify viable units that are too small to ever be translated into a perceptible improvement in systolic function. Since both nuclear and echocardiographic viability studies are critically dependent on the quality of the personnel and equipment available for the test, the selection of the most appropriate test for a given patient should be based on the quality of the services available.

STRESS ECHOCARDIOGRAPHY IN THE EVALUATION OF PATIENTS UNDERGOING NONCARDIAC SURGERY

As many as one third of the patients undergoing noncardiac surgical procedures have increased cardiovascular risk. Over 1 million cardiac events complicate the more than 25 million noncardiac procedures that take place annually in the United States with an attendant cost of over 10 billion dollars. Noncardiac surgery may stress the heart in a number of ways, including fluid shifts, hypothermia, the adverse effects of anesthetic agents on loading conditions, myocardial contractility,

and perturbations of cardiac rhythm as well as risks specific to the surgery itself such as aortic cross-clamping.

It is hoped that the preoperative identification of patients at high risk for cardiac events might alter their management in ways that minimize their risk. Indeed the American Heart Association and American College of Cardiology have issued comprehensive *Guidelines for Perioperative Cardiovascular Evaluation for Noncardiac Surgery* (28). Since a detailed discussion of this document is beyond the scope of this chapter, it is strongly recommended that the reader review the *Guidelines* in their entirety. However, several general points must be made in order to put the following discussion of the role of echocardiography in context. First, the most important elements of the preoperative assessment are the clinical evaluation of the patient (history, physical examination, and ECG) and an assessment of the risk posed by the planned surgery. The clinical evaluation is directed toward an identification of major, intermediate, and minor predictors of cardiovascular events as well as an assessment of the patient's functional capacity.

Stress testing plays no immediate role in the assessment of patients with major clinical predictors that include unstable coronary syndromes, decompensated heart failure, significant arrhythmias, or severe valve disease. These patients must have their surgery postponed or canceled while they undergo coronary angiography and/or aggressive treatment of their heart disease. Similarly, stress testing plays no role in the setting of emergency life-saving surgery. These patients must go directly to the operating room. In general, stress echocardiography is reserved for patients undergoing high-risk surgery who have at least minor clinical predictors of cardiovascular risk. High-risk procedures are those that carry a greater than 5% risk of a cardiac event and include aortic and other major vascular surgery, peripheral vascular surgery, and prolonged procedures associated with major blood loss or fluid shifts.

With this as a background, let us address some specifics concerning stress echocardiography. First, it should be acknowledged that most patients undergoing high-risk vascular or orthopedic surgery are not capable of adequate exercise stress. Therefore, the preoperative stress literature is restricted to patients undergoing pharmacologic (primarily dobutamine) stress echocardiography.

One of the first considerations in evaluating stress echocardiography in this setting is that of safety. It has previously been stated that dobutamine stress echocardiography has an excellent safety record, and it should be noted that many of the large reported series include not only patients undergoing preoperative evaluation but those with known coronary disease. Of particular interest is the study of Pellikka and coworkers (60) who studied 98 patients with abdominal aortic aneurysm undergoing preoperative dobutamine stress echo. In that series, there were no instances of aortic rupture or hemodynamic instability.

Studies addressing the utility of dobutamine stress echo in evaluating patients prior to noncardiac surgery are listed in Table 14. Several points deserve emphasis. First, it is

TABLE 14. *Use of dobutamine in preoperative risk-stratification[a]*

Author	Design	N total (going to OR)	Protocol	Criteria for positive test	Surgery	PPV peri-op MI or death	NPV peri-op MI or death	Comments	Results used in decision making	Event rates AMI death
Lane et al. (84)	Retro	57 (38)	2.5–40 no atropine	New WMA ≥2 seq	Vascular (2/3) Major Ortho (1/6) Other (1/6)	4/19 (20%)	100% (19/19)	24/57 pts had prior MI	Y	4 (10%)
Lalka et al. (85)	Prospective	76 (60)	2.5–40 5–50 ± atropine	New or worsening WMA ≥2 seq	Aortic	9/30 (30%)	93% (28/30)	30 day peri-op period WMA at HR>120 especially bad prognosis	Y	9 (15%)
Eichelberger et al. (86)	Prospective double-blind	75	5–40 + atropine	New or worsening RWMA ≥2 seq	Peripheral vasc or aortic	5/27 (19%)	100% (48/48)		N	5 (7%)
Davila-Roman et al. (87)	Prospective	93 (88)	5–40 + atropine	New or worsening RWMA	Peripheral vasc or aortic	2/20 (10%)	100% (68/68)	13 pts had coronary revasc. prior to vasc surgery	Y	2 (2%)
Poldermans et al. (18)	Prospective/ blended	131	10–40 + atropine	New or worsening RWMA	Peripheral vasc or aortic	14/35 (40%)	100% (96/96)		—	—

[a] Individual studies considered other endpoints such as silent CK elevation, CHF, and ECG changes as positive cardiac events.
RWMA, regional wall motion abnormalities.

notable that a large majority of the patients studied were those undergoing peripheral vascular or aortic surgery. This is important since angiographically significant coronary disease has been reported in up to 75% of consecutive patients undergoing coronary angiography prior to vascular surgery (28). Thus, the pretest probability of coronary disease is high. Second, the echo criteria for a positive test (new or worsening regional wall motion abnormalities) are those that identify ischemia not simply the presence of coronary disease. Patients whose dobutamine stress test demonstrated only resting wall motion abnormalities that did not worsen with stress were not considered positive even though these patients likely had coronary disease. Using these criteria, roughly one third of patients had a positive dobutamine stress study. Third, hard cardiac event rates (perioperative myocardial infarction and death) were low even in patients with positive stress studies. The bottom line is that the positive predictive value of stress echocardiography in this setting is low (only 10 to 0%), while the negative predictive value is very high (93 to 100%).

Since the individual study groups are all small, it is worth reviewing the metaanalysis of Shaw et al., which combines data from 5 studies and 445 patients. This reaffirms the low perioperative event rate in patients with negative dobutamine stress studies (0.37%). In contrast, patients with positive studies who did not undergo revascularization had a cardiac event rate of 26.3%. In these studies, the risk was eliminated with revascularization. The collective positive predictive value was 13% for cardiac death or myocardial infarction and 26% for any cardiac event. The overall negative predictive value was 99%.

While it is true that data are available for a smaller number of patients evaluated preoperatively with dobutamine stress than with dipyridamole thallium, it appears that the two tests provide comparable information. There is limited data concerning the role of dipyridamole stress echocardiography in risk stratification prior to vascular surgery. However, Sicari et al. (29) used high-dose dipyridamole to evaluate 121 patients undergoing vascular surgery and reported a positive predictive value of 25% and negative predictive value of 98%. There were no complications during the stress test.

In summary, it must be noted that stress testing is only one element of the preoperative evaluation of patients undergoing noncardiac surgery. However, it plays an important role in patients who are undergoing high-risk surgery.

STRESS ECHOCARDIOGRAPHY IN VALVULAR HEART DISEASE

Stress echocardiography may be very helpful in the assessment of patients with valvular heart disease. Although much of its use in this setting is anecdotal, there is a growing literature on the subject. In general terms, stress echocardiography is helpful when it is difficult to reconcile symptoms with the clinical and resting echocardiographic assessment of the severity of valve disease, in decision-making concerning the need for intervention and in patients where an assessment of ischemic mitral regurgitation is important. Native and prosthetic aortic and mitral valvular stenotic and regurgitant lesions have been evaluated by this modality. In mitral stenosis, the Doppler-measured mean transvalvular pressure gradient has been demonstrated to increase with exercise (30) and to correlate highly with simultaneous left heart manometric gradients. A concurrent rise in pulmonary artery pressures has also been demonstrated. Similar exercise-induced increases in Doppler-assessed mitral valve gradients have been reported in patients with mitral prostheses (31). Doppler stress echocardiography has also been used to demonstrate improved mitral flow hemodynamics both at rest and with stress following successful percutaneous balloon mitral valvuloplasty (32). This study also reported a fall in postvalvuloplasty peak exercise heart rate suggesting that the same degree of tachycardia was no longer required to augment cardiac output.

STRESS ECHOCARDIOGRAPHY VERSUS NUCLEAR STRESS

Nuclear stress techniques are widely used clinically and are discussed in detail elsewhere. In individual patients, there may be advantages to the use of one imaging modality over another, although, in aggregate, the two techniques appear to have equivalent diagnostic capabilities. The principal advantages of echocardiography are its ability to provide ancillary information, such as valve function, and to monitor the ventricular response to stress in a continuous fashion. Currently, cost considerations also favor stress echocardiography. The lack of radiation exposure is a minor consideration in most patients. The principal disadvantage of stress echocardiography is the inability to obtain diagnostic images in some patients. With harmonic imaging and contrast agents, this number should fall. Stress echocardiography has a shorter history and there is a larger literature on nuclear imaging especially in the areas of prognosis and risk stratification. Since both techniques are critically dependent on the availability of skilled personnel and good equipment, the choice of imaging modality for a given patient should be heavily influenced by the relative quality of the services that are available.

CONCLUSION

Since the introduction of stress echocardiographic concepts in the era of M-mode echocardiography, the technique has evolved dramatically, thanks in large part to the technical advances in ultrasound imaging and digital image manipulation. It is now a mainstay of clinical cardiology. Its utility in the diagnosis of coronary artery disease is well established and there is a growing body of data supporting its use in other settings. The future of stress echocardiography is bright with the potential for the incorporation of real-time three-dimensional displays and myocardial contrast perfusion imaging.

REFERENCES

1. Wann LS, Faris JV, Childress RH, et al. Exercise cross-sectional echocardiography in ischemic heart disease. *Circulation* 1979;60: 1300–1308.
2. Schiller NB, Shah PM, Crawford M. Recommendations for quantitation of the left ventricle by two-dimensional echocardiography. *J Am Soc Echocardiogr* 1989;2:358–367.
3. Arnese M, Cornel JH, Salustri A, et al. Prediction of improvement of regional left ventricular function after surgical revascularization. *Circulation* 1995;91:2748–2752.
4. Presti CF, Armstrong WF, Feigenbaum H. Comparison of echocardiography at peak exercise and after bicycle exercise in the evaluation of patients with known or suspected coronary artery disease. *J Am Soc Echocardiogr* 1988;1:119–126.
5. Cohen JL, Chan KL, Jaarsma W, et al. Arbutamine echocardiography: Efficacy and safety of a new pharmacologic stress agent to induce myocardial ischemia and detect coronary artery disease. *J Am Coll Cardio* 1995;26(5):1168–1175.
6. Shehata AT, Travin MI, Miller D, et al. Multicenter evaluation of the relationship between myocardial perfusion defect localization and defect size in the prediction of cardiac death. *Circulation* 1996;94(I):656.
7. Kelsey AM, Shaw LJ, Donovan CL, et al. Fifteen years of exercise echocardiography: a meta-analysis. *Circulation* 1998;96(8):1-276.
8. Hecht HS, DeBord L, Shaw R, et al. Digital supine bicycle stress echocardiography: A new technique for evaluating coronary artery disease. *J Am Coll Cardiol* 1993;21:950–956.
9. Barrett-Connor E, Wilcosky T, Wallace RB. Resting and exercise electrocardiography abnormalities associated with sex hormone use in women: the Lipid Research Clinics Program Prevalence Study. *Am J Epidemiol* 1985;123:81–88.
10. Clark PI, Glasser SP, Lyman GH. Relation of results of exercise stress tests in young women to phases of the menstrual cycle. *Am J Cardiol* 1988;61:197–199.
11. Heinsimer JA, Dewitt CM. Exercise testing in women. *J Am Coll Cardiol* 1989;14:1448–1449.
12. Gibbons RJ, Balady GJ, Beasley JW, et al. ACC/AHA Guidelines for exercise testing: a report of the American College of Cardiology/American Heart Association Task Force on Practice Guidelines (Committee on Exercise Testing). *J Am Coll Cardiol* 1997;30(1): 260–315.
13. Crouse LJ, Harbrecht JJ, Vacek JL, et al. Exercise echocardiography as a screening test for coronary artery disease and correlation with coronary arteriography. *Am J Cardiol* 1991;67:1213–1218.
14. Armstrong WF, O'Donnell J, Dillon JC, et al. Complementary value of two-dimensional exercise echocardiography to routine treadmill exercise testing. *Ann Intern Med* 1986;105:829–835.
15. Marwick TH, Nemec JJ, Pahkow FJ, et al. Accuracy and limitations of exercise echocardiography in a routine clinical setting. *J Am Coll Cardiol* 1992;19:74–81.
16. Ryan T, Segar DS, Sawada SG, et al. Detection of coronary artery disease using upright bicycle exercise echocardiography. *J Am Soc Echocardiogr* 1993;6:186–197.
17. Sawada SG, Ryan T, Conley M, et al. Prognostic value of a normal exercise echocardiogram. *Am Heart J* 1990;120:49–55.
18. Poldermans D, Arnese M, Fioretti PM, et al. Sustained prognostic value of dobutamine stress echocardiography for late cardiac events after major noncardiac vascular surgery. *Circulation* 1997;95:53–58.
19. Williams MJ, Odabashian J, Lauer MS, et al. Prognostic value of dobutamine echocardiography in patients with left ventricular dysfunction. *J Am Coll Cardiol* 1996;27:132–139.
20. Jaarsma W, Visser C, Funke Kupper A. Usefulness of two-dimensional exercise echocardiography shortly after myocardial infarction. *Am J Cardiol* 1986;57:86–90.
21. Applegate RJ, Dell'Italia LJ, Crawford MH. Usefulness of two-dimensional echocardiography during low-level exercise testing early after uncomplicated myocardial infarction. *Am J Cardiol* 1987;60:10–14.
22. Ryan T, Armstrong WF, O'Donnell JA, et al. Risk stratification following acute myocardial infarction during exercise two-dimensional echocardiography. *Am Heart J* 1987;114:1305–1316.
23. Sawada SG, Judson WE, Ryan T, et al. Upright bicycle exercise echocardiography after coronary artery bypass surgery. *Am J Cardiol* 1989; 64:1123–1127.
24. Pirelli S, Massa D, Faletra F, et al. Exercise electrocardiography versus dipyridamole echocardiography testing in coronary angioplasty. *Circulation* 1991;83[Suppl]:III-38–III-42
25. Dagianti A, Rosanio S, Penco M, et al. Clinical and prognostic usefulness of supine bicycle exercise echocardiography in the functional evaluaton of patients undergoing elective percutaneous transluminal coronary angioplasty. *Circulation* 1997;95:1176–1184.
26. Chen C, Li L, Chen LL, et al. Incremental doses of dobutamine induce a biphasic response in dysfunctional left ventricular regions subtending coronary stenoses. *Circulation* 1995;92:756–766.
27. Afridi I, Kleiman NS, Raizner AE, et al. Dobutamine echocardiography in myocardial hibernation: optimal dose and accuracy in predicting recovery of ventricular function after coronary angioplasty. *Circulation* 1995;91:663–670.
28. Eagle KA, Brundage BH, Chaitman BR, et al. Guidelines for perioperative cardiovascular evaluation for noncardiac surgery: report of the American College of Cardiology/American Heart Association Task Force on practice guidelines. *Circulation* 1996;93:1278–1317.
29. Sicari R, Picano E, Lusa A.M., et al. The value of dipyridamole echocardiography in risk stratification before vascular surgery. A multicenter study. The EPIC (Echo Persantine International Study) Group-Subproject: risk stratification before major vascular surgery. *Eur Heart J* 1995;16(6):842–847.
30. Voelker W, Jacksch R, Dittman H, et al. Validation of continuous-wave Doppler measurements of mitral valve gradients during exercise: a simultaneous Doppler-catheter study. *Eur Heart J* 1989;10:737–746.
31. Leavitt JI, Coats MH, Falk RH. Effects of exercise on transmitral gradient and pulmonary artery pressure in patients with mitral stenosis or a prosthetic mitral valve: a Doppler echocardiographic study. *J Am Coll Cardiol* 1991;17:1520–1526.
32. Tamai J, Nagata S, Akaike M. Improvement in mitral flow dynamics during exercise after percutaneous transvenous mitral commisurotomy: noninvasive evaluation using continuous wave Doppler technique. *Circulation* 1990;81:46–51.
33. Bonow RO. Identification of viable myocardium. *Circulation* 1996;94: 2674–2680.
34. Pingitore A, Picano E, Colosso MQ, et al. The atropine factor in pharmacologic stress echocardiography. *J Am Coll Cardiol* 1996;27: 1164–1170.
35. Aboul-Enein H, Bengtson JR, Adams DB, et al. Effect of the degree of effort on exercise echocardiography for the detection of restenosis after coronary artery angioplasty. *Am Heart J* 1991;122:430–437.
36. Amanullah AM, Lindvall K. Predischarge exercise echocardiography in patients with unstable angina who respond to medical treatment. *Clin Cardiol* 1992;15:417–423.
37. Armstrong WF, O'Donnell J, Ryan T, et al. Effect of prior myocardial infarction and extent and location of coronary artery disease on accuracy of exercise echocardiography. *J Am Coll Cardiol* 1987;10: 531–538.
38. Cohen JL, Ottenweller JE, George AK, et al. Comparison of dobutamine and exercise echocardiography for detecting coronary artery disease. *Am J Cardiol* 1993;72:1226–1231.
39. Dagianti A, Penco M, Agati L, et al. Stress echocardiography: comparison of exercise, dipyridamole and dobutamine in detecting and predicting the extent of coronary artery disease. *J Am Coll Cardiol* 1995;26: 18–25.
40. Galanti G, Sciagrà R, Comeglio M, et al. Diagnostic accuracy of peak exercise echocardiography in coronary artery disease: comparison with thallium-201 myocardial scintigraphy. *Am Heart J* 1991;122: 1609–1616.
41. Hecht HS, DeBord L, Shaw R, et al. Supine bicycle stress echocardiography versus tomographic thallium-201 exercise imaging for the detection of coronary artery disease. *J Am Soc Echocardiogr* 1993;6: 177–185.
42. Iliceto S, D'Ambrosio G, Sorino M, et al. Comparison of postexercise and transesophageal atrial pacing two-dimensional echocardiography

for detection of coronary artery disease. *Am J Cardiol* 1986;57: 547–553.

43. Kafka H, Leach AJ, Fitzgibbon GM. Exercise echocardiography after coronary artery bypass surgery: correlation with coronary angiography. *J Am Coll Cardiol* 1995;25:1019–1023.

44. Limacher MC, Quiñones MA, Poliner LR, et al. Detection of coronary artery disease with exercise two-dimensional echocardiography: description of a clinically applicable method and comparison with radionuclide ventriculography. *Circulation* 1983;67:1211–1218.

45. Marangelli V, Iliceto S, Piccinni G, et al. Detection of coronary artery disease by digital stress echocardiography: comparison of exercise, transesophageal atrial pacing and dipyridamole echocardiography. *J Am Coll Cardiol* 1994;24:117–124.

46. Marwick TH, D'Hondt AM, Mairesse GH, et al. Comparative ability of dobutamine and exercise stress in inducing myocardial ischaemia in active patients. *Br Heart J* 1994;72:31–38.

47. Quinones MA, Verani MS, Haichin RM, et al. Exercise echocardiography versus 201Tl single-photon emission computed tomography in evaluation of coronary artery disease. Analysis of 292 patients. *Circulation* 1992;85(3):1217–1218.

48. Ryan T, Vasey CG, Presti CF, et al. Exercise echocardiography: detection of coronary artery disease in patients with normal left ventricular wall motion at rest. *J Am Coll Cardiol* 1988;11:993–999.

49. Cohen JL, Greene TO, Ottenweller J, et al. Dobutamine digital echocardiography for detecting coronary artery disease. *Am J Cardiol* 1991; 67:1311–1318.

50. Previtali M, Lanzarini L, Ferario M, et al. Dobutamine versus dipyridamole echocardiography in coronary artery disease. *Circulation* 1991; 83:27–31.

51. Sawada SG, Segar DS, Ryan T, et al. Echocardiographic detection of coronary artery disease during dobutamine infusion. *Circulation* 1991; 83:1605–1614.

52. Mazeika PK, Nadazdin A, Oakley CM. Dobutamine stress echocardiography for detection and assessment of coronary artery disease. *J Am Coll Cardiol* 1992;19:1203–1211.

53. Marcovitz PA, Armstrong WF. Accuracy of dobutamine stress echocardiography in detecting coronary artery disease. *Am J Cardiol* 1992;69: 1269–1273.

54. Marwick T, D'Hondt AM, Baudhuin T, et al. Optimal use of dobutamine stress for the detection and evaluation of coronary artery disease: combination with echocardiography or scintigraphy, or both? *J Am Coll Cardiol* 1993;22:159–167.

55. Marwick TH, Willemart B, D'Hondt A, et al. Selection of the optimal nonexercise stress for the evaluation of ischemic regional myocardial dysfunction and malperfusion. *Circulation* 1993;87:345–354.

56. Hoffmann R, Lethen H, Kleinhaus E, et al. Comparative evaluation of bicycle and dobutamine stress echocardiography with perfusion scintigraphy and bicycle electrocardiogram for identification coronary artery disease. *Am J Cardiol* 1993;72:555–559.

57. Forster T, McNeill AJ, Salustri A, et al. Simultaneous dobutamine stress echocardiography and technetium-99m isonitrile single-photon emission computed tomography in patients with suspected coronary artery disease. *J Am Coll Cardiol* 1993;21:1591–1696.

58. Gunalp B, Dokumaci B, Uyan C, et al. Value of dobutamine technetium-99m-sestamibi SPECT and echocardiography in the detection of coronary artery disease compared with coronary angiography. *J Nucl Med* 1993;34(6):889–894.

59. Belesin BD, Ostojic M, Stepanovic J, et al. Stress echocardiography in the detection of myocardial ischemia: head-to-head comparison of exercise, dobutamine, and dipyridamole tests. *Circulation* 1994;90: 1168–1176.

60. Ling LH, Pellikka PA, Mahoney DW, et al. Atropine augmentation in dobutamine stress echocardiography: role and incremental valve in a clinical practice setting. *J Am Coll Cardiol* 1996;28:551–557.

61. McNeill AJ, Fioretti PM, El-Said EM, et al. Dobutamine stress echocardiography before and after coronary angioplasty. *Am J Cardiol* 1992; 69:740–745.

62. Picano E, Distante A, Masini M, et al. Dipyridamole-echocardiography test in effort angina pectoris. *Am J Cardiol* 1985;56:452–456.

63. Labovitz AJ, Pearson AC, Chaitman BR. Doppler and two-dimensional echocardiographic assessment of left ventricular function before and after intravenous dipyridamole stress testing for detection of coronary artery disease. *Am J Cardiol* 1988;62:1180–1185.

64. Picano E, Lattanzi F, Masini M, et al. High dose dipyridamole echocardiography test in effort angina pectoris. *J Am Coll Cardiol* 1986;8: 848–854.

65. Zoghbi WA, Cheirif J, Kleiman NS, et al. Diagnosis of ischemic heart disease with adenosine echocardiography. *J Am Coll Cardiol* 1991;18: 1271–1279.

66. Edlund A, Conradsson T, Sollevi A. A role for adenosine in coronary vasoregulation in man. Effects of theophylline and enprofylline. *Circulation* 1995;15(6):623–636.

67. Amanullah AM, Bevegard A, Lindvall K, et al. Assessment of left ventricular wall motion in angina pectoris by two-dimensional echocardiography and myocardial perfusion by technetium-99m sestamibi tomography during adenosine-induced coronary vasodilation and comparison with coronary angiography. *Circulation* 1993;72(14):983–989.

68. Tawa CB, Baker WB, Kleiman NS, et al. Comparison of adenosine echocardiography with and without isometric handgrip, to exercise echocardiography in the detection of ischemia in patients with coronary artery disease. *J Am Soc Echocardiogr* 1996;9:33–43.

69. Bjornstad K, Al Amri M, Lingamanaicker J, et al. Interobserver and intraobserver variation for analysis of left ventricular wall motion at baseline and during low- and high-dose dobutamine stress echocardiography in patients with high prevalence of wall motion abnormalities at rest. *J Am Soc Echocardiogr* 1996;9:320–328.

70. Rallidis L, Cokkinos P, Tousoulis D, et al. Comparison of dobutamine and treadmill exercise echocardiography in inducing ischemia in patients with coronary artery disease. *J Am Coll Cardiol* 1997;30: 1660–1668.

71. Sawada SG, Ryan T, Fineberg NS, et al. Exercise echocardiographic detection of coronary artery disease in women. *J Am Coll Cardiol* 1989; 14:1440–1447.

72. Williams MJ, Marwick T, O'Gorman D, et al. Comparison of exercise echocardiography with an exercise score to diagnose coronary artery disease in women. *Am J Cardiol* 1994;74(5):435–438.

73. Roger VL, Pellikka PA, Miller FA. Stress echocardiogrpahy for the detection of coronary artery disease in women. *Circulation* 1993;88 (Suppl I):1–403.

74. Masini M, Picano E, Lattanzi F, et al. High dose dipyridamole-echocardiography test in women: correlation with exercise-electrocardiography test and coronary arteriography. *J Am Coll Cardiol* 1988;12:682–685.

75. Marwick TH, Anderson T, Williams MJ, et al. Exercise echocardiography is an accurate and cost efficient technique for detection of coronary artery disease in women. *J Am Coll Cardiol* 1995;26(2):335–341.

76. Pierard LA, de Landsheere CM, Berthe C, et al. Identification of viable myocardium by echocardiography during dobutime infusion in patients with myocardial infarction after thrombolytic therapy: comparison with positron emission tomography. *J Am Coll Cardiol* 1990;15:1021–1031.

77. Smart SC, Sawada S, Ryan T, et al. Low-dose dobutamine echocardiography detects reversible dysfunction after thrombolytic therapy of acute myocardial infarction. *Circulation* 1993;88:405–415.

78. Watada H, Ito H, Oh H, et al. Dobutamine stress echocardiography predicts reversible dysfunction and quantitates the extent of irreversibly damaged myocardium after reperfusion of anterior myocardial infarction. *J Am Coll Cardiol* 1994;24:624–630.

79. Barilla F, Gheorghiade M, Alam M, et al. Low-dose dobutamine in patients with acute myocardial infarction identifies viable but not contractile myocardium and predicts the magnitude of improvement in wall motion abnormalities in response to coronary revascularization. *Am Heart J* 1991;122:1522–1531.

80. Cigarroa CG, DeFilippi CR, Brickner ME, et al. Dobutamine stress echocardiography identifies hibernating myocardium and predicts recovery of left ventricular function after coronary revascularization. *Circulation* 1993;88:430–436.

81. LaCanna G, Alfieri O, Giubbini R, et al. Echocardiography during infusion of dobutamine for identification of reversible dysfunction in patients with chronic coronary artery disease. *J Am Coll Cardiol* 1994; 23:617–626.

82. Perrone-Filardi P, Pace L, Prastaro M, et al. Dobutamine echocardiography predicts improvement of hypoperfused dysfunctional myocardium after revascularization in patients with coronary artery disease. *Circulation* 1995;91:2556–2565.

83. Perrone-Filardi P, Pace L, Prastaro M, et al. Assessment of myocardial viability in patients with chronic coronary artery disease. *Circulation* 1996;94:2712–2719.

84. Lane RT, Sawada SG, Segar DS, et al. Dobutamine stress echocardiography for assessment of cardiac risk before noncardiac surgery. *Am J Cardiol* 1991;68:976–977.

85. Lalka SG, Sawada SG, Dalsing MC, et al. Dobutamine stress echocardiography as a predictor of cardiac events associated with aortic surgery. *J Vasc Surg* 1992;15:831–841.

86. Eichelberger JP, Schwarz KQ, Black ER, et al. Predictive value of dobutamine echocardiography just before noncardiac vascular surgery. *Am J Cardiol* 1993;72:602–609.

87. Davila-Roman VG, Waggoner AD, Sicard GA, et al. Dobutamine stress echocardiography predicts surgical outcome in patients with an aortic aneurysm and peripheral vascular disease. *J Am Coll Cardiol* 1993;21: 957–963.

CHAPTER 6

Contrast Echocardiography

Thomas R. Porter and Jucyléa M. Cwajg

HISTORICAL DEVELOPMENT

The observation of an echo contrast coming out from blood was first described in 1968, when Gramiak and Shah (1) were studying M-mode echocardiograms of the aortic valve to estimate stroke volume at the catheterization laboratory. They incidentally depicted an intense contrast effect within the normally echo-free lumen of that vessel after injection of indocyanine green into the left atrium. In the early 1980s, several investigators began observing myocardial contrast following intracoronary or aortic root injections of microbubbles. DeMaria et al. (2) were able to visualize myocardial perfusion territories after intracoronary injections of either carbon dioxide or 30-micron diameter microballoons. In 1982, Armstrong et al. (3) reported that regions of poorly perfused myocardium following coronary artery occlusion could be identified after aortic root injections of gelatin-encapsulated microbubbles containing nitrogen. These contrast defects were correlated to the extent of wall motion abnormality, and found to better define the true risk area. Numerous contrast-producing materials, such as hand-agitated normal saline, hand-agitated indocyanine green, gelatin, or even hydrogen peroxide, were utilized in these early studies (4). Because of their size and poor survival time in blood, these ultrasound contrast agents could only be used in an experimental setting. Indeed, the size of the bubbles led to air embolizations, hemodynamic instability, and myocardial depression (5).

The large size and brief survival in blood of these bubbles precluded their utilization for intravenous contrast, but these problems were overcome by the advent of the sonication

technique patented by Feinstein et al. (6). This process consists in exposing a liquid medium containing air to a high energy source of ultrasound, thus creating smaller particles that were in general less than 10 microns. Sonication was first utilized for intracoronary injection of sonicated radiographic contrast agents like Renografin. Immediately following sonication, the bubbles were injected directly into the coronary artery (4). In 1984, Tei et al. (7) created different degrees of coronary stenosis in a dog model and observed that the wash out of sonicated Renografin analyzed by video densitometry correlated with known reductions in luminal diameters. More stable agents were produced when albumin was sonicated instead of Renografin. Despite the excitement of these findings, intravenous microbubbles made by sonication were not capable of surviving long enough to reach the left ventricular cavity on a consistent basis because of the rapid diffusion of air out of the microbubble. This led to extensive research to study what physical and chemical factors would be needed to optimize microbubbles for intravenous use.

ULTRASOUND CONTRAST AGENT DEVELOPMENT

Physical Principles

To achieve the main goal of left heart and myocardial opacification through an intravenous injection, some basic knowledge on physical properties of an ideal agent was necessary. First, a method of prolonging microbubble survival following intravenous injection was required. The persistence of a bubble is directly proportional to the square power of its radius, and its scattering cross section (i.e., its ability to produce ultrasound contrast) is related to the sixth power of its radius. Although this suggests that microbubbles should be large, they must be less than 8 microns in order to pass through the pulmonary capillary bed (8). Sonication reliably produces smaller size particles, but the partial pres-

T. R. Porter: Department of Internal Medicine, Section of Cardiology, University of Nebraska Medical Center; Department of Internal Medicine, Section of Cardiology, Nebraska Health System/University Hospital, Omaha, Nebraska 68198.

J. M. Cwajg: Department of Cardiology, Echocardiography Laboratory, Hospital Barra d'Or, Rio de Janeiro, 22793-000 Brazil.

sure of gases inside these microbubbles increases significantly as its size decreases, leading to more rapid diffusion out of the microbubble.

Microbubbles have subsequently been formulated to reduce this rate of diffusion of gas out of the microbubble. One way to do this is to increase shell thickness. A second method employed has been to use high molecular weight gases with low saturation concentration and low solubility.

The first-generation contrast agents were manufactured with room air. Sonicated albumin microbubbles containing room air were the first intravenous agent to pass the pulmonary circulation, but achieved variable degrees of left ventricle (LV) opacification. This agent was termed Albunex, and was the first commercially available contrast agent approved by the Food and Drug Administration (FDA) for LV opacification from a venous injection (9,10). In no cases was visually evident myocardial opacification ever observed with Albunex. Since the albumin shell is thin and the gas inside the microbubble (room air) is rapidly diffusible, its survival in blood has been shown to be brief. Nonetheless, intravenous delivery of large quantities of these microbubbles was clinically safe and without hemodynamic alterations. Levovist is another air-containing bubble widely used in Europe. It is manufactured as a powder of galactose and palmitic acid and needs water for reconstitution. Similar to Albunex, it is mainly used for LV opacification.

Fluorocarbon Ultrasound Contrast

Second-generation bubbles have incorporated higher molecular weight gases into the microbubble, such as perfluorocarbons (molecular weight range 188 to 338 g/mol). These gases are much less diffusible than room air and therefore persist longer following venous injection. This leads to greater left ventricular cavity and even myocardial contrast (Fig. 1). A large variety of microbubbles containing fluorocarbons are undergoing clinical trials (Table 1) with the hope of achieving FDA approval. The different formulations have different sizes and concentrations. Shell composition of the different fluorocarbon products varies from no shell at all to albumin, lipid, surfactant, or cyanoacrylate-coated. The microbubble formulations that have been successful in achieving left ventricular opacification and myocardial contrast from a venous injection have been those containing a fluorocarbon and having a large concentration of smaller (<7 microns) microbubbles.

Perfluorocarbon-exposed sonicated dextrose albumin (PESDA) microbubbles are a formulation that can be produced on site (11); several investigators have used this agent extensively in animal and human studies. It contains decafluorobutane (molecular weight, 238g/mol) and its mean size is 4.7 ± 0.2 microns. Optison (formerly known as FS069) is a second-generation contrast agent composed of perfluoro-

TABLE 1. *Ultrasound contrast agents*

Name	Manufacturer/U.S. Distributor	Size (μ)	Conc.	Shell composition	Gas content
Albunex*†	Molecular Biosystems/Mallinckrodt Medical	3–5‡	3–5 × 10§	Denatured albumin	Air
Optison (FS069)	Molecular Biosystems/Mallinckrodt Medical	2–4.5‡	5–8 × 10§	Denatured albumin	Perfluoropropane
PESDA	Thomas Porter, M.D.	4–5.0‡	1.2 × 10§	Denatured albumin	Perfluorobutane
Aerosomes (MRX-115)	ImaRx Pharmaceutical/DuPont-Merck	2.5‖	1–2 × 10^9§	Phospholipids	Perfluoropropane
MRX 408	ImaRX Pharmaceutical/DuPont-Merck	2.1‖	1.4 × 10^9§	Phospholipids	Perfluorobutane
Imagent (AF0150)	Alliance/Schering	5.0‖	5 × 10^8§	Surfactant stabilized	Perfluorohexane
Sonovist (SHU 568A)	Schering	1.0‖	2 × 10^19§	Cyanacrylate polymer	Air
EchoGen (QW3600)	Sonus Pharmaceutical/Abbott Laboratories	2–4‡	1.0 × 10^12§	Surfactant stabilized	Dodecafluoropentane
QW 7437	Sonus Pharmaceutical	—		Surfactant stabilized (anionically charged)	Dodecafluoropentane
Acusphere	Acusphere Inc.	2.0‖	—	Polyethylene glycol	Air
BiSphere	Point BioMedical	4.0‖	—	Polymer (composite shell)	Air
SonoVue (BR1)	Bracco/Bracco	2.5‖	1–5 × 10^8§	Phospholipids and surfactants	Sulfur hexafluoride
Levovist	Schering	2–4‡	200–400¶	Galactose matrix and palmitic acid	Air
Echovist	Shering	—	200–400¶	Galactose matrix	Air
NC100100	Nycomed Imaging/Nycomed	3–5‡	7.5 × 10^6§	Not disclosed at present time	
Quantison	Andaris/Advanced Magnetics, Inc.	3.2‖		Spray-dried albumin	Air
Quantison Depot	Andaris	12‖	1–2 × 10^9§	Spray-dried albumin	Air
BY963	Byk Gulden/Bracco	3.8‖	1.7 × 10^8§	Saccharide and phospholipid	Air
BR14	Bracco	2.0–2.5‡	4–7 × 10^8§	Phospholipid	Perfluorobutane
OUC 82755	Otsuka	5.5‖	?	Lactate polymer	Perfluoropropane

* FDA approved for LV opacification.

† Indicated for LV cavity opacification only. Produces myocardial opacification from direct coronary and aortic root injections but rarely from venous injections.

‡ Range of *in vitro* measurements.

§ Concentration (mean + standard deviation *in vitro* measurements).

‖ Mean *in vitro* measurements.

¶ mg/mL (powder).

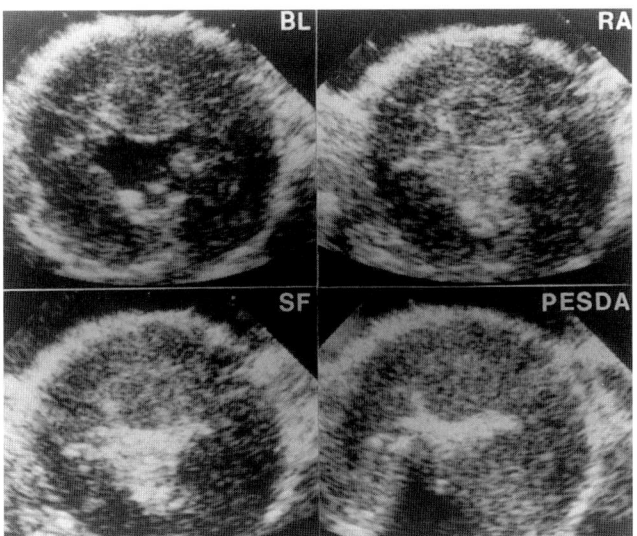

FIG. 1. Differences in myocardial contrast produced by sonicating dextrose albumin with gases of different molecular weights. There is clear myocardial opacification after intravenous injection of the gas with the highest molecular weight: perfluorocarbon exposed sonicated dextrose albumin (*PESDA*). *BL*, baseline; *RA*, room air-exposed sonicated dextrose albumin; *SF*, sulfurhexafluoride-exposed sonicated albumin. (From ref. 11, with permission.)

propane-filled albumin microspheres. Both PESDA and Optison produce no changes in hemodynamic function, myocardial blood flow, left ventricular thickening, or pulmonary gas exchange when injected intravenously and are capable of consistent and reproducible myocardial opacification. Optison is the first second-generation microbubble to be approved by the FDA for LV opacification from a venous injection (12). As can be seen in Table 1, several other second-generation agents are on the pathway to FDA approval.

ULTRASOUND INSTRUMENTATION CHANGES

Harmonic Imaging

As we know, bubbles containing compressible gas represent strong scatterers. Whenever submitted to low incident pressures (below 100 K Pa) they manifest a linear behavior in terms of backscatter enhancement, but these low levels of pulse pressure cannot practically be used for transthoracic imaging.

At higher peak incident pressures (above 0.1 megapascals) bubbles respond in a nonlinear fashion, which means they no longer respond equally to the negative and positive portions of the sound wave. They can easily expand but they get smaller with more difficulty because of the increased partial pressure of gas inside the bubble during compression. The consequence of this nonlinear radial oscillation is that

the sound emitted by the bubbles and received by the ultrasound scanner contain resonant frequencies or harmonics (13). The harmonic response depends not only on incident pressures but also on incident frequency and on the physical characteristics of the bubble, e.g., its size and shell thickness. Thicker shells may increase its rigidity and might, therefore, attenuate the nonlinear behavior.

The principle of harmonic technology is that the transmitted fundamental frequency is separated from the received signal by using bandpass filters. Current ultrasound systems are able to transmit at one frequency and to listen to its second multiple, known as second harmonic (Fig. 2). This results in an improved signal-to-noise ratio in the general ultrasound image as well as increased sensitivity to microbubble presence in the myocardium (15).

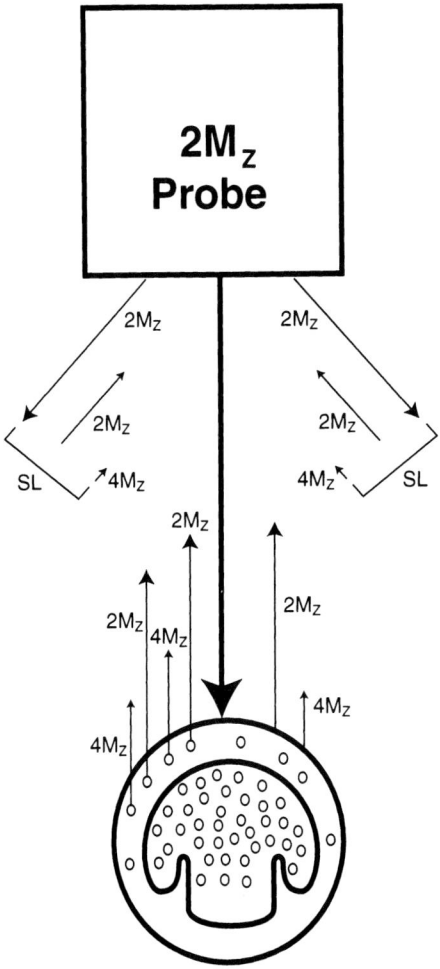

FIG. 2. The cartoon illustrates the returning signal intensity (indicated by *arrow length*). Microbubbles have the greatest harmonic signal intensity (*longest arrow*), but myocardium also has a harmonic response. Fortunately, side lobe (*SL*) artifacts have very little harmonic signal intensity and thus, do not reduce the image quality of a harmonic image as they do in fundamental images. *Mz*, megahertz. (From ref. 14, with permission.)

Intermittent Imaging Combined with Harmonic Imaging

Porter et al. (16) described how significantly greater myocardial contrast can be produced with very small doses of intravenous microbubbles when diagnostic ultrasound is transmitted in an interrupted manner instead of conventional 30 Hz frame rate (Fig. 3). This strategy is called transient response imaging (TRI) or intermittent imaging (17). The myocardial contrast intensity produced with TRI correlates with coronary blood flow changes and quantifies the spatial extent of ischemia (16). In humans, myocardial contrast can be consistently produced when using TRI and can accurately identify regional perfusion abnormalities (18).

Although it is evident that TRI is a remarkable method of producing myocardial contrast from a small intravenous injection of microbubbles, there are still questions on how to optimally apply this technique to detect myocardial perfusion abnormalities. For example, what would be the most appropriate timing for triggering? End-diastolic frames seem a logical approach since coronary perfusion occurs mainly in diastole. On the other hand, systolic frames offer better resolution in part because of a partial volume effect (the thicker the segment, the better the distinction between two points) and because the LV cavity is at its smallest size (resulting in the least posterior wall attenuation) (19). Besides this question, several new modifications of TRI have been introduced by investigators or manufacturers that are designed to improve image quality and ease of acquisition of perfusion data.

Power Doppler

Doppler is an effective way of making distinction between scatterers with high velocity and tissue. Myocardial blood flow cannot be ideally studied with frequency shift Doppler. Power Doppler, however, examines the amplitude of the Doppler signal, which presumably represents the concentration of scatterers at one spatial location. Theoretically, then, this should be the most sensitive tool for contrast-enhanced studies. Unfortunately, it suffers from moving wall interference or clutter artifact. The addition of harmonic imaging and TRI to power Doppler has further improved the signal-to-noise ratio and can be used to detect myocardial blood flow.

Accelerated Intermittent Imaging

One of the limiting factors with TRI or intermittent harmonic imaging (IHI) is that image acquisition requires trig-

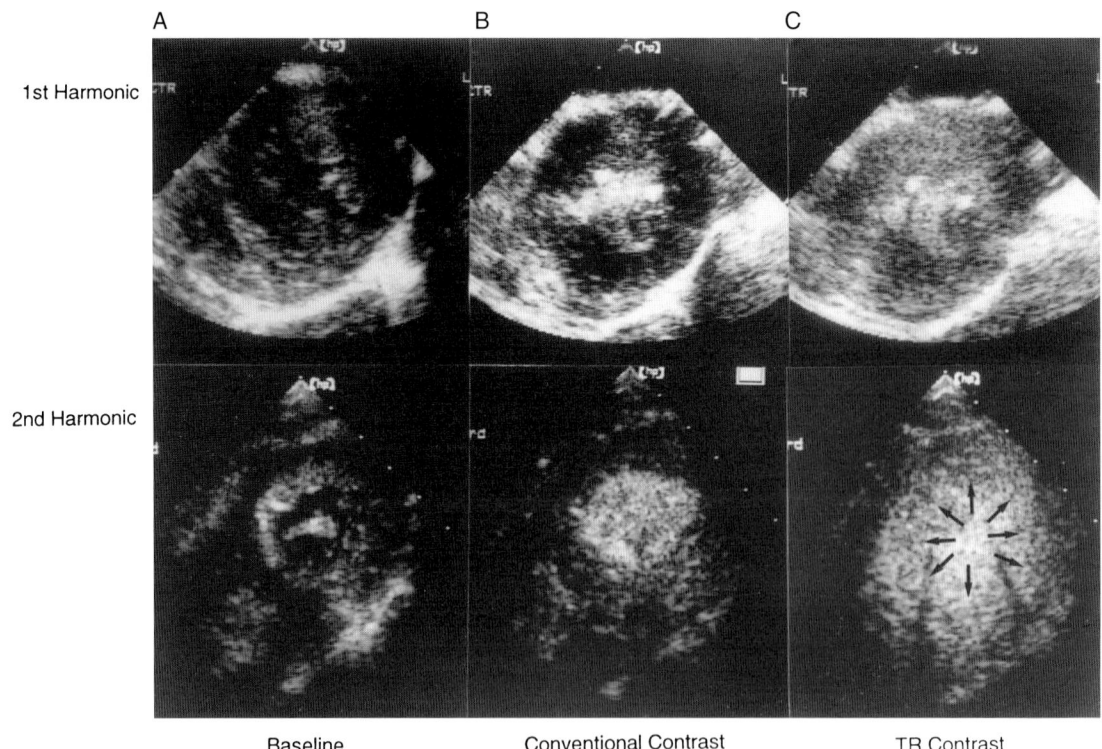

FIG. 3. The improvement in myocardial contrast produced with transient response imaging (TRI) versus conventional imaging with use of first-harmonic and second-harmonic imaging is demonstrated. **A:** Before intravenous injection of perfluorocarbon-exposed sonicated dextrose albumin. **B, C:** myocardial opacification seen with conventional 30 Hz frame rate imaging (**B**) compared with TRI. The second-harmonic transient myocardial contrast is the brightest (*arrows*) and occurs without posterior wall attenuation. (From ref. 16, with permission.)

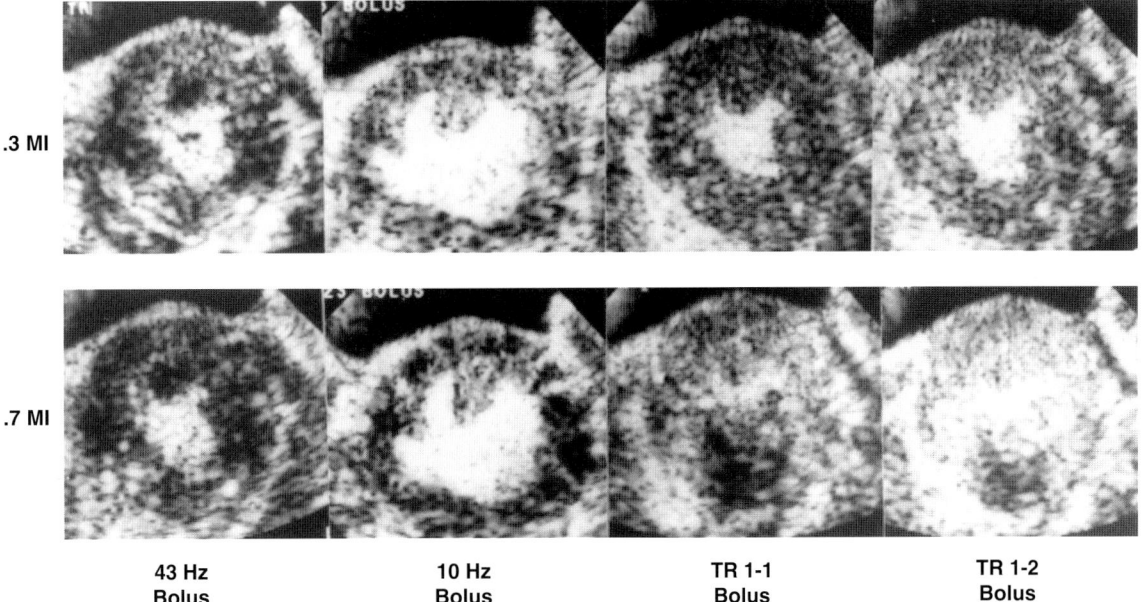

.3 MI

.7 MI

43 Hz	10 Hz	TR 1-1	TR 1-2
Bolus	Bolus	Bolus	Bolus

FIG. 4. The increase in myocardial contrast depiction as a function of pulsing interval at the 0.3 mechanical index (MI) and 0.7 MI as seen in one dog. Note that at 10 Hz frame rate, there is an increase in myocardial contrast that is not seen at the 0.7 MI.

gering at once every one or more cardiac cycles, thus preventing the simultaneous analysis of wall thickening and prolonging the time required to obtain perfusion data. Based on evidence that both reduced microbubble destruction and enhanced cavitational activity are responsible for the myocardial contrast seen during IHI, Porter et al. (20) showed that a lower mechanical index (0.3) that still elicits harmonic behavior in microbubbles without significant bubble destruction can detect myocardial perfusion at more rapid frame rates (Fig. 4). This methodology has already been applied during stress echocardiography in humans, where rapid analysis of wall thickening and perfusion within 30 to 50 seconds at peak stress can be obtained with this accelerated form of intermittent imaging (AIHI) (21).

Stimulated Acoustic Emissions/Other Imaging Modalities

At high diagnostic peak incident pressures (or power outputs), microbubbles tend to burst. Whenever that happens, they emit very strong sound-wave signals, which have been described as stimulated acoustic emission. This has been observed immediately following resumption of ultrasound in dogs when using a high acoustic output (16). Its extent may also depend on physicochemical properties of different microbubbles (22). Another measurement is pulse inversion, which utilizes characteristics specific to microbubble vibrations to subtract rather than filter out the fundamental signal. In pulse-inversion harmonic imaging, two pulses are transmitted down each ray line, instead of only a single pulse as in "conventional harmonic." The first one is a normal pulse, the second is an identical copy of the first, but inverted. In

other words, if there was a positive pressure on the first pulse, there will be an equal negative pressure on the second. Linear targets will respond equally to positive and negative pressures and thus cancel each other, while nonlinear targets (e.g., microbubbles) will not respond equally to positive and negative pressures. Instead, they will give twice the harmonic level of a single pulse. Although this may lead to increased sensitivity to contrast and improved resolution, tissue motion artifacts may still be a problem.

CLINICAL APPLICATIONS OF MICROBUBBLES

Detection of Intracardiac Shunts

Contrast echocardiography (transthoracic and transesophageal) has been used to diagnose intracardiac and intrapulmonary shunts by observing the presence of contrast echoes in cardiac chambers after intravenous hand-agitated saline injection. The greatest current utility for this is in the detection of a patent foramen ovale.

Doppler Enhancement

Doppler echocardiography provides a noninvasive assessment of intracardiac flows, velocities, and pressure gradients. However, its diagnostic accuracy can be partially limited by increased absorption and scattering of ultrasound. Transpulmonary contrast agents have been shown to increase the signal-to-noise ratio by improving the spectral Doppler evaluation of aortic stenosis, pulmonary venous flow, mitral and tricuspid regurgitation, and prosthetic aortic flows (23–25).

Endocardial Border Resolution

One recent surprising discovery is that tissue is also able to produce harmonics, at least in part due to nonlinear propagation of ultrasound through its pathway. Although this response is small, newer ultrasound systems are able to filter this signal and to display this portion of the received information. This phenomenon, described as tissue harmonic imaging, has improved endocardial border definition, especially in technically difficult cases, even without contrast use.

Additional use of a contrast agent to provide left ventricular opacification (LVO) can further enhance endocardial visualization. The improved border detection has improved the determination of left ventricular volumes and ejection fraction, but has yet to be more extensively validated (26).

Recently, data has been presented that intravenous contrast can further improve endocardial echoes when using harmonic imaging during stress echocardiography (14). This has led to an increase in the number of interpretable segments at rest and during stress. It is still to be determined how improved LVO with intravenous microbubbles will impact the accuracy of stress echo in detecting significant coronary artery disease.

PERFUSION IMAGING

The utilization of microbubbles to study myocardial blood flow with contrast echocardiography has been examined and validated both for intracoronary, aortic root, and intravenous ultrasound contrast.

Intracoronary and Aortic Root Contrast Echocardiography

One of the most clinically relevant areas where intracoronary ultrasound contrast has been useful is defining viability after coronary reperfusion in acute myocardial infarction. After reperfusion, contractile and microvascular reserve seem to be comparable in defining extent of viable myocardium within the infarct bed in the absence of residual coronary stenosis. Whereas contractile reserve in this scenario provides an indirect assessment of the extent of viability, microvascular reserve delineated with ultrasound contrast defines the topography of the infarct, thus assisting in a more direct evaluation of infarct size and viability. In the presence of a residual stenosis, the degree of contractile reserve is attenuated depending on coronary stenosis severity.

When anterograde epicardial flow is restored to an occluded coronary artery, it was previously assumed that microvascular flow is also restored. However, as characterized by Kloner et al. (27), in terms of its pathology, the presence of no-reflow phenomenon proved that this assumption is not always the truth. Ito et al. (28) utilized intracoronary ultrasound contrast to demonstrate that myocardial perfusion is absent in about one-fourth of patients with anterior myocardial infarction (AMI), despite an angiographically open-infarct artery following intracoronary thrombolysis or coronary angioplasty. Detection of this no-reflow phenomenon with intracoronary contrast has prognostic implications since these patients had comparatively poor regional and global left ventricular function 1 month after AMI (28–30).

Another area where intracoronary contrast has been useful is in defining collateral blood flow in acute myocardial infarction. Coronary angiography, the most frequently used technique for studying coronary circulation in humans, is inadequate in the detection of collateral vessels less than 100 μm in diameter. Identification of collateral blood flow by myocardial contrast echocardiography is superior to angiography and is accurate in identifying viability in segments supplied by occluded arteries (31). Regions supplied by collaterals are less likely to exhibit the no-reflow phenomenon after reperfusion (32). There even seems to be a potential benefit from late revascularization, as long as collateral blood flow by myocardial contrast echocardiography (MCE) is present within the infarct bed (31).

Another clinical scenario where intracoronary contrast echocardiography has been tested is in identifying viable myocardium in chronic coronary artery disease. DeFilippi et al. (33) compared intracoronary Renographin and low-dose dobutamine stress echo in predicting recovery of function after coronary revascularization in patients with chronic coronary artery disease (CAD). There were no significant differences between the two methods in predicting functional recovery of hypokinetic segments. In akinetic segments, however, contractile reserve by dobutamine had better specificity and positive predictive value than MCE. Nagueh et al. (34) assessed the comparative accuracy of intracoronary MCE with Albunex, rest-redistribution Tl-201 scintigraphy, and dobutamine stress echo in identification of patients with hibernating myocardium. Methods evaluating rest perfusion (MCE and Tl-201) or contractile reserve (sustained improvement plus biphasic response) had a similar sensitivity but a low specificity for predicting functional recovery. The presence of ischemia represented by a biphasic response increased dobutamine specificity. With our current knowledge about the relevance of outcome data, it would be a misconception to define viability merely as recovery of function.

Intraaortic injections of ultrasound contrast have found their most important application in the operating room, where ultrasound contrast has been injected with the cardioplegic solution to determine adequacy of cardioplegic delivery. Adequate delivery of both anterograde and retrograde cardioplegia can be assisted with MCE and hence guide the sequence of graft placement and its success on-line (35,36).

Intravenous Ultrasound Contrast and the Physiologic Concept of Microbubbles: Deposit Agents versus True Intravascular Tracers

Intravenous ultrasound contrast agents that act as deposit tracers are known to have prolonged myocardial persistence, even after LV cavity dissipation. Similar to microspheres, they seem to induce some microvascular plugging. One of them, Echogen, can be injected as a liquid emulsion that is converted to gas at body temperature. Inside the circulation, these bubbles tend to become larger due to inward diffusion of nitrogen and oxygen. Since these microbubbles would be larger when they reach the left ventricular cavity, bubbles that reach the left side of the heart will nicely opacify the myocardium even with fundamental imaging. High doses of Echogen have resulted in pulmonary hypertension, hypoxia, and hemodynamic collapse in dogs. A modification of Echogen called QW7427 (anionically charged 2% dodecafluoro-pentane) has been used in animal studies without derangements in hemodynamics or LV function and also in normal volunteers with apparently no serious adverse effects so far. Preliminary images in humans have demonstrated dramatic left ventricular myocardial opacification with QW7427.

Intravascular tracers represent the majority of second-generation agents. They follow closely the red blood cells rheology and have a mean size around 5 μm and a nonrelevant percentage of larger bubbles. For this reason, their myocardium contrast enhancement is transitory and does not cause changes in hemodynamic profile.

Conceptual Differences between Intravascular Tracer Microbubbles and Radionuclide Tracers

Different from microbubbles that follow red blood cell rheology and thus act as a pure flow tracer (37), radioisotopes penetrate the myocyte. Radioactive thallium (Tl-201) is a potassium analog that enters the cell and undergoes continuous exchange across its membrane in a process involving the Na$^+$/K$^+$ ATPase pump. Tc-99m sestamibi enters the myocyte by passive diffusion and binds with relative stability to plasma and mitochondria membranes; unlike Tl-201, it undergoes less redistribution. Interpretation of perfusion scintigraphy assumes that segments with maximum tracer uptake have normal flow and that any region with an apparent reduction of flow tracer uptake is underperfused. Therefore, its analysis provides only relative differences in flow distribution between different regions. The accuracy of nuclear techniques is also affected by its limited spatial resolution, which for SPECT (38) varies from 12 to 20 mm (depending on many factors) and, for positron emission tomography (PET), is 6 mm (39). A phenomenon known as partial volume effect explains how counts measured from a region with reduced thickness will underestimate true regional activity concentrations. PET has better resolving power compared to other nuclear techniques and corrects for attenuation and, to some extent, for the partial volume effect described above, but it is still limited by its inability to accurately measure true tissue tracer concentrations when the thickness of the imaged object is less than twice the spatial resolution of the imaging device (40). Conversely, echocardiography spatial resolution in the axial direction is between 1 and 2 mm depending on the transducer frequency.

Quantification of Myocardial Perfusion Abnormalities with Intravenous Contrast

During continuous infusion of a contrast agent, the power output on a transducer can be increased so that each pulse of ultrasound destroys a sufficient number of microbubbles to remove any contrast enhancement from the myocardium. Shorter pulsing intervals will allow partial replenishment of microbubbles within the capillary cross-sectional area of the beam width, while longer pulsing intervals will approach a plateau or peak myocardial videointensity (MVI). The rate at which MVI reappears (slope) is proportional to blood velocity and the peak background subtracted MVI is proportional to capillary cross-sectional area. Therefore, slope times peak MVI is an index of myocardial blood flow (41) (Fig. 5).

While bolus injections of intravenous contrast cannot be used to detect rates of myocardial contrast replenishment, the peak MVI ratio (ratio of peak contrast enhancement in one region divided by the region with greatest enhancement) has been utilized to quantify myocardial perfusion abnormalities (18).

Despite these quantification techniques, myocardial contrast echocardiography (MCE) has to overcome several problems if it is to be able to quantify myocardial blood

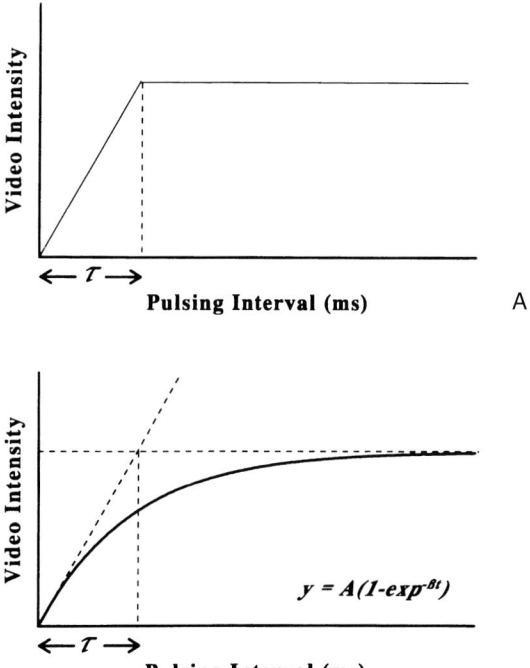

FIG. 5. The pulsing interval (*x* axis) versus myocardial contrast video intensity (*y* axis) relation as (**A**) predicted by the model and (**B**) observed experimentally during a continuous infusion of perfluorocarbon containing microbubbles. The function is used to derive parameters *A* (plateau) and β (slope). τ, time to plateau myocardial videointensity. (From ref. 41, with permission.)

flow. First, it must deal with attenuation artifacts that vary from patient to patient. Although attenuation due to microbubbles has been partially corrected with continuous infusions, it will not overcome the different regional variations we see in contrast enhancement between individuals.

Stress Echocardiography

Canine experimentations have demonstrated that during hyperemic stimulus MCE can be used to visualize and quantitate the amount of jeopardized myocardium due to moderate to severe degrees of coronary stenosis, and that this correlates with Tl-201 SPECT (42). During dipyridamole vasodilation of coronary microcirculation, relative videointensity ratios within different myocardial regions have been shown to reflect relative ratios of both myocardial blood volume and flow. Accordingly, Kaul et al. (43) demonstrated that MCE can define the presence of abnormal perfusion at rest and during dipyridamole stress in humans. The location and physiological relevance (reversible or irreversible) of perfusion defects was similar to that provided by Tc-99m sestamibi SPECT. Porter et al. (18) demonstrated that regional peak myocardial videointensity (PMVI) correlated closely with regional tracer uptake (dual isotope protocol) in patients both at rest ($r = 0.84$) and following dipyridamol stress ($r = 0.88$). A PMVI ratio (abnormal region divided by the region with the highest videointensity) of less than 0.6 had a sensitivity of 92% and a specificity of 84% in identifying abnormally perfused segments by SPECT (Fig. 6).

More recently, it has been observed that myocardial contrast enhancement obtained with intermittent harmonic imaging during PESDA bolus injection or continuous infusion can evaluate myocardial perfusion in the setting of a dobutamine stress echo. In this setting, MCE better defined the extent of coronary artery disease and also improved the sensitivity for single-vessel disease diagnosis when compared to wall motion analysis (44). Contrast defects were seen in 21% of regions with normal wall motion at peak stress. These findings are strikingly similar to comparative nuclear perfusion studies, where Elhendy et al. found that 26% of perfusion abnormalities identified with Tc-99m sestamibi SPECT and supplied by angiographically significant stenosis were in regions with normal wall motion responses during dobutamine stress. Accelerated intermittent imaging as a method of assessing perfusion and function simultaneously can depict the same finding (Fig. 7). Further studies will be needed to better define sensitivity and specificity of this new methodology in diagnosis of CAD, as well as its role in patient outcome.

Acute Myocardial Infarction

As stated previously, animal studies have indicated that MCE tends to underestimate infarct size early after reperfu-

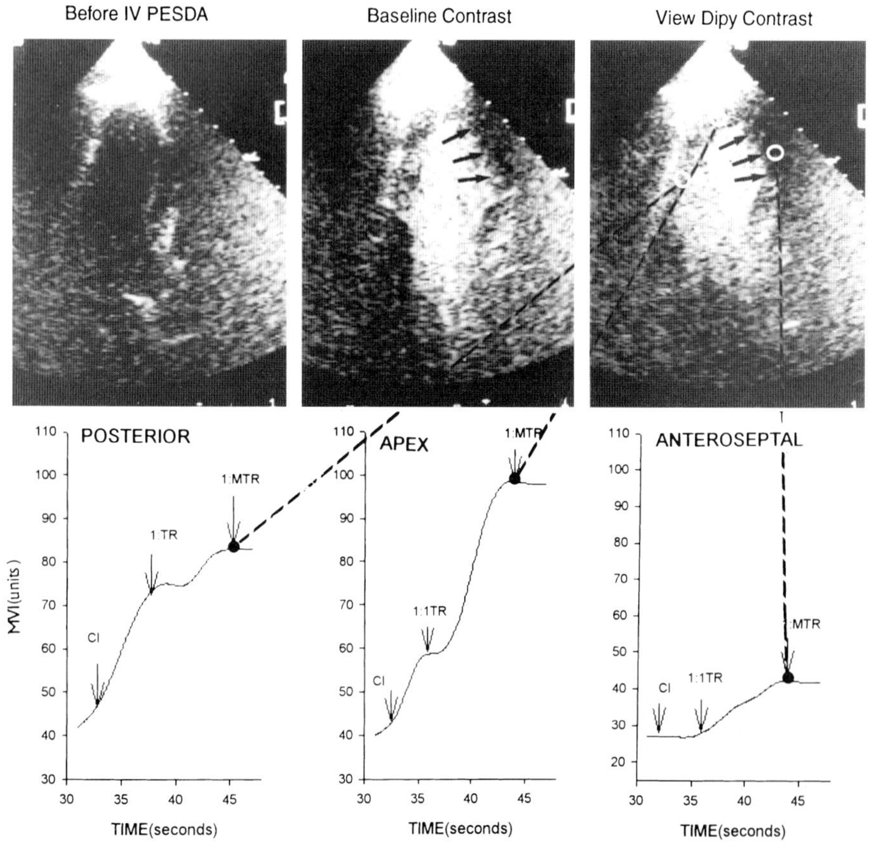

FIG. 6. Apical long-axis view in a patient who had both visual and quantitative evidence of an anteroseptal contrast defect (*arrows*) at rest and during dipyridamol (*Dipy*) stress when an extended time interval between frame rates was used. Note the abnormal enhancement in myocardial video intensity (*MVI*) in the anteroseptal region when switching triggering ultrasound frame rates from one point every cardiac cycle (1:1TR) to one point every multiple cardiac cycles (1:MTR) with that in the apical and posterior regions. This patient also had an anteroseptal defect during dipyridamol stress with Tc-99m sestamibi. (From ref. 18, with permission.)

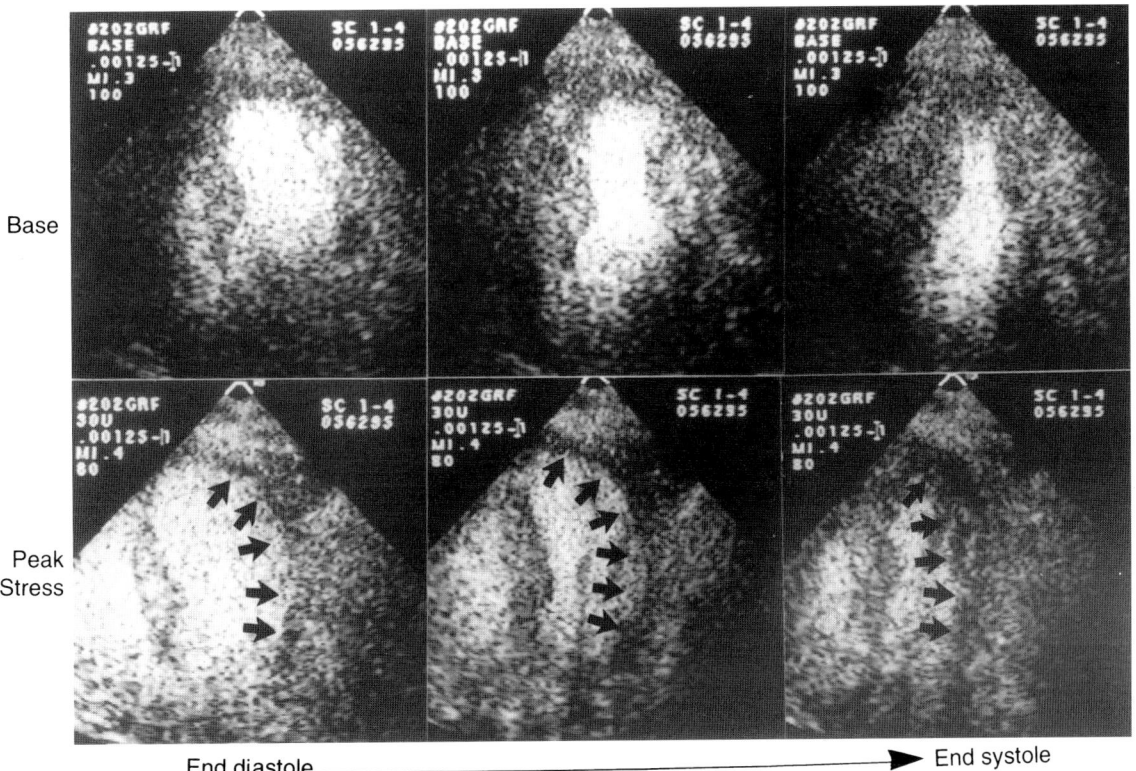

Base

Peak
Stress

End diastole ⟶ End systole

FIG. 7. This example of accelerated intermittent imaging during dobutamine stress shows normal wall motion at peak stress with a lateral perfusion defect. This patient had a 70% lesion in the circumflex by quantitative angiography.

sion. Since it is the microcirculatory reserve that is impaired, a coronary vasodilator is necessary to unmask the actual topography in the early infarct period (45). At longer time intervals following reperfusion (24 hours), the resting contrast defect size does correlate closely with infarct size. Recently, intravenous ultrasound contrast agents have been able to identify the same no reflow zones that have previously been described only with intracoronary ultrasound contrast (30) (Fig. 8).

Future Utilization of Intravenous Microbubbles

Evaluation of Acute Chest Pain

With the advent of accelerated intermittent harmonic imaging, MCE has become a rapid noninvasive method that can be used at the bedside, in the emergency room, or in the coronary care unit. Its role as a gatekeeper in the setting of chest pain at the emergency department is yet to be clarified. The detection of perfusion abnormalities with radionuclide imaging in patients with chest pain and nondiagnostic ECGs in the emergency department has been shown to not only identify high-risk patients, but a negative study has been useful in detecting patients who do not require admission. The future for MCE in this setting, therefore, is very bright.

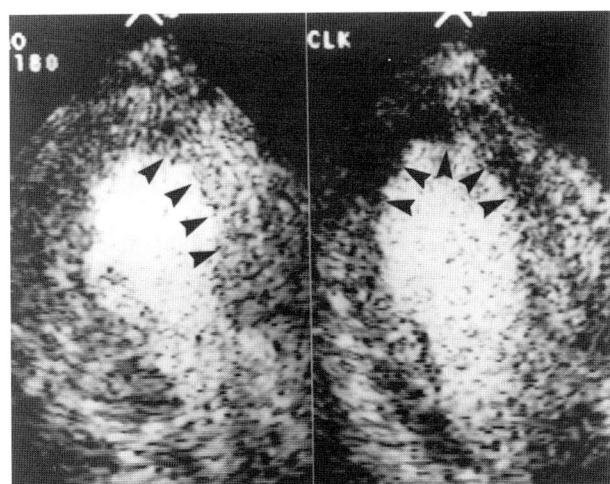

FIG. 8. Examples from two different patients who had anteroseptal myocardial infarctions and similar wall motion score indexes following restoration of epicardial flow in the left anterior descending artery. **Right:** The patient had a persistent perfusion defect (no reflow; *arrows*) following intravenous PESDA. **Left:** The patient demonstrated reflow in the same regions (reflow; *arrows*). (From ref. 30, with permission.)

Enhanced Intraarterial and Intracoronary Thrombus Imaging

A tissue-targeted ultrasound contrast agent can be designed to specifically enhance the acoustic reflectivity of a certain tissue and better differentiate it from surrounding structures. Lanza et al. (46) demonstrated the usefulness of an antifibrin-targeted biotinylated contrast agent for detecting thrombus *in vitro* and *in vivo*. Takeuchi et al. (47,48) demonstrated that MRX 408 microbubbles increase the acoustic reflectivity of acute experimentally induced intravascular and intracardiac thrombus, improving its delineation. The reason for its efficiency in binding fresh thrombus comes from a ligand that binds to GPIIb-IIIa receptor of activated platelets.

Therapeutic Uses of Perfluorocarbon Microbubbles

PESDA microbubbles have been shown to have the capability of disrupting thrombus *in vitro* in similar quantities to that achieved with urokinase (49). The size of the residual particles appear to be larger than that seen with fibrinolysis, but not of sufficient size to cause significant macroscopic distal embolization (50). Based on these *in vitro* observations, it has been demonstrated that ultrasound plus intravenous PESDA are capable of producing iliac artery recanalization following acute arterial thrombosis in rabbits (50). This exciting approach might turn into an alternative to thrombolytic therapy and a pioneering improvement in the treatment of acute coronary artery occlusion. Ultrasound induced recanalization with microbubbles does not appear to activate the fibrinolytic system and, therefore, may be safer than thrombolytics.

Intimal proliferation of smooth muscle cells is one of the mechanisms of restenosis. Intraarterial delivery of antisense to the c-myc protooncogene has been shown to inhibit neointimal hyperplasia following balloon injury. PESDA microbubbles bind large quantities of this synthetic antisense oligodeoxynucleotide (ODN) and deposit them within the vascular wall in the presence of ultrasound (51). Recently, intravenous ODN-PESDA and transcutaneous low frequency ultrasound have been shown to inhibit carotid stenosis formation in a manner similar to direct application of antisense to the vessel wall after balloon injury (52). This would be a powerful, noninvasive method to inhibit restenosis and in-stent restenosis.

In the field of endothelial function, this may imply in noninvasive assessment of endothelial integrity and preclinical coronary atherosclerotic disease.

Image Processing and Analysis

It is yet to be defined what would be the correct way to process and analyze data. It has become increasingly evident that processing is important to acquire accurate and reproducible data on myocardial perfusion with intravenous ultrasound contrast.

During the cardiac cycle the heart contracts, relaxes, rotates, translates, as well as changes its myocardial thickness and its cavity size. Therefore correct alignment of images to compare before and after contrast, as well as to compare rest with stress images would be an important goal. This can be achieved automatically by a computer algorithm or manually by identification of borders and landmarks rather than pixel intensity. A different strategy that has been useful is the flash echo technique, which means imaging first in real time in order to destroy bubbles and then holding ultrasound for a certain pulsing interval allowing the beam width to be replenished with microbubbles. This gives us a much better aligned picture that can be used as a background "precontrast" baseline image.

Another tool to increase accuracy of the data is averaging several contrast-enhanced images at peak intensity. This consists of adding gray-scale values for the same pixels in each of the selected images and then dividing by the number of images averaged. The next step is to subtract the precontrast frame from the contrast-enhanced one, a process known as background subtraction. Areas of interest are then placed between endocardium and epicardium, and videointensity in this region can be measured. Videointensity data can also be rescaled to a dynamic range of 256 gray levels, where all regions will be assigned proportional levels to what was considered the "hottest pixel." Normalization can also be done using color code, which enables the human eyes to perceive several hues of colors, assisting in better detection of perfusion abnormalities.

Regional heterogeneity of myocardial videointensity at baseline and in the increment in videointensity with a constant infusion of microbubbles has recently been described. These regional variations have led to a compensated digital subtraction technique that corrects for the heterogeneity in contrast enhancement due to differences in baseline pixel intensity and regional variations in contrast enhancement. In conjunction with Dr. Caio Medeiros in Brazil, we are formulating a normal database, which will determine what normal regional contrast enhancement is for a wide range of ages and body habitus. These methodologies have the potential to improve the accuracy of detecting myocardial perfusion defects.

CONCLUSION

Over the past three years, tremendous advances in both ultrasound contrast agents and in ultrasound imaging techniques have led to the application of intravenous ultrasound contrast agents to study myocardial perfusion. In the near future, ultrasound may become the most widely used technique to study myocardial perfusion because of its accuracy, cost-effectiveness, and ease of use in a clinical setting.

REFERENCES

1. Gramiak R, Shah PM. Echocardiography of the aortic root. *Invest Radiol* 1968;3:356–366.
2. DeMaria AN, Bommer WJ, Rigg SK, et al. Echocardiographic visualization of myocardial perfusion by left heart and intracoronary injection of echo contrast agents. *Circulation* 1980;60[Suppl III]:III-143(abst).
3. Armstrong WF, West SR, Mueller TM, et al. Assessment of myocardial perfusion abnormalities with contrast-enhanced two-dimensional echocardiography. *Circulation* 1982;66:166–173.
4. Tei C, Sakamaki T, Shah PM, et al. Myocardial contrast echocardiography. A reproducible technique of myocardial opacification for identifying regional perfusion deficits. *Circulation* 1983;67:585–593.
5. Kemper AJ, O'Boyle JE, Sharma S, et al. Hydrogen peroxide contrast enhanced two-dimensional echocardiography: real-time *in-vivo* delineation of regional myocardial perfusion. *Circulation* 1983;68:603–611.
6. Feinstein SB, TenCate F, Zwehl W, et al. Two-dimensional contrast echocardiography, I: *in vitro* development and quantitative analysis of echo contrast agents. *J Am Coll Cardiol* 1984;3:14–20.
7. Tei C, Kondo S, Meerbaum S, et al. Correlation of myocardial echo contrast disappearance rate ("washout") and severity of experimental coronary stenosis. *J Am Coll Cardiol* 1984;3:39–40.
8. Meltzer RS, Tickner EG, Popp RL. Why do the lungs clear ultrasonic contrast? *Ultrasound Med Biol* 1980;263–269.
9. Feinstein SB, Cheirif J, TenCate FJ, et al. Safety and efficacy of a new transpulmonary ultrasound contrast agent: initial multicenter clinical results. *J Am Coll Cardiol* 1990;16:316–324.
10. TenCate FJ, Widimsky P, Cornel JH, et al. Intracoronary Albunex: its effects on left ventricular hemodynamics, function, and coronary sinus flow in humans. *Circulation* 1993;88:2123–2127.
11. Porter TR, Xie F, Kilzer K. Intravenous perfluoropropane-exposed sonicated dextrose albumin produces myocardial ultrasound contrast that correlates with coronary blood flow. *J Am Soc Echocardiogr* 1995;8:710–718.
12. Skyba DM, Camarano G, Goodman NC, et al. Hemodynamic characteristics, myocardial kinetics, and microvascular rheology of FS-069, a second-generation echocardiographic contrast agent capable of producing myocardial opacification from a venous injection. *J Am Coll Cardiol* 1996;28:1292–1300.
13. Burns PN, Powers JE, Simpson DH, et al. Harmonic imaging: principles and preliminary results. *Clin Radiol* 1996;51(Suppl I):50–55.
14. Porter TR. Harmonic ultrasound imaging during routine and contrast-enhanced echocardiography. *Cardiac Ultrasound Today* 1998;4:121–136.
15. Mulvaugh SL, Foley DA, Aeschbacher BC, et al. Second harmonic imaging of an intravenously administered echocardiographic contrast agent: visualization of coronary arteries and measurement of coronary blood flow reserve. *J Am Coll Cardiol* 1996;27:1519–1525.
16. Porter TR, Xie F. Transient myocardial contrast following initial exposure to diagnostic ultrasound pressures with minute doses of intravenously injected microbubbles: demonstration and potential mechanisms. *Circulation* 1995;92:2391–2395.
17. Porter TR, Xie F, Kricsfeld D, Armbruster RW. Improved myocardial contrast with second harmonic transient ultrasound contrast response imaging in humans using intravenous perfluorocarbon-exposed sonicated dextrose albumin. *J Am Coll Cardiol* 1996;27:1497–1501.
18. Porter TR, Li S, Kricsfeld D, Armbruster RW. Detection of myocardial perfusion in multiple echocardiographic windows with one intravenous injection of microbubbles using transient response second harmonic imaging. *J Am Coll Cardiol* 1997;29:791–799.
19. Firschke C, Camarano G, Lindner JR, Wei K, Goodman NC, Kaul S. Myocardial perfusion imaging in the setting of coronary artery stenosis and acute myocardial infarction using venous injection of FS-069, a second-generation echocardiographic contrast agent. *Circulation* 1997;96:959–967.
20. Porter T, Li S, Hiser W, et al. Simultaneous assessment of wall motion and myocardial perfusion using a rapid acquisition Intermittent harmonic imaging pulsing interval of 5–15 hertz following acute myocardial infarction and during stress echocardiography. *J Am Coll Cardiol* 1998;30:123A.
21. Porter T, Li S, Oster R, Deligonul U. Comparison of accelerated intermittent imaging with standard triggering to detect perfusion and wall motion during stress echocardiography in humans. *J Am Soc Echocardiogr* 1998;11:498.
22. Porter TR, Xie F, Li S, et al. Increased ultrasound contrast and decreased microbubble destruction rates with triggered ultrasound imaging. *J Am Soc Echocardiogr* 1996;9:599–605.
23. Nakatani S, Imanishi T, Terasawa A, et al. Clinical application of transpulmonary contrast-enhanced Doppler technique in the assessment of severity of aortic stenosis. *J Am Coll Cardiol* 1992;20 (4):973–978.
24. Byrd BF, O'Kelly BF, Schiller NB. Contrast echocardiography enhances tricuspid but not mitral regurgitation. *Clin Cardiol* 1991;11 [Suppl 5]:10–14.
25. Okura H, Yoshida K, Akasaka T, et al. Improved transvalvular continuous-wave Doppler signal intensity after intravenous albunex injection in patients with prosthetic aortic valves. *J Am Soc Echocardiog* 1997;10:608–612.
26. Porter TR, Xie F, Kricsfeld A, et al. Improved endocardial border resolution during dobutamine stress echocardiography with intravenous sonicated dextrose albumin. *J Am Coll Cardiol* 1994;23:1440–1443.
27. Kloner RA, Ganote CE, Jennings RB. The "no-reflow" phenomenon after temporary coronary occlusion in the dog. *Clin Invest* 1974;54:1496–1508.
28. Ito H, Tomooka T, Sakai N, et al. Lack of myocardial perfusion immediately after successful thrombolysis: a predictor of poor recovery of left ventricular function in anterior myocardial infarction. *Circulation* 1992;85:1699–1705.
29. Kenner MD, Zajac EJ, Kondos JT, et al. Ability of the no reflow phenomenon during an acute myocardial infarction to predict left ventricular dysfunction at one-month follow-up. *Am J Cardiol* 1995;76:861–868.
30. Porter TR, Li S, Oster R, et al. The clinical implications of no-reflow demonstrated with intravenous perfluorocarbon containing microbubbles following restoration of TIMI 3 flow in patients with acute myocardial infarction. *Am J Cardiol* 1998;82:1173–1177.
31. Sabia PJ, Powers ER, Ragosta M, et al. An association between collateral blood flow and myocardial viability in patients with recent myocardial infarction. *N Engl J Med* 1992;372:1825–1831.
32. Sabia PJ, Powers ER, Jayaweera AR, et al. Functional significance of collateral blood flow in patients with recent acute myocardial infarction: a study using myocardial contrast echocardiography. *Circulation* 1992;85:2080–2089.
33. DeFilippi CR, Willett DL, Irani WN, et al. Comparison of myocardial contrast echocardiography and low-dose dobutamine stress echocardiography in predicting recovery of left ventricular function after coronary revascularization in chronic ischemic heart disease. *Circulation* 1995;92:2863–2868.
34. Nagueh SF, Vaduganathan P, Ali N, et al. Identification of hibernating myocardium: comparative accuracy of myocardial contrast echocardiography, rest-redistribution thallium-201 tomography and dobutamine echocardiography. *J Am Coll Cardiol* 1997;29:985–993.
35. Spotnitz WD, Keller MW, Watson DD, et al. Success of internal mammary artery bypass grafting can be assessed intraoperatively using myocardial contrast echocardiography. *J Am Coll Cardiol* 1988;12:196–201.
36. Villanueva FS, Kaul S, Glasheen WP, et al. Intraoperative assessment of the distribution of retrograde cardioplegia using myocardial contrast echocardiography. *Surg Forum* 1990;41:252–255.
37. Jayaweera AR, Edwards N, Glasheen WP, et al. *In-vivo* myocardial kinetics of air-filled albumin microbubbles during myocardial contrast echocardiography: comparison with radiolabeled red blood cells. *Circ Res* 1994;74:1157–1165.
38. Iskandrian AS, Verani MS. Instrumentation and technical considerations in planar and SPECT imaging. In: *Nuclear cardiac imaging: principles and applications*, 2nd ed. Philadelphia: FA Davis Co, 1996:29–45.
39. Beller GA. Instrumentation in nuclear cardiology. In: *Clinical nuclear cardiology*. Philadelphia: WB Saunders, 1995:1–36.
40. Hoffman EJ, Huang SC, Phelps ME. Quantitation in positron emission computed tomography I: effect of object size. *J Comput Assist Tomogr* 1979;3:299–308.
41. Wei K, Jayaweera AR, Firoozan S, et al. Quantification of myocardial blood flow with ultrasound-induced destruction of microbubbles administered as a constant venous infusion. *Circulation* 1998;97:473–483.
42. Cheirif J, Desir RM, Bolli R, et al. Relation of perfusion defects observed with myocardial contrast echocardiography to the severity of

coronary stenosis: correlation with thallium-201 single-photon emission tomography. *J Am Coll Cardiol* 1992;19:1343–1349.

43. Kaul S, Senior R, Dittrich H, et al. Detection of coronary artery disease using myocardial contrast echocardiography: comparison with Tc-99m-sestamibi single photon emission computed tomography. *Circulation* 1997;96:785–792.

44. Porter TR, Xie F, Kilzer K, et al. Detection of myocardial perfusion abnormalities during dobutamine and adenosine stress echocardiography with transient myocardial contrast imaging after minute quantities of intravenous perfluorocarbon-exposed sonicated dextrose albumin. *J Am Soc Echocardiogr* 1996;9:779–786.

45. Firschke C, Lindner JR, Goodman NC, et al. Myocardial contrast echocardiography in acute myocardial infarction using aortic root injections of microbubbles: potential application in the cardiac catheterization laboratory. *J Am Coll Cardiol* 1997;29:207–216.

46. Lanza GM, Wallace KD, Scott MJ, et al. A novel site-targeted ultrasonic contrast agent with broad biomedical application. *Circulation* 1996;94:3334–3340.

47. Takeuchi M, McCreery TP, Avelar E, et al. Enhanced visualization of intravascular thrombus with the use of a thrombus targeting ultrasound contrast agent (MRX408): Evidence from *in vivo* experimental echocardiographic studies. *J Am Coll Cardiol* 1998;31:57A.

48. Takeuchi M, McCreery TP, Ogunyankin K, et al. A new tissue targeted contrast agent, MRX408 improves visualization and delineation of left atrial appendage clot with conventional 2-dimensional echocardiography. *J Am Coll Cardiol* 1998;31:400A.

49. Porter TR, LeVeen RF, Fox R, et al. Thrombolytic enhancement with perfluorocarbon-exposed sonicated dextrose albumin microbubbles. *Am Heart J* 1996;132:964–968.

50. Birnbaum Y, Luo H, Nagai T, et al. Noninvasive *in vitro* clot dissolution without a thrombolytic drug: recanalization of thrombosed iliofemoral arteries by transcutaneous ultrasound combined with intravenous infusion of perfluorocarbon-exposed sonicated dextrose albumin microbubbles (PESDA). *Circulation* 1998;97:130–134.

51. Porter TR, Iversen PL, Li S, et al. Interaction of diagnostic ultrasound with synthetic oligonucleotide-labeled perfluorocarbon-exposed sonicated dextrose microbubbles. *J Ultrasound Med* 1996;15:577–584.

52. Hiser W, Deligonul U, Xie F, et al. The effects of transcutaneous low frequency ultrasound and an intravenous microbubble delivery system on inhibiting stenosis formation following carotid and coronary artery balloon injury. *Circulation* 1998;98:1-291.

CHAPTER 7

Intravascular Echocardiography

Shaul Atar and Robert J. Siegel

The ability to correctly diagnose and quantify coronary and vascular pathology has substantially improved since the introduction of intravascular ultrasound (IVUS). Although coronary angiography, introduced by Sones in 1958, is still the predominant imaging method for the diagnosis of coronary artery disease and for guiding coronary interventions, it is limited for accurate quantification of the severity of coronary pathology and the identification of intraluminal morphology.

Traditional methods for studying human coronary artery disease, such as angiography and histological evaluation of autopsy material, are problematic for evaluating atherosclerosis. Angiography evaluates only a two-dimensional projection of the three-dimensional geometry of the arterial lumen and does not provide information on the arterial wall, which is essential to evaluate the detailed mechanistic processes of plaque progression, regression, and arterial wall remodeling. Although histological analysis directly addresses the question of atherosclerotic plaque structure, it cannot be used in longitudinal studies in patients, as the necessary tissue specimens are only available at autopsy. Intravascular ultrasound (IVUS), one of the more recent innovations of medical imaging technology, provides substantial assistance in guiding drug or interventional therapy, as well as insight into the pathogenesis and progression or regression of coronary atherosclerosis.

Due to the recent developments in IVUS equipment and techniques, with miniaturization of the imaging catheters and real-time simultaneous acquisition of IVUS and angiographic images, IVUS has become an important daily tool for both the clinician and the researcher. IVUS permits a greater understanding and quantification of plaque size and morphology and its response to various coronary interventions, and it adds information regarding reference segments believed to be "normal" by angiography. In addition to valuable information regarding intraluminal structures, IVUS identifies the vessel wall morphology, lesion size—i.e., diameter and length, as well as reference vessel size prior to coronary interventions. Recently the prognostic implications of IVUS findings after coronary interventions have been studied and have been shown to aid the clinician in choosing an effective modality for each lesion, as well as being able to predict which lesions are more prone to restenose and should be further treated.

Future advances and technical improvements in image quality, catheter miniaturization, automatic lumen tracking, and three-dimensional lumen reconstruction will enhance the diagnostic accuracy as well as the utility of IVUS for improving clinical decision-making in the catheterization laboratory.

EQUIPMENT AND TECHNICAL ASPECTS

Three types of IVUS catheters are currently available:

1. A single ultrasound element rotating at a rate of 1800 rpm yielding 30 images per minute, with a fixed ultrasound-reflecting "mirror" angled at 45 degrees (Sonicath, Boston Scientific, Watertown, MA).
2. A rotating "mirror" (1500 to 3000 rpm) with a fixed ultrasound element (Ultracross, Boston Scientific, Sunnyvale, CA).
3. A solid-state catheter with multiple circular ultrasound piezoelectric elements—currently up to 64 (Endosonics, Rancho Cordova, CA).

The first two catheters are mechanical transducers, and the third is based on the solid-state technique. Both types of catheters generate a 360 degree-, cross-sectional image plane

S. Atar: Cardiology Division, Cedars-Sinai Medical Center, Los Angeles, California 90048.

R. J. Siegel: Department of Medicine, University of California–Los Angeles School of Medicine, Los Angeles, California 90095; Cardiac Noninvasive Laboratory, Department of Cardiology, Cedars-Sinai Medical Center, Los Angeles, California 90048.

perpendicular to the transducer. Since the catheter is placed in very near proximity to the vessel wall, high frequencies (20 to 50 MHz) can be used for imaging with a strongly expected axial resolution of 100 μm (1.0 mm) at 30 MHz. Current ultrasound catheters used for coronary imaging have distal-tip diameters of 0.92 to 1.7 mm (2.9 French to 5.1 French); therefore, only vessels with a diameter greater than 0.92 mm can be readily visualized. Most IVUS catheters are braided polyethylene and require a sheath for introduction. Guiding catheters may help facilitate the use of IVUS in the peripheral circulation at the expense of upsizing the sheath size. Penetration is very important in large vessels such as the aorta, where a coronary-type probe will not penetrate to the wall of the aorta. Probes with a frequency of 20 MHz will generally penetrate up to 2 cm from the catheter.

The solid-state catheters contain 64 transducer elements arranged radially near the catheter tip and transmit at a frequency of 25 MHz. The elements receive the backscattered ultrasound waves and transmit the signals to a computer system that reconstructs the image in a near real-time mode. These elements contain highly miniaturized integrated circuits responsible for the timing and integration of the configuration. The system employs a reconstruction algorithm known as the "synthetic aperture array." With this approach, radial scans are reconstructed using data derived from the multiple transducer elements, using fewer numbers of elements for pixels in the far-field. The image quality throughout the near and far fields as well as the focus are improved. The solid-state catheters are produced with both a rapid exchange monorail design and a coaxial over-the-wire design. Current catheter size is 3.2F (1.07 mm diameter), which can be introduced through a 7F (2.3 mm) guiding catheter. The advantages of the solid-state design include the absence of any moving parts and the ability to manipulate the ultrasound beam electronically, allowing the operator to manipulate the depth and focus of the images. The solid-state catheter is connected to a remote unit, which is connected to the system cart containing a monitor, a videotape recorder, and a digital storage system.

A disadvantage of the solid-state system is the "ring-down" artifact that encircles the catheter. In order to overcome the artifact, a mask needs to be created near the catheter and, later on, subtracted from the image. This is done by disengaging the guiding catheter from the coronary ostium and positioning the tip of the imaging catheter free in the aorta.

The most commonly used mechanical imaging catheters create the IVUS image by rotating a single piezoelectric transducer element attached to a flexible torque cable inside the tip of the catheter. The transducer usually transmits at a frequency of 20 to 40 MHz (mostly 30 MHz). Increasing imaging frequency will increase resolution, at the expense of increased attenuation and backscatter from red blood cells and reduced image penetration. The two basic designs of catheter delivery are either the short monorail system with a short lumen for the guidewire at the tip of the catheter, causing the guidewire to be seen adjacent to the catheter, or

the longer monorail system. The latter catheter has a longer "tunnel" (sheath-type) for the guidewire (approximately 30 cm), which provides better catheter tracking as a result of the longer guidewire engagement. The distal portion of the catheter has a common lumen that alternately houses the guidewire and the imaging transducer. Once the catheter is in place, the guidewire is retracted backwards, eliminating the appearance of the guidewire in the imaging field as well as allowing a lower catheter profile.

The short monorail systems are currently available with a distal dimension of 3.2F or 3.5F (1.07 and 1.17 mm diameter), while the longer monorail system (sheath-type) allows a profile of 2.9F (0.92 mm diameter), compatible with a 7F guide catheter. Soon these catheters will have a 2.6F (0.8 mm diameter) profile, that will allow them to be inserted through a 6F (2 mm diameter) guiding catheter.

The operation of the mechanical systems is the same as the solid-state. However, the mechanical system requires flushing prior to insertion in order to eliminate any air microbubbles in the path of the ultrasound beam that can significantly reduce image quality. Certain mechanical catheter systems are deployed within a sheath. This allows retracting and advancing the imaging transducer within a sheath without traumatizing the vessel. This kind of system permits effective use of an automatic pullback device, which maintains the pullback velocity at a constant speed (usually 0.5 mm/ses). The automatic pullback device is a useful tool for measuring lesion length and thus helps in the selection of the appropriate device for intervention and the correct length of stent to be deployed. It may also help in correctly aligning cross-sectional images for repeat future studies, as well as providing a method for three-dimensional reconstruction of vessels in the future.

IMAGE INTERPRETATION

Morphology of Plaques and Vessel Wall

Arterial Wall

As demonstrated in Figure 1, the inner arterial layer as seen by the IVUS image is relatively bright compared to the blood speckle surrounding the catheter and represents the intima and internal elastic lamina (IEL). The IEL has a normal thickness of up to 200 μm. Muscular arteries—e.g., coronary and peripheral arteries—have a medial layer by IVUS. However, elastic arteries like the carotid arteries do not have a medial layer. The outer layer as seen by IVUS is echogenic and represents the external elastic lamina (EEL), the adventitia and periadventitial tissue. Distinct separation between the intimal and medial layers may sometimes be absent, due to a higher collagen content of the media relative to the intima or due to a small medial thickness in atherosclerotic coronary arteries.

Atherosclerotic Plaques

Atherosclerotic plaques can be categorized by IVUS into three groups: calcific, fibrous, and fatty. Calcific plaque is

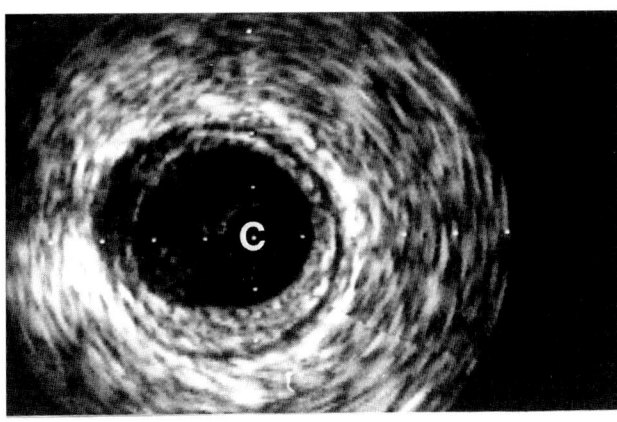

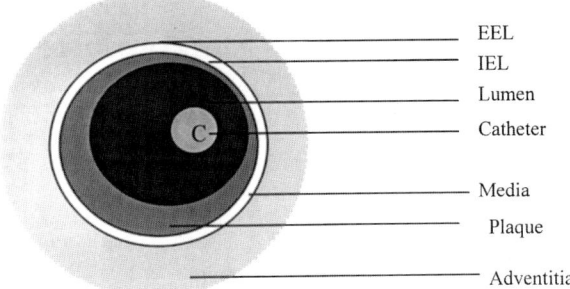

FIG. 1. **Top:** IVUS image of a human coronary artery with mild atherosclerosis. **Bottom:** The external elastic lamina (*EEL*), internal elastic lamina (*IEL*), lumen, ultrasound catheter (*C*), media, plaque, and adventita are identified. (From ref. 9, with permission.)

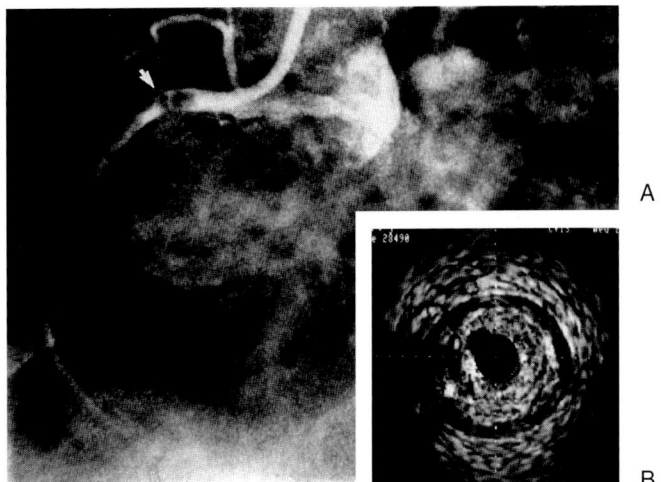

FIG. 2. **A:** Right coronary artery angiogram (left anterior oblique projection) after one pass of excimer laser and adjunctive balloon dilatation. There is a prominent residual filling defect in the right coronary artery (*arrow*). **B:** Intravascular ultrasound imaging showing the catheter surrounded by specular echoes that fill the lumen of the vessel; the dark black circle in the center of the cross-sectional image is the catheter. The grid marks are at 0.5 mm intervals. (From ref. 1, with permission.)

the simplest to identify. It is characterized by a bright reflection with intense attenuation and shadowing beyond. The calcium deposits may be deep, superficial, or intermixed within a fibrous plaque. Calcification may also cause concentric ''ghost arcs'' or reverberations beyond it, which are multiplications of the echo signal. Coronary calcification is recognized twice as often by IVUS compared to fluoroscopy or angiography. The presence or absence of calcium deposits has been used to divide plaques into ''soft'' and ''hard'' plaques (however, this classification has no histopathologic validation).

Fibrous plaques are less bright than calcium, but have higher echogenicity than muscle or fat tissue due to their higher content of collagen and elastin. Fatty, lipid-rich plaques are relatively echolucent compared to the vessel wall and calcified or fibrotic plaques. Lipid-rich plaques are hypoechoic and do not induce acoustic shadowing since the ultrasound signal can travel through this tissue without encountering a high impedance mismatch. The adventitia and perivascular structures can more easily be seen than when calcified or fibrous plaques are present. Echolucent areas that can be demonstrated within the plaque often represent lipid accumulations, but must be differentiated from intramural hematoma and/or a dissection site.

False Lumen

False lumens can either occur spontaneously or mostly due to dissections in postintracoronary interventions. IVUS can help locate the site of entry and exit of dissections, thus preventing further manipulations within the false arterial lumen that may lead to catastrophic results (Fig. 2A). The recognition of a false lumen can be facilitated by a careful inspection of the artery for the three-layer morphology; by looking for a slower blood flow in the false lumen; and by identification of side-branches emerging from the true lumen. The injection of agitated saline or angiographic contrast agent can be helpful in these cases.

Aneurysm

IVUS may also help discriminate between coronary true and false aneurysms. In true aneurysms the media encompasses the perimeter of the aneurysm, although it is thinned. In false aneurysms on the other hand, the damaged media cannot be appreciated, and the vessel is contained by the adventitia and perivascular structures only. In cases where the discrimination of blood and vessel wall is difficult, a contrast or saline intracoronary injection may be helpful.

Intraluminal Structures

Slowly flowing blood can be recognized due to a characteristically speckled pattern within the arterial lumen. Its backscatter increases in systole, when blood flow is slower, and decreases in diastole. In segments with severe stenosis the backscatter from the red blood cells increases dramatically because of rouleaux formation, making it resemble a fresh thrombus. A flush of contrast or normal saline from the guiding catheter can help distinguish between the two.

Thrombus

Thrombus may be hard to identify by IVUS. It often looks like a granular mass (1) on real-time imaging, as shown in Figure 2. Other helpful characteristics may be the presence of microchannels within the thrombus, small amplitude vibrations or mobility with the cardiac cycle of the intraluminal mass, and an echodensitiy that is approximately half that of the adventitia. The appearance of thrombus in stented segments, mainly immediately postprocedure, is often easier to detect due to clearer delineation of the border between the stent struts and the lumen. Nevertheless, the discrimination of a thrombus from fatty (soft) plaques (which are within the arterial wall versus the intraluminal thrombus) or low-flowing stagnant blood proximal to a high-grade stenosis is often difficult.

Quantitative Measurements

IVUS image measurements have been validated in histologic studies, and were found to strongly correlate in vessel and lumen cross-sectional area, and mean percent narrowing, respectively (r = 0.94, 0.85, 0.84). IVUS has also been proved to be more accurate than quantitative coronary angiography (QCA) for quantification of lumen and vessel dimension, as well as for a better appreciation of plaque area and volume before and after various coronary interventions. The principal method of measurement is manual planimetry, and is usually accurate according to reproducibility studies. As demonstrated in Figure 1, the parameters frequently measured with IVUS are the following:

- Minimal and maximal luminal diameters.
- Lumen eccentricity ratio, which is equal to (maximal lumen diameter − minimal lumen diameter) × 100 / maximal lumen diameter. A value smaller than 1 indicates an increased lumen eccentricity.
- Lumen area, which is equal to the area delineated manually by the blood-intimal border.
- Vessel area, which is equal to the area circumscribed by the external elastic lamina (EEL).
- Internal elastic lamina (IEL) area.
- Intimal area, which is equal to IEL area minus the lumen area.
- Medial area, which is equal to EEL area minus IEL area. (Since in many cases it is extremely difficult to discriminate plaque border from medial border, due to medial thinning, plaque area and medial area are referred to as a single entity in atherosclerotic vessels.)
- Plaque area stenosis, which is equal to: (EEL − lumen area) × 100 / EEL.

- Plaque eccentricity ratio, which is equal to (maximal plaque thickness − minimal plaque thickness) × 100 / maximal plaque thickness.

As in QCA, lesion sites are compared to reference sites. These are located either proximally or distally within 10 mm from the lesion and are the most normal-appearing segments and should ideally have no major side branches.

Histopathologic Correlation

The correlation of IVUS interpretation and measurements has been studied both qualitatively and quantitatively in artificial vascular models and in histopathologic specimens *in vitro*, as well as by *in vivo* correlation with angioscopy. These studies have provided an insight to the pathophysiology of acute coronary syndromes (2). The three-layered appearance of the human muscular artery is normally present only in late adulthood, as was demonstrated by Fitzgerald and colleagues (3). In that study hearts of previously healthy patients ranging in age from 13 to 55 were autopsied and correlated with IVUS findings. A three-layered appearance of the arterial wall was detected in cases when the intimal thickness was greater than 178 μm. The average age of the group with nonlayered appearance was 27 years, whereas the average age of the patients with three-layered appearance was 42 years. Medial thickness was not different between the groups.

Siegel and colleagues (4) correlated the morphology of muscular arteries in normal human adults with IVUS findings. They examined grossly normal femoropopliteal arteries obtained at autopsy and removed the intima, the internal elastic lamina, the media, and the external elastic lamina in several steps, using microsurgical techniques. The removal of the intima and/or internal elastic lamina resulted in the creation of an acoustic interface by the media (which is normally echolucent). Removal of the external elastic lamina and/or adventitia resulted in an outer acoustic interface, while the removal of the media did not alter the three-layered appearance of the vessel. Since the media is echolucent, it is often difficult to measure its thickness in an atheromatous vessel. Therefore it has been suggested that the intimal and medial thickness would be measured as the sum of the inner echogenic and echolucent layers.

IVUS is more sensitive for the detection of intraarterial calcium than fluoroscopy. The accuracy of IVUS in detecting calcium depositions in the coronary vessel wall as demonstrated by IVUS has been correlated with histopathologic specimens. IVUS correctly detected 89% of the dense and deep calcium deposits (sensitivity and specificity of 90% and 100%, respectively), but only 17% of the microcalcifications.

Coronary atherosclerosis often results in disruption of the normal vascular morphology resulting from deposition of lipid, calcium, and collagen in the vascular wall layers. Porter and colleagues (5) evaluating atheromatous vessels by IVUS showed that the echogenic reflectivity increases with greater histologic levels of calcium and collagen and lesser amounts of lipid. The correlation of medial thickness was higher with higher contents of intimal and medial collagen ($r = 0.89$). In a study done by Di Mario and colleagues (6), histologically proved fibrous intimal thickening was detected by IVUS in 67% of specimens, while calcium deposits were correctly detected in 97%. IVUS has been shown to be accurate in distinguishing between lipid-rich, fibrous, and calcified lesions. In a study by Potkin et al. (7) IVUS correctly identified 91% of fibrous plaques, 78% of lipid deposits, and 100% of calcified plaques.

In saphenous vein bypass grafts, IVUS studies have demonstrated an increase in wall thickness in vein grafts after long-term implantation, which correctly correlated histologically with vein wall fibrosis.

The detection of dissections, intimal flaps and intraluminal thrombi by IVUS was studied *in vitro* and *in vivo* compared to angioscopy. In a study by Weintraub et al., IVUS had a sensitivity and specificity of 92% for the detection of thrombi, while Siegel et al. (8) found IVUS to have only 57% sensitivity. The detection and estimation of length of dissections was found to be 80% accurate compared to histopathologic findings in two studies.

Quantitative IVUS measurements have also been shown to correspond well with histologic specimens. The quantitative analysis by Di Mario (6) and colleagues revealed a significantly smaller vessel area as measured by IVUS, probably due to vessel shrinkage during preparations, while lumen area as well as plaque area and medial thickness correlated well with histology ($r = 0.96, 0.87, 0.93$, respectively). In other studies, the correlation coefficients were similar and ranged from 0.76 to 0.98 for lumen diameter and area, wall thickness cross-sectional area stenosis, and plaque area.

CURRENT IVUS LIMITATIONS AND ARTIFACTS

Catheter size is a limitation of all the available IVUS systems. It is currently impossible to image vessels smaller than 1 mm in diameter without causing vessel and lesion distortion. Reducing catheter size has been limited by decreasing lateral resolution, but may be overcome in part by imaging at higher frequencies, e.g., 40 and 50 MHz.

Qualitative and quantitative IVUS imaging has several limitations, which depend in part on the type of imaging system. The mechanical systems are superior in penetration and resolution with respect to image quality compared to the solid-state systems. One common artifact to both systems is the "ring-down" artifact, seen as a bright halo surrounding the catheter. It is caused by the oscillation of the transducer, and it makes the area immediately adjacent to the catheter unavailable for imaging. As a consequence, the catheter may appear larger than its actual size.

Another artifact that occurs with the mechanical systems

is nonuniform rotational distortion (NURD), caused by exposing the catheter to frictional forces, often due to multiple bends and/or tight stenosis as well as tortuous vessels, leading to nonuniform rotation and distortion of the ultrasound catheter and image. NURD can sometimes be solved by catheter manipulation. NURD is not present in the solid-state systems.

Quantitative measurements may be affected by several factors: (i) Catheter position within the lumen is often off center, causing structures near the catheter to appear brighter than structures in the far field, mainly in large vessels (aorta and peripheral arteries) or ostial segments. (ii) Catheter angulation may alter vessel geometry, making it more elliptical and eccentric. (iii) The "ghost" phenomenon, caused by high-intensity reflections from structures such as a metal stents' struts or calcium, and result in a mirror-image of the lesser intense reflections. These occur on the vessel wall on the opposite side of the catheter.

CLINICAL UTILITY AND APPLICATIONS

Comparative Value

The three methods used for coronary imaging—angiography, IVUS, and angioscopy are compared in Table 1 for their potential use and limitations. They all provide valuable complementary information regarding the vessel wall and intraluminal structures. Yet their simultaneous use in every patient would be unnecessary and not cost-effective. They have different capabilities for selecting the appropriate intervention (Table 2) and for identifying complications of different interventions (Table 3). Therefore wise usage of each of the methods can assist the cardiologist in selecting the appropriate treatment and monitoring the results and complications of treatment. Doppler flow wire as well as the pressure wire are not imaging modalities and are currently the only transcatheter methods providing physiologic information on vascular blood flow.

Angiography

During the last four decades, angiography has been the "gold standard" and the principal method used by clinicians and investigators to determine the anatomic severity of vascular disease. Yet, angiography has several limitations that make the interpretation of the angiographic images strongly subject to both interobserver and intraobserver variability; to magnification errors; to an inability to detect or accurately estimate disease at the reference sites; and to the limited number of the angiographic projections (Table 4). Moreover, several studies have shown a large discrepancy between lesion severity by angiography and postmortem examinations or physiologic measurements of coronary flow impairment.

Since the angiographic images are made of a longitudinal cross section of a contrast-filled lumen, they do not provide

TABLE 1. *Coronary imaging—potential and limitations of different imaging techniques*

	Angiography	Angioscopy	IVUS
Lumen Quantification:	+ +	—	+ + +
Intraluminal flaps/dissection	+	+ + +	+ +
Thrombus			
Red	+	+ + +	—
White	—	+ +	—
Endoluminal Lining			
Smooth/complex	+	+ +	+
Color	—	+ + +	—
Plaque Composition			
Calcific	+	—	+ + +
Fibrous (dense)	—	—	+
Lipid	—	yellow	+ ?
Plaque Quantification			
Lumen encroachment	+ +	—	+ + +
Intraluminal	—	—	+ + +
Total Vessel Area: Quantification	—	—	+ + +
Plaque Topography			
Eccentric/concentric	+	+	+ + +
Feasibility	+ + +	+	+ +
Safety	+ +	+	+
Applicability			
Segments	Entire coronary tree	Mid-straight	Pro-mid
Structure	Lumen	Lumen/lining	Lumen/wall
Severe lesions	+ + +	—	—
Coronary Flow	+	–	–
Collaterals	+ +	—	—
Ischemia during Imaging	—	+ +	+ (wedge imaging)
Functional Field	Contrast-filled	Flush-filled	Blood-filled
Vasomotion	+	—	+
Cost	Low	High	High

(Adapted from ref. 20, with permission.)

detailed information on the intraluminal structures or the true cross-sectional vessel dimensions. This limitation mostly affects the interpretation of postintervention results. The disruption of the atherosclerotic plaque allows the contrast media to enter into the fractures beneath the plaque. This "hazy" appearance may be misinterpreted as an enlarged lumen. The assessment of intracoronary stent-to-wall apposition and expansion may also be misinterpreted due to

the inability of angiography to provide intraluminal information.

IVUS is the only diagnostic method that is able to overcome the limitations of angiography; it achieves this due to its ability to provide cross-sectional tomographic images of the vessel lumen and intraluminal structures and to provide

TABLE 2. *Comparison of imaging methods for mechanisms of coronary interventions*

	Angiography	IVUS	Angioscopy
Plaque Removal	—	+ +	+
Vessel Wall Stretching	—	+ +	—
Dissection			
Intraluminal	+	+	+ + +
Intramural	+	+ + +	+
Normal Vessel Wall Involvement	—	+ + +	+
Plaque Distribution	—	+ + +	—
Plaque Compression	—	+ +	—
Lumen Enlargement	+ + +	+ + +	+

(Adapted from ref. 20, with permission.)

TABLE 3. *Postintervention findings: relative merits of the different imaging techniques*

	Angiography	Angioscopy	IVUS
Intraluminal			
Smooth/hazy	+	—	—
Thrombus	+	+ + +	+
Flaps/dissection	+	+ + +	+
Stent	+	+ +	+ + +
Endoluminal Lining			
Disruption	+	+ +	+
Discoloration	—	+	—
Bleeding	—	+	—
Lesion Wall			
Dissection	+	+	+ + +
Lumen Enlargement	+ + +	+	+ + +
"Run-off"	+ + +	—	—

(Adapted from ref. 20, with permission.)

TABLE 4. *Factors contributing to coronary arteriographic lesion*

Technical	Biologic
Intra- and Interobserver Variability (u,o)	Vasospasm (o)
Inadequate Filling of Artery with Contrast (u,o)	Diffuse Atherosclerotic Narrowing (u)
Inadequate Angiographic Projections (u)	Concentric Short Stenosis (u)
Foreshortening of Artery (u)	Crescentic, Slit-like, and Star-shaped Lumens (u)
Overlap or Superimposition of Arterial Branches (u,o)	Poststenotic Dilatation (o)
	Recanalized Segments with
	Multiple Channels (u)
	Distal Obstruction (u)
	Arterial Remodeling (Glagov phenomenon) (u)

u, underestimation; o, overestimation.
(Adapted from ref. 2, with permission.)

information on the vessel wall. IVUS enables the operator to measure the maximal and minimal lumen diameters, quantify plaque burden, consistency, and eccentricity, and quantify ''reference site'' disease and the presence of vascular remodeling (a phenomenon that cannot be detected by angiography).

The severity and extent of coronary stenoses are usually calculated to be greater by IVUS than by angiography. This is a consequence of the inability of angiography to detect the ''normal'' reference site that is diseased and has undergone vascular remodeling. The correlation of IVUS and angiography is somewhat better in vessels with concentric plaques than in those with a high eccentricity index. Nevertheless, most atherosclerotic plaques are eccentric by IVUS, with an eccentricity index greater than 2 to 1. Plaque calcification has major implications for choosing the right device for intervention. In a study by Tuzcu et al. (9) angiography was able to detect plaque calcification in only 45% of patients in whom calcification was detected by IVUS and only 63% of calcifications greater than 180 degrees were detected by angiography.

Angioscopy

Angioscopy provides the operator with real-time visualization of intraluminal structures and the endoluminal surface by using optic fibers. This method has been in use since the early 1980s, and was used mostly in research of acute coronary syndromes. Unlike IVUS, its greatest potential is the ability to detect flaps, dissections, and intraluminal thrombi and differentiate red from white thrombi, thus allowing the cardiologist to select treatment with thrombolytic agents or with an antithrombotic agent. The procedure is expensive and technically more difficult, as well as more time-consuming, than IVUS. In order to get a clear image of the vessel, it is necessary to occlude any forward blood flow with an inflated balloon that potentially increases the risk of procedural complications in patients with acute coronary syndromes. Thus, the use of angioscopy in the routine daily work of a catheterization laboratory has been limited.

Doppler Flow Wire

The Doppler flow wire provides functional and physiologic information regarding blood flow and blood flow reserves in coronary arteries. The intracoronary flow velocity is measured with a Doppler ultrasound piezoelectric transducer integrated at the tip of an angioplasty guidewire connected to a real-time spectral analyzer. The primary indication for its use is the evaluation of epicardial coronary artery blood flow in arteries with an intermediate grade angiographic stenosis. Doppler flow wire is also used for the assessment of coronary flow reserve (CFR) in the microvasculature (vessels smaller than 0.9 mm in diameter as well as collaterals), that cannot be assessed by IVUS or angiography.

The measurements are done at baseline (without the use of nitroglycerin before the procedure) and after stimulation with various agents such as adenosine, acetylcholine, nitroglycerin, etc. The flow is calculated at baseline and at peak, and the ratio of peak to baseline flow velocity is the CFR, with a normal value of 6 to 8. An impaired response at the site of an intermediate-grade stenosis compared to an angiographically normal vessel implies that the lesion is physiologically significant. Differentiation of endothelial-dependent from nonendothelial-dependent vasodilation can also be made using this system. Doppler flow wire is also being used for the evaluation and monitoring of different coronary interventions.

Since the Doppler flow wire does not provide any information on the anatomy and morphology of the coronary stenosis as provided by IVUS, these two methods can be used in a complementary manner to precisely determine the anatomy and physiologic significance of coronary lesions.

INDICATIONS FOR IVUS IMAGING

The indications for IVUS imaging may vary in different institutions, and are based on the number of coronary interventions performed in the catheterization laboratory, the devices and technology available in the institution, and the skills and degree of confidence of the interventional cardiol-

TABLE 5. *Information currently obtained from IVUS imaging*

Diagnostic Evaluation
Lesion Characteristics—Quantitative Information
Vessel and lumen area and diameter
Plaque circumference and burden
Percent stenosis
Lesion Characteristics—Qualitative Information
Location of branch/vessels bifurcations
Plaque calcification and lipid content
Tissue characterization
Plaque vs. thrombus
Vessel wall analysis
Perivascular tissue analysis
Evaluation of angiographic findings
Therapeutic Evaluation
Transluminal angioplasty—peripheral and coronary
Stent implantation
Rotational and directional atherectomy
Vascular remodeling and restenosis
Evaluation of fibrinolysis
Confirming Aortic Dissection, Pseudoaneurysm,
Coarctation

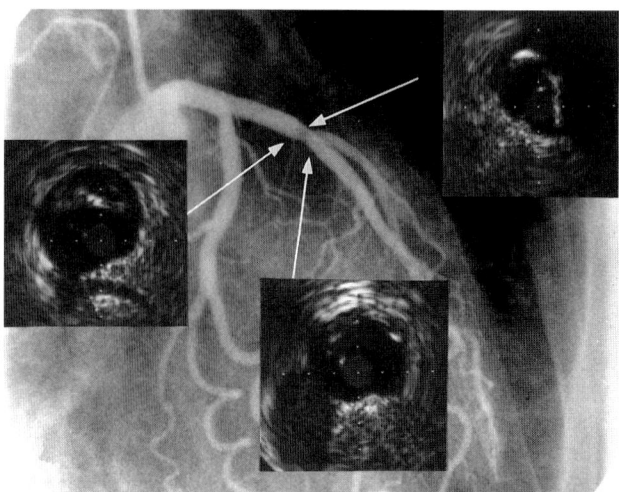

FIG. 3. A: An angiographic projection (right anterior oblique) demonstrating an intermediate-grade stenosis of the proximal segment of the left anterior descending artery (*arrows*). **B:** An IVUS image of the proximal portion of the stenosis demonstrating a fibrocalcific plaque (9 to 3 o'clock). **C:** An IVUS image of the midportion of the lesion, demonstrating a calcified plaque (10 to 5 o'clock, 210 degree arc, producing acoustic shadowing), causing a severe stenosis unidentified accurately by the angiogram. **D:** An IVUS image at the distal portion of the lesion, at the origin of the diagonal branch, demonstrating the fibrofatty plaque.

ogist. In institutions with a large number of procedures, there is often a dedicated group of echocardiographers and/or interventional cardiologists who are responsible for performing and interpreting the images, as well as maintenance of equipment and storage and archiving of the studies. The indications and possible applications of IVUS are presented in Table 5.

Coronary Artery Disease

Evaluation of Stenosis Severity

Stenosis severity is usually evaluated by angiography alone. Due to its superior imaging ability, IVUS can be used when stenosis severity is not clearly determined by angiography, such as in ostial stenosis (e.g., left main coronary artery, right coronary artery and left anterior descending artery). IVUS can also be used for the assessment of overlapping vessels (especially when there is a discrepancy between the angiographic findings and the clinical manifestations or noninvasive studies). As demonstrated in Figure 3, IVUS can identify a high-grade stenosis that is borderline by angiography. IVUS may also exclude the presence of a significant stenosis and the procedure can thus be terminated at that stage.

Selection of the Optimal Therapy

In cases where a significant stenosis is identified by angiography and/or IVUS, the lesion can be evaluated for the appropriate treatment—catheter intervention, surgery (espe-

cially in the case of left main coronary artery lesion and three-vessel disease), or medical treatment.

Selection of the Type and Size of Device When Catheter Intervention Is Preferred

In cases where the interventional cardiologist decides to perform catheter intervention, the type of interventional therapy [percutaneous transluminal coronary angioplasty (PTCA), stent deployment, directional coronary atherectomy, rotational coronary atherectomy, excimer laser coronary ablation] and the size of the interventional devices can be better selected by the IVUS findings. If preintervention IVUS imaging reveals severe endoluminal calcification of the plaque, rotational coronary atherectomy or excimer laser coronary angioplasty is often preferred over PTCA or directional coronary atherectomy.

Evaluation of the Results of Intervention

The procedural results can be readily evaluated by IVUS for the cross-sectional lumen area, the presence of flaps or dissections, stent-to-wall apposition, and the presence of additional stenoses. The procedure can thus be terminated due to achieving optimal results, or the need for further intervention (increase in device size or balloon inflation pressure) can be decided immediately. The need for different devices or procedural failure can also be evaluated.

Impact of IVUS Imaging on Clinical Decision-Making

In a study done at a center in which a selective use of IVUS imaging is being done (10), interventional decisions based on IVUS findings were made in 84% (133/158) of all cases in which IVUS was used. IVUS imaging was considered significantly more useful for decision-making in stent cases (97%) than in balloon angioplasty cases (64%, $P <$ 0.001) and plaque ablation cases (75%, $P = 0.0015$). Preintervention or diagnostic IVUS imaging was defined as useful in 72% of the cases. In this group, IVUS was used for the detection of significant stenoses (43%), exclusion of significant stenoses (20%), and selection or sizing of interventional devices (15%).

Postintervention imaging was defined as useful in 77% of cases. In this group, IVUS was used for the detection of inadequate interventional results (31%), for the need of additional interventional therapy, and for confirmation of adequate stent deployment (45%). Balloon angioplasty results were deemed inadequate in one third of cases in which post-PTCA IVUS imaging was performed and the patients needed further various interventions. Stent deployment in a series of studies was judged as inadequate in 25 to 85% of cases in which poststent IVUS imaging was performed, and all stents needed redilation by balloons with larger diameters or higher inflation pressures.

There is an ongoing controversy whether IVUS imaging should be routinely performed after stent deployment and high-pressure inflations with noncompliant balloons. Clinical trials to answer this question are currently being performed.

Saphenous Vein Graft Disease

IVUS can be used for the evaluation and follow-up of saphenous vein graft disease and for monitoring of therapeutic interventions in the same way it is used in de novo coronary artery disease. Implanted saphenous vein bypass grafts frequently undergo major morphologic changes after surgery. The reported patency of the grafts is 50% 10 to 15 years after surgery, suggesting that vein grafts undergo either an acute or progressive atherothrombotic occlusion.

Newly implanted saphenous vein bypass grafts and those with no evidence of atherosclerotic disease at 6 months after surgery usually demonstrate a single-layered vessel wall morphology by IVUS. An arterialized triple-layered appearance is normally found in 75% of grafts 5 and 10 years after operation, and it can be related to the marked intimal proliferation and degeneration found by histologic studies. IVUS studies have shown a significant increase in intimal thickness and intimal area 1 month and 1 year postsurgery, as well as a doubling of vessel-wall thickness that correlated histologically with vessel wall fibrosis.

IVUS has also provided an insight into vascular remodeling and the formation of vessel stenosis in saphenous vein grafts. The absence of focal compensatory enlargement or constriction in stenotic areas was demonstrated *in vivo* by IVUS.

Peripheral Vascular Disease

As in coronary artery disease, IVUS has been found to be a useful imaging tool for both pre- and postintervention assessment. While most endovascular surgeons and radiologists still use pre- and postintervention angiography and measurements of pressure gradients across the lesion to determine the success of intervention, IVUS will undoubtedly have an incremental diagnostic role in the future.

In carotid artery disease, IVUS may be better for the detection of stenoses at the origin of the common carotid artery, an area often masked by the aortic arch in angiography. IVUS can also provide information on lesion calcification that is not easily visible by angiography. Balloon angioplasty and stent deployment is currently being evaluated as a substitute for endarterectomy. The IVUS procedure is technically performed the same way as in the coronary arteries, and can obtain images that are useful for both a correct evaluation of lumen and vessel size and selection of the correct stent length and size. Postintervention results, stent expansion, and stent-to-wall apposition are readily evaluated.

In subclavian and innominate artery disease, IVUS is most useful in determining the anatomic relations of the vascular stenosis to the vertebral arteries, which might be compromised during intervention. For the evaluation of aortic disease, a 6F, 12.5 MHz catheter is most suitable. Three-dimensional IVUS has been found useful in the evaluation of abdominal aneurysms prior to surgery. The assessment of the shape of the proximal and distal necks often gives an indication of how well an endoluminal graft will exclude the aneurysm. The role and feasibility of IVUS imaging in evaluation of the renal, iliac, superficial femoral, popliteal and distal arteries has also been described.

The advent of three-dimensional IVUS, as well as improvements in imaging catheters in the future will likely improve the diagnostic aspects of peripheral vascular interventions.

IVUS Postheart Transplantation

Although short-term survival after heart transplantation has dramatically improved in the last decade, long-term survival remains limited mostly due to the early development of cardiac allograft vasculopathy (CAV) in 30 to 50% of patients 5 years after transplantation. The nature of CAV is different from native coronary artery atherosclerosis—CAV is more diffuse and involves smaller vessels as well as epicardial vessels. The lesions in CAV are more concentric, do not usually have ulcerations or calcifications, and the patients do not develop collaterals in occluded segments.

Moreover, due to cardiac denervation, the patients do not have the ischemic type of chest pain in the presence of ischemia.

The detection of CAV by noninvasive testing is particularly difficult due to the diffuse nature of the disease. Most of the current noninvasive methods (conventional stress testing, nuclear perfusion studies, and stress echocardiography) have a very low sensitivity and low positive predictive value rates of 25%, and a specificity and negative predictive value of 86%. Therefore, a policy of yearly angiograms has been adopted in many transplantation centers.

The limitations of angiography in detecting coronary disease is more pronounced in CAV than in atherosclerotic cardiovascular disease. Since CAV is a diffuse process, the reference segments are also involved, and, thus, the severity of disease may be underestimated. Comparing yearly angiograms with previous ones may be an insensitive method due to the subtle changes invisible to the angiographer.

IVUS imaging may, therefore, be superior to angiography in detecting CAV. IVUS studies have shown that IVUS imaging can be done annually without an increase in procedural risk. Other IVUS studies have shown that intimal thickening in angiographically normal arteries begins to appear 1 month after transplantation in 65% of patients and is found in 100% of patients 1 year after transplantation. While intimal thickening progresses rapidly, calcification of the lesions starts usually after year 6. The grading of intimal thickening to mild (less than 0.3 mm), moderate, and severe has prognostic implications, regardless of the presence of angiographic evidence of CAV. The patients with intimal thickening greater than 0.3 mm had decreased survival and were prone to retransplantation. Another striking IVUS study found the left anterior descending artery to be the most frequently affected coronary artery, and the proximal segments were found to be more affected than the distal segments. IVUS has also shown that vascular remodeling is present in CAV as in native coronary atherosclerosis.

The possible risk factors for CAV were evaluated by several IVUS studies. Independent risk factors or predictors for CAV by IVUS were total and LDL cholesterol levels, elevated triglycerides levels, body mass index and weight gain, as well as the donor age greater than 35 and a history of smoking. These studies also allowed a quantification of the effect of different preventive therapies on the progression of CAV.

The question of whether IVUS imaging should be performed in every transplant recipient with annual IVUS follow-up studies still remains unanswered, and multicenter trials are currently addressing these questions. It has been suggested that IVUS imaging be performed at baseline and at 1 year after transplantation. If both these studies show no significant intimal thickening, the next IVUS imaging has been recommended to be at 5 years. If the initial studies are abnormal, the patients should be treated aggressively by calcium antagonists and lipid-lowering therapies and fol-

lowed annually with IVUS of the affected epicardial coronary arteries.

IVUS AS AN ADJUNCT TO VASCULAR INTERVENTIONS

IVUS in PTCA

Since the introduction of PTCA by Gruentzig in 1977, the procedure has become a major therapeutic tool in cardiology all over the world. It has continuously been modified and with the use of improved balloons, adjunctive therapies, and bail-out procedures (e.g., stents) the current immediate success rates are greater than 90%. Although angiography is still the major imaging modality for PTCA in most catheterization laboratories, the advent of IVUS during the late 1980s has made a major contribution for better guidance of coronary interventions. IVUS has contributed to the improvement of the immediate and late procedural results, as well as to a better understanding of the mechanisms of the actions of balloon angioplasty, and to an emergence of new definitions of pathologic processes both pre- and postangioplasty.

Three different mechanisms for luminal enlargement by PTCA have been defined by IVUS imaging (11). The mechanisms of action of balloon angioplasty are different in various plaque morphologies, and, thus, awareness and recognition of these mechanisms may allow the interventional cardiologist to optimize the selection of equipment, inflation pressures, and duration of treatment. The first mechanism attributed to PTCA was plaque fracture and dissection, which was later confirmed by histopathologic studies. While these fractures and dissections were not readily recognized by angiography, they have been found by IVUS in 50 to 80% of patients with successful angiographic results. An example of the type of plaque disruption or fracture that occurs postballoon PTCA is demonstrated in Figure 4. The plaque fracturing occurs mostly in calcified lesions, and is greatest in plaques occupying a large luminal circumference. The site of fracturing is usually the junction of a calcified plaque and a normal or less calcified tissue (''soft plaque''). Plaque eccentricity (defined as the ratio of maximal to minimal plaque thickness ≥ 2) is also a major risk factor for fracturing and dissection at the juncture of a large plaque and a segment with lesser plaque burden.

The second mechanism for lumen enlargement by balloon angioplasty is vessel stretching, defined as the enlargement of the EEL area (vessel area). This mechanism is probably the major contributing mechanism for lumen enlargement in about 20% of angioplasties, mostly in areas with a smaller plaque burden, or lesions with eccentric atheromas and ''softer'' plaques. In these lesions the stretching occurs mostly in the side opposite to the atheroma. Vessel stretching has also been suggested as a possible mechanism for lumen en-

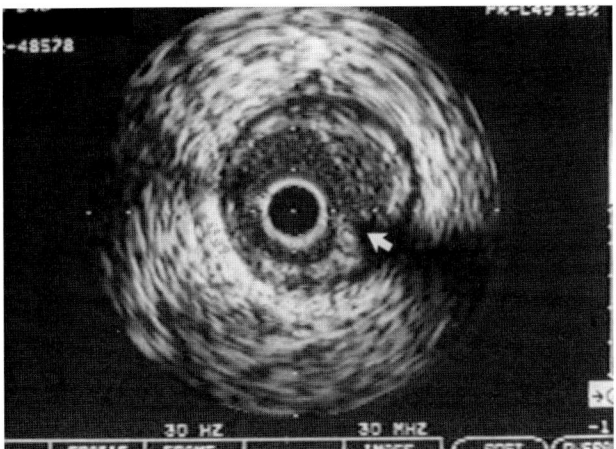

FIG. 4. A plaque rupture and an intimal dissection (*arrow*) at the proximal site of a lesion following PTCA of a left anterior descending artery. The dissection was successfully treated with subsequent stent deployment. (Courtesy of Tomoo Nagai, M.D., Division of Cardiology, Cedars-Sinai Medical Center, Los Angeles, California.)

largement in lesions with focal constriction and "negative remodeling" (11).

The third mechanism for lumen enlargement after balloon angioplasty is the redistribution of the atheroma along the axial axis of the vessel. Studies using an IVUS automatic pullback device have confirmed this mechanism of "plaque compression" at the intervention site, usually at the expense of an increase of the plaque plus media volume both proximally and distally to the target lesion. This mechanism is thought to be most frequent in patients with clinically unstable coronary syndromes, due to a "softer" plaque composition and/or a higher incidence of thrombus at the target lesion.

The quantification of PTCA results by angiography correlates poorly with IVUS measurements. Preprocedural measurements are somewhat better correlated than postprocedural measurements due to the inability of angiography to delineate all the fractures and fissures created by PTCA. Therefore, angiography usually overestimates luminal diameter at the target site, and underestimates luminal diameter at the reference site because of reference site disease. Thus an angiographic "stent-like" result or a residual diameter stenosis of 10%, may be associated with 60% of the vessel area still occupied by plaque on IVUS imaging.

Balloon sizing by IVUS may be crucial for better acute and long-term outcomes of the procedure. This can be done more accurately by IVUS than by angiography due to the diffuse nature of the atherosclerotic process involving also angiographically "normal-looking" reference segments. The selection of balloons with a balloon/artery ratio of 1.1 to 1, as determined by angiography in the CLOUT trial (Clinical Outcomes with Ultrasound Trial) (12), did not significantly improve the immediate postprocedural results. Thus, additional inflations with bigger balloons to a ratio of 1.3

to 1 were needed in 73% of the lesions. This resulted in an average increase in lumen area from 3.16 to 4.52 mm^2 ($P < 0.0001$). Thus a selection of balloon size based only on angiographic criteria may be insufficient, while IVUS appears to provide a simple tool for improvement of procedural results.

The evaluation of immediate PTCA results has major implications both medically and economically, since stenting or the use of other devices can be time-consuming as well as expensive. IVUS may be extremely helpful for evaluating therapeutic PTCA results and identifying acute procedural complications (e.g., dissections). It has thus been suggested that stenting is clearly indicated when the dissection: (i) encompasses an arc of more than 180 degrees (type D dissection); (ii) is more than 1 cm in length; (iii) is more than 1.5 mm thick; (iv) has long false channels (greater than 5 mm); (v) results in the flap reaching the opposite vessel wall or when the flap is more than 5 mm in length. The flaps that are pushed against the wall by the IVUS catheter in small vessels should also be stented. On the other hand, it has been previously demonstrated by the BENESTENT-I substudy, that an angiographic "stent-like" result has a favorable long-term outcome, comparable with those of stent deployment; thus, IVUS may not be helpful in this group.

Acute or abrupt vessel closure can be better evaluated with IVUS than with angiography. IVUS facilitates the identification of dissections, thrombi, or vasospasm and guides the operator in selecting the best treatment, especially if preprocedure IVUS has been performed. Angiographically "hazy" lesions can be better evaluated, as IVUS can help determine whether the haziness is due to dissection, thrombus, irregularly shaped lumen, residual plaque, or any combination of the above.

IVUS in Stent Deployment

The rapid increase in the frequency of stent deployment in the last decade has been a major factor in the development of IVUS imaging. IVUS, on the other hand, has contributed significantly to reducing the rate of stent-related acute and subacute complications and restenosis, as well as facilitating the understanding of the mechanisms underlying luminal area gain and loss. While angiographically "acceptable" results still provide a rapid method for on-line decision-making in the catheterization laboratory, 25 to 85% of implanted stents (in different studies) are suboptimally expanded as assessed by IVUS imaging. A case example of suboptimal stent deployment with an apparently satisfactory angiographic result is shown in Figure 5. After further subsequent balloon dilatation the stent is adequately deployed by IVUS imaging (and angiography). IVUS can therefore be used both before and after stent implantation, and can provide information on: (i) lesion length and vessel size—for the selection of the appropriate stent and balloon sizing (by using vessel size, bordered by EEL, and not lumen size); (ii) lesion morphology—for the selection of the proper device; (iii) severe

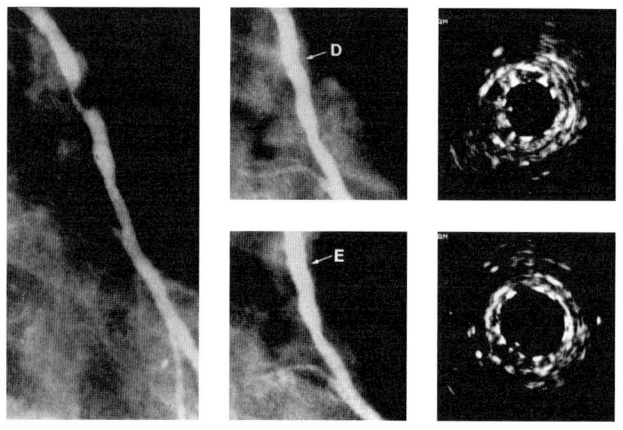

A
B,D
C,E

FIG. 5. IVUS imaging for stent deployment. **A:** Coronary angiogram of a saphenous bypass graft to left anterior descending artery revealed eccentric subtotal occlusion at the middle portion of the graft. After stent deployment, angiography revealed widely patent vein graft (**B**), but IVUS imaging showed inadequate expansion of stent with lumen diameter of only 2.4 mm (**D**). After larger (4.0 mm) PTCA balloon was used for dilatation, follow-up angiogram revealed no significant change (**C**), but subsequent IVUS imaging showed expansion of stent with increasing lumen diameter to 3.5 mm (**E**). (From ref. 21, with permission.)

lesions distally and proximally to the target lesion that appear moderate in severity by angiography; (iv) evaluation of stent implantation results.

Acute Complications

IVUS is helpful in identifying acute complications resulting from PTCA, such as dissections and elastic recoil, necessitating the need for stent implantation. Acute stent thrombosis is related to the thrombogenicity of the stent material, as well as to turbulence of blood within the stent. Both are augmented when the stent is not well apposed to the vessel wall. Heparin-coated stents (BENESTENT I and II trials), high-pressure balloon inflations, and IVUS imaging have all contributed to a significant reduction in acute stent complications. Now, with the use of aspirin in combination with ticlopidine or plavix, and without anticoagulation, acute stent thrombosis occurs in fewer than 1% of cases.

Studies published recently have determined that the factors increasing the risk of subacute stent thrombosis are low ejection fraction, intraprocedural complications leading to deployment of several stents (particularly of different designs), suboptimal final result (i.e., small lumen area by angiography and IVUS), dissections, and intraluminal low flow. In patients with acute myocardial infarction who have undergone emergent PTCA, an IVUS finding of low echogenicity and bright speckled material that was partially enhanced with the injection of ultrasound contrast agent, was suspected to be a combination of plaque disruption and thrombus. This was associated with abrupt vessel closure

post-PTCA, indicating the need for a more aggressive and prolonged antithrombotic treatment. Thus, in patients with acute myocardial infarction, IVUS may be safely performed and may reduce possible acute post-PTCA complications.

Optimal Stent Expansion

The criteria for optimal stent expansion (Fig. 4) include:

1. Full strut to vessel wall apposition to avoid turbulent flow through the stent struts;
2. A round-looking stent with symmetric dimensions equal to the "symmetric index" (minimal/maximal diameter greater than 0.7);
3. In-stent lumen cross-sectional area as large as proximal and distal (taking into consideration vessel tapering) "normal appearing" reference segments. Trials have shown that optimal stent expansion in-stent cross-sectional area is 90% of the average of the proximal and distal reference lumen area or achieving in-stent cross-sectional area of a minimum of 9.0 mm^2;
4. Absence of a significant (angiographically occult) dissection that exposes the deep elements of the media of a native vessel or a vein graft, which are thought to be highly thrombogenic.

IVUS in Directional Coronary Atherectomy

Due to a relatively high rate of restenosis after PTCA, directional coronary atherectomy (DCA) was introduced in the early 1980s in an attempt to reduce the restenosis rate. The first trials with DCA demonstrated a success rate of approximately 90%, with a reduction of percent area stenosis as measured by quantitative coronary angiography from 70 to 90% to 15 to 30%. However, IVUS studies post-DCA have shown that debulking was not as complete as demonstrated by quantitative coronary angiography (QCA) and plaque cross-sectional area was reduced by only 18%, while percent area stenosis decreased by only 22%. Several IVUS studies have shown that even though angiography demonstrates complete debulking, 35 to 70% of the cross-sectional vessel area is still occupied by atheroma (13). The mechanism underlying these differences was also discovered by IVUS imaging. It appears that the acute gain in lumen area comes not only from debulking, but also from plaque displacement as the vessel stretches. Although procedural success results primarily from debulking, only 25 to 60% of lesions experience plaque reduction alone. IVUS studies have shown that vessel stretching contributes between 15 and 50% to the increase in lumen area following DCA. This may provide an insight into the results of studies such as the Coronary Angioplasty Versus Excisional Atherectomy Trial (CAVEAT) and the Canadian Coronary Atherectomy Trial (CCAT) in which no IVUS guiding was used. These major trials were unable to show a substantial benefit of DCA over PTCA with regard to the need for repeat revascularization, rates of restenosis, death, and myocardial infarction at 6 months and 1 year of follow-up.

The results of DCA and the rate of procedural complications depend primarily on plaque composition and architecture. Calcification of a coronary lesion significantly reduces the effectiveness of DCA plaque removal. IVUS has been previously demonstrated to identify calcium deposits better than angiography (50 to 70% versus 20 to 30%). It has been shown that the preintervention arc of calcium as measured by IVUS was the most consistent negative predictor of residual lumen area, percent of cross-sectional narrowing, and degree of plaque volume removal by DCA. Plaque removal was also lowest in lesions with superficial calcium deposits as compared to deep or subendothelial calcium, while it was highest in lesions with no calcium deposits.

Lesions with eccentric plaque were considered better suited for DCA than concentric plaques. Studies have not demonstrated any advantage of DCA in those lesions with angiographic guidance only, and it may well be necessary to use IVUS guidance with DCA to improve results in both eccentric and concentric lesions.

IVUS-guided DCA trials such as the Balloon versus Optimal Atherectomy Trial (BOAT) and the Optimal Atherectomy Restenosis Study (OARS) have shown that both the extent of lumen gain and the postprocedure minimal lumen size following DCA predict the degree of late lumen loss (the "bigger the better" theory). They have shown that a more aggressive resection of plaque with DCA resulted in an improved postprocedural lumen diameter and percent stenosis measured by QCA, as well as lower rates of angiographic restenosis, without an increase in procedural complications as compared to the CAVEAT trials. Although the DCA in the OARS trial was guided by IVUS, adjunctive PTCA was required in 87% of patients, and the average residual cross-sectional stenosis post-DCA was 57%. This suggests that more aggressive plaque resection would have been feasible in the OARS study population.

In order to improve procedural outcome, IVUS should be performed at both the reference and lesion sites to determine the extent, architecture, and composition of the plaque. Superficial calcium greater than 180 degrees at the lesion site is generally a contraindication for DCA. Plaque eccentricity should be appreciated and anatomic landmarks should direct the cut away from the normal vessel wall. Catheter sizing is essential for the prevention of medial and adventitial damage. IVUS imaging should be repeated after the initial DCA cuts to determine whether additional or deeper atherectomy is necessary. If residual plaque is still excessive despite maximal balloon inflations, a larger atherotome may be needed. A reasonable goal for DCA is to reduce the percent plaque area to 20% or less. Resection beyond this point has not been demonstrated to provide additional benefit and may lead to excessive subintimal tissue resection or even perforation. IVUS should also be used to identify any possible procedural complications and determine the presence, extent, and orientation of intimal dissection. Coronary dissection should be treated by salvage DCA directed toward the dissection flap or by stent implantation.

IVUS in Excimer Laser Angioplasty

The application of new devices such as excimer laser in interventional cardiology approximately a decade ago has not yet caused a dramatic change in either the immediate or long-term procedural results. The current devices emit laser in pulses at a wavelength of 308 nm. The laser tissue effects are three: (i) thermal ablation; (ii) photoacoustic ablation; (iii) photodecomposition that results in direct molecular bond breaking. These effects are very precise and do not cause damage to tissues adjacent to the laser beam.

Excimer laser is indicated and was shown to be valuable in saphenous vein graft stenoses, long lesions, ostial lesions, total occlusions, and as an adjunct to partially successful PTCA. The procedure has reported success rates of 90%, with a complication rate of 6.4 to 7.6%.

The major mechanisms of laser effect on coronary atherosclerotic lesions is by both tissue ablation and vessel expansion, as shown in several *in vivo* studies. The proposed mechanism for vessel expansion was laser-induced shock waves and forceful expansion of vapor bubbles into tissue. Nevertheless, in these studies the plaque burden was still substantial, and most lesions needed adjunctive therapy (e.g., balloon angioplasty).

Preintervention IVUS is helpful in deciding whether excimer laser should be performed or if another device would be more appropriate. Since excimer laser is indicated in totally occluded vessels or mildly calcified plaques, IVUS imaging should focus on: (i) estimating the amount of lesion calcification; (ii) evaluating lesion eccentricity (in eccentric lesions it is preferable to use eccentric laser catheters); (iii) determining vessel size accurately, since the laser catheter should be larger than the lumen size preintervention to maximize plaque ablation.

Postintervention IVUS can determine residual plaque burden, lumen cross-sectional area, and procedural complications. Since excimer laser angioplasty usually necessitates the use of adjunctive therapy, IVUS can help in the sizing of stents and balloons.

IVUS in Rotational Coronary Atherectomy

The high-speed, diamond-coated metal burr of the rotational atherectomy device rotates at a speed of 160,000 to 190,000 rpm. It is used mostly in highly calcified plaques, and abrades the atheroma to microparticles 5 to 10 μm in size. The damage to the arterial wall is confined to the intima with no evidence of medial injury.

The mechanisms of rotational atherectomy in coronary lesions have been studied by IVUS. The main increase in lumen cross-sectional area resulted from a decrease in plaque-plus-media area, while vessel size (EEL area) did not change. Nevertheless, a remaining average plaque burden of

74% still remained postintervention (14). The rate of plaque dissections post–rotational atherectomy was reported to be 26%, in contrast to 50 to 80% plaque dissections post successful PTCA.

VASCULAR REMODELING AND RESTENOSIS

It has long been appreciated that the severity of coronary artery disease is solely determined by the accumulation of plaque along the arterial wall, regardless of the effects on the arterial wall itself. It was assumed, therefore, that there is a linear relation between the plaque area size and coronary stenosis. IVUS imaging has provided an accurate and feasible method for assessment of the effects of atherosclerosis on the coronary artery wall and its response to plaque accumulation. Since first published in human postmortem histopathologic examinations by Glagov et al. in 1987 (15), the concept of arterial remodeling, also known now as the "Glagov effect," has been studied thoroughly in animals and humans. It is now clear that the vessel cross-sectional area is not constant and reacts differently to different degrees of plaque burden and to arterial injury as well as to other stimuli.

The concept of vascular remodeling suggests that coronary and peripheral arteries enlarge in parallel with the accumulation of atherosclerotic plaque, thus preserving the lumen size ("positive" or compensatory remodeling). When the progressive accumulation of plaque exceeds the compensatory mechanism of the artery, the luminal cross-sectional vessel area (EEL area) starts to decrease. Figure 6 illustrates the "Glagov effect" on the arterial wall and lumen during the remodeling process. Positive remodeling is arbitrarily defined as a vessel cross-sectional area at the lesion site being larger than the proximal reference site. Negative remodeling is defined as a cross-sectional area at the lesion site smaller than the distal reference site. Intermediate remodeling is defined as a CSA at the lesion site in an intermediate size between the two reference sites (16).

IVUS allows quantitative *in vivo* assessment of the arterial lumen and wall size and shape. It permits delineation of the intima, media, and adventitia, and the presence of calcification, lipid pools, and fibrous regions. In a study of vascular remodeling, IVUS imaging was performed in coronary arteries with an angiographic diameter stenosis of greater than 70%. A comparison of the stenosis site with a proximal reference site that had less than a 25% diameter narrowing by angiography and less than a 50% cross-sectional area stenosis by IVUS was done. Compensatory enlargement was defined as being present when the total coronary arterial cross-sectional area at the stenotic site was greater than that at the proximal nonstenotic site. It was documented that the majority of stenotic lesions had compensatory enlargement and thus exhibited "positive" remodeling. Of note, however, is that in 26% of arteries there was "inadequate" remodeling in that the total cross-sectional area at the stenotic site was less than that in both the proximal and distal reference sites. Unfortunately, vascular remodeling is variable

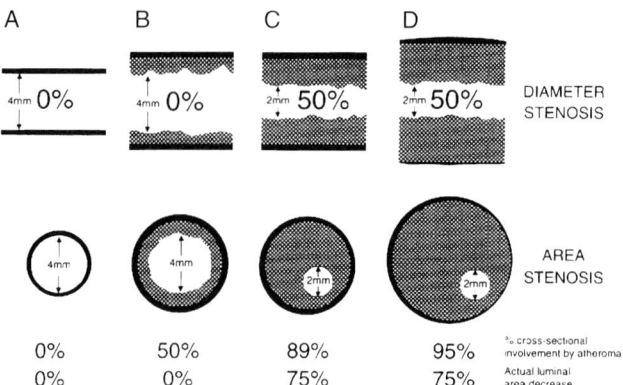

FIG. 6. Top row: Angiographic views. **Bottom row:** Pathological views. **Column A:** Normal artery. **Column B:** Artery with "moderate" atherosclerosis. Because of remodeling with consequent enlargement of the vessel, the angiographer sees a normal lumen. A pathologist viewing the same artery would see the same lumen, but 50% of the cross-sectional area would be occupied by plaque. Since the pathologist has no way of knowing that this lumen is of normal size, he or she concludes that this artery has a 50% cross-sectional area narrowing. **Column C:** More involved artery. The angiographer sees that the lumen is 50% less in diameter than the adjacent "normal" (**B**) segment. This would translate into a 75% cross-sectional area narrowing, but the angiographer might conclude that there is mild to moderate disease. The pathologist sees the 2-mm lumen but a larger plaque and measures the stenosis as an 89% narrowing. **Column D:** Same situation, but with even more remodeling present. The angiographer still sees a 50% diameter narrowing, even though the plaque is much larger than in column C, and would still conclude that this is not severe disease. Because of the greater enlargement of the artery, the pathologist now measures the stenosis as a 95% cross-sectional narrowing, even though the lumen size is actually the same as in column C. The pathologist is left with no other explanation than that the angiographer has grossly underestimated the degree of stenosis in the patient's coronary artery. (Adapted from ref. 2, with permission.)

and inconsistent. This finding indicates that clinically significant coronary arterial narrowing by atherosclerosis may be a function of not only the amount of atherosclerosis but also the degree of remodeling present. Thus the most stenotic area is not necessarily the one with the largest plaque burden.

The vascular response to plaque accumulation can vary not only in the same patient but also in a single coronary vessel and is not confined to a certain vessel or segment or to a specific spatial relation to the maximum stenosis. While there may be an adequate compensatory enlargement in a certain lesion, there might be an inadequate ("negative") remodeling in another lesion in the same vessel. Moreover, it was demonstrated by IVUS that vascular remodeling is a highly localized process and can affect only a portion of the vessel wall occupied by plaque. There are three major types of vascular response to plaque accumulation: (i) a concentric plaque with round lumen and round EEL (20% of lesions); (ii) an eccentric plaque with round lumen and an ovoid, expanded EEL (40%); and (iii) a concentric plaque with an ovoid lumen and a round EEL (30%). A round lumen was preserved in 66% of the lesions, which had a significantly larger lumen area than those with an ovoid lumen. A failure to preserve a rounded lumen may indicate a greater tendency to develop coronary stenosis in the future at the lesion site. The mechanisms underlying the differential patterns of vascular remodeling may be related to locally mediated endothelial factors, which still remain to be determined.

Saphenous vein grafts implanted during coronary artery bypass surgery undergo major morphologic changes, which include intimal thickening and intimal fibromuscular hyperplasia, and increases in fibrous tissue in the adventitia with replacement of the elastic fibers. The denervation and loss of vasa vasorum may also affect vessel properties, even though their ability to dilate in response to nitroglycerin is not affected (17). The implanted saphenous vein grafts cannot thus be considered to be passive conduits. It has also been demonstrated that vascular remodeling in vein grafts is usually absent in response to atherosclerosis, with loss of the grafts' ability either to constrict or enlarge locally. The loss of compensatory enlargement may be a contributing factor in the progression of stenoses in saphenous vein bypass grafts.

FUTURE DIRECTIONS

Combined Imaging and Therapeutic Devices

Combined imaging and therapeutic catheters are being introduced and probably will have an increased use in the future. One system (Endosonics, Rancho Cordova, CA) has already received Food and Drug Administration approval. The imaging element is mounted immediately proximal to the balloon, enabling the operator to image the lesion and then to use the same catheter to deliver a stent and check the results immediately. A combined imaging and directional atherectomy catheter is also in development. This system has the transducer mounted on the cutting device, and the operator can determine on-line whether there is any residual plaque to be removed and then assess the results immediately.

Imaging Guidewires

Imaging guidewires are also an appealing future development. Currently there are imaging wires that are actually rotating cores that can be substituted for a guidewire once a catheter is in place. One prototype uses a wire size of 0.014″ with the transducer rotating at 40 MHz. They can image through most balloon materials, but the image is disrupted by stents or air bubbles. Another factor limiting image quality is the imaging element size, since the image quality depends on the size of the transducer. A 0.035-inch imaging core wire is now commercially available for peripheral artery disease imaging.

Therapeutic Intravascular Ultrasound

A possible future therapeutic aspect of IVUS is the treatment of total coronary occlusions, either acute or chronic (18). Revascularization of total coronary occlusions that cannot be readily crossed with the guiding wire can be facilitated by using an intravascular ultrasound catheter (Sonicross, Advanced Cardiovascular Systems, Temecula, CA) that creates a channel for the wire sufficient for crossing the occlusion. This is followed by either simple balloon angioplasty or by stenting the lesion. Real-time imaging of the procedure can theoretically be done by forward-looking devices currently being developed. These devices have the ability to direct the ultrasound beam forward in a sector fanning out from the catheter tip, with the imaging plane in an approximately flat projection.

Tissue Characterization

One of the current limitations of IVUS is its reduced ability to correctly identify and diagnose intraluminal thrombi or lipid accumulations within coronary plaques. Tissue characterization techniques are currently in development for this purpose. The different radiofrequency signals backscattered from the different intravascular tissues are being identified and quantified in an attempt to characterize each tissue by its own typical frequency. A possible major application of tissue characterization by IVUS is in diagnosing unstable, or vulnerable, plaque with a large lipid pool and a thin fibrous cap. These plaques have a major potential for rupture and can lead to acute coronary syndromes. Color visualization is another feature of IVUS that has a potential for detecting intraluminal blood flow. It may allow a better definition of intimal–lumen border and improve identification of intraluminal structures such as thrombi.

Forward-viewing Catheters

The ability to image forward with the IVUS catheter can have major implications for the treatment of chronic or acute total occlusions without disrupting the plaque by passing the catheter distally. Although it is usually considered to be a safe procedure, distal embolization and vasospasm occur in 5% of IVUS procedures and may be prevented by using forward viewing catheters. A combination of forward-and-side Doppler imaging may be used for real-time flow measurements and quantification. However, the technical difficulties in developing the catheters and their miniaturization are still significant.

Three-dimensional Reconstruction

The utility of IVUS in visualizing and quantifying coronary morphology has been limited by its two-dimensional tomographic nature. IVUS imaging lacks the ''angiography-like'' longitudinal visualization of the coronary vessel. It is therefore appealing to try to create a three-dimensional configuration of the vessel lumen and its wall, in order to get a better insight into the complex plaque architecture and to facilitate serial IVUS studies. However, limiting problems for a more routine clinical use of these systems are uneven pullback velocity of the catheter, the tortuousity of vessels, and movement of the catheter with each cardiac cycle, as well as respiration (19).

Performance of a three-dimensional IVUS study is basically the same as for two-dimensional IVUS. The catheters are sheath-type catheters, with either a monorail short lumen or a longer lumen. The transducer is moved freely within the sheath, allowing a smoother forward and backward motion. An automated continuous pullback system is most commonly used for a better image reconstruction. This is best combined with an automated echocardiogram- or ECG-gated image acquisition, but is more time-consuming than conventional acquisition. This allows measurements of vascular and segmental dimensions at any time of the cardiac cycle. After the upper and lower limits of the cardiac cycle are defined, up to 25 cardiac cycles can be sampled and displayed later as a continuous motion. Digitization of the images can be done either on-line or off-line. Dedicated algorithms that identify structures by their gray-scale scheme, discriminate between the blood pool inside the lumen and the vessel wall. Sophisticated algorithms, such as acoustic quantification (which uses statistical pattern recognition) and contour detection algorithm (which is able also to detect the EEL), may further improve image quality.

The three-dimensional images are displayed either longitudinally or in a cylindrical format, and tangential and oblique sections are also available. The ECG-gated acquisition allows dynamic visualization. Reconstruction of a 30 mm segment may take 3 minutes with the acoustic quantification algorithm and can be done on-line in the catheterization laboratory. However, this algorithm depends on IVUS image quality, while the contour detection algorithm does not. With the contour detection systems, 25 to 40 mm segments can be reconstructed on-line or off-line.

Validation of three-dimensional IVUS images was reported in both *in vitro* and *in vivo* studies. High correlation with histopathologic sections of aortic segments and with quantitative angiographic measurements or two-dimensional IVUS was reported ($r = 0.97, 0.93, 0.81$, respectively) with the acoustic quantification system. The contour detection system has nearly the same results.

The advantage of three-dimensional IVUS may be greater mostly in long, complex lesions with eccentric plaque. The results of balloon angioplasty can be better evaluated for the presence of deep fissures and dissections of the plaque and vessel wall, which may necessitate the deployment of stents. The relation between the plaque and side branches permits improved sizing of stent length and diameter. In addition, it may also improve procedural results by avoiding unnecessary high-pressure inflations and increase the cross-sectional lumen area by improving stent-to-wall apposition, stent symmetry, and stent geometry.

Many technical obstacles still delay the applicability of three-dimensional IVUS in routine daily use. Image quality limited by the lateral resolution is still crucial for the reconstruction; the speed of automated pullback devices is still affected by cardiac motion, catheter angulations, and bends; and the long acquisition time may cause problems in patients with severe stenoses. A solution introduced lately was the utilization of information about the catheter trajectory from the angiographic pullback biplane images. Performing cineangiography during pullback provides points of reference for an accurate catheter position as a function of time. Typical three-dimensional reconstruction techniques of coronary arteries from IVUS images have assumed that the artery was straight and disregarded the angular orientation of IVUS slices. Accurate three-dimensional reconstruction of coronary arteries by following the transducer in real-time with the aid of biplane angiograms can now be achieved. Simultaneously acquired IVUS images are then placed perpendicular to the transducer path, using angiography to aid in determining the correct rotational orientation. A novel three-dimensional method (automated morphometry analysis) that automatically identifies the luminal and medial-adventitial borders is currently being developed and can be used for better visualization and morphometry. This method can provide an accurate reconstruction, without any of the possibly inaccurate assumptions or mechanical aids required by other methods.

Thus, although three-dimensional intravascular reconstruction may seem a promising on-line imaging tool for the interventional cardiologist, it is uncertain how soon it is likely to become a part of the routine practice in the catheterization laboratory.

Other Future Applications

Pulmonary artery imaging has been reported as an additional possible future application of IVUS. It has been performed with a 6F catheter inserted under fluoroscopic guidance, and the IVUS findings were highly correlated with histopathologic findings in patients with pulmonary hypertension. Recently a 4.8F flow-directed, balloon-tipped ultrasound catheter with a 20-MHz transducer has been developed that can be passed transvenously to the pulmonary artery without fluoroscopic guidance at the bedside. The catheter may be used for documentation and evaluation of pulmonary artery size and wall morphology in patients with pulmonary hypertension, chronic pulmonary embolism, and congenital heart disease, and for monitoring and evaluation of the effects of drug therapy. IVUS imaging has also been used to document pulmonary artery thrombi in patients with pulmonary embolism. The flow-directed, balloon-tipped IVUS catheters can also be used for imaging the right atrium and ventricle as well as the tricuspid and pulmonic valves.

Improvement of the catheters could make IVUS a useful future bedside imaging method for right heart disease.

Intracardiac ultrasound imaging using 10- to 20-MHz transducers has been reported to successfully assist in evaluation and monitoring of left ventricular function, assessment of valve morphology, and guidance of transseptal catheterization, as well as the monitoring and guidance of balloon mitral valvuloplasty and the closure of patent ductus arteriosus. Another promising future application of IVUS is for the guidance and monitoring of electrophysiologic studies and radiofrequency ablations. This is a method likely to greatly facilitate catheter placement for localized tissue ablation.

SUMMARY

Although angiography still remains the major diagnostic and therapy-guiding imaging modality in most catheterization laboratories throughout the world, IVUS imaging is superior to angiography for the detailed evaluation of coronary morphology. IVUS is no longer an experimental modality, but a feasible and accurate tool for a variety of indications and applications. IVUS provides visual and quantitative information not only on the vessel lumen, but on the vessel wall as well. This information has contributed immensely to the newly emerging concept of vascular remodeling. IVUS has been proved to be safe and feasible in clinically stable patients as well as in patients with acute coronary syndromes. IVUS has become a standard method for the diagnosis and evaluation of the severity and extent of coronary stenoses, for guiding various therapeutic modalities, and for follow-up and assessment of short- and long-term results. IVUS has, therefore, both clinical and research applications.

The increase in time, required technical expertise, and cost have hindered the universal adoption of IVUS technology in the cardiac catheterization laboratory. With future improvements in image quality and resolution, catheter miniaturization, and combined therapeutic devices, and with additional features (three-dimensional, forward imaging, Doppler and color imaging) of the catheters, IVUS is likely to have an increasing role as an imaging modality in the catheterization laboratory.

REFERENCES

1. Lee DY, Eigler NL, Fishbein MC, et al. Identification of intracoronary thrombus and demonstration of thrombectomy by intravascular ultrasound imaging. *Am J Cardiol* 1994;73:522–523.

2. Fishbein MC, Siegel RJ. How big are coronary artery atherosclerotic plaques that rupture? *Circulation* 1996;94:2662–2666.

3. Fitzgerald PJ, St Goar FG, Connolly AJ, et al. Intravascular ultrasound imaging of coronary arteries. Is three layers the norm? *Circulation* 1992;86:154–158.

4. Siegel RJ, Chae JS, Maurer G, et al. Histopathologic correlation of the three-layered intravascular ultrasound appearance of normal adult human muscular arteries. *Am Heart J* 1993;126:872–878.

5. Porter TR, Radio SJ, Anderson JA, et al. Composition of coronary atherosclerotic plaque in the intima and media affects intravascular ultrasound measurements of intimal thickness. *J Am Coll Cardiol* 1994; 23:1079–1084.

6. Di Mario C, The SH, Madretsma S, et al. Detection and characterization of vascular lesions by intravascular ultrasound: an *in vitro* study correlated with histology. *J Am Soc Echocardiogr* 1992;5:135–146.

7. Potkin BN, Bartorelli AL, Gessert JM, et al. Coronary artery imaging with intravascular high-frequency ultrasound. *Circulation* 1990;81: 1575–1585.

8. Siegel RJ, Ariani M, Fishbein MC, et al. Histopathologic validation of angioscopy and intravascular ultrasound. *Circulation* 1991;84: 109–117.

9. Tuzcu EM, Berkalp B, Defranco AC, et al. The dilemma of diagnosing coronary calcification: angiography versus intravascular ultrasound. *J Am Coll Cardiol* 1996;27:832–838.

10. Nishioka T, Luo H, Eigler NL, et al. Clinical application of IVUS imaging in a center with selective use of IVUS imaging. In: Siegel RJ, ed. *Intravascular ultrasound imaging in coronary artery disease.* New York: Marcel Dekker, 1998;75–94.

11. De Franco AC, Tuzcu EM, Ziada K, et al. Intravascular ultrasound assessment of PTCA results: Mechanisms and clinical implications. In: Siegel RJ, ed. *Intravascular ultrasound imaging in coronary artery disease.* New York: Marcel Dekker, 1998;205–243.

12. Stone GW, Hodgson JM, St Goar FG, et al. Improved procedural results of coronary angioplasty with intravascular ultrasound-guided balloon sizing. The CLOUT pilot trial. *Circulation* 1997;95:2044–2052.

13. Matar FA, Mintz GS, Farb A, et al. The contribution of tissue removal to lumen improvement after directional coronary atherectomy. *Am J Cardiol* 1994;74:647–650.

14. Mintz GS, Potkin BN, Keren G, et al. Intravascular ultrasound evaluation of the effect of rotational atherectomy in obstructive atherosclerotic coronary artery disease. *Circulation* 1992;86:1383–1393.

15. Glagov S, Weisenberg E, Zarins CK, et al. Compensatory enlargement of human atherosclerotic coronary arteries. *N Engl J Med* 1986;316: 1371–1375.

16. Birnbaum Y, Fishbein MC, Luo H, et al. Regional remodeling of atherosclerotic arteries: A major determinant of clinical manifestations of disease. *J Am Coll Cardiol* 1997;30:1149–1164.

17. Berglund H, Luo H, Nishioka T, et al. Preserved vasodilatory response to nitroglycerin in saphenous bypass vein grafts. *Circulation* 1996;94: 2871–2876.

18. Siegel RJ, Gunn J, Ashan J, et al. Use of therapeutic ultrasound in percutaneous coronary angioplasty. Experimental *in vitro* studies and initial clinical experience. *Circulation* 1994;89:1587–1592.

19. Von Birgelen C, Mintz GS, de Feyter PJ, et al. Reconstruction and quantification with three-dimensional intracoronary ultrasound: an update on techniques, challenges, and future directions. *Eur Heart J* 1997; 18:1056–1067.

20. de Feyter PJ, von Birgelen C, Serruys PW. Coronary imaging: angiography, angioscopy, and ultrasound. In: Siegel RJ, ed. *Intravascular ultrasound imaging in coronary artery disease.* New York: Marcel Dekker, 1998:111–131.

21. Lee DY, Eigler NL, Luo H, et al. Effect of intracoronary ultrasound imaging on clinical decision making. *Am Heart J* 1995;129:1084–1093.

CHAPTER 8

Myocardial Tissue Characterization

An Extension of Echocardiography

Julio E. Pérez and James G. Miller

Ultrasonic cardiac tissue characterization entails the identification and delineation of the physical or physiologic state of myocardium based on the analysis of the interactions between ultrasound and the tissue itself. The rationale for this approach is that sufficient information is contained in the ultrasound signal returning from myocardial tissue *per se* to permit the classification of the tissue as normal or abnormal and to indicate the nature of the abnormality (1).

INTERACTION BETWEEN ULTRASOUND AND MYOCARDIUM

Acoustic Properties of Tissue

One of the principal features of ultrasound that makes it powerful as a diagnostic tool is its property of being reflected when the waves reach a boundary between tissues (or areas within the same tissue) with different acoustic impedance values. When the incident wavelength is smaller than the dimension of the boundary, the reflection occurring is *specular* (e.g., conventional echocardiography).

On the other hand, when the boundary (between the different tissues or components of a given tissue) is smaller than the wavelength of the incident wave, the type of reflection that takes place is called *scattering*. As opposed to specular reflections, scattering is multidirectional, but the waves that

are redirected back to the transmitting transducer are defined as being *backscattered* from myocardium. Both the backscatter as well as the extent of attenuation of a given tissue can be expressed in quantitative terms and are useful parameters for its ultrasonic characterization. Backscatter can be expressed as a function of frequency over the useful bandwidth of frequencies for a particular transducer.

To derive the ultrasonic backscatter measurement of tissue, the insonifying transducer is first excited with an electrical voltage. The power spectrum corresponding to the backscattered signal received from tissue is referenced to the power spectrum obtained from a reference perfect reflector (which might be a steel plate or might be a known reflector such as a specific concentration of a well-characterized contrast agent) to obtain the backscatter transfer function. Power spectrum refers to the plot of the ultrasonic energy returned from the tissue or reflector, with power as ordinate and frequency as abscissa. *Integrated backscatter* (2) is defined as the frequency average of the backscatter transfer function (over the bandwidth of the transmitting/receiver transducer).

Our remarks will be limited here to the use of radiofrequency data to generate real-time integrated backscatter imaging.

Analysis of Radiofrequency Data

The analysis of unprocessed radio-frequency signals returning from myocardium has been used to quantify the extent of ultrasonic backscatter. Measurements of backscatter have been developed by detecting the signals reflected from a selected segment of myocardium. An electronic gate (typi-

J. E. Pérez: Department of Medicine, Washington University; Barnes-Jewish Hospital, St. Louis, Missouri 63110.

J. G. Miller: Department of Physics, Washington University, St. Louis, Missouri 63130.

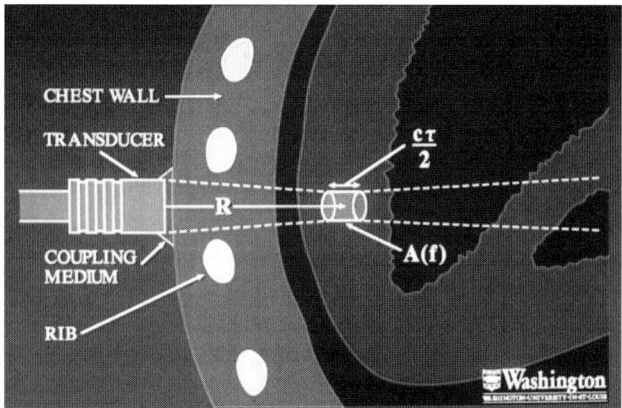

FIG. 1. Idealized model of midmyocardial segment analyzed for backscatter, with the segment defined by the duration of the pulse (CT/2) and the beam width (A(f)) at that point (R).

cally, 3 μsec in duration) and the beam width define the volume of tissue of interest for measurements, avoiding specular reflections from endocardial and epicardial surfaces (Fig. 1). Although integrated backscatter can be estimated in both the frequency and the time domain, the time domain approach provides a real-time estimate of tissue scattering by simply squaring and summing the time-domain signal to obtain an approximate value of integrated backscatter for clinical applications (3).

Integrated Backscatter Imaging

To obtain measurements of segmental ventricular myocardial quantitative acoustic properties contained in the image (M-mode or two-dimensional) a commercially available system computes in real time by a time-domain approach the integrated backscatter along each individual line of sight in the field of view. The dynamic range of the integrated backscatter processor is approximately 60 dB. The full dynamic range of the integrated backscatter data is mapped in 0.5-dB increments into the approximately 30-dB dynamic range available in the displayed video images. Thus, the image is created on the basis of integrated backscatter, and the image resolution is adequately preserved. This results in the creation of a quantitative, parametric image in which each picture element represents the value of relative integrated backscatter from data obtained in real time. The magnitude (in decibels) of the *cyclic* (diastolic-to-systolic) *variation of integrated backscatter* of a specific myocardial site is given by the logarithm of the ratio of the maximum to minimum backscattered energy (4). Over the range of transmit power employed in the system, the magnitude of cyclic variation of integrated backscatter is approximately independent of transmit power. Studies by investigators at Osaka University (5) have employed an approach to obtain fully calibrated integrated backscatter images that should facilitate longitudinal clinical investigations in groups of patients,

or serial observations in a single patient. In this approach, myocardial integrated backscatter is referenced to the backscatter power from the blood in the cavity in the vicinity of the myocardial tissue of interest.

Tissue Determinants of Ultrasonic Parameters

Various structural components of myocardium can influence its acoustic properties under physiologic and pathologic conditions. Tissue elements responsible for scattering (i.e., scatterers) represent local regions of acoustic impedance mismatch. The intensity of scattering depends on (i) the size, shape, and concentration of scatterers; (ii) the difference in intrinsic acoustic impedance of the scatterers relative to the medium in which they reside; and (iii) the spatial distribution of individual scatterers (e.g., random versus highly ordered). Intramyocardial elements responsible for scattering are much smaller than the wavelengths of ultrasound used for clinical imaging.

Extracellular Matrix

Collagen is a primary determinant of both scattering and attenuation of myocardial tissue (6). The relationship between collagen content and ultrasonic attenuation and backscatter in dogs after myocardial infarction has been determined. Backscatter, attenuation, and collagen content increased significantly in infarcted myocardium. Studies of human hearts at autopsy from patients with previous infarction demonstrated a monotonic relationship between integrated backscatter and collagen content. The myocardial echo amplitude measured in patients after cardiac transplantation significantly correlate with tissue collagen content, even within the physiologic range of collagen content.

Based on measurements of the frequency-dependence of scattering for normal myocardium, myocardial scatterers are thought to be comparable in size to cardiac myocytes. The relationship between scattering and the frequency (f) of insonification can be expressed by a power law in which backscatter increases approximately as f^3 for normal myocardium. Theoretically, scatterers that are much smaller than a wavelength of sound are characterized by f^4 (Rayleigh scattering), and scatterers much larger than the wavelength by f^0 (specular scattering). The reduction of the frequency dependence from approximately f^m to f^n, where $n < m$ in previously infarcted myocardium, indicates that the dominant myocardial scatterers are larger for infarcted than for normal myocardium consistent with pathologic replacement of normal myocytes by scar (7).

Electron microscopy studies of myocardium have shown that cardiac myocytes are invested externally by a complex collagen matrix that provides structural support. This microstructural arrangement of cells embedded in a collagen matrix may provide a sufficient local acoustic impedance mismatch to account for the ultrasonic scattering from normal myocardium.

Myocardial Fiber Orientation

Myocardial acoustic properties also are influenced by the predominant orientation of ventricular muscle fibers. Studies have demonstrated that transmural ventricular muscle fiber bands spiral from endocardium to epicardium such that the predominant orientation of endocardial fiber bands is nearly perpendicular to the orientation of epicardial fibers. The middle portion of the ventricular wall comprises mainly circumferentially oriented fiber bands. Studies have demonstrated that the magnitude of both ultrasonic attenuation and backscatter in excised heart tissue is highly dependent on the angle of insonification. Attenuation is maximal when sound waves propagate parallel to the major fiber orientation, and minimal if perpendicular to the fiber orientation. Ultrasonic backscatter, on the other hand, is maximal perpendicular to the fibers and minimal when parallel to the fiber axis.

Myocardial Blood Flow/Water Content

It has been well established that tissue water content and blood content both influence myocardial scattering and attenuation. Integrated backscatter increased by 200 percent after a brief washout with buffer solution in isolated heart preparations and returned to normal after perfusion with whole blood. Perfusion with buffer promoting tissue edema resulted in increased tissue wet weight that paralleled increases in integrated backscatter. Other studies reported minimal changes in integrated backscatter immediately following restoration of coronary artery blood flow after 1 hour of occlusion in dogs, associated with a lack of recovery of wall thickening after reperfusion. In other studies, myocardial blood flow was varied and cyclic variation showed little relationship to tissue blood flow. If reduction in coronary blood flow rate results in early manifestations of tissue ischemia, these can be detected by alterations in backscatter. Blunting of integrated backscatter cyclic variation occurs by reducing coronary flow rate by 50% in open-chest dogs, despite the absence of wall motion abnormalities. These results have been confirmed in clinical studies of transient ischemia where ultrasonic parameters became altered before mechanical dysfunction was evident.

Dynamic Scattering Properties

In intact hearts, there is a dynamic contribution of myocytes to the scattering process. As previously described, backscatter intensity varies throughout the cardiac cycle. For ultrasound incident approximately perpendicular to myofibers, maximal levels of scattering occur at end-diastole and minimal levels at end-systole (i.e., *cardiac cycle–dependent variation of integrated backscatter*). This has been widely confirmed in both experimental animals and human studies, with an average magnitude of approximately 5 dB for normal

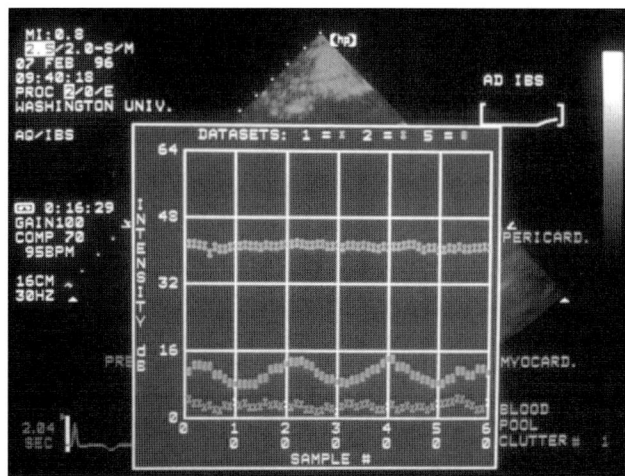

FIG. 2. Results of integrated backscatter (expressed in dB in the ordinate) versus time (60 frames, or 2.04 seconds in the abscissa) of data measured from the pericardium (strongest reflector in the heart), myocardium (showing the diastolic-to-systolic cyclic variation—higher near end-diastole), and blood pool signal clutter (close to zero dB).

myocardium (Fig. 2). Cyclic variation of backscatter decreases within seconds as a result of myocardial ischemia injury and recovers after reperfusion of injured but viable myocardial tissue in both experimental animals and humans. The magnitude and rate of change of cyclic variation of backscatter are related to intrinsic myocardial contractile performance, and they are greater in subendocardial than in subepicardial regions. Others have described a quantitative relationship between the cyclic variation of echo amplitude and the degree of segmental myocardial shortening in normals and patients with cardiomyopathy.

These observations indicate that acoustic properties of myocardium are influenced, but are not entirely determined by, the tissue mechanical function.

Integrated Backscatter Imaging for Endocardial Detection

Cardiac Function

Because quantitative characterization of myocardial acoustic properties via the measurement of tissue integrated backscatter entails the measurement (in dB) of the power along each radiofrequency line employing a relatively long integration time (3.2 μs) the images exhibit considerable reduction in noise (speckle). This property lends itself for facilitating the recognition between blood pool (very low scattering) and endocardium boundary (relatively much higher scattering) in each frame of the image (8) to allow on-line differentiation of blood pool cavity areas or volumes in real time (i.e., Acoustic Quantification, Hewlett-Packard, Andover, MA). Thus, the implementation of this approach opened a new line for investigations and clinical applications in echocardiography by removing the subjectivity of the visual interpretation of chamber size and function (ventricular

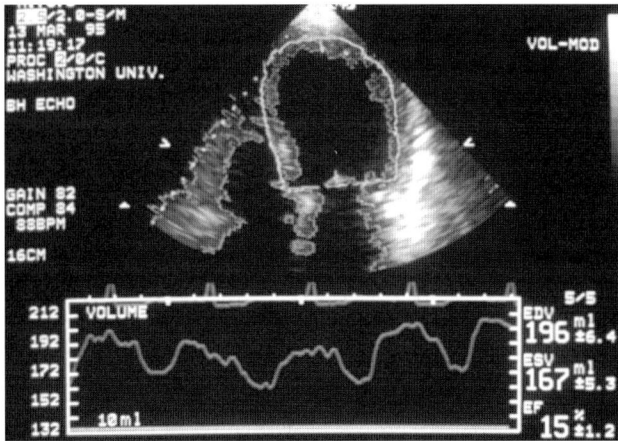

FIG. 3. On-line measurement of left ventricular volumes and ejection fraction (*EF*) by the method of Acoustic Quantification (Hewlett-Packard, Andover, MA), measuring the differences in scattering between blood pool and endocardium in real-time. The physiologic signal of the left ventricular volume over time is displayed for the apical four-chamber view in a patient with depressed function. *EDV*, end-diastolic volume; *ESV*, end-systolic volume.

and atrial) solely from the opinion of the echocardiographer, and incorporating the role of the sonographer in the laboratory acquiring the images under optimal conditions to obtain the physiologic cardiac measurements (volumes, ejection fraction) on-line beat-by-beat at the time of the examination (Fig. 3).

TISSUE ACOUSTIC PROPERTIES IN PATHOLOGY AND PATHOPHYSIOLOGY

Myocardial Ischemia/Infarction/Reperfusion

Early increases in regional echo amplitude are noted within seconds after coronary artery occlusion. Other investigators describe differences in regional echo amplitude by color encoding during the evolution of myocardial infarction in experimental animals.

In a series of studies utilizing quantitative analysis of radio-frequency signals, various aspects of the acoustic characteristics of ischemia in experimental animals have been delineated. The cyclic variation of ultrasonic integrated backscatter has been employed as a variable to assess ischemic tissue damage. Initial studies, subsequently confirmed, demonstrated that the pattern of cyclic variation of backscatter is promptly blunted by ischemia. The role of the absolute myocardial wall thickness after myocardial ischemia in the measured integrated backscatter suggested that increase in backscatter after ischemia was primarily related to decreases in wall thickness.

Transient blunting (during stress testing) and subsequent recovery of the septal backscatter power in patients with known anterior descending coronary artery disease has been documented. In addition, the phase (analogous to the delay

of cyclic variation) in the septum was increased transiently with subsequent normalization. Other studies have demonstrated that patients with acute myocardial infarction studied early after admission to a coronary care unit exhibit characteristic alterations in acoustic properties. A parameter closely related to the magnitude of cyclic variation was significantly reduced in infarcted as compared to normal myocardium and the phase was significantly delayed. The sensitivity, specificity, and accuracy of the tissue characterization criteria were comparable to those of conventional echocardiographic detection of wall motion abnormalities. Marked reduction of the cyclic variation of integrated backscatter induced by reduction of coronary blood flow rate by 50% was associated with regional asynergy in only 33% of the dogs. Ischemia induced by adenosine infusion in dogs with 75% reduction in coronary flow caused significant reductions in cyclic variation of integrated backscatter and increases in phase before any segmental dysfunction was evident. Transient, short-lasting myocardial ischemia was detected in patients with vasospastic angina provoked by ergonovine, in patients with coronary artery disease subjected to dipyridamole stress, and also in patients studied during coronary angioplasty. During transient ischemia, the myocardial region at risk exhibited increased mean echo amplitude that was not related to the degree of segmental myocardial dyssynergy induced. During angioplasty, elevation in myocardial gray levels (analogous to increased backscatter) was evident 10 seconds after occlusion at a time when no dyssynergy was detectable. In another study, myocardial gray levels were analyzed by transesophageal echocardiography in patients in whom myocardial ischemia occurred spontaneously and transiently during surgery. Ischemia was characterized by acute regional increases in echodensity and blunting of the cyclic variation of gray levels. Furthermore, there was no correlation between the extent of dyssynergy and the degree of blunting of the cyclic variation. Thus, alterations in myocardial acoustic properties due to acute ischemia actually precede, or, are more sensitive than, the attendant mechanical dysfunction.

Echocardiographic tissue characterization data suggest that viable myocardium can also be correctly identified based on acoustic analysis of the tissue (9). Initial experiments in dogs showed alterations in ultrasound backscatter following 20 minutes of coronary artery occlusion were reversed after 30 minutes of reperfusion. In other studies, viable myocardium demonstrated differences in mean echo amplitudes and skewness of gray level distributions compared to regions that were infarcted. The cardiac cycle-dependent variation in backscatter blunted by ischemia returns toward normal after reperfusion. Reversible myocardial injury was differentiated from irreversible injury measuring integrated backscatter dogs subjected to either 15 or 90 minutes of coronary artery occlusion. Ischemia of short duration increased values of integrated backscatter transiently with normalization after reperfusion. Thus, the degree of alterations in the cyclic variation of backscatter resulting from ischemia and the magnitude of subsequent recovery after reperfusion are not merely related to the level of segmental wall thickening. Similarly, studies have demonstrated in dogs and in patients that the cyclic variation of backscatter may recover after reperfusion at a time when wall motion and thickening abnormalities persist. Persistently dysfunctional myocardium after 10 minutes of coronary artery occlusion followed by reperfusion exhibits normalization of the cyclic variation pattern but not the phase, despite restoration of myocardial blood flow. In clinical studies, a causal relationship between coronary artery occlusion and blunting of myocardial echo amplitude cyclic variation has been found in patients undergoing coronary angioplasty. The reduction in the variation was completely reversed following balloon deflation. Thus, reperfused, viable, but "stunned" myocardium can be differentiated from necrotic tissue and myocardial viability can be assessed (Fig. 4) by ultrasound tissue characterization.

Progressive increases in echo image amplitude as displayed by a color-encoding technique have been noted during evolving infarction. Color encoding has been employed to detect regions of fibrosis in patients with remote myocardial infarction. Regions of myocardial infarction exhibit a decrease in the kurtosis (peakedness) of the echo amplitude distribution as compared to normal myocardium. Furthermore, integrated backscatter showed a substantial increase in remote experimental myocardial infarction. Fibrotic human myocardium is associated with both increased collagen content and also increased ultrasound integrated backscatter. Scarred myocardium lacks cyclic variation of integrated backscatter and exhibits relatively higher values of backscatter. In regions of completed infarction the cyclic variation of integrated backscatter is significantly diminished as compared to values from normal segments.

Cardiomyopathy

Experimental

Anthracycline-induced experimental cardiomyopathy is characterized by increases in ultrasound integrated backscatter associated with fibrosis. Acoustic abnormalities occur also in the spontaneous cardiomyopathy of the Syrian hamster, characterized as increased regional ultrasound backscatter within regions of calcification and fibrosis.

Dilated

Myocardial tissue in patients with dilated cardiomyopathy is characterized by increased time-averaged ultrasound backscatter and a reduction in the cyclic variation of backscatter. Others have noted increased echo brightness in patients with endomyocardial involvement due to hypereosinophilic cardiomyopathy. Patients with suspected dilated cardiomyopathy underwent endomyocardial biopsies that showed a significant correlation between percent integrated backscatter index and percent connective tissue area.

Hypertrophic

Patients with hypertrophic cardiomyopathy exhibit an unusual ("ground-glass") texture or bright echoes in the ventricular septal images. Studies with on-line radiofrequency analysis to obtain tissue reflectivity (analogous to integrated backscatter) of the septum and the posterior wall demonstrated that patients with hypertrophic cardiomyopathy had significantly higher values of backscatter than those of normals in the septum and in the posterior wall, independent of left ventricular wall thickness. In addition, patients with hypertrophic cardiomyopathy exhibit decreased values of cyclic variation of integrated backscatter in the septum as compared to normal controls. Myocardial integrated backscatter was increased in the endocardial half as compared to the epicardial half of the wall in patients with hypertrophic cardiomyopathy.

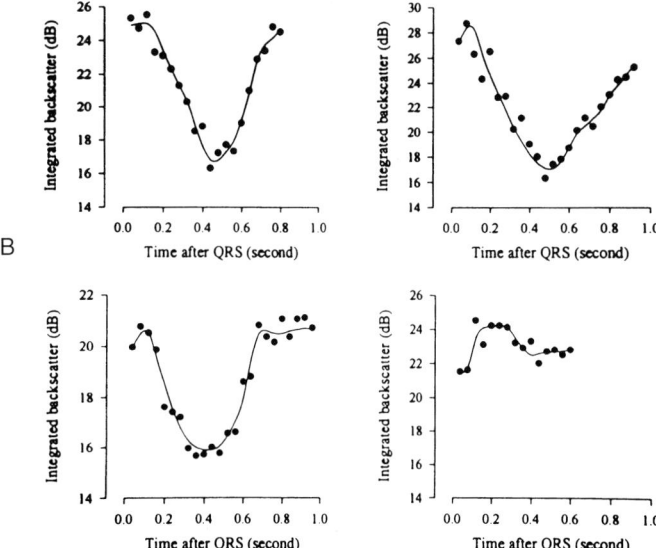

A,B

C,D

FIG. 4. Backscatter power curves obtained in control myocardial segment (**A**), in remote normally contracting segment from a coronary patient (**B**), from a dysfunction segment showing improvement after dobutamine (**C**), and from a persistently dysfunctional segment despite dobutamine (**D**). (From ref. 9, with permission.)

Diabetes Mellitus

In patients with insulin-dependent diabetes, ultrasonic tissue characterization detects changes possibly indicative of occult cardiomyopathy (10). In spite of normal ventricular systolic function cyclic variation of integrated backscatter was significantly reduced and its delay was prolonged in the patients with diabetes as compared to controls. Reduction of cyclic variation was greatest in these patients who had associated neuropathy, retinopathy and nephropathy. Independent reanalysis of this data has confirmed the validity of these results with excellent values of receiver-operator-characteristic area under the curve of approximately 0.9 for all acoustic parameters.

Arterial Hypertension

In hormotensive athletes, despite increases in left ventricular mass, there were no abnormalities in echo intensity or diastolic function. The cyclic variation of myocardial integrated backscatter was reduced in the septum of patients with uncomplicated pressure overload ventricular hypertrophy to a comparable extent, as was the case for patients with hypertrophic cardiomyopathy. The relation between wall thickness and tissue reflectivity has also been studied in open-chest pigs, but in the context of coronary artery occlusion and reperfusion. An inverse relationship was found between the value of end-systolic integrated backscatter and myocardial wall thickness in the experimental preparation in which tissue collagen content would not play a role.

In contrast, several studies suggest that increased myocardial thickness *per se* does not alter the acoustic properties of the tissue unless there are concomitant alterations in tissue composition or histology. Integrated backscatter of myocardium in athletes and in control subjects with sedentary lifestyle showed that in spite of significantly greater wall thickness in the athletes, values for myocardial integrated backscatter were similar for both groups. Athletes and patients with hypertrophic cardiomyopathy with similar wall thickness exhibited different values of myocardial backscatter. In elite senior athletes, as compared with normal age-matched controls with sedentary lifestyle, there were no significant differences with respect to tissue integrated backscatter, in spite of greater left ventricular mass in the athletes. In other patients with uncomplicated arterial hypertension, hypertrophy *per se* does not affect tissue acoustic parameters as indicators of myocardial structure (11). Integrated backscatter of the myocardium in patients with hypertension was similar to that of controls in spite of higher values of mean blood pressure and left ventricular mass index.

In summary, studies suggest that in the absence of ischemia or other confounding events, myocardial wall thickness may influence tissue acoustic properties only when as-

sociated with alterations in collagen content or gross morphologic alterations, such as in hypertrophic cardiomyopathy or arterial hypertension associated with aging.

CONCLUSIONS

Abundant experimental and clinical evidence supports the concept that ultrasound interacts differently with normal and abnormal cardiovascular tissue. Ultrasonic tissue characterization techniques have been shown by a variety of methods and different groups of investigators to be accurate in identifying acute myocardial ischemia, reperfusion, infarction, and tissue scar formation. Cardiomyopathies, intracardiac masses, and atherosclerotic plaque also can be characterized with quantitative ultrasonic tissue analysis. Clinical results published in a sustained fashion over the last 20 years support the potential applicability of noninvasive ultrasonic tissue characterization in the clinical setting.

REFERENCES

1. Miller JG, Pérez JE, Wickline SA, et al. Backscatter imaging and myocardial tissue characterization. *Proc IEEE Ultrason Symp* 1999;98: 1373–1383.
2. Miller JG, Pérez JE, Mottley JG, et al. Myocardial tissue characterization: an approach based on quantitative backscatter and attenuation. *Proc IEEE Ultrason Symp* 1983;1:782–793.
3. Pérez JE, Madaras EI, Sobel BE, et al. Quantitative myocardial characterization with ultrasound. *Automedica* 1984;5:201–218.
4. Miller JG, Yuhas DE, Mimbs JW, Dierker SB, et al. Ultrasonic tissue characterization: correlation between biochemical and ultrasonic indices of myocardial injury. *Proc IEEE Ultrason Proc* 1976;5:33–43.
5. Takiuchi S, Ito H, Iwakura K, et al. Ultrasonic tissue characterization predicts myocardial viability in early stage of reperfused acute myocardial infarction. *Circulation* 1998;97:356–362.
6. O'Donnell M, Mimbs JW, Miller JG. The relationship between collagen and ultrasonic backscatter in myocardial tissue. *J Acoust Soc Am* 1981;69:580–588.
7. Wear KA, Milunski MR, Wickline SA, et al. Differentiation between acutely ischemic myocardium and zones of completed infarction on the basis of frequency dependent backscatter. *J Acoust Soc Am* 1989; 85:2634–2641.
8. Pérez JE, Waggoner AD, Barzilai B, et al. On-line assessment of ventricular function by automatic boundary detection and ultrasonic backscatter imaging. *J Am Coll Cardiol* 1992;19:313–320.
9. Pasquet A, D'Hondt AM, Melin JA, et al. Relation of ultrasonic tissue characterization with integrated backscatter to contractile reserve in chronic left ventricular ischemic dysfunction. *Am J Cardiol* 1998;81: 68–74.
10. Pérez JE, McGill JB, Santiago JV, et al. Abnormal myocardial acoustic properties in diabetic patients and their correlation with the severity of disease. *J Am Coll Cardiol* 1992;19:1154–1162.
11. DiBello V, Talarico L, Picano E, et al. Increased myocardial echo density in left ventricular pressure and volume overload in human aortic valvular disease: An ultrasonic tissue characterization study. *J Am Soc Echocardiogr* 1997;10:320–329.

CHAPTER 9

Three-dimensional Echocardiography

Jiefen Yao, H. Joachim Nesser,
and Natesa G. Pandian

Major advances have occurred in the discipline of echocardiography both in technology and applications during the past three decades (1,2). With the use of two-dimensional and Doppler echocardiographic techniques, better delineation of cardiac pathology and precise determination of hemodynamic and flow abnormalities have become possible. Every part of the heart and every facet of its function and flow, however, are three-dimensional; with two-dimensional evaluation the examiner has to mentally reconstruct three-dimensional images of the specific regions of the heart in order to evaluate its overall performance or abnormalities. The realization that optimal examination of the heart should be done in a multidimensional mode led to efforts directed toward three-dimensional echocardiography.

The development of three-dimensional echocardiography dates back to the early 1970s and great progress has been achieved since then (3–6). In its early stage, three-dimensional echocardiography was mainly applied to volume measurement of the ventricles. By manually tracing the cardiac borders from multiple two-dimensional images, static wireframe images are reconstructed that demonstrated the shape of the ventricles and provided volume information (7–9). Recent developments in sequential and real-time image acquisition and employment of computer interpolation algorithms now allow volume-rendered data collection, three-dimensional image reconstruction, and dynamic display of images of the heart. Such advances allow for depiction of cardiac structures in their full dimensions and accurate quantification of volumes, areas, and dimension of any part of the heart (6).

METHODS

Real-time Three-dimensional Echocardiography

The ideal technique for three-dimensional echocardiography would be to view the heart in all its dimensions on-line. A real-time volumetric ultrasound imaging system is under development that aids in on-line three-dimensional data acquisition. This system consists of a phase array transducer steered in a pyramidal volumetric format and an image processing unit (10,11). With the use of this system, multiple orthogonal cross-sectional views of the heart can be displayed simultaneously on-line (Fig. 1). A dynamic volumetric data set of the heart can be achieved at one heartbeat from a given acoustic window. Reconstruction of three-dimensional images is performed off-line after postprocessing of the data. Quantitative measurement of chamber volume or myocardial mass is also carried out off-line. This mode of three-dimensional echocardiography could be especially useful in pharmacologic or exercise stress tests when ischemic wall motion abnormalities are often transient. If harmonic imaging mode is incorporated, this approach could also be optimal for myocardial perfusion study in combination with ultrasound contrast agent administration. The disadvantages of this technique at the present time include suboptimal image quality and lack of Doppler facilities. So far, this method has been applied in surface examination only. The size of the probe needs to be minimized for transesophageal use.

J. Yao: Cardiology Division, Department of Medicine, New England Medical Center; Tufts University School of Medicine, Boston, Massachusetts 02111.
H. J. Nesser: Department of Medicine, Division of Cardiology, KH d. Elisabethinen Hospital, A-4010 Linz, Austria.
N. G. Pandian: Tufts University School of Medicine; Cardiovascular Imaging and Hemodynamic Laboratory, Tufts-New England Medical Center, Boston, Massachusetts 02111.

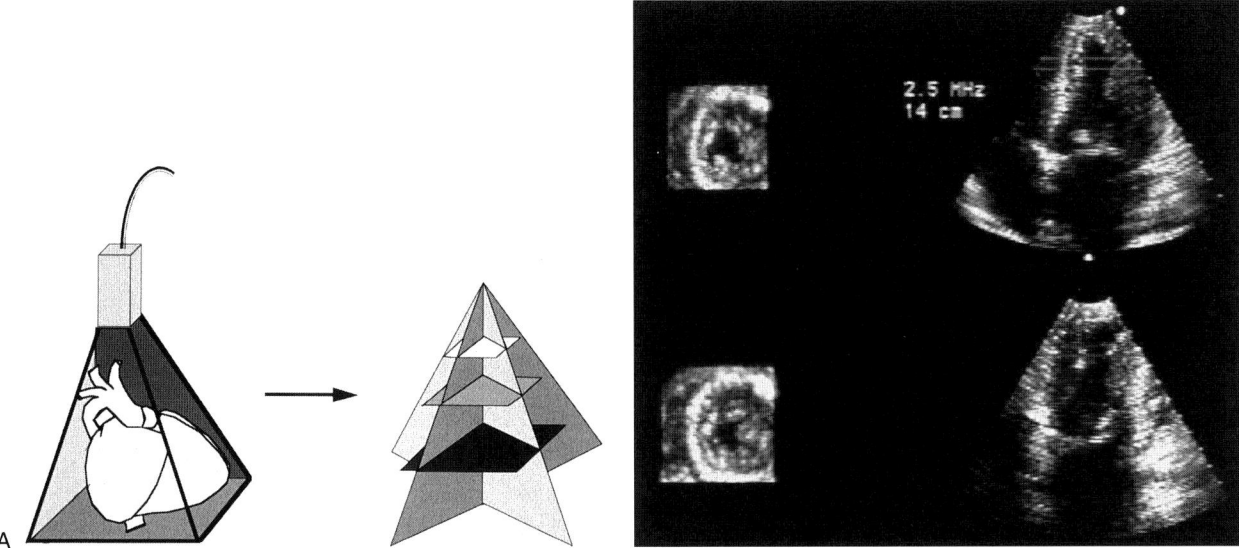

FIG. 1. A: Schematic showing the basic principle of real-time three-dimensional echocardiography and on-line display of orthogonal two-dimensional views derived from the volumetric scanning of the heart. **B:** An example of multiple two-dimensional display using real-time three-dimensional echocardiography. With the volumetric probe at the apical window, two short-axis views (**left**), apical four-chamber view (**upper right**) and apical two-chamber view (**lower right**) are displayed simultaneously. (Courtesy of Masood Ahmad, M.D., University of Texas at Galveston, Galveston, Texas.)

Three-dimensional Echocardiography Using Sequential Data Collection

Using conventional ultrasound machines, two-dimensional images of the heart are collected to derive three-dimensional data sets. Though various methods have been employed, the essential steps of three-dimensional reconstruction are as follows: (i) data acquisition, (ii) data processing, and (iii) three-dimensional image rendering and display.

Data Acquisition Methods

Three-dimensional reconstruction requires accurate location of each two-dimensional imaging plane to its spatial position in the heart. Temporal information has to be considered for correct registration of the images collected through sequential cardiac phases. Images can be collected either randomly or sequentially.

Random data acquisition, also known as free-hand imaging, requires a spatial sensing device (magnetic or acoustic sensors) to detect and register the location of the transducer and, thus, the imaging plane (12,13). Images can be obtained either at one acoustic window (by tilting the probe) or from different acoustic windows. Therefore, limitation by restricted or suboptimal acoustic windows is minimized. However, care must be taken to avoid big gaps between imaging planes for accurate three-dimensional reconstruction. This mode of data acquisition has yielded accurate measurements of chamber volumes. By contouring the two-dimensional images, wire-frame or surface-rendered three-dimensional images can be reconstructed. Recently, volume-rendered three-dimensional image reconstruction from free-hand imaging has been realized.

Sequential data acquisition obviates the need of a spatial sensor by acquiring images at equally paced intervals. The intervals between acquired views can be controlled manually, mechanically, or by computer. A simple approach is manually controlled data acquisition of the left ventricle from three apical views (apical four-chamber, two-chamber, and long-axis views) for volume and function analysis. With a mechanical caliber device, images of the heart are obtained in a rotational manner at predefined angles (14). The most sophisticated mode of sequential data acquisition is controlled by computer, in which the transducer or the imaging plane is moved at equal intervals in a predetermined fashion, such as linear, rotational, or fan-like scanning modes (Fig. 2). Using linear scanning, parallel equidistant images of the heart are collected. This can be done by mounting a surface probe or a transesophageal probe onto a computer-controlled carriage device. The total range of scanning and the distance between the scan planes can be predefined according to the region of interest and the requirement of spatial resolution of the three-dimensional data set (15,16). Using rotational scanning, images of the heart are collected by rotating the transducer in a semicircle of 180 degrees around the central axis of the imaging plane. This can be realized either with a computer-controlled rotational device adapted to a conventional surface transducer or with a multiplane transesophageal or transthoracic probe (6,17–20). This mode of data acquisition needs a relatively smaller acoustic window. Using fan-like scanning, images of the heart are collected by moving the ultrasound transducer in a fan-like arc at prescribed angles, in surface or transesophageal approaches. Both the total angles of the arc and the intervals between the scan planes can be prescribed (21). Se-

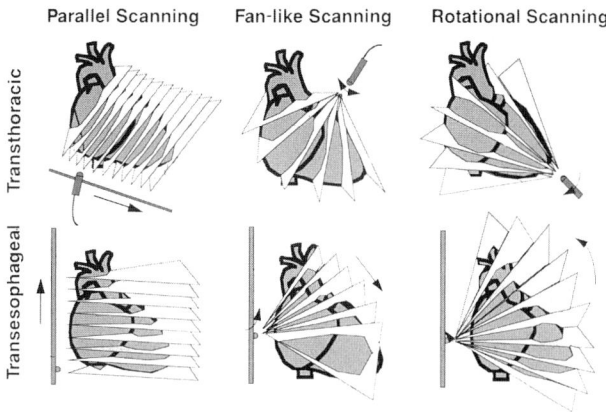

Parallel Scanning   Fan-like Scanning   Rotational Scanning

Transthoracic

Transesophageal

FIG. 2. Schematic drawing showing various modes of three-dimensional echocardiographic data acquisition (*parallel, fan-like,* and *rotational scanning*) with transthoracic (**upper row**) and transesophageal (**lower row**) approaches.

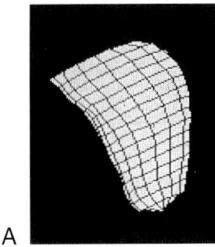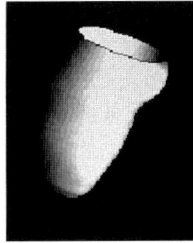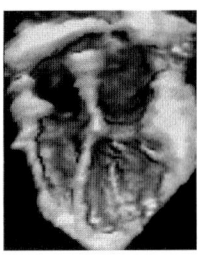

A   B,C

FIG. 4. Examples of three-dimensional reconstruction in (**A**) wire-frame, (**B**) surface-rendered, and (**C**) volume-rendered image formats.

quential data acquisition employs both electrocardiogram and respiration gating (Fig. 3). The former is useful in temporal registration of the cardiac images by excluding images with irregular R-R intervals on the electrocardiogram. Respiration gating is used to minimize the artifacts caused by respiration-related movement of the heart. In most patients, image acquisition takes only about 3 minutes.

Image Processing and Three-dimensional Reconstruction

Two-dimensional images collected in the above mentioned fashion need to be processed before three-dimen-

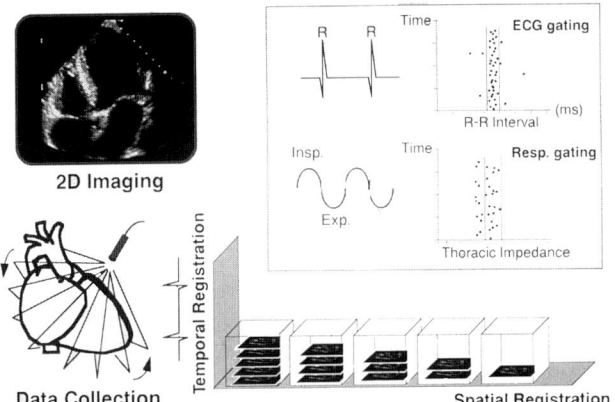

2D Imaging

Data Collection

Temporal Registration

Spatial Registration

Time   ECG gating
R   R
R-R Interval   (ms)

Insp.   Time   Resp. gating

Exp.

Thoracic Impedance

FIG. 3. Schematic description of spatial and temporal registration of images acquired in a rotational scanning format using electrocardiographic (ECG) and respiratory gating. Two-dimensional images are acquired sequentially with the probe steered through 0 degrees to 180 degrees (**left**). Acquisition of images is determined by ECG gating and respiratory gating using thoracic impedance (**upper right**). The acquired images from each phase of the cardiac cycle are then registered temporally as represented on *y* axis and images from each step of the acquisition are registered spatially as shown on *x* axis (**lower right**).

sional image reconstruction is realized (Fig. 4). Wire-frame images are derived from reconstruction of manually traced cardiac borders. Although it has been used in structures like the mitral valve or vegetation, it is mainly used for cardiac chambers during volume quantitation (22,23). A surface can be applied to the wire-frame image. While this method displays the shape of the subject of interest, it does not provide anatomical detail of the cardiac structures. Manual tracing of the two-dimensional images can be time-consuming and inaccurate.

Surface-rendered images are formed by extracting the contour of the structure from three-dimensional data and are displayed, in a solid appearance, as the surface of the object that faces the observer. Shadowing techniques are used to create a three-dimensional perspective (24). Information about the tissue beneath the surface is missing.

Volume-rendered three-dimensional image reconstruction engages all the information of the cardiac structures within the data set (6). This mode of reconstruction usually employs three-dimensional data collected from computer-controlled sequential imaging or from real-time volumetric imaging. Postprocessing includes digitization (if video signals are acquired instead of digital signals), spatial and temporal registration, and geometric transformation (when images are acquired in nonlinear fashion, e.g., data from rotational or fan-like scanning needs to be converted into an isotropic cubic data set). The computer fills gaps between two-dimensional images with different interpolation algorithms for different acquisition modes. Then the pixels in two-dimensional images are transformed into voxels in a three-dimensional data set. These volumetric data can be electronically dissected in any orientation, and, therefore, the anatomy of the heart can be studied comprehensively in a dynamic mode. Three-dimensional projections of the heart in either conventional or unconventional orientations employed in two-dimensional echocardiography or those mimicking the surgeons' views are easily obtained (25,26). Using cutting planes away from the structure to be observed, *en face* views that are unavailable by conventional two-dimensional echocardiography, can be reconstructed and displayed.

Anyplane Two-dimensional Imaging

Besides three-dimensional images, novel two-dimensional views can be extracted as well from the volumetric data set (27). Limitations in acoustic access to optimal cutting planes and spatial registration of individual images with conventional two-dimensional echocardiography are overcome by three-dimensional echocardiography. It is possible to select any desired cutting plane of the heart from a volumetric three-dimensional data set. Innumerable cross-sectional views of the heart, which could be difficult or physically impossible to obtain from conventional precordial or transesophageal acoustic windows, can be computed from three-dimensional data set and be displayed dynamically. These images can be reconstructed individually or collectively using various reconstruction algorithms, such as parallel, equidistant tomographic views, orthogonal views, or revolving views (e.g., multiple longitudinal views of the left ventricle). These secondarily derived cross-sectional images aid in a systematic review of the cardiac structures, better evaluation of morphology and function of a given region, and selection of optimal cutting planes as well as accurate quantitation of the volume of a selected region.

CLINICAL APPLICATIONS OF THREE-DIMENSIONAL ECHOCARDIOGRAPHY

Valvular Diseases

Visualization of Valve Morphology

Three-dimensional echocardiography provides unique views useful in delineating the morphologic changes in diseased cardiac valves (25,28–32). Without cutting through a valve, three-dimensional reconstruction may provide *en face* views of the valve as if it is being observed from a distance, unlike two-dimensional methods in which the imaging plane has to cut through the valve. All leaflets and their commissures can be visualized simultaneously in a dynamic mode. Each valve can be observed from above or below, e.g., mitral and tricuspid valves can be observed from the atria and the ventricles, while aortic and pulmonary valves can be observed from the ventricles and the aorta or pulmonary artery. In case of mitral or aortic valve stenosis, not only the thickening of the leaflets, but also fusion of the commissures, the opening area of the valve, and the shape of the opening are well appreciated (Fig. 5). In addition to

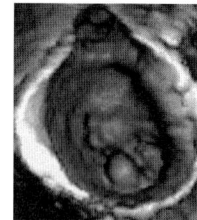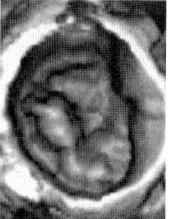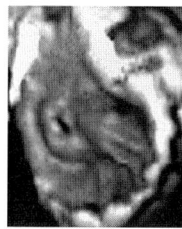

FIG. 6. Various examples of mitral valve prolapse viewed from the left atrium. **Left:** The image on the left shows a prolapse located at the posterior scallop of the posterior mitral leaflet. **Middle:** The image in the middle demonstrates a more severe prolapse of the posterior mitral leaflet that involves posterior and middle scallops. **Right:** The image on the right shows a flail posterior mitral leaflet. The regurgitant orifice can also be seen.

such views, the valvular apparatus can be visualized in any orientation including longitudinal and tangential projections. Such an examination serves to define the pathology better, especially when the shape of a valvular opening is irregular and needs to be measured. In case of mitral valve prolapse, it is sometimes difficult to decide the exact location of the prolapsing portion of the valve using two-dimensional echocardiography. This is overcome by three-dimensional reconstruction, which demonstrates the prolapse as a depression on the ventricular side and a protrusion on the atrial side, the latter similar to the surgeon's view (Fig. 6). By providing accurate information of the location and extension of the prolapse, it can be helpful to the surgeon in choosing patients for valve repair and designing specific repair procedures. Not only the valves, but also the subvalvular abnormalities and the annulus of the valves can be better evaluated with three-dimensional echocardiography (33–36). Three-dimensional echocardiographic study of the dynamic movement and shape changes of the mitral and tricuspid annuli has provided insights into the mechanism of functional mitral and tricuspid regurgitation. The physiological properties of the annuli learned from these studies could be valuable for improving the design of artificial annular rings. Three-dimensional image reconstruction and display of prosthetic valves may provide useful information on their performance (Fig. 7). Three-dimensional echocardiography correlates

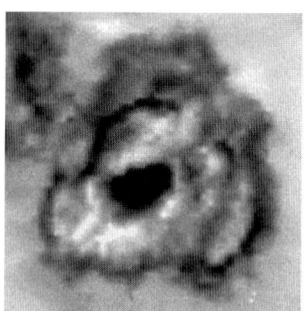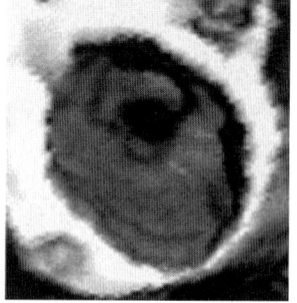

FIG. 5. Three-dimensional images of a stenotic mitral valve viewed from left ventricle (**left**) and left atrium (**right**).

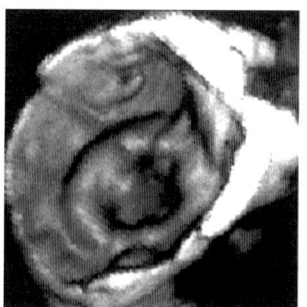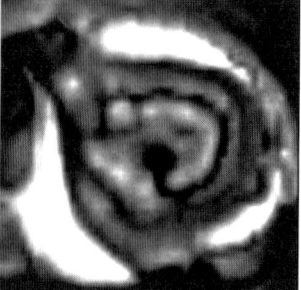

FIG. 7. Three-dimensional echocardiographic images as viewed from the left atrium obtained from patients with St. Jude (**left**) and Bjork-Shiley (**right**) prosthetic mitral valves.

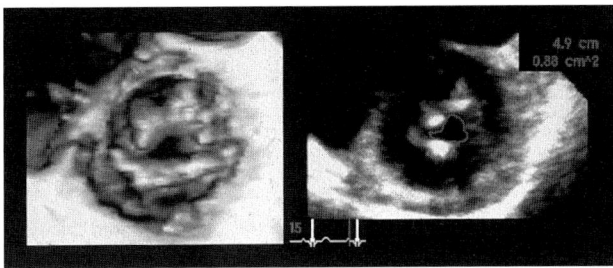

FIG. 8. Side-by-side display of a three-dimensional image (**left**) and tomographic two-dimensional image (**right**) is useful in guiding the placement of the optimal cutting plane within a three-dimensional data set and planimetry of the valve area.

closely with surgical findings of valvular endocarditis in recognition of number, site, and size of vegetations, perforations of valvular leaflets, and perivalvular abscesses. Importantly, three-dimensional imaging delineates the extent of valve abscesses and their relation to adjacent structures.

Quantitation of Valve Area

The accuracy of planimetry in obtaining valve areas using two-dimensional echocardiography could be limited by difficulties in aligning the imaging plane properly, due to physical constraints by the acoustic windows and the probe orientation and in the setting of deformed orifices (35). However, a cutting plane can be placed anywhere or in any direction within a volumetric data set, free of the position and orientation of the imaging probe. For example, short-axis views of the mitral valve or aortic valve can be reconstructed from data acquired at the apical window. Side-by-side display of an *en face* three-dimensional image of a stenotic valve can be used as guidance for accurate selection of the cutting plane at the tip of the valve for planimetry of the orifice area (Fig. 8). When the level of the smallest opening of a stenotic valve is difficult to decide, such as in a severely calcified valve or a tunnel-shaped stenotic valve, multiple parallel cutting planes at different levels of the valve provide data on valve narrowing. Measurements are taken at various levels to obtain the correct area (Fig. 9) (37,38).

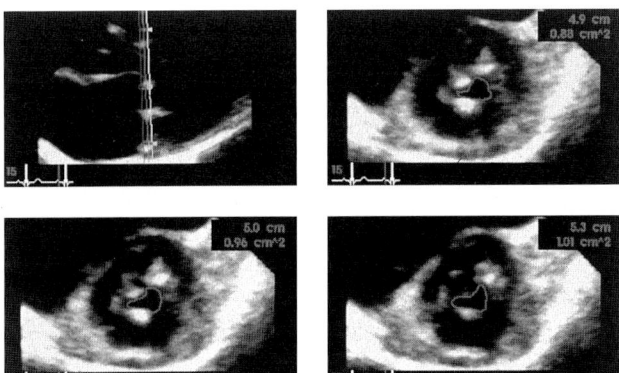

FIG. 9. Multiple paraplane images of a stenotic mitral valve for selection of the optima measurement of the valve area.

Three-dimensional Reconstruction of Color Doppler Flow Jets

When combined with color Doppler flow imaging, intracardiac flow jets with relatively high velocities, such as regurgitant jets or intracardiac shunt, can be reconstructed and displayed in three dimensions (39–43). Acquisition of color Doppler flow images is similar to that of B-mode images. The original two-dimensional color Doppler images can be transferred as video signals or digital signals and postprocessed for three-dimensional reconstruction. Video signals of color Doppler flow imaging are digitized in gray-scale or in color-encoded format during postprocessing. If images are digitized in gray-scale format only, three-dimensional images of blood flow jets are reconstructed and displayed in gray-scale or in pseudocolor formats (encoded by video intensity). Three-dimensional data of color Doppler flow images acquired in digital format do not need color transformation, so the voxels may contain the original colors of red, green, blue, yellow, and orange seen in two-dimensional color Doppler images. Thus, the flow jets within such a volumetric data set also retain the original digital information of its velocity and direction (Fig. 10; see also Color Plate 8 following page 294). The dynamic three-dimensional display of an intracardiac jet helps in better appreciation and understanding of its site of origin, spatial distribution, and morphology, especially in cases of eccentric jets, multiple jets from one origin, or interactive jets from different origins (Fig. 11). It also provides a unique view of the proximal flow convergence of a given jet and an opportunity to study the shape and real surface area of the flow convergence zone (Fig. 12) (39). Since a three-dimensional data set of a flow jet obtained with the imaging planes parallel to the flow direction can be used to reconstruct cross-sectional images perpendicular to the flow, cross-sectional area of the vena contracta of a flow can be measured accurately from three-dimensional echocardiography. Coupled with continuous-wave Doppler data for time velocity integrals, flow rate can be calculated more accurately than when obtained by two-dimensional examination, which requires many assumptions about the shape of flow jets. Using multiple tomographic cutting planes, the volume of a regurgitant jet can be measured as well (Fig. 13). Three-dimensional echocardiography has the potential to improve accuracy in the assessment of the severity of valvular regurgitation and in quantitation of the regurgitant volume.

Ischemic Heart Disease

Two-dimensional echocardiography is already playing an important role in the diagnosis and evaluation of coronary artery disease. Limitations exist in two-dimensional methods in that geometric assumptions have to be employed for measurements of chamber volumes (and thus ventricular function), and difficulty exists in some patients in getting true longitudinal and short-axis views of the left ventricle (2).

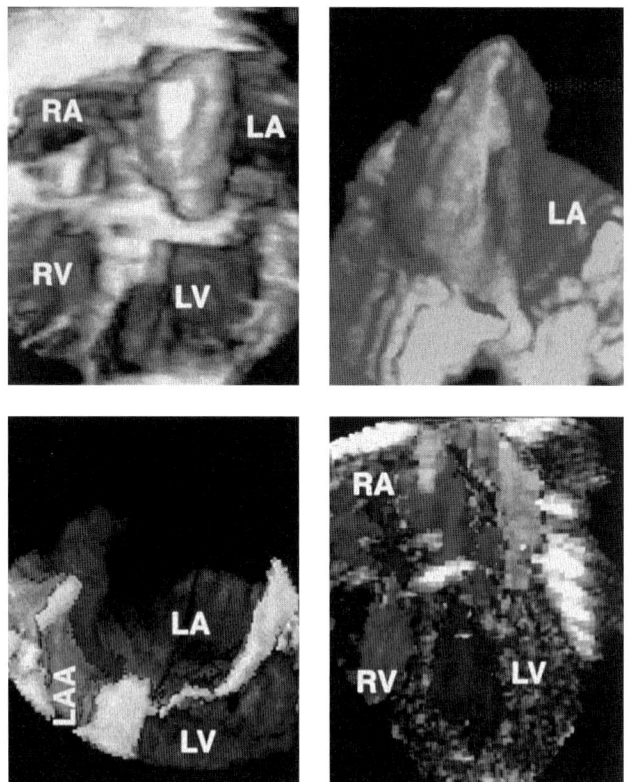

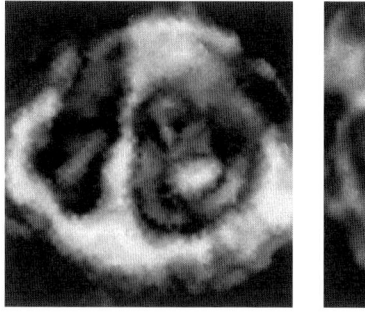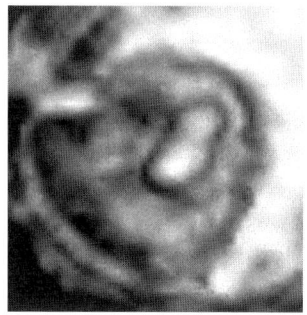

FIG. 12. Three-dimensional reconstruction of proximal flow convergence zones demonstrates various shapes of the flow convergence zones of mitral regurgitation flow when viewed from the left ventricle.

Three-dimensional echocardiography overcomes these limitations and has been shown to be accurate not only in measurements of ventricular volumes and global function, but also in evaluation and quantitation of regional wall motion abnormalities and myocardial perfusion defects. Incremental information may be obtained from three-dimensional data in patients with complications of myocardial infarction on location and size of aneurysm, pseudoaneurysm, necrotic ventricular septal defect, or mural thrombus and on the mechanism of mitral or tricuspid regurgitation caused by

FIG. 10. Images demonstrating various display formats of three-dimensional color Doppler data obtained in patients with mitral regurgitation. Images acquired with video signals can be transferred into gray-scale images (**upper left**). The gray-scale images can also be encoded with pseudo-colors depending on their video intensity (**upper right**). Video signals of color Doppler images transferred and digitized can be used to reconstruct three-dimensional images in gray-scale (for cardiac tissue) and red or blue (for flow jets) colors. Images in different colors can be displayed simultaneously or individually. In this example (**lower left**), the blue flow signals were discarded to highlight the mitral regurgitation jet in red. Three-dimensional color Doppler flow reconstruction from digital data retains all the original color in the image (**lower right**). *RA*, right atrium; *LA*, left atrium; *RV*, right ventricle; *LV*, left ventricle; *LAA*, left atrial appendage. (See also Color Plate 8 following page 294.)

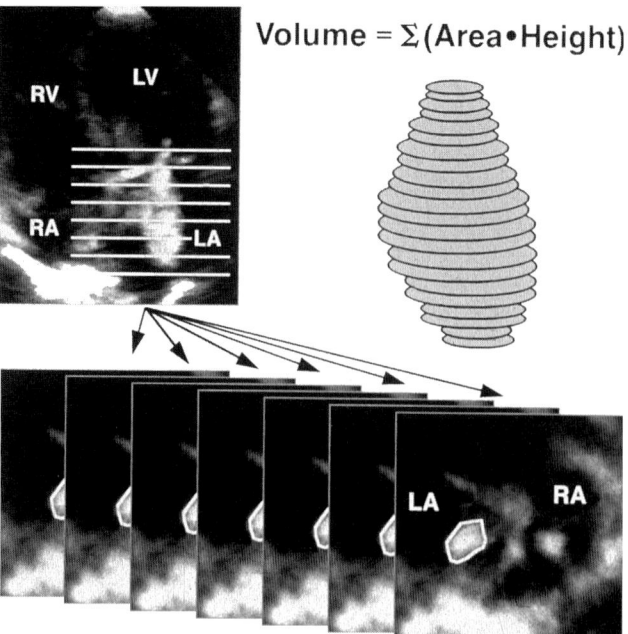

Volume = Σ(Area•Height)

FIG. 13. Schematic display of volume measurement of a mitral regurgitant jet from a three-dimensional data set. The **upper left** is a reference image in a four-chamber format showing a mitral regurgitant jet and placement of the cutting planes. The regurgitant jet on each cross-sectional view is traced (**bottom**). With known slice thickness, the volume of the jet on each slice is obtained. The summation of volumes on all slices yields in the total volume of the jet (**upper right**).

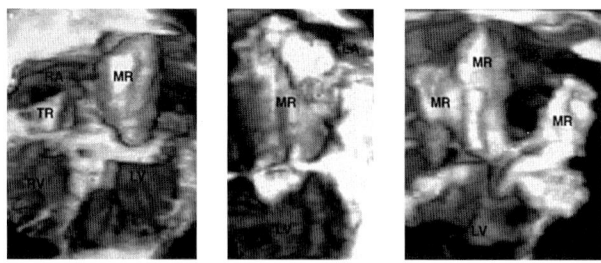

FIG. 11. Three-dimensional images of mitral regurgitant jets: central jet (**left**), eccentric jet (**middle**), and multiple jets (**right**). *RA*, right atrium; *LA*, left atrium; *RV*, right ventricle; *LV*, left ventricle; *MR*, mitral regurgitant jet; *TR*, tricuspid regurgitant jet.

dysfunction or rupture of papillary muscles or chordae tendinae.

Ventricular Volume and Function

Three-dimensional echocardiographic measurements of the left and right ventricular volumes and function have shown good correlations with angiography, magnetic resonance imaging, established two-dimensional methods, and anatomical measurements (12,13,22,23,44–47). A ventricle within a three-dimensional data set can be sectioned into multiple parallel, equidistant shot-axis slices of prescribed thickness at end-systole and end-diastole. Its volume is calculated by endocardial tracing of each slice and summation of the voxels included in the traced area, either manually or automatically by border detection methods. Stroke volume and ejection fraction is derived from the end-systolic and end-diastolic volumes of the ventricle (48). Since no geometric assumption is involved in volume measurement from three-dimensional echocardiography, distorted shapes of the ventricle do not affect the accuracy of the measurement. Therefore, it is particularly useful in volume and function evaluation of aneurysmal left ventricle and right ventricle.

Regional Wall Motion

Regional wall motion abnormality is a hallmark of ischemic heart disease. The geometric distribution of regional wall motion abnormalities varies from patient to patient because of the variation in coronary artery anatomy and in the location of the obstructive lesions. Two-dimensional echocardiography employs only a few standard-cutting planes of the left ventricle. The global extent of wall motion abnormalities has to be extrapolated from these incomplete views of the ventricle. In order to assess the location and extension of regional wall motion abnormalities, the left ventricle has to be arbitrarily divided into a number of segments or representative territories of the major coronary arteries. Therefore, the exact mass of ischemic or infarct myocardium cannot be accurately quantified.

When a volumetric data set of the whole left ventricle is acquired, three-dimensional echocardiography is able to demonstrate the true extent of global and regional contraction abnormalities by reconstruction of either dynamic three-dimensional images or multiple cross-sectional views of the left ventricle (Fig. 14) (49,50). Regional myocardial mass and the total left ventricular mass can be quantified without any geometric assumption. The principle for quantifying myocardial mass is similar to that for quantifying chamber volumes. After the left ventricle is sectioned into multiple parallel, equidistant short-axis slices, the extent of dysfunctional myocardium on each slice is examined in a dynamic mode. The 'myocardial region with abnormal wall motion is traced. The volume of the myocardium with wall motion abnormalities is summed up from all slices, and its mass is calculated from the volume and the specific gravity of the

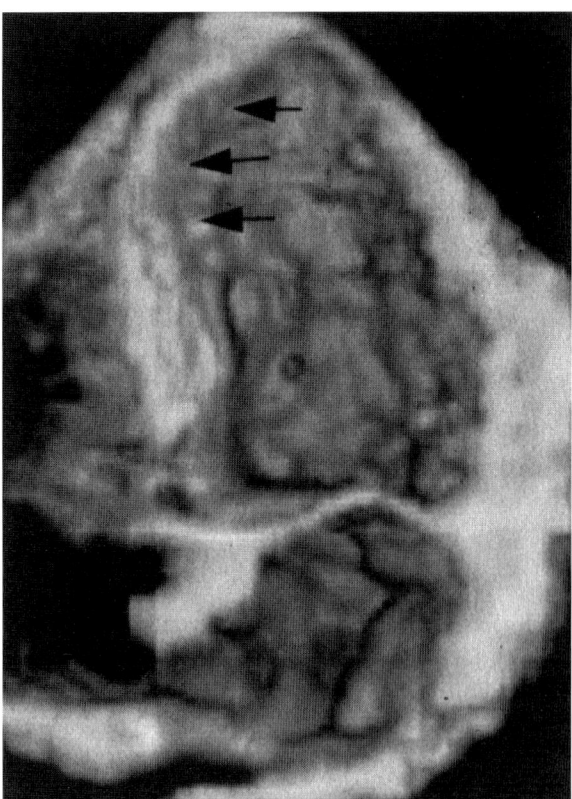

FIG. 14. Three-dimensional reconstruction of left ventricle for visual evaluation of global and regional wall motion abnormalities (*arrows*).

myocardium. If the total myocardial mass of the left ventricle is measured, the percent of left ventricle involved in wall motion abnormalities can be calculated as well. Being able to display multiple cross-sectional views of the left ventricle on-line simultaneously, real-time three-dimensional echocardiography can be very useful in stress echocardiography in studying regional wall motion in a real synchronized manner and in detecting transient ischemia. It has the potential to shorten the duration of the test.

Myocardial Perfusion

A recent advance in echocardiography, due to rapid developments in transpulmonary contrast agents (microbubbles) and innovations in ultrasound imaging modalities (such as harmonic imaging, power Doppler tissue imaging, pulse inversion harmonic imaging, etc.), is myocardial perfusion imaging using intravenous ultrasound contrast (51). Three-dimensional reconstruction has been used successfully in experimental studies of myocardial perfusion abnormalities during acute ischemia and after reperfusion therapy (52,53). Three-dimensional contrast echocardiographic data are acquired during cavity opacification and myocardial enhancement following intravenous administration of contrast microbubbles. Real-time three-dimensional imaging could be useful in detecting transient perfusion abnormalities with a single bolus of contrast agent. More experience has been gained with reconstructed three-dimensional echocardiography in which the images are usually acquired using transient imaging with trigger intervals of every cardiac cycle at end-systole or end-diastole. Depending on data acquisition time, slow single bolus administration, multiple bolus injections, or continuous infusion of intravenous contrast agent may be necessary. Harmonic imaging is used to improve the signal-to-noise ratio of the contrast enhanced myocardial perfusion images.

There are various ways to display and quantify contrast-enhanced three-dimensional myocardial perfusion abnormalities (54). One way is to reconstruct secondary cross-sectional views of the left ventricle, using anyplane, para-plane or revolving-plane methods to display contrast enhancement of the myocardium in free views, tomographic short-axis views or longitudinal views. The hypoperfused myocardium demonstrates lack of signal enhancement by contrast or remains dark, while the normally perfused myocardium becomes brighter (Fig. 15). The hypoperfused myocardial mass can be quantified by contouring the hypoperfused region on short-axis views of the left ventricle, similar to quantitation of dysfunctional mass. A traced region can be applied with a volumetric label and can be extracted from

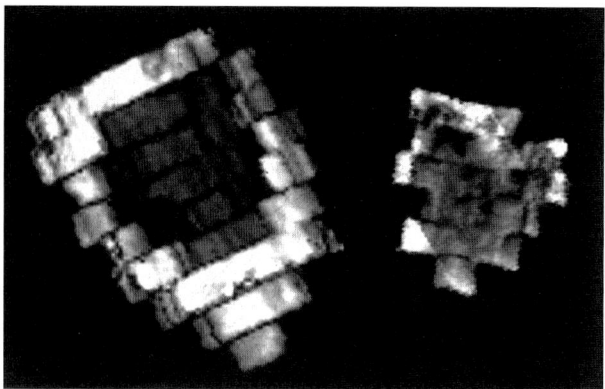

FIG. 16. Three-dimensional reconstruction and display of the normally perfused (**left**) and hypoperfused (**right**) myocardial regions extracted from a three-dimensional data set.

the whole data set. The extracted region can be reconstructed in a three-dimensional image. By applying different labels, the perfused and nonperfused myocardium can be extracted and reconstructed separately in three-dimensional images, facilitating visual appraisal of the location, shape, and size of the hypoperfused zone (Fig. 16). By aligning the tomographic short-axis views of the left ventricle in a "bulls-eye" format, with the apex in the center and the basal region in the periphery, perfusion abnormalities of the whole left ventricle can be portrayed in a single image. Not only can the site, size, and shape of the hypoperfused region be easily appreciated, the mass of the hypoperfused myocardium can be rapidly quantified. This is done by laying a grid over the bulls-eye image to divide the left ventricular myocardium into numerous segments (Fig. 17). The percentage of the left ventricle involved in hypoperfusion is obtained simply by counting the number of sectors with perfusion abnormalities and dividing it by the known total number of sectors of the left ventricle (55). Three-dimensional echocardiography has shown accurate measurement of the myocardial mass at risk during accurate ischemia and infarct mass with or without reperfusion procedures (52,56).

Three-dimensional Reconstruction of Coronary Arteries

Proximal lesions in the coronary arteries are responsible for many major cardiac events. Reconstruction of the proxi-

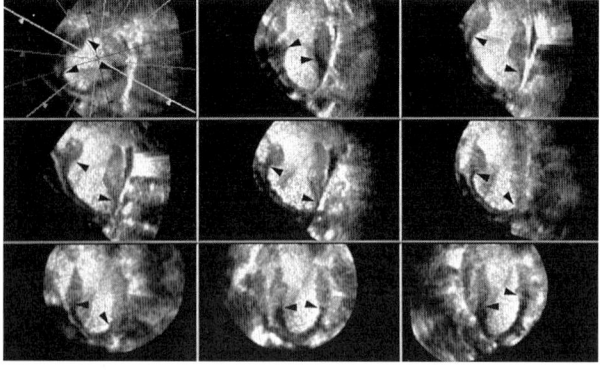

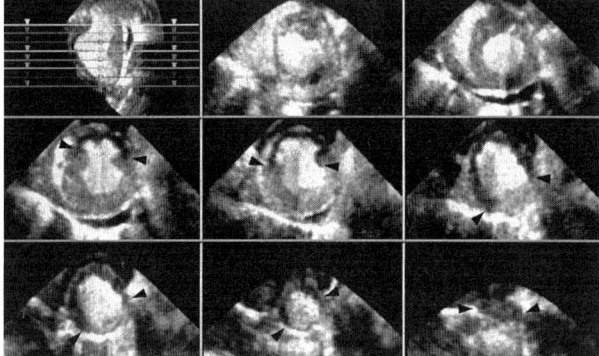

A

B

FIG. 15. Longitudinal (**A**) and short-axis (**B**) views of the left ventricle reconstructed from a three-dimensional contrast echocardiographic data set obtained from an experimental study following occlusion of the anterior descending coronary artery, demonstrating the location and extension of myocardial perfusion abnormalities (*arrows*).

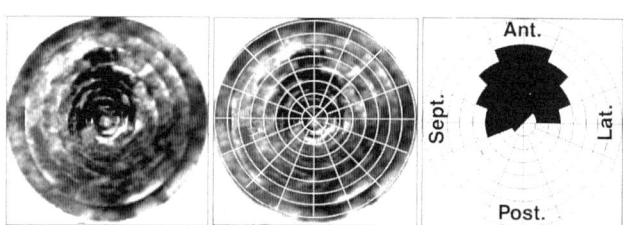

FIG. 17. Bulls-eye display and quantitation of left ventricular myocardial perfusion abnormalities, with the use of three-dimensional contrast echocardiography.

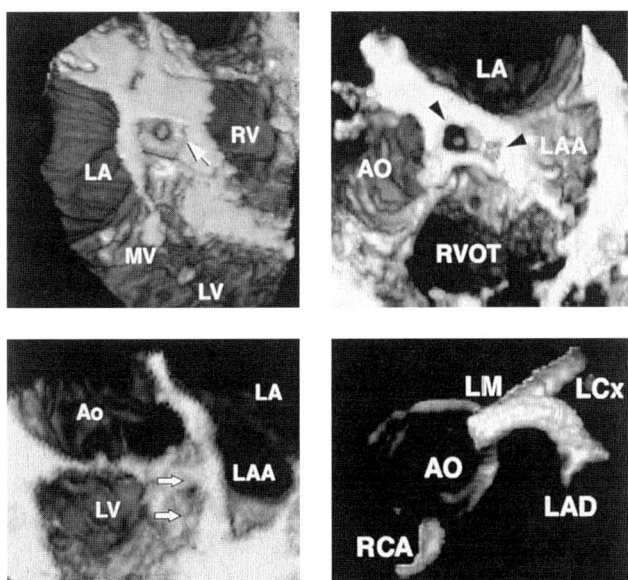

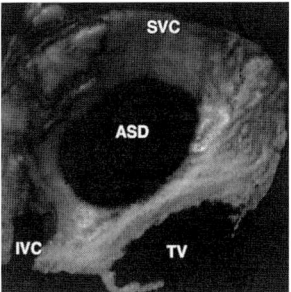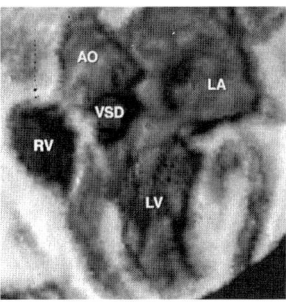

FIG. 19. *En face* projections of three-dimensional images obtained from one patient with atrial septal defect (ASD) viewed from the right atrium (**left**) and another patient with membranous ventricular septal defect (VSD) viewed from the left ventricle (**right**). *AO*, aorta; *IVC*, inferior vena cava; *LA*, left atrium; *LV*, left ventricle; *RV*, right ventricle; *SVC*, superior vena cava; *TV*, tricuspid valve.

FIG. 18. Three-dimensional image reconstruction of proximal coronary arteries in various projections including an *en face* view of the ostium of left main coronary artery (**upper left**), a longitudinal view of the left main coronary artery (**upper right**), a longitudinal view of the left anterior descending coronary artery showing two plaques (*arrows*) (**lower left**) and an image of the extracted proximal segments of the right and left coronary arteries (**lower right**). *AO*, aorta; *LA*, left atrium; *LAA*, left atrial appendage; *LAD*, left anterior descending; *LCx*, left circumflex; *LM*, left main; *LV*, left ventricle; *MV*, mitral valve; *RCA*, right coronary artery; *RV*, right ventricle; *RVOT*, right ventricular outflow tract.

mal coronary segments and detection and evaluation of stenotic lesions using three-dimensional echocardiography has proved feasible and reliable (Fig. 18) (57,58). Three-dimensional data obtained by transesophageal approach appears superior to that obtained by transthoracic imaging. Good agreement on the presence and severity of stenotic lesions in the proximal segments of coronary arteries were obtained between three-dimensional echocardiography and coronary angiography. With ongoing refinements in ultrasound instrumentation, it may become possible to perform three-dimensional reconstruction of proximal coronary arteries using transthoracic approaches.

Congenital Heart Diseases

In patients with congenital heart diseases, the alterations in morphology and spatial relationship of the cardiac structures can be complex. The ability of three-dimensional echocardiography to generate anyplane or sequential cross-sectional views and three-dimensional images has proven valuable in studying congenital heart diseases for better delineation of the complex anatomy of abnormally developed hearts and special features after surgical repair or correction (59–65).

Septal Defects

The location, size, shape, and number of atrial or ventricular septal defects can be difficult to evaluate with two-dimensional echocardiography, especially in patients with multiple defects or defects of irregular shape. Three-dimensional visualization of *en face* views of the atrial or ventricular septum can be helpful in these cases, increasing diagnostic confidence and quantitative accuracy (Fig. 19) (60,61). Three-dimensional echocardiography also demonstrates dynamic changes in the size of septal defects. The maximum dimension of the defects as well as the size of the rims can be measured directly from three-dimensional *en face* view images. Three-dimensional imaging has been applied in patients with atrial septal defects for selection of candidates for catheter-based device closure (62). Follow-up studies of these patients using three-dimensional echocardiography provides information of the seating and functioning of the implanted device.

Ventricular Inflow and Outflow Abnormalities

Three-dimensional echocardiography can be used in studying left and right ventricular inflow and outflow tracts including the valves, subvalvular structures, and supravalvular structures by providing morphologic and quantitative information on these structures. In patients with Ebstein's anomaly, the degree of displacement of each leaflet of the tricuspid valve, the coaptation and freedom of movement of the leaflets and the volume and function of the right ventricle (the true right ventricle and the atrialized right ventricle) can be evaluated comprehensively. In patients with atrioventricular septal defect, the existence and extension of mitral valve cleft are better visualized from three-dimensional images than from two-dimensional views (Fig. 20). Three-dimensional echocardiography has provided a better understanding of the relationship between the morphology and dynamics of the cleft mitral valve and the severity of mitral valve regurgitation in patients before and after surgical repair of

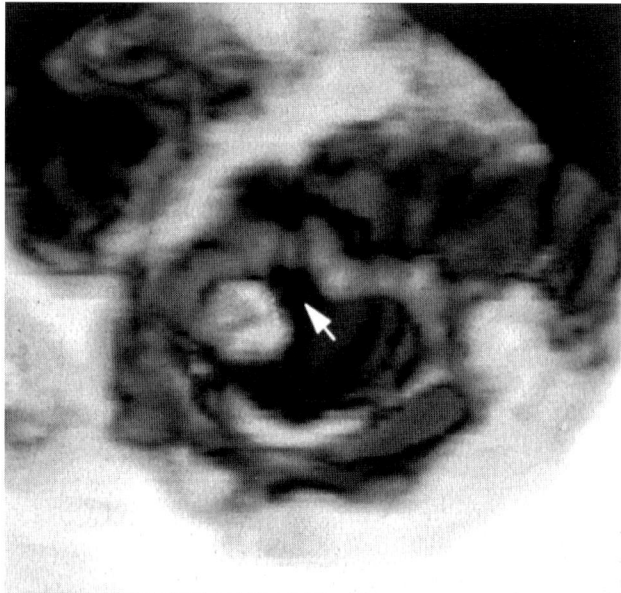

FIG. 20. Three-dimensional image of a cleft mitral valve (*arrow*) viewed from the left ventricle.

the cleft (63). Bicuspid aortic valve is not an uncommon finding, but it can sometimes be difficult to differentiate from a normal aortic valve by two-dimensional imaging, especially when the raphe is prominent. Three-dimensional *en face* view images of the valves allows for better evaluation of the number of cusps or leaflets in a valve (Fig. 21). Diagnosis of subvalvular or supravalvular stenosis, especially the membranous type, can also be facilitated by three-dimensional echocardiographic analysis using anyplane

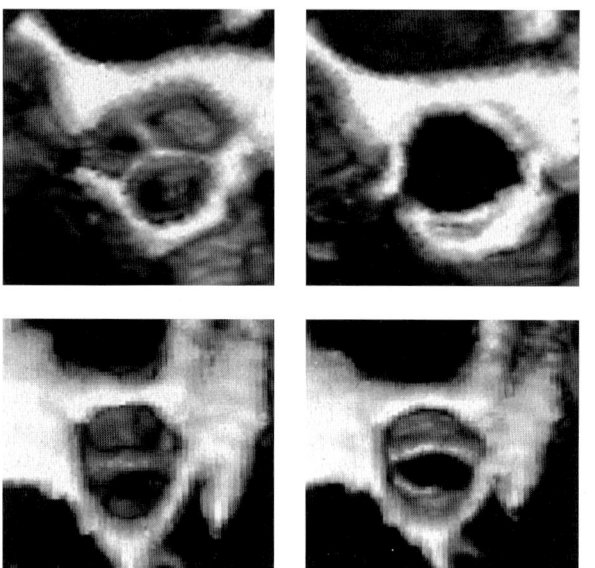

FIG. 21. Three-dimensional images of a normal aortic valve (**top**) and a bicuspid aortic valve (**bottom**) in diastole (**left**) and systole (**right**). The number of cusps and their commissures are clearly displayed in these *en face* projections.

cross-sectional reconstruction or three-dimensional image reconstruction in multiple projections (64). Other congenital inflow or outflow abnormalities, such as parachute valves or valvular atresia, can also be studied by three-dimensional echocardiography adjuvant to two-dimensional imaging to obtain incremental information.

Other Congenital Heart Diseases

In patients with complex congenital heart diseases such as transposition of great arteries, the relationship between, and the position of, the cardiac chambers and great arteries can sometimes be difficult to decide from two-dimensional echocardiography. Three-dimensional echocardiography provides an easier understanding of the anatomic relationships of the cardiac structures. A cutting plane can be placed freely within a volumetric data set, able to generate novel two-dimensional views that are inaccessible from conventional imaging. Cardiac structures can be observed in three-dimensions from many vantage projections (65). In patients with tetralogy of Fallot, the size of the ventricular septal defect and the severity of right ventricular outflow stenosis can be assessed from three-dimensional images or reconstructed cross-sectional views. Also, the volume and function of the right and left ventricles can be evaluated accurately before the surgery and in follow-up studies postoperatively. In patients with coarctation of aorta, the site, severity, and extension of stenosis may affect clinical decision-making. The segment of coarctation may not be symmetrical and regular. Measurements from two-dimensional echocardiography on limited views may not be accurate. Three-dimensional echocardiography has the potential to improve these measurements. Benefit may also be gained from three-dimensional echocardiography in other complex congenital defects as well as in patients following compound surgical repairs.

Other Applications

Three-dimensional imaging provides incremental information in almost all forms of cardiac disorders. Evaluation of intracardiac or intravascular masses including vegetations, tumors, thrombi, or plaques is facilitated by three-dimensional display of their site, size, attachment, and mobility and by accurate measurement of their dimensions and volumes (66). Aortic diseases such as dilatation, dissection, aneurysm, and coarctation have been studied with three-dimensional echocardiography (67). Insights were gained from three-dimensional echocardiographic study of the shape of left ventricular outflow tract on the mechanism of flow obstruction in patients with outflow abnormalities (68,69). With its ability to accurately quantify myocardial mass, three-dimensional echocardiography could be a reliable method of studying progression and regression in patients with hypertrophied myocardium (70).

Three-dimensional Imaging of Physiology

To date, three-dimensional echocardiography has been primarily applied to the evaluation of morphologic abnormalities. Current interest focuses on examination of physiologic events in a multidimensional mode. As outlined earlier, intracardiac flow abnormalities can be interrogated by volumetric data collection of color Doppler signals. Contrast three-dimensional echocardiography provides information of myocardial flow abnormalities. With the use of tissue velocity imaging in a three-dimensional mode, global depiction of myocardial motion velocity images can be reconstructed. Velocity of any myocardial region through a cardiac cycle can be extracted from the volumetric tissue velocity recordings. In addition, measurement of velocity at adjacent sites yields indices of regional myocardial strain. When coupled with intracardiac pressure data, regional myocardial stress could then be obtained as well. Such capabilities could serve to strengthen the technique of three-dimensional echocardiography—not only as a diagnostic tool but also as an investigative vehicle to study cardiac physiology.

FUTURE DIRECTIONS

Three-dimensional echocardiography is likely to become a standard examination in the future. For daily clinical application, further development and improvement are necessary to ease data acquisition, accelerate data processing, and facilitate image reconstruction. To increase the image resolution and to employ on-line analysis, digital data should be acquired instead of video signals. On-line quantitation of chamber volumes and function and display of three-dimensional images is likely to become a reality. Three-dimensional shape analysis programs currently in development could yield newer avenues to understand the relation between form and function. Digital data acquisition of color Doppler flow data could enable off-line analysis of flow and more accurate assessment of flow volume and flow rate. Efforts are being made to merge three-dimensional echocardiography with other imaging modes such as mapping of electrical events, radionuclide study of perfusion and metabolic indices derived by magnetic resonance imaging. The three-dimensional data set displayed in a virtual reality format could serve in teaching and in the rehearsal of therapeutic procedures. This approach may also provide accurate guidance to surgical repairs and reconstructions and thus aid in developing innovative approaches. Holograms, stereolithograms and solid models have been built from three-dimensional echocardiography (71,72). These techniques could improve communication between cardiologists and nonspecialists as well as with patients. Such advances should make three-dimensional echocardiography even more versatile—at the bedside as well as in training theaters.

REFERENCES

1. Tajik AJ, Seward JB, Hagler DJ, et al. Two-dimensional real-time ultrasonic imaging of the heart and great vessels: technique, image orientation, structure identification, and validation. *Mayo Clin Proc* 1978;53:271–303.
2. Feigenbaum H. *Echocardiography: The echocardiographic examination.* 5th ed. Philadelphia: Lea & Febiger, 1994: 68–133,
3. Dekker DL, Piziali RL, Dong E Jr. A system for ultrasonically imaging the human heart in three dimensions. *Comput Biomed Res* 1974;7: 544–553.
4. Moritz WE, Shreve PL. A microprocessor based spatial locating system for use with diagnostic ultrasound. *Proc IEEE* 1976;64:966–974.
5. Matsumoto M, Matsuo H, Kitabatake A, et al. Three-dimensional echocardiograms and two-dimensional echocardiographic images at desired planes by a computerized system. *Ultrasound Med Biol* 1977;3: 163–178.
6. Pandian NG, Roelandt J, Nanda NC, et al. Dynamic three-dimensional echocardiography: methods and clinical potential. *Echocardiography* 1994:11:237–259.
7. Ariet M, Geiser EA, Lupkiewicz SM, et al. Evaluation of a three-dimensional reconstruction to compute left ventricular volume and mass. *Am J Cardiol* 1984;54:415–420.
8. Linker DT, Mortiz WE, Pearlman AS. A new three-dimensional echocardiographic method of right ventricular volume measurement: *in vitro* validation. *J Am Coll Cardiol* 1986;8:101–106.
9. King DL, Harrison MR, King DL Jr, et al. Improved reproducibility of left atrial and left ventricular measurements by guided three-dimensional echocardiography. *J Am Coll Cardiol* 1992;20:1238–1245.
10. von Ramm OT, Smith SW. Real time volumetric ultrasound imaging system. *J Digit Imaging* 1990;3:261–266.
11. Sheikh KH, Smith SW, von Ramm OT, et al. Real-time, three-dimensional echocardiography: feasibility and initial use. *Echocardiography* 1991;8:119–125.
12. Handschumacher MD, Lethor JP, Siu SC, et al. A new integrated system for three-dimensional echocardiographic reconstruction: development and validation for ventricular volume with application in human subjects. *J Am Coll Cardiol* 1993;21;743–753.
13. Gopal AS, King DL, Katz J, et al. Three-dimensional echocardiographic volume computation by polyhedral surface reconstruction: *in vitro* validation and comparison to magnetic resonance imaging. *J Am Soc Echocardiogr* 1992;5:115–124.
14. Ghosh A, Nanda NC, Maurer G. Three-dimensional reconstruction of echocardiographic images using the rotation method. *Ultrasound Med Biol* 1982;8:655–661.
15. Pandian NG, Nanda NC, Schwartz SL, et al. Three-dimensional and four-dimensional transesophageal echocardiographic imaging of the heart and aorta in humans using a computed tomographic imaging probe. *Echocardiography* 1992;9:677–687.
16. Fulton DR, Marx GR, Pandian NG, et al. Dynamic three-dimensional echocardiographic imaging of congenital heart defects in infants and children by computer-controlled tomographic parallel slicing using a single integrated ultrasound instrument. *Echocardiography* 1994;11: 155–164.
17. Ludomirsky A, Vermilion R, Nesser J, et al. Transthoracic real-time three-dimensional echocardiography using the rotational scanning approach for data acquisition. *Echocardiography* 1994;11:599–606.
18. Sugeng L, Cao QL, Delabays A, et al. Three-dimensional echocardiographic evaluation of aortic disorders with rotational multiplanar imaging: experimental and clinical studies. *J Am Soc Echocardiogr* 1997; 10:120–132.
19. Salustri A, Roelandt J. Three-dimensional reconstruction of the heart with rotational acquisition: methods and clinical applications. *Br Heart J* 1995;73:10–15.
20. Yao J, Cao QL, Pandian NG, et al. Multiplane transthoracic echocardiography: Image orientation, anatomic correlation, and clinical experience with a prototype phased array multilane surface probe. *Echocardiography* 1997;14(6):559–588.
21. Delabays A, Pandian NG, Cao QL, et al. Transthoracic real-time three-dimensional echocardiography using a fan-like scanning approach for data acquisition: methods, strength, problems, and initial clinical experience. *Echocardiography* 1995;12:49–59.
22. Gopal AS, Keller AM, Rigling R, et al. Left ventricular volume and endocardial surface area by three-dimensional echocardiography: comparison with two-dimensional echocardiography and nuclear magnetic imaging in normal subjects. *J Am Coll Cardiol* 1993;22:258–270.
23. Jiang L, Siu SC, Handschumacher MD, et al. Three-dimensional echo-

cardiography: *in vivo* validation for right ventricular volume and function. *Circulation* 1994;89:2342–2350.

24. Cao QL, Pandian NG, Azevedo J, et al. Enhanced comprehension of dynamic cardiovascular anatomy by three-dimensional echocardiography with the use of mixed shading techniques. *Echocardiography* 1994; 11:627–633.

25. Schwartz SL, Cao QL, Azevedo J, et al. Simulation of intraoperative visualization of cardiac structures and study of dynamic surgical anatomy with real-time three-dimensional echocardiography. *Am J Cardiol* 1994;73:501–507.

26. Vogel M, Ho SY, Lincoln C, et al. Three-dimensional echocardiography can simulate intraoperative visualization of congenitally malformed hearts. *Ann Thorac Surg* 1995;60:1282–1288.

27. Roelandt JRTC, Yao J, Kasprzak KD. Three-dimensional echocardiography. *Cur Opin Cardiol* 1998;13:386–396.

28. Ge S, Warner JG Jr, Fowle KM, et al. Morphology and dynamic change of discrete subaortic stenosis can be imaged and quantified with three-dimensional transesophageal echocardiography. *J Am Soc Echocardiogr* 1997;10(7):713–716.

29. Otsuji Y, Handschumacher MD, Schwammenthal E, et al. Insights from three-dimensional echocardiography into the mechanism of functional mitral regurgitation: direct *in vivo* demonstration of altered leaflet tethering geometry. *Circulation* 1997;96:1999–2008.

30. Trocino G, Salustri A, Roelandt JR, et al. Three-dimensional echocardiography of a flail tricuspid valve. *J Am Soc Echocardiogr* 1996;9: 91–93.

31. Pai RG, Tanimoto M, Jintapakorn W, et al. Volume-rendered three-dimensional dynamic anatomy of the mitral annulus using a transesophageal echocardiographic technique. *J Heart Valve Dis* 1995;4:623–627.

32. Salustri A, Becker AE, Van Herwerden L, et al. Three-dimensional echocardiography of normal and pathologic mitral valve: a comparison with two-dimensional transesophageal echocardiography. *J Am Coll Cardiol* 1996;27:1502–1510.

33. Levine RA, Handschumacher MD, Sanfilippo AJ, et al. Three-dimensional echocardiographic reconstruction of the mitral valve, with implications for the diagnosis of mitral valve prolapse. *Circulation* 1989; 80:589–598.

34. Cheng TO, Wang XF, Zheng LH, et al. Three-dimensional transesophageal echocardiography in the diagnosis of mitral valve prolapse. *Am Heart J* 1994;128:1218–1224.

35. Kasprzak JD, Nosir YF, Dall'Agata A, et al. Quantification of the aortic valve area in three-dimensional echocardiographic data sets: analysis of orifice overestimation resulting from suboptimal cut-plane selection. *Am Heart J* 1998;135:995–1003.

36. Hozumi T, Yoshikawa J, Yoshida K, et al. Assessment of flail mitral leaflets by dynamic three-dimensional echocardiographic imaging. *J Am Cardiol* 1996;79:223–225.

37. Chen Q, Nosir YF, Vletter WB, et al. Accurate assessment of mitral valve area in patients with mitral stenosis by three-dimensional echocardiography. *J Am Soc Echocardiogr* 1997;10:133–140.

38. Menzel T, Mohr-Kahaly S, Kolsch B, et al. Quantitative assessment of aortic stenosis by three-dimensional echocardiography. *J Am Soc Echocardiogr* 1997;10:215–223.

39. Delabays A, Sugeng L, Pandian NG, et al. Dynamic three-dimensional echocardiographic assessment of intracardiac blood flow jets. *Am J Cardiol* 1995;76:1053–1058.

40. Yao J, Masani N, Cao QL, et al. Clinical application of transthoracic volume-rendered three-dimensional echocardiography in the assessment of mitral regurgitation. *Am J Cardiol* 1998;82:189–196.

41. Laskari CV, Masani ND, Pandian NG. Three-dimensional echocardiography in mitral regurgitation. *Coron Artery Dis* 1996;7:206–210.

42. Belohlavek M, Foley DA, Gerber TC, et al. Three-dimensional reconstruction of color Doppler jets in the human heart. *J Am Soc Echocardiogr* 1994;7:553–560.

43. De Simone R, Glombitza G, Vahl CF, et al. Three-dimensional color Doppler: a clinical study in patients with mitral regurgitation. *J Am Coll Cardiol* 1999;33:1646–1654.

44. Zoghbi WA, Buckey JC, Massey MA, et al. Determination of left ventricular volumes with use of a new nongeometric echocardiographic method: Clinical validation and potential application. *J Am Coll Cardiol* 1990;15:610–617.

45. Handschumacher MD, Lethor JP, Siu SC, et al. A new integrated system

for three-dimensional echocardiographic reconstruction: development and validation for ventricular volume with application in human subjects. *J Am Coll Cardiol* 1993;21;743–753.

46. Siu SC, Rivera JM, Guerrero JL, et al. Three-dimensional echocardiography: *in vivo* validation for left ventricular volume and function. *Circulation* 1993;88[Part 1]:1715–1723.

47. Sapin PM, Schroder KM, Gopal AS, et al. Comparison of two- and three-dimensional echocardiography with cineventriculography for measurement of left ventricular volume in patients. *J Am Coll Cardiol* 1994;24:1054–1063.

48. Nosir YF, Lequin MH, Kasprzak JD, et al. Measurements and day-to-day variabilities of left ventricular volumes and ejection fraction by three-dimensional echocardiography and comparison with magnetic resonance imaging. *Am J Cardiol* 1998;82:209–214.

49. Yao J, Cao QL, Masani N, et al. Three-dimensional echocardiographic estimation of infarct mass based on quantification of dysfunctional left ventricular mass. *Circulation* 1997;96:1660–1666.

50. De Castro S, Yao J, Magni G, et al. Three-dimensional echocardiographic assessment of the extension of dysfunctional mass in patients with coronary artery disease. *Am J Cardiol* 1998;81:103G–106G.

51. Kaul S. Myocardial contrast echocardiography in coronary artery disease: potential applications using venous injections of contrast. *Am J Cardiol* 1995;75(11):61D–68D.

52. Linka AZ, Ates G, Wei K, et al. Three-dimensional myocardial contrast echocardiography: validation of *in vivo* risk and infarct volumes. *J Am Coll Cardiol* 1997;30(7):1892–1899.

53. Kasprzak JD, Vletter WB, Roelandt JRTC, et al. Visualization and quantification of myocardial mass at risk using three-dimensional contrast echocardiography. *Cardiovasc Res.* 1998;40:314–321.

54. Yao J, Masani N, Pandian NG. Three-dimensional echocardiographic assessment of myocardial perfusion abnormalities. In: Nanda NC, Schlief R, Goldberg BB, eds. *Advances in echo imaging using contrast enhancement,* 2nd ed. Boston: Kluwer Academic Publishers, 1997: 465–477.

55. Yao J, Delabays A, Masani N, et al. Tomographic "bulls-eye" display and quantitation of myocardial perfusion defects using 3-dimensional contrast echocardiography. *Circulation* 1998;17:I–503(abst).

56. Yao J, Takeuchi M, Teupe C, et al. 3-Dimensional contrast echocardiography can delineate and quantify residual infarct mass and salvaged myocardial mass in reperfused myocardium following acute ischemia: experimental studies using a new contrast agent—SHU 563A. *Circulation* 1998;17:I–194(abst).

57. El-Rahman SMA, Khatri G, Nanda N, et al. Transesophageal three-dimensional echocardiographic assessment of normal and stenosed coronary arteries. *Echocardiography* 1996;13:503–510.

58. Yao J, Taams MA, Kasprzak JD, et al. Usefulness of three-dimensional transesophageal echocardiographic imaging for evaluating narrowing in the coronary arteries. *Am J Cardiol* 1999;84:41–45.

59. Vogel M, Ho SY, Buhlmeyer K, et al. Assessment of congenital heart defects by dynamic three-dimensional echocardiography: methods of data acquisition and clinical potential. *Acta Paediatr* 1995;410[Suppl]: 34–39.

60. Marx G, Fulton DR, Pandian NG, et al. Delineation of site, relative size and dynamic geometry of atrial septal defects by real-time three-dimensional echocardiography. *J Am Coll Cardiol* 1995;25:482–490.

61. Kardon RE, Cao QL, Masani N, et al. New insights and observations in three-dimensional echocardiographic visualization of ventricular septal defects: experimental and clinical studies. *Circulation* 1998;98(13): 1307–1314.

62. Magni G, Hijazi ZM, Pandian NG, et al. Two- and three-dimensional transesophageal echocardiography in patient selection and assessment of atrial septal defect closure by the new Das-Engel Wings device: initial clinical experience. *Circulation* 1997;96:1722–1728.

63. Acar P, Laskari C, Rhodes J, et al. Three-dimensional echocardiographic analysis of valve anatomy as a determinant of mitral regurgitation after surgery for atrioventricular septal defects. *Am J Cardiol* 1999; 83(5):745–749.

64. Dall'Agata A, Cromme-Dijkhuis AH, Meijboom FJ, et al. Use of three-dimensional echocardiography for analysis of outflow obstruction in congenital heart disease. *Am J Cardiol* 1999;83(6):921–925.

65. Bartel T, Muller S. Corrected transposition of the great arteries: dynamic three-dimensional echocardiography and volumetry. A new diagnostic tool in intensive care management. *Jap Heart J* 1995;36: 819–824.

66. Borges AC, Witt C, Bartel T, et al. Preoperative two- and three-dimensional transesophageal echocardiographic assessment of heart tumors. *Ann Thorac Surg* 1996;61:1163–1167.

67. Ross JJ Jr, D'Adamo AJ, Karalis DG, et al. Three-dimensional transesophageal echo imaging of the descending thoracic aorta. *Am J Cardiol* 1993;71:1000–1002.

68. Fyfe DA, Ludomirsky A, Sandhu S, et al. Left ventricular outflow tract obstruction defined by active three-dimensional echocardiography using rotational transthoracic acquisition. *Echocardiography* 1994;11:607–615.

69. Salustri A, Kofflard MJ, Roelandt JR, et al. Assessment of left ventricular outflow in hypertrophic cardiomyopathy using anyplane and paraplane analysis of three-dimensional echocardiography. *Am J Cardiol* 1996;78:462–468.

70. Franke A, Schondube FA, Kuhl HP, et al. Quantitative assessment of the operative results after extended myectomy and surgical reconstruction of the subvalvular mitral apparatus in hypertrophic obstructive cardiomyopathy using dynamic three-dimensional transesophageal echocardiography. *J Am Coll Cardiol* 1998;31(7):1641–1649.

71. Vannan MA, Cao QL, Pandian NG, et al. Volumetric multiplexed transmission holography of the heart with echocardiographic data. *J Am Soc Echocardiogr* 1995;8:567–575.

72. Gilon D, Cape EG, Handschumacher MD, et al. Insights from three-dimensional echocardiographic laser stereolithography. Effect of leaflet funnel geometry on the coefficient of orifice contraction, pressure loss, and the Gorlin formula in mitral stenosis. *Circulation* 1996;94:452–459.

CHAPTER 10

The Future of Echocardiography

Vincent L. Sorrell and Navin C. Nanda

The future of echocardiography appears very bright. Advances in all fields of echo: transthoracic, exercise, and transesophageal echocardiography are being made at extraordinary rates. Ultrasound images of the heart have only been utilized since the inception of M-mode echocardiography in the mid-1960s. It was nearly 10 years later that two-dimensional scanning revolutionized this technique and catapulted echocardiography into the cardiology community. Doppler techniques allowed echocardiography to expand from an anatomic laboratory to a hemodynamic laboratory in the late 1970s. For many subsequent years, it was necessary to focus research efforts on the clinical impact of these powerful diagnostic tools. The last 15 years have allowed echocardiography to become one of the most commonly employed techniques in the mainstream medical community, utilized by general internists, internal subspecialists, family practitioners, and surgeons alike. Recently, with the development of second harmonic imaging and the increasing use of transesophageal echocardiography, the limitations of poor ultrasonic image has been even further reduced.

With its strengths now clinically well defined, newer research developments have focused on imaging techniques, using the rapid advances in computer technology to its advantage. Contrast echocardiography is currently being utilized to enhance endocardial definition and significantly improve our assessment of ventricular function. Such an approach is especially helpful in stress echocardiography. Second harmonic imaging was specifically developed for this and has markedly helped in the area. Utilizing electrocardiography or ECG-gating techniques, intermittent ultra-sound imaging, continuous intravenous infusions of newer, more sophisticated contrast agents and multiple harmonic transducers, imaging of myocardial perfusion may be possible. Thus, extensive research is ongoing in this area. Power pulse inversion imaging is an important investigational technique that may overcome the limitation that intermittent imaging offers (loss of simultaneous assessment of function) and may allow real-time myocardial perfusion assessment.

Since the advent of two-dimensional echo, development of a three-dimensional system has been attempted and various devices that reconstruct two-dimensional images are available. More recently, a novel real-time three-dimensional system (Volumetrics) has been developed that provides an advanced transducer with extensive parallel processing capabilities offering a pyramidal scanning plane. By instantly obtaining three-dimensional data, images can either be displayed in the usual two-dimensional format, or in frontal planes (C-scans) that are parallel to the transducer's surface, or eventually, displayed as a three-dimensional image.

Other important areas of continued development include color M-mode and tissue Doppler techniques that are focused primarily on furthering our understanding of diastolic function, intravascular and intracardiac transducers that utilize very high frequencies for direct, concentrated images of specific anatomic regions, and overseeing all of these developments, the advancement of the digital echo laboratory. The application of digital technology will allow more comprehensive examinations to be completed more quickly. Such digital methods will lead to improved clinical interpretation using direct side-by-side comparisons. Finally, images may be transmitted to distant locations instantly through the Internet for interpretations, to assist the managing physician, or to obtain expert consultations.

It is impossible to accurately predict the clinical impact that any new technique will eventually provide, but it seems likely that these new developments will expand our diagnos-

V. L. Sorrell: Section of Cardiology, East Carolina University Brody School of Medicine; Graphics and Exercise Physiology Laboratories, Greenville, North Carolina 27858.

N. C. Nanda: Department of Medicine, Heart Station, Echocardiography Laboratories, University of Alabama at Birmingham, Birmingham, Alabama 35249.

tic acumen. These newer tools are being developed to limit the necessity for additional testing and to make echocardiography even more comprehensive for evaluation of the cardiovascular system. In time, it is felt that echocardiography should be able to provide a detailed, three-dimensional anatomic description of the heart, a more complete, noninvasive, hemodynamic evaluation, a quantitative interrogation of systolic and diastolic performance, and even a portrait of the coronary perfusion. Thus, the future of echocardiography appears very bright.

Imaging in Cardiovascular Disease, edited by Gerald M. Pohost et al., Lippincott Williams & Wilkins, Philadelphia © 2000

CHAPTER 11

Basic Principles, Techniques, Camera/ Computer Systems, and Safety

Guido Germano and Daniel S. Berman

Nuclear cardiology is based on the intravenous injection of small quantities of radioactive materials (radiopharmaceuticals). In most applications the radioactivity is preferentially absorbed by the myocardium (myocardial perfusion imaging, infarct-avid imaging), whereas in other applications it remains in the blood pool (blood pool imaging). Examples of agents used for perfusion imaging are Tl-201, Tc-99m-sestamibi, and Tc-99m-tetrofosmin, while Tc-99m-pertechnetate labeled to red blood cells is generally used for blood pool imaging. Whether the radioactive materials are "taken up" by the myocardium or just pass through the cardiac chambers during the cardiac cycle, their localization and measurement is most commonly accomplished using an Anger scintillation camera, referred to as gamma camera. A gamma camera consists of one or more high-density scintillation detectors (typically, sodium iodide or NaI), whose function is that of converting incoming gamma rays into light photons. The photons are in turn converted into electrons by a photocathode and amplified into an electric current by a set of contiguous photomultiplier tubes (PMTs) directly coupled to the scintillation crystal (Fig. 1) (1,2). When the incoming gamma ray's radiation is completely absorbed by the detector, the current generated is directly proportional to the energy of the gamma ray. A collimator allows the

G. Germano: Department of Radiological Sciences, University of California–Los Angeles School of Medicine, Los Angeles, California 90024; Department of Medicine, Cedars-Sinai Medical Center, Los Angeles, California 90048.

D. S. Berman: University of California–Los Angeles School of Medicine, Los Angeles, California 90025; Department of Imaging/ Nuclear Medicine, Cedars-Sinai Medical Center, Los Angeles, California 90048.

determination of the x and y coordinates of where a gamma ray arose in the patient. Collimators are metal devices (usually lead, sometimes tungsten) that sit on top of the detector and let pass only a small part of the incoming radiation (2). The reason for this is that most radiation is scattered inside the patient, and therefore must be eliminated because it carries inaccurate information as to the location of the emitting isotope. Since the assumption is that the unscattered radiation's path is perpendicular to the plane of the detector, a "parallel hole" collimator is the standard collimator used in nuclear cardiology. The exact location where the gamma ray interacted with the detector is typically derived by analysis of the fraction of light photons collected by different PMTs, according to the Anger scheme reproduced in Fig. 2 (1,3,4). The gamma camera's specialized electronics analyzes the energy from each gamma ray interaction (generally referred to as an "event") to determine whether the ray was a primary event or was attenuated or scattered, and accumulates the event coordinates in an image matrix. Typical image matrix sizes in nuclear cardiology are 64×64 pixels^2 and 128×128 pixels^2.

IMAGE ACQUISITION

Generally, more than one image of the radioactivity inside the patient is acquired for the purposes of a nuclear cardiology study. The first reason for acquiring multiple images is spatial: the activity distribution is three-dimensional, while a single image matrix is two-dimensional. In order to alleviate the fact that three-dimensional information is compressed into a two-dimensional (planar) image, several planar images (from different spatial directions or "views") are acquired.

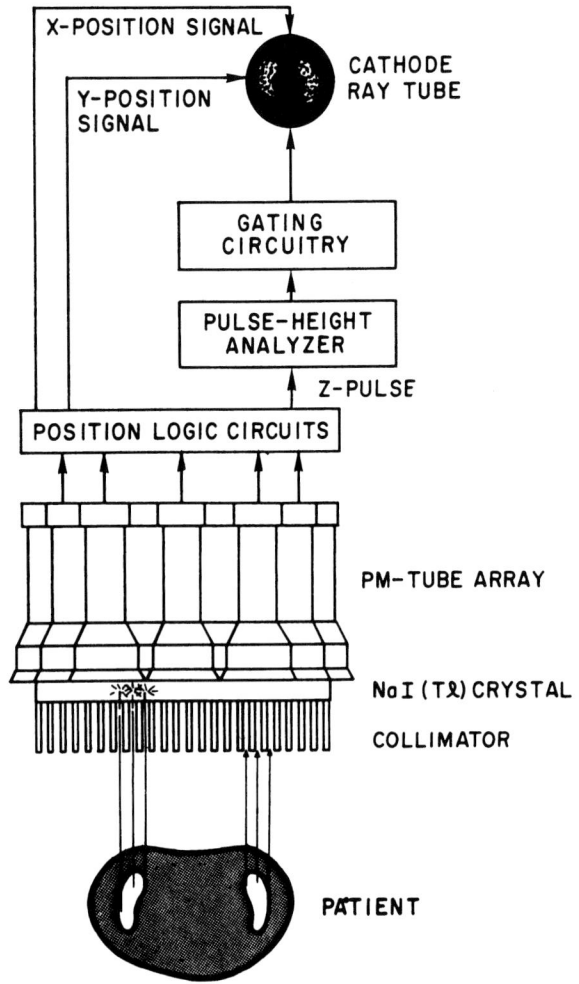

FIG. 1. Basic components of the Anger camera. (From ref. 2, with permission.)

in the structure of interest, blurring structure definition and decreasing defect contrast. These problems are a direct consequence of the three-dimensional (volumetric) to two-dimensional (planar) image data compression inherent in planar imaging (5). As a result, planar perfusion imaging has been demonstrated in multicenter trials to be lacking in sensitivity for the detection of coronary artery disease (CAD), particularly in patients with single vessel disease, as well as lacking in sensitivity for the localization of CAD in patients with left circumflex disease (6). Figure 3 shows a series of planar images (from the mid-right anterior oblique RAO 45 degrees to the mid-left posterior oblique RPO 45 degrees) from a patient with coronary artery disease of the left anterior descending territory.

Planar imaging of the myocardium generally involves acquiring two or three images at different angles (views): typical views are the anterior, the LAO 45 degrees, and a left lateral view. These planar images are often evaluated at the same time, but are not digitally combined. SPECT (single photon emission computed tomography) imaging extends the planar approach by rotating the gamma camera detector around the patient and acquiring a series of planar images separated by a constant angular displacement (Fig. 3). A key word in SPECT is ''tomography'': the tomographic process, originally developed by Bracewell for astronomic applications and successively modified by Shepp and Logan for use

The second reason is temporal: the activity distribution may vary with time, but the detector ''integrates'' information from all the events that hit it during the acquisition. In order to alleviate the fact that intrinsically dynamic information is pooled into a static image, several images (each corresponding to a portion of the acquisition time) are acquired.

Planar versus Single Photon Emission Computed Tomography Imaging

A planar image is a single ''snapshot'' acquired with the detector plane parallel to the patient's long axis. A problem of the planar approach is that an imaging angle may not be found that allows different structures of interest to be clearly separated in the image, as they are in the actual three-dimensional patient body: for example, the lateral myocardial wall is foreshortened and is visualized only in the mid-left anterior oblique (LAO 45 degrees) view typically used in planar perfusion imaging, and right and left ventricular as well as right and left atrial cavities are partly overlapping in planar blood pool imaging. Another problem is that underlying and overlying activity contribute ''background'' counts to those

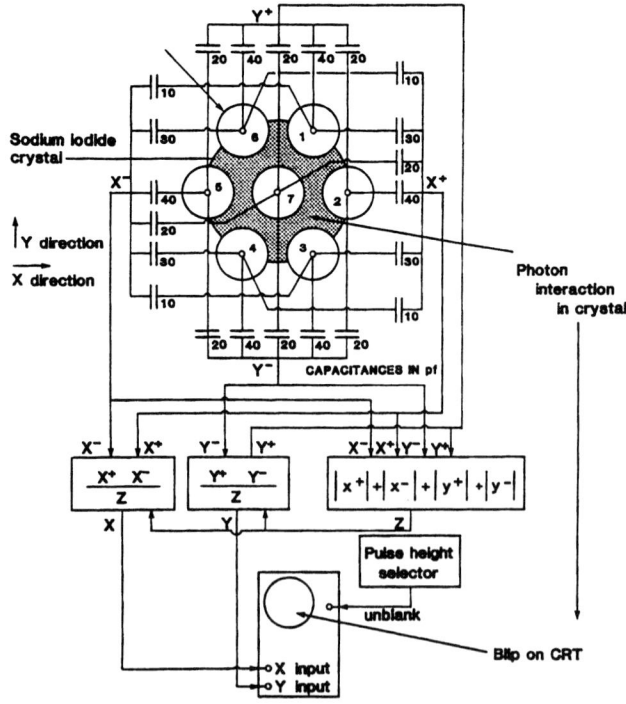

FIG. 2. Anger positioning scheme: the exact location (*x, y*) of each gamma ray interaction in the detector is derived from weighted analysis of the outputs of the various photomultiplier tubes or PMTs. The global summed output *Z*, if within the preset energy window, enables collection of the interaction's coordinates in the image matrix. (From ref. 57, with permission.)

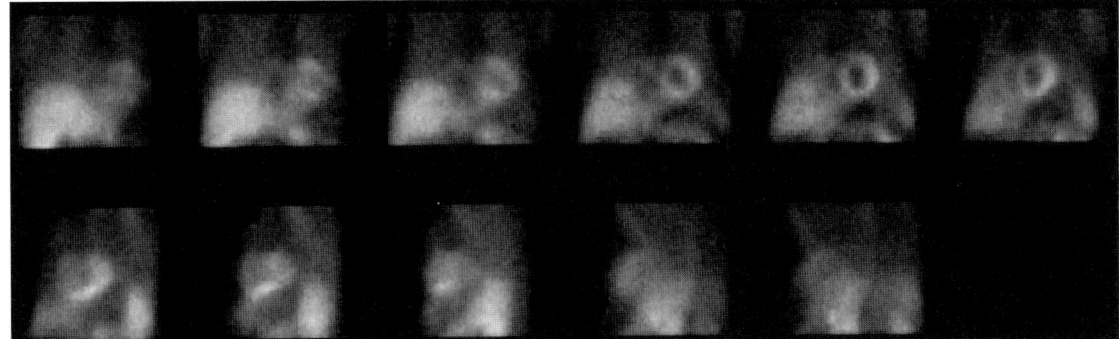

FIG. 3. Series of planar (projection) images (**left** to **right** and **top** to **bottom** show right anterior oblique 45 degrees to right posterior oblique 45 degrees, 6 degrees apart) for a patient with a severe perfusion defect in the left anterior descending coronary territory.

in the medical field (7), is based on the theory that a three-dimensional object can be "reconstructed" into a three-dimensional image volume from a set of planar images, each representing a "projection" of the object in the two-dimensional space. This is why planar images are also referred to as "projection images." Tomographic reconstruction in nuclear cardiology is accomplished by filtered backprojection or iterative techniques.

Single Photon Emission Computed Tomography Reconstruction

Figure 4 illustrates the practical implementation of single photon emission computed tomography (SPECT) reconstruction by backprojection. The two-dimensional projection images (perpendicular to the plane of the page, and parallel to the patient) yield a series of "activity profiles" (also termed count profiles or scan profiles) for each plane of interest (Fig. 4**A**). Each profile represents the integrated sum of the activity underneath the detector along a given angle in that particular plane, and all profiles are used to "reconstruct" the image representing the activity in that plane (transaxial image). Since no information is available concerning the depth of the activity responsible for a peak in a profile, the assumption is made that it was uniformly distributed. Thus, the counts in each profile are uniformly redistributed (back-projected) onto the transaxial image, following the linear superimposition of back projections (LSBP) scheme (Fig. 4**B**). A drawback of this approach is that LSBP results in loss of resolution, loss of contrast and creation of the characteristic "star artifact." To alleviate this problem, count profiles can be altered (filtered) before reconstruction using an oscillating function that has both positive and negative values, so as to cancel out the star's "rays" (Fig. 4**C**). This latter approach is termed linear superimposition of filtered backprojections (LSFBP), or filtered backprojection with short notation, and represents the current standard for reconstruction of tomographic images in nuclear cardiology. Transaxial images resulting from filtered backprojection reconstruction of the projection images in Figure 3 are shown in Figure 5.

A different reconstruction technique that is gaining wider acceptance, fueled by increases in computer speed and increased use of attenuation correction protocols, is iterative reconstruction (8). Iterative reconstruction is based on the algebraic reconstruction technique (ART), which sees each count profile as an equation with a number of unknowns equal to the dimension of the image matrix (9). If enough equations are provided (enough projection images are acquired), the system can be solved and the mathematically exact values for all pixels in the transaxial image can be derived (Fig. 6). System solving is practically implemented using an iterative process, whose convergence is generally achieved in 10 to 15 iterations starting with an "educated guess" represented by the filtered backprojection output.

In addition to the "ramp filter" used to eliminate the star artifact in filtered backprojection reconstruction, "low pass" filters are used to slightly blur the projection images before reconstruction. This is usually necessary to improve the statistical quality and interpretability of the final tomo-

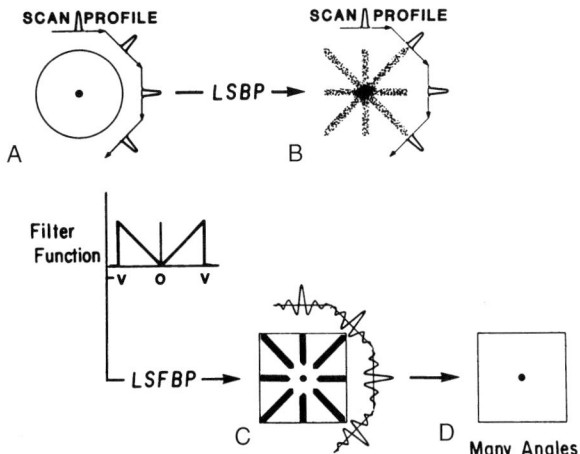

FIG. 4. Implementation of tomographic reconstruction of a point source (**A**) by linear superimposition of backprojections (*LSBP*) (**B**) and filtered backprojections (*LSFBP*) (**C, D**). (From ref. 2, with permission.)

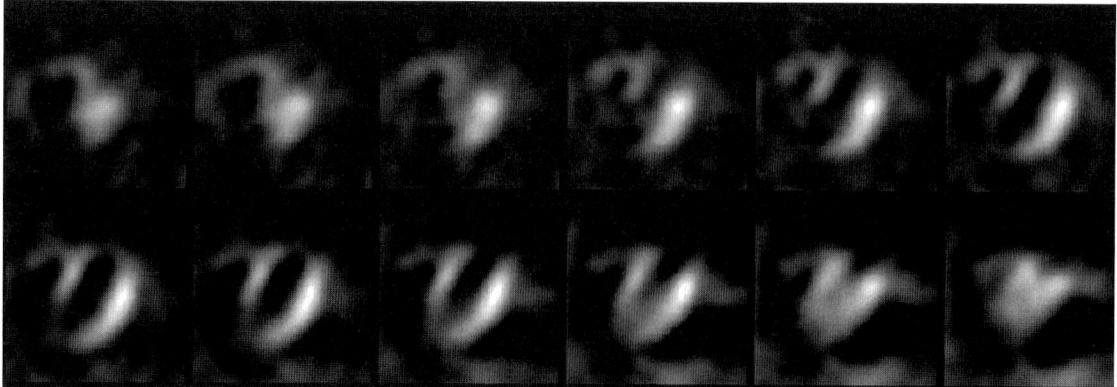

FIG. 5. Transaxial images reconstructed from the projection images in Figure 3.

graphic images; it is accomplished using ''families'' of filters (such as the Hanning or the Butterworth) able to produce finely controlled smoothing of the images by varying appropriate mathematical parameters. A comprehensive discussion on the structure and role of low pass filters in nuclear medicine can be found in (10).

Single Photon Emission Computed Tomography Acquisition Variables

There are many different strategies to consider when acquiring a SPECT sudy. Given that projection images need to be distributed over a minimum of 180 degrees in order not to introduce severe artifacts during reconstruction (2), a much-debated issue has been whether data should be acquired over 180 degrees, 360 degrees, or intermediate length orbits (11–14). The almost unanimous current consensus appears to be that 180-degree orbits spanning from the right anterior oblique (RAO) to the left posterior oblique (LPO) view are preferred because they result in images of the heart with the best resolution and the best defect contrast. The remaining posterior views are greatly affected by attenuation and Compton scatter, and thus would contribute ''lower quality'' counts, as well as blur the reconstructed

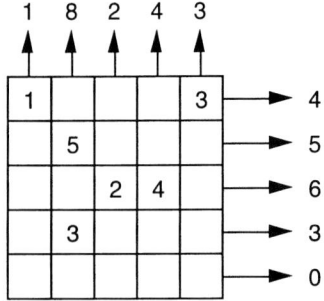

FIG. 6. Algebraic reconstruction of tomographic images. Each point in each count profile is the sum of a row, a column, or a diagonal distribution of pixels (two profiles are shown here). If enough profiles are acquired, a system of equations can be built and solved for the exact count values in those pixels.

image. Moreover, acquiring 360-degrees worth of data takes longer than 180 degrees, unless one uses a triple-detector camera or a dual-detector camera with opposing detectors. Today, the overwhelming majority of all clinical nuclear cardiology studies are reconstructed over 180 degrees, even when 360 degrees of data are acquired. Little published data exists on the effect of less conventional orbit lengths, like 240 degrees or 270 degrees, on image quality.

A more controversial issue is whether circular or noncircular orbits (also referred to as elliptical, peanut-shaped, or patient-contoured orbits) should be employed (15). The traditional rationale for using circular orbits has been that all projection images have approximately the same resolution with this approach, given their fairly constant distance from the imaged heart (source-to-collimator distance is the main determinant of resolution). On the other hand, noncircular orbits, which aim at achieving the best possible resolution at each view by bringing the detector as close to the patient as practical, may introduce artifacts when they combine these projection images of widely different resolutions during reconstruction (16). As a result of the recent introduction of attenuation correction protocols requiring the use of noncircular acquisition orbits, as well as the development of software to compensate for distance-dependent resolution in noncircular orbits, no universal guideline can be given as to whether circular or noncircular orbits should be preferred in cardiac SPECT.

The traditional way of acquiring projection images at different angles as the detector rotates around the patient follows the ''step-and-shoot'' approach. In this approach, the detector steps through a discrete number of views along the orbit, and the camera electronics temporarily stop data collection while the detector advances from one angle to the next. This causes a ''dead time'' of a few seconds per view. Conversely, in the continuous acquisition approach the detector rotates continuously and at constant speed around the patient. The acquisition orbit is divided in a number of subarcs, and data collected along each arc is assigned to a projection image. Pseudo-continuous (also called modified step-and-shoot) acquisition is a hybrid approach: the detector moves as in step-and-shoot, but data collection continues during the stepping period. Since it has been demonstrated that continuous acquisition does not appreciably decrease image resolution if the spacing between projections is, at most, 6 degrees (10), acquisitions should preferrably be performed in the continuous or pseudo-continuous mode, to avoid dead time-related inefficiencies. The number of projection images acquired over a 180-degree orbit is not critical: as long as their angular spacing is constant and does not exceed 6 degrees, neither perfusion nor function assessment will likely be affected (17). Standard numbers of projections in current camera systems are 30, 32, 60, and 64 for 180-degree acquisitions.

Collimators vary according to the energy of the radiopharmaceutical and the count rate observed in a particular type of study. There is a direct trade-off between resolution (distance required to distinguish two radioactive sources as separate) and sensitivity (proportion of the emitted radioactivity detected) with parallel hole collimators, and substantial differences can be achieved by varying the number, bore, shape, and length of the holes. As with prereconstruction filters, the choice of collimators can have a major effect on image quality; therefore, care should be taken to use collimators that have been established as appropriate for a given study with a specific camera/computer system. A more radical way to increase sensitivity is to map the organ of interest (the myocardium) to a larger portion of the detector by using a fan beam or cone beam collimator (18). These collimators focus to a point (cone beam) or to a line parallel to the axis of rotation of the camera and beyond the patient (fan beam). The increase in sensitivity produced by these collimators is not associated with a loss of resolution; however, the data volume may not be adequately sampled at all angles due to truncation artifacts (19), and fan beam/cone beam collimators are not widely used in clinical practice.

Single Photon Emission Computed Tomography Multidetector Cameras

Although single-detector cameras were introduced first and still represent the majority of all gamma cameras worldwide, multidetector cameras have been consistently outselling them over the past few years. The main reason for the success of dual- and triple-detector cameras is their ability to produce images of higher statistical quality in the same (or shorter) acquisition time compared to the single-detector approach. Standard gamma cameras configurations are shown in Figure 7 (20). The dual-detector, 90-degree con-

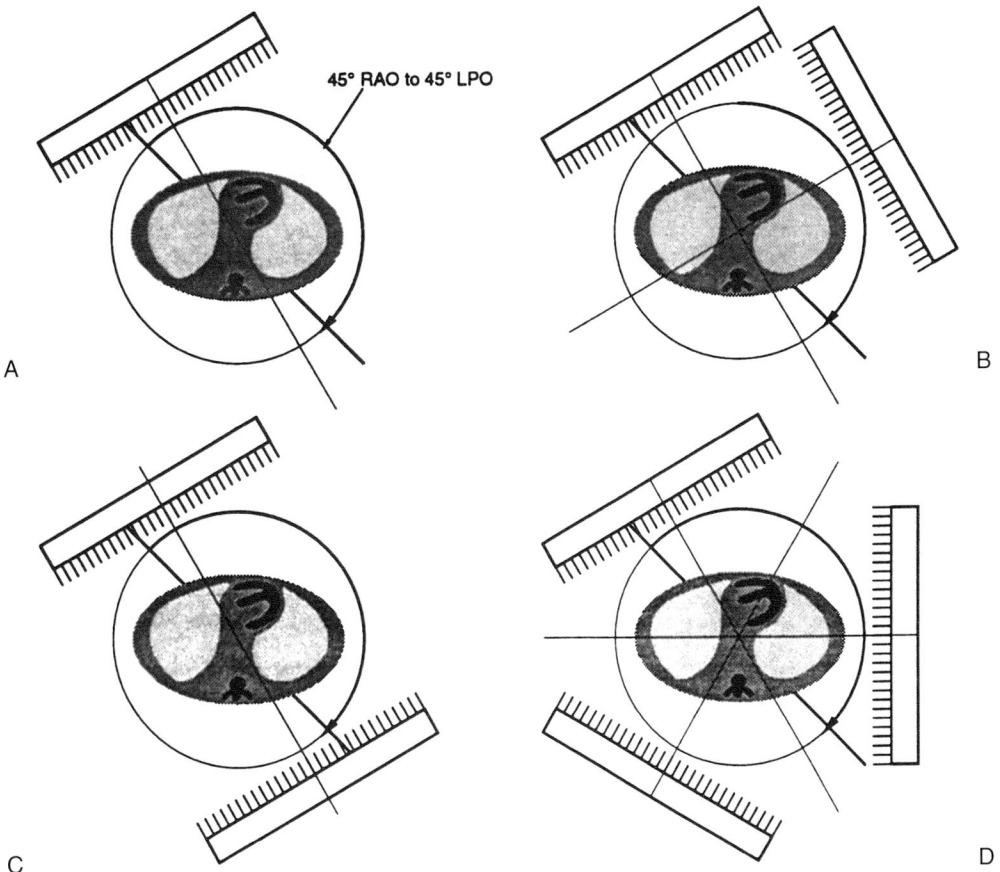

FIG. 7. Common detector configurations in SPECT cameras: (**A**) basic single-detector camera, (**B**) dual-detector, 90-degree configuration camera, (**C**) dual-detector, 180-degree configuration camera, and (**D**) triple-detector camera. *LPO*, left posterior oblique; *RAO*, right anterior oblique. (From ref. 20, with permission.)

figuration camera is possibly the best fit for cardiac imaging, because it is allowed to complete 180-degree acquisitions in half the time as with a single-detector camera, and three quarters of the time as with a triple-detector camera. The need for imaging flexibility has also led to variable-angle cameras that can be optimally configured for different types of studies. The most popular are dual-detector systems whose detectors can be positioned at 90 degrees for cardiac applications and at 180 degrees for general nuclear medicine applications, or at an intermediate angle. Recently, a triple-detector system has been developed whose detectors can be arranged in the traditional triangular scheme as well as in a U configuration.

Single Photon Emission Computed Tomography Attenuation Correction

Photon attenuation refers to the partial absorption of radioactivity arising in the patient by the tissue structure of the body. In cardiac imaging, attenuation affects different areas of the heart differently, thus preventing an accurate measurement of the relative amount of radioactivity in a given myocardial region, and has long been recognized as a fundamental limitation of myocardial perfusion SPECT (21). A recently developed approach to attenuation correction that has quickly become commercially applied in nuclear cardiology is the "simultaneous emission/transmission" technique. Transmission images can be acquired using a modified x-ray tube (22), a flood source (23), or a line source (24,25) positioned opposite the detector, and their goal is that of providing pixel-specific tissue attenuation information from which spatially-varying correction coefficients can be derived and used to modify the related emission images. Line sources are the most widely employed means of generating transmission images. In one approach, a tightly collimated line source (containing the same or a different isotope as was injected in the patient) is moved across the detector and electronically synchronized with a "scanning window" designed to acquire transmission information (transmitted through the patient), while the remainder of the detector acquires the emission data (emitted by the patient) (24). In another approach, a stationary line source is positioned between two of a triple-detector camera's detectors, and transmission data is collected by the third detector, equipped with a fan-beam collimator (25). Whatever the method, it is generally accepted that attenuation correction ought to be performed in conjunction with scatter correction, downscatter correction (if the isotope used to generate transmission information has higher energy that the injected isotope), and compensation for resolution nonuniformities (26,27). It is hoped that these corrections will eliminate or minimize differences between images of normal male and female patients, as well as nonuniformities in a given patient study caused by nonuniform tissue attenuation. To date, however, the implementation of attenuation correction with SPECT has not led to complete, accurate attenuation correction. Since the ability to perform attenuation correction based on simultaneously acquired transmission/emission data requires considerable expense to purchase the transmission hardware, in some systems may be incompatible with simultaneous gated SPECT imaging and is, to some extent, manufacturer-specific, its success will ultimately depend on standardization, full clinical validation of its incremental diagnostic and prognostic value, and clear demonstration of its cost-effectiveness compared to alternative approaches and techniques.

Positron Emission Tomography Imaging

Positron emission tomography (PET), although similar to SPECT, presents some conceptually unique features (28). To start with, PET commonly uses positron-emitting isotopes of elements naturally occurring in the human body. These isotopes are 15-O, 13-N, 11-C, and 18-F, the latter a hydrogen analog. The obvious advantage of this approach is that substrates and drugs can be labeled with those radioisotopes without having their chemical or biological properties altered. The second unique feature associated with PET imaging is the fact that not one, but two 511 keV gamma rays are emitted simultaneously as a result of the positron annihilation. For most purposes, the two gamma rays can be considered to be perfectly collinear and traveling in opposite directions. Thus, a "line of response" (LOR) is defined as the result of each annihilation, and collimation can be implemented electronically by looking at the temporal coincidence of gamma rays detected by directly opposing detectors (29). Being able to do away with a conventional collimator leads to higher sensitivity with PET compared to SPECT. Moreover, the total attenuation for the two gamma rays is constant along a given LOR, regardless of the activity's depth within the patient's body (Fig. 8); this phenomenon facilitates the measurement of attenuation using an external transmission source.

PET imaging has traditionally been performed using circular rings of bismuth germanate (BGO) detectors (28),

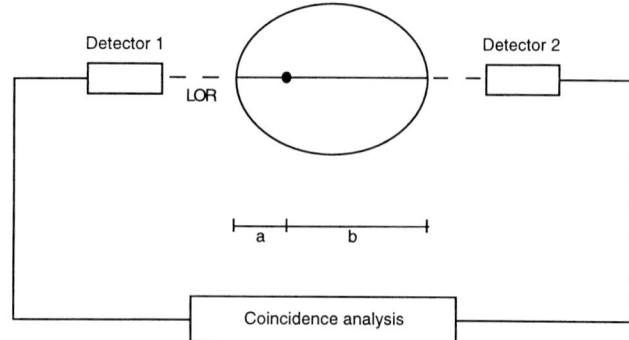

FIG. 8. Photon attenuation in positron emission tomography. Assuming (for ease of discussion) that the object being imaged has uniform attenuation coefficient μ, attenuation along the line of response (LOR) is always $e^{-a\mu} e^{-b\mu} = e^{-(a+b)\mu}$, no matter what the values for a and b (i.e., the depth of positron annihilation within the object).

TABLE 1. *Radioisotopes commonly used in position emission tomography*

Radioisotope	Half-life (min)
18-F	109.7
11-C	20.4
13-N	9.96
15-O	2.07
68-Ga	68.3
82-Rb	1.25

which are extremely dense and capable of most effectively stopping the 511 keV gamma rays. Alternative designs also exist that utilize NaI detectors arranged in a poligonal configuration (30). More recently, dual detector cameras in the 180-degree setting have been equipped with coincidence circuitry to unable them to perform both SPECT and PET imaging (31).

Most PET isotopes are cyclotron-produced, and can be divided into flow tracers (13-N ammonia, 11-C acetate) and metabolic markers (18-F fluorodeoxyglucose). A generator-produced flow tracer also exists (82-Rb), allowing facilities without cyclotrons to perform clinical myocardial perfusion SPECT. A classic way to utilize PET imaging for viability in nuclear cardiology is that of acquiring a flow study as well as a metabolic study. Myocardial areas that have impaired flow but preserved metabolism (''mismatch'' pattern) are deemed viable and are good candidates for revascularization, while areas with matching defects are likely infarcted (32).

It is interesting to note that virtually all PET isotopes have half lives that are quite short compared to their SPECT counterparts, as shown in Table 1. While this means that most of the dose to the patient is delivered during image acquisition, thus minimizing unnecessary exposure, it also implies that regional distribution of PET isotopes to imaging centers without a cyclotron can only be possible for 18-F, or possibly 68-Ga. This limitation, coupled with the fact that flow/metabolism studies using positron-emitting isotopes must be acquired sequentially (no energy discrimination is possible), has led to the suggestion that a hybrid PET/SPECT approach be used. In one of its most popular implementations, Tc-99m-sestamibi (flow) and 18F-FDG (metabolism) are imaged simultaneously employing a 511 keV collimator (33).

Because PET imaging is inherently transaxial, its basic raw data is stored in sinogram format, rather than projection image format. A sinogram is a typically nonsquare image matrix, containing a number of rows equal to the number of views from which the data was acquired, and a number of pixels per row equal to the number of parallel LORs acquired along a particular view (29). The relationship between sinograms and projection images is demonstrated in Figure 9, using familiar concepts from the SPECT world. The fact that the sinogram is a hybrid matrix containing both angular and positional information requires some care when pre-reconstruction filtering is applied (by comparison, a projection image is parallel to the patient's axis and contains only *x* and *y* positional information). Nevertheless, tomographic transaxial images are reconstructed analogously to SPECT, mainly using the filtered backprojection technique.

Tomographic Image Reorientation

The reorientation of transaxial images into short-axis images is a common practice in myocardial perfusion SPECT and PET. As explained earlier, transaxial images are perpen-

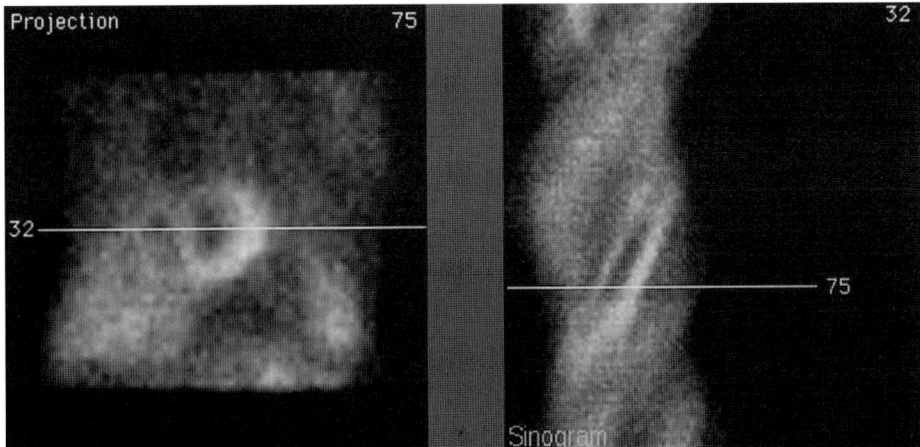

FIG. 9. Projection images and sinograms. If one imagines stacking all projection images collected in a single photon emission computed tomography acquisition on top of one another, so as to generate a "projection image volume," sinograms are obtained by "reslicing" that volume perpendicularly to the projection images. The left anterior oblique 45-degree image (which happens to be projection number 75 in a 120-deep stack) is shown on the **left**, and sinogram number 32 (which cuts through the projections' 32nd row) is shown on the **right**. In other words, there are as many sinograms as there are pixel rows in the projection images, and the number of rows in any sinogram is equal to the number of projection images collected.

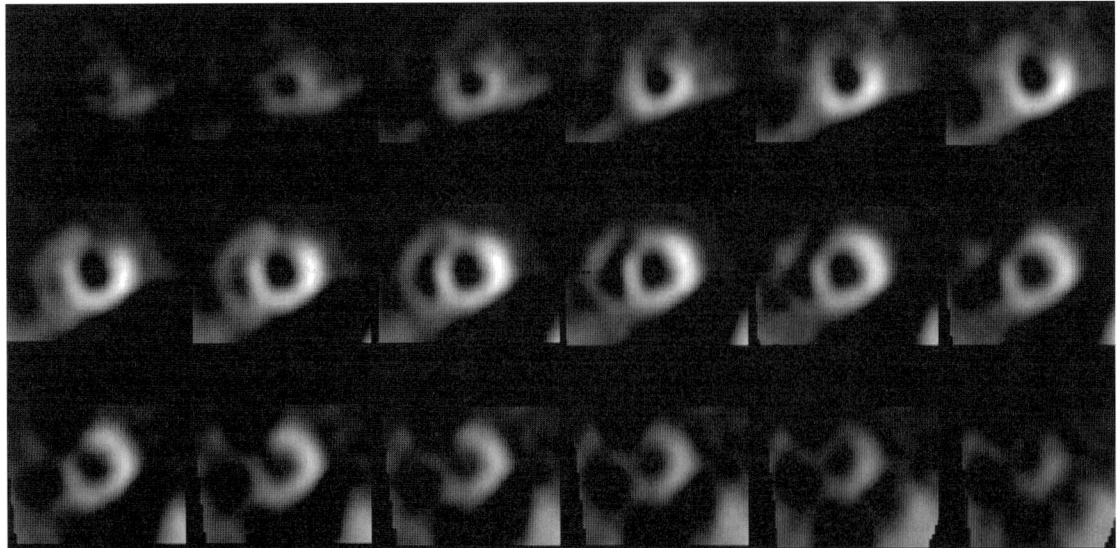

FIG. 10. Series of short-axis images (**left** to **right** and **top** to **bottom** show apical to basal) for the same patient as in Figures 3 and 5.

dicular to the patient's long axis, but not to the long axis of the patient's left ventricle. The fact that they cut through the myocardium at an oblique angle leads to regional differences in the apparent myocardial thickness, which, in turn, causes artifactual inhomogeneities in regional perfusion due to the partial volume effect phenomenon (34). Another limitation of transaxial images is that the heart's orientation within the thorax is patient-specific, thus making it difficult to compare transaxial perfusion patterns across patients.

Short-axis images, which are perpendicular to the left ventricle's long axis, allow standardization of display and interpretation by "reorienting" data from different patients to a common coordinate system. Reorientation typically requires manual selection of a midventricular transaxial and a sagittal image, as well as manual drawing of the left ventricle's (LV) long axis in those two images. The long-axis orientation in the three-dimensional space is derived based on those two

determinations, and the image volume resliced perpendicularly to it, generating short-axis, horizontal long-axis and vertical long-axis images (35). Figures 10, 11, and 12 show full sets of short-axis, horizontal long-axis, and vertical long-axis images generated from the transaxial images in Figure 5, for the patient with coronary artery disease of the left anterior descending territory.

The manual reorientation procedure is not only time consuming, but it is also subjective. In fact, manual selection of the LV's long axis for reorientation is probably the most variable step in processing myocardial perfusion SPECT data. It has been shown that if reorientation is not performed correctly, artifacts may result (36). Various software algorithms have aimed at implementing automatic reorientation as a means of promoting standardization and eliminating or reducing inter- and intraobserver variability (35,37,38), as shown in Figure 13.

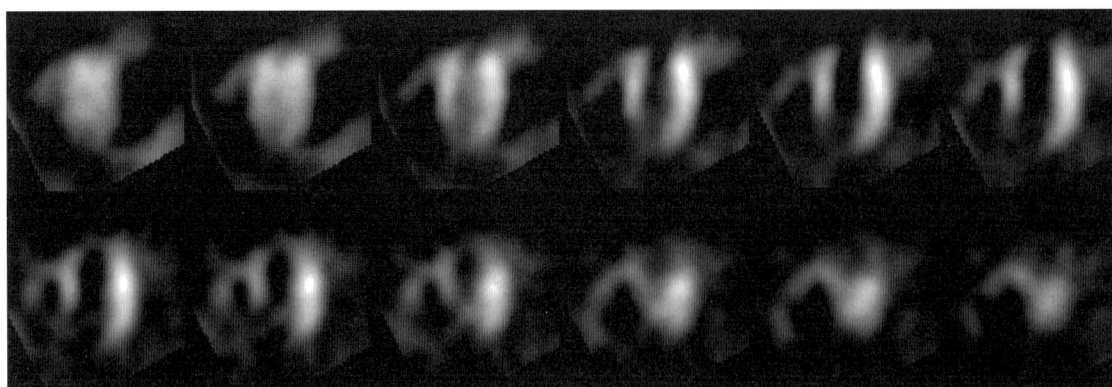

FIG. 11. Series of horizontal long-axis images (**left** to **right** and **top** to **bottom** show inferior to anterior) for the patient in Figure 10.

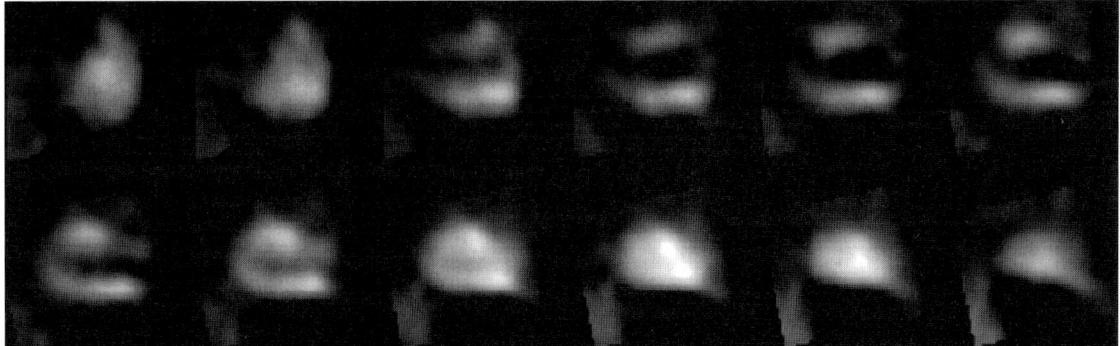

FIG. 12. Series of vertical long-axis images (**left** to **right** and **top** to **bottom** show medial to lateral images) for the patient in Figure 10.

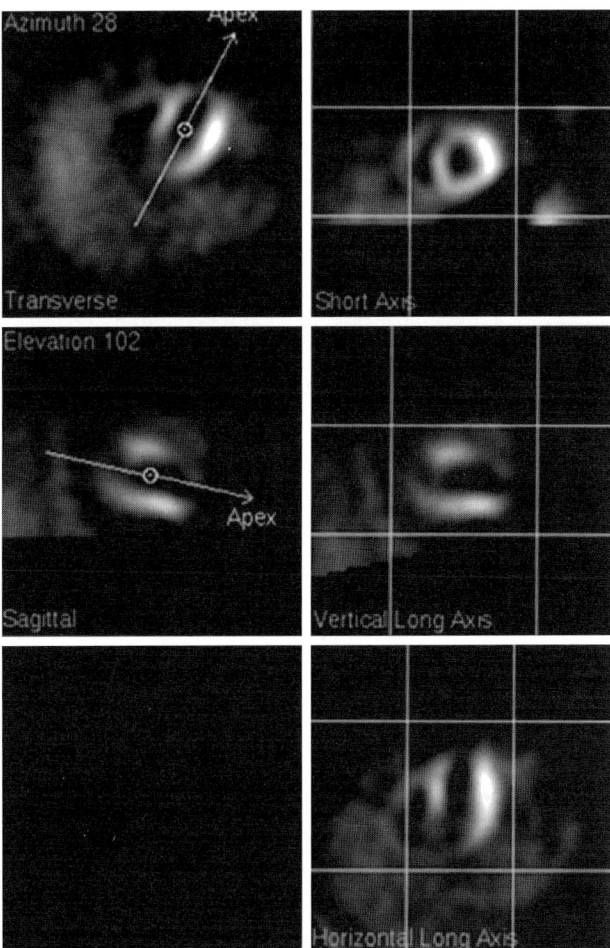

FIG. 13. Automatic reorientation of transaxial images. Determination of the left ventricle long axis in a transverse and a sagittal midventricular plane yields two angular values (azimuth and elevation), that together define the three-dimensional location of the long axis and allow reformatting of the transaxial data set into short-axis, horizontal, and vertical long-axis images.

Dynamic Planar Imaging

Dynamic acquisitions are targeted following the evolution of a dynamic process, such as the change in the location of injected activity over time. For ease of visualization, a dynamic planar acquisition can be thought of as a series of planar images, each corresponding to a specific time interval (hence the notation of "frames" for these images, analogously to cinematography).

The first-pass technique is a type of dynamic acquisition that uses very fine temporal sampling (20 to 100 frames per second) to look at the initial transit of a radionuclide bolus through the central circulation, as shown in Figure 14 (39). In principle, the radionuclide should remain in the vascular space for the duration of the study. In practice, since the duration of first-pass studies is very short, virtually all non-particulate technetium-labeled radiopharmaceuticals are appropriate for this study. With 99m technetium-labeled myocardial perfusion agents, a minor error in first-pass studies is introduced by the small fraction of the injected dose that is taken up in the initial transit by the myocardium. However, this fraction is minimal, and the perfusion agents Tc-99m-sestamibi and Tc-99m-tetrofosmin have been used with success in first-pass studies. First-pass acquisition often immediately precedes standard SPECT imaging in single-injection protocols aimed at measuring true stress cardiac function (left and right ventricular ejection fraction, emptying/filling rates, and regional wall motion) as well as stress myocardial perfusion.

Key to the successful application of the first-pass technique is the administration of the bolus, which should be extremely compact (less than 1 ml in volume). Acquisition is completed in less than 1 minute, and can be performed in any desired view, since distinct temporal relationships in the transit of radioactivity through the various cardiac chambers allow their separation with first pass studies.

Electrocardiographically (ECG)-gated planar acquisitions are another form of dynamic imaging. With this approach, each image corresponds to a specific portion (also termed interval, gate, or frame) of the cardiac cycle, identified rela-

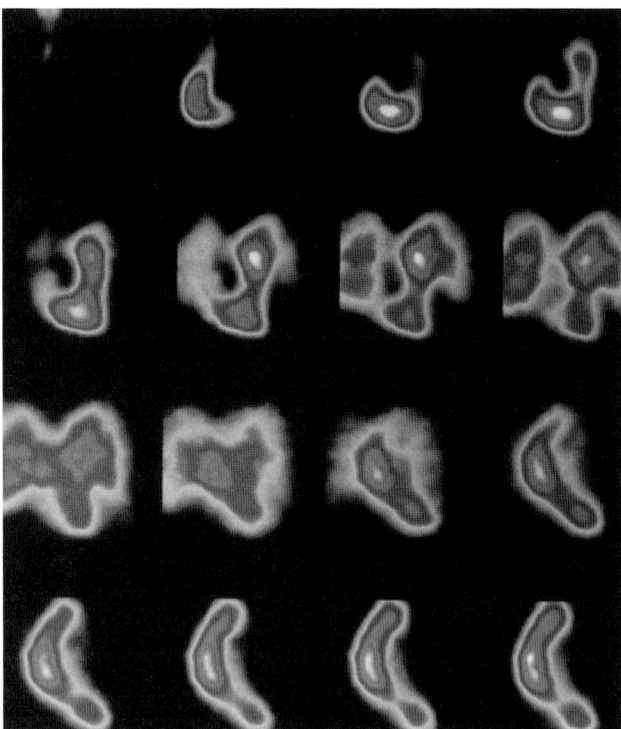

FIG. 14. First pass data grouped into 1-second images to show the transit of the injected radioactive bolus through (**left** to **right**, **top** to **bottom**) the superior vena cava, right atrium and ventricle, pulmonary artery and lungs, and left ventricle and ascending aorta. (From ref. 58, with permission.)

tive to the R wave of the patient's ECG. Because the cardiac cycle is divided in as many as 8 to 64 intervals, data from many different cycles (up to several hundreds of them) must be averaged to ensure adequate count statistics. In brief, counts collected during the nth interval from the occurrence of each R-wave trigger are accumulated in the same planar image (frame n). Acquisition stops when a preset number of counts has been collected, or when a predetermined period of time has elapsed.

Although ECG-gating can be employed in conjunction with first-pass imaging, it is more commonly used with equilibrium blood pool imaging (40,41). Unlike first-pass scintigraphy, equilibrium-gated blood pool scintigraphy requires that the injected radiopharmaceutical remain within the vascular compartment for a prolonged period. Although labeled proteins, such as Tc-99m-albumin, could be employed for blood pool imaging, labeled red blood cells are most commonly employed, labeled through either *in vivo* or *in vitro* methods. The latter provides the highest target to background ratio.

In conventional ECG-gated acquisition (also referred to as "fixed temporal resolution"), there is a fixed number of gating intervals, all of which have the same length (generally between 10 to 20 msec or 50 to 100 msec), as shown in Figure 15. Since in reality all cardiac cycles do not have the same length, some problems may ensue. In the "forward

gating" mode, where intervals are assigned to adjacent locations starting at the R-wave, (i) the final portion of the cycle may not be adequately sampled when the time between two consecutive R-wave triggers is longer than average (Fig. 15**A**), or (ii) the later intervals may consistently collect fewer counts when the R-wave triggers are closer than average. Because of these intrinsic limitations to the forward gating approach, alternative gating methods have been developed (42). In the "backward gating" mode, the gating intervals are synchronized from the R wave backwards (Fig. 15**B**), while in the "hybrid forward-backward" mode a combination of the two modes is used (Fig. 15**C**). The "variable temporal resolution" method is a more complex approach in which the R–R duration is dynamically adjusted to match the average length of the latest few cardiac cycles, and the length of the gating intervals, which remain constant in number, changes accordingly (Fig. 15**D**). This method is, of course, computationally more intensive, since it requires the alteration of the intervals' length on a beat-by-beat basis.

Gated Single Photon Emission Computed Tomography/Positron Emission Tomography Imaging

Gated acquisitions can also be employed when collecting tomographic data with either myocardial perfusion SPECT (43,44), myocardial perfusion PET (45), or blood pool SPECT (46). Most of the considerations previously described for gated planar imaging apply to the individual projection images acquired in gated-SPECT imaging. Projection

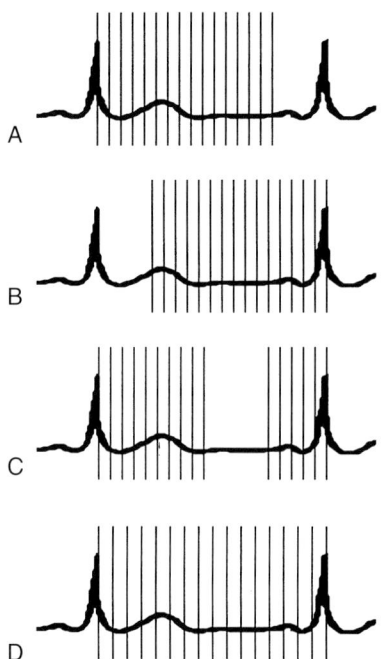

FIG. 15. Examples of a 16-interval, fixed temporal (**A**) forward-gated, (**B**) backward-gated, and (**C**) forward/backward-gated (²⁄₃ of the intervals forward-gated, ⅓ backward-gated) acquisition, as well as (**D**) a 16-interval, variable temporal acquisition, all for a cardiac cycle of longer than average duration. (From ref. 10, with permission.)

TABLE 2. *Dimensionality of common nuclear cardiology protocols*

Study	Dimensions	Variables	Number of images
Standard planar	2	X, Y	1–4
First pass	3	X, Y, time	500–5000
Gated planar	3	X, Y, time	14–100
Standard SPECT or PET	3	X, Y, Z	30–120
Gated SPECT or PET	4	X, Y, time	240–1920

images corresponding to the same interval of the cardiac cycle are typically reconstructed to yield a three-dimensional representation of the LV and/or cavity in that interval. After iterating this process, the various three-dimensional datasets (usually 8 to 16) can be displayed in cinematic loop, to better allow the visual and quantitative assessment of global ejection fraction and regional wall motion and wall thickening. Gated SPECT or PET imaging produces four-dimensional datasets (X, Y, Z, and time), but not necessarily a larger number of images than a three-dimensional technique like first-pass imaging (X, Y, and time). Table 2 illustrates the dimensionality associated with various nuclear cardiology protocols.

All other factors being equal, one would want to acquire data using the highest number of dimensions possible, since additional information can be gathered in this manner. However, Table 2 clearly shows that higher dimension acquisitions produce a greater number of images. Since the injected dose is limited by dosimetry constraints and the acquisition time is limited by patients' tolerance and motion, a higher-dimension acquisition must distribute approximately the same number of counts amongst more images. Thus, a compromise is usually sought between image dimensions and image statistics. (It should be noted that first-pass and blood pool studies have intrinsically more available counts than perfusion studies for an equal injected dose, because radioactivity concentration in the blood with blood pool tracers is much higher than in the myocardium with myocardial perfusion tracers.)

CAMERA/COMPUTER SYSTEMS

Gamma cameras are usually equipped with an acquisition computer (used to control the motion of the detector and the initial sorting of the data into projection images) and a processing/display workstation (used to reconstruct, analyze, and display the data). Acquisition computers are typically not very powerful, but are "dedicated" to the specific camera with which they interface. Processing workstations, on the other hand, can be extremely powerful, and have been trending toward incorporating fewer and fewer proprietary graphic display boards or camera-specific "accelerator" hardware. The ultimate goal should be to allow end-users to purchase processing/analysis/display workstations "off

the shelf" and to connect them (over a local or a wide area network) to any gamma camera. The main impediment to this approach is the proprietary image format employed by camera manufacturers. In order to process, analyze, or display an image file, the proprietary database that contains that file must be queried, the file retrieved, and (in many cases) transferred to the polling workstation. If the file is altered or new files are created as a result of processing, the processed file(s) must be written back to the originating database. Since image formats are widely considered "trade secrets," manufacturers usually tend to provide a software "server" that will query, read from and write to the database, but will make all data available in a converted, nonproprietary format. A very popular nonproprietary format for nuclear medicine is Interfile (47), while most imaging-wide approaches (incorporating nuclear medicine as well as x-ray, computerized tomography, and magnetic resonance images) are based on the DICOM standard (48).

At the current time, different manufacturers' implementations of DICOM often have a small number of noncorresponding or incompatible fields, and some of the original fields may be lost in the conversion process (49). This situation, however, is expected to improve in the near future. In addition, processing, analysis, and display software used on nonacquisition workstations is increasingly being developed by academic institutions and licensed to various camera manufacturers. This presents the dual advantage of speeding up clinical validation of the software and promoting a more standardized approach.

SAFETY

The most commonly used isotopes in nuclear cardiology are listed in Table 3, together with their photon energy and half-life. Table 4 summarizes typical nuclear cardiology procedures that employ those isotopes, together with the injected dose and procedure duration. Radiation exposure to either patients or staff of a nuclear cardiology laboratory is relatively low, and certainly much less than that associated with other radiation-rich environments, such as a catheterization laboratory (50). In addition, strict regulations have been developed that control and limit the amount of radioactivity administered as well as establishing clear procedures for

TABLE 3. *Radioisotopes commonly used in nuclear cardiology*

Isotope	Half-life (min)	Energy (keV)
Thallium-201 (Tl-201)	4,380	68–83, 162
Indium-111 (111-In)	4,032	171, 246
Iodine-123 (123-I)	780	159
Technetium-99m (Tc-99m)	360	140
Fluorine-18 (18-F)	110	511
Nitrogen-13 (13-N)	10	511
Rubidium-82 (82-Rb)	1.3	511

(From ref. 50, with permission.)

TABLE 4. *Common nuclear cardiology protocols**

	Isotope	Injected dose (mCi)	Duration (min)
First-pass Radionuclide Angiography	Tc-99m	25	1–2
Planar/SPECT equilibrium-gated blood Pool	Tc-99m	20–30	2–30
Planar/SPECT Perfusion	Tl-201	2.5–3.5	10–40
Planar/SPECT Perfusion (with Reinjection)	Tl-201	3 + 1.5 @ 2–4 hr	10–40 + 10–40 @ 2–4 hr
Planar/SPECT Perfusion	Tc-99m-MPA	20–25	10–30
Planar/SPECT Perfusion (2-day stress-rest)	Tc-99m-MPA	20–30 + 20–30 next day	10–30 + 10–30 next day
Planar/SPECT Perfusion (1-day stress-rest with Reinjection)	Tc-99m-MPA	10–15 + 25–30 @ 2–4 hr	10–30 + 10–30 @ 2–4 hr
Planar/SPECT Perfusion (1-day rest-stress with Reinjection)	Tc-99m-MPA	8–12 + 22–25 @ 2–4 hr	10–30 + 10–30 @ 2–4 hr
Dual isotope SPECT Perfusion (rest-stress)	Tl-201 + Tc-99m-MPA	2.5–3 + 22–25 @ <1 hr	15–30 + 20–40 @ <1 hr
Technetium-99m pyrophosphate	Tc-99m	15	10–40
Metabolic FDG imaging (SPECT or PET)	18-FDG	10	15–45
Indium-111 antimyosin antibodies	111-In	2	10–40

*Study duration depends on the use of single or multidetector camera, as well as on the number of views acquired (planar studies). *MPA*, myocardial perfusion agent (usually Tc-99m-sestamibi or Tc-99m-tetrofosmin).
(From ref. 50, with permission.)

handling and monitoring it. In the United States, regulatory jurisdiction is provided (i) by the Nuclear Regulatory Commission (NRC) under the Atomic Energy Act, or (ii) by state radiation regulatory agencies. The NRC can agree to transfer most regulatory authority to the individual states ("Agreement States"), if their regulatory program is deemed compatible with that of the NRC. NRC regulations are codified in the Code of Federal Regulations (CFR), Title 10 of which (civilian use of radioactivity) has special relevance for nuclear medicine. In particular, 10 CFR, Part 19, covers instructions to radiation workers and the right of the regulatory agency to conduct inspections and investigations, while 10 CFR, Part 20, defines the standards for protection against radiation, including (i) occupational dose limits for adults, minors, and pregnant women, (ii) determination of internal exposure, (iii) individual monitoring of occupational dose, and (iv) labeling, waste disposal, and reporting requirements. In practice, radioactive materials licenses of various scope are issued to hospitals, research universities, and private practice clinics that can demonstrate to have an adequate radiation safety program in place. Once the license has been granted, the Radiation Safety Committee or the Radiation Safety Officer at the licensed institution issues radioactive materials use permits to individuals. At the present time, nuclear physicians and radiologists who need a license to possess radioactive materials in order to perform nuclear cardiology procedures must be board certified and other physicians (such as cardiologists) must receive a minimum of (i) 200 hours of didactic instruction on the basics of radioisotope handling, and (ii) 500 hours of clinical preceptorship focused on the performance and interpretation of actual nuclear procedures.

As far as radiation delivered to the patient is concerned, the standard method for performing internal radiation dosimetry calculation from injected radioisotopes is the *absorbed fraction method* (2). The assumption underlying this method

is that the radiation dose delivered to a "target organ" can be reasonably estimated from the radioactivity contained in a number of "source organs" (including the target organ) in the patient body. Variables to be considered are the type, amount, and physical and biological half-life of the radioisotope(s) used, the pattern of uptake in the various source organs, and the spatial and geometric relationship of the source organs to the target organ in each specific patient. To simplify matters, dose calculations are performed for an "average patient," using the data published by the Medical Internal Radiation Dosimetry (MIRD) committee of the Society of Nuclear Medicine (51). Maximum admissible dose to a critical target organ (or to the patient's body as a whole) limits the amount of radioactive material that can be injected into a patient. Thus, radioisotopes with a longer half-life are injected in smaller quantities (see Tables 3 and 4).

As far as exposure to technologists and physicians performing nuclear procedures is concerned, the maximum allowable radiation limits for medical radiation workers are summarized in Table 5 (50). In addition, the National Council on Radiation Protection and measurements (NCRP) has

TABLE 5. *Maximum allowable radiation limits for medical radiation workers, from all sources*

Organ	Maximum allowable radiation	
	rem/yr	mSv/yr
Whole body	5	50
Skin	30–50	300–500
Hands, feet	50–75	500–750
Lens of the eye	5–15	50–150
Fetus (pregnant worker)	0.5	5
Other, including thyroid	15	150
Cumulative exposure	1 rem × age	10 mSv × age

mSv, milliSievert; yr, year.
(From refs. 54, 55, and 56, with permission.)

recommended the use of the "As Low As Reasonably Achievable" (ALARA) principle (52). ALARA is based on the three fundamental rules of (i) increasing distance from the radioactive source (including the patient), (ii) decreasing time of exposure to radiation, and (iii) use of shielding. Exposure from a radioactive source is inversely proportional to the square of the distance from the source ("inverse square law"), implying that exposure can be reduced by 75% if only one doubles one's distance from the source (53). Also, working quickly and/or behind leaded glass when preparing injectable doses will greatly reduce exposure. Shielding a radiation worker's body with a lead apron is effective and practical when the radiation's energy is relatively low (140 keV or less); conversely, gamma rays of 511 keV or above are highly penetrating, and a wearable lead shield would unduly slow down the operator while not providing adequate protection.

REFERENCES

1. Knoll GF. *Radiation detection and measurement.* New York: Wiley, 1979.
2. Sorenson JA, Phelps ME. *Physics in nuclear medicine,* 2nd ed. Orlando: Grune & Stratton; 1987.
3. Anger H. Scintillation camera. *Rev Sci Instr* 1958;29(1):27–33.
4. Simmons G. Gamma camera imaging systems. In: RE Henkin, ed. *Nuclear medicine.* St. Louis: Mosby, 1996:85–95.
5. Cullom S. Principles of cardiac SPECT. In: EG DePuey, DS Berman, and EV Garcia, eds. *Cardiac SPECT imaging.* New York: Raven Press, 1995:1–19.
6. Kiat H, Berman DS, Maddahi J. Comparison of planar and tomographic exercise thallium-201 imaging methods for the evaluation of coronary artery disease. *J Am Coll Cardiol* 1989;13(3):613–616.
7. Shepp LA, Logan BF. The Fourier reconstruction of a head section. *IEEE Trans. Nucl. Sci.* 1974-21(3):21–43.
8. Brooks RA, Di Chiro G. Theory of image reconstruction in computed tomography. *Radiology* 1975;117(3 Pt 1):561–572.
9. Herman GT, Meyer LB. Algebraic reconstruction techniques can be made computationally efficient (positron emission tomography application). *IEEE Trans. Med. Imaging* 1993;12(3):600–609.
10. Germano G, Van Train K, Kiat H, et al. Digital techniques for the acquisition, processing, and analysis of nuclear cardiology images. In: MP Sandler, ed. *Diagnostic nuclear medicine.* Baltimore: Williams & Wilkins, 1995:347–386.
11. Maublant JC, Peycelon P, Kwiatkowski F, et al. Comparison between 180 degrees and 360 degrees data collection in technetium-99m MIBI SPECT of the myocardium. *J Nucl Med* 1989;30(3):295–300.
12. Eisner RL, Nowak DJ, Pettigrew R, et al. Fundamentals of 180 degree acquisition and reconstruction in SPECT imaging. *J Nucl Med* 1986; 27(11):1717–1728.
13. Knesaurek K, King MA, Glick SJ, et al. Investigation of causes of geometric distortion in 180 degrees and 360 degrees angular sampling in SPECT. *J Nucl Med* 1989;30(10):1666–1675.
14. Go RT, MacIntyre WJ, Houser TS, et al. Clinical evaluation of 360 degrees and 180 degrees data sampling techniques for transaxial SPECT thallium-201 myocardial perfusion imaging. *J Nucl Med* 1985; 26(7):695–706.
15. Todd-Pokropek A. Non-circular orbits for the reduction of uniformity artefacts in SPECT. *Phys Med Biol* 1983;28(3):309–313.
16. Maniawski PJ, Morgan HT, Wackers FJ. Orbit-related variation in spatial resolution as a source of artifactual defects in thallium-201 SPECT [Comments]. *J Nucl Med* 1991;32(5):871–875.
17. Germano G, Kavanagh PB, Berman DS. Effect of the number of projections collected on quantitative perfusion and left ventricular ejection fraction measurements from gated myocardial perfusion single-photon emission computed tomographic images. *J Nucl Cardiol* 1996;3(5): 395–402.

18. Moore SC, Kouris K, Cullum I. Collimator design for single photon emission tomography. *Eur J Nucl Med* 1992;19(2):138–150.
19. Gregoriou GK, Tsui BM, Gullberg GT. Effect of truncated projections on defect detection in attenuation-compensated fanbeam cardiac SPECT. *J Nucl Med* 1998;39(1):166–175.
20. Galt J, Germano G. Advances in instrumentation for cardiac SPECT. In: EG DePuey, DS Berman, and EV Garcia, eds. *Cardiac SPECT imaging.* New York, Raven Press, 1995:91–102.
21. Chang L-T. A method for attenuation correction in radionuclide computed tomography. *IEEE Trans. Nucl. Sci.* 1978-25(1):638–643.
22. Hasegawa BH, Lang IF, Brown JK, et al. Object-specific attenuation correction of SPECT with correlated dual-energy X-ray CT. *IEEE Trans. Nucl. Sci.* 1993;40(4, Part 2):1242–1252.
23. Bailey DL, Hutton BF, Walker PJ. Improved SPECT using simultaneous emission and transmission tomography. *J Nucl Med* 1987;28(5): 844–851.
24. Tan P, Bailey DL, Meikle SR, Eberl S, Fulton RR, Hutton BF. A scanning line source for simultaneous emission and transmission measurements in SPECT. *J Nucl Med* 1993;34(10):1752–1760.
25. Tung CH, Gullberg GT, Zeng GL, et al. Nonuniform attenuation correction using simultaneous transmission and emission converging tomography. *IEEE Trans. Nucl. Sci.* 1992;39(4):1134–1143.
26. Cullom S, Hendel R, Liu L, et al. Diagnostic accuracy and image quality of a scatter, attenuation and resolution compensation method for Tc-99m cardiac SPECT: preliminary results. *J Nucl Med* 1996;37(5): 81P(abst).
27. Cullom S, Liu L, White M. Compensation of attenuation map errors from Tc-99m-sestamibi downscatter with simultaneous Gd-153 transmission scanning. *J Nucl Med* 1996;37(5):215P(abst).
28. Hoffman E, Phelps M. Positron emission tomography: principles and quantitation. In: ME Phelps, JC Mazziotta, and HR Schelbert, eds. *Positron emission tomography and autoradiography: principles and applications for the brain and heart.* New York: Raven Press, 1986: 237–286.
29. Germano G. "An investigation of deadtime and count rate limitations for high resolution, multiplane PET systems." Ph.D. thesis, UCLA, 1991.
30. Muehllehner G, Karp JS, Mankoff DA, et al. Design and performance of a new positron tomograph. *IEEE Trans. Nucl. Sci.* 1988;35(1, pt.1): 670–674.
31. Jarritt PH, Acton PD. PET imaging using gamma camera systems: a review. *Nucl Med Commun* 1996;17(9):758–766.
32. Schelbert H, Schwaiger M. PET studies of the heart. In: ME Phelps, JC Mazziotta, and HR Schelbert, eds. *Positron emission tomography and autoradiography: principles and applications for the brain and heart.* New York: Raven Press, 1986:581–661.
33. Sandler MP, Patton JA. Fluorine 18-labeled fluorodeoxyglucose myocardial single-photon emission computed tomography: an alternative for determining myocardial viability. *J Nucl Cardiol* 1996;3(4): 342–349.
34. Hoffman EJ, Huang SC, Phelps ME. Quantitation in positron emission computed tomography: 1. Effect of object size. *J Comput Assist Tomogr* 1979;3(3):299–308.
35. Germano G, Kavanagh PB, Su HT, et al. Automatic reorientation of three-dimensional, transaxial myocardial perfusion SPECT images [Comments]. *J Nucl Med* 1995;36(6):1107–1114.
36. DePuey E. Artifacts in SPECT myocardial perfusion imaging. In: EG DePuey, DS Berman, EV Garcia, eds. *Cardiac SPECT imaging.* New York: Raven Press, 1995:169–200.
37. Cauvin JC, Boire JY, Maublant JC, et al. Automatic detection of the left ventricular myocardium long axis and center in thallium-201 single photon emission computed tomography. *Eur J Nucl Med* 1992;19(12): 1032–1037.
38. Slomka PJ, Hurwitz GA, Stephenson J, et al. Automated alignment and sizing of myocardial stress and rest scans to three-dimensional normal templates using an image registration algorithm [Comments]. *J Nucl Med* 1995;36(6):1115–1122.
39. Port S. First-pass radionuclide angiography. In: ML Marcus and E Braunwald, eds. *Marcus cardiac imaging: a companion to Braunwald's heart disease.* Philadelphia: WB Saunders, 1996:923–941.
40. Strauss HW, Zaret BL, Hurley PJ, et al. A scintiphotographic method for measuring left ventricular ejection fraction in man without cardiac catheterization. *Am J Cardiol* 1971;28(5):575–580.
41. Berman DS, Salel AF, DeNardo GL, et al. Clinical assessment of left

ventricular regional contraction patterns and ejection fraction by high-resolution gated scintigraphy. *J Nucl Med* 1975;16(10):865–874.

42. Bacharach SL, Bonow RO, Green MV. Comparison of fixed and variable temporal resolution methods for creating gated cardiac blood-pool image sequences. *J Nucl Med* 1990;31(1):38–42.

43. Mannting F, Morgan-Mannting MG. Gated SPECT with technetium-99m-sestamibi for assessment of myocardial perfusion abnormalities. *J Nucl Med* 1993;34(4):601–608.

44. Berman DS, Kiat H, Van Train K, et al. Technetium 99m sestamibi in the assessment of chronic coronary artery disease [Comments]. *Semin Nucl Med* 1991;21(3):190–212.

45. Yamashita K, Tamaki N, Yonekura Y, et al. Quantitative analysis of regional wall motion by gated myocardial positron emission tomography: validation and comparison with left ventriculography. *J Nucl Med* 1989;30(11):1775–1786.

46. Moore ML, Murphy PH, Burdine JA. ECG-gated emission computed tomography of the cardiac blood pool. *Radiology* 1980;134(1):233–235.

47. Todd-Pokropek A, Cradduck TD, Deconinck F. A file format for the exchange of nuclear medicine image data: a specification of Interfile version 3.3. *Nucl Med Commun* 1992;13(9):673–699.

48. Horii SC, Bidgood WD, Jr. PACS mini refresher course. Network and ACR-NEMA protocols. *Radiographics* 1992;12(3):537–548.

49. Eichelberg M, Baljion M, Gerritsen M, Jensch P. Interoperability of DICOM implementations can be enhanced significantly by a QC approach using automated validation tools. *J Am Coll Cardiol* 1999;33(2)[Suppl.A]:8A (Abst).

50. Limacher MC, Douglas PS, Germano G, et al. ACC expert consensus document. Radiation safety in the practice of cardiology. *J Am Coll Cardiol* 1998;31(4):892–913.

51. Loevinger R, Budinger TF, Watson EE. MIRD primer for absorbed dose calculations, New York: Society of Nuclear Medicine, 1991.

52. Implementation of the as low as reasonably achievable (ALARA) for medical and dental personnel. NCRP Report No. 107. 1990.

53. Johns HE, Cunningham JR. *The physics of radiology,* 4th ed, Springfield, IL: Charles C Thomas, 1983.

54. Radiation protection for medical and allied health personnel. NCRP Report No. 105. 1989.

55. Johnson LW, Moore RJ, Balter S. Review of radiation safety in the cardiac catheterization laboratory. *Cathet Cardiovasc Diagn* 1992;25(3):186–194.

56. Judkins MP. Guidelines for radiation protection in the cardiac catheterization laboratory. *Cathet Cardiovasc Diagn* 1984;10(1):87–92.

57. Henkin RE. *Nuclear medicine.* St. Louis: Mosby, 1996.

58. Marcus ML, Braunwald E. *Marcus cardiac imaging: a comparison to Braunwald's heart disease*, 2nd ed. Philadelphia: W. B. Saunders, 1996.

CHAPTER 12

Stress Approaches

Techniques

Mario S. Verani

Resting myocardial perfusion is often normal in patients with coronary artery disease (CAD), because arterial coronary vasodilation distal to coronary stenosis may be sufficient to preserve myocardial blood flow within the baseline levels. Thus, imaging during stress is required to demonstrate abnormalities in myocardial perfusion. Contrary to intuitive reasoning, the putative mechanism of stress-induced perfusion abnormalities is not the provocation of myocardial ischemia but rather the creation of heterogeneous myocardial perfusion in different myocardial vascular territories. The mechanism of stress-induced perfusion abnormalities is essentially the same, regardless of the type of stress—a maximal or near maximal increase in coronary blood flow through the normal coronary arteries and a lesser increase, or no increase through stenotic coronary arteries. As originally demonstrated by Gould et al. (1–5), the normal coronary flow reserve is an increase of four- to fivefold above the baseline flow values. In arteries with significant coronary stenosis, the coronary flow reserve is reduced in proportion to the stenosis severity and is essentially abolished when the degree of stenosis reaches 80 to 90%.

Within limits, the myocardial uptake of radioactive tracers is linearly related to the myocardial blood flow (6–8). This is certainly true when the myocardial blood flow is normal, decreased, or moderately increased (Fig. 1). However, when the coronary blood flow increases above 2 to 2½ times the baseline values, the increase in myocardial tracer is less than the increase in flow (the so-called "roll-off effect") (9). This roll-off effect is more severe during pharmacologic coronary vasodilation than during exercise, presumably because the uptake falls when the coronary flow velocity is very rapid and the myocardial oxygen demand is not increased propor-

tionately. The roll-off effect is also more severe for tracers with lower myocardial extraction; consequently, it is less with Tc-99m teboroxine (10) and thallium-201 (11) than with the other available Tc-99m labeled compounds, such as sestamibi (11–13) and tetrofosmin (14).

EXERCISE STRESS

Exercise remains the most common type of stress used in association with myocardial perfusion imaging. In the United States, approximately 70% of all stress perfusion imaging is performed with exercise stress. Moderately severe exercise elicits major hemodynamic, respiratory, and metabolic adaptations in sedentary young subjects (15). Under resting conditions, the fraction of the cardiac output that perfuses the coronary arteries is approximately 5%. During moderately severe exercise, the cardiac output increases by approximately threefold, largely due to a marked increase in heart rate, with a smaller increase in stroke volume. In well-conditioned athletes, the increase in heart rate is of less magnitude, whereas the increase in stroke volume is more substantial (15).

Exercise affects all of the factors that control the myocardial oxygen consumption producing large increases in heart rate, contractility, and systolic blood pressure with smaller increases in left ventricular end-diastolic volume. In normal individuals, the increase in myocardial oxygen demand is paralleled by an increase in myocardial oxygen supply, which is achieved by an increase in coronary blood flow (dominant) and a widening of the arteriovenous oxygen difference across the coronary bed (secondary).

Exercise, however, does not preferentially increase the myocardial blood flow; thus, the increase in coronary flow is directly dependent on the increase in cardiac output. The fraction of the cardiac output perfusing the coronary arteries

M. S. Verani: Department of Medicine/Cardiology, Baylor College of Medicine; Department of Nuclear Cardiology, The Methodist Hospital, Houston, Texas 77030.

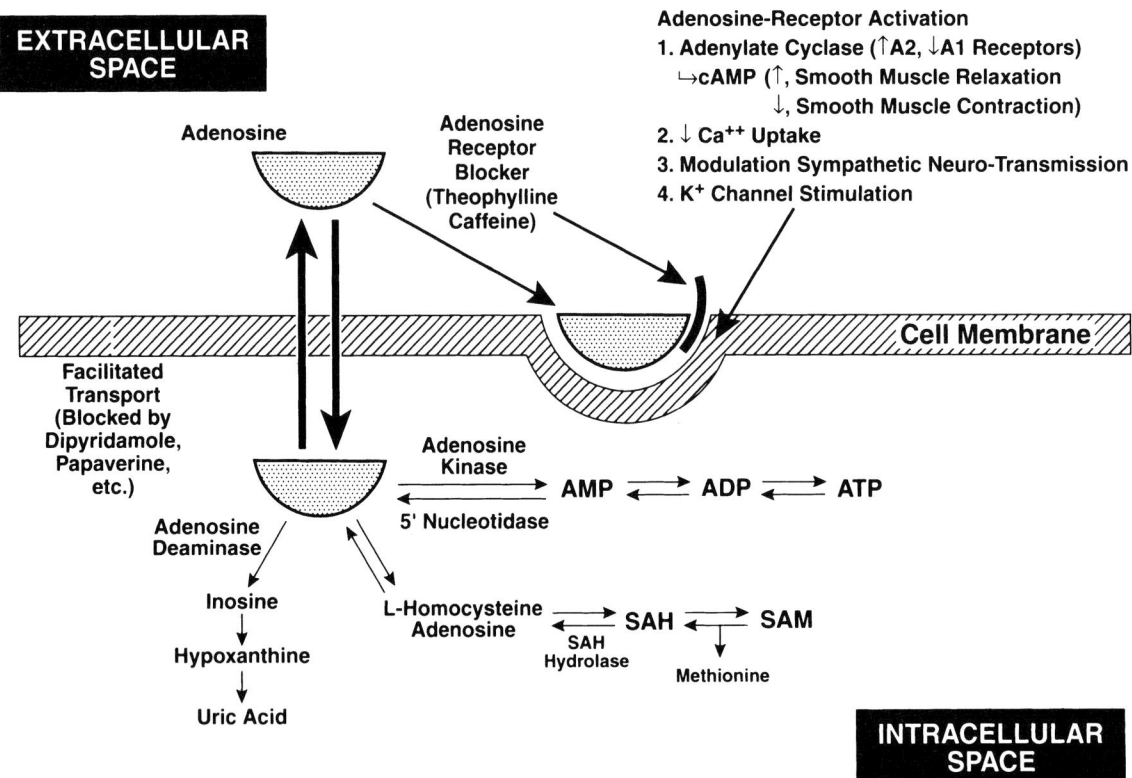

FIG. 1. Mechanism of pharmacologic coronary vasodilation by adenosine and dipyridamole.

is the same during exercise as that during rest conditions. For a threefold increase in cardiac output, the coronary blood flow will also increase approximately threefold. Thus, even maximal exercise does not fully stress the coronary flow reserve. Importantly, the lower the intensity of the exercise, the less the increase in coronary blood flow. The corollary is that if the coronary flow increases only minimally during a low-intensity exercise, flow heterogeneity between normal and abnormal coronary arteries may not be achieved and therefore even a relatively severe stenosis with very limited flow reserve may not be identifiable.

There is an approximate linear relationship between peak exercise heart rate or peak heart rate times peak systolic blood pressure and myocardial oxygen demands (16). Thus, the peak exercise heart rate, or the product of the peak systolic pressure and heart rate ("double product"), are used as surrogate measures of the increase in oxygen demand.

EXERCISE PROTOCOLS

In the United States, exercise is usually performed on a treadmill, during which the speed and the inclination are progressively increased at 3-minute intervals. In European and other countries, bicycle exercise is more popular. For persons not particularly experienced in bicycling, the treadmill is an easier approach. The Bruce protocol is most often utilized and has stood the test of time. Other protocols are preferred in certain institutions (17). The exercise test proceeds until a target is achieved, which is usually the maximal

predicted heart rate, calculated by the formula "220−age in years." A test is considered "maximal" when the heart rate reaches 100% of the age and gender maximal predicted rates. A commonly used target heart rate is 85% of the maximal predicted heart rate; by definition, this is a submaximal test although attainment of 85% of this target is considered evidence of "sufficient" exercise. Other targets may be selected, such as a "symptom-limited" test where the termination of the test is dictated by the physical inability of the patient to proceed; i.e., exercise would be carried even beyond maximal predicted heart rate until limiting symptoms develop.

The effect of a maximal versus a submaximal exercise test on the sensitivity of myocardial perfusion imaging is controversial (18–20). In the author's laboratory, the preferred target is either 100% of the maximal heart rate or a symptom-limited test. The 85% target heart rate is viewed as the minimal rate to consider the test adequate. Obviously, certain exercise end-points may be reached before achieving the target heart rate. For example, strongly positive ischemic ST-segment changes, severe angina, severe dyspnea, or a fall in systolic blood pressure are all traditional indications to terminate the test, regardless of the peak heart rate achieved. However, one should always keep in mind that the goal of the exercise stress is to induce the largest possible discrepancy in blood flow because the larger the discrepancy achieved, the more likely it is that a perfusion defect will be identified.

MONITORING THE EXERCISE TESTS

At the present time, most laboratories monitor the standard 12-lead electrocardiogram (ECG) and the blood pressure during exercise. Measurements of actual oxygen consumption are largely restricted to exercise physiology or pulmonary laboratories, the one exception being evaluation of patients for cardiac transplant, where a very low maximal oxygen consumption is usually regarded as one of the indications for transplantation (<10 mL/kg/min) (21). The 12-lead ECG is typically recorded at baseline with the patient supine, then in the upright position and subsequently toward the completion of each exercise stage. In most systems, two or three leads are continuously monitored throughout the exercise testing. The blood pressure, likewise, is measured by cuff or Doppler toward the end of each exercise stage.

DIAGNOSTIC AND PROGNOSTIC VALUE OF EXERCISE TESTING

A recent review of the published literature indicates an overall sensitivity of 67%, with a specificity of 72% for the exercise treadmill test. The sensitivity appears to be lower in women. Although the specificity of the treadmill test is often regarded as lower in females, the ACC/AHA Guidelines on Exercise Testing found the specificity not to be uniform in women (22).

Because the exercise treadmill test is often performed in patients with a low prevalence of coronary artery disease, the positive predictive value of the test may be low. For this reason, in accordance with the Baye's theorem, the treadmill test is not generally considered indicated in totally asymptomatic, low-risk patients (22).

The treadmill test is often interpreted on a dichotomous fashion (positive or negative). A positive test is one with ≥0.1 millivolts (or 1 mm) ST-segment depression measured 0.08 seconds after the J point. It has become clear over the years that the mere evaluation of the ST-segment changes is unsatisfactory. One needs to consider also the maximal amount, the time of onset, and the total duration of ST-depression in the recovery phase. Although the presence of angina during exercise does not necessarily make the test a positive one, it certainly suggests that ischemia occurred irrespective of concomitant ST-segment changes. This is particularly true when the exercise reproduces the usual chest pain that the patient has experienced during other types of exertion. Exertional chest discomfort or exertional hypotension are often referred to as ischemic clinical responses and are reported separately from the ECG response to stress. In order to calculate the prognostically important Duke Treadmill Score, it is also important to distinguish more mild chest discomfort simply occurring during stress from that which actually limits the exercise procedure.

Although the severity and time of onset of ST-segment depression have some prognostic value, other variables such as the total duration of the exercise test, the number of METS achieved, the maximal heart rate achieved, and the response of the blood pressure during exercise are even more important prognostically. Patients who can reach a stage III of the Bruce protocol without ST-segment changes have an exceedingly low risk for future cardiac events (estimated annual mortality less than 1%). Likewise, those who can achieve 100% of the maximal predicted heart rate without clinical evidence of myocardial ischemia, have a very benign prognosis. In patients undergoing an exercise treadmill test for risk stratification after a myocardial infarction, these variables are also the ones most importantly related to prognosis, as opposed to the mere presence or absence of ST-segment depression (22). For a comprehensive evaluation of the exercise test, the reader is referred to the ACC/AHA Guidelines on Exercise Testing (22).

INDICATIONS FOR EXERCISE RADIONUCLIDE IMAGING

Table 1 lists indications for radionuclide imaging. The most frequent reason to perform an exercise test is the evaluation of suspected or documented coronary artery disease. Although it is still controversial whether most patients benefit from an imaging modality in association with the exercise test, at least in certain patient groups perfusion imaging should definitely be combined with the exercise test. This includes patients with an abnormal resting ECG, which may compromise the interpretation during stress. For patients with a left bundle branch block (23,24) and those with a ventricular paced rhythm (25), in whom the exercise ECG cannot reliably demonstrate the presence of myocardial ischemia, and in

TABLE 1. *Indications for exercise perfusion scintigraphy*

I. Diagnosis of CAD
  • Stable angina or chest pain of uncertain origin
  • Unstable angina after initial stabilization
  • Positive exercise ECG without symptoms
  • Screening of high-risk, asymptomatic patients
  • Patients referred for exercise ECG test but with abnormal test ECG that hampers evaluation of ischemia
  • Prior nondiagnostic exercise ECG test
II. Assessment of functional importance of known coronary stenosis
  • "Borderline" stenoses (40–70%) by coronary angiography
  • Assessment of "culprit lesion" prior to coronary angioplasty
  • Stenoses of small branches or of distal location
III. Assessment of therapeutic benefits
  • After coronary angioplasty
  • After coronary artery bypass surgery
  • After medical therapy
IV. Risk stratification
  • Stable angina
  • Unstable angina
  • Postmyocardial infarction
  • Prior to major vascular surgery
V. Demonstration of myocardial ischemia in patients with angiographically normal coronary arteries

(From ref. 26, with permission.)

27. Amanullah AM, Kiat H, Friedman JD, et al. Adenosine technetium-99m sestamibi myocardial perfusion SPECT in women: diagnostic efficacy in detection of coronary artery disease. *J Am Coll Cardiol* 1996; 27:803–809.

28. Friedman J, Van Tain K, Maddahi J, et al. "Upward creep" of the heart: a frequent source of false-positive reversible defects during thallium-201 stress-redistribution SPECT. *J Nucl Med* 1989;30:1718–1722.

29. Pennell DJ, Mavrogeni SI, Forbat SM, et al. Adenosine combined with dynamic exercise for myocardial perfusion imaging. *J Am Coll Cardiol* 1995;25:1300–1309.

30. Parikh A, Kiat H, Kang X, et al. Addition of low level treadmill exercise to adenosine stress Tc-99m sestamibi myocardial perfusion SPECT allows for early post-stress imaging. *J Nucl Med* 1996;37:59P(abst).

31. Leppo JA. Dipyridamole-thallium imaging: the lazy man's stress test. *J Nucl Med* 1989;30:281–287.

32. Verani MS. Adenosine thallium-201 myocardial perfusion scintigraphy. *Am Heart J* 1991;122:269–278.

33. Leppo J, Rosenkrantz J, Rosenthal R, et al. Quantitative thallium-201 redistribution with a fixed coronary stenosis in dogs. *Circulation* 1981; 63:632–639.

34. Verani MS, Mahmarian JJ, Hixson JB, et al. Diagnosis of coronary artery disease by controlled coronary vasodilation with adenosine and thallium-201 scintigraphy in patients unable to exercise. *Circulation* 1990;82:80–87.

35. O'Keefe JH Jr, Bateman TM, Handlin LR, et al. Four-versus 6-minute infusion protocol for adenosine thallium-201 single photon emission computed tomography imaging. *Am Heart J* 1995;129:482–487.

36. Villegas BJ, Hendel RC, Dahlberg ST, et al. Comparison of 3-versus 6-minute infusions of adenosine in thallium-201 myocardial perfusion imaging. *Am Heart J* 1993;126:103–107.

37. Ranhosky A, Kempthorne-Rawson J, and the Intravenous Dipyridamole Thallium Imaging Study Group. The safety of intravenous dipyridamole thallium myocardial perfusion imaging. *Circulation* 1990;81: 1205–1209.

38. Cerqueira MD, Verani MS, Schwaiger M, et al. Safety profile of adenosine stress perfusion imaging: results from the adenoscan multicenter trial registry. *J Am Coll Cardiol* 1994;23:384–389.

39. Abreu A, Mahmarian JJ, Nishimura S, et al. Tolerance and safety of pharmacologic coronary vasodilation with adenosine in association with thallium-201 scintigraphy in patients with suspected coronary artery disease. *J Am Coll Cardiol* 1991;18:730–735.

40. Wilson RF, Wyche K, Christensen GV, et al. Effects of adenosine on human coronary arterial circulation. *Circulation* 1990;82:1595–1606.

41. Amanulla AM, Berman DS, Kiat H, et al. Usefulness of hemodynamic changes during adenosine infusion in predicting the diagnostic accuracy of adenosine technetium-99m sestamibi single-photon emission computed tomography (SPECT). *Am J Cardiol* 1997;79:1319–1322.

42. Matzer L, Kiat H, Friedman JD, et al. A new approach to the assessment of tomographic thallium-201 scintigraphy in patients with left bundle branch block. *J Am Coll Cardiol* 1991;17:1309–1317.

43. DePuey EG, Guertler-Krawczynska E, Robbins WL. Thallium-201 SPECT in coronary disease patients with left bundle branch block. *J Nucl Med* 1988;29:1479–1485.

44. Hirzel HO, Msenn N, Nuesch K, et al. Thallium-201 scintigraphy in complete left bundle branch block. *Am J Cardiol* 1984;53:764–769.

45. Larcos G, Gibbons RJ, Brown, ML. Diagnostic accuracy of exercise thallium-201 single photon emission computed tomography in patients with left bundle branch block. *Am J Cardiol* 1991;68:756–760.

46. Burns RJ, Galligan L, Wright LM, et al. Improved specificity of myocardial thallium-201 single-photon emission computed tomography in patients with left bundle branch block by dipyridamole. *Am J Cardiol* 1991;68:504–508.

47. Larcos G, Brown ML, Gibbons RJ. Role of dipyridamole thallium 201 imaging in left bundle branch block. *Am J Cardiol* 1991;68:1097–1098.

48. Jukema JW, Van der Wall E-E, Van der VisMeesen MJ, et al. Dipyridamole thallium-201 scintigraphy for improved detection of left anterior descending coronary artery stenosis in patients with left bundle branch block. *Eur Heart J* 1993;14:53–56.

49. O'Keefe JH, Bateman TM, Barnhart CS. Adenosine thallium-201 is superior to exercise thallium-201 for detecting coronary artery disease in patients with left bundle-branch block. *J Am Coll Cardiol* 1993;21: 1332–1338.

50. O'Keefe JH Jr, Bateman TM, Silvestri R, et al. Safety and diagnostic accuracy of adenosine thallium-201 scintigraphy in patients unable to exercise and those with left bundle branch block. *Am Heart J* 1992; 124:614–621.

51. Samuels B, Kiat H, Friedman J, et al. Adenosine pharmacologic stress myocardial perfusion tomographic imaging in patients with significant aortic stenosis. *J Am Coll Cardiol* 1995;25:99–106.

52. Mahmarian JJ, Pratt CM, Nishimura S, et al. Quantitative adenosine thallium-201 single-photon emission computed tomography for the early assessment of patients surviving acute myocardial infarction. *Circulation* 1993;87:1197–1210.

53. Mahmarian JJ, Mahmarian AC, Marks GF, et al. Role of adenosine thallium-201 tomography for defining long-term risk in patients after acute myocardial infarction. *J Am Coll Cardiol* 1995;25:1333–1340.

54. Brown KA, O'Meara J, Chambers CE, et al. Ability of dipyridamole-thallium-201 imaging one to four days after acute myocardial infarction to predict in-hospital and late recurrent myocardial ischemic events. *Am J Cardiol* 1990;65:160–167.

55. Jain A, Hicks RR, Frantz DM, et al. Comparison of early exercise treadmill test and oral dipyridamole thallium-201 tomography for the identification of jeopardized myocardium in patients receiving thrombolytic therapy for acute Q-wave myocardial infarction. *Am J Cardiol* 1990;66:551–555.

56. Dakik HA, Kleiman NS, Farmer JA, et al. Intensive medical therapy versus coronary angioplasty for suppression of myocardial ischemia in survivors of acute myocardial infarction: a prospective, randomized pilot study. *Circulation* 1998;98:2017–2023.

57. Brown KA. Prognostic value of thallium 201 myocardial perfusion imaging in patients with unstable angina who respond to medical treatment. *J Am Coll Cardiol* 1991;17:1053–1057.

58. Johnston DL, Scanlon PD, Hodge DO, et al. Pulmonary function monitoring during adenosine myocardial perfusion scintigraphy in patients with chronic obstructive pulmonary disease. *Mayo Clinic Proc* 1999; 74:339–346.

59. Mason JR, Palac RT, Freeman ML, et al. Thallium scintigraphy during dobutamine infusion: Nonexercise-dependent screening test for coronary diease. *Am Heart J* 1984;107:481–485.

60. Pennell DJ, Underwood SR, Swanton RH, et al. Dobutamine thallium myocardial perfusion tomography. *J Am Coll Cardiol* 1991;18: 1471–1479.

61. Hays JT, Mahmarian JJ, Cochran AJ, et al. Dobutamine thallium-201 tomography for evaluating patients with suspected coronary artery disease unable to undergo exercise or vasodilatory pharmacologic testing. *J Am Coll Cardiol* 1993;21:1583–1590.

62. Krivokapich J, Huang S-C, Schelbert HR. Assessment of the effects of dobutamine on myocardial blood flow and oxidative metabolism in normal human subjects using nitrogen-13 ammonia and carbon-11 acetate. *Am J Cardiol* 1993;71:1351–1356.

63. Dakik HA, Vempathy H, Verani MS. Tolerance, hemodynamic changes, and safety of dobutamine stress perfusion imaging. *J Nucl Cardiol* 1996;3:410–414.

64. Dakik HA, Mahmarian JJ, Kimball KT, et al. Prognostic value of exercise thallium-201 tomography in patients treated with thrombolytic therapy during acute myocardial infarction. *Circulation* 1996;94: 2735–2742.

65. Kiat H, Iskandrian AS, Villegas BJ, et al. Arbutamine stress thallium-201 single-photon emission computed tomography using a computerized closed-loop delivery system. Multicenter trial for evaluation of safety and diagnostic accuracy. The International Arbutamine Study Group. *J Am Coll Cardiol* 1995;26:1159–1167.

CHAPTER 13

Myocardial Perfusion
Single Photon Approaches

Daniel S. Berman and Guido Germano

This chapter explores the currently most commonly used nuclear cardiology imaging technique: myocardial perfusion single photon emission computed tomography (SPECT). In comparison to the planar scintigraphic method, myocardial perfusion SPECT increases contrast resolution and leads to improved ability to localize coronary artery disease. It is estimated that by 1997 over 90% of myocardial perfusion scintigraphy in the United States was performed using SPECT. At the present time, approximately 20% of these procedures are performed with thallium-201 alone, 40% with technetium-99m sestamibi alone, 20% with rest thallium-201/stress technetium-99m sestamibi in a dual isotope protocol, and 20% using technetium-99m tetrofosmin (Tc-99m tetrofosmin, tetrofosmin), either alone or in combination with thallium-201.

With the recent widespread availability of powerful computer systems as well as multidetector SPECT, gated myocardial perfusion scintigraphy has now become routine, providing additional objective assessments of global and regional myocardial function (see Chapter 19). The technique of gated myocardial perfusion SPECT provides a powerful clinical tool for a variety of clinical questions arising in assessment of patients with known or suspected coronary artery disease (CAD). This chapter is divided into the three following sections: radiopharmaceuticals and acquisition protocols, interpretation and reporting, and clinical applications.

D. S. Berman: University of California–Los Angeles School of Medicine, Los Angeles, California 90025; Department of Imaging/Nuclear Medicine, Cedars-Sinai Medical Center, Los Angeles, California 90048.

G. Germano: Department of Radiological Sciences, University of California–Los Angeles School of Medicine, Los Angeles, California 90024; Department of Medicine, Cedars-Sinai Medical Center, Los Angeles, California 90048.

RADIOPHARMACEUTICALS

Thallium-201

The Anger scintillation camera, the type of imaging device most commonly used today in nuclear cardiology, became clinically available in the late 1960s. Shortly thereafter, this camera was used with rubidium-81, a positron-emitting radiopharmaceutical, in conjunction with thick lead shielding necessitated by the high energy of this positron-emitting radioisotope (1). The physiologic basis for the use of rubidium-81 as a myocardial perfusion imaging agent was that it was a potassium analog, potassium and rubidium being cationic elements that are efficiently extracted by the myocardium during the initial transit, thereby being tracers of regional myocardial perfusion. Zaret et al. (2) had first demonstrated with the rectilinear scanner that exercise-induced regional myocardial perfusion defects could be visualized with potassium-43. In 1973, Liebowitz et al. (3) introduced thallium-201 for medical use. Due to its more favorable imaging characteristics compared to potassium-43 and rubidium-81 (lower energy allowing imaging with technetium-99m collimators), following its commercial availability, thallium-201 quickly became the myocardial perfusion imaging agent of choice, a position it maintained until the Tc-99m perfusion agents became widely accepted.

Physical Characteristics

Thallium-201 is a cyclotron-generated radionuclide with a half-life of 73 hours, which emits characteristic x-rays from 68 to 80 kev (94% abundant) and thallium-201 gamma rays at 167 kev (10% abundant). Due to its relatively long half-life, the absorbed radiation dose is higher than that associated with technetium-99m myocardial perfusion agents, resulting in recommended doses between 2 and 4 mCi.

Physiologic Characteristics

Despite the less than ideal physical properties, thallium-201 has excellent physiological properties for myocardial perfusion imaging.

Initial Distribution

Assuming no significant early washout of radioactivity, conceptually the regional myocardial concentration of a perfusion tracer is equal to the product of the delivery of the tracer to the myocardium (regional blood flow) and the ability of the myocardium to extract the tracer from the blood (extraction fraction). With thallium-201, early studies documented a linear relationship between uptake and myocardial blood flow from resting baseline levels down to zero (4). Importantly for stress myocardial perfusion scintigraphy, the linear relationship between blood flow and thallium-201 uptake is maintained during exercise (5). At very high levels of flow, such as those achieved with vasodilator stress (in excess of 3 mL/min/g), a "roll-off" in uptake occurs. This is because the extraction fraction, which is estimated to be about 85% (6), up to flow levels of 2 to 3 mL/min/g, is reduced at very high flow rates. This roll-off is characteristic of myocardial perfusion tracers in general, either single photon or positron emitting, with the exception of oxygen-15 water (see Chapter 14).

Redistribution

Although it was initially expected that Tl-201 would remain fixed in the myocardium for a prolonged period after initial myocardial update (7), Pohost and associates (8) demonstrated in an ischemic animal model that delayed imaging revealed disappearance of initial perfusion defects. This change from initial myocardial distribution is referred to as "redistribution." Subsequently, redistribution was also observed following resting injection in patients with severe fixed coronary defects without infarction (9–11). Redistribution appears to result from both accumulation of thallium in previously underperfused zones (washin) and more rapid washout of radioactivity from the normal myocardium than from hypoperfused zones (11).

After intravenous injection, thallium is rapidly extracted, roughly in proportion to the distribution of cardiac output (12). Since the myocardium receives approximately 5% of the cardiac output, given the high myocardial extraction, approximately 4% of the injected dose goes to the heart, with greater than 95% of the injected dose going to the other body organs, which serve as a large systemic reservoir of thallium. While the initial distribution of thallium-201 is proportional to regional myocardial blood flow, the equilibrium distribution of thallium is proportional to the regional potassium pool, reflecting the amount of viable myocardium. Like potassium, thallium is not bound in the myocardial cell, but equilibrates following the same electrochemical gradient

as applies to potassium. Following intravenous injection, approximately half of the thallium washes out from the normal myocardium over 5 to 8 hours (7). Differential washout rates between hypoperfused but viable myocardium and normal zones and washin to initially hypoperfused zones are the fundamental mechanisms of Tl-201 redistribution.

Washout Rates of Thallium-201

A factor governing the "washout rate" of thallium-201 is the concentration gradient between the myocardial cell and the blood. A variety of factors can affect this concentration gradient. One factor is the patient's physiologic state at the time of injection (e.g., rest, minimal exercise, maximal exercise). Following injection, at rest, or with only low-level exercise, there is slower blood clearance of thallium. Therefore, after a resting or low-level exercise injection, the myocardial/blood gradient is not as high, and the washout rate is lower than after injection at maximal exercise. For this reason, diffuse slow washout rates, mimicking diffuse ischemia, may be observed in normal patients who do not achieve adequate levels of stress. From a practical standpoint, these considerations are important if one tries to use thallium-201 analysis in a spatially nonrelative manner; i.e., to evaluate the rate of washout of thallium as an indicator of normal perfusion (13). In general, if exercise normal limits for washout rates are to be applied clinically, patients must achieve maximal exercise.

The other process involved in redistribution-accumulation or "washin" of radioactivity in the underperfused zone-can also have a variable rate. Typically, redistribution occurs over a few hours, but in certain circumstances this process can be delayed. For example, if the thallium blood levels are very low, less thallium is available to be delivered to previously ischemic myocardium in the redistribution phase. Budinger and colleagues (14,15) showed that rapid blood clearance of thallium could eliminate the appearance of defect reversibility and could lead to an underestimation of viable myocardium. In a study with clear relevance to current thallium-201 protocol design, Angello et al. (16) demonstrated that carbohydrate loading can obscure potential defect reversibility with thallium-201. The mechanism involved appears to be related to a fall in circulating potassium (and thallium) levels that occur with rising plasma insulin levels following carbohydrate meals. Because hyperinsulinemic states can slow the redistribution process, it is recommended that patients fast prior to and for 4 hours following thallium-201 injection, with either rest or stress acquisitions.

Late Redistribution

The time to completed redistribution of thallium-201 (at which true equilibrium concentration is reached) is variable. In 1978, our laboratory first reported the inverse relationship between the degree of coronary stenosis and subsequent redistribution of thallium-201 (17). Previously, Maseri et al.

(18) had demonstrated in the setting of variant angina that redistribution of thallium-201 could occur as early as 45 minutes after resting injection. Since medically relieved variant angina would be expected to be associated with local hyperemia to the ischemic zone, we reasoned that the blood flow to the ischemic zone (and thus the thallium delivery) could influence the rate of redistribution. Testing this hypothesis, we studied patients undergoing coronary angiography at 1 hour, 4 hours, and 24 hours after stress injection. We found that redistribution was frequently rapid in areas with minor stenoses (where hyperemia postexercise would be expected), and was frequently delayed in regions with critical stenoses (in which not only would poststress hyperemia be unlikely, but resting hypoperfusion might slow the delivery of thallium to the region) (19). These initial findings with planar imaging were confirmed subsequently with thallium-201 SPECT. The application of this concept improved the ability of thallium-201 stress/redistribution myocardial perfusion scintigraphy to detect viable myocardium (20,21). It is likely that the two major factors governing the time to equilibration of thallium-201 are circulating blood levels of thallium (in turn influenced by carbohydrate ingestion and insulin levels) and the status of the coronary stenosis responsible for the initial perfusion defect. Thus, some of the failure of Tl-201 redistribution to detect viable myocardium (some ''fixed'' defects improve after revascularization) may be related to carbohydrate ingestion prior to or early following injection of Tl-201 or to inadequate time between injection and redistribution imaging.

Reverse Redistribution

The pattern of reverse redistribution refers to the finding of normal or nearly normal initial uptake of thallium, followed in the redistribution phase by the development of an uptake defect. Although the finding was first reported on stress/redistribution studies (22,23), it has been observed to be frequent on rest/redistribution imaging in patients who had undergone thrombolytic therapy for acute myocardial infarction, occurring in 75% of these patients (24). Weiss et al. (24) from our laboratory made several observations that appear to explain the phenomenon of reverse redistribution. In comparison with regions demonstrating fixed defects, reverse redistribution was more likely to be associated with normal or near normal wall motion on 10-day postinfarction radionuclide ventriculography. Reverse redistribution was also more common in areas with extensive myocardial salvage as documented by resting Tl-201 myocardial perfusion scintigraphy performed pre- and ten-day postthrombolytic therapy and was associated with a more rapid washout rate of thallium than in the contralateral normal zones. The pattern was also more commonly associated with patent infarct-related coronary artery. These authors postulated that the mechanism most commonly producing the pattern is higher than normal blood flow to the noninfarcted tissue in a reperfused zone of nontransmural myocardial infarction (a failure

of autoregulation). Conceptually, for consideration of the extent of myocardial viability, the late image, reflecting the potassium pool, may be more accurate than the early image in patients with this pattern. Another possible mechanism creating the pattern of reverse redistribution is artifact, as suggested in the initial description of the pattern (23). Artifacts of the acquisition associated with the redistribution image (e.g., patient motion) and not present on the initial image could produce this pattern. The findings initially observed in planar scintigraphy have been confirmed with myocardial perfusion SPECT (25). Since the differential washout rates between ischemic and normal myocardium of the technetium-99m myocardial perfusion imaging agents sestamibi and tetrofosmin are minimal, the pattern of reverse redistribution with these agents usually represents an artifact occurring during the rest acquisition.

Diffuse Slow Washout of Thallium

Bateman et al. (26) from our laboratory documented an additional clinically relevant but rare pattern, which might be detected by quantitative thallium-201 imaging. As noted above, the disappearance of defects over time with thallium-201 myocardial perfusion scintigraphy is due in part to slower washout rate of thallium from the ischemic zone than from the normal zone. If all zones are equally ischemic, conceptually a pattern of diffuse slow washout of thallium could occur in which the globally ischemic myocardium may show no initial perfusion defect. The study of Bateman et al. demonstrated that 72% of 32 patients manifesting patterns of diffuse slow washout of thallium and undergoing coronary angiography had triple vessel or left main coronary artery disease. The authors noted, however, that the pattern is extremely rare, being observed with planar imaging in only 3% of patients. The authors also noted that the pattern was at times unrelated to myocardial ischemia. As noted earlier, patients injected at rest have slower myocardial washout than those injected during exercise. Thus, a common source of an ''artifactual'' pattern of diffuse slow washout is submaximal exercise (26). Another cause of an artifactual diffuse slow washout pattern is partial infiltration of the injected dose. Despite problems associated with the specificity of the diffuse slow washout pattern, the concept of detecting additional disease in regions without perfusion defects manifesting slow washout of thallium deserves further exploration. It is of note that most of the work dealing with thallium-201 washout rates was performed on planar rather than SPECT imaging (13,27) and that this potentially valuable concept has not yet been widely applied to SPECT.

Acquisition Protocols

With thallium-201, a variety of SPECT acquisition protocols are available. When thallium-201 alone is employed as the radiopharmaceutical, the most common acquisition protocol uses some combination of stress with redistribution and/or reinjection imaging. The latter, as initially described, involved obtaining an additional image in patients with non-reversible (''fixed'') perfusion defects following reinjection of one half of the dose used at stress, with imaging performed immediately thereafter (28). This protocol has been shown to improve the ability to detect viable myocardium over standard stress/4-hour redistribution imaging (29). Since it requires three image acquisitions and a decision as to whether the reinjection is needed, a two-acquisition sequence with stress and redistribution/reinjection imaging is commonly performed. If no fixed defects are noted with this approach, further imaging is not required. If, on the other hand, following the 4-hour reinjection/redistribution image, fixed defects are present, 24-hour imaging results in a small but significant improvement in detection of viable myocardium (29). An alternate protocol that is gaining popularity is to give sublingual nitroglycerin prior to the reinjection of thallium-201. With this approach, the frequency of further improvement at 24-hour imaging may be substantially reduced, i.e., we consider it likely that a stress and nitrate augmented early reinjection protocol will reduce the benefit of, and thus the need for, 24-hour imaging (30). The other form of thallium imaging in frequent use is the rest/redistribution protocol, considered to be the most effective thallium-201 protocol for the assessment of viable myocardium (8,31). Figures 1 and 2 illustrate thallium-201 SPECT acquisition protocols.

From a technical standpoint, several considerations are important. With pure Tl-201 SPECT protocols, most investigators utilize all-purpose collimators rather than high-resolution collimators (32), although some suggest the use of high-resolution collimators (33,34). If high-resolution collimators are used, consideration should be given to lengthening the time of acquisition for thallium-201 SPECT, compared to

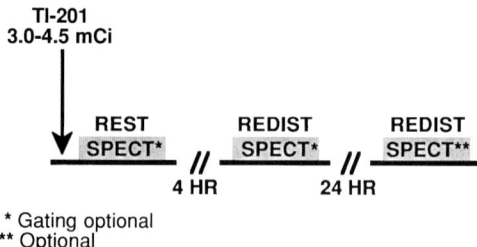

FIG. 2. Rest-redistribution thallium 201 SPECT acquisition protocol. *SPECT*, single photon emission computed tomography.

technetium-99m-based SPECT protocols, so as to provide adequate SPECT count statistics. This lengthening of the acquisition time is particularly important for late redistribution imaging, due to the lower count rate due to radioactive decay. The timing of the initial poststress acquisition is particularly important with thallium, since, as noted earlier, excessive delay could result in decreased sensitivity for detection of coronary artery disease, due to early redistribution of the radiopharmaceutical. On the other hand, SPECT acquisition of either thallium-201 or the technetium-99m myocardial perfusion agents should generally not begin less than 10 minutes following exercise injection; this is due to ''upward creep of the heart'' (35), a frequent observation of an artifactual perfusion defect. This phenomenon is related to the increased depth of respiration that occurs very early postexercise, which is associated with an average lower position of the diaphragm (and consequently of the heart) in the chest, compared to the normal ventilatory state. This causes the heart to gradually move cephalad during the early portion of SPECT acquisition, resulting in a form of motion artifact in reconstruction. By delaying acquisition until 10 to 15 minutes after exercise stress, this ''upward creep'' artifact is avoided.

Although initially described with technetium-99m sestamibi, gated SPECT can also be performed with thallium-201, particularly with multidetector system. Left ventricular ejection fraction measurement with gated thallium-201 SPECT correlates highly with that of technetium-99m sestamibi SPECT (36). If adequate myocardial counts can be obtained with a given camera/computer/collimator system, we advocate the routine use of gated SPECT with thallium-201, since it provides additional useful information regarding ventricular function. However, the necessity of employing acquisition protocols that provide an adequate total number of myocardial counts in each frame of the gated SPECT study must be emphasized.

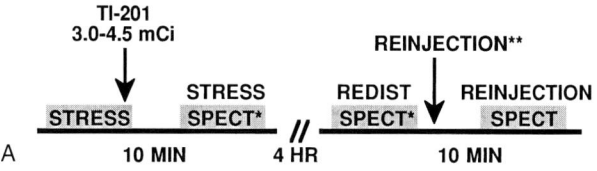

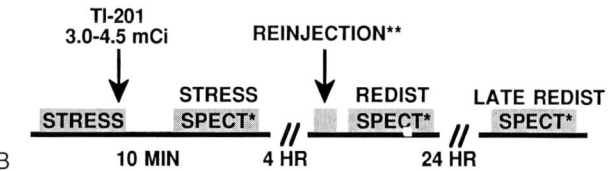

FIG. 1. Common Tl-201 SPECT acquisition protocols: **A:** stress, redistribution, reinjection; **B:** stress, reinjection, with 24-hour imaging if fixed defects found. *REDIST*, redistribution; *NTG*, nitroglycerin; *SPECT*, single photon emission computed tomography.

Technetium-99m Myocardial Perfusion SPECT

Physical Characteristics

Technetium-99m is produced from a molybdenum-99m generator, has a half-life of 6 hours, and emits monoenergetic

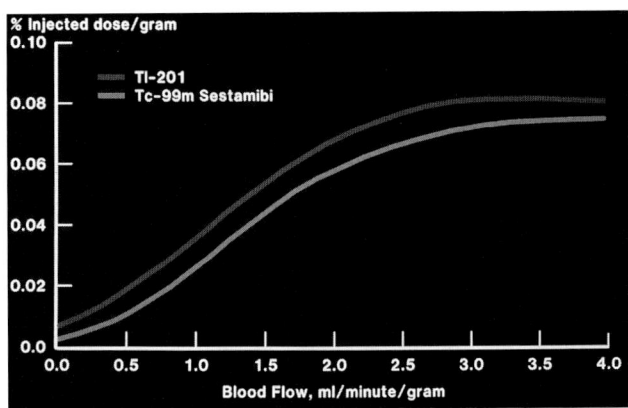

FIG. 3. Relationship between blood flow and percent injected dose per gram for TI-201 and Tc-99m sestamibi. (See also Color Plate 9 following page 294.) (Courtesy of DuPont Medical Imaging, Billerica, Massachusetts.)

gamma rays at 140 kev. The whole body radiation dose is estimated to be 16 mrad/mCi, in contrast to the higher radiation dose associated with thallium-201, 240 mrad/mCi. Due to this more favorable dosimetry, larger doses of technetium-99m myocardial perfusion imaging agents are used than with thallium-201, usually in the range of 30 mCi.

Technetium-99m Sestamibi

Physiologic Properties

The strengths and weaknesses of technetium-99m sestamibi compared to thallium-201 for myocardial perfusion imaging are understood by comparing their relative physiologic characteristics.

Figures 3 and 4 (see also Color Plates 9 and 10 following page 294) illustrate the comparative kinetics of thallium-

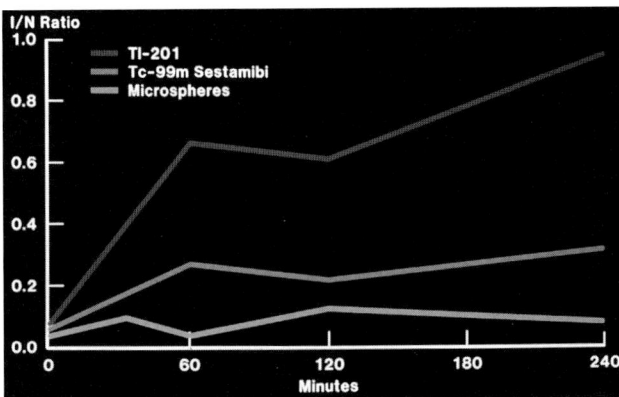

FIG. 4. Redistribution characteristics of TI-201, Tc-99m sestamibi, and microspheres. The ischemic/normal zone (I/N) ratio for the three tracers was measured in a swine model following injection (intravenous for TI-201 and Tc-99m sestamibi, left atrial for microspheres) during a 10-minute coronary occlusion followed by 4 hours of reflow. (See also Color Plate 10 following page 294.) (Courtesy of DuPont Medical Imaging, Billerica, Massachusetts.)

201 and technetium-99m sestamibi, as initially observed in a swine model. Techetium-99m sestamibi belongs to a class of compounds called isonitriles and is a complex organic compound that behaves physiologically as a monovalent cation. Following its extraction from the blood, technetium sestamibi is bound by mitochondria so that there is a limited amount of technetium-99m sestamibi myocardial washout (or washin) over time (37,38). As with thallium-201, the initial uptake of technetium-99m sestamibi is a function of myocardial perfusion to viable tissue. As shown in Figure 3, there is a linear relationship between intravenously injected dose per gram of myocardium and myocardial blood flow, from the very low range up to approximately 2 to 2.5 mL/min/g (39). These latter levels are those characteristically associated with maximal treadmill exercise (40). At very low levels of flow, extraction of these tracers appears to increase, affecting technetium-99m sestamibi more than thallium-201 (41). At very high levels of flow, there is a progressive decline in the degree by which the uptake of radioactivity increases as a function of flow; i.e., the linear relationship between uptake and flow no longer is observed. Since pharmacologic stress testing with adenosine or dipyridamole frequently results in flow rates in the range of 4 mL/min/g (42), on a theoretical basis one would expect that either thallium-201 or technetium-99m sestamibi imaging would have difficulties in distinguishing myocardial regions in which the flow increased to 3 mL/min/g from regions in which flow increased to 4 mL/min/g. In other words, both tracers may be limited in detecting coronary lesions with mild hemodynamic significance, as might be expected of lesions causing 50 to 70% luminal diameter narrowing of the coronary artery. Figure 3 further demonstrates that thallium-201 has a higher myocardial uptake (as measured by the percent injected dose/gram of myocardium) throughout the range of flow, secondary to a higher extraction fraction than technetium-99m sestamibi (approximately 85% compared to 65%) (43,44). Technetium-99m tetrofosmin (see below) has an uptake curve with similar shape; however, its uptake is lower than that of technetium-99m sestamibi throughout the medium to higher flow ranges, due to an even lower extraction fraction (approximately 50%) (45,46).

Figure 4 provides insight into the change of myocardial thallium-201 and technetium-99m sestamibi distribution over time. An ischemic swine model was studied with a coronary occlusion of 10 minutes duration, during which thallium-201, technetium-99m sestamibi, and labeled microspheres were injected. Following the release of the coronary occlusion, changes in tracer distribution or "redistribution" were observed over several hours, with sacrifice of the animals at various times. Differences in the ischemic-to-normal-zone uptake ratios over time between the agents were assessed. Since microspheres "stick" to their initial distribution in the coronary capillary bed, there was no significant change in the ischemic-to-normal-zone ratio of microspheres over time. As noted above, since thallium-201 is a potassium analogue, it redistributed in this ischemic model, so that the ischemic-to-normal-zone ratio of thallium-201 became unity over time. As noted in Figure 4, this ratio became ≃0.7 at only 60 minutes after injection. These data fit well with the clinical observation that approximately 20% of thallium-201 defects observed immediately after stress would not be observed on repeat imaging 45 minutes later (17,19). Technetium-99m sestamibi, on the other hand, demonstrates minimal change in distribution over time. Although reduction in defect contrast over time can occur with technetium-99m sestamibi (47,48), for practical clinical purposes this phenomenon is considered of minimal significance, and technetium-99m sestamibi imaging is thought to be nearly as accurate when performed up to 2 hours after as when performed 10 to 15 minutes after a stress injection. As with technetium-99m sestamibi, there is very little change in the myocardial distribution of technetium-99m tetrofosmin over time (45).

On theoretical grounds, the implications of Figures 3 and 4 are that thallium-201 could be more effective in defining mild coronary stenosis and may be associated with a "deeper" defect contrast (more count reduction compared to normal) than technetium-99m sestamibi, while technetium-99m sestamibi may show greater defect contrast on stress studies than technetium-99m tetrofosmin (49). On the other hand, from a practical standpoint, the technetium agents provide greater flexibility than thallium-201, since they do not require that imaging be accomplished soon after the stress injection for maximal sensitivity. With thallium-201, imaging must be performed very close to the stress testing, and if soft tissue attenuation or patient motion compromises a study, the benefit of repeating the acquisition is questionable. In contrast, technetium-99m sestamibi or tetrofosmin, permit stress testing and tracer injection to take place at a location remote from the imaging laboratory, and image acquisition can simply be repeated when patient motion, soft tissue attenuation, or other artifact is considered to be responsible for the production of a perfusion defect.

The benefit of being able to repeat images is illustrated in Figure 5, which shows resting technetium-99m sestamibi acquisition performed with the patient in the supine and prone positions. Although the supine images show an apparent perfusion defect, the prone images are normal, demonstrating that the inferior wall defect observed in the supine position was simply secondary to soft tissue attenuation. Our laboratory and others have previously shown that prone imaging is associated with less patient motion and less inferior wall attenuation than supine imaging (50–52). The combination of supine and prone images is also helpful in identifying breast attenuation and attenuation due to excessive lateral

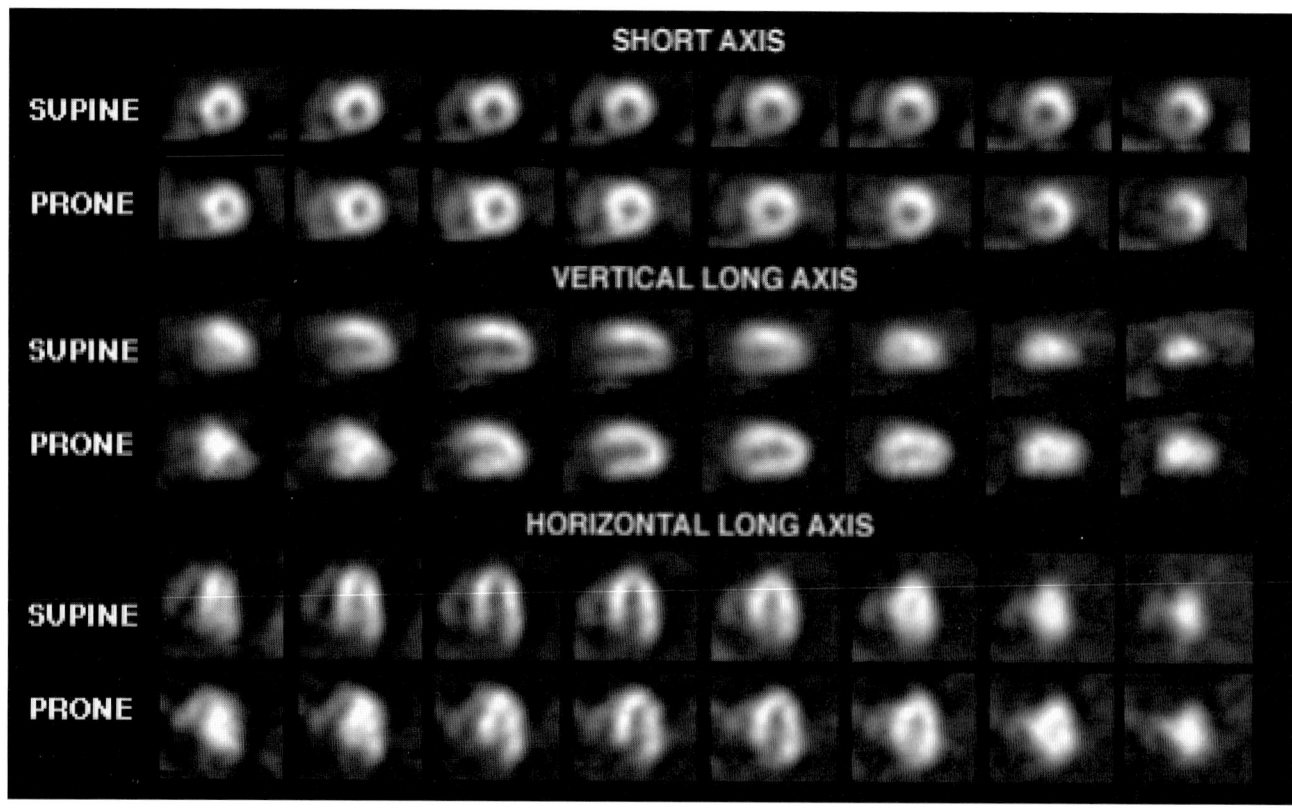

FIG. 5. Rest sestamibi (MB) SPECT images in the supine position (**top**) and prone position (**bottom**) in a 55-year-old patient with a low likelihood of coronary artery disease. Prone images are normal, demonstrating that the apparent inferior wall perfusion defect on the supine images is secondary to soft tissue attention. Normal wall motion was noted on gated SPECT. *SPECT,* single photon emission computed tomography.

chest-wall fat, due to the shift in position of the attenuating structures that occur in the prone position. However, since the prone position frequently causes an artifactual anteroseptal defect secondary to increased sternal attenuation in this position, prone imaging is used as an adjunct to, not a replacement for, supine imaging.

Acquisition Protocols

Due to the absence of clinically significant redistribution, separate rest and stress injections are standard with technetium-99m sestamibi SPECT (53,54). A variety of protocols can be used with this agent, including 2-day stress/rest, same-day rest/stress, same-day stress/rest, and dual isotope. From the standpoint of defect contrast and optimal image quality, the 2-day stress/rest protocol is ideal (Figure 6). With the 2-day stress/rest protocol, both the stress and the rest study are obtained following the injection of high doses of technetium-99m sestamibi, allowing the acquisition of high quality, high count images for the accurate assessment of perfusion and function. The principal drawback of this protocol is its requirement for two imaging days, resulting in a delay in the delivery of final information to be used in patient management. The same-day low-dose rest/high-dose stress protocol (55) (Fig. 6), perhaps the most commonly employed technetium-99m sestamibi protocol, has the disadvantage of causing a reduction in stress defect contrast, as approximately 15% of the radioactivity observed at the time of stress imaging comes from the preexisting resting myocardial distribution. The same-day low-dose stress/high-dose rest sequence (56,57) (Fig. 6), on the other hand, has the advantage of requiring image acquisition times essentially identical to those used for thallium-201 imaging, making it easy for a laboratory to alternate between stress/

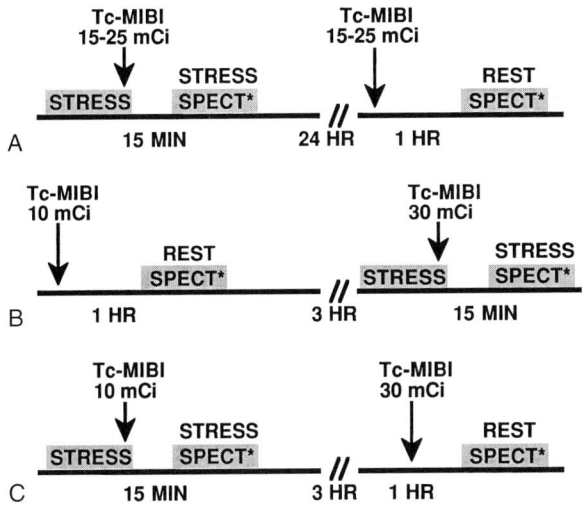

FIG. 6. A: Two day; B: same day rest-stress; and C: same day stress-rest: Tc-99m sestamibi protocols. Tc-MIBI, technetium-99m sestamibi.

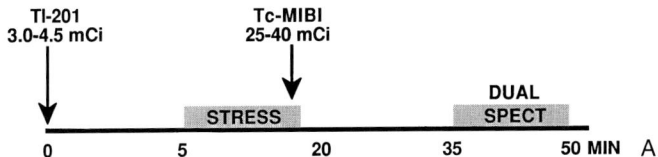
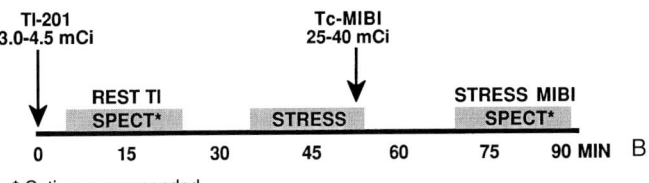

* Gating recommended

FIG. 7. Simultaneous (A) and separate acquisition (B) dual isotope rest thallium-201/stress technetium 99m sestamibi SPECT protocols.

redistribution thallium-201 and stress/rest technetium-99m sestamibi protocols. The principal drawback of this approach is that less than ideal count rates are associated with the most important stress image set, and it is difficult to accurately assess defect reversibility (58). With respect to the assessment of myocardial viability, all stress/rest or rest/stress technetium-99m sestamibi imaging protocols have theoretical limitations in separating severely hibernating myocardium from infarction. These constraints do not apply to thallium-201, because of its redistribution properties (59,60). Viability assessment with technetium-99m sestamibi may be improved by the administration of nitroglycerin prior to the rest-injection study (61).

Given the limitations of standard technetium-99m sestamibi protocols, our group has developed a rest thallium-201/ stress technetium-99m sestamibi dual isotope SPECT approach that has been in place in our institution since 1990 (62), essentially unmodified with the exception of the addition of gated SPECT. Dual isotope imaging takes advantage of the Anger camera's ability to collect data in different energy windows. The two fundamental types of dual isotope protocols are referred to as "simultaneous" or "separate" dual isotope SPECT (Fig. 7).

Simultaneous dual isotope imaging would have many theoretical advantages, compared with conventional stress and rest protocols (60,63). It would halve camera acquisition time and substantially abbreviate the overall study duration for the patient. Furthermore, the inherent registration of stress and rest image sets would reduce the frequency of unrecognized artifacts associated with separate stress and rest image acquisitions. This protocol, however, rests on unproven assumptions, the most important being that the effects of radioisotope cross-talk between the two energy acquisition windows is insignificant, or can be accounted for. Kiat et al. (63) demonstrated in a report of patient studies that the downscatter of technetium-99m sestamibi into the lower energy thallium-201 acquisition window causes substantial (approximately 20%) reduction in thallium-201 defect contrast, leading to an overestimation of defect reversibility. Interesting preliminary data regarding downscatter correction methods has been reported by Kamphuis et al. (64), as well as other groups (65). Until an approach to downscatter correction is validated clinically, however, we do not recommend general use of the simultaneous dual isotope protocol.

Because of the negligible (2.9%) contribution of thallium-201 into the technetium-99m energy acquisition window (63) and the fact that the thallium-201 image dataset is acquired before technetium-99m administration, the separate acquisition approach using rest thallium-201/stress technetium-99m sestamibi provides an alternative that does not require correction for cross contamination between the two radioisotopes. The sensitivity and specificity of this protocol have been shown to be approximately 90% (62). We believe that, for purposes of detecting coronary artery disease, all of the sestamibi protocols are likely to be very similar, with possible minimal reduction in sensitivity in the same-day rest/stress protocol due to the resting activity background. Of note, with this protocol, if defects are present on the rest Tl-201 study, redistribution Tl-201 SPECT can be performed before or 24 hours after the technetium-99m sestamibi injection (Figs. 8 and 9).

An additional advantage of the technetium-99m myocardial perfusion imaging agents is the ease with which ventricular function can be assessed at the time of myocardial perfusion SPECT. As discussed in Chapter 19, gated SPECT has become routine in the performance of myocardial perfusion SPECT, particularly with the technetium-99m agents ses-

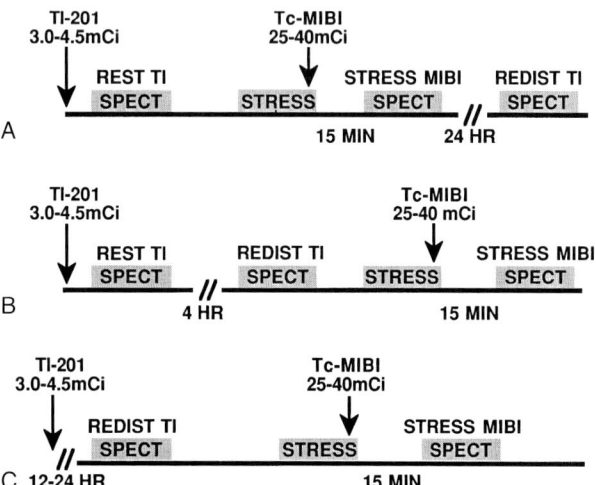

FIG. 8. Common protocols for combining redistribution thallium-201 imaging with rest thallium-201/stress technetium 99m sestamibi SPECT. **A:** protocol for 24-hour imaging after standard dual isotope acquisition; **B:** protocol for 4-hour redistribution imaging prior to stress; **C:** protocol for injection the day or night before with redistribution Tl-201 SPECT as first acquisition sequence.

tamibi and tetrofosmin. With this approach, the poststress and even the resting phases of the examination can be acquired with ECG gating, allowing the assessment of regional wall motion, left ventricular ejection fraction, and ventricular volumes, in addition to the assessment of regional myocardial perfusion. With the technetium-99m myocardial perfusion imaging agents, the additional ability to perform first-pass radionuclide angiography at rest or at peak exercise is present. However, the technique of first-pass radionuclide ventriculography as an adjunct to myocardial perfusion SPECT has not become widely utilized due to the expense of the additional equipment needed and the added complexity of routine use of first-pass exercise radionuclide ventriculography in busy laboratories. Our current protocol for rest thallium-201/technetium-99m myocardial perfusion SPECT, which includes gating both at rest and poststress and the routine acquisition of both supine and prone poststress studies, is shown in Figure 10.

Tc-99m Tetrofosmin

A recently Food and Drug Administration (FDA)-approved technetium-99m myocardial perfusion imaging agent is technetium-99m tetrofosmin, which is extracted by the myocardium and accumulated in mitochondria in a manner similar to that observed with technetium-99m sestamibi. As noted above, the extraction fraction of this agent is slightly lower than that of technetium-99m sestamibi. In the canine model, the compound has been shown to have a linear relationship to flow from levels of 2 mL/min/g to near zero, but a marked plateau appears to occur in the relationship between flow rate and uptake above 2 mL/min/g (66). There is less hepatic uptake with this tracer than with technetium-99m sestamibi, resulting in more favorable heart/liver ratios early following resting injection (67,68). Despite this difference, optimal imaging following rest injection is at 1 hour after injection. The various acquisition protocols recommended for technetium-99m tetrofosmin are the same as those for technetium-99m sestamibi.

Other Tc-99m Myocardial Perfusion Agents

Technetium-99m teboroxime belongs to another class of technetium-99m myocardial perfusion agents, which are neutral lipophilic complexes of boronic acid called BATO compounds. Unlike technetium-99m sestamibi and tetrofosmin, which have lower extraction fractions than thallium-201, technetium-99m teboroxine appears to have a higher extraction fraction than thallium-201. Additionally, it appears that the high extraction fraction with this agent plateaus at a higher flow rate than the other agents (69,70). These highly desirable extraction characteristics of teboroxime are counterbalanced by prominent backdiffusion related to its neutral, lipophilic properties and to the fact that this agent is not bound intracellularly; i.e., teboroxime washes out very

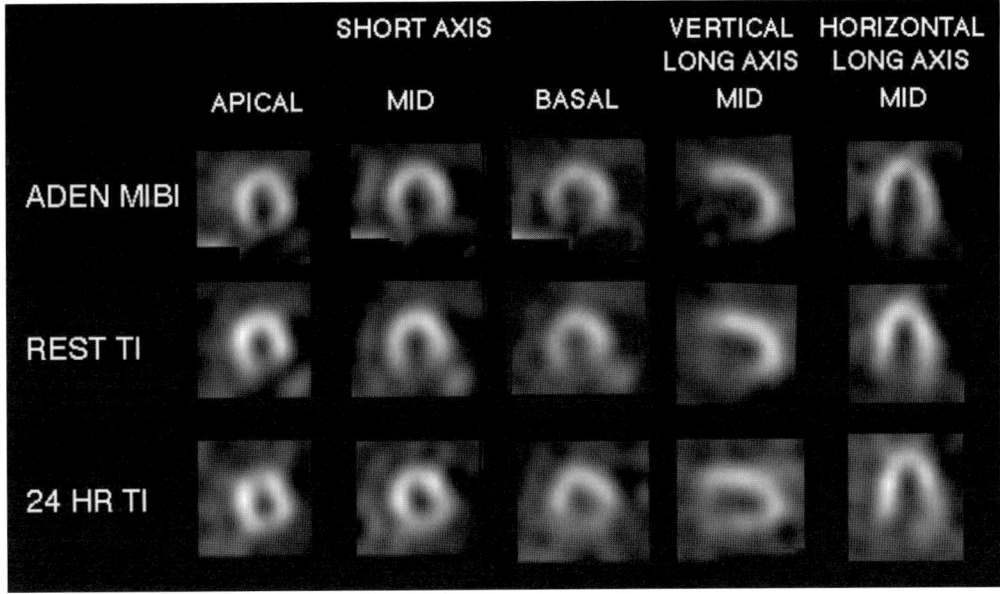

FIG. 9. Patient BB: Adenosine stress Tc-99m sestamibi (**top**), rest thallium-201 (**middle**), and 24-hour thallium-201 (**bottom**) SPECT images in a patient with small Q waves in leads II, III, and ABF and no history of prior myocardial infarction. By stress/rest imaging, the findings suggested an inferior wall myocardial infarction; the 24-hour images, however, demonstrate reversibility in the inferior wall. A rest technetium 99m sestamibi study (not shown), performed following the 24-hour thallium study, showed an inferior wall perfusion defect. The findings of the 24-hour thallium study are consistent with severe hibernation of the inferior wall. (From ref. 78, with permission.)

rapidly from the myocardium (71). Although the myocardium can be visualized with this tracer for approximately 20 minutes after injection, the kinetic properties of Tc-99m teboroxime require that initial imaging be completed within the first few minutes after tracer injection in order to reflect blood flow distribution at the time of injection. Single detector SPECT imaging and gated SPECT imaging are essentially not feasible with this agent; however, with multiple detector systems, rapid SPECT imaging is feasible. Data from our laboratory demonstrated that a rapid back-to-back

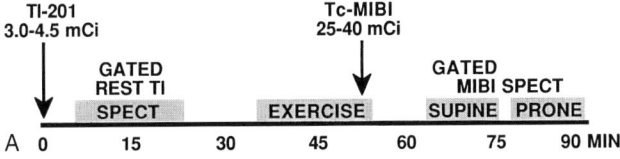

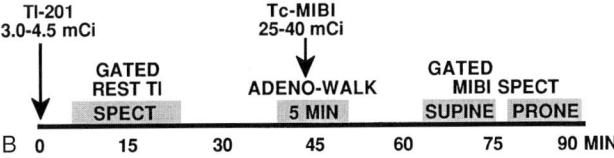

FIG. 10. Current Cedars-Sinai Medical Center exercise (**A**) and pharmacologic stress (**B**) protocols demonstrating combined supine and prone, separate acquisition dual isotope gated SPECT acquisition. *ADENO,* adenosine.

adenosine stress/rest technetium-99m myocardial perfusion SPECT protocol using a triple detector camera could be accomplished in approximately 30 minutes and demonstrated high sensitivity and specificity for coronary artery disease (72).

Due to the requirement for very rapid imaging, Tc-99m teboroxime is the most technically demanding of the available myocardial perfusion tracers. On the other hand, its excellent extraction and washout kinetics provide opportunities not present with the other agents. The high extraction across the full range of flow suggests the possibility that this tracer would be more sensitive for detecting mild coronary stenoses than the other available perfusion agents. Furthermore, an even greater potential and greater challenge would be to take advantage of the relationship between regional myocardial washout of technetium-99m teboroxime and coronary flow to further enhance detection of individual stenoses (71). Previous work from our laboratory has documented that there is slower washout of teboroxime from areas of coronary stenoses than in others supplied by normal vessels, suggesting that the spatially nonrelative regional washout approach to detecting coronary stenosis mentioned above for thallium-201 could be applicable to teboroxime imaging. Interesting work in this regard was reported by Stewart et al. (73), who demonstrated the potential of dynamic SPECT imaging of washout rates of this tracer for quantitation of regional myocardial blood flow. Accumulation of Tc-99m teboroxime appears to be purely related to blood flow and is not to be dependent on myocardial viability (74). Thus, unlike Tc-99m sestamibi or tetrofosmin, Tc-99m teboroxime could be used as a pure marker of reperfusion.

Technetium-99m-NOET is a neutral lipophilic myocardial perfusion imaging agent (75). This agent demonstrates excellent extraction fraction across a wide range of flow. Extraction fraction of 85% with this tracer has been observed under hyperemic conditions (76). There appears to be redistribution over time with this tracer, related in part to the absence of intracellular binding and in part to higher circulating blood levels of radioactivity with this tracer compared to technetium-99m sestamibi (76). It has been suggested that Tc-99m-NOET overall may have kinetic properties and imaging properties very similar to Tl-201, with the advantage of the higher photon flux associated with the higher injected dose, which is possible with a Tc-99m agent. The redistribution of Tc-99m-NOET appears to be almost complete after 90 minutes of reflow, potentially shortening the clinical protocols applicable for assessment of myocardial viability with this tracer. A disadvantage compared to Tc-99m sestamibi or tetrofosmin, however, is the relatively rapid redistribution of this tracer, like that of Tl-201; this makes the agent less forgiving in terms of the ability to repeat imaging should questions arise after the initial acquisition.

Technetium-99m furifosmin appears to be very similar to Tc-99m tetrofosmin (77). Its extraction fraction is lower than that of Tc-99m sestamibi. Neither Tc-99m-NOET nor Tc-99m furifosmin have been approved for clinical use in the United States at this time.

Optimizing Stress Protocols

Most of the above discussion dealt with exercise stress protocols. For all of the radiopharmaceuticals discussed above, pharmacologic stress approaches can also be applied (see Chapter 12). One of the fundamental advantages of myocardial perfusion SPECT over stress echocardiography is the ability to obtain diagnostic studies in virtually all patients. To this end, appropriate patient preparation is necessary. In order to derive optimal diagnostic and prognostic information from a study, it is important that a maximal hyperemic state be achieved with myocardial perfusion SPECT. Thus we recommend that, when clinically feasible, beta blocking medications be withheld for 48 hours prior to exercise stress to increase the likelihood of achieving greater than or equal to 85% of maximal predicted heart rate. We also recommend that all patients scheduled for exercise SPECT not ingest caffeine-containing compounds for 24 hours prior to exercise testing. Thus, if a patient fails to achieve greater than 85% of maximal predicted heart rate during exercise, the radioactive tracer would not be injected. Rather, pharmacologic stress with adenosine or dipyridamole would be immediately substituted, allowing for diagnostic test results. The sensitivity and specificity and risk stratification information of pharmacologic stress myocar-

dial perfusion SPECT are essentially the same as those observed with exercise stress with all of the available tracers.

INTERPRETATION AND REPORTING

A systematic approach to the interpretation and reporting of myocardial perfusion SPECT is essential to the optimal utilization of this modality (78). Since the assessments of perfusion and function are intimately related, this section will address the interpretation and reporting of the combination of perfusion and function in gated myocardial perfusion SPECT. As with myocardial perfusion SPECT in general, careful attention to all aspects of camera/computer system quality control is essential to ensure the adequacy of gated myocardial perfusion SPECT studies (79). These quality control measures include, among others, verification of camera peaking, detector(s) uniformity, alignment, center of rotation, and closeness to the patient. With regard to the injected radiopharmaceuticals, care must be taken to document that the radiopharmaceutical tagging was appropriate, an adequate dose was injected, and no infiltration of radioactivity occurred.

Initial Patient Information

Due to the subjective nature of a scan interpretation, it is generally recommended that all scans first be interpreted without knowledge of the patient's clinical state. It is important, however, to know the patient's height, weight, gender, and, if female, bra size, in order to best recognize possible soft tissue artifacts. If the study is an exercise study, the exercise heart rate achieved and the exercise duration should be known.

Inspection of the Raw Projection Data

One of the most important steps in SPECT interpretation is the review of the raw data, consisting of the projection images prior to filtering and reconstruction. The most useful method for such review is the endless loop "cinematic" display of the rotating projection images. This review ensures that the images were acquired over the appropriate acquisition arc [generally right anterior oblique (RAO) 45 degrees to left posterior oblique (LPO) 45 degrees] and that the heart was within the field of view throughout the entire acquisition. These images also provide useful information regarding count statistics.

Patient Motion

Inspection of the rotating projection images is also important for detecting patient motion as well as "upward creep" of the heart (35). Careful attention should be paid to patient motion in the vertical (craniocaudal) and lateral (horizontal) direction, since either can be associated with an artifactual defect that may go undetected by simple inspection of the tomographic slices. Moderate motion is frequently associated with artifactual defects (80). When Tc-99m sestamibi or tetrofosmin are employed, scans in which motion is observed can be repeated, preferably in the prone position, since these agents are associated with insignificant redistribution between two datasets obtained in close temporal proximity (52). If a validated motion correction algorithm is available, it could be applied to projection datasets in which motion is observed; however, to date, most such algorithms have not been adequately validated. Figure 11**A** illustrates an apparent perfusion defect in typical SPECT images reconstructed from projection images, corresponding to moderate motion on visual inspection. Figure 11**B** represents the reconstructed SPECT images from this same patient's study when the acquisition was repeated in the prone position. No motion was associated with the second acquisition, and the reconstructed images demonstrate no perfusion defect.

It is worthy of note that while most efficient from the standpoint of acquisition time (81), the dual detector 90-degree configuration may accentuate the problems associated with patient motion. In a 64-projection acquisition with a dual detector 90-degree camera, 32 projections would be obtained by each detector. With most types of motion, the greatest difference between projections is noted between the first and last (1 and 32 for the first detector). Since the first projection of the first detector (projection 1) and the first of the second detector (projection 33) are acquired at the same time and with the patient in exactly the same position, if the patient moved, motion is most evident between projections 32 and 33. Unfortunately, this greatest discrepancy between datasets occurs in a portion of the acquisition that is highly sensitive to motion—at approximately a 45 degree-LAO view of the heart, a view associated with relatively high myocardial count rates. Because of this problem, cameras with dual detectors oriented at 90 degrees are more subject to motion artifacts than single detector or triple detectors, and require a higher degree of vigilance for motion (and perhaps a lower threshold for repeating the acquisition) than the other types of cameras. The accentuation of patient mo-

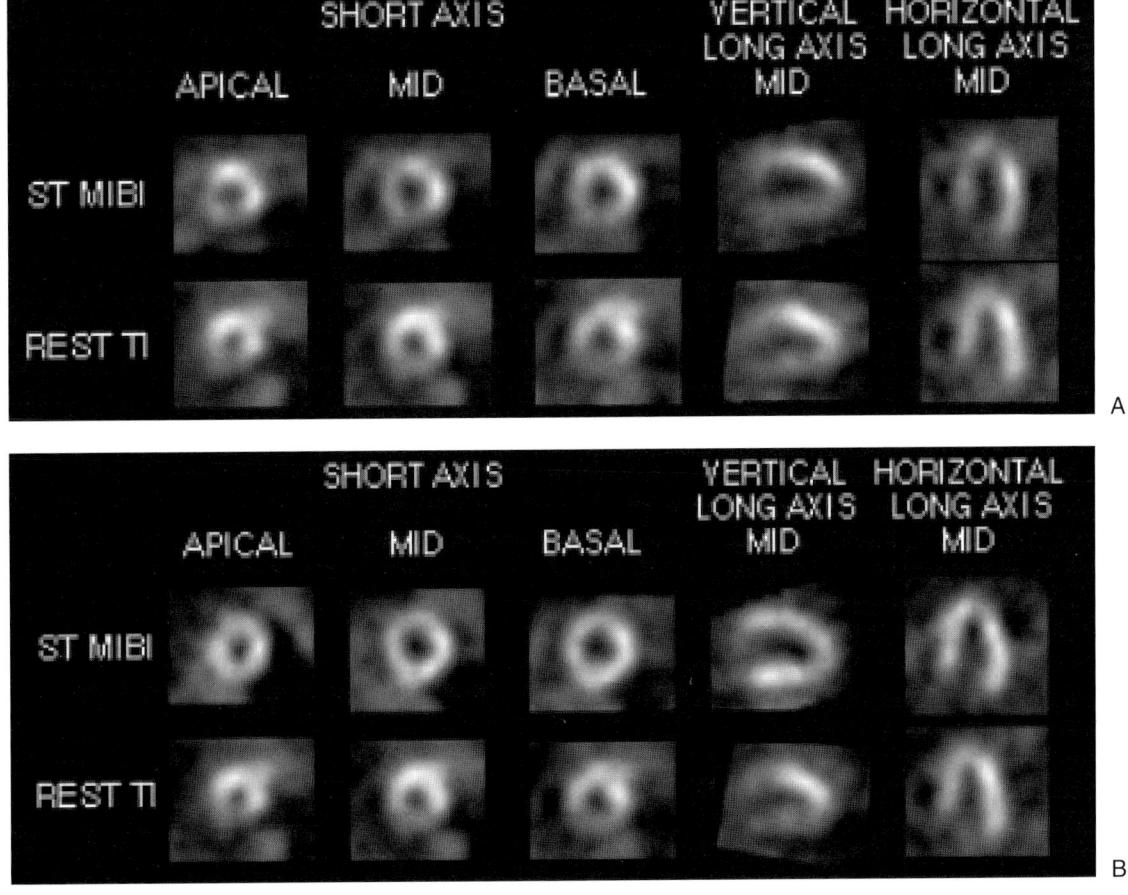

FIG. 11. A: Stress sestamibi (ST MIBI), rest thallium-201 (TI) images in a patient with a low likelihood of coronary artery disease. An apparent septal and apical reversible perfusion defect is present, as well as an apparent nonreversible inferior wall defect. Patient motion was noted during acquisition. Compare Figure 11**B. B:** Stress technetium-99m sestamibi/rest thallium-201 myocardial perfusion SPECT images with stress SPECT in the prone position in the patient illustrated in Figure 11**A**. Diaphragmatic artifacts were eliminated by prone imaging, allowing the study to be correctly interpreted as normal.

tion between frames 32 and 33 was associated with the artifactual defect in the patient study presented in Figure 11**A**.

Attenuation Artifacts

Inspection of the rotating projection images provides a convenient method for detecting sources of attenuation artifacts. In female patients, for example, the degree of breast attenuation can be estimated with reasonable accuracy by an experienced observer looking at the projection data. Special attention should be paid, when comparing differing datasets (e.g., stress/rest, stress/redistribution, supine/prone) side-by-side, to determining whether the position of the attenuating structure changed between acquisitions. Although most artifactual attenuation perfusion defects are nonreversible on inspection of the tomographic slices, breast attenuation artifacts may appear to be reversible if the breast moved between acquisitions. Other sources of attenuation artifacts observed with the help of the rotating image display include the arms, diaphragm, subdiaphragmatic structures, and general obesity. Many of the attenuation artifacts can be eliminated by repeating the acquisition in the prone position (52), as noted above. An example of supine/prone imaging's ability to clarify diaphragmatic attenuation is shown in Figure 12.

Extra Cardiac Uptake

The raw projection data should also be examined for evidence of extra cardiac radioactivity uptake, perhaps the most important example of this occurring with occult cancer. Given the reduced reliance on standard chest x-rays as routine procedures, it is not uncommon for the first evidence of cancer in the thorax to come from an incidental observation at the time of myocardial perfusion scintigraphy. Indeed, Tc-99m sestamibi and Tl-201 have been utilized for cancer detection as well as for myocardial perfusion imaging (82,83). An example of a patient with an undiagnosed lung cancer detected by the rotating projection images of a myocardial perfusion SPECT study is shown in Figure 13**A**, with the tomographic images shown in Figure 13**B**. Lung cancer, lymphoma, and breast cancer are the most common kinds of cancers detected through this approach.

Lung Uptake

The degree of lung uptake of myocardial perfusion tracers should be noted from visual inspection of the raw projection images. In addition, the lung/heart ratio can also be quantified by automatically or manually placing a region of interest over the most normal cardiac zone as well as a representative pulmonary region of an anterior or LAO 45-degree projection image, and by making a ratio of the average or maximum pixel counts in the lung and heart regions. In general, quantitative lung/heart ratios for Tl-201 have been shown to have an upper limit of normal of 0.54 (84–86), while preliminary data for Tc-99m sestamibi suggests an upper limit of 0.44 (87). In general, there is a strong linear correlation relationship between the degree of lung uptake and the pulmonary capillary wedge pressure at the time of injection (88,89).

Hepatic/Gastrointestinal Uptake

The degree of myocardial perfusion tracer uptake in the liver and the gastrointestinal tract adjacent to the heart should be noted. If excessive, consideration should be given to repeating image acquisition after a delay of 1 hour, if Tc-99m sestamibi or tetrofosmin are used. The increased uptake in structures adjacent to the heart can be a source of artifacts on the reconstructed tomograms. In particular, either artifactual decrease in severity of true perfusion defects may occur (due to scatter from the adjacent "hot" source) or an artifactual myocardial perfusion defect may be created by the mathematics of the reconstruction process (cancellation of counts in regions immediately adjacent to "hot" objects) (90).

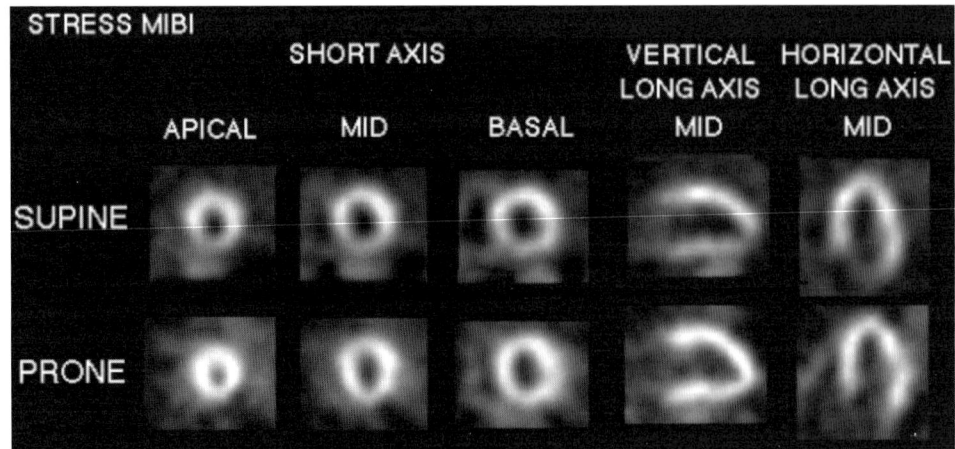

FIG. 12. This is in a patient with a low likelihood of angiographically significant coronary artery disease. Stress sestamibi images in the supine (**top**) and prone (**bottom**) positions from a patient with diaphragmatic attenuation. The normal appearance of the inferior wall in the prone acquisition allowed the study to be correctly interpreted as normal.

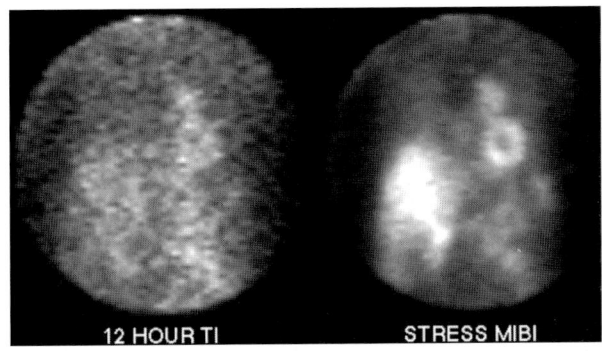

FIG. 13. A: Stress sestamibi/12-hour redistribution thallium-201 SPECT acquisitions in a patient with a malignant thymoma. Careful inspection of the extra cardiac area reveals the increased uptake in the tumor. **B:** Selected anterior view projections from the raw data of the SPECT acquisition from the patient illustrated in Figure 12. *SPECT*, single photon emission computed tomography; *ST MIBI*, stress sestamibi; *TI*, thallium-201.

Assessment of Myocardial Perfusion from SPECT Images

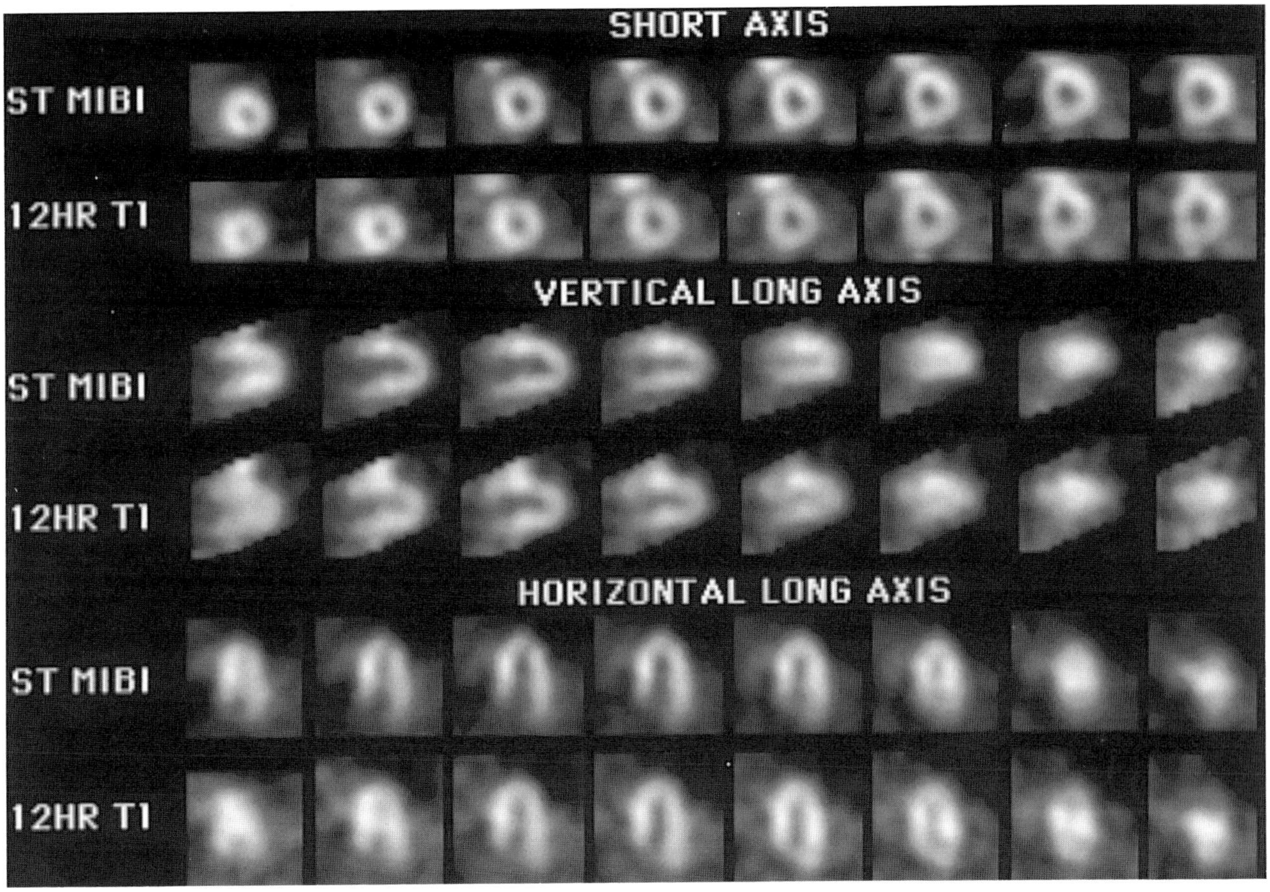

Display

A uniform approach to SPECT image display is recommended, based on the reorientation of images (slices) relative to the axis of orientation of the heart in the chest (91). The reoriented slices are termed the short-axis, vertical long-axis, and horizontal long-axis-images. Images from different acquisitions (e.g., stress/rest, rest/redistribution, stress/redistribution) should be appropriately aligned and displayed simultaneously in interleaved fashion. As for image normalization, there are two widely used approaches. Each series (short-axis, vertical long-axis, and horizontal long-axis images) can be normalized to the pixel with the highest count in the entire series (series normalization). This approach provides the most intuitively accurate assessment of the presence, extent, and severity of perfusion defects, although it presents the drawbacks of lack of ideal display for each individual slice, sensitivity to focal hot spots, and insensitivity to basal perfusion defects. Alternatively, each tomographic slice can be normalized to the brightest pixel within that slice ("frame normalization"). This approach provides ideal display of each individual slice and is less sensitive to the problem of basal attenuation.

Twenty-segment Visual Analysis

The use of a semiquantitative scoring system in which each of 20 segments is scored according to a 5-point scheme

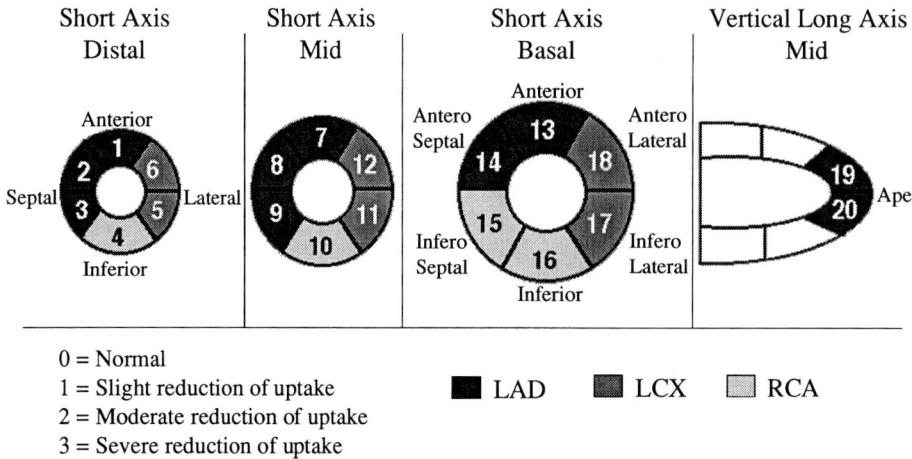

0 = Normal
1 = Slight reduction of uptake
2 = Moderate reduction of uptake
3 = Severe reduction of uptake
4 = Absent radioactive uptake

■ LAD   ▨ LCX   ▢ RCA

FIG. 14. Diagrammatic representation of the segmental division of the SPECT slices and assignment of individual segments to individual coronary arteries using the 20-segment model. LAD, left anterior descending coronary artery; LCX, left circumflex coronary artery; RCA, right coronary artery. (From ref. 78, with permission.)

provides an approach to interpretation that is more systematic and reproducible than simple qualitative evaluation. The 20-segment scoring system is based on three short-axis slices (distal or apical, mid, and basal) to represent the entire left ventricle, with the apex represented by two segments visualized in a mid-vertical long-axis image. Each of the 20 segments has a distinct name and number, as indicated in Figure 14. Since the anteroapical and inferoapical segments are visualized in the midventricular vertical long-axis image, the distal short-axis slice is chosen as one that is a few slices into the left ventricle; i.e., not the first slice to contain the ventricular cavity. Each segment is scored as follows: 0 = normal; 1 = slight reduction of uptake (equivocal); 2 = moderate reduction of uptake (usually implies a significant abnormality); 3 = severe reduction of uptake; 4 = absence of radioactive uptake (92). Perfusion defects with scores of 3 or 4 can be reported as consistent with a critical (greater than or equal to 90%) coronary stenosis (93,94).

The 20-segment, 5-point scoring system standardizes the visual interpretation of scans, reduces the likelihood of overlooking significant defects, and provides an important semiquantitative global index that can be used for overall assessment of extent and severity of abnormality. Each segment roughly corresponds to 5% of the left ventricle (LV). The system has been utilized for approximately 15 years at Cedars-Sinai Medical Center, and forms the basis for the diagnostic and prognostic publications that have emanated from our laboratory.

Recently, a 17-segment scoring system has been proposed as illustrated in Figure 15. With this system, the smaller size of the apical short-axis slice is accounted for by dividing the slice into four segments, and the apex is considered a single segment. The advantage of the 17-segment model is that each segment is more accurately weighted as a proportion of LV mass. Furthermore, the 17-segment model may be preferred over the 20-segment model for use in other imaging modalities (e.g., two-dimensional echo, magnetic resonance imaging), facilitating cross modality comparisons. The drawbacks of the 17-segment approach are that it has been less well documented for diagnostic and prognostic applications. Although we prefer the 20-segment model because of this documentation, we believe that in practical applications it will not be of major consequence which of these protocols is used.

Summed Scores

In addition to the segmental visual scores, the 20-segment 5-point scoring system lends itself to the derivation of summed scores, which can be considered global indices of perfusion (95). The summed stress score (SSS) is defined as the sum of the stress scores for the 20 segments. The summed rest score (SRS) is defined as the sum of the rest scores or redistribution scores, and the summed differences score (SDS), measuring the degree of reversibility, is defined as the difference between the summed stress score and the summed rest score. These summed scores are to perfusion what the ejection fraction index is to ventricular function. Specifically, the SSS is the perfusion analog of the peak exercise ejection fraction, the SRS is the perfusion analog of the resting ejection fraction, and the SDS is the perfusion analog of the change in ejection fraction with stress. Of note, it is essential that the observer take into account the normal regional variation of count distribution typical of myocardial

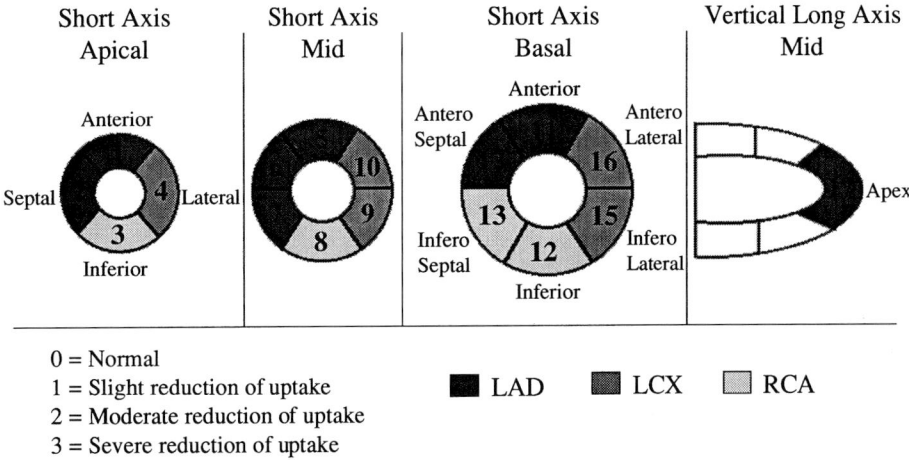

0 = Normal
1 = Slight reduction of uptake
2 = Moderate reduction of uptake
3 = Severe reduction of uptake
4 = Absent radioactive uptake

■ LAD   ▨ LCX   ☐ RCA

FIG. 15. Diagrammatic representation of segmental division of the SPECT slices and assignment of the individual segments of the individual coronary arteries using the 17-segment model. Abbreviations as in Figure 14.

perfusion scintigraphy, before assigning a perfusion score. For example, the basal interventricular septum (membranous septum) has reduced blood flow, and (because of its depth) is subject to greater attenuation than other portions of the myocardium. This ''normal septal dropout,'' frequently observed as an apparent defect on the basal septal slices, should be assigned a score of 0 rather than a score suggesting the presence of abnormality. Based on our previous prognostic work (96,97), summed stress scores less than 4 are considered normal or nearly normal, summed stress scores of 4–8 are considered mildly abnormal, summed stress scores of 9–13 moderately abnormal, and summed stress scores greater than 13 severely abnormal. An example of a patient

with a moderately abnormal scan (summed stress score of 10) is illustrated in Figure 16.

Ascribing Abnormalities to Coronary Vascular Territories

As illustrated in Figures 14 and 15, the 20 myocardial segments can be ascribed to individual coronary territories (62,98). Specifically, the inferior and basal septal segments are ascribed to the posterior descending coronary artery (Figs. 16 and 17), the lateral segments to the left circumflex coronary artery (Fig. 18), and the mid and distal septal as well as all anterior slices to the left anterior descending coronary artery (LAD) (Figs. 19 and 20). Although isolated api-

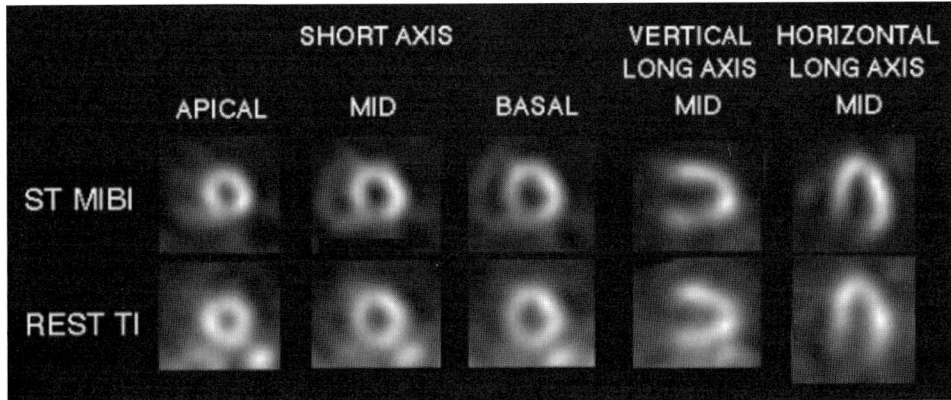

FIG. 16. Stress sestamibi/rest thallium-201 myocardial perfusion SPECT images of a 63-year-old patient with nonanginal chest pain. The study demonstrates a summed stress score of 10 with scores of 2 in the 3 inferior segments and the mid- and basal inferoseptal segments, all corresponding to the right coronary artery territory. ST MIBI, stress sestamibi; TI, thallium-201.

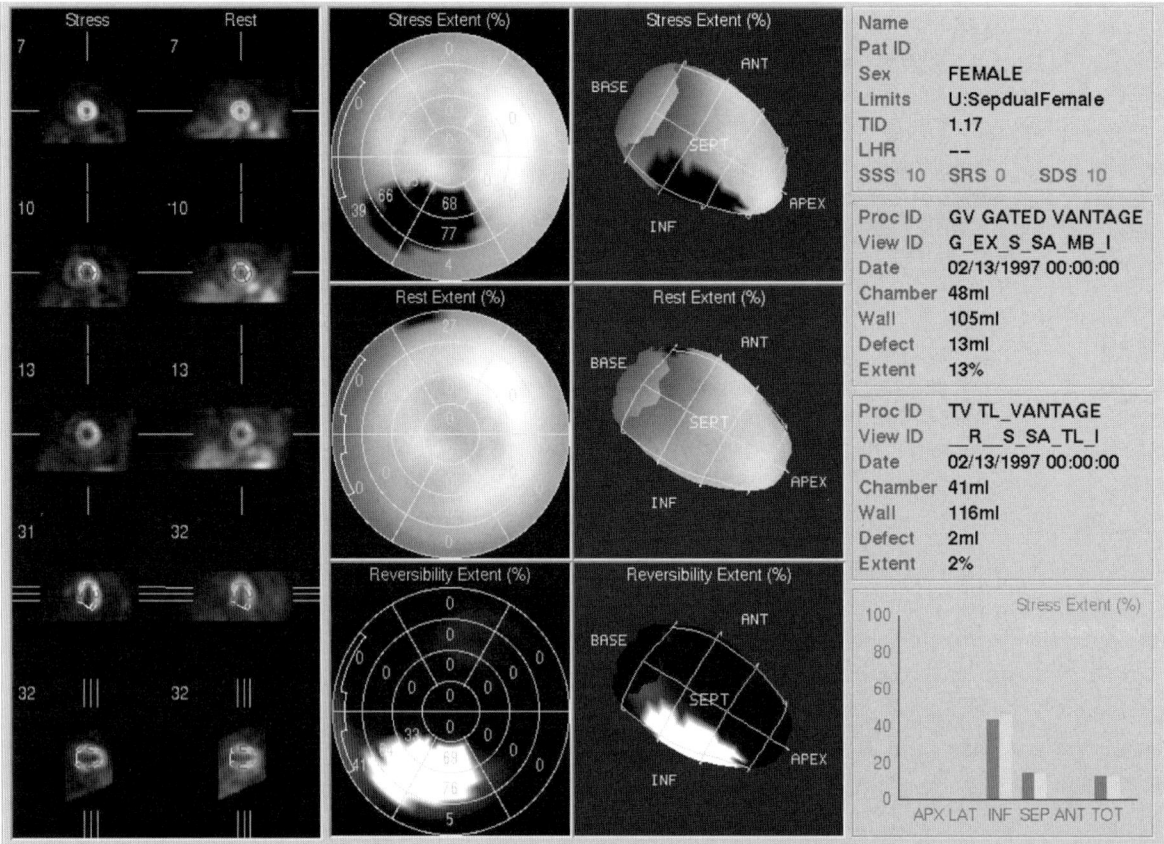

FIG. 17. Quantitative perfusion SPECT (QPS) of the patient shown in Figure 16 indicating the presence of a moderate-sized perfusion defect in the distribution of the proximal right coronary artery.

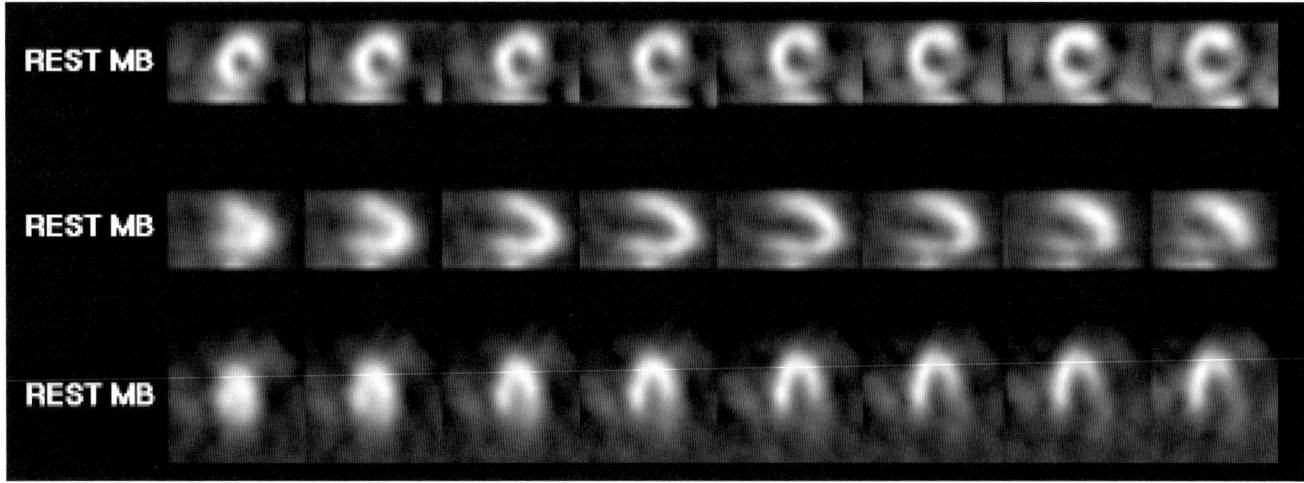

FIG. 18. Rest sestamibi/myocardial perfusion SPECT study in a 54-year-old patient with 5 hours of resting chest pain and a normal ECG. A severe defect (with scores of 3) is seen throughout the lateral wall, the territory of the left circumflex coronary artery. The summed rest score was 15. Immediate catherization revealed an occluded left circumflex coronary artery, which was successfully dilated. MB, technetium-99m sestamibi.

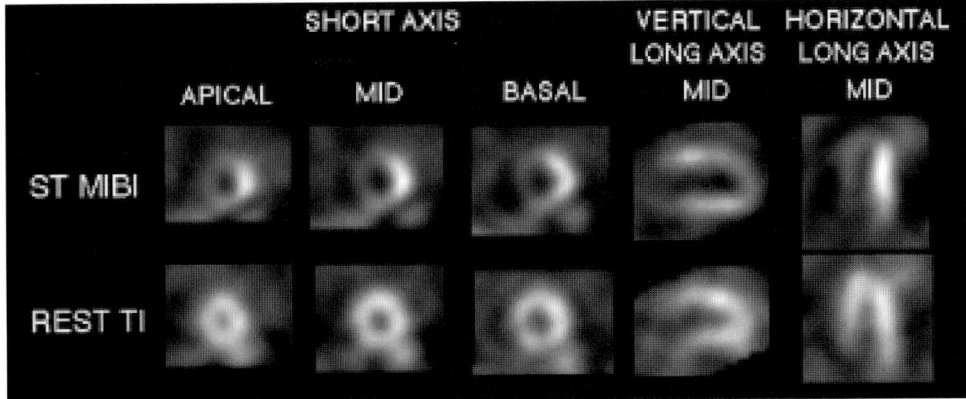

FIG. 19. Exercise sestamibi/rest thallium-201 myocardial perfusion SPECT in a 60-year-old patient with atypical angina. The summed stress score is 35. A severe and extensive reversible perfusion defect is seen throughout the left anterior descending coronary artery territory. There is additional evidence of transient ischemic dilation of the left ventricle.

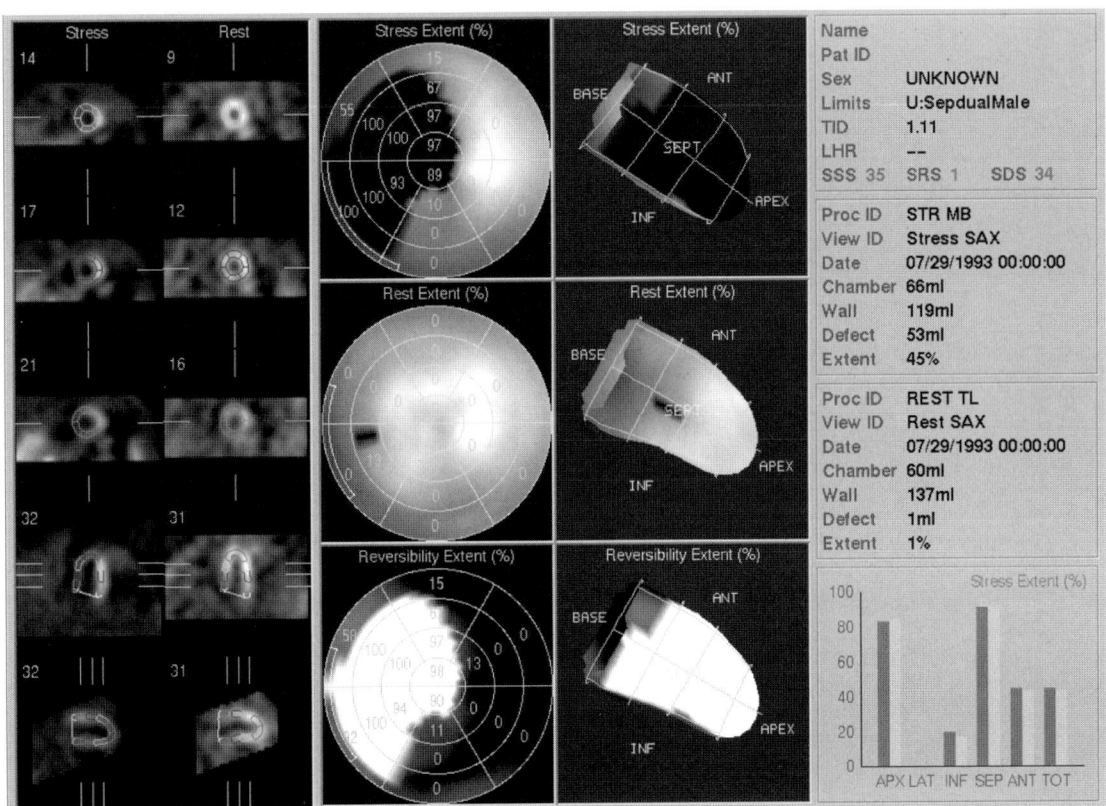

FIG. 20. Quantitative perfusion SPECT (QPS) of the patient shown in Figure 19 demonstrating the prevalence of a large perfusion defect in the distribution of the proximal left anterior descending coronary artery.

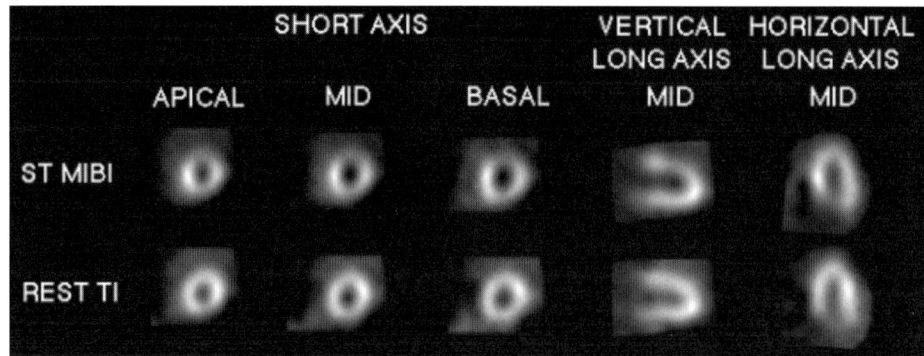

FIG. 21. Exercise stress (ST) technetium 99m sestamibi/rest thallium-201 myocardial perfusion SPECT in a 60-year-old male patient with atypical angina. A small reversible defect is seen in the diagonal territory, with scores of 2 in the 3 anterior segments but no abnormality in the apex. The summed stress score was 6.

cal abnormalities are usually associated with left anterior descending artery disease, the apex can also be supplied by the left circumflex or right coronary arteries. If only anterior wall segments are abnormal, sparing the apex and the septum, the abnormalities are usually considered to represent disease of the diagonal branch of the left anterior descending coronary artery (Fig. 21).

The coronary assignment is altered for regions at the border between specific vessels territories, depending on the pattern of perfusion defect abnormality in the adjacent segments. When defects cross the usual coronary territories, judgment is required to determine whether to report multivessel disease as being likely. At times, a dominant perfusion defect in a specific vascular territory will "tail" into a contiguous territory generally assigned to another vessel. In these circumstances, the defect would generally be attributed to the vessel associated with the dominant defect. This pertains most commonly to the inferoseptal and inferolateral walls, but also applies to the anterolateral wall. Regarding the septum, if an inferoseptal defect is present (excluding the basal inferoseptal segment, which is generally a right coronary artery territory), the septal abnormalities would be assigned to the left anterior descending or right coronary artery, depending on which of these vessels had a perfusion defect. Similarly, if an inferolateral or anterolateral defect, but not both, were present in patients with adjacent defects in either the anterior or inferior wall, the lateral wall defect would be assigned to the vessel attributed to the neighboring defect. In general, isolated septal defects (without anterior wall or inferior wall involvement) are rare; isolated lateral wall defects (in the absence of anterior wall or inferior wall defects) would be attributed to the left circumflex coronary artery (98). These are general associations, which may vary in an individual patient based on variations in coronary anatomy.

For purposes of reporting, ascribing a perfusion defect to a specific coronary artery is influenced by the specific pattern of abnormality observed, and, of course, by the specifics of a patient's coronary anatomy, if known. For example,

involvement of the midinferoseptum in the patient shown in Figures 16 and 17 is considered to be part of a right coronary artery territory abnormality, due to the presence of a clear abnormality in the more specific right coronary artery segments in the inferior wall and no abnormality in the other LAD territory segments.

In determining the overall interpretation (from definitely normal to definitely abnormal), the degree to which an apparent perfusion defect corresponds to a known coronary vascular territory is taken into account. Perfusion defects that fail to correspond to a standard vascular territory are more likely to be artifacts than those corresponding to typical vascular distributions.

Attenuation Corrected Images

Recently, several camera manufacturers have provided hardware and software implementation of attenuation correction protocols (99,100). In general, these attenuation corrections are imperfect, reducing but not eliminating apparent perfusion defects due to soft tissue attenuation in normal patients. In addition, at times, true perfusion defects might be obscured or eliminated by application of these approaches. The artifactual elimination of perfusion defects is usually due to filtering or to scatter from adjacent organs, which becomes more apparent after attenuation correction. Because of these limitations, it is currently recommended that attenuation-corrected tomographic datasets be visualized simultaneously with noncorrected datasets. The interpreter should be aware that, because of the imperfection in present day attenuation correction algorithms, a uniform distribution of radioactivity throughout the myocardium cannot be expected. Furthermore, the normal regional distribution of counts on a segment-by-segment basis may be different in attenuation-corrected images than in nonattenuation corrected images. Thus, the normal regional distribution of counts in the attenuation-corrected images should be taken into account prior to segmental scoring.

Quantitative Analysis

It is recommended that semiquantitative visual analysis and quantitative analysis be assessed simultaneously. A variety of quantitative approaches have been developed, most of which compute myocardial counts in the various myocardial segments and display these counts using a two-dimensional or three-dimensional polar map (55,101). Most commonly, abnormalities are then defined by comparison of a patient's polar map to the polar maps derived from gender-matched normal patients. Due to the objective nature of the analyses, quantitative assessments are more reproducible than visual assessments and are particularly useful in assessing interval change when patients are evaluated serially. Examples of quantitative analyses, employing Quantitative Perfusion SPECT (a system developed at Cedars-Sinai Medical Center), are illustrated in Figures 17 and 20. For relatively inexperienced readers, the quantitative analysis is helpful in teaching the regional variation associated with myocardial perfusion SPECT and improving interpretive skills. For experienced readers, quantitation serves as a second expert observer, frequently causing a more careful inspection of a regional abnormality that may have been overlooked. Despite the advantages of quantitative analysis, visual analysis is still an integral part of myocardial perfusion SPECT interpretation, since the quantitative analyses have not yet been refined to detect a variety of artifactual patterns easily recognized by visual inspection (e.g., breast attenuation, motion artifact, noncoronary patterns).

Assessment of Myocardial Viability

The presence of myocardial viability is implied with the myocardial perfusion tracers if the degree of uptake at rest, redistribution, or following nitrate-augmented rest injection is normal or nearly normal. If a region has severely reduced or absent uptake of radioactivity in these settings, it is considered to be nonviable. Areas with moderate reduction of counts in these conditions (score 2 at redistribution or nitrate-augmented rest) are usually partially viable, and patients in this group have a variable response in terms of postoperative improvement. Although some have suggested that a single cutoff point (chosen as a percentage of maximal counts in the myocardium) is predictive of viability in a region in question (102,103), we would prefer the use of the number of standard deviations below normal, since the latter would take into account the rather marked normal reduction in counts that occurs in the inferior wall and nonattenuation-corrected myocardial perfusion SPECT images.

"Nonperfusion" Abnormalities

In addition to perfusion defects, several nonperfusion abnormalities should be observed and, when present, described. They include size of the left ventricle, transient ischemic dilation of the left ventricle (TID) (104,105), right ventricle myocardial uptake pattern, and right ventricular size. As noted before, a note should also be made of abnormalities of lung uptake or other abnormal extra-cardiac activity.

Transient ischemic dilation is considered present when the left ventricular cavity appears to be significantly larger in the poststress images than in the resting images. The degree of enlargement needed depends on the imaging protocol used. For example, with dual-isotope protocols, the greater Compton scatter associated with Tl-201 causes the myocardial walls to appear intrinsically thicker (and the cavity smaller) in Tl-201 rest images compared to poststress Tc-99m sestamibi images (105). Therefore, a greater degree of transient enlargement must be evident for a dual-isotope study to be considered to demonstrate transient ischemic dilation. Transient ischemic dilation can easily be measured by slight modifications of the quantitative gated SPECT algorithms described in Chapter 19. We have found that the upper limits of normal for the transient ischemic dilation ratio in dual-isotope imaging is 1.22. Patients who have transient ischemic dilation of the left ventricle (TID greater than 1.22) are likely to have severe and extensive coronary artery disease (greater than 90% stenosis of the proximal left anterior descending coronary artery, or of multiple vessels) (105). It should be noted that the term "transient ischemic dilation" is imprecise. What is referred to as transient ischemic dilation may actually be an apparent cavity dilation secondary to diffuse subendocardial ischemia (obscuring the endocardial border). This phenomenon is likely to explain why "transient ischemic dilation" may be seen for several hours following stress, when true cavity dilation is probably no longer present. The pattern of transient and ischemic dilation of the left ventricle has similar clinical implications whether it is observed on exercise or pharmacologic stress studies (106). An example of a patient illustrating transient ischemic dilation of the left ventricle is shown in Figure 19.

Overall Assessment of Myocardial Perfusion

We recommend that the interpreter form an overall interpretation of the myocardial perfusion scan, prior to incorporation of the clinical information. To minimize the use of an equivocal category, we advocate using a 5-point scoring system (normal, probably normal, equivocal, probably abnormal, abnormal), based predominantly on the segmental score, but also on other considerations, including the degree to which the scan abnormality conforms to a known vascular coronary territory, the presence of transient ischemic dilation or lung uptake, and the heart rate achieved (on exercise studies). This overall interpretation is subjective, but guidelines are provided by the factors listed in Table 1.

Assessment of Ventricular Function from Gated SPECT Images

As with the assessment of myocardial perfusion, a systematic approach to the assessment of ventricular function from

TABLE 1. *Overall interpretation of myocardial perfusion SPECT*

Visual criteria for abnormality (exercise or pharmacologic testing)	
• Normal:	All segments = 0
• Probably normal:	Few segments = 1
• Equivocal:	Multiple reversible 1
	1 Segment = 2
• Probably abnormal:	2 Segments = 2
• Definitely abnormal:	≥3 Segments = 2
	≥1 Segments ≥ 3

Weighing toward abnormal if defects are reversible, conform to a standard coronary territory, are associated with transient ischemic dilation, or lung uptake.

the gated SPECT portion of the study is recommended. The use of a systematic approach greatly reduces the chances of misinterpretation.

Quality Control

As with myocardial perfusion, assessment of adequacy of the technical quality of the data is, of course, an integral part of the interpretation of gated SPECT. Inspection of the rotating "summed" projection images is frequently a source of information regarding inadequacy of the data. Observation of "flashing" usually indicates that a gating error has occurred, resulting in the acquisition of a widely different number of cardiac cycles at the different angles along the acquisition arc. Inadequacy of the gating process can also be detected by inspection of the time-volume curve. This curve is derived from quantitative gated SPECT algorithms (107), and provides an assessment (see Chapter 19) of the left ventricular cavity size at the various phases of the cardiac cycle. Figure 22 illustrates an example of quantitative gated SPECT results, including the time-volume curve. Note that the frame with the largest volume is the first frame, corresponding to end-diastole, and that the overall curve has a characteristic U-shape. When the time activity curve is clearly inappropriately timed, the gated SPECT data is generally considered nondiagnostic. The rotating summed projection images should also be evaluated for count statistics; at times, the count density in the overall summed images may be adequate for the interpretation of perfusion SPECT data, but is inadequate for the assessment of wall motion and wall thickening from the individual gated frames.

Display

Because each image is obtained over eight or sixteen frames of the cardiac cycle, we have found that displaying all myocardial slices simultaneously results in too much information to easily interpret. We therefore recommend a five-slice display in which three representative short-axis slices (apical, midventricular and basal), as well as one vertical long-axis and one horizontal long-axis midventricular

tomogram, are displayed. The five-slice display is viewed in a "cine" format, alternating between the "contours on" and the "contours off" mode of the quantitative algorithm. When appropriate software is available, this alternation is a quality control measure to verify that the endocardial and epicardial surfaces determined by the algorithm were appropriate for computation of left ventricular ejection fraction and left ventricular volumes, and also provides assistance in the accurate scoring of regional function.

Twenty-segment Wall Motion Analysis

We recommend that the same 20 or 17 segments utilized for perfusion assessment be used for the visual assessment of regional ventricular function. A diagrammatic representation of the five slices chosen for analysis and the 6-point motion scoring system is illustrated in Figure 23. As noted, the assignment of the segmental regional wall motion scores is based on what is "normal" for a given region. This approach assumes that the observer is familiar with the range of motion that is normal for a given segment, just as he/she would be expected to be familiar with the range of "normal" perfusion in a given segment. Wall motion analysis is performed by visualizing the endocardial edge of the left ventricle, a process that is aided by the alternation between "contours on" and "contours off." As a general rule, most experts recommend the use of a gray scale for the interpretation of regional wall motion.

Twenty-segment Wall Thickening Analysis

Visual assessment of wall thickening takes advantage of the direct relationship between the increase in the apparent brightness of a wall during the cardiac cycle (partial volume effect (108)) and the actual increase in its thickness. For purposes of wall thickening evaluation, many investigators recommend the use of a 10-step color scale as opposed to a gray scale. The degree of all thickening is similarly scored with a 4-point system (0 = normal, 3 = absent thickening). In general, for a given short-axis slice, there is greater uniformity of "absolute" thickening than there is of wall motion, due to the greater effect of translational motion of the heart's long axis during systole on perceived regional wall motion than on thickening.

Discordance between Wall Motion and Wall Thickening

In general, abnormalities of regional wall motion and wall thickening accompany each other. We have thus found it most convenient to score function in combined fashion for the 20 segments, only making note of whether wall motion and wall thickening are found to be discordant. The most common cause of discordance between wall motion and wall thickening is found in patients who have undergone bypass surgery; in these cases, "abnormal" wall motion with pre-

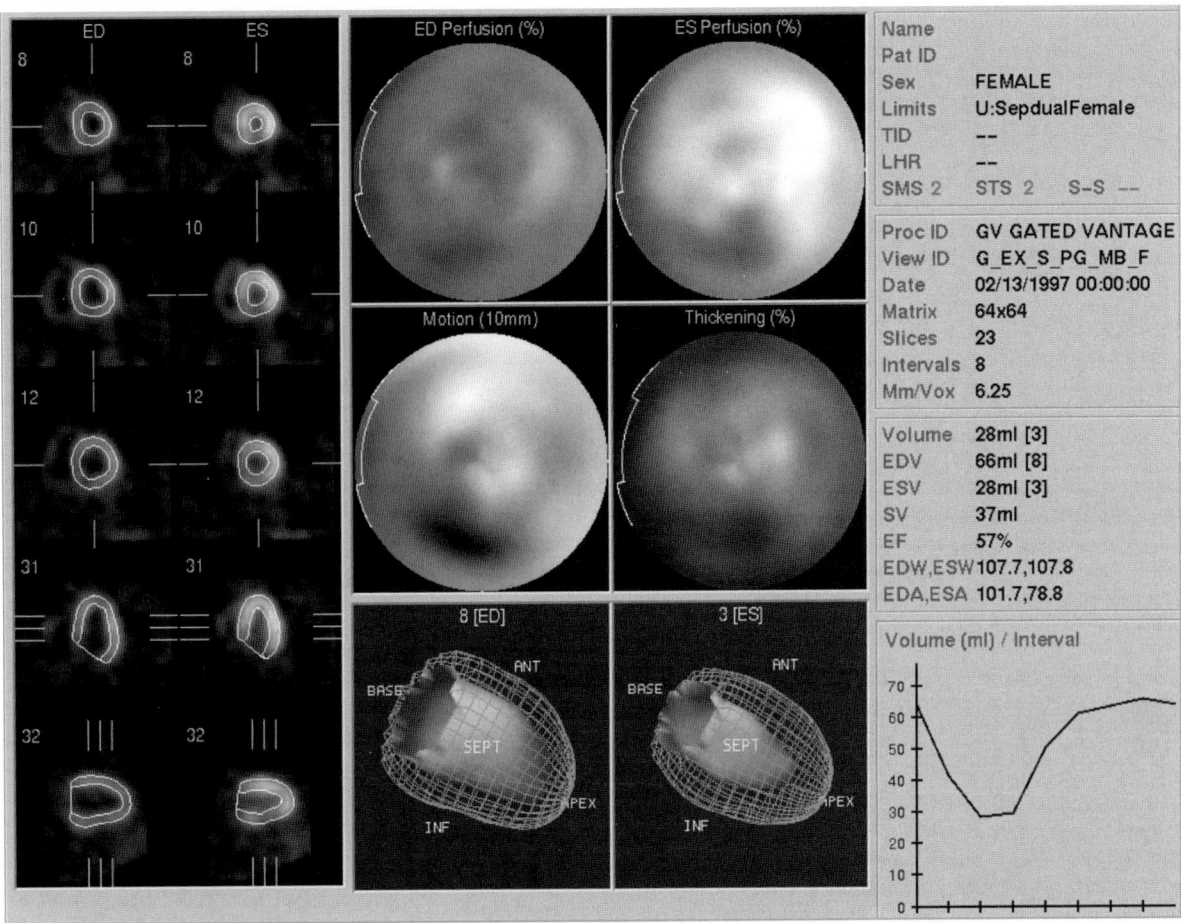

FIG. 22. Quantitative gated SPECT (QGS) analysis of the poststress study from the patient illustrated in Figures 16 and 17. The left ventricular ejection fraction is normal at 57%. There is evidence of normal left ventricular wall motion.

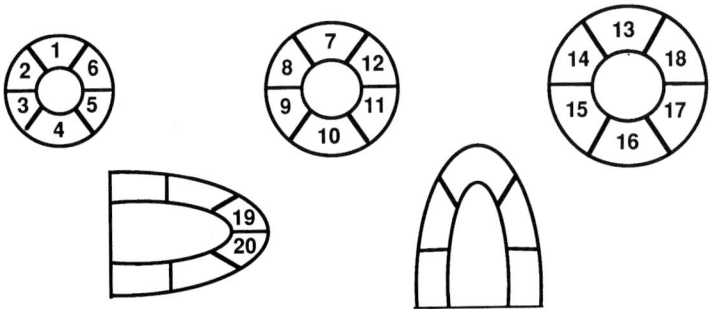

6- or 4-POINT SCORING*

WALL MOTION

    0 = NORMAL   3 = SEVERE HYPOKINESIS
    1 = MILD HYPOKINESIS   4 = AKINESIS
    2 = MODERATE HYPOKINESIS   5 = DYSKINESIS

WALL THICKENING

    0 = NORMAL   2 = MODERATE-SEVERE (DEFINITE) REDUCTION
    1 = MILD (EQUIVOCAL) REDUCTION   3 = NO DETECTABLE THICKENING

* Based on what is "normal" for a region

FIG. 23. Diagrammatic representation of the 20-segment model utilized for analysis of wall motion and wall thickening from gated myocardial perfusion SPECT.

served thickening of the interventricular septum is an expected normal variant. Similar discordance between wall motion and wall thickening also occur in left bundle-branch block, where preserved thickening with abnormal motion of the interventricular septum is also a common variant. At the edges of a large infarct, normal thickening with minimal or absent motion may be observed in the periinfarction zone, with reduced motion being due to the adjacent infarct. The presence of thickening is considered to be indicative of viable myocardium; conversely, "normal" wall motion of an abnormally perfused segment that does not thicken could be associated with passive inward motion of a nonviable myocardial region (tethering), due to hypercontractility of adjacent noninfarcted segments.

Combined Rest/Poststress Regional Function Analysis

When available, the rest and poststress gated images should be compared to identify the development of new wall motion abnormality. Wall motion abnormalities that occur on poststress images but are not seen on resting images imply the presence of ventricular stunning, and are highly specific for the presence of coronary artery disease (109,110). If resting gated SPECT studies are not available, a note should still be made of discrete regional wall motion or wall thickening abnormalities, since these can often be indicators of the presence of a severe coronary stenosis (greater than 90% diameter narrowing). This finding might be missed by perfusion defect assessment alone, particularly in patients with a greater degree of ischemia in a region other than that demonstrating the wall motion abnormality (110). As a general rule, it is important to routinely report the patient's state at the time of gated SPECT acquisition; i.e., rest, 30-minute poststress, 1-hour poststress, etc. Of interest in protocol design, the earlier this acquisition is performed after stress, the more likely that the poststress wall motion abnormality will be observed.

Quantitative Wall Motion/Wall Thickening Assessment

Ideally, quantitative methods for comparing the degree of wall motion and wall thickening of each segment of the left ventricle to the lower limit of normal would be available and would augment the visual analysis of ventricular function from gated SPECT data. Algorithms for the automatic quantitative measurement of absolute endocardial motion and relative myocardial thickening between end-diastole and end-systole have been developed and validated at our laboratory (111), and the determination of segment-specific normal limits is currently underway.

Left Ventricular Volume

It has recently been demonstrated that quantitative assessments of absolute left ventricular cavity volumes correlate well with echocardiography (112–116), thermal dilution catheterization methods (117,118), and magnetic resonance imaging (119). We have also found the absolute measurements of left ventricular volume to be essentially perfectly reproducible (repeated assessment in a given dataset) (120) and highly repeatable (repeated data acquisition) (121,122). If a validated method for measuring left ventricular volumes is available on a particular camera-computer system, it is recommended that this measurement be reported as a standard component of gated SPECT analysis. Volume measurements are helpful in prognostication (123), as well as in guiding the use of ACE-inhibitors (124). Absolute LV volumes tend to be underestimated in patients with very small hearts.

Overall Interpretation of Ventricular Function

An overall interpretation of the ventricular function component of the gated SPECT examination is recommended, as discussed earlier for myocardial perfusion, and can be accomplished using the same scale with five gradations (from definitely normal to definitely abnormal). In general, a study is considered to show abnormal function if a severe wall motion abnormality is present. If only a moderate wall motion abnormality is present, the determination as to whether the ventricular function portion of the study should be considered abnormal depends on the ejection fraction.

Modification of the Interpretation of Perfusion and Function Based on Clinical Information

Having analyzed the perfusion and function portions of the gated perfusion SPECT examination without knowledge of the patient's clinical state, the observer should incorporate knowledge of all clinically relevant data, including symptoms, risk factors, the results of treadmill testing, and the results of coronary angiography into the final interpretation. By convention, modification of the nuclear interpretation should not change the initial assessment by more than one category of abnormality, using the 5-point scale from normal to abnormal (Table 2). For example, if the initial inter-

TABLE 2. *Interpretation of myocardial perfusion SPECT showing the convention for modification based on clinical information*

Modify interpretation based on clinical information				
Convention: shift by a maximum of 1 degree				
Normal	Probably normal	Equivocal	Probably abnormal	Abnormal

TABLE 3. *Nonscintigraphic information that should be incorporated into the final report*

Incorporate all clinical information and other test results into the final report
- Risk factors
- Presenting symptoms
- Nonnuclear exercise test results
  —Duration
  —Heart rate and blood pressure response
  —Symptoms
  —ST response
- Coronary angiography
- Other imaging tests

pretation was equivocal, the study could be considered probably normal in a patient with a low prescan likelihood of coronary artery disease. Conversely, the equivocal study could be reported as probably abnormal in a high prescan likelihood setting (e.g., typical angina pectoris with multiple risk factors and an abnormal treadmill test). The modification has the effect of improving the overall concordance of information sent to clinicians (a type of "smoothing" function). It is of critical importance to exercise restraint, so that the maximal shift is one category in the 5-point scale. Shifting by a greater extent would be confusing, in that it would no longer provide data representative of the scintigraphic study.

Integration of Information

Table 3 lists the items of information that an ideal nuclear cardiology report would contain in addition to the scintigraphic information. The final comprehensive report should represent a synthesis of nuclear and nonnuclear information. We recommend that several summary statements be included as components of the final report, including the following:

1. In patients who are not known to have coronary artery disease, the postscan likelihood of angiographically significant coronary artery disease should be expressed. This likelihood can be calculated by using commercially available programs such as Cadenza (125), or look-up tables (126,127). Table 4 lists the adjectives that we

TABLE 4. *Percentages and adjectives used to describe the likelihood of angiographically significant coronary artery disease*

(%)	Adjective
<5–14	Low
15–29	Low intermediate
30–69	Intermediate
70–85	High intermediate
85–94	High
95–98	Very high
≥99	Virtually diagnostic

associate with the various postscan likelihoods of angiographically significant coronary artery disease.

2. In patients with known disease [postangiography, postmyocardial infarction, postcoronary artery bypass graft (CABG) surgery, postpercutaneous transluminal coronary angioplasty (PTCA)] undergoing exercise studies, the postscan likelihood is referred to as the "likelihood of exercised-induced ischemia." In patients with known disease undergoing pharmacological stress, the term "likelihood of jeopardized myocardium" is used. This distinction between "exercised-induced ischemia" and "jeopardized myocardium" is used since the large majority of patients demonstrating reversible defects (evidence of jeopardized myocardium) with vasodilator stress (dypridamole/adenosine) develop a perfusion imbalance during stress but have not actually developed "ischemia" (128).

3. The extent, severity, and location of reversible defects should be reported and related to the likely coronary anatomy.

4. The extent and location of fixed defects (which might be referred to as "apparent scarring" or "prior myocardial infarction") should be described. In general, the terms "myocardial infarction" or "scarring" should be avoided unless late redistribution imaging is performed, since nonreversible defects may still be seen in areas with hibernating, viable myocardium.

5. It is important that the final summation should answer the specific question being asked by the referring physician.

6. Using the combined clinical information and scintigraphic scores, it is also recommended that a statement regarding the patient's risk of subsequent cardiac event be considered for inclusion in the final report. We routinely ascribe an expected risk of death or myocardial infarction based on the summed stress score, with the categories less than 1% per year considered low, 1% to 5% per year, intermediate, and greater than 5% per year, high.

7. If myocardial viability is being questioned, specific statements regarding the viability of abnormally contracting segments should be included.

Integration of Information about Perfusion and Function from Gated SPECT

As noted above, data relative to perfusion and function are usually similar. The classic examples of discordance that occur in the interventricular septum in patients who have undergone bypass surgery or in patients with left bundle-branch block are expected, but should still be reported.

Unexpected discordance of data should be accompanied by a specific description of the discordance at the end of the final report. In our experience, the most common occurrences of discordance are in patients with cardiomyopathy. For example, if a patient has a very reduced left ventricular ejection fraction, a large left ventricle and no perfusion defect (the myocardial perfusion SPECT study is normal, but its gated SPECT component is abnormal) we categorize this type of study as "abnormal, with left ventricular enlargement, but no perfusion defects." We would then add a statement such as "the findings of severe left ventricular enlargement and severe depression of left ventricular ejection fraction with no associated perfusion defect are most consistent with a dilated nonischemic cardiomyopathic process." In our laboratory, many patients with a report such as this will not undergo subsequent cardiac catherization.

A somewhat less common but important additional source of discordance between perfusion and function data occurs in patients with ventricular remodeling following myocardial infarction. These patients will typically have large nonreversible perfusion defects with no reversible perfusion defects, but marked left ventricular enlargement and reduction of left ventricular ejection fraction and regional ventricular function out of proportion to the size of the perfusion defect. In those circumstances, a statement such as the following is included in the final summation: "The left ventricular enlargement and marked left abnormality of ventricular function are out of proportion to the size of the perfusion defect. These findings are most compatible with ventricular remodeling." Depending on the clinical situation, we may add, "Less likely, but still possible, the patient may have an ischemic cardiomyopathic process with balanced reduction in flow." To make the latter statement, there would usually be further evidence of exercise-induced ischemia or jeopardized myocardium, such as marked chest discomfort, ST-segment depression or unexpected akinesis/dyskinesis in zones with normal resting motion or normal resting perfusion (110).

In dilated nonischemic cardiomyopathic processes and in ventricular remodeling, the portions of the left ventricle demonstrating normal perfusion but abnormal function are usually hypokinetic. When frank akinesis or dyskinesis is noted in zones that appear to have normal perfusion, the final report is weighted toward the possibility of an ischemic cardiomyopathy with balanced reduction in flow, since stress-induced stunning in an ischemic cardiac myopathy would be more likely to explain this discordance than ventricular remodeling or a nonischemic cardiomyopathic process.

The overall interpretation of gated myocardial perfusion SPECT remains an art. Following the systematic approach recommended in this section allows this art to be refined, and makes the results more reproducible from observer to observer and from center to center.

CLINICAL APPLICATIONS

Detection of Coronary Artery Disease

Tables 5 and 6 present sensitivities and specificities of myocardial perfusion SPECT for the detection of angiographically significant (greater than 50% stenosis) coronary artery disease. It should be noted that published reports have consistently demonstrated that the sensitivity of exercise electrocardiography is significantly lower than that of myocardial perfusion SPECT (129). Despite the noted differences in the initial extraction characteristics of these tracers, to date there have been few clinical reports documenting lower sensitivity of the technetium-99m tracers compared to thallium-201 for the detection of coronary artery disease. With respect to specificity, the main difference between thallium-201 and technetium-99m sestamibi or tetrofosmin SPECT is considered to be the slightly-to-moderately reduced susceptibility to artifact due to lower attenuation of technetium-99m, greater use of gated SPECT with the Tc-99m perfusion agents, and, most importantly, the ability to repeat the SPECT acquisition with these agents when either attenuation or motion artifacts are suspected.

In estimating the true sensitivity and specificity of noninvasive testing, referral or work-up bias needs to be taken into account (54,130). In cardiology, this work-up bias has been shown to be very powerful. Once a noninvasive test is accepted as being clinically effective, its results strongly influence the performance of subsequent coronary angiography. Referral bias results in an overestimation of test sensitivity, and an underestimation of test specificity. In the extreme case, where the noninvasive test result becomes the "gatekeeper" to the performance of angiography, its observed sensitivity and specificity will become 100% and 0%, respectively. This occurs due to the basic definitions of sensitivity and specificity. Sensitivity is the proportion of patients with disease who are correctly detected as abnormal by the test, and specificity is the proportion of patients without disease who are correctly detected as normal by the test. Once the test becomes used as the "gatekeeper" to catheterization, sensitivity and specificity can no longer be accurately measured. Even if the test in question had a true sensitivity of 50% and a true specificity of 99%, the observed sensitivity and specificity would still by definition be 100% and 0%, respectively, since only positive test responders are catheterized. This extreme example illustrates the care with which current medical literature needs to be interpreted in respect to sensitivity and specificity rates.

Due to the profound impact of the referral bias on specificity, we advocate the concept of the normalcy rate and have applied it in multiple different clinical studies. First applied in 1981 (131) and named in 1986 (132), the normalcy rate refers to patients with a low likelihood of coronary artery disease, based on sequential Bayesian analysis of age, sex, symptom classification and the results of noninvasive stress testing (other than the test in question). We have used the term normalcy rate to describe the frequency of normal test results in these patients with a low likelihood of coronary artery disease, to differentiate it from specificity, which as noted above refers to the frequency of normal test results in patients with normal coronary angiograms. "Low-likelihood" patients are chosen since they are closer in age and risk factors to patients with known coronary artery disease

TABLE 5. *Sensitivity and specificity of exercise myocardial perfusion SPECT for detecting CAD (≥ 50% stenosis)*

Year	Author	Isotope	Previous MI (%)	Sensitivity	%	Specificity	%
1990	Kiat et al. (165)	MIBI	45	45/48	94	4/5	80
1990	Mahmarian et al. (166)	Tl	43	192/221	87	65/75	87
1990	Nguyen et al. (167)	Tl	N/R	19/25	75	5/5	100
1990	Van Train et al. (168)	Tl	35	291/307	95	30/64	47
1991	Coyne et al. (169)	Tl	N/R	38/47	81	39/53	74
1993	Berman et al. (62)	MIBI Tl	0	50/52	96	9/11	82
1993	Forster et al. (170)	MIBI	0	10/12	83	8/9	89
1993	Chae et al. (171)	Tl	42	116/163	71	52/80	65
1993	Minoves et al. (172)	MIBI Tl	42	27/30	90	22/24	92
1993	Van Train et al. (173)	MIBI	16	30/31	97	6/9	67
1994	Sylven et al. (174)	MIBI	37	41/57	72	5/10	50
1994	Van Train et al. (175)	MIBI	19	91/102	89	8/22	36
1995	Palmas et al. (176)	MIBI	30	60/66	91	3/4	75
1995	Rubello et al. (177)	MIBI	57	100/107	93	8/13	61
1996	Hambye et al. (178)	MIBI	0	75/91	82	28/37	75
1997	Yao et al. (179)	MIBI	55	34/36	94	14/15	93
1997	Heiba et al. (180)	MIBI	31	28/30	93	2/4	50
1997	Ho et al. (181)	Tl	33	29/38	76	10/13	77
1997	Taillefer et al. (182)	MIBI	17	23/32	72	13/16	81
1997	Van Eck-Smit et al. (183)	Tetrofosmin	N/R	46/53	87	6/7	86
1998	Budoff et al. (184)	MIBI	0	12/16	75	12/17	71
1998	Santana-Boado et al. (185)	MIBI	0	92/101	91	56/62	90
1998	Acampa et al. (186)	MIBI	47	23/25	92	5/7	71
1998	Acampa et al. (186)	Tetrofosmin	47	24/25	96	6/7	86
1998	Ho et al. (187)	Tl	22	19/24	79	15/20	75
	Total			1515/1739	87	431/589	73

Based on English language manuscripts providing data with ≥ 50% stenosis criterion.
CAD, coronary artery disease; *N/R*, not reported; *MIBI*, Tc-99m-sestamibi; *Tl*, Tl-201; *≥ 50% MI*, myocardial infarction; *SPECT*, single photon emission computed tomography.

undergoing testing than are normal volunteers (in fact, low-likelihood patients are part of a population of patients with suspected coronary artery disease prior to their referral). The normalcy rate has been reported to be in the 80 to 90% range with thallium-201 testing, generally greater than 90% with technetium-99m sestamibi SPECT and would be expected to be similar to the latter for Tc-99m tetrofosmin SPECT. As noted earlier, the better normalcy rate and likely better specificity of the Tc-99m agents is most likely secondary to the ability to repeat imaging in case of suspected artifactual abnormality. The reported normalcy rates for myocardial perfusion SPECT are illustrated in Table 7.

TABLE 6. *Sensitivity and specificity of vasodilator stress SPECT for detecting CAD (≥ 50% stenosis)*

Year	Author	Drug	Isotope	Previous MI (%)	Sensitivity	%	Specificity	%
1990	Nguyen et al. (167)	adenosine	Tl	37	49/53	92	7/7	100
1990	Verani et al. (188)	adenosine	Tl	N/R	24/29	83	15/16	94
1991	Iskandrian et al. (189)	adenosine	Tl	25	121/132	92	14/16	88
1991	Coyne et al. (169)	adenosine	Tl	N/R	39/47	83	40/53	75
1991	Nishimura et al. (190)	adenosine	Tl	13	61/70	87	28/31	90
1995	Aksut et al. (191)	adenosine	Tl	24	358/398	90	38/45	84
1995	Miyagawa et al. (192)	adenosine	Tl	15	67/76	88	35/44	80
1996	Amanullah et al. (193)	adenosine	MIBI	21	87/94	93	28/36	78
1997	Watanabe et al. (194)	adenosine	Tl	19	40/46	87	21/24	88
1997	Watanabe et al. (194)	dipyridamole	Tl	23	34/41	83	21/29	72
1997	Taillefer et al. (182)	dipyridamole	MIBI	11	23/32	72	5/5	100
1997	He et al. (195)	dipyridamole	Tetrofosmin	52	41/48	85	6/11	55
1997	Amanullah et al. (196)	adenosine	MIBI	0	159/171	93	37/51	73
1997	Cuocolo et al. (197)	adenosine	Tetrofosmin	23	22/25	88	1/1	100
1998	Takeishi et al. (198)	adenosine	Tetrofosmin	17	39/44	89	17/21	81
	Total				1164/1306	89	313/390	80

Based on English language manuscripts providing data with ≥ 50% stenosis criterion.
CAD, coronary artery disease; *N/R*, not reported; *MIBI*, Tc-99m-sestamibi; *Tl*, Tl-201; *MI*, myocardial infarction; *SPECT*, single photon emission computed tomography.

TABLE 7. *Normalcy rate for myocardial perfusion*

Year	Author	Stress	Isotope	Normalcy rate	%	Subjects
1989	Maddahi et al. (199)	exercise	Tl	24/28	86	low likelihood (< 5%) of CAD
1989	Iskandrian et al. (200)	exercise	Tl	123/131	94	low likelihood (< 5%) of CAD
1990	Kiat et al. (165)	exercise	MIBI	7/8	88	low likelihood (< 5%) of CAD
1990	Van Train et al. (168)	exercise	Tl	62/76	82	low likelihood (< 5%) of CAD
1992	Kiat et al. (52)	exercise	Tl	49/55	89	low likelihood (< 5%) of CAD
1993	Berman et al. (62)	exercise	Tl/MIBI	102/107	95	low likelihood (< 5%) of CAD
1994	Heo et al. (201)	exercise or adenosine	Tl/MIBI	33/34	97	low pretest probability (< 5%) of CAD
1994	Van Train et al. (202)	exercise	MIBI	30/37	81	low likelihood (< 5%) of CAD
1995	Zaret et al. (203)	exercise	Tetrofosmin	56/58	97	low likelihood (< 3%) of CAD
1995	Kiat et al. (204)	arbutamine	Tl	52/58	90	low likelihood (< 5%) of CAD
1996	Hendel et al. (205)	exercise	Furifosmin	39/39	100	low likelihood (< 5%) of CAD
1996	Amanullah et al. (193)	adenosine	MIBI	66/71	93	low likelihood (< 10%) of CAD
1997	Heo et al. (206)	exercise	MIBI	58/61	95	low pretest probability (< 5%) of CAD
	Total			701/763	92	

Based on English language manuscripts.
CAD, coronary artery disease; *MIBI*, Tc-99m-sestamibi; *Tl*, Tl-201; *Tetrofosmin*, Tc-99m-tetrofosmin; *Furifosmin*, Tc-99m-furifosmin; *SPECT*, single photon emission computed tomography.

Simple detection of coronary artery disease remains one of the most common indications for performing myocardial perfusion SPECT. It is particularly important in certain patients with high-risk occupations, as well as in younger patients in whom the definitive diagnosis of coronary artery disease, with its life-long implications for therapy, may be important, regardless of the likelihood of cardiac events over a 1- to 3-year period. The basis for the practical diagnostic application of nuclear testing lies in the concept of sequential Bayesian analysis of disease probability. This analysis requires knowledge of the pretest likelihood of disease, as well as of the sensitivity and specificity of the test. The pretest likelihood of disease or prevalence of disease varies according to age, sex, symptoms, and risk factors, and can be directly derived from the work of Diamond and Forrester (133), as well as other sources (125–127).

Our clinical algorithm for the purpose of simple detection of coronary artery disease is illustrated in Figure 24 (134). Patients with a low probability (<0.15) of having angio-graphically significant (>50% stenosis) CAD can be identified, even before standard exercise tolerance test (ETT) is performed. Patients with a low pre-ETT likelihood of CAD do not require further diagnostic testing, although continued medical follow-up or a "watchful waiting" approach is recommended. Patients with a low-intermediate pre-ETT likelihood of CAD (0.15 to 0.50) would undergo standard ETT as the next diagnostic step. Those who continue to have an intermediate likelihood of CAD after ETT (or those with an indeterminate ETT) and those whose pre-ETT likelihood of CAD was in the 0.50 to 0.85 range (in these patients, even a negative ETT would not result in a low likelihood of CAD) will benefit from exercise nuclear testing. Patients with a high pre-ETT likelihood of CAD (greater than 0.85) are generally considered to have an established diagnosis of CAD and would not need nuclear stress testing for diagnostic purposes. As described later, however, nuclear stress testing may be very effective in risk stratification of such patients.

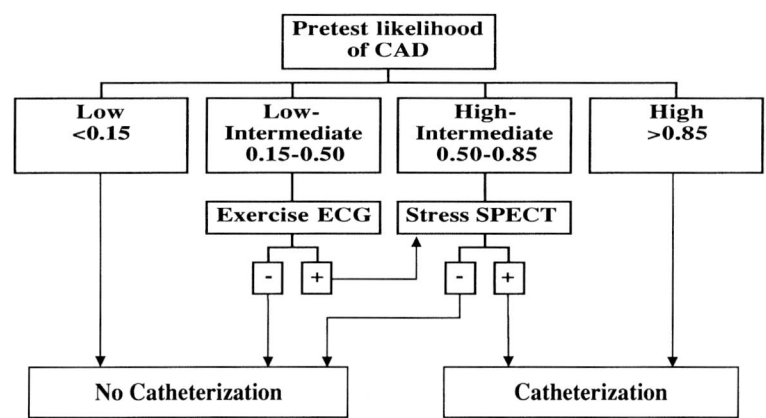

FIG. 24. Role of myocardial perfusion SPECT in detection of coronary artery disease. (From ref. 134, with permission.)

Risk Stratification/Patient Management

The most rapidly growing area of application of myocardial perfusion SPECT is risk stratification based on increased acceptance of a new paradigm in patient management. A risk-based approach to patients with suspected coronary artery disease appears better suited to the modern environment of cost containment and dramatic improvements in medical therapy than the approach focusing on simple diagnosis, in which the patient with disease undergoes coronary angiography and then frequently is revascularized. With the risk-based approach, the focus is not on predicting who has coronary artery disease, but on identifying and separating patients at risk for cardiac death, patients at risk for nonfatal myocardial infarction, and patients at low risk for either event. The advantage of this prognostic endpoint in noninvasive testing is that it defines who has disease *and* is at risk for an adverse event, thus needing to be treated.

The basic concept in the use of nuclear tests for risk stratification is that they are best applied to patients with an intermediate risk of a subsequent cardiac event, analogous to the optimal diagnostic application of nuclear testing of patients with an intermediate likelihood of having coronary artery disease. For prognostic testing, patients known to be at high risk or low risk would not be appropriate patients for cost-effective risk stratification, since they are already risk stratified. For purposes of risk assessment, we have proposed that low risk be defined as a less than 1% cardiac mortality rate per year, high risk as a greater than 3–5% cardiac mortality rate per year, and intermediate risk as referring to the 1% to 3–5% cardiac mortality rate per year range (88–90).

The basis for the power of nuclear testing for risk stratification is found in the fact that the major determinants of prognosis in coronary artery disease can be assessed by measurements of stress-induced perfusion or function. These measurements include the amount of infarcted myocardium, the amount of jeopardized myocardium (supplied by vessels with hemodynamically significant stenosis), and the degree of jeopardy (tightness of the individual coronary stenosis). An additional important factor in prognostic assessment is the stability (or instability) of the coronary artery disease process. This last consideration may help interpret what appears to be a paradox: nuclear tests, which in general are expected to be positive only in the presence of hemodynamically significant stenosis, are associated with a very low risk of either cardiac death or nonfatal myocardial infarction when normal; in contrast, it has been observed that most myocardial infarctions occur in regions with premyocardial infarction lesions causing less than 50% stenosis (136,137). It has been postulated that this paradox may be explained by the different response to stress of mild stenoses associated with stable and unstable plaque. For example, it has been shown that unstable plaque is associated with abnormal endothelial function, resulting in a vasoconstrictive response to acetylcholine stimulation, whereas stable mild coronary lesions respond with vasodilation to acetylcholine (138). It is

possible that factors released during exercise or vasodilator stress may be similar to acetylcholine in terms of stimulation of a differential endothelial response in stable and unstable plaque. Thus, beyond the ability to define anatomic stenosis, nuclear tests (by virtue of their physiologic assessments) may be able to discern abnormalities of endothelial function associated with high risk, even in the absence of significant stenosis.

To maximally extract the information regarding these prognostic determinants in coronary artery disease, it is necessary to consider the full extent and severity of abnormality, either quantitatively (139,140) or semiquantitatively (62) (as discussed earlier), rather than simply determining that the nuclear study is normal or abnormal. Furthermore, as described more fully in Chapter 19, there appears to be incremental value in measuring both perfusion and function for the purposes of risk stratification, thus leading to increased prognostic utility of gated cardiac SPECT over standard myocardial perfusion SPECT.

Suspected Chronic Coronary Artery Disease

Ladenheim et al. from our group (141) have previously documented that the extent and severity of ischemia, as reflected by nuclear variables, are independent prognostic markers and that, for prognostic purposes, exercise myocardial perfusion SPECT provides incremental information over clinical and exercise variables (142).

The most remarkable aspect of this work was that the greatest incremental information for prognosis was provided not in the patients with intermediate likelihood of disease, but in those with a high likelihood of coronary disease (when this method is not useful for detection of coronary artery disease). Exercise thallium-201 SPECT was subsequently shown by Iskandrian et al. (143) to provide significant information over clinical information alone or clinical plus exercise information. Furthermore, these authors demonstrated that, once the SPECT information was known, there was no further incremental prognostic information provided by catheterization data (144).

After converting to the use of stress sestamibi imaging as part of the dual isotope protocol, we felt it important to investigate whether the previous prognostic experience using thallium-201 was also applicable to technetium-99m sestamibi imaging. This was considered to be of particular importance, since it was known that technetium-99m sestamibi had a lower extraction fraction than thallium-201, potentially causing mild perfusion defects to be missed and perhaps affecting prognostic assessment. In a study of 1,702 patients, of whom 1,131 had normal scan results, we demonstrated that a normal technetium-99m sestamibi scan is associated with a very low (0.2%) likelihood of cardiac death or myocardial infarction over a 20-month period (Fig. 25) (95). Concordant with the results of Ladenheim et al. (141), this study also documented that the greatest separation in event

important to determine whether noninvasive test results can be cost effective. To this end, Shaw et al. (160) have evaluated a patient population of 11,249 consecutive stable angina patients, gathered in a large multicenter trial comprising many laboratories around the United States, including our own. In a matched cohort study comparing direct catherization to myocardial perfusion SPECT with selective catheterization in patients with chronic stable angina, for all levels of pretest clinical risk, there was a substantial reduction (31 to 50%) in costs using the myocardial perfusion SPECT plus selective catheterization approach. This cost reduction was seen in both the diagnostic (early) and follow-up (late) costs, which included costs of revascularization (Figure 28). The rates of subsequent nonfatal myocardial infarction and cardiac death were virtually identical, when comparing the direct catheterization and myocardial perfusion imaging with selective catheterization approaches in all patient risk subsets. What was significantly different was the rate of revascularization, which was reduced by nearly 50% in the myocardial perfusion imaging with selective catheterization cohort (Fig. 29).

Assessing patients by noninvasive testing at one particular point in time does not imply that no follow-up testing is necessary. There can be progression of coronary disease over time, particularly in the absence of aggressive medical therapy. In that regard, our group has preliminarily evaluated the "warranty period" for a normal scan. It appears that for patients who are appropriately referred to testing in the first place (patients with intermediate-to-high likelihood of coronary artery disease), a normal scan result is associated with

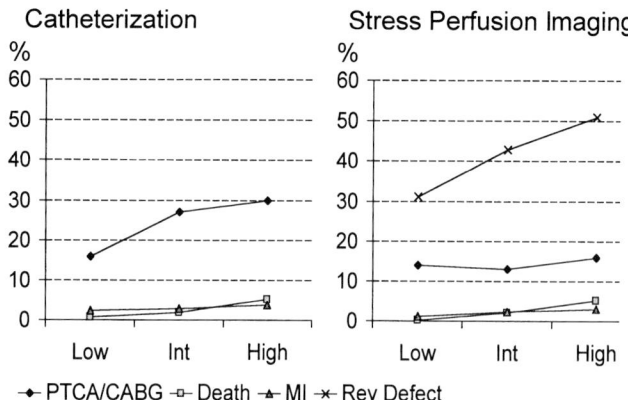

FIG. 29. Subsequent event rates in the patient populations illustrated in Figure 28. The rates of myocardial infarction and cardiac death were identical between the populations. What was different was an approximate 50% reduction in revascularization rate in the group approached with myocardial perfusion imaging and selective catheterization. Abbreviated terms, Low, Int, High, as defined in Figure 28. *CABG*, coronary artery bypass graft; *PTCA*, percutaneuous transluminal coronary angioplasty; *Death*, cardiac death; *MI*, myocardial infarction; *REV* defect, reversible defect. (From ref. 160, with permission.)

a very low risk for approximately 2 years. After that time, the risk rises, suggesting that repeat testing after 2 years should be considered in most patients for prognostic purposes (161).

The foregoing information provides compelling evidence that myocardial perfusion SPECT is effective in the prognostic stratification of patients. It would appear, however, that current data on risk stratification by myocardial perfusion SPECT may actually underestimate the strength of this modality. In all the manuscripts quoted earlier, patients referred for early revascularization following nuclear testing were excluded (censored) from consideration in the prognostic studies. While there is a reason for this censorship, namely that the event rate may have been altered by the revascularization procedure, the exclusion results in the published data's inability to reflect the prognostic information data derived from scans performed in the highest risk patient subset. A similar effect occurs to the extent that physicians and patients alter therapy and modify risk factors on the basis of the scan information, thereby likely reducing the event rate that might be observed for a given abnormal scan pattern in a natural history study.

In addition, recent technical advances in the field of myocardial perfusion SPECT have typically not been included in the prognostic assessments. For example, the impact of quantitative analysis on prognosis has not been studied in any detail, although it has been reported to be equal to semiquantitative analysis, potentially improving the ability to generalize the findings to less experienced laboratories (162). Furthermore, the potent information contained in the ejection fraction and ventricular volumes assessed from gated

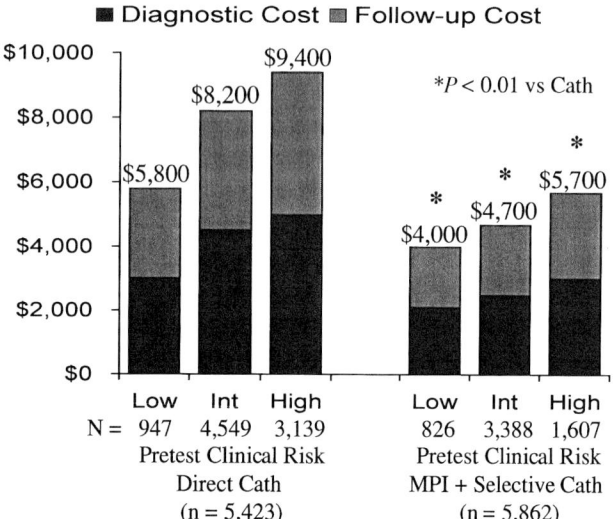

FIG. 28. Comparative cost between screening strategies employing direct catheterization (Cath) and myocardial perfusion imaging (MPI) with selective Cath. Low, Int, and High represent low-, intermediate-, and high-risk subsets of the patients with stable angina. Shown are the initial diagnostic costs (*solid bars*) and follow-up costs, including costs of revascularization (*gray bars*). A 30 to 41% reduction in costs was noted in each category. (From ref. 160, with permission.)

SPECT is likely to enhance the prognostic content of myocardial perfusion SPECT (163), as explained in detail in Chapter 19. A similar gain may occur through consideration of poststress wall motion abnormalities on gated SPECT (110). In addition to the ejection fraction, other important information that can be derived from nuclear studies has not been included in the prognostic assessment, including transient ischemic dilation of the left ventricle (104,105), pulmonary uptake of radioactivity as determined by the measurement of lung/heart ratios of radioactivity, and absolute left ventricular volumes (87,164).

In summarizing this section, one of the principal strengths of nuclear cardiology is that a very large database has been accumulated, far larger than for any other noninvasive modality, documenting clear effectiveness of myocardial perfusion SPECT in risk stratification of appropriately selected patients with suspected coronary artery disease. These applications of myocardial perfusion SPECT in risk stratification are discussed further in Chapters 37 through 40. It is of note that, based on the large database of patients followed up after nuclear testing, data now exists documenting the efficacy of risk stratification with this modality in the management of patients with intermediate risk of cardiac death on the basis of all available information in each of the following categories: suspected chronic CAD prior to discharge in acute myocardial infarction, uncertain findings at the time of catheterization, before vascular surgery, and after interventions, as well as in patients with ischemic cardiomyopathy in whom the question of myocardial viability is central to patient management.

ACKNOWLEDGMENTS

The authors gratefully acknowledge the assistance of Xingping ("Connie") Kang, M.D., and Naoya Matsumoto, M.D., in the preparation of this manuscript, as well as the expert editorial assistance provided by Suzanne Ridgway.

REFERENCES

1. Berman DS, Salel AF, DeNardo GL, et al. Non-invasive detection of regional myocardial ischemia using rubidium-81 and the scintillation camera: Comparison with stress electrocardiography in patients with arteriographically documented coronary stenosis. *Circulation* 1975;52:619–626.
2. Zaret, BL, Strauss, HW, Martin, ND, et al. Noninvasive regional myocardial perfusion with radioactive potassium. *N Engl J Med* 1973;288:809.
3. Lebowitz, E, Greene, M, Bradley-Moore, P, et al. Tl-201 for medical use. *J Nucl Med* 1973;14:421(abst).
4. Weich, HF., Strauss, HW, Pitt, B, The extraction of Tl-201 by the myocardium. *Circulation* 1977;56:188.
5. Nielsen AP, Morris KG, Murdock BS, et al. Linear relationship between the distribution of thallium-201 and blood flow in ischemic and nonischemic myocardium during exercise. *Circulation* 1980;61:797–801.
6. L'Abbate A, Biagin A, Michelassic, et al. Myocardial kinetics of thallium and potassium in man. *Circulation* 1979;60:776.
7. Bradley-Moore PR, Lebowitz E, Greene M, et al. Tl-201 for medical use: II. Biologic behavior. *J Nucl Med* 1975;16:156.
8. Pohost GM, Zir LM, Moore RH, et al. Differentiation of transiently ischemic from infarcted myocardium by serial imaging after a single dose of thallium-201. *Circulation* 1977;55(2):294–302.
9. Berger BC, Watson DD, Sipes JN, et al. Redistribution of thallium at rest in patients with coronary artery disease. *J Nucl Med* 1978;19:680.
10. Pohost GM, O'Keefe DD, Gewirtz H, et al. Thallium redistribution in the presence of severe fixed coronary stenosis. *J Nucl Med* 1978;19:680.
11. Beller GA, Pohost GM. Mechanism for Tl-201 redistribution after transient myocardial ischemia. *Circulation* 1977;56:141.
12. Strauss HW, Harrison BS, Pitt B. Thallium-201: Noninvasive determination of the regional distribution of cardiac output. *J Nucl Med* 1977;18:1167.
13. Garcia E, Maddahi J, Berman D, et al. Space/time quantitation of thallium-201 myocardial scintigraphy. *J Nucl Med* 1981;22(4):309–317.
14. Budinger TF, Knittel BL. Cardiac thallium redistribution and model. *J Nucl Med* 1987;28:588(abst).
15. Budinger TF, Pohost GM, Bichoff P. Tl-201 integral blood concentration over 2 hours explains persistent defects in patients with no evidence of MI by ECG. *Circulation* 1987;76(IV):64(abstr).
16. Angello DA, Wilson RA, Palac RT, Effect of eating on thallium-201 myocardial redistribution after myocardial ischemia. *Am J Cardiol* 1987;60(7):528–533.
17. Berman D, Maddahi J, Charuzi Y, et al. Rate of redistribution in Tl-201 exercise myocardial scintigraphy: inverse relationship to degree of coronary stenosis. *Circulation* 1978;58[Suppl 2]:II–63(abst).
18. Maseri A, Parodi O, Severi S, et al. Transient transmural reduction of myocardial blood flow demonstrated by thallium-201 scintigraphy, as a cause of variant angina. *Circulation* 1976;54(2):280–288.
19. Gutman J, Berman DS, Freeman M, et al. Time to completed redistribution of thallium-201 in exercise myocardial scintigraphy: relationship to the degree of coronary artery stenosis. *Am Heart J* 1983;106(5 Pt 1):989–995.
20. Kiat H, Berman DS, Maddahi J, et al. Late reversibility of tomographic myocardial thallium-201 defects: an accurate marker of myocardial viability. *J Am Coll Cardiol* 1988;12(6):1456–1463.
21. Yang LD, Berman DS, Kiat H, et al. The frequency of late reversibility in SPECT thallium-201 stress-redistribution studies. *J Am Coll Cardiol* 1990;15(2):334–340.
22. Hecht HS, Hopkins JM, Rose JG, et al. Reverse redistribution: worsening of thallium-201 myocardial images from exercise to redistribution. *Radiology* 1981;140(1):177–181.
23. Tanasescu D, Berman D, Staniloff H, et al. Apparent worsening of thallium-201 myocardial defects during redistribution—what does it mean? *J Nucl Med* 1979;20:688(abst).
24. Weiss AT, Maddahi J, Lew AS, et al. Reverse redistribution of thallium-201: a sign of nontransmural myocardial infarction with patency of the infarct-related coronary artery. *J Am Coll Cardiol* 1986;7(1):61–67.
25. Popma JJ, Smitherman TC, Walker BS, et al. Reverse redistribution of thallium-201 detected by SPECT imaging after dipyridamole in angina pectoris. *Am J Cardiol* 1990;65(18):1176–1180.
26. Bateman TM, Maddahi J, Gray RJ, et al. Diffuse slow washout of myocardial thallium-201: a new scintigraphic indicator of extensive coronary artery disease. *J Am Coll Cardiol* 1984;4(1):55–64.
27. Abdulla A, Maddahi J, Garcia E, et al. Slow regional clearance of myocardial thallium-201 in the absence of perfusion defect: Its contribution to detection of individual coronary artery stenoses and mechanisms for its occurrence. *Circulation* 1985;71(1):72–79.
28. Dilsizian V, Rocco TP, Freedman NM, et al. Enhanced detection of ischemic but viable myocardium by the reinjection of thallium after stress-redistribution imaging. *N Engl J Med* 1990;323(3):141–146.
29. Dilsizian V, Smeltzer WR, Freedman NM, et al. Thallium reinjection after stress-redistribution imaging. Does 24-hour delayed imaging after reinjection enhance detection of viable myocardium? *Circulation* 1991;83(4):1247–1255.
30. Basu S, Senior R, Raval U, et al. Superiority of nitrate-enhanced 201Tl over conventional redistribution 201Tl imaging for prognostic evaluation after myocardial infarction and thrombolysis. *Circulation* 1997;96(9):2932–2937.
31. Ragosta M, Beller GA, The noninvasive assessment of myocardial viability. *Clin Cardiol* 1993;16(7):531–538.

32. Bateman TM, Nuclear cardiology in private practice. *J Nucl Cardiol* 1997;4(2 Pt 2):S184–188.

33. Mahmarian JJ, Boyce TM, Goldberg RK, et al. Quantitative exercise thallium-201 single photon emission computed tomography for the enhanced diagnosis of ischemic heart disease. *J Am Coll Cardiol* 1990; 15(2):318–329.

34. Mahmarian J. State of the art for coronary artery disease detection: thallium-201. In: *Nuclear cardiology: state of the art and future directions*, 2nd ed. Zaret BL, Beller G, eds. St. Louis: Mosby, 1998: 237–272.

35. Friedman J, Van Train K, Maddahi J, et al. "Upward creep" of the heart: a frequent source of false-positive reversible defects during thallium-201 stress-redistribution SPECT. *J Nucl Med* 1989;30(10): 1718–1722.

36. Germano G, Erel J, Kiat H, et al. Quantitative LVEF and qualitative regional function from gated thallium-201 perfusion SPECT. *J Nucl Med* 1997;38(5):749–754.

37. Li Q-S, Frank TL, Franceschi D, et al. Technetium-99m methoxyisobutyl isonitrile (RP30) for quantification of myocardial ischemia and reperfusion in dogs. *J Nucl Med* 1988;29:1539.

38. Sinusas AJ, Bergin JD, Edwards NC, et al. Redistribution of ^{99m}Tc-sestamibi and ^{201}Tl in the presence of a severe coronary artery stenosis. *Circulation* 1994;89:2332.

39. Nielsen AP, Morris KG, Murdock R, et al. Linear relationship between the distribution of thallium-201 and blood flow in ischemic and nonischemic myocardium during exercise. *Circulation* 1980;61(4): 797–801.

40. Krivokapich J, Smith GT, Huang SC, et al. 13N ammonia myocardial imaging at rest and with exercise in normal volunteers. Quantification of absolute myocardial perfusion with dynamic positron emission tomography. *Circulation* 1989;80(5):1328–1337.

41. Udelson JE. Choosing a thallium-201 or technetium 99m sestamibi imaging protocol. *J Nucl Cardiol* 1994;1(5 Pt 2):S99–108.

42. Chan SY, Brunken RC, Czernin J, et al. Comparison of maximal myocardial blood flow during adenosine infusion with that of intravenous dipyridamole in normal men. *J Am Coll Cardiol* 1992;20(4): 979–985.

43. Leppo JA, Meerdink DJ, Comparison of the myocardial uptake of a technetium-labeled isonitrile analogue and thallium. *Circ Res* 1989; 65(3):632–639.

44. Hurwitz GA, Blais M, Powe JE, et al. Stress/injection protocols for myocardial scintigraphy with 99Tcm-sestamibi compared with 201Tl: implications of early post-stress kinetics. *Nucl Med Commun* 1996; 17(5):400–409.

45. Takahashi N, Reinhardt CP, Marcel R, et al. Myocardial uptake of 99mTc-tetrofosmin, sestamibi, and 201Tl in a model of acute coronary reperfusion. *Circulation* 1996;94(10):2605–2613.

46. Arbab AS, Koizumi K, Toyama K, et al. Technetium-99m-tetrofosmin, technetium-99m-MIBI and thallium-201 uptake in rat myocardial cells. *J Nucl Med* 1998;39(2):266–271.

47. Taillefer R, Primeau M, Costi P, et al. Technetium-99m-sestamibi myocardial perfusion imaging in detection of coronary artery disease: comparison between initial (1-hour) and delayed (3-hour) postexercise images. *J Nucl Med* 1991;32(10):1961–1965.

48. Maurea S, Cuocolo A, Soricelli A, et al. Myocardial viability index in chronic coronary artery disease: technetium-99m-methoxy isobutyl isonitrile redistribution. *J Nucl Med* 1995;36(11):1953–1960.

49. Soman P, Taillefer R, DePuey EG, et al. Improved detection of reversible ischaemia by Tc-99m sestamibi compared to Tc-99m tetrofosmin SPECT imaging in mild to moderate coronary artery disease. *J Nucl Cardiol* 1999;6(1)[Pt 2]:S35(abst).

50. Esquerré JP, Coca FJ, Martinez SJ, et al. Prone decubitus: a solution to inferior wall attenuation in thallium-201 myocardial tomography. *J Nucl Med* 1989;30(3):398–401.

51. Segall GM, Davis MJ. Prone versus supine thallium myocardial SPECT: a method to decrease artifactual inferior wall defects. *J Nucl Med* 1989;30(4):548–555.

52. Kiat H, Van Train KF, Friedman JD, et al. Quantitative stress-redistribution thallium-201 SPECT using prone imaging: methodologic development and validation. *J Nucl Med* 1992;33(8):1509–1515.

53. Berman DS, Kiat H, Maddahi J. The new 99mTc myocardial perfusion imaging agents: 99mTc-sestamibi and 99mTc-teboroxime. *Circulation* 1991;84(3 Suppl):I7–21.

54. Berman D, Kiat H, Germano G, et al. 99m Tc-sestamibi SPECT. In: DePuey EG, Berman DS, EV Garcia, eds. *Cardiac SPECT imaging.* New York: Raven Press, 1995:121–146.

55. Van Train KF, Areeda J, Garcia EV, et al. Quantitative same-day rest-stress technetium-99m-sestamibi SPECT: definition and validation of stress normal limits and criteria for abnormality. *J Nucl Med* 1993; 34(9):1494–1502.

56. Buell U, Dupont F, Uebis R, et al. 99Tcm-methoxy-isobutyl-isonitrile SPECT to evaluate a perfusion index from regional myocardial uptake after exercise and at rest. Results of a four hour protocol in patients with coronary heart disease and in controls. *Nucl Med Commun* 1990; 11(2):77–94.

57. Heo J, Kegel J, Iskandrian AS, et al. Comparison of same-day protocols using technetium-99m-sestamibi myocardial imaging. *J Nucl Med* 1992;33(2):186–191.

58. Taillefer R, Gagnon A, Laflamme L, et al. Same day injections of Tc-99m methoxy isobutyl isonitrile (hexamibi) for myocardial tomographic imaging: comparison between rest-stress and stress-rest injection sequences. *Eur J Nucl Med* 1989;15(3):113–117.

59. Marzullo P, Parodi O, Reisenhofer B, et al. Value of rest thallium-201/technetium-99m sestamibi scans and dobutamine echocardiography for detecting myocardial viability. *Am J Cardiol* 1993;71(2): 166–172.

60. Berman DS, Kiat HS, Van Train KF, et al. Myocardial perfusion imaging with technetium-99m-sestamibi: comparative analysis of available imaging protocols. *J Nucl Med* 1994;35(4):681–688.

61. Sciagrà R, Bisi G, Santoro GM, et al. Comparison of baseline-nitrate technetium-99m sestamibi with rest-redistribution thallium-201 tomography in detecting viable hibernating myocardium and predicting postrevascularization recovery. *J Am Coll Cardiol* 1997;30(2): 384–391.

62. Berman DS, Kiat H, Friedman JD, et al. Separate acquisition rest thallium-201/stress technetium-99m sestamibi dual-isotope myocardial perfusion single-photon emission computed tomography: a clinical validation study. *J Am Coll Cardiol* 1993;22(5):1455–1464.

63. Kiat H, Germano, G, Friedman J, et al. Comparative feasibility of separate or simultaneous rest thallium-201/stress technetium-99m-sestamibi dual-isotope myocardial perfusion SPECT. *J Nucl Med* 1994;35(4):542–548.

64. Kamphuis C, Beekman FJ, van Rijk PP, et al. Dual matrix ordered subsets reconstruction for accelerated 3D scatter compensation in single-photon emission tomography. *European J Nucl Med* 1998;25(1): 8–18.

65. Cullom S, Liu L, White M. Compensation of attenuation map errors from Tc-99m-sestamibi downscatter with simultaneous Gd-153 transmission scanning. *J Nucl Med* 1996;37(5):215P(abst).

66. Sinusas AJ, Shi Q, Saltzberg MT, et al. Technetium-99m-tetrofosmin to assess myocardial blood flow: experimental validation in an intact canine model of ischemia. *J Nucl Med* 1994;35(4):664–671.

67. Jain D, Wackers FJ, Mattera J, et al. Biokinetics of technetium-99m-tetrofosmin: myocardial perfusion imaging agent: implications for a one-day imaging protocol. *J Nucl Med* 1993;34(8):1254–1259.

68. Wackers FJ, Berman DS, Maddahi J, et al. Technetium-99m hexakis 2-methoxyisobutyl isonitrile: human biodistribution, dosimetry, safety, and preliminary comparison to thallium-201 for myocardial perfusion imaging. *J Nucl Med* 1989;30(3):301–311.

69. Meerdink DJ, Leppo JA. Experimental properties of technetium-99m agents: myocardial transport of perfusion imaging agents. *Am J Cardiol* 1990;66:9E–15E.

70. Leppo JA, Meerdink DJ, Comparative myocardial extraction of two technetium-labeled BATO derivatives (SQ30217,SQ30214) and thallium. *J Nucl Med* 1990;31:67–74.

71. Chua T, Kiat H, Germano G, et al. Technetium-99m teboroxime regional myocardial washout in subjects with and without coronary artery disease. *Am J Cardiol* 1993;72(9):728–734.

72. Chua T, Kiat H, Germano G, et al. Rapid back to back adenosine stress/rest technetium-99m teboroxime myocardial perfusion SPECT using a triple-detector camera. *J Nucl Med* 1993;34(9):1485–1493.

73. Stewart RE, Schwaiger M, Hutchins GD, et al. Myocardial clearance kinetics of technetium-99m-SQ30217: a marker of regional myocardial blood flow. *J Nucl Med* 1990;31:1183–1190.

74. Kronauge JF, Chiu ML, Cone JS, et al. Comparison of neutral and cationic myocardial perfusion agents: characteristics of accumulation and cultured cardiac cells. *Int J Rad Appl Instrum [B]* 1992;19: 141–148.

75. Pasqualini R, Duatti A, Bellande E, et al. Bis(dithiocarbamato) nitrido

technetium-99m radiopharmaceuticals: A class of neutral myocardial imaging agents. *J Nucl Med* 1994;35:334.

76. Ghezzi C, Fagret D, Arvieux CC, et al. Myocardial kinetics of TcN-NOET: a neutral lipophilic complex tracer of regional myocardial blood flow. *J Nucl Med* 1995;36(6):1069–1077.

77. Gerson MC, Lukes J, Deutsch E, et al. Comparison of technetium 99m Q12 and thallium 201 for detection of angiographically documented coronary artery disease in humans. *J Nucl Cardiol* 1994;1(6):499–508.

78. Berman DS, Germano G. An approach to the interpretation and reporting of gated myocardial perfusion SPECT. In: *Clinical gated cardiac SPECT.* Germano G, Berman DS, eds. Armonk, NY: Futura Publishing, 1999.

79. DePuey EG. Artifacts clarified by and caused by gated myocardial perfusion SPECT. In: *Clinical gated cardiac SPECT.* Germano G, Berman DS, eds. Armonk, NY: Futura Publishing, 1999.

80. Prigent FM, Hyun M, Berman DS, et al. Effect of motion on thallium-201 SPECT studies: a simulation and clinical study. *J Nucl Med* 1993. 34(11):1845–1850.

81. Germano G, Van Train K, Kiat H, et al. Digital techniques for the acquisition, processing, and analysis of nuclear cardiology images. In: *Diagnostic nuclear medicine.* Sandler MP, ed. Baltimore: Williams & Wilkins: 1995:347–386.

82. Piwnica-Worms D, Holman,BL. Noncardiac applications of hexakis(alkylisonitrile) technetium-99m complexes [comment]. *J Nucl Med* 1990;31(7):1166–1167.

83. Waxman AD. The role of (99m)Tc methoxyisobutylisonitrile in imaging breast cancer. *Semin Nucl Med* 1997;27(1):40–54.

84. Aksut SV, Mallavarapu C, Russell J, et al. Implications of increased lung thallium uptake during exercise single photon emission computed tomography imaging. *Am Heart J* 1995;130(2):367–373.

85. Jain D, Thompson B, Wackers FJ, et al. Relevance of increased lung thallium uptake on stress imaging in patients with unstable angina and non-Q wave myocardial infarction: results of the thrombolysis in myocardial infarction (TIMI)-IIIB study. *J Am Coll Cardiol* 1997; 30(2):421–429.

86. Vaccarino RA, Johnson LL, Antunes ML, et al. Thallium-201 lung uptake and peak treadmill exercise first-pass ejection fraction. *Am Heart J* 1995;129(2):320–329.

87. Bacher-Stier C, Kavanagh P, Sharir, T, et al. Post-exercise tc-99m sestamibi lung uptake determined by a new automatic technique. *J Nucl Med* 1998;39(5):104P(abst).

88. Liu P, Kiess M, Okada RD, et al. Increased thallium lung uptake after exercise in isolated left anterior descending coronary artery disease. *Am J Cardiol* 1985;55(13 Pt 1):1469–1473.

89. Martinez EE, Horowitz,SF, Castello HJ, et al. Lung and myocardial thallium-201 kinetics in resting patients with congestive heart failure: correlation with pulmonary capillary wedge pressure. *Am Heart J* 1992;123(2):427–432.

90. Germano G, Chua T, Kiat, H, et al. A quantitative phantom analysis of artifacts due to hepatic activity in technetium-99m myocardial perfusion SPECT studies. *J Nucl Med* 1994;35(2):356–359.

91. Standardization of cardiac tomographic imaging. The Cardiovascular Imaging Committee, American College of Cardiology; The Committee on Advanced Cardiac Imaging and Technology, Council on Clinical Cardiology, American Heart Association; and Board of Directors, Cardiovascular Council, Society of Nuclear Medicine. *J Am Coll Cardiol* 1992;20(1):255–256.

92. Berman DS, Kiat H, Van Train, K, et al. Technetium 99m sestamibi in the assessment of chronic coronary artery disease. *Semin Nucl Med* 1991;21(3):190–212.

93. Reisman S, Berman D, Maddahi J, et al. The severe stress thallium defect: an indicator of critical coronary stenosis. *Am Heart J* 1985; 110(1)[Pt 1]:128–134.

94. Matzer L, Kiat H, Van Train K, et al. Quantitative severity of stress thallium-201 myocardial perfusion single-photon emission computed tomography defects in one-vessel coronary artery disease. *Am J Cardiol* 1993;72(3):273–279.

95. Berman DS, Hachamovitch R, Kiat H, et al. Incremental value of prognostic testing in patients with known or suspected ischemic heart disease: a basis for optimal utilization of exercise technetium-99m sestamibi myocardial perfusion single-photon emission computed tomography. *J Am Coll Cardiol* 1995;26(3):639–647.

96. Hachamovitch R, Berman DS, Kiat, H, et al. Exercise myocardial

perfusion SPECT in patients without known coronary artery disease: incremental prognostic value and use in risk stratification. *Circulation* 1996;93(5):905–914.

97. Hachamovitch R, Berman DS, Shaw LJ, et al. Incremental prognostic value of myocardial perfusion single photon emission computed tomography for the prediction of cardiac death: differential stratification for risk of cardiac death and myocardial infarction. *Circulation* 1998; 97(6):535–543.

98. Matzer L, Kiat H, Friedman JD, et al. A new approach to the assessment of tomographic thallium-201 scintigraphy in patients with left bundle branch block. *J Am Coll Cardiol* 1991;17(6):1309–1317.

99. Ficaro EP, Fessler JA, Shreve PD, et al. Simultaneous transmission/emission myocardial perfusion tomography. Diagnostic accuracy of attenuation-corrected 99mTc-sestamibi single-photon emission computed tomography. *Circulation* 1996;93(3):463–473.

100. Cullom S, Hendel R, Liu L, et al. Diagnostic accuracy and image quality of a scatter, attenuation and resolution compensation method for Tc-99m cardiac SPECT: preliminary results. *J Nucl Med* 1996; 37(5):81P(abst).

101. Germano G, Kavanagh P, Waechter P, et al. A new automatic approach to myocardial perfusion SPECT quantitation. *J Nucl Med* 1998; 39(5):62P(abst).

102. Bonow R. Assessment of myocardial viability with thallium-201 In: *Nuclear cardiology: state of the art and future directions,* 2nd ed. Zaret BL, Beller G, eds. St. Louis: Mosby, 1998:503–512.

103. Udelson JE, Coleman PS, Metherall J, et al. Predicting recovery of severe regional ventricular dysfunction. Comparison of resting scintigraphy with 201Tl and 99mTc-sestamibi. *Circulation* 1994;89(6): 2552–2561.

104. Weiss AT, Berman DS, Lew AS, et al. Transient ischemic dilation of the left ventricle on stress thallium-201 scintigraphy: a marker of severe and extensive coronary artery disease. *J Am Coll Cardiol* 1987; 9(4):752–759.

105. Mazzanti M, Germano G, Kiat H, et al. Identification of severe and extensive coronary artery disease by automatic measurement of transient ischemic dilation of the left ventricle in dual-isotope myocardial perfusion SPECT. *J Am Coll Cardiol* 1996;27(7):1612–1620.

106. Chouraqui P, Rodrigues EA, Berman DS, et al. Significance of dipyridamole-induced transient dilation of the left ventricle during thallium-201 scintigraphy in suspected coronary artery disease. *Am J Cardiol* 1990;66(7):689–694.

107. Germano G, Kiat H, Kavanagh PB, et al. Automatic quantification of ejection fraction from gated myocardial perfusion SPECT. *J Nucl Med* 1995;36(11):2138–2147.

108. Smith WH, Kastner RJ, Calnon DA, et al. Quantitative gated single photon emission computed tomography imaging: a counts-based method for display and measurement of regional and global ventricular systolic function. *J Nucl Cardiol* 1997;4(6):451–463.

109. Johnson LL, Verdesca SA, Aude WY, et al. Postischemic stunning can affect left ventricular ejection fraction and regional wall motion on post-stress gated sestamibi tomograms. *J Am Coll Cardiol* 1997; 30(7):1641–1648.

110. Sharir T, Bacher-Stier C, Dhar S, et al. Postexercise regional wall motion abnormalities detected by Tc-99m sestamibi gated SPECT: a marker of severe coronary artery disease. *J Nucl Med* 1998;39(5): 87P–88P(abst).

111. Germano G, Erel J, Lewin H, et al. Automatic quantitation of regional myocardial wall motion and thickening from gated technetium-99m sestamibi myocardial perfusion single-photon emission computed tomography. *J Am Coll Cardiol* 1997;30(5):1360–1367.

112. Zanger D, Bhatnagar A, Hausner E, et al. Automated calculation of ejection fraction from gated Tc-99m sestamibi images—comparison to quantitative echocardiography. *J Nucl Cardiol* 1997;4(1)[Pt 2]: S78(abst).

113. Bateman T, Magalski A, Barnhart C, et al. Global left ventricular function assessment using gated SPECT-201: comparison with echocardiography. *J Am Coll Cardiol* 1998;31(2)[Suppl A]:441A(abst).

114. Cwajg E, Cwajg J, He Z, et al. Comparison between gated-SPECT and echocardiography for the analysis of global and regional left ventricular function and volumes. *J Am Coll Cardiol* 1998;31(2)[Suppl A]:440A–441A(abst).

115. Mathew D, Zabrodina Y, Mannting F. Volumetric and functional analysis of left ventricle by gated SPECT: a comparison with echocardio-

graphic measurements. *J Am Coll Cardiol* 1998;31(2)[Suppl A]: 44A(abst).

116. Akinboboye O, El-Khoury Coffin L, Sciacca R, et al. Accuracy of gated SPECT thallium left ventricular volumes and ejection fractions: comparison with three-dimensional echocardiography. *J Am Coll Cardiol* 1998;31(2)[Suppl A]:85A(abst).

117. Germano G, Vandecker W, Mintz R, et al. Validation of left ventricular volumes automatically measured with gated myocardial perfusion SPECT. *J Am Coll Cardiol* 1998;31(2)[Suppl A]:43A(abst).

118. Iskandrian A, Germano G, VanDecker W, et al. Validation of left ventricular volume measurements by gated SPECT Tc-99m sestamibi imaging. *J Nucl Cardiol* 1998;5(6):574–578.

119. He Z, Vick G, Vaduganathan P, et al. Comparison of left ventricular volumes and ejection fraction measured by gated SPECT and by cine magnetic resonance imaging. *J Am Coll Cardiol* 1998;31(2)[Suppl A]:44A(abst).

120. Germano G, Berman D. On the accuracy and reproducibility of quantitative gated myocardial perfusion SPECT. *J Nucl Med* 1999;40(5): 810–813.

121. Berman D, Germano G, Lewin H, et al. Comparison of post-stress ejection fraction and relative left ventricular volumes by automatic analysis of gated myocardial perfusion single-photon emission computed tomography acquired in the supine and prone positions. *J Nucl Cardiol* 1998;5(1):40–47.

122. Germano G, Kavanagh P, Kavanagh J, et al. Repeatability of automatic left ventricular cavity volume measurements from myocardial perfusion SPECT. *J Nucl Cardiol* 1998;5(5):477–483.

123. White HD, Norris RM, Brown MA, et al. Left ventricular end-systolic volume as the major determinant of survival after recovery from myocardial infarction. *Circulation* 1987;76(1):44–51.

124. Pfeffer MA, Braunwald E, Moye LA, et al. Effect of captopril on mortality and morbidity in patients with left ventricular dysfunction after myocardial infarction. Results of the survival and ventricular enlargement trial. The SAVE Investigators. *N Engl J Med* 1992; 327(10):669–677.

125. Diamond GA, Staniloff HM, Forrester, JS, et al. Computer-assisted diagnosis in the noninvasive evaluation of patients with suspected coronary artery disease. *J Am Coll Cardiol* 1983. 1(2)[Pt 1]:444–455.

126. Staniloff HM, Diamond GA, Freeman MR, et al. Simplified application of Bayesian analysis to multiple cardiologic tests. *Clin Cardiol* 1982;5(12):630–636.

127. Pryor DB, Shaw L, Harrell, FE Jr, et al. Estimating the likelihood of severe coronary artery disease. *Am J Med* 1991;90(5):553–562.

128. Iskandrian AS, Verani MS, Heo J, Pharmacologic stress testing: mechanism of action, hemodynamic responses, and results in detection of coronary artery disease. *J Nucl Cardiol* 1994;1(1):94–111.

129. Fleischmann KE, Hunink MG, Kuntz KM, et al. Exercise echocardiography or exercise SPECT imaging? A meta-analysis of diagnostic test performance. *JAMA* 1998;280(10):913–920.

130. Rozanski A, Diamond GA, Berman, D, et al. The declining specificity of exercise radionuclide ventriculography. *N Engl J Med* 1983;309(9): 518–522.

131. Maddahi J, Garcia EV, Berman DS, et al. Improved noninvasive assessment of coronary artery disease by quantitative analysis of regional stress myocardial distribution and washout of thallium-201. *Circulation* 1981;64(5):924–935.

132. Van Train KF, Berman DS, Garcia EV, et al. Quantitative analysis of stress thallium-201 myocardial scintigrams: a multicenter trial. *J Nucl Med* 1986;27(1):17–25.

133. Diamond GA, Forrester JS. Analysis of probability as an aid in the clinical diagnosis of coronary-artery disease. *N Engl J Med* 1979; 300(24):1350–1358.

134. Berman D, Hachamovitch R, Lewin H, et al. Risk stratification in coronary artery disease: implications for stabilization and prevention. *Am J Cardiol* 1997;79(12B):10–16.

135. Comparison of coronary bypass surgery with angioplasty in patients with multivessel disease. The Bypass Angioplasty Revascularization Investigation (BARI) Investigators. [published erratum appears in *N Engl J Med* 1997;9;336(2):147]. *N Engl J Med* 1996;335(4):217–225.

136. Little WC, Constantinescu M, Applegate RJ, et al. Can coronary angiography predict the site of a subsequent myocardial infarction in patients with mild-to-moderate coronary artery disease? *Circulation* 1988;78(5)[Pt 1]:1157–1166.

137. Ambrose JA, Tannenbaum MA, Alexopoulos D, et al. Angiographic

138. Hasdai D, Gibbons RJ, Holmes DR Jr, et al. Coronary endothelial dysfunction in humans is associated with myocardial perfusion defects. *Circulation* 1997;96(10):3390–3395.

139. Garcia EV. Quantitative myocardial perfusion single-photon emission computed tomographic imaging: quo vadis? (Where do we go from here?). *J Nucl Cardiol* 1994;1(1):83–93.

140. Sharir T, Germano G, Kavanagh P, et al. A novel method for quantitative analysis of myocardial perfusion SPECT: validation and diagnostic yield. *J Nucl Med* 1998;39(5):103P(abst).

141. Ladenheim ML, Pollock BH, Rozanski A, et al. Extent and severity of myocardial hypoperfusion as predictors of prognosis in patients with suspected coronary artery disease. *J Am Coll Cardiol* 1986;7(3): 464–471.

142. Ladenheim M, Kotler T, Pollock B, et al. Incremental prognostic power of clinical history, exercise electrocardiography and myocardial perfusion scintigraphy in suspected coronary artery disease. *Am J Cardiol* 1987;59:270–277.

143. Iskandrian AS, Chae,SC, Heo, J, et al. Independent and incremental prognostic value of exercise single-photon emission computed tomographic (SPECT) thallium imaging in coronary artery disease. *J Am Coll Cardiol* 1993;22(3):665–670.

144. Hachamovitch R, Berman, DS, Kiat, H, et al. Effective risk stratification using exercise myocardial perfusion SPECT in women: gender-related differences in prognostic nuclear testing. *J Am Coll Cardiol* 1996;28:34–44.

145. Mark DB, Hlatky MA, Harrell FE Jr, et al. Exercise treadmill score for predicting prognosis in coronary artery disease. *Ann Intern Med* 1987;106(6):793–800.

146. Hachamovitch R, Berman, DS, Kiat H, et al. Gender-related differences in clinical management after exercise nuclear testing. *J Am Coll Cardiol* 1995;26(6):1457–1464.

147. Bateman TM, O'Keefe JH Jr, Dong VM, et al. Coronary angiographic rates after stress single-photon emission computed tomographic scintigraphy. *J Nucl Cardiol* 1995;2(3):217–223.

148. Nallamothu N, Pancholy SB, Lee KR, et al. Impact on exercise single-photon emission computed tomographic thallium imaging on patient management and outcome. *J Nucl Cardiol* 1995;2(4):334–338.

149. Randomised trial of cholesterol lowering in 4,444 patients with coronary heart disease: the Scandinavian Simvastatin Survival Study (4S). *Lancet* 1994;344(8934):1383–1389.

150. Kjekshus J, Pedersen TR. Reducing the risk of coronary events: evidence from the Scandinavian Simvastatin Survival Study (4S). *Am J Cardiol* 1995;76(9):64C–68C.

151. Shepherd J, Cobbe SM, Ford I, et al. Prevention of coronary heart disease with pravastatin in men with hypercholesterolemia. West of Scotland Coronary Prevention Study Group. *N Engl J Med* 1995; 333(20):1301–1307.

152. Pfeffer MA, Sacks FM, Moyé LA, et al. Cholesterol and recurrent events: a secondary prevention trial for normolipidemic patients. CARE Investigators. *Am J Cardiol* 1995;76(9):98C–106C.

153. Pasternak RC, Brown LE, Stone PH, et al. Effect of combination therapy with lipid-reducing drugs in patients with coronary heart disease and "normal" cholesterol levels. A randomized, placebo-controlled trial. Harvard Atherosclerosis Reversibility Project (HARP) Study Group. *Ann Intern Med* 1996;125(7):529–540.

154. Borzak S, Cannon CP, Kraft PL, et al. Effects of prior aspirin and anti-ischemic therapy on outcome of patients with unstable angina. TIMI 7 Investigators. Thrombin inhibition in myocardial ischemia. *Am J Cardiol* 1998;81(6):678–681.

155. Køber L, Torp-Pedersen C, Carlsen JE, et al. A clinical trial of the angiotensin-converting-enzyme inhibitor trandolapril in patients with left ventricular dysfunction after myocardial infarction. Trandolapril Cardiac Evaluation (TRACE) Study Group. *N Engl J Med* 1995; 333(25):1670–1676.

156. Haim M, Shotan A, Boyko V, et al. Effect of beta-blocker therapy in patients with coronary artery disease in New York Heart Association classes II and III. The Bezafibrate Infarction Prevention (BIP) Study Group. *Am J Cardiol* 1998;81(12):1455–1460.

157. de Lorgeril M, Salen P, Caillat-Vallet E, et al. Control of bias in dietary trial to prevent coronary recurrences: The Lyon Diet Heart Study. *Eur J Clin Nutr* 1997;51(2):116–122.

158. Ornish D, Brown SE, Scherwitz LW, et al. Can lifestyle changes

reverse coronary heart disease? The Lifestyle Heart Trial. *Lancet* 1990;336(8708):129–133.

159. Berman D, Hachamovitch, R, Shaw L, et al. Prognostic risk stratification with SPECT imaging: results from a 20,340 patient multicenter registry. *J Am Coll Cardiol* 1998;31(2)[Suppl A]:410A(abst).

160. Shaw L, Hachamovitch R, Berman D, et al. The economic consequences of available diagnostic and prognostic strategies for the evaluation of stable angina patients. *J Am Coll Cardiol* 1999;33(3): 661–669.

161. Hachamovitch R, Berman D, Kiat H, et al. What is the warranty period for a normal scan? Temporal changes in risk in patients with normal exercise sestamibi SPECT. *Circulation* 1995;92(8):I–130(abst).

162. Berman D, Kang X, Van Train K, et al. Comparative prognostic value of automatic quantitative analysis versus semiquantitative visual analysis of exercise myocardial perfusion single-photon emission computed tomography. *J Am Coll Cardiol* 1998;32(7):1987–1995.

163. Hachamovitch R, Berman D, Lewin H, et al. Incremental prognostic value of gated SPECT ejection fraction in patients undergoing dual-isotope exercise or adenosine stress SPECT. *J Am Coll Cardiol* 1998; 31(2)[Suppl A]:441A(abst).

164. Morise AP. An incremental evaluation of the diagnostic value of thallium single-photon emission computed tomographic imaging and lung/heart ratio concerning both the presence and extent of coronary artery disease. *J Nucl Cardiol* 1995;2(3):238–245.

165. Kiat H, Van Train KF, Maddahi J, et al. Development and prospective application of quantitative 2-day stress-rest Tc-99m methoxy isobutyl isonitrile SPECT for the diagnosis of coronary artery disease. *Am Heart J* 1990;120:1255–1266.

166. Mahmarian JJ, Boyce TM, Goldbert RK, et al. Quantitative exercise thallium-201 single photon emission computed tomography for the enhanced diagnosis of ischemic heart disease. *J Am Coll Cardiol* 1990; 15:318–329.

167. Nguyen T, Heo J, Ogilby JD, et al. Single photon emission computed tomography with thallium-201 during adenosine induced coronary hyperemia: correlation with coronary arteriography, exercise thallium imaging and two-dimensional echocardiography. *J Am Coll Cardiol* 1990;16:1375–1383.

168. VanTrain KF, Maddahi J, Berman DS, et al. Quantitative analysis of tomogrpahic stress thallium-201 myocardial scintigrams: a multicenter trial. *J Nucl Med* 1990;31:1168–1179.

169. Coyne E, Belvedere D, Vande Streek PR, et al. Thallium-201 scintigraphy after intravenous infusion of adenosine compared with exercise thallium testing in the diagnosis of coronary artery disease. *J Am Coll Cardiol* 1991;17:1289–1294.

170. Forster T, McNeill AJ, Salustri A, et al. Simultaneous dobutamine stress echocardiography and technetium-99m isonitrile single-photon emission computed tomography in patients with suspected coronary artery disease. *J Am Coll Cardiol* 1993;21:1591–1596.

171. Chae SC, Heo J, Iskandrian A, et al. Identification of extensive coronary artery disease in women by exercise single-photon emission computed tomography (SPECT) thallium imaging. *J Am Coll Cardiol* 1993;21:1305–1311.

172. Minoves M, Garcia A, Magrina J, et al. Evaluation of myocardial perfusion defects by means of ''bull's eye'' images. *Clin Cardiol* 1993;16:16–22.

173. Van Train KF, Areeda J, Garcia EV, et al. Quantitative same-day rest-stress technetium-99m-sestamibi SPECT: definition and validation of stress normal limits and criteria for abnormality. *J Nucl Med* 1993; 34:1494–1502.

174. Sylven C, Hagerman I, Ylen M, et al. Variance ECG detection of coronary artery disease—a comparison with exercise stress test and myocardial scintigraphy. *Clin Cardiol* 1994;17:132–140.

175. Van Train KF, Garcia EV, Maddahi J, et al. Multicenter trial validation for quantitative analysis of same-day rest-stress technetium-99m-sestamibi myocardial tomograms. *J Nucl Med* 1994;35(4):609–618.

176. Palmas W, Friedman JD, Diamond GA, et al. Incremental value of simultaneous assessment of myocardial function and perfusion with technetium-99m sestamibi for prediction of extent of coronary artery disease. *J Am Coll Cardiol* 1995;25:1024–1031.

177. Rubello D, Zanco P, Candelpergher G, et al. Usefulness of Tc-99m-MIBI stress myocardial SPECT bull's eye quantification in coronary artery disease. *Q J Nucl Med* 1995;39:111–115.

178. Hambye AS, Vervaet A, Lieber S, et al. Diagnostic value and incremental contribution of bicycle exercise, first-pass radionuclide angi-

ography, and 99mTc-labeled sestamibi single-photon emission computed tomography in the identification of coronary artery disease in patients without infarction. *J Nucl Cardiol* 1996;3(6)[Pt 1]:464–474.

179. Yao Z, Liu XJ, Shi R, et al. A comparison of 99m Tc-MIBI myocardial SPET with electron beam computed tomography in the assessment of coronary artery disease. *Eur J Nucl Med* 1997;24(9).

180. Heiba SI, Hayat NJ, Salman HS, et al. Technetium-99m-MIBI myocardial SPECT: supine versus right lateral imaging and comparison with coronary arteriography. *J Nucl Med* 1997;38(10):1510–1514.

181. Ho Y, Wu C, Huang P, et al. Dobutamine stress echocardiography compared with exercise thallium-201 single-photon emission computed tomography in detecting coronary artery disease—effect of exercise level on accuracy. *Cardiology* 1997;88:379–385.

182. Taillefer R, DePuey EG, Udelson JE, et al. Comparative diagnostic accuracy of Tl-201 and Tc-99m sestamibi SPECT imaging (perfusion and ECG-gated SPECT) in detecting coronary artery disease in women. *J Am Coll Cardiol* 1997;29(1):69–77.

183. Van Eck-Smit BLF, Poots S, Zwinderman AH, et al. Myocardial SPET imaging with 99Tc m-tetrofosmin in clinical practice: comparison of a 1 day and a 2 day imaging protocol. *Nucl Med Commun* 1997;18: 24–30.

184. Budoff MJ, Gillespie R, Georgiou D, et al. Comparison of exercise electron beam computed tomography and sestamibi in the evaluation of coronary artery disease. *Am J Cardiol* 1998;81(6):682–687.

185. Santana-Boado C, Candell-Riera J, Castell-Conesa J, et al. Diagnostic accuracy of technetium-99m-MIBI myocardial SPECT in women and men. *J Nucl Med* 1998;39:751–755.

186. Acampa W, Cuocolo A, Sullo P, et al. Direct comparison of technetium 99m-sestamibi and technetium 99m-tetrofosmin cardiac single photon emission computed tomography in patients with coronary artery disease. *J Nucl Cardiol* 1998;5(3):265–274.

187. Ho Y, Wu C, Huang P, et al. Assessment of coronary artery disease in women by dobutamine stress echocardiography: comparison with stress thallium-201 single-photon emission computed tomography and exercise electrocardiography. *Am Heart J* 1998;135:655–662.

188. Verani MS, Mahmarian JJ, Hixson JB, et al. Diagnosis of coronary artery disease by controlled coronary vasodilation with adenosine and thallium-201 scintigraphy in patients unable to exercise. *Circulation* 1990;82:80–87.

189. Iskandrian AS, Heo J, Nguyen T, et al. Assessment of coronary artery disease using single-photon emission computed tomography with thallium-201 during adenosine-induced coronary hyperemia. *Am J Cardiol* 1991;67:1190–1194.

190. Nishimura S, Mahmarian JJ, Boyce TM, et al. Quantitative thallium-201 single-photon emission computed tomography during maximal pharmacologic coronary vasodilation with adenosine for assessing coronary artery disease. *J Am Coll Cardiol* 1991;18:736–745.

191. Aksut SV, Pancholy S, Cassel D, et al. Results of adenosine single photon emission computed tomography thallium-201 imaging in hemodynamic nonresponders. *Am Heart J* 1995;130:67–70.

192. Miyagawa M, Kumano S, Sekiya M, et al. Thallium-201 myocardial tomography with intravenous infusion of adenosine triphosphate in diagnosis of coronary artery disease. *J Am Coll Cardiol* 1995;26: 1196–1201.

193. Amanullah AM, Kiat H, Friedman JD, et al. Adenosine technetium-99m sestamibi myocardial perfusion SPECT in women: diagnostic efficacy in detection of coronary artery disease. *J Am Coll Cardiol* 1996;27(4):803–809.

194. Watanabe K, Sekiya M, Ikeda S, et al. Comparison of adenosine triphosphate and dipyridamole in diagnosis by thallium-201 myocardial scintigraphy. *J Nucl Med* 1997;38(4):577–581.

195. He ZX, Iskandrian AS, Gupta NC, et al. Assessing coronary artery disease with dipyridamole technetium-99m-tetrofosmin SPECT: a multicenter trial. *J Nucl Med* 1997;38(1):44–48.

196. Amanullah AM, Berman DS, Kiat H, et al. Usefulness of hemodynamic changes during adenosine infusion in predicting the diagnostic accuracy of adenosine technetium-99m sestamibi single-photon emission computed tomography (SPECT). *Am J Cardiol* 1997;79(10): 1319–1322.

197. Cuocolo A, Sullo P, Pace L, et al. Adenosine coronary vasodilation in coronary artery disease: technetium-99m tetrofosmin myocardial tomography versus echocardiography. *J Nucl Med* 1997;38(7): 1089–1094.

198. Takeishi Y, Takahashi N, Fujiwara S, et al. Myocardial tomography

with technetium-99m-tetrofosmin during intravenous infusion of adenosine triphosphate. *J Nucl Med* 1998.

199. Maddahi J, Van Train K, Prigent F, et al. Quantitative single photon emission computed thallium-201 tomography for detection and localization of coronary artery disease: optimization and prospective validation of a new technique. *J Am Coll Cardiol* 1989;14(7):1689–1699.
200. Iskandrian AS, Heo J, Kong B, et al. Effect of exercise level on the ability of thallium-201 tomographic imaging in detecting coronary artery disease: analysis of 461 patients. *J Am Coll Cardiol* 1989;14:1477–1486.
201. Heo J, Wolmer I, Kegel J, et al. Sequential dual-isotope SPECT imaging with thallium-201 and technetium-99m-sestamibi. *J Nucl Med* 1994;35:549–553.
202. Van Train KF, Garcia EV, Maddahi J, et al. Multicenter trial validation for quantitative analysis of same-day rest-stress technetium-99m-sestamibi myocardial tomographs. *J Nucl Med* 1994;35:609–618.
203. Zaret BL, Rigo P, Wackers FJT, et al. Myocardial perfusion imaging with 99mTc tetrofosmin. *Circulation* 1995;91:313–319.
204. Kiat H, Iskandrian AS, Villegas BJ, et al. Arbutamine stress thallium-201 single-photon emission computed tomography using a computerized closed-loop delivery system. *J Am Coll Cardiol* 1995;26:1159–1167.
205. Hendel RC, Verani MS, Miller DD, et al. Diagnostic utility of tomographic myocardial perfusion imaging with technetium 99m furifosmin (Q12) compared with thallium 201: results of a phase III multicenter trial. *J Nucl Cardiol* 1996;3(4):291–300.
206. Heo J, Powers J, Iskandrian AE, Exercise-rest same-day SPECT sestamibi imaging to detect coronary artery disease. *J Nucl Med* 1997;38(2):200–203.

CHAPTER 14

Assessment of Myocardial Blood Flow with Positron Emission Tomography

Markus Schwaiger, Sibylle I. Ziegler, and
Frank M. Bengel

Measurement of regional myocardial perfusion under physiologic and pathophysiologic conditions remains an important and challenging methodologic task in the evaluation of patients with various cardiovascular diseases. Numerous approaches have been introduced ranging from qualitative assessment of relative perfusion to absolute quantification of myocardial perfusion reserve (1). Invasive procedures require the introduction of especially equipped catheters, which provide estimates of blood flow velocities (Doppler wire) or blood flow (dye or thermodilution techniques). The major limitation of such techniques is the regional measurement of these parameters in a coronary artery or coronary vein, which does not allow estimate of amount of tissue supplied or drained by these vessels. Therefore, these techniques are most suitable for evaluating relative changes of flow following interventions such as intracoronary injection of papaverin or acetylcholine (2).

Measurement of tissue perfusion (mL/min/g) requires the employment of contrast agents that display myocardial retention or washout kinetics proportional to blood flow. Experimentally, the most successful method represents the use of radiolabeled or colored microspheres that are trapped in the capillaries as a function of myocardial perfusion. Com-

parison of microspheres trapped in the heart with the number of microspheres in an arterial reference sample with a known flow rate allows simple and accurate determination of absolute flow (3). However, these measurements are invasive requiring microspheres application in the left atrium or ventricle and, therefore, applicable only in the experimental setting.

Tracer methods in combination with scintigraphic imaging devices have been shown to provide sensitive detection of radiolabeled flow markers retained in the myocardium following intravenous injection. In combination with gamma camera technology, myocardial perfusion scintigraphy has gained wide clinical acceptance. With the advent of tomographic imaging devices, the principle of relating myocardial tracer kinetics to arterial tracer input can be applied to the *in vivo* situation. Improving spatial and temporal resolution of modern scintigraphic techniques such as positron emission tomography (PET) have led to a variety of methodologic strategies to quantitatively evaluate myocardial perfusion. The accuracy of noninvasive flow measurements is dependent on three important methodologic principles: First, the radiotracer used must behave in a predictable pattern under physiologic and pathophysiologic conditions in order to relate measured radioactivity to myocardial blood flow. Second, the imaging device used should provide accurate representation of myocardial radioactivity distribution, and acquisition times have to match the biological behavior of the tracer. Third, tracer kinetic modeling needs to be developed to relate tracer kinetics within blood and myocardium, resulting in regional flow measurements.

M. Schwaiger: Klinikum rechts der Isar, Technical University of Munich, D-81675 Munich, Germany.

S. I. Ziegler: Nuklearmedizinische Klinik, Technical University of Munich, D-81675 Munich, Germany.

F. M. Bengel: Nuklearmedizinische Klinik, Technical University of Munich, D-81675 Munich, Germany.

PET in combination with positron emitting flow tracers fulfills most of these requirements and, at the present time, represents the most accurate noninvasive approach to quantitate regional blood flow at the level of myocardial tissue in mL/min/g. This chapter will review methodologic aspects in using PET for myocardial blood flow measurements and describe the current state of clinical applications of PET in various cardiovascular diseases.

TECHNICAL CONSIDERATIONS

Advantages of Positron Emission Tomography

State-of-the-art positron emission tomographs consist of ring systems of several thousand small detectors, yielding an axial field of view of more than 10 cm, appropriate for simultaneous volumetric acquisition of radioactivity distribution within the entire heart. The spatial resolution of the modern instrumentation is 4 to 6 mm, which compares favorably with a left ventricular wall thickness of 10 to 15 mm. The advantage of coincidence detection as employed in PET versus single photon technology is that spatial resolution is highest in the center of the field of view, whereas in the case of single photon detection the spatial resolution deteriorates as a function of distance from the detector. Since the heart is located in the center of the thorax, PET systems offer distinct advantages in spatial resolution, which is important for accurate determination of radioactivity distribution in the myocardium. Although PET cameras allow gated data acquisition, most dynamic studies require nongated data collection, which limits the final spatial resolution achievable for quantitative measurements (4).

Besides high spatial resolution, which reduces the partial volume effect, attenuation correction is mandatory for quantification of regional tracer distribution. Estimates of relative myocardial blood flow are significantly affected by attenuation artifacts using single photon emission computed tomography (SPECT) imaging. Transmission scans determining regional attenuation factors have been developed for PET and SPECT and are used to correct the emission data. Attenuation is applied routinely to cardiac imaging. The acquisition of emission data, however, standardly requires separate imaging that prolongs the time of the PET study. A number of new approaches are currently under investigation to shorten the acquisition time for the transmission scan. Methods will be developed that allow simultaneous acquisition of emission and transmission data. Such improvements are likely to succeed and minimize artifacts caused by misalignment of transmission and emission data. The combination of CT and PET technology in one imaging instrument represents an interesting alternative approach. This would allow highly accurate measurements of tissue attenuation using brief CT scans.

PET imaging is about 100 times more sensitive than SPECT for detection of radioactivity. The newer generation of positron emission tomographs acquire data in two- and three-dimensional modes. Two-dimensional acquisition em-

ploys interleaved septa, which collimate the coincidence planes, thus reducing the contamination by scattered radiation. Without septa, a large number of coincidence lines can be used to obtain volumetric information about radiotracer distribution. This so-called three-dimensional acquisition mode is electronically more demanding, resulting in a significantly larger data set. Correction methods have been introduced to compensate for the intrinsically higher sensitivity in the center of the axial field of view as well as minimize the contribution of scattered radiation. The advantage of three-dimensional data acquisition is increased sensitivity, which reduces the required dose of radiopharmaceuticals, but also shortens the acquisition time. Three-dimensional data acquisition is routinely employed in brain imaging, but is also increasingly being extended to whole-body applications with improved scatter correction algorithms. Both rapid attenuation correction and short three-dimensional acquisition protocols will considerably reduce the duration of cardiac PET studies and, thus, improve throughput in a cardiac imaging laboratory (4).

Coincidence Gamma Cameras

With the wide availability of dual-head gamma cameras, several companies have introduced the concept of "coincidence gamma cameras." The advantage of such a system is the use of standardized gamma cameras, which can be used for imaging of low-energy single photons as well as 511 keV photons produced by positron annihilation. Most systems employ three-dimensional coincidence data acquisition (5). In contrast to ring PET cameras that use BGO crystals, the lower sensitivity of the sodium iodide detector material limits the sensitivity of this approach for coincidence events. Therefore, these cameras usually employ thicker sodium iodide crystals and special electronic approaches to compensate for the slow light response of the sodium iodide crystal and improve count rate performance. Modern coincidence gamma camera systems are also equipped with attenuation correction, which allows quantitative determination of regional myocardial activity using such devices. Because data acquisition requires 180-degree rotation of the dual head SPECT system, the temporal resolution is limited to about 15 minutes per tomographic data set.

RADIOPHARMACEUTICALS

Flow Tracers

The currently available radiopharmaceuticals for the assessment of myocardial blood flow using PET can be divided into two groups (Table 1). The first group consists of freely diffusable tracers that accumulate and wash out from tissue as a function of myocardial blood flow. The most commonly used representative of this group is O-15-labeled water. The second group of tracers is characterized by the retention of the radiopharmaceutical in tissue as a function of myocardial

TABLE 1. *PET flow tracers*

Radioisotope	Pharmaceutical	Half-life	Positron energy (MeV)	Mean range (mm)
O-15	Water	20 sec	1.72	3.8
N-13	Ammonia	10 min	1.19	2.5
Rb-82	Rubidium	76 sec	3.15	7.5
K-38	Potassium	7.6 min	2.7	6.4
Cu-62	PTSM	9.8 min	2.94	7.1
C-11	Acetate	20 min	0.96	1.9

PET, positron emission tomography.

blood flow (chemical microspheres). The most commonly used tracer of this group is N-13 ammonia.

Physiologic Properties

For both groups of radiopharmaceuticals the extraction of the tracer by myocardial tissue is important. O-15 water diffuses freely across membranes resulting in a rapid exchange of radioactivity between vascular and extravascular space. The relative distribution of the tracer in vascular and extra-vascular space depends on the partition coefficient. This partition coefficient for O-15 water is about 0.8, which is stable over a range of physiologic and pathophysiologic conditions (6). The comparison of the uptake of O-15 water in myocardial tissue and microsphere blood flow has shown that even at high flow rate the uptake of O-15 water is not diffusion-limited (6). Therefore, O-15 water has unique physiologic properties to reflect changes in myocardial blood flow. However, the rapid myocardial clearance of a freely diffusable tracer demands rapid imaging protocols in order to obtain adequate counting statistics.

The extraction fraction of nondiffusable tracers decreases with increasing blood flow, since the extraction or retention process is saturable (Fig. 1). Schelbert et al. (7) have shown that the initial exchange of the N-13 ammonium ion displays an extraction fraction exceeding 90%, which is quite stable over wide flow range. Metabolic trapping of N-13 in the

form of N-13 glutamine by the glutamine synthetase reaction, however, determines the retention fraction of this tracer in the myocardium. Comparison of N-13 ammonia retention fraction and microsphere blood flow demonstrates decreasing retention fraction as a function of increasing blood flow (8). The same applies for rubidium-82 (9), which is considered a potassium analog, and for potassium-38 (10). The extraction fraction of these tracers is lower than that of N-13 ammonia and rapidly decreases with increasing blood flow. Since the resulting radioactivity of a flow tracer in the myocardium (CM) depends on the product of extraction (E) and flow (F) ($CM = E \times F$), decreasing extraction fraction with increasing flow leads to underestimation of flow based on the measurement of radioactivity in the tissue.

Copper-62-pyruvaldehyde bis (n-methy-thio-semicarbazonado) (PTSM) and manganese-52m are alternate blood flow tracers retained in myocardial tissue that are currently under investigation (11,12). Both are generator-produced radioisotopes, which offer practical advantages for clinical use. However, the physiologic properties of these compounds are not well characterized yet.

C-11 acetate has been proposed as radiopharmaceutical for simultaneous evaluation of flow and metabolism. Early myocardial C-11 acetate uptake has been shown to reflect blood flow, while the washout of the tracer can be used to estimate myocardial oxygen consumption. Comparison with microsphere blood flow measurement and clinical studies indicate that C-11 acetate can be used as blood flow marker (13,14).

Application of Flow Tracers

As mentioned above, O-15 water represents the most physiologic tracer that requires dynamic data acquisition and sophisticated data analysis (discussed later). In addition, the short physical half-life of O-15 water limits the widespread clinical use, since a cyclotron in close proximity to the PET scanner is required. Therefore, O-15 water has been used almost exclusively in academic institutions.

N-13 ammonia is widely used for the clinical application of PET. This tracer has been extensively validated as flow tracer experimentally and clinically (15,16). The physical half-life of N-13 ammonia is 10 minutes, thus also restricting its use to PET centers with on-site cyclotron. The physical properties, on the one hand, provide sufficient count statis-

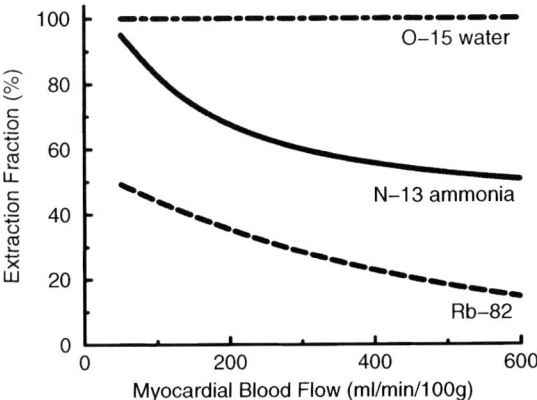

FIG. 1. Myocardial extraction fraction for O-15 water, N-13 ammonia, and Rb-82 as a function of myocardial blood flow in the canine heart (see text).

tics yielding excellent image quality, and, on the other hand, allow the combination with other tracers, such as F-18 deoxyglucose for comparison of blood flow and metabolism. Following injection, the tracer is rapidly extracted by myocardium and cleared from blood, providing good myocardial contrast as early as 3 minutes after injection. Studies in normal volunteers revealed a slight heterogeneity of regional tracer retention. N-13 ammonia retention is about 8 to 10% lower in the lateral wall of the left ventricle as compared to the septum. The underlying physiologic mechanism of this phenomenon is poorly understood. Visual and semiquantitative interpretation of N-13 ammonia images have to consider this inhomogeneity of tracer distribution (12).

Rubidium-82 is a commercially available generator-produced flow tracer. The 82-strontium and rubidium generator system provides application of this tracer independent of an on-site cyclotron facility. The short physical half-life of Rb-82 of 76 seconds is ideal for repeated injections under rest and stress conditions, as well as for the combination with other radiopharmaceuticals. Rubidium-82 has a high positron energy (3.2 MeV) that determines the range a positron travels before it interacts with an electron. The positron range averages 7.5mm for Rb-82 as compared to 2.5 mm for N-13, thus lowering the resolution of the imaging.

The practical advantages of rubidium-82 as short-lived generator-produced radiopharmaceutical are somewhat offset by the less optimal physiologic properties. The myocardial extraction fraction is lower than that of N-13 ammonia and O-15 water (9,17). However, for the qualitative assessment of myocardial blood flow, this tracer may provide practical advantages over cyclotron-produced compounds (18, 19). A small and mobile generator-infusion system is available that guarantees eluation of Rb-82 every 10 to 15 minutes with low radiation exposure to personnel or patient. Such a system is easy to handle by technologists and provides 24-hour availability of a myocardial blood flow tracer, which is most attractive for busy cardiac laboratories and for use of this tracer in acute ischemic syndromes. The relatively high costs associated with the use of rubidium-82 require a high volume of cardiac studies in order to justify the use of such generator with a shelf life of only 6 weeks (20).

Qualitative Assessment of Myocardial Perfusion

For clinical questions such as detection and localization of coronary artery disease (CAD), the evaluation of relative perfusion and perfusion reserve has been shown to be of diagnostic and prognostic value. N-13 ammonia and Rb-82 are the tracers of choice for this purpose. Similar rest and stress protocols as for SPECT perfusion scintigraphy are employed. Since attenuation correction requires close alignment of transmission and emission data, exercise studies in the PET scanner are difficult to perform. In addition, repositioning of the patient following exercise is difficult, especially in view of the short physical half-life of the tracers involved. Therefore, most PET studies use pharmacologic stress procedures to evaluate coronary flow reserve. Resting perfusion studies are commonly followed by the pharmacologic stress and subsequent second tracer injection (Fig. 2). Due to the short physical half-life of rubidium-82, rest/stress imaging protocols can be completed in about 60 minutes, while about 90 minutes are required for N-13 ammonia with a waiting period of about 60 minutes between rest and stress necessary for decay of N-13 activity.

Image analysis commonly involves visual inspection of tracer distribution of the myocardium in standard views eval-

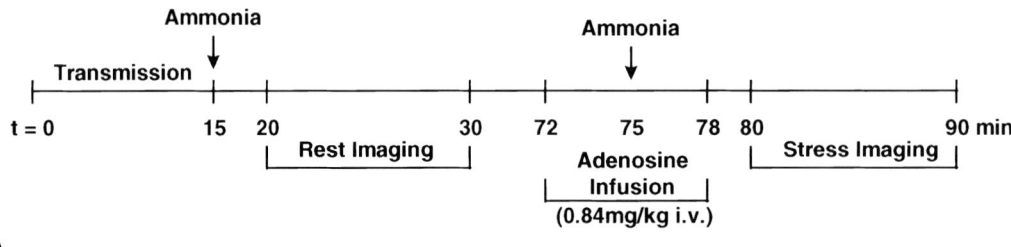

A

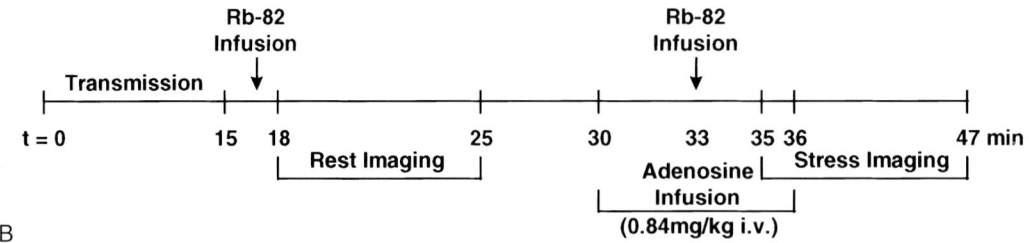

B

FIG. 2. Acquisition protocols for N-13 ammonia (A) and Rb-82 (B) PET studies at rest and during stress by pharmacological vasodilation with adenosine. *PET*, positron emission tomography.

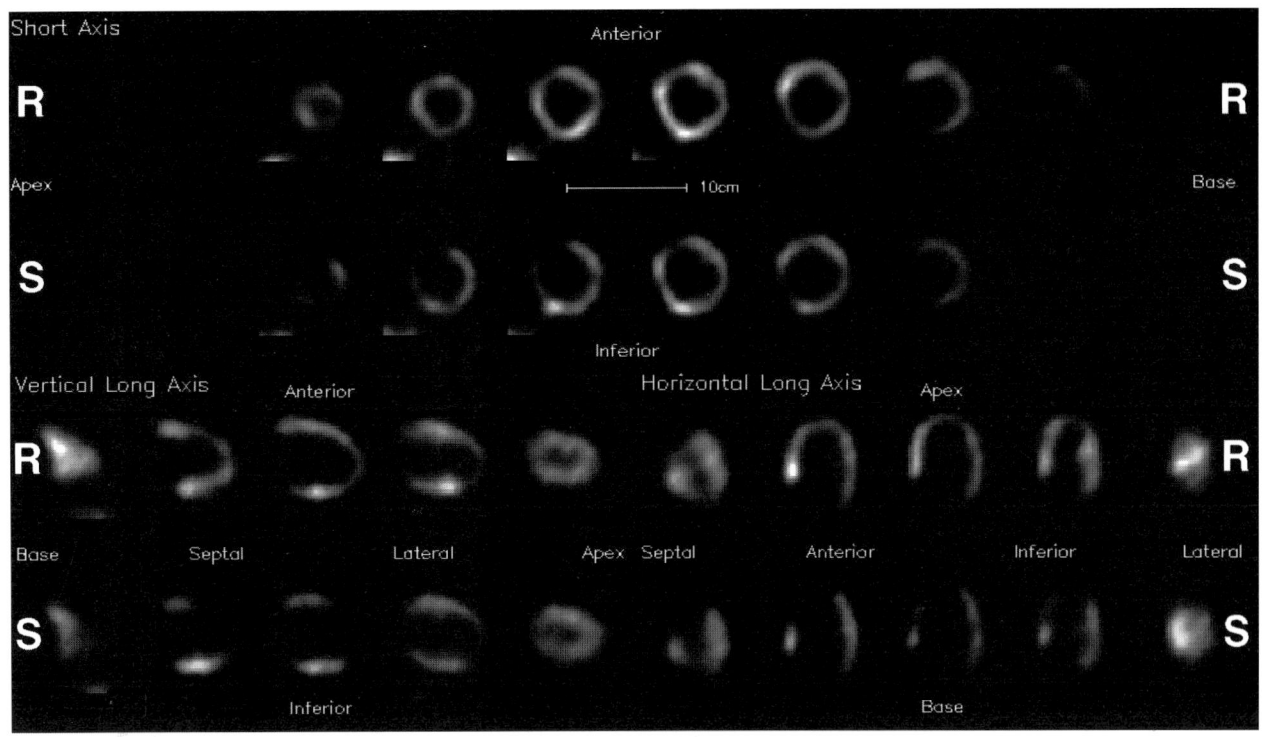

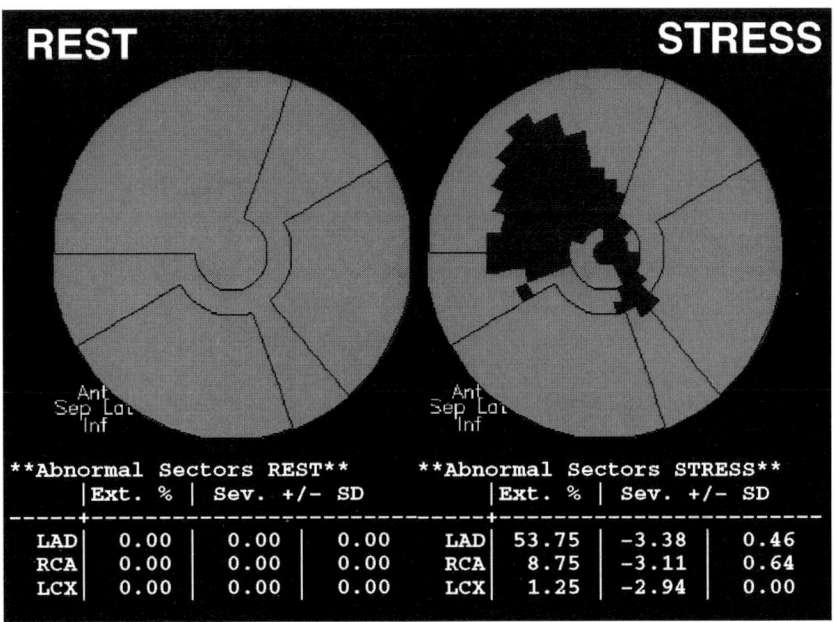

FIG. 3. Images (**top**) and polar maps (**bottom**) of regional N-13 ammonia distribution of a patient with repeated episodes of angina pectoris. Short- and long-axis images depict an adenosine-induced defect in the apex and distal anteroseptal wall. For the polar map analysis, regional perfusion is compared to a normal data base. Normal areas are shown in *light gray*, while the abnormal area during pharmacologic stress (shown in *dark gray*) covers 54% of the LAD territory. In summary, results in this patient suggest a hemodynamic relevant stenosis of the LAD. (See also Color Plate 11 following page 294.)

uating relative perfusion distribution (Fig. 3; see also Color Plate 11 following page 294). In addition, semiquantitative analysis similar to that used in SPECT imaging is employed to define perfusion abnormalities in comparison to a normal control data base. This approach yields extent and severity of perfusion abnormalities in individual patients. Comparison with a data base reflecting normal myocardial distribution of a given flow tracer can be used to objectively define regional perfusion abnormalities and express the degree of abnormalities in standard deviations of 'normal distribution.' Several analysis software has been validated for detection and localization of CAD (21–23).

Quantitative Assessment of Myocardial Perfusion

Absolute quantification of myocardial perfusion requires the dynamic definition of radioactivity concentration in blood and myocardium. Based on this information, tracer kinetic models representing the physiologic behavior of the tracer must be applied to derive values of myocardial perfusion in mL/min/gm tissue. The definition of acquisition parameters has to incorporate the kinetic behavior of the tracer as well as the performance of the camera system. This applies especially to short-lived radioisotopes that are injected as bolus. The administered bolus may deliver radioactivity to the field of view that exceeds the linear counting range of the camera system, while at later time points the count statistics may be limited due to the rapid decay of radioactivity. Therefore, the frame duration for dynamic studies has to be variable with short sampling intervals during the initial bolus phase followed by longer duration during retention or wash-out phase. Prolonged bolus injection using an infusion pump provides a distributed bolus activity profile and reduces variability of input function (24).

It is of utmost importance to minimize patient motion during dynamic studies since the generation of time curves of myocardial and left ventricular activity requires the serial application of regions of interest over these structures. Patient motion leads to artifacts in the time activity curves, which affect the flow estimates by tracer kinetic modeling. Recent software developments also include motion correction, which can retrospectively realign single frames to ensure proper definition of time activity curves with reduced motion artifacts (24–26).

TRACER KINETIC MODELING

O-15 Water

As discussed earlier, O-15 water is a diffusible tracer that rapidly equilibrates between the vascular and extravascular space (Fig. 4A). Therefore, the kinetics can be modeled with a one-tissue compartment based on the work of Kety (27). The time course of radioactivity concentration in the tissue is described by:

$$C_t(t) = K_1 \cdot C_a(t) \otimes e^{-k2t}$$

The two model parameters K_1 and k_2 represent the transport of tracer from arterial blood into tissue and the washout from tissue back in the blood, respectively. Measured time-activity curves, $Ct(t)$ in the tissue and $C_a(t)$ in the arterial blood, are used in the dynamic fitting process ($\otimes$ mathematical convolution) to determine K_1 and k_2. Delivery to the tissue is defined by myocardial blood flow and first pass extraction E ($K_1 = E \times MBF$). Since E can be assumed to be 100% for water, K_1 equals MBF. The washout parameter

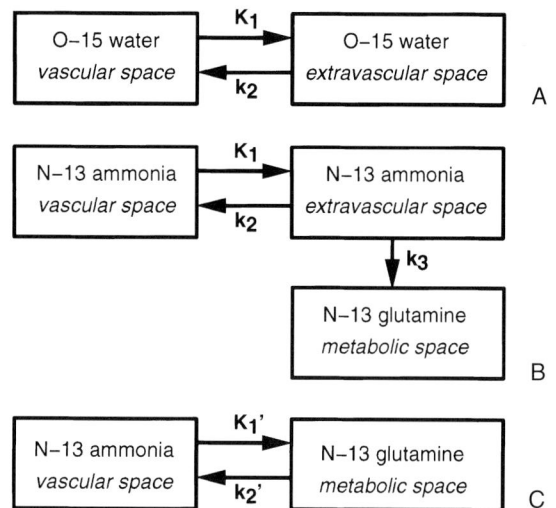

FIG. 4. Compartmental scheme representing distribution of O-15 water and N-13 ammonia in blood and tissue: (**A**) O-15 water model, (**B**) three-compartmental model for N-13 ammonia, and (**C**) two-compartmental model for N-13 ammonia.

k_2 is related to MBF in the case of freely diffusible tracers by the partition coefficient p: $k_2 = K_1/p = MBF/p$ (28).

Sequences of short frames are acquired for the determination of the time course of radioactivity in a given region of the myocardial wall. Simultaneously, the arterial input function $C_a(t)$ is measured from the PET images by using a region-of-interest (ROI) inside the left ventricular cavity. Image contrast between myocardial wall and blood pool can not be reached because of the fast exchange of O-15 water between vascular and extravascular space. Therefore, estimates of blood pool activity from separate scans with O-15 CO are subtracted to enhance contrast for improved delineation of myocardium. For this purpose, O-15 CO gas is inhaled. O-15 CO binds to hemoglobin labeling red blood cells and, hence, can be used to determine vascular space. The O-15 CO data are used to correct O-15 water studies.

Due to limited image resolution and motion during the cardiac cycle, the measured data do not exactly represent the tissue and blood O-15 concentrations. Thus, reduction of tissue activity by partial volume effect and spillover from the blood pool into the tissue are included in the operational equation by introducing correction terms for these effects. Several different approaches to either treat these as additional fitting parameters or include predetermined values, are in use (29–31). In general, estimation of myocardial blood flow based on wash-out kinetics k_2 is more stable since it is not affected by scaling or partial volume effects, in contrast to extraction parameter K_1.

Various administration protocols for myocardial O-15 water studies have been used in the past: direct intravenous bolus injection or slow infusion of O-15 water (6,31), or inhalation of C-15O-2 with subsequent rapid conversion to O-15 water in the lungs (29,32). The advantages of the inhalation method are lower count rate load and less spillover from right to left ventricular cavity. However, compared to bolus injection of O-15 water, radiation exposure, especially to lung tissue, during inhalation is higher.

Using a region-of-interest inside the left ventricular cavity to measure the arterial input function proved to be feasible if a tissue-to-blood spillover term is included in the model (33). A region-of-interest in the left atrial cavity yields the highest agreement with the true input function (31), but care has to be taken in including an estimate of time delay in order to reduce bias in flow values (34).

Recently, a study comparing different administration protocols (35) showed that the bolus injection of O-15 water and a model including spillover from right ventricular cavity yields the best results for simultaneous determination of myocardial blood flow and perfusable tissue fraction (see below) in all regions of left ventricular myocardium.

Perfusable Tissue Index

Since scar tissue in patients with CAD causes tissue heterogeneity in the myocardium, methods have been developed to separate viable from nonviable tissue based on O-15 water kinetics. The perfusable tissue fraction is the fraction of tissue that can rapidly exchange O-15 water within a tissue region. Tissue that rapidly exchanges water is assumed to be viable. Thus, the perfusable tissue index (PTI), defined as the fraction of perfusable tissue within the total, anatomical tissue fraction in the region, is used as index for viability (30,36,37). Since water is a freely diffusible tracer, a one-tissue compartment model is used to describe the time course of activity in the myocardial region-of-interest. The operational equation includes a parameter PTF (perfusable tissue fraction) defining the fraction of tissue in the region that is perfused:

$$C_t(t) = PTF \cdot K_1 \cdot C_a(t) \otimes e^{-k_2} + bv \cdot C_a(t)$$

PTF includes partial volume effect as well as the physiologic property of the myocardial tissue to exchange water. Assuming a constant partition coefficient for water, flow, *PTF* and arterial blood volume (*bv*) are determined by nonlinear least squares fitting of measured time-activity curves. The flow value is interpreted as myocardial blood flow in the perfusable tissue. It is different from the average blood flow in the volume of the region-of-interest or the average blood flow in the anatomical tissue. The anatomical fraction of tissue (ATF), representing the extravascular tissue space, can be determined from density and blood volume images. While transmission images yield the distribution of density, blood volume is determined by inhalation of O–15 labeled carbon monoxide. Subtraction of blood volume density (mL blood per mL ROI) from the normalized transmission image (tissue density) delineates extravascular tissue. Since both PTF and ATF are affected by partial volume effects in the same way, the ratio is independent of this scanner parameter. This water perfusable index (PTI) may be a marker of tissue

viability, assuming that irreversibly damaged tissue cannot exchange water rapidly. Thus, viable tissue is expected to show a PTI of 1.0. It has been shown that a reduced PTI does not necessarily mean diminished capability of O-15 water exchange in tissue but can also be attributed to heterogeneous flow (38). Tissue heterogeneity in infarcted areas can cause underestimation of PTI in these regions (38,39), suggesting a PTI threshold for viability of less than unity. Pixel-by-pixel analysis reduces this effect, although it does not eliminate it and may suffer from limited count statistics.

N-13 Ammonia

A schematic display of the model for physiologic behavior of N-13 ammonia in myocardium is depicted in Figure 4**B** and **C**. As mentioned above, the initial extraction of the N-13 ammonium ion from vascular into tissue space is approaching 100% while the retention of N-13 as N-13-glutamine represents the rate limiting step. Assuming compartments such as a vascular, extravascular, and metabolic space allows the mathematical description of the behavior of this tracer in the myocardium.

The mathematical description of the tissue time-activity curve includes the rate constants K_1, k_2, k_3, and the time course of radioactivity in the arterial blood (16,40). From time sequences of PET measurements and region-of-interest analysis ($C_t(t)$ tissue and $C_a(t)$ arterial input function), the model parameters can be determined by fitting the operational equation:

$$C_t(t) = \frac{K_1 k_2}{k_2 + k_3} \cdot e^{-(k_2 + k_3)t} \otimes C_a(t)$$
$$+ \frac{K_1 k_3}{k_2 + k_3} \int_0^t C_a(\tau)d\tau$$

Assuming a 100% first-pass extraction, K_1 serves as estimate of myocardial blood flow.

This model can be further reduced to a two-compartment model comprising the pool of free ammonia and the pool of metabolically trapped glutamine (15,41). The exchange between the two compartments is described by the new rate constants K_1' and k_2' (Fig. 4**C**). Assuming conversion from glutamine back to free ammonia to be negligible, k_2' can be set to 0, leaving one fitting variable K_1'. A functional relation for K_1' and myocardial blood flow was derived from equating the net extraction fraction of this two-compartment model to the previously measured first-pass extraction in dogs (7,8). Fixing the volume of distribution in the free space to 0.8, model fitting to the time-activity curves results in an estimate of myocardial blood flow.

Further simplification of data analysis is reached with a graphical approach similar to the one that is used in FDG imaging (42). With a reduced scan protocol and data analysis that does not require nonlinear fitting, it was shown that the results using this approach correlated very well with the results from compartmental fitting (43). Quantitative blood

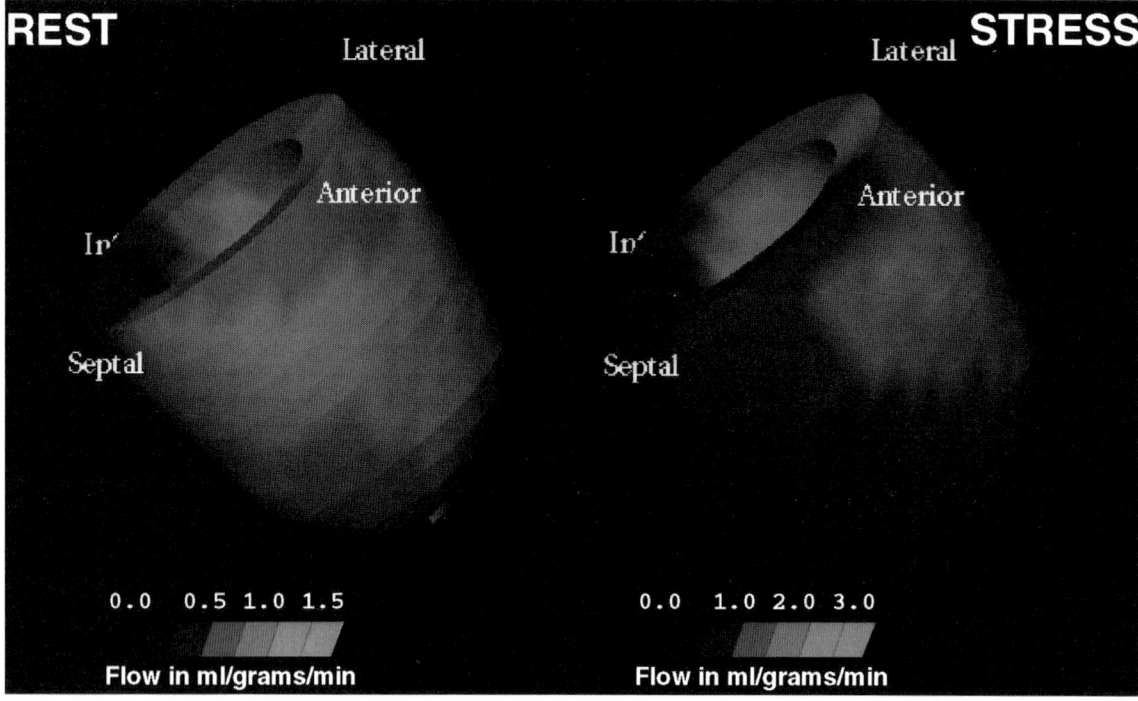

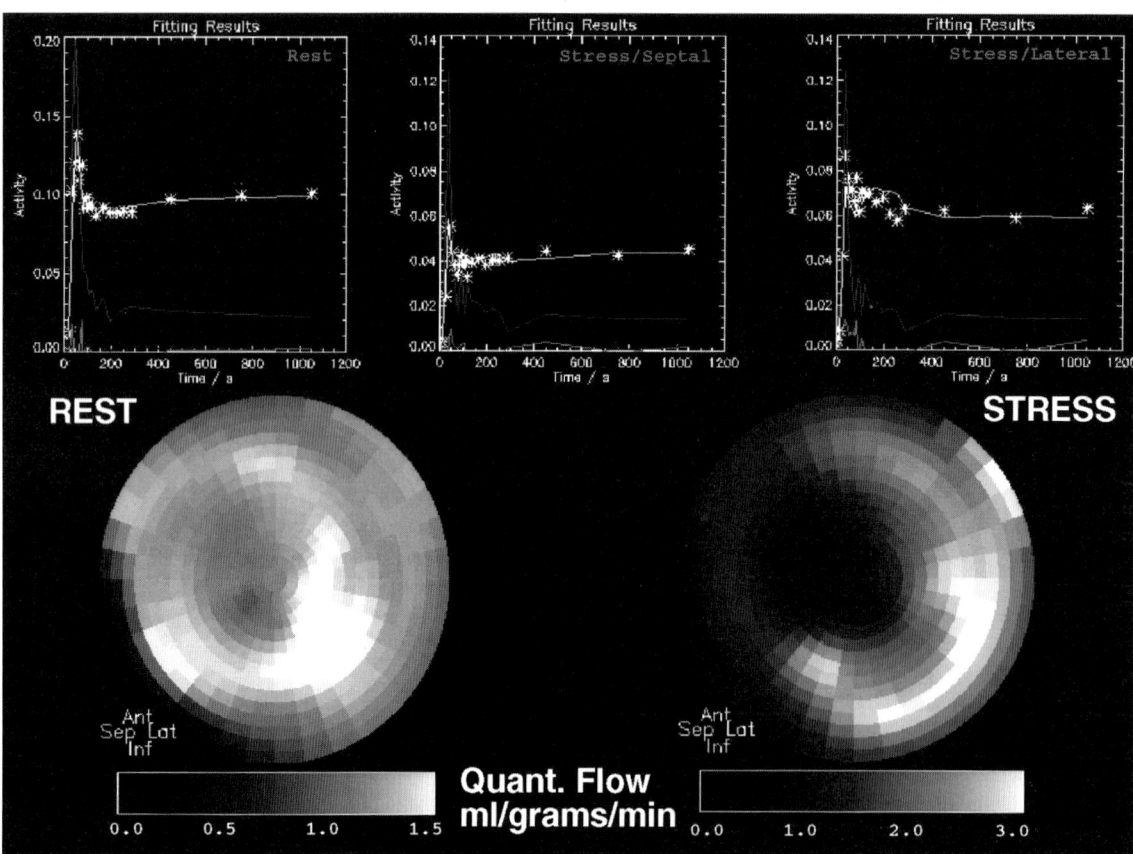

FIG. 5. Quantitative analysis of myocardial blood flow using N-13 ammonia. Depicted is the three-dimensional distribution of myocardial blood flow at rest and during stress (**top**) showing reduced stress flow and thus reduced flow reserve in the septal wall. The **bottom** part shows representative time activity curves for blood (*red lines*) and myocardium (*white lines*) at rest and during stress in septum and lateral wall along with two-dimensional polar maps of quantitative flow. (See also Color Plate 12 following page 294.)

flow values from this analysis may be affected by the acquisition protocol, and careful scan paradigms have to be designed such that the inherent assumption ($k_2' = 0$) of the method is fulfilled (44).

Independent of the model, i.e., of a three- or two-compartment model, several methods for correcting partial volume effect and/or spillover of blood radioactivity have been implemented. For this purpose, additional fit parameters are included taking into account the fraction of blood volume and tissue f_t in the region-of-interest (*ROI*):

$$C_{ROI}(t) = f_t\, C_t(t)\, +\, f_a\, C_a(t)$$

To improve fitting, strategies for the definition of regions-of-interest have been developed (45) that minimize bias in myocardial blood flow.

N-13 ammonia imaging yields high contrast between myocardial wall and blood pool. The main drawback in using ammonia as a perfusion tracer is the fact that due to metabolism, myocardial perfusion is not always the rate-limiting step, and there is a nonlinear relationship between blood flow and N-13 tissue tracer retention. Thus, kinetic modeling is needed to analyze dynamic data sets yielding estimates of K_1 corrected for extraction fraction variations at higher flow states. Software approaches have been introduced that allow rapid fitting of regional time activity curves and parametric display of flow values at rest and during pharmacologic vasodilation. Figure 5 (see also Color Plate 12 following page 294) shows regional tissue activity curves, parametric display of flow values in polar map and three-dimensional mode. Resting blood flow is homogeneous while maximal blood flow and flow reserve is reduced in anteroseptal regions.

Rubidium-82 and Other Flow Tracers

Quantitation of myocardial blood flow is more difficult using rubidium-82 or potassium-38. Extraction of these tracers is lower and nonlinearly related to blood flow. Therefore the quantitation of myocardial blood flow, especially in the high flow range is limited. However, there are several experimental studies indicating the potential of quantitative

blood flow measurements using rubidium-82. From first-pass measurements, a relationship between extraction and flow has been established (9) that can be used to quantify blood flow from a model that includes a tissue and a blood pool compartment (46). This approach facilitates estimation of blood flow from tissue uptake curves without measuring extraction directly. The relation between flow and extraction causes the tissue uptake of Rb-82 to change very little for high flow values, thus identification of these flow values is not possible by this method. In comparison to ammonia, the scan sequence using Rb-82 is much shorter, reducing the total time, e.g., a rest/stress study.

CLINICAL APPLICATION

Because of the improved image quality associated with the use of PET, several groups propagated the clinical application of PET for noninvasive detection and localization of CAD (47–50). In combination with pharmacologic vasodilation, the regional coronary reserve can be qualitatively evaluated. Studies evaluating the sensitivity and specificity in comparison to the gold standard coronary angiography revealed an excellent accuracy of this technique for the detection of CAD. Table 2 summarizes published results on the sensitivity and specificity of rubidium-82 or N-13 ammonia PET imaging for detection of CAD. In over 700 patients, the sensitivity and specificity averaged 94% and 95%, respectively. The experience of dedicated PET centers evaluating a large number of patients for the presence or absence of CAD documents the usefulness of this approach in clinical practice (19,49). Studies comparing PET and SPECT perfusion imaging in the same patient population indicated a significant improvement of diagnostic accuracy as a consequence of the better image quality (49,51,52) . It needs to be pointed out, however, that attenuation correction for SPECT has not been applied in these studies. In addition to visual analysis, automated image analysis can be easily applied to assist the visual observer and to reduce interobserver variability, as has been proposed for SPECT imaging (22,23). Using this approach, Laubenbacher et al. (21) observed a diagnostic accuracy of 91%, 79%, and 88% for localization of disease in the left anterior descending (LAD),

TABLE 2. *Diagnostic performance of PET in combination with N-13 ammonia and Rb-82 in detection of CAD*

Reference	N	Tracer	Sens. (%)	Spec. (%)	Acc. (%)
Gould et al. (20)	50	Rb-82	95	100	—
Yonekura et al. (92)	49	N-13 ammonia	97	100	—
Williams et al. (47)	146	Rb-82	98	100	96
Schelbert et al. (7)	32	N-13 ammonia	97	100	98
Demer et al. (53)	193	Rb-82	82	95	88
Stewart et al. (93)	81	Rb-82	84	88	85
Go et al. (49)	135	Rb-82	95	82	92
Tamaki et al. (94)	46	N-13 ammonia	98	—	—
Total	732		94	95	92

Acc., accuracy; *CAD*, coronary artery disease; *PET*, positron emission tomography; *Sens.*, sensitivity; *Spec.*, specificity.

SECTION I / TECHNOLOGY OF CARDIOVASCULAR IMAGING

204

circumflex (LCX), and right coronary artery (RCA), respectively. Demer et al. (53) indicated that the extent and severity of perfusion abnormalities assessed by PET correlated with the severity of CAD. Gould and colleagues (54) extended this observation by measuring the changes of perfusion defect size and severity before and 5 years following intense risk factor modification in patients with CAD. In a randomized trial, they were able to demonstrate that the quantitative assessment of regional perfusion abnormalities yields important information about the functional regression or progression of CAD. While a group of patients randomized to risk factor modification consisting of low-fat diet, exercise training, and stress management demonstrated improvement of perfusion defects, those who were randomized to usual care showed worsening of defects. The PET findings were substantially more sensitive in detecting such changes in response to therapy as compared to angiographic criteria in the same patient population.

The potential of myocardial perfusion PET for prognostic assessment of suspected or known CAD has been demonstrated in a recent study by Marwick and colleagues. Using rubidium-82 and dipyridamole stress in a large series of 685 patients, they found that PET results were independent predictors of cardiac death and total cardiac events. Within a mean follow-up period of 41 months, patients with a normal scan had an event-free survival of 90%. Those with a mild (less than 15% of left ventricular myocardium) defect had a survival rate of 87% compared to 75% for patients with moderate (15 to 30%) and 76% for patients with severe (greater than 30%) defects (Fig. 6). The results of perfusion PET yielded incremental prognostic information in comparison to clinical and angiographic findings alone (48).

The higher costs of PET studies compared to SPECT and echocardiography raise questions about the cost-effectiveness of PET for detection of CAD. Patterson et al. (55) recently applied a mathematical model to compare various diagnostic strategies for the detection of CAD. The results of the decision-tree analysis suggested that stress perfusion PET may be cost-effective for the primary diagnosis of CAD in patients with a pretest likelihood for CAD of less than 70%. The relative saving in diagnostic costs were based largely on the improved specificity of attenuation corrected PET flow images reducing the costs and risks of unnecessary cardiac catheterizations. In addition, the costs of PET studies were based on Rb-82 as radiotracer and high daily throughput (8 studies) in the cardiac laboratory. Further studies are needed to compare PET with SPECT protocols designed to improve specificity, such as attentuation correction, gating, and combined prone and supine imaging that would be expected to change this cost-effective analysis in favor of SPECT. These further considerations are necessary so that the calculations can be made applicable to the routine clinical work-up of patients with suspected CAD.

Quantitative Assessment of Coronary Artery Disease

PET represents the most accurate noninvasive technique currently available to quantitate regional myocardial blood flow. Numerous animal studies demonstrated the accuracy of PET flow measurements in comparison with radiolabeled microspheres (8,15,16). A few investigators have performed O-15 water and N-13 ammonia studies in the same animal model. The results indicate excellent agreement of both techniques over a wide flow range (16). Following the experimental validation, several laboratories have employed PET with O-15-water and N-13-ammonia to establish ''normal'' values of resting as well as stress perfusion in healthy volunteers. Despite varying methodology, the relative increase of myocardial blood flow during pharmacologic stress is reproducible (Table 3) among different laboratories, documenting the feasibility of this approach.

The coronary flow values obtained at rest and vasodilatory

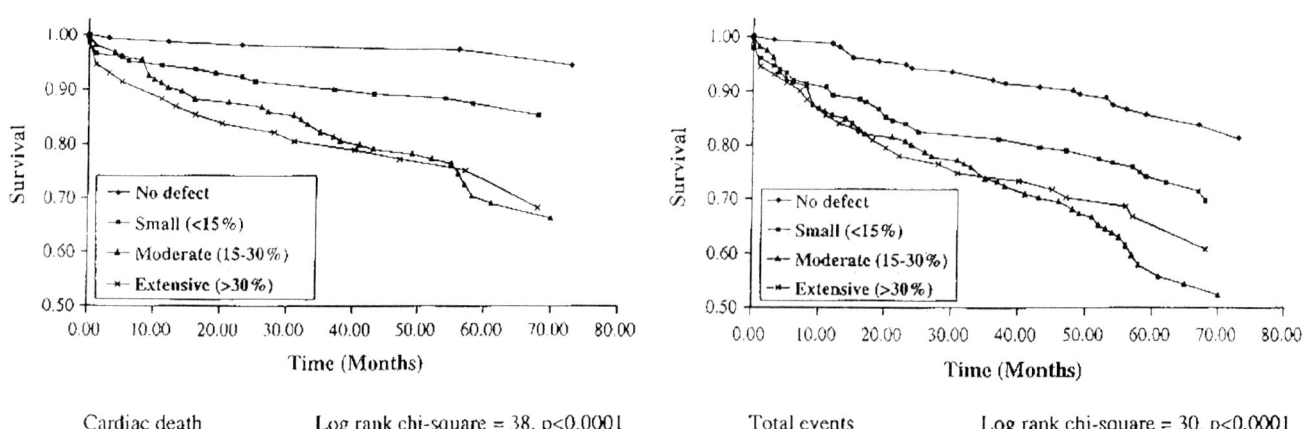

FIG. 6. Kaplan-Meier curves describing the correlation between mortality (**left**) and total events (**right**) with the extent of abnormally perfused myocardium defined by Rb-82 PET. *PET*, positron emission tomography. (From ref. 48, with permission.)

TABLE 3. *PET measurements of myocardial blood flow in normal volunteers*

Study	Tracer	No. of volunteers	Rest flow (mL/100 g/min)	Intervention	Stress flow (mL/100 g/min)	Coronary flow reserve
Araujo et al. (29)	O-15 water	11	84 ± 9	Dipyridamole	352 ± 112	4.0 ± 1.6
Bergmann et al. (6)	O-15 water	11	90 ± 22	Dipyridamole	355 ± 115	3.9 ± 2.2
Camici et al. (95)	O-15 water					4.0 ± 1.6
Chan et al. (89)	N-13 ammonia	20	110 ± 20	Dipyridamole	430 ± 130	3.9 ± 0.8
				Adenosine	440 ± 90	4.0 ± 1.5
Czemin et al. (61)	N-13 ammonia	30	76 ± 17	Dipyridamole	300 ± 80	3.9 ± 1.9
Geltman et al. (96)	O-15 water	16	125 ± 26	Dipyridamole	460 ± 158	3.7 ± 2.1
Hutchins et al. (40)	N-13 ammonia	7	88 ± 17	Dipyridamole	417 ± 110	4.7 ± 2.2
Krivokapich et al. (41)	N-13 ammonia	13	70 ± 17	Exercise	135 ± 22	1.9 ± 0.8
Krivokapich et al. (87)	N-13 ammonia	11	79 ± 17	Dobutamine	227 ± 25	2.9 ± 0.8
Sambuceti et al. (97)	N-13 ammonia	14	103 ± 25	Dipyridamole	366 ± 92	3.5 ± 1.7

stress as well as estimates of coronary reserve agree well with invasive measurements derived from Doppler wire estimates (1,56). The vasodilatory reserve is homogeneous throughout the left ventricle in healthy volunteers. Hutchins et al. (40) demonstrated that the observed heterogeneity of N-13 ammonia retention is not present when tracer kinetic modeling is performed. Muzik et al. (57) studied 20 individuals with low likelihood of CAD, reporting a specificity of 97% for a coronary reserve threshold of 2.7. In addition, several groups investigated the reproducibility of this technique as well as the interobserver variability of the processing software (Fig. 7). Data by Sawada and Nagamachi (58,59) indicate that differences of blood flow measurements obtained up to 2 weeks apart in patients at rest and during pharmacologic stress vary less than 20%. Myocardial blood flow data in CAD patients displayed high segmental reproducibility documenting the robustness of this technique to detect regional changes in myocardial perfusion, e.g., following therapeutic interventions (58).

Chan et al. (60) compared the coronary flow reserve values with dipyridamole and adenosine infusions. They reported a similar increase of myocardial blood flow with both

vasodilating substances, although interindividual variability has been observed in response to these drugs. Little experience exists with the quantitative PET flow measurements during physical exercise using bicycle ergometry. Krivokapich et al. (41) demonstrated that the coronary flow reserve in healthy normal volunteers undergoing bicycle exercise during PET imaging revealed coronary flow reserve of about 2.5, indicating the lower coronary reserve values associated with physical exercise as compared to pharmacologic vasodilation.

PET flow studies in asymptomatic patients of varying age without evidence for CAD showed that coronary flow reserve measurements decrease with increasing age. This finding is controversially discussed but most likely reflects changes in hemodynamic parameters as defined by blood pressure and heart rate with increasing age. Czernin et al. (61) observed increased resting blood flow associated with increased blood pressure and heart rate with increasing age as explanation of decreasing coronary flow reserve values in elderly patients. On the other hand, considering the sensitivity of flow reserve measurements for detection of early vascular abnormalities associated with the atherosclerotic

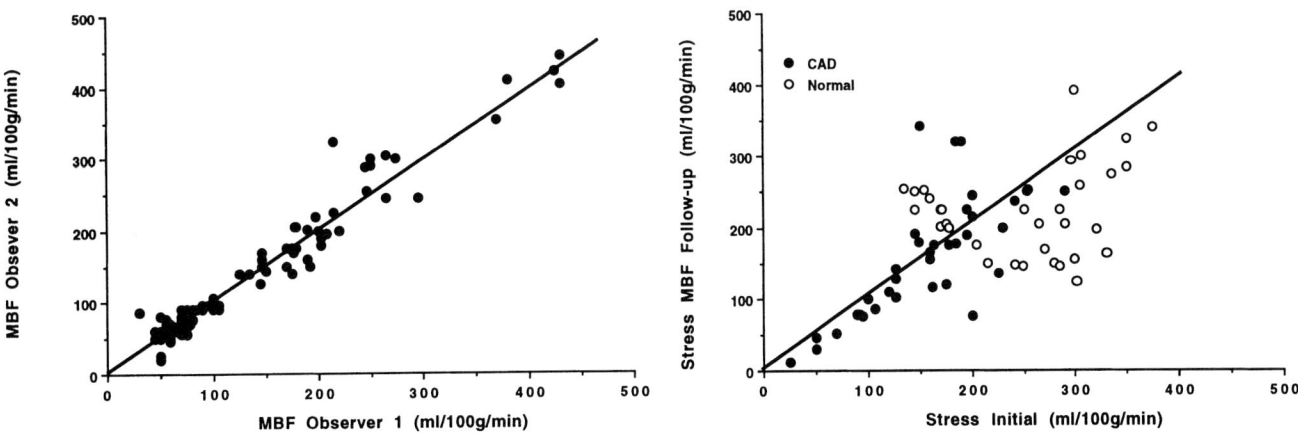

FIG. 7. Scatter plots demonstrating high inter-observer (**left**) and inter-study (**right**) concordance for quantitative measurements of myocardial blood flow using N-13 ammonia. (From ref. 58, with permission.)

process, the observed changes with increasing age may reflect increasing prevalence of artherosclerosis in patients with advanced age (62). Alternatively, there may be a reduction in peak achievable flow with increasing age due to changes in vascular reactivity and stiffness.

Comparison of Quantitative Flow Measurements with Coronary Angiography

Quantitative flow measurements with PET provide noninvasive means to estimate functional severity of a given coronary artery stenosis. In contrast to coronary angiography, which defines stenosis severity based on morphologic alterations, the measurement of perfusion at a cellular level represents a parameter that not only reflects antegrade flow through a stenosed vessel but also incorporates possible collateral circulation (63). In addition, by providing three-dimensional information, the extent of perfusion abnormalities associated with a given coronary stenosis can be evaluated. Therefore, quantitative regional blood flow measurements complement morphologic characterization of disease by angiographic findings and are useful in the clinical decision-making process as well as serve as endpoints in clinical research evaluating coronary physiology.

This complementary role of perfusion imaging to angiography has been addressed by several groups. Uren et al. (64) demonstrate a linear relationship between the severity of CAD as defined by lumen diameter stenosis and coronary flow reserve assessed by O-15-water PET studies. These data were confirmed by similar work of the University of California at Los Angeles and University of Michigan groups, which again showed a significant correlation between angiographic and functional measurements (65,66). Common to all the studies—despite the correlation of both measurements—was considerable scattering of the data, indicating the limitation of angiographic criteria in predicting the functional significance of CAD in individual patients. The mean values of flow reserve as a function of stenosis severity indicate relatively little difference in stenosis from 50 to 90%, defined angiographically. The relationship to angiographic data improved if absolute lesion diameter was compared to flow reserve instead of percentage luminal narrowing (Fig. 8).

Other studies comparing PET results with angiographic findings have reported that patients with CAD in one vessel displayed abnormal coronary flow reserve values in otherwise angiographically normal vessels. In one study, 11 patients with CAD had a vascular territory without significant angiographic disease. Flow and flow reserve in these regions were compared to results obtained in healthy volunteers. Flow reserve and maximal stress flow were significantly lower suggesting flow impairment in the absence of angiographic stenosis. Based on these findings, Beanlands et al. (67) postulated that quantitative flow measurements in combination with pharmacologic stress provide more sensitive techniques than angiography to detect altered flow dynamics in patients with CAD and to describe the extent of vascular

involvement. Muzik et al. (68) demonstrated that applying a threshold of abnormal flow reserve of 2.7 provides a highly sensitive method of detecting CAD, but only moderate specificity as compared to the presence or absence of coronary stenosis documented by angiography.

These data, confirmed by several groups, indicate that perfusion abnormalities may be much more extensive than angiographic documentation of regional CAD. This observation confirms previous pathologic studies that suggest larger extent of disease based on histologic examination and intravascular ultrasound as compared to coronary angiography and suggests the potential of functional flow measurements with PET to detect vascular alterations early and to monitor response to therapy. Based on this hypothesis, several groups have investigated the relationship of coronary flow reserve and risk factors for CAD (69,70). Dayanikli et al. (69) first described the linear relationship between coronary flow measurements and cholesterol levels in asymptomatic patients at high risk for developing CAD. In comparison to a lower-risk patient population with neither family history of CAD nor elevated cholesterol levels, the patients displayed a significantly reduced coronary flow reserve. Yokayama et al. (70) confirmed these results in patients with familial hypercholesterolemia. Coronary flow reserve was reduced in asymptomatic patients with familial hypercholesterolemia. The reduction was more prominent in male than in female patients for the same increase in cholesterol levels. Symptom-limited treadmill testing was performed in all patients without any electrocardiographic abnormalities or symptoms. This study also revealed a significant relationship between total cholesterol and coronary flow reserve measurements in individual patients (r-value: 0.59, $P < 0.01$) Pitkanen et al. (71) studied young patients with familial hypercholesterolemia (under 40 years of age). Coronary flow reserve was significantly reduced in comparison to an age-matched control population. The baseline blood flow was similar in both groups, but flow at maximal vasodilation was 29% lower in patients compared to healthy control subjects. Coronary flow reserve was inversely associated with serum total cholesterol concentration, raising the question if cholesterol has a direct effect on vasodilatory reserve. This notion is supported by the recent observation that acute changes of cholesterol levels by LDL apheresis are associated with improved myocardial perfusion reserve (72). However, these results are not confirmed by pharmacologic studies.

Güthlin et al. (73) evaluated the effect of lipid-lowering medication on the coronary flow reserve in patients with hypercholesterolemia and CAD. Thirteen patients were followed with PET at 3 and 6 months after initiation of therapy with Fluvastatin. All patients demonstrated significant reduction of cholesterol, LDL, and triglycerides early after onset of therapy. However, cardiac flow reserve did not show a significant increase at 3 months but increased significantly only after 6 months of therapy. These findings are in agreement with data evaluating endothelial function by injecting acetylcholine into the coronary arteries (74). This study dem-

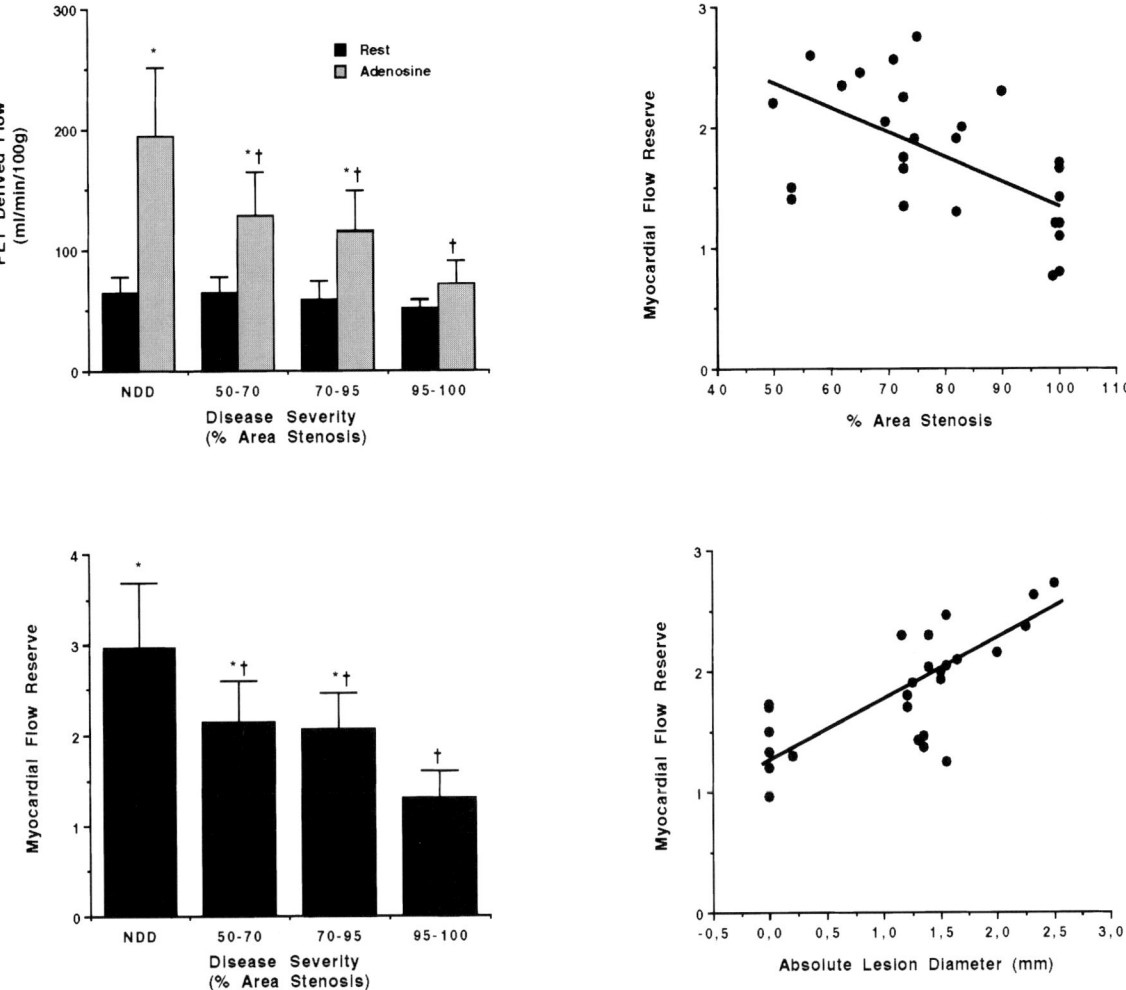

FIG. 8. Bar charts and scatter plots indicating a close relationship between regional myocardial flow reserve determined by N-13 ammonia PET and percentage of stenosis and diameter of the supplying vessel determined by coronary angiography. *PET*, positron emission tomography. (From ref. 67, with permission.)

onstrates the beneficial effect of cholesterol lowering medication on coronary microcirculation after 6 months of therapy and indicates the potential of flow measurement to assess the effect of risk factor modification. A few patients who did not respond to lipid lowering medication showed clinical deterioration of symptoms and exercise tolerance. Quantitative flow measurements may be suitable for following patients under lipid lowering therapy and for identifying nonresponders with higher risk for progression of CAD. This hypothesis needs to be tested prospectively in a larger patient population in order to define the prognostic value of decreased coronary flow reserve in patients with documented CAD.

Other studies indicate that the combination of lipid lowering medication and lifestyle modification may improve coronary flow reserve. Czernin et al. (75) defined the effect of short-term cardiovascular conditioning and low-fat diet on myocardial blood flow and flow reserve. Thirteen patients were studied before and upon completion of a 6-week program of cardiovascular conditioning and low-fat diet. Exer-

cise capacity and serum lipid profiles were assessed at the start of and at the end of the program. Eight normal volunteers of similar age, not participating in the conditioning program served as control group. Cardiovascular conditioning resulted in an improved myocardial flow reserve by lowering resting blood flow and increasing coronary vasodilatory capacity. These changes were associated with improved exercise capacity—again demonstrating the potential of PET for follow-up in such interventions.

Besides cholesterol, other risk factors, such as diabetes mellitus, smoking, and hypertension, are known to affect coronary vasculature. Czernin et al. (76) investigated the acute effect of smoking on myocardial vascular reactivity to vasodilatory stimulation. Short-term smoking markedly reduced coronary flow reserve (3.4 ± 0.8 to 2.3 ± 0.3). In contrast, Campisi et al. (77) reported that vasodilatory reserve is unaltered in long-term smokers, whereas an abnormal response to cold exposure was observed, suggesting altered endothelial function as an early marker of vascular injury by smoking.

Hypertension and Myocardial Hypertrophy

Arterial hypertension is a well-known risk factor for coronary artery disease and cardiac death. Even without the presence of coronary artery disease, hypertension may result in reduced coronary flow reserve by an interaction between myocardial hypertrophy, increasing perfusion pressure, and changes of the microvasculature.

In a recent report by Gimelli et al. (78), hyperemic flow and coronary reserve in 50 untreated hypertensive patients without evidence of coronary disease were reduced compared to healthy patients. The authors also investigated the relationship between flow alterations and myocardial hypertrophy: impairment of flow reserve was not directly correlated to ventricular mass. Additionally, there were no differences of myocardial blood flow and coronary reserve between patients with hypertrophy and those with normal left ventricular mass. However, an association between increased regional heterogeneity of myocardial perfusion and ventricular hypertrophy was observed.

In addition to myocardial hypertrophy, other pathophysiologic factors seem to influence coronary flow in hypertensive patients. To gain further insights into the effect of hypertrophy itself on myocardial blood flow, Radvan et al. (79) recently investigated myocardial blood flow at rest and during dipyridamole vasodilation in elite rowing athletes with physiologic ventricular hypertrophy and did not find significant differences compared to age-matched healthy individuals.

An improved understanding of the relationship between hypertrophy, hypertension, vascular resistance, and coronary flow may be of clinical and therapeutic importance. In addition to studies of pathophysiology, measurements of myocardial blood flow by PET may also be used to investigate the effects of antihypertensive drugs. Parodi et al. (80) demonstrated that coronary flow reserve can be improved by treatment with verapamil, while enalapril appears to reduce regional heterogeneity but not to alter overall flow reserve.

PET may be an important tool in future efforts to elucidate the effects of therapeutic approaches and to determine the prognosis of patients with hypertension.

Syndrome X

The presence of chest pain together with ischemia-like changes during exercise ECG in the absence of angiographic coronary stenosis has been defined as syndrome X. Several studies applying PET methodology focused on the investigation of coronary microcirculation and vasoreactivity in these patients.

While Camici et al. (81) found a blunted flow reserve in approximately 30% of patients with syndrome X, myocardial blood flow and flow reserve did not correlate with electrocardiographic signs of ischemia in this study. A further study by Rosen et al. (82) compared coronary flow reserve in 29 patients with syndrome X with 20 age- and gender-matched normal controls; after normalization of resting flow to the rate pressure product, they did not find a difference between the two groups. Thus, controversy remains about the pathophysiologic role of microvascular dysfunction in patients with syndrome X.

Hypertrophic Cardiomyopathy

Hypertrophic cardiomyopathy is a genetically transmitted disease and results in abnormal hypertrophy of the myocardium, which often is regionally heterogeneous and especially pronounced in the septum.

Camici et al. (83) found an impaired global flow reserve not only in hypertrophied, but also in nonhypertrophied areas of 23 patients with hypertrophic cardiomyopathy and concluded that the observed results are due to primary changes rather than regional hypertrophy. Their results are further supported by a study by Radvan et al., (79) who observed impaired coronary vasodilatory reserve in patients with hypertrophic cardiomyopathy, but not in athletes with physiologic myocardial hypertrophy. PET has also been used to measure the effect of verapamil treatment on myocardial blood flow. Gistri et al. (84) found reduced regional heterogeneity but no changes in absolute flow during therapy with verapamil in 20 patients with hypertrophic cardiomyopathy.

Dilated Cardiomyopathy

Few studies have investigated myocardial blood flow in patients with idiopathic dilated cardiomyopathy. In 6 patients with overt heart failure and depressed left ventricular function and normal coronary arteries, dipyridamole flow was substantially reduced compared to healthy individuals and correlated with intracoronary Doppler flow measurements (56).

Impaired ventricular hemodynamics and cardiovascular changes secondary to heart failure may have influenced these results. Thus, Neglia et al. (85) investigated a larger series of 22 patients with dilated cardiomyopathy, but without overt heart failure in order to minimize the influence of secondary hemodynamic factors. Compared to normal volunteers, myocardial blood flow was significantly lower at rest, during atrial pacing tachycardia and during dipyridamole vasodilation (Fig. 9). Additionally, flow at rest and during pacing was significantly correlated with left ventricular end-diastolic pressure and degree of fibrosis, suggesting that progression of disease was associated with more severe depression of perfusion. The authors concluded that the observed flow abnormalities in the absence of overt heart failure may be explained by microvascular alterations as a part of the pathogenetic mechanism of dilated cardiomyopathy.

The Transplanted Human Heart

Various studies using dipyridamole vasodilation (86) or physical exercise (87) indicated that coronary flow reserve

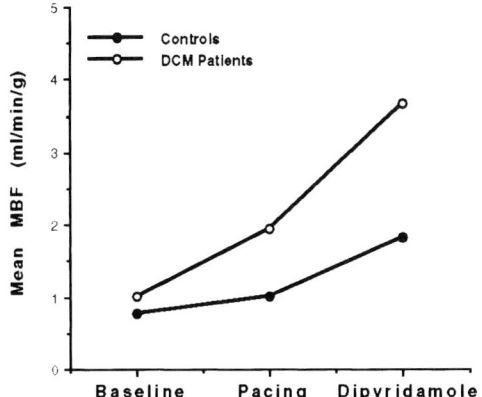

FIG. 9. Myocardial blood flow in patients with idiopathic dilated cardiomyopathy and normal controls at rest, during pacing-induced tachycardia and during dipyridamole-induced maximal vasodilation. (From ref. 85, with permission.)

remains normal after orthotopic heart transplantation in the absence of angiographic transplant vasculopathy or rejection, if baseline flow is corrected for a higher rate pressure product. Impaired exercise performance, a well-known phenomenon after transplantation, does not, therefore, seem to be related to altered vasoreactivity or limited coronary flow reserve.

The relationship between myocardial blood flow and transplant vasculopathy has been investigated by Kofoed et al. (88). The authors found that myocardial blood flow during dipyridamole vasodilation was reduced in 32 patients with transplant vasculopathy and inversely correlated with intimal thickness measured by intravascular ultrasound. These results support the deleterious effect of progressive graft vessel disease on myocardial blood flow and flow reserve of the transplanted heart.

Chan et al. (89) demonstrated a reduction of hyperemic flow and an increase of resting flow during acute allograft rejection in 10 patients. During a follow-up study after successful treatment, however, the authors found significant improvement, pointing toward reversible alterations, e.g., of endothelial function, local coagulation, or edema during acute rejection. The authors suggested that serial noninvasive flow measurements may therefore be used to guide immunosuppressive therapy.

Pediatric Cardiology

Recently, PET flow measurements have also been applied for investigation of heart disease in children since noninvasive measurements are attractive in this patient population.

In patients with a history of Kawasaki disease but normal epicardial coronary arteries, Muzik et al. (90) found reduced hyperemic flow and flow reserve, suggesting residual damage of coronary microcirculation after this inflammatory process.

Myocardial blood flow has also been studied in children

late after arterial switch operation for transposition of great arteries. This surgical procedure includes excision of the coronary trunks and reinsertion into the neo-aorta. A reduced coronary flow reserve was found, suggesting impaired vasoreactivity as a consequence of either surgical manipulations or congenital heart disease (91).

In both studies, results in children were compared to healthy young adults. Although the conclusiveness of these studies was limited due to the lack of age-matched normal individuals, it has been demonstrated that PET technology can be successfully applied in patients with congenital heart disease. PET may hold promise for an improved understanding of pathophysiology of various cardiac diseases in childhood, but ethical constraints due to radiation exposure in childhood have to be considered.

CONCLUSION

PET represents the most advanced scintigraphic approach for qualitative and quantitative evaluation of myocardial flow and flow reserve. It is currently the best validated imaging modality for the quantitative assessment of absolute blood flow. Although clinical studies document the high diagnostic and prognostic value of PET in proven and suspected CAD, its limited availability and high cost prevent widespread clinical application at the current time. Less costly PET instrumentation and increasing reimbursement of cardiac PET will support wider clinical application in the future. The use of PET as a research tool has provided unique new insights into the pathophysiology of various disease processes. The noninvasiveness and high reproducibility of the technique allows longitudinal study protocols for evaluating new therapeutic strategies. Coronary flow measurements may serve as endpoint in clinical study protocols investigating new cardiovascular drugs. Technical improvements, broader access to PET technology in the future, and increasing acceptance of functional imaging in cardiology may foster further development of PET as an important diagnostic and prognostic tool in the management of patients with cardiovascular diseases.

REFERENCES

1. Marcus M. Methods of measuring coronary blood flow. In: *The coronary circulation in health and disease.* New York: McGraw-Hill, 1983.
2. Wilson RF, Marcus ML, White CW. Prediction of the physiologic significance of coronary arterial lesions by quantitative lesion geometry in patients with limited coronary artery disease. *Circulation* 1987;75(4): 723–732.
3. Heymann M, Payne B, Hoffman J, Rudolph A. Blood flow measurements with radionuclide-labeled particles. In: *Principles of cardiovascular nuclear medicine.* Holman B, Sonnenblick E, Lesch M, eds. New York: Grune & Stratton, 1977:135–159.
4. Spinks T, Jones T. Trends in instrumentation. In: *Cardiac positron emission tomography.* Schwaiger M, ed. New York: Kluwer Academic Publishers, 1996, 3–47.
5. Schwaiger M, Ziegler S. PET using a coincidence camera versus ring tomography, progress or recession? (editorial). *Nuklearmedizin* 1997; 26(6):3–5.

6. Bergmann SR, Fox K, Rand A, et al. Quantification of regional myocardial blood flow *in vivo* with H215-0. *Circulation* 1984;70:724–733.

7. Schelbert H, Phelps M, Huang S, et al. N-13 ammonia as an indicator of myocardial blood flow. *Circulation* 1981;63:1259–1272.

8. Shah A, Schelbert HR, Schwaiger M, et al. Measurement of regional myocardial blood flow with N-13 ammonia and positron emission tomography in intact dogs. *J Am Coll Cardiol* 1985;5:92–100.

9. Mullani N, Goldstein R, Gould K, et al. Perfusion imaging with rubidium-82: I. Measurement of extraction and flow with external detectors. *J Nucl Med* 1983;24:898–906.

10. Melon P, Brihaye C, Degueldre C, et al. Myocardial kinetics of potassium-38 in man and comparison with copper-62-PTSM. *J Nucl Med* 1994;35(7):1122–1124.

11. Buck A, Nguyen N, Burger C, et al. Quantitative evaluation of manganese-52m as a myocardial perfusion tracer in pigs using positron emission tomography. *Eur J Nucl Med* 1996;23(12):1619–1627.

12. Beanlands R, Muzik O, Hutchins G, et al. Heterogeniety of regional nitrogen 13-labeled ammonia tracer distribution in the normal heart: Comparison with rubidium 82 and copper 62-labeled PTSM. *J Nucl Cardiol* 1994;1:225–235.

13. Wolpers H, Burchert W, van den Hoff J, et al. Assessment of myocardial viability by use of C-11 acetate and positron emission tomography. Threshold criteria of reversible dysfunction. *Circulation* 1997;95(6):1417–1424.

14. van den Hoff J, Burchert W, Wolpers H, et al. A kinetic model for cardiac PET with (1-carbon-11) acetate. *J Nucl Med* 1996;37(3):521–529.

15. Kuhle W, Porenta G, Huang S, et al. Quantification of regional myocardial blood flow using 13N-ammonia and reoriented dynamic positron emission tomographic imaging. *Circulation* 1992;86:1004–1017.

16. Muzik O, Beanlands RSB, Hutchins GD, et al. Validation of nitrogen-13-ammonia tracer kinetic model for quantification of myocardial blood flow using PET. *J Nucl Med* 1993;34:83–91.

17. Goldstein R, Mullani N, Marani S, et al. Myocardial perfusion with rubidium-82: II. Effects of metabolic and pharmacologic interventions. *J Nucl Med* 1983;24(10):907–915.

18. Yoshida K, Mullani N, Gould K. Coronary flow and flow reserve by PET simplified for clinical applications using rubidium-82 or nitrogen-13-ammonia. *J Nucl Med* 1996;37(10):1701–1712.

19. Williams BR, Mullani NA, Jansen DE, et al. A retrospective study of the diagnostic accuracy of a community hospital-based PET center for the detection of coronary artery disease using rubidium-82. *J Nucl Med* 1994;35(10):1586–1592.

20. Gould K, Goldstein R, Mullani N. Economic analysis of clinical positron emission tomography of the heart with rubidium-82. *J Nucl Med* 1989;30(5):707–717.

21. Laubenbacher C, Rothley J, Sitomer J, et al. An automated analysis program for the evaluation of cardiac PET studies: Initial results in the detection and localization of coronary artery disease using nitrogen-13 ammonia. *J Nucl Med* 1993;34:968–978.

22. Hicks K, Ganti G, Mullani N, et al. Automated quantitation of three-dimensional cardiac positron emission tomography for routine clinical use. *J Nucl Med* 1989;30:1787–1797.

23. Porenta G, Kuhle W, Czernin J, et al. Semiquantitative assessment of myocardial blood flow and viability using polar map displays of cardiac PET images. *J Nucl Med* 1992;33(9):1628–1636.

24. Muzik O, Beanlands RSB, Wolfe E, et al. Automated region definition for cardiac nitrogen-13-ammonia PET imaging. *J Nucl Med* 1993;34(2):336–344.

25. Hoh C, Dahlbom M, Harris C, et al. Automated iterative three-dimensional registration of positron emission tomography images. *J Nucl Med* 1993;34:2009–2018.

26. Turkington T, DeGrado T, Hanson M, et al. Alignment of dynamic cardiac PET images for correction of motion. *IEEE Trans Nucl Sci* 1997;44:235–242.

27. Kety S, The theory and applications of the exchange of inert gas at the lungs and tissues. *Pharmacol Rev* 1951;3:1–41.

28. Hutchins G, Schwaiger M. Quantitative evaluation of myocardial perfusion. In: Schwaiger M, ed. *Cardiac positron emission tomography.* New York: Kluwer Academic Publishers, 1996, 97–118.

29. Araujo LI, Lammertsma AA, Rhodes CG, et al. Noninvasive quantification of regional myocardial blood flow in coronary artery disease with oxygen-15-labeled carbon dioxide inhalation and positron emission tomography. *Circulation* 1991;83(3):875–885.

30. Iida H, Kanno I, Takahashi A, et al. Measurement of absolute myocardial blood flow with H215O and dynamic positron emission tomography. Strategy for quantification in relation to the partial-volume effect. *Circulation* 1988;78:104–115.

31. Bergmann SR, Herrero P, Markham J, et al. Non-invasive quantitation of myocardial blood flow in human subjects with oxygen-15 labeled water and positron emission tomography. *J Am Coll Cardiol* 1989;14:639–652.

32. Lammertsma A, DeSilva R, Araujo L, et al. Measurement of regional myocardial blood flow using C15O2 and positron emission tomography: comparison of tracer models. *Clin Phys Physiol Meas* 1991;13:1–20.

33. Iida H, Rhodes C, DeSilva R, et al. Use of left ventricular time-activity curve as a noninvasive input function in dynamic oxygen-15-water positron emission tomography. *J Nucl Med* 1992;33:1669–1677.

34. Herrero P, Hartmann J, Senneff M, et al. Effects of time discrepancies between input and myocardial time-activity curves on estimates of regional myocardial perfusion with PET. *J Nucl Med* 1994;35:558–566.

35. Hermansen F, Rosen S, Fath-Ordoubadi F, et al. Measurement of myocardial blood flow with oxygen-15 labelled water: comparison of different administration protocols. *Eur J Nucl Med* 1998;25(7):751–759.

36. Iida H, Rhodes CG, DeSilva R, et al. Myocardial tissue fraction—correction for partial volume effects and measure of tissue viability. *J Nucl Med* 1991;32:2169–2175.

37. Yamamoto Y, DeSilva R, Rhodes C, et al. A new strategy for the assessment of viable myocardium and regional myocardial blood flow using 15O-water and dynamic positron emission tomography. *Circulation* 1992;86:167–178.

38. Herrero P, Staudenherz A, Walsh JF, et al. Heterogeneity of myocardial perfusion provides the physiological basis of perfusable tissue index. *J Nucl Med* 1995;36(2):320–327.

39. Iida H, Kanno I, Miura S, et al. A determination of the regional brain/blood partition coefficient of water using dynamic positron emission tomography. *J Cereb Blood Flow Metab* 1989;9(6):874–885.

40. Hutchins G, Schwaiger M, Rosenspire K, et al. Noninvasive quantification of regional myocardial blood flow in the human heart using N-13 ammonia and dynamic positron emission tomographic imaging. *J Am Coll Cardiol* 1990;15:1032.

41. Krivokapich J, Smith GT, Huang SC, et al. 13N ammonia myocardial imaging at rest and with exercise in normal volunteers. Quantification of absolute myocardial perfusion with dynamic positron emission tomography. *Circulation* 1989;80(5):1328–1337.

42. Patlak C, Blasberg R, Fenstermacher J. Graphical evaluation of blood-to-brain transfer constants from mulitple-time uptake data. *J Cereb Blood Flow Metab* 1983;3:1–7.

43. Choi Y, Huang SC, Hawkins RA, et al. A simplified method for quantification of myocardial blood flow using nitrogen-13-ammonia and dynamic PET. *J Nucl Med* 1993;34(3):488–497.

44. Kitsukawa S, Yoshida K, Mullani N, et al. Simple and Patlak models for myocardial blood flow measurements with nitrogen-13-ammonia and PET in humans. *J Nucl Med* 1998;39:1123–1128.

45. Hutchins GD, Caraher JM, Raylman RR. A region of interest strategy for minimizing resolution distortions in quantitative myocardial PET studies. *J Nucl Med* 1992;33:1243–1250.

46. Herrero P, Markham J, Shelton ME, et al. Noninvasive quantification of regional myocardial perfusion with rubidium-82 and positron emission tomography. *Circulation* 1990;82:1377–1386.

47. Williams B, Jansen D, Wong L, et al. Positron emission tomography for the diagnosis of coronary artery disease: a non-university experience and correlation with coronary angiography. *J Nucl Med* 1989;30:845.

48. Marwick T, Shan K, Patel S, et al. Incrementai value of rubidium-82 positron emission tomography for prognostic assessment of known or suspected coronary artery disease. *Am J Cardiol* 1997;80(7):865–870.

49. Go RT, Marwick TH, MacIntyre WJ, et al. A prospective comparison of rubidium-82 PET and thallium-201 SPECT myocardial perfusion imaging utilizing a single dipyridamole stress in the diagnosis of coronary artery disease. *J Nucl Med* 1990;31:1899–1905.

50. Gould K. New concepts and paradigms in cardiovascular medicine: the noninvasive management of coronary artery disease. *Am J Med* 1998;104(6A):2S–17S.

51. Stewart RE, Popma J, Gacioch GM, et al. Comparison of thallium-201 SPECT redistribution patterns and rubidium-82 PET rest-stress myocardial blood flow imaging. *Int J Card Imaging* 1994;10:15–23.

52. Marwick T, Go R, MacIntyre W, et al. Myocardial perfusion imaging with positron emission tomography and single photon emission computed tomography: frequency and causes of disparate results. *Eur Heart J* 1991;12(10):1064–1069.

53. Demer LL, Gould KL, Goldstein RA, et al. Assessment of coronary artery disease severity by positron emission tomography. Comparison with quantitative arteriography in 193 patients. *Circulation* 1989;79: 825–835.

54. Gould KL, Ornish D, Scherwitz L, et al. Changes in myocardial perfusion abnormalities by positron emission tomography after long-term, intense risk factor modification. *JAMA* 1995;274(11):894–901.

55. Patterson RE, Eisner RL, Horowitz SF. Comparison of cost-effectiveness and utility of exercise ECG, single photon emission computed tomography, positron emission tomography, and coronary angiography for diagnosis of coronary artery disease. *Circulation* 1995;91(1):54–65.

56. Merlet P, Mazoyer B, Hittinger L, et al. Assessment of coronary reserve in man: comparison between positron emission tomography with oxygen-15-labeled water and intracoronary Doppler technique. *J Nucl Med* 1993;34(11):1899–1904.

57. Muzik O, Duvernoy C, Beanlands R, et al. Assessment of diagnostic performance of quantitative flow measurements in normal subjects and patients with angiographically documented coronary artery disease by means of nitrogen-13 ammonia and positron emission tomography. *J Am Col Cardiol* 1998;31(3):534–540.

58. Sawada S, Muzik O, Beanlands RSB, et al. Interobserver and interstudy variability of myocardial blood flow and flow-reserve measurements with nitrogen 13 ammonia-labeled positron emission tomography. *J Nucl Cardiol* 1995;2:413–422.

59. Nagamachi S, Czernin J, Kim A, et al. Reproducibility of measurements of regional resting and hyperemic myocardial blood flow assessed with PET. *J Nucl Med* 1996;37(10):1626–1631.

60. Chan SY, Brunken RC, Czernin J, et al. Comparison of maximal myocardial blood flow during adenosine infusion with that of intravenous dipyridamole in normal men. *J Am Coll Cardiol* 1992;20(4):979–985.

61. Czernin J, Muller P, Chan S, et al. Influence of age and hemodynamics on myocardial blood flow and flow reserve. *Circulation* 1993;88(1): 62–69.

62. Uren NG, Camici PG, Melin JA, et al. Effect of aging on myocardial perfusion reserve. *J Nucl Med* 1995;36(11):2032–2036.

63. Gould KL, Kirkeeide RL, Buchi M. Coronary flow reserve as a physiologic measure of stenosis severity. *J Am Coll Cardiol* 1990;15(2): 459–474.

64. Uren NG, Melin JA, De-Bruyne B, et al. Relation between myocardial blood flow and the severity of coronary-artery stenosis. *N Engl J Med* 1994;330(25):1782–1788.

65. Beanlands R, Melon P, Muzik O, et al. N-13 ammonia PET identifies reduced perfusion reserve in angiographically normal regions of patients with CAD. *Circulation* 1992;86(4):1–184.

66. DiCarli M, Czernin J, Hoh CK, et al. Relation among stenosis severity, myocardial blood flow, and flow reserve in patients with coronary artery disease. *Circulation* 1995;91(7):1944–1951.

67. Beanlands RS, Muzik O, Melon P, et al. Noninvasive quantification of regional myocardial flow reserve in patients with coronary atherosclerosis using nitrogen-13 ammonia positron emission tomography. Determination of extent of altered vascular reactivity. *J Am Coll Cardiol* 1995;26(6):1465–1475.

68. Muzik O, Beanlands RSB, Dayanikli F, et al. Quantification of myocardial blood flow reserve using PET and [N-13]ammonia in patients with angiographically documented CAD. *J Nucl Med* 1993;34(5):35P.

69. Dayanikli F, Grambow D, Muzik O, et al. Early detection of abnormal coronary flow reserve in asymptomatic men at high risk for coronary artery disease using positron emission tomography. *Circulation* 1994; 90(2):808–817.

70. Yokoyama I, Murakami T, Ohtake T, et al. Reduced coronary flow reserve in familial hypercholesterolemia. *J Nuc Med* 1996;37(12): 1937–1942.

71. Pitkanen O, Raitakari O, Niinikoski H, et al. Coronary flow reserve is impaired in young men with familial hypercholesterolemia. *J Am Coll Cardiol* 1996;28(7):1705–1711.

72. Mellwig K, Baller D, Gleichmann U, et al. Improvement of coronary vasodilatation capacity through single LDL apheresis. *Atherosclerosis* 1998;139(1):173–178.

73. Güthlin M, Kasel A, Coppenrath K, et al. Delayed response of myocardial flow reserve to lipid lowering therapy with fluvastatin. *Circulation* 1999;99:475–481.

74. Treasure C, Klein J, Weintraub W, et al. Beneficial effects of cholesterol-lowering therapy on the coronary endothelium in patients with coronary artery disease. *N Engl J Med* 1995;332:481–487.

75. Czernin J, Barnard R, Sun K, et al. Effect of short-term cardiovascular conditioning and low-fat diet on myocardial blood flow and flow reserve. *Circulation* 1995;92(2):197–204.

76. Czernin J, Sun K, Brunken R, et al. Effect of acute and long-term smoking on myocardial blood flow and flow reserve. *Circulation* 1995; 91(12):2891–2897.

77. Campisi R, Czernin J, Schoder H, et al. Effects of long-term smoking on myocardial blood flow, coronary vasomotion, and vasodilator capacity. *Circulation* 1998;98(2):119–125.

78. Gimelli A, Schneider-Eicke J, Neglia D, et al. Homogeneously reduced versus regionally impaired myocardial blood flow in hypertensive patients: two different patterns of myocardial perfusion associated with degree of hypertrophy. *J Am Coll Cardiol* 1998;31(2):366–373.

79. Radvan J, Choudhury L, Sheridan D, et al. Comparison of coronary vasodilator reserve in elite rowing athletes versus hypertrophic cardiomyopathy. *Am J Cardiol* 1997;80(12):1621–1623.

80. Parodi O, Neglia D, Palombo C, et al. Comparative effects of enalapril and verapamil on myocardial blood flow in systemic hypertension. *Circulation* 1997;96(3):864–873.

81. Camici PG, Gistri R, Lorenzoni R, et al. Coronary reserve and exercise ECG in patients with chest pain and normal coronary angiograms. *Circulation* 1992;86(1):179–186.

82. Rosen SD, Uren NG, Kaski JC, et al. Coronary vasodilator reserve, pain perception, and sex in patients with syndrome X. *Circulation* 1994; 90(1):50–60.

83. Camici P, Chiriatti G, Lorenzoni R, et al. Coronary vasodilation is impaired in both hypertrophied and nonhypertrophied myocardium of patients with hypertrophic cardiomyopathy: a study with nitrogen-13 ammonia and positron emission tomography. *J Am Coll Cardiol* 1991; 17(4):879–886.

84. Gistri R, Cecchi F, Choudhury L, et al. Effect of verapamil on absolute myocardial blood flow in hypertrophic cardiomyopathy. *Am J Cardiol* 1994;74(4):363–368.

85. Neglia D, Parodi O, Gallopin M, et al. Myocardial blood flow response to pacing tachycardia and to dipyridamole infusion in patients with dilated cardiomyopathy without overt heart failure. A quantitative assessment by positron emission tomography. *Circulation* 1995;92(4): 796–804.

86. Rechavia E, Araujo L, DeSilva R, et al. Dipyridamole vasodilator response after human orthotopic heart transplantation: quantification by oxygen-15-labeled water and positron emission tomography. *J Am Coll Cardiol* 1992;19(1):100–106.

87. Krivokapich J, Stevenson LW, Kobashigawa J, et al. Quantification of absolute myocardial perfusion at rest and during exercise with positron emission tomography after human cardiac transplantation. *J Am Coll Cardiol* 1991;18(2):512–517.

88. Kofoed K, Czernin J, Johnson J, et al. Effects of cardiac allograft vasculopathy on myocardial blood flow, vasodilatory capacity, and coronary vasomotion. *Circulation* 1997;95(3):600–606.

89. Chan SY, Kobashigawa J, Stevenson LW, et al. Myocardial blood flow at rest and during pharmacological vasodilation in cardiac transplants during and after successful treatment of rejection. *Circulation* 1994; 90(1):204–212.

90. Muzik O, Paridon S, Singh T, et al. Quantification of myocardial blood flow and flow reserve in children with a history of Kawasaki disease and normal coronary arteries using positron emission tomography. *J Am Coll Cardiol* 1996;28(3):757–762.

91. Bengel F, Hauser M, Duvernoy C, et al. Myocardial blood flow and coronary flow reserve late after anatomical correction of transposition of the great arteries. *J Am Coll Cardiol* 1998;32:1955–1961.

92. Yonekura Y, Tamaki N, Senda M, et al. Detection of coronary artery disease with 13N-ammonia and high-resolution positron-emission computed tomography. *Am Heart J* 1987;113:645–654.

93. Stewart R, Schwaiger M, Molina E, et al. Comparison of rubidium-82

positron emission tomography and thallium-201 SPECT imaging for detection of coronary artery disease. *Am J Cardiol* 1991;67:1303–1310.

94. Tamaki N, Yonekura Y, Senda M, et al. Myocardial positron computed tomography with 13N-ammonia at rest and during exercise. *Eur J Nucl Med* 1985;11:246–251.

95. Camici P, Marracini P, Marzilli M. Coronary hemodynamics and myocardial metabolism during and after pacing stress in normal humans. *Am J Physiol* 1989;257:E309.

96. Geltman E, Henes C, Senneff M, et al. Increased myocardial perfusion at rest and dimished perfusion reserve in patients with angina and angiographically normal coronary arteries. *J Am Coll Cardiol* 1990;16(3): 586–595.

97. Sambuceti G, Parodi O, Marcassa C, et al. Alteration in regulation of myocardial blood flow in one-vessel coronary artery disease determined by positron emission tomography. *Am J Cardiol* 1993;72: 538–543.

CHAPTER 15

Myocardial Viability

Radionuclide-based Methods

James A. Arrighi and Vasken Dilsizian

Substantial data now exist to indicate that under certain conditions, when viable myocytes are subjected to ischemia, prolonged alterations in regional left ventricular function may occur, which may lead to global left ventricular dysfunction (1–7). The concepts of stunning and hibernation, represent two pathophysiologic states that may alone or in combination result in reversible left ventricular dysfunction (2,4). The goal of myocardial viability assessment, is to differentiate, prospectively, patients with potentially reversible (hibernating or stunned) from irreversible (scarred or fibrotic) left ventricular dysfunction whose prognosis may be favorably altered with revascularization. This may result in more appropriate utilization of health care resources.

Currently, there are a number of diagnostic techniques for assessing myocardial viability. Among them, evaluation of regional perfusion, cell membrane integrity, and metabolism using nuclear techniques, as well as contractile reserve with low-dose dobutamine echocardiography, have proven to be fairly accurate in the clinical setting. Newer modalities include the use of metabolic tracers with single photon emission tomography (SPECT), more precise quantitative metabolic evaluations with positron emission tomography (PET), echocardiographic assessment of perfusion with contrast agents, and the use of magnetic resonance imaging. This chapter will focus on the assessment of myocardial viability using radionuclide-based methods (SPECT and PET).

J. A. Arrighi: Section of Cardiovascular Medicine, Yale University, New Haven, Connecticut 06520; Section of Nuclear Medicine, Veterans Administration Healthcare System, West Haven, Connecticut 06516.

V. Dilsizian: Georgetown University School of Medicine, Washington, District of Columbia 20007; Department of Cardiology and Nuclear Medicine, National Institutes of Health, Bethesda, Maryland 20892.

THALLIUM-201 IMAGING

Thallium has been a clinically important tracer with which to assess both regional blood flow and myocardial viability. The biological properties of thallium (a group IIIA metallic element) is similar to potassium. Because potassium is the major intracellular cation in muscle and is essentially absent in scar tissue, potassium analogs such as thallium are particularly well suited for differentiating viable from nonviable, scarred myocardium. Like potassium, thallium crosses the cell membrane via the active Na-K ATPase transport system and by facilitative diffusion (8,9). There are a number of thallium protocols that are clinically used for assessing myocardial viability (Fig. 1). Strengths and weaknesses of these various protocols are discussed below.

Stress Redistribution

The initial distribution of thallium in the myocardium (during stress or at rest) is dependent on regional blood flow and the extraction fraction of the tracer by the myocardium. Peak myocardial concentration of thallium generally occurs within 5 minutes of intravenous injection. At normal (physiologic) flow rates, the first-pass extraction fraction of thallium is in the range of 85% with rapid clearance of thallium from the intravascular compartment to the peripheral, extracardiac compartments. At high (nonphysiologic) flow rates, which may occur during the infusion of coronary vasodilators such as adenosine or dipyridamole, thallium extraction rises proportionally less. Thus, the linear relationship between blood flow and thallium uptake is preserved except for very high flow rates. Experimental studies with thallium have shown that the cellular extraction of the tracer across the sarcolemma membrane is unaffected by hypoxia unless irreversible injury is present (10,11). Similarly, pathophysio-

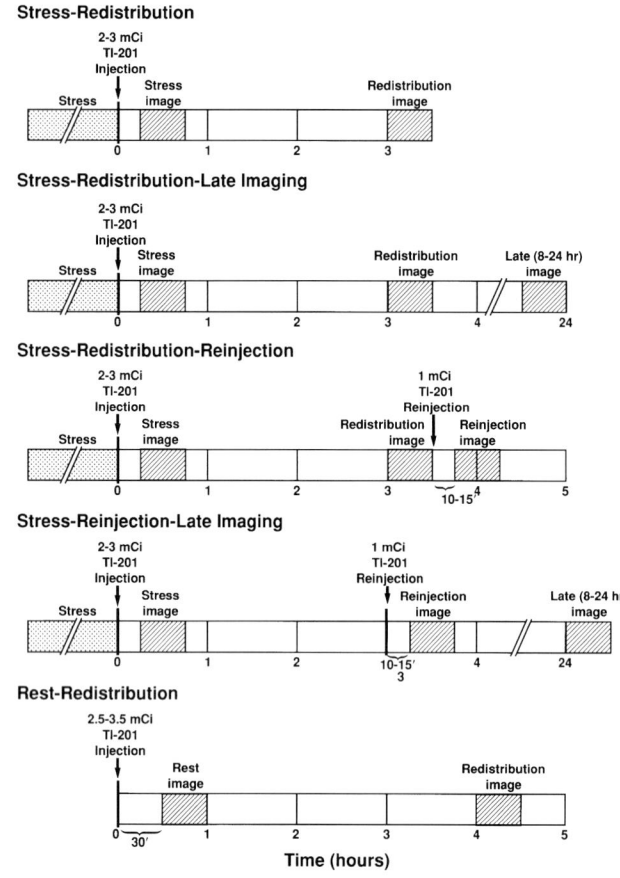

FIG. 1. Thallium protocols that are used clinically for assessing myocardial viability. (From ref. 117, with permission.)

logic conditions in which regional contractile function is impaired in the presence of myocardial viability (as in hibernation and stunning), do not adversely alter thallium extraction (12–14). Therefore, decreased myocardial thallium uptake on the initial images implies reduced myocardial perfusion that could be caused either by reduced regional blood flow or infarction.

The delayed (3 to 4 hour) redistribution phase of thallium reflects the continued balance of myocardial extraction of thallium (from the intravascular compartment) and myocar-

dial washout of thallium (to the extracardiac compartments). In animal studies, redistribution phase was shown to represent reduced thallium activity in normal regions along with increased thallium activity in ischemic regions (15–17). Thus, during redistribution, there is continuous exchange of thallium between the myocardium and the extracardiac compartments, driven by the concentration gradient of thallium and myocyte viability.

The extent of defect resolution from the initial to redistribution images, termed reversible defect, reflects viable myocardium. If the initial defect was produced during exercise or pharmacologic stress, then the reversible defect indicates ischemic but viable myocardium. When the extent of initial thallium defect (with stress or at rest) persists over time without redistribution, it is termed irreversible or fixed defect, which connotes scarred myocardium. Partial reversibility from the initial to redistribution images may represent an admixture of both viable and scarred myocardium (Table 1).

In clinical studies, stress-induced thallium defects that redistribute on 3-to-4 hour delayed images are accurate indicators of ischemic but viable myocardium. However, the converse, abnormal thallium defects during stress that persist on 3-to-4 hour redistribution images, does not necessarily indicate myocardial scar. Many patients with persistent thallium defects on stress-redistribution imaging may have no history of prior myocardial infarction (18–23). When quantitative analysis was applied, 45% of segments with irreversible thallium defects on conventional stress-redistribution studies showed improved or normal thallium uptake after revascularization (19). Segments that were likely to improve had thallium activity that was greater than 50% of the activity in normal reference regions. Thus, in patients with chronic coronary artery disease, stress-redistribution imaging may underestimate the presence of ischemic but viable myocardium.

Late (8-to-24 Hour) Redistribution

Because defect resolution of thallium from the initial to redistribution images is dependent on the equilibrium be-

TABLE 1. *Assessment of myocardial viability with SPECT: stress protocols*

Scintigraphic interpretation	Clinical interpretation	Probability of functional recovery after revascularization
I. Reversible defects		
• Complete	Ischemic, viable myocardium	High
• Partial	Ischemic, mixed viable/scarred myocardium	Likely
II. Irreversible defects		
• Mild–Moderate	Nonischemic, mixed viable/scarred myocardium	Low
• Severe	Nonischemic, scarred myocardium	Unlikely

(From ref. 172, with permission.)

tween myocardial extraction and washout of thallium with the extracardiac compartments, it is possible that in some patients the 3-to-4 hour time interval for redistribution is too short. Thus, if a greater time is allowed for redistribution the identification of viable myocardium may be improved.

In a series of patients with coronary artery disease, 21% of regions with fixed thallium defects on the 3-to-4 hour redistribution images showed defect reversibility when late (18-to-24 hours) redistribution images were obtained after exercise (18). Myocardial regions demonstrating such late redistribution were usually supplied by critically stenosed coronary arteries. In a subsequent prospective study, late redistribution was observed in 22% of the regions with fixed 4-hour defects, representing 53% of the patients (19). However, despite implementing 50% longer image acquisition time, a number of late redistribution studies had suboptimal count statistics at 24 hours.

Among regions demonstrating late redistribution, 95% showed improved thallium uptake after revascularization (24). However, 37% of regions that remained irreversible on both 3-to-4 hour and 24-hour studies also showed improved thallium uptake after revascularization. These data suggest that although late redistribution improves the identification of viable myocardium when compared to 3-to-4 hour redistribution imaging, it remains an inaccurate marker for scarred myocardium.

Thallium Reinjection

In 1990, we introduced the concept that reinjection of a second dose of 1 mCi (37 MBq) of thallium at rest immediately after stress-3-to-4 hour redistribution imaging improves the detection of viable myocardium (20,21). Among 100 patients with coronary artery disease studied using thallium SPECT, 49% of fixed defects on 3-to-4 hour redistribution images demonstrated improved or normal thallium uptake after reinjection (20). A patient example demonstrating the thallium reinjection effect is shown in Figure 2. Among regions that were identified as viable by thallium reinjection (and successfully revascularized), 87% showed normal thallium uptake and improved regional wall motion after revascularization. In contrast, all regions with irreversible defects on reinjection imaging before revascularization had abnormal thallium uptake and regional wall motion after revascularization. These results were confirmed subsequently in other medical centers (22,23,25–29), as well as in a multicenter trial (30).

To determine whether delaying the redistribution period between reinjection and repeat imaging from 10 minutes to 24 hours may identify additional viable regions, 50 patients with chronic coronary artery disease underwent four sets of images (stress, 3-to-4 hour redistribution, reinjection, and 24-hour redistribution images) (31). In this study, only 11% of myocardial regions (involving 6% of patients) that re-

Stress

Redistribution

Reinjection

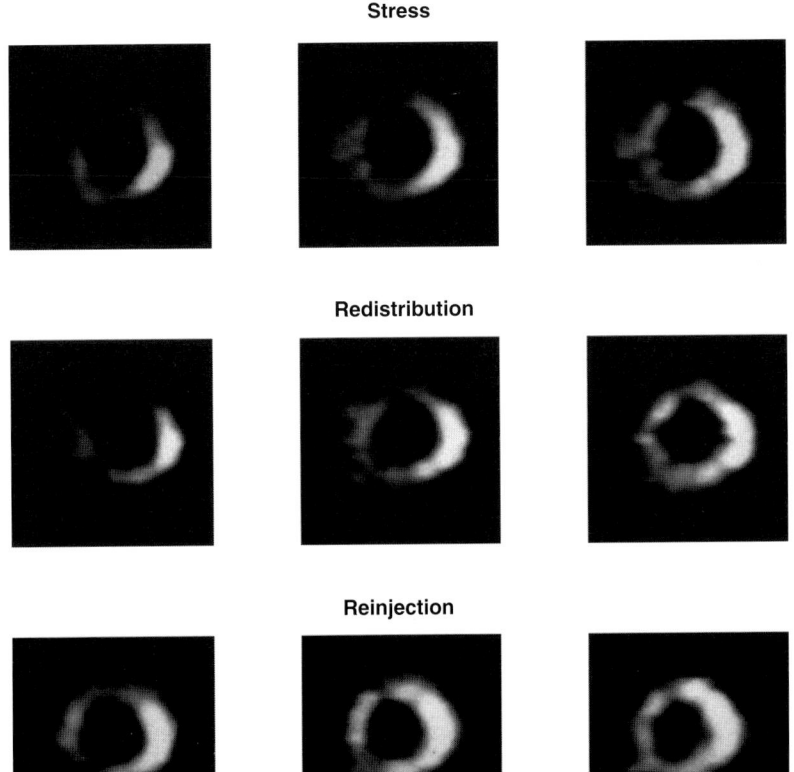

FIG. 2. Short-axis Tl-201 tomograms during stress, redistribution, and reinjection imaging in a patient with coronary artery disease. There are extensive Tl-201 abnormalities in the anterior and septal regions during stress that persist on redistribution images but improve markedly on reinjection images. (From ref. 20, with permission.)

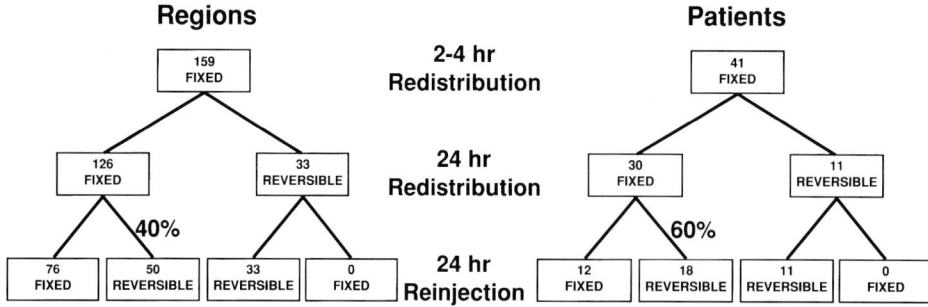

FIG. 3. Flow diagram displaying the fate of "fixed" thallium defects on the 2- to 4-hour standard redistribution studies, 24-hour redistribution, and after reinjection of thallium at 24 hours. (From ref. 38, with permission.)

mained irreversible after both 3-to-4 hour redistribution and reinjection showed evidence of late redistribution. It was concluded that all clinically relevant information pertaining to viability was obtained by a stress-redistribution-reinjection protocol. The data also showed that reinjection of thallium without acquiring 3-to-4 hour redistribution images could be confounded by underperfusion at rest, such that some stress-induced thallium defects that become reversible with redistribution will seem to worsen after thallium reinjection (32). Thus, for most accurate assessment of myocardial viability, three sets of images should be acquired, either stress-redistribution-reinjection or stress-reinjection-late redistribution imaging.

Explanation for the Salutary Results of Thallium Reinjection

The initial (poststress) myocardial distribution of thallium reflects regional blood flow while the subsequent redistribution of thallium in a given stress-induced defect may depend not only on the severity of the initial defect but also on the presence of viable myocytes (33), the concentration of the tracer in the blood (34,35), and the rate of decline of thallium levels in the blood (36). If the blood-thallium level remains the same (or increases) during the period between stress and 3-to-4 hour redistribution imaging, then an apparent defect in a region with viable myocytes that can retain thallium should improve. On the other hand, if the thallium concentration in the blood is low or decreases during the imaging interval, the delivery of thallium may be insufficient, and stress-induced defect may remain irreversible even though the underlying myocardium is viable (37). This suggests that some ischemic but viable regions may never redistribute, even with late (24-hour) imaging, unless blood levels of thallium are increased. This hypothesis is supported by a study where thallium reinjection was performed immediately after 24-hour redistribution images were obtained (38). Improved thallium uptake after reinjection occurred in 40% of defects (representing 60% of patients) that appeared irreversible on late (24-hour) redistribution images (Fig. 3). This

percentage is remarkably similar to the 37% of irreversible defects at 24 hours that improve after revascularization, as previously reported (24).

Prognostic Value of Thallium Reinjection

Currently, there are three studies in the literature that have assessed the prognostic value of thallium reinjection; all using planar technique (39–41). In patients with coronary artery disease and left ventricular dysfunction, thallium reinjection provided incremental prognostic information to clinical, exercise, and thallium stress-redistribution data (Fig. 4) (39). In another study of similar patient population, the scintigraphic variable that was the strongest predictor of cardiac death or myocardial infarction was the presence of more than three irreversible defects that remained fixed after thallium reinjection (40). In a retrospective study, when the prognostic value of thallium reinjection was assessed among patients

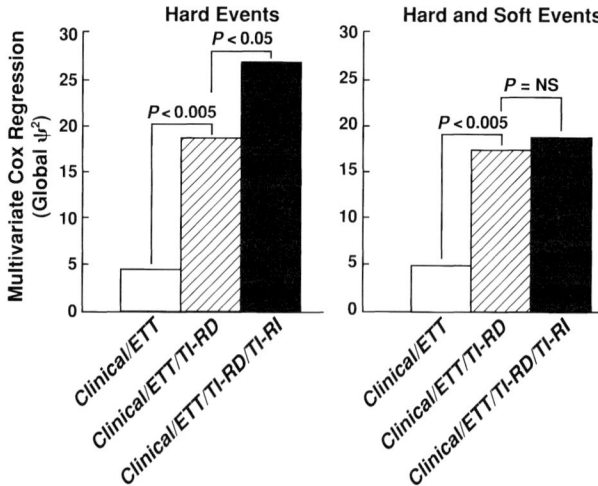

FIG. 4. Incremental prognostic value (global chi-squared values on y-axis) of clinical, electrocardiogram stress test (*ETT*), thallium stress-redistribution (*Tl-RD*) and reinjection (*Tl-RI*) data for hard events (**left**) and for hard and soft events combined (**right**). (From ref. 39, with permission.)

not selected for left ventricular dysfunction or prior myocardial infarction, the number of reversible thallium defects was not predictive of future cardiac events on either redistribution or reinjection studies (41). Whether the application of SPECT imaging (with quantitation of defect severity) in patients with chronic coronary artery disease and left ventricular dysfunction (in whom the assessment of myocardial viability is pertinent) will reinforce the prognostic value of thallium reinjection is a subject of ongoing investigation.

Rest-redistribution Imaging

Stress thallium protocols provide important information regarding both inducible ischemia and myocardial viability. However, among patients with known coronary artery disease, if the clinical question is one of the presence or absence of viable myocardium within dysfunctional regions, then it is reasonable to perform only rest-redistribution thallium imaging.

Thallium defects on resting images have been observed in patients with severe coronary artery disease in the absence of an acute ischemic process or previous myocardial infarction (42). In addition, it has been recognized that many of these defects on the resting images may redistribute over the next 3 to 4 hours. Since these initial reports, several studies have evaluated the utility of rest-redistribution thallium studies in predicting recovery of asynergic myocardial regions after revascularization (43–45). Using quantitative analysis,

when myocardial viability was defined as thallium activity greater than 50% of peak activity in normal regions, 57% of asynergic regions that were viable by thallium showed improved wall motion after surgery, compared to only 23% of asynergic regions that were considered to be nonviable by thallium (46). Moreover, the number of asynergic but viable myocardial regions correlated well with postoperative improvement in global left ventricular function. Recent studies confirm the utility of quantitative analysis of rest-redistribution studies for predicting recovery of function after revascularization (47–50).

In another study, quantitative thallium findings obtained from patients undergoing both stress-redistribution-reinjection and rest-redistribution SPECT imaging were compared (Fig. 5) (51). Beyond classifying regions as reversible or irreversible, when the severity of thallium defects was assessed (mild-to-moderate versus severe) within irreversible defects, the concordance between stress-redistribution-reinjection and rest-redistribution imaging regarding myocardial viability was 94% (51). These data suggest that while the pattern of defect reversibility on rest-redistribution thallium imaging may be important in some patients, the final thallium content of rest-redistribution images also provides insight into viability and recovery of function after revascularization.

If the clinical question is one of myocardial viability within dysfunctional myocardial regions, then a rest-redistribution thallium protocol may suffice. On the other hand, if

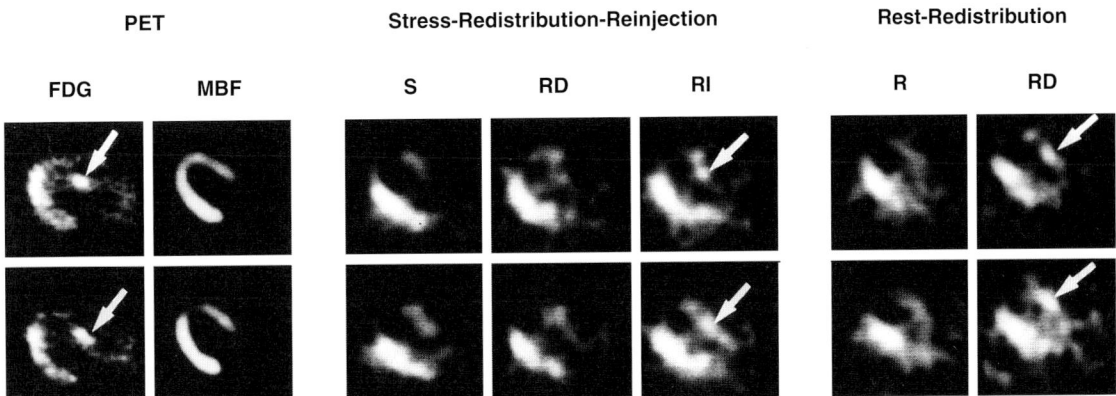

FIG. 5. Concordance between positron emission tomography (*PET*), stress-redistribution-reinjection, and rest-redistribution imaging is demonstrated in this patient example. Two consecutive transaxial tomograms are displayed for fluorodeoxyglucose (*FDG*) and myocardial blood flow (*MBF*) by PET, with corresponding thallium tomograms of stress (*S*), redistribution (*RD*), reinjection (*RI*) and rest(*R*)-redistribution. On the PET study, myocardial blood flow is reduced in the anteroapical, anteroseptal, and posteroseptal regions. FDG uptake in the corresponding regions demonstrate a *mismatch* in the posteroseptal region (*arrow*) and a *match* between FDG uptake and blood flow in the anteroapical and anteroseptal regions. Corresponding SPECT thallium images reveal extensive perfusion abnormalities involving the apical and septal regions during stress, which persist on redistribution images. However, thallium reinjection images show improved thallium uptake in the posteroseptal region (*arrow*), while the apical region remains fixed. On rest-redistribution images, the apical region has severely reduced thallium activity, which remains fixed, while the posteroseptal region that was abnormal on the initial rest study shows significant improvement on 3-to-4 hour redistribution study, suggesting viable myocardium. (From ref. 51, with permission.)

the clinical question is one of ischemia and viability, then reasonable options include stress-redistribution-reinjection imaging, stress-reinjection-late redistribution imaging, or stress-redistribution imaging with separate-day rest-redistribution study.

ISSUES REGARDING INTERPRETATION OF THALLIUM STUDIES THAT MERIT EMPHASIS

Functional Outcome after Revascularization Is Critically Dependent on the Adequacy of Revascularization

For an asynergic region to improve function after revascularization, it must not only retain viable myocardium but also be adequately revascularized (20,26). When taking into consideration regions with reversible thallium defects (demonstration of myocardial ischemia) and success of revascularization (reexamining regional perfusion or vessel patency after revascularization), stress-redistribution-reinjection thallium imaging yields excellent positive and negative predictive accuracy (80 to 90% range) for recovery of function after revascularization (20,52). Most recent comparative studies utilizing thallium reinjection technique with dobutamine echocardiography do not reexamine regional perfusion or vessel patency after revascularization. Although functional studies are acquired before and after the revascularization (usually echocardiography), repeat thallium studies or coronary angiography are not performed postoperatively (22,25,27,28,30). Furthermore, application of the same imaging modality (echocardiography) to both "test" and "confirm" myocardial viability before and after revascularization raises the potential for unintentional yet important bias against thallium scintigraphy, favoring more accurate anatomic alignment of corresponding echocardiographic regions before and after revascularization (53). This may explain, in part, the greater specificity achieved with dobutamine echocardiography when compared to thallium in recent publications.

Defect Severity: Mild-to-moderate versus Severe Irreversible Defects

There is ample evidence for thallium as well as other radiotracers that, in general, the degree of radiotracer uptake on resting or redistribution images correlates with myocardial viability. From comparative metabolic PET and thallium SPECT studies, among regions considered "irreversible" on redistribution images, the severity of reduction in thallium activity correlated with the degree of metabolic activity as assessed by F-18 fluorodeoxyglucose (FDG) uptake. FDG uptake was preserved in 91% of mildly reduced (60 to 84% of peak activity) and 84% of moderately reduced (50 to 59% of peak activity) irreversible thallium defects (54). The concordance of stress-redistribution-reinjection thallium and FDG PET imaging is excellent (up to 88%) when quantitative image analysis is employed (54,55).

In a comparative clinicopathological study, the magnitude of thallium activity within irreversible preoperative stress-redistribution-reinjection thallium images correlated with the extent of interstitial fibrosis determined from intraoperative transmural left ventricular biopsies (56). There was a good overall inverse correlation between percent thallium activity on redistribution and reinjection images and percent interstitial fibrosis in biopsy specimens (Fig. 6). However, it is important to point out that the presence of viable tissue in regions with mild-to-moderately reduced thallium defects does not necessarily imply the potential of such regions to improve function after revascularization. Thus, a potential limitation inherent in many comparative studies of thallium reinjection with echocardiography is in the grouping of stress-induced reversible and mild-to-moderately reduced ir-

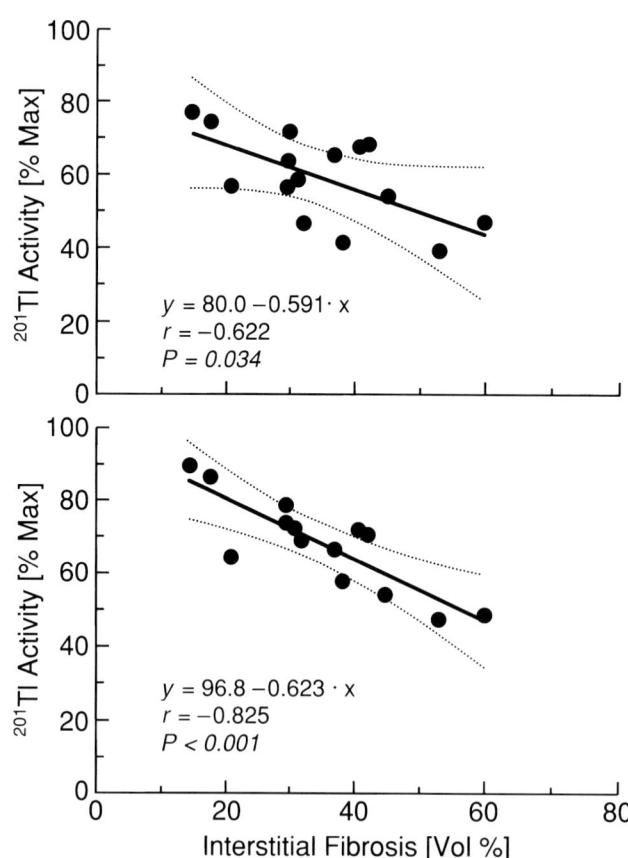

FIG. 6. Graphs showing the relation between regional Tl-201 activity on redistribution (**top panel**) and reinjection (**bottom panel**) images and regional volume fraction of interstitial fibrosis in patients with chronic stable coronary artery disease undergoing coronary artery bypass surgery. Two transmural biopsy specimens were taken during surgery and volume fraction of interstitial fibrosis was assessed by use of light microscopic morphometry. *Dotted lines* indicate 95% confidence limits for the regression line. Percentage of maximum normal activity is indicated by *% Max*. When compared to redistribution images, regression analysis reveals a significantly improved correlation (*P* < 0.01) between Tl-201 reinjection and regional volume fraction of interstitial fibrosis. (From ref. 56, with permission.)

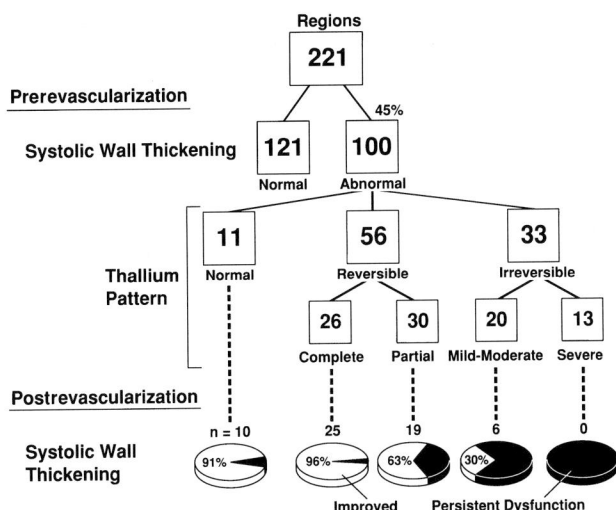

FIG. 7. Flow diagram of prerevascularization systolic wall thickening and thallium pattern and postrevascularization functional outcome of the 221 revascularized regions. (From ref. 52, with permission.)

reversible thallium defects. When performing rest-redistribution studies, mild-to-moderate irreversible thallium defects represent viable myocardium with the potential of recovery after revascularization. On the other hand, most mild-to-moderate irreversible thallium defects on stress studies represent an admixture of viable (nonischemic) and scarred myocardium, and therefore, may not recover function after revascularization (Fig. 7).

Stress-induced Ischemia

Inasmuch as we now believe that the left ventricular dysfunction in coronary artery disease could result from prior myocardial infarction and/or a combination of hibernation and repetitive stunning, it is intuitive to think that stress-induced reversible defects may be a stronger predictor of functional recovery after revascularization than mild-to-moderate irreversible defects. In patients who underwent exercise-redistribution-reinjection thallium SPECT before and after revascularization, regional contraction improved in 79% of asynergic regions with reversible thallium defects, compared with 30% of regions with irreversible defects ($P < 0.001$) (52). Importantly, when all asynergic regions were grouped according to the final thallium content (maximum tracer uptake on redistribution-reinjection images), functional recovery was observed in 83% of regions with reversible defects compared to 33% of regions with irreversible defects ($P < 0.001$). These data suggest that the identification of reversible thallium defects (inducible ischemia) in asynergic regions more accurately predicts functional recovery after revascularization than does final thallium content (severity of defect) alone. Thus, a more accurate noninvasive determination of myocardial viability requires the demonstration of myocardial ischemia (Fig. 7).

TECHNETIUM-99m LABELED PERFUSION TRACERS

While the physiologic properties of thallium make it ideally suited for viability imaging, its physical properties are less ideal from an imaging standpoint. Its low-energy gamma emission and long half-life limits the injected dose and makes it particularly prone to effects of attenuation. As such, much interest has emerged in developing Tc-99m-based tracers of myocardial perfusion and viability. The physical advantages of Tc-99m over thallium include a shorter half-life, which permits a larger injected dose, and an energy spectrum (140keV) that is better suited for most imaging systems, resulting in better image resolution and count statistics. Although the physical properties of Tc-99m-based tracers are identical, the physiologic properties vary depending on the particular ligand. While each compound displays different kinetics, the concepts that their uptake is related to myocardial perfusion and that some aspect of their kinetics is related to cell membrane integrity and thus to viability, is common to each of them. Currently, three Tc-99m-based tracers have received United States Food and Drug Administration approval for myocardial perfusion imaging in the United States: sestamibi, tetrofosmin, and teboroxime. Among these, sestamibi is the tracer that has accumulated the most experience in the literature. Multicenter trials are currently underway for other Tc-99m-based tracers, such as Tc-99m-furifosmin (Q12) and TcN-99m-NOET.

Tc-99m-sestamibi

Tc-99m-sestamibi is a lipophilic cationic complex that is taken up by myocytes across mitochondrial membranes, but at equilibrium it is retained within the mitochondria due to a large negative transmembrane potential (57). Like thallium, initial uptake of sestamibi reflects both regional blood flow and myocardial extraction. Its extraction fraction is considerably less than that of thallium, and its uptake appears to reflect its lipophilicity rather than active transport processes. The dependence of sestamibi retention on intact mitochondrial membranes suggest that this agent may be a useful marker of myocardial viability, a concept that has been born out in clinical and experimental studies (58–60). In animal models of acute myocardial infarction, sestamibi uptake correlated closely with blood flow and postmortem angiographic risk area (59). However, when sestamibi was injected after reperfusion, its uptake tracked infarct size but not myocardial blood flow (Fig. 8). A good correlation between scintigraphic infarct size with sestamibi and pathologic infarct size has been demonstrated by other investigators (61). These findings in experimental animals were confirmed in patients studied in the setting of acute myocardial infarction and reperfusion (thrombolysis or acute angioplasty) (62,63). However, clinical studies examining the role of sestamibi for viability assessment in patients with chronic coronary artery disease have yielded mixed results.

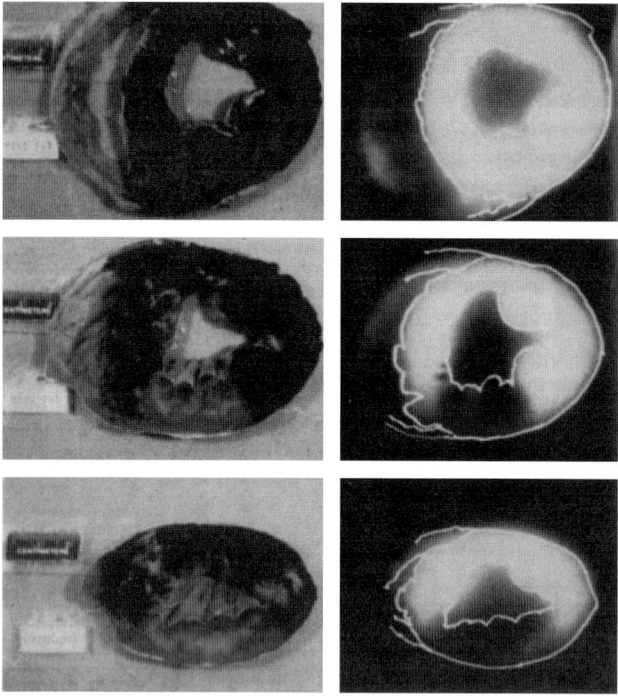

FIG. 8. Postmortem dual perfusion maps (**left panels**) and sestamibi autoradiographs (**right panels**) from a representative dog injected with sestamibi after reperfusion. Shown, on the **left,** are three slices oriented with the right ventricle on the **left** and the anterior wall of the left ventricle on the **bottom.** Infarct area is the pale unstained region within the risk area. Defects seen on unenhanced autoradiographs with superimposed overlay (**right**) correlate closely with the area of infarction defined by TTC staining. No significant sestamibi activity is seen in the central necrotic region, whereas some activity is seen in the perinecrotic area. Figure is reduced. (From ref. 59, with permission.)

Chronic Coronary Artery Disease

Using planar imaging and qualitative analysis, Cuocolo and coworkers (64) reported that 29% of reversible myocardial regions by thallium reinjection were underestimated as irreversible on a 2-day stress-rest sestamibi protocol. These initial observations were confirmed both with planar and SPECT imaging (65–78). Consequently, a number of approaches have emerged in order to optimize the utility of sestamibi, and other Tc-99m-based tracers, for viability assessment. The most important of these is quantitation of regional radiotracer activity within irreversible defects (65). Among patients undergoing stress-rest sestamibi and stress-redistribution-reinjection thallium SPECT, 36% of myocardial regions that were classified as ischemic and viable by thallium were misclassified as irreversible defects by sestamibi (65). However, quantitative analysis of relative tracer activity within the irreversible sestamibi defects increased the concordance between the two tracers to 93%. However, despite the application of quantitative techniques, other studies have reported that rest sestamibi imaging underestimates

myocardial viability when compared to PET (70,72, 74,76–78). In patients with chronic coronary artery disease undergoing rest sestamibi SPECT and FDG PET studies, Altehoefer et al. (70,74) reported a significant discordance in regions with severe sestamibi defects (less than 50% of peak activity) and FDG uptake (Fig. 9). Using similar threshold quantitative values for viability, Sawada et al. (72) studied patients with previous myocardial infarction and found that 47% of segments with severe sestamibi defects had preserved metabolic activity as assessed by FDG PET.

In an attempt to delineate potential factors affecting accuracy of sestamibi in assessing viability, the results of sestamibi SPECT and FDG PET were compared in patients with varying degrees of left ventricular dysfunction. The concordance between sestamibi and FDG was 64% in patients with severe left ventricular dysfunction and 78% in patients with mild-to-moderate left ventricular dysfunction (78). In particular, only 42% of regions with blood flow:metabolism mismatch pattern by PET (the pattern most predictive of functional recovery after revascularization), were identified as viable by quantitative sestamibi SPECT. These data suggest a potential influence of both left ventricular function and regional perfusion on the ability of sestamibi to track myocardial viability.

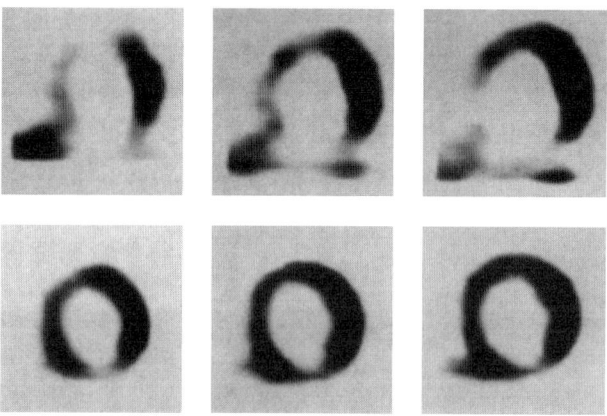

FIG. 9. Discordance between positron emission tomography (PET) and rest sestamibi single photon emission computed tomography (SPECT) imaging is demonstrated in this patient with three-vessel coronary artery disease. Three consecutive short-axis tomograms are displayed for technetium-99m sestamibi (**top**), with corresponding fluorodeoxyglucose (FDG) PET tomograms (**bottom**). Rest sestamibi images reveal extensive perfusion abnormalities involving the anteroapical, septal, and inferior regions with preserved viability in the posterolateral region and mixed viable and scarred myocardium in the septal region. FDG uptake in the corresponding regions demonstrate preserved metabolic activity and viability in all three coronary artery vascular territories. The patient had totally occluded but collateralized left anterior descending and right coronary arteries and severe stenosis of the left circumflex artery. (From ref. 70, with permission.)

Delayed Sestamibi Images (Redistribution)

Another potential method to enhance viability detection with sestamibi is by acquisition of delayed (redistribution) images. Unlike thallium, the extent of sestamibi redistribution over a 2-to-4 hour period, postinjection, is significantly less. Nonetheless, redistribution of sestamibi has been demonstrated both in animals (79–82) and in human subjects (65–67,83,84). Using an experimental model of sustained low-flow ischemia, as one might expect to be present clinically in hibernation, Sinusas et al. (81) detected significant sestamibi redistribution over 2.5 hours both by gamma well counting and high-resolution postmortem imaging of myocardial slices. In patients with scintigraphic or angiographic evidence of coronary artery disease, significant differences in clearance rates between normal and ischemic myocardium were observed approximately 6 hours after sestamibi injection at peak stress (83). These differences in clearance rates were clinically relevant in up to 31% of regions with stress studies (66) and 44% of regions with rest-injected studies (Fig. 10) (65,67).

Functional Improvement after Revascularization

There are a number of studies in the literature that have examined the ability of sestamibi imaging to predict functional improvement after revascularization (47,67–69,75). The initial experience with sestamibi performed at rest, using quantitative analysis, resulted in favorable positive (80 to 82%) and negative (78% to 96%) predictive accuracies for functional recovery after revascularization (47,85) (Fig. 11). However, there are a number of other studies in the literature that suggest that sestamibi may underestimate myocardial viability, particularly in patients with severe left ventricular dysfunction (67–69,75). Whether the factors contributing to impaired sestamibi uptake and defect reversibility when compared to thallium relate to differences in extraction frac-

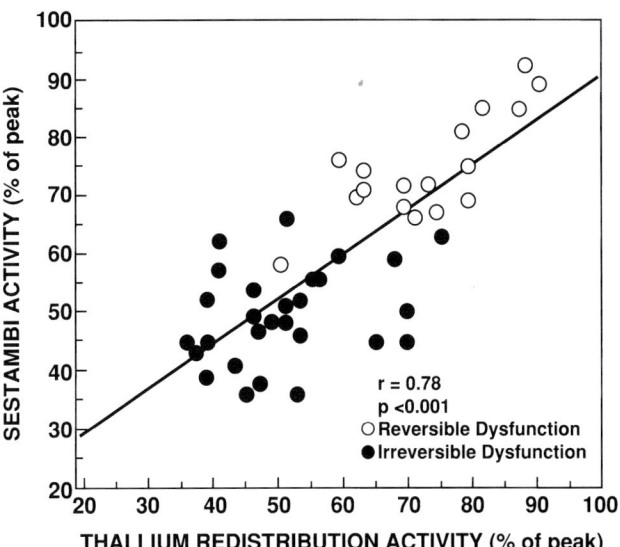

FIG. 11. Scatterplot showing correlation of quantitative regional activities of thallium (at redistribution imaging after rest injection) on the abscissa and regional activities of sestamibi (at rest) on the ordinate among segments with signficant regional dysfunction in patients undergoing revascularization. (From ref. 47, with permission.)

tion and/or redistribution remains unknown. Perhaps many of the potential limitations of sestamibi may be due to limitations in instrumentation rather than radiotracer. If so, emerging strategies such as gated SPECT perfusion (combined sestamibi perfusion and functional imaging) (86,87) and attenuation correction (88,89) may further enhance the utility of this radiotracer to detect myocardial viability. Other proposed strategies include combined stress sestamibi with rest-redistribution thallium (dual-isotope) imaging (90), administration of nitrate before sestamibi injection at rest (physiologic manipulation) (91,92), and acquisition of delayed (redistribution) images (65–67,79–84).

Tc-99m-tetrofosmin

Tc-99m-tetrofosmin is a lipophilic, cationic diphosphine that is distributed within the myocardium in proportion to regional blood flow (93,94). Like sestamibi, redistribution of tetrofosmin is minimal over time (95,96). Myocardial uptake and blood clearance kinetics of tetrofosmin are similar to sestamibi, but the clearance of tetrofosmin from the liver is faster than sestamibi, which may improve the resolution of early cardiac images. Experimental studies of low-flow ischemia and reperfused myocardial infarction suggest that both initial uptake and retention of tetrofosmin are reflective of myocardial viability (95,97,98).

In a multicenter trial, when the efficacy of tetrofosmin was compared with thallium (applying the standard stress-redistribution protocol), the overall concordance between the two tracers for defining normal or abnormal regions was approximately 80% using a stress protocol (99). However,

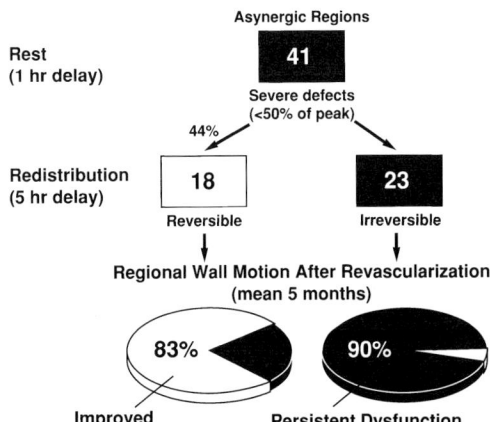

FIG. 10. Flow diagram displaying the prevalence of sestamibi redistribution and recovery of function after revascularization in asynergic regions with severe reduction in resting sestamibi images. (From ref. 67, with permission.)

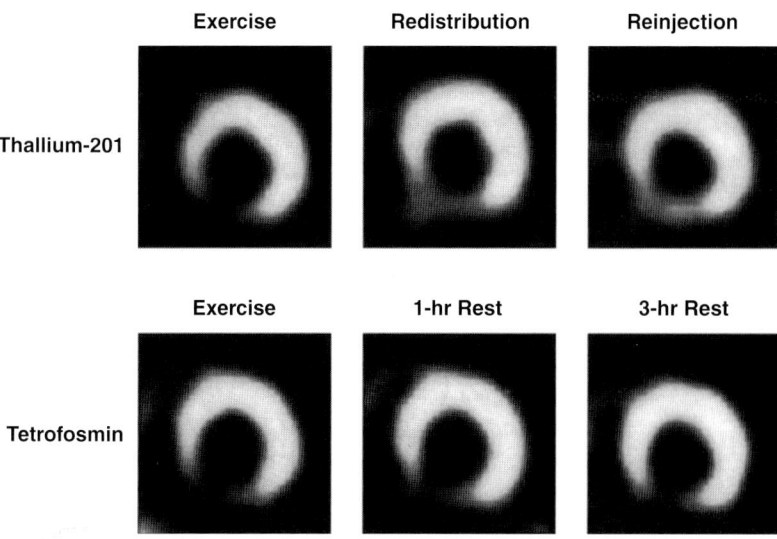

Exercise   Redistribution   Reinjection

Thallium-201

Exercise   1-hr Rest   3-hr Rest

Tetrofosmin

FIG. 12. An example of a patient with reversible thallium and irreversible tetrofosmin defects. Short-axis tomograms are displayed for thallium stress, redistribution, and reinjection with corresponding tetrofosmin stress, 1-hour delayed rest, and 3-hour delayed rest injected tomograms. Thallium tomograms reveal a severe inferior perfusion defect during stress with partial reversibility on redistribution and further improvement on reinjection images. Stress, 1-hour delayed rest and 3-hour delayed rest tetrofosmin images show a severe irreversible defect in the inferior region. (From ref. 100, with permission.)

when the data were further analyzed in the following subgroups: normal, ischemia, infarction, or mixed (infarction and viable) myocardium, the concordance between tetrofosmin and thallium decreased to only 59%. Among patients with coronary artery disease and left ventricular dysfunction, when the 2-day stress-rest tetrofosmin protocol was compared with thallium (utilizing the stress-redistribution-reinjection protocol), tetrofosmin and thallium provided discordant information in 40% of segments, 88% of which appeared irreversible on tetrofosmin images but reversible on thallium reinjection images (Fig. 12) (100). Approaches to enhance the diagnostic accuracy of tetrofosmin have developed and are analogous to those used for sestamibi (101,102).

Tc-99m-teboroxime

Tc-99m-teboroxime is a neutral, lipophilic compound with first-pass extraction fraction of 88% at rest and 91% under hyperemic conditions (103,104). After the initial uptake, teboroxime washes out rapidly from the myocardium at a rate proportional to regional blood flow. Both uptake and washout of teboroxime seem to depend predominantly upon regional myocardial blood flow and not by tissue metabolism or other binding characteristics within the myocardium (105,106). The rapid washout of teboroxime from myocardial cells makes SPECT imaging technically difficult. In clinical studies, teboroxime was shown to underestimate myocardial ischemia and viability when compared to thallium imaging (107–109). However, larger series are needed to define the utility of teboroxime for the assessment of myocardial viability.

Tc-99m-furifosmin

Tc-99m-furifosmin (Q12) is a mixed-ligand cationic complex that is linearly extracted by the myocardium for blood

flows up to 2 mL/gm/min (110). However, for blood flows above 2 mL/gm/min, as with pharmacologic stress studies, Q12 activity does not increase proportionately. Unlike thallium, Q12 does not redistribute significantly from the time of injection (110). In a pilot study, in which Q12 and thallium imaging were compared for detection of 50% or greater coronary artery stenosis by coronary angiography, the two tracers had comparable sensitivities and specificities (111). Although the overall concordance of Q12 and thallium were good in normal and irreversible regions, the concordance between stress-redistribution-reinjection thallium and rest-stress Q12 for detecting myocardial ischemia and viability (defect reversibility) was poor. Larger clinical trials are needed to better define the role of Q12 in assessing myocardial ischemia and viability.

TcN-99m-NOET

TcN-99m-NOET is a new Tc-99m-based perfusion tracer that redistributes significantly over time, with myocardial kinetics similar to thallium. In experimental models of sustained low-flow and transient coronary occlusion, serial NOET images showed significant defect resolution over several hours (112). Quantitative assessment showed that NOET redistribution resulted primarily from a greater clearance of tracer from normal areas compared with abnormal areas (differential washout) (112). Thus, NOET is a promising agent for assessing patients with coronary artery disease, and may have a role in viability assessment in the future (113). However, data regarding the utility of NOET in the clinical setting is limited.

POSITRON EMISSION TOMOGRAPHY

Positron emission tomography (PET) is a powerful noninvasive method that has been used to assess myocardial perfusion and metabolism, and, as such, has contributed much to our understanding of myocardial viability. From an instrumentation aspect, PET has several advantages over SPECT, including an accepted method to correct for attenuation effects, increased spatial resolution, and higher count densities. These factors, combined with the ability to synthesize unique radiotracers, have made it possible to use PET for absolute quantification of regional myocardial blood flow and metabolism. Such quantitative methods, however, primarily have been limited to the research arena. Clinical PET imaging is generally performed using assessments of relative radiotracer uptake, much like SPECT. A variety of radiotracers are available, and fall within two broad categories, those that track specific metabolic pathways and those that track blood flow. Like SPECT, most PET flow tracers possess dual characteristics in that while initial uptake relates to flow, some aspect of their kinetics reflects cell membrane integrity and thus viability. While SPECT development initially focused primarily on combined flow/metabolism tracers, initial PET development for viability assessment focused on metabolic tracers, particularly F-18 fluorodeoxyglucose (FDG).

Metabolic Imaging with PET

The assessment of myocardial metabolism is the most well established means by which to assess viability, and is based on the principle that scarred myocardium is relatively metabolically inactive compared to normal or ischemic myocardium. FDG is the primary radiotracer used for this purpose, and is capable of being imaged with high-energy SPECT imaging or new hybrid gamma/SPECT cameras. Other PET metabolic radiotracers include [11]carbon acetate and [11]carbon palmitate, which are used in selected centers primarily as research tools.

[18]F-2-fluoro-2-deoxyglucose

[18]F-2-fluoro-2-deoxyglucose, or FDG, is a metabolic marker for glucose uptake that competes with glucose for hexokinase and tracks transmembranous exchange of glucose (114). FDG is phosphorylated by hexokinase into FDG-6-phosphate, a form of deoxyglucose that cannot be metabolized further (115). Thus, myocardial uptake of FDG reflects the overall rate of transmembrane exchange and phosphorylation of glucose, but its uptake does not selectively track any of the potential metabolic pathways of glucose metabolism such as glycolysis, glycogen synthesis, or the fructose-pentose shunt. Because the dephosphorylation rate of glucose is slow, FDG becomes essentially trapped in the myocardium, and measurement of its uptake reflects regional glucose flux.

In the fasting state, free fatty acids are the preferred substrate for cardiac metabolism, and glucose uptake is relatively low. In the fed state, insulin levels increase and lead to a number of metabolic alterations in the heart, including stimulation of glucose metabolism and inhibition of tissue lipolysis. With ischemia, metabolic alterations include lac-

tate production, enhanced glucose uptake, and a shift toward increased glucose utilization through enhanced glycolysis. While the energy produced by enhanced glycolysis may be sufficient to maintain cellular viability, it may be inadequate to maintain mechanical work, i.e., cellular contraction. The signature of viable myocardium with FDG imaging thus is preserved or *enhanced* regional FDG uptake.

Clinical Assessment of the Viability of Using FDG

For the clinical assessment of myocardial viability, FDG imaging usually is combined with resting perfusion imaging. This is partly due to the fact that FDG uptake may be increased in abnormal, ischemic regions. Stated in other terms, normalization of an FDG study to the "hottest" pixel within the myocardium may not be appropriate, since this region may, in fact, have above normal FDG uptake. Thus, FDG images usually are compared to resting perfusion images, and regions with normal resting perfusion are generally considered viable by perfusion criteria alone. If semiquantitative methods are used (e.g., circumferential analysis), FDG images may be normalized to the perfusion images. Studies are usually performed after oral glucose loading (50 gm) in nondiabetic patients, or after administration of insulin with or without glucose in diabetic patients.

Several patterns of perfusion and FDG uptake have been recognized (Fig. 13) (116,117). As noted above, if perfusion is normal, regions are considered viable on the basis of perfusion criteria alone. Among regions with resting hypoperfusion, two patterns of radiotracer uptake have been recognized: a concordant decrease in both perfusion and metabolism (termed flow-metabolism "match") and a discordant increase in FDG uptake compared with decreased perfusion (termed flow-metabolism "mismatch"). Flow-metabolism mismatch is considered to represent viable, ischemic myocardium. Flow-metabolism match may be severe (that is, considered to represent scar) or mild-to-moderate in severity (that is, considered to represent an admixture of scar and viable myocardium).

Initial studies evaluated the utility of resting N-13 ammonia/FDG PET for determination of whether enhanced or preserved FDG uptake was capable of predicting function improvement after revascularization (116,118). These studies indicated positive predictive accuracies of 78 to 85% and negative predictive accuracies of 78 to 92%. Subsequent studies have confirmed similar predictive accuracies for functional recovery (or lack thereof) (119–123).

Strengths and Limitations of FDG Metabolic Imaging

Several concepts regarding viability assessment with FDG PET warrant emphasis. First, the predictive value of FDG PET for functional improvement is highest among regions with more severe resting dysfunction (severe hypokinesis or akinesis) (124). This underscores the importance of appropriate patient selection for viability assessment. Second, the

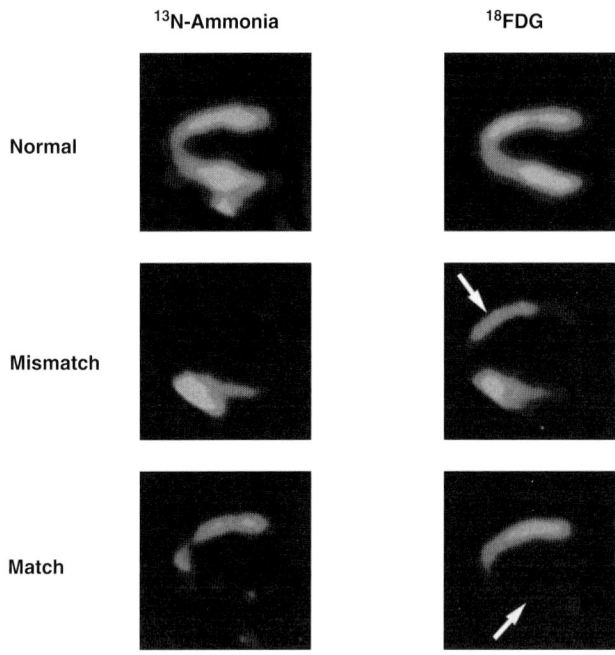

¹³N-Ammonia   ¹⁸FDG

Normal

Mismatch

Match

FIG. 13. Cross-sectional vertical long-axis PET images are shown for ¹³N-ammonia and ¹⁸F-FDG. **Top panel** shows examples of *normal* ¹³N-ammonia and ¹⁸F-FDG uptake. **Middle panel** shows discordance between ¹⁸F-FDG uptake and ¹³N-ammonia uptake (FDG-blood flow *mismatch*) in the anterior region indicative of viable myocardium (*arrow*). **Lower panel** shows concordant severely reduced ¹³N-ammonia and ¹⁸F-FDG uptake (FDG-blood flow *match*) in the inferior region indicative of myocardial scar (*arrow*). (From ref. 117, with permission.)

specific pattern of flow-metabolism mismatch, which represents a subset of all viable myocardium, is associated with the greatest likelihood of functional improvement after revascularization (125). Third, approximately 10% of patients with clinical or subclinical diabetes mellitus will have unintelligible FDG studies, due to poor radiotracer uptake. An insulin clamp procedure may reduce this incidence. Fourth, the utility of FDG imaging early (within 1 week) after infarction is unclear, and studies suggest an overestimation of viability based on FDG uptake in this setting (126). Finally, although it is technically feasible to quantify regional myocardial glucose uptake with PET, regional uptake values vary considerably from patient to patient, and have not been shown to improve assessment of viability over the measurement of normalized FDG uptake values (127).

FDG SPECT

Because of the relatively long physical half-life of ¹⁸F (110 minutes), offsite production of FDG and subsequent transport to satellite nuclear cardiology laboratories has recently been proposed. This, combined with the advent of SPECT technology, has made possible the use of FDG

SPECT for detection of myocardial viability (Fig. 14) (128–131). This can be accomplished by using either high-energy collimation (true single-photon imaging) or with coincidence detection (hybrid PET-SPECT) systems. In general, the resolution of these systems (particularly with high-energy collimated SPECT) is lower than that of dedicated PET systems, and attenuation correction is often not available or not yet validated. Therefore, large scale clinical trials comparing dedicated PET to these FDG SPECT or hybrid PET SPECT systems are needed prior to clinical extrapolation of these results of clinical studies using dedicated PET compared to these less expensive systems.

¹¹Carbon Acetate

¹¹Carbon acetate is taken up by the myocardium in proportion to blood flow, and its washout rate is directly related to oxidative metabolism. In theory, acetate may thus be used to assess both perfusion and metabolism, although considerable rolloff of extraction fraction at high flows may limit its utility during hyperemia (132). The clinical utility of acetate imaging has been limited by the necessity of acquiring images dynamically and generating regional time-activity curves for analysis. Potential advantages over FDG include a shorter imaging time, shorter radioisotope half-life (20 minutes for ¹¹C), and lower incidence of unintelligible studies in patients with diabetes. The major disadvantage is the need for an onsite cyclotron. In contrast, a nationwide distribution system for the 110 minute half-life fluorine 18 of FDG has already been established.

Although the data for acetate are fewer compared with FDG, the data that do exist are promising. Analysis of the initial portion of the time-activity curve correlates well with regional myocardial blood flow assessed by O-15 water, and thus may serve as a means for assessment of myocardial perfusion at rest (133). Analysis of the rate of clearance of acetate, however, reflects myocardial oxygen consumption. Several clinical studies indicate that preservation of oxidative metabolism as measured by acetate clearance is a good predictor of myocardial viability and correlates well with FDG imaging (134). Unlike FDG, preliminary studies indicate that the utility of acetate is preserved in patients studied soon after myocardial infarction (135). More recently, reports from two different centers have indicated that measurement of relative perfusion by acetate is a very accurate predictor of functional recovery after revascularization, in some cases outperforming measurements of resting oxidative metabolism (136,137). Whether this reflects the importance of perfusion in the maintenance of viability, or the dual properties of acetate as a perfusion and metabolic tracer, is unclear. Finally, assessment of acetate clearance at baseline and after low-dose dobutamine infusion allows measurement of an "oxidative reserve," which may be more accurate than baseline measurements alone (137).

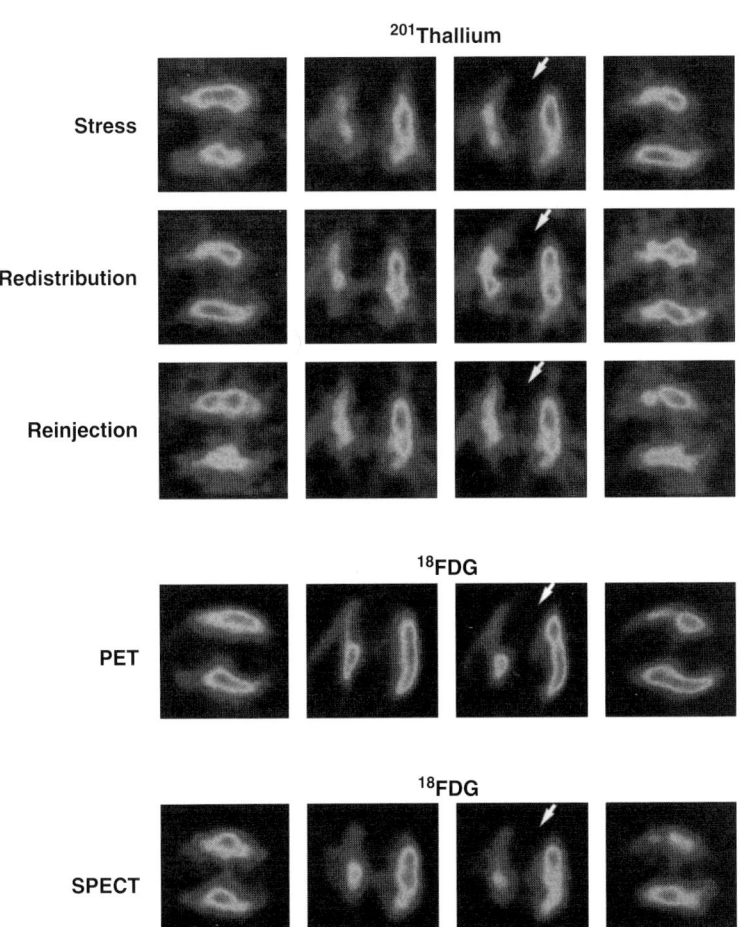

FIG. 14. Concordance between [18]FDG SPECT, [18]FDG positron emission tomography (PET), and stress-redistribution-reinjection thallium single photon emission computed tomography (SPECT) is demonstrated in this patient example. Four radial long-axis tomograms are displayed for [18]FDG SPECT, [18]FDG PET, with corresponding thallium tomograms of stress, redistribution, and reinjection. On the [18]FDG SPECT and PET studies, [18]FDG uptake is severely reduced in the apical region (shown by the *arrowheads*), suggestive of scarred myocardium. As in the findings on [18]FDG SPECT and PET, thallium images show severe perfusion defect in the apical region during stress, which persist on redistribution and reinjection images (scarred by thallium). (From ref. 131, with permission.)

[11]Carbon Palmitate

Like acetate, multicompartmental quantitative analysis of [11]carbon palmitate kinetics may be used to gain insight into myocardial oxidative metabolism and the turnover of palmitate into the endogenous pool of phospholipids and triglycerides (138,139). While in theory, the analysis of myocardial palmitate uptake should be a useful marker of viability, in practice this has not been realized. Major limitations to its use include conflicting animal data concerning its behavior under ischemic conditions and the potential alteration in its kinetics as a result of arterial substrate concentration, myocardial ischemia, and hormonal milieu (140–142).

PET Perfusion Tracers and Viability

Myocardial perfusion tracers used in PET include ^{15}O-water and ^{13}N-ammonia, which are cyclotron-produced, and [82]rubidium and [62]Cu-PTSM, which are generator-produced. As noted above, the early uptake of acetate also provides information on perfusion. The ability of a particular perfusion tracer to give information on viability depends partly on the properties of the tracer itself, and partly on understanding the underlying pathophysiologic concepts that link viability to perfusion.

Myocardial perfusion tracers can be divided into two broad categories, those that are freely diffusible (^{15}O-water), and those whose uptake and/or retention are dependent not only on flow but also on intact cellular viability (^{13}N-ammonia, [82]rubidium). [62]Cu-PTSM remains investigational at this time. Thus, two approaches can be considered to use these tracers for viability assessment. In the first approach, the goal is to obtain an accurate assessment of perfusion using any of the tracers. The presence of myocardial viability is then determined on the basis of parameters of perfusion (e.g., absolute myocardial blood flow, perfusion reserve). In the second approach, the goal is to analyze some aspect of the radiotracer's kinetics (e.g., its retention, volume of distribution), and to relate this kinetic analysis to intact viability.

The concept that parameters of perfusion may be used as markers of myocardial viability emerged from two lines of investigation: (i) that a threshold of flow exists below which viability is not sustainable and (ii) that intact coronary flow reserve translates into intact viability.

Threshold Value for Absolute Blood Flow

Gewirtz et al. (143) reported that regions with blood flow <0.25 mL/g/min were unlikely to be viable by FDG PET or recover function after revascularization (144). While such studies support the concept of a threshold value for absolute myocardial blood flow as it relates to viability, several questions remain. First, there is considerable overlap in perfusion values between viable and nonviable segments in most studies. Second, the accuracy to predict functional recovery in intermediate flow defects is unclear. Third, the comparability of radiotracers utilized for assessment of absolute myocardial blood flow (^{15}O-water and ^{13}N-ammonia) is unproven. In a direct comparison of these two radiotracers in patients with coronary artery disease and left ventricular dysfunction, differences in estimates of regional myocardial blood flow were noted (145). Regional blood flow estimates using ^{13}N-ammonia, but not using ^{15}O-water, correlated with intact viability. When ^{15}O-water studies were analyzed to determine the perfusible tissue fraction (see below), however, the two tracers compared favorably. Finally, it remains to be determined whether relative measures of perfusion are accurate markers of viability. Several studies using assessment of relative ^{13}N-ammonia activity have indicated that asynergic regions with resting ^{13}N-ammonia activity less than 40% are unlikely to improve function after revascularization (146,147).

Coronary Flow Reserve

Recent data have begun to explore the issue of whether reversible perfusion defects, as defined by visual assessment and/or circumferential profiles, are predictive of functional recovery. The relationship between coronary flow reserve and viability has been demonstrated in experimental and preclinical studies, and several groups of investigators have shown that functionally impaired myocardium may retain residual vasodilating capacity (148,149). Clinical studies seem to support this concept. Using analysis of Tc-99m microsphere uptake, a persistent vasodilating capacity has been demonstrated after papaverine infusion in patients with coronary artery disease, regional left ventricular dysfunction, and resting hypoperfusion (150). Marzullo and colleagues (151), using rest and dipyridamole ^{13}N-ammonia and FDG PET, demonstrated that regions with metabolic activity had preserved coronary flow reserve, whereas regions that were metabolically inactive showed virtually absent flow reserve. Investigators from the NIH recently reported that exercise-induced reversible thallium defects were predictive of functional recovery after revascularization (52). These preliminary data indicate that intact coronary flow reserve is an accurate marker of myocardial viability.

Assessment of Myocardial Viability Using Parameters of Radiotracer Kinetics

Similar to perfusion tracers utilized for SPECT, analysis of certain parameters of radiotracer uptake and retention may be used with PET perfusion tracers as indices of myocardial viability. Such methods include perfusible tissue index (PTI)

with ^{15}O-water, analysis of ^{82}rubidium retention, and analysis of late uptake or volume of distribution of ^{13}N-ammonia.

Perfusible Tissue Index

Studies have explored the ability of ^{15}O-water to assess myocardial viability through modification of the blood flow information. This method is based on measurement of perfusable tissue fraction (PTF), which was first introduced by Iida et al. (152) as a method to correct for the partial volume effects in ^{15}O-water studies. These investigators defined PTF as the fractional volume of a given region of interest occupied by myocardium that is capable of rapidly exchanging water. Using transmission and C^{15}O blood pool images, a quantitative estimate of extravascular tissue density, called anatomical tissue fraction (ATF), is derived. The ratio of PTF/ATF, called the perfusable tissue index (PTI), thus represents the proportion of the extravascular tissue that is perfusable by ^{15}O-water. The ratio should be unity in normal myocardium and reduced in scar.

Yamamoto and colleagues (153) applied this technique to patients with acute and chronic ischemic heart disease and in healthy volunteers. In healthy volunteers, PTI was 1.08 plus or minus 0.07 g (perfusable tissue)/g (total anatomical tissue). Among patients who were treated successfully with thrombolysis after an acute myocardial infarction, no segment with a PTI less than 0.7 exhibited functional recovery. The same investigators subsequently reported their experience in 12 patients with chronic ischemic heart disease and prior myocardial infarction who were undergoing revascularization (154). The data showed that regions in which functional recovery was observed after revascularization always had a PTI greater than 0.7, whereas functional recovery was not observed in regions with PTI less than 0.7. As noted above, assessment of PTI may be more accurate than myocardial blood flow estimates alone (155). While these results are promising, at present the application of this technique has been limited to a few selected academic centers.

Rubidium Retention

The potential utility of rubidium as a marker of myocardial viability is based upon its similarities to potassium (as with Tl-201) with regard to membrane transport, trapping, and extraction characteristics. Experimental studies have demonstrated that rubidium initially distributes in relation to blood flow, and is trapped in normal cells (156). In necrotic cells, however, the tracer washes out rapidly, and the rate of washout may reliable identify necrotic from viable myocardium (156). Hence, rubidium is taken up by both viable and necrotic myocardium, but is not retained by necrotic myocardium. Based on these observations, Gould et al. (157) have suggested that the kinetics of rubidium washout may be used clinically as an index of myocardial viability

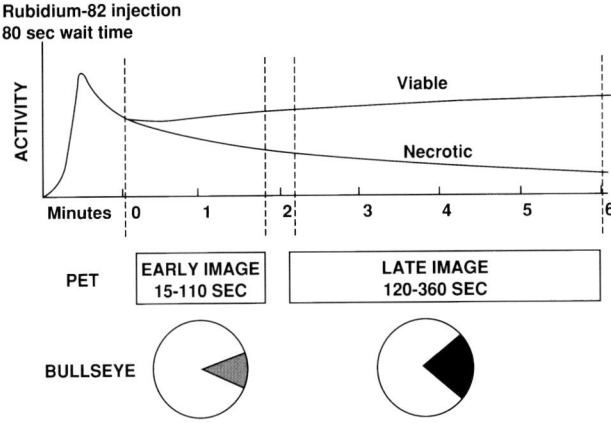

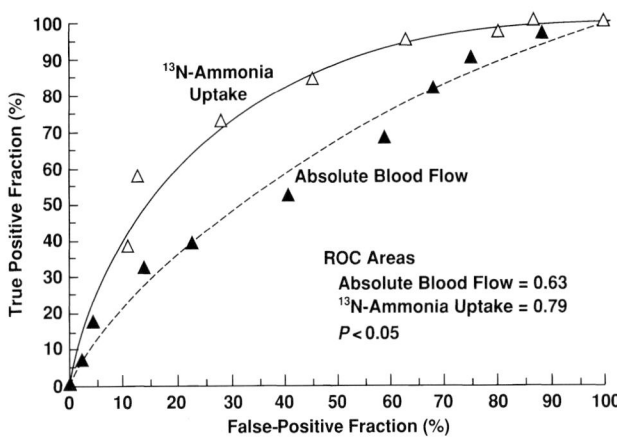

FIG. 15. Schematic protocol utilizing the kinetic changes of rubidium-82 after intravenous injection to assess myocardial viability. As illustrated on the bullseye diagram, a new or worsening defect on the late image compared to the early image indicates washout or failure to trap rubidium, and, therefore, necrosis. *PET*, positron emission tomography. (From ref. 157, with permission.)

FIG. 16. Plots of receiver operator characteristic (*ROC*) curves for late ¹³N-ammonia uptake and absolute blood flow to predict functional improvement after revascularization in asynergic regions. Area under ROC curve for absolute blood flow and late ¹³N-ammonia uptake is displayed. Late ¹³N-ammonia uptake was significantly better predictor of functional improvement when compared to absolute blood flow. (From ref. 160, with permission.)

(Fig. 15). Using a simple, background-corrected ratio of rubidium activity in the late to early image, the authors estimated that a ratio of 0.825 represented the threshold below which less than 50% of viable tissue was present in any given transmural segment. Using this method in patients after recent myocardial infarction, infarct size assessed by analysis of rubidium kinetics correlate well to infarct size by FDG PET, independent of infarct age (157). Utilizing dynamic data acquisition, good agreement has also been shown between washout of rubidium (after only a single injection) and FDG uptake (158). Thus, preliminary data suggest that assessment of cell membrane integrity using rubidium-82 kinetics compares favorably to FDG, and additional studies are warranted to investigate the predictive value of this approach.

¹³N-ammonia Uptake

Studies have also investigated whether analysis of ¹³N-ammonia kinetics may improve viability detection over perfusion parameters alone. Using kinetic modeling of ¹³N-ammonia dynamic PET data, measurements of myocardial blood flow and volume of distribution were compared to FDG parameters of viability in patients with previous myocardial infarction (159). While each parameter of ¹³N-ammonia kinetics has a reasonable accuracy to detect viability alone, the combination of the two variables (flow greater than or equal to 0.45 mL/min/g and volume of distribution greater than 2.0 mL/g) yielded superior positive and negative predictive values (86% and 100%, respectively). More recently, analysis of late N-13 ammonia uptake was compared to absolute myocardial blood flow in patients with chronic coronary artery disease and left ventricular dysfunction who underwent revascularization (160). In this study, late ¹³N-

ammonia uptake was a significantly better predictor of functional improvement after revascularization than was absolute myocardial blood flow (Fig. 16). Thus, additional methods are emerging that may enhance, and perhaps simplify, the assessment of viability using PET perfusion tracers.

Clinical and Prognostic Impact of PET Viability Assessment

Despite the preponderance of literature using improvement in ventricular function as a clinical endpoint, the real purpose of revascularization is to improve patient outcome, as assessed by morbidity and mortality. The prognostic significance of viability assessment has been addressed in several studies. The importance of perfusion-metabolism mismatch on PET imaging has been demonstrated in four studies comprising over 300 total patients and an average follow-up of at least 1 year (161–164). Despite nonrandomization of therapy and certain methodological flaws, the studies have shown remarkably consistent findings. Patients with perfusion-metabolism mismatch have very high mortality if medically managed and much lower mortality if revascularized. Patients with matched defects, indicating scar, displayed no such difference in outcomes between medical and surgical management. Furthermore, preoperative PET viability assessment may be useful in identifying a subgroup of high-risk patients who would benefit from early revascularization (165). The relationship of viability assessment to morbidity and functional capacity deserves further study (166–168).

Several studies are emerging that suggest an important role of viability assessment in decision-making in patients with chronic coronary artery disease. In particular, assessment of viability with PET in patients with severe ischemic cardiomyopathy who are being considered for transplantation may alter the therapeutic strategy by identification of a subset of patients who may be suitable for bypass surgery (169,170). Auerbach and colleagues (170) examined 283 patients with ischemic cardiomyopathy (mean left ventricular ejection fraction of 26%) with ^{13}N-ammonia/FDG PET studies. In this study, 55% of patients had evidence of viable myocardium in at least one region, and 27% had viable myocardium in at least five regions. Preliminary data suggest that such patients may have a good outcome with revascularization (169), although additional studies are needed to confirm this concept. Finally, a retrospective study suggested that, among patients undergoing bypass surgery, those in whom a preoperative PET study was part of the clinical evaluation may have better short-term survival than those who are assessed by clinical and angiographic parameters alone (171). In this study, 1-year survival was 97% in the former group, compared with 79% in the latter group. Likewise, the risk of postoperative complications was reduced in the group studied with PET. These intriguing data suggest a potential role for PET viability imaging in the decision-making process in patients with ischemic left ventricular dysfunction.

FUTURE PERSPECTIVES

A number of important questions still remain operative in the clinical arena. Perhaps the most important questions relate to the definition of myocardial viability itself, in addition to questions related to the impact of the extent of viability as it relates to improvement in function, the degree to which hibernation and stunning are operative clinically, the standardization of approaches to viability assessment, and the need for data on how such assessment affects clinical outcomes. While assessment of ventricular function seems to be a reasonable surrogate for studies of outcome, given the relationship between left ventricular function and outcome, this relationship may not be as relevant after revascularization.

In the future, large clinical trials are needed that evaluate not only recovery of left ventricular function after revascularization but also left ventricular cavity dilatation, episodes of clinical heart failure, arrhythmias, recurrent ischemic events, and long-term survival. Such trials will need large populations and will likely require multicenter approaches with standardization of methodology. Important questions to be answered from such studies include: (i) Is revascularization beneficial to clinical outcome even in the absence of improvement in ventricular function and/or in the absence of viable myocardium? (ii) Which patients are most appropriate candidates for viability assessment? (iii) Is viability assessment cost-effective?

REFERENCES

1. Heyndrickx GR, Baig H, Nelkins P, et al. Depression of regional blood flow and wall thickening after brief coronary occlusions. *Am J Physiol* 1978;234:H653–H659.
2. Braunwald E, Kloner RA. The stunned myocardium: prolonged, postischemic ventricular dysfunction. *Circulation* 1982;66:1146–1149.
3. Matsuzaki M, Gallagher KP, Kemper WS, et al. Sustained regional dysfunction, produced by prolonged coronary stenosis: Gradual recovery after reperfusion. *Circulation* 1983;68:170–182.
4. Rahimtoola SH. A perspective on the three large multicenter randomized clinical trials of coronary bypass surgery for chronic stable angina. *Circulation* 1985;72[Suppl V]:V-123–V-135.
5. Braunwald E, Rutherford JD. Reversible ischemic left ventricular dysfunction: evidence for the "hibernating myocardium." *J Am Coll Cardiol* 1986;8:1467–1470.
6. Dilsizian V, Cannon RO, Tracy CM, et al. Enhanced regional left ventricular function after distant coronary bypass via improved collateral blood flow. *J Am Coll Cardiol* 1989;14:312–318.
7. Ross J Jr. Myocardial perfusion-contraction matching: implications for coronary heart disease and hibernation. *Circulation* 1991;83:1076–1082.
8. Mullins LJ, Moore RD. The movement of thallium ions in muscle. *J Gen Physiol* 1960;43:759–773.
9. Gehring PJ, Hammond PB. The interrelationship between thallium and potassium in animals. *J Pharmacol Exp Ther* 1967;155:187–201.
10. Leppo JA, Macneil PB, Moring AF, Apstein CS. Separate effects of ischemia, hypoxia, and contractility on thallium-201 kinetics in rabbit myocardium. *J Nucl Med* 1986;27:66–74.
11. Leppo JA. Myocardial uptake of thallium and rubidium during alterations in perfusion and oxygenation in isolated rabbit hearts. *J Nucl Med* 1987;28:878–885.
12. Moore CA, Cannon J, Watson DD, et al. Thallium-201 kinetics in stunned myocardium characterized by severe postischemic systolic dysfunction. *Circulation* 1990;81:1622–1632.
13. Sinusas AJ, Watson DD, Cannon JM, et al. Effect of ischemia and postischemic dysfunction on myocardial uptake of technetium-99m-labeled methoxyisobutyl isonitrile and thallium-201. *J Am Coll Cardiol* 1989;14:1785–1793.
14. Granato JE, Watson DD, Flanagan TL, et al. Myocardial thallium-201 kinetics and regional flow alterations with 3 hours of coronary occlusion and either rapid reperfusion through a totally patent vessel or slow reperfusion through a critical stenosis. *J Am Coll Cardiol* 1987;9:109–118.
15. Pohost GM, Zir LM, Moore RH, et al. Differentiation of transiently ischemic from infarcted myocardium by serial imaging after a single dose of thallium-201. *Circulation* 1977;55:294–302.
16. Beller GA, Watson DD, Ackell P, et al. Time course of thallium-201 redistribution after transient myocardial ischemia. *Circulation* 1980;61:791–797.
17. Okada RD, Pohost GM. Effect of decreased blood flow and ischemia on myocardial thallium clearance. *J Am Coll Cardiol* 1984;3:744–750.
18. Gutman J, Berman DS, Freeman M, et al. Time to completed redistribution of thallium-201 in exercise myocardial scintigraphy: relationship to the degree of coronary artery stenosis. *Am Heart J* 1983;106:989–995.
19. Yang LD, Berman DS, Kiat H, et al. The frequency of late reversibility in SPECT thallium-201 stress-redistribution studies. *J Am Coll Cardiol* 1989;15:334–340.
20. Dilsizian V, Rocco TP, Freedman NM, et al. Enhanced detection of ischemic but viable myocardium by the reinjection of thallium after stress-redistribution imaging. *N Engl J Med* 1990;323:141–146.
21. Rocco TP, Dilsizian V, McKusick KA, et al. Comparison of thallium redistribution with rest "reinjection" imaging for the detection of viable myocardium. *Am J Cardiol* 1990;66:158–163.
22. Ohtani H, Tamaki N, Yonekura Y, et al. Value of thallium-201 reinjection after delayed SPECT imaging for predicting reversible ischemia after coronary artery bypass grafting. *Am J Cardiol* 1990;66:394–399.
23. Lekakis J, Vassilopoulos N, Germanidis J, et al. Detection of viable tissue in healed infarcted myocardium by dipyridamole thallium-201 reinjection and regional wall motion studies. *Am J Cardiol* 1993;71:401–404.
24. Kiat H, Berman DS, Maddahi J, et al. Late reversibility of tomographic myocardial thallium-201 defects: An accurate marker of myocardial viability. *J Am Coll Cardiol* 1988;12:1456–1463.
25. Tamaki N, Ohtani H, Yamashita K, et al. Metabolic activity in the areas of new fill-in after thallium-201 reinjection: Comparison with

positron emission tomography using fluorine-18-deoxyglucose. *J Nucl Med* 1991;32:673–678.

26. Bartenstein P, Hasfeld M, Schober O, et al. Tl-201 reinjection predicts improvement of left ventricular function following revascularization. *Nucl Med* 1993;32:87–90.

27. Haque T, Furukawa T, Takahashi M, et al. Identification of hibernating myocardium by dobutamine stress echocardiography: Comparison with thallium-201 reinjection imaging. *Am Heart J* 1995;130:553–563.

28. Vanoverschelde JJ, D'Hondt AM, Gerber BL, et al. Head-to-head comparison of exercise-redistribution-reinjection thallium SPECT and low-dose dobutamine echocardiography for prediction of the reversibility of chronic left ventricular dysfunction. *J Am Coll Cardiol* 1996;28:432–442.

29. Gursurer M, Pinarli AE, Aksoy M, et al. Assessment of viable myocardium and prediction of postoperative improvement in left ventricular function in patients with severe left ventricular dysfunction by quantitative planar stress-redistribution-reinjection Tl-201 imaging. *Int J Cardiol* 1997;58:179–184.

30. Inglese E, Brambilla M, Dondi M, et al. Assessment of myocardial viability after thallium-201 reinjection or rest-redistribution imaging: a multicenter study. *J Nucl Med* 1995;36:555–563.

31. Dilsizian V, Smeltzer WR, Freedman NMT, et al. Thallium reinjection after stress-redistribution imaging: does 24-hour delayed imaging following reinjection enhance detection of viable myocardium? *Circulation* 1991;83:1247–1255.

32. Dilsizian V, Bonow RO. Differential uptake and apparent thallium-201 "washout" after thallium reinjection: options regarding early redistribution imaging before reinjection or late redistribution imaging after reinjection. *Circulation* 1992;85:1032–1038.

33. Goldhaber SZ, Newell JB, Alpert NM, et al. Effects of ischemic-like insult on myocardial thallium-201 accumulation. *Circulation* 1983;67:778–786.

34. Budinger TF, Pohost GM. Indication for thallium reinjection by 3-hour plasma levels. *Circulation* 1993;88:I–534(abst).

35. Budinger TF, Pohost GM. Thallium "redistribution"—an explanation. *J Nucl Med* 1986;27:996(abst).

36. Grunwald A, Watson D, Holzgrefe H, Irving J, Beller GA. Myocardial thallium-201 kinetics in normal and ischemic myocardium. *Circulation* 1981;64:610–618.

37. Budinger TF, Knittel BL. Cardiac thallium redistribution and model. *J Nucl Med* 1987;28:588(abst).

38. Kayden DS, Sigal S, Soufer R, et al. Thallium-201 for assessment of myocardial viability: quantitative comparison of 24-hour redistribution imaging with imaging after reinjection at rest. *J Am Coll Cardiol* 1991;18:1480–1486.

39. Petretta M, Cuocolo A, Bonaduce D, et al. Incremental prognostic value of thallium reinjection after stress-redistirbution imaging in patients with previous myocardial infarction and left ventricular dysfunction. *J Nucl Med* 1997;38:195–200.

40. Tisselli A, Pieri P, Moscatelli G, et al. Prognostic value of persistent thallium-201 defects that become reversible after reinjection in patients with chronic myocardial infarction. *J Nucl Cardiol* 1997;4:195–201.

41. Zafrir N, Leppo JA, Reinhardt CP, et al. Thallium reinjection versus standard stress/delay redistribution imaging for prediction of cardiac events. *J Am Coll Cardiol* 1998;31:1280–1285.

42. Gewirtz H, Beller GA, Strauss HW, et al. Transient defects of resting thallium scans in patients with coronary artery disease. *Circulation* 1979;59:707–713.

43. Berger BC, Watson DD, Burwell LR, et al. Redistribution of thallium at rest in patients with stable and unstable angina and the effect of coronary artery bypass surgery. *Circulation* 1979;60:1114–1125.

44. Iskandrian AS, Hakki A, Kane SA, et al. Rest and redistribution thallium-201 myocardial scintigraphy to predict improvement in left ventricular function after coronary artery bypass grafting. *Am J Cardiol* 1983;51:1312–1316.

45. Mori T, Minamiji K, Kurogane H, Ogawa K, Yoshida Y. Rest-injected thallium-201 imaging for assessing viability of severe asynergic regions. *J Nucl Med* 1991;32:1718–1724.

46. Ragosta M, Beller GA, Watson DD, et al. Quantitative planar rest-redistribution ^{201}Tl imaging in detection of myocardial viability and prediction of improvement in left ventricular function after coronary

artery bypass surgery in patients with severely depressed left ventricular function. *Circulation* 1993;87:1630–1641.

47. Udelson JE, Coleman PS, Metherall JA, et al. Predicting recovery of severe regional ventricular dysfunction: comparison of resting scintigraphy with ^{201}Tl and Tc-99m-sestamibi. *Circulation* 1994;89:2552–2561.

48. Perrone-Filardi P, Pace L, Prastaro M, et al. Assessment of myocardial viability in patients with chronic coronary artery disease: Rest-4-hour-24-hour ^{201}Tl tomography versus dobutamine echocardiography. *Circulation* 1996;94:2712–2719.

49. Sciagra R, Bisi G, Santoro GM, et al. Comparison of baseline-nitrate techetium-99m sestamibi with rest-redistribution thallium-201 tomography in detecting viable hibernating myocardium and predicting post-revascularization recovery. *J Am Coll Cardiol* 1997;30:384–391.

50. Bax JJ, Cornel JH, Visser FC, et al. Comparison of fluorine-18 FDG with rest-redistribution thallium-201 SPECT to delineate viable myocardium and predict functional recovery after revascularization. *J Nucl Med* 1998;39:1482–1486.

51. Dilsizian V, Perrone-Filardi P, Arrighi JA, et al. Concordance and discordance between stress-redistribution-reinjection and rest-redistribution thallium imaging for assessing viable myocardium: comparison with metabolic activity by PET. *Circulation* 1993;88:941–952.

52. Kitsiou AN, Srinivasan G, Quyyumi AA, et al. Stress-induced reversible and mild-to-moderate irreversible thallium defects: Are they equally accurate for predicting recovery of regional left ventricular function after revascularization? *Circulation* 1998;98:501–508.

53. Dilsizian V. Myocardial viability: contractile reserve or cell membrane integrity? *J Am Coll Cardiol* 1996;28:443–446.

54. Bonow RO, Dilsizian V, Cuocolo A, et al. Identification of viable myocardium in patients with coronary artery disease and left ventricular dysfunction: Comparison of thallium scintigraphy with reinjection and PET imaging with ^{18}F-fluorodeoxyglucose. *Circulation* 1991;83:26–37.

55. Dilsizian V, Freedman NMT, Bacharach SL, et al. Regional thallium uptake in irreversible defects: Magnitude of change in thallium activity after reinjection distinguishes viable from nonviable myocardium. *Circulation* 1992;85:627–634.

56. Zimmermann R, Mall G, Rauch B, et al. Residual Tl-201 activity in irreversible defects as a marker of myocardial viability: clinicopathological study. *Circulation* 1995;91:1016–1021.

57. Piwnica-Worms D, Kronauge JF, Chiu ML. Uptake and retention of hexakis (2-methoxyisoobutyl isonitrile) technetium in cultured chick myocardial cells: mitochondrial and plasma membrane potential dependence. *Circulation* 1990;82:1826–1838.

58. Maublant JC, Gachon P, Moins N. Hexakis (2-methoxyisobutyl isonitrile) technetium-99m and thallium-201 chloride: uptake and release in cultured myocardial cells. *J Nucl Med* 1988;29:48–54.

59. Sinusas AJ, Trautman KA, Bergin JD, et al. Quantification of area at risk during coronary occlusion and degree of myocardial salvage after reperfusion with technetium–99m methoxyisobutyl isonitrile. *Circulation* 1990;82:1424–1437.

60. Beanlands R, Dawood F, Wen WH, et al. Are the kinetics of technetium-99m methoxyisobutyl isonitrile affected by cell membrane metabolism and viability? *Circulation* 1990;82:1802–1814.

61. Verani MS, Jeroudi MO, Mahmarian JJ, et al. Quantification of myocardial infarction during coronary occlusion and myocardial salvage after reperfusion using cardiac imaging with technetium-99m hexakis 2-methoxybutyl isonitrile. *J Am Coll Cardiol* 1988;12:1573–1581.

62. Christian TF, Behrenbeck T, Pellikka PA, et al. Mismatch of left ventricular function and infarct size demonstrated by technetium–99m isonitrile imaging after reperfusion therapy for acute myocardial infarction: identification of myocardial stunning and hyperkinesis. *J Am Coll Cardiol* 1990;16:1632–1638.

63. Gibbons RJ, Verani MS, Behrenbeck T, et al. Feasibility of tomographic 99mTc–hexakis–2–methoxy–2–methylpropyl–isonitrile imaging for the assessment of myocardial area at risk and the effect of acute treatment in myocardial infarction. *Circulation* 1989;80:1277–1286.

64. Cuocolo A, Pace L, Ricciardelli B, et al. Identification of viable myocardium in patients with chronic coronary artery disease: comparison of thallium-201 scintigraphy with reinjection and technetium-99m methoxyisobutyl isonitrile. *J Nucl Med* 1992;33:505–511.

65. Dilsizian V, Arrighi JA, Diodati JG et al. Myocardial viability in patients with chronic coronary artery disease: comparison of Tc-99m-

sestamibi with thallium reinjection and ^{18}F-fluorodeoxyglucose. *Circulation* 1994;89:578–587.

66. Richter WS, Cordes M, Calder D, et al. Washout and redistribution between immediate and two-hour myocardial images using technetium-99m sestamibi. *Eur J Nucl Med* 1995;22:49–55.

67. Maurea S, Cuocolo A, Soricelli A, et al. Myocardial viability index in chronic coronary artery disease: Technetium-99m-methoxy isobutyl isonitrile redistribution. *J Nucl Med* 1995;36:1953–1960.

68. Marzullo P, Sambuceti G, Parodi O. The role of sestamibi scintigraphy in the radioisotopic assessment of myocardial viability. *J Nucl Med* 1992;33:1925–1930.

69. Lucignani G, Paolini G, Landoni C, et al. Presurgical identification of hibernating myocardium by combined use of technetium-99m-hexakis-2-methoxyisobutylisonitrile single photon emission tomography and fluorine-18-fluoro-2-deoxy-D-glucose positron emission tomography in patients with coronary artery disease. *Eur J Nucl Med* 1992; 19:874–881.

70. Altehoefer C, Kaiser HJ, Dorr R, et al. Fluorine-18 deoxyglucose PET for assessment of viable myocardium in perfusion defects in 99mTc-MIBI SPET: a comparative study in patients with coronary artery disease. *Eur J Nucl Med* 1992;19:334–342.

71. Maurea S, Cuocolo A, Pace L, et al. Left ventricular dysfunction in coronary artery disease: comparison between rest-redistribution thallium-201 and resting technetium-99m methoxyisobutyl isonitrile cardiac imaging. *J Nucl Cardiol* 1994;1:65–71.

72. Sawada SG, Allman KC, Muzik O, et al. Positron emission tomography detects evidence of viability in rest technetium-99m sestamibi defects. *J Am Coll Cardiol* 1994;23:92–98.

73. Maurea S, Cuocolo A, Nicolai E, et al. Improved detection of viable myocardium with thallium-201 reinjection in chronic coronary artery disease: comparison with technetium-99m-MIBI imaging. *J Nucl Med* 1994;35:621–624.

74. Altehoefer C, vom Dahl J, Biedermann M, et al. Significance of defect severity is technetium-99m-MIBI SPECT at rest to assess myocardial viability: comparison with fluorine-18-FDG PET. *J Nucl Med* 1994; 35:569–574.

75. Marzullo P, Sambucetti G, Parodi O, et al. Regional concordance and discordance between rest thallium-201 and sestamibi imaging for assessing tissue viability: comparison with postrevascularization functional recovery. *J Nucl Cardiol* 1995;2:309–316.

76. Soufer R, Dey HM, Ng CK, Zaret BL. Comparison of sestamibi single-photon emission tomography with positron emission tomography for estimating left ventricular myocardial viability. *Am J Cardiol* 1995;75:1214–1219.

77. Rossetti C, Landoni C, Lucignani G, et al. Assessment of myocardial perfusion and viability with technetium-99m methoxybutylisonitrile and thallium-201 rest redistribution in chronic coronary artery disease. *Eur J Nucl Med* 1995;22:1306–1312.

78. Arrighi JA, Ng CK, Dey HM, et al. Effect of left ventricular function on the assessment of myocardial viability by 99mTc-sestamibi and correlation with positron emission tomography in patients with healed myocardial infarcts or stable angina pectoris or both. *Am J Cardiol* 1997;80:1007–1013.

79. Canby RC, Silber S, Pohost GM. Relations of the myocardial imaging agents 99mTc–MIBI and 201–Tl to myocardial blood flow in a canine model of ischemic insult. *Circulation* 1990;81:286–296.

80. Li QS, Solot G, Frank TL, et al. Myocardial redistribution of technetium-99m-methoxyisobutyl isonitrile (sestamibi). *J Nucl Med* 1990; 31:1069–1076.

81. Sinusas AJ, Bergin JD, Edwards NC, et al. Redistribution of 99mTc-sestamibi and 201Tl in the presence of a severe coronary artery stenosis. *Circulation* 1994;89:2332–2341.

82. Sansoy V, Glover DK, Watson DD, et al. Comparison of thallium-201 resting redistribution with technetium-99m-sestamibi uptake and functional response to dobutamine for assessment of myocardial viability. *Circulation* 1995;92:994–1004.

83. Franceschi M, Guimond J, Zimmerman RE, et al. Myocardial clearance of Tc-99m hexakis-2-methoxy-2-methylpropyl isonitrile (MIBI) in patients with coronary artery disease. *Clin Nucl Med* 1990;15: 307–312.

84. Taillefer R, Primeau M, Costi P, et al. Technetium-99m-sestamibi myocardial perfusion imaging in detection of coronary artery disease: Comparison between initial (1-hour) and delayed (3-hour) postexercise images. *J Nucl Med* 1991;32:1961–1965.

85. Maes AF, Borgers M, Flameng W, et al. Assessment of myocardial viability in chronic coronary artery disease using technetium-99m sestamibi SPECT. Correlation with histologic and positron emission tomographic studies and functional follow-up. *J Am Coll Cardiol* 1997;29:62–68.

86. Shehata AR, Mitchell J, Heller GV. Use of gated SPECT imaging in the prediction of myocardial viability. *J Nucl Cardiol* 1997;4:99–100.

87. Levine MG, McGill CC, Ahlberg AW, et al. Functional assessment with electrocardiographic gated single-photon emission computed tomography improves the ability of technetium-99m sestamibi myocardial perfusion imaging to predict myocardial viability in patients undergoing revascularization. *Am J Cardiol* 1999;83:1–5.

88. Corbett JR, Ficaro EP. Clinical review of attenuation-corrected cardiac SPECT. *J Nucl Cardiol* 1999;6:54–68.

89. Matsunari I, Boning G, Ziegler SI, et al. Attenuation-corrected 99mTc-tetrofosmin single-photon emission computed tomography in the detection of viable myocardium: comparison with positron emission tomography using 18F-fluorodeoxyglucose. *J Am Coll Cardiol* 1998;32:927–935.

90. Berman DS, Kiat H, Friedman JD, et al. Separate acquisition rest thallium-201/stress technetium-99m sestamibi dual-isotope myocardial perfusion single-photon emission computed tomography: a clinical validation study. *J Am Coll Cardiol* 1993;22:1455–1464.

91. Galli M, Marcassa C, Imparato A, et al. Effects of nitroglycerin by technetium-99m sestamibi tomoscintigraphy on resting regional myocardial hypoperfusion in stable patients with healed myocardial infarction. *Am J Cardiol* 1994;74:843–848.

92. Bisi G, Sciagra R, Santoro GM, et al. Sublingual isosorbide dinitrate to improve technetium-99m-teboroxime perfusion defect reversibility. *J Nucl Med* 1994;35:1274–1278.

93. Kelly JD, Forester AM, Higley B, et al. Technetium-99m Tetrofosmin as a new radiopharmaceutical for myocardial perfusion imaging. *J Nucl Med* 1993;34:222–227.

94. Sinusas AJ, Shi QX, Saltzberg MT, et al. Technetium-99m tetrofosmin to assess myocardial blood flow: experimental validation in an intact canine model of ischemia. *J Nucl Med* 1994;35:664–671.

95. Koplan BA, Beller GA, Ruiz M, et al. Comparison between thallium-201 and technetium-99m-tetrofosmin uptake with sustained low flow and profound systolic dysfunction. *J Nucl Med* 1996;37:1398–1402.

96. Jain D, Wackers FJ, Mattera J, et al. Biokinetics of 99m Tc-tetrofosmin, a new myocardial perfusion imaging agent: implications for a one day imaging protocol. *J Nucl Med* 1993;34:1254–1259.

97. Glover DK, Ruiz M, Koplan BA, et al. 99mTc-tetrofosmin assessment of myocardial perfusion and viability in canine models of coronary occlusion and reperfusion. *J Nucl Med* 1999;40:142–149.

98. Takahashi N, Reinhardt CP, Marcel R, et al. Myocardial uptake of 99mTc-tetrofosmin, sestamibi, and 201Tl in a model of acute coronary reperfusion. *Circulation* 1996;94:2605–2613.

99. Zaret BL, Rigo P, Wackers FJT, et al. Myocardial perfusion imaging with Tc-99m tetrofosmin: comparison to thallium imaging and coronary angiography in a phase III multicenter trial. *Circulation* 1995; 91:313–319.

100. Matsunari I, Fujino S, Taki J, et al. Myocardial viability assessment with technetium-99m-tetrofosmin and thallium-201 reinjection in coronary artery disease. *J Nucl Med* 1995;36:1961–1967.

101. Galassi AR, Tamburino C, Grassi R, et al. Comparison of technetium 99m-tetrofosmin and thallium-201 single photon emission computed tomographic imaging for the assessment of viable myocardium in patients with left ventricular dysfunction. *J Nucl Cardiol* 1998;5: 56–63.

102. Matsunari I, Fujino S, Taki J, et al. Quantitative rest technetium-99m tetrofosmin imaging in predicting functional recovery after revascularization: comparison with rest-redistribution thallium-201. *J Am Coll Cardiol* 1997;29:1226–1233.

103. Weinstein H, Reinhardt CP, Leppo JA. Teboroxime, sestamibi and thallium-201 as markers of myocardial hypoperfusion: comparison by quantitative dual-isotope autoradiography in rabbits. *J Nucl Med* 1993;34:1510–1517.

104. DiRocco RJ, Rumsey WL, Kuczynski BL, et al. Measurement of myocardial blood flow using a coinjection technique for technetium-99m teboroxime, technetium-99m sestamibi and thallium-201. *J Nucl Med* 1992;33:1152–1159.

105. Stewart RE, Schwaiger M, Hutchins GD, et al. Myocardial clearance

kinetics of technetium-99m SQ30217: a marker of regional myocardial blood flow. *J Nucl Med* 1990;31:1183–1190.

106. Maublant JC, Moins N, Gachon P, et al. Uptake of technetium-99m teboroxime in cultured myocardial cells: comparison with thallium-201 and technetium-99m sestamibi. *J Nucl Med* 1993;34:255–259.

107. Seldin DW, Johnson L, Blood DK, et al. Myocardial perfusion imaging with technetium-99m SQ30217: comparison with thallium-201 and coronary anatomy. *J Nucl Med* 1989;30:312–319.

108. Fleming RM, Kirkeeide RL, Taegtmeyer H, et al. Comparison of technetium-99m teboroxime tomography with automated quantitative coronary arteriography and thallium-201 tomographic imaging. *J Am Coll Cardiol* 1991;17:1297–1302.

109. Hendel RC, Dahlberg ST, Weinstein H, et al. Comparison of teboroxime and thallium for the reversibility of exercise-induced myocardial perfusion defects. *Am Heart J* 1993;126:856–862.

110. Gerson MC, Millard RW, Roszell NJ, et al. Kinetic properties of 99mTc-Q12 in canine myocardium. *Circulation* 1994;89:1291–1300.

111. Gerson MC, Lukes J, Deutsch E, et al. Comparison of technetium-99m Q12 and thallium-201 for detection of angiographically documented coronary artery disease in humans. *J Nucl Cardiol* 1994;1:499–508.

112. Vanzetto G, Calnon DA, Ruiz M, et al. Myocardial uptake and redistribution of Tc-99m-N-NOET in dogs with either sustained coronary low flow or transient coronary occlusion: comparison with ^{201}Tl and myocardial blood flow. *Circulation* 1997;96:2325–2331.

113. Fagret D, Marie PY, Brunotte F, et al. Myocardial perfusion imaging with technetium-Tc-99m-NOET: comparison with thallium-201 and coronary angiography. *J Nucl Med* 1995;36:936–943.

114. Sokoloff L, Reivich M, Kennedy C, et al. The [14C]-deoxyglucose method for the measurement of local cerebral glucose utilization: theory, procedure and normal values in the conscious and anesthetized albino rat. *J Neurochem* 1977;28:897–916.

115. Phelps ME, Schelbert HR, Mazziotta JC. Positron computer tomography for studies of myocardial and cerebral function. *Ann Intern Med* 1983;98:339–359.

116. Tillisch JH, Brunken R, Marshall R, et al. Reversibility of cardiac wall-motion abnormalities predicted by positron tomography. *N Engl J Med* 1986;314:884–888.

117. Dilsizian V, Arrighi JA. Myocardial viability in chronic coronary artery disease: perfusion, metabolism and contractile reserve. In: Gerson MC, ed. *Cardiac nuclear medicine*, 3rd ed. New York: McGraw-Hill, 1996:143–191.

118. Tamaki N, Yonekura Y, Yamashita K, et al. Positron emission tomography using fluorine-18 deoxyglucose in evaluation of coronary artery bypass grafting. *Am J Cardiol* 1989;64:860–865.

119. Luciganani G, Paolini G, Landoni C, et al. Presurgical identification of hibernating myocardium by combined use of technetium-99m hexakis 2-methoxyisobutylisonitrile single photon emission tomography and fluorine-18-fluoro-2-deoxy-D-glucose positron emission tomography in patients with coronary artery disease. *Eur J Nucl Med* 1992;19:874–881.

120. Carrel T, Jenni R, Haubold-Reuter S, et al. Improvement of severely reduced left ventricular function after surgical revascularization in patients with preoperative myocardial infarction. *Eur J Cardiothorac Surg* 1992;6:479–484.

121. Nienaber CA, Brunken RC, Sherman CT, et al. Metabolic and functional recovery of ischemic human myocardium after coronary angioplasty. *J Am Coll Cardiol* 1991;18:966–978.

122. Tamaki N, Ohtani H, Yamashita K, et al. Metabolic activity in the areas of new fill-in after thallium-201 reinjection: comparison with positron emission tomography using fluoro-18-deoxyglucose. *J Nucl Med* 1991;32:673–678.

123. Marwick TH, MacIntyre WJ, LaFont A, et al. Metabolic responses of hibernating and infarcted myocardium to revascularization: a follow-up study of regional perfusion, function, and metabolism. *Circulation* 1992;85:1347–1353.

124. von Dahl J, Eitzman DT, Al-Aouar ZR, et al. Relation of regional function, perfusion, and metabolism in patients with advanced coronary artery disease undergoing surgical revascularization. *Circulation* 1994;90:2356–2366.

125. Flameng WJ, Shivalkar B, Spiessens B, et al. PET scan predicts functional recovery of left ventricular function after coronary artery bypass operation. *Ann Thorac Surg* 1997;64:1694–1701.

126. Schwaiger M, Brunken R, Grover-McKay M, et al. Regional myocardial metabolism in patients with acute myocardial infarction assessed by positron emission tomography. *J Am Coll Cardiol* 1986;8:800–808.

127. Knuuti MJ, Nuutila P, Ruotsalainen U, et al. The value of quantitative analysis of glucose utilization in detection of myocardial viability by PET. *J Nucl Med* 1993;34:2068–2075.

128. Hoflin F, Ledermann H, Noelpp U, et al. Routine ^{18}F-2-deoxy-2-fluoro-D-glucose (^{18}F-FDG) myocardial tomography using a normal large field of view gamma camera. *Angiology* 1989;140:1058–1064.

129. Drane WE, Abbott FD, Nicole MW, et al. Technology for FDG SPECT with a relatively inexpensive gamma camera. *Radiology* 1994;191:461–465.

130. Huitink JM, Visser FC, van Lingen A, et al. Feasibility of planar fluorine-18-FDG imaging after recent myocardial infarction to assess myocardial viability. *J Nucl Med* 1995;36:975–981.

131. Srinivasan G, Kitsiou AN, Bacharach SL, et al. ^{18}F-fluorodeoxyglucose single photon emission computed tomography: can it replace PET and thallium SPECT for the assessment of myocardial viability? *Circulation* 1998;97:843–850.

132. Armbrecht JJ, Buxton DB, Schelbert HR. Validation of [1-^{11}C] acetate as a tracer for noninvasive assessment of oxidative metabolism with positron emission tomography in normal, ischemic, postischemic, and hyperemic canine myocardium. *Circulation* 1990;81:1594–1605.

133. Gropler RJ, Siegel BA, Sampathkumaran K, et al. Dependence of recovery of contractile function on maintenance of oxidative metabolism after myocardial infarction. *J Am Coll Cardiol* 1992;19:989–997.

134. Gropler RJ, Geltman EM, Sampathkumaran K, et al. Functional recovery after coronary revascularization for chronic coronary artery disease is dependent on maintenance of oxidative metabolism. *J Am Coll Cardiol* 1992;20:569–577.

135. Gropler RJ, Siegel BA, Sampathkumaran K, et al. Dependence of recovery of contractile function on maintenance of oxidative metabolism after myocardial infarction. *J Am Coll Cardiol* 1992;19:989–997.

136. Wolpers HG, Burchert W, van den Hoff J, et al. Assessment of myocardial viability by use of 11C-acetate and positron emission tomography. Threshold criteria of reversible dysfunction. *Circulation* 1997;95:1417–1424.

137. Hata T, Nohara R, Fujita M, et al. Noninvasive assessment of myocardial viability by positron emission tomography with 11C acetate in patients with old myocardial infarction. Usefulness of low-dose dobutamine infusion. *Circulation* 1996;94:1834–1841.

138. Rosamond TL, Abendschein DR, Sobel BE, et al. Metabolic fate of radiolabeled palmitate in ischemic canine myocardium: implications for positron emission tomography. *J Nucl Med* 1987;28:1322–1329.

139. Bergmann SR, Weinheimer CJ, Markham J, et al. Quantitation of myocardial fatty acid metabolism using PET. *J Nucl Med* 1996;37:1723–1730.

140. Schelbert HR, Henze E, Schon HR, et al. Carbon-11 palmitate for the noninvasive evaluation of regional myocardial fatty acid metabolism wtih positron computed tomography, III: *in vivo* demonstration of the effects of substrate availability on myocardial metabolism. *Am Heart J* 1983;105:492–504.

141. Fox KAA, Abendschein D, Ambos HD, et al. Efflux of metabolized and nonmetabolized fatty acid from canine myocardium. Implications for quantifying myocardial metabolism tomographically. *Circ Res* 1985;57:232–243.

142. Myears DW, Sobel BE, Bergmann SR. Substrate use in ischemic and reperfused canine myocardium: quantitative considerations. *Am J Physiol: Heart Circ Physiol* 1987;253:H107–H114.

143. Gewirtz H, Fischman AJ, Abraham S, et al. Positron emission tomographic measurements of absolute regional myocardial blood flow permits identification of nonviable myocardium in patients with chronic myocardial infarction. *J Am Coll Cardiol* 1994;23:851–859.

144. Grandin C, Wijns W, Melin JA, et al. Delineation of myocardial viability with PET. *J Nucl Med* 1995;36:1543–1552.

145. Gerber BL, Melin JA, Bol A, et al. Nitrogen-13 ammonia and oxygen-15-water estimates of absolute myocardial perfusion in left ventricular ischemic dysfunction. *J Nucl Med* 1998;39:1655–1662.

146. Duvernoy C, Rothley J, Sitomer J, et al. Relationship of blood flow and functional outcome after coronary revascularization. *J Nucl Med* 1993;34:155P(abst).

147. Tamaki N, Kawamoto M, Tadamura E, et al. Prediction of reversible ischemia after revascularization: Perfusion and metabolic studies with positron emission tomography. *Circulation* 1995;91:1697–1705.

148. Aversano T, Becker LC. Persistence of coronary vasodilator reserve

despite functionally significant flow reduction. *Am J Physiol* 1985; 248:H403–H411.

149. Gallagher KP, Folts JP, Shebuski RJ, et al. Subepicardial vasodilator reserve in the presence of critical coronary stenosis in dogs. *Am J Cardiol* 1980;46:67–73.

150. Parodi O, Sambuceti G, Roghi A, et al. Residual coronary reserve despite decreased resting blood flow in patients with critical coronary lesions: A study by technetium-99m human albumin microsphere myocardial scintigraphy. *Circulation* 1993;87:330–344.

151. Marzullo P, Parodi O, Sambuceti G, et al. Residual coronary reserve identifies segmental viability in patients with wall motion abnormalities. *J Am Coll Cardiol* 1995;26:342–350.

152. Iida H, Kanno I, Takahashi A, et al. Measurement of absolute myocardial blood flow with O-15 water and dynamic positron emission tomography. *Circulation* 1988;78:104–115.

153. Yamamoto Y, DeSilva R, Rhodes CG, et al. A new strategy for the assessment of viable myocardium and regional myocardial blood flow using 15O-water and dynamic positron emission tomography. *Circulation* 1992;86:167–178.

154. DeSilva R, Yamamoto Y, Rhodes CG, et al. Preoperative prediction of the outcome of coronary revascularization using positron emission tomography. *Circulation* 1992;86:1738–1742.

155. Gerber BL, Melin JA, Bol A, et al. Nitrogen-13 ammonia and oxygen-15-water estimates of absolute myocardial perfusion in left ventricular ischemic dysfunction. *J Nucl Med* 1998;39:1655–1662.

156. Goldstein RA. Kinetics of rubidium-82 after coronary occlusion and reperfusion: assessment of patency and viability in open-chested dogs. *J Clin Invest* 1985;75:1131–1137.

157. Gould KL, Yoshida K, Hess MJ, et al. Myocardial metabolism of fluorodeoxyglucose compared to cell membrane integrity for the potassium analogue rubidium-82 for assessing infarct size in man by PET. *J Nucl Med* 1991;32:1–9.

158. von Dahl J, Muzik O, Wolfe ER, et al. Myocardial rubidium-82 tissue kinetics assessed by dynamic positron emission tomography as a marker of myocardial cell membrane integrity and viability. *Circulation* 1996;93:238–245.

159. Beanlands RS, deKemp R, Scheffel A, et al. Can nitrogen-13 kinetic modeling define myocardial viability independent of fluorine-18 fluorodeoxyglucose? *J Am Coll Cardiol* 1997;29:537–543.

160. Kitsiou AN, Bacharach SL, Bartlett ML, et al. ^{13}N-Ammonia myocardial blood flow and uptake: Relation to functional outcome of asynergic regions after revascularization. *J Am Coll Cardiol* 1999;33:678–686.

161. Eitzman D, Al-Aouar Z, Kanter HL, et al. Clinical outcome of patients with advanced coronary artery disease after viability studies with positron emission tomography. *J Am Coll Cardiol* 1992;20:559–565.

162. DiCarli MF, Davidson M, Little R, et al. Value of metabolic imaging with positron emission tomography for evaluation prognosis in patients with coronary artery disease and left ventricular dysfunction. *Am J Cardiol* 1994;73:527–533.

163. Lee KS, Marwick TH, Cook SA, et al. Prognosis of patients with left ventricular dysfunction, with and without viable myocardium after myocardial infarction: relative efficacy of medical therapy and revascularization. *Circulation* 1994;90:2687–2694.

164. Di Carli MF, Maddahi J, Rokhsar S, et al. Long-term survival of patients with chronic coronary artery disease and left ventricular dysfunction: implications for the role of myocardial viability assessment in management decisions. *J Thorac Cardiovasc Surg* 1998;116:997–1004.

165. Beanlands RS, Hendry PJ, Masters RG, et al. Delay in revascularization is associated with increased mortality rate in patients with severe left ventricular dysfunction and viable myocardium on fluorine-18 fluorodeoxyglucose positron emission tomography imaging. *Circulation* 1998;98:II51–56.

166. Marwich TH, Zuchowski C, Lauer MS, et al. Functional status and quality of life in patients with heart failure undergoing coronary bypass surgery after assessment of myocardial viability. *J Am Coll Cardiol* 1999;33:750–758.

167. Di Carli MF, Maddahi J, Rokhsar S, et al. Long-term survival of patients with chronic coronary artery disease and left ventricular dysfunction: implications for the role of myocardial viability assessment in management decisions. *J Thorac Cardiovasc Surg* 1998;116:997–1004.

168. Pagano D, Townend JN, Littler WA, et al. Coronary artery bypass surgery as treatment for ischemic heart failure: the predictive value of viability assessment with quantitative positron emission tomography for symptomatic and functional outcome. *J Thorac Cardiovasc Surg* 1998;115:791–799.

169. Akinboboye OO, Idris O, Cannon PJ, et al. Usefullness of positron emission tomography in defining myocardial viability in patients referred for cardiac transplantation. *Am J Cardiol* 1999;83:1271–1274.

170. Auerbach MA, Schoder H, Hoh C, et al. Prevalence of myocardial viability as detected by positron emission tomography in patients with ischemic cardiomyopathy. *Circulation* 1999;99:2921–2926.

171. Haas F, Haehnel CJ, Picker W, et al. Preoperative positron emission tomographic viability assessment and perioperative and postoperative risk in patients with advanced ischemic heart disease. *J Am Coll Cardiol* 1997;30:1693–1700.

172. Dilsizian V. Myocardial viability: a clinical and scientific treatise. In: Dilsizian V, ed. *Thallium-201 scintigraphy: experience of two decades.* Armonk, NY: Futura Publishing Co., 2000:265–313.

CHAPTER 16

Myocardial Infarct Imaging

Ban-An Khaw

There are approximately 8 million emergency room visits associated with various forms of chest pain in the United States annually (1). One and a half million of these chest pain patients have acute myocardial infarction. Diagnosis of the usual acute myocardial infarction (MI) is relatively easy utilizing the classical clinical symptoms, electrocardiogram and serum enzyme assessments. However, of the 1.5 million acute myocardial infarct patients, approximately one third are initially misdiagnosed by the existing traditional methods (2). Therefore, there is a need for a better, very accurate method for early diagnosis of acute MI.

There are two general gamma-imaging approaches for diagnosis of acute myocardial infarction; myocardial perfusion (3–5) and infarct avid imaging techniques (6–8). Although myocardial perfusion assessment methods can result in diagnostic end-point relatively early after administration of the radiotracers, their primary function is to assess the perfusion status of the myocardium. Therefore, they cannot differentiate necrotic from nonnecrotic but compromised myocardial tissues. Difficulties also exist in differentiating acutely infarcted myocardium from scar tissues based solely on perfusion scans. Therefore, a positive indicator of acute, irreversible myocardial injury would be highly useful if the sensitivity and specificity were high, providing an unequivocal diagnostic end-point within the very acute phases of the evolving myocardial infarction.

Among the infarct-avid imaging agents, three stand apart: Tc-99m labeled pryophosphate (6,9–11), In-111 labeled

B.-A. Khaw: Department of Pharmaceutical Sciences, Bouvé College of Health Sciences/Northeastern University, Boston, Massachusetts 02115; Department of Cardiac/Nuclear Medicine, Massachusetts General Hospital, Boston, Massachusetts 02114.

antimyosin (7, 12–14), and Tc-99m labeled glucaric acid (15,16). Tc-99m pyrophosphate has been commercially available for over two decades. In-111 antimyosin was recently approved by the FDA for commercialization but is not currently available. The last reagent, Tc-99m glucarate is still in its initial clinical trail stages. The utility of each radiopharmaceutical will be presented in this chapter.

Tc-99m PYROPHOSPHATE

Tc-99m pyrophosphate was initially developed for diagnosis of bone lesions. It was serendipitously observed to also localize in acute myocardial infarction. Due to its avidity for bones, the mechanism of localization of Tc-99m pyrophosphate was initially believed to be binding to hydroxyapatite. Buja et al. (17) observed that the quantity of Tc-99m pyrophosphate binding to the necrotic myocardium correlated to the amount of calcium deposited in the tissue. However, Dewanjee and Kahn (18) found that Tc-99m pyrophosphate localization occurred primarily in the cytosolic fraction and that hydroxyapatite was not the primary target. Irrespective of the exact mechanism of localization of Tc-99m pyrophosphate, experimental and clinical reports support the assertion that this radiopharmaceutical localizes in infarcted (9–11) or severely injured myocardium (19,20). Optimal localization of Tc-99m pyrophosphate in the infarcted myocardium occurs 1 to 5 days after the acute coronary event (21). Nonreperfused MIs, studied by Kondo and colleagues (22), were not visualized by gamma imaging with Tc-99m pyrophosphate on day 1 when the radiotracer was injected 5 to 8 hours after the onset of acute myocardial infarction. When these same patients were reimaged at 22 to 57.7 hours, positive gamma images were obtained in 5 out of the 6 patients with persistent coronary artery occlusion. In reperfused MI patients, visualization of the infarcts was possible in 19 out of 22. Of the 19 positive reperfused patients, Tc-99m pyrophosphate uptake averaged only 2.42 ± 0.61 on a scale of 0 to 4 +, where less than 2 + is considered normal. Nevertheless, the utility of Tc-99m pyrophosphate for diagnosis of acute myocardial infarction at 2 to 3 days is well established.

Whether Tc-99m pyrophosphate is exclusively specific for delineation of irreversibly damaged myocardium is however, not certain. Tc-99m pyrophosphate has been observed to be sequestered by viable but severely injured myocardium (19,20). It is also taken up in patients with stable angina without clinical evidence of myocardial necrosis (23), in unstable angina (24) as well as in patients several months (25) to 1 year (26) after the acute event. These observations suggest that there could be an ongoing process of myocyte necrosis hitherto not appreciated under certain circumstances or alternatively, that pyrophosphate binds to both severely ischemic and necrotic myocardium. Since elevation of intracellular calcium is a common denominator in both ischemic and infarcted myocardium (27), localization of Tc-99m pyrophosphate in severely ischemic and infarcted myocardium is not surprising.

Irrespective of the exact mechanism of Tc-99m pyrophosphate localization, if this reagent can delineate severely ischemic or necrotic myocardium very acutely, pyrophosphate would be extremely useful clinically. In this regard, however, pyrophosphate appears to be a useful radiopharmaceutical agent only in reperfused myocardial infarctions. In nonreperfused MIs, Tc-99m pyrophosphate is useful as a confirmatory diagnostic reagent only 2 to 3 days after the acute event. Thus, even though Tc-99m pyrophosphate is very easy to use and requires only a delay of 2 to 3 hours after intravenous administration for image acquisition, its disadvantage resides in the inability to delineate the infarcted myocardium very acutely, prior to reperfusion.

ANTIMYOSIN ANTIBODIES

The use of antibodies for *in vivo* targeting started with the demonstration by Pressman and Keighley (28) in 1948 using radiolabeled antibodies to kidneys to specifically target the kidneys in rats. Since that seminal demonstration, oncologic applications dominated the field of *in vivo* antibody imaging. It was not until 1976 that the use of polyclonal antimyosin antibody F(ab′)₂ labeled with I-125 radioisotope was reported for *in vivo* localization of the antibody in acute canine myocardial infarction (29).

PRECLINICAL STUDIES

Localization of antimyosin antibody in the necrotic myocardium is based on the following hypothesis: normal myo-

cardial cells with intact cell membrane will not permit extracellular macromolecules to gain access into the cytosol (in any appreciable concentrations), whereas myocardial cells with sarcolemmal disruption cannot prevent entry of extracellular macromolecules nor egress of intracellular components. Since myosin exists as insoluble components of the intracellular contractile myofibrils, myosin will not be washed out but remain in the compromised cell with cell membrane lesions (29). If a specific antibody, such as antimyosin, were introduced into the extracellular milieu, the antibody should be able to interact with the once privileged intracellular cardiac myosin. If this antimyosin antibody were appropriately radiolabeled, then the regions of cell membrane disruption should be visualizable by identifying the region of accumulation of the radiolabeled antimyosin antibody (29). Such an *in vivo* application is shown in Figure 1A, where the experimentally infarcted canine myocardium was visualized by gamma imaging within 3 to 5 hours after intravenous administration of In-111-labeled monoclonal antimyosin Fab (30). However, no delineation of the infarct was seen when In-111-labeled nonspecific Fab was used (Fig. 1B). Similarly, when antimyosin antibody was administered to sham-operated dogs, no myocardial activity was observed. *In vitro* demonstration of the specificity of antimyosin for the necrotic myocytes was established using hypoxic neonatal murine myocytes in primary culture treated with antimyosin antibody attached covalently to 1 micron diameter polystyrene beads (31). Normal myocytes with intact sarcolemma prevented accumulation of the antimyosin beads (Fig. 2A), whereas hypoxic myocytes with sarcolemmal lesions showed specific targeting of the antimyosin beads at the lesions sites (Fig. 2B). Higher magnification

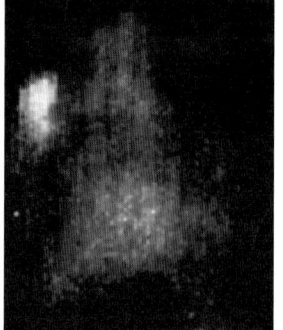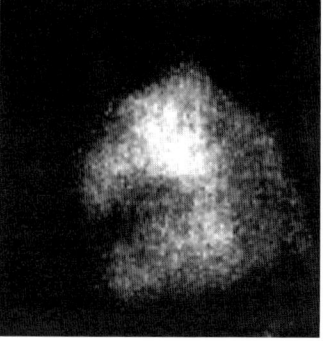

A,B

FIG. 1. A: Left lateral gamma image of a dog with acute experimental myocardial infarction imaged with In-111-labeled monoclonal antimyosin Fab. The image was obtained 5 hours after intravenous administration of the radiolabeled antimyosin Fab. **B:** Left lateral gamma image of a dog with acute experimental myocardial infarction injected with In-111-labeled nonspecific antibody Fab. Image also was acquired at 5 hours after intravenous administration. (From ref. 32, with permission.)

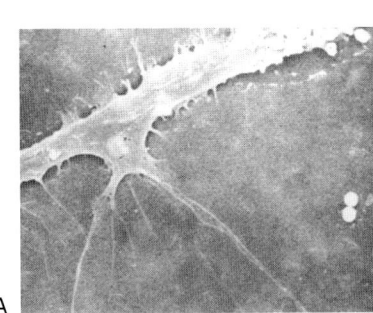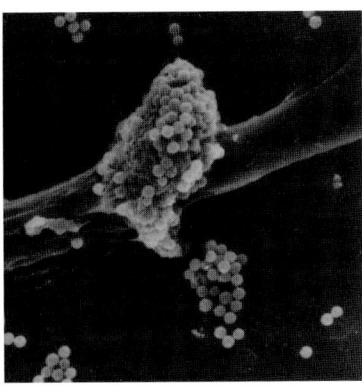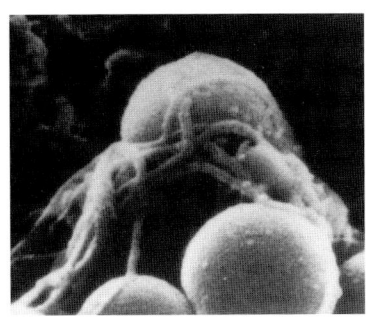

A   B,C

FIG. 2. Scanning electron micrographs of murine neonatal primary myocytes in culture treated with antimyosin linked 1 μ diameter fluorescent polystyrene beads. **A:** A normal myocyte showing the intact cell membrane and a lack of antimyosin-bead binding. **B:** A necrotic myocyte with a region of sarcolemmal disruption showing antimyosin-bead binding in that region. **C:** Magnification of 100,000 times showing binding of antimyosin beads with myofilaments containing myosin. (From ref 17, with permission.)

at 100,000x enabled visualization of the interaction of the antimyosin bead with the myofilaments containing the cardiac myosin (Fig. 2C).

Irrefutable demonstration of the exquisite specificity of antimyosin antibody for irreversibly damaged myocardium was provided by using three monoclonal antimyosin antibodies with different apparent affinities. Fab fragments of R11D10 (Ka = 1.5–2.5 × 10^9 liters/mole), 2G42D7 (Ka = 3 × 10^9 liters/mole), and 3H31E6 (Ka = 3–6 × 10^5 liters/mole) (32) were prepared by papain digestion (32). Fab fragments were either modified with DTPA as previously described (33) and labeled with In-111, or labeled with I-123 by the lactoperoxidase radioiodination method (34). As shown in Figure 3, dogs injected with radiolabeled R11D10 and 2G42D7 Fab all showed unequivocal delineation of the infarcted myocardium *in vivo*. However, dogs injected with radiolabeled 3H31E6 Fab showed only blood pool activity similar to that obtained with nonspecific Fab (Fig. 1). These studies proved that despite the specificity

of all three antimyosin antibodies for the cardiac myosin, only the high affinity antimyosin monoclonal antibodies localized in the infarct to a concentration high enough to develop a target-to-nontarget ratio consistent with visualization by *in vivo* gamma imaging. Thus, the above studies demonstrated that not only is antimyosin specific for the delineation of the necrotic myocardium, but also that high enough affinity is required to enable development of sufficiently high target to background ratios for *in vivo* visualization.

CLINICAL STUDIES

Localization of In-111-labeled monoclonal antimyosin in patients with acute myocardial infarction with and without reperfusion provides accurate delineation of irreversible myocardial injury. In most cases, interpretation of the antimyosin images is quite simple if the images are obtained 18 to 24 hours after intravenous administration. The

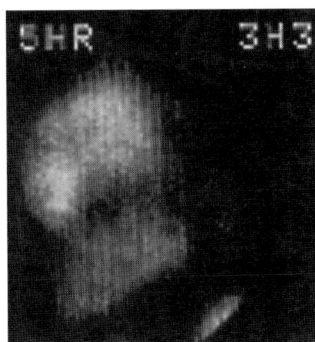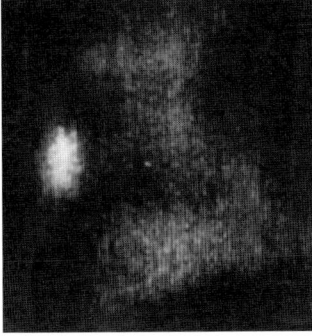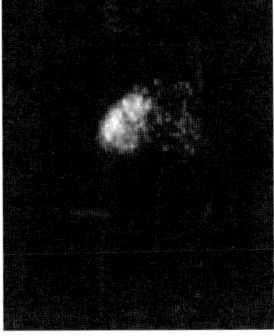

FIG. 3. Left lateral gamma images of three dogs with experimental myocardial infarction injected intravenously with ^{111}In-labeled 3H31E6 antimyosin Fab (Ka = 5 × 10^6 L/M) (**left panel**) and ^{111}In-labeled R11D10 antimyosin Fab (Ka = 1.5 − 2.5 × 10^9 L/M) (**middle panel**) and I-123 labeled 2G42D7 antimyosin Fab (Ka = 3.0 × 10^9 liters/mole) (**right panel**) obtained at 5 hours postinjection. The infarcts in all three animals were approximately the same size but unequivocal visualization was possible only with R11D10 Fab and 2G42D7 Fab; whereas, with 3H3 Fab it was not.

radioactivity is localized to discrete regions corresponding to the territories of the culprit coronary vessels. Figure 4 shows the anterior and left anterior oblique gamma images of patients with anterior (left panels) and inferior (right panels) MIs with (bottom panels) and without (top panels) successful thrombolytic therapy obtained at about 24 hours after intravenous injection of the radiolabeled antibody preparations (20). However, infarct visualization can be problematic in patients with minimal myocardial injury due to residual blood pool activity even at 24 hours. In such cases, repeated imaging at 48 hours normally resolves the dilemma (Fig. 5).

Despite the ability of antimyosin Fab to specifically delineate acute myocardial infarction, its clinical utility is hampered by the slow blood clearance of the Fab fragments. If, on the other hand, a qualitative diagnostic endpoint is the desired result, infarcts may be detected earlier than 18 to 24 hours. Infarcts can often be visualized over blood pool activity from 6 to 14 hours after intravenous administration.

Clinical studies have reported the sensitivity of antimyosin for diagnosis of Q-wave acute myocardial infarction to be between 87 and 98% (20,35–38). In a multicenter trial of 50 patients, Johnson et al. (39) reported positive antimyosin delineation of the infarcts in 46 patients (92% sensitivity). In a larger phase III trial of 492 patients, undertaken

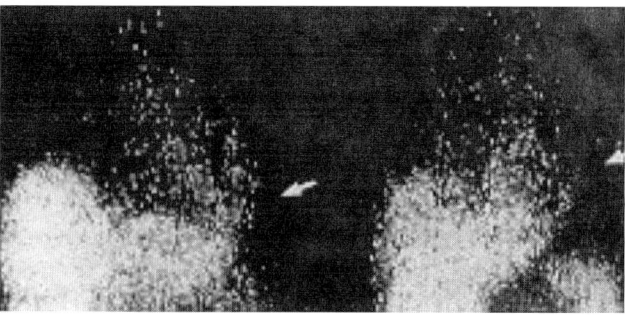

FIG. 5. Anterior and LAO 45-degree gamma images of a patient with minimal myocardial injury in the anterior myocardium visualizable only at 48 hours after intravenous administration of ^{111}In-antimyosin Fab.

at 26 centers (40), 190 out of 202 patients with Q-wave MI were positive by antimyosin imaging (94% sensitivity) and 48 of 57 patients (84% sensitivity) with non-Q-wave MI. A specificity of 93% was reported in patients with chest pain but no clinical evidence of infarction. Specificity of In-111-antimyosin imaging for detection of acute myocardial infarction was further demonstrated by Jain and collegues (41,42) and Hendel et al. (43) in case reports of antimortem confirmation of antimyosin infarct delineation to the postmortem histochemically and histologically demarcated infarction (Fig. 6A–C; see also Color Plate 13 following page 294).

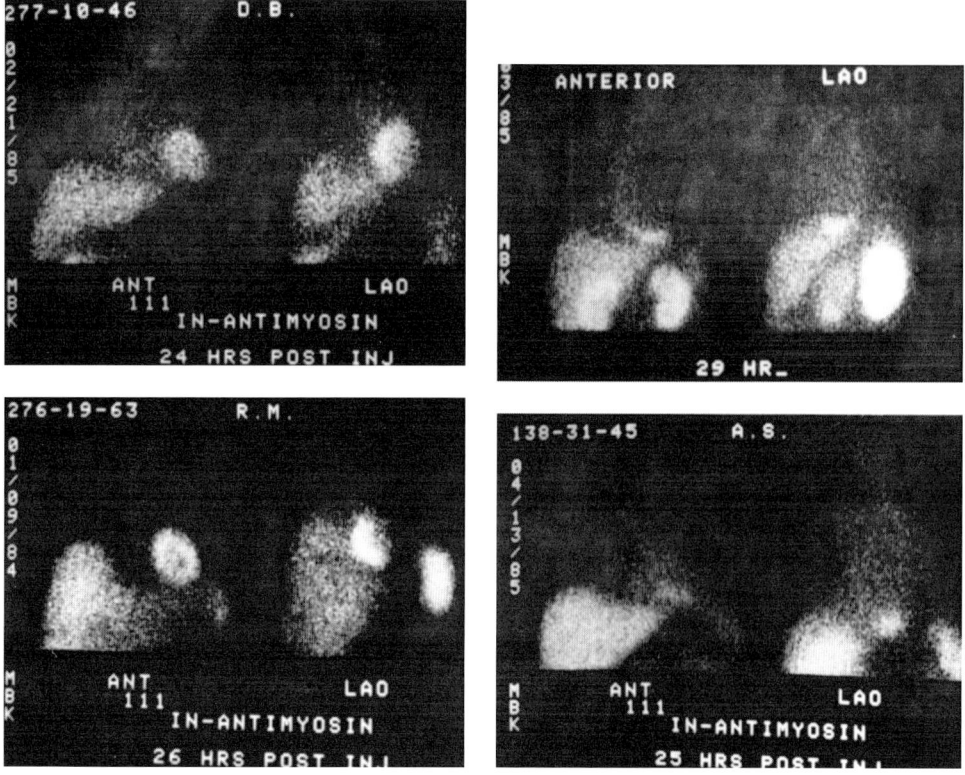

FIG. 4. Anterior and 45-degree LAO images of two patients (**left panels**) with anterior MI and two patients with inferior MIs (**right panels**). The **top panels** were from patients with persistently occluded coronary vessels and the **bottom panels** were from patients with successful reperfusion.

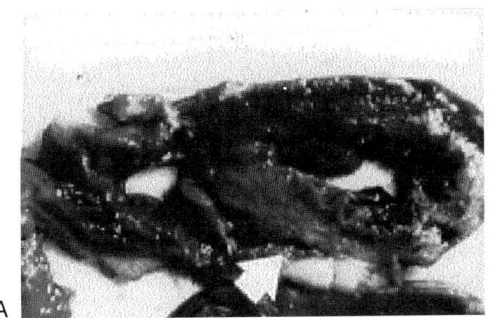

A

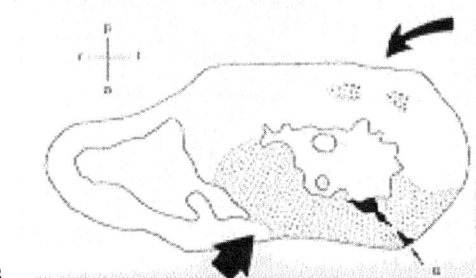

B

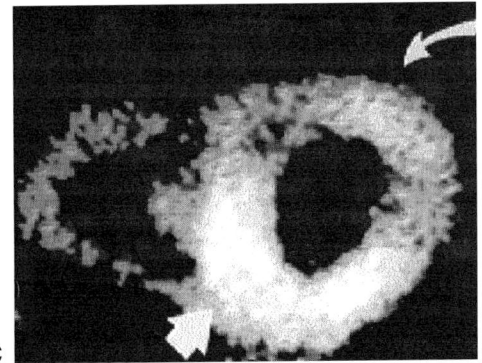

C

FIG. 6. Slice of the heart (**A**) showing anterior wall infarction with rupture of the free anterior wall; schematic representation of the histologically identified region of infarction (**B**); and the gamma image of the above slice showing antimyosin delineation of the infarct (**C**). (From ref. 41, with permission.) **D:** Anterior and LAO views of ^{111}In-antimyosin Fab images of a patient with acute myocardial infarction with no ECG changes. Serum CK showed typical rise and fall on serial estimation. Tracer uptake was seen in two areas (*arrows*) in each view. Coronary angiography showed minor plaques in the left main and right coronary arteries. Embolization from the lesion in the left main may have produced myocardial necrosis at the two sites. (See also Color Plate 13 following page 294.) (From ref. 44, with permission.)

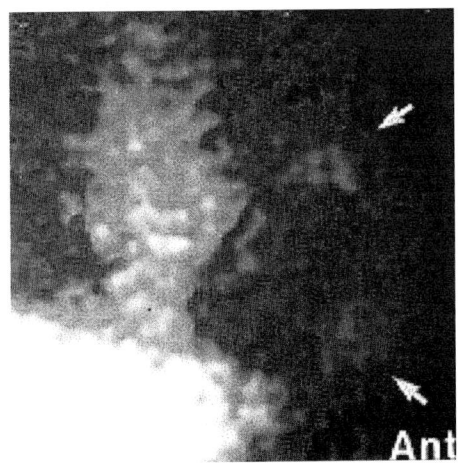

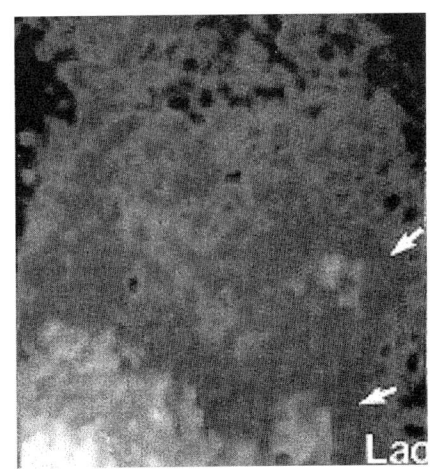

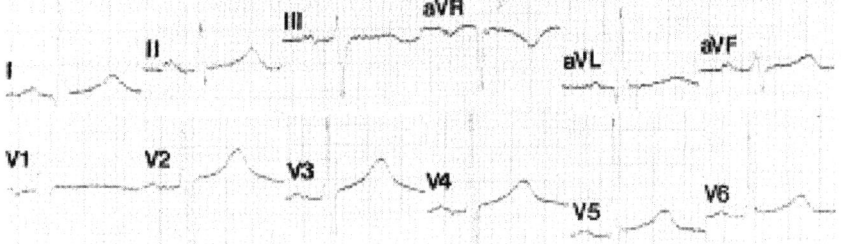

D

Because of the high sensitivity and specificity of antimyosin imaging for diagnosis of acute myocardial infarction, antimyosin imaging can be highly useful for definitive diagnosis of equivocal MI. In a study by Jain et al. (44), 75 patients with suspected acute MI were evaluated. Of the 75 patients, 7 had no electrocardiographic (ECG) changes diagnostic of acute MI. However, all 7 were positive for presence of myocardial necrosis by antimyosin imaging criteria. Figure 6**D** shows one such example.

Due to the high specificity and sensitivity of antimyosin immunoscintigraphy for detection of acute myocardial necrosis, antimyosin has also been used for detection of right ventricular (RV) infarction. Right ventricular infarction is reported to occur in up to 50% of patients dying of inferior MI. Since diagnosis of right ventricular infarction is often difficult unless severe right ventricular dysfunction occurs from extensive RV MI or unless ST-segment elevation occurs in right ventricular precordial leads, Tc-99m-labeled pyrophosphate scintigraphy has been assessed as a diagnostic test. Although a positive study may confirm presence of right ventricular infarction, a negative pyrophosphate scan does not necessarily exclude diagnosis of RV MI (45). Johnson et al. (46) studied 34 patients with posteroinferior MI with In-111 antimyosin and Tl-201 simultaneous imaging by single photon emission computed tomography (SPECT). RV MI was detected in 12 patients; only three had ECG evidence of right ventricular MI. In one patient, diagnosis of RV MI was made solely on the basis of the antimyosin scans. This patient was misdiagnosed as an anterior wall ischemia due to ST-segment elevation in leads V1-3.

Antimyosin imaging has also been used to diagnose postoperative MIs (47). The reported incidence of postoperative MI is based on the appearance of new Q-waves in 5% and ST-T changes in 40% of patients undergoing coronary bypass surgery (48). In a study by Bulkley and Hutchins (49), of the 58 patients who died within 30 days after coronary bypass grafting, 48 had evidence of subendocardial contraction band necrosis in the areas of the patent bypass grafts. van Vlies et al. reported on 23 patients who had undergone coronary bypass surgery for stable angina, had no history of MI, and were evaluated by antimyosin scintigraphy. Antimyosin uptake was observed in 19 with diffuse uptake in 7, and localized uptake in 12. Although 14 of the 19 patients had ST segment changes, no postoperative pathologic Q-waves were observed.

It appears that antimyosin is highly specific for delineation of irreversibly injured myocardium with a sensitivity averaging in the range of 95%. As an agent for very early diagnosis of acute myocardial infarction for directing revascularization therapy, however, antimyosin is not adequate since it requires a minimum of 6 to 7 hours just to ascertain that there is myocardial injury superimposed on the blood pool activity. Revascularization therapy is most effective if initiated within 6 hours from the time of the onset of chest pain, and if initiated within 2 hours, left ventricular function can be preserved and mortality reduced by 50% (50,51). Therefore, an agent that can delineate the infarcted myocardium within a few hours after intravenous administration and whose diagnostic images can be used to direct revascularization could be of clinical use.

Tc-99m GLUCARATE

Glucaric acid is a 6-carbon dicarboxylic acid sugar that can be labeled with Tc-99m (52). It was initially developed as an intermediary transchelator of Tc-99m for radiolabeling of antibody Fab' fragments. However, we observed that it localized in canine reperfused experimental myocardial infarcts very quickly after intravenous administration (Fig. 7**A**) (53). Glucaric acid being a small molecule clears from the blood with a very short $T_{1/2}$. This may permit development of target to background ratios consistent with the ability to visualize acute myocardial infarcts very early by gamma scintigraphy. Preliminary results of Fornet et al. (8) suggested that Tc-99m glucaric acid identified both zones of reversible and irreversible myocardial injury. However, subsequent studies by Orlandi and coworkers (16) as well as by us (54), established unequivocally that Tc-99m glucarate is not sequestered by ischemic tissues in the absence of restenosis. Orlandi et al. (16) showed that in dogs subjected to 20 minutes of ischemia (no TTC infarction) no Tc-99m glucarate localization was obtained. Narula et al. (54) using 5 and 15 minutes of left anterior descending coronary artery (LAD) occlusion in a rabbit model of ischemia also were not able to demonstrate uptake of Tc-99m glucarate in the ischemic tissues.

In canine reperfused myocardial infarction, Orlandi et al. observed that Tc-99m glucarate uptake was positive as early as after 3 hours of reperfusion and was significantly higher at 48 hours. However, uptake assessed at 10 days was near baseline. We, on the other hand, found that in reperfused canine acute myocardial infarction, infarcts can be visualized within in 4 to 10 minutes after intravenous administration of Tc-99m glucarate (Fig. 7**B**) (53). In nonreperfused rabbit acute myocardial infarction, delineation of the infarcts were visualized within 1 hour. Reperfused rabbit MIs were visualized within 30 minutes. Similarly, Ohtani et al. (55) reported that in nonreperfused acute MI in rats, optimal uptake occurred acutely at 4 hours of persistent coronary artery occlusion, with diminishing localization after 24 hours; no localization of Tc-99m glucarate was seen when assessed at 75 hours and 7 days. These studies all indicate that glucarate may be useful as a hyperacute diagnostic reagent in reperfused as well as nonreperfused acute myocardial infarction.

In another study, Yaoito et al. (56) compared Tc-99m glucaric acid uptake to tritiated deoxyglucose uptake in acute myocardial infarcts and multiple episodes of ischemia in rabbits. In the multiple episode model of ischemia where the left anterior descending coronary artery (LAD) was occluded for 20 minutes followed by 5 minutes of reperfusion × 3, uptake ratios of Tc-99m glucaric acid and ^{3}H-deoxy-

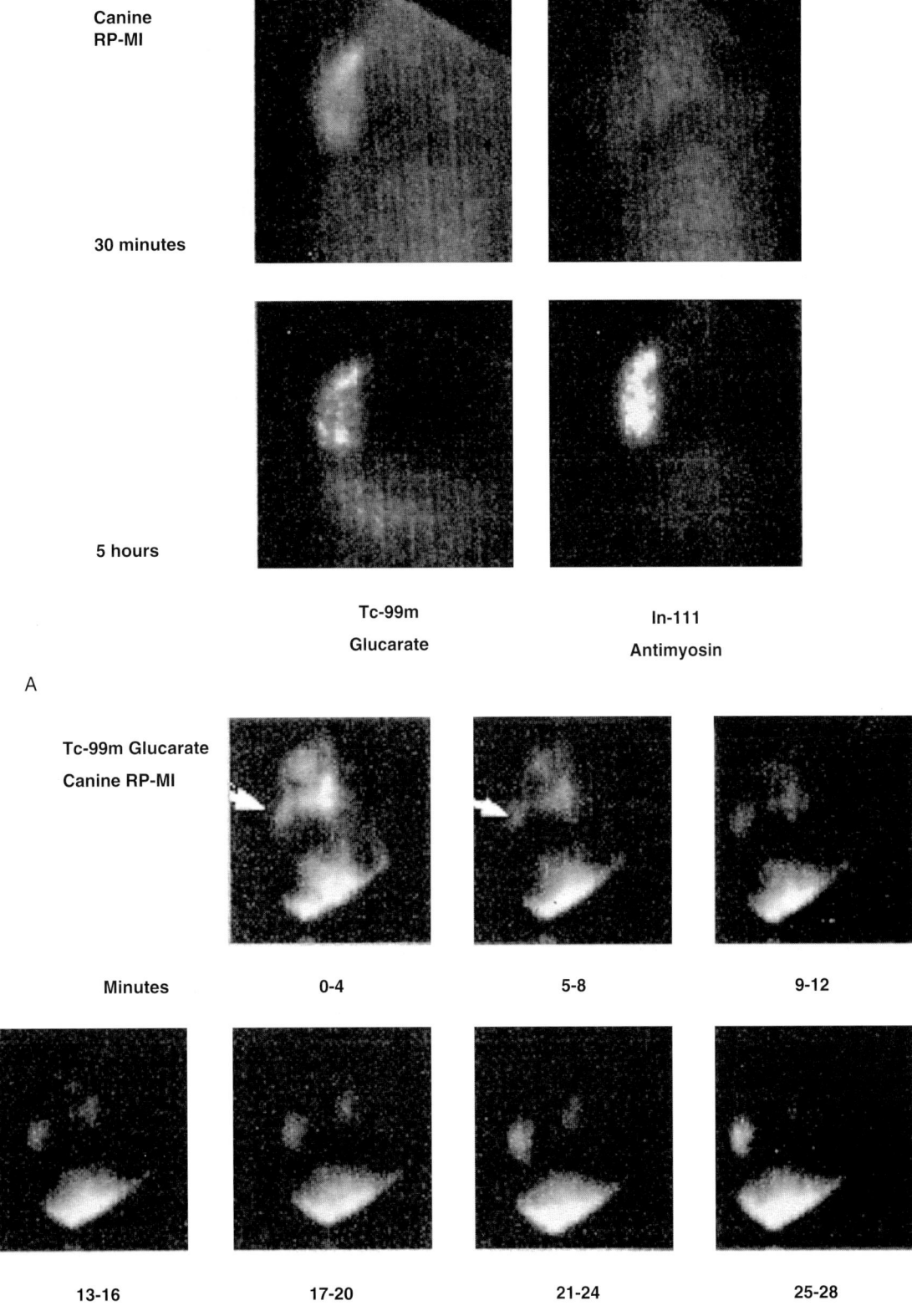

Canine
RP-MI

30 minutes

5 hours

Tc-99m
Glucarate

In-111
Antimyosin

A

Tc-99m Glucarate
Canine RP-MI

Minutes   0-4   5-8   9-12

13-16   17-20   21-24   25-28

B

FIG. 7. A: Left lateral gamma images of a dog with reperfused MI imaged at 30 minutes after intravenous administration of Tc-99m glucarate (**left top panel**) and the corresponding In-111 antimyosin image (**right top panel**). By 5 hours after radiotracer administration, the infarct delineated by both Tc-99m glucarate and In-[111] antimyosin is the same. **B**: Serial left lateral gamma images of a dog with acute myocardial infarction injected with Tc-99m glucarate. The infarct can be visualized as early as 4 to 8 minutes (*arrows*) after intravenous administration of the radiotracer. (From ref. 53, with permission.)

glucose in the normal myocardium, and in the surrounding, margin, and center of the ischemic myocardium were similar, whereas, in the infarcted myocardium, the Tc-99m glucaric acid activity in the infarct center was the greatest. ^{3}H-deoxyglucose uptake in the infarct center was similar but less than that in the margin of the infarct. Although Tc-99m glucaric acid accumulated in mildly damaged myocardium, only severe myocardial injury would be visualized by *in vivo* imaging at 1 hour after intravenous administration. Therefore, it appears that only infarcts can be visualized by gamma imaging, whereas tissue counting can show areas of radiotracer uptake in the ischemic zones.

Recently, Narula et al. (54) reported that Tc-99m glucarate can be used for hyperacute localization and visualization of experimental myocardial infarcts in reperfused and nonreperfused rabbit infarct models. When uptake of Tc-99m glucarate and In-111 antimyosin Fab, administered simultaneously into rabbits with acute MI, were compared, a direct correlation was obtained in either nonreperfused or reperfused infarcts. Target to nontarget ratios of Tc-99m glucarate were substantially higher than the corresponding In-111 antimyosin-Fab uptake ratios in the same tissue samples. This difference was more pronounced in nonreperfused MIs. When uptake ratios of Tc-99m glucarate were compared to In-111 antimyosin-Fab uptake ratios in canine reperfused myocardial infarction, a direct correlation was also obtained ($r^2 = 0.98$) (53). Since antimyosin is highly specific for delineation of myocardial necrosis, and a direct correlation is obtained between Tc-99m glucarate and In-111 antimyosin Fab, the former must also be delineating acute myocardial necrosis. Since the correlation coefficient is almost 1, the two infarct avid agents appear to be delineating the same infarcted tissues. However, since Tc-99m glucarate generated higher target-to-nontarget ratios than In-111 antimyosin Fab within the same time period, it stands to reason that visualization of the infarct should occur faster with Tc-99m glucarate than with In-111 antimyosin Fab. Figure 6**A** shows that Tc-99m glucaric acid already delineated the infarct as early as 30 minutes postradiotracer administration, whereas the simultaneously administered In-111 antimyosin Fab showed only blood pool activity at the same time. By 5 hours, both radiotracers showed equivalent infarct delineation in canine reperfused myocardial infarcts (53).

The mechanism for the necrotic tissue specificity of Tc-99m-labeled glucarate is due to its affinity for targeting the histone of the necrotic myocytes. Figure 8 (see also Color Plate 14 following page 294) shows that when infarcted tissues at 1 and 3 hours after intravenous administration of Tc-99m glucarate were fractionated into nuclear, mitochondrial, and cytosolic fractions, greater than 75% of the infarct radioactivity was associated with the nuclear fraction. Further fractionation of the nuclear activity into nucleoproteins and DNA demonstrated that the predominant radioactivity was associated with the nucleoproteins, which consist primarily of histones. Therefore, it appears that when acute myocardial necrosis occurs, the nucleohistones become accessible to Tc-

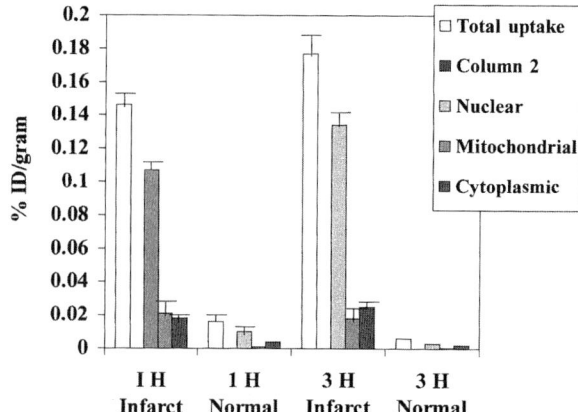

FIG. 8. Subcellular distribution of Tc-99m glucarate activity in the infarcted rabbit myocardium at 1 and 3 hours postintravenous administration of the radiotracer. Total uptake as well as activities in the nuclear, mitochondrial, and cytoplasmic fractions are shown. (See also Color Plate 14 following page 294.)

99m glucaric acid. The initial entry of Tc-99m glucaric acid into the infarct zone appears to be via collateral circulation and or diffusion. However, the highly basic nucleohistones may act as a sink for concentrating the acidic glucaric acid once the integrity of the sarcolemma has been lost. This high avidity for the nucleo-histones together with the fast blood clearance should allow development of target to background ratios that permit early visualization of the infarcted myocardium.

This very acute localization capability of Tc-99m glucarate has also been seen in patients. Figure 9 shows the anterior and left anterior oblique (LAO) images of a patient who underwent successful thrombolysis within 3.5 hours of chest pain. Tc-99m glucaric acid was administered at 4.5 hours (57). To date, studies from Europe have demonstrated that hyperacute visualization of acute MI is feasible with Tc-99m glucaric acid. Large MIs can be visualized earlier than small MIs. Nevertheless, diagnostic results of small nonreperfused MIs can be obtained within 3 hours of intravenous

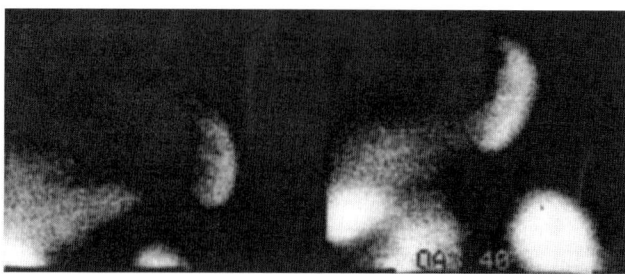

FIG. 9. Anterior and LAO (40 degrees) gamma image of a patient with reperfused anterior MI injected with Tc-99m glucarate. The image was obtained at about 3.5 hours after intravenous administration of the radiotracer. (From ref. 57, with permission.)

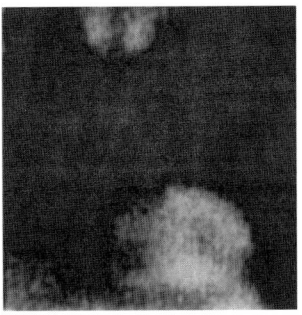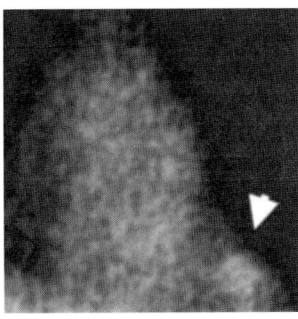

FIG. 10. Tc-99m glucarate anterior gamma image of a patient with nonreperfused apical MI (**right panel**, *arrowhead*). Note the focal apical activity corresponding to the region of Tl-201 defect (**right panel**). (From ref. 57, with permission.)

administration of this reagent (Fig.10). Furthermore, it appears that Tc-99m glucaric acid is highly sensitive and specific for acute MI but not sensitive for MI older than 2 to 3 days. This observation is consistent with the avidity of Tc-99m glucarate for the nucleoproteins, since it appears that at 2 to 3 days, the targets of Tc-99m glucarate would no longer be present due to autolysis in the infarct. However, the exact duration for Tc-99m glucarate positivity is not known. Mariani et al. (57) observed that, in reperfused MIs, positivity waned after peak serum creatine kinase levels have been reached. Whether the same time frame will hold for nonreperfused MI must await additional studies.

Therefore, it appears that Tc-99m glucarate may provide a method for a very acute myocardial infarct imaging. Large MIs should be visualizable by gamma imaging in about 1 hour after intravenous administration and small MIs should be detectable by 3 hours. This time frame may be compatible with diagnostic utility for directing reperfusion therapy in the emergency department in situations where the diagnosis of acute MI is uncertain.

SUMMARY

Tc-99m pyrophosphate imaging is abnormal in the setting of acute myocardial necrosis and often in the setting of severe myocardial ischemia. Antimyosin provides exquisite specificity for the detection of myocardial necrosis, irrespective of the cause of the injury. Therefore, diagnosis of equivocal MI or confirmation of diffuse myocardial necrosis could be achieved with In-111-labeled antimyosin Fab. Tc-99m glucaric acid, on the other hand, may fulfill the original role envisioned for antimyosin, which was to enable hyperacute diagnosis of acute myocardial infarction. However, the window for Tc-99m glucaric acid appears to be about 2 to 3 days. Therefore, there is a potential utility of using both Tc-99m glucaric acid and In-111 antimyosin in tandem, which would not only permit hyperacute detection and diagnosis of acute myocardial infarction and diagnosis of equivocal MI, but would also permit stratification of the infarct age.

REFERENCES

1. Pasternak RC, Braunwald E. Acute myocardial infarction. In: Isselbacher KJ, Braunwald E, Wilson JD, et al., eds. *Harrison's principles of internal medicine,* 13th ed. New York: McGraw-Hill, 1994:1066.
2. McCarthy BD, Beshansky JR, D'Agostino RB, et al. Missed diagnosis of acute myocardial infarction in the emergency department: results from a multicenter study. *Ann Emerg Med* 1993;22:579–582.
3. Bailey IK, Griffith LSC, Rouleau J, et al. Thallium-201 myocardial perfusion imaging at rest and during exercise: Comparative sensitivity to electrocardiography in coronary artery disease. *Circulation* 1977; 55:79–87.
4. Van Train KF, Garcia EV, Maddahi J, et al. Multicenter trial validation for quantitative analysis of same-day rest-stress technetium-99m-sestamibi myocardial tomograms. *J Nucl Med* 1994;35:609–618.
5. Kelly JD, Forster AM, Higley B, et al. Technetium-99m-tetrofosmin as a new radiopharmaceutical for myocardial perfusion imaging. *J Nucl Med* 1993;34:222–227.
6. Parkey RW, Bonte FJ, Meyer SL, et al. A new method for radionuclide imaging of acute myocardial infarction in humans. *Circulation* 1974; 50:540–546.
7. Khaw BA, Gold HK, Yasuda T, et al. Scintigraphic quantification of myocardial necrosis in patients after intravenous injection of myosin specific antibody. *Circulation* 1986;74:501–508.
8. Fornet B, Yasuda T, Wilkinson R, et al. Detection of acute cardiac injury with technetium-99m glucaric acid. *J Nucl Med* 1989;30:1743.
9. Kronenberg MW, Wooten NE, Friesinger GC, et al. Scintigraphic characterisics of experimental myocardial infarct extension. *Circulation* 1979;60:1130–1140.
10. Cowley MJ, Mantle JA, Rogers WJ, Russell RO, Jr., Rackley CE, Logic JR. Technetium-99m stannous pyrophosphate myocardial scintigraphy: Reliability and limitations in assessment of acute myocardial infarction. *Circulation* 1977;56:192–198.
11. Willerson JT, Parkey RW, Bonte FJ, et al. Acute subendocardial myocardial infarction in patients: its detection by technetium-99m stannous pyrophosphate myocardial scintigrams. *Circulation* 1975;51:436–441.
12. Khaw BA, Strauss HW, Moore R, et al. Myocardial damage delineated by In-111 antimyosin Fab and Tc-99m-pyrophosphate. *J Nucl Med* 1987;28:76–82.
13. Khaw BA, Yasuda T, Gold HK, et al. Acute myocardial infarct imaging with Indium-111-labeled monoclonal antimyosin Fab. *J Nucl Med* 1987;28:1671–1678.
14. Khaw BA, Fallon JT, Strauss HW, et al. Myocardial infarct imaging with Indium-111-diethylene triamine pentaacetic acid-anticanine cardiac myosin antibodies. *Science* 1980;209:295–297.
15. Yaoita H, Juweid M, Wilkinson R, et al. Detection of myocardial reperfusion injury with Tc-99m glucarate. *J Nucl Med* 1990;31(5):795(abst).
16. Orlandi C, Crane PD, Edwards DS, et al. Early scintigraphic detection of experimental myocardial infarction in dogs with technetium-99m-glucaric acid. *J Nucl Med* 1991;32:263–268.
17. Buja LM, Tofe AJ, Kulkarni PV, et al. Sites and mechnaisms of localization of technetium-99m phosphorus radiopharmaceuticals in acute myocardial infarcts and other tissues. *J Clin Invest* 1977;60: 724–740.
18. Dewanjee MK, Kahn PC. Mechanism of localization of Tc-99m-labeled pyrophosphate and tetracycline in infarcted myocardium. *J Nucl Med* 1976;17:639–646.
19. Bianco JA, Kemper AJ, Taylor A, et al. Technetium-99m (Sn^{2+}) pyrophosphate in ischemic and infarcted dog myocardium in early stages of acute coronary occlusion: histochemical and tissue-counting comparisons. *J Nucl Med* 1983;24:485–491.
20. Khaw BA, Strauss HW, Moore R, et al. Myocardial damage delineated by In-111 antimyosin Fab and Tc-99m-pyrophosphate. *J Nucl Med* 1987;28:76–82.
21. Parkey RW, Kulkarni PV, Lewis SE, et al. Effect of coronary blood flow and site of injection on Tc-99m Ppi detection of early canine myocardial infarction. *J Nucl Med* 1981;22:133–137.
22. Kondo M, Takahashi M, Matsuda T, et al. Clinical significance of early myocardial Tc-99m-pyrophosphate uptake in patients with acute myocardial infarction. *Am Heart J* 1987;113:250–256.
23. Mason JW, Myers RW, Alderman EL, et al. Technetium-99m pyrophosphate myocardial uptake in patients with stable angina pectoris. *Am J Cardiol* 1977;40:1–5.
24. Jaffe AS, Klein MS, Patel BR, et al. Abnormal technetium-99m pyro-

phosphate images in unstable angina: ischemia versus infarction? *Am J Cardiol* 1979;44:1035–1039.

25. Olson HG, Lyons KP, Aronow WS, et al. Follow-up technetium-99m stannous pyrophosphate myocardial scintigrams after myocardial infarction. *Circulation* 1977;56:181–187.

26. Olson HG, Lyons KP, Aronow WS, et al. Prognostic value of a persistently positive technetium-99m stannous pyrophosphate myocardial scintigram after myocardial infarction. *Am. J. Cardiol* 1979;43:889–898.

27. Schwartz A, Wood JM, Allen JC, et al. Biochemical and morphologic correlates of cardiac ischemia. I. Membrane systems. *Am J Cardiol* 1973;32:46–61.

28. Pressman D, Keighley G. Zone of activity of antibodies as determined by the use of radioactive tracers; zone of activity of nephrotoxic antikidney serum. *J Immunol* 1948;59:141–146.

29. Khaw BA, Beller GA, Haber E, et al. Localization of cardiac myosin-specific antibody in myocardial infarction. *J Clin Invest* 1976;58:439–446.

30. Khaw BA, Mattis JA, Melincoff G, et al. Monoclonal antibody to cardiac myosin; sintigraphic imaging of experimental myocardial infarction. *Hybridoma* 1984;3:11–23.

31. Khaw BA, Scott J, Fallon JT, et al. Myocardial injury: quantitation by cell sorting initiated with anti-myosin fluorescent spheres. *Science* 1982;217:1050–1053.

32. Khaw BA, Petrov A, Narula J. Complementary roles of antibody affinity and specificity in *in vivo* diagnostic cardiovascular targeting: how specific is antimyosin for irreversible myocardial damage? *J Nucl Cardiol* 1999;6:316–323.

33. Khaw BA, Mattis JA, Melincoff G, et al. Monoclonal antibody to cardiac myosin; Scintigraphic imaging of experimental myocardial infarction. *Hybridoma* 1984;3:11–23.

34. Khaw BA, Beller GA, Haber E. Experimental myocardial infarct imaging following intravenous administration of Iodine-131 labeled antibody (Fab')₂ fragments specific for cardiac myosin. *Circulation* 1978;57:743–750.

35. Braat SH, de Zwaan C, Teuke J, et al. Value of indium-111 monoclonal antimyosin antibody for imaging in acute myocardial infarction. *Am J Cardiol* 1987;60:725–726.

36. Cox PH, Schonfeld D, Remme WF, et al. A comparative study of myocardial infarct detection using Tc-99m–pyrophosphate and In-111 antimyosin. *Int J Card Imaging* 1987;2:197–198.

37. Volpini M, Giubbini R, Gei P, et al. Diagnosis of acute myocardial infarction by indium-111 antimyosin antibody and correlation with traditional techniques for the evaluation of extent and localization. *Am J Cardiol* 1989;63:7–13.

38. Antunes ML, Seldin DW, Wall RM, et al. Measurement of acute Q-wave myocardial infarct size with SPECT imaging of In-111 antimyosin. *Am J Cardiol* 1989;63:777–783.

39. Johnson LL, Seldin DW, Becker LC, et al. Antimyosin imaging in acute transmural myocardial infarction: results of a multicenter clinical trial. *J Am Coll Cardiol* 1989;13:27–35.

40. Berger H, Lahiri A, Leppo J, et al. Antimyosin imaging in patients with ischemic chest pain: initial results of phase III multicenter trial. *J Nucl Med* 1988;28:805(abst).

41. Jain D, Lahiri A, Crawley JCW, et al. Indium-111 antimyosin imaging in a patient with acute myocardial infarction: postmortem correlation between histopathologic and autoradiographic extent of myocardial necrosis. *Am J Card Imaging* 1988;2:158–161.

42. Jain D, Crawley JC, Lahiri A, et al. Indium-111-antimyosin images compared with TTC staining in a patient six days after myocardial infarction. *J Nucl Med* 1990;31:231–233.

43. Hendel RC, McSherry BA, Leppo JA. Myocardial uptake of indium-111-labeled antimyosin in acute subendocardial infarction: clinical, histochemical and autoradiographic correlation of myocardial necrosis. *J Nucl Med* 1990;31:1851–1853.

44. Jain D, Lahiri A, Raftery E. Immunoscintigraphy for detecting acute myocardial infarction without electrocardiographic changes. *Br Med J* 1990;300:151–153.

45. Khaw BA, Narula J. Antimyosin scintigraphy in cardiovascular diseases. *Trends Cardiovasc Med* 1992;2:197–204.

46. Johnson LL, Seldin DW, Tresgallo ME, et al. Right ventricular infarction and function from dual isotope indium-111 antimyosin/thallium-201 SPECT and gated blood pool scintigraphy. *J Nucl Med* 1991;32:1018(abst).

47. van Vlies B, van Royen ED, Visser CA, et al. Frequency of myocardial indium-111 antimyosin uptake after uncomplicated coronary bypass surgery. *Am J Cardiol* 1990;66:1191–1195.

48. Hultgren HN, Shettigar UR, Pfeifer JF, et al. Acute myocardial infarction ischemic injury during surgery for cornary artery disease. *Am Heart J* 1977;94:146–153.

49. Bulkley BH, Hutchins GM. Myocardial consequences of coronary artery bypass graft surgery: the paradox of necrosis in areas of revascularization. *Circulation* 1977;56:906–913.

50. Califf RM, Topol EJ, George BS, et al. One-year outcome after therapy with tissue plasminogen activator: report from the Thrombolysis and Angioplasty in Myocardial Infarction trial. *Am Heart J* 1990;119:777–785.

51. The TIMI Study Group. Comparison of invasive and conservative strategies after treatment with intravenous tissue plasminogen activator in acute myocardial infarction: Results of the Thrombolysis in Myocardial Infarction (TIMI) Phase II trial. *N Engl J Med* 1989;320:618–627.

52. Pak KY, Nedelman MA, Kanke M, et al. An instant method for labeling antimyosin Fab' with technetium-99m: evaluation in an experimental myocardial infarct model. *J Nucl Med* 1992;33(1):144–149.

53. Khaw BA, Nakazawa A, O'Donnell, et al. Avidity of Tc-99m-glucarate for the necrotic myocardium: *in vivo* and *in vitro* assessment. *J Nucl Cardiol* 1997;4:283–290.

54. Narula J, Petrov A, Pak KY, et al. Very early noninvasive detection of acute experimental nonreperfused myocardial infarction with technetium-99m-labeled glucarate. *Circulation* 1997;95:1577–1584.

55. Ohtani H, Callahan RJ, Khaw BA, et al. Comparison of technetium-99m-glucarate and thallium-201 for the identification of acute myocardial infarction in rats. *J Nucl Med* 1992;33:1988–1993.

56. Yaoito H, Fischman AJ, Wilkinson R, et al. Distribution of deoxyglucose and technetium-99m-glucarate in the acutely ischemic myocardium. *J Nucl Med* 1993;34:1303–1308.

57. Mariani G, Villa PF, Rosettin C, et al. Direct scintigraphic imaging of acute myocardial infarction with Tc-99m-glucaric acid in humans. *Eur J Nucl Med* 1996;23(9):1045(abst).

CHAPTER 17

Assessment of Ventricular Function by Equilibrium Blood Pool Scintigraphy

Stephen L. Bacharach

Radionuclide-based techniques have been used to measure ventricular function for over two decades (1–5). Either of two fundamentally different approaches can be used. The most recently developed method involves labeling the myocardial walls with a radiotracer, and then examining how those walls thicken and/or translate and rotate throughout the cardiac cycle. This method will be discussed in detail in Chapter 19. The second, and older, method involves imaging the blood itself and then examining how this blood is moved by the thickening and motion of the myocardial walls. The two methods are to some degree complementary. Motion of the endocardial wall of the ventricular chambers must cause the blood adjacent to that wall to move. Despite this, the two methods give somewhat different information regarding ventricular function. By examining the motion of the endo- and epicardial walls of the myocardium, one could in principle determine the degree to which the ventricular wall is thickening (and how thick it actually is) at every location in the myocardium. In theory, one could integrate the endocardial component of this information over the entire chamber to determine, indirectly, how much and how rapidly blood will be ejected as a result of that motion. On the other hand, by labeling the blood with a radiotracer one can directly determine the relative volume of blood ejected from or filling the chamber, and the rates at which that ejection and filling occur. By observing the motion of the blood at the endocardial borders one can, indirectly, infer the regional endocar-

dial wall motion that must have caused that movement of blood. However, since direct observation of the blood does not give any information about the epicardial wall, one can infer only the absolute endocardial motion, not the relative thickening of that wall. Why then would one choose the second technique (the direct observation of the blood pool) over the first (the direct observation of the myocardial wall)? The answer is that it may not be easy to make accurate and reproducible measurements of thickening or regional LV function from direct observations of the wall itself (6–8). Even with high-resolution imaging methods, such as echocardiography or magnetic resonance imaging, accurate measurements of the motion of the epicardial and endocardial walls is at times problematic. The problem is further compounded if, as often is the case for echocardiography, one can not image the entire myocardial cavity of interest. Both first-pass radionuclide angiography and equilibrium gated blood pool (GBP) imaging avoid the necessity for accurate determination of myocardial edges. The first pass method is described in Chapter 18. For the more commonly used method of equilibrium gated blood pool imaging, if one can label the blood (and several tracers are available to do so), the number of photons emitted by the left ventricular cavity will be directly proportional to the volume of blood within it. In principle, then, one does not need to precisely define the surface of the endocardium. Instead, all one need do is to separate the blood pool from other structures, for example by drawing a region of interest (ROI) that encompasses the blood pool (preferably without including other structures that contain large volumes of blood). The counts within this

S. L. Bacharach: Imaging Science Program, National Institutes of Health, Bethesda, Maryland 20892.

region are then proportional to the blood volume in the region. Even if one does not know the proportionality factor, relative changes in the number of photons emitted will be directly proportional to relative changes in blood volume. With single photon emission computed tomography (SPECT) or planar imaging, as has been described in Chapter 11, such relative measurements are all one can currently obtain (although the possibility of absolute measurements may not be far off). With positron emission tomography (PET), however, absolute measurements of activity are quite readily obtained, and the proportionality factor between activity and blood volume can easily be determined by drawing and counting a small venous blood sample. This permits accurate absolute blood volume measurements.

For all the above reasons, measurement of ventricular function by labeling and imaging the blood pool remains an accurate, reproducible tool of considerable clinical importance. This chapter will review those parameters that are useful in describing global and regional function, and discuss how the techniques of blood pool imaging, both planar and tomographic, can be used to measure these parameters.

PLANAR GATED BLOOD POOL IMAGING

The principal measures of ventricular function, which can be determined from radionuclide blood pool imaging (or, in fact, from nearly any imaging modality), are measures extracted from the ventricular volume curve–that is from the curve of ventricular volume as a function of time (9–11). Since the primary clinical interest is most frequently the functioning of the left ventricle, this chapter will focus on this chamber, although the right ventricle and the left atrium will also be considered briefly. Figure 1 illustrates a typical left ventricular (LV) volume curve. The shape and informa-

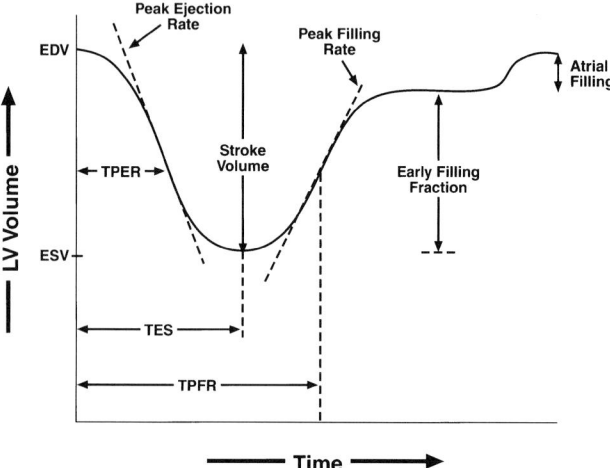

FIG. 1. Left ventricular volume curve, showing parameters one can extract from it. *TES* is time to end-systole, *TPER* and *TPFR* are the times to peak ejection and filling rates. *EDV* and *ESV* are the end diastolic and end systolic volumes, respectively.

tion extracted from this curve is independent of whether it was produced from imaging using radionuclide techniques, ultrasound, or magnetic resonance imaging (MRI). In the sections that follow, how one produces such a curve using radionuclide blood pool imaging will be explained. In addition, how one analyzes such a curve (independent of the modality used to produce it) will be described.

Planar Gated Blood Pool Image Acquisition

One of the simplest and earliest radionuclide methods to image global ventricular function is the method of planar gated blood pool imaging (GBP). To use this method, one first labels the blood pool itself—preferably the red blood cells, rather than the plasma—with a radioisotope suitable for gamma camera imaging. As described in a previous chapter, Tc-99m, which emits 140 keV photons, is the most commonly used tracer for this purpose. Several methods are available for performing the blood pool labeling, all with quite high labeling efficiencies (12). Activities of between 10 and 20 mCi are usually used, although if short acquisitions are desired (e.g., for imaging during exercise or pharmacological stress), even higher activities can be employed. A gamma camera is placed over the patient's chest, with the LV chamber near the center of the field of view. A general purpose, medium resolution, low energy collimator is usually used (often called an all-purpose collimator), although again for short duration studies, one may wish to use a higher sensitivity collimator. In this latter case, great care must be taken to keep the collimator close to the chest wall, as resolution falls off far more dramatically with distance from the chest with high sensitivity collimators than with other collimators. Typically a left anterior oblique (LAO) view (approximately 35 degrees), with a slight caudal tilt (5 to 15 degrees) is used. The LAO angle is adjusted to give the optimum left/right heart separation, as judged visually. The long axis of the heart is usually tilted not just left and right (which can be compensated for with the LAO angle), but also is tilted in the anterior-posterior direction. This means that the gamma camera should ideally be given a caudal tilt in order to view the LV chamber perpendicular to the long axis (a desirable view, so as to maximize the area of LV wall visible on the image, as well as to reduce atrial overlap). Unfortunately, the amount of caudal tilt required to achieve a true long-axis view has been shown (13) to be on the order of 60 degrees. In practice, the physical constraints of the patient's chest result in being able to tilt the planar gamma camera caudally only about 5 to 15 degrees. Thus even in the best of circumstances the LV is quite foreshortened, with the apex overlapping the lower and mid-ventricular cavity, and there is also usually considerable overlap between the left atrium and the base of the LV cavity. Figure 2 shows a typical end diastolic (ED) image obtained with a planar gamma camera in the LAO view. In this figure, brightness is proportional to the number of photons detected. More detailed guidelines describing the optimal recommended

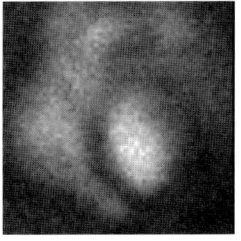 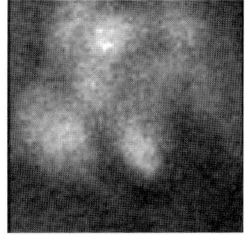

End Diastole   **End Systole**

FIG. 2. Typical end diastolic and end systolic images from a planar gated blood pool study. The left ventricle is on the right hand side of each image, and the right ventricle is to the left.

methods for data acquisition, camera positioning, radiopharmaceuticals, etc. are available elsewhere (12).

Gating the Data

In order to image the heart throughout the cardiac cycle, the image acquisition is gated to the patient's electrocardiographic (ECG) signal (11). A "trigger" pulse is derived from the R-to-S transition of the ECG signal to perform this gating. The gamma camera is connected to a computer, as described in Chapter 11. The computer sets aside a user selectable number of images, used to span the cardiac cycle. For example, 40 images might be used to span a cardiac cycle that had, on average, a 1 second R-to-R time (i.e., 60 beats per minute). Each image is of a user selected matrix size. Typically, the matrix size is selected so as to give about 2-to-3 mm/pixel. Since one is interested only in the heart, the computer may be used to "zoom" the images, in which case a 64*64 matrix may be sufficient. At each trigger pulse, the computer begins sorting the incoming data into each of the images in sequence, each for a preset period of time. For example, if the user had selected 40 images to span a 1 second R-R interval, each image would be acquired sequentially for 1sec/40 = 25 msec. Each of the 40 images would accumulate very few counts in a single 25 msec time period—far too few to create an image of useable statistical quality. Therefore at the end of the first heart beat (i.e., the occurrence of the next R-wave trigger), the computer would "reset" to the first image in the 40-image sequence, and the next 25 msec of data would be added to that already present. Then, during the next 25 msec interval, data would be added to the second image in the sequence, etc. Thus, for example, after 100 beats, the first image in the sequence would contain all the data that had occurred during the first 25 msec following each of the 100 R waves (therefore, 25msec*100 = 2.5 seconds), the next image would contain the next 25 msec of data, etc. The process is illustrated schematically in Figure 3, and is often referred to as "frame mode" or "gated frame mode" acquisition. A typical gated set of blood pool images are shown in Figure 4. Typically for a rest study, one might acquire data for 6 to 10 minutes in the LAO view. There is an assumption implicit in the gating process—namely, that

the heart beats in exactly the same way (i.e., it has the same contraction and relaxation pattern) from one beat to the next. If the subject is in normal sinus rhythm (NSR), this approximation holds quite well (14), except at the end of the cycle (due to sinus arrhythmia). The end of the cycle has to be handled somewhat differently, because not all beats will be of the same length. In fact, fluctuations in R-to-R interval times can be quite large—as much as 100 msec or more for a normal subject in NSR at rest. This means that for beats shorter than average, the last few of the 40 frames will not accumulate additional counts, while for beats longer than average, the 40-frame limit will be exceeded, and data will be thrown away. Both of these circumstances can easily be accounted for by keeping accurate account of the actual length of each beat (and therefore the actual acquisition time for each of the frames that span the cardiac cycle). Of course, such beat length fluctuations may degrade the ability of the gated data to portray events occurring very late in the cycle (e.g., the volume increase due to atrial contraction). Not all computer systems make the compensation for varying beat lengths described above. If it is not made, then the images at the end of the cycle will have an artificially reduced intensity and quantitative data extracted from these images may be subject to error.

At first one might think that a shorter than average beat might be a "condensed" version of an average length beat—i.e., that a long beat is simply a uniformly stretched version of a short beat, scaled temporally, and having a shorter than average time to end-systole, etc. If this were true, then the assumption that all beats are identical would be violated. Fortunately, for subjects in NSR, it has been shown that at rest, fluctuations in heart rate are caused primarily by fluctuations in the initiation of the next beat. That is, a "short" beat is shorter only because the next beat begins slightly earlier than average. Thus, at rest, in normal individuals, it is only diastole that is shorter, and the earlier parts of the cycle remain unaltered. This is not true at higher heart

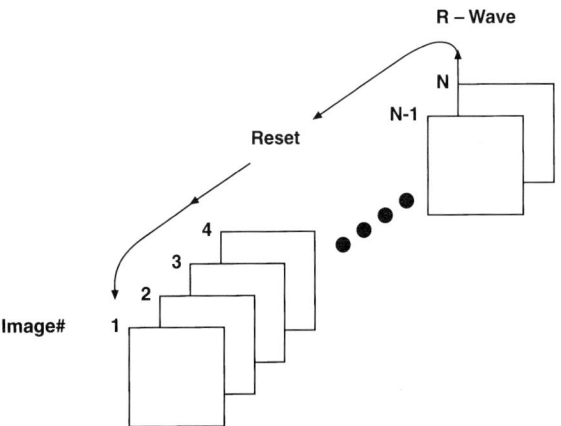

FIG. 3. Schematic illustration of the gating process. Here N images are shown. Data is acquired into each image sequentially, starting at image 1, until an R wave in the electrocardiogram signal occurs, which resets the entire process.

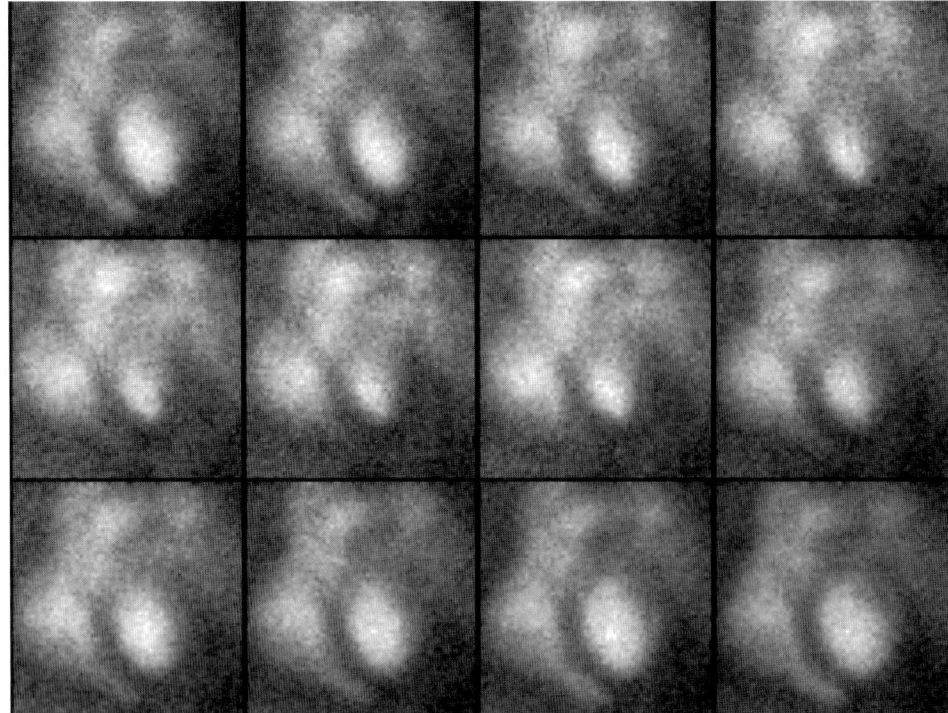

FIG. 4. A series of 12 gated images from end diastole (**upper left**), to end systole (second from left on middle row), to end diastole (**bottom right**). This figure shows only 12 images spanning the cardiac cycle, but usually many more images are used.

rates (where there is no diastasis period), nor is it necessarily true for subjects who are not in NSR, or for subjects in whom the filling portion of the LV volume curve is so distorted that there is no discernable diastasis period. In these situations, a technique known as "beat length windowing" could be used for optimal accuracy, in which beats shorter or longer than some predetermined length are not included in the data. Since in the method described for data acquisition, the length of a beat is only known *after* the data have been added to the images, a somewhat more elaborate computer acquisition scheme is required in which the event data are initially placed in a holding buffer. There are several options available for beat length windowing. If a beat is too long or too short, one may simply choose to reject that particular beat. However, this may not make physiological sense. The short beat itself functioned like all other beats up until the time it was terminated. That is, it was too short simply because the next beat began too early. If the next beat began prior to complete LV filling, the beat following the short beat would NOT be identical to all the other beats. It would have a different preload and, therefore, a different pattern of contraction and filling (15,16). The differences are most marked if the early beat is a premature ventricular beat, as compared to a super ventricular contraction. Therefore, one may wish to reject the beat following the short beat, not just the short beat itself (in fact, there may be no reason to reject the short beat itself). The user of the computer program for gated acquisition is usually permitted to choose not simply what

length beats are unsuitable, but also what to do about the succeeding (or even previous) beats.

For resting studies, two additional views are also usually acquired. These are most frequently an anterior view and a left lateral view. These other two views are used to provide additional visual information concerning wall motion. Generally, only the LAO view is used to compute quantitative indices of LV function, since that view is the one thought to be most free from overlapping structures.

For purposes of visually assessing wall motion, the series of gated images is displayed sequentially as a movie. The number of gated images may be condensed (by averaging) to 12 to 16 images for optimal cine display purposes although the full set of images is usually kept as well, for computational purposes, as described below.

There are two other methods for performing gating that are available on many commercial gamma camera/computer systems. The first of these is called "list mode" acquisition. In this mode of operation, the computer simply records on disk (i.e., makes a "list" of), the timing and location of every photon that is recorded by the camera. Since typically many million counts make up a gated blood pool cardiac study, many million words of disk storage are required. On older systems this was a serious problem, as disk space was often both limited and expensive, and reconstruction times required to reformat the data into images were long. With the marked changes in computer power, this is no longer an issue. Once the data have been recorded, one can read it back from disk and perform the gating just as previously described. Why should this more complex process be preferred? There are several reasons. First, in frame mode, selecting the beat length window (i.e., the range of beats to accept and reject) is often problematic. One has to make this decision prior to beginning the acquisition, and it is quite possible (and common) for the heart rate to change during the course of the study (e.g., if the patient becomes more comfortable on the table, or even falls asleep, or conversely, becomes uncomfortable). Thus, the heart rate may slowly shift as the study progresses. Similarly, during exercise studies, it is often not possible to accurately predict the heart rate—and to hold it stable. In a list mode study such difficulties are easily overcome, because one is processing the data after the fact, and the computer can first display the progression of heart rates that occurred during the study to the user, who can select whichever range of heart rates seem most suitable. This method also permits multiple levels of exercise to be studied easily. One can select any combination of heart rates and time periods desired. Finally, list mode acquisition allows the very end of the cycle (e.g., atrial contraction) to be reproduced. Again, since processing is retrospective, one can gate "backwards" in time from the R-wave trigger. If the P-wave-to-R-wave interval is relatively constant from beat to beat, one can then faithfully reproduce the volume increases due to atrial contraction.

A second variant on frame mode acquisition has also been employed and is available on many computer systems. This method is quite similar to the frame mode method already described. One first divides the cycle into some predefined number of images (e.g., 40, as in the example above). However, instead of fixing the time duration of each frame (e.g., 25 msec in the example), one lets the duration of acquisition for each frame vary depending on the beat length. For example, if the user has decided to use 40 frames and if the current beat is exactly 1 second long, then 25 msec duration per frame is used, just as in the frame mode example. If, however, the next beat is shorter (e.g., only 0.92 seconds long), then 23 msec (0.92 sec/40 frames = 0.023 sec/frame) acquisition time per frame is used. Each frame's acquisition duration is therefore expanded or contracted so that the entire series of 40 frames exactly fits the length of the beat. This method is often called "phase mode" acquisition (17). Since the length of the beat is not known until *after* the cycle is over, one must either process the data retrospectively from a list (as is acquired in list mode), or maintain a "buffer" of one beat worth of data in the computer's memory. The latter method permits acquisition to be performed in real time, without the need for retrospective processing.

Phase mode has the advantage of having every frame acquired for the same length of time (i.e., the same number of beats). That is, there is no "drop off" at the end of the cycle due to fluctuations in heart rate. However, the phase mode method's underlying assumption is that shorter beats are not just like longer ones that have been truncated (the frame mode assumption), but rather that short beats are temporally compressed long beats. This latter assumption has been shown to be true at higher heart rates, and, in this case, it will accurately portray all parts of the cardiac cycle—even the late diastolic portion. As with the other acquisition modes, one can "beat length window" to reject beats that are longer or shorter than desired. The assumption is not quite true at low heart rates, but the resulting errors have been shown to be fairly small (18).

It should be pointed out that severe heart rate fluctuations—e.g., as occur during atrial fibrillation—cannot really be "corrected" by any of the methods previously described. In atrial fibrillation, the underlying assumption that all beats have the same or very similar mechanical function is violated. One can perform a gated study on such subjects (with windowing), but the results will simply portray the average behavior of the cycles selected, which may or may not be indicative of the true cardiac function (16).

Producing the LV Volume Curve

In addition to providing a cinematic display from which LV function can be assessed visually, planar gated blood pool images can be analyzed to extract quantitative indices of ventricular function. As mentioned, this analysis is most often based on producing a plot of relative LV volume versus time. The most obvious way to produce such a plot from images like those in Figure 4 would be to proceed just as with LV contrast ventriculography. That is, to trace the edges of the LV chamber at each time point and compute volume by making some sort of assumption about the geometric shape of the ventricle (e.g., that it is an ellipsoid of revolution, as has occasionally been assumed in single-plane contrast ventriculography). This method was indeed used in the past, but it has two significant drawbacks. First, as mentioned, the LAO view does not reflect a true long-axis view of the heart, so the geometric assumption made for single-view contrast ventriculography may not be valid (and, in fact, this assumption is often not valid even when the view *is* correct). Note that acquiring additional views, e.g., anterior and lateral views, does not solve this problem, since there are too many overlapping structures in the images. Second, the resolution of the nuclear technique is considerably poorer than in x-ray studies, and the pixel size is much coarser. This means that it is likely that one may make errors in determining the geometric boundaries of the LV chamber. Even when such errors in tracing are small, they can cause much larger errors in volume calculations. This problem is accentuated because, since the images are two-dimensional projections of the photons emitted by the heart, definition of the "edge" is quite difficult—counts fall off slowly as the projection lines through the LV chamber get shorter and shorter toward the edges of the ventricle. For all these reasons, another, nongeometric, approach has usually been used to extract quantitative information from planar gated blood pool studies. This approach makes use of the fact that the number of photons emitted from the LV cavity is directly

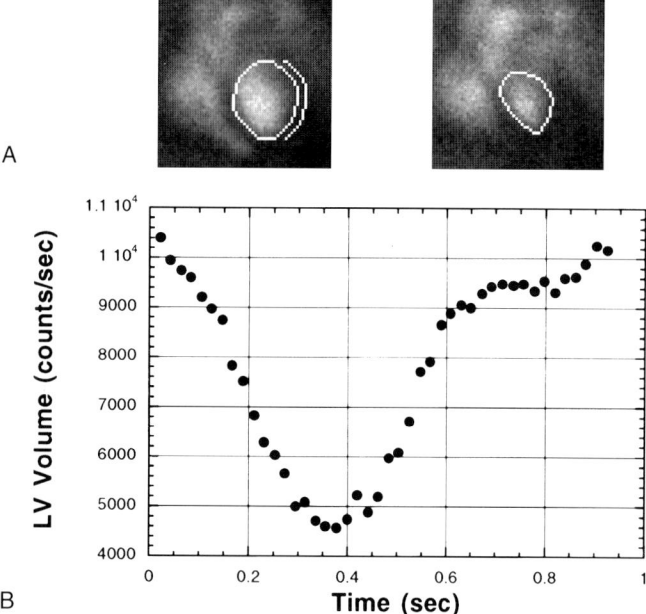

FIG. 5. **A** shows an ED and ES image (just as in Fig. 2), with regions of interest drawn over the left ventricle at ED (**left**) and ES (**right**). Also shown is a typical background region of interest (**left**). **B**: The bottom curve shows the relative left ventricular volume plotted as a function of time over the cardiac cycle. This plot was obtained by acquiring a gated set of 44 images (just as in Fig. 4, but with 44 images instead of 12), and computing the count rate in the ED region of interest at every point, and then correcting for background. Compare this actual measured curve to that shown in Figure 1. *ED*, end diastole; *ES*, end systole.

proportional to the blood volume in that cavity. As mentioned previously, one advantage of this method is that the results no longer depend critically on an exact definition of the endocardial border. Instead, one must simply be able to trace an outline on the image that includes all (or most) of the LV cavity, while excluding other structures. This methodology has proven quite powerful, and has played an important clinical role over the years, often being accepted as a more reliable standard for measurement of left ventricular ejection fraction (EF) than even contrast ventriculography. A typical method of producing an LV volume curve from a planar gated blood pool study is illustrated in Figure 5. In Figure 5**A**, an end diastolic (ED) region of interest has been drawn and is shown superimposed on the ED image. Figure 5**B** shows the counts within that region plotted as a function of time.

Parameters of LV Function

The ordinate values of the LV curves in Figures 1 or 5 may be in arbitrary, relative units, or, in some cases, in absolute units (i.e., milliliters), depending on the particular technique used to produce the curve. The most widely used parameter describing global LV function is EF, the fraction of

blood at ED that is ejected during systole. This is defined as

$$EF = \{(ED\ volume) - (ES\ volume)\} / (ED\ volume)$$

or as

$$EF = (stroke\ volume) / ED\ volume$$

Since the units of the volume measurement (e.g., mL) appear in both the denominator and the numerator, the units cancel out. That is, EF is independent of whether the units of ED and ES volume are measured in mL, liters, or gallons. In fact, since the units cancel, one may make the measurement of ED and ES volume using units that are proportional to volume, but for which the proportionality factor is unknown. Thus, if a value proportional to the number of photons emitted by the LV cavity can be measured (e.g., counts in a gamma camera), then this will permit measurement of EF. There is a a huge body of literature describing the clinical utility of measuring EF (4,19–22). There are several radionuclide imaging methods available to measure EF (as well as methods using several other modalities). Each method has its own limitations in terms of accuracy and reproducibility. To determine the optimum method to use in a particular situation it is necessary to consider how the value of EF will be used. Depending on the particular clinical circumstance, it may be necessary in some cases to have a measure of EF that is absolutely accurate. More commonly, however, multiple measurements of EF are made, and the quantity of greatest interest is how EF has changed from one measurement to the next. The change in EF from rest to stress (e.g., with exercise or pharmacological stress) has been of great use in evaluating a large number of cardiac diseases (4,20). Similarly, accurate measurements of the change in resting EF over time has had wide application, ranging from making decisions regarding aortic valve replacement, to the monitoring of cardiotoxic cancer chemotherapy drugs, for example. It is important, therefore, to consider the factors that influence a particular method's ability to measure such changes reproducibly (even if the absolute values at any one time point are not themselves accurate).

While ejection fraction is a very important clinical determinant of ventricular function, several other parameters describing global function have also proven useful, which can be computed from the curve of relative volume versus time (e.g., Fig. 5). These parameters include:

Time to end systole (TES): The time at which the volume curve has reached its minimum.
Peak ejection rate (PER): The maximum down slope of the LV volume curve, indicative of the maximal rate at which blood is ejected from the heart.
Time to peak ejection (TPER): The time at which peak ejection rate occurs.
Peak filling rate (PFR): The maximum up-slope of the LV volume curve, indicative of the maximal rate at which blood fills the relaxing ventricle.

Time to peak filling rate (TPFR): The time at which PFR occurs.

Atrial contribution to filling: The fraction of the stroke volume that is due to blood filling the ventricle during atrial contraction.

All of these parameters are illustrated in Figure 1, and they could be calculated from any method that produces a global plot of relative ventricular volume versus time. The volume curve must be sampled at sufficient density (i.e., the number of time points per cardiac cycle must be large enough) to accurately compute the parameters shown in Figure 1. Some parameters can be computed using only a few time points per cardiac cycle, while others require a large number of frames per cardiac cycle. Typically, EF requires at least one time point (and therefore 1 image) every 50 to 60 msec, while parameters based on slopes of the curve (e.g., PFR and PER) require more finely sampled curves (as rapidly as 20 msec per frame). The exact number of time points required for a particular parameter, as well as the error incurred by sampling the cardiac cycle too coarsely, have been previously determined (23,24).

The parameters mentioned above are often difficult to measure unless the LV volume curve is "smooth"—i.e., unless it has no statistical fluctuations. This is certainly not the case for LV volume curves derived from nuclear techniques and is probably not the case for data derived from any imaging modality. Parameters dependent on measurement of slopes (e.g., PFR, PER) are especially susceptible to error in the presence of the statistical fluctuations that are always present in LV volume curves (e.g., Fig. 5). One common method to reduce these statistical fluctuations, is to "smooth" the data. This can be done in a number of different ways. The two most often used are "temporal smoothing," and "Fourier filtering" (25). Temporal smoothing is performed by averaging (perhaps with weighting factors) one point on the LV time activity curve (TAC) with its neighbors. Each point on the TAC is replaced with the average (weighted or not) of itself and its neighbors. While temporal smoothing makes the LV curve look smoother, it also has the adverse effect of reducing its effective temporal resolution—that is, a curve that has been smoothed is similar to a curve that has coarser sampling. For example, consider a curve with 50 msec per time point. This resolution is considered good enough to make an accurate computation of EF. If, however, this curve is smoothed too heavily, it can no longer be used to give an accurate computation of EF. The adverse effects of excessive smoothing have been discussed in detail elsewhere (26). Smoothing, then, requires a tradeoff between reducing statistical fluctuations and reducing accuracy.

Fourier filtering is an alternative to smoothing. It is based on the fact (discovered by Jean Baptiste Fourier) that any curve (such as an LV volume curve) can be described as a constant value plus the sum of many sine and cosine waves (called harmonics) each of higher and higher frequency. The lowest frequency sine wave is one cycle per cardiac cycle, the next highest is two cycles per cardiac cycle, etc. The process is illustrated in Figure 6. A large number of harmonics may be required to faithfully reproduce a curve. As fewer than the maximum required number of harmonics are used, the curve no longer faithfully reproduces the original data. The first features to be lost are those involving rapid changes—i.e., point-to-point fluctuations, caused primarily by statistical fluctuations or "noise." This is just the effect one desires. As fewer still harmonics are used, noise continues to drop, but also fewer and fewer of the rapid changes present in the original curve (changes presumably of physiologic origin) are reproduced. A more detailed explanation of Fourier filtering as it applies to nuclear cardiology is available elsewhere (25). Just as with smoothing, selecting the optimum number of harmonics to use involves a trade-off between reduction of statistical fluctuations and loss of faithful reproduction of the original data. The optimal number of harmonics required in order to compute a particular parameter of LV function has been previously investigated (27).

Limitations of the Counts Based Method

There are several important limitations of the counts based method when it is used to quantify planar gated blood pool studies. First, note that it was stated above that the number of photons *emitted* by the LV chamber is directly proportional to LV blood volume. While this is indeed true, the number of photons *detected* by the gamma camera (i.e., the "counts" detected) are not precisely proportional to the number of photons emitted, due to the effects of photon attenuation and, to a lesser extent, scatter. For very low EFs, where ES and ED volumes are quite similar, photon attenuation is nearly unchanged across the cardiac cycle. Patients with low EFs, however, tend to have large left ventricular volumes in which there is more attenuation from the blood furthest from the camera than from those parts of the LV chamber closest to the camera. These effects, while real and measureable, produce only small errors in relative measurements of volume such as EF (13). The effects of attenuation do, however, prevent one from knowing the exact proportionality factor between detected photons and volume. This means that methods based on "counts" have not been readily used to measure absolute volumes (e.g., in mL). Although several attempts have been made to overcome this limitation (e.g., by estimating the attenuation from the heart), none has been widely adopted in clinical practice. Fortunately, a great number of important clinical parameters are dependent only on relative volume changes, and therefore do not require knowledge of absolute volumes.

Another limitation of the counts based method of analysis is caused by the planar (i.e., the two-dimensional) nature of the data. The counts emitted from the LV are a superimposition of the counts from the blood in the LV chamber, and the blood in the tissue in front of and behind the LV chamber.

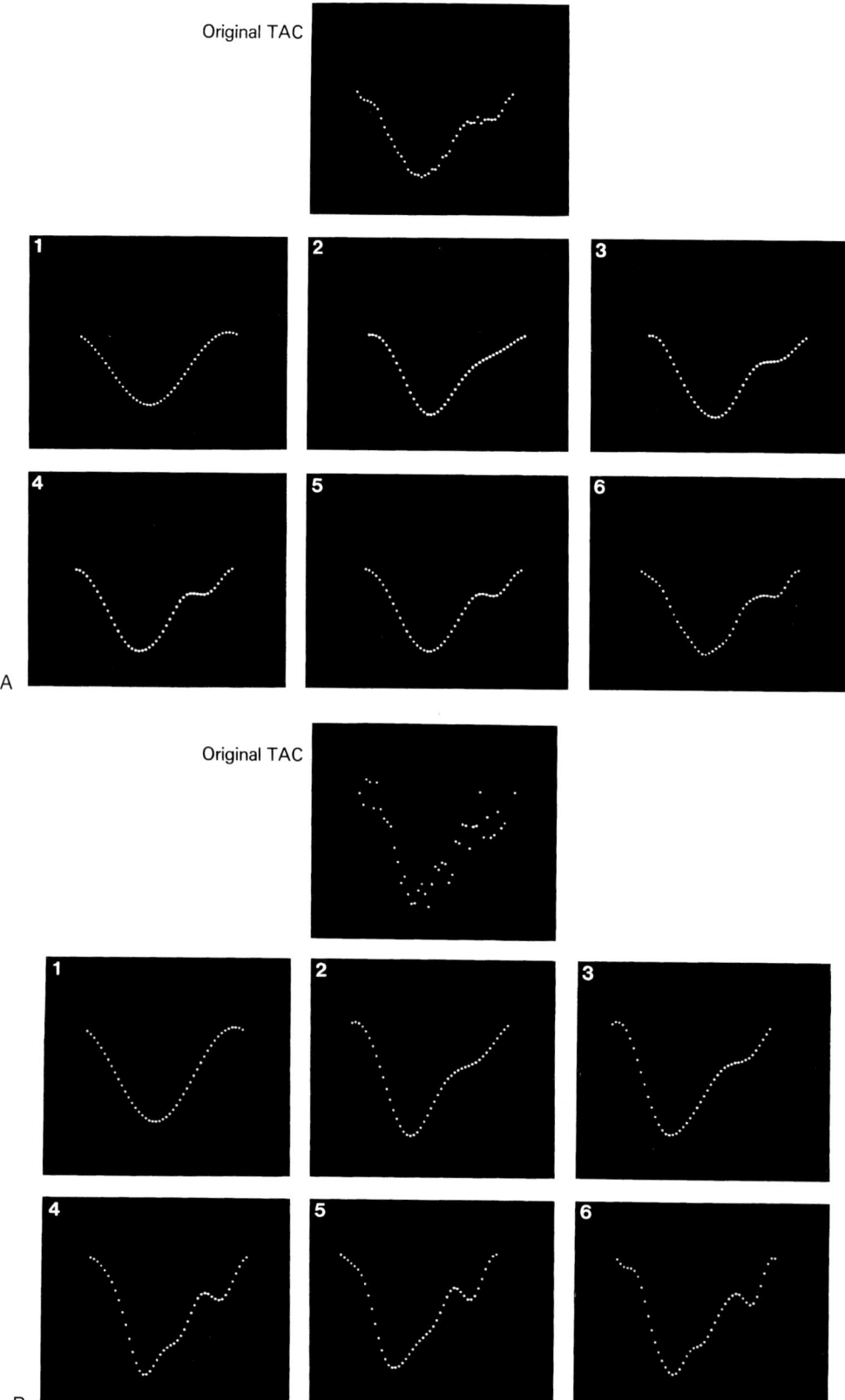

FIG. 6. A: **Top panel** shows the original volume curve (a relatively noise free curve), while **panels 1** through **6** show 1 through 6 harmonic fits. Increasing number of harmonics appears to better reproduce the fine detail in the original curve. **B**: This curve is a very noisy curve. Again the top panel shows the original volume curve while **panels 1** through **6** show 1 through 6 harmonics. As the number of harmonics increases, the noise in the original data begins to be reproduced in the fits. One would probably limit the fit to 3 harmonics to produce the best compromise between noise and reproduction of the physiologic data. *TAC*, time activity curve.

As noted earlier, it is difficult to avoid some degree of overlap from chambers other than left ventricle. In the optimized LAO view, one attempts to correct for these extraneous "background" counts by drawing a region of interest adjacent to the LV chamber (usually along the free wall), and assuming the number of photons emitted by that region is a measure of this background activity (Fig. 5). While this assumption may be fairly accurate, the number of background counts is rather large (typically 40 to 60% of the total counts at ED). Therefore, small errors in the measurement of background can cause significant errors in EF (typically when EF is 0.5, a 10% error in background measurement can cause up to a 20% error in EF—i.e., 10 EF points). It has been shown that the error in EF due to errors in background determination can be reduced by drawing not simply one ROI at ED, but instead two ROIs—one at ED and one at ES, as shown in Figure 5.

Measurement of Regional Function

Regional function is most often assessed by cinematic display of the GBP images, as already described. However, several methods have been employed successfully to compute quantitative indices of regional function from planar GBP images. One method involves dividing the LV cavity into several pie-shaped sectors, and then computing an LV volume curve from the change in counts in each of the sectors (28). From this collection of LV curves, one can compute "regional" EF values, as well as regional values of all the other parameters of global function described earlier. Since the curves from each sector are derived from planar images, the change in counts (and, therefore, volume) within the sector arises from two sources. Counts change both due to motion of the endocardial wall at the edge of the sector, as well as from changes in blood volume produced by the motion of the myocardial walls that lay above and below the portion of the ventricular cavity being examined. A visual assessment of wall motion, on the other hand, depends primarily on observation of the endocardial border of the sector. Quantitative indices of regional function, therefore, may sometimes disagree with the visual assessment of wall motion in the sector.

Another simple approach to the analysis of regional function is to compute a "functional map"—i.e., a pixel by pixel computation of some parameter of ventricular function. For example, by subtracting the ES image from the ED image one produces an image of regional stroke counts (proportional to stroke volume). Each pixel within such a functional image has an intensity proportional to the value of the functional parameter. Similarly, other parameters can be computed on a pixel by pixel basis, although image noise often makes such calculations problematic.

One quite useful set of functional maps are the so-called Fourier phase and amplitude maps. In this analysis scheme, one assumes that each pixel by pixel LV volume curve can be described by a single cosine curve with amplitude A and phase P (i.e., by a single Fourier harmonic). The amplitude image (i.e., the image of A values) is very similar to a stroke volume map, while the phase image gives information as to regional synchrony of contraction. The method has often been employed for the clinical assessment of conduction abnormalities (29–32). Again, it must be emphasized that if one derives regional ventricular function parameters from planar images, the under- and overlying portions of the heart both contribute to what is observed as regional ventricular function.

TOMOGRAPHIC GATED BLOOD POOL IMAGING

Single Photon Emission Computed Tomography

Despite the great utility of planar GBP imaging, it suffers from one serious drawback—namely, it produces images that are only two dimensional projections of a three-dimensional object. This problem can be overcome by the use of gated single photon emission computed tomography (GBP SPECT), which produces gated tomographic images of the cardiac blood pool (33–38). While the technology of SPECT has been available for many years, recent decreases in computer costs and increases in computer speeds, as well as the application of the multiheaded SPECT camera have made the technique clinically practical. Performing GBP SPECT acquisition opens the possibility for true three-dimensional qualitative and quantitative assessment of ventricular function.

Acquiring a Gated Blood Pool SPECT Image Sequence

The blood pool is labeled just as in planar gated blood pool imaging. Typically, 25 mCi of Tc99m labeled red blood cells are used, with either *in vitro* or *in vivo* labeling techniques. Forty mCi doses have been suggested for rapid SPECT imaging (e.g., for pharmacologic stress imaging), but, in this case, care has to be taken to account for camera dead time. Imaging during exercise has been attempted, but has proven difficult.

With two gamma cameras, with the cameras 90 degrees apart, typically at least 60 projections (in 3-degree steps) should be taken over 180 degrees. The optimal 180-degree span is usually considered to be 45 degrees RAO to 45 degrees LPO. As in all SPECT imaging, artifacts will result unless care is taken to make sure that all regions in the organ of interest remain in the field of view throughout the data acquisition. If a three-headed camera is used, the same minimum 3-degree steps are recommended, giving 120 projections. There is little data about the relative advantages of 360- versus 180-degree imaging for GBP SPECT. This issue has been investigated much more thoroughly for perfusion SPECT imaging (see Chapter 11), but, even in that case, there is still controversy as to which methodology is better. Several facts are agreed upon, however: that 180-degree SPECT is most efficiently performed with a 90-degree, two-headed camera while 360-degree SPECT is most efficiently done with a three-headed camera. Obviously, if the same number of angles and time-per-angle were used for three-headed, 360-degree versus two-headed, 180-degree imaging, then three-headed, 360-degree imaging would require 30% more total imaging time than two-headed, 180-degree imaging. The extra 30% acquisition time does not necessarily produce 30% more counts, however, because the posterior views of the heart have very reduced count rates (from the heart) due to attenuation. Also, two-headed, 180-degree imaging, because all views are relatively close to the heart, can in theory produce images with slightly better spatial resolution. However, the resolution in 180-degree imaging is often less uniform than with 360-degree imaging—i.e., for 180-degree imaging, the resolution is poorer in some angles of acquisition than in others. Although this factor may cause small artifacts in perfusion imaging, it is probably not a significant factor for GBP imaging. The resolution is more homogeneous with 360-degree imaging, especially when conjugate view averaging is used (i.e., a view from one side of the body is averaged with the view taken 180 degrees apart), as is typical. Finally, artifacts caused by inconsistent projections (which in turn are caused primarily by not performing corrections for attenuation and scatter) may be slightly more pronounced for 180 degrees than for 360 imaging. Again, it is unclear whether any of these differences are of clinical importance for GBP blood pool SPECT, and both 180 and 360 acquisitions have been used successfully in clinical situations.

Imaging time is comparable for GBP SPECT and planar imaging, when one accounts for the fact that three views are usually acquired for planar imaging. If each planar view takes approximately 6 to 10 minutes, then a total of 18 to 30 minutes are required for a complete set of planar images. This is quite similar to the 20 to 30 minutes required for a SPECT acquisition with a single detector camera. All the gating issues mentioned above for planar imaging also apply to SPECT imaging. At least one additional gating choice must be made for GBP SPECT imaging, however—whether to acquire for a fixed time at each projection angle or for a fixed number of beats. In the latter case, if the heart rate has shifted out of the beat length window, acquisition time can increase intolerably. Some method should be available to circumvent this problem (e.g., automatically varying the window width as the heart rate shifts—although this in turn may violate the assumption of all beats being identical). On the other hand, if a fixed time is set, and again heart rate has shifted, some projections may have very few total beats (and hence very few counts). Methods are available to minimize these problems on many (but not all) commercially available computer systems.

The high temporal resolution (i.e., large number of frames per cardiac cycle) easily achieved with planar imaging is usually not possible with GBP SPECT imaging. This is because each time point requires the image space associated with a complete ungated SPECT study. So, for example, a 16-image gated SPECT sequence, acquired with 60 projections, 3 degrees apart, as recommended above, requires 16*60 = 960 projection images. Not only does image storage space become a difficulty, so too does reconstruction time. Sixteen gates means that reconstruction time increases by a factor of 16 as well, often resulting in quite long reconstruction times. Nonetheless, increases in computer speed have made reconstruction times clinically practicable, even for gated studies.

The SPECT projection data are usually first reconstructed into a set of gated transaxial slices. In the past, these in turn have been reoriented into short-axis images. While this makes some quantitative analysis schemes easy to implement (since each slice is approximately a circular disk), there is some advantage to be gained in being able to display the gated images in the long-axis, rather than the short-axis projection (Fig. 7). In particular, the long-axis view makes visualization of the apex and the base of the heart (often a problematic region for short-axis displays) quite easy, while preserving the ability to perform quantitative analysis. Long-axis display of the data can also facilitate comparisons between other physiologic measures made with SPECT (e.g., comparisons between function and perfusion). In Figure 7, four long-axis slices are shown, rather than the usual two. By the use of three or four, rather than only two long-axis slices, the long-axis slices can be made to correspond one-to-one to the six or eight sectors often used in analysis of short-axis images, as shown in the figure.

As with other tomographic modalities, our ability to acquire three-dimensional data has outpaced our ability to display such data. Ideally, one would be able to display the three-dimensional data describing the beating heart using some sort of pseudo three-dimensional display, and some progress has been made to this end (39–44). In theory, displaying the data in this fashion would improve the ability of a reader to detect and grade wall motion, but much work remains before such displays are adopted clinically.

Global Function from GBP SPECT

One of the principal advantages of SPECT imaging is its ability to portray accurate regional information. However, many decades of experience with measures of global function (e.g., ejection fraction), make it essential that one be able to extract such global quantitative measures from the SPECT data as well. At first, one might think the best way to do this would be to analyze the data slice by slice. This has indeed been tried, with both geometric "coin stacking" methods, as well as with counts based methods (38,45,46). However, slice-by-slice approaches are often both tedious and subject to variabilities caused by having to draw large numbers of regions of interest—one on each of the slices and time points, if a left ventricular volume curve is desired. An alternative method has been described (13) to compute global information from the tomographic data. In this method, one reprojects the tomographic data back into a

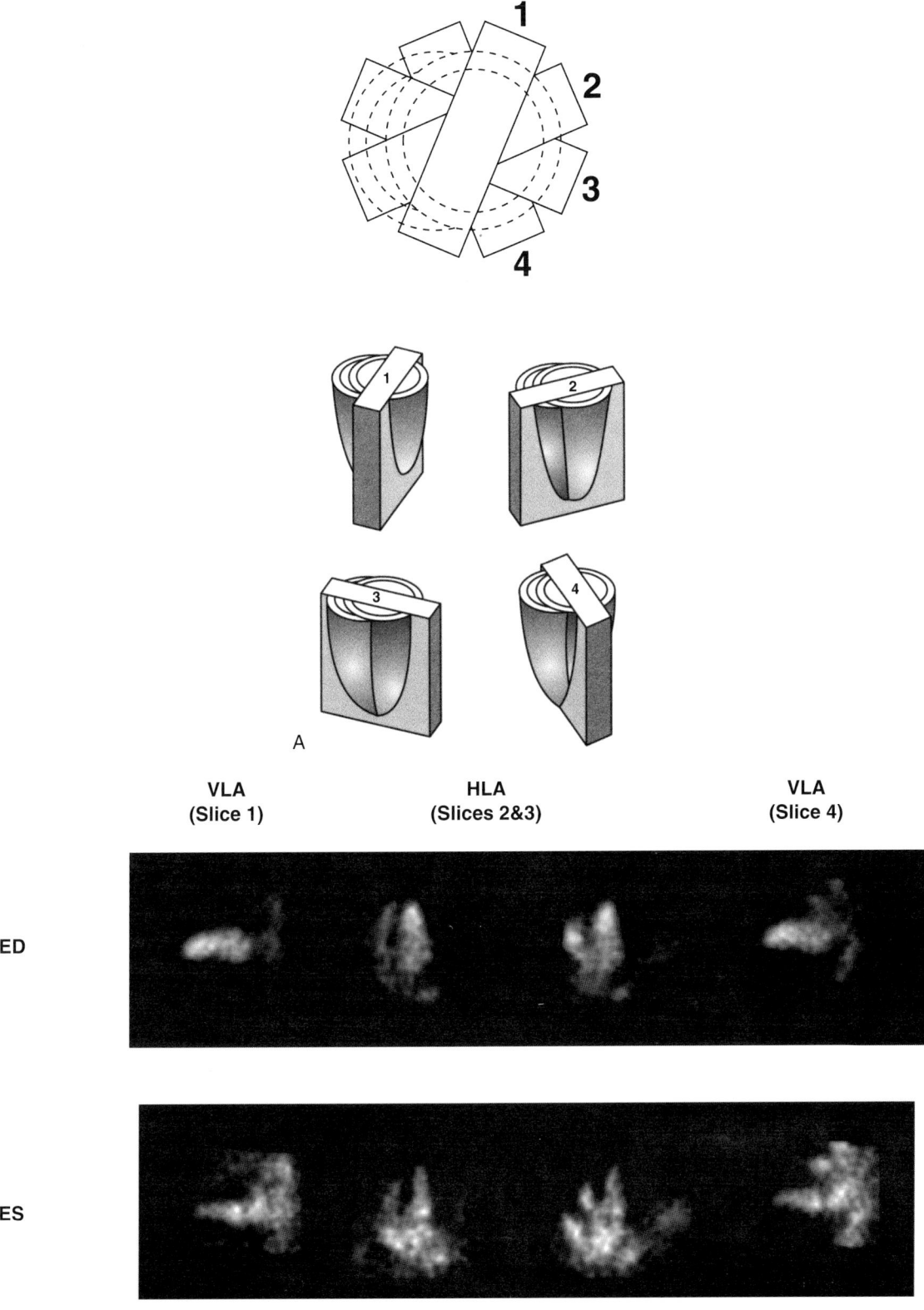

FIG. 7. A: Illustrating how the 4 long-axis slices are made from a set of short-axis images. **B**: An actual set of 4 long-axis slices (oriented as in **A**) at end diastole (*ED*) and end systole (*ES*). Slices 1 and 4 are verticle long-axis (*VLA*) slices, while slices 2 and 3 are horizontal long-axis (*HLA*) slices.

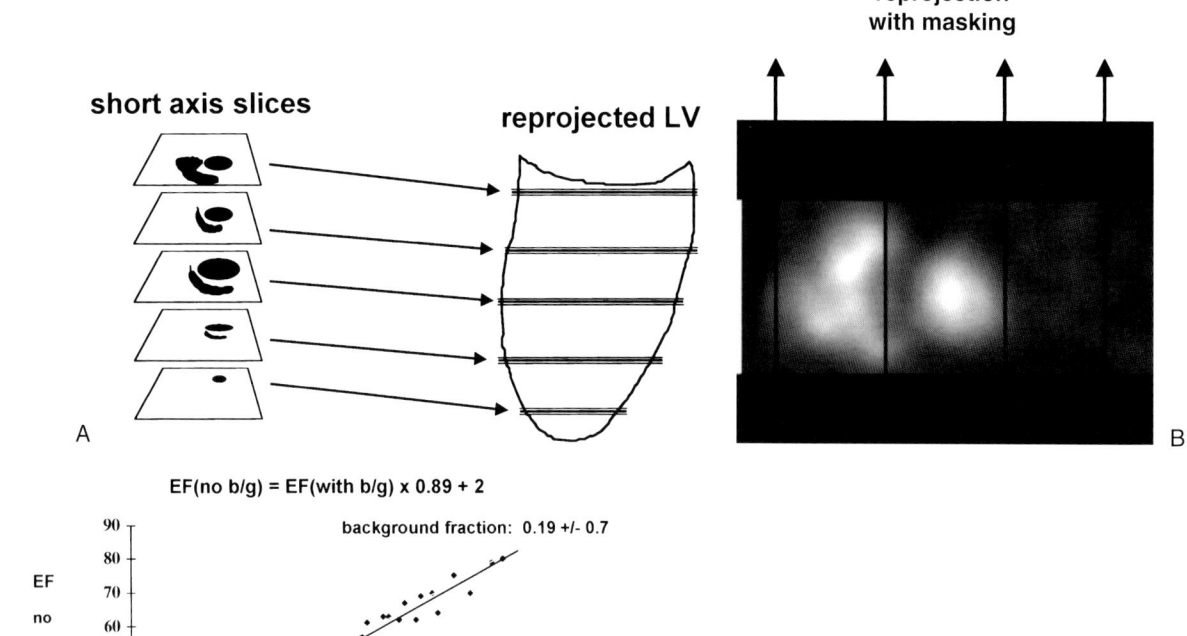

FIG. 8. A: Illustrating how short-axis tomographic slices can be "reprojected" back into a pseudo-planar image. B: The reprojection process shown on 1 short axis slice, with a mask to reduce background. C: Ejection fraction (*EF*) *without* a background correction (on ordinate) versus ejection fraction *with* a background correction (abscissa). Note high degree of linear correlation and low standard estimate of the error.

pseudo-planar set of gated images (Fig. 8), and then analyzes them just as with a planar blood pool study. This approach greatly simplifies analysis, while avoiding many of the limitations associated with true planar imaging. Since the full three-dimensional set of data is available for projection, any viewing angle may be selected for projection, including the true long-axis view (a view that is physically impossible to acquire with actual gamma camera planar imaging). In this view, overlap with the atrium is minimized, and the apex can be clearly separated from the rest of the ventricle. Since the data that one projects is tomographic, it is relatively easy at least to reduce the contribution of background activity—i.e., activity that over- and underlies the ventricle—by appropriate masking. Even a simple rectangular mask can be used to greatly reduce the superimposition problem encountered in true planar imaging. It has been shown that background counts can be reduced by a factor of between 2 and 3 by this method (13). At this level of reduction, correction for background is no longer a significant source of error in EF calculations, and, in fact, recent results have shown that it might be possible to completely ignore background. Although ignoring background results in a slightly lowered value of EF, Figure 8 shows that one could easily correct for this by using a correction based on a simple linear correlation to produce the "true" EF from the background un-corrected value. If a similar comparison between EF with

and without background correction were made for an actual planar study, the variability would be expected to be prohibitively large. As mentioned, by reprojecting the SPECT data, global analysis is considerably simplified. Only two ROIs need be drawn (at ED and ES), and because of the improved noise characteristics due to lower background in the reprojected images, automatic methods of region drawing may behave much more reliably with reprojected images than with true planar images.

Ejection fractions computed from reprojected SPECT have been shown to be about 30% higher than EFs computed from planar studies (13) (i.e., a 50% EF by planar translates to about 65% EF by reprojected SPECT). These reprojected SPECT EF values are consistent with the EF values that have been reported from other modalities (e.g., MRI, echo and biplane ventriculography).

Regional Function from Gated Blood Pool SPECT

Just as with planar imaging, regional function is most commonly evaluated visually from GBP SPECT. Visual analysis can be performed by examining gated short-axis images, gated long-axis images, or even multiview gated reprojection images. Each approach has its own advantages and disadvantages. Short-axis images are useful because they portray function around the circumference of the LV chamber all at once, but since all short-axis slices look similar in shape, one needs some way to know where (from base to apex) each gated short-axis set comes from. Short-axis images are poor at visualizing apical contraction. In addition, much of the LV contraction involves shortening along the long-axis direction (i.e., decrease in the distance from valve plane to apex), and this also is not appreciated well from short-axis images. Long-axis imaging appears to overcome many of these disadvantages because the entire length of the LV chamber can be viewed simultaneously. The reprojection method for EF computation from GBP SPECT may also be useful for visualization of regional wall motion. At first one might think that reprojected SPECT images would not be a suitable method for determining regional wall motion because such images contain the sum of all counts along the projection lines through the heart. The edges of such images, however, are usually the regions used to assess wall motion, and these edges only include counts from a relatively small volume of blood. Since many views can be produced without worrying about superimposing structures, the technique may prove to be advantageous, especially in limited counts situation (e.g., pharmacologic stress imaging) when standard SPECT studies have high noise.

When visualization of cine images acquired from a planar camera are compared with those from GBP SPECT, regional defects seen as being only mild on the planar images may often be perceived as severe defects with GBP SPECT imaging. Which analysis is correct? By reprojecting the SPECT study into the equivalent planar view at the same angle as used by the planar gamma camera (13), it quickly becomes obvious that wall motion abnormalities can easily be masked in planar imaging, by over- and underlying activity in the ventricle. The superimposition of regions of the LV with normal counts-changes on top of regions with abnormal counts-changes can transform a truly severe defect into an apparently mild one when planar imaging is used. This quite commonly occurs with defects at the apex, since in the foreshortened view used in planar studies, the apex is superimposed on the lower portion of the ventricular cavity. It also frequently occurs with anterior or inferior wall defects. Gated blood pool SPECT avoids these difficulties. This is probably one of the reasons that several studies have indicated that tomographic blood pool imaging may have increased sensitivity for LV wall motion detection (33,47,48).

Gated blood pool SPECT imaging produces images that are not affected by overlying or underlying activity. This removes one of the principal difficulties associated with quantifying regional function from planar images. Nearly all the same techniques of measuring regional function mentioned above for planar imaging can be applied as well to single slices (long or short axis) from a GBP SPECT study. Many of these techniques did not find widespread application when applied to planar imaging. It is quite possible that this situation will change when the methods are used for SPECT. These methods of analyzing regional function made several assumptions, which were severely violated in the

planar case, but are at least partially satisfied in the SPECT case. Many of the quantitative methods used to determine regional function in both SPECT perfusion imaging and planar gated blood pool imaging have been successfully adopted for gated blood pool SPECT. These methods include Fourier phase analysis for detection of wall motion and conduction abnormalities (29,31,32,49,50), use of "polar maps" to evaluate regional parameters of function (51,52), as well as others. In general, it has been found that quantitative analysis of gated blood pool SPECT data improves its clinical utility (37,47,48,53).

LV Function from Gated Blood Pool Positron Emission Tomography

There is an alternative tomographic approach to SPECT gated blood pool imaging—namely, the use of positron emission tomography (PET) (33,54). The advantages of PET for this purpose are several fold. First, the resolution of modern PET scanners is about twice as high (~7mm) as that achieved with SPECT. Second, the sensitivity (i.e., the fraction of photons emitted by the heart that are detected by the scanner) of PET is considerably greater than multiheaded gamma camera SPECT, so, for a given dose of radioactivity, PET can achieve better noise characteristics than SPECT in the same time. Third, the blood pool agent used for PET is usually ^{11}CO (or sometimes $C^{15}O$). This agent (which is administered by breathing the CO at very low—lower than found on many city streets—concentrations) is an exception-

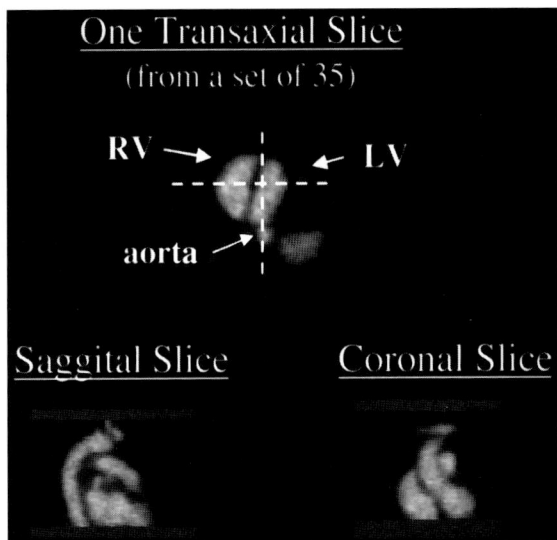

FIG. 9. An example of a ^{11}CO gated positron emission tomography study. **Top:** a single transaxial slice is shown (one of 35). This slice is 4.25 mm thick and has a resolution of about 6 mm in plane. **Bottom left:** Saggital slice produced from the transaxial slices at the location shown by the *dotted lines* in the transaxial slice. Again, this slice is 4.25 mm thick. **Bottom right:** Coronal slice (4.25 mm thick). *LV*, left ventricle; *RV*, right ventricle.

ally good blood pool label, yielding plasma counts (i.e., non red blood cell labeled radioactivity) of less than 0.1%. This results in exceptional image quality and in very low background activity (Fig. 9). Finally, because PET can correct for the effects of attenuation, the PET CO scan can yield accurate absolute concentrations of blood, and, therefore, accurate estimates of absolute ventricular volumes. The principal disadvantage of PET CO blood pool imaging is its expense and lack of availability. A cyclotron is required to produce the radiopharmaceutical. This cost coupled with that of the PET scanner itself makes it unclear whether this technique will be of clinical use outside of centers that already have PET and cyclotron capabilities.

REFERENCES

1. Strauss HW, Zaret BL, Hurley PJ. A scintiphotographic method for measuring left ventricular ejection fraction in man without cardiac catheterization. *Am J Cardiol* 1971;28:575–580.
2. Zaret BL, Strauss HW, Hurley PJ. A noninvasive scintiphotographic method for detecting regional ventricular dysfunction in man. *N Engl J Med* 1971;284:1165–1170.
3. Parker JA, Secker-Walker R, Hill R. A new technique for the calculation of left ventricular ejection fraction. *J Nucl Med* 1972;13:649–651.
4. Borer JS, Bacharach SL, Green MV. Real-time radionuclide cineangiography in the noninvasive evaluation of global and regional left ventricular function at rest and during exercise in patients with coronary-artery disease. *N Engl J Med* 1977;296:839–844.
5. Bacharach SL, Green MV, Borer JS. A real-time system for multiimage gated cardiac studies. *J Nucl Med* 1977;18:79–84.
6. Bartlett ML, Buvat I, Vaquero JJ, et al. Measurement of myocardial wall thickening from PET/SPECT images: comparison of two methods. *J Comput Assist Tomogr* 1996;20:473–481.
7. Mok DY, Bartlett ML, Bacharach SL, et al. Can partial volume effects be used to measure myocardial thickness and thickening? *IEEE Comput Cardiol* 1992;19:195–198.
8. Cooke CD, Garcia EV, Cullom SJ, et al. Determining the accuracy of calculating systolic wall thickening using a fast Fourier transform approximation: a simulation study based on canine and patient data. *J Nucl Med* 1994;35:1185–1192.
9. Bacharach SL, Green MV. Data processing in nuclear cardiology: measurement of ventricular function. *IEEE Trans Nucl Sci* 1982;29:1343–1354.
10. Green MV, Ostrow HG, Douglas MA, et al. High temporal resolution ECG-gated scintigraphic angiocardiography. *J. Nucl Med* 1975;16:95–98.
11. Bacharach SL, Green MV, Borer JS. Instrumentation and data processing in cardiovascular nuclear medicine: evaluation of ventricular function. *Semin Nucl Med* 1979;IX:257–274.
12. Garcia E, Bacharach SL, Mahmarian JJ, et al. Imaging guidelines for nuclear cardiology procedures: Part 1. *J Nucl Cardiol* 1996;3:G3–G46.
13. Bartlett ML, Srinivasan G, Barker WC, et al. Left ventricular ejection fraction: comparison of results from planar and SPECT gated blood-pool studies. *J Nucl Med* 1996;37:1795–1799.
14. Bacharach SL, Green MV, Borer JS, et al. Beat-by-beat validation of ECG gating. *J Nucl Med* 1980;21:307–313.
15. Braunwald E, Frye RL, Aygen MM, et al. Studies on Starling's law of the heart. *J Clin Invest* 1960;39:1874–1884.
16. Bacharach SL, Green MV, Bonow RO, et al. Measurement of ventricular function by ECG gating during atrial fibrillation. *J Nucl Med* 1981;22:226–231.
17. deGraaf CN, van Rijk PP. High temporal and high phase resolution construction techniques for cardiac motion imaging. *Proceedings, IAEA International Symposium on Medical Radionuclide Imaging* 1978;IAEA-SM:201–229.
18. Bacharach SL, Bonow RO, Green MV. Comparison of fixed and variable temporal resolution methods for creating gated cardiac blood-pool image sequences. *J Nucl Med* 1990;31:38–42.
19. Borer JS, Miller D, Schreiber T, et al. Radionuclide cineangiography in acute myocardial-infarction: role in prognostication. *Semin Nucl Med* 1987;17:89–94.
20. Borer JS, Herrold EM, Hochreiter C, et al. Natural history of left ventricular performance at rest and during exercise after aortic valve replacement for aortic regurgitation. *Circulation* 1991;84:133–139.
21. Weissler AM, Miller BI, Granger CB, et al. Augmentation of mortality risk discriminating power of left ventricular ejection fraction by measures of nonuniformity in systolic emptying on radionuclide ventriculography. *J Am Coll Cardiol* 1990;16:387–395.
22. Mock MB, Ringvist I, Fisher LD, et al. Survival of medically treated patients in the Coronary Artery Surgery Study (CASS) registry. *Circulation* 1982;66:562.
23. Bacharach SL, Green MV, Borer JS, et al. Left-ventricular peak ejection rate, filling rate, and ejection fraction: frame rate requirements at rest and exercise. *J Nucl Med* 1979;20:189–193.
24. Hamilton GW, Williams DL, Caldwell JH. Frame rate requirements for recording time-activity curves by radionuclide angiocardiography. In: *Nuclear cardiology: selected computer aspects.* New York: Society of Nuclear Medicine 1978:75–83.
25. Bacharach SL. Image analysis. In: Wagner HN, ed. *Principles of nuclear medicine.* Philadelphia: WB Saunders 1995:393–404.
26. Bonow RO, Bacharach SL, Crawford-Green C, et al. Influence of temporal smoothing on quantitation of left ventricular function by gated blood pool scintigraphy. *Am J Cardiol* 1989;64:921–925.
27. Bacharach SL, Green MV, Vitale D, et al. Optimum Fourier filtering of cardiac data: a minimum-error method. *J Nucl Med* 1983;24:1176–1184.
28. Vitale DF, Green MV, Bacharach SL, et al. Assessment of regional left ventricular function by sector analysis: a method for objective evaluation of radionuclide blood pool studies. *Am J Cardiol* 1983;52:112–119.
29. Lucas JR, O'Connell JW, Lee RJ, et al. First Harmonic (Fourier) analysis of gated SPECT blood pool scintigrams provides refined assessment of the site of initial activation of accessory pathways in patients with the Wolf-Parkinson-White syndrome. *J Nucl Med* 1993;34:P151.
30. Weismuller P, Clausen M, Weller R, et al. Noninvasive three-dimensional localization of arrhythmogenic foci in Wolff-Parkinson-White syndrome and in ventricular tachycardia by radionuclide ventriculography: phase-analysis of double-angulated integrated single photon emission computed tomography (SPECT). *Br Heart J* 1993;69:201–210.
31. Dormehl IC, Vangelder AL, Hugo N et al. Gated blood-pool SPECT and phase-analysis to assess simulated Wolff-Parkinson-White syndrome in the baboon. *Nuklearmedizin* 1993;32:222–226.
32. Bontemps L, BenBrahim H, Kraiem T et al. Gated blood-pool SPECT assessment of Wolff-Parkinson-White syndrome before and after radiofrequency ablation of accessory pathways. *Med Nucl* 1997;21:299–308.
33. Cross SJ, Lee HS, Metcalfe MJ, et al. Assessment of left-ventricular regional wall-motion with blood-pool tomography: comparison of 11co PET with Tc-99m SPECT *Nucl Med Commun* 1994;15:283–288.
34. Eilles C, Gaudron P, Ertl G, et al. SPECT radionuclide ventriculography: results in patients with myocardial infarction. *Nuklearmediziner* 1991;14:122–128.
35. Fischman AJ, Moore RH, Gill JB, et al. Gated blood pool tomography: a technology whose time has come. *Semin Nucl Med* 1989;19:13–21.
36. Gill JB, Moore RH, Tamaki N, et al. Multigated blood-pool tomography: new method for the assessment of left ventricular function. *J Nucl Med* 1986;27:1916–1924.
37. Groch MW, Marshall RC, Erwin WD, et al. Quantitative gated blood pool SPECT for the assessment of coronary artery disease at rest. *J Nucl Cardiol* 1998;5:567–573.
38. Stadius ML, Williams DL, Harp G. Left ventricular volume determination using single-photon emission computed tomography. *Am J Cardiol* 1985;55:1185–1191.
39. Indovina AG. 3-Dimensional surface display in blood-pool gated SPECT. *Angiology* 1994;45:861–866.
40. Honda N, Machida K, Takishima T, et al. Cinematic 3-dimensional surface display of cardiac blood pool tomography. *Clin Nucl Med* 1991;16:87–91.
41. Links JM, Devous MD. 3-Dimensional display in nuclear medicine: a more useful depiction of reality, or only a superficial rendering. *J Nucl Med* 1995;36:703–704.
42. Honda N, Machida K, Takishima T, et al. Cinematic three-dimensional surface display of cardiac blood pool tomography. *Clin Nucl Med* 1991;16:87–91.

43. Indovina AG. Three-dimensional surface display in blood pool gated SPECT. *Angiology* 1994;45:861–866.

44. Miller TR, Starren JB, Grothe RA. Three-dimensional display of positron emission tomorgraphy of the heart. *J Nucl Med* 1988;31:2064–2068.

45. Ziada G, Mohamed MM, Hayat N, et al. Quantitative analysis of cardiac function: comparison of electrocardiogram dual gated single photon emission tomography, planar radionuclide ventriculogram and contrast ventriculography in the determination of LV volume and ejection fraction. *Eur J Nucl Med* 1987;12:592–597.

46. Underwood SR, Walton S, Laming PJ, et al. Left ventricular volume and ejection fraction determined by gated blood pool emission tomography. *Br Heart J* 1985;53:216–222.

47. Groch MW, Marshall RC, Erwin WD, et al. Quantitative gated blood pool SPECT imaging: enhanced sensitivity for noninvasive assessment of coronary artery disease. *J Nucl Med* 1993;34:P35.

48. Botvinick EH, O'Connell JW, Glickman SL, et al. The potential added clinical value of gated SPECT blood pool imaging. *Clin Res* 1992;40:A119.

49. Casset-Senon D, Cosnay P, Philippe L, et al. Gated blood pool tomography with Fourier analysis in diagnosis of arrhythmogenic right ventricular cardiomyopathy. *Arch Malad Coeur Vaiss* 1997;90:935–944.

50. Casset-Senon D, Philippe L, Babuty D, et al. Diagnosis of arrhythmogenic right ventricular cardiomyopathy by Fourier analysis of gated blood pool single-photon emission tomography. *Am J Cardiol* 1998;82:1399–1404.

51. Neumann DR, Go RT, Myers BA, et al. Parametric phase display for biventricular function from gated cardiac blood pool single photon emission tomography. *Eur J Nucl Med* 1993;20:1108–1111.

52. Honda N, Machida K, Mamiya T, et al. Two-dimensional polar display of cardiac blood pool SPECT. *Eur J Nucl Med* 1989;15:133–136.

53. Eilles C, Borner W. Clinical results of SPECT radionuclide ventriculography (Gaspect). *Nuklearmediziner* 1989;12:35–51.

54. Freedman NMT, Bacharach SL, Cuocolo A, et al. ECG gated PET C-11 monoxide studies: an answer to the "background" question in planar Tc-99m gated blood pool imaging. *J Nucl Med* 1992;33:938.

CHAPTER 18

Assessment of Ventricular Function

First-pass Methods

Steven C. Port

First-pass radionuclide angiography (FPRNA) occupies a unique niche in cardiovascular radionuclide imaging. The abbreviation FPRNA is used because all the data to be used for image processing and quantitation are acquired during the initial transit of a radionuclide bolus through the central circulation. The technique relies more on the *temporal* separation of the cardiac chambers as the radionuclide bolus makes its way from one chamber to the next rather than on the spatial separation of chambers as is the case with equilibrium radionuclide angiography. Since relatively few heart beats will occur during that short time, both the dose of a radionuclide and the count rate capability of the imaging system must be adequate to provide and extract the count statistics necessary for image generation and quantitation.

Despite a total history of over 70 years (1), and a modern history of 30 years (2), FPRNA is currently practiced in a small minority of clinical laboratories. Barriers to its more widespread application include: (i) a lack of widely available commercial systems with the count rate capability required for FPRNA; (ii) the lack of appropriate software for acquisition and processing of first-pass data in many commercial gamma camera systems, and (iii) the lack of experience with FPRNA amongst physicians and technologists.

First-pass RNA has several unique advantages over gated equilibrium imaging. Since only the initial transit of a radionuclide bolus is required for imaging, the acquisition time is very short, on the order of seconds. That makes FPRNA ideal for the evaluation of ventricular function during exercise or during other transient phenomena. FPRNA has the inherent ability to analyze the transit of an injected tracer

through the central circulation, which permits detection and quantitation of left-to-right shunts and valvular insufficiency and identification of congenital abnormalities. Since individual beat information is stored, arrhythmic beats can be excluded easily or analyzed separately. Lastly, there is no dependence upon red blood cell labeling.

Recently, there has been a resurgence of interest in first-pass imaging because of the widespread application of the technetium-based myocardial perfusion imaging agents that allow combined FPRNA and single photon emission computed tomography (SPECT) perfusion imaging from the same injection.

In this chapter, the details of acquisition and processing, the results of the procedure, and the clinical applications of FPRNA will be discussed.

ACQUISITION

To ensure the temporal separation of cardiac chambers, the radionuclide must be injected as a discrete compact bolus into a large bore vein as close to the central circulation as possible. For routine clinical practice, two sites are typically used, the antecubital and the external jugular veins. Injection into any veins distal to the elbow is likely to result in a fractured or delayed bolus. Delayed or split boluses are likely to yield suboptimal images and inaccurate quantitation. To ensure a rapid bolus injection, the radionuclide dose and a saline flush syringe should be attached to a three-way stopcock, which is placed at the end of a short length of tubing connected to an intravenous cannula.

An exception to the general rule of rapidly injecting the bolus is the injection technique for right ventricular studies. In this situation, reducing the speed of injection slows the

S. C. Port: Department of Medicine, University of Wisconsin, Madison, Wisconsin 53792; Department of Medicine, St. Luke's Medical Center, Milwaukee, Wisconsin 53215.

transit through the right heart, providing more right ventricular beats for analysis. Unfortunately, that approach may compromise left ventricular analysis, and, if results for both ventricles are equally important, some compromise is necessary.

For first-pass studies, the radionuclide must remain in the intravascular space for the duration of the transit through the central circulation, and it must be safe enough to inject in an amount sufficient to generate the high count rates required. Although those requirements can actually be met by a wide variety of agents, technetium-99m is the radionuclide used in almost all clinical studies. Virtually any Tc-99m radiopharmaceutical can be used for FPRNA, with the exception of the particulate agents that are used for lung scanning, since they are trapped in the pulmonary capillary bed. In addition to the previous generation standard agents of technetium-99m pertechnetate and Tc-99m DTPA, FPRNA has now been performed with Tc-99m sestamibi (3,4), Tc-99m teboroxime (5,6), and Tc-99m tetrofosmin (7). Unfortunately, the 6-hour half-life of Tc-99m is relatively long for this purpose, since it limits the dose in 1 day. It is virtually impossible to perform more than three technetium first-pass studies in 1 day and, typically, only two are performed. There are very short-lived radionuclides that have been used for FPRNA that permit multiple sequential studies. For example, iridium-191m has an extremely short half-life of 4.9 seconds that minimizes radiation exposure and lends itself to sequential studies. This agent is particularly well suited to pediatric imaging. However, the ultra-short half-life requires that the patient be directly connected to a portable generator. Treves et al. (8) have demonstrated its application for assessment of left ventricular function and for detection and quantitation of left-to-right shunts.

Gold-195m has a half-life of 30.5 seconds. It can be produced with a portable generator that uses a mercury parent. First-pass left ventricular ejection fractions (LVEFs) have been validated with gold-195m (9), and multiple studies in rapid sequence with this agent have been performed. Unfortunately, multiple technical problems precluded clinical approval of the portable generator.

Tantalum-178m has a half-life of 9.3 minutes, making it easier to use than either iridium or gold. However, its primary photopeak energy of 55–65 keV makes it unsuitable for standard gamma cameras. The development of a proportional wire detector that is well suited to such low energies and approval of a portable generator have led to clinical validation of FPRNA using tantalum (10–12). None of these short-lived tracers, however, has gained widespread acceptance.

The required dose for a given injection depends upon the size of the individual, the sensitivity of the detector, the number of injections to be made that day, and the specific radionuclide being used. With the high sensitivity of the multicrystal gamma camera, doses as low as 8 to 10 millicuries (mCi) of technetium may be used. However, 20 to 25 mCi are recommended to guarantee adequate count rates, especially in large individuals or when few beats are expected to be available for analysis, such as in an exercise study. If two studies are being performed, such as rest and exercise studies, then two doses of 20 to 25 mCi are appropriate. In general, in order to minimize radiation exposure, the resting study can be performed with about 10 mCi and the exercise study with about 20 mCi. However, a 10 mCi dose may be suboptimal in large individuals, even with a multicrystal camera. For single-crystal systems with lower sensitivity, doses of 20 to 25 mCi are generally recommended for all injections. If an ultra-short-lived radionuclide is used, then the dose may be considerably higher.

During the initial transit of a radionuclide bolus through the left ventricle, there are, on average, only 6-to-10 beats at rest and 4-to-8 beats during exercise that may be used for data analysis. Consequently, the imaging devices used for FPRNA must be capable of recording very high count rates in order to extract as much data as possible from each beat. Although ejection fraction (EF) may be calculated with total count rates as low as 100,000 cts/sec, the error of the measurement will be high and the image quality will be marginal to unacceptable. Count rates should exceed 150,000 cts/sec for the whole-field-of-view during the right ventricular phase and ideally should be greater than 200,000 cts/sec. Few single crystal gamma cameras can reliably deliver such count rates.

The multicrystal gamma camera was the first instrument specifically designed for high count rate FPRNA. The first generation of multicrystal cameras was able to record count rates in excess of 250,000 cts/sec while maintaining enough spatial resolution to produce clinically adequate images. It should be noted, however, that there is always a trade-off between count rates and resolution, and earlier instruments dedicated to FPRNA were therefore inadequate for other types of clinical imaging. To some degree, the latest generation of multicrystal camera has improved upon the spatial resolution while, at the same time, improving the count rate capability as well. However, the spatial resolution is still not equivalent to that of a single crystal camera. The newer multicrystal systems are smaller, more maneuverable, and truly portable.

The multicrystal camera remains the instrument of choice for FPRNA, especially for exercise studies. Single-crystal gamma cameras were designed more for resolution than for count rate capability, and, until recently, most examples of the genre were able to count linearly up to about 60,000 cts/sec. At higher count rates, there was substantial loss of data due to system dead time, and peak count rates rarely exceeded 100,000 cts/sec. As such, those systems were inadequate for high count rate FPRNA. However, a new generation of single-crystal cameras has evolved that takes advantage of both integrated digital detector-computer technology and newer collimation to reduce system dead time and enhance count rates. Count rates of up to 200,000 cts/sec have been recorded, and clinically adequate FPRNA has been performed and validated with these new single-crystal cameras (13,14). High or ultra-high sensitivity collimators must be used on the single-crystal gamma cameras to achieve the requisite count rates, which results in lower spatial resolution. Although not commercially available, the proportional wire camera has been used in clinical research to acquire FPRNA with tantalum-178, an ultra-short-lived radionuclide (10–12). The images appear to be of diagnostic quality, although no prospective trial is available that has tested the sensitivity and specificity of the results.

The first-pass study can theoretically be acquired in any view due to the temporal separation of the cardiac chambers. However, either the anterior or a shallow right anterior oblique (RAO) view is recommended. Since FPRNA was widely applied to bicycle exercise for many years, the straight anterior view was very popular because it was a simple matter to stabilize the subject's chest against the detector while exercise continued. Because of its similarity to contrast angiographic ventriculography, a shallow RAO view was also popular. The shallow RAO view enhances separation between the atria and ventricles and between the left ventricle and the descending aorta. For right ventricular studies, the 30-degree RAO view is best for separating the right atrium from the right ventricle. The left anterior oblique (LAO) view may be used for interrogating the circumflex coronary distribution. However, left atrial activity tends to be rather high in a first-pass study, more so than during an equilibrium study, and, therefore, LAO views of 30 degrees to 60 degrees may result in considerable left atrial–left ventricular overlap that may compromise analysis of regional ventricular function and spuriously lower the left ventricular ejection fraction. The left lateral view is better in that regard. For left-to-right shunt detection and quantitation, the anterior view is preferred and as much of the lung fields as possible, especially the right lung, should be in the field of view.

Once the desired imaging angle is established, the detector must be positioned so that the entire heart is well within the field of view. Unlike an equilibrium study, where the angle can be adjusted repeatedly, positioning for a first-pass study must be correct before the bolus is injected. Use of a uniform flood source or a dose syringe moved behind the subject allows identification of the lungs and mediastinum (Fig. 1) and aids in positioning.

Alternatively, a test dose of 1 mCi may be injected for positioning. When two or more studies are performed, the background from the previous injection may be used for identifying the location of the heart.

For most studies, the subject should be in the upright position. That is true for both rest and exercise acquisitions. The upright position minimizes pulmonary blood volume and therefore background activity, which results in better quality images. Supine studies can certainly be performed and may be particularly appropriate for studies acquired during inotropic or vasodilatory stress.

First-pass studies are acquired by arbitrarily assigning timing intervals and then storing whatever image information appears in each interval. This is distinctly different from a typical frame-mode gated equilibrium study in which each

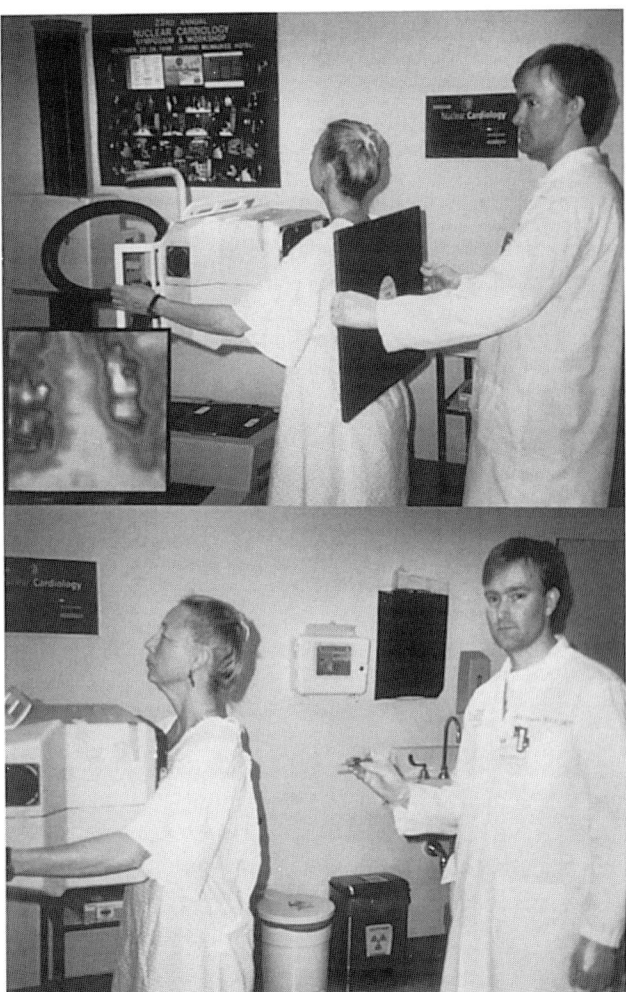

FIG. 1. Positioning for a first-pass study must be accurate prior to injection. It is, therefore, helpful to use a uniform flood source (**top**) or a syringe source (**bottom**) to identify the mediastinum and lungs (**insert**).

cardiac cycle is divided into a number of frames with each frame containing data from all beats so that no individual beat information is retained. The first-pass study is more like a list-mode equilibrium acquisition (see Chapter 17), but, unlike the list-mode acquisition, the temporal resolution of the first-pass study is predetermined by the time assigned to each interval, the so-called frame time. In general, the frame time should vary inversely with the heart rate. At resting rates of 50 to 100 beats/min, 50 msec (20 frames/sec) is adequate to measure systolic and diastolic events. At heart rates of 100 to 150 beats/min, as occurs during exercise, frame times of 25 msec are necessary to adequately characterize the physiology of emptying and filling. When heart rates approach 200 beats/min, 10 msec frame times may be optimal (15). For practical reasons, most laboratories have compromised on a single frame of 20 to 25 msec for all heart rates in order to avoid errors from repeatedly changing the acquisition parameters.

The duration of the acquisition must also be determined

prior to initiating the study. Enough time should be allowed for the bolus to completely clear the left ventricle, which at rest is 20 to 30 seconds and during exercise or inotropic stimulation is 10 to 20 seconds. Since there are occasional, unintentional delays between starting the gamma camera and injecting the radionuclide and since some patients will have markedly prolonged transit times, it is customary to acquire at least 30 seconds for all studies. Unnecessary frames may be discarded prior to data processing.

When operating at very high count rates, the time activity curves displaying the cyclic change in counts in the ventricle have sufficient resolution to be able to clearly identify end-diastole and end-systole without the aid of an electrocardiographic signal. When count rates are consistently lower, as occurs with single-crystal gamma camera acquisitions, it is particularly helpful to record an electrocardiographic signal with the image data. The ECG can be used during processing to aid in identification of end-diastolic frames and to facilitate the generation of a preliminary representative cycle.

EXERCISE PROTOCOLS

Bicycle Exercise

For many years, FPRNA and bicycle exercise were virtually synonymous. With so few heart beats available for analysis during exercise, it was mandatory that any cardiac motion during the study be eliminated. During bicycle exer-

cise, it is relatively easy to stabilize the chest against the detector while the subject continues to exercise. Initial work with FPRNA actually used supine exercise, but upright bicycle ergometry proved better for stabilizing the chest, and, as indicated above, the upright position decreased background activity (16,17). Upright exercise is also better tolerated, especially in deconditioned individuals. Bolus injection of radioactivity is made at peak exercise, and exercise is continued with the chest stabilized against the detector until the radionuclide bolus has been seen to clear the left ventricle. For most clinical studies, resting and peak exercise acquisitions are sufficient. If additional exercise data are required or if a postexercise study is necessary, the doses are adjusted accordingly. Acquisitions may be repeated almost immediately as long as the computer software has the capability of correcting for background activity from a previous injection.

Treadmill Exercise

Until recently, FPRNA was virtually never performed during treadmill exercise because there was so much chest motion. Now, however, there are methods for detection and correction of cardiac motion during FPRNA. The simpler of the two is a postacquisition method, in which a center-of-mass calculation is applied to the representative left ventricular cycle and tracks the center of mass for each frame of data during the left ventricular transit. The center is reposi-

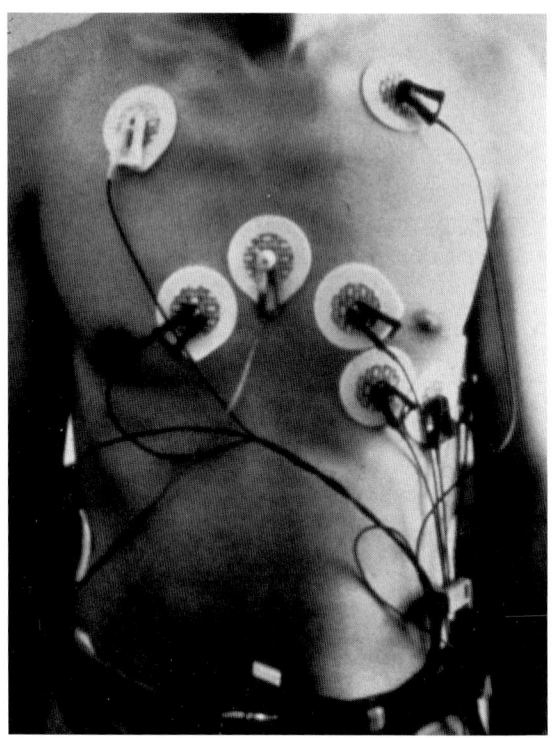
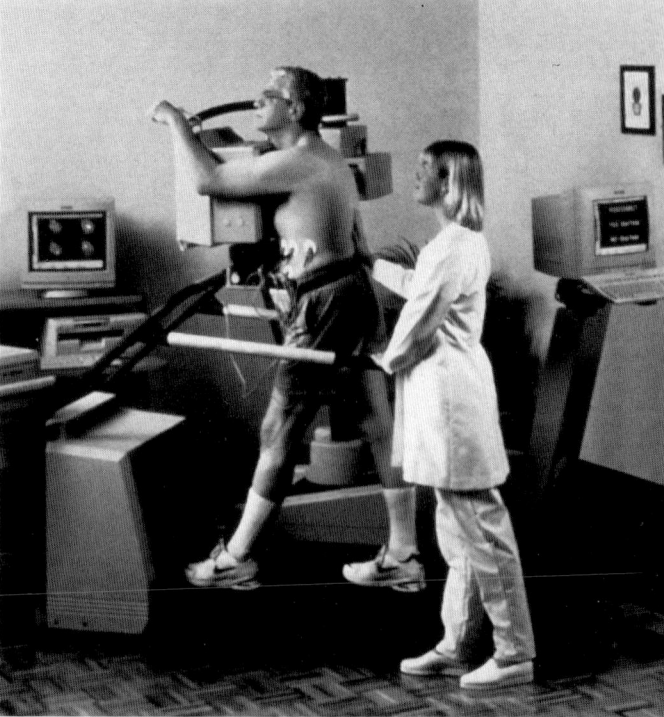

FIG. 2. First-pass imaging has been adapted to treadmill exercise with the aid of a motion detection and correction scheme. One such approach uses a sealed source of Americium-241 (attached like an electrode over the sternum) that can be tracked throughout the study and subsequently used to reregister data according to its motion.

tioned to a theoretical "true" location, which is defined as the average x,y location of the center-of-mass during the left ventricular phase. The more rigorous approach involves the use of an external radioactive source attached to the chest (Fig. 2).

The external marker must contain a gamma emitter with an energy that can be distinguished from the 140 keV photon of the technetium study. Americium-241 is most commonly used for this purpose. When the first-pass study is acquired, the gamma camera is set for a dual energy acquisition. In essence, two first-pass studies are acquired simultaneously, one of the marker and one of the Tc-99m bolus traveling through the central circulation. The movement of the marker is determined in each frame, and the technetium study is then spatially reregistered on a frame-by-frame basis according to the direction and magnitude of the marker motion. Clinically satisfactory FPRNA can be performed during treadmill exercise using such a scheme (4,5). It should be noted that this approach to motion correction does result in some image distortion. As a result, chamber volumes during treadmill exercise are larger than the volumes recorded in the same subjects during bicycle exercise. The ejection fraction measurements, however, are not significantly different (18,19).

Regardless of the type of exercise protocol, it is paramount that images be acquired at the peak of exercise, not immediately after exercise is terminated. It is clear from the experience of laboratories performing first-pass or gated equilibrium imaging, that once exercise is terminated, there are rapid changes in ventricular function. The first-pass literature suggests that exercise ejection fraction rapidly increases

within seconds of stopping exercise in both normal individuals and in those with ischemic exercise responses (20).

DATA PROCESSING

First-pass data processing for ventricular function involves four basic routines; the creation of a time activity curve displaying the cyclic changes in radioactivity within the ventricle, the selection of the beats to be included in the analysis, background correction, and, lastly, the creation of the final representative cycle from which all quantitative data and wall motion data are derived (13,21–27). A fifth routine is that of motion correction, which is essential to treadmill exercise studies and occasionally necessary during bicycle exercise studies.

Time Activity Curve

The changes in the radionuclide concentration of each beat during the ventricular phase of the study are displayed as a time activity curve (Fig. 3).

The curve is generated by drawing a region of interest (ROI) around the ventricle on a frame of raw data and then displaying the count changes within that ROI during the ventricular phase of the study. An initial representative cycle can be created by cyclically adding together each beat of the time activity curve. The initial representative cycle can then be displayed, and the preliminary ventricular region of interest may be modified on the statistically now stronger image of the chamber. The updated ventricular region of

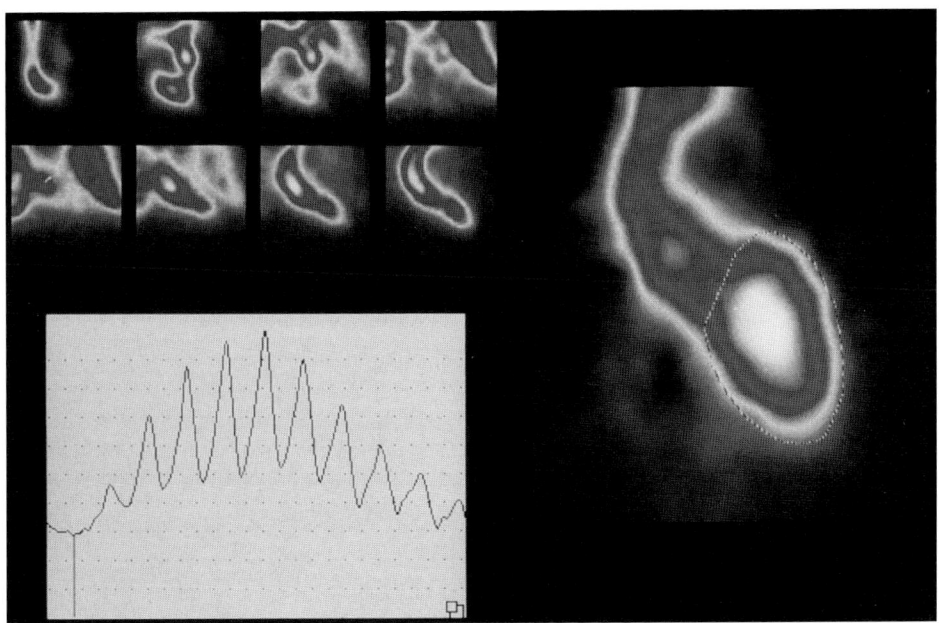

FIG. 3. Processing of first-pass data begins with the identification of a frame of data (**upper left**) in which the left ventricle is clearly defined. An initial region of interest is then drawn (**right**) to create a time activity curve (**lower left**), which, after correction for background, will be used to calculate the ejection fraction and all quantitative information about left ventricular function.

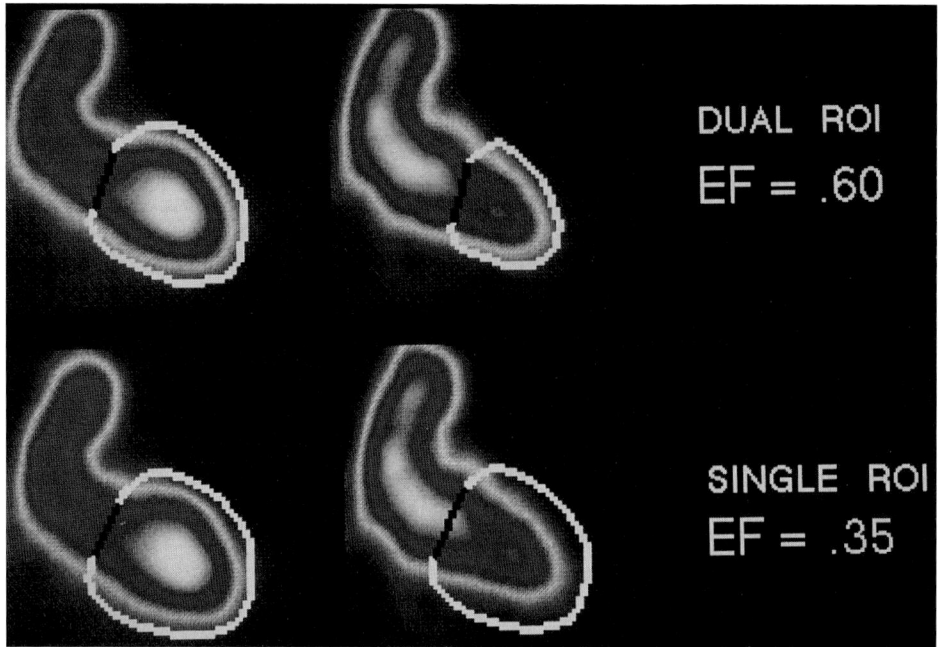

FIG. 4. To calculate the left ventricular ejection fraction (*EF*), it is most accurate to use both end-diastolic and end-systolic regions of interest (*ROI*) (**upper**) as opposed to a single end-diastolic region of interest (**lower**). This case, chosen because of the magnitude of the discrepancy, emphasizes the underestimation of ejection fraction using a single region of interest. The lower ejection fraction results from inclusion of left atrial and aortic counts at end-systole with the single region of interest (**lower right**).

interest is then used to regenerate a ventricular time-activity curve. Various parametric images, such as phase and stroke volume images, may be used to facilitate drawing of the ventricular region of interest. Automated and semiautomated methods are also available for that purpose. Either a single end-diastolic region of interest or both end-diastolic and end-systolic regions of interest may be used for the final representative cycle. For studies acquired in the anterior view, left atrial and aortic root activity are frequently contained within a single end-diastolic region of interest at end-systole and a separate end-systolic region of interest is therefore preferred (28) (Fig. 4).

For studies acquired in the RAO view, a single ROI may suffice, but movement of the aortic valve plane during systole may still make the dual ROI approach preferred.

Beat Selection

All beats whose counts are sufficient may be included in the final representative cycle. Any beat whose end-diastolic counts equal 50 to 70% of the highest end-diastolic count in the left ventricular (LV) phase should be selected. Beats below that threshold should probably not be used unless there is a paucity of beats for analysis. Premature ventricular (PVC) beats should be excluded as should post-PVC beats. The latter will have an ejection fraction that is significantly higher than that of a sinus beat. One has the ability to generate separate ejection fractions for sinus, premature, and post-premature beats, if necessary. If there are frequent PVCs or

ventricular bigeminy, an accurate ejection fraction cannot be determined. If frequent PVCs or bigeminy is noted prior to acquisition, the study should be postponed or the arrhythmia treated. Atrial fibrillation may also be problematic during FPRNA, more so than during an equilibrium study. If atrial fibrillation is present, the calculated ejection fraction will obviously represent an average of the ejection fractions of the individual beats. If the atrial fibrillation is very irregular, the study should probably not be performed.

Background Correction

The purpose of correcting the data for background activity is to isolate the true ventricular counts from those counts adjacent to the left ventricle so that an accurate quantitative analysis of left ventricular function may be performed. All background methods are approximations and no one method will work in all situations. Of all the steps in data processing, the operator can exert the most influence on ejection fraction by varying the background. The ejection fraction is calculated as follows:

$$LVEF = \frac{(ED\ cts\ -\ bkgd\ cts)\ -\ (ES\ cts\ -\ bkgd\ cts)}{(ED\ cts\ -\ bkgd\ cts)}$$

Since the calculated background is virtually the same for *ED* and *ES*, the background term (*bkgd cts*) cancels out of the numerator and the above equation simplifies to:

$$LVEF = \frac{ED\ cts\ -\ ES\ cts}{ED\ cts\ -\ bkgd\ cts}$$

where *LVEF* is left ventricular ejection fraction; *ED cts*, end-diastolic counts; *ES cts*, end-systolic counts; and *bkgd cts*, background counts.

The ejection fraction will, therefore, vary directly with the background activity since the higher the background, the smaller the denominator and the higher the LVEF. Although several approaches to background correction of FPRNA have been described, the most accurate appears to be the lung-frame method (25). The distribution of the activity in a frame in which the counts are largely in the lung and not yet in the LV is taken as representative of the true background activity present during the LV phase of the study. Ideally, it only includes activity in the pulmonary circulation and left atrium. Since the actual background activity is changing throughout the LV phase as the radionuclide clears the lungs and left atrium, a correction for washout must be made. At the same time, the background activity is increasing in the myocardium itself due to the coronary circulation, but the latter is a very small component compared to the amount of activity in the lungs or the ventricle. The selection of the background frame is probably the most important operator intervention other than the drawing of the final ventricular ROI.

Representative Cycle

Once the background correction has been performed, it becomes easier to redraw the ventricular ROI, and, in particular, to identify the aortic valve plane on both the ED and ES frames of the background-corrected representative cycle. These ROI are then used to generate a final representative cycle from which all quantitative data are derived.

The LVEF calculated from this final representative cycle has correlated closely with the LVEF measured during cardiac catheterization (24,25,27). The accuracy of the first-pass LVEF is directly related to the statistical content of the data. The error of the measurement increases as the end-diastolic counts in the representative cycle decreases (Table 1).

The percent error also increases as the LVEF decreases, since small changes in counts result in relatively large

changes in low-ejection fractions (29). Fortunately, as the LVEF decreases, counts within the LV tend to be high due to the large volumes at ED and ES. There is no absolute count rate limit below which first-pass data are guaranteed to be unacceptable, but the statistical error for measurement of an LVEF of 0.40 is almost 10% at an end-diastolic count rate of 2000 counts/frame, which means that the true LVEF could be anywhere from 0.36 to 0.44. If one considers the fact that 2-year survival of a patient with stable coronary artery disease is approximately 83% at an exercise LVEF of 0.36 compared to 93% at an LVEF of 0.44, it is of considerable clinical importance to reduce the statistical error of the measurement to as low a level as reasonably achievable. By increasing the end-diastolic count rate to 5000 counts/frame, the true LVEF in the same situation would range from 0.38 to 0.42 and the 2-year survival would be predicted to be in a narrower range from 85 to 90%. Variability in counts from study to study will also affect the reproducibility of the measurement. When the same subjects were studied on two separate occasions and under similar hemodynamic conditions, the mean differences in ejection fractions measured using the processing scheme described above were 0.04 and 0.03 ejection fraction units at rest and at peak exercise respectively (30,31). Interobserver variability was 2.0% at rest and 2.1% at peak exercise (31).

Left Ventricular Volume

The volume of the ventricle may be calculated on a first-pass study using either geometric or count-proportional methods. The geometric technique is similar to the standard contrast angiographic approach and requires measurement of the area of the left ventricle at end diastole and the length of the longest axis. The modified Sandler-Dodge equation can then be used to generate the end-diastolic volume. Since the LV border is not as statistically reliable at end systole, the end-systolic volume is typically derived from the end-diastolic volume and the stroke volume, the latter being calculated as the product of the end-diastolic volume and the ejection fraction. Although reasonable correlations with contrast angiographic volumes have been obtained with that approach (32), the geometric method is dependent upon the accuracy of the edge detection scheme. Since the spatial resolution of the first-pass study is lower than that of other types of radionuclide imaging, geometric approaches are prone to error.

The count proportional approach relies upon the principle that when completely mixed in a chamber, the radioactivity recorded from the chamber is directly proportional to its volume. The main problem with that approach is that the constant of proportionality differs for each individual because of differences in tissue attenuation, attenuation within the chamber, background activity, and the contribution of scattered activity. Several investigators have proposed a count proportional method that obviates the need to directly measure the constant of proportionality. First proposed by

TABLE 1. *Percent statistical error in calculation of ejection fraction*

ED counts	Ejection fraction						
	0.20	0.30	0.40	0.50	0.60	0.70	0.80
500	30	24	17	13	10	8	6.5
2000	20	12	9	6	5	4	3
10,000	9	5	4	3	2	1.5	1.5

ED, end-diastolic.
(From ref. 29, with permission.)

Nickel et al. (33) and modified by Massaro et al. (34) and Levy et al. (35), the method uses the ratio of the total counts recorded in the chamber and the peak count recorded in any single pixel within the chamber and has been applied to both equilibrium and first-pass data (36). Application of the ratio between total counts and peak pixel counts eliminates the need to calculate or estimate attenuation since the attenuation would affect both the numerator and denominator, thereby canceling out. In addition to the total chamber and peak pixel counts, one must also know the area of a pixel for the acquisition system being used. The method has been rigorously validated using both spherical and ellipsoidal phantoms and in clinical comparisons to contrast angiographic volumes. Using the formula:

$$V = 1.8 \left(\frac{total\ LV\ cts}{peak\ pixel\ cts} - 3.5 \right)^{3/2}$$

where V is volume and LV cts are observed counts in the entire LV phase, the mean biplane contrast ED volume was 162 ± 57 compared to 150 ± 62 ($P = NS$) using FPRNA and a multicrystal camera in 25 patients with contrast end-diastolic volumes ranging from 94 to 453 mL. Using a single crystal camera and FPRNA, the radionuclide ED volume (EDV) averaged 202 ± 88mL compared to 210 ± 92 mL ($P = NS$) for the biplane contrast study.

Standard errors of the estimate (SEE) using that technique compare favorably to methods that attempt to measure attenuation by blood sampling. For EDV, the SEE was 23 mL or 14% of the average EDV. For ESV, calculated from EDV and LVEF, the SEE was 16 mL or 18% of the mean ESV (36).

Normal values from our laboratory for ventricular volumes measured in the upright position using the count proportional technique described above are presented in Table 2.

As one might expect, the end-diastolic volumes tend be be significantly lower in the upright compared to the supine position at rest and show a much greater increase during exercise than is typically seen during supine exercise.

Right Ventricular Function

The first-pass method is the nuclear technique of choice for the measurement of right ventricular ejection fraction (RVEF) but the acquisition technique requires some modification. When a bolus is rapidly injected into a vein close to the central circulation, it arrives in the right ventricle (RV) without much time for mixing and clears the RV quickly. Consequently, there are few beats available, all of which have a rapidly changing concentration of the radionuclide. It is, therefore, helpful to delay the bolus injection when the evaluation of RV function is the main indication for the study. That will increase the number of RV beats available for processing and provide a more stable radionuclide concentration during the RV phase. It is also helpful to acquire the study in a 30-degree RAO view, which maximizes separation of the right atrium and the right ventricle.

Early attempts at measuring the RVEF with the first-pass technique yielded values that were frequently as low as those reported with the equilibrium technique (37). That was primarily due to the use of a single ROI. Both atrial and pulmonary activity encroach upon the end-diastolic RV ROI at end-systole and spuriously lower the RVEF. Use of separate end-diastolic and end-systolic ROI obviates this problem (Fig. 5).

Various types of background correction schemes have been proposed for processing the RV study (37,38).

RV regional wall motion is generally better evaluated with the higher resolution-gated equilibrium method than it is with FPRNA. It is, therefore, often beneficial to acquire both types of studies sequentially. A first-pass study may be acquired during the injection of technetium-99m for an equilibrium-gated blood pool study. After the first-pass study is acquired, a multiview gated study can be acquired.

Gated First-pass Technique

Another approach to the measurement of RVEF, which is popular with single crystal cameras, is the so-called gated first-pass technique. In this case, the acquisition is set up as if a standard gated equilibrium study was to be performed. A bolus of technetium is injected, and the acquisition is started as soon as the bolus is seen to reach the RV and stopped as soon as the majority of the bolus has cleared the RV. In that way, one generates a gated study that includes the data from only those RV beats that occurred while the camera was turned on. Although the resolution of the image is not as good as a standard gated study due to the paucity

TABLE 2. *Normal values for first-pass radionuclide angiography upright acquisitions*

	Heart rate	Ejection fraction	End-diastolic volume index (mL/m²)	End-systolic volume index (mL/m²)	Cardiac index (L/m²)
Female:					
Rest	76 ± 11	0.67 ± 0.04	61 ± 11	21 ± 4	3.0 ± 0.7
Exercise	168 ± 10	0.76 ± 0.04	88 ± 24	22 ± 6	11.0 ± 3.2
Male:					
Rest	75 ± 12	0.66 ± 0.06	60 ± 12	21 ± 6	2.0 ± 0.6
Exercise	163 ± 18	0.76 ± 0.06	83 ± 17	22 ± 7	9.9 ± 1.8

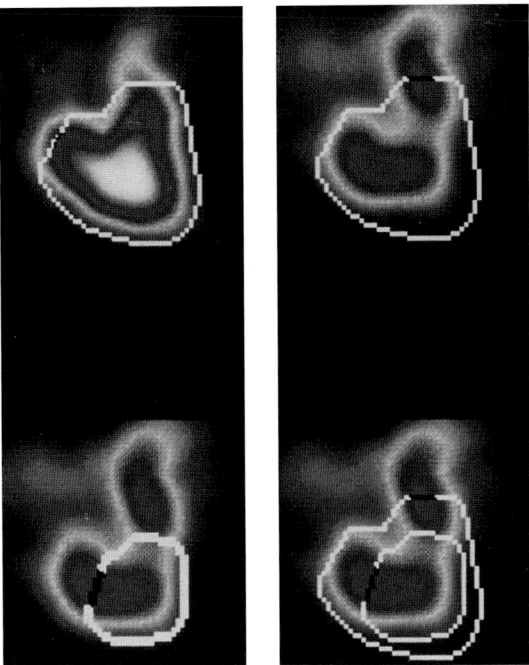

FIG. 5. The concept described in Figure 4 is equally valid for right ventricular processing where a single region of interest for both end-diastole and end-systole (**upper**) underestimates the ejection fraction generated from separate end-diastolic and end-systolic regions of interest (**lower**). As can be seen in the **upper right** image, a single end-diastolic region of interest includes both right atrial and pulmonary activity at end-systole.

of beats, the resolution may be comparable to a standard RV first-pass study and the statistics are usually adequate for calculation of RVEF. The RVEF measured with the gated first-pass technique is systematically higher than that calculated by the standard gated equilibrium method in subjects with normal right ventricles and in those with valvular heart disease (39). Morrison et al. (40) showed that the linear correlation between gated first-pass RVEF and angiographic RVEF was significantly better than that obtained using standard gated equilibrium RVEF.

Chamber-to-chamber Transit Times

The temporal separation of chambers in a first-pass study allows the calculation of the time required for the bolus to travel from one chamber to another or through a given chamber. This capability has not received much clinical application. However, the pulmonary blood volume may be calculated from the product of the pulmonary mean transit time and the cardiac output. Estimates of the pulmonary blood volume have been shown to be of diagnostic value in the detection of coronary artery disease (41,42). In addition, the lung uptake of thallium on exercise or dipyridamole perfusion scans is of important prognostic value. It is conceivable, therefore, that the pulmonary blood volume during exercise

may also be of prognostic importance. This hypothesis has never been tested.

To calculate the mean transit time through the lung, time activity curves are generated from ROI over the left atrium and the pulmonary artery. The pulmonary transit time is then calculated as the left atrial mean transit time-pulmonary arterial mean transit time.

DATA ANALYSIS AND INTERPRETATION

Tracer Transit

The normal sequential appearance of the radionuclide bolus in the superior vena cava, right atrium, right ventricle, pulmonary circulation, left side of the heart, and the aorta should be confirmed in every study. It is helpful to format the data into 1.0 second images in order to easily visualize the entire transit through the central circulation in 16 to 20 images.

Occasionally, deviations from the normal sequence are encountered suggesting a congenital or acquired anatomical abnormality. From time to time there are variations in the sequence of tracer transit that cannot be easily assessed using a display of serial static images; in those situations, it is particularly helpful to create a cinematic display of the raw data. In addition to confirming the normal anatomical sequence of the bolus, the duration of tracer transit through the right heart and left heart phases should be noted. Tracer transit times will vary with the heart rate, to some degree with the rhythm (atrial fibrillation may prolong transit), with the strength of contraction (severely depressed ejection fractions result in prolonged transit), and with the injection technique. In the presence of a good injection bolus, prolongation of tracer transit through the right heart phase may occur because of pulmonary hypertension or tricuspid or pulmonary valve insufficiency. A left-to-right intracardiac shunt will cause early reappearance of tracer in the right heart, but the initial clearance should be normal. If tracer transit through the right heart phase is normal, then prolongation of tracer transit through the left heart suggests mitral or aortic insufficiency or a left-to-right shunt.

Cardiac Rhythm

If there is no ECG signal recorded during the first-pass acquisition, then the interpreting physician must evaluate the time activity curve to determine if regular rhythm was present throughout the study. Atrial fibrillation, ventricular ectopy, or very premature supraventricular ectopy can alter the ejection fraction. One must be certain that the final representative cycle does not contain data from post-PVC or PVC beats unless there is no alternative due to a paucity of beats. In the latter situation, one should note that the reported ejection fraction and wall motion may be over- or underestimated, as the case may be. If ventricular bigeminy is present during the ventricular phase of the study, there is no way to accurately evaluate ventricular function, and one is obliged to report the results for the post-PVC beats.

Assessment of Regional Systolic Function

The interpreting physician should first confirm the integrity of the time activity curve, the appropriateness of the final ventricular ROI, proper beat selection, and the timing of the background frame. In the case of an exercise study, the time activity curve should also be inspected for evidence of cardiac motion.

Regional wall motion may be evaluated using the cinematic display of the representative cycle, in which case, abnormalities of regional wall motion should be characterized using the conventional terms indicating hypokinesia of varying degrees, akinesia, and dyskinesia. In addition, one should comment on the extent of wall motion abnormality.

In the anterior view first-pass left ventricular study, the anterolateral, apical, and inferoseptal walls are defined by the perimeter of the image. In the RAO view, the anterior, apical, and inferior walls are visible. In the LAO view, the septal, inferoapical, and lateral or true posterior walls may be evaluated. The semiquantitative assessment of regional wall motion using the cinematic display of the representative cycle acquired in the RAO view has been compared to the results of contrast angiography in the same subjects (13). The correlation between the anterior and apical walls was quite good. The weakest correlation was noted in the inferior wall, which is probably due to oversubtraction of inferior wall activity as a result of persistent RV activity in the background frame. Since the first-pass study is typically acquired in only one view, and resolution is somewhat limited, it may be difficult to separate regional wall motion abnormalities in contiguous or overlapping segments. A typical example of that shortcoming is the appearance of ''anterior'' hypokinesia on a study acquired in the anterior view in a subject whose actual dysfunction involves the circumflex territory. In that case, the three-dimensional effect of the posterior wall dysfunction is misinterpreted in two dimensional analysis as a problem with the overlying anterior wall. Visual assessment of regional function is obviously subjective. To improve interobserver variability, several parametric images may be generated that aid in the detection and characterization of regional dysfunction.

These parametric images can be as simplistic as displaying the superimposed end-diastolic and end-systolic perimeters after an edge-defining threshold has been applied to the data, or they may be complex as in the case of the mean systolic transit time images (43). One of the most commonly used parametric image is the regional ejection fraction image in which the ejection fraction of each pixel within the ventricular ROI is calculated and color coded. Based on reproducibility data, changes in regional ejection fraction of 0.25 have been considered indicative of a true change in regional function. The amplitude image is similar except that its output reflects the amplitude of the cosine function applied to each

pixel after a Fourier transform has been performed. Phase images are typically used to characterize the timing of events during the cardiac cycle but may also help in detecting regional dysfunction since the latter is typically accompanied by altered timing as well as altered magnitude of contraction.

In contrast angiography, regional wall motion has been quantified by calculating regional shortening fractions applied to an arbitrary number of radii drawn from the center of the ventricle to the perimeter of the chamber at both ED and ES (44,45). The same approach has been taken with gated equilibrium scintigraphy (46). Due to the more limited spatial resolution of the first-pass study, that type of quantitation has not been reliably applied to FPRNA.

Analysis of right-ventricular systolic function is not nearly as straightforward as that of the left ventricle because of its unique geometry. Furthermore, little clinical attention has been paid to regional RV function and no commonly accepted norms are available. Review of the cinematic display of the RV representative cycle is perhaps the best way to evaluate regional RV function and application of the conventional terms, hypokinesia, akinesia, and dyskinesia are appropriate. The gated equilibrium study is better suited for description of regional RV function because of its better spatial resolution.

Ejection Fraction

Normal values for the left-ventricular ejection fraction will vary somewhat according to the exact type of processing used. At rest, an LVEF of 0.50 is generally accepted as the lower limit of normal for untrained individuals. Our most recent results (Table 2) using anterior view acquisitions, dual-ROI processing, and the latest generation of multicrystal gamma camera showed that the resting LVEF, measured in the upright position, was 0.66 ± 0.06 in a group of healthy male volunteers (n = 33) with an average age of 47. The lowest resting LVEF was 0.55. For healthy female volunteers (n = 13) with an average age of 44, the resting LVEF was 0.67 ± 0.04, and the lowest LVEF was 0.55. At peak exercise, the males had an LVEF of 0.76 ± 0.06 with the lowest value being 0.64 while the females had an average exercise LVEF of 0.76 ± 0.04 with the lowest value at 0.69. The exercise measurements were acquired during upright bicycle exercise and may not be applicable to either supine, semisupine, or treadmill exercise.

Left Ventricular Diastolic Function

The temporal resolution of a first-pass study acquired at 25 msec/frame is comparable to a 32-frame/cycle gated acquisition at a heart rate of 60 where the frame time is 31 msec (Fig. 6).

The peak diastolic filling rate, time-to-peak filling rate and filling fractions have been calculated (47,48). In two separate reports, the normal peak diastolic filling rates were 3.13 ± 0.85 in one (47) and 2.14 ± 0.63 in the other (48).

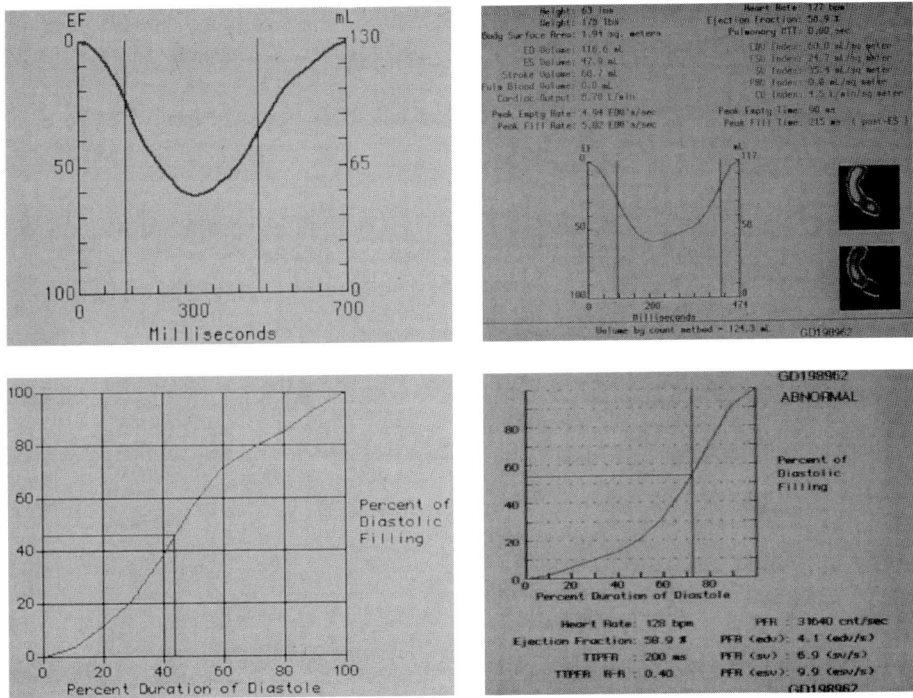

FIG. 6. Diastolic function may be quantified using the conventional indices of time-to-peak filling rate and peak filling rate. The curves on the left are normal and those on the right display a gross abnormality of diastolic filling with a delayed and reduced peak-filling rate. An alternative graphic display (**bottom curves**) shows that 45% of filling has occurred after 45% of diastole in the normal curve, whereas less than 20% of filling has taken place at 45% of diastole in the abnormal curve.

Measurement of diastolic filling rates and intervals may vary with beat selection due to the changing radionuclide concentration throughout the ventricular phase of a first-pass study. Beats occurring early in the LV phase tend to have higher peak-filling rates than beats at the end of the LV phase. It is, therefore, advisable only to include beats that closely surround the beat with the peak end-diastolic count rate since those beats contain the best mixed concentration of radionuclide. If diastolic function is the primary reason for a radionuclide study being performed, then it may be more appropriate to perform a gated equilibrium study to ensure an adequate number of beats and to screen out ectopic beats. The clinical utility of the first-pass study in evaluating diastole has been recently underscored by a study that used such data to distinguish between constrictive and restrictive disease (49), two entities that are difficult to distinguish invasively.

Assessment of Valvular Insufficiency

Prolongation of ventricular tracer transit, when not due to a technical problem, is usually due to valvular insufficiency. As indicated previously, prolonged tracer transit may be identified by an excessive number of beats during the ventricular phase. To quantify left-sided valvular insufficiency, it has been suggested that the pulmonary time-activity curve be used as a monoexponential input function to deconvolute

the left-ventricular time-activity curve. In that way, the contribution of regurgitation to the LV curve can be isolated and quantified using standard curve analysis techniques. The correlation of that approach with results from invasive data has been favorable (50). Tricuspid insufficiency has also been quantified using a curve analysis method (51). Another approach is to calculate the total stroke output of the two ventricles, which would differ by a degree proportional to the amount of regurgitation (52). When left-sided tracer transit is prolonged, the left ventricular image should be examined for the presence of a dilated left atrium (Fig. 7) or dilated aortic root, the former suggesting mitral and the latter aortic insufficiency.

Left-to-right Shunts

The quantitation of left-to-right shunts using radionuclides is an extension of classical indicator dilution theory. Any measurable, nondiffusable indicator injected into the central circulation has a finite circulation time and a typical monoexponential appearance and disappearance when sampled downstream from the injection site. In the catheterization laboratory, the traditional indicator was indocyanine green, which was sampled by drawing downstream blood through a densitometer (53). In FPRNA, the indicator is Tc-99m, and the sampling is performed externally with the gamma camera. In the presence of a left-to-right shunt, the

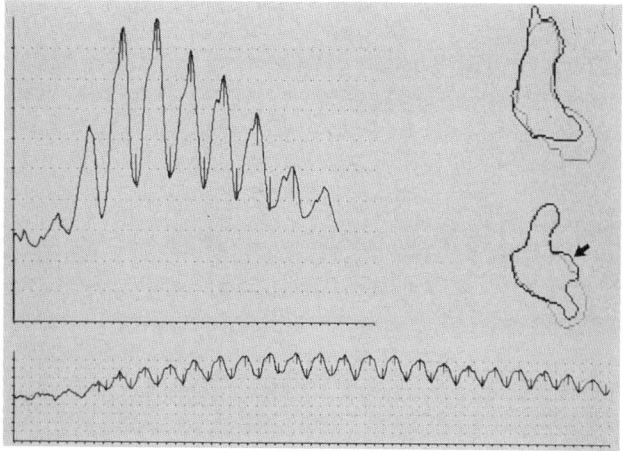

FIG. 7. First-pass studies allow the analysis of tracer transit through the cardiac chambers, the left ventricle being shown here. A normal study (**upper curve** and **image**) contrasts with the markedly prolonged left ventriclular tracer transit due to mitral valve disease (**bottom curve** and **image**). Note the enlarged left atrium (*arrow*), which allows the interpreter to distinguish mitral from aortic valve disease.

curve described by sampling the indicator downstream from the shunt is no longer monoexponential because of the early recirculation of the indicator via the shunt. The radionuclide injection is performed as usual in a peripheral vein. The appearance in and clearance from the lungs is then recorded and graphed.

Standard curve analysis techniques, such as exponential and gamma variate fitting, are then used to separate the observed curve into primary and shunt components. The areas of these two components are proportional to the systemic and shunt flows and allow calculation of the ratio of pulmonary to systemic flow or Qp/Qs. The Qp/Qs is directly proportional to the magnitude of the shunt. Using FPRNA, shunts with a Qp/Qs greater than or equal to 1.2/1 can usually be detected. The early reports using this technique showed excellent correlations with invasive oximetric data (54,55). The pulmonary time-activity curves are usually generated from ROI over both the right and left lung. The right lung is most important since it is spatially more separate from the LV and aorta whose cyclic changes in activity can contaminate the pulmonary curve analysis. The Qp/Qs calculated from the two lungs are rarely identical due to statistical fluctuations in the curves, which influence the identification

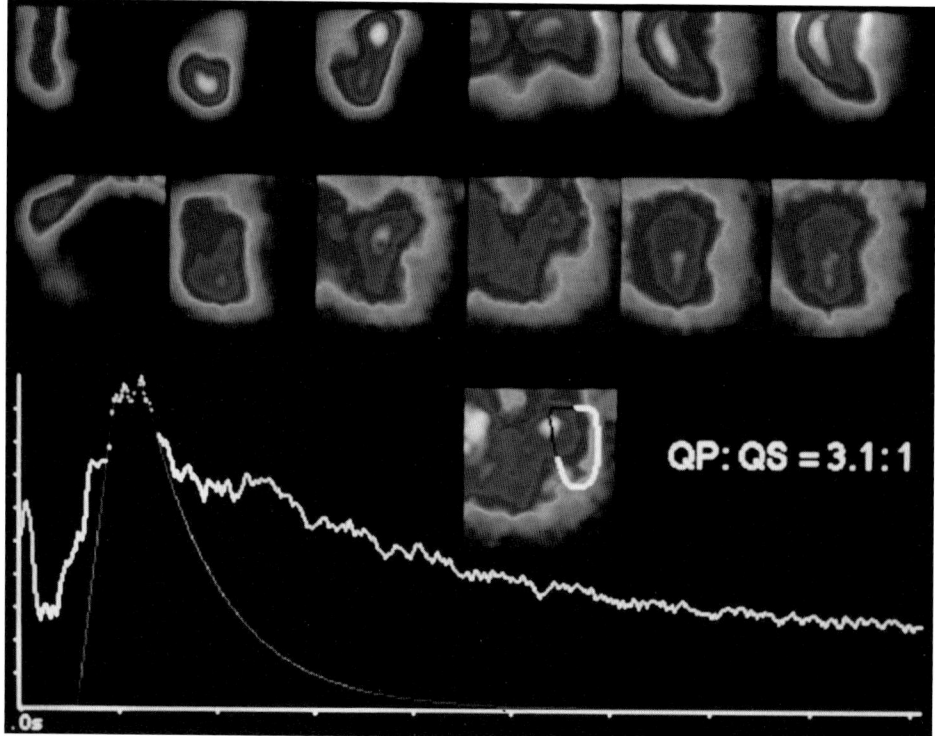

FIG. 8. Analysis of tracer transit permits detection and quantitation of left-to-right shunts. The image set on **top** shows normal tracer transit through the central circulation. The **lower row** of images shows the case of a left-to-right shunt. Note that one cannot distinguish a clear left ventricular image in the **lower row** due to simultaneous appearance of tracer in both ventricles during the left ventricular phase. A region of interest drawn around the lung (**lowest image**) is used to generate the pulmonary time-activity curve seen **below**. The superimposed gamma-variate fit emphasizes the difference between a theoretical monoexponential washout and the patient's actual curve and is used to calculate the Qp/Qs.

of the break point in the curve analysis. The raw pulmonary time-activity curves should be adequately smoothed to minimize the effect of the high frequency statistical noise that can cause incorrect curve fitting.

It is important to remember that the application of monoexponential curve analysis is dependent upon the integrity of the input function, i.e., the bolus entering the pulmonary circulation. A delayed bolus or prolonged right-sided tracer transit, as may occur with tricuspid or pulmonary insufficiency, may preclude accurate quantitation of a shunt. The presence of a shunt, however, may almost always be confirmed visually. The sequential appearance of the radionuclide in the right atrium, right ventricle, pulmonary circulation, and left ventricle is obvious in a normal study, and the left ventricle is free of any right ventricular activity. When there is a significant intracardiac left-to-right shunt, the bolus initially transits the right heart normally, but, upon reaching the left heart, it reappears in the right heart at the same time so a clear LV phase cannot be identified (Fig. 8).

Consequently, simple visual confirmation of a clearly identifiable LV that is not contaminated by RV activity excludes the presence of a significant left-to-right intracardiac shunt. That is not the case with an extracardiac shunt such as a patent ductus arteriosus in which the right heart does not participate in the shunt.

Attempts at quantitation of right-to-left shunts have been made with FPRNA. By placing an ROI over a systemic vessel that is uncontaminated by the pulmonary artery, early appearance of a radionuclide bolus in the systemic circulation following intravenous injection is consistent with a right-to-left shunt (56). A more commonly used approach, however, is to inject radiolabeled macroaggregated albumin. The activity that bypasses the lung through the right-to-left shunt and arrives in systemic organs is compared to the activity that is trapped in the lung, resulting in a semiquantitative estimate of the shunt magnitude (57).

CLINICAL APPLICATIONS OF FIRST-PASS RNA

First-pass RNA can theoretically be applied to any clinical situation in which the evaluation of ventricular function is important or in which the assessment of tracer transit (as in the case of shunts) is necessary. Practically, however, the technique is best applied to situations in which the unique characteristics of FPRNA make it superior to other modalities such as gated equilibrium imaging, gated SPECT imaging, or echocardiography. As such, FPRNA is not typically the procedure of choice when one is evaluating ventricular function at rest. In that situation, the availability of enough acquisition time, the ability to acquire multiple views, and the superior spatial resolution make alternative imaging methods preferable. However, the extremely short acquisition time makes the first-pass method the nuclear technique of choice for the evaluation of ventricular function during exercise. The diagnostic and prognostic applications of exercise ventricular function imaging are, therefore, the main indications for first-pass studies.

DIAGNOSIS OF CORONARY ARTERY DISEASE

Screening

In order for a test to be successfully used as a screening tool for a condition, several criteria must be met, only a few of which actually pertain to the test itself. First, the goal of the screening must be very focused. Many conditions exist in dichotomous states, i.e., one either has it or one doesn't, as would be the case if one were screening for blue eyes in the population. Unfortunately, many conditions, with coronary disease being a perfect example, exist in a wide range of severity. If the goal is to detect any coronary artery disease, regardless of severity, then perhaps electron-beam computed tomography scanning, with its ability to detect small amounts of calcium in arterial walls, is appropriate. If the goal is to detect only physiologically significant stenoses (which could be as mild as a 50%-diameter stenosis), then a form of perfusion imaging that is very sensitive for small reductions in peak coronary blood flow would be more appropriate. In its current form, FPRNA cannot be advocated as a screening tool for the presence or absence of physiologically significant stenoses because its sensitivity and specificity are inadequate for that purpose. If the goal is to detect only prognostically high-risk coronary artery disease (CAD), it is possible that either exercise ECG testing, myocardial perfusion imaging, exercise ventricular function imaging, or some combination of the three might be appropriate.

Since prognosis in stable CAD has a very quantitative relationship with exercise LVEF, exercise first-pass ventricular function imaging could have a role in screening for prognostically high-risk coronary disease (58–61). However, in one direct comparison, it did not perform significantly better than stress ECG for the detection of left main or severe three-vessel disease (62).

Diagnosis-regional Dysfunction

Since radionuclide ventriculography can detect both regional and global ventricular dysfunction, it has been applied to the diagnosis of coronary artery disease. The sensitivity of FPRNA for the detection of exercise-induced regional wall motion abnormalities in patients with known coronary artery disease has been reported to be as low as 53% (63). In contrast, the specificity of a new regional wall motion abnormality in the same study was over 90%. The test appeared to perform more poorly in women than in men (Table 3), but the disease prevalence was much lower in the women than in the men.

As one would expect, the sensitivity for detection of regional LV dysfunction did increase as the disease became more extensive. Regional wall motion abnormalities were detected in 40% of patients with single-vessel CAD, 50% of those with two-vessel CAD, 60% of those with three-

TABLE 3. *Sensitivity and specificity of exercise FPRNA for detection of CAD*

Criteria	173 men		56 women		All	
	Sensitivity	Specificity	Sensitivity	Specificity	Sensitivity	Specificity
ΔEF < 5%	82%	73%	78%	46%	81%	60%
Ex EF at least 6% less than predicted	85%	81%	50%	71%	79%	76%
Ex wall motion abnormality	56%	96%	38%	88%	53%	92%

CAD, coronary artery disease; Δ, exercise minus rest; *EF*, left ventricular ejection fraction; *Ex*, exercise; *FPRNA*, first-pass radionuclide angiography.
(From ref. 63, with permission.)

vessel CAD, and 65% of those with left main disease. The low sensitivity of FPRNA for detection of exercise-induced regional wall motion abnormalities occurs for at least two important reasons. First, the exercise FPRNA is typically acquired in only one view, which precludes detection of disease in nonvisualized segments. Second, the spatial resolution of the first-pass technique is inadequate for detection of subtle changes in regional function. Unfortunately, no large trials of sensitivity or specificity are available that take advantage of the new generation of first-pass cameras, which have much better energy and spatial resolution than did the cameras of the 1970s that were used to generate most of the data we have on this subject. As indicated previously, various parametric images that are more sensitive to three-dimensional count changes and, are therefore, conceivably more sensitive than the standard visual assessment of the beating chamber, have been advocated to improve the sensitivity of the first-pass method (43); however, such approaches have not been rigorously tested.

Diagnosis-global LV Function

The left ventricular ejection fraction response to exercise has long been advocated as a criterion for the diagnosis of coronary artery disease. Early experience suggested that the LVEF would increase by at least 0.05 during dynamic exercise in normal subjects. Failure to increase the LVEF by 0.05 became a diagnostic criterion with early claims of very high sensitivity (64–67). Unfortunately, the early work in this area was skewed by the fact that the majority of subjects in the studies had extensive CAD, which would typically lead to global LV dysfunction during exercise. However, if localized ischemia occurs that does not involve enough myocardium, there may be no changes in global LV function; therefore, it is inconceivable that the LVEF alone would have a high sensitivity for detection of a wide range of CAD extent and severity. In addition, after much more experience with RNA, it has become clear that there are many reasons for the LVEF failing to increase by 0.05 during exercise. Females seem to rely more on an increase in end-diastolic volume than upon an increase in LVEF (68,69). Healthy older subjects have been shown to have a blunted LVEF response to exercise (70). Isometric exercise results in an acute drop in LVEF (71), and the exact exercise protocol itself may influence the LVEF response (20). Both the resting LVEF (72) and the change in EDV during exercise (68) appear to influence the change in LVEF during exercise. The ejection fraction response may also be altered by hypertension or valvular heart disease.

Given all the factors that can affect the LVEF response to exercise, it is not surprising that the use of an LVEF criterion (whether failure to increase by 0.05, failure to increase at all, or even a drop in LVEF) has a poor specificity for the diagnosis of CAD (41,63) (Table 3). In the largest study of the subject, the specificity of a failure to increase the LVEF by 0.05 was only 60% while the sensitivity was 81% (63). Because of that, some investigators have suggested using an equation to predict the LVEF response based upon age, sex, change in end-diastolic volume, etc. (68). If the observed LVEF response was lower than that predicted by the model, CAD could be diagnosed with an improved specificity of 76% while sensitivity remained at 79%. Sensitivity is further increased if one restricts the analysis to those subjects achieving an adequate exercise endpoint. A widely accepted alternative approach is to use an absolute exercise LVEF based upon the lowest exercise LVEF of an age-matched, normal reference population. That value may vary from one laboratory to another because of differences in data processing, but an exercise LVEF of approximately 0.55 is a reasonable cutoff.

Although ejection fraction criteria do not perform very well for the detection of all coronary disease, peak exercise LVEF does vary inversely with the extent and severity of coronary disease (58). As such, it has been used to identify patients with a large ischemic burden, i.e., those most likely to have multivessel or left main disease (59–61), who are those most likely to benefit from revascularization (73).

Other indicators of global LV function that may be of value in the diagnosis of CAD include the end-diastolic and end-systolic volumes and changes in diastolic LV function. None of those is specific for CAD and may occur in valvular and hypertensive heart disease. Typically, end-diastolic and end-systolic volumes increase during ischemia. The peak rate of early left ventricular diastolic filling may be decreased and the time to peak filling prolonged during ischemia. Quantitation of diastolic function is, however, difficult at exercise heart rates using standard FPRNA.

Pharmacologic Interventions

There is ample evidence to support the diagnostic use of myocardial perfusion imaging following pharmacological coronary vasodilatation with dipyridamole (74,75) and adenosine (76). There is also evidence that myocardial perfusion imaging can be linked to catecholamine administration for the diagnosis of CAD (77). There is less evidence that ventricular function imaging during pharmacologic stress is useful diagnostically. Some investigators have reported a high sensitivity for the detection of CAD by using transthoracic echocardiography during coronary vasodilatation (78,79) or during dobutamine infusion (80,81). Gated equilibrium blood pool imaging has been found to be modestly sensitive but quite specific for the diagnosis of coronary disease when performed after a dipyridamole infusion (82) and has recently been used with some success during dobutamine infusion as well (83). We have tested the value of adding a first-pass acquisition to both dipyridamole and dobutamine myocardial perfusion imaging and have not found it to be incrementally useful. Our preliminary experience from a study comparing exercise to dobutamine first-pass LV function suggests that the two types of stress produce very different results.

Combined Function and Perfusion Imaging

The combination of rest and exercise ventricular function imaging with rest and exercise tomographic myocardial perfusion imaging provides the most comprehensive noninvasive assessment of the patient with known or suspected coronary artery disease. Most of the important diagnostic and prognostic variables ever described noninvasively can be assessed or quantified with this approach.

Several attempts to perform both ventricular function and myocardial perfusion imaging during a single exercise test have been made in the past. The rationale, of course, was to improve the diagnostic sensitivity of either test alone as well as add the well-recognized prognostic value of the exercise LVEF to the perfusion data. The early work used the simultaneous injection of short-lived radionuclides, such as gold-195m (84), iridium-191 (85), along with thallium-201. A first-pass study was acquired during the exercise by imaging the gold or the iridium; perfusion scanning then followed the decay of the short-lived isotope. Use of technetium-based myocardial perfusion imaging agents has made it possible to routinely acquire first-pass studies at peak exercise and subsequently perform myocardial perfusion imaging of the same agent (3–7). Preliminary evidence suggests that the diagnostic sensitivity is improved over that of perfusion imaging alone for both the detection of ischemia (4) and for the detection of multivessel disease (86). In a study of 86 patients with documented coronary artery disease, a stepwise analysis showed that the perfusion data contained two thirds of the diagnostic information and the first-pass exercise function data added an independent one third of the total

diagnostic information (4). More recently, it was shown that the addition of the first-pass wall motion analysis increased the detection of multivessel coronary artery disease from 64 to 83% (86). Since regional perfusion abnormalities, by definition, must be present before regional dysfunction can occur, one must question why functional imaging would improve the detection of multivessel disease. The answer is most likely related to the fact that all single-photon perfusion imaging methods look at relative perfusion, i.e., comparing uptake in one segment to that of an adjacent segment. When perfusion is more homogeneously reduced, as may occur in multivessel disease, it may be more difficult to appreciate all the abnormalities of perfusion. In contrast, ventricular dysfunction becomes progressively more extensive as the ischemia increases in extent, even if it is "balanced."

From the standpoint of clinical practice and interpretation, we have found that the addition of functional imaging to perfusion imaging greatly enhances diagnostic confidence. By performing a stress function-perfusion study first, we are much more confident of our results, especially normal studies, and, as a result, fewer patients return for resting imaging, thus saving time, radiation exposure, and cost. Two groups of patients tend to fall into this category. One is the group of patients whose stress perfusion scans are equivocal. The second group includes patients whose exercise perfusion scans are abnormal but whose exercise function is either so well preserved that further testing may not be necessary or so abnormal as to mandate catheterization.

Preliminary comparisons of exercise LVEF to quantitative perfusion defect size suggests a linear correlation (4). In general, subjects with small perfusion defects have exercise ejection fractions above 0.50, which would put them in a very favorable prognostic category while subjects, with large perfusion defect scores tend to have exercise LVEF below 0.35, which would put them in an unfavorable prognostic category. Thus, for patients at the extremes of exercise perfusion defect sizes, the addition of functional data may not be prognostically helpful. However, for those individuals with exercise perfusion defect scores in the intermediate range, the exercise LVEF varies widely suggesting an important prognostic role in this patient subset.

Prognosis in Stable Coronary Artery Disease

The prognosis of patients with stable coronary artery disease is directly related to the contractile state of the left ventricle. Large series of both medically and surgically treated patients have been followed for several years, and the data from different investigators confirm that the resting LVEF measured either invasively or noninvasively is a powerful predictor of subsequent outcome (87,88). Follow-up data are now available that address the prognostic roles of the resting LVEF, exercise LVEF, and the change in LVEF from rest to exercise (ΔLVEF) in a cohort of patients with coronary artery disease followed during medical management subsequent to baseline catheterization. As noted in ear-

TABLE 4. *Comparison of prognostic information from clinical, radionuclide, and catheterization variables*

	Total model chi square	
	CV death	CV events
Clinical	71	48
Catheterization	102	64
Exercise LVEF	104	66
Clinical + Nuclear	120	78
Clinical + Cath	124	82
Clinical + Cath + Nuclear	138	93

Cath, catheterization; *CV*, cardiovascular; *LVEF*, left ventricle ejection fraction.
(From ref. 90, with permission.)

lier work, the resting LVEF proved to be a powerful predictor of prognosis; however, the peak-exercise LVEF proved to be even more powerful in predicting subsequent mortality (89,90). The ΔLVEF was of little prognostic significance when the exercise LVEF was included in a multivariable model. That finding has been confirmed by another group using gated equilibrium data (91). Furthermore, when the radionuclide data were compared to the clinical and catheterization-derived variables, it was shown that the combination of the exercise LVEF and the clinical data contained as much or more prognostic information available from a catheterization (Table 4).

As such, the noninvasive evaluation of patients with coronary disease, when an exercise LVEF is included, may be used as a surrogate for cardiac catheterization for predicting outcome.

Patients with an exercise LVEF of greater than 0.50 have an excellent long-term outlook. Mortality increases sharply once the exercise LVEF drops below 0.35. Other investigators, using gated equilibrium RNA have suggested that there is prognostic information in the ΔLVEF. In a study of mildly symptomatic patients with three-vessel disease, those subjects whose LVEF fell during exercise had more subsequent events than those subjects whose LVEF increased during exercise (92). All deaths in that study occurred in the subgroup with a drop in LVEF and greater than or equal to 1 mm ST segment depression during exercise. The differences between study results is certainly related, at least in part, to differences in the populations included. Although some controversy exists regarding which of the three variables, rest, exercise, or ΔLVEF is most important in a particular population, there is certainly universal agreement that the LVEF can be used to stratify patients according to their likelihood of subsequent mortality. Although most of the data on prognosis and ejection fraction relates to patients with stable coronary artery disease, similar results have been demonstrated for patients soon after acute myocardial infarction (93). There are also data to suggest that the same relationship is true for predicting outcome in patients after surgical revascularization.

No prospective study has been performed that has exam-

ined the outcome of patients randomized to treatment strategies based upon the results of noninvasive testing. In a nonprospective, nonrandomized study of subjects with normal resting LV function, it was shown that those subjects with the greatest fall in LVEF during exercise preoperatively showed the most benefit in terms of pain relief and longevity following bypass surgery (73).

Evaluation of Patients with Chronic Obstructive Pulmonary Disease

As with the left ventricle, the function of the right ventricle function is related to the afterload presented to it, which, in turn, is related to the pulmonary arterial pressure or pulmonary vascular resistance. When pulmonary hypertension is present, right ventricular ejection fraction (RVEF) may be decreased. Using first-pass data, RVEF has been shown to vary inversely with pulmonary pressure in patients with chronic obstructive pulmonary disease (COPD) (94). Patients with clinical cor pulmonale tend to have lower RVEF than those with COPD without heart failure. In addition, an abnormal resting RVEF in the presence of COPD may be predictive of the subsequent appearance of cor pulmonale (95). Patients with COPD and a normal resting RVEF may have an abnormal RVEF response to exercise (96).

REFERENCES

1. Blumgart HL, Weiss M. Studies on the velocity of blood flow. VII The pulmonary circulation time in normal resting individuals. *J Clin Invest* 1927;4:399–425.
2. Mason DT, Ashburn WL, Harbert JC, et al. Rapid sequential visualization of the heart and great vessels in man using the wide-field anger scintillation camera. *Circulation* 1969;39:19–28.
3. Jones RH, Borges-Neto S, et al. Simultaneous measurement of myocardial perfusion and ventricular function during exercise from a single injection of technetium-99m sestamibi in coronary artery disease. *Am J Cardiol* 1990;66:68E–71E.
4. Borges-Neto S, Coleman RE, Potts JM, et al. Combined exercise radionuclide angiocardiography and single photon emission computed tomography perfusion studies for assessment of coronary disease. *Semin Nucl Med* 1991;21:223.
5. Johnson LL, Rodney RA, Vaccarino RA, et al. Left ventricular perfusion and performance from a single radiopharmaceutical and one camera. *J Nucl Med* 1992;33:1411–1416.
6. Williams KA, Taillon LA, Draho JM, et al. First-pass radionuclide angiographic studies of left ventricular function with technetium-99m-teboroxime, technetium-99m sestamibi and technetium-99m-DTPA. *J Nucl Med* 1993;34:394–399.
7. Takahashi N, Tamaki N, Tadamura E, et al. Combined assessment of regional perfusion and wall motion in patients with coronary artery disease with technetium-99m-tetrofosmin. *J Nucl Cardiol* 1994;1:29–38.
8. Treves S, Cheng C, Samuel A, et al. Iridium-191 angiocardiography for the detection and quantitation of left-to-right shunting. *J Nucl Med* 1980;21:1151–1157.
9. Mena I, Narahara KA, de Jong R, et al. Gold-195-m, an ultra-short-lived generator-produced radionuclide: clinical application in sequential first pass ventriculography. *J Nucl Med* 1983;24:139–144.
10. Adams R, Lacy JL, Ball ME, et al. The count rate performance of a multiwire gamma camera measured by a decaying source method with 9.3-minute Tantalum-178. *J Nucl Med* 1990;31:1723–1726.
11. Lacy JL, Layne WW, Guidry GW, et al. Development and clinical performance of an automated, portable Tungsten-178/Tantalum-178 generator. *J Nucl Med* 1991;32:2158–2161.

12. Verani MS, Lacy JL, Guidry GW, et al. Quantification of left ventricular performance during transient coronary occlusion at various anatomic sites in humans: a study using tantalum-178 and a multiwire gamma camera. *J Am Coll Cardiol* 1992;297–306.

13. Gal R, Grenier RP, Carpenter J, et al. High count rate first-pass radionuclide angiography using a digital gamma camera. *J Nucl Med* 1986; 27:198–206.

14. Nichols K, DePuey EG, Gooneratne N, et al. First-pass ventricular ejection fraction using a single-crystal nuclear camera. *J Nucl Med* 1994;35:1292–1300.

15. Bowyer KW, Konstantinow G, Rerych SK, et al. Optimum counting intervals in radionuclide cardiac studies: In: *Nuclear cardiology: selected computer aspects.* New York: Society of Nuclear Medicine, 1978:85.

16. Rerych SK, Scholz PM, Newman GE, et al. Cardiac function at rest and during exercise in normals and in patients with coronary heart disease. Evaluation by radionuclide angiocardiography. *Ann Surg* 1978; 187:449.

17. Berger HI, Reduto LA, Johnstone DE, et al. Global and regional left ventricular response to bicycle exercise in coronary artery disease. *Am J Med* 1979;66:13–21.

18. Potts JM, Borges-Neto S, Smith LR, et al. Comparison of bicycle and treadmill radionuclide angiocardiography. *J Nucl Med* 1991;32: 1918–1922.

19. Friedman JD, Berman DS, Kiat H, et al. Rest and treadmill exercise first-pass radionuclide ventriculography: validation of left ventricular ejection fraction measurements. *J Nucl Cardiol* 1994;4:382–388.

20. Foster C, Dymond DS, Anholm JD, et al. Effect of exercise protocol on the left ventricular response to exercise. *Am J Cardiol* 1983;51: 859–864.

21. Rerych SK, Scholz PM, Newman GE, et al. Cardiac function at rest and during exercise in normals and in patients with coronary heart disease. Evaluation by radionuclide angiocardiography. *Ann Surg* 1978; 187:449.

22. Berger HI, Reduto LA, Johnstone DE, et al. Global and regional left ventricular response to bicycle exercise in coronary artery disease. *Am J Med* 1979;66:13–21.

23. Jengo MA, Mena I, Blaufuss A, et al. Evaluation of left ventricular function (ejection fraction and segmental wall motion) by single pass radioisotope angiography. *Circulation* 1978;57:326.

24. Marshall RC, Berger HJ, Costin JC, et al. Assessment of cardiac performance with quantitative radionuclide angiocardiography. *Circulation* 1977;56:820–829.

25. Gal R, Grenier RP, Schmidt DH, et al. Background correction in first-pass radionuclide angiography: comparison of several approaches. *J Nucl Med* 1986;27:1480–1486.

26. Scholz PM, Rerych SK, Moran JF, et al. Quantitative radionuclide angiocardiography. *Cathet Cardiovasc Diagn* 1980;6:265–283.

27. Bodenheimer MM, Banka VS, Fooshee CM, et al. Quantitative radionuclide angiography in the right anterior oblique view: comparison with contrast ventriculography. *Am J Cardiol* 1978;41:718–725.

28. Williams KA, Bryant TA, Taillon LA. First-pass radionuclide angiographic analysis with two regions of interest to improve left ventricular ejection fraction accuracy. *J Nucl Med* 1998;39:1857–1861.

29. Wackers FJTh. First-pass radionuclide angiocardiography. In: Gerson MC, ed. *Cardiac nuclear medicine.* New York: McGraw-Hill, 1991: 67–80.

30. Marshall RC, Berger HJ, Reduto LA, et al. Variability in sequential measures of left ventricular performance assessed with radionuclide angiocardiography. *Am J Cardiol* 1978;41:531.

31. Upton MT, Rerych SK, Newman GE, et al. The reproducibility of radionuclide angiographic measurements of LV function in normal subjects at rest and during exercise. *Circulation* 1980;62:126–132.

32. Anderson PAW, Rerych SK, Moore TE, et al. Accuracy of left ventricular end-diastolic dimension determinations obtained by radionuclide angiocardiography. *J Nucl Med* 1981;22:500.

33. Nickel O, Schad N, Andrews EJ, et al. Scintigraphic measurement of left ventricular volumes from the count-density distribution. *J Nucl Med* 1982;23:404–410.

34. Massardo T, Gal RA, Grenier RP, et al. Left ventricular volume calculations using a count based ratio method applied to multigated radionuclide angiography. *J Nucl Med* 1990;31:450–456.

35. Levy WC, Cerqueira MD, Matsuoka DT, et al. Four radionuclide methods for left ventricular volume determination: comparison of a manual and an automated technqiue. *J Nucl Med* 1992;33:763–770.

36. Gal R, Grenier RP, Port SC, et al. Left ventricular volume calculation using a count-based ratio method applied to first-pass radionuclide angiography. *J Nucl Med* 1992;33:2124–2132.

37. Berger HJ, Matthay RA, Loke J, et al. Assessment of cardiac performance with quantitative radionuclide angiocardiography: right ventricular ejection fraction with reference to findings in chronic obstructive pulmonary disease. *Am J Cardiol* 1978;41:897–905.

38. Huang PJ, Su CT, Lee YT, et al. Right ventricular ejection fraction: validation of first-pass radionuclide studies by contrast angiography. *Jpn Heart J* 1984;25:533–546.

39. Winzelberg GG, Boucher CA, Pohost GM, et al. Right ventricular function in aortic and mitral valve disease. *Chest* 198;79:520–528.

40. Morrison DA, Turgeon J, Ouitt T. Right ventricular ejection fraction measurements: contrast ventriculography versus gated blood pool and gated first-pass method. *Am J Cardiol* 1984;54:651–653.

41. Osbakken MD, Boucher CA, Okada RD, et al. Spectrum of global left ventricular responses to supine exercise: limitation in the use of ejection fraction in identifying patients with coronary artery disease. *Am J Cardiol* 1983;51:28.

42. Hanley PC, Gibbons RJ. Value of radionuclide-determined changes in pulmonary blood volume for the detection of coronary artery disease. *Chest* 1990;97:7–11.

43. Schad N, Andrews ES, Fleming JW. *Colour atlas of first-pass functional imaging of the heart.* Hingham, MA: MTP Press Ltd., 1985.

44. Sheehan FH, Dodge HT, Mathey DG, et al. Application of the centerline method: analysis of change in regional left ventricular wall motion in serial studies. *IEEE Comput* 1982;9–12.

45. Sheehan FH, Mathey DG, Schofer J, et al. Effect of interventions in salvaging left ventricular function in acute myocardial infarction: a study of intracoronary streptokinase. *Am J Cardiol* 1983;52:431–438.

46. Zaret BL, Wackers FJ. Radionuclide methods for evaluating the results of thrombolytic therapy. *Circulation* 1987;76(II):1117–1118.

47. Reduto LA, Wickemeyer WJ, Young JB, et al. Left ventricular diastolic performance at rest and during exercise in patients with coronary artery disease. *Circulation* 1981;63:1228–1237.

48. Polak JF, Kemper AJ, Bianco JA, et al. Resting early peak diastolic filling rate: a sensitive index of myocardial dysfunction in patients with coronary artery disease. *J Nucl Med* 1982;23:471–478.

49. Aroney CN, Ruddy TD, Dighero H, et al. Differentiation of restrictive cardiomyopathy from pericardial constriction: assessment of diastolic function by radionuclide angiography. *J Am Coll Cardiol* 1989;13: 1007–1014.

50. Philippe L, Mena I, Darcourt J, et al. Evaluation of valvular regurgitation by factor analysis of first-pass angiography. *J Nucl Med* 1988;29: 159–167.

51. Kanishi Y, Tatsuta N, Hikasa Y, et al. Assessment of tricuspid regurgitation by analog computer analysis of dilution curves recorded by scintillation camera. *Jpn Circulation* 1982;6:1147.

52. Janowitz WR, Fester A. Quantitation of left ventricular regurgitant fraction by first pass radionuclide angiocardiography. *Am J Cardiol* 1982;49:85–92.

53. Braunwald E, Tannenbaum HL, Morrow AG. Localization of left-to-right cardiac shunts by dye-dilution curves following injection into the left side of the heart and into the aorta. *Am J Med* 1958;24:203.

54. Maltz DL, Treves S. Quantitative radionuclide angiocardiography: determination of Qp:Qs in children. *Circulation* 1973;47:1048–1056.

55. Askenazi J, Ahnberg DS, Korngold E, et al. Quantitative radionuclide angiocardiography: detection and quantitation of left to right shunts. *Am J Cardiol* 1976;37:382–387.

56. Peter CA, Armstrong BE, Jones RH. Radionuclide quantitation of right-to-left intracardiac shunts in children. *Circulation* 1981;64:572.

57. Dogan AS, Rezai K, Kirchner PT, et al. A scintigraphic sign for detection of right-to-left shunts. *J Nucl Med* 1993;34:1607–1611.

58. DePace NL, Iskandrian AS, Hakki A, et al. Value of left ventricular ejection fraction during exercise in predicting the extent of coronary artery disease. *J Am Coll Cardiol* 1983;1:1002.

59. Johnson SH, Bigelow C, Lee KL, et al. Prediction of death and myocardial infarction by radionuclide angiocardiography in patients with suspected coronary artery disease. *Am J Cardiol* 1991;67:919–926.

60. Weintraub WS, Schneider RM, Seelaus PA, et al. Prospective evaluation of the severity of coronary artery disease with exercise radionuclide angiography and electrocardiography. *Am Heart J* 1986;111:537.

61. Gibbons RJ, Fyke FE III, Clements IP, et al. Noninvasive identification of severe coronary artery disease using exercise radionuclide angiography. *J Am Coll Cardiol* 1988;11:28–34.

62. Campos, CT, Chu HW, D'Agostino HJ Jr, et al. Comparison of rest and exercise radionuclide angiocardiography and exercise treadmill testing for diagnosis of anatomically extensive coronary artery disease. *Circulation* 1983;67:1204–1210.

63. Jones RH, McEwen P, Newman GE, et al. Accuracy of diagnosis of coronary artery disease by radionuclide measurement of left ventricular function during rest and exercise. *Circulation* 1981;64:586–601.

64. Rerych SK, Scholz PM, Newman GE, et al. Cardiac function at rest and during exercise in normals and patients with coronary artery disease. *Ann Surg* 1978;187:449.

65. Borer JS, Kent KM, Bacharach SL, et al. Sensitivity, specificity and predictive accuracy of radionuclide cineangiography during exercise in patients with coronary artery disease. *Circulation* 1979;60:572.

66. Berger H, Reduto L, Johnstone D, et al. Global and regional left ventricular response to bicycle exercise in coronary artery disease: assessment by quantitative radionuclide angiocardiography. *Am J Med* 1979;66: 13.

67. Jengo JA, Oren V, Conant R, et al. Effects of maximal exercise stress on left ventricular function in patients with coronary artery disease using first pass radionuclide angiocardiography. A rapid noninvasive technique for determining ejection fraction and segmented wall motion. *Circulation* 1979;59:60–65.

68. Gibbons RJ, Lee KL, Cobb F, et al. Ejection fraction response to exercise in patients with chest pain and normal coronary arteriograms. *Circulation* 1981;64:952–957.

69. Higginbotham MB, Morris KB, Coleman RE, et al. Sex-related differences in the normal cardiac response to upright exercise. *Circulation* 1984;70:357.

70. Port SC, Cobb FR, Coleman E, et al. Effect of age on the response of the left ventricular ejection fraction to exercise. *N Engl J Med* 1980; 303:1133–1137.

71. Peter CA, Jones RH. Effects of isometric handgrip and dynamic exercise on left ventricular function. *J Nucl Med* 1980;21:1131.

72. Port SC, McEwan P, Cobb FR, et al. Influence of resting left ventricular function on the left ventricular response to exercise in patients with coronary artery disease. *Circulation* 1981;63:856.

73. Jones RH, Floyd RD, Austin EH, et al. The role of radionuclide angiocardiography in the preoperative prediction of pain relief and prolonged survival following coronary artery bypass grafting. *Ann Surg* 1983; 197:743.

74. Leppo J, Boucher CA, Okada RD, et al. Serial thallium-201, myocardial imaging after dipyridamole infusion:diagnostic utility in detecting coronary stenoses and relationship to regional wall motion. *Circulation* 1982;66:649–657.

75. Leppo JA. Dipyridamole-thallium imaging: the lazy man's stress test. *J Nucl Med* 1989;30:281–287.

76. Verani MS, Mahmarian JJ, Hixson JB, et al. Diagnosis of coronary artery disease by controlled coronary vasodilation with adenosine and thallium-201 scintigraphy in patients unable to exercise. *Circulation* 1990;82:80–87.

77. Pennell DJ, Underwood SR, Swanton RH, et al. Dobutamine thallium myocardial perfusion tomography. *J Am Coll Cardiol* 1991;18: 1471–1479.

78. Picano E, Lattanzi F, Masini M, et al. Usefulness of the dipyridamole-exercise echocardiography test for diagnosis of coronary artery disease. *Am J Cardiol* 1988;62(1):67–70.

79. Masini M, Picano E, Lattanzi F, et al. High dose dipyridamole-echocardiography test in women: correlation with exercise-electrocardiography test and coronary arteriography. *J Am Coll Cardiol* 1988;12:682.

80. Cohen JL, Greene TO, Ottenweller J, et al. Dobutamine digital echocardiography for detecting coronary artery disease. *Am J Cardiol* 1991; 67:1311–1318.

81. Baudhuin T, Marwick T, Melin J, et al. Diagnosis of coronary artery disease in elderly patients: safety and efficacy of dobutamine echocardiography. *Eur Heart J* 1993;14:799–803.

82. Cates CU, Kronenberg MW, Collins HW, et al. Dipyridamole radionuclide ventriculography: a test with high specificity for severe coronary artery disease. *J Am Coll Cardiol* 1989;13:841–851.

83. Bahl VK, Vasan RS, Malhotra A, et al. A comparison of dobutamine infusion and exercise during radionuclide ventriculography in the evaluation of coronary artery disease. *Int J Cardiol* 1992;35:49–55.

84. Narahara KA, Mena I, Maublaut JC, et al. Simultaneous maximum exercise radionuclide angiography and Thallium stress perfusion imaging. *Am J Cardiol* 1984;53:812.

85. Verani MS, Lacy JL, Ball ME, et al. Simultaneous assessment of regional ventricular function and perfusion utilizing iridium-191m and thallium-201 during a single exercise test. *Am J Cardiol Imaging* 1988; 2:206.

86. Palmas W, Friedman JD, Diamond G, et al. Incremental value of simultaneous assessment of myocardial function and perfusion with technetium 99m sestamibi for prediction of extent of coronary artery disease. *J Am Coll Cardiol* 1995;25:1024–1031.

87. Harris PJ, Harrell FE Jr, Lee KL, et al. Nonfatal myocardial infarct in medically treated patients with coronary artery disease. *Circulation* 1980;62:240–248.

88. CASS Principal Investigators. Coronary artery surgery study (CASS): a randomized trial of coronary bypass surgery. Survival date. *Circulation* 1983;68:989.

89. Pryor DB, Harrel FE, Lee KL, et al. Prognostic indicators from radionuclide angiography in medically treated patients with coronary artery disease. *Am J Cadiol* 1984;53:18.

90. Lee KL, Pryor DB, Pieper KS, et al. Prognostic value of radionuclide angiography in medically treated patients with coronary artery disease. *Circulation* 1990;82:1705–1717.

91. Iqbal A, Gibbons RJ, Zinmeister AR, et al. Prognostic value of exercise radionuclide angiography in a population-based cohort of patients with known or suspected coronary artery disease. *Am J Cardiol* 1994;74: 119–124.

92. Bonow RO, Kent KM, Rosing DR, et al. Exercise-induced ischemia in mildly symptomatic patients with coronary artery disease and preseved left ventricular function: identification of subgroups at risk of death during medical therapy. *N Engl J Med* 1984;311:1339.

93. Morris KG, Palmeri ST, Califf RM, et al. Value of radionuclide angiography for predicting specific cardiac events after acute myocardial infarction. *Am J Cardiol* 1985;55:318–324.

94. Brent BN, Mahler D, Matthay RA, et al. Noninvasive diagnosis of pulmonary arterial hypertension in chronic obstructive pulmonary disease: right ventricular ejection fraction at rest. *Am J Cardiol* 1984;53: 1349–1353.

95. Berger HJ, Matthay RA, Loke J, et al. Assessment of cardiac performance with quantitative radionuclide angiography: right ventricular ejection fraction with reference to findings in chronic obstructive pulmonary disease. *Am J Cardiol* 1978;41:897.

96. Matthay RA, Berger HJ, Davies RA, et al. Right and left ventricular exercise performance in chronic obstructive pulmonary disease: radionuclide assessment. *Ann Intern Med* 1980;93:234.

CHAPTER 19

Assessment of Ventricular Function

Gated-perfusion Methods

Guido Germano and Daniel S. Berman

Cardiac function has long been studied for its diagnostic and prognostic value (1–3). To give just one example of its importance, low-rest left ventricular ejection fraction (LVEF) has been associated with increased cardiac death events in patients after myocardial infarction, the event rate being directly proportional to the degree of LVEF abnormality (4). Cardiac function is increasingly being assessed using nonnuclear techniques, most notably echocardiography (5) and contrast ventriculography (6), neither one of which is intrinsically digital or three-dimensional in their most common clinical implementation. Determination of cardiac function parameters from two-dimensional datasets requires certain geometric assumptions and, if performed manually, leads to intrinsic nonreproducibilities. When nuclear techniques have been used for the analysis of cardiac function, the traditional methods of choice have been planar-gated blood pool (7,8) or first-pass studies (9).

The recent increase in the utilization of gated single photon emission computed tomography (SPECT) protocols has led to the development of software and algorithms for the quantitation of global and regional parameters of cardiac function from gated SPECT data. While the different approaches vary in their degree of automation and validation and are based on different mathematical operators, their common goal is to standardize the measurement of cardiac

G. Germano: Department of Radiological Sciences, University of California–Los Angeles School of Medicine, Los Angeles, California 90024; Department of Medicine, Cedars-Sinai Medical Center, Los Angeles, California 90048.

D. S. Berman: University of California–Los Angeles School of Medicine, Los Angeles, California 90025; Department of Imaging/ Nuclear Medicine, Cedars-Sinai Medical Center, Los Angeles, California 90048.

function and make it more reproducible, similar to what was done for myocardial perfusion quantitation (10,11). This chapter will cover some key technical aspects of the acquisition and processing of gated SPECT studies, present a review of the different gated cardiac SPECT methods published in the literature, and outline ways in which gated SPECT imaging can be clinically utilized. For those interested in further information on these subjects, a recent textbook devoted to gated cardiac SPECT may be of interest (12).

ACQUISITION AND PROCESSING

A gated SPECT acquisition is similar to a standard SPECT acquisition, since in both cases the camera detector(s) rotate around the long axis of the patient, acquiring a number of planar ("projection") images at regular angular intervals (see Chapter 11). What distinguishes the gated from the nongated technique is that, in the former, a number (8 or 16) of projection images is acquired at each projection angle, with each image (also called interval or frame) corresponding to a specific portion of the cardiac cycle. All projection images for a given interval are reconstructed into a SPECT image volume using standard filtered backprojection or iterative reconstruction, and the SPECT volumes relative to the various acquisition intervals can be displayed in four-dimensional format (x, y, z, and time) allowing for the assessment of dynamic cardiac function. In addition, summing all individual intervals' projections at each angle before reconstruction is essentially equivalent to having acquired a static perfusion SPECT study and results in what are generally referred to as the "ungated" or summed gated SPECT image volume. Thus, a gated myocardial perfusion SPECT acquisition results in a standard SPECT data set ("summed" gated

SPECT), from which perfusion is assessed, and a larger gated SPECT data set, from which function is evaluated.

Isotopes

It is the authors' belief that, as long as adequate count statistics are achieved, there is no limitation as to the specific perfusion agent that can be imaged with the gated SPECT technique. Gated Tc-99m-sestamibi and Tc-99m-tetrofosmin SPECT imaging is routinely performed at a steadily increasing number of institutions, totaling over 40% of all Tc-99m-based SPECT studies in 1997. Gated Tl-201 SPECT imaging, originally considered not feasible, is now commonly performed, especially in sites with multidetector cameras, with quantitative results not substantially different from gated Tc-99m-based SPECT (13,14). The basic idea is that, no matter what radiopharmaceutical is used, the quality of the gated SPECT study will be closely and directly related to the number of counts in its individual frames. Count statistics are influenced by numerous factors, including injected dose, acquisition time, patient size, camera configuration and sensitivity, collimation, number of frames, and count acceptance criteria. In the context of our standard gated SPECT acquisition protocols (13; see Chapter 13), we have found that, with a 60-to-64 angle acquisition, if one creates a composite image by adding together the eight gated projection images for the seven angles within ± 10.5 degrees of LAO 45 degrees and one isolates the myocardium in that composite image, the average number of myocardial counts/pixel is around 789 ± 237 for gated Tc-99m-sestamibi, and 306 ± 81 for gated Tl-201. In our experience, these count statistics are adequate. Ideally, this number should be greater if, in a given individual, the target-to-background ratio is lower than usual.

Single-detector versus Multidetector Cameras

As explained in Chapter 11, multidetector cameras have consistently outsold single-detector systems over the past few years, and their increasing diffusion is an important factor supporting the increasing utilization of gated SPECT imaging. In particular, dual-detector cameras with the two detectors positioned at 90 degrees allow completion of 180-degree SPECT acquisitions in half the time as with a single detector system for the same count level, or collection of twice the counts in the same time, and are, therefore, highly efficient for gated cardiac SPECT imaging.

Length of Acquisition

Ideally, the length of acquisition (expressed in seconds per projection) for a gated Tc-99m-based SPECT study need not exceed that traditionally employed for a nongated SPECT study, as it has been suggested that the latter may consistently provide more counts than are needed (15). For gated Tl-201 SPECT, extending the acquisition time may be

necessary, especially for gated redistribution analysis. As a general rule, 25 sec/projection (Tc-99m-sestamibi or Tc-99m-tetrofosmin) or 35 sec/projection (Tl-201) are appropriate for low-energy-high-resolution (LEHR) collimation, 3-degree projection spacing and 8-frame gating. It is clear that, although in principle any type of acquisition can be gated, practical considerations on patient tolerance and avoidance of motion limit some acquisitions to multidetector cameras.

Number of Frames

While it is obvious that the cardiac cycle can be more accurately described if the acquisition process involves frequent temporal sampling (more gating intervals or frames), 8-frame gating has become the practical standard in gated perfusion SPECT imaging. This is due to a number of factors, including shorter processing and analysis times, reduced storage requirements, and better image count statistics. Eight-frame gating leads to quantitative ejection fraction results that are slightly lower than those obtained from 16-frame gating, but the relationship between the two is predictable and quite uniform (3 to 4 LVEF points) over a wide ejection fraction range (16). The considerations contained in this book relative to acquisition, processing, and quantitation of gated perfusion SPECT data are most likely the same for 8- or 16-frame gated acquisitions.

Collimators

The standard collimator used in nuclear cardiology is a parallel hole collimator. Specifically, virtually all manufacturers offer a parallel hole collimator that favors resolution—the low-energy high-resolution (LEHR) collimator—and one that favors sensitivity—the low-energy all-purpose (LEAP) collimator. When acquiring SPECT images using different radiopharmaceuticals [for example, rest Tl-201 and poststress Tc-99m-sestamibi in the separate dual isotope protocol developed at our institution (17)], it is important to minimize intrinsic resolution differences by using the same collimator, and our preference is the LEHR. While the dual isotope approach was developed for perfusion imaging, we do believe it is also valid for gated SPECT imaging, and much of the published literature on gated Tl-201 SPECT is in fact based on the use of a LEHR collimator (13,14,18). Using a LEAP collimator in conjunction with gated Tl-201 SPECT imaging may be a viable approach for maximizing sensitivity with "Tl-201-only" protocols (19,20), especially if implemented on single-detector systems. Focusing collimators (21,22), which increase system sensitivity by mapping the myocardium to a larger portion of the detector, are still not widely used in clinical practice, due principally to compromise in perfusion image quality.

Gating

The gating of a SPECT acquisition is easily implemented using the QRS complex of the electrocardiographic (ECG) signal, since its principal peak (R wave) corresponds to end-diastole. The gating hardware interfaces with the acquisition computer controlling the gantry, and sorting of the data corresponding to each frame into the appropriate image matrix is automatically accomplished by the camera. In essence, data from each cardiac beat or "R–R interval" are sorted into 8 or 16 temporal bins, based on their time of occurrence relative to the R wave. The R–R interval duration can be modeled as being constant (fixed temporal resolution mode) or be dynamically adjusted to match the actual heart rhythm (variable temporal resolution mode), each approach having their own advantages and disadvantages (11).

Beat Length Acceptance Window

The usual variation of the cardiac beat length during gated acquisitions has led to building tolerances into the gating process. The beat length acceptance window aims at eliminating data from beats that are "too short" or "too long," while still accepting a sensible range of durations. For example, a beat length acceptance window of 20% allows accumulation of data from cardiac beats having a duration within ± 10% of the expected duration, while an acceptance window of 100%, somewhat counterintuitively, allows accumulation of data from beats of duration within ± 50% of the expected. This is *not* equivalent to accepting 100% of the beats, which is, instead, consistent with having a window of infinite width. Accepting data from all beats in a gated perfusion SPECT study makes sense in order not to compromise the perfusion SPECT data, which is derived by summing the various intervals of the gated study. This is not an issue if all rejected counts are automatically accumulated in an extra frame (a 9th frame in 8-frame gated SPECT imaging), and added back during generation of the "summed" perfusion SPECT study. In that case, summed perfusion SPECT data will be exactly the same as if it had been acquired as nongated perfusion SPECT. Our advice is to use as wide an acceptance window as possible if no extra frame is available to "save" rejected counts, or a 20 to 30% acceptance window if the extra frame feature is available. These issues are important so that the use of ECG gating with SPECT does not compromise the quality of the perfusion SPECT examination.

Image Reconstruction and Filtering

Gated SPECT images are reconstructed and reoriented similarly to nongated SPECT images, as described in Chapter 11. Prereconstruction low-pass filtering of gated projection images is more intense compared to nongated projection images, due to the lower statistical quality of the former. If a Butterworth filter is used (11), a general rule can be to use the same order but a 10 to 20% lower cutoff frequency for the gated projection filter, so as to achieve adequate "smoothing" and good signal-to-noise in the final gated short-axis images.

QUANTITATION

Gated SPECT parameters that can be quantitatively measured by gated SPECT techniques include global (left ventricular ejection fraction, end-diastolic and end-systolic volume) and regional (myocardial wall motion and thickening) measurements of function. The following is a review of published data on the accuracy and reproducibility of quantitative methods with regard to the measurement of global and regional cardiac function from gated SPECT.

Cedars-Sinai Method

The Cedars-Sinai Quantitative Gated SPECT (QGS) approach was originally described in an abstract by Moriel et al. (23) and a subsequent paper by Germano et al. (16). The software operates in the three-dimensional space and utilizes the gated short-axis datasets after stacking them together to form a three-dimensional image volume. The software's first step involves the automatic segmentation of the left ventricular (LV) myocardium, based on initial heuristic thresholding, binarization, and clusterification of the three-dimensional image, followed by iterative cluster refinement using pixel erosion and pixel growing. The iterative process is terminated when a mask consistent with the expected size, shape, and location of the LV is obtained. Once the LV has been isolated, its center of mass is automatically determined, and rays are drawn from it according to a spherical sampling model. The local maxima along all rays define a first estimate of the three-dimensional midmyocardial surface, which is then fitted to an ellipsoid. The best-fit ellipsoid defines a new sampling coordinate system, along which new rays are drawn and count profiles measured normally to the myocardium. These count profiles are fitted to asymmetric Gaussian curves. The Gaussians' maxima represent the final estimate of the midmyocardial surface, while the endocardial and epicardial surfaces are determined based on the Gaussians' standard deviations, and the valve plane is determined by fitting a plane to the most basal myocardial points. Endocardium, epicardium, and valve plane are calculated for each gating interval. LV cavity volumes are calculated by multiplying the individual voxel volume by the number of voxels contained in the three-dimensional space bound by the endocardium and the valve plane. The largest and the smallest LV cavity volumes correspond to end diastole and end systole, from which the ejection fraction is derived. The algorithm further measures regional motion as the excursion of the three-dimensional endocardial surface from end diastole to end systole, using a modification of the centerline method (24). Segmental thickening is calculated using both geometric (distance between epicardium and endocardium) and count considerations (apparent count increase from end diastole to end systole, due to the partial volume effect). Figure 1 shows three representative end-diastolic and end-systolic midventricular slices (short-axis, horizontal long-axis, and vertical long-axis) for a normal patient undergoing gated Tc-

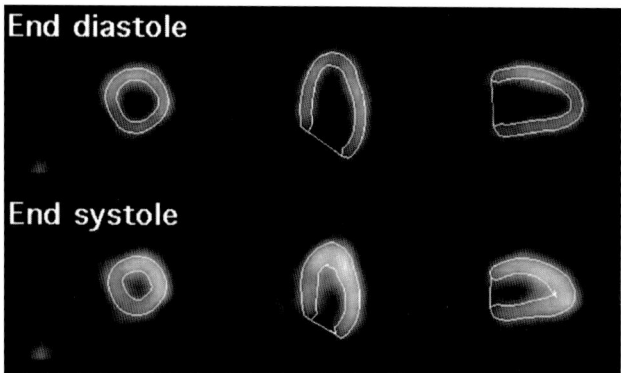

FIG. 1. Myocardial contours overlayed by Cedars-Sinai's quantitative gated SPECT algorithm onto three midventricular slices (short-axis, horizontal and vertical long-axis) for a normal patient, at end diastole and end systole.

99m-sestamibi SPECT, together with the overlayed, QGS-derived contours. Figure 2 shows the same slices and overlays for a gated Tc-99m-sestamibi patient with substantial perfusion defects, an enlarged left ventricle, and poor myocardial motion.

LVEFs measured by Cedars-Sinai's QGS have been validated by a number of independent institutions by comparison to a variety of gold standards: first pass (16,25), planar blood pool (23,26), two-dimensional echocardiography (20, 27–29), contrast ventriculography (30), three-dimensional echocardiography (19), magnetic resonance imaging (MRI) (31), and thermodilution (32). Published results include 496 patients and, overall, show very good correlation ($r = 0.86$) between QGS and gold standard measurements, quite inde-

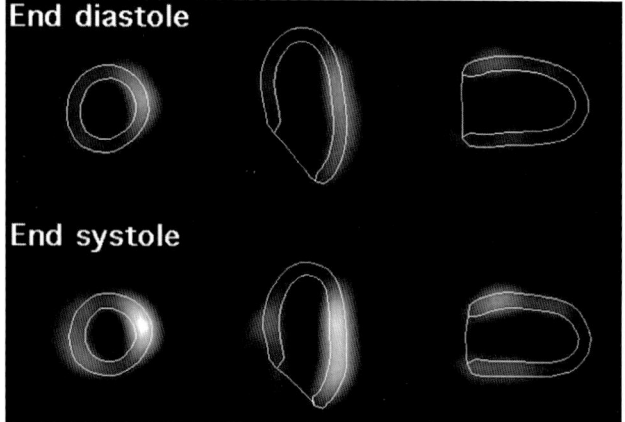

FIG. 2. Myocardial contours overlayed by Cedars-Sinai's quantitative gated SPECT algorithm QGS onto three midventricular slices (short-axis, horizontal and vertical long-axis) for a patient with left anterior descending coronary artery disease, at end diastole and end systole.

pendent of isotope (Tl-201, Tc-99m-sestamibi, and Tc-99m-tetrofosmin) or type of camera used. QGS's LVEF measurements are virtually perfectly reproducible when performed twice on the same patient data (because of QGS's automatic approach and extremely low failure rate), resulting in intraobserver and interobserver reproducibility of 1. They are also extremely reproducible when applied to separate studies acquired on the same patient population, as was verified in a group of 15 patients who underwent rest-gated SPECT on 2 consecutive days ($r = 0.99$) (33), as well as in a group of 180 patients who underwent two immediately consecutive gated SPECT acquisitions, one in the supine and the other in the prone position ($r = 0.93$) (34).

Validation of QGS-derived absolute end-systolic and end-diastolic volume measurements (ESV and EDV, respectively) has also been performed using a variety of gold standards, such as two-dimensional echocardiography (20, 27–29), three-dimensional echocardiography (19), magnetic resonance imaging (31), and thermodilution (32). Published results include 242 patients, and again show very good average correlation ($r = 0.84$ for EDV, $r = 0.88$ for ESV) between QGS and gold standard measurements, regardless of isotope or camera used. The interstudy reproducibility of QGS's volume measurements (again, intra- and interobserver reproducibility are essentially equal to 1) has also been assessed in a group of 926 patients who underwent consecutive SPECT acquisitions, the second of which gated with excellent correlation ($r = 0.99$). Regional quantitative measurements of myocardial wall motion and thickening by QGS have been validated, in 79 patients, by comparison to a semiquantitative visual standard based on a 20-segment, 6-point model (for motion—0 to 5, with 0 equal to normal and 5 equal to dyskinesia) or on a 5-point model (for thickening—0 to 4 with 0 equal to normal and 4 equal to absent), with very good correlation ($r = 0.97$ for motion, $r = 0.95$ for thickening) (35).

Figures 3 and 4 show the new QGS's result pages for the same normal and abnormal patients as in Figures 1 and 2. The left two columns display five ventricular images (three short-axis, two long-axis) at end diastole and end systole, while the rightmost portion contains the time-volume curve, various quantitative measurements and patient information. The center portion of the page contains four regional polar maps and two three-dimensional parametric images. The two regional perfusion polar maps refer to end-diastolic and end-systolic perfusion and are normalized to the maximum myocardial pixel count at end-diastole and end-systole, respectively. Absolute endocardial motion is polar-mapped following a linear model from 0 to 10 mm. Motion greater than 10 mm is displayed as if it were equal to 10 mm, while motion less than 0 mm (dyskinesia) is displayed as if it were equal to 0 mm. Polar mapping of thickening is relative and follows a linear model from 0 to 100% (with 0% indicating no thickening and 100% indicating doubling of the myocardial thickness from end diastole to end systole). Thickening

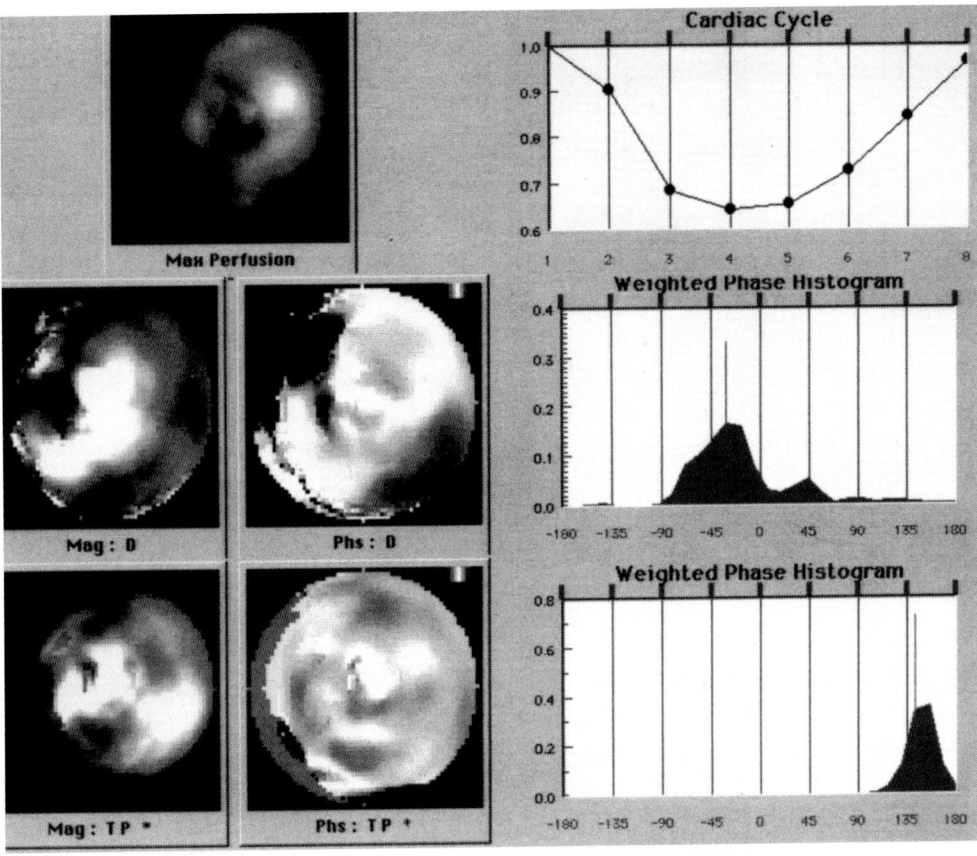

FIG. 8. Stanford method: polar maps representing end-diastolic perfusion (**upper left**), amplitude and phase of wall motion (**middle left**) and wall thickening (**bottom left**) in a patient. The time-volume curve from which the LVEF is derived (**upper right**) and two amplitude-weighted phase histograms (**middle** and **bottom right**) are also shown. (From ref. 39, with permission.)

mal studies. The initial probabilities or likelihoods that the various points belong to a myocardial surface are then iteratively revised using a relaxation labeling technique and the previously described constraints, the goal being to "label" points as "surface" or "not surface" and to assign to each sampling angle in each cardiac interval, the radius corresponding to the LV endocardium and epicardium. Since the iterative process is computationally intensive, and there is a possibility that it may not converge (44), the maximum number of iterations is set to 10. An indication of convergence is the fact that all points labeled as surface are "compatible" with their neighbors, compatibility being related to positive cross-correlation in space and time. Figure 9 shows an example of contours generated by the algorithm before and after relaxation labeling. Once the surface points for every cardiac frame have been determined, regional motion can be calculated as the absolute distance between an endocardial point and its position at end-systole, this distance being measured perpendicularly to the surface midway between the endocardium at end diastole and end systole (modified centerline method). In this approach, either perfusion or endocardial motion are usually mapped onto a three-dimensional parametric image, as shown in Figure 10 for a normal patient.

Endocardial and epicardial volumes measured using the model-based relaxation labeling method have been validated against an MRI standard (44) in 4 patients, with extremely good correlation ($r = 0.99$ and $SEE = 3.4$ mL, $r = 0.98$ and $SEE = 12.7$ mL, respectively). These volume measurements also have good intraobserver reproducibility (average absolute difference equals 0.67 mm) and interobserver reproduc-

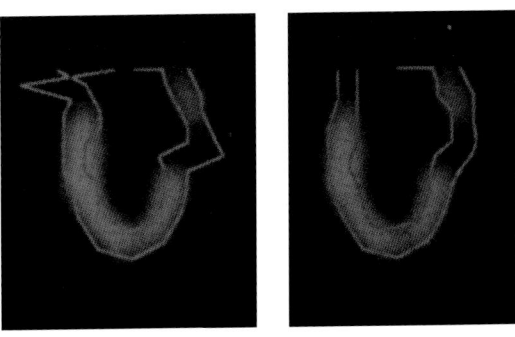

FIG. 9. Model-based relaxation labeling method: contours determined by the algorithm before (**left**) and after (**right**) relaxation labeling, in a midventricular long-axis image of a gated Tc-99m-sestamibi study. (From ref. 44, with permission.)

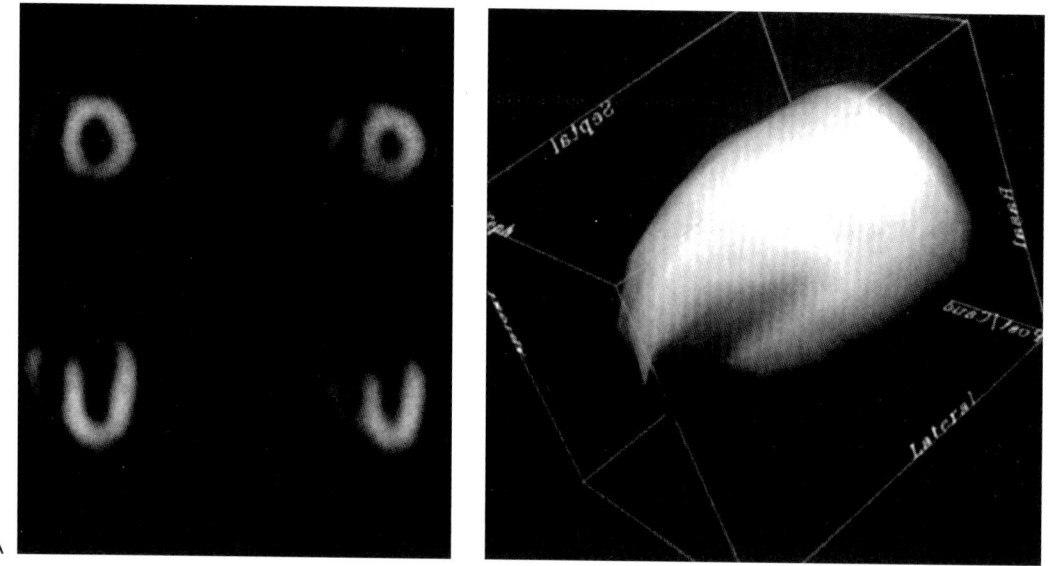

FIG. 10. Model-based relaxation labeling method: (**A**) end-diastolic (**left**) and end-systolic (**right**) mid-ventricular short-axis (**top**) and long-axis (**bottom**) images from a gated Tc-99m-sestamibi study; (**B**) endocardial motion coded onto the three-dimensional epicardial surface for the same study. (From ref. 42, with permission.)

ibility (average absolute difference equals 0.93 mm), as demonstrated in the same 4 patients, whose gated images were processed twice. Validation of regional motion measurements has been performed using the MRI standard in the same 4 patients, with average errors ranging from −2.53 ± 2.93 mm (in the basal septum) to 1.58 ± 2.91 mm (in the basal lateral region).

A variation of the model-based relaxation labeling has also been developed, which (i) estimates three-dimensional endocardial and epicardial surfaces based on count gradients, (ii) assigns binary weights to surface points based on region analysis and least square fitting, and (iii) aims at iteratively converging to the "true" myocardial surfaces (45). LVEFs, endocardial and epicardial volumes measured using this method have been validated against a contrast ventriculography standard (45) in 27 patients, with very good correlation ($r = 0.93$ for LVEF; $r = 0.95$ for EDV and ESV).

Partial Volume Methods

The University of Virginia method is based on partial volume effect that has been described in a paper by Smith et al. (46). The algorithm requires manual placement of search boundaries for the diastolic and systolic short-axis images, and is not based on endocardial/epicardial detection. Rather, it estimates relative myocardial thicknesses using the partial volume effect, then determines the global LVEF from the regional myocardial thickening values. The partial volume effect was initially described by Hoffman et al. (47) in regard to positron emission tomography (PET), pointing out the fact that, in nuclear medicine imaging, the average counts measured in a structure or organ are not only proportional to the amount of activity contained in that structure, but

also proportional to the size of the structure itself, this latter dependence being particularly strong for structures less than twice the "full width half maximum" (FWHM) resolution of the imaging system. The result of this phenomenon is that a "recovery coefficient curve" can be built that links the average counts contained in a region of interest (ROI) centered on various sections of the myocardium and the thickness of that section, as shown in Figure 11. Quantitation approaches like those by the University of Virginia, Cooke et al. (48) and Mochizuki et al. (18) assume a linear relationship between the increase in maximal counts in a myocardial segment from diastole to systole and the physical thickening of that segment in the same time interval. The LVEF can then be calculated by modeling the LV as an ellipsoid with constant myocardial volume and measuring an average "index of myocardial thickening" (46).

LVEFs measured using the University of Virginia method as applied to gated 99m-Tc sestamibi SPECT have been validated against a planar blood pool standard (49) in 23 patients with very good correlation ($r = 0.91$). These LVEF measurements also have very good intraobserver and interobserver reproducibility, as demonstrated in the same 23 patients whose gated images were processed twice ($r = 0.97$). No validation of regional thickening measurements has been reported, but those measurements enjoy very good intraobserver reproducibility ($r = 0.91$ in the same 23 patients).

A variation of the partial volume approach has been described in a paper by Buvat et al. (50) from the National Institutes of Health group. The algorithm uses the segmental count increase from diastole to systole as a proxy for wall thickening, but integrates it with a geometric estimate of the actual wall thickness at diastole and systole (hybrid method).

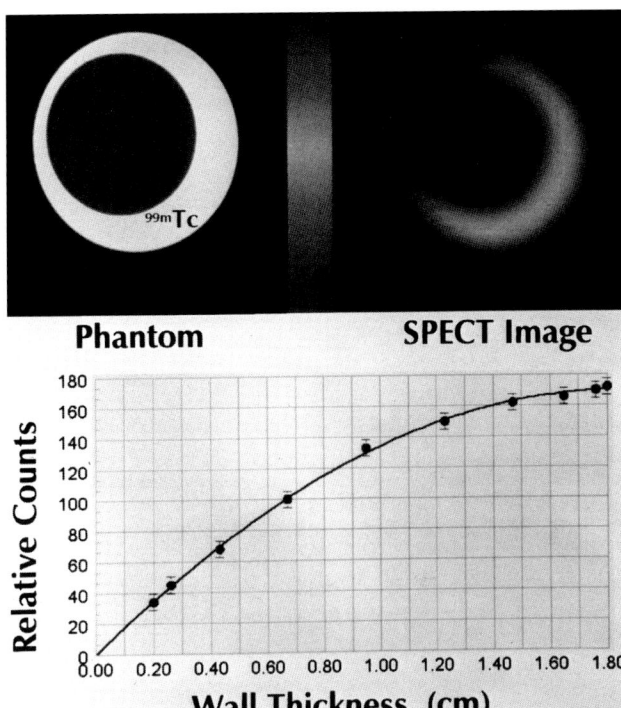

FIG. 11. Partial volume effect methods: (**top left**) section of an asymmetrical phantom containing a uniform concentration of Tc-99m, and (**top right**) transaxial SPECT image of the phantom obtained using a standard gamma camera: the thinner regions of the phantom appear to contain a lower concentration of activity. The relationship between "wall thickness" and corresponding maximum count value is shown in the graph, and has been previously referred to as the "recovery coefficient curve" (47). (From ref. 46, with permission.)

In brief, after manual selection of the LV cavity center in the end-diastolic frame, count profiles are computed across the myocardium in the short-axis images, each of which is divided into a number of sectors. The portion of each profile that falls within the profile's FWHM, rather than just the profile's maximum, is used in the count-based thickening calculation. Since, in most cases, the profile FWHM is not symmetric about the profile maximum (mainly due to "count spillover" in the LV cavity and extracardiac activity), the smaller of the two "half-FWHMs" is doubled for each profile. This "hybrid" approach (HYB) proved superior to the geometric approach alone (FWHM) and the maximal count-based approach alone (MAX) in 5 patients undergoing both a gated MRI and a gated 18F-FDG PET study, using receiver operating characteristic (ROC) curve analysis of semiquantitative visual thickening scores on a three-point scale (Fig. 12).

Image Inversion Method

The myocardial perfusion image inversion method has been described in a paper by Williams et al. (51). This approach's basic principle is that the activity in the perfused

walls of the myocardium is in contrast with the absence of activity in the LV cavity blood, and this contrast is preserved when the perfusion image is digitally inverted. Image inversion can be performed by first reformatting a gated SPECT volume into one horizontal and one vertical long-axis image per interval, each of which is the sum of the central region of the LV, preferably from endocardial edge to edge. The resulting images, containing the myocardium and the cavity in gated biplane fashion, are normalized to a maximum pixel value of 255, which typically occurs at end-systole. All frames are then subtracted from a mask image containing 255 counts per pixel. This will result in at least one myocardial pixel with a value of zero for each axis (again, usually occurring at end systole), with high counts in the LV chamber and low counts throughout the myocardium. In essence, with this technique, counts are produced within the LV chamber, and the change in these counts reflects the volumetric alterations occurring in the LV during systole (Fig. 13). If a master region of interest is manually placed around the LV chamber counts at end diastole, regions of interest can be automatically generated for each frame of the cardiac cycle using a center-of-mass, combination derivative-threshold border detection technique (Fig. 14). Tracking of the valve plane frequently requires additional operator intervention, since there is no contrast between the LV chamber, the valve plane, and the left atrial cavity. The ejection fraction is then calculated for each long-axis data set as the end-diastolic counts minus the end-systolic counts, divided by the end-diastolic counts. The biplane ejection fraction is the numerical average of the horizontal and vertical long-axis ejection fractions. This method of edge detection and ejection fraction determination is commonly employed for gated planar blood pool equilibrium analysis, except that no background correction is utilized here.

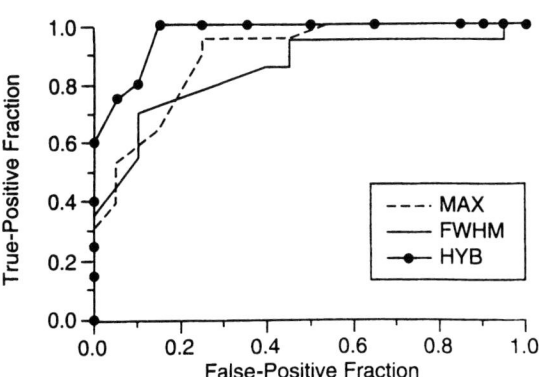

FIG. 12. National Institues of Health method: comparison of ROC curves reflecting a count-based (*MAX*), a geometric (*FWHM*), and a "hybrid" (*HYB*) approach in 40 data points from 5 patients undergoing gated MRI and gated 18F-FDG studies. The hybrid approach appeared to significantly improve sensitivity and specificity for the detection of wall thickening abnormalities. *FWHM*, full width, half maximum; *MAX*, maximal. (From ref. 50, with permission.)

Planar Projections   Transaxial Slices

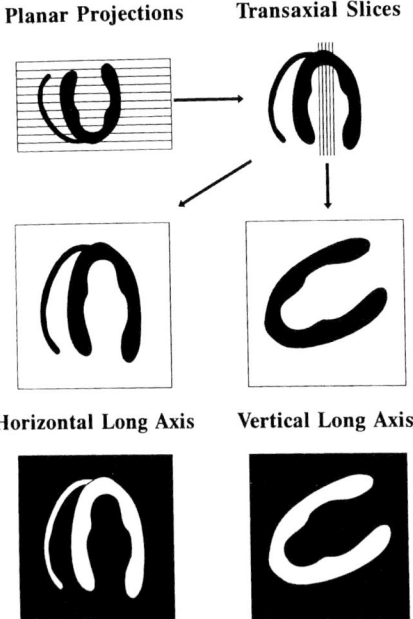

Horizontal Long Axis   Vertical Long Axis

Inverted Perfusion Images

FIG. 13. Image inversion method: horizontal and vertical transaxial images (**middle row**) from a perfusion SPECT study are normalized to a maximum pixel value of 255. Pixel-by-pixel subtraction of count values from 255 creates "inverted perfusion images" (**bottom row**), which can be considered pseudo-blood pool images and analyzed as such. (From ref. 51, with permission.)

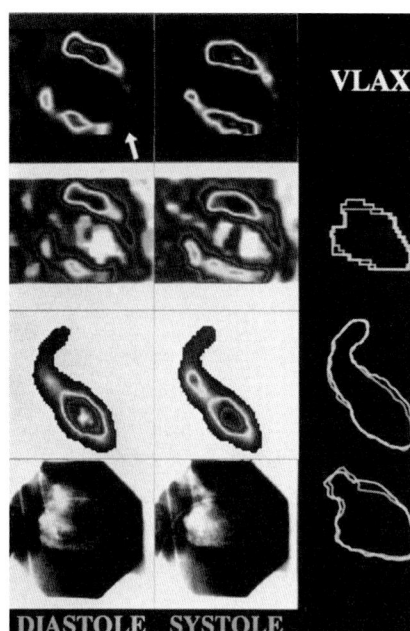

FIG. 14. Image inversion method: end-diastolic frames (**left column**), end-systolic frames (**middle column**), and quantitative measurements (**right column**) for (**A**) gated perfusion SPECT and (**B**) "inverted" gated perfusion SPECT vertical long axis (*VLAX*) images, (**C**) first pass images, and (**D**) contrast ventriculography images, in a patient with coronary artery disease and a LVEF = 16%. (From ref. 51, with permission.)

LVEFs measured using the image inversion method applied to gated Tc-99m sestamibi SPECT have been validated against a contrast ventriculography standard (51) in 54 patients, with very good correlation ($r = 0.90–0.93$), as well as against a first pass standard in 38 of those 54 patients ($r = 0.83$). These LVEF measurements also have very good intraobserver reproducibility ($r = 0.98–0.99$, *SEE* = 3.1%–3.6%) and interobserver reproducibility ($r = 0.93–0.95$, *SEE* = 6.1%–7.8%), as demonstrated in 14 patients whose gated images were processed twice.

Quantitation of Gated Blood Pool SPECT

Although gated blood pool SPECT (blood pool SPECT) imaging presents some advantages compared to gated perfusion SPECT (among them, the ability to assess both left and right ventricular function and the virtual absence of partial volume effects), algorithms for the quantitation of gated blood pool SPECT are not as widely diffused or validated as their gated perfusion SPECT counterparts. While this is obviously a reflection of the fact that cardiac perfusion studies outnumber blood pool studies by more than 10:1 and that blood pool imaging has been steadily losing out to echocardiography, some suggest that many more blood pool studies would be performed if accurate and reproducible quantitative blood pool SPECT algorithms were available to replace planar blood pool techniques (52).

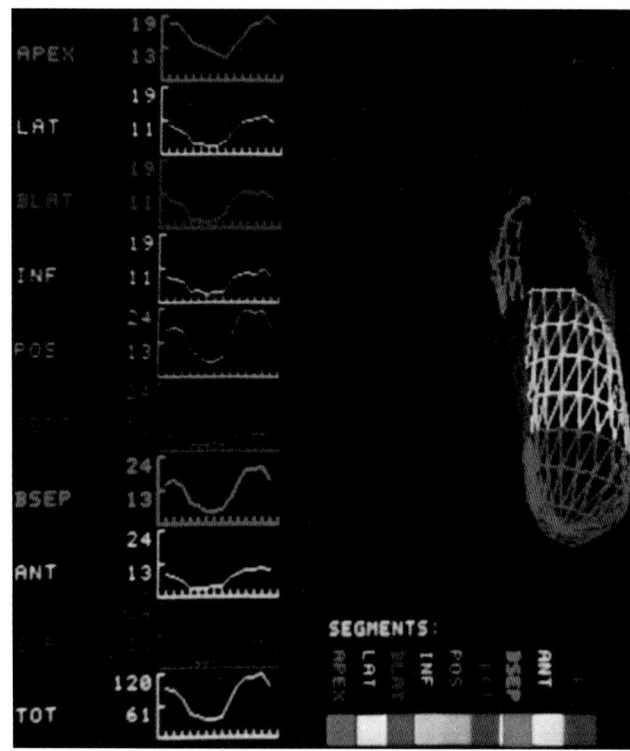

FIG. 15. Gated blood pool SPECT quantitation: color-coded three-dimensional LV wire mesh and time-volume curves corresponding to its different segmental regions, in a patient with 100% stenosis of the left anterior descending coronary artery. (From ref. 41, with permission.)

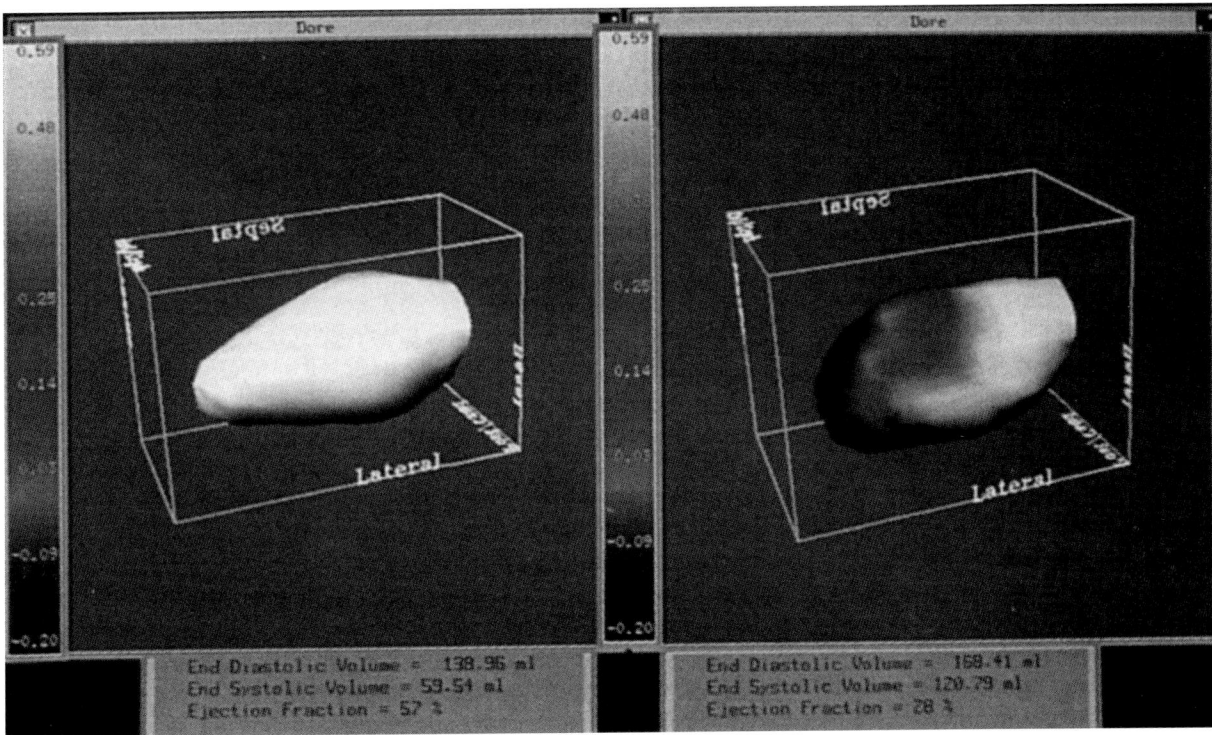

FIG. 16. Gated blood pool SPECT quantitation: endocardial motion coded onto the three-dimensional epicardial surfaces of (**left**) a healthy volunteer, and (**right**) a patient with a large apical anterior septal and lateral infarct. (From ref. 57, with permission.)

Parameters of cardiac function that can be measured by gated blood pool SPECT include endocardial wall motion, cavity volumes, and ejection fraction. Identification of the three-dimensional endocardial surface offers the opportunity to (i) assess motion from the difference in the endocardium's location at diastole and systole, and (ii) measure cavity volumes as the number of voxels encompassed by the endocardium and the valve plane, multiplied by the individual voxel's volume. While this approach to determining cavity volumes (and the related ejection fraction) is similar to that used in gated perfusion SPECT, the cavity diameter is generally larger than the myocardium's thickness, and, consequently, the accuracy of quantitative gated blood pool SPECT measurements is expected to be less compromised by partial volume effects (47). Endocardial surfaces can be estimated from operator-guided or semiautomatic thresholding (41), where the threshold has been reported to vary from 37% (53) to as much as 70% (54) of the peak ventricular counts. Alternatively, the maximum steepness of the count profiles (the point where the second derivative of each profile equals zero) can be used as a proxy for the location of the endocardial edge. This latter approach, initially proposed by Faber et al. (44), is the basis for the most widely used quantitative gated blood pool SPECT software today, and it is essentially the same as the model-based relaxation labeling method described above for gated perfusion SPECT. Regional wall motion is measured by creating a midsurface as the locus of the points equidistant from the location of the endocardial surface at end systole and end

diastole. The lengths of the segments perpendicular to the midsurface, and connecting the end-diastolic and end-systolic surfaces, are taken as a measure of regional wall motion (42) (Fig. 15). This data can also be coded onto the three-dimensional representation of the endocardium, for easier parametric assessment of regional function (Fig. 16).

Phase analysis has been used in the quantitative assessment of gated blood pool SPECT images (55), as an extension of pixel-by-pixel approaches common in planar blood pool imaging. Regional ejection fractions, too, have been proposed based on regional volumes obtained by connecting the vertexes of endocardial surface "patches" to the LV's long axis (41,56). A comprehensive review of the published range of quantitative gated blood pool SPECT approaches and their validation can be consulted for further information (57). As with gated perfusion SPECT, one should be aware that the two-dimensional gold standards used to validate gated blood pool SPECT measurements may, in some cases, be less accurate than the three-dimensional technique they seek to sanction (58).

CLINICAL VALUE OF GATED SPECT

Increasing Specificity

One of the principal applications of gated SPECT is in patients without known coronary artery disease. In this group, gating is useful in improving the specificity of SPECT imaging. Taillefer et al. (59) compared the sensitivity and specificity of thallium 201, nongated technetium 99m sestamibi, and gated technetium 99m sestamibi SPECT for detection of coronary artery disease in 115 women. A significant improvement in specificity was observed through the use of gated technetium sestamibi SPECT compared to thallium 201 SPECT, using criteria of 50% stenosis or 70% stenosis for significant coronary artery disease. No significant differences in sensitivity for detection of disease were noted. In a preliminary report from our laboratory, Erel et al. (60) compared the normalcy rate in 50 patients with a low likelihood of angiographically significant coronary artery disease. The overall normalcy rate rose from 78% with nongated technetium 99m sestamibi SPECT to 98% with gated SPECT. Thus, gated SPECT is frequently useful in determining whether nonreversible defects in regions of possible attenuation artifact (e.g., breast, diaphragm) are artifactual or real. This improvement in specificity, however, is largely limited to the situation where questionable nonreversible defects are found. When a questionable reversible defect is found, a normal motion pattern on gated SPECT would be consistent with either ischemia or artifact. In this circumstance, our group has found that a preferred manner for improving specificity is to combine supine and prone imaging with the technetium 99m-perfusion agents rather than to simply rely on gating (see Chapter 13).

Ejection Fraction for Risk Stratification

Gated SPECT allows the routine reporting of LVEF, still considered the single-most important measurement of cardiac performance and a parameter of major prognostic importance. This extra information may be useful in appropriate risk stratification of patients. For example, it is known that the prognosis of patients with depressed ventricular function and two- or three-vessel coronary artery disease improves with bypass surgery. By measuring LVEF from gated SPECT, it is now possible to add further to the risk stratification of patients provided by perfusion SPECT by determining whether depressed global ventricular function is present. However, whether the routine measurement of resting LVEF augments the prognostic power of myocardial perfusion SPECT has not yet been documented and is currently under study. Preliminary analysis of the first 1,032 patients from our laboratory undergoing a gated poststress myocardial perfusion SPECT has demonstrated that, in patients with abnormal myocardial perfusion scans, the rate of death or myocardial infarction is significantly higher in patients with ejection fractions less than 50% compared to those with poststress gated SPECT ejection fractions greater than 50% (61). In that same report, we documented that there was a significant increase in information provided by the addition of poststress ejection fraction information over the most powerful prognostic variable from nongated SPECT, the summed perfusion stress score. In a subsequent preliminary report, our group evaluated a larger population of 2,315

patients who were followed for more than 1 year for cardiac events (19.6 ± 4.8 months). In this study, left ventricular ejection fraction was found to be a superior predictor of cardiac death than the summed stress score by SPECT, but the summed stress score was a better predictor of nonfatal myocardial infarction and late clinical worsening. These preliminary studies provide promising data supporting the incremental prognostic value of the assessment of ejection fraction as well as myocardial perfusion on gated SPECT studies (62). We have also demonstrated that the gated SPECT results appear to be affecting catheterization referrals. In patients with small amounts of ischemia, those with ejection fractions greater than 50% were less commonly referred to catheterization compared to those with ejection fraction less than 50%. Similarly, in patients with moderate amounts of ischemia, patients with ejection fractions less than 50% had a high catheterization rate compared to patients with ejection fractions greater than 50% (63). Thus, the early information suggests that there is clinically useful incremental prognostic information gained from the use of gated SPECT over standard myocardial perfusion SPECT. In the first manuscript on this subject, Sharir et al. (67), studying 1,680 patients, demonstrated that poststress LVEF, as measured by gated SPECT, provided significant information over the extent and severity of perfusion defect as measured by the summed stress score. Another source of incremental value from gated SPECT is provided from assessment of the difference between resting ejection fraction and poststress ejection fraction (33). These authors noted that patients with reversible perfusion defects frequently had a lower left ventricular ejection fraction poststress than at rest, which the authors attributed to postischemic stunning. Sharir et al., from our institution, further evaluated this concept by determining the angiographic correlates of postexercise regional wall motion abnormalities detected by technetium-99m sestamibi gated SPECT in patients with normal resting myocardial perfusion SPECT (64). These investigators reported that postexercise wall motion abnormality had a 77% sensitivity and an 85% specificity for detection of a ≥90% stenosis. Sharir et al. further documented that the additional assessment of poststress wall motion abnormality allowed greater detection of severe and extensive coronary artery disease than was possible from nongated perfusion SPECT alone. These preliminary observations regarding the additional value of regional wall motion abnormalities suggest that this assessment may also be of prognostic value in the assessment of patients with coronary artery disease.

In the setting of recovery from acute myocardial infarction, Mahmarian et al. (65) demonstrated that there is incremental value in knowing the left ventricular ejection fraction as well as the extent of jeopardized myocardium as determined by equilibrium blood pool scintigraphy and adenosine thallium-201 myocardial perfusion SPECT. These parameters can now be obtained with a single poststress gated myocardial perfusion SPECT study.

Finally, with respect to risk stratification, it has been known in the cardiologic literature that absolute left ventricular volumes provide incremental information over ejection fraction. White et al. (66) have demonstrated that left ventricular end systolic volume is the major determinant of survival after myocardial infarction. In patients with mildly or severely reduced left ventricular ejection fraction, further information regarding survival was provided by knowledge of absolute end systolic volumes. Since, as noted, absolute volumes can now be accurately measured by gated myocardial perfusion SPECT, it is likely that the addition of absolute volume assessments to the assessment of myocardial perfusion and function by gated SPECT will provide incremental prognostic information. In this regard, Sharir and colleagues from our institution have shown, in the setting of suspected chronic coronary artery disease, that end systolic volume provided incremental information over ejection fraction in the prediction of cardiac death in patients undergoing gated myocardial perfusion SPECT (67).

Viability Assessment

In patients in whom the clinical question is myocardial viability, gated SPECT may also provide incremental information in addition to perfusion defect analysis. If left ventricular walls move, it can be assumed that they are viable. If gated SPECT indicates that the left ventricular wall associated with regions of moderate to severe nonreversible defects are still moving, these regions can be considered viable. If, however, walls with stress perfusion defects fail to move, further assessment may be needed to determine whether they may be hibernating.

COST-EFFECTIVENESS

More Information for Minimal Added Cost

Improvements in the processing rates of recent generations of nuclear medicine computer systems have markedly reduced the overall processing time of gated SPECT studies. Furthermore, algorithms that automatically perform filtering, reconstruction, and reorientation of the gated SPECT data can reduce or eliminate the need for manual intervention, allowing batch processing of several gated studies, and thereby effectively decreasing the time for generation of the final images while improving the reproducibility of the results (68). Time needed for the interpretation of the gated SPECT data can be reduced and accuracy of interpretation enhanced by software that automatically calculates the endocardial and epicardial surfaces from the data in each gating interval, displays these surfaces in cinematic mode as contours overlaid on the images in the two-dimensional or three-dimensional space, and derives global ejection fraction values from the end systolic and end diastolic intervals (16). With these hardware and software improvements, the extra information provided by gated SPECT can be provided for modest added cost.

Potential for Reducing Costs with a Stress-only Protocol

Gating may even reduce the costs of SPECT imaging by making stress-only procedures feasible in some patients. Gated SPECT can effectively provide an assessment of defect reversibility from the stress study alone, based on whether the myocardium in a perfusion defect zone contracts or thickens (69), assuming that the defect is real and not an attenuation artifact. The implementation of successful attenuation correction programs with gated SPECT imaging should allow the stress gated SPECT study to be assessed for perfusion defect presence and type.

In short, if a defect is present (and can be assumed to be real because of attenuation correction) and if the defect area contracts on gated SPECT, the defect can be considered to be reversible. In this scenario, (that is, gated SPECT with attenuation correction), only patients with stress defect areas that do not contract would need to return for resting perfusion measurements.

Reducing Unnecessary Catheterization

Another area in which gated SPECT imaging may have an impact on costs is in reducing unnecessary catheterization associated with false/positive (nongated) SPECT studies. Increasing the specificity of SPECT leads to more effective risk stratification than is achieved by myocardial perfusion SPECT alone, as suggested by the preliminary work of Lewin et al. (70).

REFERENCES

1. Shah PK, Pichler M, Berman DS, et al. Left ventricular ejection fraction determined by radionuclide ventriculography in early stages of first transmural myocardial infarction. Relation to short-term prognosis. *Am J Cardiol* 1980;45(3):542–546.
2. European Coronary Surgery Study Group. Long-term results of prospective randomised study of coronary artery bypass surgery in stable angina pectoris. *Lancet* 1982;2(8309):1173–1180.
3. Lee KL, Pryor DB, Pieper KS, et al. Prognostic value of radionuclide angiography in medically treated patients with coronary artery disease. A comparison with clinical and catheterization variables. *Circulation* 1990;82(5):1705–1717.
4. Risk stratification and survival after myocardial infarction. *N Engl J Med* 1983;309(6):331–336.
5. Katz A, Force T, Folland E, et al. Echocardiographic assessment of ventricular systolic function. In: Marcus ML, Braunwald E, eds. *Marcus cardiac imaging: a companion to Braunwald's Heart disease.* Philadelphia: WB Saunders, 1996:297–324.
6. Sheehan F. Principles and practice of contrast ventriculography. In: Marcus ML, Braunwald E, eds. *Marcus cardiac imaging: a companion to Braunwald's heart disease.* Philadelphia: WB Saunders, 1996:164–187.
7. Strauss HW, Zaret BL, Hurley PJ, et al. A scintiphotographic method for measuring left ventricular ejection fraction in man without cardiac catheterization. *Am J Cardiol* 1971;28(5):575–580.
8. DePuey E. Evaluation of cardiac function with radionuclides. In: Gottschalk A, ed. *Diagnostic nuclear medicine.* Baltimore: Williams & Wilkins, 1988:355–398.
9. Port S. First-pass radionuclide angiography. In: Marcus ML, Braunwald E, eds. *Marcus cardiac imaging: a companion to Braunwald's heart disease.* Philadelphia: WB Saunders, 1996:923–941.

10. Garcia EV, Van Train K, Maddahi J, et al. Quantification of rotational thallium-201 myocardial tomography. *J Nucl Med* 1985;26(1):17–26.

11. Germano G, Van Train K, Kiat H, et al. Digital techniques for the acquisition, processing, and analysis of nuclear cardiology images. In: Sandler MP, ed. *Diagnostic nuclear medicine.* Baltimore: Williams & Wilkins, 1995:347–386.

12. Germano G, Berman DS, eds. *Clinical gated cardiac SPECT.* Armonk, NY: Futura Publishing, 1999.

13. Germano G, Erel J, Kiat H, et al. Quantitative LVEF and qualitative regional function from gated thallium-201 perfusion SPECT. *J Nucl Med* 1997;38(5):749–754.

14. Maunoury C, Chen CC, Chua KB, et al. Quantification of left ventricular function with thallium-201 and technetium-99m-sestamibi myocardial gated SPECT. *J Nucl Med* 1997;38(6):958–961.

15. DePuey EG, Nichols KJ, Slowikowski JS, et al. Fast stress and rest acquisitions for technetium-99m-sestamibi separate-day SPECT. *J Nucl Med* 1995;36(4):569–574.

16. Germano G, Kiat H, Kavanagh PB, et al. Automatic quantification of ejection fraction from gated myocardial perfusion SPECT. *J Nucl Med* 1995;36(11):2138–2147.

17. Berman DS, Kiat H, Friedman JD, et al. Separate acquisition rest thallium-201/stress technetium-99m sestamibi dual-isotope myocardial perfusion single-photon emission computed tomography: a clinical validation study. *J Am Coll Cardiol* 1993;22(5):1455–1464.

18. Mochizuki T, Murase K, Fujiwara Y, et al. Assessment of systolic thickening with thallium-201 ECG-gated single-photon emission computed tomography: a parameter for local left ventricular function. *J Nucl Med* 1991;32(8):1496–1500.

19. Akinboboye O, El-Khoury Coffin L, Sciacca R, et al. Accuracy of gated SPECT thallium left ventricular volumes and ejection fractions: comparison with three-dimensional echocardiography. *J Am Coll Cardiol* 1998;31(2)[Suppl A]:85A(abst).

20. Bateman T, Magalski A, Barnhart C, et al. Global left ventricular function assessment using gated SPECT-201: comparison with echocardiography. *J Am Coll Cardiol* 1998;31(2)[Suppl A]:441A(abst).

21. Everaert H, Vanhove C, Hamill JJ, et al. Cardiofocal collimators for gated single-photon emission tomographic myocardial perfusion imaging. *Eur J Nucl Med* 1998;25(1):3–7.

22. Everaert H, Vanhove C, Franken P. Gated SPECT myocardial perfusion acquisition within 5 minutes using focussing collimators and a three-head gamma camera. *Eur J Nucl Med* 1998;25(6):587–593.

23. Moriel M, Germano G, Kiat H, et al. Automatic measurement of left ventricular ejection fraction by gated SPECT Tc-99m sestamibi: a comparison with radionuclide ventriculography. *Circulation* 1993;88(4):I-486(abst).

24. Sheehan FH, Dodge HT, Mathey D, et al. Application of the centerline method: analysis of change in regional left ventricular wall motion in serial studies. In: *Computers in cardiology.* Ninth Meeting of Computers in Cardiology. Seattle, WA: IEEE Computer Society Press, 1983.

25. He Z, Mahmarian J, Preslar J, et al. Correlations of left ventricular ejection fractions determined by gated SPECT with thallium and sestamibi and by first-pass radionuclide angiography. *J Nucl Med* 1997;38(5):27P(abst).

26. Everaert H, Bossuyt A, Franken PR. Left ventricular ejection fraction and volumes from gated single photon emission tomographic myocardial perfusion images: comparison between two algorithms working in three-dimensional space. *J Nucl Cardiol* 1997;4(6):472–476.

27. Zanger D, Bhatnagar A, Hausner E, et al. Automated calculation of ejection fraction from gated Tc-99m sestamibi images—comparison to quantitative echocardiography. *J Nucl Cardiol* 1997;4(1)[Prt 2]:S78(abst).

28. Cwajg E, Cwajg J, He Z, et al. Comparison between gated-SPECT and echocardiography for the analysis of global and regional left ventricular function and volumes. *J Am Coll Cardiol* 1998;31(2)[Suppl A]:440A–441A(abst).

29. Mathew D, Zabrodina Y, Mannting F. Volumetric and functional analysis of left ventricle by gated SPECT: a comparison with echocardiographic measurements. *J Am Coll Cardiol* 1998;31(2)[Suppl A]:44A(abst).

30. Di Leo C, Bestetti A, Tagliabue L, et al. Tc-99m-tetrofosmin gated-SPECT LVEF: correlation with echocardiography and contrastographic ventriculography. *J Nucl Cardiol* 1997;4(1)[Prt 2]:S56.

31. He Z, Vick G, Vaduganathan P, et al. Comparison of left ventricular volumes and ejection fraction measured by gated SPECT and by cine magnetic resonance imaging. *J Am Coll Cardiol* 1998;31(2)[Suppl A]:44A(abst).

32. Germano G, Vandecker W, Mintz R, et al. Validation of left ventricular volumes automatically measured with gated myocardial perfusion SPECT. *J Am Coll Cardiol* 1998;31(2)[Suppl A]:43A(abst).

33. Johnson LL, Verdesca SA, Aude WY, et al. Postischemic stunning can affect left ventricular ejection fraction and regional wall motion on post-stress gated sestamibi tomograms. *J Am Coll Cardiol* 1997;30(7):1641–1648.

34. Berman D, Germano G, Lewin H, et al. Comparison of post-stress ejection fraction and relative left ventricular volumes by automatic analysis of gated myocardial perfusion single-photon emission computed tomography acquired in the supine and prone positions. *J Nucl Cardiol* 1998;5(1):40–47.

35. Germano G. Study of cardiac function with PET or SPECT. In: van der Wall EE, Blanksma PK, Niemeyer MG, et al., eds. *Advanced imaging in coronary artery disease.* Dordrecht, The Netherlands: Kluwer Academic Publishers, 1998:273–287.

36. DePuey EG, Nichols K, Dobrinsky C. Left ventricular ejection fraction assessed from gated technetium-99m-sestamibi SPECT. *J Nucl Med* 1993;34(11):1871–1876.

37. Nichols K, DePuey EG, Rozanski A. Automation of gated tomographic left ventricular ejection fraction. *J Nucl Cardiol* 1996;3(6)[Prt 1]:475–482.

38. Nichols K, DePuey EG, Rozanski A, et al. Image enhancement of severely hypoperfused myocardia for computation of tomographic ejection fraction. *J Nucl Med* 1997;38(9):1411–1417.

39. Goris ML, Thompson C, Malone LJ, et al. Modelling the integration of myocardial regional perfusion and function. *Nucl Med Commun* 1994;15(1):9–20.

40. Everaert H, Franken PR, Flamen P, et al. Left ventricular ejection fraction from gated SPET myocardial perfusion studies: a method based on the radial distribution of count rate density across the myocardial wall. *Eur J Nucl Med* 1996;23(12):1628–1633.

41. Faber TL, Stokely EM, Templeton GH, et al. Quantification of three-dimensional left ventricular segmental wall motion and volumes from gated tomographic radionuclide ventriculograms. *J Nucl Med* 1989;30(5):638–649.

42. Faber TL, Akers MS, Peshock RM, et al. Three-dimensional motion and perfusion quantification in gated single-photon emission computed tomograms. *J Nucl Med* 1991;32(12):2311–2317.

43. Faber TL, McColl RW, Opperman RM, et al. Spatial and temporal registration of cardiac SPECT and MR images: methods and evaluation. *Radiology* 1991;179(3):857–861.

44. Faber TL, Stokely EM, Peshock RM, et al. A model-based four-dimensional left ventricular surface detector. *IEEE Trans Med Imaging* 1991;10(3):321–329.

45. Adiseshan P, Corbett J. Quantification of left ventricular function from gated tomographic perfusion imaging: development and testing of a new algorithm. *Circulation* 1994;90(4):I-365(abst).

46. Smith WH, Kastner RJ, Calnon DA, et al. Quantitative gated single photon emission computed tomography imaging: a counts-based method for display and measurement of regional and global ventricular systolic function. *J Nucl Cardiol* 1997;4(6):451–463.

47. Hoffman EJ, Huang SC, Phelps ME. Quantitation in positron emission computed tomography: 1. Effect of object size. *J Comput Assist Tomogr* 1979;3(3):299–308.

48. Cooke CD, Garcia EV, Cullom SJ, et al. Determining the accuracy of calculating systolic wall thickening using a fast Fourier transform approximation: a simulation study based on canine and patient data. *J Nucl Med* 1994;35(7):1185–1192.

49. Calnon DA, Kastner RJ, Smith WH, et al. Validation of a new counts-based gated single photon emission computed tomography method for quantifying left ventricular systolic function: comparison with equilibrium radionuclide angiography. *J Nucl Cardiol* 1997;4(6):464–471.

50. Buvat I, Bartlett ML, Kitsiou AN, et al. A ''hybrid'' method for measuring myocardial wall thickening from gated PET/SPECT images. *J Nucl Med* 1997;38(2):324–329.

51. Williams KA, Taillon LA. Left ventricular function in patients with coronary artery disease assessed by gated tomographic myocardial perfusion images. Comparison with assessment by contrast ventriculography and first-pass radionuclide angiography. *J Am Coll Cardiol* 1996;27(1):173–181.

52. Corbett JR. Tomographic radionuclide ventriculography: opportunity ignored? [editorial; comment]. *J Nucl Cardiol* 1994;1(6):567–570.

53. Gill JB, Moore RH, Tamaki N, et al. Multigated blood-pool tomography: new method for the assessment of left ventricular function. *J Nucl Med* 1986;27(12):1916–1924.

54. Yamashita K, Tanaka M, Asada N, et al. A new method of three dimensional analysis of left ventricular wall motion. *Eur J Nucl Med* 1988; 14(3):113–119.

55. Graf G, Mester J, Clausen M, et al. Reconstruction of Fourier coefficients: a fast method to get polar amplitude and phase images of gated SPECT. *J Nucl Med* 1990;31(11):1856–1861.

56. Cerqueira MD, Harp GD, Ritchie JL. Quantitative gated blood pool tomographic assessment of regional ejection fraction: definition of normal limits. *J Am Coll Cardiol* 1992;20(4):934–941.

57. Corbett J. Gated blood-pool SPECT. In: DePuey EG, Berman DS, Garcia EV, eds. *Cardiac SPECT imaging.* New York: Raven Press, 1995:257–273.

58. Bartlett ML, Srinivasan G, Barker WC, et al. Left ventricular ejection fraction: comparison of results from planar and SPECT gated bloodpool studies. *J Nucl Med* 1996;37(11):1795–1799.

59. Taillefer R, DePuey EG, Udelson JE, et al. Comparative diagnostic accuracy of Tl-201 and Tc-99m sestamibi SPECT imaging (perfusion and ECG-gated SPECT) in detecting coronary artery disease in women. *J Am Coll Cardiol* 1997;29(1):69–77.

60. Erel J, Kiat H, Friedman JD, et al. The added diagnostic value of gating to exercise Tc-99m sestamibi SPECT for detection of coronary artery disease (abs). In: *Journal of Nuclear Medicine.* Proceedings of the 43rd Annual Meeting, Society of Nuclear Medicine, Denver, CO, 1996.

61. Hachamovitch R, Berman DS, Shaw LJ, et al. Incremental prognostic value of myocardial perfusion single photon emission computed tomography for the prediction of cardiac death: differential stratification for risk of cardiac death and myocardial infarction. *Circulation* 1998;97(6): 535–543.

62. Hachamovitch R, Berman D, Lewin H, et al. Relative prognostic value of post-stress left ventricular ejection fraction and stress myocardial perfusion for prediction of outcomes. *Circulation* 1998;98(17):I-654(abst).

63. Lewin H, Hachamovitch R, Germano G, et al. The impact of gated SPECT on the rate of early referral to catheterization following myocardial perfusion SPECT. *J Nucl Med* 1998;39(5):87P(abst).

64. Sharir T, Bacher-Stier C, Dhar S, et al. Post exercise regional wall motion abnormalities detected by Tc-99m sestamibi gated SPECT: a marker of severe coronary artery disease. *J Nucl Med* 1998;39(5): 87P–88P(abst).

65. Mahmarian JJ, Mahmarian AC, Marks GF, et al. Role of adenosine thallium-201 tomography for defining long-term risk in patients after acute myocardial infarction. *J Am Coll Cardiol* 1995;25(6):1333–1340.

66. White HD, Norris RM, Brown MA, et al. Left ventricular end-systolic volume as the major determinant of survival after recovery from myocardial infarction. *Circulation* 1987;76(1):44–51.

67. Sharir T, Germano G, Kavanagh P, et al. Incremental prognostic value of post-stress left ventricular ejection fraction and volume by gated myocardial perfusion single photon emission computed tomography. *Circulation* 1999;100:1035–1042.

68. Germano G, Kavanagh PB, Su HT, et al. Automatic reorientation of three-dimensional, transaxial myocardial perfusion SPECT images [comments]. *J Nucl Med* 1995;36(6):1107–1114.

69. Chua T, Kiat H, Germano G, et al. Gated technetium-99m sestamibi for simultaneous assessment of stress myocardial perfusion, postexercise regional ventricular function and myocardial viability. Correlation with echocardiography and rest thallium-201 scintigraphy. *J Am Coll Cardiol* 1994;23(5):1107–1114.

70. Lewin H, Hachamovitch R, Germano G, et al. The impact of gated SPECT on the rate of early referral to catheterization following myocardial perfusion SPECT. *J Nucl Med* 1998;39(5):87P(abst).

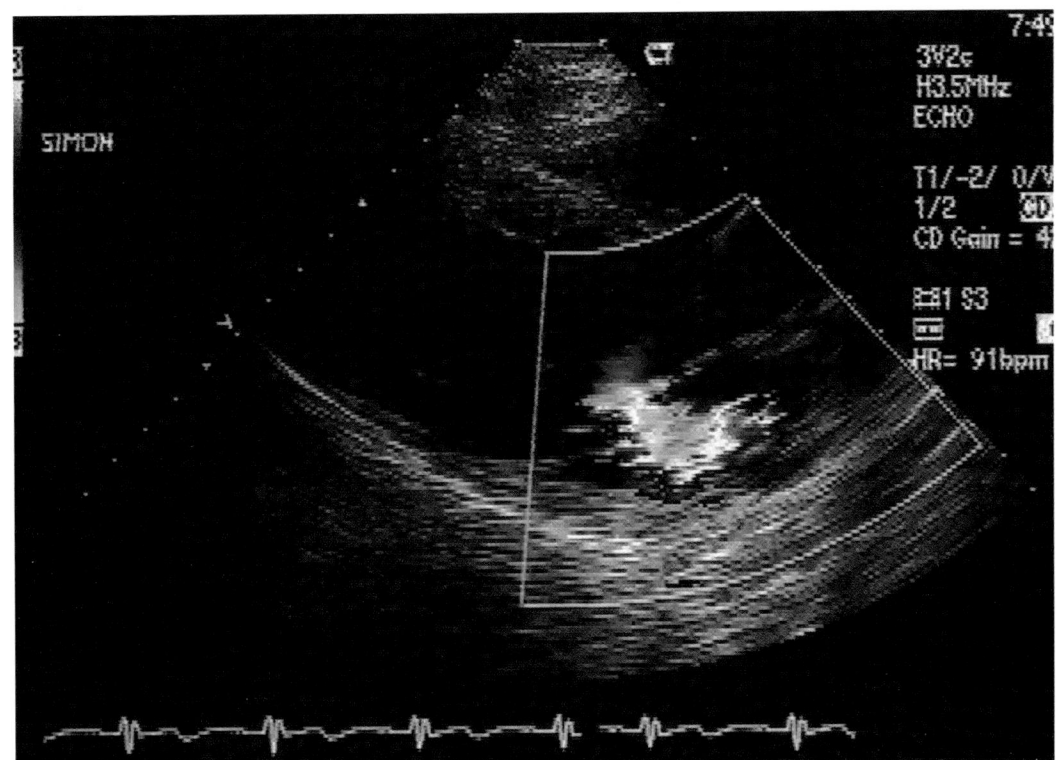

COLOR PLATE 1. Color flow Doppler of mitral regurgitation.

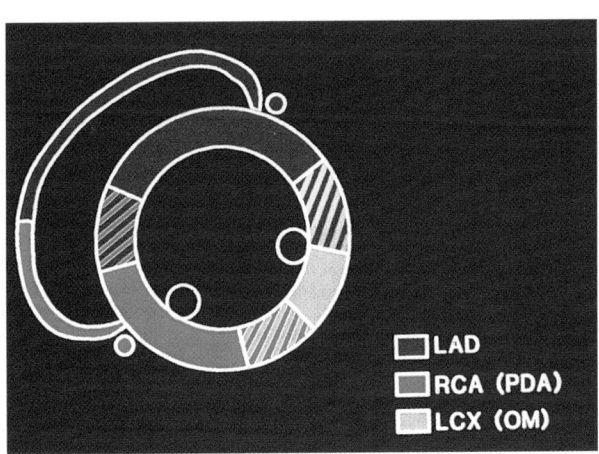

COLOR PLATE 2. Wall segments at papillary muscle level and expected coronary distribution. The crosshatched areas in this and subsequent five figures represent overlapping perfusion territories. *LAD*, left anterior descending artery; *LCX*, left circumflex; *OM*, obtuse marginal; *PDA*, posterior descending artery; *RCA*, right coronary artery.

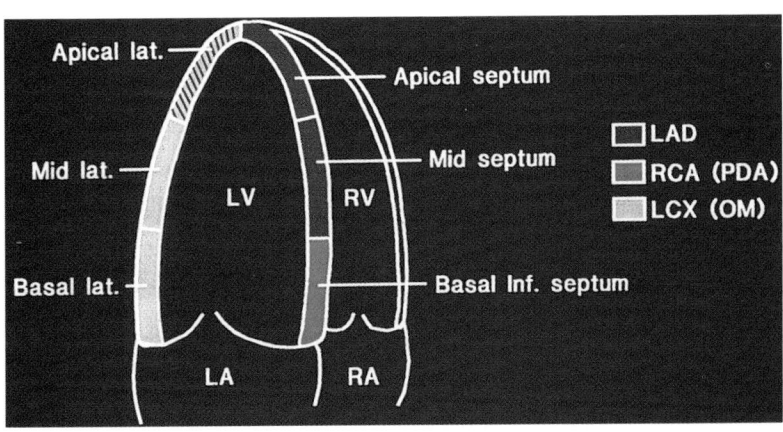

COLOR PLATE 3. Four-chamber view with left ventricle and atrium positioned to the viewer's left, showing coronary distribution. *LA*, left atrium; *LAD*, left anterior descending artery; *LCX*, left circumflex; *LV*, left ventricle; *OM*, obtuse marginal; *PDA*, posterior descending artery; *RA*, right atrium; *RCA*, right coronary artery.

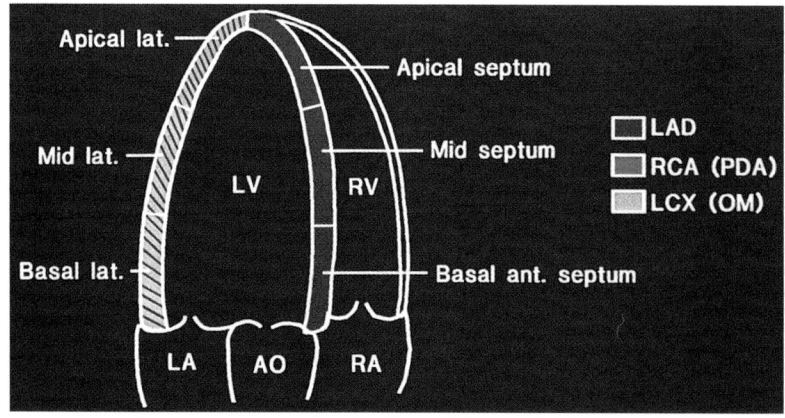

COLOR PLATE 4. Five-chamber view with anterior angulation of the transducer. *AO*, aorta; *LA*, left atrium; *LAD*, left anterior descending artery; *LCX*, left circumflex; *LV*, left ventricle; *OM*, obtuse marginal; *PDA*, posterior descending artery; *RA*, right atrium; *RCA*, right coronary artery.

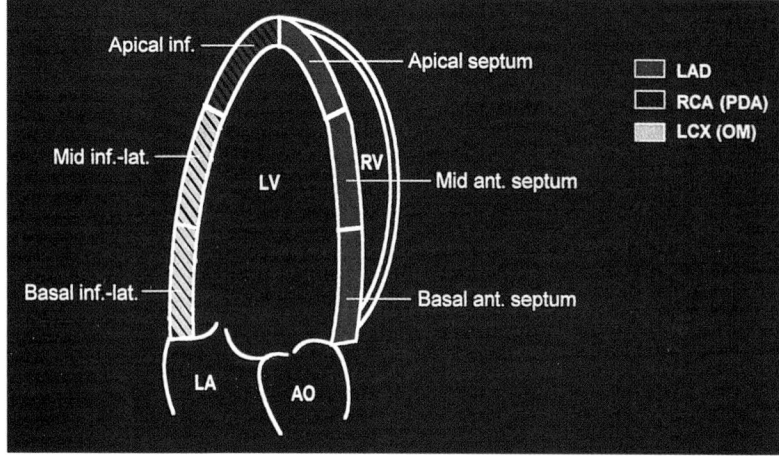

COLOR PLATE 5. Long-axis view with wall segments and coronary distribution. This view will have a similar cross section of segments, whether obtained from parasternal window or the apex. *LA*, left atrium; *LAD*, left anterior descending artery; *LCX*, left circumflex; *LV*, left ventricle; *OM*, obtuse marginal; *PDA*, posterior descending artery; *RCA*, right coronary artery.

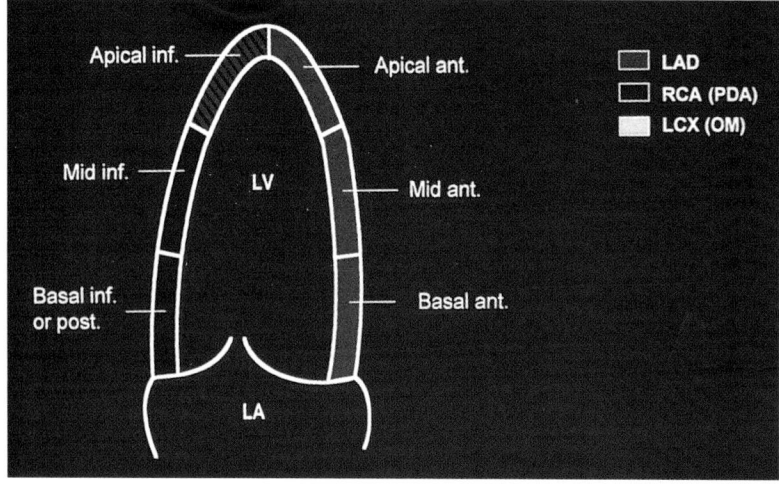

COLOR PLATE 6. Two-chamber view with wall segments and coronary distribution. *LA*, left atrium; *LAD*, left anterior descending artery; *LCX*, left circumflex; *LV*, left ventricle; *OM*, obtuse marginal; *PDA*, posterior descending artery; *RCA*, right coronary artery.

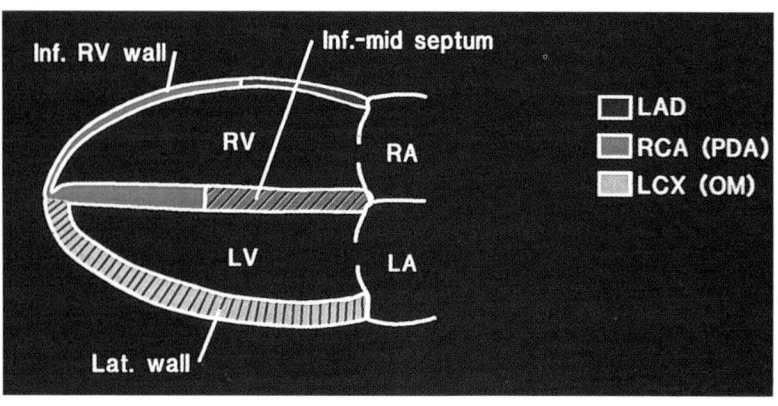

COLOR PLATE 7. Subcostal four-chamber view with appropriate coronary distribution. This view is frequently useful for assessment of right ventricular ischemic dysfunction. *LA*, left atrium; *LAD*, left anterior descending artery; *LCX*, left circumflex; *LV*, left ventricle; *OM*, obtuse marginal; *PDA*, posterior descending artery; *RA*, right atrium; *RCA*, right coronary artery.

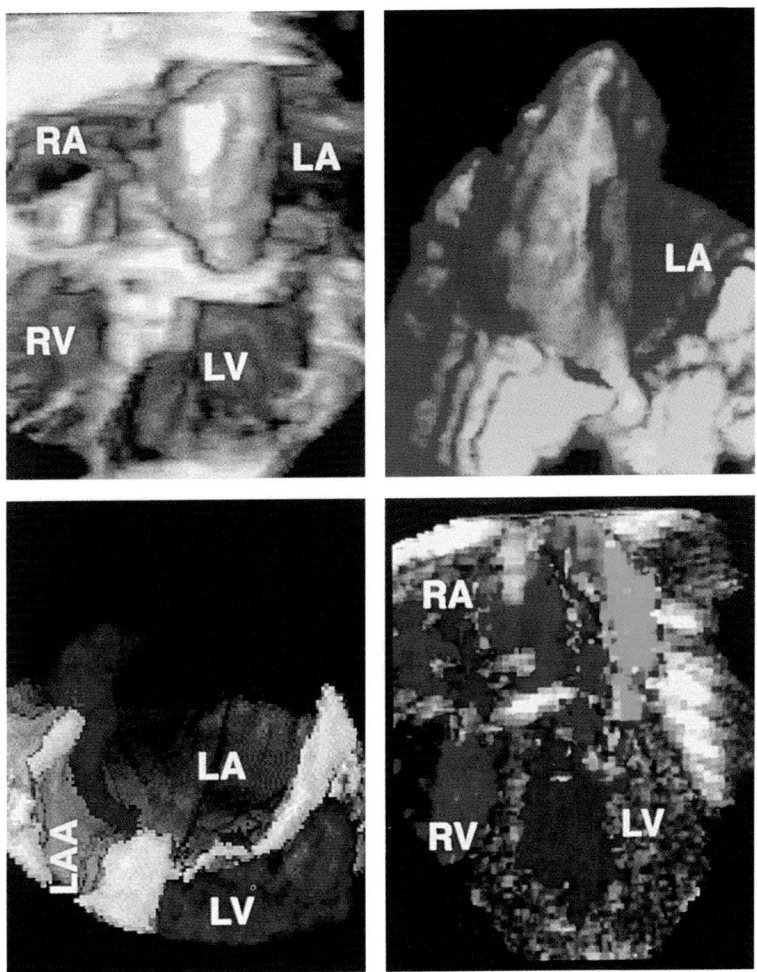

COLOR PLATE 8. Images demonstrating various display formats of three-dimensional color Doppler data obtained in patients with mitral regurgitation. Images acquired with video signals can be transferred into gray-scale images (**upper left**). The gray-scale images can also be encoded with pseudo-colors depending on their video intensity (**upper right**). Video signals of color Doppler images transferred and digitized can be used to reconstruct three-dimensional images in gray-scale (for cardiac tissue) and red or blue (for flow jets) colors. Images in different colors can be displayed simultaneously or individually. In this example (**lower left**), the blue flow signals were discarded to highlight the mitral regurgitation jet in red. Three-dimensional color Doppler flow reconstruction from digital data retains all the original color in the image (**lower right**). *RA*, right atrium; *LA*, left atrium; *RV*, right ventricle; *LV*, left ventricle; *LAA*, left atrial appendage.

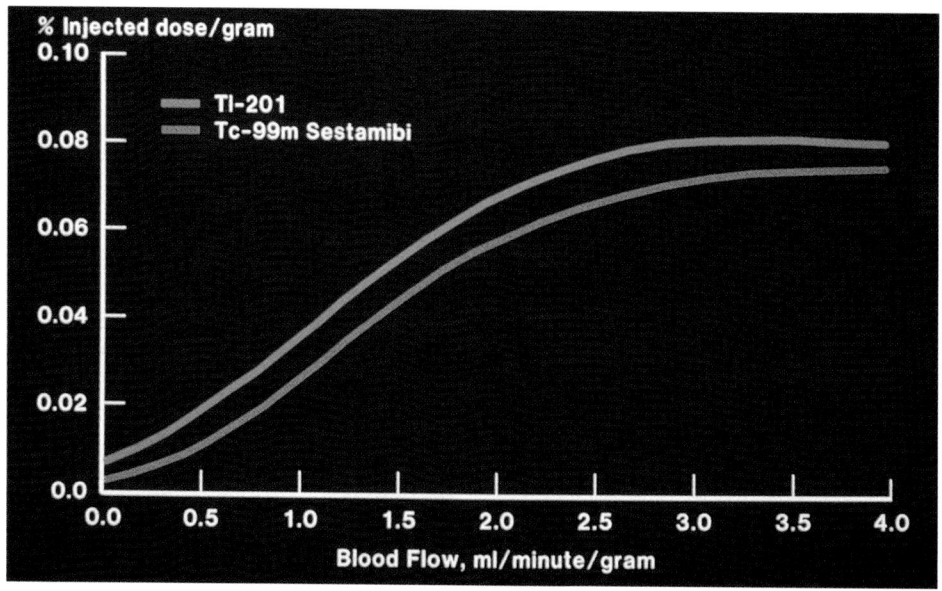

COLOR PLATE 9. Relationship between blood flow and percent injected dose per gram for Tl-201 and Tc-99m sestamibi. (Courtesy of DuPont Medical Imaging, Billerica, Massachusetts.)

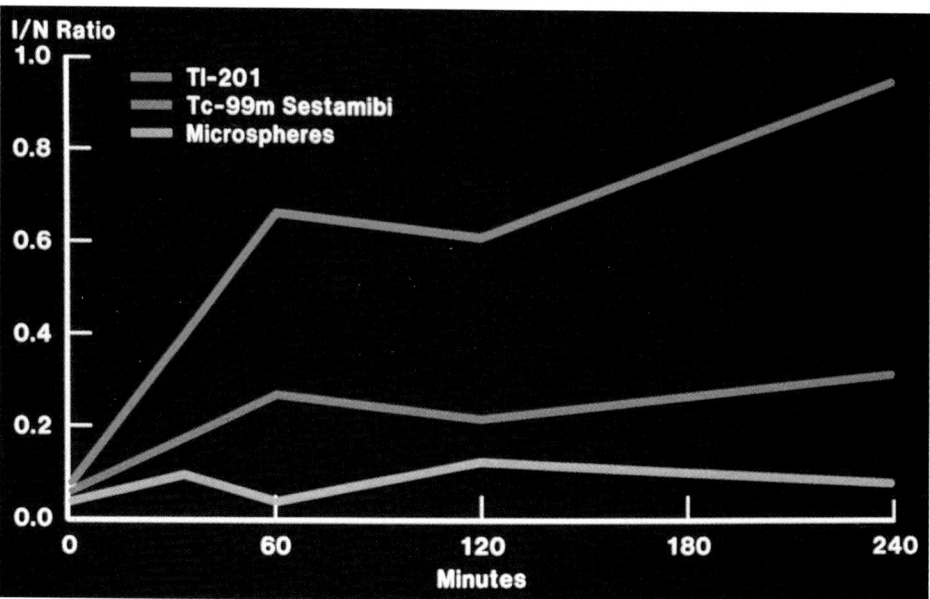

COLOR PLATE 10. Redistribution characteristics of Tl-201, Tc-99m sestamibi, and microspheres. The ischemic/normal zone (*I/N*) ratio for the three tracers was measured in a swine model following injection (intravenous for Tl-201 and Tc-99m sestamibi, left atrial for microspheres) during a 10-minute coronary occlusion followed by 4 hours of reflow. (Courtesy of DuPont Medical Imaging, Billerica, Massachusetts.)

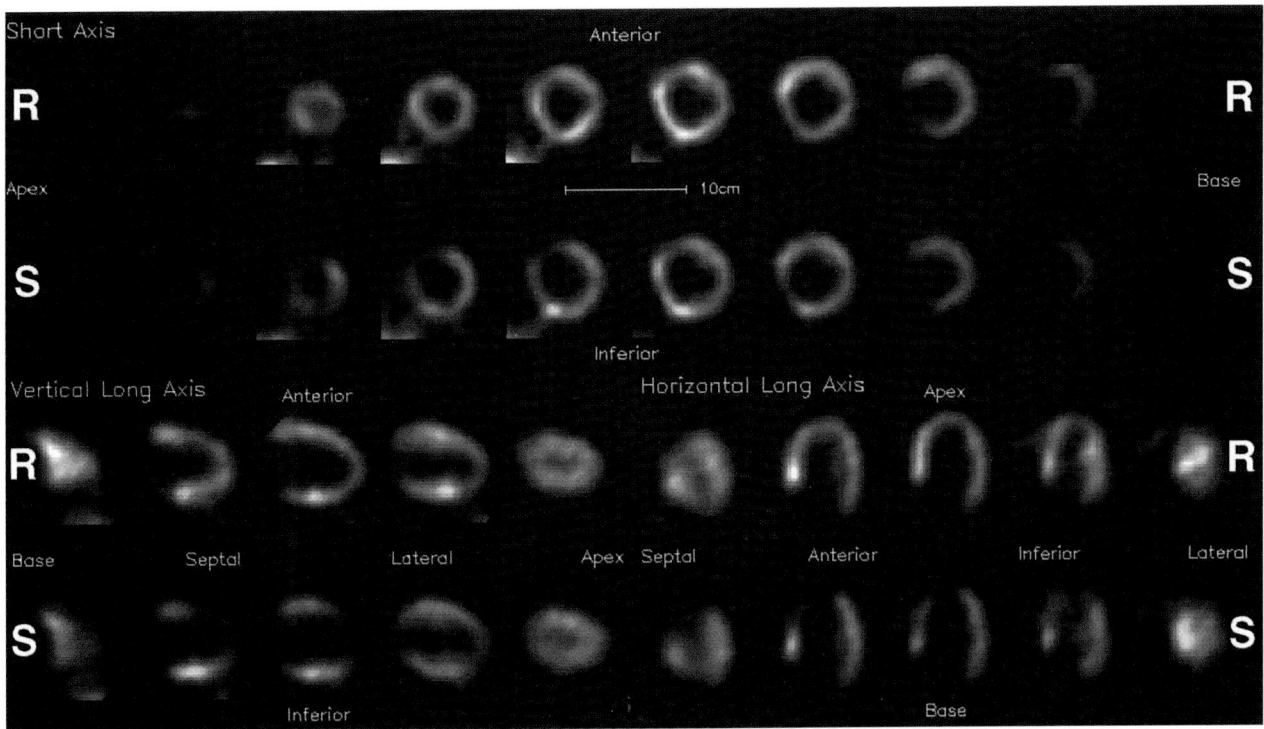

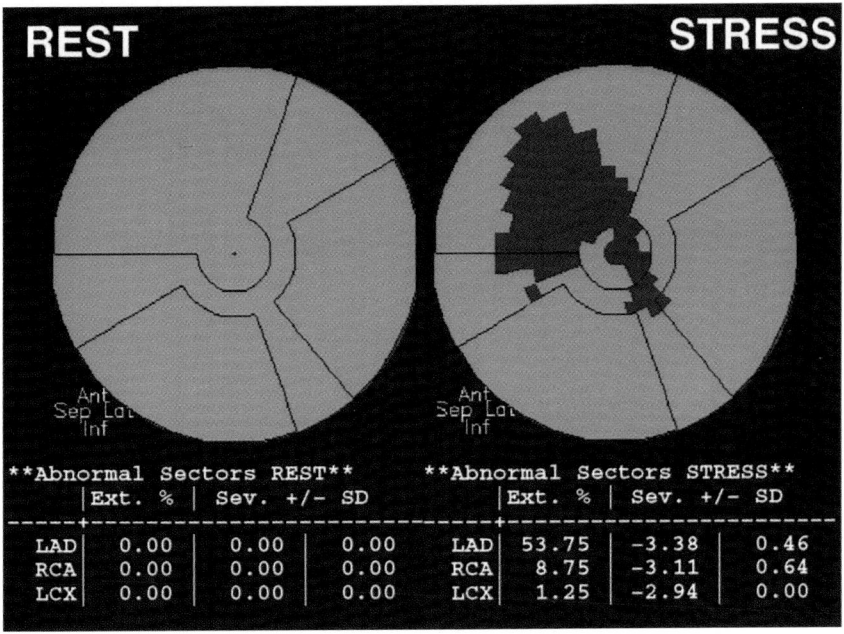

| **Abnormal Sectors REST** | | | **Abnormal Sectors STRESS** | | |
Ext. %	Sev.	+/- SD	Ext. %	Sev.	+/- SD
LAD 0.00	0.00	0.00	LAD 53.75	-3.38	0.46
RCA 0.00	0.00	0.00	RCA 8.75	-3.11	0.64
LCX 0.00	0.00	0.00	LCX 1.25	-2.94	0.00

COLOR PLATE 11. Images (**top**) and polar maps (**bottom**) of regional N-13 ammonia distribution of a patient with repeated episodes of angina pectoris. Short- and long-axis images depict an adenosine-induced defect in the apex and distal anteroseptal wall. For the polar map analysis, regional perfusion is compared to a normal data base. Normal areas are shown in *light gray*, while the abnormal area during pharmacologic stress (shown in *dark gray*) covers 54% of the LAD territory. In summary, results in this patient suggest a hemodynamic relevant stenosis of the LAD.

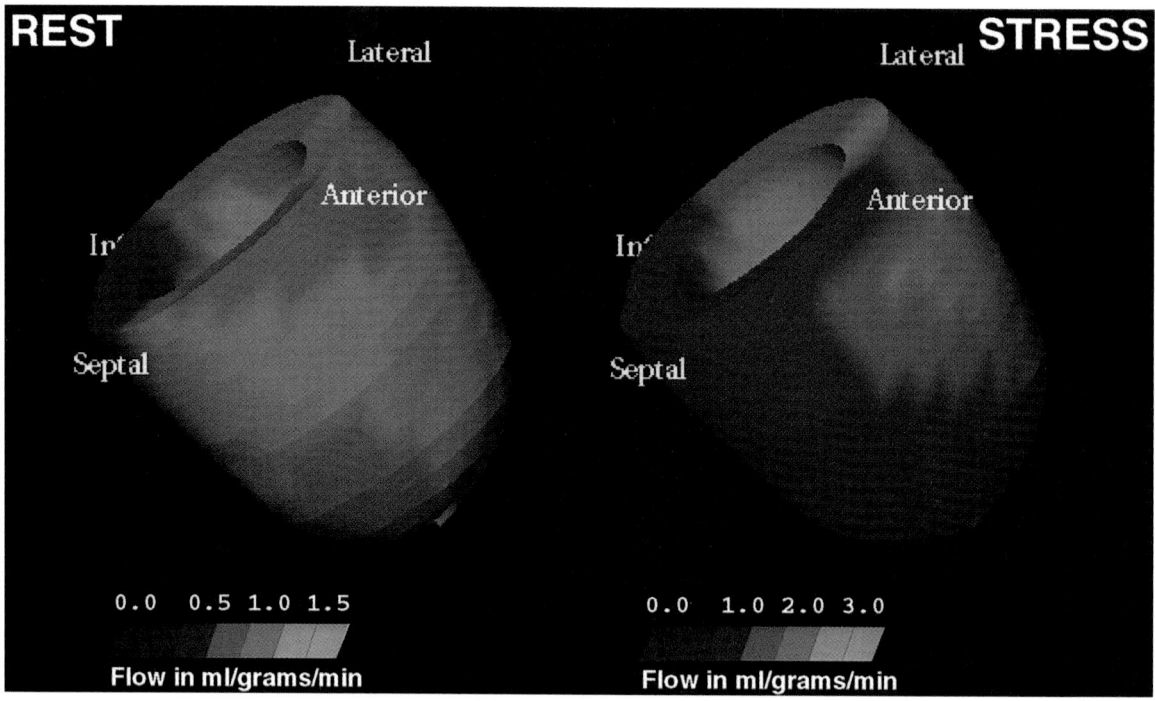

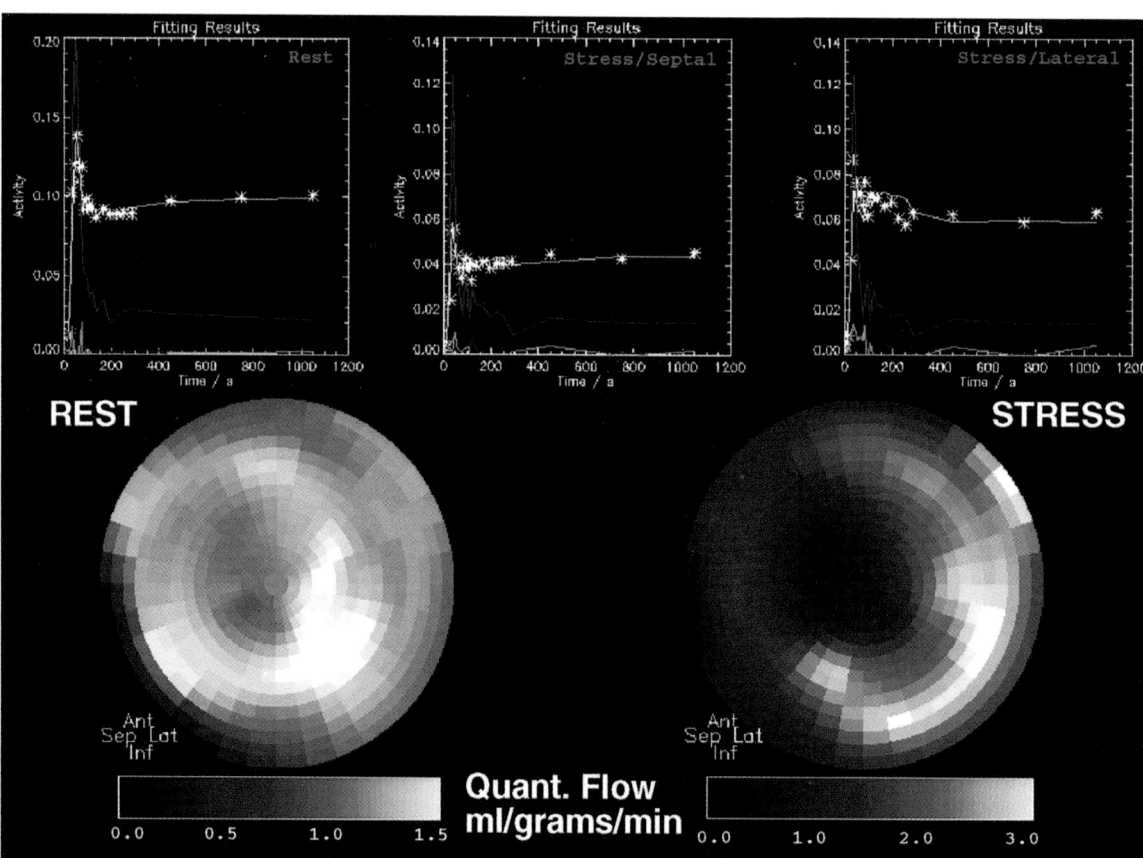

COLOR PLATE 12. Quantitative analysis of myocardial blood flow using N-13 ammonia. Depicted is the three-dimensional distribution of myocardial blood flow at rest and during stress (**top**) showing reduced stress flow and thus reduced flow reserve in the septal wall. The **bottom** part shows representative time activity curves for blood (*red lines*) and myocardium (*white lines*) at rest and during stress in the septum and lateral wall, along with two-dimensional polar maps of quantitative flow.

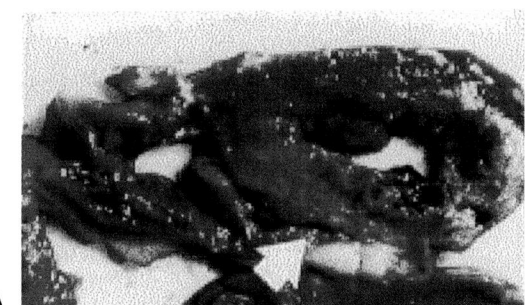

A

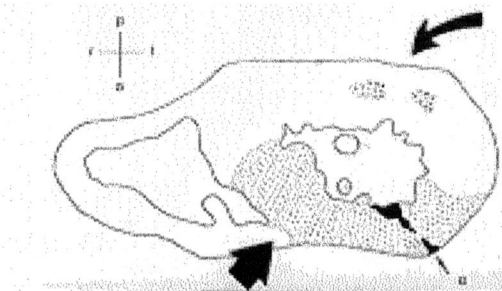

B

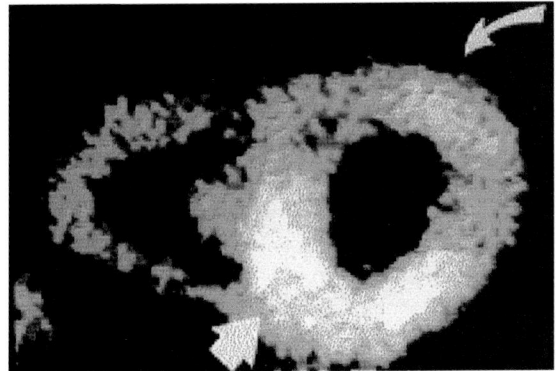

C

COLOR PLATE 13. Slice of the heart (A) showing anterior wall infarction with rupture of the free anterior wall; schematic representation of the histologically identified region of infarction (B); and the gamma image of the above slice showing antimyosin delineation of the infarct (C). (From ref. 41, with permission.) D: Anterior and LAO views of ^{111}In-antimyosin Fab images of a patient with acute myocardial infarction with no ECG changes. Serum CK showed typical rise and fall on serial estimation. Tracer uptake was seen in two areas (arrows) in each view. Coronary angiography showed minor plaques in the left main and right coronary arteries. Embolization from the lesion in the left main may have produced myocardial necrosis at the two sites. (From ref. 44, with permission.)

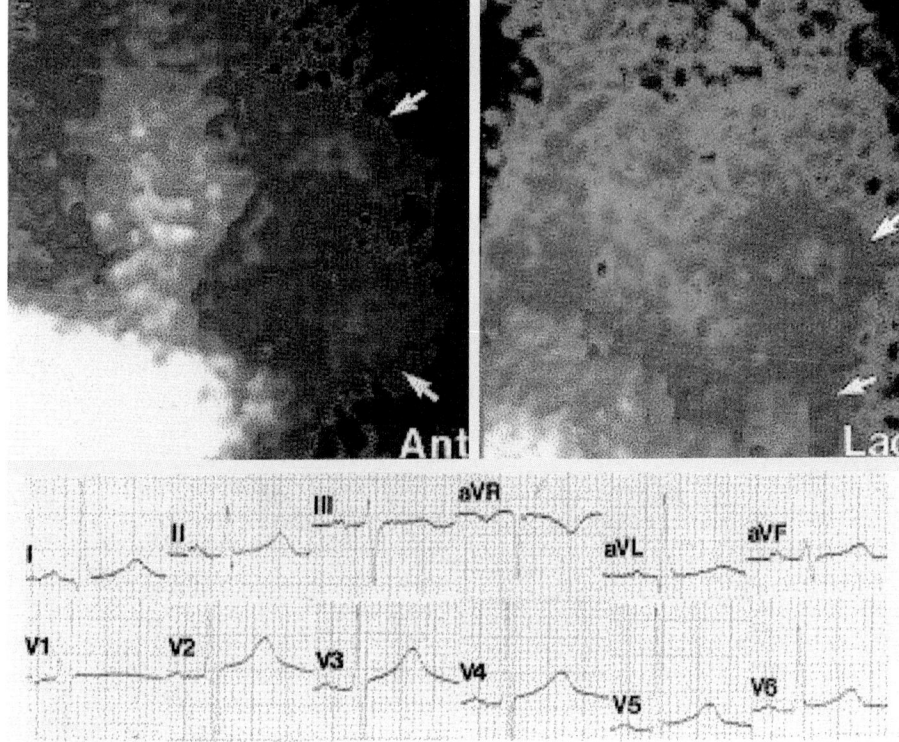

D

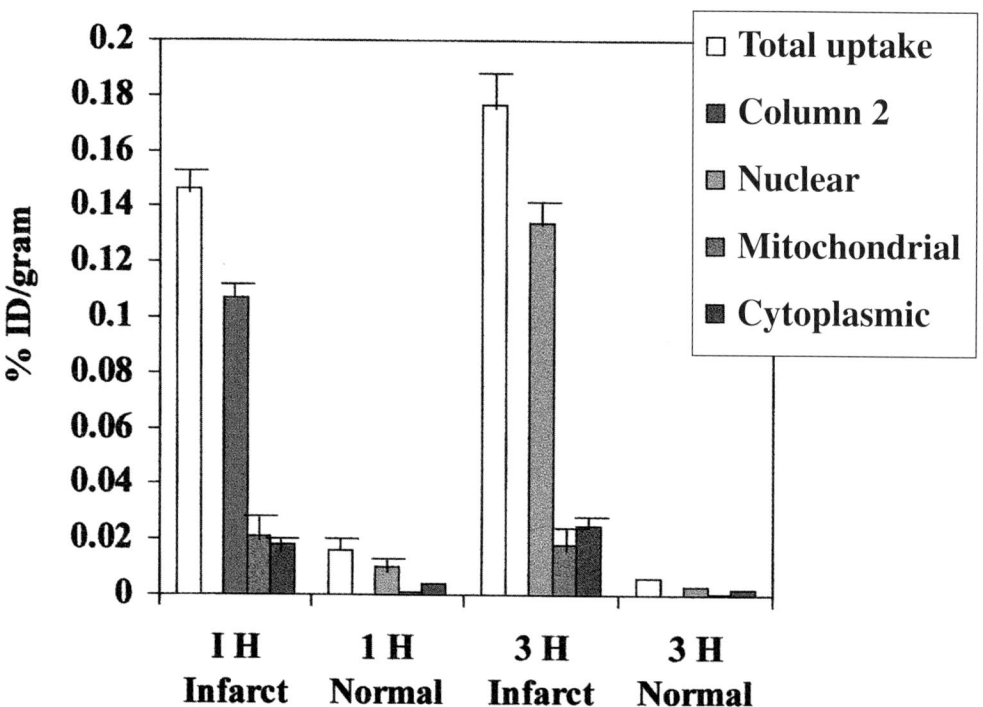

COLOR PLATE 14. Subcellular distribution of Tc-99m glucarate activity in the infarcted rabbit my-ocardium at 1 and 3 hours postintravenous administration of the radiotracer. Total uptake as well as ac-tivities in the nuclear, mitochondrial, and cytoplasmic fractions are shown.

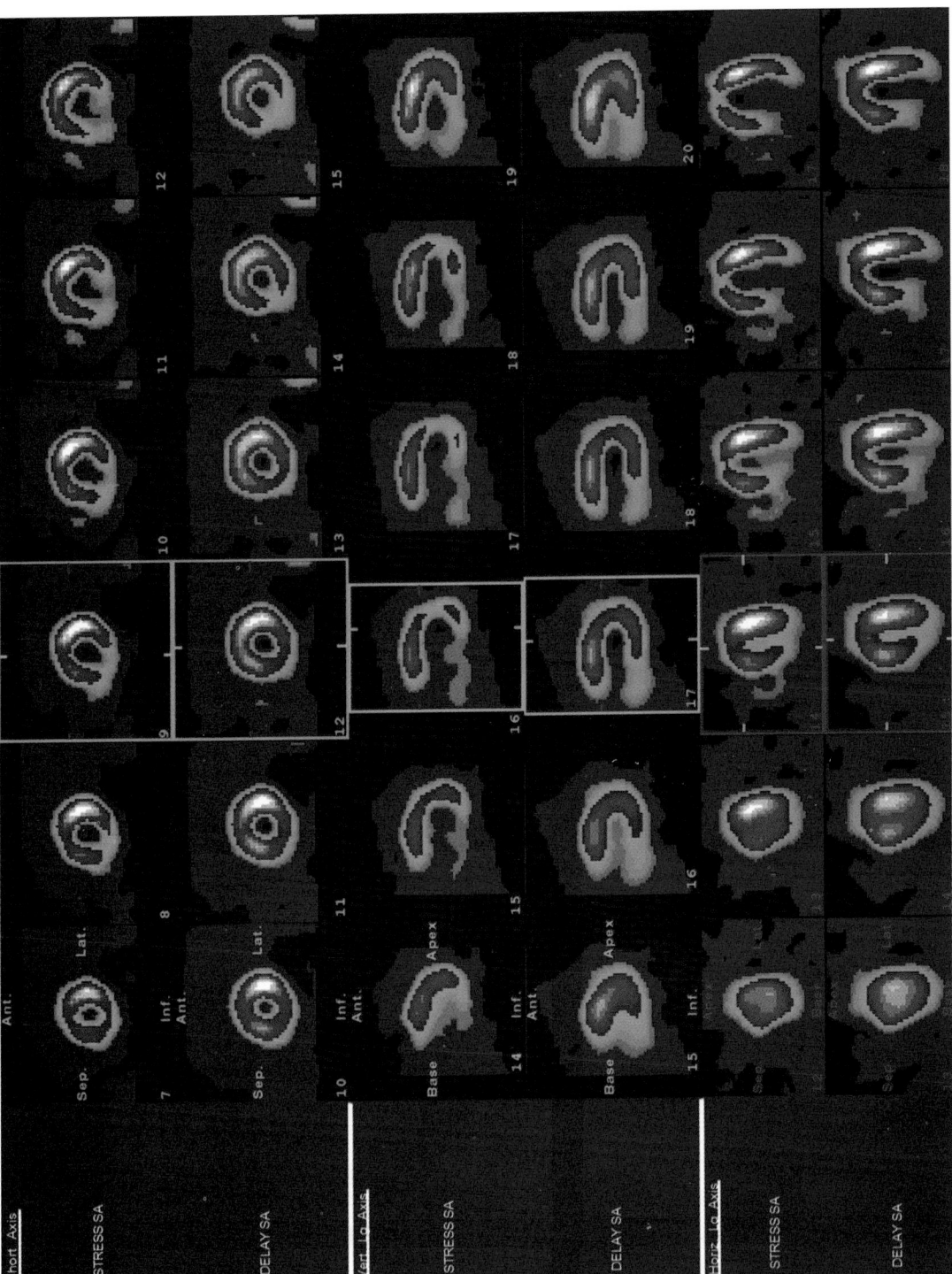

COLOR PLATE 15. Unstable angina with extensive myocardium at ischemic risk. Shown are the stress Tl-201 single-photon emission computed tomography myocardial perfusion images in a 74-year-old male with unstable angina and severe coronary artery disease. Short-axis slices (**top**), vertical long-axis slices (**middle**), and horizontal long-axis slices (**bottom**) are shown. In each view, the postexercise images are shown above, while those acquired after Tl-201 at rest are displayed below. A severe reversible perfusion defect is evident in the apical, inferior, and posterior-septal left ventricular walls. Coronary angiography demonstrated severe coronary artery disease in the right coronary artery and left circumflex artery vessels.

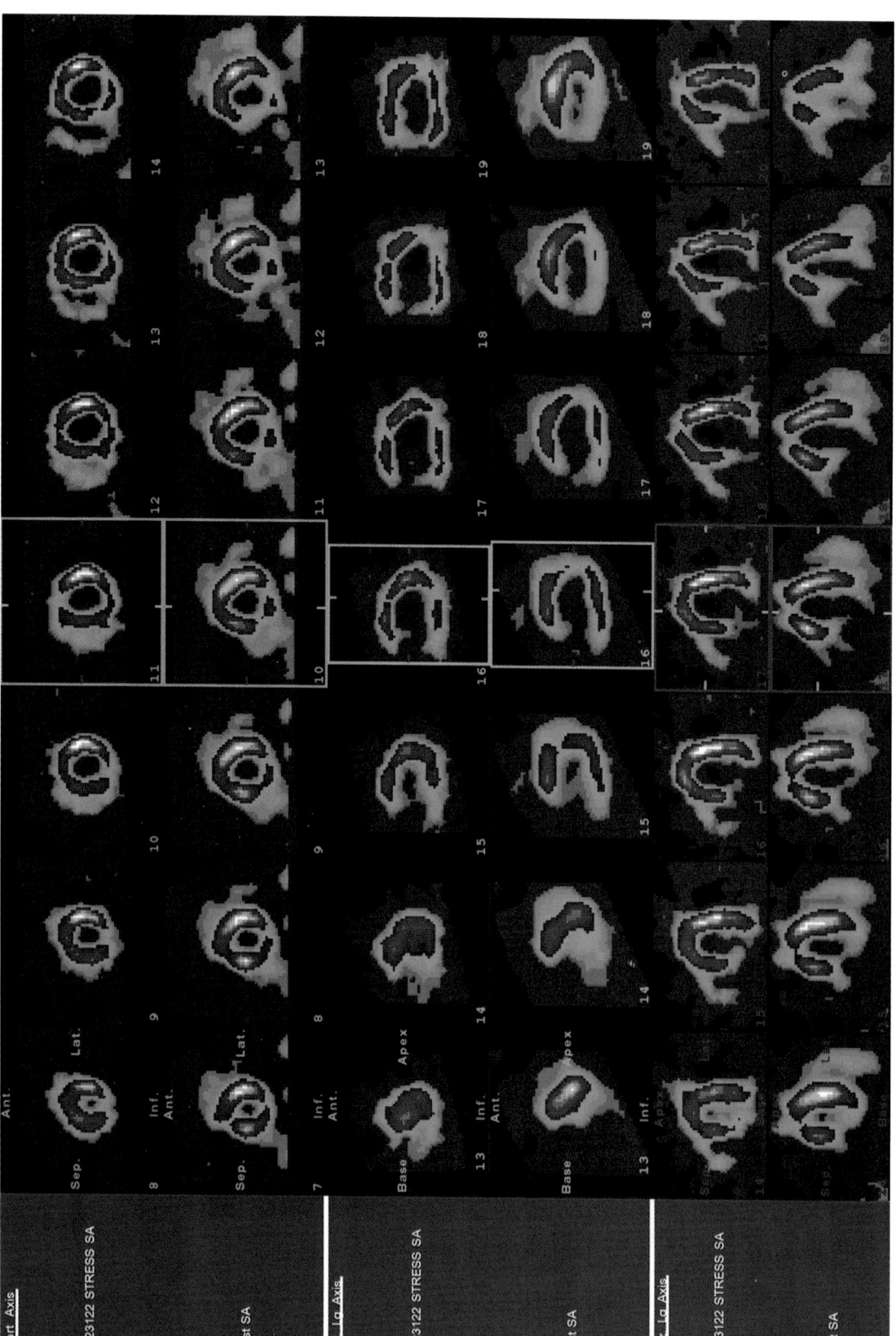

COLOR PLATE 16. Non-Q-wave myocardial infarction with extensive myocardium at ischemic risk: electrocardiogram (ECG). Shown in the same format as Color Plate 15 are the dual-isotope stress-gated single-photon emission computed tomography myocardial perfusion images that belong to the 72-year-old man whose ECG is shown in Figure 37-3. In each view, the postdipyridamole images are shown **above**, while those acquired earlier, after Tl-201 at rest, are displayed **below**. Evident are left ventricular dilatation associated with inferior, anterior, and septal perfusion defects that show partial reversibility. Concomitant gated images reveal a dilated left ventricle with global left ventricular dysfunction and an ejection fraction of 28%. (From Pharmacologic stress in nuclear medicine self study III: cardiology, with permission.)

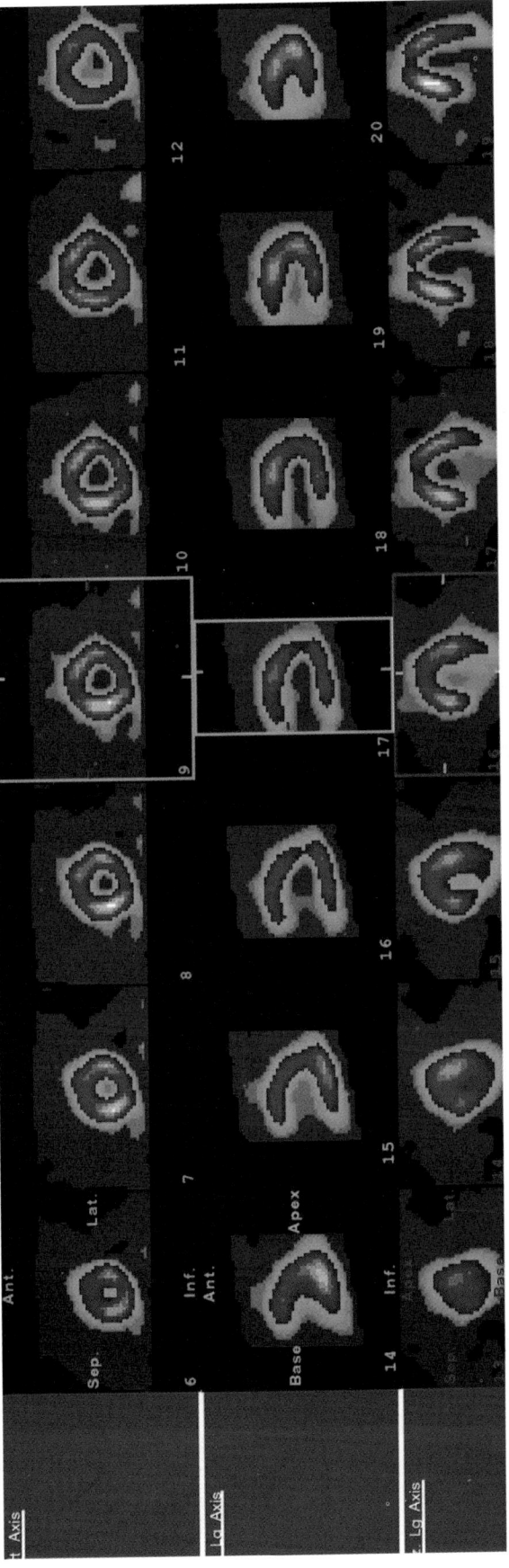

COLOR PLATE 17. Non-Q-wave myocardial infarction with extensive myocardium at ischemic risk. Shown are the 24-hour delayed 201-TL images performed in the patient presented in Color Plate 16. The myocardial perfusion is completely normal. The evidence of complete redistribution, viability, and widespread left ventricular dysfunction brought aggressive evaluation and management, with a strong likelihood of functional improvement after revascularization. (From Pharmacologic stress in nuclear medicine self study III: cardiology, with permission.)

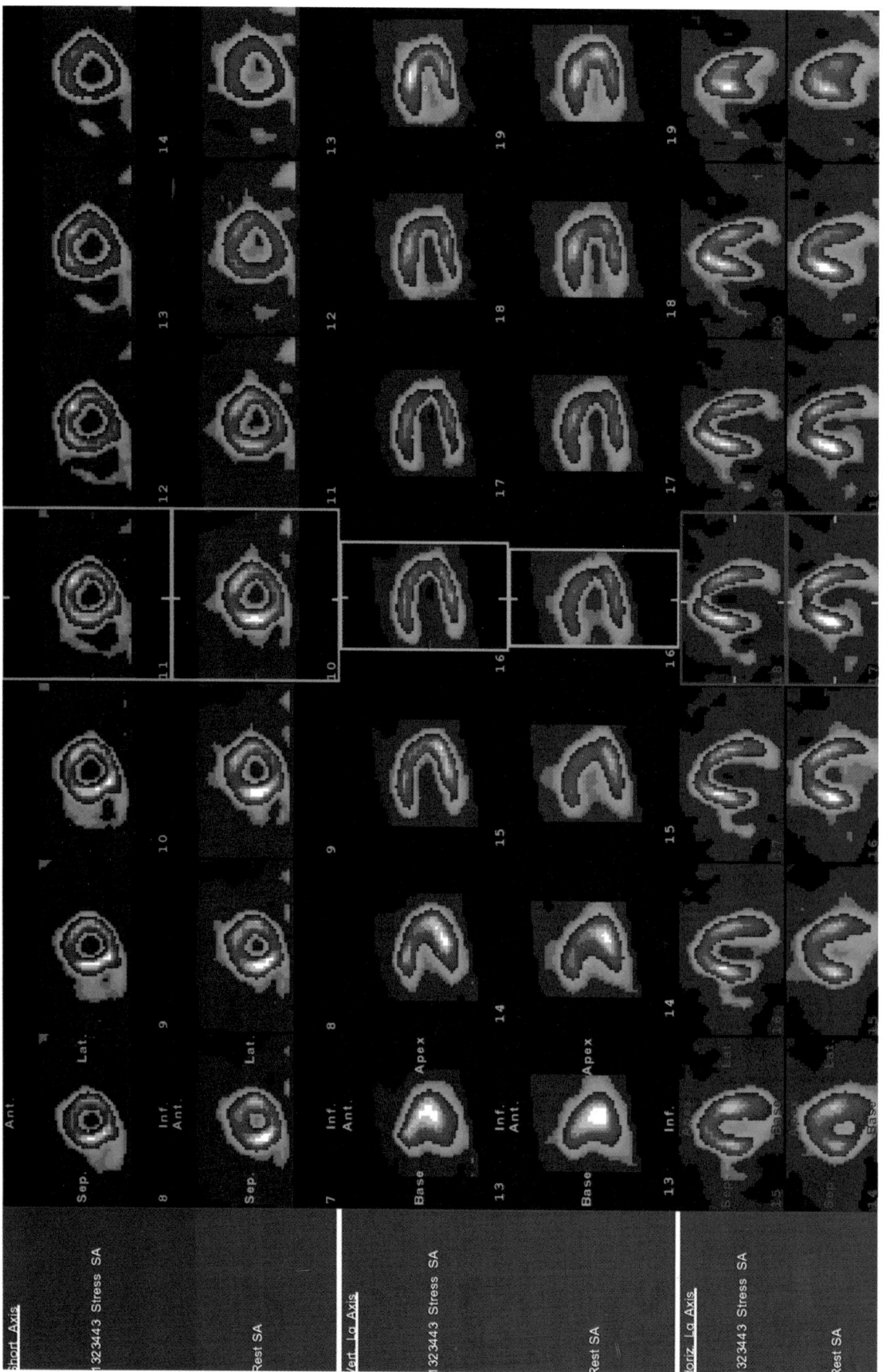

COLOR PLATE 18. Non-Q-wave myocardial infarction with extensive myocardium at ischemic risk after revascularization procedure. Shown in the same format as Color Plate 15 are the dual isotope stress-gated single-photon emission computed tomography (SPECT) myocardial perfusion images obtained 8 weeks after surgery in the same 72-year-old man presented in Color Plates 16 and 17. The left ventricle is reduced in size, myocardial perfusion is normal, and the calculated ejection fraction by gated SPECT is 50%. The images were acquired at Stage IV of the Bruce protocol. (From Pharmacologic stress in nuclear medicine self study III: cardiology, with permission.)

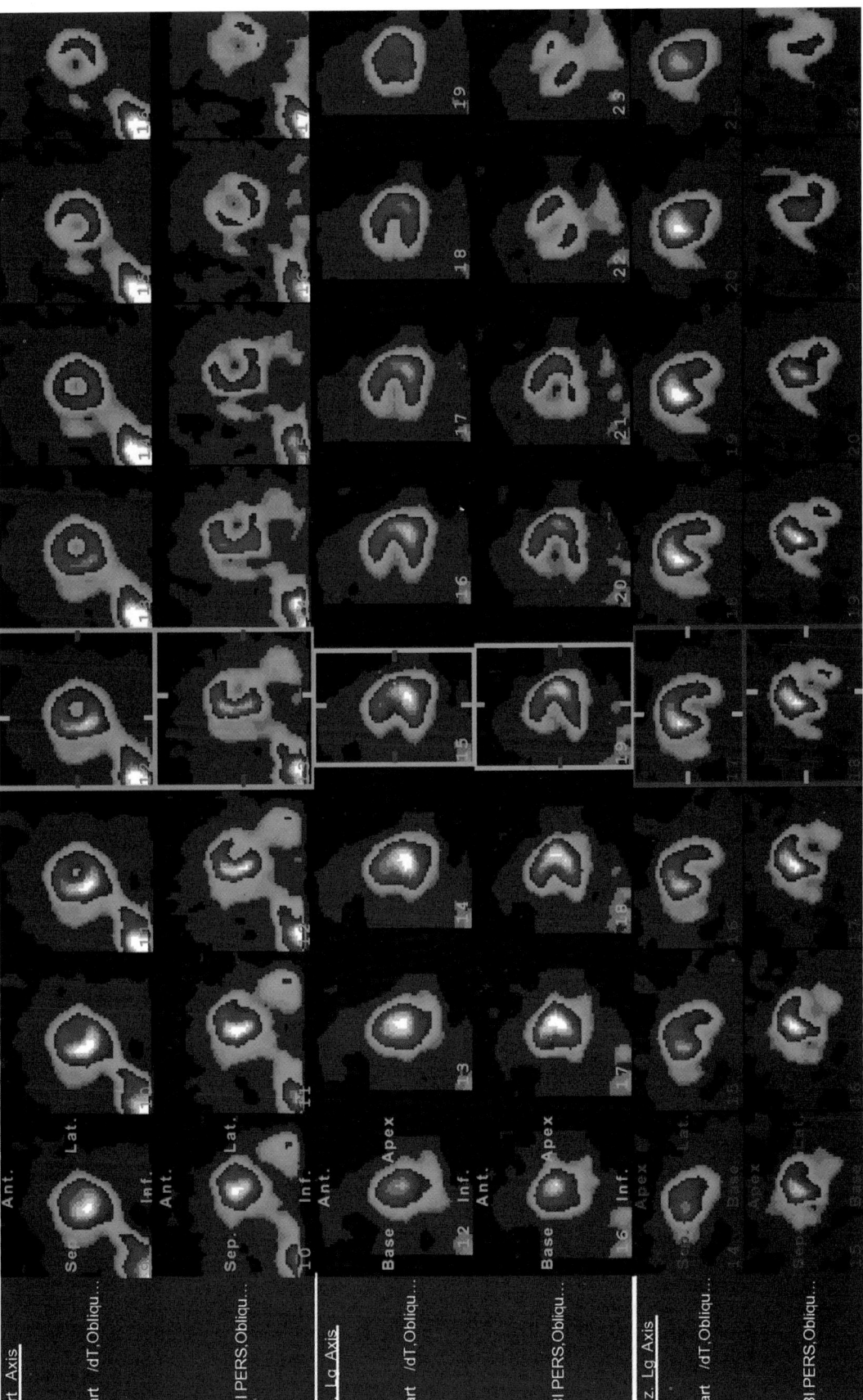

COLOR PLATE 19. End-diastolic (ED) chest pain. Shown in the same display as Color Plate 15 are rest and dipyridamole-gated Tc-99m MIBI myocardial perfusion images in an obese 84-year-old woman with chest pressure. Her electrocardiogram shows right bundle-branch block. In each view, rest Tc-99m MIBI images at presentation to the emergency department are shown above while those acquired after dipyridamole are shown below. There is evidence of subtle decreased uptake of the tracer in the lateral wall on rest ED images. Gated single-photon emission computed tomography images showed normal global and regional wall motion. These findings suggest myocardial ischemia as the cause of the perfusion defect. The dipyridamole images show a dense and extensive myocardial perfusion defect in the same lateral wall region. These findings demonstrate the presence of myocardium at ischemic risk, likely in the distribution of the left circumflex coronary artery. Coronary angiography showed a tight proximal lesion of the left circumflex coronary artery. (From Pharmacologic stress in nuclear medicine self study III: cardiology, with permission.)

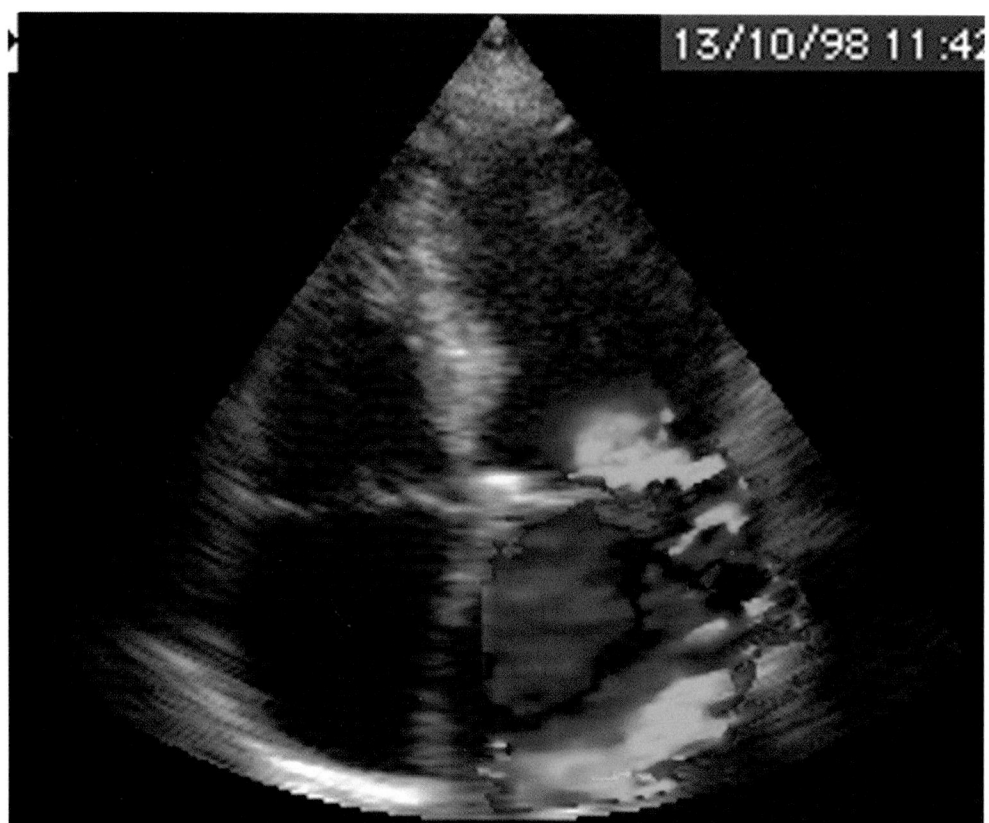

COLOR PLATE 20. Proximal convergence of the mitral regurgitation jet on the left ventricular side of the mitral valve is shown. A schematic is presented for determining the area of the jet at the site of aliasing. When this area is multiplied by the aliasing velocity, flow can be obtained.

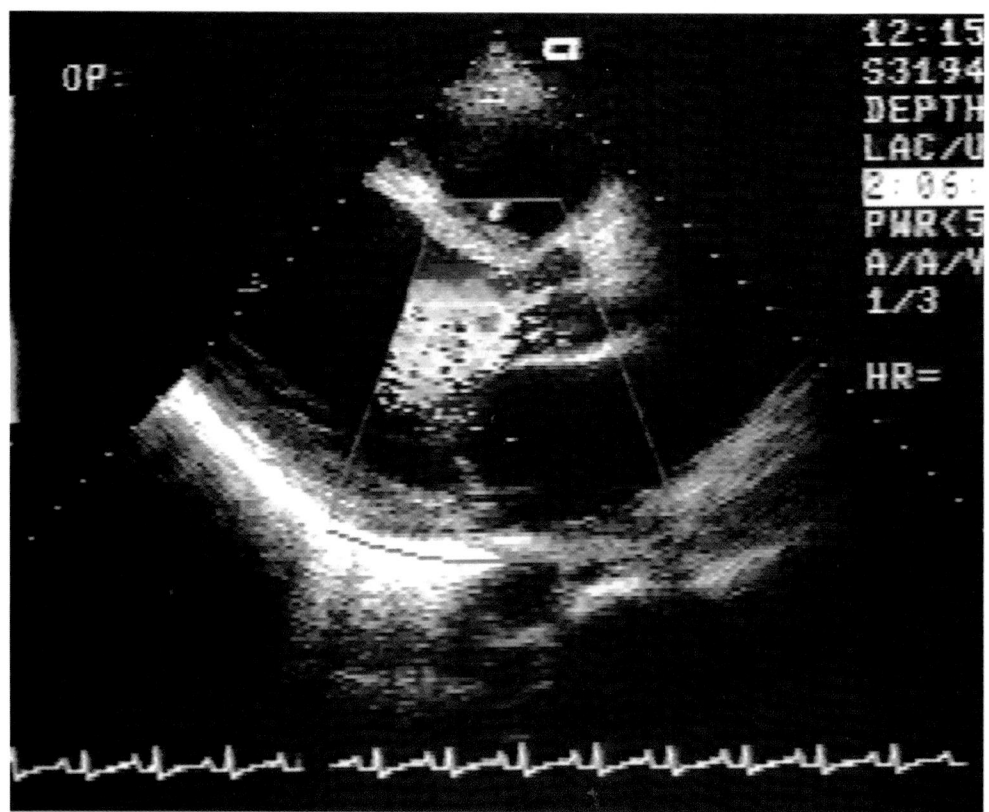

COLOR PLATE 21. Color flow Doppler with severe aortic regurgitation. The color flow signal occupies the majority of the left ventricular outflow tract and has a lot of turbulence, as witnessed by mosaicism.

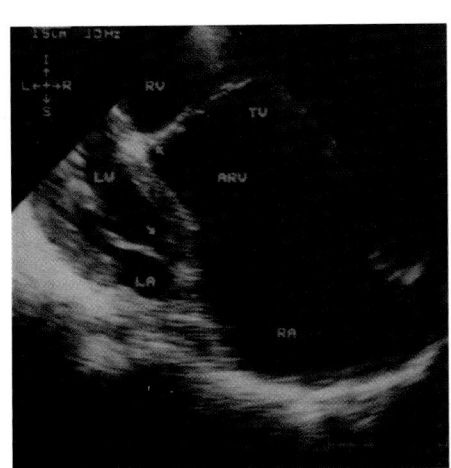

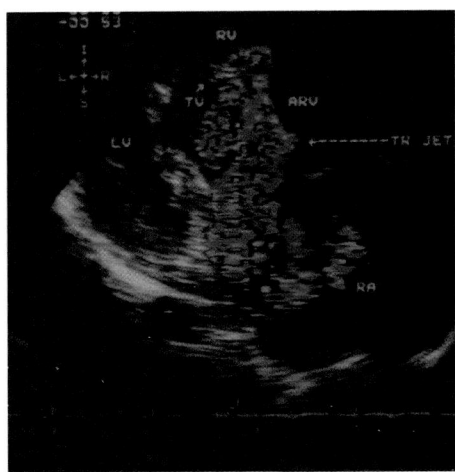

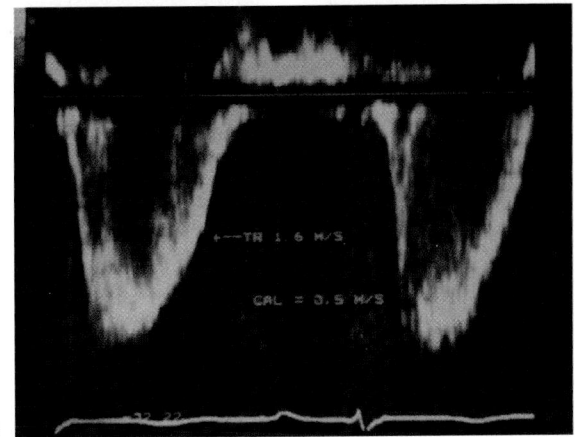

COLOR PLATE 22. Two-dimensional echocardiograph of the right ventricular inflow view without color (**A**) and with color flow (**B**), showing marked inferior displacement of the tricuspid valve diagnostic of Ebstein's anomaly. Color flow imaging shows severe tricuspid regurgitation (TR). **C:** Image shows color-wave Doppler signal of the TR jet, showing feature of high "V" wave pressure in the right atrium. *RA*, right atrium; *RV*, right ventricle; *TV*, tricuspid valve. (Courtesy of Ramesh Bansal, M.D.)

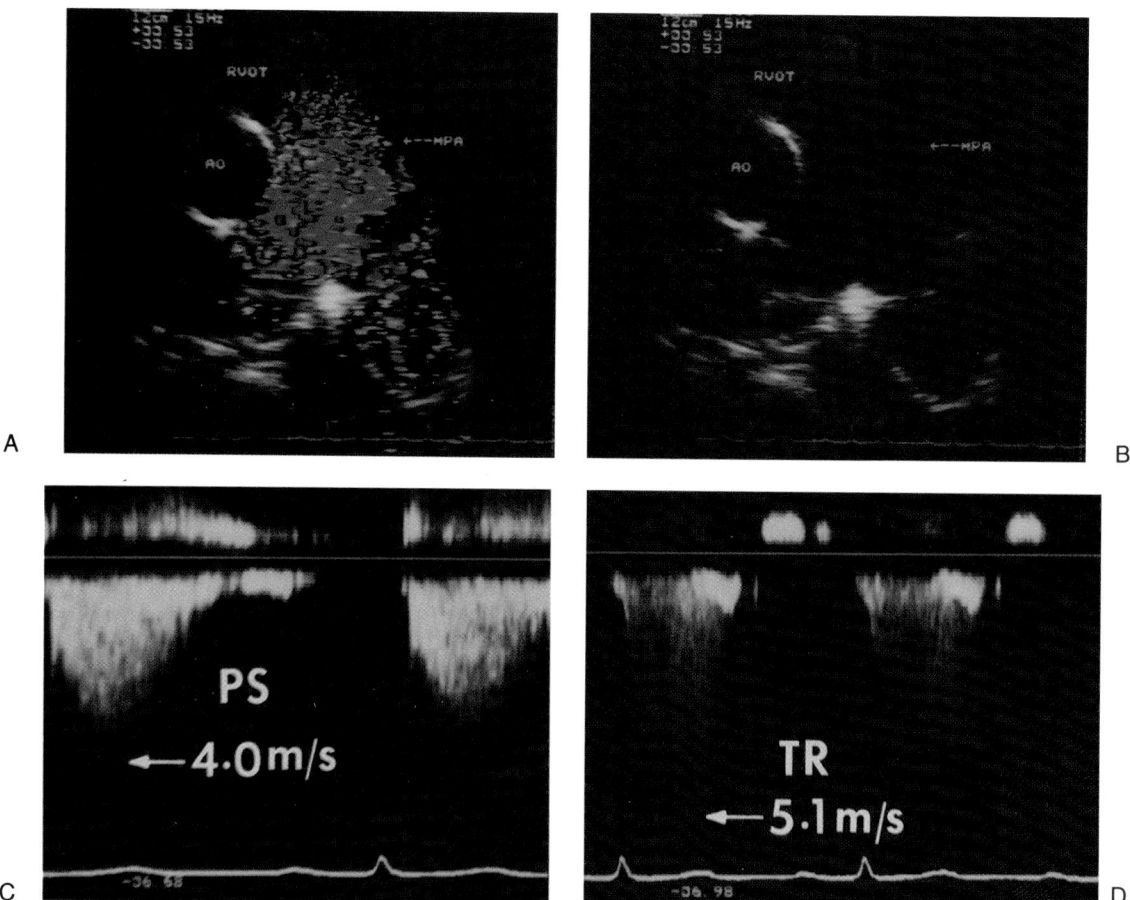

COLOR PLATE 23. Parasternal two-dimensional echocardiographic study from a patient with severe valvular pulmonic stenosis (*PS*): **A:** Panel shows the mosaic-like color flow jet of PS during systole in the main pulmonary artery (MPA). **B:** Panel of the same image without color, showing dilated MPA. **C:** Panel of continuous-wave Doppler (CWD) study of the PS jet showing velocity of 4 m/sec, consistent with a peak gradient of 64 mm Hg. **D:** Image shows trace of *TR*, using CWD. The TR velocity is 5.1 m/sec, consistent with right ventricular systolic pressure of 110 mm Hg. *TR*, tricuspid regurgitation. (Courtesy of Ramesh Bansal, M.D.)

CHAPTER 20

Fatty Acid Imaging

Nagara Tamaki and Eiji Tadamura

Among various imaging modalities, radionuclide imaging has an advantage for imaging physiological and biochemical information. It has a great sensitivity so that even concentrations of nanomoles per milliliter can be measured to assess various biological and biochemical processes without any pharmacological effects, compared with other imaging modalities, which may require tracer concentrations of micro- or even millimoles. Thus, nuclear medicine has been progressed in conjunction with the growth of molecular medicine.

Myocardial energy function can easily be assessed *in vivo* with nuclear medicine techniques. Long-chain fatty acids are the principal energy source for the normoxic myocardium and are rapidly metabolized by beta-oxidation. Approximately 60 to 80% of adenosine 5'-triphosphate (ATP) produced in aerobic myocardium derives from fatty acid oxidation, whereas the remaining ATP is obtained from glucose and lactate metabolism. In ischemia, glucose plays a major role for residual oxidative metabolism, while oxidation of long-chain fatty acid is greatly suppressed (1,2). Thus, alteration of fatty acid oxidation is considered to be a sensitive marker of both ischemia and myocardial damage. Radiolabeled fatty acid tracers represent potential probes to evaluate differences in oxidative metabolism, which is present in a variety of cardiac disorders.

POSITRON EMISSION TOMOGRAPHY

Positron emission tomography is uniquely suited for *in vivo* assessment of physiologic and biochemical functions using

N. Tamaki: Department of Radiology, Hokkaido University School of Medicine; Department of Nuclear Medicine, Hokkaido University Hospital, Sapporo 060-8638, Japan.
E. Tadamura: Department of Nuclear Medicine and Diagnostic Imaging, Kyoto University Graduate School of Medicine; Department of Nuclear Medicine, Kyoto University Hospital, Sakyo, Kyoto 606-8507, Japan.

various carbon-11-(C-11), oxygen-15-(O-15), nitrogen-13-(N-13), or fluorine-18- (F-18) labeled compounds. C-11 palmitate is a radiolabeled long-chain saturated fatty acid compound and is the fatty acid most commonly used for PET studies. After intravenous administration, C-11 palmitate is rapidly cleared from the blood, incorporated to palmitate-CoA in the cytoplasm, and is further metabolized via beta-oxidation in the mitochondria or stored in triglyceride pool in the cytoplasm. Initial uptake of C-11 palmitate correlates well with regional myocardial blood flow (3). However, the single-pass extraction fraction is not constant. It is influenced by both residence time in the capillary bed and the rate of metabolism extracted into myocyte (4). In ischemic myocardium, fatty acid utilization is suppressed with a reduction of beta-oxidation. Single-pass extraction fraction of C-11 palmitate decreases, probably due to the increase in the shunt into the triglyceride pool and back diffusion into coronary venous circulation (5). Thus, regional uptake of C-11 palmitate is reduced in the severely ischemic myocardium. In the clinical setting, quantitative estimation and characterization of myocardial infarction has been evaluated by the defect size of the early C-11 palmitate images (6–8).

Schon et al. (9) nicely demonstrated the clearance of the radioactivity from the myocardium following intravenous administration of C-11 palmitate. The clearance of C-11 palmitate showed two components consistent with incorporation of the tracer into at least two pools with different turnover rates. Because the clearance rate of the fast component is closely correlated with C-11 carbon dioxide clearance, this component is considered to represent beta-oxidation of C-11 palmitate. On the other hand, the slow component of the tracer washout may reflect slow turnover of the triglycerides and phospholipid. Schon et al. (10), in their study of ischemia, showed the significant reduction of the size and the rate of the fast clearance component of the activity, indicating reduced beta-oxidation. For better differentiation of metabolic alteration in the ischemic myocardium, metabolic studies under certain interventions are often required. Grover-McKay et al. (4) used atrial pacing for delineating ischemic myocardium. Tamaki et al. (11) used dobutamine infusion, which enhanced separation of ischemia from normal myocardium based on the difference in clearance of C-11 palmitate (Fig. 1). The abnormal response (delayed clearance of C-11 palmitate) was more often observed in patients with severe coronary artery stenosis (Fig. 2). On a theoretical basis, the metabolic response under various types of stress may play a role in differentiating reversible ischemia from irreversible scar tissue, similar to that applied to low-dose dobutamine echocardiography; however, this has not been fully validated with use of C-11 palmitate.

C-11 acetate has been used to assess pathophysiologic conditions in patients with coronary artery disease and cardiomyopathy. Following intravenous administration, C-11 acetate is activated to acetyl CoA, oxidized in mitochondria by the tricarbonic acid (TCA) cycle, and washed out from the myocardium as C-11 CO_2 and H_2O. The early clearance rate in the myocardium measured by PET corresponds closely to release of C-11 CO_2, indicating oxidative metabolism (12). The major advantage of this study is that, unlike glucose or fatty acid metabolism, the oxidative metabolism is not influenced by plasma substrate levels. Gropler et al. (13) showed that left ventricular dysfunctional areas with preserved oxidative metabolism by C-11 acetate represents reversibly ischemic myocardium in which regional function improved after revascularization. The predictive value of C-11 acetate was slightly higher than that of F-18 fluorodeoxyglucose (FDG). Weinheimer et al. (14) in an experimental

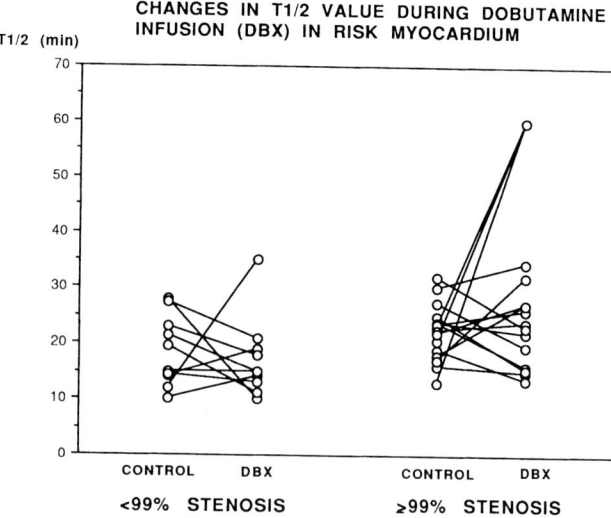

CHANGES IN T1/2 VALUE DURING DOBUTAMINE INFUSION (DBX) IN RISK MYOCARDIUM

FIG. 2. The clearance rate (T1/2) of C-11 palmitate at rest (control) and during dobutamine infusion (DBX) in the risk myocardium in patients with coronary artery disease with less than 99% stenosis (**left**) or 99% or more stenosis (**right**) on coronary angiogram. Although T1/2 value was reduced during dobutamine infusion, indicating enhanced beta-oxidation in the majority areas with <99% stenosis, this was scattered in the areas with >99% stenosis, indicating abnormal fatty acid oxidation in many of these segments.

study also supported the idea that the functional recovery after reperfusion was associated with the recovery of oxidative metabolism. Hata et al. (15) studied oxidative metabolism both at rest and under low-dose dobutamine infusion. The oxidative metabolic responses measured by C-11 acetate PET were similar to the functional responses assessed by echocardiography. They concluded that the metabolic response was a better marker of the recovery of regional function than the resting metabolism alone.

Because of limited availability, only a relatively small number of sites are equipped with both a PET camera and cyclotron, which are needed to study myocardial energy metabolism *in vivo*. With PET, on the other hand, a variety of iodine-123-(I-123)-labeled fatty acid compounds have been introduced to probe myocardial energy metabolism *in vivo* in routine clinical nuclear medicine facilities.

SINGLE PHOTON EMISSION COMPUTED TOMOGRAPHY

I-123-labeled Straight-chain Fatty Acids

Compounds

Iodine-123 is an excellent radionuclide for labeling metabolic substrates because it is easily incorporated into a wide variety of compounds by a halogen exchange reaction in which the iodine replaces a methyl group. Additionally, I-123 has a monoenergetic gamma emission with an energy appropriate for gamma camera imaging (159 keV) and a

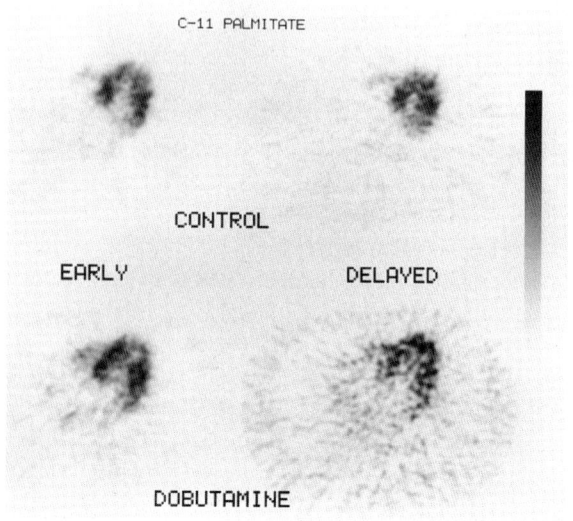

FIG. 1. The early and the delayed images of one representative PET tomogram after C-11 palmitate administration at control state (**top**) and during dobutamine infusion (**bottom**) in a patient with coronary artery disease. (From ref. 11, with permission.)

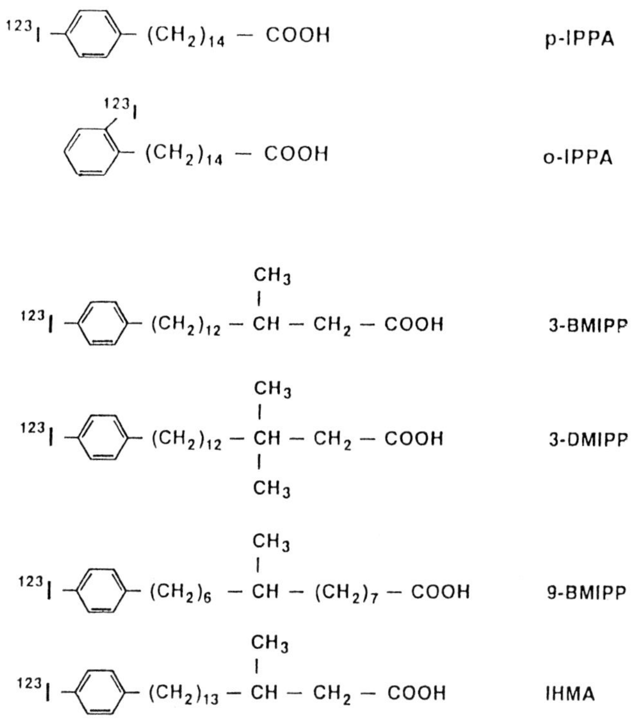

FIG. 3. Structures of various iodinated fatty acid compounds.

half-life of 13 h, which is practical for routine imaging studies and allows relatively favorable radiation dosimetry. Thus, I-123 has found widespread clinical application in a variety of clinical settings and I-123-labeled fatty acids have received great attention for assessing myocardial metabolism in vivo (16–18) (Fig. 3) Unfortunately, none of the I-123-labeled fatty acids are currently available for routine use in the United States.

There are two fundamental groups of iodinated fatty acid compounds, including straight-chain fatty acids and modified branched fatty acids (Table 1). The straight-chain fatty acids are generally metabolized via beta-oxidation and released from the myocardium. Therefore, fatty acid utilization can be directly assessed by the washout kinetics of these tracers, similar to C-11 palmitate. However, rapid washout from the myocardium often requires a fast dynamic acquisition for imaging following tracer administration. This may become a critical problem applied with SPECT using a rotating gamma camera. Furthermore, inadequate image quality due to low target-to-background ratio may often be observed

with these tracers. In addition, back diffusion and metabolites need to be considered in kinetic modeling for quantitative analysis of fatty acid metabolism with the straight-chain fatty acids.

The modified fatty acids have been introduced principally based on the concept of myocardial retention due to metabolic trapping (19). Therefore, the myocardial retention provides higher target-to-background ratios for a longer period of time than observed with the metabolized straight-chain fatty acids, allowing myocardial images to be obtained over as long an acquisition time as is required for good count statistics. On the other hand, the uptake of these agents may not directly reflect fatty acid oxidation. With these agents, the combined imaging of the iodinated fatty acid and perfusion is required to demonstrate perfusion-metabolism mismatch and to characterize fatty acid utilization.

An early example of a straight-chain iodinated fatty acid is 17-iodohexadecanoic acid (HDA), the iodoalkyl substituted series (20). The tissue clearance of the tracer is prolonged in ischemic myocardium, suggesting ischemia-induced impairment of fatty acid oxidation (21). Experimental studies have indicated that transmembraneous exchange of iodine rather than oxidation determines the rate of radioiodine clearance from myocardium with this agent (22,23). In addition, the difficulty of performing tomography due to rapid washout is a factor that would limit the clinical use of HDA (24,25).

To eliminate rapid deiodination, Machulla et al. (26) introduced the terminally phenylated iodinated straight-chain fatty acid: 15(p-(^{123}I)-iodophenyl) pentadecanoic acid (IPPA). Reske et al. (27–30) demonstrated rapid accumulation of this tracer in the heart following administration of IPPA with fast clearance from the myocardium in biexponential fashion as previously observed with C-11 palmitate. Early imaging studies showed a high myocardial uptake with decreased distribution in the areas supplied with occluded coronary artery (30). Caldwell et al. (31) subsequently compared the IPPA uptake with perfusion during exercise and found a linear correlation of IPPA uptake with myocardial blood flow during exercise.

Clinical Applications of IPPA

IPPA imaging has been applied for identifying ischemia in patients with coronary artery disease. A segmental reduction of IPPA correlated well with a regional perfusion defect

TABLE 1. *Characteristics of straight-chain and branched-chain fatty acids*

	Straight-chain fatty acids	Branched-chain fatty acids
PET tracers	^{11}C-palmitate	^{11}C-β-methyl heptadecanoic acid
SPECT tracers	^{123}I-hexadecenoic acid (IHA)	^{123}I-βmethyl iodophenylpentadecanoic acid (BMIPP)
	^{123}I-iodophenylpentadecanoic acid (IPPA)	^{123}I-dimethyl iodophenylpentadecanoic acid (DMIPP)
Measurement	Uptake and clearance	Uptake (metabolic trapping)
Advantages	β-oxidation assessment	Suitable for SPECT imaging
		Excellent image quality

on thallium scan (32,33). Reske et al. (28) showed the IPPA defects to be generally more prominent than thallium defects, probably due to lower extraction fraction of IPPA in ischemic areas. Wieler et al. (34,35) suggested that the IPPA study at rest could be useful for the detection of coronary artery disease.

For viability assessment, Kuikka et al. (36) described that IPPA uptake was identified in 39% of the segments with persistent methoxyisobutyl isonitrile (MIBI) defect and normalized in 25% of these segments, indicating its value over the resting MIBI perfusion study. Murray et al. (37,38) compared the dynamic IPPA study data using a multicrystal camera with viability information from those of transmural biopsies and thallium scans, and concluded that the IPPA viability findings were quite similar to those of the biopsy findings and that viability was more often seen with IPPA than with thallium scans. A recent study showed the clinical value of IPPA SPECT imaging at rest for viability assessment based on the prediction of functional recovery after revascularization. Hansen et al. (39) identified the areas showing intermediate range IPPA washout (less than the normal range but more than the infarcted areas) as an ischemic but viable myocardium in which contraction improves after revascularization. Iskandrian et al. (40) indicated that the reversible defects were more often seen with IPPA SPECT than the rest-redistribution thallium SPECT (Fig. 4). These investigators suggested that semiquantitative analysis of IPPA kinetics had advantages over rest-redistribution thallium imaging in viability assessment.

Because of the unique property of I-123 IPPA for tracing perfusion and fatty acid turnover, this tracer has been used for the detection of coronary lesions and viability assessment. On the other hand, the rapid washout from the myocardium may present difficulty for high-quality SPECT imaging because of low count statistics. Nonetheless, IPPA could play an important future role for precise evaluation of fatty acid turnover in the assessment of pathophysiology in ischemic heart disease and other myocardial diseases.

I-123-labeled Modified Fatty Acids

Compounds

A number of attempts have been made to decrease the washout rate of fatty acid tracers from the myocardium so as to provide better imaging characteristics (Fig. 3). The ortho-IPPA (o-IPPA) is a product from the synthesis of para-IPPA (p-IPPA) with different isomer (41). It has a unique character having long retention in the myocardium because of metabolic trapping by binding to coenzyme A. Henrich et al. (42) showed high retention of this compound in the ischemic myocardium in a manner similar to F-18 FDG.

Another approach to increased myocardial retention is methyl branching of the fatty acid chain, which is thought to protect these compounds against metabolism by beta-oxidation (43) while allowing them to retain some of the physiologic properties of straight-chain fatty acids, such as initial uptake and turnover rate of triglyceride pool. The degree of branching and the chain length appear to be the main determinants of myocardial uptake of these tracers.

A number of iodinated branched-chain fatty acids have been introduced to assess fatty acid utilization. These are particularly useful for SPECT imaging with a conventional gamma camera, because they are retained in the myocardium for long time (metabolic trapping). One example is iodine-123-iodophenyl-9-methyl-pentadecanoic acid ([^{123}I] 9MPA). Chouraqui et al. (44), in a small clinical study, indicated a high uptake and retention in the myocardium shortly after 9MPA administration. However, the early postexercise and delayed imaging studies showed comparable findings with stress/redistribution thallium studies. Recently clinical trials of [^{123}I] 9MPA have been performed in Japan. The results seem to be comparable or even better than 15-(p-iodophenyl)-3R,S-methyl pentadecanoic acid (BMIPP) findings in terms of identifying ischemic myocardium. In addition, there is some washout from the myocardium, and the washout rate seem to differ in various myocardial disorders (45,46). Because the washout rate of this compound was

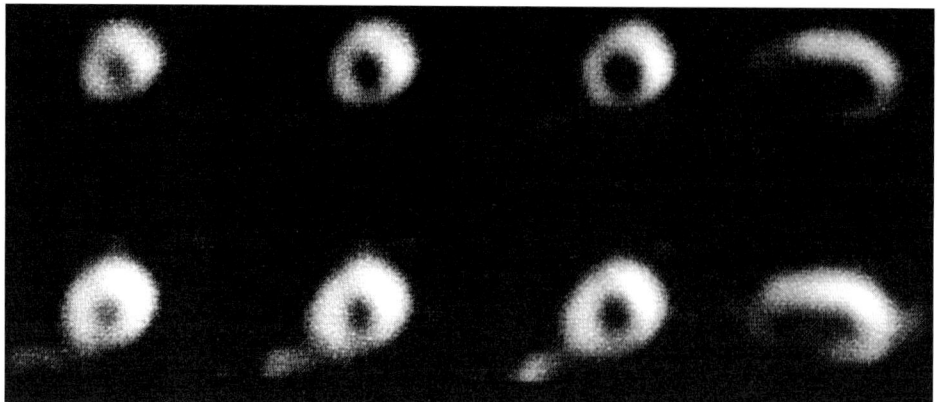

FIG. 4. The early (**top**) and late (**bottom**) scans after administration of I-123 IPPA in a patient with coronary artery disease. Initial decrease in tracer uptake with partial fill-in in inferoseptal regions indicating decreased fatty acid uptake and oxidation. (Courtesy of Dr. E. Iskandrian.)

slower than the straight-chain fatty acid, IPPA, high-quality SPECT imaging is feasible with this agent. The final reports are expected to be seen within a year or two.

16-[^{123}I]-iodo-3-methylhexadecanoic acid (IMHA) is another example of a methyl-branched analog. Marie et al. (47) showed that reversible IMHA defects were more often observed than reversible rest-reinjection thallium defects, suggesting the superiority of IMHA over thallium-201 in identifying ischemic myocardium.

Methyl-branched fatty acid imaging is based on the expected inhibition of beta-oxidation by the presence of methyl group in the β-position. Knapp et al. (49) first introduced BMIPP and 15-(p-iodophenyl)-3,3-dimethyl pentadecanoic acid (DMIPP). The animal experiments showed approximately 25% clearance of BMIPP in 2 h, whereas DMIPP showed no clearance. The fractional distribution of these compounds at 30 min after tracer injection in rats indicated 65 to 80% of the total activity resided in the triglyceride pool. Sloof et al. (50) compared these two compounds in the human subjects to conclude that BMIPP was more favorable because of lower liver counts.

BMIPP has been the most widely used fatty acid, particularly in Japan and Europe (51). In the last half of this chapter, the most commonly used iodinated fatty acid compound, BMIPP is described.

Basic Analysis of BMIPP

A number of experimental studies have focused on the BMIPP distribution in the myocardium. Fujibayashi et al. (52,53) indicated that BMIPP uptake correlated with ATP concentration in acutely damaged myocardium treated with dinitrophenol or tetradecylglycidic acid, an inhibitor of mitochondrial carnitine acyltransferase I. They also showed a high retention and slow washout of the myocardium due to α and β oxidation in the open chest dog model (54–56). Fujibayashi et al. (54) showed the enhanced rapid washout from the myocardium by long-chain fatty acid transporter inhibitor, etomoxir, which may produce similar conditions as myocardial ischemia. Similarly, Hosokawa et al. (57) showed that BMIPP uptake correlated with ATP levels in an occlusion and reperfusion canine model and concluded that BMIPP may be useful to differentiate ischemic from infarcted myocardium in their model. These results support the importance of ATP levels for the retention of BMIPP, probably because of cytosolic activation of BMIPP into BMIPP-CoA. In the ischemic canine model, Miller et al. (59) studied the BMIPP uptake and clearance with planar imaging and demonstrated higher BMIPP uptake than thallium uptake. Similar findings were observed *ex vivo* in an occlusion-reperfusion model (59). These data indicate BMIPP may provide some aspect of metabolic function independent from myocardial perfusion. However, such BMIPP/perfusion mismatch (more BMIPP uptake than perfusion) is in direct conflict with the clinical findings, in which less BMIPP than perfusion is often observed. Such conflicting results may be partly explained by the fatty acid uptake, which is influenced by both residence time in the capillary bed and the rate of metabolism of the myocyte. In acute ischemia, prolonged residence time may cause higher retention of the fatty acid analog in the myocardium. In chronic prolonged ischemia, on the other hand, the single-pass extraction fraction of the tracer decreases probably due to the increase in the shunt into triglyceride pool and backdiffusion into coronary venous circulation (57,61). Thus, regional uptake of fatty acid analog may be reduced in the severely and chronically ischemic myocardium. The BMIPP uptake is usually injected under fasting conditions and SPECT imaging is obtained approximately 20 to 30 min after tracer administration. The BMIPP uptake in the myocardium does not appear to be greatly influenced by the plasma substrate levels in humans (62), although BMIPP extraction has been shown to decrease and backdiffusion to increase during lipid infusion in the canine model (63).

In approximately 0.2 to 1% of clinical BMIPP studies, there is no evidence of accumulation of BMIPP in the myocardium (64). In these cases, the clearance of the blood pool activity is reduced. The finding does not appear to be related to any disease entity or to plasma substrate levels. Comparative studies have indicated a reduction of C-11 palmitate uptake with enhanced FDG uptake in the myocardium in these patients, consistent with a metabolic shifting from free fatty acid to glucose utilization (64). Hwang et al. (65) reported absent myocardial uptake of BMIPP in a family, suggestive of a hereditary myocardial metabolic abnormality. Tanaka et al. (66) in a recent experimental study indicated the presence of membrane fatty acid binding protein, @CD-36, which might possibly relate to the absence of BMIPP uptake in these familial cases. However, the pathophysiological conditions and clinical significance of such metabolic shifts remain to be clarified.

Clinical Applications of BMIPP

The phase 1 clinical trials demonstrated a rapid myocardial uptake with long retention after BMIPP administration. There was high myocardial uptake, with low blood background, and low uptake in the liver and lung at 60 min after BMIPP injection (Fig. 5) (67). High-quality SPECT images can be obtained with collecting myocardial images for approximately 20 min. Generally, BMIPP uptake was similar to thallium perfusion (Fig. 6). On the other hand, less BMIPP uptake than thallium perfusion is often observed in patients with various cardiac disorders (68,69). Sequential dynamic SPECT imaging, performed using a triple-head camera, demonstrated very early that the initial distribution was similar to perfusion and that 20–30-min images may reflect more metabolic function (70,71). Therefore, a single injection of BMIPP might possibly provide both perfusion and metabolism without use of perfusion tracer. However, the image quality of initial BMIPP images 2 to 5 min following BMIPP administration is not as good as that of the slightly delayed images.

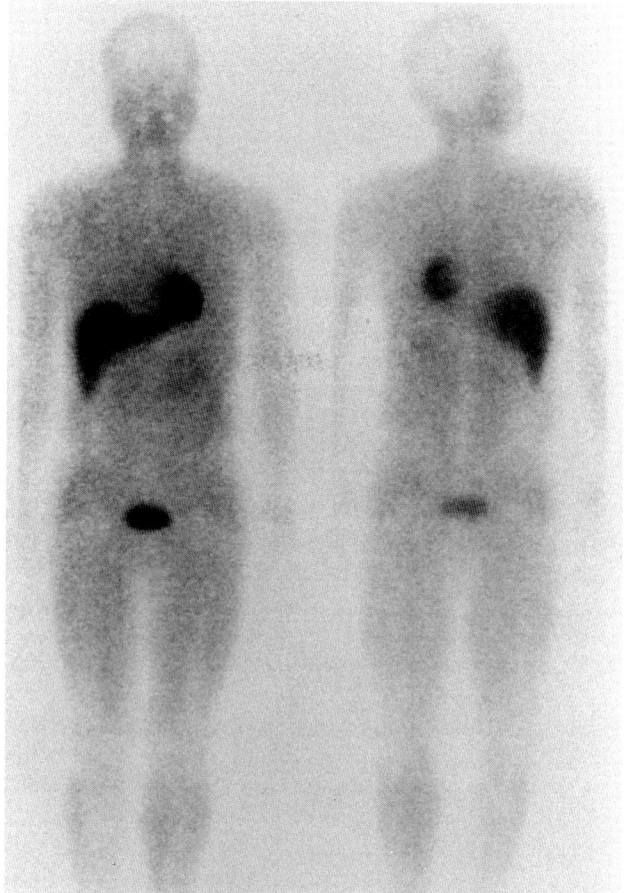

FIG. 5. Whole-body images taken at 60 min following BMIPP administration at rest of a normal subject. A high myocardial uptake of the tracer is seen.

In a study of myocardial infarction, Tamaki et al. (72) reported less BMIPP uptake than thallium perfusion in the areas of myocardial infarction (Fig. 7). Such discordance with BMIPP uptake less than thallium was seen most often in areas of infarction, areas with recanalized arteries, and areas with severe wall motion abnormalities, in comparison with what would be expected by the degree of the thallium perfusion abnormality. Saito et al. (73) also showed that iodinated branched-chain fatty acid uptake was lower than thallium perfusion in patients with unstable angina, and in patients with acute myocardial infarction who are acutely revascularized.

Many other papers have been published in patients with ischemic heart disease showing that regions with less BMIPP uptake than perfusion also have regional wall motion abnormalities (71,74–82). The findings are considered to represent a persistent metabolic abnormality that is out of proportion to the perfusion abnormality at the time of the study. Matsunari et al. (77) indicated that this metabolic abnormality may be reversible after revascularization therapy and that this reversibility is associated with improvement in regional wall motion abnormality. Taki et al. (83) showed that the

improvement in BMIPP uptake was closely related to the functional recovery after revascularization. On the other hand, Tsubokura et al. (84) illustrated a feature of stunned myocardium in which perfusion was normalized but metabolic abnormalities of glucose and fatty acid persisted even after there was recovery of regional wall motion. A careful follow-up study may identify the differences of the sequential improvement of regional blood flow, function, and metabolism.

A recent study by Furutani et al. (85) suggests that BMIPP uptake permits determination of the amount of myocardium at risk identified by contrast ventriculography in the subacute phase of myocardial infarction. Kawai et al. (86), in another recent study of patients with acute myocardial infarction, also indicated that the size of a BMIPP defect after revascularization may reflect the area at risk as measured by Tc-99m perfusion imaging before revascularization therapy. Thus, the BMIPP imaging may identify prior ischemic insult as an area of reduced tracer uptake even after successful revascularization therapy. The latter authors concluded that the combined imaging of BMIPP and perfusion at 1 week after myocardial infarction may identify the areas at risk and salvaged myocardium. Because the approach could elimi-

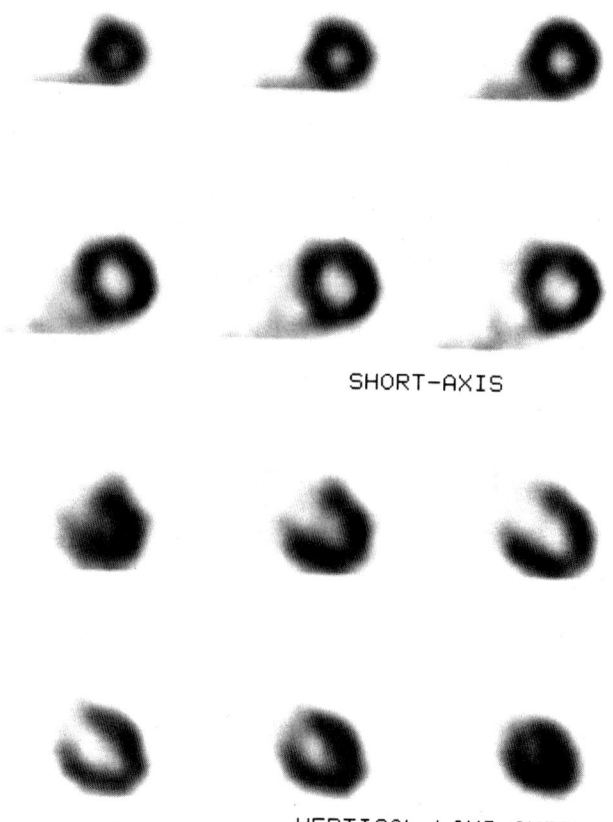

FIG. 6. A series of short-axis (**top**) and vertical long-axis (**bottom**) images obtained 20 min following BMIPP administrations of a normal subject. Homogeneous distribution of BMIPP in the left ventricular myocardium is noted.

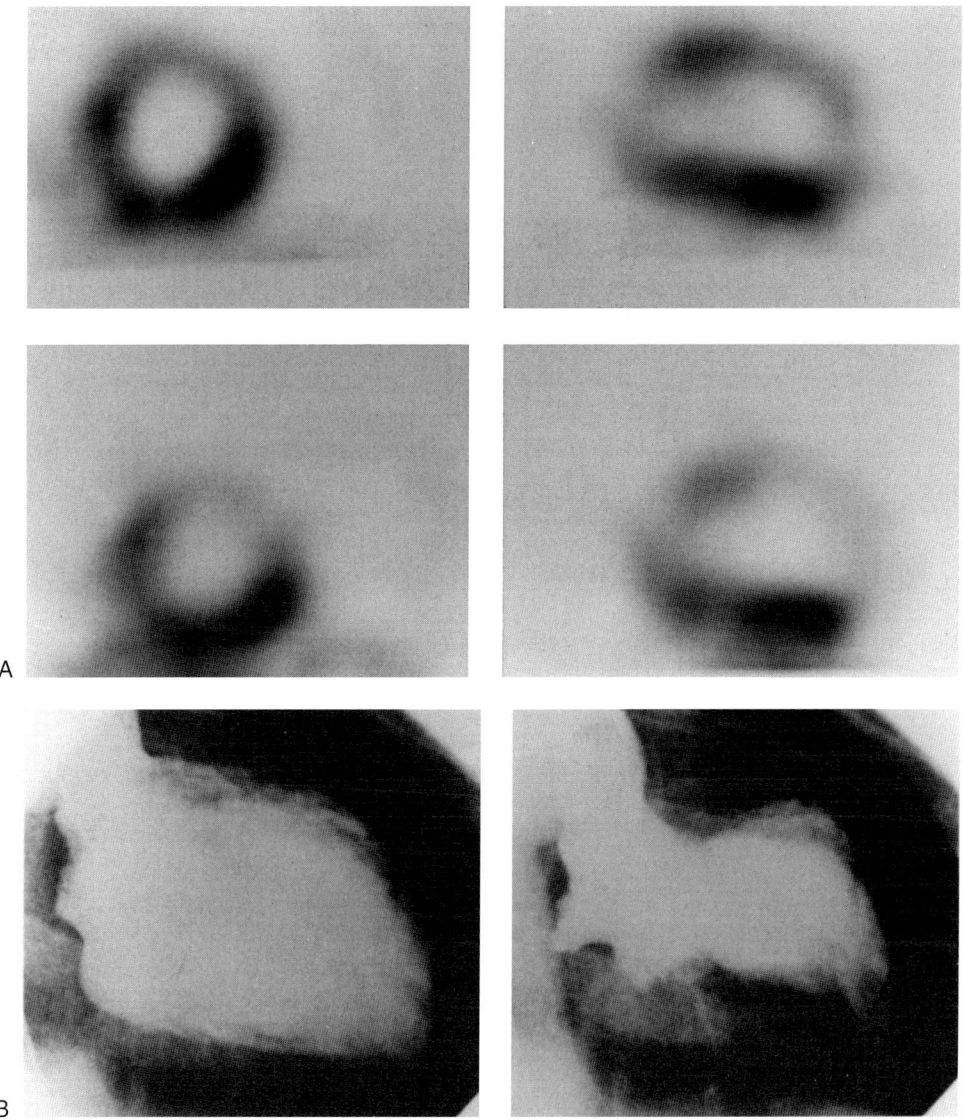

FIG. 7. **A:** Representative short-axis (**left**) and vertical long-axis (**right**) slices of thallium (**top**) and BMIPP (**bottom**) images of a patient with anterior wall myocardial infarction after successful revascularization in acute stage of infarction. These images show a significant decrease in both thallium and BMIPP uptake in anterior and apical regions, but the BMIPP decrease is greater than thallium decrease indicating discordant BMIPP decrease relative to thallium perfusion. **B:** End diastolic (**left**) and end systolic (**right**) images of contrast ventriculography of the same patients show severe wall motion abnormality in anterior and apical regions. (From ref. 18, with permission.)

nate the practical difficulties associated with the need for imaging before intervention when assessing areas at risk and myocardial salvage in acute ischemic syndromes, these results are quite promising; however, the optimum threshold for comparing the area at risk and the ultimate infarct size should be further defined for quantitative measurement.

In the study of patients with angina without prior myocardial infarction, a decrease in BMIPP uptake has often been seen at rest despite normal perfusion, particularly in those with unstable and vasospastic angina associated with regional wall motion abnormality, indicating presence of metabolic impairment in stunned and/or hibernating myocardium

(Fig. 8). Takeishi et al. (87) reported a decrease in BMIPP uptake in resting conditions despite normal perfusion in patients with chronic stable angina. In unstable angina, these investigators demonstrated that this discordant abnormal BMIPP uptake was more often seen in severe coronary stenosis in the presence of coronary collaterals and that patients with abnormal BMIPP were more likely to undergo percutaneous transluminal coronary angioplasty (PTCA) therapy (88). Nakajima et al. (78) showed a decrease in BMIPP uptake with normal perfusion in patients with vasospastic angina. Tateno et al. (89) showed that a decrease of BMIPP was related to the presence of severe coronary stenosis and

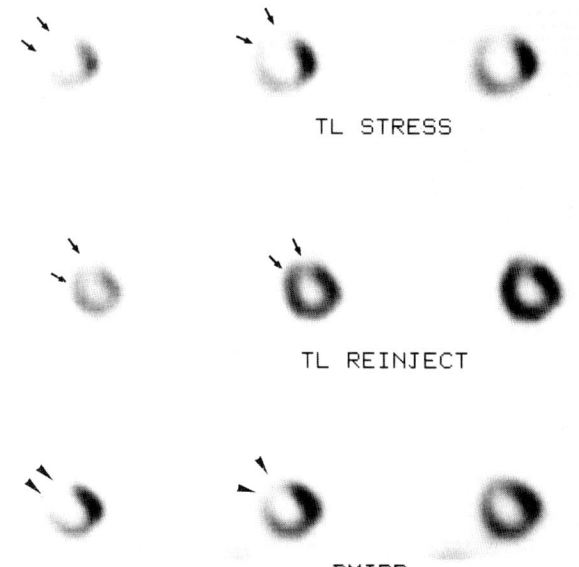

FIG. 8. A series of short-axis slices of stress (**top**) and rein-jection (**middle**) thallium scans and resting BMIPP scan (**bottom**) of a patient with unstable angina. Decreased BMIPP uptake is observed in anteroseptal region (*arrowheads*) where stress-induced hypoperfusion with redistribution is seen on thallium study (*arrows*). (From ref. 81, with permission.)

concordant decrease both in BMIPP and thallium uptake is associated with no increase in FDG uptake (PET scar). Hambye et al. (91) showed that BMIPP and perfusion study correlated well with response to the dobutamine by echocardiography.

A number of reports now indicate that regions demonstrating this discordant BMIPP uptake represent areas that frequently demonstrate improvement in regional function after revascularization. Franken et al. (92) first showed that the areas of less BMIPP uptake than Tc-99m sestamibi improved in cardiac function shortly after myocardial infarction. Ito et al. (93) also showed the recovery of regional dysfunction and perfusion after myocardial infarction in the areas with discordant defect size by BMIPP and thallium images (Fig. 9). Furthermore, Hashimoto et al. (94) nicely showed that the degree of perfusion-metabolism mismatch may reflect subsequent improvement from postischemic dysfunction. More recently, Taki et al. (83) showed that the areas of discordant BMIPP uptake less than reinjection thallium uptake before revascularization was a good predictor of improvement of ejection fraction. All of these reports indicate that the discordant BMIPP uptake less than perfusion may represent reversible ischemic myocardium in which it is expected that regional function will improve either spontaneously or in response to revascularization, depending on the clinical setting in which it is observed.

regional asynergy. In addition, such abnormality was more often seen in patients with unstable rather than stable angina. Although the sensitivity of BMIPP imaging for detecting coronary artery lesions may be low compared to the conventional stress perfusion imaging (40–60%), this metabolic imaging does not require a provocative test and appears to be providing unique information. Therefore, BMIPP imaging may be suitable for patients with unstable angina or severe coronary artery disease. Metabolic alterations may be seen with this agent, possibly as a result of repetitive ischemic episodes, even when perfusion imaging may not identify regional perfusion abnormalities. Thus, BMIPP imaging is considered by many to be a method of choice to identify regions of recent severe ishemia through providing an "ischemic memory" noninvasively.

A number of reports indicate that the discordance shown by BMIPP uptake less than perfusion also represents reversible ischemic myocardium. Matsunari et al. (71) and Kawamoto et al. (76) both reported that the areas with reduced uptake of BMIPP showed thallium redistribution on stress-delayed scan (Fig. 8). Tamaki et al. (17,90) showed that such discordant BMIPP uptake was observed in the areas with an increase in FDG uptake as a marker of exogenous glucose utilization (PET ischemia). In ischemic myocardium, fatty acid oxidation is easily suppressed and glucose metabolism serves as a major energy source. Furthermore, areas of discordant BMIPP uptake showed preserved oxidative metabolism assessed by C-11 acetate PET studies. In contrast, the

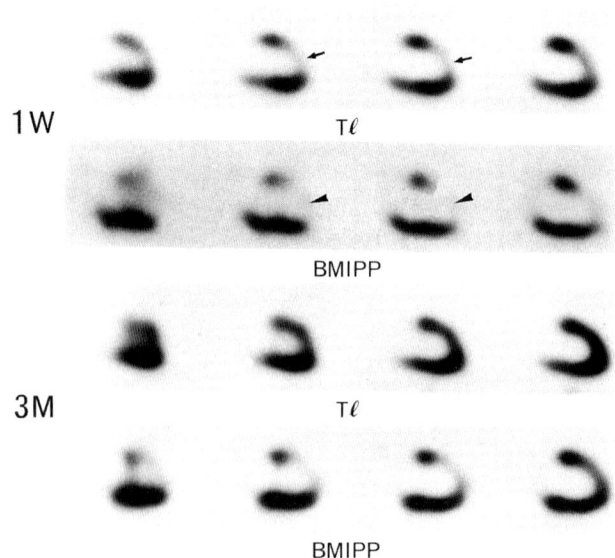

FIG. 9. A series of vertical long-axis slices of thallium and BMIPP images in 1 week (**top**) and 3 months (**bottom**) after anterior wall myocardial infarction. A large defect in anterior and apical regions is noted in both thallium and BMIPP scans, but note that the decrease in BMIPP (*arrowheads*) is greater than thallium defect (*arrows*), indicating discordant BMIPP decrease relative to thallium. The thallium perfusion is significantly improved in the chronic state in the areas of discordant BMIPP uptake. The improvement in BMIPP uptake is less prominent than that of perfusion, indicating improvement in fatty acid metabolism may be delayed compared to the perfusion improvement.

Because the discordant BMIPP uptake less than thallium may represent previously ischemic myocardium, combined BMIPP and thallium imaging has been tested for prognostic value (95,96). Tamaki et al. (95) surveyed 50 consecutive patients with myocardial infarction who received BMIPP and thallium scans and who are followed up for a mean interval of 23 months. Among various clinical, angiographic, and scintigraphic indices, discordant BMIPP uptake was the best predictor of future cardiac events followed by a number of coronary stenosis. Although these data remain preliminary, combined BMIPP and thallium imaging may hold prognostic value for identifying high-risk subgroups among patients with coronary artery disease.

CONCLUSIONS

Although fatty acid is a major energy source in the normal myocardium, fatty acid oxidation is easily suppressed in ischemic and postischemic myocardium. Therefore, assessment of fatty acid metabolism by the radionuclide technique can play an important role for early detection of myocardial ischemia and assessment of severity of ischemic heart disease. PET C-11 palmitate is a well-established tracer to probe myocardial fatty acid metabolism. For SPECT, on the other hand, a variety of iodinated fatty acid compounds have been introduced for assessment of fatty acid metabolism, including straight-chain and branched-chain fatty acid compounds. Straight-chain fatty acids have advantages for measuring fatty acid oxidation on the basis of clearance of the tracer from the myocardium. Modified fatty acid can be trapped in the myocardium without further wash-out from the myocardium. Among them, a branched-chain fatty acid compound, BMIPP, provides excellent images of the left ventricular myocardium and may probe myocardial energy metabolism *in vivo*. In addition, this tracer appears to uncover an ''ischemic memory'' and may have unique capabilities for the assessment of previously severely ischemic myocardium. The segments with discordant BMIPP uptake less than thallium, often seen in patients with severe coronary artery disease, may represent previously ischemic but viable myocardium. Therefore, the combined imaging using BMIPP and thallium may permit detection of ischemic but viable myocardium on the basis of alteration of myocardial energy metabolism. Hopefully, this agent, which has proven so useful in other countries, will be approved in the near future in the United States, where nuclear cardiology plays such an important role.

REFERENCES

1. Liedke AJ. Alterations of carbohydrate and lipid metabolism in the acutely ischemic heart. *Prog Cardiovasc Dis* 1981;23:321–336.
2. Neely JR, Rovetto M, Oram J. Myocardial utilization of carbohydrate and lipids. *Prog Cardiovasc Dis* 1972;15:289–329.
3. Schelbert HR, Henze E, Keen R, et al. C-11 palmitate for the noninvasive evaluation of regional myocardial fatty acid metabolism with positron computed tomography. IV. *In vivo* evaluation of acute demand-induced ischemia in dogs. *Am Heart J* 1983;106:736–750.
4. Grover-McKay M, Schelbert HR, Schwaiger M, et al. Identification of impaired metabolic reserve by atrial pacing in patients with significant coronary stenosis. *Circulation* 1986;74:281–292.
5. Weiss ES, Hoffman EJ, Phelps ME, et al. External detection and visualization of myocardial ischemia with C-11 substrates *in vivo* and *in vitro*. *Circ Res* 1976;39:24–32.
6. Geltman EM, Biello D, Welch MJ, et al. Characterization of nontransmural myocardial infarction by positron emission tomography. *Circulation* 1982;65:747–755.
7. Lerch RA, Ambos HD, Bergmann SR, et al. Localization of viable, ischemic myocardium by positron emission tomography with C-11 palmitate. *Circulation* 1981;64:689–699.
8. Sobel BE, Weiss ES, Welch MJ, et al. Detection of remote myocardial infarction in patients with positron transaxial tomography and intravenous C-11 palmitate. *Circulation* 1977;55:853–857.
9. Schon HR, Schelbert HR, Robinson G, et al. C-11 labeled palmitic acid for the noninvasive evaluation of regional myocardial fatty acid metabolism with positron computed tomography. I. Kinetics of C-11 palmitic acid in normal myocardium. *Am Heart J* 1982;103:532–547.
10. Schon HR, Schelbert HR, Nahaji A, et al. C-11 labeled palmitic acid for the noninvasive evaluation of regional myocardial fatty acid metabolism with positron computed tomography. II. Kinetics of C-11 palmitic acid in acutely ischemic myocardium. *Am Heart J* 1982;103:548–561.
11. Tamaki N, Kawamoto M, Takahashi N, et al. Assessment of myocardial fatty acid metabolism with positron emission tomography at rest and during dobutamine infusion in patients with coronary artery disease. *Am Heart J* 1993;125:702–710.
12. Brown M, Marshall DR, Sobel BE, et al. Delineation of myocardial utilization with carbon-11-labeled acetate. *Circulation* 1987;76: 687–696.
13. Gropler RJ, Geltman EM, Sampathkumaran K, et al. Functional recovery after coronary revascularization for chronic coronary artery disease is dependent on maintenance of oxidative metabolism. *J Am Coll Cardiol* 1992;20:69–77.
14. Weinheimer CJ, Brown MA, Nohara R, et al. Functional recovery after reperfusion is predicated on recovery myocardial oxidative metabolism. *Am Heart J* 1993;125:939–949.
15. Hata T, Nohara R, Tamaki N, et al. Noninvasive assessment of myocardial viability by positron emission tomography with 11C-acetate in patients with old myocardial infarction. *Circulation* 1996;94: 1834–1841.
16. Knapp FF Jr, Kropp J. Iodine-123-labelled fatty acids for myocardial single-photon emission tomography:current status and future perspectives. *Eur J Nucl Med* 1995;22:361–381.
17. Tamaki N, Kawamoto M. The use of iodinated free fatty acids for assessing fatty acid metabolism. *J Nucl Cardiol* 1994;1:S72–78.
18. Tamaki N, Fujibayashi Y, Magata Y, et al. Radionuclide assessment of myocardial fatty acid metabolism by PET and SPECT. *J Nucl Cardiol* 1995;2:256–266.
19. Livni E, Elmaleh DR, Levy S, et al. Beta-methyl (1-C-11)-heptadecanoic acid: a new myocardial metabolic tracer for positron emission tomography. *J Nucl Med* 1982;23:169–176.
20. Poe ND, Robinson GD Jr, Graham LS, et al. Experimental basis for myocardial imaging with I-123-labeled hexadecanoic acid. *J Nucl Med* 1976;17:1077–1082.
21. van der Wall EE, Heidendal GAK, Den Hollander W, et al. Metabolic myocardial imaging with I-123 labeled heptadecanoic acid in patients with angina pectoris. *Eur J Nucl Med* 1981;6:391–396.
22. Cuchet P, Demaison L, Bontemps L, et al. Do iodinated fatty acids under a nonspecific deiodination in the myocardium? *Eur J Nucl Med* 1985;10:505–510.
23. Visser FC, van Eenige J, Westera G, et al. Metabolic fate of radioiodinated heptadecanoic acid in the normal canine heart. *Circulation* 1985; 72:565–571.
24. Dudczak R, Kletter K, Frichauf H, et al. The use of I-123-labelled heptadecanoic acid (HDA) as a metabolic tracer. *Eur J Nucl Med* 1984; 9:81–85.
25. Railton R, Rogers JC, Small DR, et al. Myocardial scintigraphy with I-123 heptadecanoic acid as a test for coronary heart disease. *Eur J Nucl Med* 1987;13:63–66.
26. Machulla HJ, Marsmann M, Dutschka K. Biochemical synthesis of a radioiodinated phenyl fatty acid for *in vivo* metabolic studies of the myocardium. *Eur J Nucl Med* 1980;5:171–173.
27. Reske SN, Machulla HJ, Winkler C. Metabolism of 15-p-(I-123-

phenyl)-pentadecanoic acid in hearts of rats. *J Nucl Med* 1982;23:10–18.

28. Reske SN, Biersack HJ, Lackner K, et al. Assessment of regional myocardial uptake and metabolism of w-(p-123I-iodophenyl)-pentadecanoic acid with serial single-photon emission tomography. *J Nucl Med* 1982;23:249–253.
29. Reske SN, Sauer W, Machulla HJ, et al. 15-(p-(123I)-iodophenyl)-pentadecanoic acid as a tracer of lipid metabolism: comparison with (1-14C) palmitic acid in murine tissues. *J Nucl Med* 1984;25:1335–1342.
30. Reske SN, Sauer W, Machulla HJ, et al. Metabolism of 15-(p-(123I)-iodophenyl)-pentadecanoic acid in heart muscle and noncardiac tissue. *Eur J Nucl Med* 1985;10:228–234.
31. Caldwell JH, Martin GV, Link JM, et al. Iodophenylpentadecanoic acid-myocardial blood flow relationship during maximal exercise with coronary occlusion. *J Nucl Med* 1990;31:99–105.
32. Hansen CL, Corbett JR, Pippin JJ, et al. Iodine-123 phenylpentadecanoic acid and single-photon emission computed tomography in identifying left ventricular regional metabolic abnormalities in patients with coronary heart disease: comparison with thallium-201 myocardial tomography. *J Am Coll Cardiol* 1988;12:78–87.
33. Kennedy PL, Corbett JR, Kulkarni PV, et al. Iodine 123-phenylpentadecanoic acid myocardial scintigraphy: usefulness in the identification of myocardial ischemia. *Circulation* 1986;74:1007–1015.
34. Wieler H, Kaiser KP, Frank J, et al. Standardized non-invasive assessment of myocardial free fatty acid kinetics by means of 15-(para-iodophenyl) petadecanoic acid (123I-pPPA) scintigraphy. I. Method. *Nucl Med Commun* 1990;11:856–878.
35. Wieler H, Kaiser KP, Frank J, et al. Standardized non-invasive assessment of myocardial free fatty acid kinetics by means of 15-(para-iodophenyl) petadecanoic acid (123I-pPPA) scintigraphy. II. Clinical results. *Nucl Med Commun* 1992;13:165–185.
36. Kuikka JT, Mussalo H, Hietakorpi S, et al. Evaluation of myocardial viability with technetium-99m hexakis-2-methoxyisonitrile isonitrile and iodine-123 phenyl-pentadecanoic acid and single photon emission tomography. *Eur J Nucl Med* 1992;19:882–889.
37. Murray G, Schad N, Ladd W, et al. Metabolic cardiac imaging in severe coronary disease: assessment of viability with iodine-123-iodophenylpentadecanoic acid and multicrystal camera, and coronary relation with biopsy. *J Nucl Med* 1992;33:1269–1277.
38. Murray G, Schad N, Magill HL, et al. Dynamic low dose I-123 iodophenyl-pentadecanoic acid metabolic cardiac imaging: comparison to myocardial biopsy and reinjection SPECT thallium in ischemic cardiomyopathy and cardiac transplantation. *Ann Nucl Med* 1993;7:SII79–SII85.
39. Hansen CL, Heo J, Oliner CM, et al. Prediction of improvement in left ventricular function with iodine-123-IPPA after coronary revascularization. *J Nucl Med* 1995;36:1987–1993.
40. Iskandrian AS, Power J, Cave V, et al. Assessment of myocardial viability by dynamic tomographic 123I-iodophenylpentadecanoic acid imaging: comparison to rest-redistribution thallium imaging. *J Nucl Cardiol* 1995;2:101–109.
41. Antar MA, Spohr G, Herzog HH, et al. 15-(ortho-123I-phenyl)-pentadecanoic acid, a new myocardial imaging agent for clinical use. *Nucl Med Commun* 1986;7:683–696.
42. Henrich MM, Vester E, von der Lohe E, et al. The comparison of 2-18F-deoxyglucose and 15-(ortho-123I-phenyl)-pentadecanoic acid uptake in persistent defects on thallium-201 tomography in myocardial infarction. *J Nucl Med* 1991;32:1353–1357.
43. Otto CA, Brown LE, Scott AM. Radioiodinated branch-chain fatty acids: substrates for beta oxidation? *J Nucl Med* 1984;25:75–80.
44. Chouraqui P, Maddahi J, Henkin R, et al. Comparison of myocardial imaging with iodine-123-iodophenyl-9-methyl pentadecanoic acid and thallium-201 chloride for assessment of patients with exercise-induced myocardial ischemia. *J Nucl Med* 1991;32:447–452.
45. Hashimoto J, Kubo A, Iwasaki R, et al. Scintigraphic evaluation of myocardial ischaemia using a new fatty acid analogue: iodine-123-labeled 15-(p-iodophenyl)-9-(R,S)-methylpentadecanoic acid (9MPA). *Eur J Nucl Med* 1999;26:887–893.
46. Fujiwara S, Takeishi Y, Tojo T, et al. Fatty acid imaging with 123I-15-(p-Iodophenyl)-9-R,S-methylpentadecanoic acid in acute coronary syndrome. *J Nucl Med* 1999;40:1999–2006.
47. Marie PY, Karcher G, Danchin N, et al. Thallium-201 rest-reinjection and iodine-123-MIHA imaging of myocardial infarction: analysis of defect reversibility. *J Nucl Med* 1995;36:1561–1568.

48. Ambrose KR, Owen BA, Goodman MM, et al. Evaluation of the metabolism in rat heart of two new radioiodinated 3-methyl-branched fatty acid myocardial imaging agents. *Eur J Nucl Med* 1987;12:486–491.
49. Knapp FF Jr, Goodman MM, Callahan AP, et al. Radioiodinated 15-(p-iodophenyl)-3,3-dimethylpentadecanoic acid: a useful new agent to evaluate myocardial fatty acid uptake. *J Nucl Med* 1986;27:521–531.
50. Sloof GW, Visser FC, Lingen AV, et al. Evaluation of heart-to-organ ratios of 123I-BMIPP and the dimethyl-substituted 123I-DMIPP fatty acid analogue in humans. *Nucl Med Commun* 1997;18:1065–1070.
51. Tamaki N, guest ed. New radionuclide metabolic imaging agent, BMIPP. *Int J Cardiac Imaging* 1999;15(1):1–89.
52. Fujibayashi Y, Yonekura Y, Takemura Y, et al. Myocardial accumulation of iodinated beta-methyl-branched fatty acid analogue, iodine-125-15-(p-iodophenyl)-3-(R,S) methylpentadecanoic acid (BMIPP), in relation to ATP concentration. *J Nucl Med* 1990;31:1818–1822.
53. Fujibayashi Y, Yonekura Y, Tamaki N, et al. Myocardial accumulation of BMIPP in relation to ATP concentration. *Ann Nucl Med* 1993;7:15–18.
54. Fujibayashi Y, Nohara R, Hosokawa R, et al. Metabolism and kinetics of iodine-123-BMIPP in canine myocardium. *J Nucl Med* 1996;37:757–761.
55. Morishita S, Kusuoka H, Yamamichi Y, et al. Kinetics of radioiodinated species in subcellular fractions from rat hearts following administration of iodine-123-labelled 15-(p-iodophenyl)-3-(R,S) methylpentadecanoic acid (123I-BMIPP). *Eur J Nucl Med* 1996;23:383–389.
56. Yamamichi Y, Kusuoka H, Morishita K, et al. Metabolism of 123I-labeled 15-p-iodophenyl-3-(R,S)-methyl-pentadecanoic acid (BMIPP) in perfused rat heart. *J Nucl Med* 1995;36:1045–1050.
57. Hosokawa R, Nohara R, Fujibayashi Y, et al. Metabolic fate of iodine-123-BMIPP in canine myocardium after administration of etomoxir. *J Nucl Med* 1996;37:1836–1840.
58. Nohara R, Okuda K, Ogino M, et al. Evaluation of myocardial viability with iodine-123-BMIPP in a canine model. *J Nucl Med* 1996;37:1403–1407.
59. Miller DD, Gill JB, Livni E, et al. Fatty acid analogue accumulation: a marker of myocyte viability in ischemic-reperfused myocardium. *Circ Res* 1988;63:681–693.
60. Nishimura T, Sago M, Kihara K, et al. Fatty acid myocardial imaging using 123I-methyl-iodophenyl pentadecanoic acid (BMIPP): comparison of myocardial perfusion and fatty acid utilization in canine myocardial infarction (occlusion and reperfusion model). *Eur J Nucl Med* 1989;15:341–345.
61. Hosokawa R, Nohara R, Fujibayashi Y, et al. Myocardial metabolism of 123I-BMIPP in a canine model with ischemia implications of perfusion-metabolism mismatch on SPECT images in patients with ischemic heart disease. *J Nucl Med* 1999;40:471–478.
62. Kurata C, Wakabayashi Y, Shouda S, et al. Influence of blood substrate levels on myocardial kinetics of iodine-123-BMIPP. *J Nucl Med* 1997;38:1079–1084.
63. Nohara R, Hosokawa R, Hirai T, et al. Effect of metabolic substrate on BMIPP metabolism in canine myocardium. *J Nucl Med* 1998;39:1132–1137.
64. Kudoh T, Tamaki N, Magata Y, et al. Metabolism substrate with negative myocardial uptake of iodine-123-BMIPP. *J Nucl Med* 1997;38:548–553.
65. Hwang E, Yamashita A, Takemori H, et al. Absent myocardial I-123 BMIPP uptake in a family. *Ann Nucl Med* 1996;10:445–448.
66. Tanaka T, Kawamura K. Isolation of myocardial membrane long-chain fatty acid-binding protein:homology with a rat long-chain fatty acids. *J Mol Cell Cardiol* 1995;27:1613–1622.
67. Torizuka K, Yonekura Y, Nishimura T, et al. The phase 1 study of methyl-p-(123I)-iodophenyl-pentadecanoic acid (123I-BMIPP). *Kaku Igaku* 1991;28:681–690.
68. Torizuka K, Yonekura Y, Nishimura T, et al. The phase 2 study of methyl-p-(123I)-iodophenyl-pentadecanoic acid, a myocardial imaging agent for evaluating myocardial fatty acid metabolism. *Kaku Igaku* 1992;29:305–317.
69. Torizuka K, Yonekura Y, Nishimura T, et al. The phase 3 study of methyl-p-(123I)-iodophenyl-pentadecanoic acid, a myocardial imaging agent for evaluating myocardial fatty acid metabolism: a multicenter trial. *Kaku Igaku* 1992;29:413–433.

70. Kobayashi H, Kusakabe K, Momose M, et al. Evaluation of myocardial perfusion and fatty acid uptake using a single injection of iodine-123-BMIPP in patients with acute coronary syndrome. *J Nucl Med* 1998; 39:1117–1122.

71. Matsunari I, Saga T, Taki J, et al. Kinetics of iodine-123-BMIPP in patients with prior myocardial infarction: assessment with dynamic rest and stress images compared with stress thallium-201 SPECT. *J Nucl Med* 1994;35:1279–1285.

72. Tamaki N, Kawamoto M, Yonekura Y, et al. Regional metabolic abnormality in relation to perfusion and wall motion in patients with myocardial infarction: assessment with emission tomography using an iodonated branched fatty acid. *J Nucl Med* 1992;33:659–667.

73. Saito T, Yasuda T, Gold HK, et al. Differentiation of regional perfusion and fatty acid uptake in zones of myocardial injury. *Nucl Med Commun* 1991;12:663–675.

74. DeGeeter F, Franken P, Knapp FF Jr, et al. Relationship between blood flow and fatty acid metabolism in subacute myocardial infarction: a study by means of Tc-99m sestamibi and iodine-123-beta-methyl iodophenyl pentadecanoic acid. *Eur J Nucl Med* 1994;21:283–291.

75. Franken P, DeGeeter F, Dendale P, et al. Abnormal free fatty acid uptake in subacute myocardial infarction after coronary thrombolysis: correlation with wall motion and inotropic reserve. *J Nucl Med* 1994; 35:1758–1765.

76. Kawamoto M, Tamaki N, Yonekura Y, et al. Combined study with I-123 fatty acid and thallium-201 to assess ischemic myocardium. *Ann Nucl Med* 1994;8:47–54.

77. Matsunari I, Saga T, Taki J, et al. Improved myocardial fatty acid utilization after percutaneous transmural coronary angioplasty. *J Nucl Med* 1995;36:1605–1607.

78. Nakajima K, Schimizu K, Taki J, et al. Utility of iodine-123-BMIPP in the diagnosis and follow-up of vasospastic angina. *J Nucl Med* 1995; 36:1934–1940.

79. Naruse H, Arii T, Kondo T, et al. Clinical usefulness of iodine-123-labeled fatty acid imaging in patients with acute myocardial infarction. *J Nucl Cardiol* 1998;5:275–284.

80. Taki J, Nakajima K, Matsunari I, et al. Impairment of regional fatty acid uptake in relation to wall motion and thallium-201 uptake in ischemic but viable myocardium. *Eur J Nucl Med* 1995;22:1385–1392.

81. Tamaki N, Tadamura E, Kudoh T, et al. Recent advances in nuclear cardiology in the study of coronary artery disease. *Ann Nucl Med* 1997; 11:55–66.

82. Tomiguchi S, Oyama Y, Nabeshima M, et al. Quantitative evaluation of BMIPP in patients with ischemic heart disease. *Ann Nucl Med* 1993; 7:SII-107–SII-112.

83. Taki J, Nakajima K, Matsunari I, et al. Assessment of improvement of myocardial fatty acid uptake and function after revascularization using iodine-123-BMIPP. *J Nucl Med* 1997;38:1503–1510.

84. Tsubokura A, Lee JD, Shimizu H, et al. Recovery of perfusion, glucose utilization and fatty acid utilization in stunned myocardium. *J Nucl Med* 1997;38:1835–1837.

85. Furutani Y, Shiigi T, Nakamura Y, et al. Quantification of area at risk in acute myocardial infarction by tomographic imaging. *J Nucl Med* 1997;38:1875–1882.

86. Kawai Y, Tsukamoto E, Nozaki Y, et al. Use of 123I-BMIPP single-photon emission tomography to estimate areas at risk following successful revascularization in patient with acute myocardial infarction. *Eur J Nucl Med* 1998;25:1390–1395.

87. Takeishi Y, Sukekawa H, Saito H, et al. Clinical significance of decreased myocardial uptake of 123I-BMIPP in patients with stable effort angina pectoris. *Nucl Med Commun* 1995;16:1002–1008.

88. Takeishi Y, Fujiwara S, Atsumi H, et al. Iodine-123-BMIPP imaging in unstable angina: a guide for interventional therapy. *J Nucl Med* 1997; 38:1407–1411.

89. Tateno M, Tamaki N, Kudoh T, et al. Assessment of fatty acid uptake in patients with ischmeic heart disease without myocardial infarction. *J Nucl Med* 1996;37:1981–1985.

90. Tamaki N, Tadamura E, Kawamoto M, et al. Decreased uptake of iodinated branched fatty acid analog indicates metabolic alterations in ischemic myocardium. *J Nucl Med* 1995;36:1974–1980.

91. Hambye ASE, Vaerenberg MM, Dobbeleir AA, et al. Abnormal BMIPP uptake in chronically dysfunctional myocardial segments; correlation with contractile response to low-dose dobutamine. *J Nucl Med* 1998; 39:1845–1850.

92. Franken PR, Dendale P, DeGeeter F, et al. Prediction of functional outcome after myocardial infarction using BMIPP and sestamibi scintigraphy. *J Nucl Med* 1996;37:718–722.

93. Ito T, Tanouchi J, Kato J, et al. Recovery of impaired left ventricular function in patients with acute myocardial infarction is predicted by the discordance in defect size on ^{123}I-BMIPP and ^{201}Tl SPECT images. *Eur J Nucl Med* 1996;23:917–923.

94. Hashimoto A, Nakata T, Tsuchihashi K, et al. Postischemic functional recovery and BMIPP uptake after primary percutaneous transluminal coronary angioplasty in acute myocardial infarction. *Am J Cardiol* 1996;77:25–30.

95. Tamaki N, Tadamura E, Kudoh T, et al. Prognostic value of iodine-123 labelled BMIPP fatty acid analogue imaging in patients with myocardial infarction. *Eur J Nucl Med* 1996;23:272–279.

96. Nakata T, Hashimoto A, Kobayashi H, et al. Outcome significance of thallium-201 and iodine-123-BMIPP perfusion-metabolism mismatch in preinfarction angina. *J Nucl Med* 1998;39:1492–1499.

CHAPTER 21

Imaging of Myocardial Innervation

Michael W. Dae

Brain-heart interactions have been acknowledged for many years (Fig. 1). The primary route of communication between the brain and the heart is through the sympathetic nervous system. The sympathetic nervous system has profound influences on myocardial function and pathophysiology. The heart is densely innervated with sympathetic nerves, which are distributed on a regional basis. Heterogeneity of myocardial sympathetic innervation, or autonomic imbalance, has long been hypothesized as a major mechanism underlying sudden cardiac death. Recent developments in cardiac imaging have led to the ability to map abnormalities in heart innervation *in vivo*, using radiolabeled metaiodobenzylguanidine (MIBG). As a result, the pathophysiologic mechanisms relating alterations in sympathetic nerve activity to disease processess are now being explored.

REGIONAL ABNORMALITIES IN MYOCARDIAL INNERVATION

Myocardial sympathetic nerves have been shown to take up exogenously administered catecholamines. Early studies in rat hearts showed rapid accumulation of tritiated norepinephrine (1) into sympathetic nerve endings by a high affinity uptake process (uptake 1). Subsequently, a low affinity, high capacity nonneuronal uptake process was also described (uptake 2) (2). Further studies showed that the neuronally bound catecholamine was retained in storage vesicles for long periods of time, whereas the nonneuronally bound compound was rapidly metabolised and subsequently washed out of the heart at a fairly rapid rate (3). Numerous

other substances with chemical structures similar to norepinephrine have also been shown to enter sympathetic nerves (false adrenergic transmitters) (4). Metaiodobenzylguanidine (MIBG), an analogue of the false adrenergic transmitter guanethidine, was initially developed at the University of Michigan, with I-131 labeling, as a potential neuronal imaging agent for detection of pheochromocytoma (5). Subsequently, MIBG was labeled with I-123, which, due to its lower energy and more favorable radiation dosimetry than I-131, enabled cardiac imaging and was an MIBG shown to localize to the heart and other organs in several animal species and in man (6).

MIBG is thought to share similar uptake and storage mechanisms with norepinephrine (7,8), but it is not metabolized by monoamine oxidase or catechol-o-methyl transferase. Hence, MIBG localizes to myocardial sympathetic nerve endings. Numerous studies have evaluated the characteristics of MIBG uptake and its distribution in experimental models designed to alter the global and regional function of myocardial sympathetic nerves (9–13). In regionally denervated myocardium, MIBG uptake was shown to be decreased, while myocardial perfusion remained intact (Fig. 2) (11). Although MIBG is *delivered* to the myocardium by perfusion, MIBG *localization* is clearly dependent on the presence of intact sympathetic nerves. Previous studies have shown that the ability of sympathetic nerves to take up radiolabeled catecolamines is a more sensitive indicator of intact neuronal function than is myocardial norepinephrine content (14). Studies in the transplanted human heart have shown an absence of MIBG uptake within the first 4 months after surgery, consistent with global denervation (10). Repeat studies at 1 year following surgery showed a return of MIBG

M. W. Dae: Department of Radiology, University of California–San Francisco, San Francisco, California 94143.

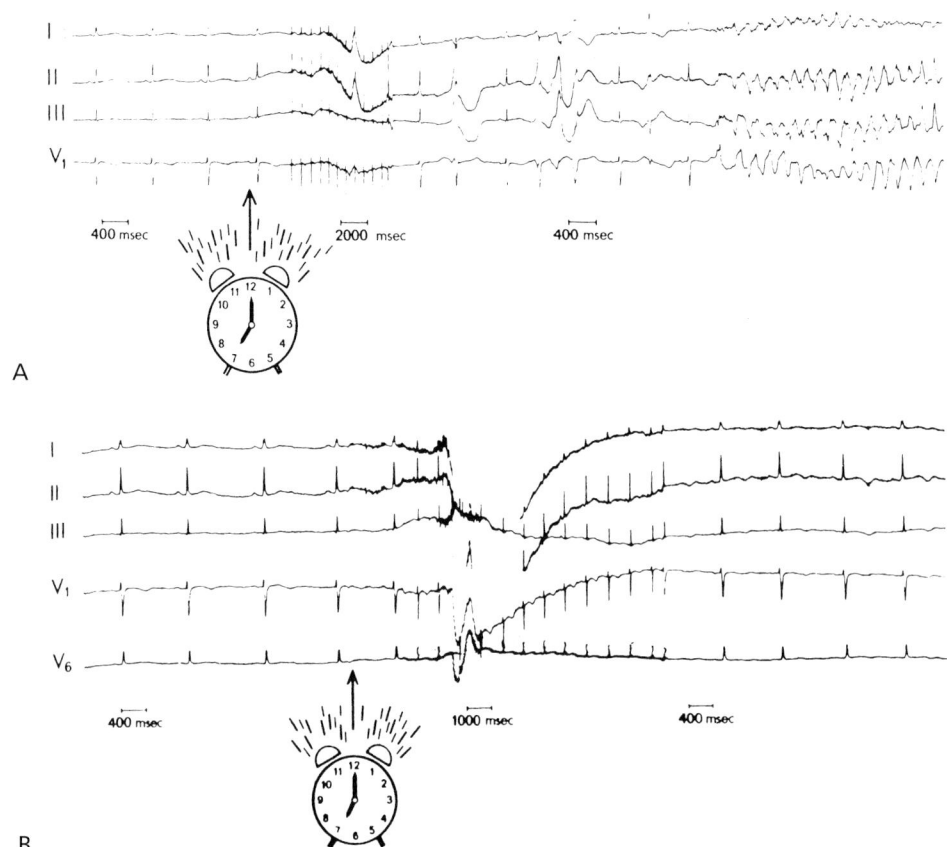

FIG. 1. A: The initiation of ventricular fibrillation in a patient following an auditory stimulus (alarm clock). **B:** After propranalol therapy, no ectopy occurs following the auditory stimulus. (From ref. 59, with permission.)

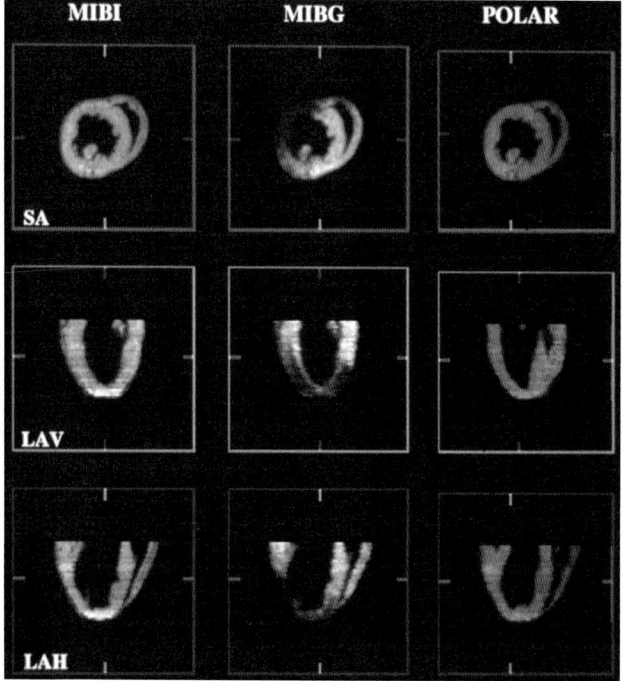

FIG. 2. Shown are autoradiographs of metaiodobenzylguanidine (*MIBG*) and sestamibi (*MIBI*) in the short axis, and vertical and horizontal long axes from a rabbit heart with regional denervation produced by the application of phenol to the epicardial surface. A defect is present in the MIBG image in a region that is well perfused in the MIBI image. The color functional map shows the reduced MIBG relative to perfusion as yellow to green. Normally innervated myocardium is shown in red. *LAH*, long axis horizontal; *LAV*, long axis vertical; *SA*, short axis.

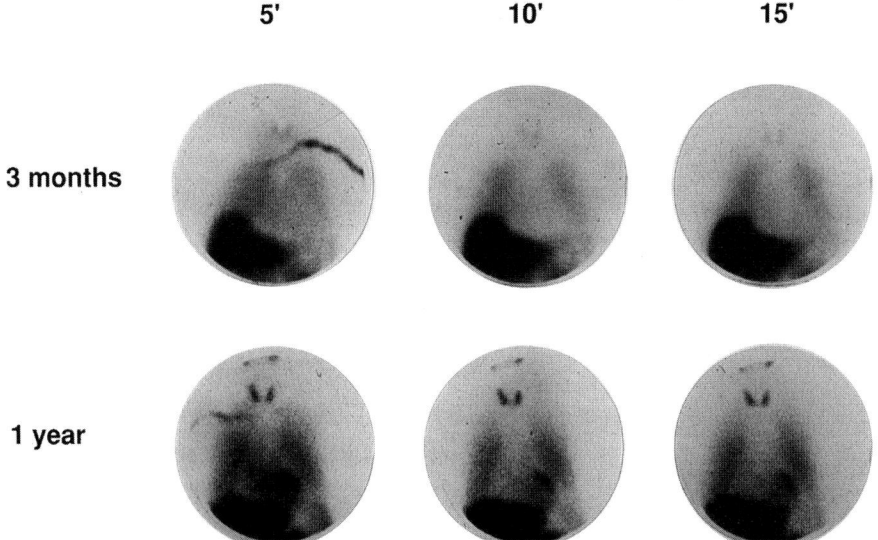

FIG. 3. Metaiodobenzylguanidine (*MIBG*) images from a patient studied at 3 months and 1 year after transplantation. There is an absence of MIBG myocardial localization at 3 months. One year after transplantation, MIBG uptake is present in the anterior wall of the left ventricle. *S/P*, status post. (From ref. 15, with permission.)

uptake in about 50% of patients, consistent with reinnervation (15) (Fig. 3).

Myocardial Ischemia

The sympathetic nerves are acutely affected in regions of myocardial ischemia. Enhanced washout of MIBG has been demonstrated from the ischemic territory. It has been shown that the release of MIBG is not due to reflex neural increases in sympathetic tone during myocardial ischemia, but to local release from sympathetic nerve endings in the ischemic bed (16). It has been demonstrated that transmural myocardial infarction can lead to a partially denervated ventricle (17), which may predispose the heart to arrhythmia (18). In experimental myocardial infarction, the relative uptake of MIBG shows a spectrum: no uptake in the center of an infarct in regions with no flow and relatively decreased (but not absent) MIBG uptake in the border zone of an infarct. This border zone with decreased uptake may be transmural or nontransmural.

The mechanisms leading to denervation in transmural and nontransmural infarction may be different. Transmural myocardial infarction has been hypothesized to produce denervation secondary to necrosis of proximal sympathetic nerve trunks, which travel in the subepicardium (17). Viable myocardium distal to the infarction but in the distribution area of a necrotic nerve trunk becomes denervated as a result of loss of proximal nerve input. In contrast to the distal denervation produced by transmural myocardial infarction, nontransmural infarction appears to lead to local ischemic damage of sympathetic nerve endings that are present within the ischemic zone, but not the nerve trunk. Studies of non-

transmural infarction produced by intracoronary balloon occlusion, which avoids denervation, due to injury of perivascular sympathetic nerves, confirmed that nontransmural myocardial infarction can produce regional denervation (Fig. 4). These studies also suggested that ischemia sufficient to cause some myocardial necrosis is necessary before regional denervation develops (16). As outlined in Figure 4, the scintigraphic pattern of regionally reduced MIBG uptake is associated with a number of biochemical, structural, and physiological changes.

Partial denervation has been shown to occur in humans after myocardial infarction (19–22). Stanton et al. (20) found a relationship between the presence of sympathetic denervation and the occurence of spontaneous ventricular tachyarrhythmias, although this relationship has not been observed in sustained ventricular tachycardia induced at electrophysiologic testing.

Diabetic Neuropathy

Recent studies have shown regional myocardial MIBG uptake abnormalities in diabetic neuropathy (23). Diabetic rats have shown reduced uptake of MIBG, which was reversed with early insulin or aldose reductase inhibitor therapy (24). The aldose reductase inhibitor improved MIBG uptake without improving glucose regulation, implying a direct neuropathy. In newly diagnosed diabetic patients, 77% have evidence of regionally reduced myocardial MIBG uptake, consistent with neuropathy (25). It is interesting that a partial restoration of MIBG abnormalities were shown at 1 year following intense metabolic control (25). In diabetic patients, assessment of MIBG uptake may be the most accurate and objective measure of autonomic dysfunction (25).

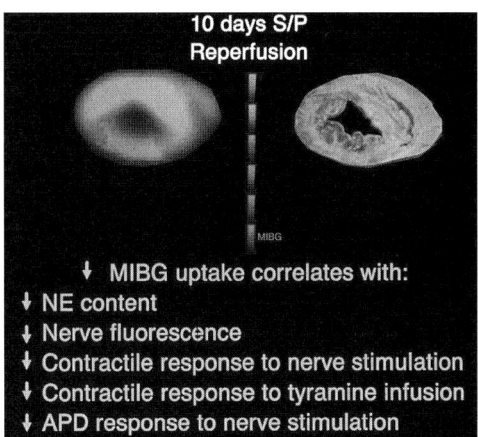

10 days S/P Reperfusion

↓ MIBG uptake correlates with:
↓ NE content
↓ Nerve fluorescence
↓ Contractile response to nerve stimulation
↓ Contractile response to tyramine infusion
↓ APD response to nerve stimulation

FIG. 4. Myocardial slice from a dog studied 10 days following intracoronary occlusion and reperfusion (**right**), and the corresponding dual-isotope functional map (**left**). There is an area of subendocardial necrosis, with morphologically normal-appearing myocardium at the mid-to-epicardial territory. This area is denervated on the functional map (yellow color). Experimental findings in regions with scintigraphic evidence of denervation are described. *APD*, action potential duration; *MIBG*, metaiodobenzylguanidine; *NE*, norepinephrine; *S/P*, status post.

Regional Innervation and Arrhythmogenesis

Schwartz (26) demonstrated that stimulation of the left stellate ganglion or removal of the right stellate ganglion lowered the ventricular fibrillation threshold. In contrast, stimulation of the right stellate ganglion or removal of the left stellate ganglion raised the ventricular fibrillation threshold (27). Randall et al. (28) demonstrated an increased incidence of spontaneous junctional and ventricular arrhythmias, particularly during exercise following partial denervation of the heart in which there was sparing of the ventrolateral cardiac nerve. These early studies led to the concept that heterogeneity of sympathetic innervation, or "sympathetic imbalance" could adversely affect the electrical stability of the heart (29).

Minardo et al. (30) correlated MIBG scintigraphy with electrophysiologic responses to sympathetic stimulation in dogs with myocardial infarction. During sympathetic stimulation, areas of viable myocardium with diminished MIBG uptake showed reduced shortening of effective refractory period compared to normal basal myocardium. However, during norepinephrine infusion, enhanced shortening of effective refractory period was found in the regions showing reduced MIBG uptake, indicating supersentivity of the denervated regions. MIBG images returned to normal a mean of 14 weeks after infarction, consistent with reinnervation. Other studies have shown increased susceptibility to induced ventricular fibrillation or ventricular tachycardia in dogs with myocardial infarction and denervation (18,31). We demonstrated dispersion of refractoriness in dogs with regional denervation following myocardial infarction (32), providing further confirmation of the electrophysiological significance of scintigraphic denervation.

Several recent clinical studies have shown regional heterogeneity of MIBG uptake in patients with ventricular tachycardia (VT) and a "clinically normal heart" (33,34). In the report by Gill et al. (34), patients with VT had a higher proportion of asymmetrical MIBG scans (47%) than subjects in the control group (0%). Sixty-two percent of patients with exercise-induced VT and clinically normal hearts had asymmetric MIBG scans with a tendency toward reduced MIBG uptake in the septum. We recently observed heterogeneous sympathetic innervation in a population of German shepherd dogs with inherited spontaneous ventricular arrhythmias and sudden death (35). In a study of patients with arrhythmogenic right ventricular cardiomyopathy (ARVC), 40 of 48 patients showed regional reductions of MIBG uptake located primarily in the basal posteroseptal left ventricle (36). All of the patients in the control group showed homogeneous innervation. Abnormalities in MIBG scintigraphy in patients with ARVC correlated with the site of origin of ventricular tachycardia, demonstrating regionally reduced uptake in 36 of 38 patients with right ventricular outflow tract tachycardia. The authors speculated that a supersensitivity related to regional sympathetic denervation may be the underlying mechanism explaining the frequent provocation of ventricular arrhythmias by exercise or catecholamine infusion. Abnormal MIBG uptake has also been found in patients with idiopathic ventricular tachycardia (37). Dispersion of regional innervation (38) and repolarization (39) have been identified in patients with dilated cardiomyopathy as well.

GLOBAL ABNORMALITIES IN MYOCARDIAL INNERVATION

One of the early physiologic responses to counteract depressed myocardial function is activation of a number of neurohumoral systems, such as the renin-angiotensin system, the sympathetic nervous system, and the arginine vasopressin system (40). It is now widely accepted that excessive stimulation of these compensatory systems eventually leads to deterioration of ventricular function and may contribute to sudden cardiac death (41). It has been suggested that sustained activation of the sympathetic nervous system plays a major role in the etiology of sudden cardiac death (42). More than 300,000 sudden cardiac deaths occur each year in the United States, accounting for 50% of all cardiac-related mortality (43). The majority of these deaths occur in patients with prior healed myocardial infarctions and left ventricular dysfunction (44). Many of these deaths originate as ventricular tachycardia, which may degenerate into ventricular fibrillation. In these circumstances, there is usually no associated evidence for either acute infarction or significant ischemia (44). Arrhythmia and sudden death are also important features of noncoronary cardiomyopathy and heart failure. Approximately 40% of patients with severe heart failure die suddenly, presumably of arrhythmia (45). The incidence of sudden death has been shown to correlate directly with both the extent of myocardial damage after infarction and the presence of complex spontaneous ventricular ectopy (46,47). Compelling evidence has emerged that implicates the sympathetic nervous system in the genesis of ventricular arrhythmias and sudden death. Beta blocker therapy has been shown to reduce the incidence of total and sudden death in patients with myocardial infarction (48). Beta blockers have been found to be particularly useful in decreasing the incidence of sudden death in patients with myocardial infarction and left ventricular dysfunction (49). Elevated plasma catecholamines have been shown to identify patients with heart failure who are also at risk for sudden death (50). Recent data showed significantly greater activation of myocardial sympathetic nerves in patients with left ventricular dysfunction and life-threatening ventricular arrhythmias compared to age-matched controls without a history of arrhythmia (42).

Dynamic Assessment of Sympathetic Nerve Activity

Myocardial MIBG imaging may play a role in detecting sympathetic nervous system activation. In experimental studies, acute changes in adrenergic nerve activity of the heart have been assessed by measuring the rates of loss of neuronally bound MIBG. Sisson et al. (51) compared rates of loss of norepinephrine and MIBG in rat and dog hearts. They used yohimbine, an alpha-2 adrenergic receptor antagonist, to increase the function of the sympathetic nerves and clonidine, an alpha-2 agonist, to decrease the activity of the sympathetic nerves. In rat hearts, yohimbine induced similar increases in rates of loss of 3H-NE and I-125 MIBG; while clonidine induced similar decreases in rates of loss of 3H-NE and I-125 MIBG. Preliminary imaging studies in dog hearts with I-123 MIBG showed similar responses to yohimbine and clonidine. These results suggest that it may be possible to assess acute changes in efferent sympathetic activity to the heart, noninvasively.

Although no studies have been reported to date in human hearts that compare MIBG washout kinetics to generally accepted standards for increased sympathetic tone, such as norepinephrine spillover (52), a number of clinical conditions thought to be associated with increased sympathetic tone have demonstrated enhanced washout of MIBG. Henderson et al. studied the myocardial distribution and kinetics of MIBG in images obtained from patients with congestive cardiomyopathy compared to normal controls (38). Patients with congestive cardiomyopathy had a 28% washout rate of MIBG from the heart over a period from 15 minutes to 85 minutes following intravenous injection, as compared to a washout rate of 6% in the controls. The differences were highly significant ($P < 0.001$). In a recent study by Nakajima et al. (53), patients with various cardiac disorders underwent planar MIBG imaging at 20 minutes and 3 hours after injection. A very high washout rate of more than 25% was frequently seen in dilated cardiomyopathy (5 of 11), hypertrophic cardiomyopathy (9 of 24), ischemic heart disease (23 of 34), essential hypertension (5 of 13), and hypothyroidism

(6 of 13). Mean washout in control patients was 9.6%. The mechanism in common in these different diseases is most likely activation of the sympathetic nervous system. It has also been shown that not all patients with the same disease have the same degree of enhanced washout

Congestive Heart Failure

Several different patterns of MIBG uptake are detectable in patients with congestive heart failure (CHF) (Fig. 5). As shown in Figure 5, patients can show good initial uptake and retention of MIBG, good initial uptake and poor retention on delayed images, or poor uptake on the initial and delayed images. The underlying mechanisms resulting in these diverse image patterns have not been well defined to date. However, enhanced washout of MIBG in congestive heart failure due to increased sympathetic tone and selective damage to sympathetic neurons in advanced disease probably play a role.

A number of studies have suggested that the degree of MIBG uptake on the delayed image carries strong prognostic information for outcome in patients with CHF. Merlet et al. (54) reported the results of a prospective study of a group of 90 patients with congestive heart failure related to idiopathic dilated cardiomyopathy. They assessed MIBG uptake, ejection fraction, cardiothoracic ratio on x-ray, and M-mode echocardiographic data and followed the patients for up to 27 months. Multivariate life-table analysis showed that MIBG uptake, as assessed by the myocardial-to-mediastinal count ratio on delayed anterior planar MIBG scans (4 hours after injection), was the best predictor for survival. Myocardial-to-mediastinal ratio on delayed MIBG images has been shown to correlate inversely with MIBG washout (53). Imamura et al. (55) recently demonstrated that the level of myocardial MIBG washout was related to the severity of heart failure, as measured by New York Heart Association classification. These interesting results suggest that there may be a significant role for MIBG imaging in the assessment of prognosis in patients with heart failure. Nakata et al. (56) evaluated the ability of MIBG imaging to predict cardiac death in failing and nonfailing hearts. They studied 414 consecutive patients—42% with symptomatic heart failure—and followed the patients for a mean period of 22 months. Among an extensive list of clinical variables that were evaluated for each patient, the late myocardial to mediastinal MIBG uptake ratio was the most powerful predictor of cardiac death. Further, the most powerful incremental prognostic variables were obtained by using MIBG imaging in combination with conventional clinical variables (56).

Other recent studies have shown the value of MIBG imaging in predicting the response to antiadrenergic therapy in patients with CHF (57,58). Suwa et al. (58) performed MIBG imaging in 45 patients with dilated cardiomyopathy before the start of bisoprolol. They measured the heart to mediastinal MIBG uptake ratio on initial and delayed images,

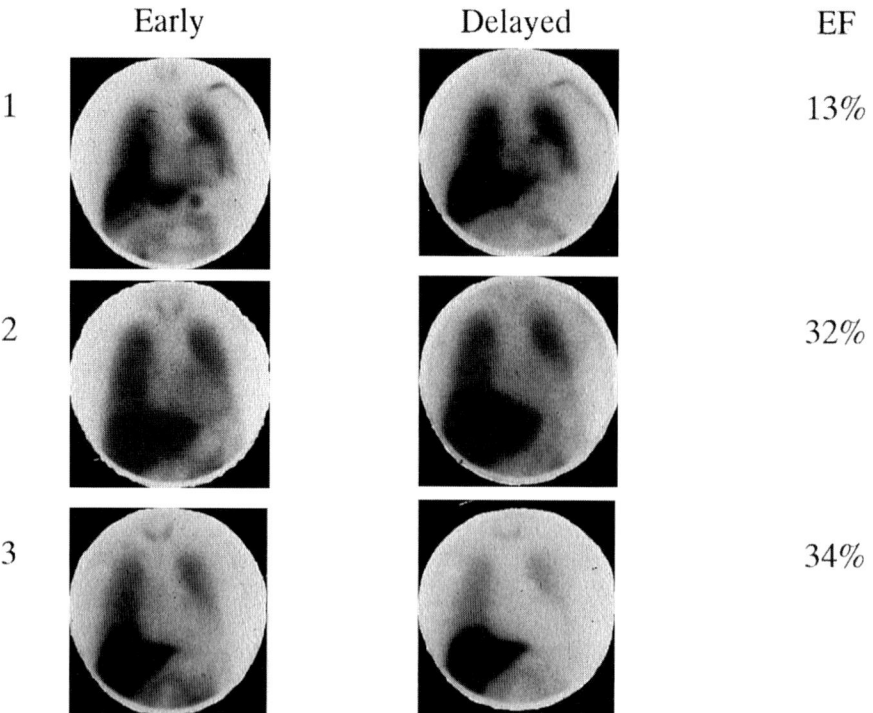

Early   Delayed   EF

1   13%

2   32%

3   34%

FIG. 5. Metaiodobenzylguanidine—congestive heart failure. Shown are *early* (15 minutes after injection) and *delayed* (3 hours after injection) images of MIBG in three patients with congestive heart failure. The corresponding ejection fractions are shown to the right.

along with MIBG washout. They showed that the heart-to-mediastinal ratio on delayed images provided a useful indication of whether patients with dilated cardiomyopathy would respond to therapy (Fig. 6). Further studies involving larger numbers of patients are needed to evaluate the prognostic utility of MIBG uptake and washout kinetics.

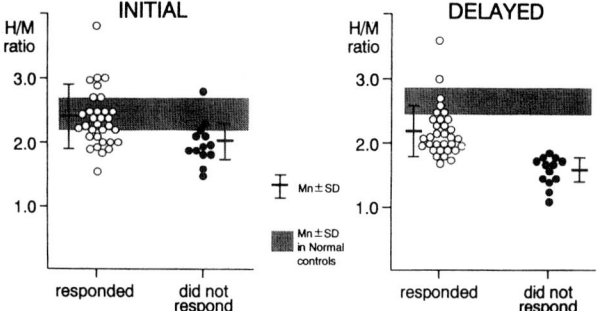

FIG. 6. Shown are heart-to-mediastinal (*H/M*) ratios from initial and delayed MIBG images in patients with dilated cardiomyopathy studied at baseline, prior to beta blocker therapy. (From ref. 58, with permission.)

CONCLUSIONS

There is an increasing body of literature confirming the clinical feasibility of imaging the sympathetic innervation of the intact heart. These early studies suggest that the numerous hypotheses relating enhanced autonomic tone and autonomic imbalance to increased risk of arrhythmia and sudden death can be successfully tested. Future studies to compare functional abnormalities of the sympathetic nerves to myocardial perfusion, metabolism, and adrenergic receptor density may provide a more comprehensive understanding of the action of the autonomic nervous system in disease states. The ability to detect the distribution of innervation scintigraphically and to correlate these imaging findings with electrophysiologic assessment of vulnerability may provide important new understanding of the interaction of the sympathetic nerves and cardiac pathophysiology. In addition, MIBG imaging may provide a noninvasive means to detect patients at risk for sudden death and possibly provide a basis for more rational approaches to therapy. For heart failure patients alone, the potential clinical utility of MIBG imaging is very significant. There are over 2 million patients with heart failure in the United States, with over 400,000 new cases diagnosed annually. These patients require costly care, and the need for rational approaches to therapy is great. A host of clinical studies are currently performed to assess prognosis in patients with heart failure, including assessments of ventricular function, exercise testing, plasma norepinephrine, serum sodium, and physical examination with only moderately effective results on patient outcomes. Given the promising preliminary data described in this chapter, MIBG imaging may become a highly effective tool for obtaining clinically useful information to assess prognosis. For these patients, this possibility, of course, is dependent on the widespread availability of the radiopharmaceutical, the use of which has not yet become a possibility in the United States.

REFERENCES

1. Whitby LG, Axelrod J, Weil-Malherbe H. The fate of 3H-norepinephrine in animals. *J Pharm Exp Ther* 1961;132:193–201.
2. Iversen LL. Role of transmitter uptake mechanisms in synaptic neurotransmission. *Br J Pharmacol* 1971;41:571–591.
3. Lightman SL, Iversen LL. The role of uptake in the extraneuronal metabolism of catecholamines in the isolated rat heart. *Br J Pharmacol* 1969;37:638–649.
4. Kopin I. False adrenergic transmitters. *Ann Rev Pharmacol* 1968;8:377–394.
5. Wieland DM, Wu JL, Brown LE, et al. Radiolabeled adrenergic neuron-blocking agents: adrenomedullary imaging with (131-I) Iodobenzylguanidine. *J Nucl Med* 1980;21:349–353.
6. Klein RC, Swanson DP, Wieland DM, et al. Myocardial imaging in man with I-123 metaiodobenzylguanidine. *J Nucl Med* 1981;22:129–132.
7. Manger WM, Hoffman BB. Heart imaging in the diagnosis of pheochromocytoma and assessment of catecholamine uptake-teaching editorial. *J Nucl Med* 1983;24:1194–1196.
8. Wieland DM, Brown LE, Rogers WL, et al. Myocardial imaging with a radioiodinated norepinephrine storage analog. *J Nucl Med* 1981;22:22–31.
9. Sisson JC, Wieland DM, Sherman P, et al. Metaiodobenzylguanidine as an index of the adrenergic nervous system integrity and function. *J Nucl Med* 1987;28:1620–1624.
10. Dae, M, De Marco T, Botvinick E, et al. Scintigraphic assessment of MIBG uptake in globally denervated human and canine hearts-Implications for clinical studies. *J Nucl Med* 1992;33:1444–1450.
11. Dae MW, O'Connell JW, Botvinick EH, et al. Scintigraphic assessment of regional cardiac adrenergic innervation. *Circulation* 1989;79:634–644.
12. Sisson JC, Lynch JJ, Johnson J, et al. Scintigraphic detection of regional disruption of adrenergic neurons in the heart. *Am Heart J* 1988;116:67–76.
13. Mori H, Pisarri T, Aldea G, et al. Usefulness and limitations of regional cardiac sympathectomy by phenol. *Am J Physiol* 1989;257:HI523–533.
14. Tyce GM. Norepinephrine uptake as an indicator of cardiac reinnervation in dogs. *Am J Physiol* 1987;235:H289–H294.
15. De Marco T, Dae M, Yuen-Green M, et al. Iodine-123 metaiodobenzylguanidine scintigraphic assessment of the transplanted human heart: evidence for late reinnervation. *J Am Coll Cardiol* 1995;25:927–931.
16. Dae M, O'Connell J, Botvinick E, et al. Acute and chronic effects of transient myocardial ischemia on sympathetic nerve activity, density, and norepinephrine content. *Cardiovasc Res* 1995;30:270–280.
17. Barber MJ, Mueller TM, Henry DP, et al. Transmural myocardial infarction in the dog produces sympathectomy in noninfarcted myocardium. *Circulation* 1983;67:787–796.
18. Herre J, Wetstein L, Lin YL, et al. Effect of transmural versus nontransmural myocardial infarction on inducibility of ventricular arrhythmias during sympathetic stimulation. *J Am Coll Cardiol* 1988;11:414–421.
19. Dae M, Herre J, O'Connell J, et al. Scintigraphic assessment of sympathetic innervation after transmural versus nontransmural myocardial infarction. *J Am Coll Cardiol* 1991;17:1416–1423.
20. Stanton MS, Tuli MM, Radtke NL, et al. Regional sympathetic denervation after myocardial infarction in humans detected noninvasively using I-123-metaiodobenzylguanidine. *J Am Coll Cardiol* 1989;14:1519–1526.
21. McGhie A, Corbett J, Akers M, et al. Regional cardiac adrenergic

function using I-123 meta-iodobenzylguanidine tomographic imaging after acute myocardial infarction. *Am J Cardiol* 1991;67:236–242.
22. Tomoda J, Yoshioka K, Shiina Y, et al. Regional sympathetic denervation detected by iodine 123 metaiodobenzylguanidine in non-W-wave myocardial infarction and unstable angina. *Am Heart J* 1994;128:452–458.
23. Langer A, Freeman M, Josse R, et al. Metaiodobenzylguanidine imaging in diabetes mellitus: assessment of cardiac sympathetic denervation and its relation to autonomic dysfunction and silent myocardial ischemia. *J Am Coll Cardiol* 1995;25:610–618.
24. Kurata C, Okayama K, Wakabayashi Y, et al. Cardiac sympathetic neuropathy and effects of aldose reductase inhibitor in streptozotocin-induced diabetic rats. *J Nucl Med* 1997;38:1677–1680.
25. Schnell O, Muhr D, Dresel S, et al. Partial restoration of scintigraphically assessed cardiac sympathetic denervation in newly diagnosed patients with insulin-dependent (type 1) diabetes mellitus at 1-year follow-up. *Diabetic Med* 1997;14:57–62.
26. Schwartz PJ, Snebold NG, Brown AM. Effects of unilateral cardiac sympathetic denervation on the ventricular fibrillation threshold. *Am J Cardiol* 1976;37:1034–1040.
27. Schwartz PJ, Stone HL, Brown AM. Effects of unilateral stellate ganglion blockade on the arrhythmias associated with coronary occlusion. *Am Heart J* 1976;92:589–599.
28. Randall WC, Kaye MP, Hageman GR, et al. Cardiac arrhythmias in the conscious dog following surgially induced autonomic imbalance. *Am J Cardiol* 1976;38:178–183.
29. Schwartz PJ. Sympathetic imbalance and cardiac arrhythmias. In: Randall WC, ed. *Nervous control of cardiovascular function*. New York: Oxford University Press, 1984:225–252.
30. Minardo JD, Tuli MM, Mock BH, et al. Scintigraphic and electrophysiologic evidence of canine myocardial sympathetic denervation and reinnervation produced by myocardial infarction or phenol application. *Circulation* 1988;78:1008–1019.
31. Inoue H, Zipes D. Results of sympathetic denervation in the canine heart: supersensitivity that may be arrhythmogenic. *Circulation* 1987;75:877–887.
32. Newman D, Munoz L, Chin M, et al. Effects of canine myocardial infarction on sympathetic efferent neuronal function: scintigraphic and electrophysiologic correlates. *Am Heart J* 1993;126:1106–1112.
33. Mitrani R, Klein L, Miles W, et al. Regional cardiac sympathetic denervation in patients with ventricular tachycardia in the absence of coronary artery disease. *J Am Coll Cardiol* 1993;22:1344–1353.
34. Gill J, Hunter G, Gane J, et al. Asymmetry of cardiac 123I metaiodobenzylguanidine scans in patients with ventricular tachycardia and a "clinically normal" heart. *Br Heart J* 1993;69:6–13.
35. Dae M, Lee R, Ursell P, et al. Heterogeneous sympathetic innervation in German shepherd dogs with inherited ventricular arrhythmia and sudden cardiac death. *Circulation* 1997;96:1337–1342.
36. Wichter T, Hindricks G, Lerch H, et al. Regional myocardial sympathetic dysinnervation in arrhythmogenic right ventricular cardiomyopathy-an analysis using 123 I-meta-iodobenzylguanidine scintigraphy. *Circulation* 1994;89:667–683.
37. Schafers M, Wichter T, Lerch H, et al. Cardiac ^{123}I-MIBG uptake in idiopathic ventricular tachycardia and fibrillation. *J Nucl Med* 1999;40:1–45.
38. Henderson, EB, Kahn JK, Corbett, et al. Abnormal I-123 metaidobenzylguanidine myocardial washout and distribution may reflect myocardial adrenergic derangement in patients with congestive cardiomyopathy. *Circulation* 1988;78:1192–1199.
39. Tomaselli G, Beuckelmann D, Calkins H, et al. Sudden cardiac death in heart failure: the role of abnormal repolarization. *Circulation* 1994;90:2534–2539.
40. Consensus Trial Study Group. Effects of enalapril on mortality in severe congestive heart failure. *N Engl J Med* 1986;316:1429–1435.
41. Eichhorn E, Hjalmarson A. Beta-blocker treatment for chronic heart failure. *Circulation* 1994;90:2153–2156.
42. Meredith I, Broughton A, Jennings G, et al. Evidence of a selective increase in cardiac sympathetic activity in patients with sustained ventricular arrhythmias. *N Engl J Med* 1991;325:618–624.
43. Myerburg R, Kessler K, Castellanos A. Sudden cardiac death: structure, function, and time-dependence of risk. *Circulation* 1992;85:I-2–10.
44. Hurwitz J, Josephson M. Sudden cardiac death in patients with chronic coronary heart disease. *Circulation* 1992;85:I-43–49.
45. Francis G. Development of arrhythmias in the patient with congestive

heart failure: pathophysiology, prevalence, and prognosis. *Am J Cardiol* 1986;57:3B–7B.

46a. Follansbe W, Michelson E, Morganroth J. Nonsustained ventricular tachycardia in ambulatory patients: characteristics and association with sudden cardiac death. *Ann Intern Med* 1980;92:741–752.

47. Gang E, Bigger J, Livell F. A model of chronic arrhythmias: the relationship between electrically inducible ventricular tachycardia, ventricular fibrillation threshold, and myocardial infarct size. *Am J Cardiol* 1982;50:469–477.

48. Yusuf S, Peto R, Lewis J, et al. Beta-blockade during and after myocardial infarction: an overview of the randomized trials. *Prog Cardiovasc Dis* 1985;25:335–371.

49. Chadda K, Goldstein S, Byington R, et al. Effect of propranalol after acute myocardial infarction in patients with congestive heart failure. *Circulation* 1986;73:503–510.

50. Cohn J, Levine T, Olivari M, et al. Plasma norepinephrine as a guide to prognosis in patients with chronic congestive heart failure. *N Engl J Med* 1984;311:819–823.

51. Sisson J, Bolgas G, Johnson J. Measuring acute changes in adrenergic nerve activity of the heart in the living animal. *Am Heart J* 1991;121:1119–1123.

52. Kingwell B, Thompson J, Kaye D, et al. Heart rate spectral analysis, cardiac norepinephrine spillover, and muscle sympathetic nerve activity during human sympathetic nervous activation and failure. *Circulation* 1994;90:234–240.

53. Nakajima K, Taki J, Tonami N, et al. Decreased 123-I MIBG uptake and increased clearance in various cardiac diseases. *Nucl Med Commun* 1994;15:317–323.

54. Merlet P, Valette H, Dubois R, et al. Prognostic valve of cardiac metaiodobenzylguanidine imaging in patients with heart failure. *J Nucl Med* 1992;33:471–477.

55. Imamura Y, Ando H, Mitsuoka W, et al. Iodine-123 metaiodobenzylguanidine images reflect intense myocardial adrenergic nervous activity in congestive heart failure independent of underlying cause. *J Am Coll Cardiol* 1995;26:1594–1599.

56. Nakata T, Miyamoto K, Doe A, et al. Cardiac death prediction and impaired cardiac sympathetic innervation assessed by MIBG in patients with failing and nonfailing hearts. *J Nucl Cardiol* 1998;5:579–590.

57. Fukukoa S, Hayashida K, Hirose Y, et al. Use of iodine-123 metaiodobenzylguanidine myocardial imaging to predict the effectiveness of β-blocker therapy in patients with dilated cardiomyopathy. *Eur J Nucl Med* 1997;24:523–529.

58. Suwa M, Otake Y, Moriguchi A, et al. Iodine-123 metaiodobenzylguanidine myocardial scintigraphy for prediction of response to β-blocker therapy in patients with dilated cardiomyopathy. *Am Heart J* 1997;133:353–358.

59. Wellens HJ, Vermeulen A, Durrer D. Ventricular fibrillation occurring on arousal from sleep by auditory stimuli. *Circulation* 1972;46:661–665.

CHAPTER 22

Future Perspectives

Guido Germano and Daniel S. Berman

Future advances in nuclear cardiology can be generically grouped in the following five categories: (i) radiopharmaceuticals, (ii) hardware and instrumentation, (iii) acquisition protocols. (iv) software, and (v) clinical applications. This chapter is meant to be a brief review of current and anticipated developments in those areas.

RADIOPHARMACEUTICALS

First introduced in the early 1970s (1), 201-thallium (Tl-201) was for many years the radionuclide of choice for clinical assessment of myocardial perfusion, with its use steadily increasing together with the number of perfusion studies performed in the United States. In the 1990s, 99m-technetium (Tc-99m) myocardial perfusion agents became available. Their use is growing, and, in 1996, the number of studies utilizing Tc-99m-based agents surpassed that of Tl-201 studies. It is expected that this trend toward increased use of the Tc-99m myocardial perfusion imaging agents will be maintained in the future. Several recently developed compounds, Tc-99m-sestamibi (2–4), Tc-99m-tetrofosmin (5), Tc-99m-furifosmin (Q12) (6), Tc-99m-Q3 (7), and Tc-99m-NOET (8) all benefit from Tc-99m's physical characteristics (i.e., higher injectable dose and higher photon energy), which make them better suited for SPECT imaging compared to Tl-201 (9). Among the Tc-99m-based agents, Tc-99m-NOET has been shown to undergo redistribution in ani-

mal models and in humans, and therefore represents a potential direct alternative to Tl-201. As noted in Chapter 13, Tc-99m teboroxime, while having very favorable initial uptake characteristics even at high flow rates, washes out very rapidly from the myocardium, making it more difficult to use on a routine clinical basis than the other Tc-99m myocardial perfusion agents or Tl-201.

It has not been clearly established that Tc-99m-based agents will eventually replace 201-Tl. With the exception of 150-H_2O and possibly Tc-99m teboroxime, Tl-201 has the highest and most linear extraction as a function of flow across the broadest flow range (Fig. 1), and is also widely considered the single-photon tracer of choice for the assessment of myocardial viability.

Regarding myocardial viability, a theoretical concern over the Tc-99m myocardial perfusion agents is related to their lack of redistribution over time (with the exception of Tc-99m NOET and teboroxime). Thus, the possibility of these agents underestimating myocardial viability in the presence of severe hibernation remains a clinical concern. In the future, broader use of nitroglycerin to reduce flow differences in the hibernating and normal zones prior to rest injection may increase the acceptance of the Tc-99m agents as excellent standards of myocardial viability measurement.

The future clinical role of positron emitting radiopharmaceuticals in nuclear cardiology is less clear. For example, 18F-FDG (fluorodeoxyglucose) is generally considered to be the "gold standard" for myocardial viability and can now be imaged with single photon emission computed tomography (SPECT) instrumentation, either utilizing 511 keV collimators (10), or modifying the SPECT camera's front end to make it capable of coincidence detection (10). To date, a systematic and comprehensive comparison of the relative clinical effectiveness of Tl-201 and 18F-FDG protocols has not been accomplished, and the potential of attenuation cor-

G. Germano: Department of Radiological Sciences, University of California–Los Angeles School of Medicine, Los Angeles, California 90024; Department of Medicine, Cedars-Sinai Medical Center, Los Angeles, California 90048.

D. S. Berman: University of California–Los Angeles School of Medicine, Los Angeles, California 90025; Department of Imaging/Nuclear Medicine, Cedars-Sinai Medical Center, Los Angeles, California 90048.

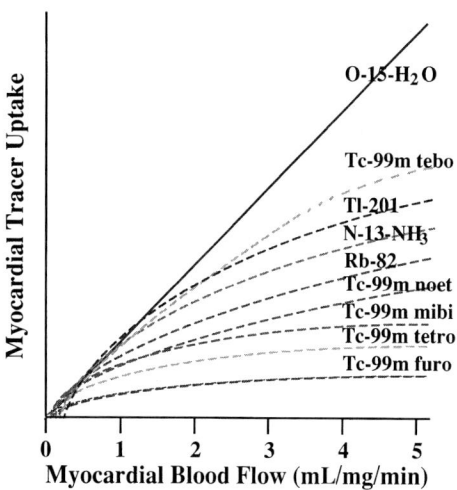

FIG. 1. Diagrammatic illustration of the theoretical relationship between myocardial tracer uptake and myocardial blood flow for the available radiopharmaceuticals.

rection, which may be of particular importance in patients with large ventricles who are commonly assessed for myocardial viability, has not yet been realized. We consider it is likely that the frequency of use of positron emitting tracers in the assessment of viability will strongly depend on availability and cost, since the differences in clinical efficacy have been small and may be reduced over time. In both those respects, 18F-FDG is at a distinct disadvantage, since it either (i) requires the presence of a cyclotron on site, or (ii) needs to be purchased from a regional distribution center within a 100-mile radius of the imaging site, at a current cost of about 10 times that of Tl-201.

As discussed in Chapter 15, rubidium-82 (Rb-82) has been proposed as a cost-effective method for detection of coronary artery disease in patients with moderate elevation of pretest likelihood of coronary artery disease. Since the extraction of positron emitting agents rolls off as a function of flow in a manner similar to that observed with Tl-201, it is likely that the reported differences in sensitivity and specificity with the PET tracers compared to SPECT are due principally to improved methods for attenuation correction with PET. As effective attenuation correction approaches with SPECT become available (see below), it is likely that these differences between PET and SPECT will diminish. While the higher costs of PET radiopharmaceuticals remain coupled to the higher costs of PET equipment, it appears unlikely that PET will displace the current or future uses of myocardial perfusion SPECT.

The ideal myocardial perfusion agent of the future should be of low cost, easy to prepare, and based on a generator-produced rather than cyclotron-produced isotope. The isotope's physical half-life should be as short or shorter and its isotopic energy as high or higher than that of Tc-99m (6 hours and 140 keV, respectively). The myocardial extraction fraction should be such that high relative concentrations in the myocardium can be achieved across the full range of

achievable flow rates. The dosimetry should be favorable, and there should be low lung and liver uptake. The tracer should be fixed in its distribution in the myocardium in proportion to flow (i.e., no back diffusion or redistribution). Although many of these characteristics are met with Tc-99m sestamibi and Tc-99m tetrofosmin, the full potential of the SPECT perfusion tracers has not been realized, due to the relatively low extraction fractions even at rest and the marked roll-off of extraction that occurs with these tracers at high flow rates, resulting in limitations in the definition of lesions of hemodynamic significance in the range of 50 to 75% obstruction. If nuclear cardiology is to compete favorably with other noninvasive imaging methods, the development of a tracer with more ideal flow-related characteristics across the spectrum of flow is needed.

A fundamental advantage of nuclear methods over all other noninvasive imaging methods is the ability to assess metabolic processes by a tracer technique in which the fundamental biologic or physiologic process being measured is not affected by the administration of the tracer. In this respect, the full advantage of the PET compounds has only begun to be explored. Since PET allows the replacement of naturally occurring elements with their radioactive analogues, oxygen-15, nitrogen-13, and carbon-11, virtually any physiologic molecule of interest can be labeled. In the commercial world of pharmaceutical development, this technology holds promise as a cost-effective tool for documenting the biodistribution and kinetics of new pharmaceuticals. For routine clinical applications, this approach may prove to be too costly to compete with SPECT methods.

For SPECT, however, there is great, unexplored promise with respect to the development of new radiopharmaceuticals for assessing clinically relevant metabolic processes. This promise is seen most notably with I-123, a radionuclide with excellent physical properties (half-life of 13 hours and monoenergetic gamma emission at 159 keV) as well as far-reaching physiologic potential. The latter is related to the ease with which I-123 can be incorporated into a wide variety of biologically active compounds without altering their physiologic behavior, through methyl substitution by the iodine. Despite great strides made with I-123 compounds in other countries, the development of lower-cost, widely available I-123 radiopharmaceutical for assessing metabolic processes has been severely retarded in the United States.

Nonperfusion tracers that are likely to play an increasingly important clinical role include (i) markers of enervation such as 123I-metaiodobenzylguanidine (11) (see Chapter 21) and (ii) markers of fatty acid metabolism such as the 123I-labeled fatty acids 123I-IPPA (12) and 123I-BMIPP (13) (see Chapter 20). I-123 labeled compounds are also potentially of interest as thrombus and plaque imaging agents. Other agents deserving further work are (iii) infarct-avid imaging agents such as 111In-antimyosin (14) and Tc-99m-glucarate (15) (see Chapter 16), and (iv) hypoxia markers such as 18F-misonidazole (16) and Tc-99m-nitroimidazole (17).

HARDWARE AND INSTRUMENTATION

The future for SPECT cameras appears to favor the multi-detector approach. Virtually every camera manufacturer offers at least a two-detector configuration, and the majority of camera purchases in the United States have been multidetector systems since 1992. Many of the two-detector cameras are either especially built for cardiac imaging (fixed detectors at 90 degrees) or can be optimized for myocardial or general nuclear medicine imaging (interdetector angle variable from 180 degrees to 90 degrees). Multidetector cameras can help overcome the main intrinsic limitation of myocardial SPECT from an image quality standpoint, i.e., limited count statistics. However, they are more commonly employed to reduce the total acquisition time for a SPECT study and consequently increase the daily patient throughput, a trend that can be expected to continue in the medical cost containment era. Fan beam collimators are also aimed at increasing count collection efficiency (sensitivity), and they do so by magnifying the principal activity distribution and mapping it to a larger portion of the camera's detector (18). Their increased acceptance will depend on cost, ease of storage and replacement, and the compensation of truncation artifacts that may affect measured perfusion (19) and function (20).

Attenuation correction hardware is provided on many of the SPECT cameras sold today, although, in general, it is not routinely used. Most current approaches to attenuation correction are based on simultaneous emission/transmission protocols (21,22). It is generally accepted that attenuation correction should be performed in conjunction with scatter correction (23) and compensation for nonuniform resolution along the noncircular acquisition orbits (24). If a transmission source is used with energy higher than that of the emission data, correction for transmission downscatter should also be implemented (25). When trying to assess the future impact of attenuation correction on the practice of nuclear cardiology, it helps to remember that the correction's ultimate goal is that of eliminating or reducing the nonuniformity of observed regional myocardial uptake due to nonuniform tissue attenuation. This nonuniformity is certainly a function of patient sex and size, as well as isotope energy and uptake pattern; after attenuation correction, hopefully, it will be eliminated and will not also turn out to depend on the specific camera vendor's implementation of the correction. In fact, since attenuation correction produces images with uptake patterns different from the "usual" ones, it is reasonable to assume that physicians will be reluctant to "relearn" to read images until they are satisfied that the process is stable and reproducible. In this respect, cross-platform validation of different attenuation/scatter/resolution correction protocols on standard patient populations should be performed, and evidence presented that they are essentially equivalent. Key evidence to provide will be documentation that the myocardial distribution patterns in males and females will be the same as has been observed with attenuation-corrected positron emission tomography (PET). When this is achieved, quantitative image interpretation will also play a facilitating role in the transition.

An interesting development in gamma camera design is the introduction of systems with totally digital front-end electronics. This approach requires digitizing the output of each photomultiplier tube rather than their summed output, and it has the potential to yield excellent energy and spatial resolution, as well as improved uniformity. Digital cameras can estimate correction factors for scatter and isotope cross-talk by analyzing information acquired from the isotope's entire energy spectrum, not just the two or three energy windows routinely used. These correction factors are likely to be of clinical importance in the implementation of attenuation/scatter correction algorithms as well as in the generation of the accurate tissue cross-talk corrections necessary for simultaneous dual-isotope acquisition (see below). Ergonomically driven modifications to the size and shape of the imaging table would also be advisable in order to make the patient more comfortable and to reduce the occurrence of motion, which currently affects up to 20% of all cardiac SPECT studies.

Finally, nuclear medicine workstations are slowly becoming less proprietary in nature: in fact, there is an established trend toward utilizing off-the-shelf computers, which do not contain custom processing, or accelerating or graphics boards. While all camera manufacturers still install their own proprietary software on these platforms and resell them at a price much higher than the off-the-shelf hardware, they have shown an increased willingness to provide access to their image databases via DICOM servers (26) and standard image formats such as Interfile (27). This approach is made necessary by the "digitalization" of the radiology or cardiology department, of which nuclear medicine is often part. Picture and Archiving Communication Systems (PACS) will eventually be integrated with the Radiology Information Systems (RIS) or cardiology information systems and permit easy generation and electronic transmission of patient reports merging images and data. A similar process is likely in the comparison of data in the catheterization lab, nuclear lab, and patient historical records, which are likely to be significant parts of future cardiology practice. As the amount of data generated increases, loss-less or minimal-loss image compression shall be required for transmission and long-term archiving. The use of telephone lines or cable to transmit image data is likely to become much more popular as a way for small or rural hospitals to gain immediate access to the expensive expertise and technology available in larger, specialized centers, and, as a way for physicians to review, from other locations, images acquired at their hospital or clinic.

PROTOCOLS

Acquisition protocols are rapidly gaining popularity (and are likely to continue to do so in the future) that provide

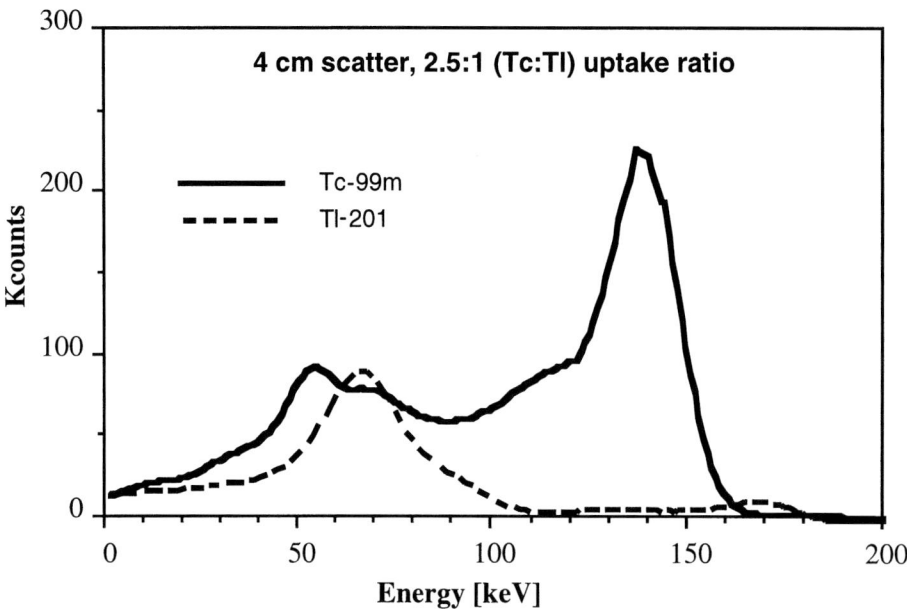

FIG. 2. Overlapping of the Tc-99m and Tl-201 energy spectra.

more information without increasing cost, or that result in time savings without a loss of accuracy. An example of this class of protocols is gated myocardial perfusion SPECT.

The attractiveness of gated SPECT lies in its ability to add accurate quantitative measurement of global and regional left ventricular function (ejection fraction, wall motion, and wall thickening) to the standard perfusion measurements, without increasing the SPECT acquisition time. While it was originally held that gated SPECT imaging would only be feasible in conjunction with Tc-99m-based agents, successful use of gated Tl-201 SPECT has been reported by many investigators, especially in conjunction with multidetector cameras (28). Moreover, the use of gated Tc-99m-sestamibi SPECT with low-dose dobutamine stress has recently been proposed as a novel and promising method to assess myocardial viability (29). The ability to perform gated SPECT acquisition in very short times has led to the investigation of protocols employing pharmacologic stressing to evaluate stress perfusion, true stress function, and poststress function using only one injection (30). In fact, in patients with no prior myocardial infarction, it may be possible to routinely forgo the resting perfusion study and simultaneously assess stress perfusion and poststress function using a single stress injection and a single tomographic acquisition (31). In summary, there is essentially no reason why most perfusion SPECT acquisitions should not be performed using the gated technique; in 1997, over 40% of all perfusion SPECT studies and over 70% of all dual-isotope perfusion SPECT performed in the United States were gated, and it is expected that these percentages will grow substantially in the future.

Separate acquisition dual isotope, rest Tl-201/stress Tc-99m-sestamibi, and Tc-99m–tetrofosmin SPECT protocols

(32) have also experienced an impressive increase in popularity; indeed, over 20% of all myocardial perfusion SPECT studies performed in the United States in 1997 used the dual isotope technique, compared to almost none in 1992. With this protocol, the entire acquisition process is completed in less than 2 hours. The Tl-201 images are uncontaminated by Tc-99m, and Tc-99m-sestamibi images are only minimally affected by the low abundance of ^{201}Tl cross-talk (33). The "simultaneous" dual isotope rest Tl-201/stress Tc-99m-sestamibi protocols would have even broader appeal, due to (i) marked increase in patient throughput (only one acquisition sequence is required), (ii) intrinsic registration of the rest and stress image sets, and (iii) reduction of motion and other artifacts (33). However, the clinical implementation of simultaneous dual-isotope studies is not currently recommended (34) due to tissue cross-talk, and will ultimately depend on the development of effective techniques to correct for Tc-99m cross-talk into the Tl-201 images (Fig. 2). These corrections will be greatly aided by truly digital cameras with full spectrum energy recording of data. To the extent that 18F-FDG achieves wider diffusion, 18F-FDG/Tc-99m-sestamibi protocols that allow to simultaneously assess cardiac perfusion and metabolism could also become more popular (10).

SOFTWARE

Current and future software developments in nuclear cardiology are likely to increase the clinical strengths of the modality. In particular, these include (i) the automation and reproducibility of processing, (ii) the ability to accurately and reproducibly quantitate a large number of cardiac parameters, and (iii) the potential for digitally merging image and

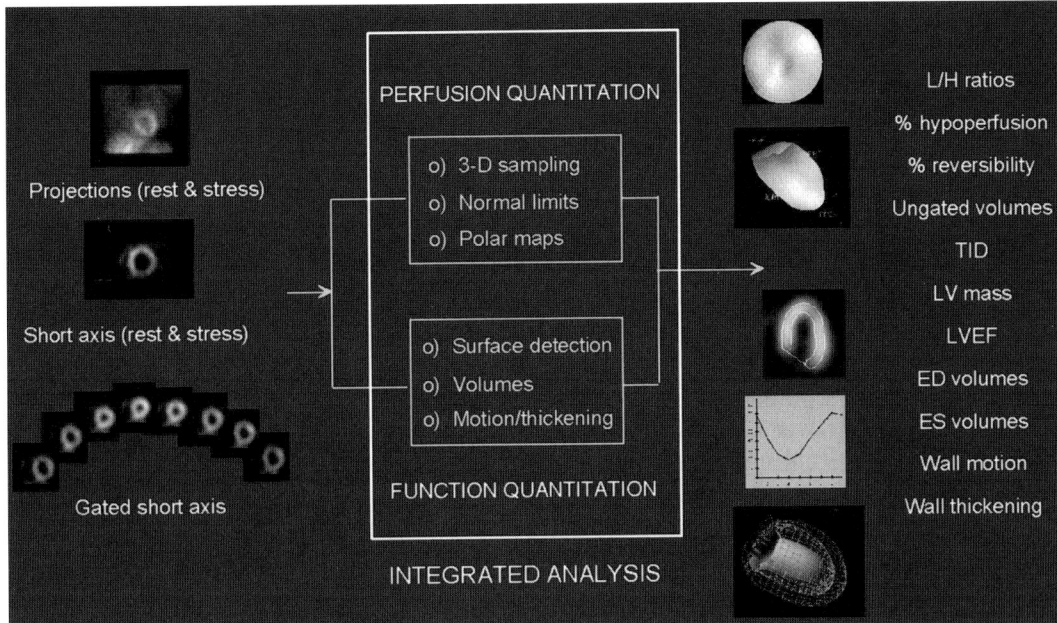

FIG. 3. Quantitative information derivable from a "separate dual isotope," rest Tl-201/stress gated Tc-99m-sestamibi SPECT protocol. *ED,* end-diastolic; *ES,* end-systolic; *H/L,* heart/lung; *LV,* left ventricle; *LVEF,* left ventricle ejection fraction; *TID,* transient ischemic dilation ratio.

text data, while at the same time automatically incorporating diagnostic and prognostic information in the final report.

The fact that automatic reconstruction and reorientation of projection images into short-axis images can promote standardization and eliminate or reduce inter- and intraobserver variability (35) is increasingly being recognized by technologists, physicians, and camera manufacturers alike. In addition, the increasing use of gated SPECT protocols has spurred the development of automatic or semiautomatic software that aims at combining several quantitative measurements of perfusion and functions (36,37). For example, quantitative cardiac parameters that are routinely, simultaneously, and automatically computed in our laboratory include lung/heart ratios (38), percent hypoperfused myocardium and percent ischemic myocardium (39–41), left ventricle (LV) cavity volumes (42), transient ischemic dilation ratios (43), LV mass (44), end-diastolic and end-systolic volumes (45), left ventricular ejection fraction (LVEF) (46), and regional myocardial wall motion and thickening (47). All these parameters are routinely available from a rest Tl-201/stress gated Tc-99m-sestamibi SPECT study within minutes of the completion of the study (Fig. 3). The development of user-friendly, widely disseminated automatic software for the quantitation of left and right ventricular function from gated blood pool SPECT may help traditional nuclear cardiology in its fight with competing modalities (48). However, it is the combination of perfusion and function that represents nuclear cardiology's brightest future.

Overall, the improved accuracy and reproducibility intrinsic to automatic processing and analysis provides the ability to generalize clinical trial results to community centers, thus promoting the diffusion and acceptance of nuclear cardiology techniques. Even at an established institution, automatic software will probably often be superior to expert assessment for the exact measurement of small interval changes in patients undergoing medical therapy and may represent a useful teaching tool in training inexperienced readers. The next frontier for computer-aided interpretation of nuclear cardiology images will be the incorporation of clinical nonnuclear data (both images and text) in the digital algorithms, so as to generate a reliable quantitative characterization of the patient's likelihood of cardiac disease, the determination of survival probability or of risk for adverse events, and the identification of the treatment strategy most likely to achieve the clinically desired goal. Artificial intelligence-based efforts in that field will surely benefit from (i) "expert systems," or software capable of accomplishing a particular task using "rules" developed by experienced clinicians (49), and (ii) "neural networks," which, by modeling neurons and dendrites with electronic nodes and connections, have the ambitious goal of emulating the behavior of the human brain as it performs specific tasks. This ability to objectively quantify nuclear cardiology results on a routine basis provides a distinct advantage for the nuclear method over other imaging techniques.

CLINICAL APPLICATIONS

Clinical requirements for application of nuclear cardiology in patient management can be broadly summarized as follows: (i) high specificity for the absence of hard events (less than 1% annual rate of cardiac death or myocardial

CHAPTER 23

Basic Principles and Safety

Edward W. Webster

This chapter has been prepared to provide essential information for the physician regarding the nature of x-rays, their application to imaging the cardiovascular system, and their safe use in a medical environment.

X-RAY IMAGE FORMATION

The Nature of X-rays

X-rays are a relatively small part of the spectrum of electromagnetic radiation that extends from radio waves and microwaves, through the several forms of light (infrared, visible, and ultraviolet), to x-rays and gamma rays. These radiations all travel through space with the velocity of light, are characterized by wave-like oscillations of electrical and magnetic (electromagnetic) forces, and are differentiated from each other by their wavelengths (distance between oscillatory crests) and their frequency of oscillations per second.

The properties of x-rays relevant to medical use are usually explained by regarding them as particles known as *photons*, each carrying a packet of energy specified in kilo-electron-volts (keV). For diagnostic imaging applications, photon energies range from 10 to 150 keV. The photons produced by an x-ray tube cover a wide range of energies from the maximum keV (which is numerically equal to the tube kV) down to much lower energies with a mean energy 30 to 50% of the maximum keV. X-ray penetration increases with photon energy and therefore the choice of tube kV for medical purposes is often determined by the thickness of the body part being examined. However, image contrast is generally lower at higher photon energies, and this factor

may cause the same kV to be used over a range of body thickness.

Geometrical Effects

Since x-rays travel in diverging straight lines from the x-ray source (tube target), two properties of an x-ray image, namely, magnification and image sharpness, are dependent on the geometry of the x-ray projection system. Magnification M as illustrated in Figure 1, depends on the distance separating the anatomic object O and the image recording plane I. The geometric blurring (or unsharpness) B depends on the x-ray source size S and again on the distance separating O and I. Apposition between the image plane and the object is therefore advantageous. The image of the anatomy closer to the x-ray source will be less sharp than the image of the distal anatomy. Therefore, geometric ''unsharpness'' is minimized when the source-object distance (x) is maximized.

X-ray Absorption and Scattering

Diagnostic x-rays entering the body are both absorbed and scattered by two different mechanisms. Both mechanisms produce some deviation of x-rays from their original direction, which is known as scattering. Both mechanisms produce high-energy electrons in the tissue; these are absorbed locally after traveling 0.1 to 0.5 mm depending on their energy, creating atomic excitation and ionization in the tissue.

The first mechanism is photoelectric absorption in which the photon transfers its energy to an atomic orbital electron, which is then ejected from the atom, followed by the emission of light or x-rays characteristic in energy for the target atom. These emissions have very low energy for tissue elements (e.g., H, C, O, Ca) and are, therefore, also locally

E. W. Webster: Department of Radiology, Harvard University, Boston, Massachusetts 02115; Department of Radiology, Massachusetts General Hospital, Boston, Massachusetts 02114.

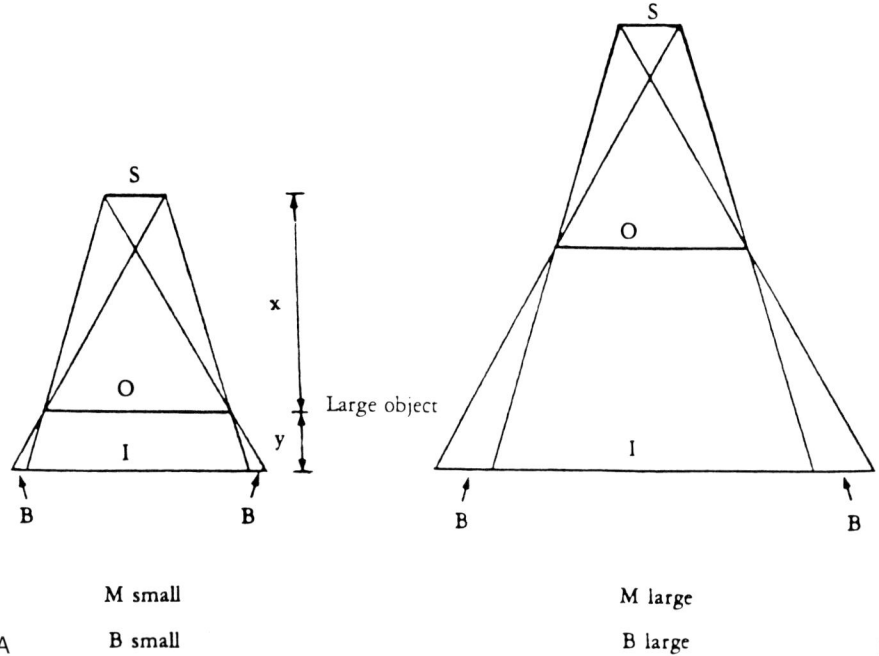

FIG. 1. Effect of distance between object and image on magnification and blurring (unsharpness or penumbra) of image. **A:** Image in close opposition to object (*y*/*x* small). **B:** Image with large separation from object (*y*/*x* large). The blurring B is proportional to *y*/*x*. (From ref. 14, with permission.)

absorbed. Photoelectric absorption of x-rays per atom of absorber increases strongly with the atomic number Z of the absorber; it is proportional to Z^3. Therefore, a heavy element such as lead (Z = 82) is a much more efficient absorber per atom than aluminum (Z = 13) by a factor of about 250; this is one reason lead is widely employed in x-ray shielding.

The second mechanism is Compton scattering, which is the most important mechanism for diverting energy (as distinct from absorbing energy) from a beam of diagnostic x-rays. In this mechanism, a photon interacts (collides) with an electron, resulting in the deflection of the photon and the transfer of some of its energy to the electron. For typical diagnostic x-ray kilovoltages there are more Compton interactions in water (i.e., in a patient) than photoelectric interactions. The scattered photons are almost as energetic as the primary radiation. They may travel in any direction: forward, sideways, or backward, and many of them escape from the body.

Compton scattering is primarily responsible for the occupational exposure of persons such as physicians and nurses near a patient during fluoroscopy. The intensity of x-rays scattered into the environment of a patient is roughly proportional to the x-ray field size.

Subject Contrast

An x-ray image of an object is created only if the x-ray transmission through the object is greater or smaller than that through the surrounding medium. The magnitude of the transmission difference is proportional to the "*subject con-*

trast" of the image. (This contrast is amplified in radiography by the photographic contrast of the recording system.) A major factor in producing subject contrast is the difference between the effective atomic number Z of the object and of its surrounding tissue. A smaller factor is the difference in the densities. The importance of the atomic number difference derives from the major role of the photoelectric absorption mechanisms for x-rays at the lower end of the diagnostic energy range 20 to 30 keV. In that range, the absorption coefficients of the elements in tissue are proportional to the cube of the atomic numbers of those elements (i.e., Z^3). For example, the absorption per gram of calcium (Z = 20) compared with oxygen (Z = 8) is 10 to 20 times greater. However, the magnitude of photoelectric absorption in water is equal to the absorption by the Compton effect at 26 keV and becomes rapidly smaller for all tissues at higher energies with consequent reduction in subject contrast. Table 1 summarizes calculations of subject contrast between tissue types each 1-cm thick with increasing photon energy, illustrating loss of contrast at higher x-ray energies. At higher energies, the photoelectric absorption in elements of higher atomic

TABLE 1. *Subject contrast between tissue types*

X-ray photon energy (keV)	Subject contrast	
	Fat/Muscle	Muscle/Bone
20	0.38	0.98
40	0.07	0.48
80	0.03	0.14

number is much greater than for elements in normal tissue, and this fact underlies the use of contrast agents in x-ray imaging. A good example is the use of iodine (Z = 53); at a photon energy of 40 keV, the absorption per gram of iodine is 44 times greater than that per gram of bone.

Image Quality

Many operating factors affect the "quality" of x-ray images. There are three principal ingredients of good image quality. These are: (i) the display of *contrast* between different objects or parts of objects, partially discussed above; (ii) the ability to exhibit the separation between details and to record an object and its internal structure sharply, i.e., *resolution*; (iii) the low level of *noise* that consists of random background image points interfering with the presentation and perception of the image.

Contrast

The "subject contrast" inherent in the image as discussed above, is degraded by the presence of scattered radiation, largely generated by Compton scattering in the patient, which reaches the recording system. The effect is analogous to that of an obscuring mist that overlaps the image and reduces both the contrast and perception of the image details. Subject contrast could be reduced by a factor of 5 or more. The intensity of scattered radiation reaching the recording system increases with the thickness of the patient, the size of the x-ray beam, and with the tube kilovoltage employed. It decreases as the distance between the patient and the recording system increases, since then some of the multidirectional scatter will "miss" the recording system. A major fraction of the scattered radiation will be removed by the use of an x-ray grid between the patient and the recording system. A grid is inserted under the x-ray table and above the recording system in radiography and is installed immediately in front of the entrance screen of the image intensifier in fluoroscopy.

The subject contrast is amplified both in radiographic and fluoroscopic recording systems by the relationship between the image display and the transmitted x-ray intensity incident on the recording system. This is true for conventional recording systems, such as the film/screen combination, and for the several types of digital systems. In the film/screen system, the radiographic film is tightly sandwiched in an x-ray cassette between two intensifying screens that have two functions: the absorption of the image-bearing x-ray beam and its conversion into light with a color matching the spectral sensitivity of the film—usually blue or green. The range of x-ray exposure received by the film/screen system is converted into a wider range of film density that enhances the original subject contrast in the x-ray beam by a "gamma

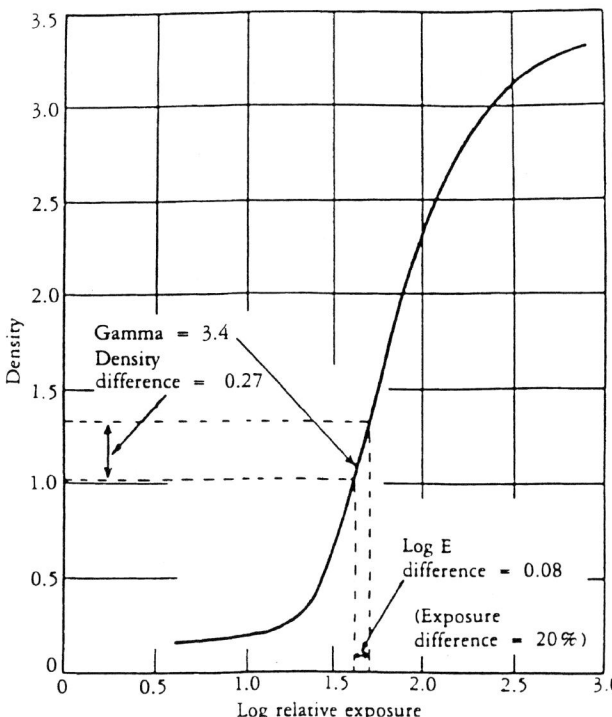

FIG. 2. Enhancement of subject contrast in radiography with intensifying screens. A logarithmic increase in x-ray exposure by 0.08 causes a film density increase of 0.27 due to the intensification factor (gamma factor) of 3.4. (From ref. 15, with permission.)

factor." This film property is illustrated in Figure 2, in which the gamma factor is 3.4 on the linear part of the curve (1). However, the use of screens in the recording system—by virtue of their thickness and granularity—degrades the image sharpness compared with that obtainable by using film alone without screens.

There are now several new digital systems for radiography where the image is formed on a new thin detector, which is scanned and read out digitally immediately after exposure (2,3). One important advantage of digital systems is the ability afforded by the digital computer to "window" regions of interest in an image and to expand the contrast of structures within a chosen region. Digital systems are also an integral part of the image receptor and storage facilities of fluoroscopic systems where digital subtraction angiography is performed (4).

Resolution

This quality factor is related to image sharpness and its converse, blur or unsharpness. It is commonly defined as the greatest number of line-pairs per millimeter in the x-ray image of a high contrast test object (bar pattern) consisting of a series of alternate bars and spaces of decreasing width, which are separately distinguishable in the image. In all x-ray imaging systems, resolution is determined by several independent system characteristics.

The first of these (discussed earlier and illustrated in Figure 1) is the "geometric" blurring due to the size of the x-ray source (the "focal spot" of the x-ray tube) and the ratio of the object-recorder distance to the source-object distance. The second is the unsharpness of the image recording system, which in conventional film/screen radiography, is mainly due to the thickness of the phosphor in the intensifying screens. In an image intensifier (see below under X-ray Imaging Equipment) the unsharpness is due to a combination of factors including the thickness of the input screen, the internal separation between the screen, and the photocathode (electron source), the electrostatic lens resolution, and the granularity of the (small) image output screen. In a cinerecording, the final resolution is always less than that of the intensifier due to the lens coupling between camera and output screen and the resolution of the miniature 35-mm cine-film frames. In digital imaging utilizing television, the principal resolution limits are due to the television line rate per frame and the matrix size for digital recording that determines the pixel size. The third source of unsharpness in the anatomic image is the motion of the object details during recording. The unsharpness is proportional to the velocity of motion and the exposure time. For pulsed cardiovascular exposures (as in cine- and digital recording), motion unsharpness is reduced by using shorter pulse widths.

Noise

The technical definition of noise is the presence of random fluctuations in the brightness of small image elements that obscure the perception of small- or low-contrast details. The most important source of noise is known as "quantum noise" and is due to the statistical nature of photon flow and absorption. The actual number of photons, N, which are absorbed in a small image element (pixel) in a specific time will be variable. A measure of the fluctuation is the standard deviation of N, which is $\sqrt{N}$ or $N^{1/2}$. The fluctuation as a fraction of the average brightness (or density) of the image will be $\sqrt{N}/N = 1/\sqrt{N}$. This random variation of the image brightness from pixel to pixel in a "uniformly" exposed image, constitutes a "noise" that overlays and prevents the identification of a recorded image with a similar contrast variation. An increase in exposure of the image receptor by a factor of 4 (to $4N$) will *decrease* the "noise" contrast by a factor of $\sqrt{4} = 2$. Thus, the necessary exposure level to perceive a detail with a certain size and contrast will *increase* as the detail size and/or its contrast decrease.

X-RAY IMAGING EQUIPMENT

X-ray imaging systems are of two types: those that capture a single static x-ray projection known as "radiography," and those that capture a dynamic continuously changing projection known as "fluoroscopy." Fluoroscopic images can be recorded by cine, television, or digital detector techniques—in which case a series of static images (radiographs known as "frames") can be obtained that can either be displayed in rapid succession, e.g., 30 frames/sec giving the illusion of motion, or as single stationary frames. Using digital computer image storage, the frames can be subtracted from each other to present the difference between them, a technique discussed later as Digital Subtraction Angiography (DSA). The great majority of cardiovascular imaging procedures employ fluoroscopy because of the dynamic nature of the cardiovascular system.

Radiographic Recording Systems

Conventional radiography has only a small role in cardiovascular imaging primarily related to the chest x-ray. The most common image receptor is the film/screen cassette discussed earlier with conventional double-coated film and two screens. There are, however, some newer commercial systems that are increasing in use that employ radically different principles including digital images. One of these (2) employs a 0.5 mm-thick layer of amorphous selenium as the image detector, the surface of which receives a uniform electrostatic charge. The absorption of the exit beam of x-rays by this layer creates a charge distribution on its surface corresponding to the x-ray image. A microelectrometer probe array advanced systematically over this surface, nondestructively reads out the charge distribution, which is digitally converted with 12-bit precision, and coupled to a laser film recorder. A chest image obtained by this process has 0.2-mm resolution and is as sensitive as photographic film/screen systems.

Another recording system using a different physical principle and a digital readout, is the photostimulable phosphor plate (3). The process is sometimes known as computed radiography (CR). It employs a photostimulable phosphor, typically a halide with an activator element that can store an x-ray image. This latent image is then released in the form of luminescent light when the plate is irradiated by a stimulating light beam. The original Japanese (Fuji) system employs barium fluoro-bromide with a europium activator (BaFBr:Eu) coated on a flat polyester plate. Before use, the plate is flooded with light (from a high-intensity sodium discharge lamp) to erase any remaining image. After exposure, the plate is transferred to a reader where it is scanned systematically line-by-line with a small (e.g., 0.1 mm $\times$ 0.1 mm) laser beam of red light. The greenish luminescence of the plate image is collected by an optical fiber bundle and converted point-by-point into an electrical analog signal that is then digitized and stored in a computer for subsequent readout. This system is notable for its high resolution and its very wide dynamic range (about 100 times greater than film/screen systems), which allows more latitude in the choice of exposure factors (kV and mAs).

A more recent development for "filmless" radiography rendered possible by digital systems, utilizes a thin cesium iodide screen deposited on a thin array of amorphous silicon photodiodes that generate electronic signals proportional to the light received from the screen (4). These are then fed into a digital computer for recording or manipulating the image. Recently, this approach has reached fruition through a joint General Electric/Edgerton, Grier and Germeshausen project, resulting in recording panels up to 41 cm × 41 cm in size with a resolution of 5 pixels/mm recorded with a 16-bit depth and therefore holding up to 4 million pixels.

The field of x-ray detectors for digital radiography has been recently comprehensively reviewed by Yaffe and Rowlands (5).

Fluoroscopic Imaging Systems

Fluoroscopy is the primary radiodiagnostic modality in cardiology practice. Since the early 1950s, the image intensifier has been the essential image receptor. In this device, the x-ray beam transmitted through the patient is absorbed by a fluorescent screen in close contact with a photocathode that converts the screen light into an electron image. These electrons, bearing the image, are then accelerated and focused onto a relatively small output screen (e.g., 1 inch in diameter), where, because of their energy gain and image minification, an image with a light gain of the order of 5,000 (compared with the input fluorescent screen) is displayed.

Over the past 50 years, the input screen has been expanded in diameter now ranging from about 9 in. for most cardiac imaging to 14 in. or more for general radiologic use. Typi-

cally also, several image magnification modes are available that allow greater image resolution. The magnification is achieved by choosing a smaller central area of the input x-ray screen for intensified display over the entire area of the output screen. For example, a 14-in. diameter intensifier yielding an output image with 4.5 line-pairs/mm resolution might have two "zoom" modes as follows: a central 10 in.-diameter mode yielding a magnified image with resolution 5.2 1p/mm, and a smaller 6 in.-diameter mode with resolution 5.8 1p/mm. These high resolutions are characteristic of the high-definition, fine-grained cesium iodide input screens and the fine-grained output screens.

The intensifier output is usually transferred by a coupling lens to a television camera for dynamic viewing or recording. The recording of a series of spot-films is another alternative. Spot film images when fed to a digital computer allow the practice of digital subtraction imaging, which displays subtle differences between successive images, sometimes including a baseline "mask" image of anatomy without contrast agent. Digital imaging is also employed in storage and rapid recall of images.

The basic elements of digital recording and digital subtraction angiography are shown in Figure 3 (6). The analog image obtained for visual display takes the form of a continuously varying voltage arriving line by line. It is converted into digital numbers on arrival by the ADC (analog-to-digital converter). Since brightness is perceived as a logarithmic (not arithmetic) process, the image signals are converted in

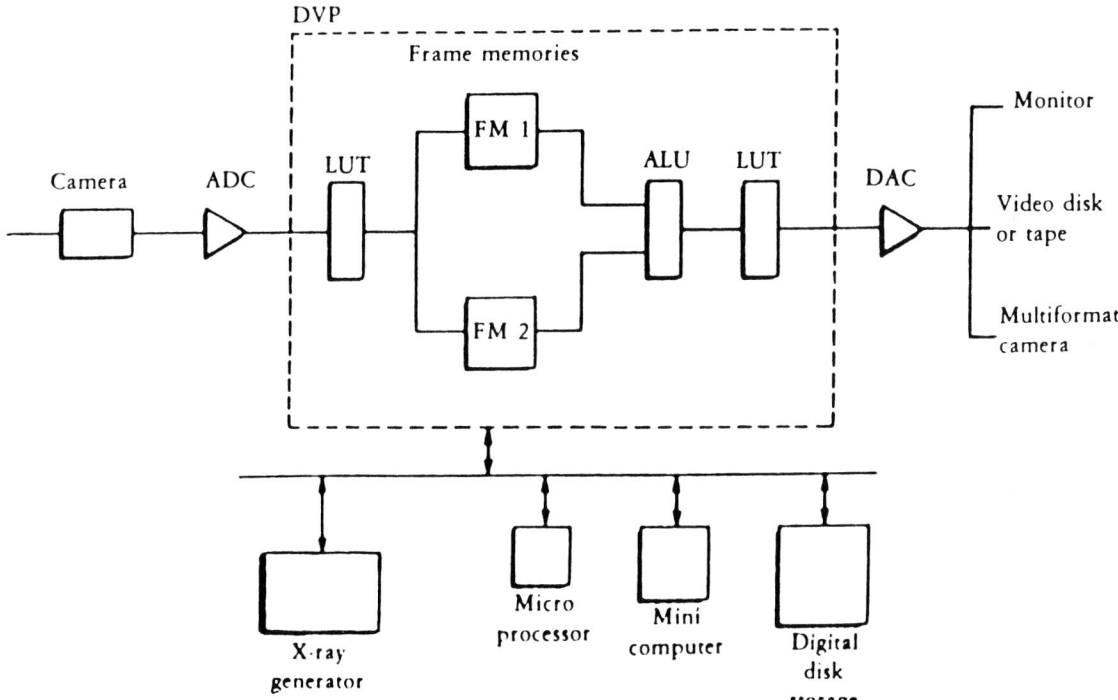

FIG. 3. Digital elements for performing digital fluoroscopy, radiography, or angiography with an intensifier-television system. The digital video processor (DVP) system shown is planned for digital subtraction angiography. (From ref. 16, with permission.)

the computer to a set of logarithms (using a "look-up table" LUT) and then stored in memory (FM). Arithmetic operations, such as averaging several images or subtraction of one frame from another or expanding the gray scale to increase contrast, are performed in the arithmetic logic unit (ALU). The processed frames to be displayed or stored are reconverted to linear form via an LUT and finally to analog form in a digital-to-analog converter (DAC).

In the past, the standard format of the television image with 525 horizontal scan lines has been used, which seriously limits the vertical image resolution to about 0.8 1p/mm with a 10 in. input image. In addition, the maximum radiofrequency (bandwidth) of the television electronic signal will limit the horizontal resolution: for example, 1.01 p/mm for a conventional television bandwidth of 5 MHz. This resolution limitation has been the primary reason for using a 35-mm cinecamera lens coupled to the intensifier output for the definitive diagnostic review of cardiac catheterization procedures.

In the most recent image intensifier systems, the severe loss of image resolution in the television image has been partially remedied by the use of television cameras operating with more than 1000 lines per frame and a higher radiofrequency bandwidth of at least 25 MHz, which provides improvement by a factor of 2 in both horizontal and vertical resolution. This technical improvement has outmoded the use of cineangiography in facilities with the most recent high quality equipment for cardiac examination.

X-rays for cardiac fluoroscopy are generated in conventional x-ray tubes operated typically at 70kVp to 80 kVp with tube currents in the 2 to 4 mA range with a total exposure time that may exceed 30 minutes. Longer exposures are frequent in interventional procedures such as practiced in electrophysiology laboratories. At the conventional focus-skin distance (FSD) of about 18 in. between the tube focal spot and the skin of the patient and a total tube filtration of 2.5 mm Al, the incident x-ray dose will range from 3.7 rads/min at 70 kVp, 2 mA up to 9.4 rads/min at 80 kVp, 4 mA (7). Thus, in 30 minutes, the entrance patient dose in a fixed fluoroscopic field (e.g., encompassing the heart) will range from 111 to 282 rads. The former dose will produce no observable skin effect, but the latter dose may produce temporary epilation (8). These and other effects are discussed in more detail in the section on radiation safety in this chapter. An important technique to reduce patient dose is to use a lower frame rate than 60 frames per second to generate images.

Grid-controlled Fluoroscopy

During the last decade, several major x-ray tube manufacturers have introduced apparatus employing grid-controlled fluoroscopy to reduce dose. In this system, a grid that is located close to the cathode in the x-ray tube is normally held at a negative potential to suppress the tube current. A short positive voltage pulse of milliseconds' duration on the grid allows a short pulse of tube current to flow with amplitude up to 50 mA. Whereas in continuous fluoroscopy, images at the rate of 60 frames/second are generated continuously, the use of a pulsed grid allows a lower frame frequency, such as 30, 15 or 7½ frames/second, with a consequent reduction in patient exposure. For example, with a 25 mA current pulse per frame at 75 kVp, the tabletop pulsed fluoroscopic exposure rate may fall from 4 roentgens per minute (R/min) to 2 R/min and 1 R/min for 30, 15, and 7½ frames/second. A flicker-free image is obtained by continuing the image display from the previous pulse until the next pulse is generated. The rectangular shape of the x-ray pulses also reduces the noise level and improves the detail sharpness in the image.

RADIATION SAFETY

The adverse effects of exposure to ionizing radiation were recognized within the first few years after the discovery of x-rays in 1895. The initial observations were skin injuries ranging from a threshold erythema to moist desquamation. Radiation-induced malignancies were not recognized until the first decade of this century because of the long latent period of about 10 years following those exposures. An excess of leukemia among practicing radiologists in the United States was noted in the 1920s, but with the introduction of safety precautions later in that decade, the excess was reduced and disappeared for radiologists entering practice after 1940. The carcinogenic effects of x-rays are due to their ability to disrupt atoms and molecules. Ionizing radiation can disrupt DNA in the cell nucleus, causing damage to genes and chromosomes, some of which are not repaired or not repaired correctly.

Among medical specialists, it is generally observed that the group receiving the highest radiation exposure is the cardiology group that is involved in cardiac catheterization and in interventional cardiology, such as angioplasty and, to a lesser extent, electrophysiologic correctional procedures. The exposure is primarily from fluoroscopy. Rooms for these activities are usually equipped with radiation shields for the personnel in addition to the provision of protective garments (lead aprons).

Radiation Dose and Units

When x-rays encounter an absorbing medium, such as the human body, the energy is gradually absorbed. A certain fraction of the incident energy is absorbed in each layer of tissue, and the fraction decreases with depth depending on the energy (keV) of the radiation. The energy absorbed by a unit mass of tissue (e.g., per gram) is referred to as the absorbed dose.

The unit of absorbed dose in international use today is the Gray (Gy), defined as an energy deposition of 1 joule per kilogram. This unit has replaced the earlier and smaller "rad" (radiation absorbed dose) unit (equal to 0.01 Gy). In the radiation protection field, the unit in common use is the Sievert (Sv) and its subunit the "rem" (equal to 0.01 Sv). For x-ray exposure, the Gray and the Sievert are identical, as are the rad and the rem. For very small doses, the subunits millirad, milligray, millirem, millisievert are in use where "milli" signifies a thousand-fold reduction.

Biological Effects

These are of two kinds. The first are those that occur only after a dose threshold has been exceeded, known as "deterministic" effects. Examples of these are skin erythema, epilation, and lens opacities (cataracts). The second are those that can occur at any dose with no threshold but with a probability proportional to the dose. These are known as "stochastic" effects (i.e., probabilistic effects) and include the more serious endpoints, such as cancer induction, which may become manifest after a latent period of several years, and genetic anomalies, which are expressed in future generations. Their likelihood is very small at the lowest doses, such as 1 rad or rem.

Table 2 reproduced from the Food and Drug Administration (FDA) (9) lists a range of deterministic skin effects with thresholds ranging from 2 to 10 Gy, which can be produced by extended fluoroscopy. The fluoroscopic exposure times at low- and high-dose rates capable of causing the effects and the times to onset of the effects are also listed.

Acute radiation doses (e.g., those delivered in a single day) of at least 3 Sv (300 rems or rads) are needed to produce a skin erythema. Much higher total doses are needed for these effects if the dose is protracted over a long period of time as occurs in occupational exposure.

For radiation protection purposes, the risk of stochastic effects in exposed patients or radiation workers is often judged by estimating a new radiation dose quantity known as the "effective dose" (10). This is the weighted sum of the doses received by up to 12 critical organs. For chest exposure (as in many cardiac procedures), the directly exposed organs considered to be at risk from stochastic effects are the lungs and the red bone marrow (both with dose weighting factors of 12%) and the female breast, the esophagus, and the thyroid gland (all with dose-weighting factors of 5%). The risk of developing late cancers after irradiation of the whole body or to an estimated effective dose based on critical organ exposure is estimated by the National Council on Radiation Protection (NCRP) and the International Commission on Radiation Protection (ICRP) to be 4% per Sievert, i.e., 1 in 2500 per rem or rad.

Maximum Permissible Doses

These limits are determined by the NCRP for two classes of exposed persons: radiation workers who are occupationally exposed and the general public exclusive of medical exposure. The policy of governmental agencies, such as the Nuclear Regulatory Commission, is guided by the NCRP recommendations. Table 3 lists the current limits in the United States. Personnel who are exposed to ionizing radiation are urged by the controlling governmental agency to maintain their exposure "as low as reasonably achievable" (ALARA).

The significant changes from recommendations published in 1971 are in the lifetime cumulative limit for radiation workers, which has been reduced by a factor of 5, and in the limit for general public exposure, also reduced by a factor of 5, reflecting an increase in the estimated cancer risk per rem.

The exposure limits in Table 3 can be compared with the unavoidable exposure to background ionizing radiation, which has an average level in the United States of 100 mrem

TABLE 2. *Radiation-induced skin injuries*

| | | Hours of fluoroscopic "on time" to reach threshold[a] at: | | |
Effect	Typical threshold absorbed dose (Gy)	Usual fluorodose rate of 0.02 Gy/min (2 rad/min)	High-level dose rate of 0.2 Gy/min (20 rad/min)	Time to onset of effect[b]
Early transient erythema	2	1.7	0.17	hours
Temporary epilation	3	2.5	0.25	3 weeks
Main erythema	6	5.0	0.50	10 days
Permanent epilation	7	5.8	0.58	3 weeks
Dry desquamation	10	8.3	0.83	4 weeks
Invasive fibrosis	10	8.3	0.83	
Dermal atrophy	11	9.2	0.92	>14 weeks
Telangiectasis	12	10.0	1.00	>52 weeks
Moist desquamation	15	12.5	1.25	4 weeks
Late erythema	15	12.5	1.25	6–10 weeks
Dermal necrosis	18	15.0	1.50	>10 weeks
Secondary ulceration	20	16.7	1.67	>6 weeks

[a] Time required to deliver the typical threshold dose at the specific dose rate; [b] time after single irradiation to observation of effect.
(Adapted from ref. 8 and reproduced from ref. 9, with permission.)

TABLE 3. *Maximum permissible radiation doses*[a]

Occupational exposures (excluding medical exposures)	
Effective dose limits	
Annual	50 mSv (5 rem)
Cumulative	10 mSv (1 rem) × age
Dose annual limits for tissues and organs	
Lens of eye	150 mSv (15 rem)
Skin, hands and feet	500 mSv (50 rem)
Public exposures (annual) (in excess of natural background exposure)	
Effective dose limit (Continuous or frequent exposure)	1 mSv (100 mrem)
Effective dose limit (Infrequent exposure)	5 mSv (500 mrem)
Embryo-fetus exposures (monthly)	
Dose limit	0.5 mSv (50 mrem)

[a] 1 mSv = 100 mrem = 0.1 rem.

(1 mSv) per year, a total contributed approximately equally by 3 sources: terrestrial radiation from buildings and the ground, cosmic radiation from outer space, and the typical body burden of naturally occurring radionuclides, such as carbon-14 and potassium-40. The actual annual level of background radiation is many times higher in some regions of the world but the few epidemiologic studies conducted have not shown a significant elevation of malignant disease. In addition to the natural background, everybody is exposed to radioactive radon gas, which, on the average in the United States, contributes 200 mrem/year effective whole-body dose and 2000 mrem/year lung dose.

Results of Epidemiological Studies of Radiation Workers

The primary data on radiation risks that underlie the exposure limits for ionizing radiation are the findings in the Japanese atomic bomb survivor study initiated in 1950. The most recent findings were published by Pierce et al. (11) in 1996. The many small epidemiologic studies of late cancer in radiation workers suffer from statistical uncertainties in the results, and, therefore, in recent years, several large studies of the combined data from one country or several countries have been made. The largest of these has combined data from the United States, the United Kingdom, and Canada for a total of more than 95,000 radiation workers employed for an average time of 21 years with total individual doses averaging about 4 rem (40 mSv) (12). There was no significant excess of all cancers, excluding leukemia. For leukemia, there was a significant elevation with a relative risk of 1.22 for a cumulative dose of 10 rem (100 mSv).

Sources of Personnel X-ray Exposure

The main source of exposure in cardiology x-ray procedures is radiation scattered from the patient during fluoroscopic and angiographic procedures. For a patient entry exposure rate of 3R/minute at 70 kVp with a field size of 10 × 10 cm, the maximum scatter exposure rate at a distance of 1 meter from the beam center will be less than 1 mR/minute, or 60 mR in 1 hour. Another potential source is the

primary x-ray beam, but this is absorbed in the patient and in the x-ray imaging system, namely, the shielded image intensifier. There is also a low permitted level of leakage radiation through the housing of x-ray tubes, namely 100 mR per hour at 1 meter when the tube is operated at its maximum rated kVp (usually 150) and maximum continuous rated current. At the lower operating kVp in cardiology facilities (e.g., 70 to 90 kVp), the leakage will be more than 1000 times smaller than the scattered radiation level.

Exposure Rates near C-arm Fluoroscopes

The C-arm fluoroscope provides a complete 360-degree range of angulation of the x-ray beam relative to the heart—or any other organ of the body. The exposure of the operator standing at a fixed location with respect to the patient is critically dependent on the angulation of the useful beam. It is well known that the exposure of the operator is much greater from an "over-table" x-ray tube than from an "under-table" tube, the eye dose for example being up to 100 times greater. Figure 4**A** and **B** illustrate the large increase in exposure rates by factors in the range of 20 to 100 when the tube is angulated at 45 degrees above the table and is close to the operator (Fig. 4**B**). The least operator exposure is received when the tube is below the table so that the exit beam and the image intensifier are adjacent to the operator (Fig. 4**A**). The reason for this result is that when the tube is below and/or behind the patient, the operator is shielded from the forward scatter by the body of the patient. Whereas, when the tube is above the patient, the backscatter from the entry portal on the patient directly irradiates the operator—particularly above the waist. The use of over-table x-ray tubes for fluoroscopy (or cine runs) is, therefore, discouraged.

Exposure Rates near the Table during Cardiac Procedures

The relatively large amounts of radiation involved in angiography and in angioplasty under fluoroscopic control cause cardiologists to be the most exposed personnel in medical practice. Figure 5 illustrates the exposure rates 50 cm from

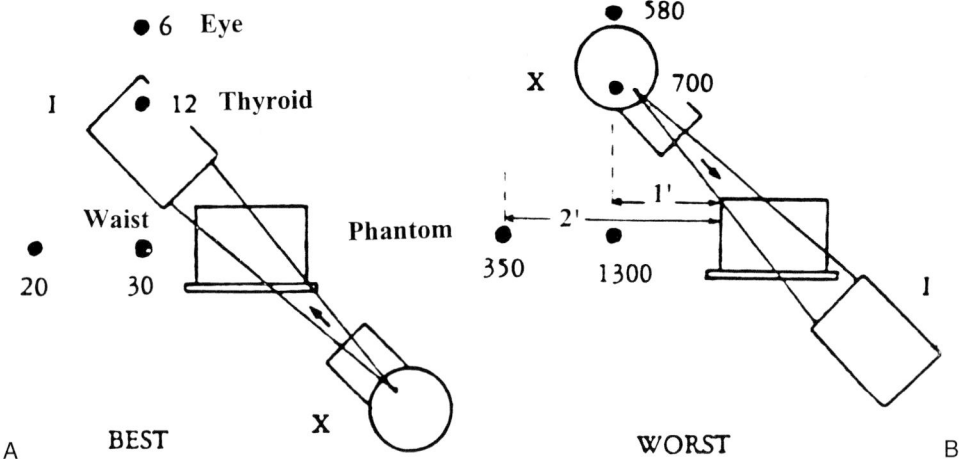

FIG. 4. Exposure rates in milliroentgens per hour at operator of a C-arm fluoroscope at the angles for lowest (**A**) and highest (**B**) rates. Phantom: 12 in. × 12 in. × 8 in. wax; x-ray factors: 110 kVp, 2 mA; field size: 6-in. diameter at intensifier. **A:** Tube under table at 45 degrees, away from operator. **B:** Tube above table at 45 degrees, next to operator.

the center of the x-ray beam during cardiac catheterization with a C-arm fluoroscope with the x-ray tube under the table. The exposure rate from scattered radiation beside the table and below the table-top level at 70 mR/hr is about three times higher than at locations above the table level. The field size should be kept to a minimum and the x-ray tube current to no more than 2 mA. If cineangiography (at 30 frames/sec) is employed, much higher tube currents, probably in short pulses, are used, and the dose rate directed at the patient is increased by a factor of about 20. The exposure rate beside the table is increased by the same factor. The duration of the cine exposure (e.g., 4 runs at 6 seconds each) is, however, much shorter than the fluoroscopy time, which may be about

10 minutes. In this case, the total exposure received by the patient and by the cardiologist is approximately equally divided between the fluoroscopy and the cine study. Lead aprons are mandatory, and lead plastic barriers should also be employed to reduce the exposure rate.

Personnel Shielding and Monitoring

As noted earlier, the protective apron is mandatory if annual exposures are to be maintained substantially below the 5 rem (50 mSv) annual limit. For many years, the conventional lead apron containing lead powder in a polyvinyl carrier with an equivalent thickness of 0.5 mm Pb has been

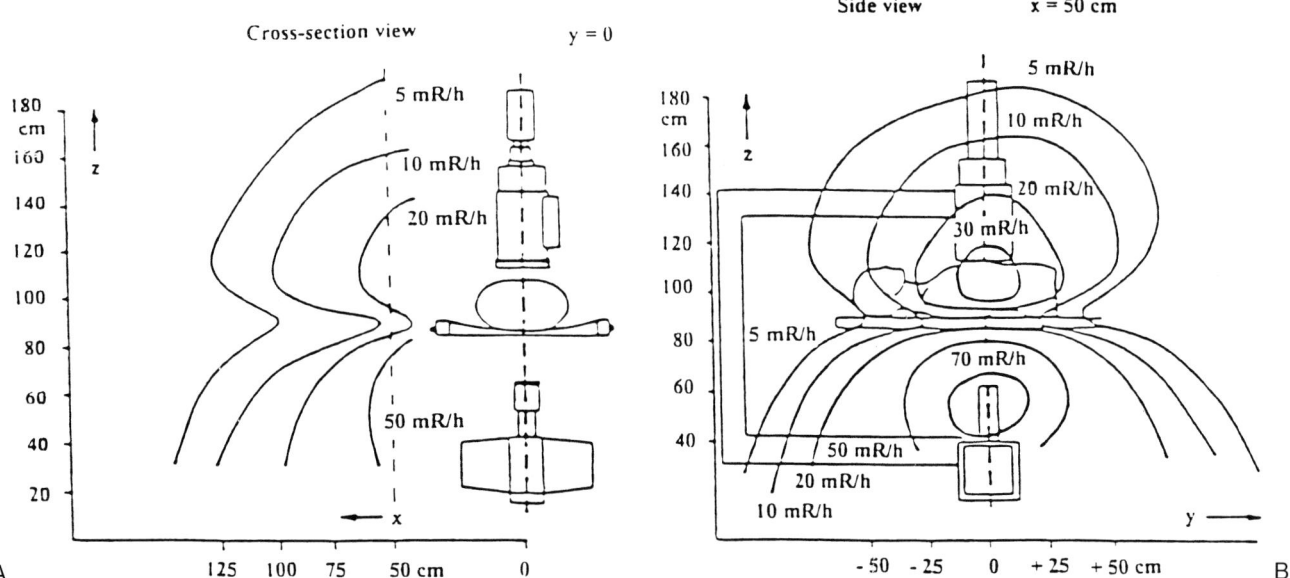

FIG. 5. Isoexposure curves in milliroentgens per hour around a cineangiographic system of the C-arm type. Fluoroscopic operational factors: 90 kVp, 1.0 mA. Entrance field size 8.5 cm × 11.0 cm. Tabletop exposure rate about 1 R/min. (Evaluation of exposure levels in cine cardiac catheterization laboratories.) (From ref. 17, with permission.)

used. This absorbs about 98.5% of scattered 80 kVp x-rays. If, for example, the workload of the cardiologist is 30 cases per month, each case involving 30 minutes of fluoroscopy and 1 minute of cinefluorography, the exposure per case arriving at the apron 75 cm from the table center would be 15 mrem from fluoroscopy and 10 mrem from cine studies. If the apron transmits 1.5%, the abdominal skin dose would be 0.375 mrem per case and 135 mrem/year. The upper arms, head, and neck are not protected by the apron and could receive about 8 mrem per case, 240 mrem/month, and 2.9 rem per year. The organs at risk outside the apron are the thyroid gland and some red bone marrow; therefore, a thyroid shield with 0.5 mm lead equivalence is strongly recommended. To reduce exposure, the cardiologist can step back from the table during cine runs.

It is, therefore, recommended that *two* personnel monitors be worn by persons performing cardiac catheterization and interventional cardiac procedures, including those in electrophysiology laboratories with extended fluoroscopic exposure. The under-apron monitor worn typically at the waist should be supplemented by a neck monitor worn typically on the *outside* of the thyroid shield. This latter monitor will register a considerably higher dose than the under-apron monitor. A recent paper (13) describes a method for deriving the effective (whole-body equivalent) dose from the two individual monitor doses. For an under-table tube, the formula for deriving effective dose is $0.5 H_1 + 0.025 H_2$, where H_1 is the under-apron monitor reading, and H_2 is the neck monitor reading.

In recent years, the typical 12-lb weight of a 0.5-mm lead apron has been reduced by about 30% by employing a mixture of one or more elements with a middle atomic number, such as antimony, tin, or barium together with a smaller amount of lead or tungsten. Originally proposed for the Picker "Litegard" apron in 1966, there are now several different lighter (but more expensive) protective aprons using the above elements.

Until recently the typical personnel monitor was a film badge containing a strip of dental film and several different filters to estimate the effective energy of the x-ray spectrum in order to assess properly the dose received. Badge films are typically changed and the photographic density measured monthly. Film badges are able to record personnel doses down to a minimum of 10 mrem. Very recently, a personnel monitor (badge) has been marketed under the trade name Luxel and is more sensitive than film. The recording material consists of Al_2O_3 crystals, which, after exposure, will fluoresce when exposed to laser light. The fluorescence intensity provides a measure of the integrated radiation exposure. The minimum dose recordable is 1 mrem. Such a badge can be changed (read-out) every 2 or 3 months.

Shielding Radiation Facilities

The shielding of a cardiology x-ray facility (e.g., for cardiac catheterization or electrophysiology) will primarily depend on the anticipated workload (cases per month) and on the distance and occupancy of adjoining space. The radiation exposure inside and potentially outside such an x-ray room is from scattered radiation leaving the patient as has been discussed earlier. As an example, assume that the room is 25 × 30 ft and holds an x-ray table, biplane C-arm x-ray equipment, and a shielded control area 12 ft from the center of the table. Fluoroscopy is used in each unit 2 hours per day with maximum of 80 kVp, maximum entrance skin dose 5R/min, and typical entrance field size 10 cm × 10 cm. The integrated skin exposure per unit will be 600 R/day. If cinefluoroscopy is used for 3 minutes per day, the entrance skin dose will be increased by 50% to 900 R/day. The scattered radiation dose at 1 meter distance from a 400 cm^2 field will be 900 mrem per day and for a 100 cm^2 field, the dose will be 225 mrem per day from each unit. At 10 ft (3 m) distance to the closest room wall, the total dose will be 50 mrem per day, 250 mrem per week, and 13 rem per year. If we now assume that each area outside the room is fully occupied by nonradiation employees, the annual dose limit is 100 mrem/year (Table 3), and the minimum thickness of the intervening wall should provide an attenuation factor of $100/13000 = 0.0077$. The available data on attenuation of x-rays through lead sheet at 80 kVp indicates that 0.7 mm of lead will be adequate. In practice, the thinnest commercial thickness of lead sheet is 1/32 in. or 0.8 mm.

It is concluded that 1/32 in. of lead carried to a height of 7 ft above the floor and included in the exposed doors will provide protection to levels well below 100 mrem/year. For observation windows, lead plastic equivalent to 1/32 in. of lead will also be more than adequate.

REFERENCES

1. Corney GM. Sensitometric properties of radiographic films. In: Haus AG, ed. *The physics of medical imaging: recording system measurements and techniques.* New York: American Institute of Physics, 1979: 72–82.
2. Chotas HG, Floyd CE, Ravin CE. Technical evaluation of a digital chest radiography system that uses a selenium detector. *Radiology* 1995;195: 264–270.
3. Sonoda M, Takano M, Miyahara J, et al. Computed radiography utilizing scanning laser stimulated fluorescence. *Radiology* 1983;148: 833–838.
4. Strotzer M, Gmeinwieser JK, Volk M, et al. Detection of simulated chest lesions with normal and reduced radiation dose: comparison of conventional screen radiography and a flat-panel x-ray detector based on amorphous silicon. *Invest Radiol* 1998;33:98–103.
5. Yaffe MJ, Rowlands JA. X-ray detectors for digital radiography. *Phys Med Biol* 1997;42:1–39.
6. Riederer SJ. Digital radiography. In: Taveras JM, Ferrucci JT, eds. *Radiology: diagnosis, imaging, intervention, vol. 1.* Philadelphia: Lippincott, 1987.
7. National Council on Radiation Protection and Measurements. *NCRP Report 102. Medical x-ray, electron beam, and gamma ray protection for energies up to 50 MeV.* Bethesda, MD: National Council on Radiation Protection and Measurements, 1989:99[Table B.3].
8. Wagner LK, Eifel PJ, Geise RA. Potential biological effects following high x-ray dose interventional procedures. *J Vasc Interv Radiol* 1994; 5:71–84.
9. Food and Drug Administration. *Information for physicians. Avoidance of serious x-ray-induced skin injuries to patients during fluoroscopically guided procedures.* Rockville, MD: Food and Drug Administra-

tion Center for Devices and Radiological Health. September 9, 1994[Table 2].
10. National Council on Radiation Protection. *NCRP Report 116. Limitation of exposure to ionizing radiation.* Bethesda, MD: National Council on Radiation Protection, 1993:23, 56.
11. Pierce D, Shimizu Y, Preston D, et al. Studies of the mortality of the atomic bomb survivors. Report 12, Part 1. Cancer: 1950–1990. *Radiat Res* 1996;146:1–27.
12. Cardis E, Gilbert ES, Carpenter L, et al. Effects of low doses and low dose rates of external ionizing radiation: cancer mortality among nuclear industry workers in three countries. *Radiat Res* 1995;142: 117–132.
13. Rosenstein M, Webster EW. Effective dose to personnel wearing protective aprons during fluoroscopy and interventional radiology. *Health Phys* 1994;67:88–89.
14. Pohost GM, O'Rourke RA, eds. *Principles and practice of cardiovascular imaging.* New York: Little, Brown and Company, 1991:332.
15. Haus AG, ed. *The physics of medical imaging: system measurements and techniques.* American Association of Physicists in Medicine. New York, 1979:78.
16. Riederer SJ. Digital radiography. In: Taveras JM, Ferrucci JT, eds. *Radiology,* Vol 1. Philadelphia: Lippincott, 1987:7.
17. American Association of Physicists in Medicine. *AAPM Report No. 12.* American Association of Physicists in Medicine.

CHAPTER 24

Chest Roentgenology and Fluoroscopy

Colleen Sanders and Benigno Soto

In these days of echocardiography, nuclear cardiology, electron beam CT, and cardiac MRI, the conventional chest film has become a forgotten stepchild in the evaluation of cardiac disease. However, it remains the least costly and frequently the most effective approach of all of the cardiac imaging examinations, yielding diagnostic information in a large variety and number of patients.

The evaluation of the chest film in the cardiac patient involves sequential logical assessment and correlation of both the anatomic and physiologic information available on the posteroanterior (PA) and lateral radiographs (1,2). Overall cardiac size as well as specific cardiac chamber enlargement can be identified based on changes in cardiac contour (3). Abnormal calcifications within the heart or its surroundings depict anatomic structures such as location of the pericardium or aortic valve and often denote the underlying disease process. Physiologic information, based on the pulmonary vasculature, provides insight into cardiac pressure, pulmonary blood flow, and degree of cardiac compensation (2,3).

Before assessing pulmonary vascularity or other findings on the chest radiograph, the overall quality of the film should be evaluated. In full inspiration, the hemidiaphragm should be approximately at the level of the 9th rib posteriorly on the right side. In suboptimal inspiration or supine radiographs, in which forced vital capacity is decreased by up to 40%, the lower lobe markings are crowded and may obscure the possibility of early pulmonary edema. Great care should be taken before assigning mild degrees of vascular abnormalities in these patients. The clavicular heads should be midline in position, because slight degrees of rotation will substantially affect the cardiac contour and may alter the apparent cardiac size as well.

ANATOMIC ASSESSMENT—CARDIOMEGALY AND CHAMBER SIZE

Cardiac Size

The cardiothoracic ratio (CT ratio), the ratio of the maximum transverse cardiac diameter compared to the widest transverse measurement of the lungs on the PA film, is a rough quantitative measurement of cardiac size. The normal CT ratio is usually 0.5 or less in adults. In the newborn, the normal ratio is approximately 0.66 due to the relatively underdeveloped lungs at this age. Elevated CT ratios usually reflect left ventricular dilatation because the left heart border is displaced laterally as the left ventricle enlarges.

Enlargement of the cardiac silhouette alone, without other information, is relatively nonspecific. Marked cardiomegaly with multichamber enlargement, seen in biventricular failure or multiple valvular insufficiency, usually represents volume overload and is associated radiographically with signs of pulmonary venous hypertension (2,3). However, severe cardiomegaly may also be seen in oligemic lesions such as pulmonary atresia without ventriculoseptal defect (VSD) or Ebstein's anomaly (4,5). Normal vascularity combined with a markedly enlarged cardiac silhouette is unusual in cardiac disease; almost all patients with dilated cardiomyopathy will

C. Sanders: Department of Radiology, University of Alabama at Birmingham; Department of Radiology, University of Alabama Hospitals, Birmingham, Alabama 35249.

B. Soto: Department of Radiology, University of Alabama at Birmingham Medical Center, Birmingham, Alabama 35233.

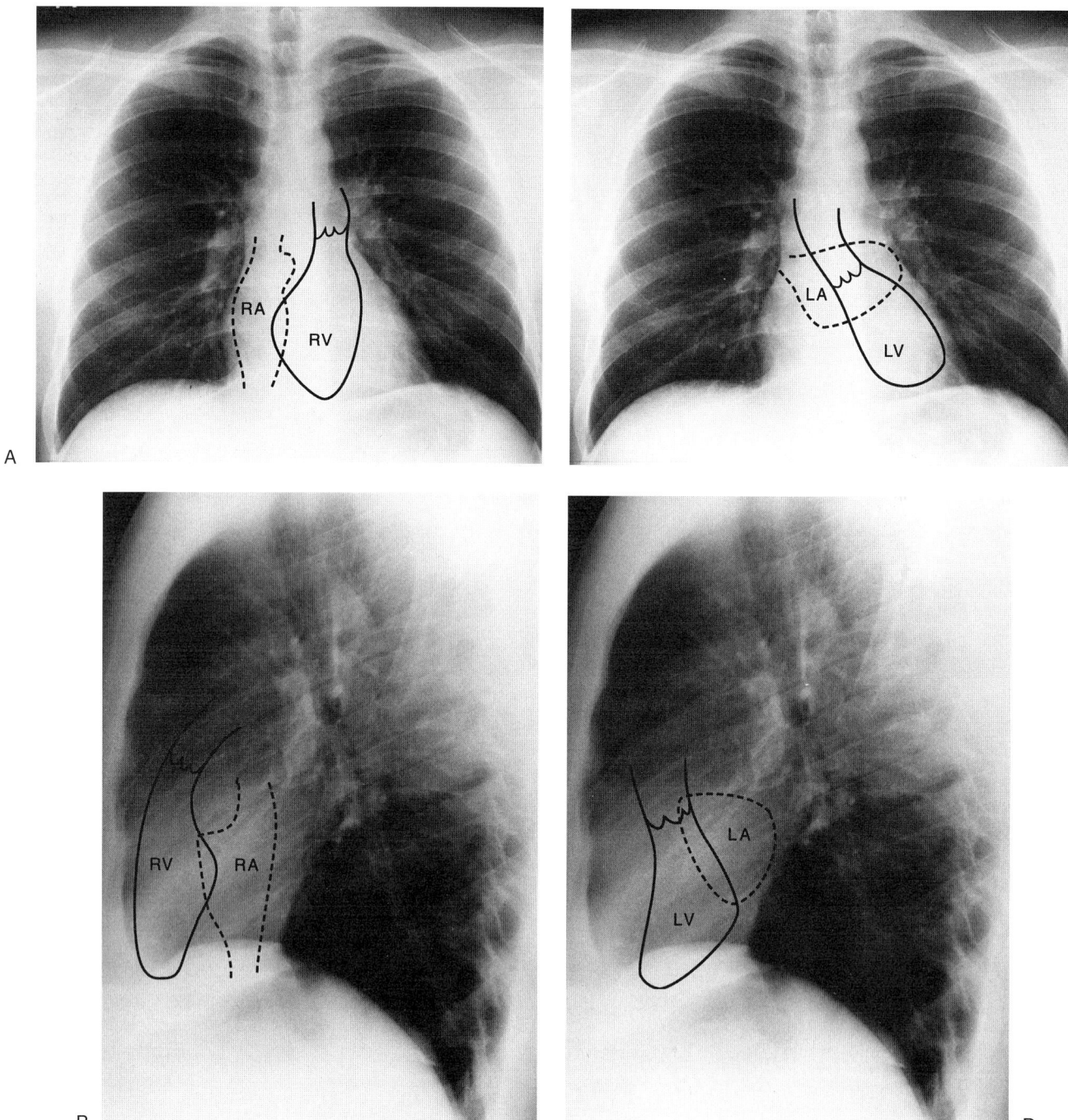

FIG. 1. Posteroanterior and lateral views of the normal heart showing major structures including cardiac chambers. **A, B:** Right heart chambers. **C, D:** Left heart chambers. *RA,* right atrium; *RV,* right ventricle; *LA,* left atrium; *LV,* left ventricle.

have some degree of pulmonary vascular hypertension (PVH) even without evidence of edema. In such a patient, pericardial effusion should be considered a possibility (6).

Cardiac size and configuration are influenced by thoracic cage abnormalities, obesity, and ventilation. A suboptimal inspiration elevates the cardiac apex and enlarges the CT ratio slightly. In patients who are extremely obese, there may be significant magnification on both the PA and lateral views causing apparent cardiomegaly. In contrast, patients with emphysema typically have a small cardiac silhouette due to their overinflated lungs; apparently normal cardiac size in these patients is often abnormal.

Specific Chamber Enlargement

Following assessment of cardiac size, the contour of the heart should be evaluated for signs of specific chamber enlargement. Individual cardiac chambers may be enlarged with or without accompanying cardiomegaly but as each chamber of the heart enlarges, the cardiac contour is altered in a logical and predictable fashion based on their location within the heart (Fig. 1). On the frontal, the right heart border is formed by the right atrium and the left border by the left atrial appendage and the lateral wall of the left ventricle. The right ventricle and the left atrium are not border-forming on the PA view except for the small area of the left atrial appendage; these chambers are best evaluated on the lateral view.

Right Atrium

Dilatation of the right atrium in adults is usually due to tricuspid insufficiency and association with right ventricular enlargement is common, especially in adults. Right atrial enlargement is often not detectable on the chest film unless moderate-to-severe in degree. Therefore, right atrial size evaluation is probably the least accurate of all the cardiac chambers. It is suggested on the posteroanterior film when the right heart border is more than 5.5 cm to the right of midline (as marked by the spinous process) or 2.5 cm to the right of the vertebral body (Fig. 2). As the right atrium enlarges, it maintains its contact with the right hemidiaphragm at the costophrenic angle. In gross right atrial dilatation, there is filling of the retrosternal space on the lateral view cephalad to the right ventricle due to enlargement of the right atrial appendage (7).

Right Ventricle

Because the right ventricle is the most anterior of the cardiac chambers, right ventricular enlargement is initially detected on the lateral view and often does not cause overt cardiomegaly. Normally, the right ventricle touches the sternum one third of the distance between the sternal angle (i.e., the junction of the sternum with the manubrium) and the diaphragm (3,7). When this contact involves one half of the sternum, the right ventricle can be confidently said to be enlarged (Fig. 3). It must be remembered that this radio-

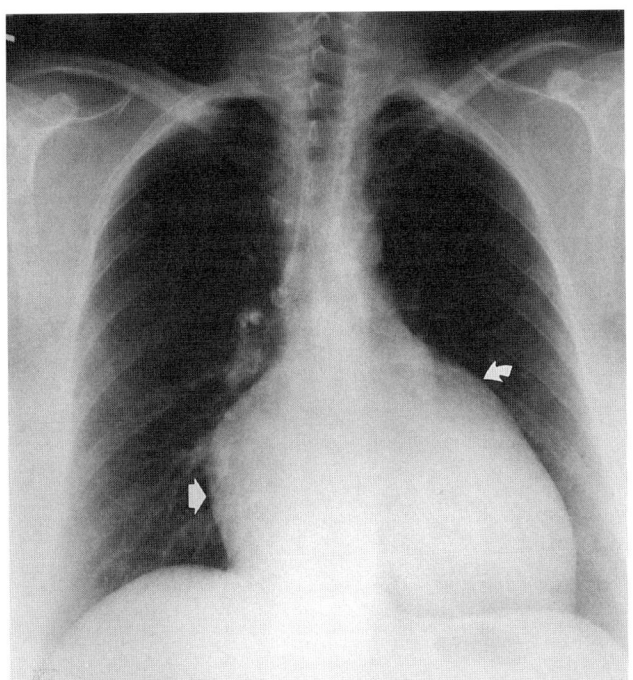

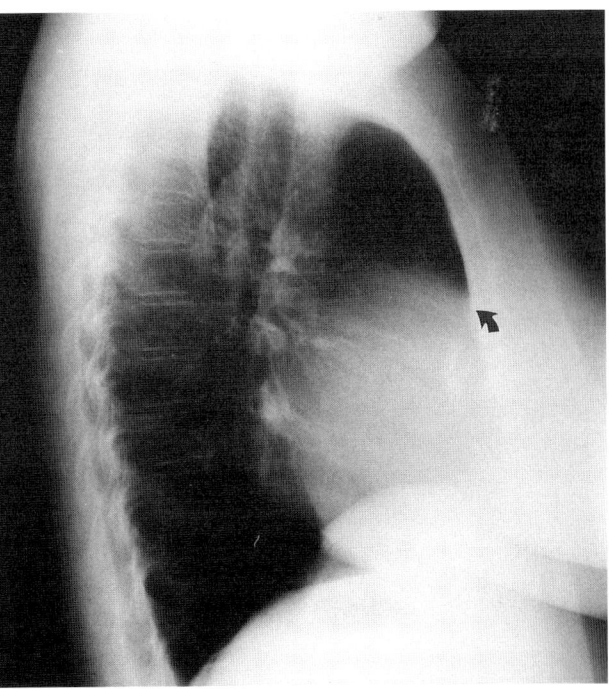

A   B

FIG. 2. A 55-year-old woman with Ebstein anomaly who presented with atrial arrhythmia. The postero-anterior view (**A**) shows marked enlargement of the right atrium (*white arrows*); the lateral view (**B**) shows retrosternal opacity (*black arrow*) due to enlargement of the right atrial appendage. Left atrial enlargement is also present (*white arrow*).

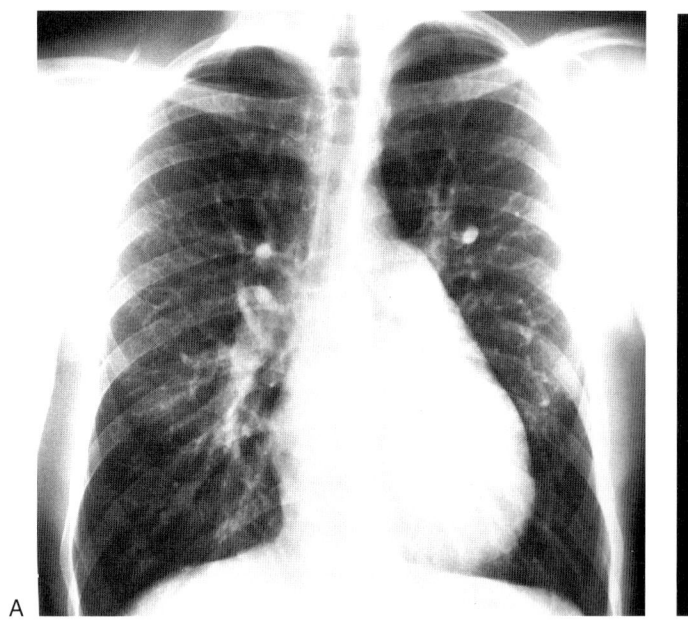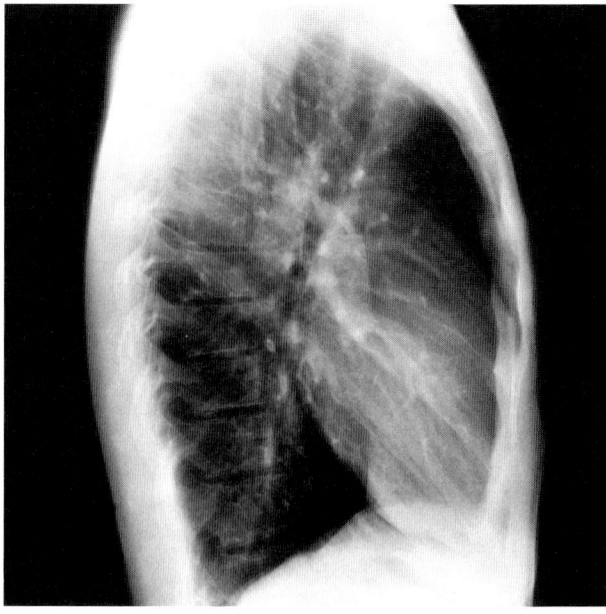

A   B

FIG. 3. An 18-year-old man with atrial septal defect and significant shunt vascularity and dilatation of the central pulmonary arteries (**A**). The overall cardiac size is within normal limits but there is increased size of the right ventricle on the lateral view, denoted by the heart of the sternal contact (**B**).

graphic sign, the filling of the retrosternal space, is based on normal sternal structure and mediastinal fat. In patients with pectus excavatum and inward curvature of the sternum, the right ventricle normally contacts the sternum for more than half its distance without right ventricular enlargement. Patients with abnormal mediastinal fat density, commonly seen following sternotomy, may lose the normally sharp interface between the fat and the right ventricle, leading to the

false diagnosis of right ventricular enlargement. As the right ventricle becomes more dilated, cardiomegaly ensues. There is displacement of the left ventricle posteriorly and rotation of the heart to the left as the right ventricle forms the left heart border (7). As a result, on the posteroanterior film, the axis of the heart, i.e., the line from the mid-right atrium to the cardiac apex, becomes relatively horizontal in its orientation (Fig. 4).

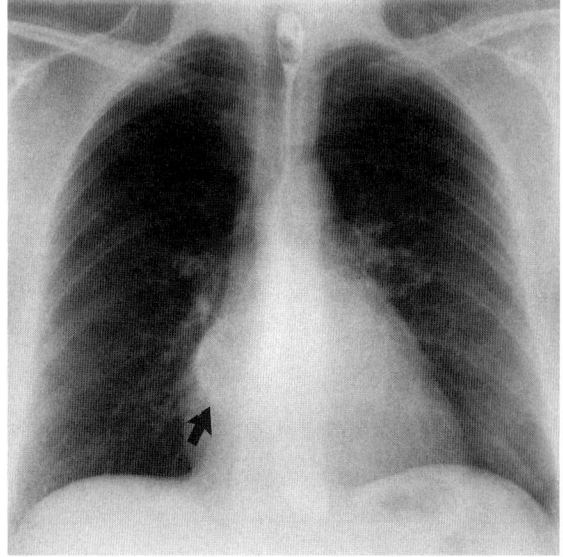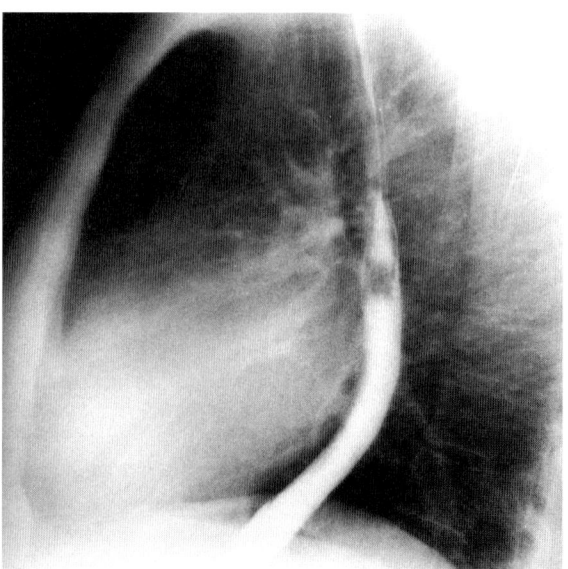

A   B

FIG. 4. A 36-year-old woman with mitral stenosis; cardiac series performed with barium swallow. The posteroanterior (PA) film (**A**) shows a double density behind the right heart border (*arrow*) with posterior deviation of the barium-filled esophagus on the lateral view (**B**). The transverse axis of the heart on the PA view is confirmed as right ventricular enlargement on the lateral exam.

Left Atrium

Left atrial enlargement can be seen in primary mitral valve disease such as mitral insufficiency or mitral stenosis, or as a reflection of left ventricular dysfunction with accompanying papillary muscle dysfunction. Radiographic assessment of left atrial enlargement is the most accurate of the specific cardiac chambers compared to echocardiographic findings (1,3,8). Because the left atrium is located most posteriorly, the earliest sign of left atrial enlargement is seen on the lateral view, with bulging of the cardiac contour immediately below the carina and left pulmonary artery but superior to that of the left ventricle (Fig. 4). If a barium swallow is performed during the chest radiograph, as previously performed for a cardiac series, the esophagus is clearly displaced in its mid-portion by a smooth bulge denoting the enlarged left atrium. The PA film is less sensitive to left atrial enlargement than the lateral view since only the left atrial appendage forms a portion of the cardiac border in this projection (Fig. 2). As the left atrium enlarges, its right wall forms a double density that may be seen just medial to the right atrium.

Bronchial displacement occurs with progressive left atrial enlargement, particularly in children because of their smaller and more pliable bronchi. On the lateral view, the left lower lobe bronchus is displaced laterally, often in a hook-like configuration, while on the PA view the carina may be widened. The carinal angle, in and of itself, is of little use since there is a wide range of normal carinal angles from 75 to 135 degrees.

As the left atrium continues to dilate, the so-called ''giant left atrium'' may develop. In this condition, almost exclu-sively seen in severe mitral insufficiency, the left atrium forms the right heart border with the right atrium seen as the double density medial to the left atrium. The atria can be distinguished based on their relationship to the hemidiaphragm. The right atrium curves slightly and maintains its contact with the right hemidiaphragm at the costophrenic angle whereas the left atrium curves inward more sharply and superiorly to attach to the center of the heart in the atrioventricular groove.

Left Ventricle

The left ventricle, based on its location, enlarges inferiorly and posteriorly. Simple left ventricle hypertrophy usually does not affect the overall cardiac size sufficiently to be detectable on the chest film, unless there is also concomitant cardiac decompensation. Left ventricular dilatation, however, results in displacement of the apex of the heart inferiorly, often resulting in an indentation on the gastric bubble. The cardiac axis, when measured from the mid-right atrium to the cardiac apex, clearly points downward in most cases of left ventricular enlargement, unlike the transverse or horizontal axis seen in isolated right ventricular enlargement (Fig. 5) (9). On the lateral view, the left ventricle is seen as a bulge in contour below the level of the left atrium, often extending more than 2 cm posterior to the inferior vena cava on a well-aligned lateral film (10).

CARDIAC CALCIFICATION

The presence and location of abnormal calcifications within the heart can be a valuable diagnostic tool. Abnormal

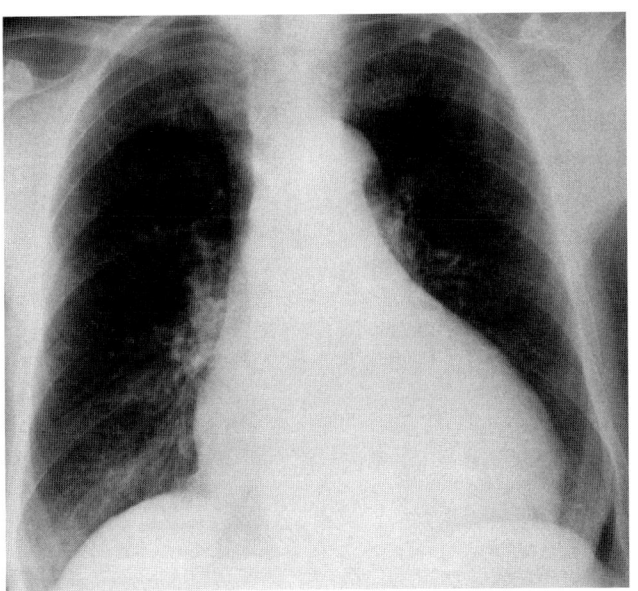
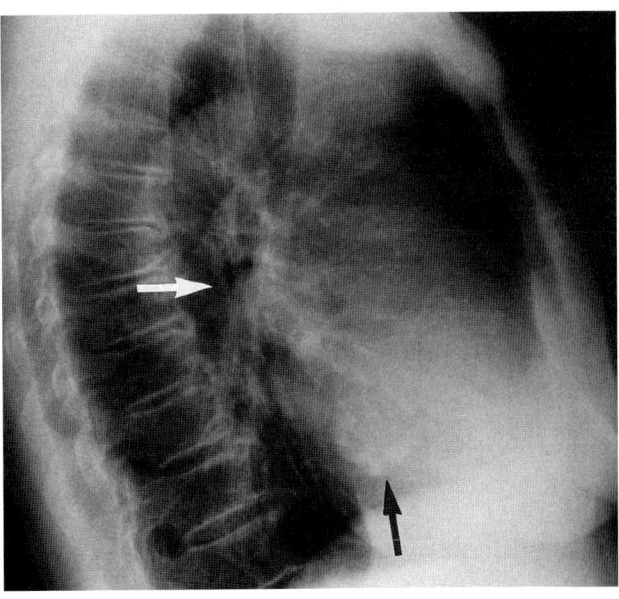

A   B

FIG. 5. A 63-year-old woman with mitral insufficiency and moderate left atrial and left ventricular enlargement. Posteroanterior (**A**) and lateral view (**B**). Dense calcification of the mitral valve annulus is seen on the lateral view (*black arrow*) with posterior displacement of the left lower lobe bronchus (*white arrow*). The cardiac axis points downward, reflecting the left ventricular dilatation.

tissue calcifications are divided into *metastatic,* caused by abnormal calcium and phosphate levels, or *dystrophic,* calcifications occurring in abnormal structures. Metastatic cardiac calcification is typically not visible on the conventional chest radiograph but may be detected by nuclear studies and, occasionally, computed tomography. Almost all cardiac calcifications visible by chest radiography or cinefluoroscopy are dystrophic in origin and occur in scars, areas of hemorrhage, or atherosclerosis.

Aortic Valve Calcification

Calcification of the aortic valve, seen best on the lateral radiograph, is highly suggestive of aortic stenosis, particularly in patients under the age of 60 (Fig. 6). In this age group, calcific tri-leaflet aortic stenosis is less common than bicuspid valvular stenosis (11). Aortic valvular calcification may be the only radiographic sign of aortic stenosis, since the associated left ventricular hypertrophy is usually not apparent. The aortic valve region can be located on the lateral view by extending the edge of the ascending aorta inferiorly to the level of the mid-portion of the left atrium.

Calcification of the Mitral Valve or Annulus

Mitral annular calcification usually is identified as a C-shaped area of dense calcification in the mitral valve region and is usually best appreciated on lateral view (Fig. 5). It is common in elderly patients and is usually of no importance (12). Mitral annular calcification is also more common in patients with calcium-phosphate abnormalities, Marfan's syndrome, and Ehlers-Danlos syndrome (13). Occasionally,

it may be associated with mitral insufficiency. Extension of the calcification and the accompanying fibrotic reaction anteriorly into the septum may result in conduction abnormalities such as first-degree heart block (13).

Identification of mitral valvular calcification is usually made by cardiac fluoroscopy rather than conventional radiography. Unlike the dense calcification seen in the annulus, the small nodules of calcification on the mitral valve leaflets caused by rheumatic heart disease are difficult to see and are further blurred by motion of the valve during the cardiac cycle.

Coronary Artery Calcification

Coronary artery calcification is easily identified on the lateral view as tubular areas of calcification along the expected course of the major coronary vessels (Fig. 7). On the posteroanterior view, coronary calcification is less readily apparent due to the density of the spine but may be seen in the region of the left atrial appendage, which overlaps the origin of the left main coronary artery (14). As with any vessel, irregular intimal calcification indicates atherosclerosis of the vessel and significant stenoses are common when the patient also has angina (4,15).

Myocardial Calcification

Calcifications in the cardiac wall are usually curved, linear and thin in their appearance. The most common site is the left ventricular wall due to previous myocardial infarction with associated scar and possible aneurysm (Fig. 8). Left

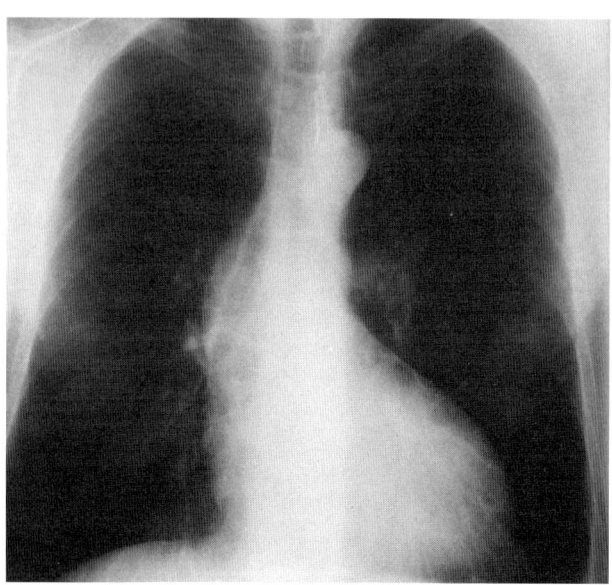
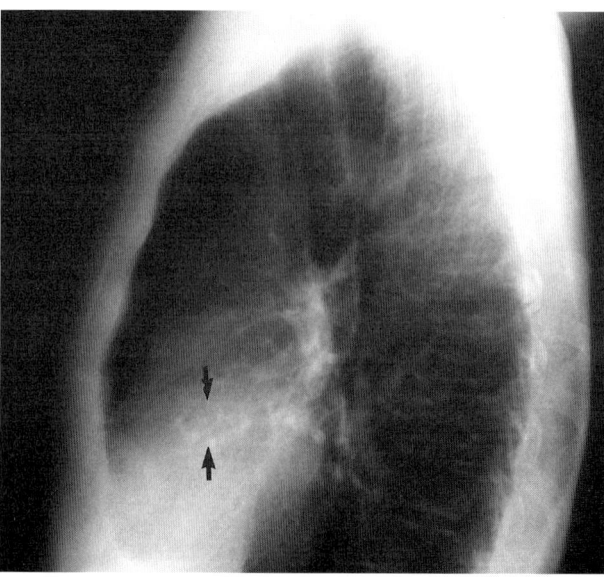

A

B

FIG. 6. A 48-year-old man with bicuspid aortic valve and aortic stenosis with 30 mm Hg pressure gradient across the aortic valve by catheterization. **A:** Posteroanterior view shows prominent ascending aorta with normal cardiac size in the patient with left ventricular hypertrophy. **B:** There is dense calcification of the aortic valve on the lateral view (*arrows*).

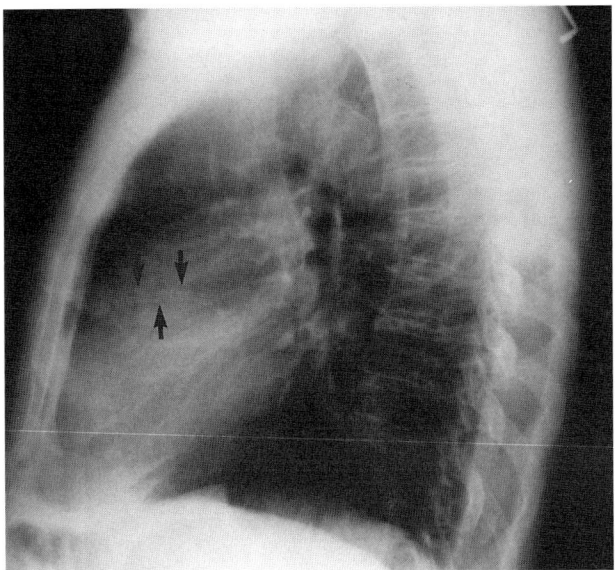

FIG. 7. A 65-year-old man with angina pectoris. There is calcification of the left anterior descending coronary artery on the lateral view (*arrows*).

ventricular aneurysms are most common in the lateral wall with a few seen posteriorly on the lateral view.

Calcification of the subendocardium of the left atrium was previously common in patients with severe rheumatic heart disease and usually associated with severe mitral stenosis. In this condition, left atrial thrombi are common and further investigation with echocardiography is recommended (16). Due to the decreasing incidence of rheumatic heart disease, this is now a rare finding in the Western world.

Pericardial Calcification

Pericardial calcification, seen as a sequelae of pericarditis, must be differentiated from myocardial calcification. Typically, the calcification is more peripheral in location than calcification within the heart itself with no significant soft tissue seen outside the calcification. Pericardial calcification is often longer, thicker, and less curved in appearance than calcification in the myocardium and favors the right ventricular surface (Fig. 9). Pericardial calcification may occur with or without constrictive pericarditis, depending on the severity and extent of the calcification (17). Associated findings

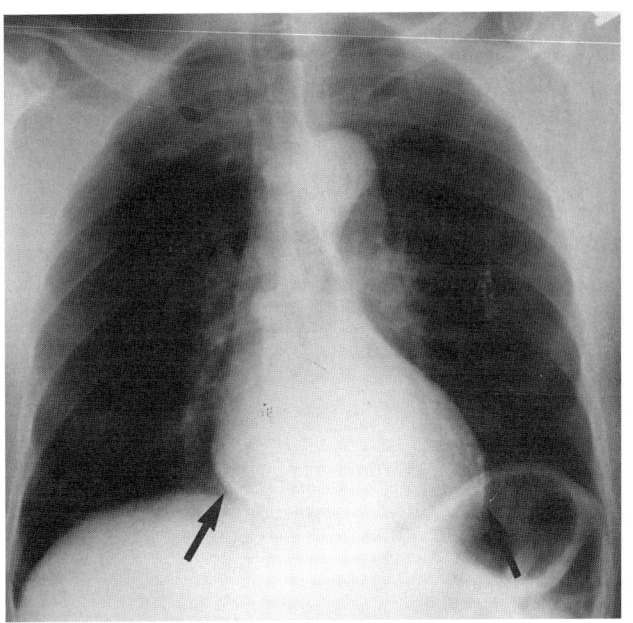

A

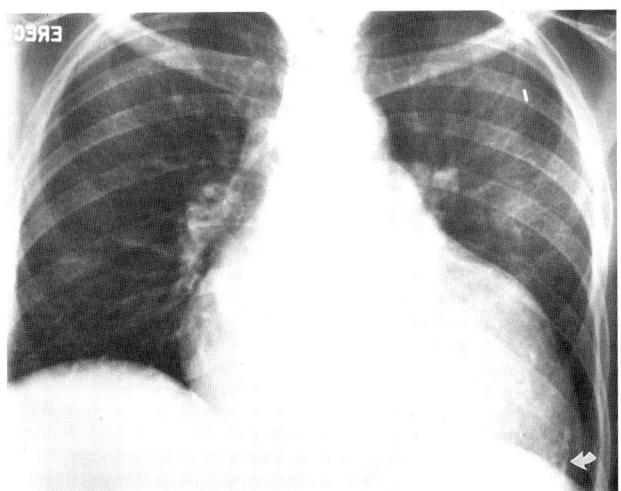

FIG. 8. A 59-year-old man with history of two myocardial infarctions with resultant ischemic cardiomyopathy. There is moderately severe cardiomegaly. At the left ventricular apex, a curvilinear calcification is present (*arrow*) due to an apical ventricular aneurysm, proven by left ventriculogram. Note the soft tissue extending lateral to the calcification due to the remainder of the left ventricular wall.

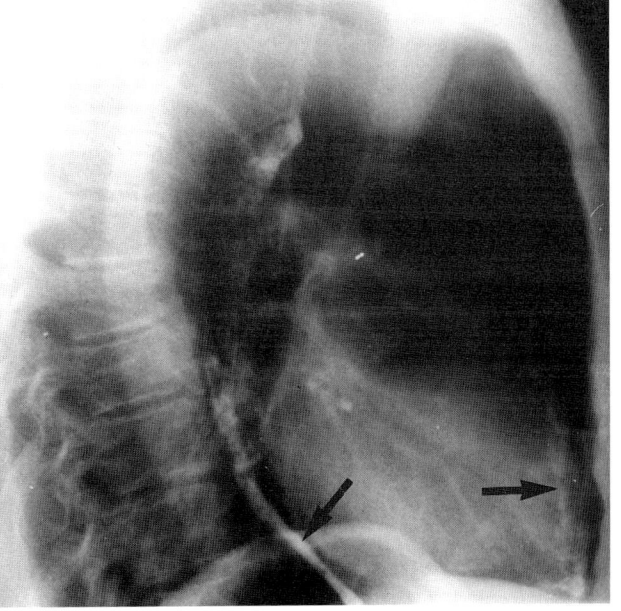

B

FIG. 9. A 54-year-old man with constrictive pericarditis and extensive pericardial calcification around both right and left ventricles (*arrows*). Posteroanterior (**A**) and lateral views (**B**).

of pulmonary oligemia, distention of the superior vena cava, or pleural effusion suggest the need for more intensive investigation to exclude constrictive pericarditis.

PHYSIOLOGIC ASSESSMENT—THE PULMONARY VESSELS

The chest film provides valuable insight into the quantity of pulmonary blood flow as well as estimates of pulmonary vascular resistance and pulmonary capillary wedge pressure. Conventionally, the pulmonary vascularity as seen on the chest film is divided into well-defined patterns: (1) normal; (2) shunt; (3) oligemia; and pulmonary hypertension, including (4) postcapillary pulmonary hypertension, also known as pulmonary venous hypertension; and (5) precapillary pulmonary hypertension, usually referred to as pulmonary arterial hypertension. The assessment and correct assignment of the vascular pattern in a given patient is the most important radiographic finding on the chest film in a patient with cardiac disease. All other findings must be correlated with this initial judgment.

Normal

Vessel margins are normally extremely well-defined because they are surrounded by lung, and gracefully and pro-

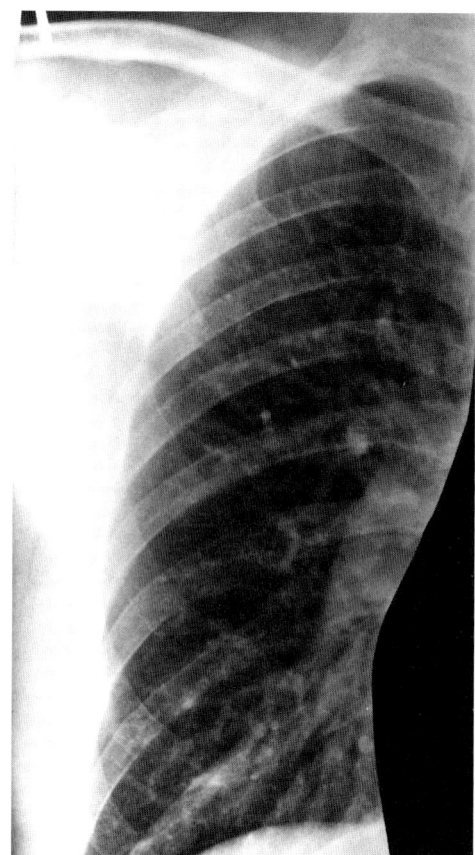

FIG. 11. Detail of right hemithorax from posteroanterior view showing a large shunt in this patient with atrial septal defect.

gressively branch toward the periphery. The right interlobar artery as measured on the PA film is up to 15-mm diameter in men and 14 mm in women (Fig. 10) (18). In the erect position, normal pulmonary vessels are clearly larger and more numerous in the larger half of the lung with approximately two to three times more blood flow in the lung bases than in the apices. This reflects that the apical blood vessels are at pulmonary reserve with little flow at rest in the erect patient. This distribution of blood flow is controlled by gravity with a 22 mm Hg apex-to-base pressure gradient in erect adults (18).

Shunt

In shunt vascularity, either due to left-to-right shunts or admixture lesions such as truncus arteriosus, the pulmonary blood vessels are increased in both size and number but retain the normal relationship of greater blood flow to the lung bases than the apices. Vessels retain their sharp margins and taper gradually but central pulmonary arteries are significantly enlarged and often exceed the 15 mm measurement considered normal for the right interlobar pulmonary artery (Fig. 11). Normally, a shunt of at least 2:1, that is twice as much blood flowing in the pulmonary bed as in the systemic circulation, is required to be visible on conventional films.

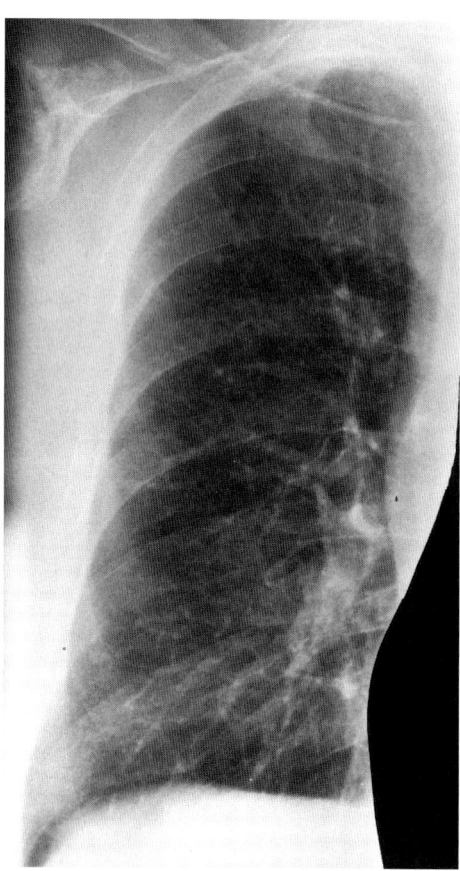

FIG. 10. Detail of right hemithorax from posteroanterior view showing normal pulmonary vascular pattern.

Therefore, circumstances of smaller increases in pulmonary blood flow, such as small shunt lesions or pregnancy, are generally not detectable by radiography (19). Identification of shunt vascularity, as in evaluation of other vascularity patterns, is generally based on experience, but large numbers of vessels seen below the level of the hemidiaphragm as well as pulmonary arteries larger than their accompanying bronchus in cross-section suggest the presence of a shunt (1,3,19,20).

Oligemia

Oligemic conditions, those with a decrease in pulmonary blood flow, include tetralogy of Fallot, Ebstein's anomaly, and tricuspid atresia (4,5). All have in common the same physiologic basis: an intracardiac defect combined with severe pulmonary outflow tract obstruction resulting in a right-to-left shunt and cyanosis. Like shunt vascularity, the vascular pattern of oligemia retains the normal 1:2 ratio of the blood flow in the upper-to-lower lungs but in this case the overall size and number of vessels is reduced (Fig. 12). Based on most readers' experience, this has proved to be

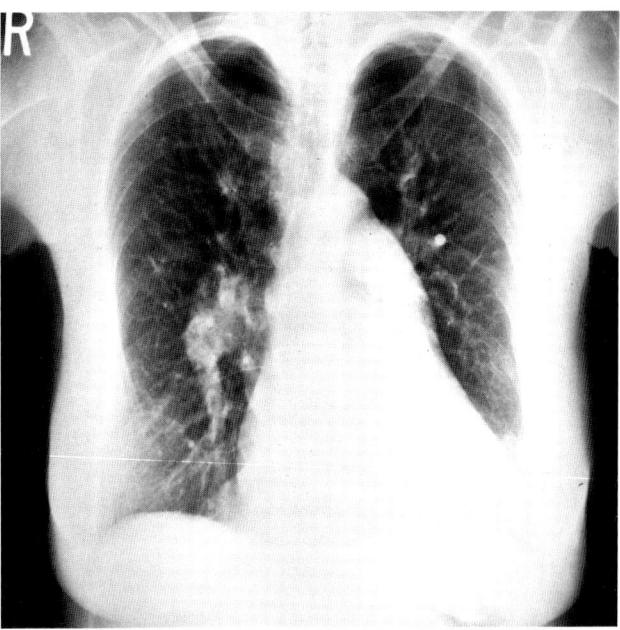

FIG. 13. Posteroanterior view of patient with long-standing large atrial septal defect with Eisenmenger syndrome and pulmonary arterial hypertension. Note the disparity in size between the large central pulmonary vessels compared to the peripheral ones compared to the uncomplicated shunt condition (see Fig. 11).

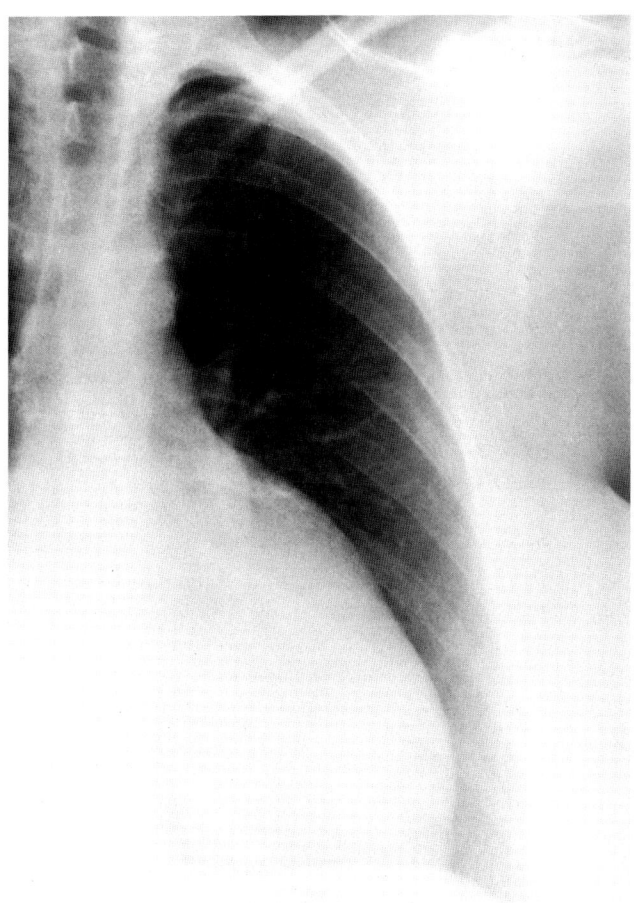

FIG. 12. Detail of left hemithorax from posteroanterior view from Figure 2 showing severe oligemia in this patient with Ebstein anomaly.

the most difficult vascular pattern to accurately identify by the plain chest film. This is due, in part, to technical considerations. The phototiming mechanism of conventional chest films and the preset parameters of most digital film systems increases the density of the lung in patients with oligemia so that the film remains within appropriate settings; this makes even small pulmonary vessels more prominent than they truly are. One helpful finding in oligemia is that the central pulmonary arteries are also extremely small on the lateral view (Fig. 2). This contrasts with the situation in pulmonary arterial hypertension, in which the central pulmonary arteries are large with small tapering peripheral vessels (Fig. 13).

Pulmonary Venous Hypertension

Pulmonary venous hypertension (PVH), also known as postcapillary pulmonary hypertension, usually results from left ventricular failure or mitral valve disease. The chest film findings reflect the rise in the pulmonary capillary wedge pressure and, by inference, the mean left atrial pressure. Initially there is dilatation of the upper zone pulmonary vessels whereas the pulmonary vessels in the lower half of the chest become relatively constricted, leading to a reversal of the normal 1:2 relationship of upper-to-lower pulmonary blood flow. This process of reversal of the normal pattern is called *cephalization* and is the earliest findings in incipient cardiac failure (Fig. 14).

The rise in pressure as measured by Swan-Ganz catheters

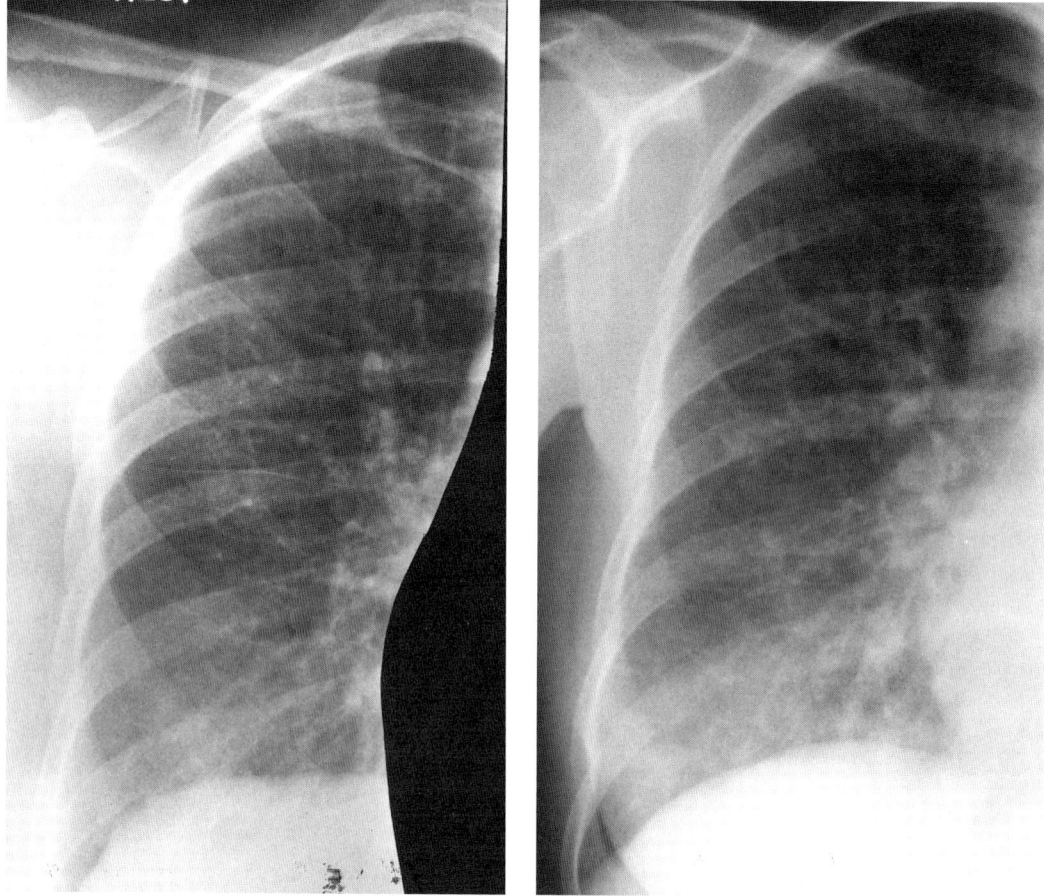

FIG. 14. Two posteroanterior chest films in patients with mitral stenosis. In early left ventricular failure, pulmonary venous hypertension occurs with distention of the upper pulmonary vessels and constriction of the vessels in the lower half of the lung (**A**). As edema develops, a basilar interstitial pattern develops and the margins of the upper lobe vessels blur due to early perivascular edema (**B**).

has been correlated by Chen (1) with the findings on the chest film in mitral stenosis. Pulmonary venous hypertension begins when pulmonary venous pressure rises to 10 to 12 mm Hg and is seen in almost all patients at 15 mm Hg (16). As the pressure in the pulmonary veins rises further to 20 to 25 mm Hg, interstitial edema can be seen in the lower lung zones with basilar interstitial pattern associated with distended ill-defined vessels in the upper lungs (Fig. 4). Further elevation of the venous pressure to 30 mm Hg or more results in progression of the findings to alveolar pulmonary edema. The physiologic basis for these findings is early development of edema of the perivascular regions of the lower lungs resulting in focal area of hypercarbia, vascular spasm, increased lower lung pulmonary vascular resistance, and redirection of flow to the lower resistance vessels of the upper lungs (21).

Not all cases of increased blood flow in the upper lungs are due to pulmonary venous hypertension. Bibasilar pulmonary or pleural disease also causes increased resistance in the basilar vessels with redirection of flow to the upper lungs. For instance, a patient with large bilateral pleural effusions will have bibasilar atelectasis and increased flow and size

and upper lung vessels with normal pulmonary venous pressures.

Pulmonary Arterial Hypertension

Pulmonary arterial hypertension (PAH), also known as precapillary pulmonary hypertension, is seen in such diseases as chronic pulmonary thromboembolism (PTE), primary pulmonary hypertension, long-standing left-to-right shunt with Eisenmenger physiology, as well as pulmonary diseases such as emphysema. Radiographically, the differentiation of this pattern appears on the detection of large central pulmonary arteries with rapid tapering and narrowing of the pulmonary arterial branches, called *pruning*, with oligemia of the distal lung (Fig. 13). Normal measurements of the transverse diameter of the right interlobar pulmonary artery are less than 15 mm in men and 14 mm in women; values greater than 17-mm diameter are indicative of moderate to severe pulmonary arterial hypertension in the absence of shunt lesions. In some patients, the pattern of the peripheral oligemia may aid in the diagnosis of the underlying condition (3). When the peripheral oligemia is patchy with areas of increased perfusion contrasting with focal oligemia, underlying lung disease or chronic PTE should be considered. In contrast, primary pulmonary hypertension usually has a uniformly distributed oligemia on the chest radiograph. Unlike the oligemia seen in congenital heart disease such as tetralogy of Fallot, there is disparity between the large central arteries and the small peripheral vessels.

CONCLUSION

The chest radiograph furnishes abundant anatomic detail in cardiac disease, such as chamber size and abnormal calcifications. Unlike most other imaging examinations, however, it also provides physiologic information on the pulmonary circulation including estimates of pulmonary blood flow and pulmonary vascular resistance as well as degree of cardiac compensation. The ability to assess and correlate both types of information is the essential value of the chest radiograph in the cardiac patient.

REFERENCES

1. Chen JT. The plain radiograph in the diagnosis of cardiovascular disease. *Rad Clin North Am* 1983;21:609–621.
2. Glover L, Baxley WA, Dodge HT. A quantitative evaluation of heart size measurements from chest roentgenograms. *Circulation* 1973;155:1289–1296.
3. Jefferson K, Rees S. *Clinical cardiac radiology*, 2nd ed. London: Butterworths, 1980.
4. Moes CAF, Freedom RH. Chest radiography In: Freedom RM, ed. *Pulmonary atresia with intact ventricular septum*. Mount Kisco, NY: Futura Publishing Company, 1989:127–132.
5. Giuliani ER, Fuster V, Branderberg RO, et al. Ebstein's anomaly. The clinical features and natural history of Ebstein's anomaly of the tricuspid valve. *Mayo Clinic Proc* 1979;54:163–173.
6. Soto B, Kasseur EG, Baxley WA. *Imaging of cardiac disorders*, vol 2. Philadelphia: JB Lippincott, 1992:184–202.
7. Miller SW. *Cardiac radiology. The requisites.* St. Louis: Mosby, 1996:3–45.
8. Higgins CB, Reinke RT, Jones NE, et al. Left atrial dimension on the frontal thoracic radiography: a method for assessing left atrial enlargement. *Am J Roentgenol* 1978;130:251–255.
9. Klatte EC, June H, Burney B. Radiographic manifestation of aortic stenosis and aortic valvular insufficiency. *Semin Roentgenol* 1979;14:122–130.
10. Rose CP, Stolberg HO. The limited utility of the plain chest film in the assessment of left ventricular structure and function. *Invest Radiol* 1982;2:139–144.
11. Szamosi A, Wassberg B. Radiographic detection of aortic stenosis. *Acta Radiologica* 1983;24:201.
12. Benjamin EJ, Plehn JE, D'Agostino RB. Mitral valvular calcification and the risk of stroke in an elderly cohort. *N Engl J Med* 1992;327:374–379.
13. Roberts WC, Honings HS. The spectrum of cardiovascular disease in the Marfan syndrome: a clinical morphologic study of 18 necropsy patients and comparison to 151 previously reported necropsy patients. *Am Heart J* 1982;104:115–135.
14. Souza AS, Bream PR, Elliott LP. Chart film detection of coronary artery calcification. The value of the CAC Triangle. *Radiology* 1978;129:7–10.
15. Margolis JR, Chen JTT, Kong YH, et al. The diagnostic and prognostic significance of coronary calcification. A report of 800 patients. *Radiology* 1980;137:609.
16. Grainger RG. An evaluation of conventional radiographs in acquired valvular disease. *Br J Radiol* 1970;43:623–684.
17. Deutsch V, Miller H, Yahini JH, et al. Angiocardiography in constrictive pericarditis. *Chest* 1974;65:379–387.
18. Simon M. The pulmonary vessels. Their hemodynamic evaluation using routine radiographs. *Rad Clin North Am* 1963;9:25–60.
19. Sanders C, Bittner V, Nath HP, et al. Atrial septal defect in older adults: atypical radiographic appearances. *Radiology* 1988;167:123–127.
20. Elliott LP. *Cardiac imaging in infants, children, and adults.* Philadelphia: JB Lippincott, 1992.
21. Milne ENC, Pistolesi M, Miniati M, et al. The radiographic distinction of cardiogenic and non-cardiogenic edema. *AJR Am J Roentgenol* 1985;144:879–894.
22. Rees S. The chest radiograph in pulmonary hypertension with central shunt. *Br Heart J* 1968;41(483):172–179.

CHAPTER 25

Cardiac Angiography

Paulo A. Ribeiro and Eileen Judkins

Coronary angiography remains at the epicenter of modern cardiology and cardiac surgery. The central dogma of clinical cardiology consists of relentlessly pursuing significant coronary stenoses to relieve angina and to improve prognosis both with interventional and surgical techniques. Coronary angiography is a unique diagnostic tool that enables the clinical cardiologist to practice evidence-based medicine, the interventionalist to "dilate," and the cardiac surgeon to "bypass." Since the original description of selective coronary angiography in 1959 by Mason Sones (1), and in 1967 by Melvin Judkins (2,3), the techniques remain virtually unchanged and unchallenged by newer imaging modalities.

HISTORICAL PERSPECTIVE

The first known cardiac catheterization was performed on a horse in 1711. Hales (4) catheterized both right and left ventricles with brass pipes via the jugular vein and carotid artery. Cardiac pressures were recorded through a long glass tube connected to a water column. Two discoveries were pivotal to the prelude of modern cardiac catheterization and cardiac angiography: the discovery of x-rays by Roentgen in 1895 and the technology for acquiring fluoroscopic images of the beating heart by Williams in 1896 (5).

Forssmann (6) was fascinated with the potential value for intracardiac drug delivery as a means for cardiac resuscitation using a uretal catheter. His initial research experiments in cadavers demonstrated the feasibility of cardiac catheterization. While a surgical resident in 1929, he performed the first human right-heart cardiac catheterization, a self-catheterization with a uretal catheter, via a left basilic vein cutdown. His superiors scorned his research work and fired him the same day. Egas Moniz (7,8) (Nobel Prize, 1949) reported

the first cerebral angiogram in 1927 and, in 1932, performed the first right-heart angiogram with contrast delivered into the right atrium (7–9). Severe joint deformities caused by arthritis onset in his early 20s prevented Moniz from actual performance of experiments. His collaborators carried out his ideas (9).

Perez Ara (10) reported his pioneering experience with pulmonary arteriography in 1931. Cournand (11) and Richards began their landmark work on right cardiac catheterization physiology and hemodynamics in 1936. They shared a 1956 Nobel Prize with Forssmann for their unique contribution to cardiac catheterization. X-ray technology advances dramatically improved angiographic image quality. The automatic cassette film changer, introduced in 1949, produced a rapid series of cut films (5,12). The image intensifier, introduced soon after, facilitated the development in the 1950s of cineangiograms recorded on roll film. Image intensifiers and cineangiography made it possible to produce better images with less radiation exposure to the patient and a smaller volume of contrast material.

Charles Dotter, a vascular radiologist, developed the first balloon-tipped angiographic catheter. Both he and Lategola as well as Rahn developed flow-directed catheters (12). These devices were the forerunners of the Swan-Ganz technique of right-sided hemodynamic monitoring. Successful human retrograde left-heart catheterization was reported by Zimmerman and Limon-Lason in 1950 (12,13). The impetus for the widespread use of cardiac catheterization took a major stride in 1953. Seldinger, a radiologist at Karolinska Institute in Sweden, devised a simple, safe technique for percutaneous insertion of catheters and guide wires (12–14). By this time, polyethylene tubing was available for custom fabrication of preformed vascular catheters. Shortly thereafter, heavy metal salts were incorporated, creating radiopaque catheter tubing.

Initial partial angiographic opacification of the coronary arteries was achieved indirectly by injection of contrast material in the aortic root by Rousthoi, Reboul, Racine, and Jonsson (12). At the time, it was believed that selective coro-

P. A. Ribeiro: Department of Cardiology, Loma Linda University Hospital, Loma Linda, California 92354.

E. Judkins: School of Medicine, Loma Linda University, Loma Linda, California 92354.

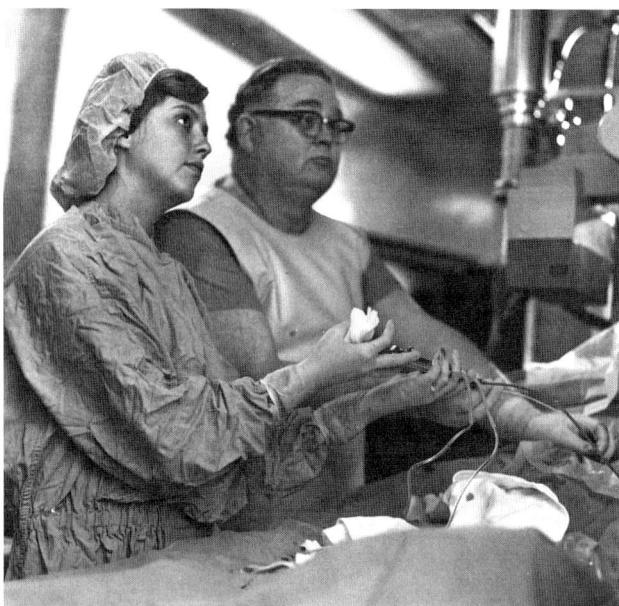

FIG. 1. Melvin P. Judkins, M.D., at Loma Linda University Medical Center in 1973.

nary angiography would cause fatal arrhythmias or an infarct. Mason Sones (1), a pediatric cardiologist at the Cleveland Clinic, had meticulously done elegant experimental dog work with semiselective coronary angiography. In 1958, Sones inadvertently performed a selective right coronary angiogram on a human with a 30-cc injection (12). To his amazement, the patient did well after a short asystolic episode that was promptly relieved by coughing. Over the next few years Sones pioneered and refined his technique of selective coronary angiography via a brachial artery cutdown using his flexible-tip radiopaque catheter.

Judkins (Fig. 1) (2,3) and Amplatz (15) revolutionized coronary angiography in 1967 when they introduced preshaped moldable catheters designed for percutaneous transfemoral insertion. Judkins had learned coronary angiography with Sones, but found his technique had limitations, particularly in patients with a large aortic root. The geniality of the Judkins technique is owed to the use and speed of transfemoral insertion and to true selective intubation with minimal manipulation of his unique preshaped catheters. He commented, ''The catheters know where to go, if not thwarted by the operator!'' Judkins (3) also introduced the ''pigtail,'' which, today, is the standard catheter for left and right ventriculography.

INDICATIONS FOR CORONARY ANGIOGRAPHY

The astute clinical cardiologist is often unsure about the presence of coronary artery disease based on the history alone and, at times, remains so even after noninvasive testing. At the other end of the spectrum, patients with frequent episodes of chest pain and multiple admissions may have normal coronary arteries. There is overwhelming evidence

of the great value of noninvasive testing, in both the diagnosis and risk stratification of patients with chest pain and coronary artery disease. Coronary angiography provides anatomical information that is complementary to the physiologic information obtained with noninvasive stress testing.

There are established indications for coronary angiography as per the American College of Cardiology/American Heart Association guidelines (16). In some cases, the indication for a coronary angiogram is a personal decision of the clinician, rather than evidence-based medicine from randomized trials, i.e., patients with multiple hospital admissions or clinic visits with chest pains and findings of normal coronary arteries. These patients can be reassured, and other causes for chest pain can be investigated. On the other hand, a patient may have unwarranted interventions to justify angiography performed for a questionable indication.

Coronary angiography is indicated for patients with angina pectoris refractory to medical therapy or at high risk for an adverse outcome such as those with: (i) angina pectoris and positive exercise stress test at low workload; (ii) greater than or equal to 2 mm ST depression; (iii) prolonged ST segment depression; (iv) decreased or flat blood pressure response; (v) exercise-induced ventricular tachycardia. However, patients with critical three-vessel coronary artery disease (CAD) or even left main stem disease with little or no chest pain may have a negative noninvasive test. A radionuclide test can be the harbinger of a high-risk subset of patients with angina: (i) low ejection fraction less than 35%; (ii) multiple defects; (iii) increase in lung uptake of thallium during exercise (14).

Patients with unstable angina are a high-risk subset and coronary angiography is indicated (13,14). For patients with acute transmural myocardial infarction, coronary angiography is performed as a prelude to percutaneous transluminal coronary angioplasty (PTCA). Results of the Primary Angioplasty in Myocardial Infarction (PAMI) and first Global Utilization of Streptokinase and Tissue plasminogen for Occluded coronary arteries (GUSTO) trials have shown the superiority of PTCA over conventional thrombolytic therapy (17,18). In patients who have had conventional conservative or thrombolytic therapy after myocardial infarction, coronary angiography is indicated in high-risk subset patients: (i) postinfarction angina; (ii) left ventricular heart failure; (iii) hemodynamic instability; (iv) mechanical complications such as ventricular septal defect or mitral regurgitation; (v) ventricular tachycardia or fibrillation; (vi) positive exercise test for ischemia.

Standard indications for coronary angiography include patients undergoing valve surgery after the age of 40, as surveillance in postcardiac transplant patients, and in screening high-risk patients undergoing noncardiac surgery.

SONES TECHNIQUE FOR CORONARY ANGIOGRAPHY

Mason Sones (1) described a brachial cutdown approach after making a small incision in the vessel wall. The catheter is introduced into the distal portion of the artery, and heparin saline is delivered to avoid thrombosis. The Sones catheter is available in a variety of lengths, diameters, bends, and compositions. The most commonly used catheter, constructed of woven Dacron or nylon with radiopaque plastic coating, has an end hole and four small side holes near the tip. Most used is a #7F or #8F catheter with a tip that tapers to a #5F.

This catheter technique requires manipulating the straight, flexible tip catheter into an open loop on the appropriate aortic cusp. A series of further maneuvers engage the tip in the target coronary sinus and ostium.

By 1967, Sones (1) and his colleagues had done coronary angiography in 8,200 patients with a 99% success rate, and he never deviated from his original brachial cutdown approach. Currently, his technique has been modified for use with a percutaneous brachial Seldinger approach. This variance of the Sones technique is less cumbersome and ideally suited for an outpatient procedure.

AMPLATZ TECHNIQUE

In 1967, Amplatz described his experience using hook-shaped coronary catheters (5) via the femoral approach (15). This technique can be used to advantage when catheterizing a patient who has a high take-off of the left main; the vessel may be difficult to engage with the Judkins technique. However, the manipulation of the catheters is more complex than in Judkins technique, and, therefore Amplatz technique is not commonly used. However, the catheters seat very well at the coronary ostia and give excellent support for coronary intervention.

MULTIPURPOSE TECHNIQUE

In 1974, Schoonmaker and King developed a technique for coronary angiography using the transfemoral approach and a multipurpose catheter (12). The main advantage of their approach is that both coronaries and the left ventricle are catheterized by a single catheter. Engaging the coronary orifices is achieved using Sones catheter manipulation technique.

JUDKINS TECHNIQUE

Melvin Judkins (2,3), a visionary cardiovascular radiologist, had the talent to develop a simple technique to perform a complex task. He had the concept of tailoring catheter configurations to aortic size by using the aortic arch to assist an appropriately shaped catheter into the target ostium. With his knowledge of aortic root anatomy and a three-dimensional spatial concept, he combined his grasp of catheter mechanics and materials to develop "coronary seeking" catheters. The unique configurations are preshaped to conform to the usual vascular anatomy, so the tip will seek the orifice regardless of aortic size if the correct catheter size configuration is chosen. Judkins advocated that safe catheterization of the coronary arteries via the femoral approach required a catheter with sensitive, positive rotary control, preferably made from a low-temperature thermoplastic. Originally, the material used was polyurethane with internal braided stainless steel wire for ultimate torque control. Radiopacity was achieved with barium salts. Catheter tips had a thinned, blunt bullet nose to reduce the chance of trauma or lumen obstruction. Several manufacturers currently market catheters patterned after the Judkins originals. Diagnostic catheter sizes available now range from 4F to 8F including thin-walled versions.

To ensure consistent successful selective catheterization, the angiographer must choose a catheter with the appropriate size configuration conforming to the anatomy of the patient to be studied (Fig. 2). The Judkins catheters are preshaped to conform to the usual aortic arch and coronary artery ostia—sinus of Valsalva anatomy. Each Judkins catheter has a primary, secondary, and tertiary curve. All catheters have a primary 90-degree initial curve. The secondary bend distinguishes the left and right catheters. The left catheter has a curve of nearly 180 degrees whereas the right is about 30 degrees. The tertiary curves are reversed in the right coronary catheter as excessive bend will jeopardize proper rotation and descent (Figs. 3 and 4).

The left and right coronary ostia configuration: The ostium of the left main arises within 15 degrees of the plane of the ascending aorta and proximal aortic root. The secondary 180-degree curve of the left Judkins provides the "spring" that maintains the catheter tip in situ. In contrast, the ostium of the right coronary artery arises between 120 to 130 degrees anterior and to the right of the plane of the aortic arch and position of the left ostium. To engage the right coronary ostium, a secondary stable fix point is achieved on the left posterior aortic wall with the right coronary catheter (Fig. 2A).

Technique for Judkins Catheterization

Percutaneous Seldinger entry is done with a #18 thin-wall needle angled 15 degrees cephaled along the sagittal plane in the common femoral artery under local anesthesia (12). A puncture should be performed 1 to 2 cm below the inguinal ligament, since high punctures can lead to inadequate post-procedure compression, hematoma, and retroperitoneal bleeding. A low femoral artery puncture increases the risk of false aneurysm formation and thrombotic occlusion by inadvertently entering the superficial femoral artery. This, anatomically, overlies the femoral vein and a low puncture can cause AV fistulas. A 0.035 to 0.038 J guidewire is introduced through the needle and threaded above the aortic bifurcation and, subsequently, a 5-8F sheath-dilator is introduced over the guidewire.

Left Coronary Artery

Radiographic aortic root size is used to assess the proper catheter configuration size to select for the patient to be

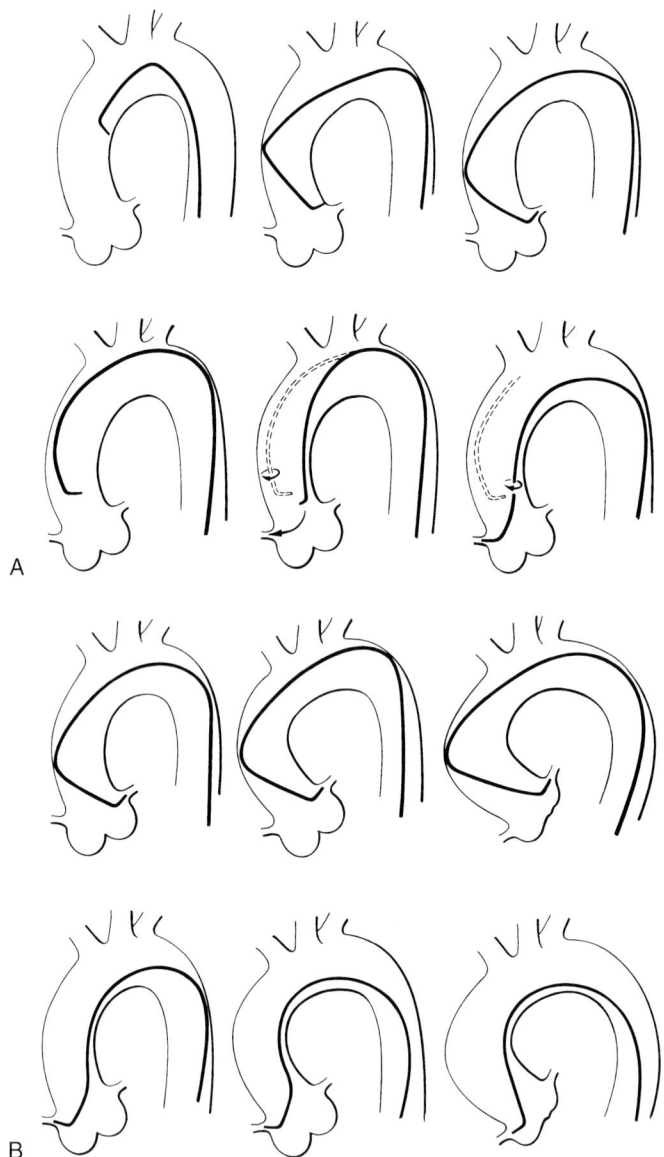

FIG. 2. A: Diagrammatic illustration of selective catheterization of a left (**top row**) and right (**bottom row**) coronary artery. **B:** Catheter mechanics for variations in aortic size and configuration. Left catheter positioned in normal, unfolded, and poststenotic aorta (**top row**) and right catheter positioned in normal, unfolded, and poststenotic aorta (**bottom row**). (From ref. 19, with permission.)

studied (Fig. 2**B**). In 80% of cases, a radiologically normal aortic root indicates the use of a 4L Judkins. For unfolded and large aortic roots, a 5 or a 6L Judkins should be selected. In children, a 3.5L is warranted (Fig. 3). Inadequate size or overinsertion may achieve a tip position near 90 degrees to the left main vessel wall, which is not acceptable. In such cases, catheter repositioning or exchange is mandatory.

With the guidewire in the distal aortic root, the left catheter is advanced to the arch beyond the neck vessels. After being flushed with heparin saline and filled with contrast, it

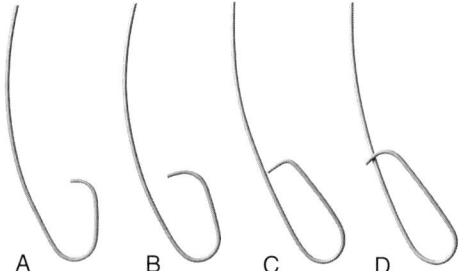

FIG. 3. Judkins left coronary catheters: (**A**) 3.5L, (**B**) 4L, (**C**) 5L, and (**D**) 6L.

is advanced gently down the medial wall of the ascending aorta. There will be a minor catheter rotation as it advances and the tip reaches the coronary ostium. At this stage, it is then advanced 2 to 4 mm to take up the slack, as the secondary catheter bend rests against the right aortic root wall. Multiple projections are imaged using 6 to 10 mL of contrast agent (Fig. 2**A**).

Right Coronary Artery

The same principles apply to suitable right catheter selection as they do for the left (Fig. 2**B**). The right catheter is introduced over the guidewire and positioned 1 to 2 cm above the left coronary ostium. In this position (2 to 4 cm above the aortic valve), the catheter is very slowly rotated clockwise. During this rotation and before reaching 60 degrees, the catheter tip will spontaneously descend about 3 cm into the right sinus of Valsalva. As clockwise rotation continues the tip will engage the right coronary artery ostium (Fig. 2**A**). Judkins specified this should be done very slowly, not like an "eggbeater" (19). Right coronary catheter configuration sizes (3.5R–5R) reflect the distance in cm between the primary catheter curve and the midpoint of the

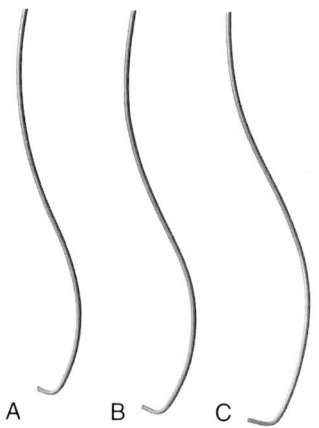

FIG. 4. Judkins right coronary catheters: (**A**) 3.5R, (**B**) 4R, and (**C**) 5R.

secondary catheter curve. In the great majority of patient cases, the 4R will do the job; the 5R is used in widened aortas. In children and in patients with very small aortas the 3.5R is recommended (Fig. 4).

Technical Tips (19)

When a single left coronary vessel is visualized, the catheter should be withdrawn to the ostium since subselective catheterization may be taking place in short left mains. Alternatively, there may be separate origins of the left anterior descending—circumflex or anomalous origin (Fig. 5). In the latter case, the suspected missing vessel often originates from the right coronary artery or right sinus of Valsalva (Fig. 6).

If rotation of the right coronary catheter is initiated too near the valve, the catheter will not descend 3 cm but rather 1 cm, and will engage deep in the sinus of Valsalva or even prolapse into the left ventricle rather than engaging in the ostium. When rotation is initiated too high, the catheter will not descend but rotate cephaled in the aortic root. Therefore, it is pivotal that the operator allow aortic flow-pulsation to contribute to the slow and steady catheter rotation, as excessive torque may lead the catheter to jump from the ostium.

When catheter pressure damping occurs, a small test injec-

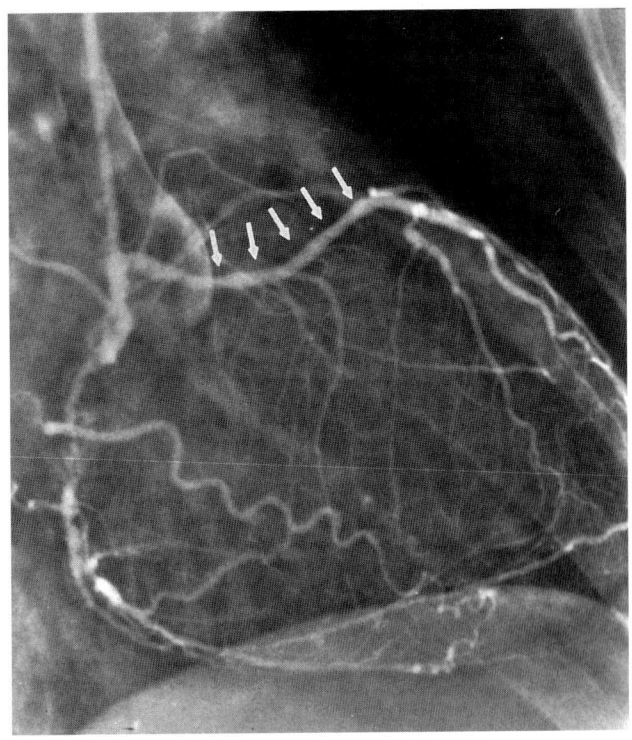

A

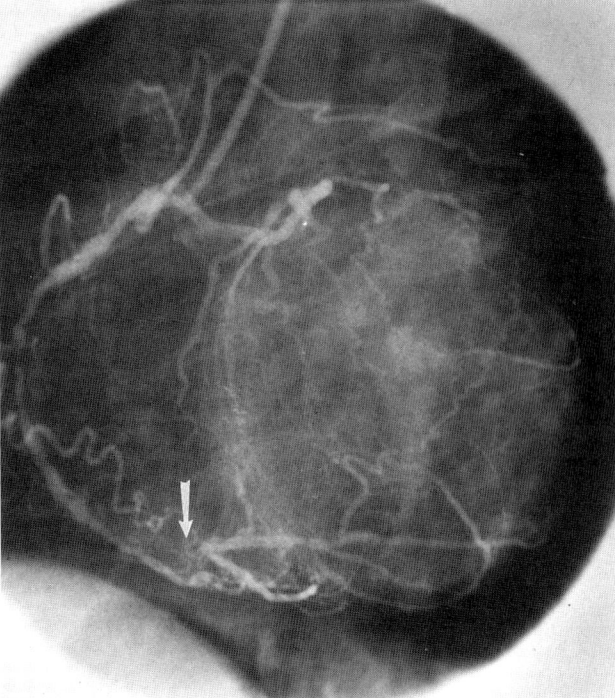

B

FIG. 6. Single coronary artery with origin from a normal situated right sinus of Valsalva. **A:** RAO view. It immediately gives rise to a large LAD branch (*arrows*) and the severely diseased RCA. **B:** LAO view. Note occlusion of RCA 3 cm proximal to the crux (*arrow*) and filling from LCA collaterals.

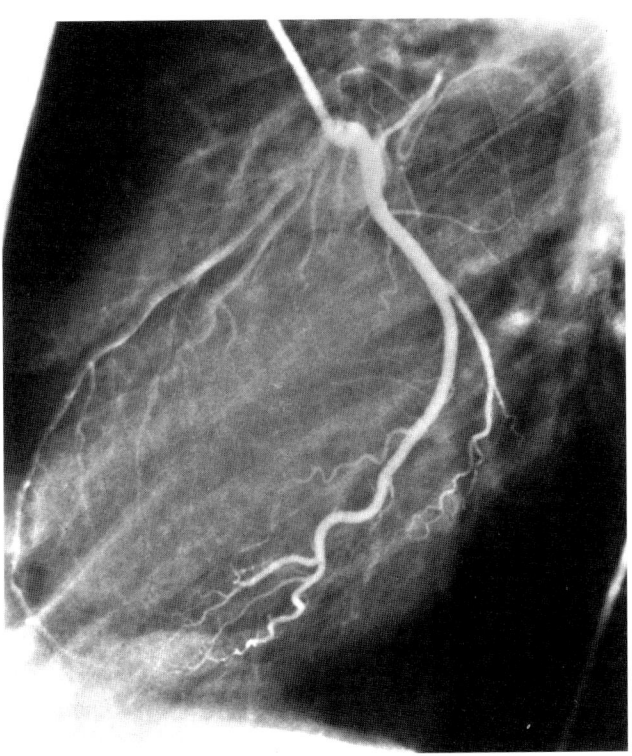

FIG. 5. Coronary angiogram showing separate origin of LCX and LAD (LCA lateral view). The catheter is selectively engaged in the LCX ostium. Note the spill of contrast in the aortic root that is faintly filling the LAD.

tion can be performed to detect the reason. Possibilities include: (i) catheter induced spasm, (ii) the presence of an ostial lesion, (iii) selective engagement of the right coronary artery (RCA) conus branch. If the right coronary catheter systematically engages the conus branch, two maneuvers can be attempted, i.e., straightening the tip of the catheter or upsizing the catheter configuration.

Rarely, catheter configuration may need to be modified to accommodate for unusual coronary anatomy, so as to engage the ostium.

Anatomical Variations

Anatomical variants of right coronary ostia origin occur more frequently than the left (19,20). Commonly, the orifice arises superior or immediately above the tip of the sinus of Valsalva. Of abnormal origins, the most common is a nondominant right coronary artery arising from the superior portion of the sinus Valsalva or tubular aorta (Fig. 7). The second most common variation is origin of the left or right coronary artery from the superior portion of the right sinus or tubular aorta (20). In this scenario, the catheter will have to probe the superior portion of the sinus of Valsalva. If the origin of the coronary ostium is from the tubular aorta, right coronary catheter manipulation will have to start from a more superior position in order to engage.

Graft Angiography

Graft catheterization is facilitated if the cardiac surgeon has marked the graft ostia with a metal ring or clip. Tradition-

ally, saphenous vein grafts (SVG) to an RCA originate from the anterolateral aorta 2 to 3 cm cephaled to the native right coronary ostium. Saphenous vein grafts to the left anterior descending (LAD) and circumflex (LCX) are attached to the anterior aspect of the aorta (Fig. 8).

To engage a right SVG, a catheter similar to a Judkins right but with a primary bend between 110 and 120 degrees is used. Alternatively, a multipurpose catheter will do the job, although this may engage too deeply, since the right SVG courses obliquely in the caudal direction. Selective engagement with a right SVG catheter requires a clockwise maneuver similar to that used for RCA engagement. This is initiated at a more cephaled level, with the catheter tip 1 cm above the ostium of the graft, and the catheter is subsequently advanced down the aorta until it engages (19).

The left bypass catheter has a primary 90-degree bend and a secondary one of 70 degrees and is ideally shaped to engage the circumflex and left anterior descending SVGs (19). Left SVGs usually originate superior and to the left of the native right ostium. The catheter should be rotated anteriorly until it passes the midway point of the ascending aorta. Circumflex grafts are traditionally inserted superior and to the left of an anterior descending SVG. The engagement maneuver is similar to that used for the LAD graft (Fig. 9). It is important to document the stump of an occluded graft and one should never rely solely on aortography (19). If the angiographer does not have a surgical report, it is crucial that he focus on the competitive flow of native coronary arteries and collateral circulation, as this may give a clue for a missed graft.

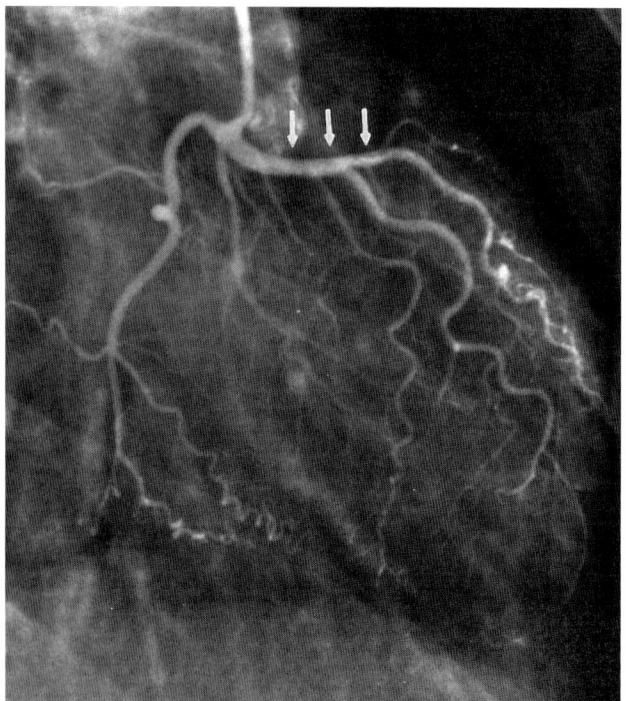 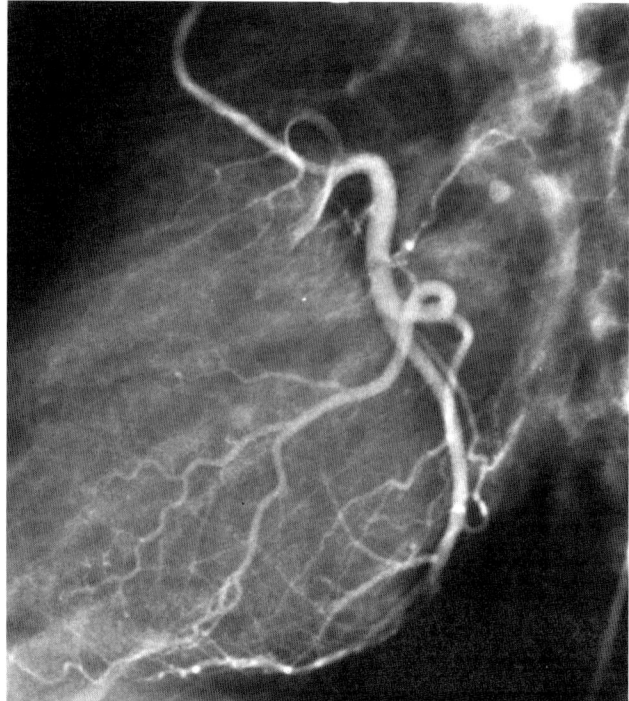

A   B

FIG. 7. A: RAO view shows origin of LAD (*arrows*) from the initial portion of the RCA vessel. **B:** Lateral view shows a separate origin of the LCX. All vessels are without disease.

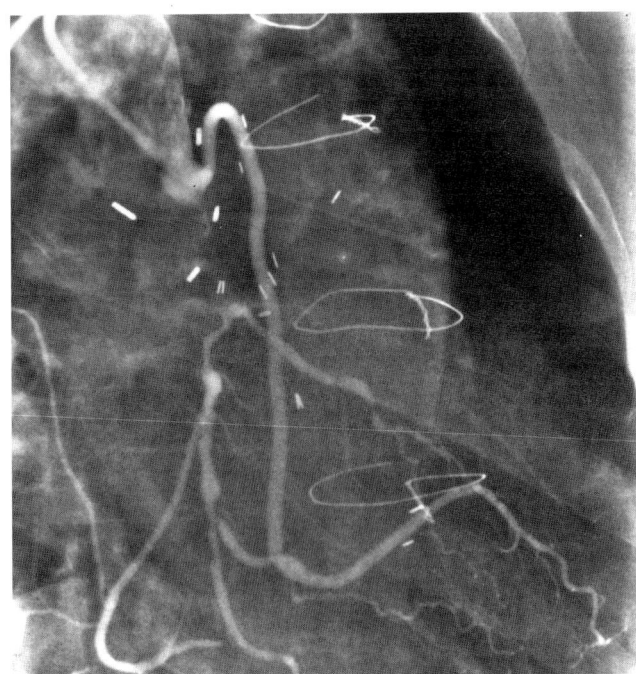 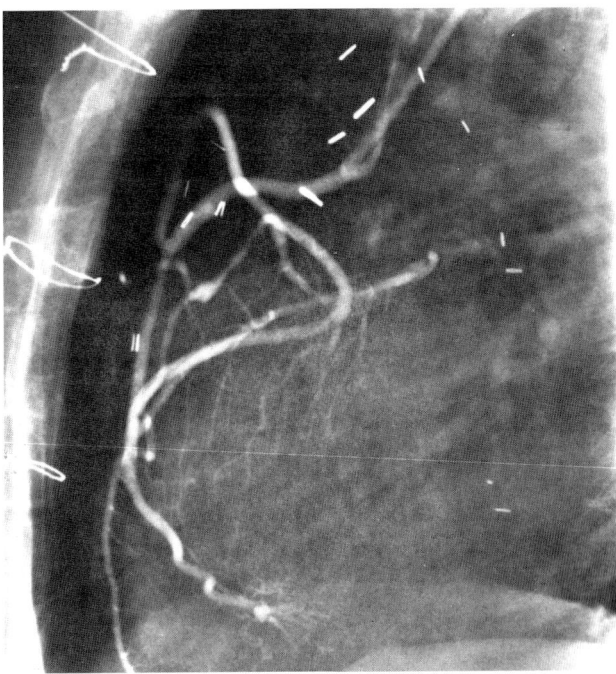

A   B

FIG. 8. Graft angiogram (**A**) showing sequential SVGs to mid-obtuse marginal and intermediate vessels. **B:** Note Y graft to principal diagonal, LAD, and RCA.

Arterial Conduit Angiography

The left internal mammary artery (LIMA) arises from the anterior inferior side of the subclavian after it curves caudad (13). An internal mammary artery (IMA) catheter is advanced distal to the origin of the left subclavian and manipulated into the vessel. A guidewire may be of help. Slow

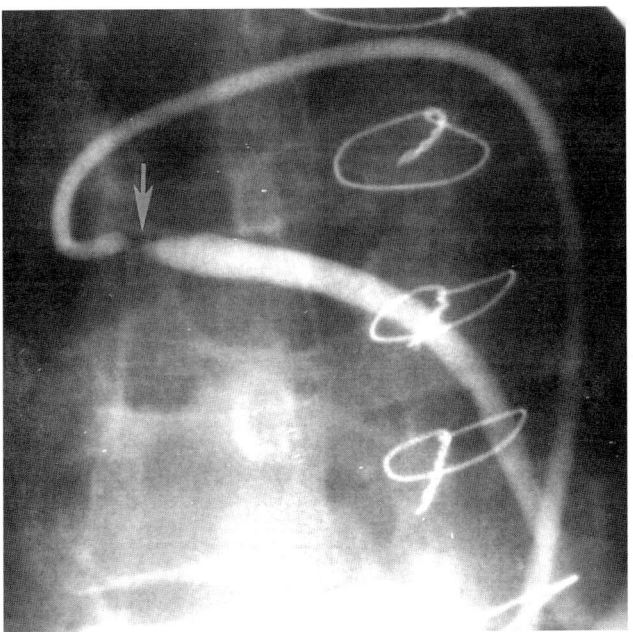

FIG. 9. RAO view of obtuse marginal SVG showing severe ostial stenosis (*arrow*).

withdrawal of the catheter, together with counterclockwise rotation, enables its entry into the subclavian artery (13). After the catheter is advanced slightly distal to the origin of the LIMA (perhaps with help from the guidewire), gently pulling back with counterclockwise rotation will direct the catheter tip inferior and selectively engage the vessel. The right anterior oblique (RAO) and left anterior oblique (LAO) with cranial views are commonly used to visualize the graft and its distal anastomosis.

The right IMA (RIMA) is catheterized after engaging the distal right subclavian artery using similar maneuvers to those described for engaging the left subclavian. The catheter is pulled back, attempting to have the catheter tip engage the origin of the RIMA, which is not always straightforward in view of the tortuosity of the right subclavian artery. The distal anastomosis of the RIMA is best visualized in the LAO or anterior posterior (AP) cranial views.

The gastroepiploic artery (GEA) is a branch of the gastroduodenal artery. Since it arises from the hepatic artery in 75% of cases, it is best to initially engage the common hepatic artery using a Cobra catheter. This is achieved with the aid of a guidewire, accessing the GEA via the gastroduodenal artery and subsequently exchanging for a Judkins right catheter for selective engagement (13).

A free radial graft is commonly anastomosed to the obtuse marginals and the aorta. In such cases, a left bypass catheter is indicated, since the aortic graft attachment is in similar anatomical position to the left circumflex SVG.

Spasm of the arterial conduits during engagement and selective angiography can be relieved with intraarterial administration of 75 to 200 mcg of nitroglycerin or 50 to 100 mcg of verapamil.

CORONARY VESSEL ANATOMY (Fig. 10)

Left Main

The left main coronary artery arises from the superior portion of the left coronary sinus (21). The diameter ranges from 3 to 6 mm; average left main stem diameter is 4.5 ± 0.5 mm in normal arteries, and 4.0 ± 0.3 mm in patients with CAD. Anatomically, the left main passes behind the right ventricular outflow tract and may extend up to 25 mm; commonly, it bifurcates into a LAD and LCX. The best angiographic projections to visualize the left main are the RAO caudal, and RAO and LAO cranial.

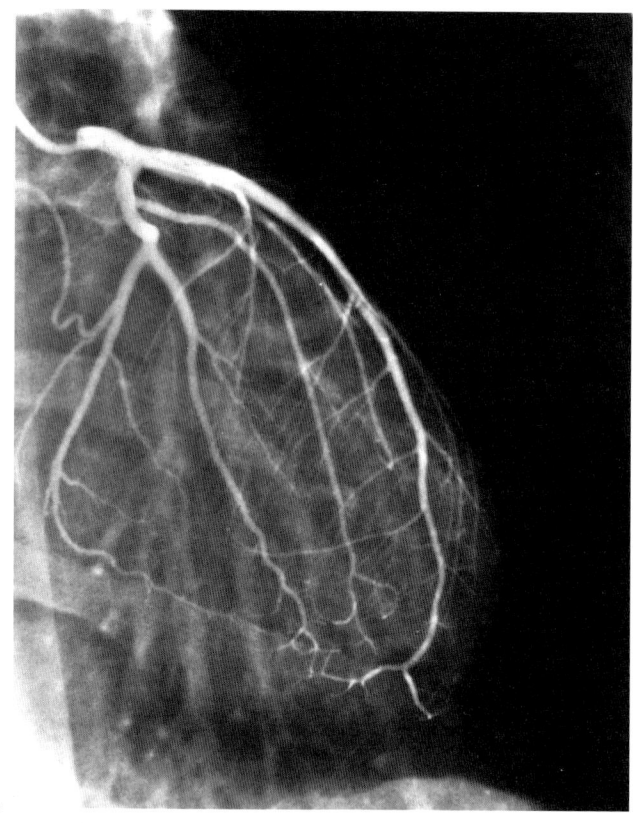

A

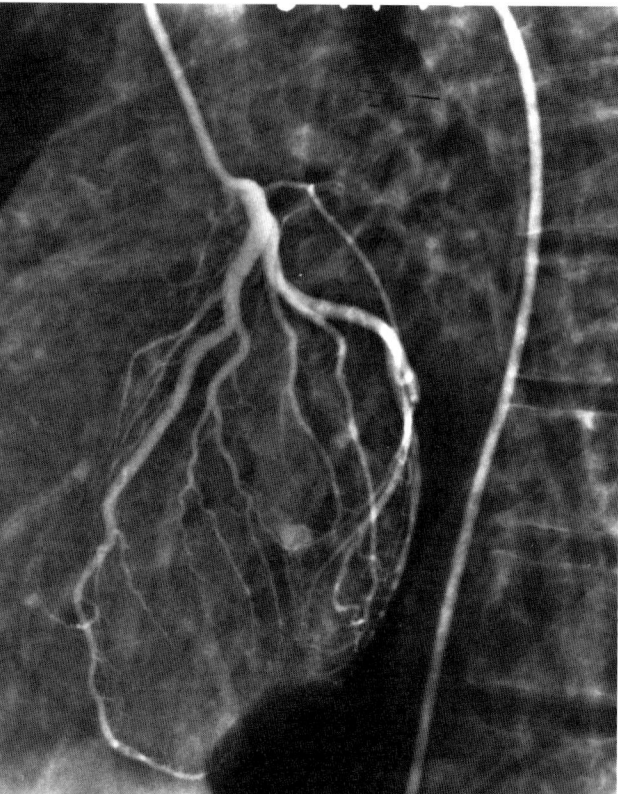

B

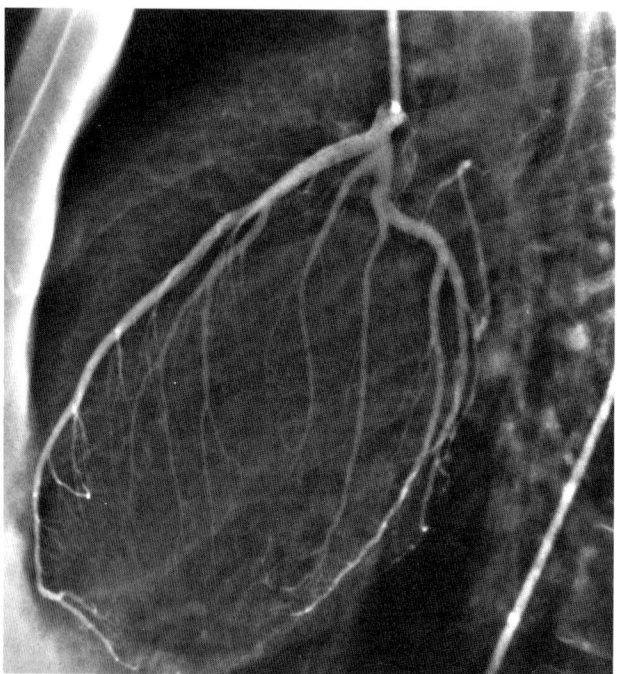

C

FIG. 10. A normal coronary angiogram. Left coronary artery: (**A**) RAO view; (**B**) LAO cranial view; (**C**) lateral view. (*continued*)

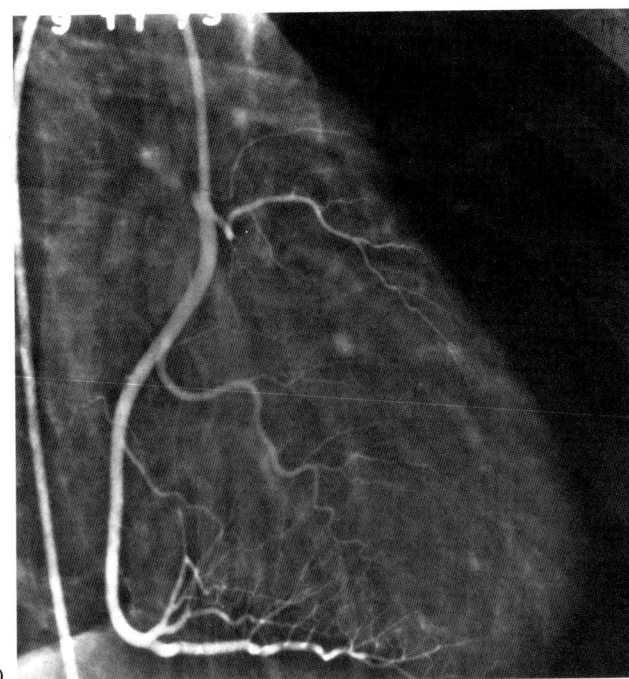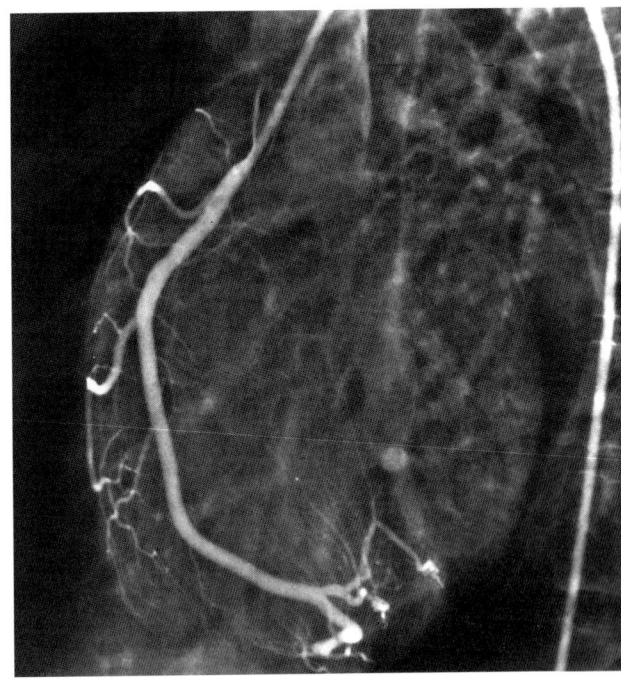

D   E

FIG. 10. *Continued.* Right coronary artery: (**D**) RAO view; (**E**) LAO view.

Left Anterior Descending

Anatomically, the LAD crosses anteriorly and inferiorly and travels in the anterior interventricular groove toward the apex and it may extend to the inferior wall in some patients (13,21). Muscular bridges may occur if the LAD courses within the myocardium. The best angiographic projections are the LAO and RAO cranial. These views separate well the diagonal vessels from the LAD, particularly at their origin. The lateral view is also helpful, particularly for mid and distal LAD lesions. An AP cranial view is often useful for visualizing the proximal and mid-left anterior descending and to separate it from the diagonal and septal vessels. Ostial LAD lesions are best seen in RAO and LAO caudal projections.

Left Circumflex

The left circumflex originates from the left main and travels down the left atrioventricular groove (21). There is a wide variation in circumflex anatomy and, in 85% of cases, it is the nondominant vessel. If it is the dominant vessel, it gives origin to the posterior descending artery (PDA). The main branches of the LCX are one to three obtuse marginals that supply the free wall of the left ventricle. The best angiographic projection to visualize the origin of the LCX is the LAO caudal. The LAO projection is also useful to show the proximal and mid-LCX. The midportion of the LCX and origin of the obtuse marginals are best imaged in the RAO caudal view. To image the posterior descending artery, the LAO cranial projection is indicated.

Right Coronary Artery

The right coronary artery (RCA) arises from the anterior portion of the right aortic sinus slightly lower than the origin of the LCA from the left aortic sinus (21). The RCA travels down in the right atrioventricular groove toward the apex. It terminates, giving origin to the PDA and several posterolateral branches. The second branch of the RCA is the sinoatrial node artery in 59% of patients. The right coronary ostium and proximal third of RCA are best visualized in a 45 to 60 degree LAO projection, whereas the distal RCA and PDA are optimally visualized in the LAO and AP cranial projections.

CORONARY ANOMALIES

Major congenital abnormalities are present in 1% of cases, commonly occurring in patients with congenital heart disease and anatomical findings that may have surgical implications (19,20). The most common congenital abnormality is a coronary artery fistula (Fig. 11). These are often asymptomatic, although some may develop ischemia, infective endocarditis, congestive heart failure, or rupture. The majority of fistulas arise from the right coronary artery and drain into the right ventricle. Aneurysms are uncommonly seen at angiography (Fig. 12).

Ischemia can be triggered by the origin of an LCA from the pulmonary artery (13,20). Only 25% of these patients survive to adulthood; they exhibit frequent episodes of congestive heart failure and ischemia. It is also important to

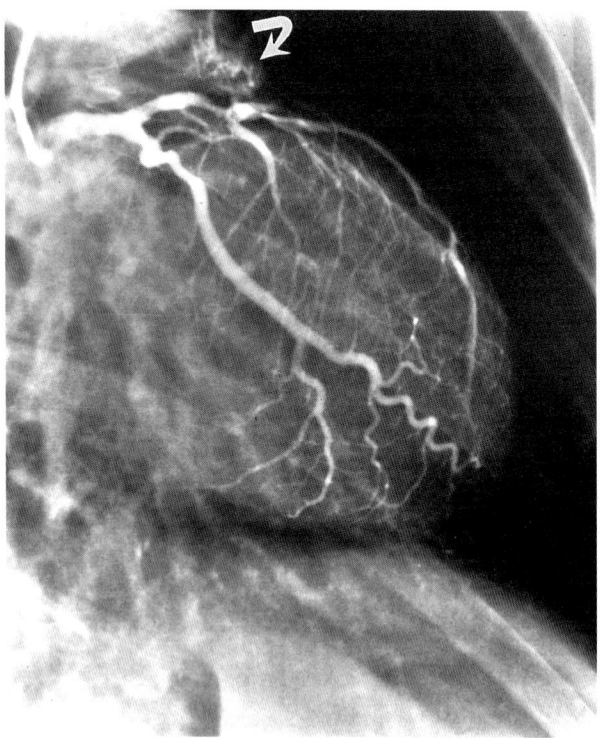

FIG. 11. Congenital A–V fistula in proximal LAD (*curved arrow*) evident in RAO view of LCA.

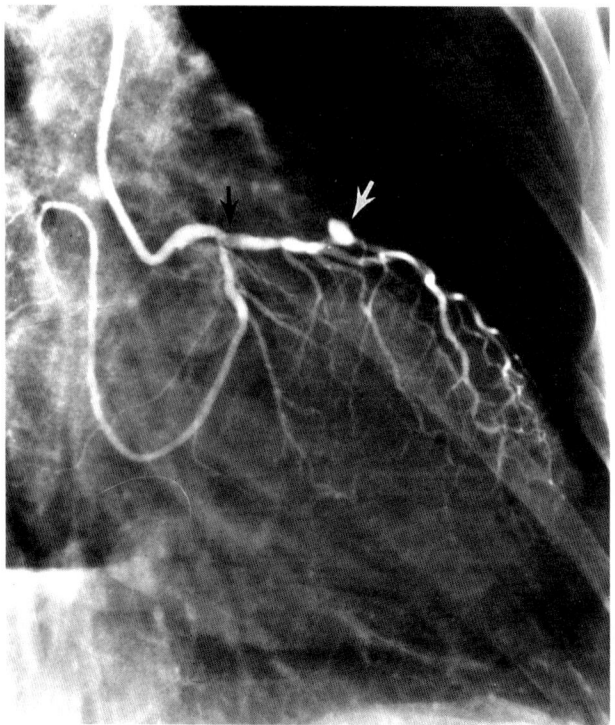

FIG. 12. Left coronary artery in RAO view. Note the saccular aneurysm (*white arrow*) of the LAD measuring 7 by 5 mm. Note the distal 50% left main stem stenosis (*black arrow*).

recognize the anomalous origin of an LCA from the RCA or right sinus, that subsequently travels in between the aorta and pulmonary artery; this variant may cause sudden death. The RAO projection is best suited to evaluate other anomalous RCA origins, such as a single coronary vessel.

COMPLICATIONS OF CORONARY ANGIOGRAPHY AND INTERVENTIONS

The advent of percutaneous coronary intervention has changed the spectrum of complications in cardiac catheterization and coronary angiography (Tables 1 and 2). Prior to the era of interventional cardiology, Bourassa and Noble (22) reported a review of 5,250 cases studied by a percutaneous femoral technique. In this series, there was a reported mortality rate of 0.23%, acute myocardial infarction of 0.09%, and coronary artery dissection of 0.07%. Data from the Coronary Artery Surgery Study (CASS) registry (23) was collected prospectively in 7,553 consecutive patients, and left main stem disease was present in all death cases. Death was 6.8 times more likely when left main stem disease was present. Multivariate statistical analysis showed that other factors, such as congestive heart failure, unstable angina, multiple premature ventricular contractions (PVCs), and hypertension also increased the risk of death (23).

The brachial artery technique increased the risk of death 3.6 times compared to the femoral approach, and the additional use of heparin did not decrease the risk of thromboembolic complications (23). The Registry of The Society for Cardiac Angiography and Interventions (24) reported the complication rates in 222,553 cases between 1984 and 1987. Death occurred in 0.1%, myocardial infarction in 0.06%, stroke in 0.07%, and vascular complications in 0.23%.

Adams and colleagues (25) reported in 1973 that the most frequently overlooked complication of coronary arteriography was an incomplete or nondiagnostic study. Melvin Judkins stated, ''We must weigh the quality of the examination versus the risk.'' Inaccurate or missing information can constitute risk and can therefore be a complication for the patient. Judkins believed that laboratories with a death rate of greater than or equal to 0.1% within 24 hours of a study should implement quality control measures in order to reduce complication rates. He further stated that cardiac catheterization laboratories with a mortality rate of greater than or equal to 0.3% should be shut down (26). Adams' survey

TABLE 1. *Complications of coronary angiography*

Complication	Percent (%)
Death	0.08–0.1
CVA	0.08–0.1
Arrhythmias	0.3–0.5
Vascular	0.2–1.6
Anaphylaxis	0.1
Cholesterol emboli	0.15

TABLE 2. *Patients clinical characteristics associated with higher mortality during coronary angiography*

Cardiogenic shock
Left main stenosis
LV ejection <30%
Diabetes mellitus
Renal failure

further established that the previously reported complication rates were directly related to the volume of the cases performed (25).

Stewart et al. (27) studied the incidence of protamine reaction used for reversing systemic heparinization in 866 consecutive patients undergoing cardiac catheterization. Of the 866 patients, 651 received protamine, with an incidence of major protamine reaction in 27% of diabetic patients treated with NPH insulin, versus 0.5% in those without a history of NPH insulin use ($p < 0.01$).

Cholesterol embolization may complicate 0.15% of cases after cardiac catheterization (28). Skin findings of purple toes or livedo reticularis and renal dysfunction are present in the majority of the cases; hypertension and eosinophilia occur frequently, together with the elevation of sedimentation rate.

Contrast Agents in Cardiac Angiography

Intracardiac administration of high osmolar agents reduces the rate of depolarization of the sinoatrial node, slows atrioventricular node conduction, and prolongs QRS and QT duration (29). High osmolar agents can cause bradycardia, sinus arrest, high-grade block, and marked ST-T changes (29,30). The electrophysiologic effects are associated with ventricular fibrillation in 0.5% of cases; these abnormalities are thought to be secondary to the calcium-chelating properties of these agents (29–31). Newer nonionic agents significantly reduce the electrophysiologic side effects and the nausea/vomiting common with high osmolar agents (30–32).

Intracoronary injection of conventional high osmolar contrast agents causes myocardial depression and vasodilatation with hypotension (29). There is a short-lived compensatory hypertensive rebound phenomenon following the immediate decrease in blood pressure. This effect may exacerbate myocardial ischemia in patients with acute ischemic syndromes. Low osmolar agents do not cause decrease in myocardial contractility and unwanted hemodynamic effects. Prospective randomized trials, in general radiographic studies, have shown a reduction in minor and major complications with the use of low osmolar agents compared to high osmolar agents (29–32).

High osmolar ionic contrast agents have anticoagulant and platelet antiaggregate properties that constitute an advantage over the newer low osmolar agents. A third new compound, ioxaglate, is ionic and low osmolar; thus, its use may consti-

tute an advantage for high-risk coronary angiography patients. Randomized angiographic and angioscopic studies have shown that nonionic, low osmolar contrast agents were associated with a significant increase in the number of visible intracoronary thrombus when compared to the cases done with an ionic low osmolar agent (ioxaglate) (32,33).

There is an overall clear advantage in using low osmolar and ionic contrast agents for both the patient and treating physician. The major drawback is the cost that spirals up to 20 times greater than ionic, high osmolar contrast agents. It is debatable that, with this staggering price tag, the current new contrast agents are cost-effective.

Anaphylactoid reactions occurred in 1 to 2% of patients, and, in 0.1% of cases, these reactions were severe. Radiographic contrast agents can cause azotemia. The risk factor predictors for renal complications are: diabetes mellitus, volume depletion, and multiple myeloma (34).

VISUAL AND QUANTITATIVE ANGIOGRAPHY: VALUE AND LIMITATIONS

Traditionally, visual analysis of coronary arteriograms is used to assess the clinical severity of coronary disease (35,36). Several studies have shown that visual assessment of the severity of coronary stenosis may be misleading, particularly when compared to quantitative coronary angiography (QCA) (35–38). Several studies have shown that visual analysis does not always correlate with the true physiologic significance of the stenosis. Quantitative coronary angiography can therefore be considered the gold standard technique to evaluate the severity of vessel stenosis in a research setting (35). The main drawback of the quantitative method is that it is time-consuming and cumbersome and therefore is not widely used in clinical decision-making.

Modern clinical cardiology practice is based on research study results based on visual estimates of severity of coronary stenosis. Mild coronary stenosis (i.e., less than 10%) and severe stenosis can be accurately assessed by visual analysis. In contrast, visual estimates of intermediate stenosis do not correlate with the physiological significance of the stenosis (35–38).

A multitude of variables influence pressure loss across the stenosis, i.e., resistance, length of the obstruction, entrance angle of the stenosis, fluid velocity and viscosity, absolute dimension, and exit angle of the stenosis (35–38). Therefore, it is not surprising that, in clinical practice, visual assessment of the degree of obstruction does not necessarily correspond to the physiologic significance of the obstruction. Furthermore, there is coronary vasomotion tone, and the percentage of stenosis may vary in different physiologic conditions. Research data indicates that in patients with multivessel disease, visual and quantitative assessment of percent stenosis do not correlate well with the physiologic significance of the lesion. In contrast, in patients with single-vessel disease, QCA correlates better with the physiologic significance of the coronary stenosis (36,37).

Since the atherosclerotic disease process is diffuse, quantifying the diameter of the localized stenosis and comparing it with the adjacent "normal segment" has limitations. Frequently, the angiographic assessment underestimates the severity of the stenosis. The use of minimal lumen diameter (MLD) may possibly resolve this pitfall in assessment of severity of coronary stenosis (13).

The edge detection method to assess severity of coronary stenosis has some methodological limitations (35–38). Lesions with plaque rupture, thrombus, and filling defects are difficult to delineate, particularly when they exhibit haziness. Geometric distortions, such as vessel shortening, can hamper edge detection. Videodensimetry methods have inherent limitations but may circumvent some of these limitations of the QCA (36,37).

Epicardial Coronary Artery System (Fig. 13)

Spatial orientation of coronary anatomy is depicted in Figure 13. The total length of the left main stem ranges from 0 to 25 mm before it bifurcates into the LAD and LCX (21) (Fig. 14). The left circumflex, when nondominant, measures 6 to 8 cm in length and has a mean diameter of 3 mm. The LAD measures between 10 to 13 cm and has a mean diameter of 3.6 mm. Ninety percent of patients have 1 to 3 diagonal branches that supply the anterolateral wall of the heart; 1% of patients have no diagonal branches. Septal branches originate at 90 degrees to the LAD and supply the interventricular

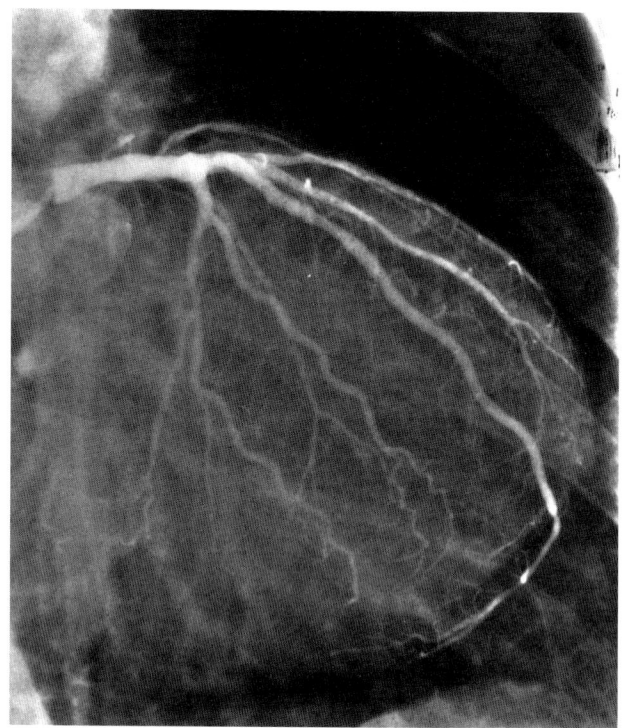

A

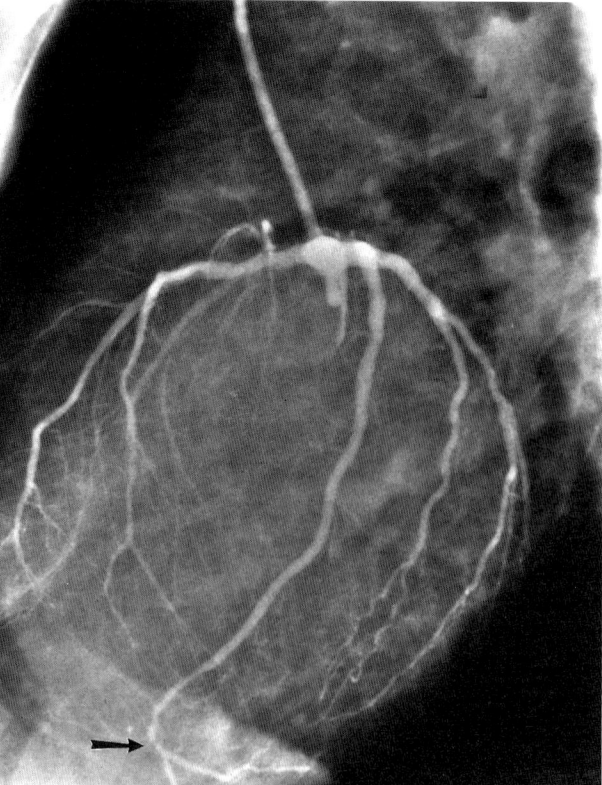

B

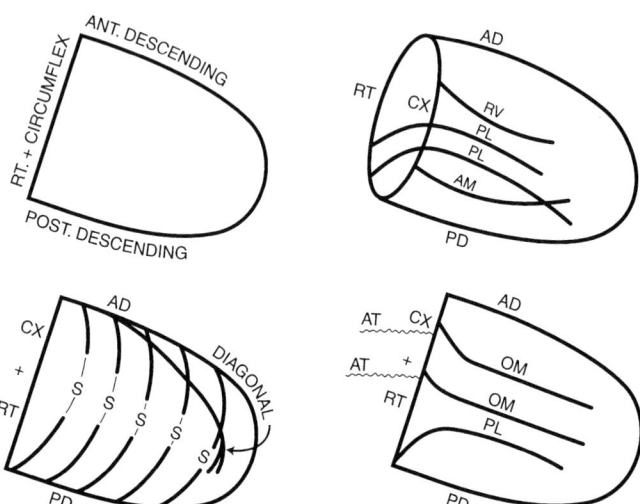

FIG. 13. Reproduction of schematic slides from Dr. Judkins personal files. He used these, and other similar schematics, in conjunction with a wire model to facilitate teaching spatial orientation of coronary anatomy (circa early 1970s). *AD*, anterior descending; *AM*, acute marginal; *AT*, atrial; *CX*, circumflex; *OM*, obtuse marginal; *PD*, posterior descending; *PL*, posterior lateral; *RT*, right; *RV*, right ventricular; *S*, septal. (Courtesy of Eileen Judkins, R.N.)

FIG. 14. Long left main stem in (**A**) RAO view. **B:** Lateral view, demonstrating a large superior obtuse marginal supplying the normal terminal LAD distribution. Note the 80% stenosis in the apical portion of this vessel (*arrow*).

septum. There is a wide spectrum of size and number of the septals. These LAD septal branches communicate with branches that originate from the posterior descending of the RCA; often these are a source of collaterals to the reciprocal vessel when one occludes. The main circumflex branches are the obtuse marginals, varying in number between 1 to 3, and supplying the free wall of the ventricle (13,21).

Commonly, the right coronary artery is the dominant vessel and measures between 12 to 14 cm in length until it bifurcates into the posterior descending and posterolateral branches (13,14,21). The mean diameter of the RCA is 3.2 mm and is usually maintained until it bifurcates distally. In contrast, the LAD and LCX diameters taper throughout their length. Epicardial coronary arteries course over the heart's surface and are embedded in the fat tissue. At times, they can dip into the myocardium, and the resulting myocardial bridges can be detected by coronary angiography.

Coronary angiography visualizes medium (greater than 200 microns) to larger epicardial coronary arteries (13,14). Therefore, a large part of the coronary circulation is not assessed with angiography.

Coronary vessels may appear to have normal morphology and vessel diameter, however, the "luminogram" may at times be misleading. In fact, coronary vessels may exhibit compensatory enlargement with preserved lumen and significant diffuse atherosclerotic plaque burden (39). Intravascular ultrasound studies (IVUS) have shown that in patients with atherosclerotic coronary disease, the great majority of angiographic "normal" reference segments are diffusely diseased (40). The average percentage of cross-sectional area stenosis of these "normal" reference segments measured by IVUS was 51%.

Several factors contribute to the incorrect quantitative assessment of vessel size in coronary angiography: vessel foreshortening; coronary ectasia; and deficient contrast opacification of the vessel. Calibration of catheter diameter for QCA calculations is hampered by x-ray attenuation of catheter material, incorrect catheter size, and also the plane of the catheter that may differ from the plane of the measured coronary segment (35–38). QCA analysis is pivotal as a research tool to study the outcome of pharmacological and percutaneous intervention trials in patients with CAD. Conversely, it has not contributed to the widespread day-to-day practice and decision-making for the clinical cardiologist.

PHYSIOLOGIC ASSESSMENT OF CORONARY STENOSIS

As discussed, there are major limitations of QCA in assessing the physiological significance of intermediate lesions, particularly in multivessel disease (41). Coronary flow has a unique phasic pattern with a high diastolic blood flow and low systolic flow. Sabiston and Gregg's (42) elegant experiments demonstrated that the systolic decrease of arterial coronary flow was due to cardiac contractility squeezing the capillary bed.

Several studies have shown the value of measuring coronary reserve flow (CRF) with the Doppler guidewire at rest and after maximal hyperemia (12 to 18 mcg intracoronary adenosine) to assess the physiological significance of the stenosis (41). More recently, FFR (fractional coronary flow reserve) was found to be superior to CFR in assessing the severity of the stenosis because it is independent of blood pressure and heart rate (41).

This preliminary data indicates that the physiological assessment of coronary stenosis may complement the anatomical information obtained with selective coronary angiography. In patients with angiographically normal coronary arteries or mild disease, a comprehensive endothelial function evaluation is warranted.

CORONARY ANGIOSCOPY

Coronary angioscopy is superior to coronary angiography in detecting coronary thrombus and dissection (43). It has proven to be a powerful research tool in differentiating different types of thrombus, i.e., white versus red in patients with acute ischemic syndromes. Angioscopy is a unique technique that permits a live three-dimensional view of the coronary lumen. The precise clinical value of this new imaging technique is yet to be defined.

PROGNOSTIC IMPLICATIONS OF CORONARY ANGIOGRAPHY

The findings of coronary angiography and left ventriculography are the strongest predictors of survival in patients with coronary artery disease (18,44–47). Left main stem stenosis is the single most important prognostic lesion (44). Conley and colleagues (44) studied the natural history of 163 medically treated patients with left main stem stenosis greater than or equal to 50%. In patients with 50–70% left main stenosis, the 3-year survival rate was 60% versus 41% for those with stenosis greater than or equal to 70% diameter, corroborating the prognostic value of coronary angiographic findings (Fig. 15).

The CASS study registry of 20,888 patients provided important prognostic information related to the extent of CAD and left ventricular systolic function (46). The extent of left ventricular (LV) dysfunction was the most powerful predictor of survival. In patients with ejection fraction (EF) less than 35%, the 4-year survival was 50% (three vessel), 57% (two vessel), and 74% (one vessel). In patients with an EF of greater than 50%, the 5-year survival was 82% (three vessel), 93% (two vessel), and 95% (one vessel).

Sanz and colleagues' (45) prospective clinical angiographic study showed that after myocardial infarction using Cox regression analysis the following were the only independent predictors of survival: ejection fraction ($p < 0.01$), number of diseased vessels ($p < 0.005$), and congestive

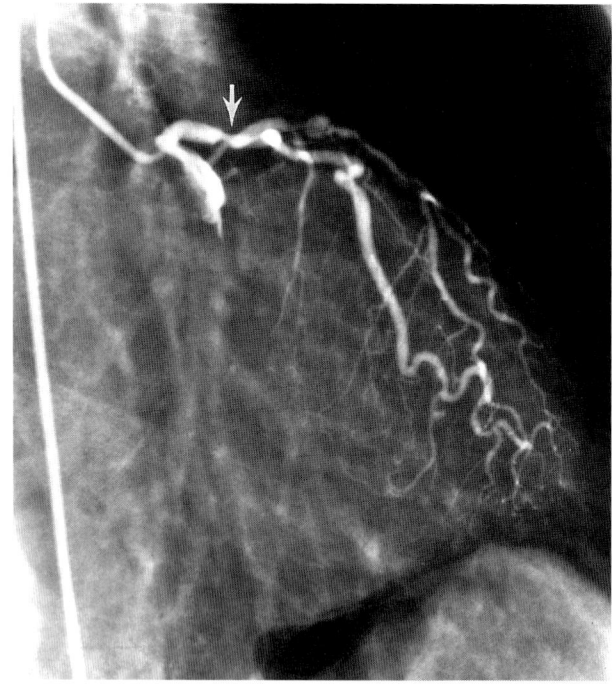

A

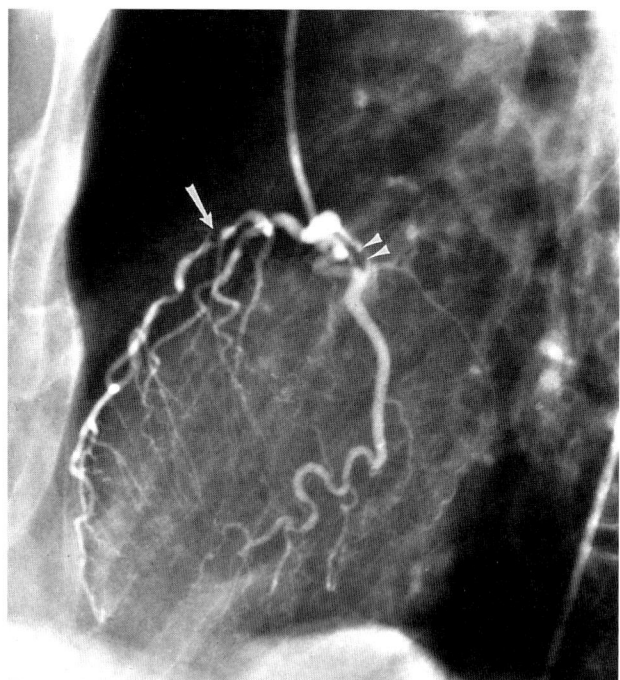

B

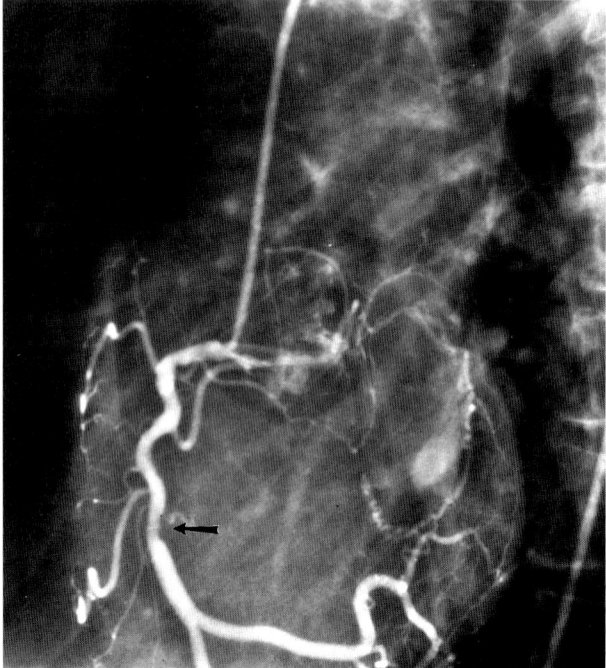

C

FIG. 15. Coronary angiogram showing three-vessel CAD. **A:** Note 90% distal left main stenosis in LCA RAO view (*arrow*). **B:** LCA lateral view showing 90% LAD proximal stenosis (*arrow*) and LCX 90% (*arrowheads*). **C:** RCA in LAO view shows a 70% mid-stenosis (*arrow*). This patient of Dr. Judkins had an exercise test achieving stage IV Bruce protocol with a peak heart rate of 143. There was 1 mm J point ST segment depression.

heart failure ($p < 0.01$). For patients with EF between 21 and 49%, the probability of survival was 78% (three vessel), and 95% (one vessel, $p < 0.01$) at 35 months of follow-up.

A normal coronary angiogram carries important prognostic information (46). The 7-year survival in patients with a normal coronary angiogram was studied in 4,051 patients from the CASS registry. There were 3,136 coronary angiograms considered normal with 915 exhibiting mild angiographic disease (less than 50% stenosis). Seven-year survival was 96% for patients with normal coronary arteries, and 92% for those patients with mild angiographic disease.

From these important studies, it is clear that the results of both left ventriculography and coronary angiography are major predictors of survival in patients with CAD. A normal coronary angiogram is a good predictor of survival, providing that left ventricular function is greater than 50%.

CHALLENGES OF INTERPRETATION

Vulnerable Plaque

The main pathophysiological mechanism underlying clinical events in patients with atherosclerotic coronary disease

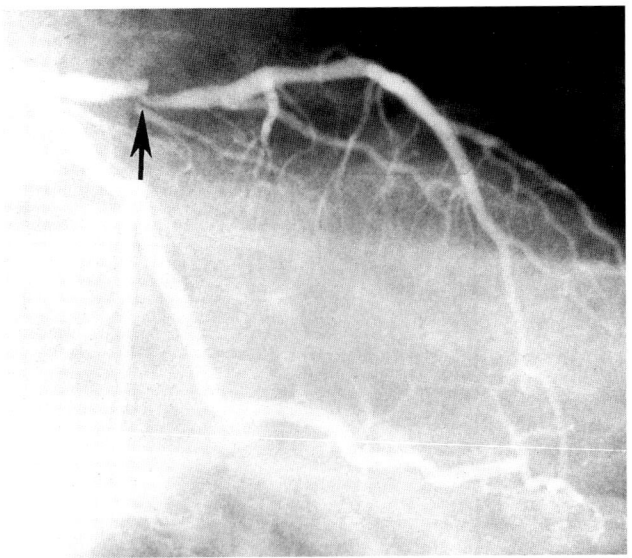

FIG. 16. LCA angiogram (RAO view) exhibiting plaque rupture in the proximal LAD (*arrow*).

is plaque rupture (48,49) (Fig. 16). Vulnerable plaques are eccentric and rich in soft lipid pool and are surrounded by macrophages that erode the thin fibrous cap (48). The majority of these vulnerable plaques occur in areas with less than or equal to 50% angiographic stenosis (49). On average, a patient with CAD has up to 30 plaques in each coronary artery (48). There is a wide spectrum of plaque composition and activity in these plaques, some of which are vulnerable (48–50). These may be present in angiographic segments that appear normal or that exhibit only mild irregularities. Coronary angiography tells us nothing about these vulnerable plaques that are prone to rupture and trigger cardiac events.

Left Main Stem Stenosis

An ostial lesion of the left main is at times an angiographic diagnostic challenge (Table 3). To exclude iatrogenic induced spasm, a catheter tip position coaxial with the left main should be achieved after an intracoronary injection of nitroglycerin. Pressure damping and absence of contrast spill into the aorta are indicators that a severe ostial lesion is present, even though the severity of the lesion may not be

TABLE 3. *Nonatherosclerotic causes of ostia narrowing*

Syphilis
Homozygous hypercholesterolemia type II
Takayasu's disease
Fibromuscular dysplasia (methysergide)
Aortic valve surgery
Ostial valve ridges
Saccular aortic aneurysm
Aortic dissection
Supravalvular aortic stenosis

angiographically apparent. Filming in an RAO oblique or an LAO cranial projection during contrast injection in the sinus of Valsalva with the catheter tip very close to the ostium may unravel the full severity of the stenosis. IVUS of the left main should also be done in these equivocal cases.

Inadequate Contrast Opacification

As Melvin Judkins (26) stated, ''The most frequent complication of cardiac catheterization is an incomplete or nondiagnostic study.'' Inadequate filling of the coronary tree may cause streaming of the contrast medium, erroneous identification of thrombus, nonvisualization of side branches, missed ostial stenosis, and over- or underestimation of the true stenosis severity. These pitfalls can be overcome with proper catheter selection and positioning and with the adequate injection of contrast material.

In a patient with a short left main coronary artery, a selective LAD, or LCX injection may give the false impression that the other vessel is occluded. Multiple filming projections are indicated during an angiographic study to accurately assess severe eccentric stenosis. These lesions need to be projected in the short-axis view so that the true narrow lumen is imaged. Two projections 90 degrees apart will prevent this pitfall of coronary angiography.

Pseudostenosis

In the field of interventional cardiology, it is important that the phenomenon of pseudostenosis be recognized. These artificial, severe coronary narrowings may be either single or multiple and are observed as a consequence of introducing a stiff guidewire through a tortuous coronary artery. Intimal coronary intussusception may be the mechanism operating in these false stenoses. Pseudostenoses do not respond to nitroglycerin and clearly should not be dilated. After the guidewire is removed, the ''stenosis'' will miraculously disappear!

Superimposed Branches

Even for the experienced angiographer, superimposition of the diagonal branches over the LAD may lead to misinterpretation of the anatomy (13). Failure to recognize obstruction of the diagonal or LAD can occur as a result of vessel overlapping. Similarly, this pitfall can occur with the LAD-septal vessels in LAO projection as the septal vessel may be misinterpreted as the occluded LAD. Caudal and cranial views with a variety of angulations may overcome this pitfall in interpreting the coronary angiogram.

Coronary Vasospasm

Variant angina was elegantly described by Myron Prinzmetal (51) in patients with episodes of spontaneous resting chest pain and ST segment elevation. Maseri (52) characterized the pathophysiology of coronary vasospasm. This can

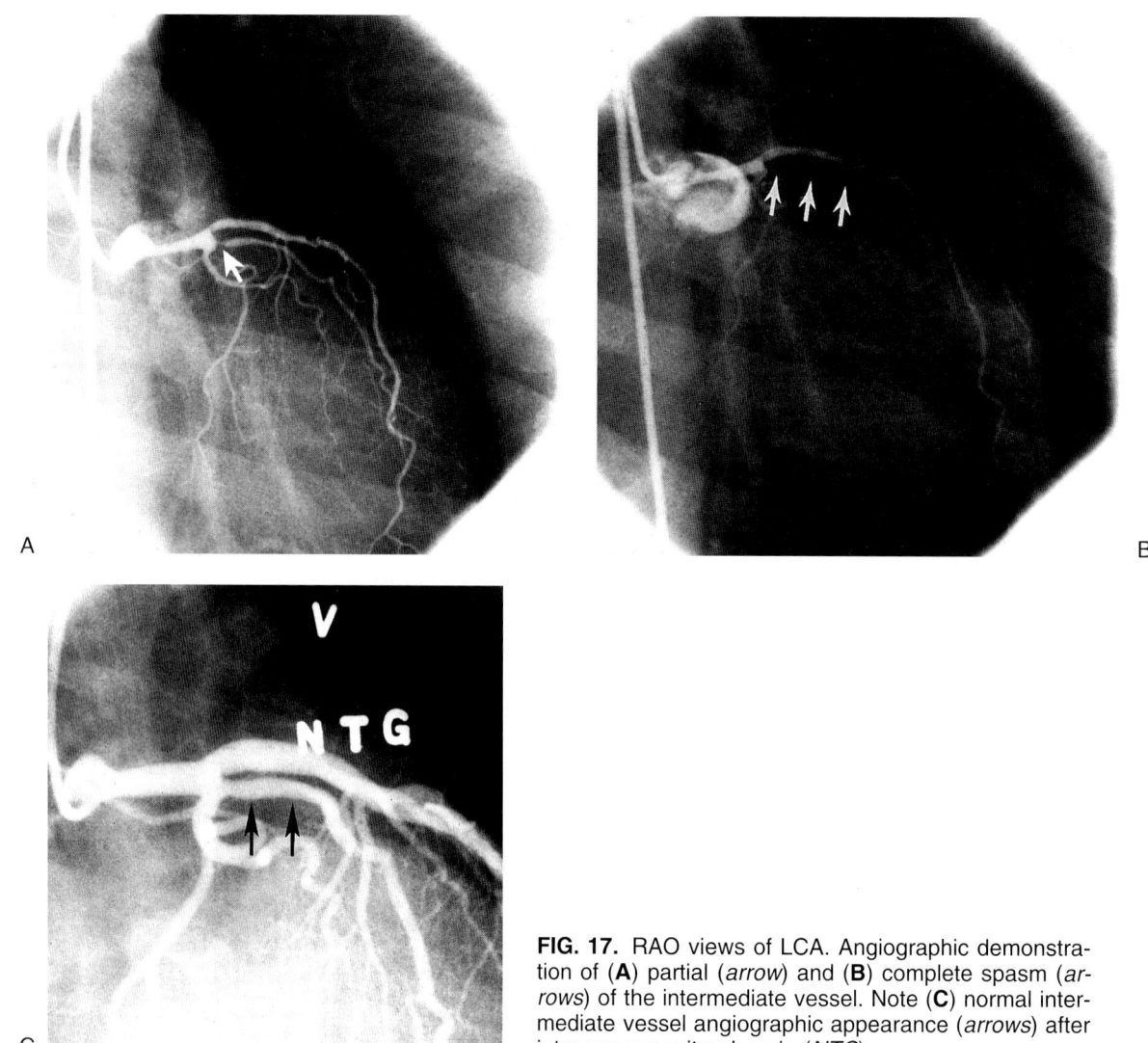

FIG. 17. RAO views of LCA. Angiographic demonstration of (**A**) partial (*arrow*) and (**B**) complete spasm (*arrows*) of the intermediate vessel. Note (**C**) normal intermediate vessel angiographic appearance (*arrows*) after intracoronary nitroglycerin (*NTG*).

occur at a site of a severe stenosis or even in angiographically normal coronary arteries. Most commonly, it occurs at the site of a nonflow limiting stenosis.

Coronary angiography, when performed during an episode of spontaneous vasospasm, may exhibit a localized or subtotal occlusion with slow contrast progression. At times, there is complete occlusion of the vessel without flow (Fig. 17). Coronary spasm can simultaneously involve two coronary arteries or two different segments of the same vessel, and, in some patients, diffuse and severe vessel constriction can involve the entire vessel. This phenomenon may be more common in Japanese patients (52). Coronary vasospasm, though uncommonly detected during coronary angiography, can be relieved with large doses of intracoronary nitrates and verapamil.

CORONARY ANGIOGRAPHY VERSUS INTRAVASCULAR ULTRASOUND IN ASSESSING PLAQUE BURDEN

There is a discrepancy between angiographic and intravascular ultrasound (IVUS) assessment of severity of athero-

sclerotic disease (40). In the majority of coronary angiograms that exhibit mild vessel irregularities, IVUS reveals diffuse atherosclerosis with a plaque burden often occupying 35% to 51% of a cross-sectional area; this is true even in some angiographic "normal" coronary segments (40). This discrepancy is explained by coronary remodeling as described by Glagov et al., i.e., a compensatory vessel enlargement due to outward plaque growth with maintenance of the initial coronary lumen (39).

Recent IVUS studies show that lesions that appear eccentric by angiography may have a concentric plaque burden and a concentric lesion (40). These findings may have implications in the management of patients with CAD.

ANGIOGRAPHIC ASSESSMENT OF CORONARY BLOOD FLOW

Assessment of coronary flow after thrombolytic therapy or coronary intervention in patients with acute myocardial infarction is important since it determines outcome. The coronary flow rate is related to the severity of the stenosis and the status of the microvasculature. The GUSTO investigators have demonstrated that improved survival after acute myocardial infarction hinges on achieving TIMI (Thrombolysis and thrombin Inhibition in Myocardial Infection trial) grade 3 flow at 90 minutes (18).

In clinical research trials, the cine frame count offers a quantitative and objective assessment of the coronary angiographic flow rate. According to the TIMI study group, angiographic coronary blood flow is classified in four grades (18): grade 0, no antegrade perfusion of contrast agent detected beyond the lesion; grade 1, contrast material that passes beyond the lesion but fails to opacify the distal coronary vessel; grade 2, contrast material reaches the distal vessel but at a lower rate than normal; grade 3, antegrade flow is complete and normal.

CORONARY LESION MORPHOLOGY

Plaque Rupture

Plaque rupture is the usual pathophysiologic mechanism of acute ischemic syndromes (48–50). Tissue thromboplastin and collagen type III within the plaque are potent stimuli that trigger platelet aggregation and thrombus that anchors at the site of plaque rupture (48). Ambrose et al. (53) described the angiographic characteristics of plaque rupture as an eccentric lesion with complex borders (narrow base on neck caused by overhanging edges) (Fig. 16). This type of angiographic lesion is present in 56% of patients with unstable angina and in only 18% of patients with stable angina (53). Several authors have reported the correlation between angiographic lesion morphology and a patient's clinical presentation and prognosis (18,53). The risk of myocardial in-

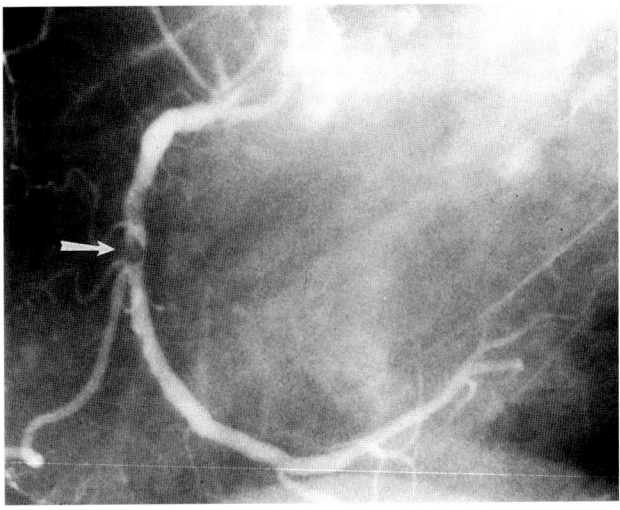

FIG. 19. LAO oblique view of a RCA showing a large filling defect that represented an immobile clot (*arrow*).

farction is higher with lesions of complex morphology than with lesions that are smooth (Fig. 18).

Coronary Thrombus

The classic angiographic finding of intracoronary thrombus includes the presence of a globular filling defect, surrounded by contrast material distal to the lesion, that, at times, moves with the blood flow (Fig. 19). Several studies reported that coronary angiography detects thrombus in 6 to 57% of patients (53,54). The difference in the reported

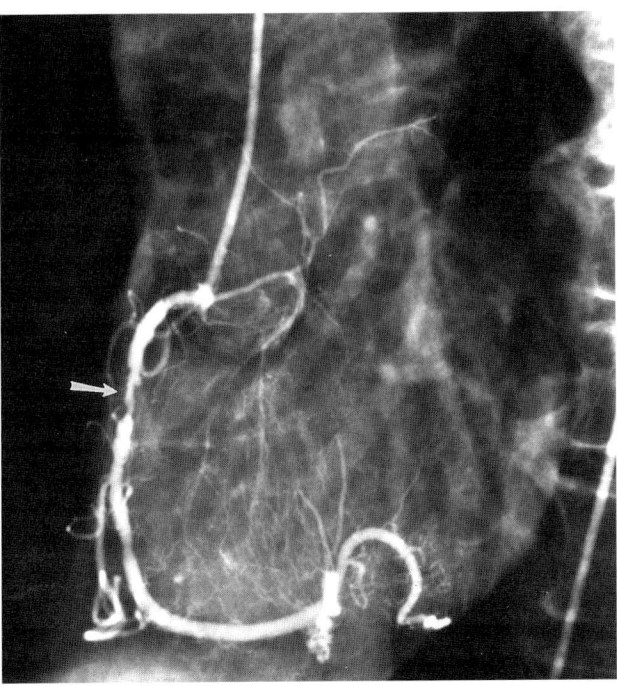

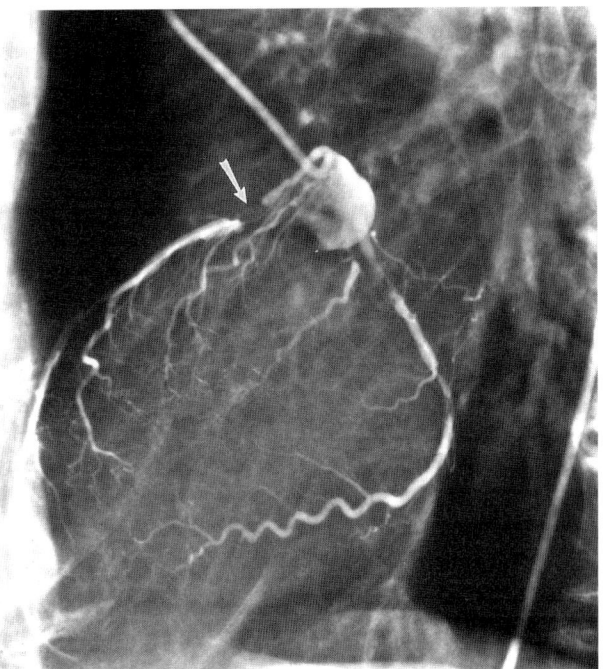

A   B

FIG. 18. Severe three-vessel coronary artery disease. **A:** LAO view RCA. **B:** Lateral view LCA. Note ulcerated plaque with severe stenosis in (**A**) RCA (*arrow*) and (**B**) LAD vessels (*arrow*).

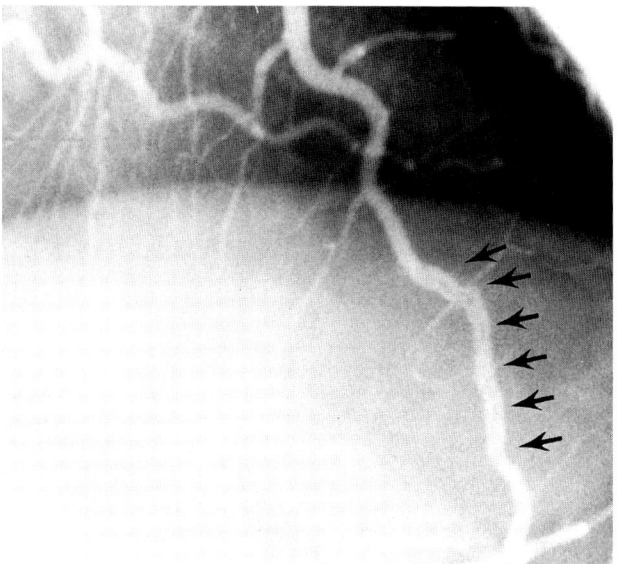

FIG. 20. Left coronary angiogram in a young female with spontaneous dissection of the distal LAD (*arrows*).

frequency is related to patient population, the clinical diagnosis, type of vessels studied, and differing definitions for thrombus. These studies have shown that the presence of a large thrombus detected at angiography is associated with a high incidence of complications and infarction during coronary intervention. Coronary angioscopy is superior to angiography for assessing the presence and type of thrombus (43).

Coronary Dissection

Spontaneous coronary dissection is a rare event that may occur in pregnant women, but commonly occurs during coronary intervention (Fig. 20). A minor dissection is frequently detected after coronary angioplasty since it is the operating pathophysiologic mechanism. In patients experiencing abrupt vessel closure following coronary intervention, coronary dissection is detected in up to 34% of cases (55,56). There is a wide spectrum of postintervention dissections, including spiral dissection that may extend the entire length of a vessel.

Myocardial Bridges

Short segments of the left anterior descending may "dip" into the myocardium. With each left ventricular contraction, the artery may narrow or even collapse (Fig. 21). Characteristically, the systolic narrowing disappears in diastole. Since coronary flow is mainly diastolic, it is not jeopardized, and there is no ischemia. These features are distinct from those observed in coronary spasm where the narrowing persists in diastole and is accompanied by chest pain along with ST segment changes (52).

Collateral Circulation

As previously discussed, resolution of modern coronary angiography is limited to vessels greater than or equal to 200 microns in diameter (13,14). Therefore, much of the extensive network of anastomotic collateral circulation

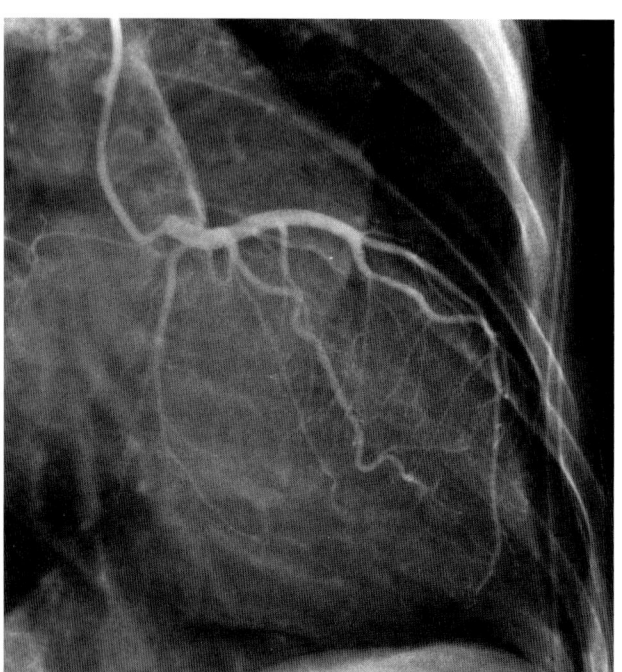

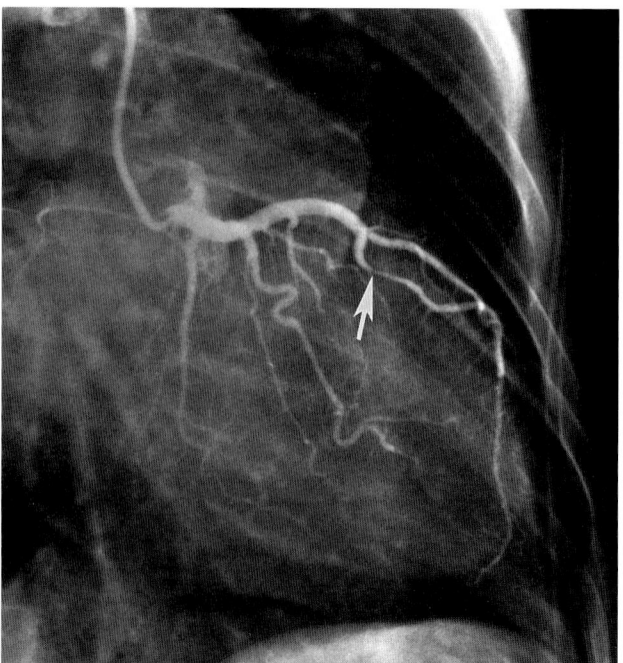

A

B

FIG. 21. Normal LCA angiogram in RAO views. Imaged in diastole (**A**) and systole (**B**). Note the LAD muscle bridge narrowing (*arrow*) in systole.

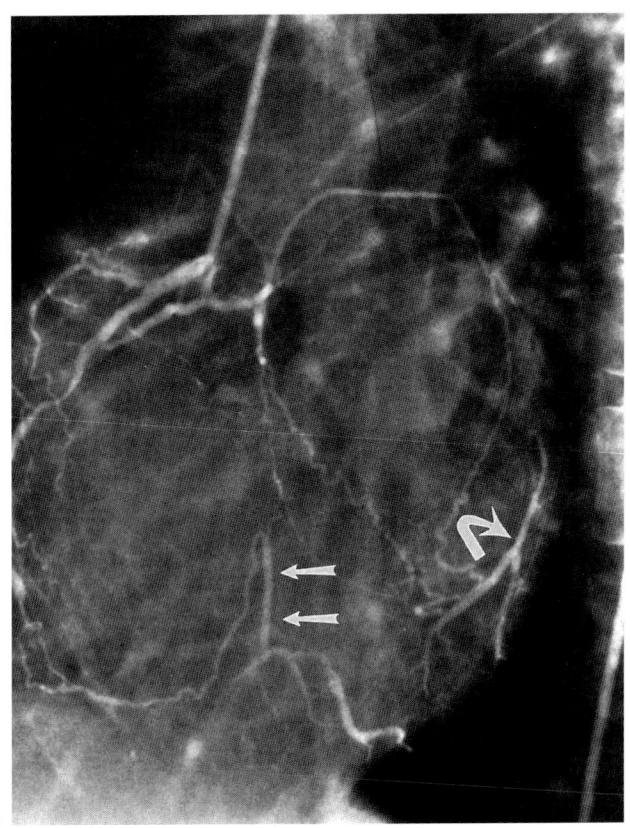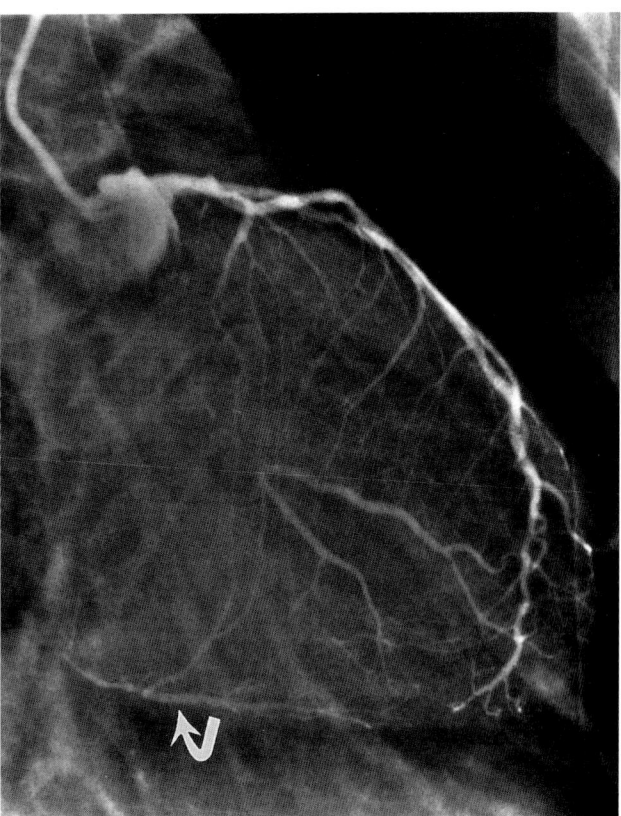

A

B

FIG. 22. Coronary angiogram exhibiting severe three-vessel diffuse coronary disease. **A:** LAO view RCA. **B:** RAO view LCA. Note collateral vessels to (**A**) LCX (*curved arrow*) and distal LAD (*arrows*) and (**B**) RCA (*curved arrow*).

among the three major coronary vessels is not visualized. A developing physiologically significant stenosis creates a gradient that propels an increasing volume of blood via small anastomatic vessels, causing them to enlarge. These enlarged collaterals become detectable by angiography when vessel stenosis is severe (i.e., 90%); their presence may be a marker of myocardial viability (Fig. 22).

Total Occlusions

The morphology and the age of a coronary occlusion are important predictors of outcome for the success of interventional procedures. To assess the length of the occlusion, it is important to simultaneously inject into the contralateral coronary artery in order to visualize the length and morphology of the total occlusion and to identify collaterals.

LEFT VENTRICULOGRAPHY

Left ventricular function evaluation is a major determinant of both prognosis and survival, providing assessment of global and segmental myocardial function (19). Biplane ventriculography facilitates a more precise evaluation of left ventricular function than does single-plane, and it often helps to identify the culprit vessel in acute ischemic syndromes (3).

Judkins introduced the "pigtail" catheter constructed of the same polyurethane material as his coronary catheters. The shaft is straight and the elongated 5-cm thinned segment is curled into a tight loop; it has four side holes (Fig. 23). Although the catheter has an end hole, it functions as a closed-end catheter. This feature coupled with its soft,

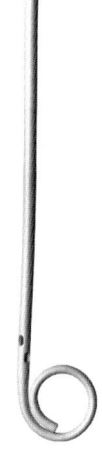

FIG. 23. Pigtail catheter for ventriculography and other mainstream injections.

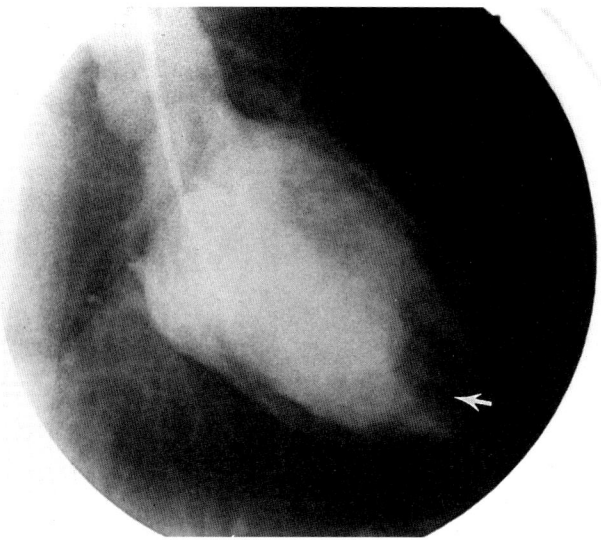

FIG. 24. Note filling defect, pedunculated clot, in RAO left ventricular angiogram (*arrow*). This clot was surgically excised and aneurysmectomy done.

rounded leading end facilitates safe ventriculography without danger of vessel or chamber injury or subendocardial injection. Evaluation of left ventricular end-diastolic pressure is done prior to angiography (3). The "pigtail" catheter can be placed in the left ventricular inflow tract or midcavity without causing arrhythmias. To introduce the "pigtail" from the ascending aorta into the left ventricle, advance the catheter onto the aortic valve structure. Gentle pressure cre-

ates a U-shaped configuration as the catheter is rolled up on the valve and rests on the medial side of the tubular aorta, the leading end no more than 2 to 3 cm above the valve. Withdraw the catheter until the leading end drops close to a transverse position in the sinus of Valsalva. As part of a continuous motion, withdraw the catheter 1 to 2 cm and advance it across the valve. Many times, this maneuver is not required, as the "pigtail" will directly enter the left ventricular cavity (19). Left ventricular contrast injection volume is 35 to 50 mL, at 12 to 15 mL per second; injections are imaged on a 9-inch mode image intensifier, using 35 mm cine with filming at 30 frames per second in 30-degree RAO and 45-degree LAO projections.

Abnormalities of ventricle contour include filling defects that commonly represent thrombus, and they are nearly always associated with regional segmental wall motion abnormalities (Fig. 24). The morphologic appearance of these filling defects may be smooth, pedunculated, or, rarely, may occupy a large portion of the left ventricular cavity. Other angiographic filling defects can be caused by tumors or by endomyocardial fibrosis, which causes the classic boxing glove left configuration. Hypertrophic cardiomyopathy can present with the classic features of cavity obliteration, grossly hypertrophied papillary muscles, and apical obliteration.

Segmental myocardial wall motion abnormalities are classified as: hypokinesis, reduced motion; akinesis, absence of systolic contraction; dyskinesis, presence of paradoxical systolic bulging. The latter is associated with left ventricular aneurysm, and it commonly involves the anteroapical seg-

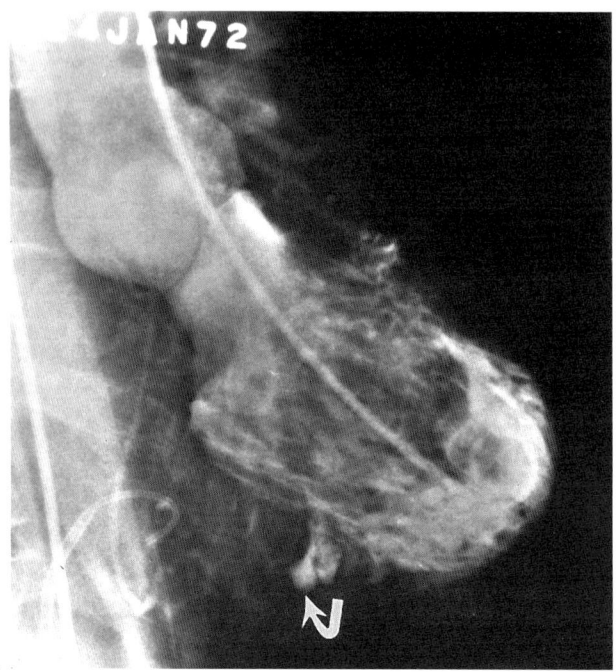

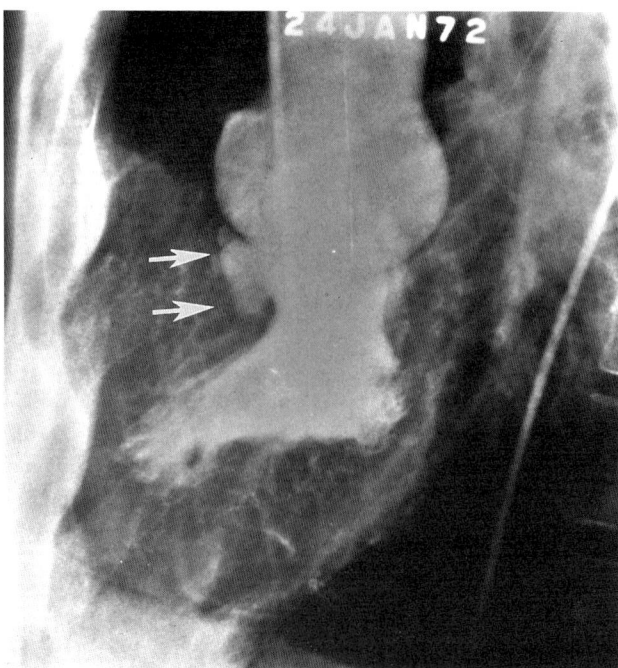

A   B

FIG. 25. Left ventriculography using Judkins pigtail catheter in (**A**) RAO view showing an inferior wall diverticulum (*curved arrow*) filling with contrast and (**B**), in lateral view, an outpouching of the ventricular membranous septum (*arrows*) extending into RV outflow tract.

ments, most often secondary to LAD occlusion. Aneurysms may be associated with ventricular arrhythmias, systemic embolism, and congestive heart failure. A true aneurysm must be distinguished from a false. Both nearly always occur as a complication of an acute myocardial infarction (18). Pathologically, a false aneurysm occurs secondary to the rupture of the ventricle free wall as the outpouch is sealed by the adherent pericardium. A false aneurysm has a narrow neck and occurs mainly in the posterolateral and inferior wall segments. Their potential for rupture mandates differentiation from true aneurysms (18). Bulging aneurysms resulting from sealed membranous ventricular septal defects (VSDs) may be detected angiographically; these are best imaged in lateral/LAO cranial views (Fig. 25**B**). Uncommonly, left ventricular diverticula may be detected at angiography (Fig. 25**A**).

For patient management, it is important to differentiate between hypokinesis and akinesis. The latter may be associated with viable or scarred myocardium. During cardiac catheterization, several maneuvers may be helpful in determining segmental myocardial viability. Nitroglycerin administration, and postextrasystolic potentiation may give important clues regarding viability. The biosystem can determine which myocardial segments are viable and may benefit from revascularization. This evaluation is based on detecting and mapping the voltage of ventricular segments, with the aid of a satellite navigation system (57).

Postmyocardial infarction left ventricular complications, such as ventricular septal defect rupture and mitral regurgitation, are currently better assessed noninvasively using two-dimensional echocardiography with Doppler (2-DE/Doppler).

RIGHT AND LEFT ATRIAL ANGIOGRAPHY

Before the advent of two-dimensional echocardiography (2-DE), atrial angiography was useful in detecting tumors, such as myxoma, and in showing leaflet thickening and doming with restricted motion in patients with mitral and tricuspid valve stenosis. Currently, these are best detected noninvasively using 2-DE techniques.

RIGHT VENTRICULAR ANGIOGRAPHY

Contrast injection into the right ventricle (RV) with a "pigtail" catheter positioned in the apex and coaxial with the tricuspid valve can assess the severity of tricuspid valve regurgitation. RV angiography is also useful in diagnosing RV infarction in the presence of regional wall motion abnormalities; this angiographic data is complementary to the hemodynamic abnormalities.

RV angiography in right ventricular endomyocardial fibrosis, exhibits the classic apical cutoff appearance (Fig. 26). It is the author's opinion that angiography is the best way to diagnose this rare disorder since it may be missed by regular transthoracic echocardiography. Right ventricular

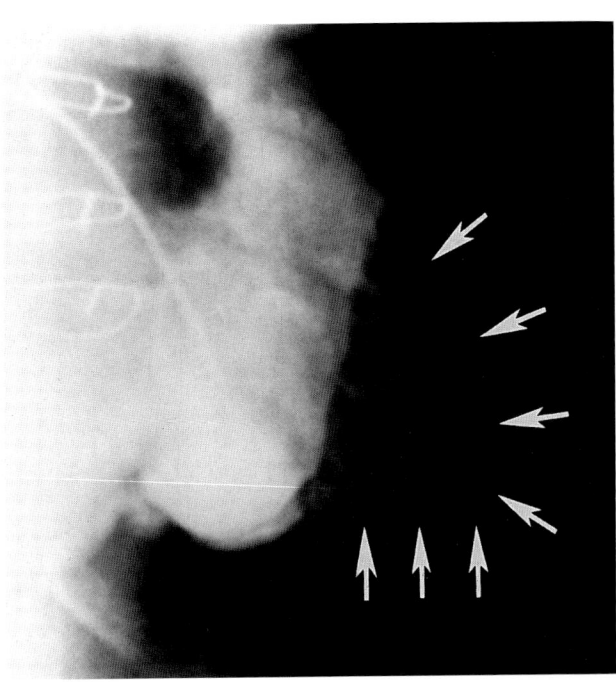

FIG. 26. Right ventriculography (RAO view) showing apex cutoff angiographic appearance (*arrows*). This is characteristic for right ventricular involvement in a patient with endomyocardial fibrosis.

angiography is useful in congenital heart disease in defining pulmonic valve morphology prior to pulmonary valve balloon valvotomy. Lateral right ventricular angiography can detect the type and level of obstruction and can differentiate between congenital stenotic and dysplastic pulmonary valves. Rare conditions, such as right ventricular cardiomyopathy, right ventricular dysplasia, and Uhl's anomaly, can be diagnosed with the aid of right ventriculography.

FUTURE OF CARDIAC ANGIOGRAPHY

It is amazing that, after 40 years, the techniques of selective coronary angiography and left ventriculography remain virtually unchanged! This fact attests to the genius of the pioneers of the techniques, Mason Sones and Melvin Judkins.

The explosion of interventional cardiac procedure assures the future of coronary angiography. However, magnetic resonance imaging (MRI) or some new imaging technology may eventually emerge as an alternative to diagnostic coronary angiography.

ACKNOWLEDGMENTS

All coronary and left ventricular radiographic illustrations (except for Figures 9, 16, 17, 19, 20, and 26) are from the Melvin P. Judkins archives of Loma Linda University and were provided by his widow, Eileen. We are grateful to James Simmons, R.T., for making the publication prints from these radiographs.

REFERENCES

1. Sones FM, Shirey EK. Cine coronary arteriography. *Mod Concepts Cardiovasc Dis* 1962;31:735–739.
2. Judkins MP. Selective coronary angiography. Part I. A percutaneous transfemoral technique. *Radiology* 1967;89:815–824.
3. Judkins MP. Percutaneous transfemoral selective coronary arteriography. *Radiologic Clinics of North America* 1968;VI:467–492.
4. Hales S. Statistical essays, containing haemastaticks, or, an account of some hydraulick and hydrostatical experiments made on the blood and blood vessels of animals, vol. 2. London: W Innys, R Manby, T Woodward, 1733.
5. Fye WB. Coronary arteriography: it took a long time! *Circulation* 1984; 7:781–787.
6. Forssmann W. *Experiments on myself: memoirs of a surgeon in Germany.* New York: St. Martin's Press, 1974;84–85.
7. Moniz E, de Carvalho L, Lima A. La visibilite des vaisseaux pulmonaires aus rayons X par injection dans l'oreillette droite de fortes solutions d'Iodure de sodium. *Bull Acad Med Paris* 1931;105:627–629.
8. Moniz E, de Carvalho L, Saldanha A. Angiopneumographie. *J Radiol d'Electrol* 1932;16:469–472.
9. Machado Macedo M. The Portuguese School of Angiography. 20 years of coronary angioplasty. *Rev Port Cardiol* 1998;18[suppl I]:9–11.
10. Perez Ara A. El sondage del corazon derechia su tecnica y aplicationes. *Rev Med Cir Habana* 1931;36:491–508.
11. Cournand AF, Lauson HD, Bloomfield RA, et al. Recording of right heart pressures in man. *Proc Soc Exp Biol Med* 1944;55:34–36.
12. Mueller RL, Sanborn TA. The history of interventional cardiology: cardiac catheterization, angioplasty and related interventions. *Am Heart J* 1995;129:146–172.
13. Levin DC, Gardiner GA. Coronary arteriography. In: Braunwald E, ed. *Heart disease,* 4th ed. Philadelphia: WB Saunders, 1992;1:235–275.
14. Pepine CJ. Coronary angiography and cardiac catheterization. In: Topol EJ, ed. *A textbook of cardiovascular medicine.* New York: Lippincott-Raven, 1998:1913–1956.
15. Amplatz K, Formanek G, Stanger P, et al. Mechanics of selective coronary artery catheterization via femoral approach. *Radiology* 1967;89: 1040–1047.
16. American College of Cardiology/American Heart Association. Guidelines for coronary angiography. A report of The American College of Cardiology/American Heart Association task force on assessment of diagnostic and therapeutic cardiovascular procedures (subcommittee on coronary angiography). *J Am Coll Cardiol* 1987;(4):935–950.
17. Grines CL, Browne UF, Marco J, et al. A comparison of immediate angioplasty with thrombolytic therapy for acute myocardial infarction. *N Engl J Med* 1993;328:673–679.
18. Topol EJ, Werf FJV. Acute myocardial infarction. Early diagnosis and management. In: Topol EJ, ed. *A textbook of cardiovascular medicine.* New York: Lippincott-Raven, 1998:395–435.
19. Judkins MP, Judkins E. Coronary arteriography and left ventriculography: Judkins technique. In: King SB III, Douglas JS Jr, eds. *Coronary arteriography and angioplasty.* New York: McGraw-Hill, 1985: 182–217.
20. Levin DC, Fellows KE, Abrams HL. Hemodynamically significant primary anomalies of the coronary arteries. Angiographic aspects. *Circulation* 1978;58:25–34.
21. Waller BF, Orr CM, Slack JD, et al. Clinical pathologic correlations. Anatomy, histology and pathology of coronary arteries: a review relevant to new interventional and imaging techniques: part I. *Clinic Cardiol* 1992;15:451–457.
22. Bourassa MG, Noble J. Complication rate of coronary arteriography. A review of 5,250 cases started by a percutaneous femoral technique. *Circulation* 1976;53:106–114.
23. Davis K, Kennedy JW, Kemp HG, et al. Complications of coronary arteriography from the collaborative study of coronary artery surgery (CASS). *Circulation* 1979;59:1105–1112.
24. Johnson LW, Lozner EC, Johnson S, et al. Coronary arteriography 1984–1987. A report of the Registry of The Society for Cardiac Angiography and Interventions. Results and complications. *Cathet Cardiovasc Diagn* 1989;17:5–20.
25. Adams DF, Fraser DB, Abrams HL. The complications of coronary arteriography. *Circulation* 1973;47:609–613.
26. Judkins MP, Gander MP. Prevention of complications of coronary arteriography. *Circulation* 1974;49:599–602.

27. Stewart WJ, Sweeney SM, Kellett MA, et al. Increased risk of severe protamine reactions in NPH—insulin-dependent diabetics undergoing cardiac catheterization. *Circulation* 1984;70:788–792.
28. Rosman HS, Davis TP, Reddy D, et al. Cholesterol embolization: clinical findings and complications. *J Am Coll Cardiol* 1990;15:1296–1299.
29. Ritchie JL, Nissen SE, Douglas JD, et al. Use of nonionic or low osmolar contrast agents in cardiovascular procedures. *J Am Coll Cardiol* 1993;21:269–273.
30. Esplugas E, Cequier A, Jara F, et al. Risk of thrombosis during coronary angioplasty with low osmolality contrast media. *Am J Cardiol* 1991; 68:1020–1040.
31. Wolf GL, Arensour L, Cross AP. A prospective trial of ionic vs. nonionic contrast agents in routine clinic practice. *Am J Roentgenol* 1989; 152:939–944.
32. Bettmann MA. Angiographic contrast agents: conventional and new media compound. *Am J Roentgenol* 1982;139:787–794.
33. Qureshi NR, Heijer P, Crijns HJGM. Percutaneous coronary angiographic comparison of thrombus formation during percutaneous coronary angioplasty with ionic and non-ionic low osmolality contrast media in unstable angina. *Am J Cardiol* 1997;80:700–704.
34. Rich MW, Crecelius CA. Incidence, risk factors and clinical course of acute renal insufficiency after cardiac catheterization in patients 70 years of age or older. A prospective study. *Arch Intern Med* 1990;150: 1237–1242.
35. Danchin N, Juilliere Y, Foley D, et al. Visual versus quantitative assessment of the severity of coronary artery stenosis: can the angiographic eye be re-educated? *Am Heart J* 1993;126:594–600.
36. Marcus ML, Skorton DJ, Johnson MR, et al. Visual estimate of percent diameter coronary stenosis. A battered gold standard. *J Am Coll Card* 1988;11:882–885.
37. White CW, Wright LB, Doty DB, et al. Does the visual interpretation of the coronary angiogram predict the physiological significance of a coronary stenosis? *N Engl J Med* 1984;310:819–824.
38. Vas R, Eigler N, Miyazono C, et al. Digital quantification eliminates intraobserver and interobserver variability in the evaluation of coronary artery stenosis. *Am J Cardiol* 1985;56:718–723.
39. Glagov S, Weisenberg E, Zarins CK, et al. Compensatory enlargement of human coronary atherosclerotic arteries. *N Engl J Med* 1987;316: 1371–1375.
40. Mintz GS, Painter JA, Pichard AD, et al. Atherosclerosis in angiographically ''normal'' coronary artery reference segments: an intravascular ultrasound study with clinical correlations. *J Am Coll Cardiol* 1995;25:1479–1485.
41. Carlier SG, DiMario C, Kern MJ, et al. Intracoronary Doppler and pressure monitoring. In: Topol EJ, ed. *Textbook of interventional cardiology.* Philadelphia: WB Saunders, 1999:748–781.
42. Sabiston DC, Gregg DE. Effect of cardiac contraction on coronary blood flow. *Circulation* 1957;15:14–20.
43. White CW, Ramee SR. Coronary angioscopy. In: Topol EJ, ed. *Textbook of interventional cardiology.* Philadelphia: WB Saunders, 1999: 783–800.
44. Conley MJ, Ely RL, Kisslo J, et al. The prognostic spectrum of left main stenosis. *Circulation* 1978;57:947–952.
45. Sanz G, Castaner A, Betriu A. Determinants of prognosis in survivors of myocardial infarction. *N Engl J Med* 1982;306:1065–1070.
46. Kemp HG, Kronmal RA, Vlietstra RE, et al. Seven year survival of patients with normal or near normal coronary arteriograms. A CASS Registry study. *J Am Coll Cardiol* 1986;7:479–483.
47. Mock MB, Ringqvist I, Fisher LD, et al. Survival of medically treated patients in the coronary artery surgery study (CASS) Registry. *Circulation* 1982;66(3):562–568.
48. Davies MJ, Thomas AC. Plaque fissuring. The cause for acute myocardial infarction, sudden ischemic death and crescendo angina. *Br Heart J* 1985;53:363–373.
49. Fuster V, Badimon L, Badimon JJ, et al. The pathogenics of coronary artery disease and acute ischemic syndromes. *N Engl J Med* 1992;326: 287–291.
50. Fuster V, Lewis A. Conner Memorial Lecture. Mechanisms leading to myocardial infarction: insights from studies of vascular biology. *Circulation* 1994;90:2126–2214.
51. Prinzmetal M, Kennamer R, Merliss R, et al. Angina pectoris. The variant form of angina pectoris. *Am J Med* 1959;27:375–383.
52. Maseri A, Severi S, Des NES, et al. Variant angina: one aspect of a

continuous spectrum of vasospastic myocardial ischemia. *Am J Cardiol* 1978;42:1019–1023.

53. Ambrose JA, Winters SL, Stern A, et al. Angiographic morphology and the pathogenesis of unstable angina pectoris. *J Am Coll Cardiol* 1985;5:609–619.

54. Gotoh K, Minamino T, Katoh O, et al. The role of intracoronary thrombus in unstable angina: angiographic assessment and thrombolytic therapy during ongoing anginal attacks. *Circulation* 1988;77:526–531.

55. Lincoff AM, Popma JJ, Ellis SG, et al. Abrupt vessel closure complicat-ing coronary angioplasty: clinical, angiographic and therapeutic profile. *J Am Coll Cardiol* 1992;19:926–935.

56. Dorros C, Cowley MJ, Simpson J, et al. Percutaneous transluminal coronary angioplasty: report of complications from the NHLBI PTCA Registry. *Circulation* 1983;67:723–727.

57. Laham RJ, Simons M, Pearlman JD, et al. Catheter myocardial revascu-larization (DMR) improves 30 day angina class, regional wall motion, and perfusion of treated zones using MRI. *J Am Coll Cardiol* 1999; 1035;138A(abst).

CHAPTER 26

Computed Tomography and Electron-beam Computed Tomography

Axel Schmermund and John A. Rumberger

TECHNICAL ASPECTS

General

The development of computed tomography (CT), that resulted in widespread clinical use of CT scanning by the early 1980s, was a major breakthrough in diagnostic imaging. Imaging a thin cross-section of the body avoided superposition of three-dimensional structures onto a planar two-dimensional representation, as seen with conventional x-ray technology. Additionally, the detection of small differences in tissue densities became feasible, spatial resolution was improved, and radiation scatter within the patient was reduced. Crucial to these developments were the perfection of mathematical algorithms needed to translate x-ray attenuation into digitized gray-scale information and the advent of adequate automated computing power.

The basic principle of CT is that a fan-shaped, thin x-ray beam passes through the body at many angles to allow for cross-sectional images. The corresponding x-ray transmission measurements are collected by a detector array. Both detector array and x-ray beam itself are collimated to produce thin sections and avoid unnecessary photon scatter. The transmission measurements recorded by the detector array are digitized in picture elements (pixels) with known dimensions. The gray-scale information contained in each individual pixel is reconstructed according to the attenuation of the x-ray beam, which it represents along its path using a standardized technique termed "filtered backprojection." Gray-scale values for pixels within the reconstructed tomogram are defined with reference to the value for water and

---

A. Schmermund: Department of Cardiology, University Clinic Essen, 45122 Essen, Germany.

J. A. Rumberger: HeartCare, Inc., Gahanna, Ohio 43230.

are called "Hounsfield Units" or simply "CT numbers." Air attenuates the x-ray less than water, and bone attenuates it more than water, so that in a given patient, Hounsfield units may range from −1000 (air) through 0 (water) to approximately +1000 (bone cortex).

Conventional and Helical Computed Tomography

CT technology has significantly improved since its first introduction into clinical practice in 1973. Current conventional scanners employ a rotating x-ray source with a circular, stationary detector array. Continuous incrementation of the patient table has enabled continuous scanning (spiral or helical CT), and "slip-ring technology" has eliminated cabling restrictions as the x-ray source rotates about the patient, allowing for scan acquisition times on the order of 0.75 to 1.0 seconds with shortened interscan delay. Algorithms have been implemented enabling volumetric imaging, and multiple high-quality reconstructions of various volumes of interest can be done in retrospect. However, precise movement of the x-ray tube, high tube currents, and the continuous x-ray exposure impose physical limits on the capacity of helical CT for short-scan acquisition times and the maximum number of scans per series. Image quality depends on patient cooperation to avoid movement and degrades considerably for the beating heart. While the recent introduction of multi-row helical CT has further shortened effective scan acquisition times to approximately 0.25 sec, the above mentioned physical restrictions also apply here, and scanning times needed for *in vivo* cardiac imaging without motion artifacts can only be achieved in patients with slow heart rates. The advantage of conventional and especially helical CT is the high image quality of nonmoving body parts; however, with respect to cardiovascular imaging, scan acquisition times equivalent to about one cardiac cycle represent a limitation.

Electron-beam Computed Tomography

Even though it has been clinically available for almost 15 years at the time of this writing, electron-beam computed tomography (EBCT) employs very progressive technology enabling ultrafast scan acquisition times of 50 to 100 msec with the potential for even faster times. This achievement is mainly accomplished by two prominent features of the scanner. As its name indicates, EBCT is distinguished from other CT scanners by the design of the electron beam. As in other body CT devices, the cathode is the source of the electron beam, which produces x-rays by striking a tungsten target (anode). However, in EBCT, the distance between cathode and anode measures approximately 9 feet (Fig. 1**A**). There are no mechanical moving parts. The electron beam is steered by an electromagnetic deflection system to sweep around the distant anode, i.e., the fixed tungsten target. Thus, as opposed to moving the x-ray tube, the electron beam is moved in EBCT. It is currently swept around the target ring in a minimum of 50 msec, and 8 more msec are required for repositioning of the electron beam for subsequent scans. The tungsten target is the second prominent feature of

EBCT. It is centered below the patient, and a stationary detector ring for measurements of transmissions that have passed through the patient is centered above. While conventional CT systems are limited by the amount of heat generated as the electron beam strikes the target, EBCT has especially large target rings and a direct water cooling system behind the targets to distribute and remove heat from the target assembly (1). Additionally, not one but four target rings are available to distribute heat depending on the scanning mode. Therefore, heating problems are avoided as the moving electron-beam design allows for ultrafast scan acquisition times.

The target rings are semicircular, forming a 210-degree arc below the patient. The detector system above the patient forms a 216-degree arc. This construction, a result of the underlying electron-beam scanning design, accounts for a nonsymmetrical geometry of the EBCT scanner as opposed to a symmetrical design of conventional CT. To allow uninhibited passage of the x-ray through the patient despite the overlap of target and detector rings, they are placed in slightly different planes. This configuration is called "cone-beam geometry" (1) (Fig. 1**B**).

As noted above, the EBCT scanner is equipped with four target rings. Further, two detector arrays are available, both having 1,728 detector elements. The two detector arrays can

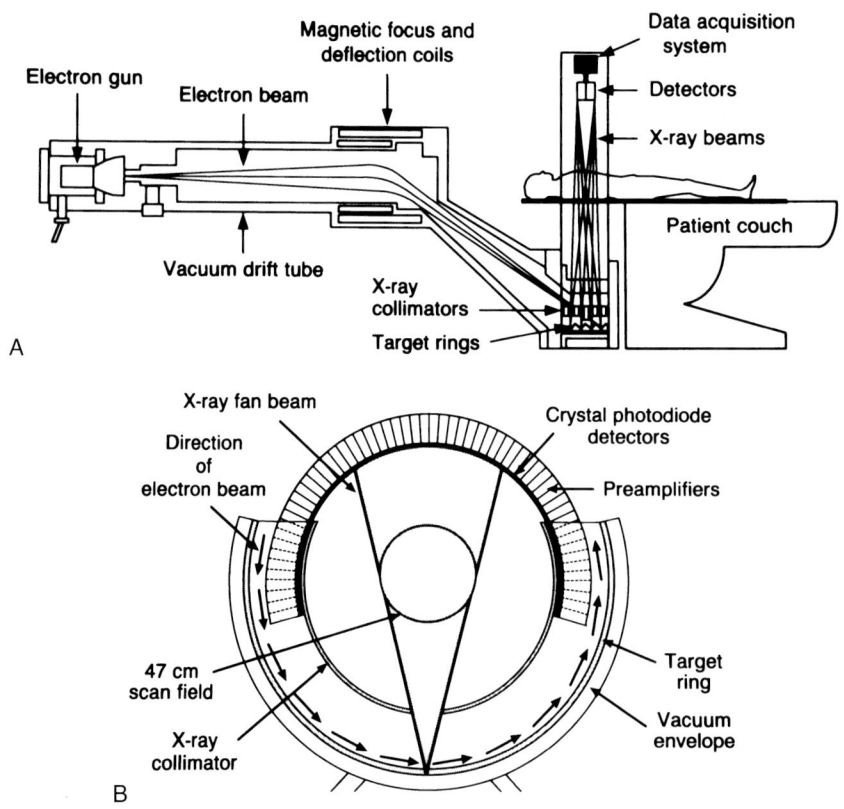

FIG. 1. Schematic design of the electron-beam computed tomography (EBCT) scanner. **A:** The electron beam is steered electromagnetically and only produces x-rays directly below the patient. **B:** The unique scanner geometry results in a cone-shaped X-ray fan. See text for details. (From ref. 1, with permission.)

be used in combination, in which case, effectively 864 detector elements are used per detector by summing the signals of two elements. Alternatively, the detector with all 1,728 elements can be used alone to achieve optimized image resolution. The latter scanning mode is called "single-slice mode" and employs only the most central of the four target rings as x-ray source. Slice thickness can be varied by collimation from 1.5 through 6 mm. The combination of both detector arrays and one through four target rings (i.e., x-ray source positions) provides for imaging of two to eight independent tomographic levels without table incrementation (1). This scanning mode is called "multislice mode" and employs a slice thickness of 8 mm.

Strengths and Limitations of Computed Tomography Techniques in Cardiovascular Imaging

The inherent strength of CT and EBCT, for cardiovascular imaging but also elsewhere, is the ability to provide for volumetric images representing a true three-dimensional display of the body. Although a series of contiguous, parallel cross-sections perpendicular to a single (longitudinal) axis are taken, a complete volume of data can be created retrospectively, lending itself to analysis of any plain or curved surface within that volume. In this fashion, noninvasive or minimally invasive techniques can be used to obtain detailed anatomical information.

CT techniques, whether conventional, spiral CT, or EBCT, are superior to most other noninvasive tomographic techniques with respect to spatial resolution. Up to 10 line-pairs per cm can be differentiated using CT techniques. The latest generation of detector array and configuration has brought EBCT scanners close to more conventional CT scanners in that respect. While the asymmetric geometry and the detector design still account for some deterioration in image quality with EBCT, this is offset by the potential for avoiding motion artifacts in cardiovascular imaging. Of note, the short scan acquisition times necessary for cardiac imaging are inherently associated with less radiation exposure and thus decreased signal-to-noise ratios. Using the EBCT single-slice ("high resolution") mode, "noise," measured as the standard deviation of pixel values in the center of a uniform object, is much greater with scan acquisition times of 100 msec than 600 msec or longer (1). However, for moving objects, such as the beating heart, only short exposure times enable imaging free of motion blurring.

The use of ionizing radiation represents an obvious disadvantage of the CT techniques. EBCT differs from other CT techniques in that the dose distribution throughout the field of view is not symmetrical. Radiation exposure to the posterior structures of a supine patient is higher than to the anterior structures (1,2). The total dose for conventional thoracic scanning is significantly less for EBCT compared to conventional or spiral CT and EBCT. A standard single slice, 100

msec EBCT examination of the chest is associated with a relatively low exposure of approximately 0.5–0.8 mSv owing to the short scan times. In women, radiation exposure to the breasts is on the order of 410 mRem, and radiation scatter to the uterus is immeasurable.

Specific limitations of EBCT relate to the more complex technology compared with conventional or spiral CT, that require more intense maintenance and quality control. Further, the current availability of EBCT is limited in North America, Europe, and Asia. Even though prospective gating of images with EBCT is of great advantage for cardiac studies, individual multilevel tomographic information may not always be acquired simultaneously but often from consecutive cardiac cycles. Thus quantitative volumetric data are generally limited to patients in normal sinus rhythm, with fairly constant electrocardiographic R–R intervals during the study.

DIAGNOSIS OF PERIPHERAL VASCULAR AND PULMONARY DISEASE

Aorta and Renal Arteries

Millisecond scan acquisition times are usually not required for CT images of the aorta and/or renal arteries. While noncontrast imaging is frequently used to delineate calcific mural atherosclerosis of the thoracic and abdominal aorta, iodinated contrast is injected to obtain a CT angiogram. Often, a spiral scanning mode (also available using EBCT) is employed to cover a large volume of interest. The "circulation time" is determined by measuring the arrival time of contrast in a specific region of interest after peripheral intravenous contrast injection.

Suspected aortic dissection and/or aneurysm are common indications for CT imaging. Dissection of the ascending aorta is acutely life-threatening, and its diagnosis is crucial for emergency surgical management. The hallmark of aortic dissection is an intimal flap floating in the vessel lumen or separating a "true" from a "false" lumen. Compared against angiography, CT imaging has been reported to be very accurate. It allows a reliable representation of the localization and extent of the dissection and the involvement of other vessels, such as the renal arteries (3). It is valuable for differentiating ascending versus descending aortic dissection and especially an involvement of the aortic arch, which is difficult to assess with transesophageal echocardiography. However, functional aspects apparent from the echocardiogram, such as the site of communication between true and false lumen or the direction of flow in the false lumen, are more difficult to assess. In some instances, discrimination between an aortic aneurysm with mural thrombus and a dissection with extensive thrombus formation in the false channel may be challenging. Intramural aortic hematoma, frequently resulting in overt dissection, can also be diagnosed

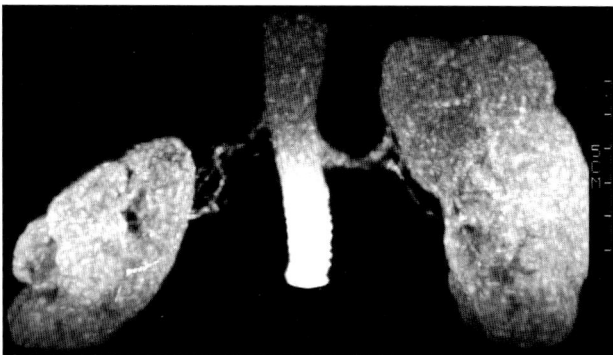

FIG. 2. High-grade, right-sided renal artery stenosis. Three-dimensional reconstruction from spiral CT (collimation 2 mm, pitch 1.5) shown as a maximum intensity projection. Note the difference in size between the two kidneys. (Courtesy of F. Schöblen, M.D., Zentralinstitut für Röntgendiagnostik, University Clinic, Essen, Germany.)

from CT images in the presence of a hyperdense rim in the aortic wall on a noncontrast enhanced scan. Formation of an aneurysm is easily detected by observation of an increase in aortic diameter and outward displacement of the often calcified aortic wall. The maximum diameter of the aneurysm can be determined to decide if and when surgery is indicated.

Spiral CT (and EBCT) have been used for three-dimensional imaging of atherosclerotic disease of the thoracic and abdominal vessels and kidneys (Fig. 2) as well as congenital abnormalities. With use of contrast enhancement, detailed assessment of renal volumes including differentiation of cortex and medulla can also be achieved. The shorter scan times available with EBCT offer the additional opportunity to examine functional aspects of renal blood flow and excretion (4).

PULMONARY EMBOLISM

Pulmonary embolism is a common consequence of deep vein thrombosis. It is associated with a mortality of up to 30% if untreated. CT imaging has recently been extensively evaluated with respect to detecting pulmonary emboli after contrast injections. Faster scan times and new reconstruction algorithms have allowed for substantially improved analysis of the volumetric data sets. Studies using spiral CT have reported reliable identification of acute and chronic central pulmonary emboli. Remy-Jardin et al. (5) found a sensitivity of 100% and a specificity of 96% in a series of 42 patients. In another study (6), preselection of cases with intermediate-probability ventilation-perfusion scans resulted in a slightly lower sensitivity and specificity of 86% and 92%, respectively, with regard to detection of central vessel emboli, whereas for all pulmonary vessels, it decreased to 63% and 89%, respectively.

The use of ultrafast CT scanning with EBCT obviates the necessity of breath holding by the patient, which is obviously difficult in hypoxic patients. Teigen et al. (7) examined EBCT images of the pulmonary vasculature in 60 patients undergoing direct pulmonary arteriography for suspicion of pulmonary embolism. The pulmonary vascular bed was divided into 12 zones, including the distal segmental vessels, and EBCT and angiographic findings were correlated on a patient-by-patient basis for each zone. Thirty-six patients had both negative EBCT and angiography, while in 15, both EBCT and angiography were positive. From these data, the sensitivity of EBCT was determined to be 65%, while the specificity was 97%. However, review of the nine discordant cases revealed that 4 patients had very small subsegmental or distal segmental emboli, 2 patients had subtle chronic emboli, and 2 patients had angiographic changes due to tumor and radiation. Thus, sensitivity and specificity of EBCT was found to approach 100% for clinically important acute pulmonary emboli. Additionally, EBCT was equally applicable to depiction of central and peripheral emboli. Figure 3 shows central pulmonary emboli in the right and left pulmonary arteries from an EBCT examination.

Potential pitfalls of CT and EBCT include inadequate imaging of horizontally oriented vessels in the right middle lobe and lingula and of peripheral areas of the upper and lower lobes, and false-positive readings in the presence of intersegmental lymph nodes. However, clinical experience is rapidly growing and strongly indicates that sensitivity and specificity for important acute emboli are excellent for both

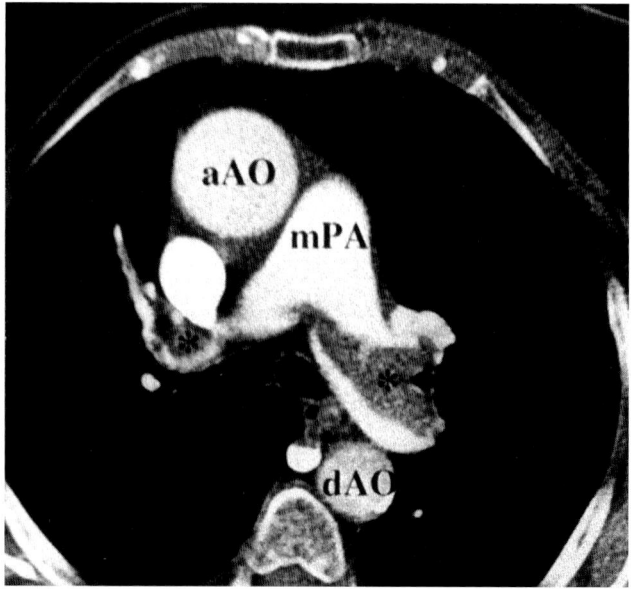

FIG. 3. EBCT section at the level of the pulmonary artery bifurcation shows visualization of extensive thrombi in the proximal right and left pulmonary arteries (*asterisk*). aAO, ascending aorta; dAO, descending aorta; mPA, main pulmonary artery. (Courtesy of Jerome F. Breen, M.D., Mayo Clinic, Rochester, Minnesota.)

spiral CT and EBCT. Because they provide a true visualization of pulmonary emboli and/or thrombi, these techniques can also be used to examine changes in thrombus burden following intervention by serial imaging.

EVALUATION OF CARDIAC MASSES AND THE PERICARDIUM

CT and EBCT have proved very useful for precise delineation of cardiac masses and the pericardium. This is based on superior spatial resolution and the inherently three-dimensional nature of the tomographic sections. EBCT, if available, is preferred, owing to the rapid scanning times to avoid motion artifacts. For intracardiac masses, contrast-enhanced scans are obtained to identify filling defects. Using EBCT, the high frame rate allows analysis of functional aspects of tumors or pericardial disease with regard to wall motion, outflow obstruction, filling and emptying dynamics, and valvular involvement throughout the cardiac cycle if the echocardiographic examination remains inconclusive. Orthogonal (short- and long-axis) EBCT contrast images can identify structures as small as 1 to 2 mm, including left atrial appendage thrombus formation.

Cardiac Tumors and Thrombi

Atrial myxoma, the most frequent primary cardiac tumor, accounts for more than 50% of all cardiac neoplasms. It is usually found in the left atrium, arising from a peduncle around the fossa ovalis of the interatrial septum. It can grow to substantial size and prolapse through the mitral valve into the left ventricle, obstructing left ventricular inflow. It is commonly associated with systemic emboli and is lethal if not eventually surgically removed. Less common primary cardiac tumors include rhabdomyomas (usually in children), fibromas, and lipomas. Fibromas are occasionally calcified, but often the CT density of fibromas and rhabdomyomas approximates that of the myocardium, which may interfere with the diagnosis if there is no obvious anatomic deformity and/or filling defect. Lipomas have lesser CT densities and are usually easily identified even if lying within the atrial septum. EBCT can demonstrate tumor size, location, attachment, morphology, and movement. It is also useful for defining cardiac involvement of metastatic tumors or cardiac extension of extracardiac carcinomas. Figure 4 shows a large cardiac lymphoma as delineated by EBCT.

In view of the accuracy with which EBCT can be used to define the right and left ventricular surfaces and left atrial anatomy, the detection of a cardiac source of cerebrovascular thromboembolism has been evaluated (8). A greater sensitivity for evaluation of left atrial thrombi by EBCT over standard transthoracic echocardiography has clearly been demonstrated, but this advantage has been somewhat obviated by the introduction of transesophageal echocardiography into accepted and widespread clinical practice. Nonetheless,

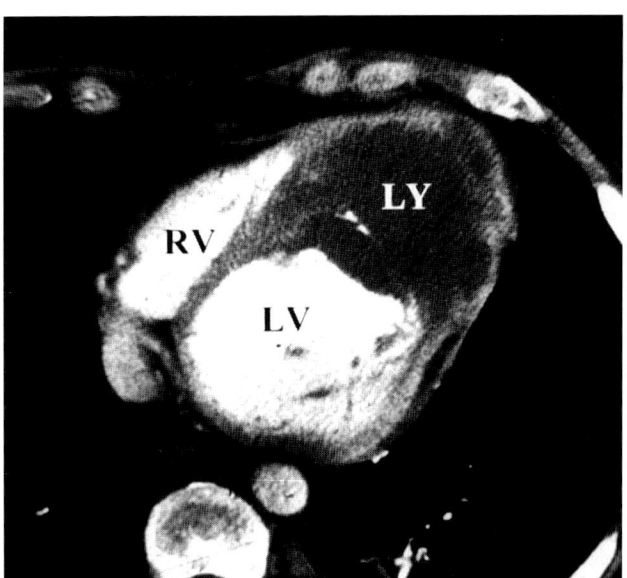

FIG. 4. Large cardiac apical lymphoma (*LY*) visualized by EBCT. *LV*, left ventricle; *RV*, right ventricle. (Courtesy of Jerome F. Breen, M.D., Mayo Clinic, Rochester, Minnesota.)

EBCT has proved very useful for delineating complex pathologies. Figure 5 shows a left ventricular thrombus (*arrows*) and a septal abscess (*asterisk*) communicating with the aortic root in a 38-year-old woman.

Diseases of the Pericardium

The pericardium is a fibroserous sac whose two serous layers are normally in close contact. The ventral pericardium is usually visualized by CT and EBCT, whereas the dorsal portions are less well appreciated. On tomographic images, the pericardium appears as a 1- to 2-mm line of a CT density comparable to the myocardium. A layer of variable thickness of epicardial fat separates this line from the epicardial aspect of the myocardium. Of note, near the inferior insertion of the pericardium into the diaphragm, its contour thickens and measures 3 to 4 mm in normal adults. By virtue of the excellent spatial and superior temporal resolution, EBCT and, to a lesser degree, spiral CT (over conventional CT) allows direct visualization of the pericardium, which is not usually feasible with other techniques. Pericardial thickening, calcification, and structural deformities are easily demonstrated.

The noninvasive first-line method to evaluate the physiologic consequences of diseases of the pericardium is two-dimensional and Doppler echocardiography. EBCT and CT can be helpful in case direct visualization of the pericardium is warranted. For example, if the differentiation between restrictive and constrictive cardiac physiology is equivocal from the echocardiogram, the detection of pericardial thickening and calcification by CT favors the diagnosis of constriction. Other scenarios where EBCT and CT can be extremely useful include pericardial cysts and tumors.

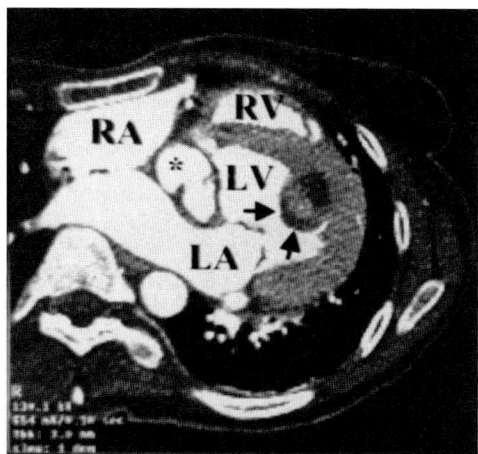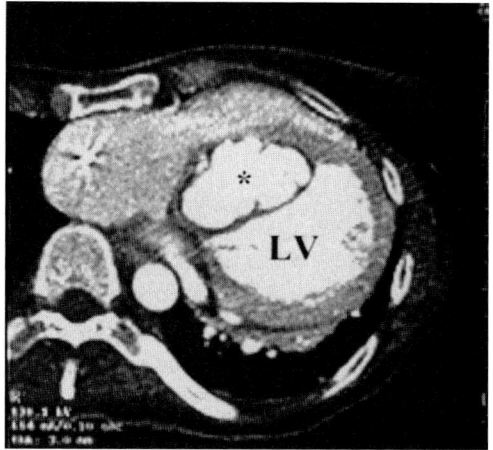

FIG. 5. EBCT sections at the base of the heart (**left panel**) and at midventricle (**right panel**). Thirty-eight-year-old woman with left ventricular thrombus (*arrows*) and a septal capsulated abcess originating from the aortic root (*asterisk*). *LA*, left atrium; *LV*, left ventricle; *RA*, right atrium; *RV*, right ventricle. (Courtesy of Jerome F. Breen, M.D., Mayo Clinic, Rochester, Minnesota.)

EVALUATION OF CARDIAC CHAMBER VOLUMES, MUSCLE MASS, AND FUNCTION

Quantitative values of ventricular volumes and muscle mass are independent predictors of cardiac morbidity and mortality. Accurate measurements are important, since diagnosis and treatment of left ventricular dysfunction and/or hypertrophy improves survival, and serial evaluation allows monitoring the impact of medical treatment in individual patients. Although estimation of left ventricular size and function is possible with several current imaging modalities, quantitation of ventricular volumes and mass often shows considerable variability and is problematic in patients with concomitant pulmonary disease, obesity, or extensive wall motion abnormalities. Due to its irregular geometric shape, the right ventricle is particularly difficult to assess using conventional angiographic, radionuclide, and ultrasonic methods.

EBCT allows for a minimally invasive means to determine high spatial, density, and temporal resolution images of the beating heart at multiple tomographic levels in a known three-dimensional registration. For functional analyses, patients are usually positioned in the short axis by slewing the scanner table 25 degrees to the patient's right and elevating it cranially by approximately 20 degrees. This results in an image orientation comparable to the parasternal echocardiographic short axis, allowing for convenient analysis of wall motion and thickening. Up to 12 contiguous tomographic levels (approximately 1.0 cm center-to-center) with 10 to 20 or more images through the cardiac cycle can be performed during a single intravenous injection of nonionic contrast

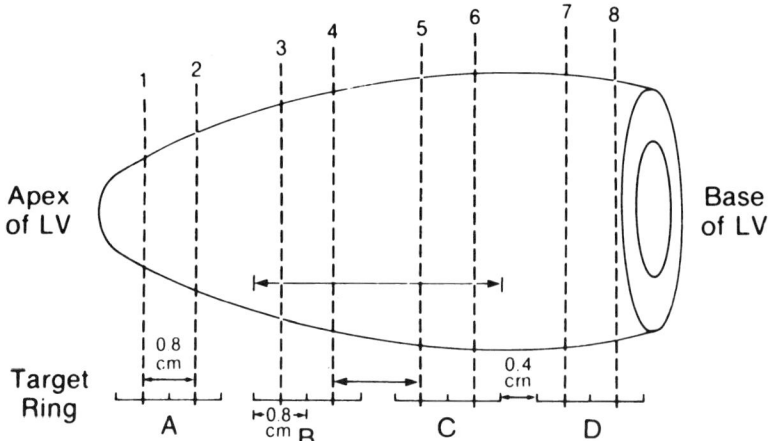

FIG. 6. Schematic representation of multislice imaging of the left ventricle using EBCT. Four target rings (*A* through *D*) and two detectors provide for a maximum of eight levels per scan series. Each level has a slice thickness of approximately 0.8 cm. Additionally, there is a space of 0.4 cm between the target rings. *LV*, left ventricle. (From ref. 10, with permission.)

media (Fig. 6). This provides for sufficient spatial resolution to define left ventricular wall thickness. Figure 7 shows diastolic and systolic frames at one tomographic level. To define right ventricular muscle mass, EBCT imaging must be done in the high spatial resolution "volume mode" due to the normally thin right ventricular wall. Composite calculations of ventricular chamber volumes and muscle mass are determined using a modified Simpson's ("stack of coins") rule. Of note, such studies are feasible not only in an optimized experimental setting, but also in the clinical environment with severely ill patients (9).

Feiring et al. (10) initially evaluated left ventricular mass using EBCT in the dog. Comparison between left ventricular mass *ex vivo* and that calculated from EBCT *in vivo* yielded an excellent correlation ($r = 0.99$) and a standard error of the mean on the order of 4.1 g (about 5% of the mean) (Fig. 8). Additionally, impressive results regarding inter- and intraobserver variability and interscan reliability (reproducibility) were found, independent of the exact position of the animals in the scanner (10). These observations were also extended to determination of left ventricular mass in a group of normal individuals, and normal values for left ventricular mass were established (98 ± 18 g/m^2) (11). The reproducibility of such means to the determination of left ventricular mass in man was shown by Roig et al. (12), who found a less than 1 to 2% difference in calculations of mass in a group of patients who had three separate EBCT scans within a 24-hour period (Fig. 9**A**). Additionally, a negligible interobserver variability with respect to analysis of the images was demonstrated (Fig. 9**B**).

Reiter et al. (13) examined the quantitation of both left and right ventricular stroke volumes in dogs using EBCT. End-diastolic (peak of R wave from the ECG) and end-systolic (smallest tomographic cavity volume during the cardiac cycle) frames were identified from left and right ventricular short-axis scans taken from apex throughout the right ventricular outflow tract. Global end-diastolic and end-systolic volumes were determined by use of Simpson's rule and the

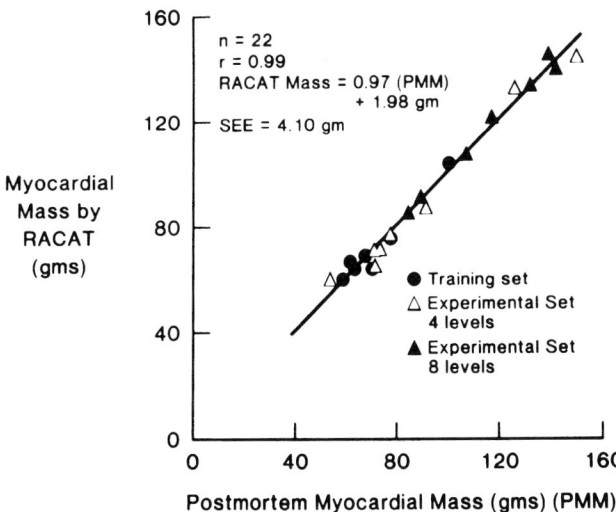

FIG. 8. Validation of EBCT measurements of left ventricular muscle mass. There is a linear, very close, and consistent correlation between postmortem determination of muscle mass (X axis) and EBCT measurements done in a blinded fashion (Y axis). *RACAT*, rapid acquisition computed tomography, i.e., EBCT. (From ref. 10, with permission.)

difference defined as the global stroke volume. Figure 10**A** shows 25 separate *in vivo* determinations of left ventricular stroke volume (determined directly from a chronically placed electromagnetic flow probe or by thermodilution) compared with stroke volume calculated from the EBCT images. These data confirm the precision of stroke volume determinations by EBCT ($r = 0.99$, standard error 1.47 mL (or less than 5% of the mean), even in the presence of experimentally induced myocardial infarction. Values for quantitation of left ventricular volumes in normal patients were later confirmed by Feiring et al. (11). Normal values were 73 ± 19 mL/m^2 for end-diastolic volume, 24 ± 8 mL/m^2 for end-systolic volume, and 48 ± 11 mL/m^2 for stroke volume. The initial study by Reiter et al. (13) also showed an excellent correlation between EBCT-derived and true right ventricular volumes (Fig. 10**B**). Whereas cardiac studies as discussed above are usually done using the multislice, cine option of the EBCT scanner, Hajduczok et al. (14) demonstrated that determinations of right ventricular mass can be done using the high resolution, single-slice mode to account for the relatively thin right ventricular wall.

Based on the highly accurate and reproducible results of the validation studies, EBCT has been used to examine physiology and pathophysiology in healthy volunteers and patients with coronary or valvular heart disease. These studies have analyzed the heterogeneity of regional ejection fraction (11), regional radius-to-wall thickness ratios (15), and diastolic function (16) with EBCT. As a logical extension, EBCT has been applied to studies of left and right ventricular remodeling after a first myocardial infarction (17,18). These studies have enabled detection of nonparallel changes in

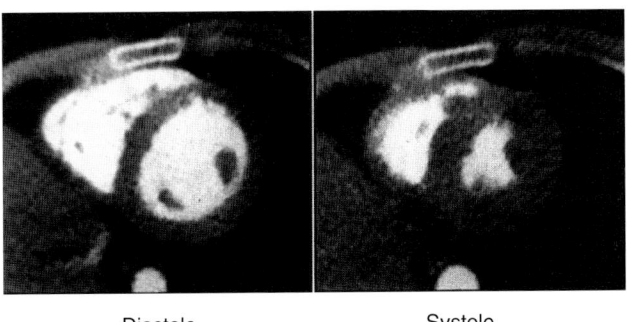

FIG. 7. Midventricular short-axis EBCT sections of diastolic (**left panel**) and systolic (**right panel**) frames. (Courtesy of Jerome F. Breen, M.D., Mayo Clinic, Rochester, Minnesota.)

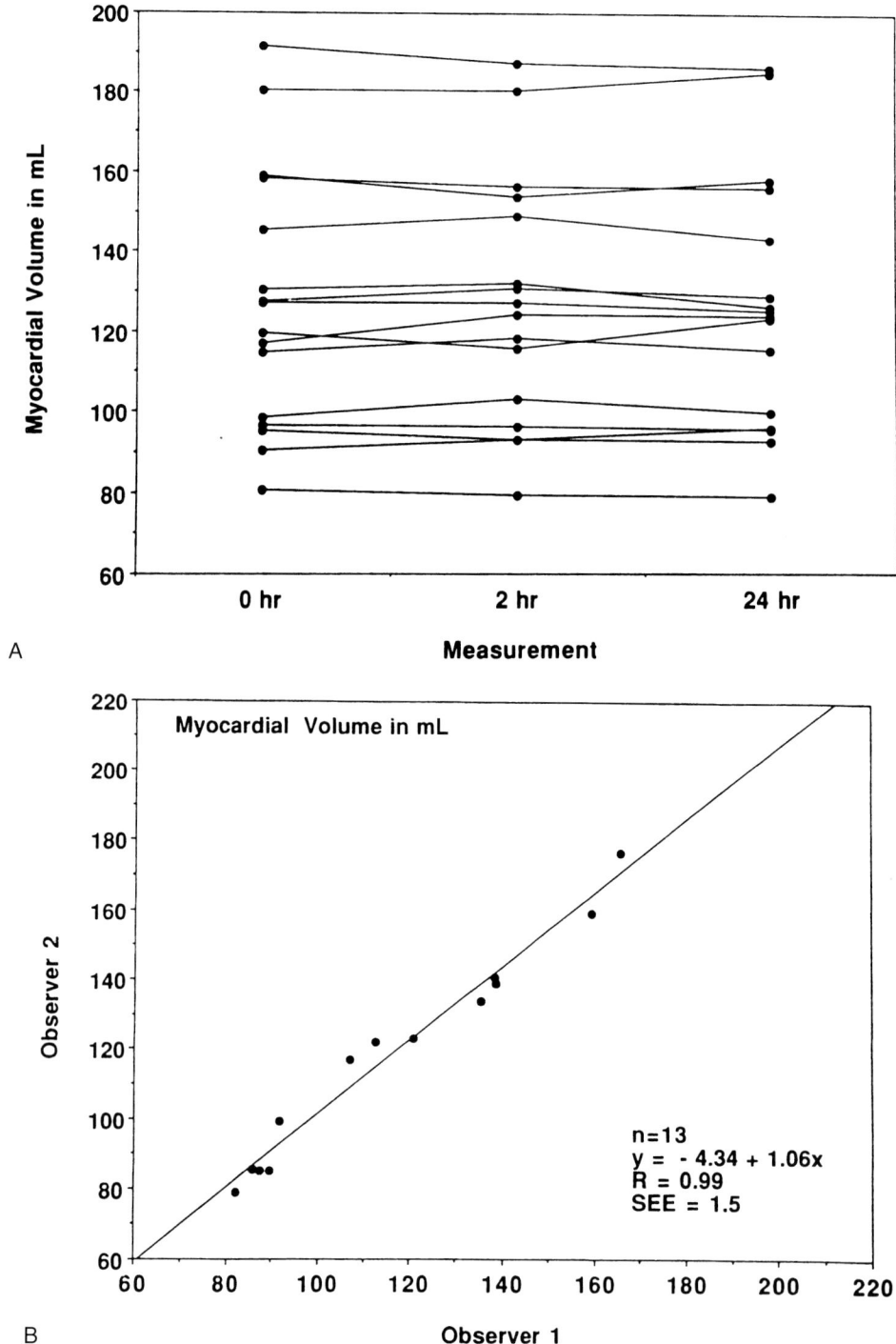

FIG. 9. Validity of EBCT measurements of left ventricular myocardial mass (or, more specifically, volume) in patients. **A:** Excellent reproducibility is shown in three serial examinations within 24 hours. **B:** Negligible interobserver variability regarding the same examination is shown. (From ref. 12, with permission.)

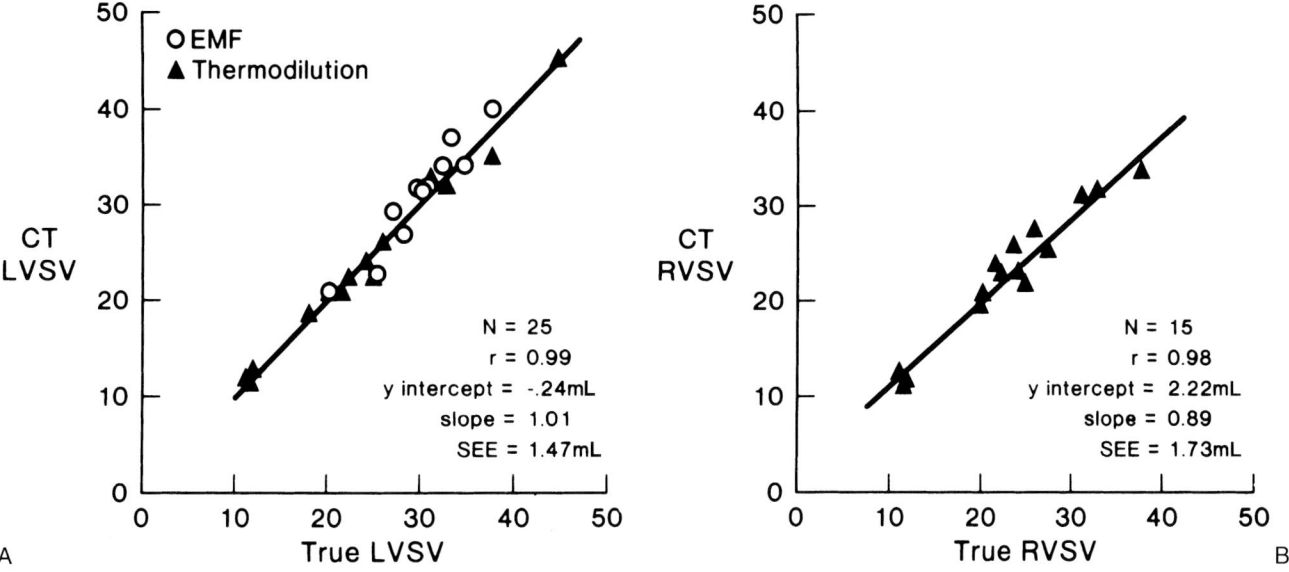

FIG. 10. Validation of EBCT measurements of left (**A**) and right (**B**) ventricular stroke volume against electromagnetic flow measurements (*EMF*) or the thermodilution method as standard. *CT*, computed tomography; *LVSV*, left ventricle stroke volume; *RVSV*, right ventricle stroke volume. (From ref. 13, with permission.)

global left ventricular chamber volume and muscle mass during the first year after myocardial infarction (Fig. 11) (17). Finally, the precision of EBCT-derived analysis of right ventricular volumes and muscle mass (13,14) has proved clinically useful for the detection and evaluation of arrhythmogenic right ventricular dysplasia (Fig. 12) (19).

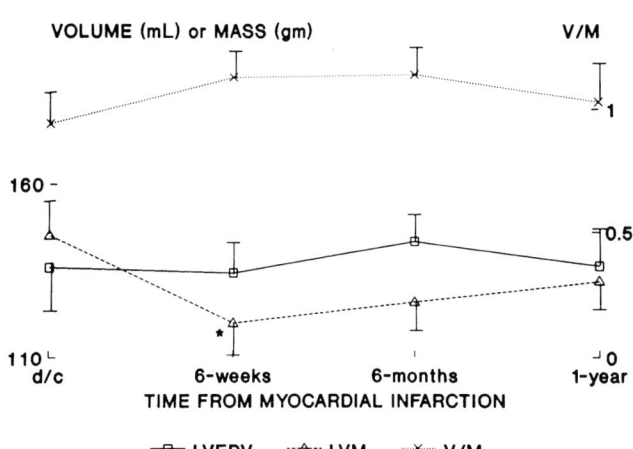

FIG. 11. EBCT-derived measurements of global left ventricular volume and muscle mass in patients during the first year after an index myocardial infarction demonstrate nonparallel changes in that the ratio of left ventricular volume to mass is decreased at 6 weeks, owing to an increase in left ventricular volume. Subsequently, with compensatory increases in muscle mass, the ratio returns to baseline values. *LVEDV*, left ventricular end-diastolic volume; *LVM*, left ventricular (muscle) mass; *V/M*, ratio of left ventricular volume to mass. (From ref. 17, with permission.)

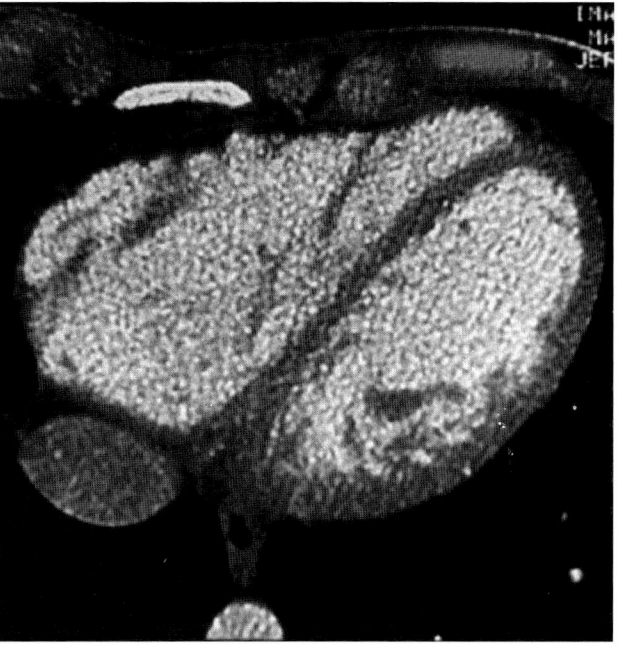

FIG. 12. EBCT representation of arrhythmogenic right ventricular dysplasia. End-diastolic frame at the midventricular level. The right ventricle is enlarged and shows multiple trabeculations. Areas of low CT density within the right ventricular free wall indicate myocardial fat deposits. In this case, the absence of abundant epicardial adipose tissue makes the diagnosis of arrhythmogenic right ventricular dysplasia more difficult using imaging modalities, and a technique as sensitive as EBCT may be required. (Courtesy of Jerome F. Breen, M.D., Mayo Clinic, Rochester, Minnesota.)

DETECTION AND DELINEATION OF CORONARY ATHEROSCLEROSIS BY QUANTIFICATION OF CORONARY CALCIUM

Among other noninvasive imaging modalities, including conventional and spiral CT, EBCT stands out in that it provides direct high-resolution images of the coronary arteries in the beating heart. Intuitively, this represents a unique opportunity for noninvasive, readily available studies of pathophysiologic and diagnostic aspects of coronary atherosclerosis. EBCT images are based on differences in CT density, and, accordingly, the analysis of coronary artery anatomy depends on the delineation of high- versus low-density structures. Therefore, two facets of atherosclerotic disease lend themselves to analysis: one is coronary calcification and the other is lumen encroachment. The latter approach requires contrast injections and is discussed in the next section of this chapter.

Noncontrast-enhanced EBCT currently represents the only noninvasive method that has undergone rigorous validation with respect to accurate quantification of coronary artery calcium (19–21). Recent developments in spiral CT technology, which allow for effectively sub-second scan times as fast as 250 msec hold promise as a viable substitute, but direct validation and clinical evaluation is pending. Open questions regarding spiral CT use relate to measurement vari-

ability and detectability of small calcified lesions. Cinefluoroscopy is of limited usefulness, because various tissues are superimposed and preclude exact analysis; there is considerable radiation exposure, the examination largely depends on the operator's skills, and lesions cannot be quantified.

Standardized methods for imaging, identification, and quantification of coronary artery calcium using EBCT have been established (20). The scanner is usually operated in the high-resolution, single-slice mode with continuous, non-overlapping slices of 3-mm thickness and an acquisition time of 100 msec. Patients are positioned supine, and, after localization of the main pulmonary artery, a sufficient number of slices is obtained to cover the complete heart through the apex (usually 36 to 40 slices). Electrocardiographic triggering is done at 80% of the R–R interval. The presence of coronary calcium is sequentially evaluated in all levels. Coronary calcium is defined as a hyperattenuating lesion above the threshold of a CT density of 130 Hounsfield units (HU) in an area of two or more adjacent pixels. Many authors currently prefer a minimum area of increased density of four adjacent pixels (roughly 1 mm^2) to diagnose coronary calcium by EBCT. Figure 13 shows representative EBCT tomograms at the base of the heart, demonstrating moderate ''ossification'' of mural arterial segments in the left anterior descending coronary artery (**upper panels**) and in the proxi-

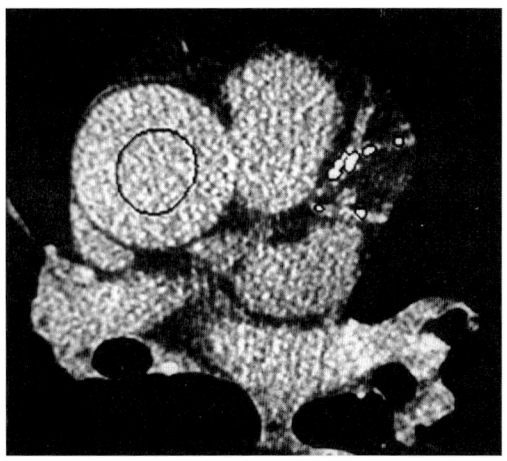
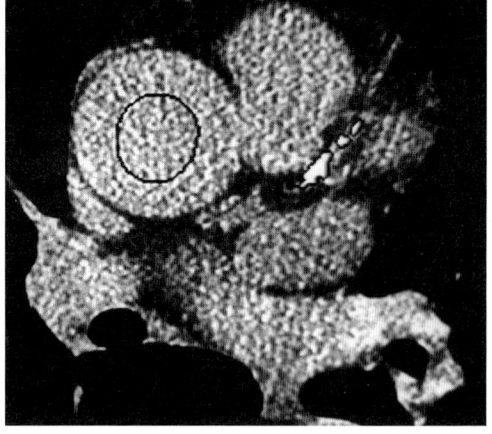
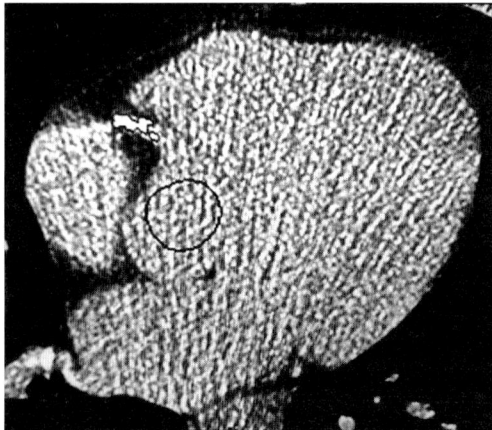

FIG. 13. Noncontrast-enhanced EBCT sections at the base of the heart showing coronary artery calcification in the proximal and mid-left anterior descending artery (**upper panels**) and the proximal right coronary artery (**lower panel**).

mal right coronary artery (**lower panel**). The "calcium score" is a product of the area of calcification per coronary segment and a factor rated 1 through 4 as dictated by the maximum calcium CT density within that segment (20). A calcium score can be calculated for a given coronary segment, a specific coronary artery, or for the entire coronary system; however, most studies have reported data related to the summed or total "score" for the entire epicardial coronary system. The total calcium score for the study shown on Figure 13 was 330. More recently, a volumetric score has been increasingly used that provides for improved reproducibility and allows the evaluation of individual calcified lesions (22,23). This volumetric score may offer significant advantages in longitudinal studies that track the progression of calcified plaque disease. However, because it does not consider CT density, the calcium score described above remains important.

Coronary artery calcium has been established as a specific expression of underlying atherosclerotic disease in pathologic-anatomic studies (24–26). It represents an active, regulated process (19,27) that can be found in stages of atherogenesis seen in young adults (25,28). Quantification of coronary calcium by EBCT provides a measure of mural atherosclerotic plaque burden (21,29,30). A linear relationship between coronary calcium area determined by EBCT and coronary plaque area has been reported (Fig. 14) (29). Thus, EBCT allows for noninvasive delineation of anatomic coronary atherosclerotic disease. In symptomatic subjects, the association of coronary calcium quantities with cardiovascular risk factors was found to be at least as strong as the association of angiographic disease severity with risk factors (Fig. 15) (31). Thus, EBCT could provide a link between coronary risk factors, preclinical disease, and susceptibility of the individual to develop symptomatic coronary artery disease. There is increasing evidence that EBCT-

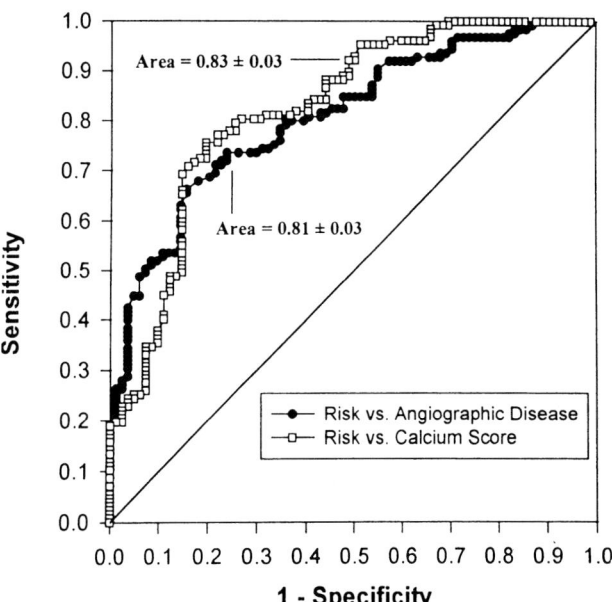

FIG. 15. Comparison of the ability of a "cardiovascular risk score" to discriminate nonobstructive angiographic coronary artery disease from obstructive angiographic coronary artery disease (*black circles*) and small amounts of coronary calcium by EBCT from great amounts of coronary calcium by EBCT (*white squares*). For this receiver operating characteristic (ROC) curve analysis, the sensitivity of the risk score with reference to coronary angiography or coronary calcium amounts is plotted as a function of {1-specificity} (equivalent to the "false-positive rate") in order to determine individual {x, y} pairs with different risk scores. The areas under the curve for coronary angiography and calcium amounts (i.e., calcium score) are presented as mean ± SE. They are not statistically different, indicating that risk factors explain a similar proportion of the variability in angiographic disease categories and amounts of coronary calcium by EBCT. (From ref. 31, with permission.)

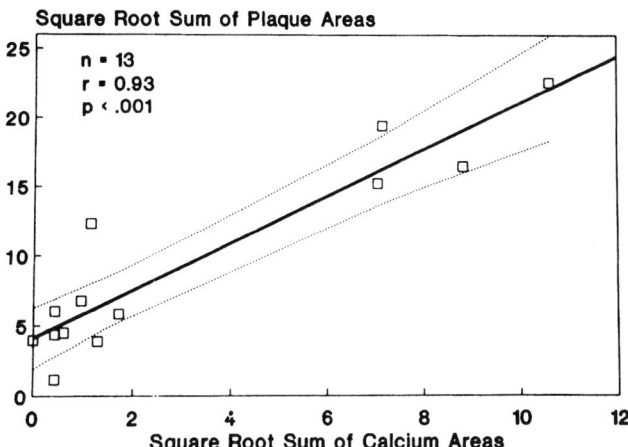

FIG. 14. Comparison of total coronary calcium area quantified by EBCT and total coronary plaque area determined by morphometry in 13 hearts examined at autopsy. A linear relationship between calcium areas by EBCT and plaque areas over a wide range of values can be appreciated. (From ref. 29, with permission.)

derived calcium quantities have prognostic value in both symptomatic and asymptomatic patients (32–34).

There are three major areas where EBCT scanning for coronary calcification is likely to prove of significant clinical value. A number of studies have confirmed that the vast majority of patients with fixed significant coronary stenoses (35,36) or those presenting with acute coronary syndromes due to significant stenoses (37) have identifiable calcium by EBCT. Subsequently, the absence of calcification by EBCT (i.e., calcium score of zero) has been shown to have negative predictive values between 90 and 100% for a greater-than-or-equal-to 50% fixed luminal coronary diameter stenosis. In view of the relatively low costs of an EBCT examination, a practical application could be realized in the patient with no prior coronary disease who presents to the emergency department with chest pain or a questionable ischemic syndrome, but has a negative or nondiagnostic electrocardiogram (ECG) and negative cardiac enzymes. Especially in a patient with a low-to-intermediate likelihood of significant fixed coronary disease, a negative EBCT could facilitate early dismissal from the emergency department or chest pain unit. Defining the presence of disease on an anatomic rather than physiologic basis, as with stress testing, has distinct clinical advantages. These principles could also apply to ambulatory patients with "atypical" cardiac symptoms in whom the pretest likelihood for ischemic disease is considered by the clinician to be low (based on age, gender, or absence of cardiovascular risk factors). Individuals with a zero calcium score could be reassured and further testing directed at noncardiac sources of chest pain. Conversely, if the calcium score is consistent with moderate or severe atherosclerotic plaque development, then additional cardiac evaluation may be appropriate. Issues specifically addressing whether the very high negative predictive value for EBCT offers economic and/or clinical advantages over other more conventional means to noninvasively diagnosis-fixed coronary disease have not been resolved. However, two reports have already provided very promising data on the performance of EBCT to identify low-risk patients in the emergency department (39,40).

Application of EBCT to define atherosclerotic plaque burden in asymptomatic individuals at risk for coronary disease, on the other hand, has received a fair amount of discussion (19,33,34,38,41) and is one of the areas of intense research. Arad and colleagues (33) followed 1,173 initially asymptomatic patients (average age 53, plus or minus 11 years) who had no known coronary disease for a mean of 19 months after a screening EBCT coronary calcium scan. Eighteen subjects had 26 cardiovascular events: 1 death, 7 nonfatal myocardial infarctions, 8 coronary bypass grafting procedures, 9 coronary angioplasties, and 1 nonhemorrhagic stroke. The magnitude of the coronary calcium score at the time of the index EBCT scan was highly predictive of subsequently developing symptomatic cardiovascular disease during follow-up. Odds ratios ranged from 20:1 for a calcium score of 100 to 35:1 for a calcium score of 160. These data along with the complementary studies by Detrano et al. (32) in symptomatic, middle-aged adults and by Secci et al. (38) in asymptomatic, elderly adults emphasize that the calcium score, as a surrogate to the total atherosclerotic plaque burden, can confer differential prognostic information. A recent study incorporating retrospective and prospective data in asymptomatic patients has reinforced the concept that the amounts of calcium (the calcium score) need to be interpreted with respect to the individual patient's age and gender (34). It appears that if this is done, high calcium scores compared to the patient's peers indicate a high risk of future "hard" events (i.e., cardiac death or myocardial infarction).

Currently, guidelines for use of EBCT as a screening test for coronary disease are under development, but broad generalizations of these opinions can be offered. The absence of identifiable coronary calcium is consistent with no, or at most, minimal atherosclerotic plaque burden. Individuals in this group are likely to fall into a favorable prognostic group (19). On the other hand, studies from our laboratory have shown that calcium scores exceeding 80 to 100 are highly consistent with at least nonobstructive coronary disease (42).

It is important to underscore that the presence of moderate, although nonobstructive, coronary disease can engender an adverse long-term prognosis. In a study of 521 patients undergoing initial diagnostic coronary angiography, Proudfit and colleagues (43) found the incidence of any cardiac events (death, arteriographic progression to obstruction, myocardial infarction) over the next 10 years was 2.1% in those with normal angiograms, increasing to 13.8% with a less than 30% stenosis, and was 33% in those with 30% to 50% maximal stenoses. Contrary to widely held beliefs, coronary calcium does not usually signify stability of individual coronary lesions. Pathologic studies of sudden coronary death have noted that the majority of ruptured plaques contain coronary calcium (44). Thus, the presence of moderate calcium scores in an otherwise asymptomatic individual suggests that further evaluations, including careful identification and aggressive treatment of modifiable risk factors, may be prudent. Individuals with significant coronary calcium (greater than 400-to-500 calcium score) have a high likelihood of at least one obstructive coronary lesion (42), have advanced plaque disease, require strict measures regarding modifiable risk factors, and, additionally, should probably be considered for further evaluations directed to determining the potential for ischemia. It is anticipated that measuring the progression of coronary calcified plaque disease will be another important application of EBCT (22,23). Although currently limited data are available, it has been suggested that progression is accelerated in high-risk patients and can be controlled by rigorous control of low-density cholesterol levels (23). EBCT is currently the only noninvasive method available to delineate the progression of coronary plaque disease, but more work is required to establish the clinical validity.

INTRAVENOUS CORONARY ANGIOGRAPHY

Direct visualization of the epicardial coronary arteries is necessary to establish the presence and focal severity of coronary luminal disease. At the moment, selective coronary angiography is the only clinical method to accurately visualize and quantify coronary artery anatomy *in vivo*. While this method provides for exceptional spatial resolution and a general "road map" of the coronary system, it is expensive, has a small but definite risk of complications, and requires at least brief hospitalization and a period of observation for several hours after the procedure. A convenient, noninvasive and safe means to perform coronary angiography clearly would be of clinical benefit.

EBCT has been studied for this purpose because of the inherently three-dimensional nature of the data set, coupled with adequate spatial and temporal image resolution. The most widely used protocol employs the single-slice, high-resolution scanning mode with a slice thickness of 3 mm and overlap to obtain a nominal slice thickness of 1 mm. Patient positioning has been varied between the neutral supine position ("modified long-axis") and some table slew

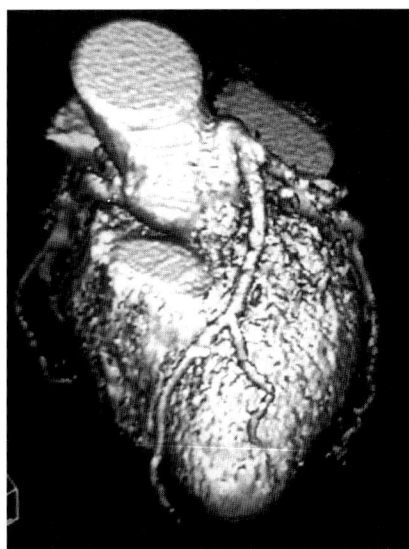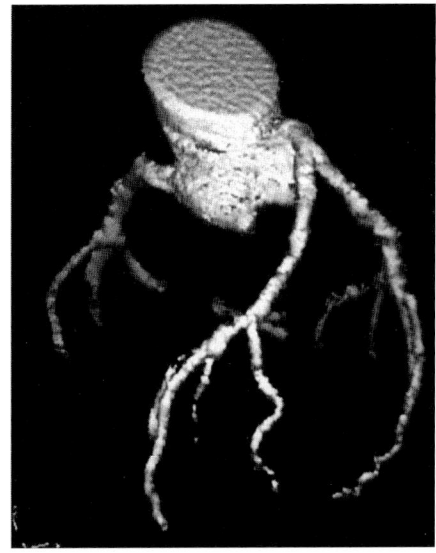

FIG. 16. Intravenous EBCT coronary angiogram, three-dimensional shaded surface representation. Ventricular cavity contrast filling is shown in the **left panel** but "edited away" in the **right panel**. The coronary arteries are widely patent, but the luminal contours are somewhat irregular, corresponding to nonobstructive coronary atherosclerotic disease.

to the patient's right and cranial elevation to obtain modified short-axis images. The patient's circulation time is determined by injection of approximately 10 mL of iodinated contrast into the same peripheral vein later used for the actual examination. A region of interest is placed in the ascending or descending aorta, and the time from injection of contrast to appearance in this region of interest is measured. For the intravenous angiogram, images are usually gated by triggering at 80% of the R–R interval, but imaging in systole may yield superior results for the right coronary artery. Depending on patient size, about 40 to 60 overlapping slices (i.e., approximately 8 to 12 cm) are necessary to cover the complete coronary tree from the aortic root caudad through the apex and inferior surface of the heart. After contrast injection has been started at a rate of 2 to 4 mL/sec, patients are asked to hold their breath, and imaging is commenced at the circulation time or somewhat later. To shorten the total breath-hold time, it may be useful to use atropine or transesophageal pacing in some patients with heart rates below 75 bpm. This and slower contrast injection rates help limit the use of contrast material to below 150 or even 100 mL without compromising image quality. Image analysis varies depending on software and personal preferences. It should involve evaluation of the original tomographic images as well as some form of volumetric (three-dimensional) data set. Figure 16 shows a three-dimensional shaded-surface display representing patent coronary arteries with some luminal irregularities.

Moshage and colleagues (45) studied 27 patients with EBCT who also underwent conventional coronary arteriography. In this preliminary study, 9 out of 11 (82%) high-grade stenoses (greater than 75% diameter stenosis) and 5 out of 5 (100%) occlusions in the proximal left anterior descending coronary artery as identified by selective arteriography were found on review of the EBCT scans by blinded observers. Five patients who underwent selective angioplasty after arteriography underwent repeat scanning with EBCT. In each case, the improvements in the arterial lumen dimensions were definable in the EBCT images. In addition, 3 of 5 (60%) high-grade stenoses were also visualized in the right coronary artery. However, recognition of stenoses of the left circumflex was more difficult, likely due to motion artifact or to difficulty in segmentation of the left atrium and appendage from the vessel's course in the atrioventricular groove. The same group has expanded their initial studies of EBCT coronary angiography to 125 patients undergoing selective coronary arteriography (46). Although only 75% of all major coronary arteries were seen using EBCT, sensitivity and specificity were good in those arteries (92% and 94%, respectively).

We have recently reported our experience in 28 patients (47). Based on quantitative (selective) coronary angiography, significant stenoses (greater-than-or-equal-to 50% diameter stenosis) were evaluated in 8 major or 12 (including side branches) coronary segments. Of the 330 segments assessable by (selective) coronary angiography, 237 (72%) were visualized by EBCT. The sensitivity for detection of significant stenoses was 82%, the specificity was 88%, positive and negative predictive values were 57% and 96%, respectively, and overall accuracy was 87%. If only 8 (major) coronary artery segments were considered, 88% (194 of 221) of segments were visualized, and the overall accuracy was 90%. The main determinant of false-negative results was substantial segmental calcification, whereas the main determinant of false-positive results was small vessel size.

Using intravenous EBCT angiography, the left main and

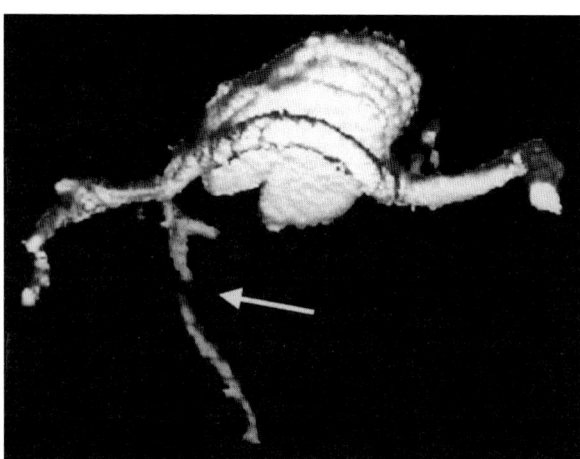

FIG. 17. Intravenous EBCT coronary angiogram, three-dimensional shaded surface representation. An abnormal origin of the left coronary artery from the right coronary artery is shown. The patient, a 65-year-old woman, became symptomatic only owing to the development of a high-grade stenosis in the midleft anterior descending artery, which was correctly diagnosed by EBCT (*arrow*).

proximal and midportions of the left anterior descending artery are generally quite well seen, but sections of the mid-to-distal right coronary artery and all but the most proximal sections of the left circumflex artery remain often problematic. Importantly, however, the negative predictive value for significant disease has been consistently in the range above 95%, suggesting that EBCT may provide for an adequate screen for individuals in which a negative EBCT would obviate the need for invasive angiography. Additionally, Achenbach et al. (48) have demonstrated the usefulness of EBCT for coronary bypass graft angiography and detection of restenosis after percutaneous balloon angioplasty (49). Intravenous EBCT coronary angiography may also be attractive for the diagnosis of congenital abnormalities of the coronary arteries. Figure 17 shows the coronary system of a woman in her mid-60s who presented with new-onset chest pain. The EBCT examination showed a midleft anterior descending coronary stenosis (*arrow*) to explain her symptoms. It also demonstrated an abnormal origin of the left coronary system from the right coronary artery. Since the left coronary artery trajectory was posterior to the aorta and thus uncompressed by the great vessels, this abnormality had remained occult.

MEASUREMENTS OF MYOCARDIAL VASCULAR BLOOD VOLUME AND PERFUSION

Pathophysiologic mechanisms at the level of the coronary microcirculation are increasingly recognized as important factors in cardiac ischemic diseases. EBCT offers the potential for direct quantitative measurements of regional myocardial vascular blood volume and perfusion. Although, generally, flow reserve (i.e., the ratio of resting and hyperemic

perfusion values) is used in clinical practice, quantitation of absolute myocardial flow values is important. This is because it may often be unclear whether a reduction in flow reserve results from increased resting blood flows (e.g., in situations of increased systolic wall stress or tachycardia) or from decreased maximal blood flows. Maximal myocardial perfusion may not only be compromised by obstruction of epicardial vessels or diseases of the coronary microcirculation, but also by an increased blood viscosity (e.g., in polycythemia), an elevated left ventricular diastolic pressure, or pronounced tachycardia.

The investigation of regional myocardial perfusion and blood volume requires evaluation of contrast clearance (or time-density) data from regions of the left ventricular myocardium and the adjacent left ventricular cavity. EBCT is used in the multislice "flow" mode with tomographic sections centered at the midleft ventricular level (papillary muscles as anatomic landmark) during the passage of contrast through the tissue and vascular regions. Scanning is performed simultaneously at two or more tomographic levels, usually on the electrocardiographic R wave ("0% of the R–R interval"). During the arrival of contrast, scanning is frequently performed with every cardiac cycle to obtain a higher sampling frequency, whereas the prolonged contrast washout phase can be covered by scanning every other, every third, or even every fourth cardiac cycle. In experimental animal studies, various protocols regarding contrast injections and positioning of the animals have been used. Good results have been obtained with central intravenous contrast injections of 0.33 mL/kg body weight over 2 seconds. Myocardial vascular blood volume (V_B) is calculated from the relation between purely intravascular and myocardial contrast-clearance curves:

$$V_B(mL/g)$$
$$= \frac{Area\ under\ intramyocardial\ contrast\ clearance\ curve}{Area\ under\ ``input''\ vascular\ contrast\ clearance\ curve}$$

Quantitative myocardial perfusion (F_M) is calculated based on the principles of indicator dilution theory:

$$F_M(mL/g/min) = \frac{V_B}{Mean\ contrast\ transit\ time}$$

Experimental validation studies have demonstrated a linear relationship between measurements of myocardial perfusion by EBCT and the standard radiolabeled microspheres technique up to absolute values of approximately 3 mL/g/min (Fig. 18) (50,51). It is important to consider the dynamic nature of myocardial vascular blood volume when calculating perfusion values. For example, blood volume increases substantially with microvascular dilation in situations of hyperemia, and myocardial perfusion is underestimated if one does not account for this. Recently, these principles have been applied to human studies in healthy volunteers (52), suggesting the feasibility of EBCT myocardial perfusion measurements in the clinical setting.

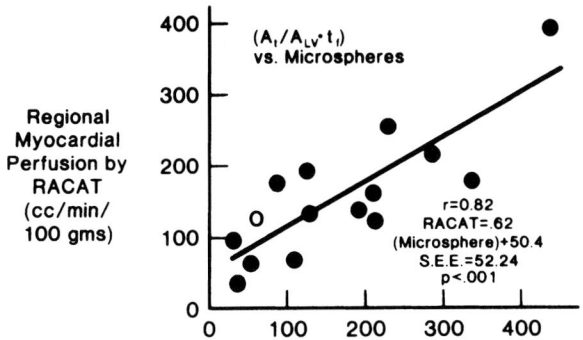

Regional Myocardial Perfusion by Microspheres (cc/min/100 gms)

FIG. 18. Validation of measurements of regional myocardial perfusion by EBCT. Comparison against the standard radiolabeled microsphere technique (X axis). *RACAT*, rapid acquisition computed tomography. (From ref. 50, with permission.)

REFERENCES

1. McCollough CH, Morin RL. The technical design and performance of ultrafast computed tomography. *Radiol Clin North Am* 1994;32:521–536.
2. McCollough CH, Zink FE, Morin RL. Radiation dosimetry for electron beam CT. *Radiology* 1994;192:637–643.
3. Small JH, Dixon AK, Coulden RA, et al. Fast CT for aortic dissection. *Br J Radiol* 1996;69:900–905.
4. Lerman LO, Taler SJ, Textor SC, et al. Computed tomography-derived intrarenal blood flow in renovascular and essential hypertension. *Kidney Int* 1996;49:846–854.
5. Remy-Jardin M, Remy J, Wattinner L, et al. Central pulmonary thromboembolism: diagnosis with spiral volumetric CT with the single-breath-hold technique—comparison with pulmonary angiography. *Radiology* 1992;185:381–387.
6. Goodman LR, Curtin JJ, Mewissen MW, et al. Detection of pulmonary embolism in patients with unresolved clinical and scintigraphic diagnosis: helical CT versus angiography. *Am J Roentgenol* 1995;164:1369–1374.
7. Teigen CL, Maus TP, Sheedy PF II, et al. Pulmonary embolism: diagnosis with contrast-enhanced electron-beam CT and comparison with pulmonary angiography. *Radiology* 1995;194:313–319.
8. Love BB, Struck LK, Stanford W, et al. Comparison of two-dimensional echocardiography and ultrafast cardiac computed tomography for evaluating intracardiac thrombi in cerebral ischemia. *Stroke* 1990;21:1033–1038.
9. Schmermund A, Rensing BJ, Sheedy PF, et al. Reproducibility of right and left ventricular volume measurements by electron-beam CT in patients with congestive heart failure. *Int J Card Imag* 1998;14:201–209.
10. Feiring AJ, Rumberger JA, Reiter SJ, et al. Determination of left ventricular mass in dogs with rapid-acquisition cardiac computed tomographic scanning. *Circulation* 1985;72:1355–1364.
11. Feiring AJ, Rumberger JA, Reiter SJ, et al. Sectional and segmental variability of left ventricular function: experimental and clinical studies using ultrafast computed tomography. *J Am Coll Cardiol* 1988;12:415–425.
12. Roig E, Georgiou D, Chomka EV, et al. Reproducibility of left ventricular myocardial volume and mass measurements by ultrafast computed tomography. *J Am Coll Cardiol* 1991;18:990–996.
13. Reiter SJ, Rumberger JA, Feiring AJ, et al. Precision of right and left ventricular volume by cine computed tomography. *Circulation* 1986;74:890–900.
14. Hajduczok ZD, Weiss RM, Stanford W, et al. Determination of right ventricular mass in humans and dogs with ultrafast cardiac computed tomography. *Circulation* 1990;82:202–212.
15. Feiring AJ, Rumberger JA. Ultrafast computed tomography analysis

16. Rumberger JA, Weiss RM, Feiring AJ, et al. Patterns of regional diastolic function in the normal human left ventricle. An ultrafast computed tomographic study. *J Am Coll Cardiol* 1989;14:119–126.
17. Rumberger JA, Behrenbeck T, Breen JR, et al. Nonparallel changes in global left ventricular chamber volume and muscle mass during the first year after transmural myocardial infarction in humans. *J Am Coll Cardiol* 1993;21:673–682.
18. Hirose K, Reed JE, Rumberger JA. Serial changes in regional right ventricular free wall and left ventricular septal wall lengths during the first 4 to 5 years after index anterior wall myocardial infarction. *J Am Coll Cardiol* 1995;26:394–400.
19. Wexler L, Brundage B, Crouse J, et al. Coronary artery calcification: pathophysiology, epidemiology, imaging methods, and clinical implications. A statement for health professionals from the American Heart Association. *Circulation* 1996;94:1175–1192.
20. Agatston AS, Janowitz WR, Hildner FJ, et al. Quantification of coronary artery calcium using ultrafast computed tomography. *J Am Coll Cardiol* 1990;15:827–832.
21. Mautner GC, Mautner SL, Froehlich J, et al. Coronary artery calcification: assessment with electron beam CT and histomorphometric correlation. *Radiology* 1994;192:619–623.
22. Callister TQ, Cooil B, Raya SP, et al. Coronary artery disease: improved reproducibility of calcium screening with an electron-beam CT volumetric method. *Radiology* 1998;208:807–814.
23. Callister TQ, Raggi P, Cooil B, et al. Effect of HMG-CoA reductase inhibitors on coronary artery disease as assessed by electron-beam computed tomography. *New Engl J Med* 1998;339:1972–1978.
24. Eggen DA, Strong JP, McGill HC. Coronary calcification: relationship to clinically significant coronary lesions and race, sex, and topographic distribution. *Circulation* 1965;32:948–955.
25. McCarthy JH, Palmer FJ. Incidence and significance of coronary artery calcification. *Br Heart J* 1974;36:499–506.
26. Sangiorgi G, Rumberger J, Severson A, et al. Arterial calcification and not lumen stenosis is correlated with atherosclerotic plaque burden in humans: a histologic study of 723 coronary artery segments using nondecalcifying methodology. *J Am Coll Cardiol* 1998;31:126–133.
27. Watson KE, Demer LL. The atherosclerosis-calcification link? *Curr Opin Lipidol* 1996;7:101–104.
28. Stary HC. The sequence of cell and matrix changes in atherosclerotic lesions of coronary arteries in the first forty years of life. *Eur Heart J* 1990;11[Suppl E]:3–19.
29. Rumberger JA, Simons DB, Fitzpatrick LA, et al. Coronary artery calcium area by electron-beam computed tomography and coronary atherosclerotic plaque area. A histopathologic correlative study. *Circulation* 1995;92:2157–2162.
30. Baumgart D, Schmermund A, Görge G, et al. Comparison of electron beam computed tomography with intracoronary ultrasound and coronary angiography for the detection of coronary atherosclerosis. *J Am Coll Cardiol* 1997;30:57–64.
31. Schmermund A, Baumgart D, Görge G, et al. Measuring the effect of risk factors on coronary atherosclerosis: coronary calcium score vs. angiographic disease severity. *J Am Coll Cardiol* 1998;31:1267–1273.
32. Detrano R, Hsiai T, Wang S, et al. Prognostic value of coronary calcification and angiographic stenoses in patients undergoing coronary angiography. *J Am Coll Cardiol* 1996;27:285–290.
33. Arad Y, Sparado LA, Goodman K, et al. Predictive value of electron beam computed tomography of the coronary arteries. 19-month follow-up of 1173 asymptomatic subjects. *Circulation* 1996;93:1951–1953.
34. Raggi P, Callister TQ, Cooil B, et al. Identification of patients at increased risk of first unheralded acute myocardial infarction by electron-beam computed tomography. *Circulation* 2000;101:850–855.
35. Rumberger JA, Sheedy PF, Breen JR, et al. Coronary calcium as determined by electron beam computed tomography, and coronary disease on arteriogram: effect of patient's sex on diagnosis. *Circulation* 1995;91:1363–1367.
36. Budoff MJ, Georgiou D, Brody A, et al. Ultrafast computed tomography as a diagnostic modality in the detection of coronary artery disease: a multicenter study. *Circulation* 1996;93:898–904.
37. Schmermund A, Baumgart D, Görge G, et al. Coronary artery calcium in acute coronary syndromes. A comparative study of electron beam computed tomography, coronary angiography, and intracoronary ultra-

sound in survivors of acute myocardial infarction and unstable angina. *Circulation* 1997;96:1461–1469.

38. Secci A, Wong N, Tang W, et al. Electron beam computed tomographic coronary calcium as a predictor of coronary events: comparison of two protocols. *Circulation* 1997;96:1122–1129.

39. Laudon DA, Vukov LF, Breen JF, et al. Use of electron-beam computed tomography in the evaluation of chest pain patients in the emergency department. *Ann Emerg Med* 1999;33:15–21.

40. McLaughlin VV, Balogh T, Rich S. Utility of electron beam computed tomography to stratify patients presenting to the emergency room with chest pain. *Am J Cardiol* 1999;84:327–328.

41. Hoeg JM. Evaluating coronary heart disease risk. Tiles in the mosaic (Grand rounds at the clinical center of the National Institutes of Health). *JAMA* 1997;277:1387–1390.

42. Rumberger JA, Sheedy PF, Breen JF, et al. Electron beam CT coronary calcium score cutpoints and severity of associated angiography luminal stenosis. *J Am Coll Cardiol* 1997;29:1542–1548.

43. Proudfit WL, Bruschke VG, Sones FM Jr. Clinical course of patients with normal or slightly or moderately abnormal coronary arteriograms: 10-year follow-up of 521 patients. *Circulation* 1980;62:712–717.

44. Farb A, Burke AP, Tang AL, et al. Coronary plaque erosion without rupture into a lipid core. A frequent cause of coronary thrombosis in sudden coronary death. *Circulation* 1996;93:1354–1364.

45. Moshage WEL, Achenbach S, Seese B, et al. Coronary artery stenoses: three-dimensional imaging with electrocardiographically triggered, contrast agent-enhanced, electron-beam CT. *Radiology* 1995;196:707–714.

46. Achenbach S, Moshage W, Ropers D, et al. Value of electron beam computed tomography for the noninvasive detection of high-grade coronary-artery stenoses and occlusions. *New Engl J Med* 1998;339:1964–1971.

47. Schmermund A, Rensing BJ, Sheedy PF, et al. Intravenous electron-beam CT coronary angiography for segmental analysis of coronary artery stenoses. *J Am Coll Cardiol* 1998;31:1547–1554.

48. Achenbach S, Moshage W, Ropers D, et al. Noninvasive, three-dimensional visualization of coronary artery bypass grafts by electron beam tomography. *Am J Cardiol* 1997;79:856–861.

49. Achenbach S, Moshage W, Bachmann K. Detection of high-grade restenosis after PTCA using contrast-enhanced electron beam CT. *Circulation* 1997;96:2785–2788.

50. Rumberger JA, Feiring AJ, Lipton MJ, et al. Use of ultrafast computed tomography to quantitate regional myocardial perfusion: a preliminary report. *J Am Coll Cardiol* 1987;9:59–69.

51. Weiss RM, Otoadese EA, Noel MP, et al. Quantitation of absolute regional myocardial perfusion using cine computed tomography. *J Am Coll Cardiol* 1994;23:1186–1193.

52. Bell MR, Lerman LO, Rumberger JA. Validation of minimally invasive measurement of myocardial perfusion using electron beam computed tomography and application in human volunteers. *Heart* 1999;81:628–635.

CHAPTER 27

The Future of X-ray Methods

Gerald M. Pohost

X-ray methods were the first of the noninvasive diagnostic imaging modalities. Due to the unique way that x-rays visualized the inside of the body and to their potentially harmful effects, a new field of medicine was born: radiology. X-rays progressed rapidly to fluoroscopy, to the chest film, to the image intensifier, and to digital methods. This progression led to the reduction of radiation dosage, improved contrast, the advent of x-ray contrast medium, cine approaches to demonstrate motion, improved image quality using digital methods, and tomographic imaging using x-ray computed tomography (CT) devices. The most recent of the CT devices is the electron beam CT and the spiral CT, both of which allow rapid image acquisition to freeze heart and respiratory motion.

The latest x-ray CT technology is very sophisticated, and the resultant images are very sharp with excellent contrast. It is not only possible to sensitively visualize coronary artery calcium (without contrast medium) indicative of atherosclerosis, but it is also possible, using a radioopaque x-ray contrast medium, to visualize regional and global contractile function, the great vessels and their branches, and even myocardial perfusion and the coronary arteries.

The future of x-ray methods as applied to the cardiovascular system must be considered in view of the future of the other imaging modalities.

Consider *ultrasound*. Ultrasound methods continue to improve. Ultrasound is nonionizing, and it generates images with high speed and with high spatial resolution. It is relatively inexpensive and it is mobile. X-ray methods will not compete with ultrasound methods as a routine cardiovascular diagnostic modality.

Consider *radionuclides*. Because of the unique properties of radionuclide imaging to visualize pathologic processes by concentrating them within normal or pathologic territories, x-ray methods cannot compete with radionuclides for the assessment of myocardial perfusion and the evaluation of myocardial viability.

Consider *magnetic resonance* methods. Magnetic resonance can generate high resolution, tomographic—three-dimensional images without ionizing radiation. The contrast agents for magnetic resonance methods do not add an osmotic burden (risking aggravating heart failure) and are not nephrotoxic. In fact, for evaluating the cardiovascular system, magnetic resonance methods can do virtually everything that x-ray CT methods can do except for visualizing coronary calcium. Magnetic resonance methods can also evaluate morphology and function without the need for contrast agents. Further, magnetic resonance methods can also display many of the metabolites within the myocardium, including the high-energy phosphates, lactic acid, and sodium.

With the advent of the other technologies, the role of the x-ray methods is uncertain. Clearly, the digital chest x-ray will remain an important x-ray approach. Certainly, x-ray CT methods for diagnosis of disease in other systems will continue to be of great importance. Clearly, cineangiography to guide coronary artery interventions will remain essential. Furthermore, the cinefluoroscopic methods will continue to improve.

However, we need to consider specifically what the future of x-ray methods is for cardiovascular disease diagnosis, and with ultrasound, radionuclide, and magnetic resonance methods, our enthusiasm regarding the future of x-ray CT

G. M. Pohost: Department of Medicine, University of Alabama at Birmingham, Birmingham, Alabama 35294.

in cardiovascular disease diagnosis must be reduced. A new innovative method was suggested using the synchrotron to generate monochromatic x-rays capable of noninvasively imaging the coronary arteries. However, such devices are enormously expensive and will never be widely available.

It is difficult to be sure about the future of x-ray methods for noninvasive diagnosis of cardiovascular disease. In conclusion, in view of the strengths of the other imaging approaches, it is unlikely that x-ray CT will occupy an important future position.

Imaging in Cardiovascular Disease, edited by Gerald M. Pohost et al., Lippincott Williams & Wilkins, Philadelphia © 2000

CHAPTER 28

Basic Principles of Cardiac Magnetic Resonance Imaging and Magnetic Resonance Spectroscopy

Robert S. Balaban

Nuclear magnetic resonance (NMR) is based on the detection of a fundamental property of matter, i.e., its intrinsic angular momentum or spin. In a nucleus with an even number of protons and neutrons, there is no net spin and these nuclides cannot be detected using NMR. Examples of these nuclides include ^{12}C and ^{16}O. However, many useful nuclides have odd numbers of protons or neutrons, resulting in a net spin that is detectable. The nuclides used in cardiac magnetic resonance imaging (MRI) and magnetic resonance spectroscopy (MRS) are presented in Table 1. The nuclide that is used for MRI is ^1H. ^1H has one proton and no neutrons. ^1H is one of the most useful nuclides for MRI, since it is a major constituent of the solvent of the body, water, as well as of fat and other important metabolites. If the nuclides possess a net spin and charge, then there will be a magnetic moment associated with this spin depending on the mass and the geometry of the nuclide. This is determined by the gyromagnetic ratio, γ, of the nuclide. Thus, the gyromagnetic ratio and the angular momentum of the nuclide determine the strength of the "molecular scale magnet" that we detect in an NMR experiment. ^1H is one of the strongest molecular magnets providing an excellent NMR signal.

When a bucket of water containing ^1H molecular magnets is placed in a large magnetic field (B_o), the ^1H magnets align with the B_o much like iron filings. In contrast to iron filings, the angular momentum of the ^1H nuclide results in a rotation around the axis of the magnetic field at a frequency determined by γ. This is why the nuclides are also referred to as "spins." The frequency of precession is a fundamental

property of the spins in a magnetic field and is given by the *Larmor equation*:

$$v = \gamma B/2\pi$$

where v is the precession frequency in cycles/sec and B is the applied magnetic field.

The *Larmor equation* is the basis of most of the unique properties of magnetic resonance imaging (MRI) and magnetic resonance spectroscopy (MRS). In MRI, the magnetic field, B, is made a linear function of position using specialized coils in the magnet. This results in v being a linear function of position in the sample. Using this information, an image can be created (1,2) as will be discussed below. In MRS, the shielding and modifications of the applied magnetic field in adjacent nuclides in a molecule causes alterations in the local magnetic field around the nuclide. This results in a near unique frequency fingerprint for molecules based on the interaction of the different molecular magnets

TABLE 1. *Nuclides used in MRI and MRS of the heart*

Nuclide	Natural abundance	Larmor frequency at 2.35T (MHz)	Sensitivity corrected for natural abundance
^1H	100	100	1
^{13}C	1.11	25.1	1.8×10^{-4}
^{14}N	99.63	7.24	1.0×10^{-3}
^{15}N	0.37	10.1	3.8×10^{-6}
^{17}O	0.04	13.6	1.2×10^{-5}
^{19}F	100	94.0	0.83
^{23}Na	100	26.5	0.093
^{31}P	100	40.5	0.066

R. S. Balaban: Laboratory of Cardiac Energetics, National Institutes of Health, Bethesda, Maryland 20892.

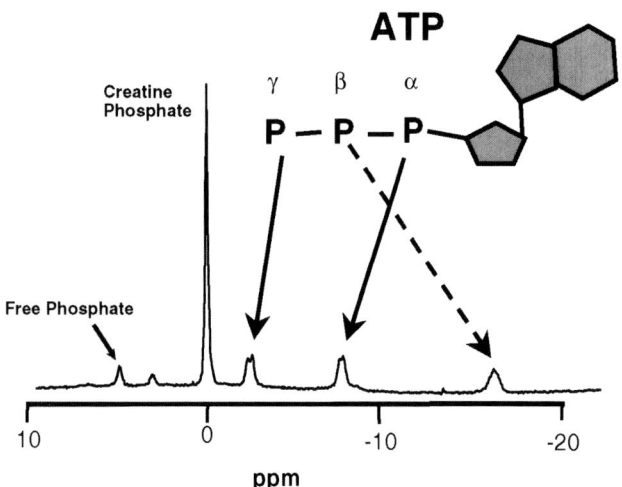

FIG. 1. ^{31}P NMR spectrum of adenosine triphosphate (*ATP*). The *arrows* indicate the phosphate resonance frequencies for the different phosphate atoms in the molecule.

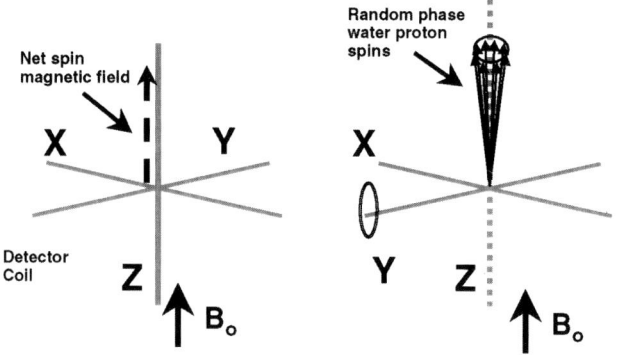

FIG. 2. Orientation of molecular spins with main magnetic field (B_o). **A:** The spins orient with the main magnetic field producing a net magnetic field aligned with B_o. **B:** The spins rotate around the B_o field axis (Z axis) in a random form resulting in no net oscillating field for detection with the coil oriented in the X-Y plane.

within the molecule. This is illustrated in Figure 1 where the frequencies of the different phosphates in adenosine triphosphate (ATP), an important metabolite in energy metabolism, are presented as a function of where these nuclides are in the ATP molecule. The phosphate at the end of the molecule (γ phosphate) is the least shielded and has a resonance frequency closest to free phosphate. The phosphate in the middle of the chain is shielded on both sides by other phosphate nuclides resulting in the largest shift from the free phosphate position (β phosphate). Finally, the phosphate closest to the adenosine ring (α phosphate) is in between the former, since it is partially shielded by the β phosphate and weakly by the sugar and adenosine ring. The chemical shifts, or frequencies of the spins in response to the chemical environment, can also be affected by the binding of ions. For example the frequency of the free phosphate peak is dependent on pH (3) while chemical shift of the β phosphate is a function of free Mg^{++} (4). This illustrates the type of molecular information, besides concentration, that is available in a simple NMR spectrum of a molecule.

DETECTION OF NMR SIGNAL

How do we detect the resonance frequency of a nuclide in NMR? It is important to realize that all of the bucket of water ^{1}H spins in a magnet are not rotating together around the axis of the magnet, but are randomly distributed around this axis. This is illustrated in three dimensions in Figure 2. The net magnetic field of the spins is aligned with the Z axis like any magnet (Fig. 2A). However, the spins rotate around the Z axis in a completely random fashion, resulting in no net signal to detect. For example, a coil placed to detect this precession in the X-Y plane will not detect a signal since the spins are all in different positions or phase, as seen in Figure 2B. The concept of phase will be further discussed

below. Thus, if a person were placed in a strong magnetic field, the rotation of the water ^{1}H spins at the Larmor frequency would not be detected by placing a coil in the X-Y plane. To get a signal, we need to get all of the water ^{1}H spins rotating together, i.e., coherent. To accomplish this task, we apply a weak magnetic field (B_1), oscillating at the Larmor frequency perpendicular to the main magnetic field, in this case along the Y axis. The frequency of the exciting field has to match the resonance frequency of the water ^{1}H to rotate the spins efficiently and to be independent of the stronger B_o field. This is much like exciting a piano string with a tuning fork, only the string with the same resonant frequency as the fork will efficiently absorb the energy from the fork and resonate. The water spins will rotate around the B_1 field following the right hand rule at a rate defined by Equation 1. Since the B_o field has a magnitude of Tesla (10,000 gauss) while the excitation field is on the order of a few gauss, the rotation frequency around the B_1 field is much lower than around the B_o field. The B_1 field is only applied transiently (milliseconds), long enough to rotate the spins into a plane perpendicular to B_o. This effect on the net magnetic field is illustrated in Figure 3A. The plane perpendicular to the B_o field is called the transverse plane or X-Y plane. Magnetization in this plane is often referred to as transverse magnetization. A B_1 pulse that drives the magnetization completely into the transverse plane is called a 90-degree pulse, referring to the angle that the net magnetization moved relative to the Z axis. Once the B_1 field is turned off, the only field causing a rotation is the B_o. However, now the net field of the spins is in the transverse plane. As the spins rotate around the B_o field axis, an oscillating field can be detected with the coil poised to detect the transverse magnetization as shown in Figure 3B. Note that, in this case, the same coil that excited the spins can be used to subsequently detect the rotating transverse magnetization. Again, the frequency of this signal detected is the Larmor frequency as defined by Equation 1.

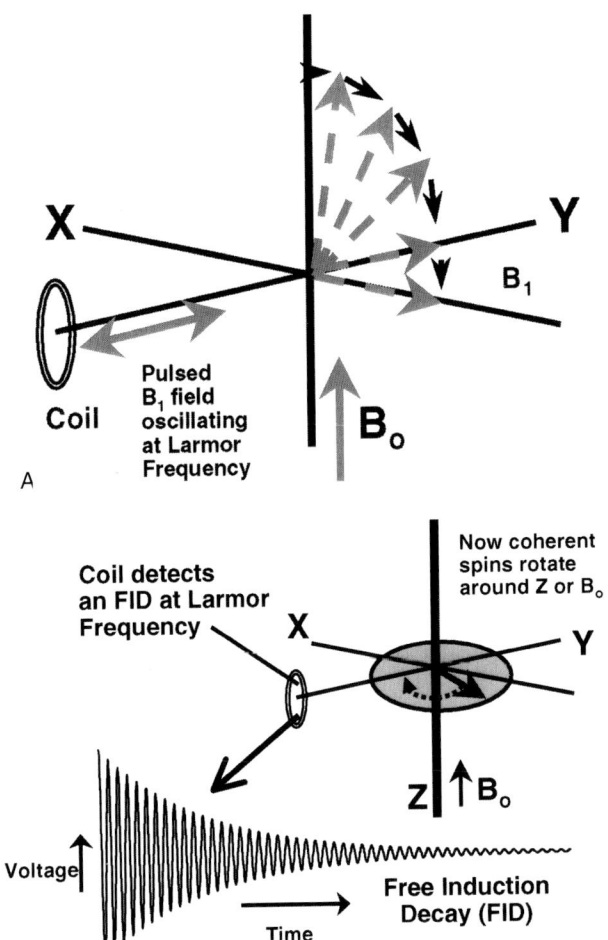

FIG. 3. Effects of a perpendicular B_1 magnetic field. **A:** The oscillating B_1 field at the Larmor frequency of the spins is absorbed by the spins and causes a rotation around the B_1 field axis (Y axis). **B:** Once the B_1 field is removed, the spins continue to rotate around the Z axis at the Larmor frequency. This results in a coherent oscillating magnetic field that is detected with the coil as the free induction decay (*FID*) illustrated. The FID is a decaying sinusoidal voltage signal with a frequency equal to the Larmor frequency of the spins.

An example of the signal detected with a coil after placing the spins in the transverse plane is also shown in Figure 3**B**. The frequency of this signal is usually determined using a Fourier transform (FT) that converts time oscillating data into its frequency components with only a few assumptions. The oscillating signal decays in amplitude with time and is called a free induction decay or FID. This decay in coherence and net magnitude in the transverse plan is what is known as magnetic relaxation. The decay must happen because the spins absorbed the energy from the B_1 field and, subsequently, must return to their original state in equilibrium with the B_o field, alone. That is, the system must revert to completely random spins aligned along the Z axis. This occurs via two processes, one is the release of the energy to the environment, or lattice, that results in the reestablishment of the magnetization along the Z axis. This is basically a

release of heat. This process is known as spin-lattice relaxation and is called T_1. The T_1 of the heart is on the order of 800 msec.

The second form of relaxation is that of the randomization of the phase of the spins. What is phase? This is reviewed in Figure 4**A** and **B**. The phase refers to the relative position, not the frequency, of the rotating net magnetic field vector of the spins in the transverse or X-Y plan. A phase diagram is used to follow the relative positions of the spin vectors. This type of phase diagram looks directly down on the X-Y plane shown in Figure 1, showing the net magnetization vector for each spin being examined (Fig. 4**A**). In Figure 4**B**, a phase diagram is used to show phase relationships for different spin vectors in different places in a sample that has different magnetic fields within it. The magnetic field

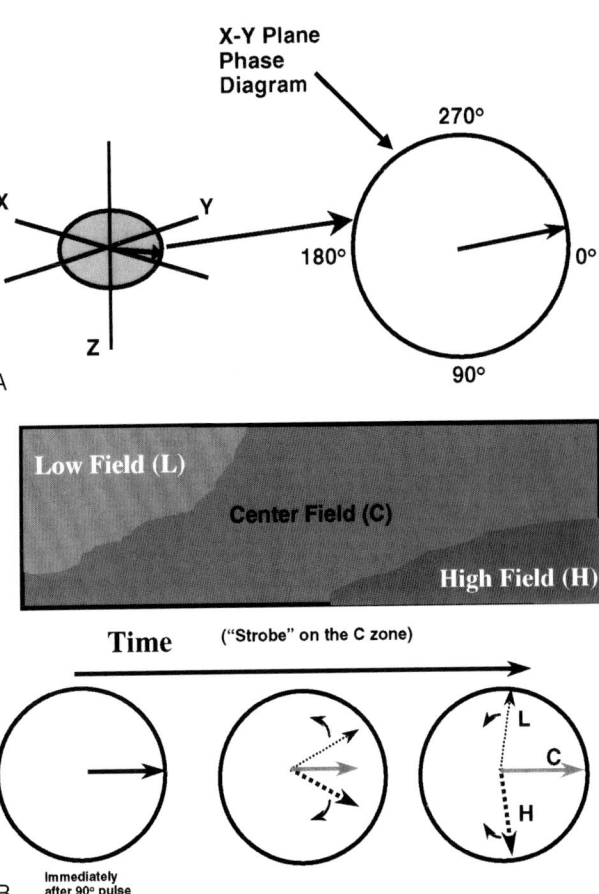

FIG. 4. The phase diagram. **A:** A phase diagram is a view of the magnetization vectors in the X-Y plane. **B:** The magnetic field is variable in the sample shown at the top. Sample spins from the low field (*L*), center field (*C*), and high field (*H*) region are followed as a function of time after a 90-degree pulse using the phase diagram. The phase diagram is set up to present the phases of the spins relative to *C*, which is always normalized to the 0-degree position. The phase diagrams at the **bottom** are presented as a function of time after the B_1 field pulse. Note that the *L* vector lags behind the *C* vector. While the *H* vector has a higher phase velocity than the other spins. This is due to the relative frequency of the spins caused by the differences in the magnetic field.

strength increases from L (low field) to C (center field) to H (high field). This is actually a common problem in MRI that will be discussed below. A phase diagram is a strobo-scopic image, since it is arbitrarily referenced to one nuclide magnetic vector, in this case, C for Figure 4**B**. This strobo-scopic effect is analogous to taking a flash picture every time the rotating C vector reaches the 0-degree position. Using this approach, the relative position of the spin vectors, or phase, of the different nuclides can be easily seen. Imme-diately after a 90-degree pulse, all of the spins have the same relative phase; however, as, with time, the different frequency of the spins causes their relative phase to change. The higher B_0 field spins, H, are advancing phase faster than C, while L, at low field, is lagging behind both. By watching the time development of this process, it is clear that phase and frequency are related. The rate of change in phase is the frequency of rotation in the X-Y plane. High frequency spins change phase rapidly, while slower frequency spins change phase more slowly. However, the initial starting points of each of these signals are independent of frequency. For ex-ample, after the 90-degree pulse, all of the spins have the same initial phase (i.e., L, C, and H all start with the same phase at 0 degrees). The initial phase can be dependent on prior conditions or on how the spin is placed in the transverse plane. Thus, despite the close relationship between phase and frequency, there is one point in the FID where the phase is independent of the frequency, namely, at the initiation point of the FID. This is information that is independent of the frequency of the spin; note that all the spins started at the same point in this example. We will find this property useful in forming a magnetic resonance image below.

Returning to relaxation, immediately after the 90-degree pulse, all of the spins have the same phase. Since nature abhors order, the randomization is necessary to minimize the energy in the system and return to equilibrium with main magnetic field, B_0. This randomization process is a spin-spin relaxation and is termed T_2. It is called spin-spin relaxa-tion since the mechanism of the relaxation process is through the interaction of spins in the sample with each other below or at the Larmor frequency, making this process dependent on the microscopic motions within the sample. In a phase diagram, this is reflected as a decrease in the magnetic vector amplitude.

We need to further develop T_2 to understand many of the problems in cardiac imaging. In general, three different processes can contribute to the dephasing of spins in the heart. The first mechanism is the true spin-spin interaction that is unavoidable and dependent on the molecular interac-tions within the tissue. This results in a decrease in the mag-nitude of the vector in the transverse plane. T_2 is on the order of 80 msec in the heart. The second process is related to the homogeneity of the main magnetic field. As illustrated in Figure 4**B**, if the B_0 field is not homogeneous through the sample, then the frequency of the spins in different re-gions will vary. In time, this results in a randomization of the spin phases as they rotate at different frequencies. This

randomization of phase also results in a decrease in the net transverse magnetization, like T_2; however, as will be dis-cussed below, this process can be reversed with B_1 field generated echo. T_2^* is an important process in the heart, since the B_0 homogeneity is very poor due to the lung cavity and deoxygenated blood in the right ventricle. Finally, the heart also moves through this inhomogeneity due to contrac-tion and respiratory motion. This also contributes to different frequencies of precession as a function of time, leading to a further dephasing of the heart water spins. All of the de-phasing processes in combination, including the molecular spin-spin interactions (T_2), are called T_2^*. The T_2^* is on the order of 30 msec at 1.5 Tesla in the human heart (5). Later in this chapter we will describe how to minimize or use these effects to make measurements in the intact heart.

In tissue, the T_2^* relaxation processes usually dominate magnetic relaxation. Thus, the decay rate of the FID is actu-ally a measure of the T_2^* in most biological tissues. Since T_2^* is a rapid process that results in a limited amount of time during which we can detect the NMR signal, there are many occasions when we would like to overcome this pro-cess. This can be accomplished using a B_1 field generated echo. This type of echo is outlined in Figure 5. Using the same convention for the behavior of the different spin fre-quencies after the 90 degree-pulse in Figure 4, we subse-quently apply another B_1 field that now rotates the magneti-zation 180 degrees around the X axis. The spins have now rotated into the opposite sector of the transverse plane. The 180-degree flip is achieved by applying the B_1 field for twice

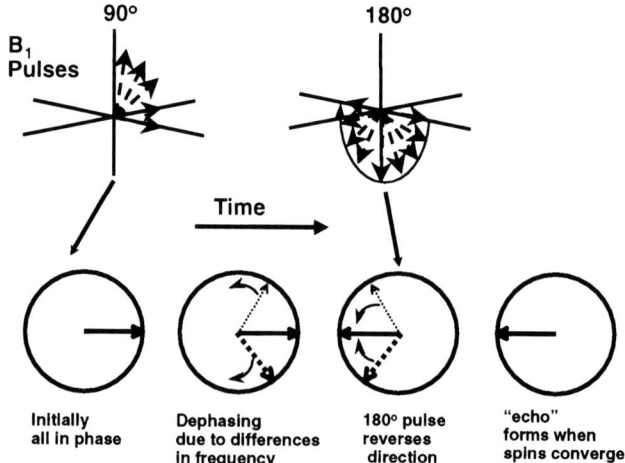

FIG. 5. Effects of a 180-degree B_1 field pulse following a 90-degree pulse. Time is running from right to left. The spins are the same populations as in Figure 4**B**. The spins are first excited by a 90-degree pulse as in Figure 3. After some time to permit dephasing due to differences in frequency as in Figure 4**B**, a 180-degree pulse is applied. The 180-degree pulse results in the spins moving toward each other due to the difference in frequency, rather than away, as was occurring before the 180-degree pulse. At a time equal to that required to dephase the spins, the spins refocus to form an echo of coherent magnetization.

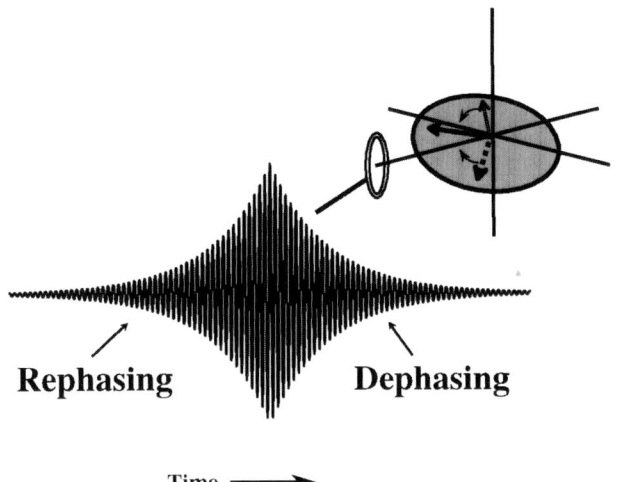

FIG. 6. The echo detected by the coil after a 90-degree to 180-degree sequence.

as long or with twice the power as the 90-degree pulse. On this side of the plane, the spins now drift together taking the same amount of time to rephase as they took to dephase. This is analogous to having two people back-to-back in a field and sending them walking apart at their own pace (i.e., the 90-degree pulse). At some time we instruct them to reverse their direction (i.e., the 180-degree pulse) and continue to walk, now toward each other, at the same pace. The time it takes them to reach each other will be precisely the same amount of time they walked apart. They will also be in the same place in the field. This is the nature of the echo that effectively recaptures all of the coherent transverse magnetization that had been destroyed by the field inhomogeneity in the sample. An example of an echo detected with a coil is shown in Figure 6. Note that the echo has known both a rephasing stage as well as a dephasing period. The spins continue to dephase after reaching the coherent echo due to the continuing field inhomogeneity; just as the people in the field will walk past each other and continue to ''dephase.'' A subsequent 180-degree B_1 pulse could be used to refocus these spins again and again. This latter method of continually refocusing the magnetization with 180-degree pulses is used in cardiac imaging as will be discussed below. However, using 180-degree pulses to refocus the spins is limited since it can not recover the spin-spin relaxation (T_2) processes occurring on the molecular level. Thus, the magnetization still dephases but at the much slower T_2 rate, when 180-degree pulses are used to refocus the magnetization.

These basic relaxation processes, T_1, T_2, and T_2^* are key in the generation of image contrast in MRI as well as guiding the optimal image sequence for gathering information on heart anatomy, function, and physiology using MRI. Heart tissue relaxation properties change with edema associated with different disease states (6). Generally, the T_1 and T_2 values increase with increasing water content. Remodeling of the myocardium or the replacement of myocytes with

connective tissue also changes the water relaxation properties, since the nature of the macromolecules in contact with water are critical for these relaxation processes. Finally, most exogenous MRI contrast agents work by enhancing either T_1 or T_2^* (7). By appropriately modifying the imaging sequences, these changes in relaxation properties due to pathology or exogenous contrast agents can be highlighted in the MRI image of the heart. How this is accomplished will be described below.

MAGNETIC RESONANCE IMAGING

Using these NMR signals, how do we create an image? Let's consider what information is needed for an image. First, information is needed on the spatial coordinates within the heart; X, Y, and Z. Next, the intensity of the NMR signal in these coordinates must be determined. Thus, for a single image, we need to collect information on X, Y, Z positions and on signal amplitude. Let's look at the echo in Figure 6, which is the fundamental signal in MRI. In this signal we can detect a frequency, amplitude, and phase that we can use to determine some spatial or amplitude information. But these are only three pieces of information and we need four. Clearly, enough information to create an image is not available in a single FID alone. As we will see, this is a major limitation of MRI, fundamentally slowing the data acquisition. This is even more of a problem with MRS, since we want to know the X,Y, and Z positions, the concentration and the frequency of the spins to identify the compound. Clearly, spatially resolved MRS will be even more difficult to collect.

The simplest imaging experiment can be divided into four stages as shown in Figure 7, which are the slice select, the phase encode, the refocusing echo, and the frequency encode/ read-out. Each of these stages will be discussed separately to describe how a simple image is created. In the slice select, one of the spatial coordinates is eliminated by only exciting magnetization in a selected slice of the sample. The slice selection process is illustrated in Figure 8. A magnetic field gradient is applied to the sample linearly along the direction in which a slice is going to be selected, the Z

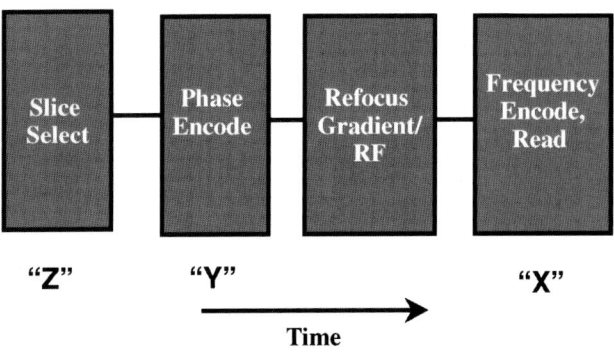

FIG. 7. General imaging scheme for collecting a simple magnetic resonance image.

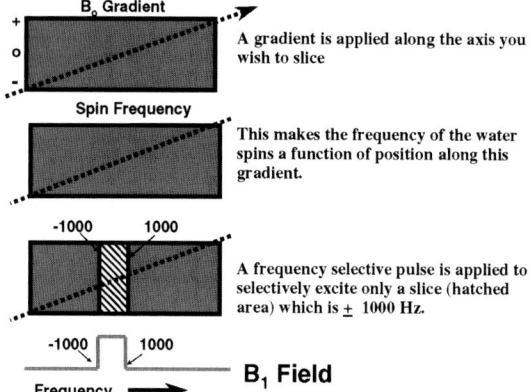

FIG. 8. Slice select. The B₀ gradient is applied from a negative to positive value with zero being near the middle of the magnet. This results in a linear distribution of frequencies as a function of position along the gradient. A frequency selective (+1000 Hz) B_1 field pulse is applied to excite those spins in that frequency bandwidth resulting in the selection of a slice to be placed in the transverse plane.

axis in this example. The magnetic field gradient causes the spins along this gradient to have different frequencies as described by Equation 1. Generally, these linear magnetic field gradients are applied plus or minus a given field strength with zero being in the center of the magnet. If only a selected band of frequencies are excited (for example −1000 to 1000 Hz), then a slice is put in the transverse plane, not affecting the rest of the sample. Thus, if a magnetic field is applied down a body from the head to the toe, the frequency of the water protons in the head will be much higher than the spins in the toe. By exciting a selected band of frequencies between the head and toe, a selective slice within the heart can be put into the transverse plan for detection.

To generate a controlled bandwidth for excitation, a sinx/x function is played out in time that results in a reasonably well-defined slice selection in frequency. This is shown in Figure 9. In summary, to selectively excite a slice, a linear magnetic field gradient is placed along the axis to be sliced; a sinx/x B_1 field pulse is then applied, and only the predefined slice within the sample will be placed in the transverse plane for further modification to create an image.

Since we have limited information in the FID, we will

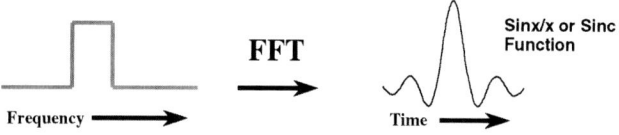

FIG. 9. The frequency selective B_1 pulse. The conversion from a frequency to a time domain is the fast Fourier transform (*FFT*). The FFT of a frequency square wave is approximated by a Sinxix function. The FFT has the desired frequency characteristics. This results in a time varying signal that has the appropriate frequency characteristics.

need to use the phase of the spins for more spatial information. Therefore, we must make sure that the slice selection process does not influence the phase of the spins. Frequency contamination is usually not a problem, since once the slice-select gradient is turned off, the frequency will almost immediately revert to the frequency driven by B₀. However, after the 90-degree pulse, the spins will dephase (depending on where they are in the slice), since a rather wide bandwidth of frequencies is excited (plus or minus 1000Hz). Thus, another magnetic field gradient of half the magnitude and of opposite direction of the slice-selection gradient must be applied to eliminate the phase introduced by the slice selection process. The amplitude is half since the spins were only in the transverse plane halfway through the slice gradient duration. By applying the gradient in the opposite direction, the spins are forced back to the same phase that they had before the slice-select gradient was applied.

Taking all of these factors together, an example of a slice selection process is presented in the imaging pulse sequence diagram shown in Figure 10. This diagram presents all of the gradients and B_1 field excitation and data collection on a time line. This permits the visual display of the sequence in a rather straightforward manner. As seen in this figure, only the slice-select portion of the sequence has been put in the diagram. The slice gradient is first brought up to a stable level by a ramp. The gradient is maintained, and the frequency selective B_1 field is applied. Subsequently, the slice gradient is ramped back down, and the dephasing gradient applied to remove the phase introduced by the slice-select gradient. The rest of the imaging sequence will be completed later. After performing the slice-select excitation, only a slice of the sample has been placed in the transverse plane with

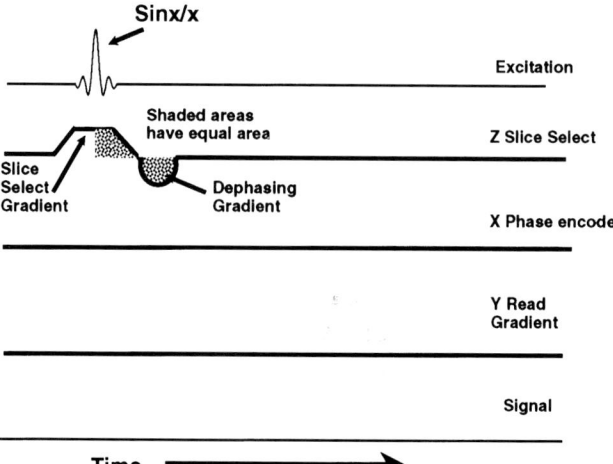

FIG. 10. Pulse sequence diagram. Each action is given a time line: the excitation, or B_1, field; the slice select; phase encode; and read-out gradient. At the bottom, the signal obtained by the coil is presented. This is the same convention used in all subsequent figures. Only the slice-select process is shown here, the other actions will be added in the later sections.

no effect on the phase or frequency of the transverse magnetization.

Now we are left with encoding spatial information in the FID for X and Y. We will skip the phase-encoding step at this point and move on to the refocusing and frequency encoding steps. We will return to the phase-encoding steps at the end of this discussion. To eliminate the effects of T_2^* on the signal, an echo is created by applying a 180-degree pulse with the excitation coil. This will result in an echo forming at a time equal to the time between the 90-degree slice select and 180-degree pulse. If a gradient is applied before the echo has formed in the direction we wish to frequency encode, X axis in this example, then the frequency of the spins will reflect the position of the spins in X. This is illustrated in Figure 11 for a simple sphere. The *arrows* from the sphere to the frequency axis indicate the frequency of these spins within the sphere. Clearly, the position of these spins along the X axis is easily detected by determining the frequency of the spins while a gradient is on along this axis. The gradient played out during this time is usually referred to as the read out gradient.

One concern we have again is the phase of the signal; since the read-out gradient is on during the acquisition of the echo, it will cause phase shifts in the data along the X axis much as the slice-select gradient could influence the phase in that stage of the acquisition. The solution is similar: an X gradient, which is half the read-out gradient and opposite in direction, is applied before the read-out gradient. This is called a dephasing gradient. The dephasing gradient causes the spins to dephase according to their position along the X axis. When the read-out gradient is applied to the spins, the frequency, relative to the X gradient, is reversed; the spins

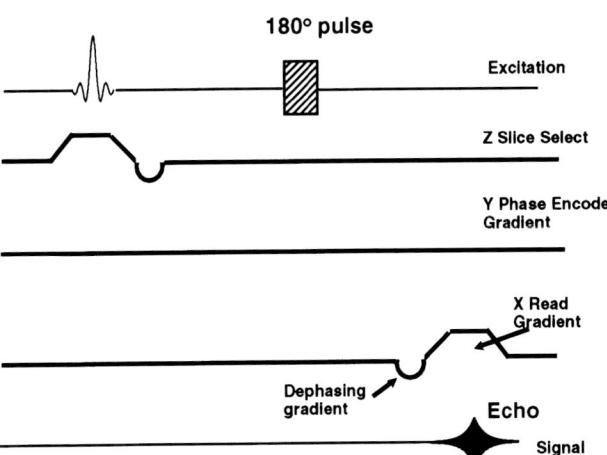

FIG. 12. Pulse sequence diagram. The read-out portion of the sequence has been added from Figure 10.

refocus to form an echo at the center of the read-out gradient at the peak of the 180-degree, pulse-generated echo. This is what is called a gradient-recalled echo since the read-out gradient is used to refocus the dephasing gradient applied before it. The gradient-recalled echo will be discussed below when we discuss fast-imaging methods. Thus, when the echo is collected, any initial phase information from the read-out gradient is removed by the gradient-recalled echo generated by the two gradients of opposing magnitude. The frequency encoding component is added to the pulse diagram in Figure 12.

We have been extremely careful to preserve the phase information for the determination of the Y spatial information. This is accomplished using a process called phase encoding. While the spins are still in the transverse plane after the slice selection process, the spins can be phase encoded by transiently applying a magnetic field gradient along the axis chosen for phase encoding, the Y axis in this case. To understand phase encoding, it is important to remember that to determine the position of a spin within the sample, a gradient is applied and the resulting frequency reports its position, and frequency is simply a measure of how fast the phase is changing in time. The complication with using a phase measurement to determine the frequency of a spin is that only one phase point, the initial point, is useful within each FID, or echo, as has been discussed above. Thus, to determine the frequency of the spin in the phase-encoding axis, a series of echos must be collected to determine how fast this initial phase of the spins is changing (i.e., frequency) with regard to the phase-encoding gradient applied. To describe phase encoding, it is best to consider three points in different Y positions in a sample through the phase-encoding process. This is illustrated in Figure 13 where three points are picked in the Y axes of our sphere. To phase encode the spins for position in the Y, a magnetic field gradient is transiently applied along the Y axis, in order to dephase the spins in proportion to their relative position in the Y axis. The spins at the center of the sphere or magnet, A, experi-

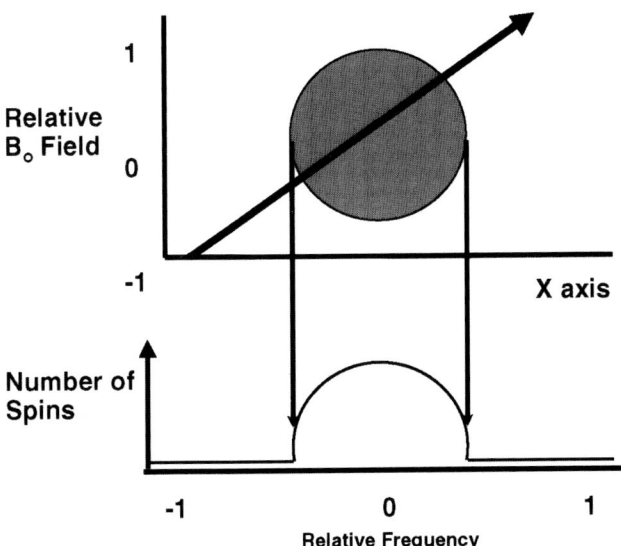

FIG. 11. Frequency encoding of position. Gradient is again applied from a negative to positive value across the sample, and the frequency of the spins is directly read out. The downward vertical *arrows* indicate the frequency of spins on either side of the sphere.

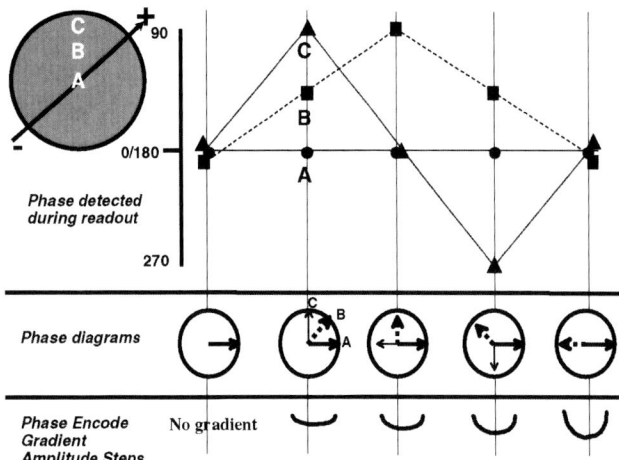

FIG. 13. Phase encoding. Across a sphere, a gradient is transiently applied as shown. The magnitude of the gradients in time are shown at the bottom of the figure. No gradient and four steps of gradient strength are being evaluated. The phase diagram showing where the spins end up after the gradient has been applied are shown directly above the gradient magnitudes. In the uppermost graph, the relative phase of the spins are plotted. *C* is shown by *triangles*; *B* is shown by *squares*, and *A* by *circles*. A is at the center of the magnet and sees no field changes. Thus, the phase of *A* is constant. *B* is further and further dephased relative to *A* by the ever increasing gradients. *C* sees the largest field difference and rapidly changes phase. The frequency of the spins is basically the rate at which the phase is changing relative to the gradient strength in this phase-encoding scheme. As seen at the **top** part of the figure, the rate of change in phase is highest for *C*, followed by *B,* and then by *A*, as they are located along the gradients direction.

ences no gradient field and, thus, continues to precess at the phase induced by the initial slice selection process. We will "strobe" our phase diagram on this position to examine what happens to the other positions along Y. The water spins in the higher field regions, *B* and *C*, have an accelerated rate of phase change due to the increase in frequency. The spins at *C* are experiencing twice the field as *B*, and, therefore, rotate twice as fast. When the gradient is turned off, the spins resume their precession rate relative to the B_o, but now they possess the "memory" of their Y position in their phase. When the echo is finally collected during the read portion of the experiment, each of the spins phase is influenced by its position in Y by the phase-encoding gradient applied. However, the frequency of the spins relative to the applied Y gradient, and, therefore, absolute position in Y, cannot be accurately determined from a single point since it is the rate of *change* in phase that determines the frequency. This relationship forces us to make repeated measurements to determine how fast the phase is changing in these different positions as a function of the Y gradient. The most obvious way of performing this task is to apply the Y gradient for different amounts of time and collect echos for each of these times. By plotting the initial phase of the spins as a function of the time the Y gradient is on, one could then determine the rate

of phase change, or frequency. Knowing the slope of the gradient, we can then determine position. Using the time the Y gradient is on is problematical, since it would require the spins to spend a great deal of time in the transverse plane, resulting in T_2 losses in signal and other complications. Thus, a more efficient system was devised in which, instead of varying time, the magnitude of the Y gradient is varied. This works, based on the simple principle that a gradient twice as strong will dephase the spins the same amount as leaving the gradient on for twice the amount of time. This results in a method of phase encoding in the Y dimension and keeping the amount of time in the transverse plane constant, but varying the magnitude of the phase encoding gradient. Five such measurements are shown in Figure 13, along with the phase diagrams and gradient transient that resulted in the phase displacement of the spins. By collecting a series of echos, all phase encoded with different gradient strengths in Y, the rate of phase change with gradient strength, or frequency, can be determined. This is shown on the top graph of Figure 13, where the phase detected in the echo is shown as a function of the gradient strength. As seen in this figure, *A* is unchanged since it always experiences no change in field at the center. The rate of change in phase of *C* is twice that of *B*, or the frequency of *C* is twice that of *B*, suggesting that *C* is further from the center position on the Y axis than *B*. The precise position of all of these spins in Y can be accurately determined if enough points are collected to accurately determine the frequency, and, as for all the encoding schemes, the precise magnitude of the gradient applied is known. This provides the last piece of information we need about the Y axis in order to create an image.

All of the steps are combined into a single acquisition scheme in Figure 14. A separate echo is collected for each phase-encode step. The precision of the determination of the phase-encode direction frequency and, therefore, position,

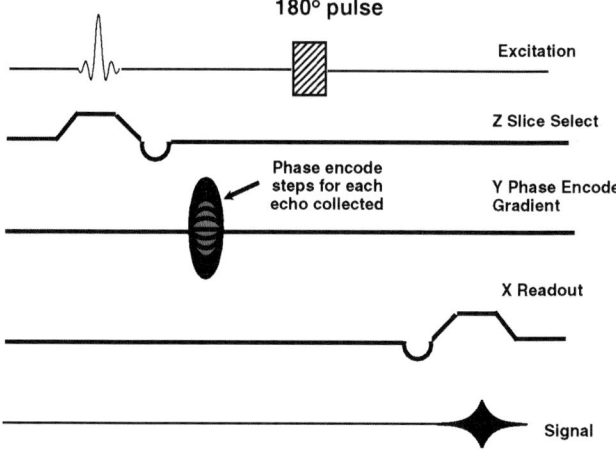

FIG. 14. Pulse sequence diagram. The phase-encoding steps are added immediately after the slice-selection process. Note that no corrections for phase are added here since this is the signal we want to persist to the read-out section.

Raw data collected in MRI:
k-space

Final image

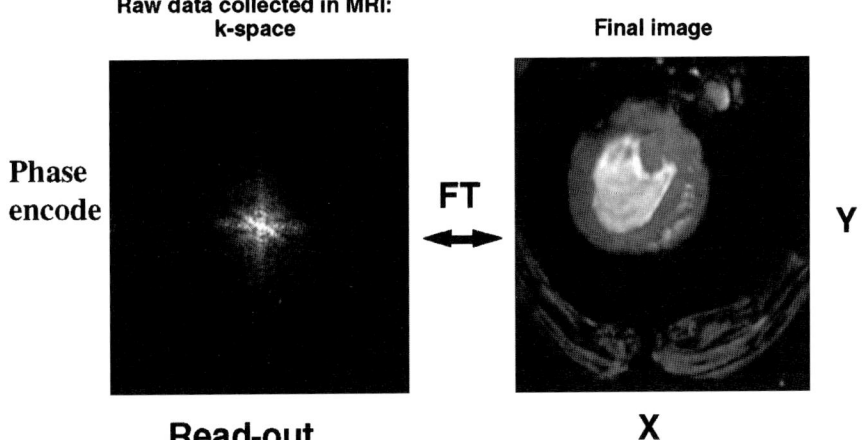

Phase
encode

FT

Y

Read-out

X

FIG. 15. Raw data, known as k-space. The image is a canine heart collected at 4T. The Fourier transform (*FT*) converts the magnetic resonance image (*MRI*) time domain data into spatial coordinates. The raw data is known as k-space and ideally represents all of the spatial spectral and intensity data in the image.

is directly proportional to the number of phase-encode steps collected. Usually this is on the order of 64 to 512 phase-encode steps.

To obtain the frequency in the read direction and phase direction, a two-dimensional Fourier transform (2-D FT) is performed on the data that extracts the frequency in both dimensions. The raw data collected in referred to as "k-space" and is shown in Figure 15. The ideal k-space model for any structure is to take an infinite resolution image and perform an FFT (fast Fourier transform) on it to generate the type of data collected in a MRI experiment. The resulting data can be viewed as the ideal k-space representation of the image that we try to attain with our pulse sequence to create the MR image. Naturally, there are limits on the amount of data that can be collected. The resolution of MRI k-space data, and the resulting image, is usually limited by the number of phase-encoded echoes that are collected, since this takes the most amount of time. As suggested earlier, in cardiac MRI, the number of phase encode steps varies from 64 to 512, depending on the speed that the data must be collected, the field of view that is being covered, and the resolution required to observe the structure of interest.

The sequence presented in Figure 14 is called a spin-echo sequence. There are several factors in this simple sequence that will change the contrast in the MRI image based on the previously described relaxation processes. Since a 180-degree refocusing pulse is used in this sequence, the total time the spins stay in the transverse plane determines the amount of T_2 relaxation that will occur. This time is called the TE and is measured from the center of the slice-select sinx/x pulse to the center of the refocused echo during the read-out or data acquisition (Fig. 16). Generally, the longer the TE, the more T_2 contrast is generated in the image. The effect of TE on normal regions (T_2 equals approximately 80

msec) and infarcted regions (T_2 equals approximately 100 msec) of the heart is shown in Figure 17A. Note that the signal in both regions decreases with TE, but the infarcted region relaxes more slowly. This results in a contrast, or difference in signal, between the normal and infarcted tissue as the TE is increased. By looking at the difference of the two tissue curves (*dotted line*), a TE of about 50 msec could be selected to optimize the contrast between these two tissue types. Thus, by simply adjusting the imaging parameters, fundamental information on the heart structure can be obtained.

Another timing parameter of the sequence has to do with T_1 relaxation. For a 90-degree excitation pulse usually used in spin echo imaging, one must wait about 5 times the T_1 value of the spin to permit it to completely relax back up the Z axis before applying another pulse to collect another phase-encode step. If adequate time for T_1 relaxation is not permitted, the spins will add up the energy applied by each excitation pulse, resulting in net saturation of the spins and a reduction in the NMR signal. The time between each slice-

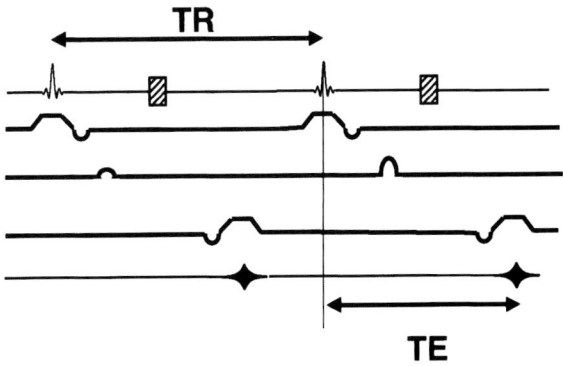

TR

TE

FIG. 16. Definitions of TR and TE in a spin-echo sequence.

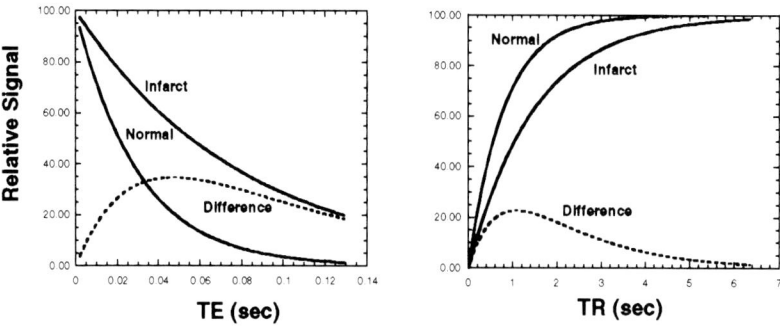

FIG. 17. Effect of time to echo (*TE*) (**A**) and time to repeat (*TR*) (**B**) on magnetic resonance image signal amplitude.

excitation pulse is the critical factor in this sequence; it is called the TR (Fig. 16). The effect of TR on signal amplitude is also shown in Figure 17**B** for a spin-echo sequence. The effect of TR is illustrated for normal myocardium with a T_1 of 0.8 sec and a severe infarct with a T_1 of 1.5 sec. Note that the shorter the T_1, the more rapidly the pulses can be applied and maintain the NMR signal. Also apparent in Figure 17**B** is that by varying the TR the contrast or difference between tissues can also be altered. Note that a TR of 1 second would be optimal in generating the largest difference (or contrast) between the normal and infarcted tissue. Thus, the TR can be used to vary the image contrast based on T_1.

The long time required for T_1 relaxation is the major reason that this approach is slow to collect an adequate number of phase-encoded data to create an image. One way around this problem is to use multiple 180-degree refocusing pulses and collect many echos per slice-selective excitation. This fast spin echo (FSE) approach is shown in Figure 18 and is an important technique in cardiac imaging (8). By applying a phase-encoding gradient between each 180-degree pulse, each echo is phase encoded with a different magnitude of gradient, providing the necessary phase data to create the image. In cardiac imaging, 16 to 64 echos can be collected per slice-selective pulse, reducing the time to collect a spin echo image by 16 to 64 times. The inherent high signal to noise of these FSE approaches provides very high resolution images of the myocardium.

To avoid the time associated with waiting for the spin relaxation from a 90-degree, slice-selective pulse, lower flip angles would be desirable. In addition, getting rid of the time required for, as well as the power deposition (to be discussed below) for, the 180-degree pulse and associated echo time might also be useful in trying to freeze the motion of the heart. Ernst showed that as the flip angle is reduced the TR can be shortened to provide the optimal signal to noise per unit time. This is because a dynamic equilibrium between the relaxation processes, T_1, and the excitation is set up to maintain a steady-state amount of magnetization to detect without saturation. This relationship is known as the Ernst angle:

$$\text{Flip angle} = \cos^{-1}(e^{-TR/T1})\,(2)$$

If you wish to collect 64 phase-encode lines to define k-space and you want to collect them in 100 msec to freeze diastolic motion of the heart, what angle should you use? The T1 of the heart is 0.8 sec, the TR is 0.1 sec/64, or appproximately 1.6 msec. Thus, the optimal angle is only about 11 degrees. Thus, data can be collected rather rapidly using a 11-degree pulse in the heart, rather than a 90-degree pulse that would require a TR of greater than 4 seconds according to Equation 2.

To use low flip angles and short TR values, the time associated with the 180-degree pulse must be removed. This is done by using the gradient-recalled echo alone to refocus

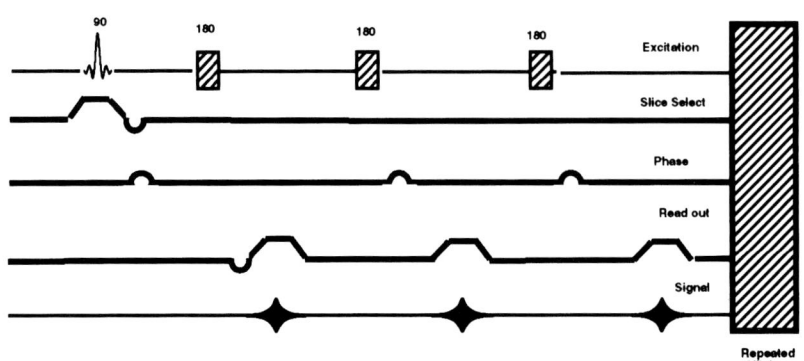

FIG. 18. Pulse sequence diagram of a fast spin echo image acquisition scheme.

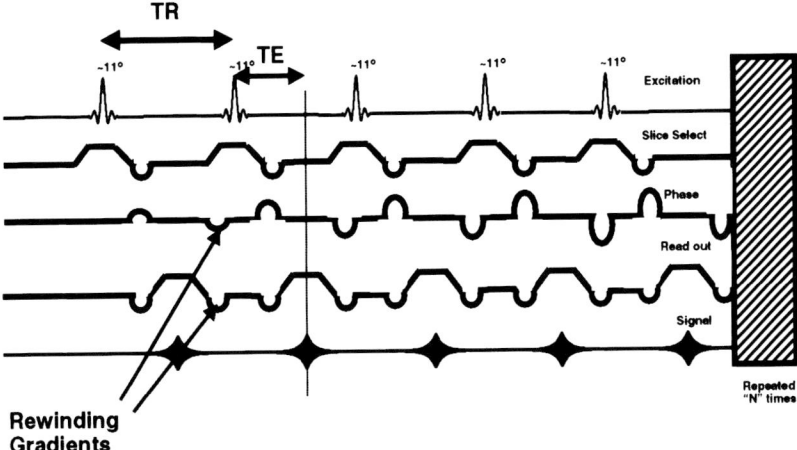

FIG. 19. Pulse sequence diagram of a gradient-recalled echo image acquisition scheme.

the magnetization at the right time for read-out. This is illustrated in Figure 19. Here the overall TR of the sequence is greatly shortened, permitting the rapid acquisition of data as long as the flip angle is appropriately adjusted. This type of data acquisition is known as a gradient-recalled echo (GRE) (9). Note that, to keep the phase information intact, the rewinding gradients are applied after each acquisition equal and opposite to the phase encoding gradient and the last half of the read-out gradient to prevent any phase information "bleeding" in to subsequent acquisitions. One of the major limitations of this approach is that the magnetization is dephasing according to T_2^* and not T_2 alone as in the spin echo approaches. This means that any field inhomogeniety within the chest could result in major decreases in signal amplitude before the echo is collected. Thus, minimizing the TE with good gradient performance is critical. The role of gradient performance will be discussed later.

The gradient-recalled echo could also be multiplied after the slice-select pulse as previously discussed for the FSE sequence. In this mode, a train of gradient-recalled echos can be collected after the slice-select pulse for as long as the T_2^* does not destroy all of the magnetization. This approach is called echo planar imaging (EPI) and was one of

the first MRI imaging methods described (2). This approach, in samples with long T_2^*, can result in a complete image collected with a single slice-select pulse and a train of gradient echos (Fig. 20). Note that, since all the data is collected in a single shot, that a 90-degree pulse is used, since T_1 is not an issue. In addition, the dephasing of the read gradient is done in a rapid ramp before the actual read gradient to minimize the time. In general, this approach is not very useful in the heart, since the T_2^* is so short at about 30 msec. This results in poor signal-to-noise and distortions of the image. However, this can be overcome by only collecting a few phase-encode steps per slice-select excitation and repeating this process at the same time in the cardiac cycle in subsequent heart beats until a complete image can be created. This is called a segmented k-space acquisition and can be expanded to cover the whole heart volume throughout the cardiac cycle. An example of a segmented EPI sequence used for imaging of the heart in shown in Figure 21. This permits a rapid acquisition of data with a minimal amount of time spent in the transverse plane. For example, eight echos can be collected per slice excitation with a TR on the order of 10 msec with modern gradient systems. Using this approach, imaging times on the order of 80 msec can be

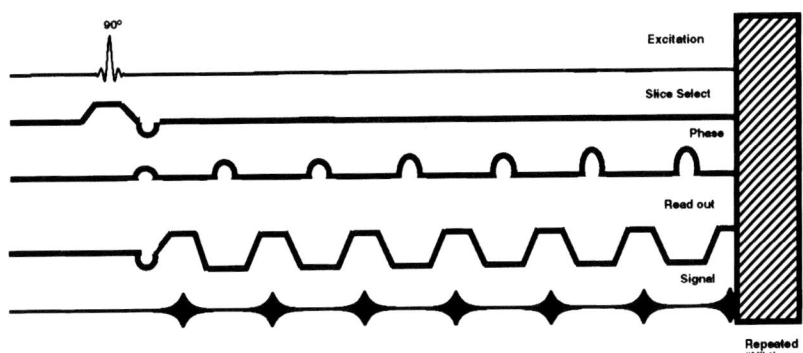

FIG. 20. Pulse sequence diagram of an echo planar image acquisition scheme.

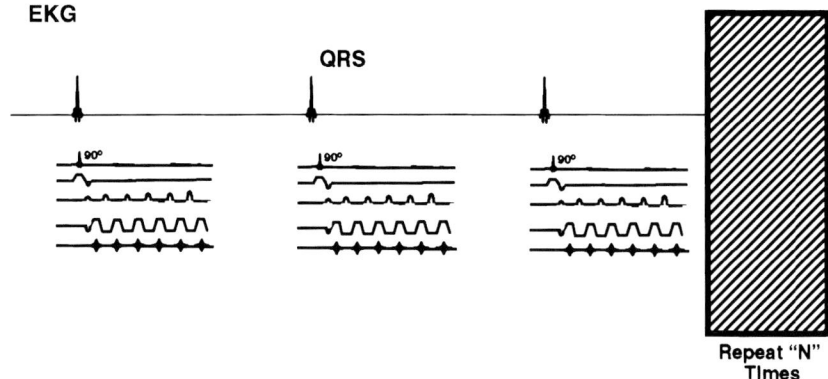

FIG. 21. Pulse sequence diagram of a segmented echo planar image acquisition scheme.

achieved in low resolution images (64 × 128 image resolution over a 15 × 32 cm field of view) without the magnetization ever spending more than 10 msec in the transverse plane. To overcome the constant motion of the heart due to respiration and contraction, but still obtain accurate high resolution images, some form of cardiac gating is required to fill in k-space over multiple heart beats, since enough data cannot be collected in a single heart beat. For most studies, a breath hold is used to eliminate the respiratory motion (10), and either prospective or retrospective gating is used to sort the data collected into the appropriate cardiac phases. Several phase-encode steps are collected per heart beat; thus, after several heart beats, enough data is collected to provide a high resolution three-dimensional image of the heart through the entire cycle (11). Naturally, this requirement results in the necessity of having good independent measures of the cardiac phase using electrocardiography (ECG). This is sometimes complicated by the interaction of moving tissue and blood in the magnetic field that will be discussed below. In addition, a steady heart rate is required that is sometimes difficult to achieve in many patients.

MAGNETIC RESONANCE SPECTROSCOPY

We have reviewed the simplest methods of collecting MRI images of water in the heart; now, what about MRS? The methods outlined above will basically not work for most MRS experiments, since the frequency information in the read-out cannot be used to determine one of the spatial coordinates. This information needs to be used to identify the chemical shift to determine the different metabolites present. For some nuclides, only one frequency is present. Thus, the straight imaging experiments will work for ^{23}Na, providing a sodium concentration image of the heart (12). However,

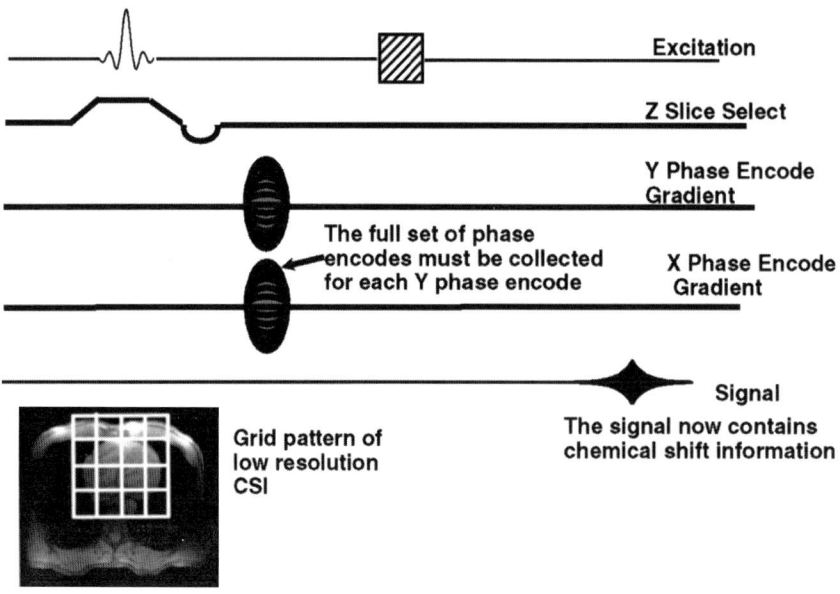

FIG. 22. Pulse sequence diagram of a chemical shift image (*CSI*) acquisition scheme. The inserted image provides a grid of the data collected. The grid is superimposed on a coronal slice of a human chest. Note that phase encoding has to occur on two planes, increasing the time of the acquisition.

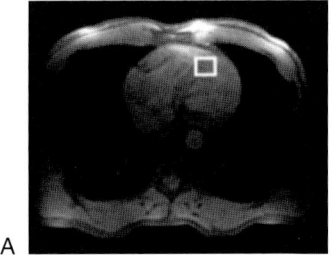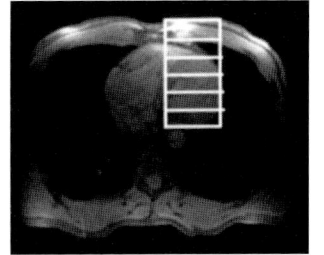

A   B

FIG. 23. Data acquisition grids for single voxel (ISIS) (**A**) and one-dimensional chemical shift image (1-D CSI) (**B**) methods. ISIS: Single voxel is selected using a series of slice selective IBO° excitation, no phase encoding. 1-D CSI: a column through the heart is selected and phase encoded along this single axis; one spatial axis is phase encoded.

in most cases we are interested in collecting ^{1}H, ^{31}P or ^{13}C spectra to identify different metabolites in the tissue (13). Since the read gradient cannot be used, it must be replaced by another phase encoding step. An example of a chemical shift image (14) is presented in Figure 22. This basically works by collecting a full series of phase encodes in X for every phase encode step in Y. This is a very inefficient process since collecting a $64 \times 64 \times 2k$ chemical shift image (CSI) requires 64×64 or 4,096 phase-encodes steps and echo acquisitions. This limitation usually results in MRS data being collected with much lower spatial resolution or using other approaches to limit the field of view. Several of these approaches are outlined in Figure 23. The first, a single voxel method or ISIS (image-selected, *in vivo* spectroscopy), where a single volume within the heart is put in the transverse plane by using the intersection of three 180-degree, slice-selective pulses (Fig. 23**A**) (15). This method is fast, but has very limited spatial coverage. The second method (Fig. 23**B**) is one-dimensional CSI, which selects or places a column of magnetization in the transverse plane and then phase encodes along the column, providing spectral information along it (16). This provides some spatial resolution without the excessive time required for two-dimensional CSI described in Figure 22.

In addition to the either limited spatial and temporal resolution of just collecting CSI data, nuclides other than ^{1}H are all weaker "magnets" with lower signal to noise/Mole of nuclide (Table 1) and the concentration of metabolites is on the order of 10^2 to 10^3 M in comparison to approximately 100 M water protons. Thus, under most circumstances, the CSI data acquisition has to be signal-averaged 8 to 64 times to get adequate signal-to-noise even in several cubic centimeter sample volumes. This signal-to-noise limitation is one reason the incorporation of MRS into clinical studies has been limited, despite the major contributions it has made to the basic understanding of cardiac metabolism and function (13).

SAFETY

In general, MRI is considered a safe and noninvasive procedure. Issues of safety can be divided into three general categories: the main magnetic field, the radiofrequency excitation for slice selection, and the gradient switching for imaging. There are several good monographs written on MRI that anyone interested in the field is encouraged to review (17). The present discussion should only be viewed as an introduction to this topic.

No clear demonstration of persistent biological effects have been documented with regard to the magnetic fields used in MRI (18). Numerous studies have demonstrated some transient effects on subjects, including vertigo, metallic taste, and magnetophosphenes, especially with movement in the field. However, all of these effects are apparently quite transient even at 4 Tesla, well below the more common clinical field of 1.5 Tesla (19). Instruments capable of studying humans at as high as 8 Tesla are now being tested at several sites around the world for bioeffects.

The major danger of the magnetic field is apparently not the effects of the field on the person, but on the objects the field might draw to, or into, the person. The literature and the folklore of NMR are full of examples of gas tanks, chairs, floor polishers, and other devices that have been attracted to and into superconducting magnets. Thus, it is critical to keep the room and the people entering the scan room free of magnetic material that could be attracted by the magnet, thus generating a possibly dangerous projectile. Several schemes, including magnetic detectors at the entry of the scan room and repeated educational programs, are used to keep inappropriate devices outside of the room.

The torque on implanted devices or embedded pieces of ferromagnetic material are also of some concern. Several lists of surgically implanted devices that are safe for MRI procedures are found in the literature (17), and anyone who is going to refer a patient or perform MRI examinations should be aware of this list. Of some concern to cardiologists are pacemakers, implanted defibrillators, or accessory pacing leads left in after surgery. In general, the cardiac pacemaker is considered to be a strict contraindication for MRI (20). The pacemakers are at risk for several reasons. The static magnetic field can alter the programming or move the whole device as well as elements within the device. The radio frequency (rf) excitation can interfere with the normal function of the device causing tachycardia. In addition, the leads can absorb large amounts of energy from the pulses that could result in burning the heart as well as the device. This latter event is a concern about any wire within the body—especially if it forms a loop that will be efficient in absorbing rf energy. There is a report of a Swan-Ganz thermodilution catheter melting in a patient, most likely due to this type of energy absorption by the wires (17). Thus, leftover wires from pacing in surgical procedures or the wires on implantable defibrillators are of concern. In addition, many defibrillators are controlled via magnetic field manipulations that clearly will be altered by the MRI magnet. In general, these magnetic field-controlled devices, such as pacemakers and defibrillators in patients should not even be close to an MR scanner's fringe field. The critical field seems to be somewhere between 5 and 15 G, which can be as much as 30 feet from an unshielded 1.5 T magnet (21,22).

It is not rare for a normal volunteer to be found with a metal shard from a lawnmower accident or BB gunfight in a leg or arm and unknown to them. In subjects who may work in a metal shop or may have been involved in a military action, an x-ray is often recommended before scanning to ensure that no metal is near a vessel or other vital area. Many times, a simple surgical procedure can remove these projectiles.

With regard to the body absorption of rf energy during the excitation of the water spins, most of the energy applied to generate the transverse magnetization in MRI is absorbed by the body and does not end up in the spins. Thus, the body absorbs energy during the pulses that causes heating. The Food and Drug Administration (FDA) has several guidelines for the limits of this heat deposition, the so-called specific absorption rate (SAR) (20,23,24), usually defined in Watts/kg. The simplest to understand is the guideline that suggests that the core temperature should not be raised more than 1 degree centigrade and localized heating should rise to no higher than 38 degrees centigrade in the head, 39 degrees centigrade in the trunk, and 40 degrees centigrade in the extremities. These guidelines only apply to subjects without compromised thermoregulatory systems (i.e., reduced cardiac output or inability to perspire). Based on the fact that many tissues can change temperature by 2 to 4 degrees centigrade with exercise or environmental extremes, this seems like a reasonable limitation. Most commercial instruments limit the power that can be delivered to a patient, depending on the weight of the individual. This is a reliable safeguard as long as customized sequences or excitation coils are being used that do not disable this safety feature. Sequences that rely on a high density of high power radiofrequency pulses, such as the train of 180-degree pulses in fast spin echo, are sometimes limited by the SAR they generate.

Finally, to create the images, gradients have to be applied across the body to encode the frequency as a function of position. To do this as fast as possible in order to freeze cardiac motion, minimize T_2^* effects, or to get the patient out of the magnet quickly, we want to be able to switch these gradients at a very high rate. However, as a time varying magnetic field is applied across a conductor, an induced voltage or electric field is generated perpendicular to the magnetic field. Since most of the tissues of the body are conductive, the rapidly switched magnetic fields result in electrical currents within the tissue. The magnitude of these currents is proportional to the rate of change in the magnetic fields as well as the magnitude and cross-sectional area through the body. These currents, if they reach an adequate magnitude and geometry, can cause nerve depolarization (25). Since the skeletal muscle motor fibers are some of the largest in the body, these fibers are the most sensitive, and, when depolarized by the field gradient switching, may result in a muscle twitch. In cardiac scans, this usually is detected in the buttocks or along the side of the torso as a mild twitching sensation. At high stimulation thresholds, smaller nerve fibers including pain receptors can be activated. All of the manufacturers have limited their instruments to avoid even the twitch threshold, as suggested by the FDA; however, some hypersensitive subjects with unfortunate geometry may still experience some sensation. Calculations have suggested that the threshold for interferring with cardiac depolarization processes are manyfold over these peripheral nerve stimulations (26).

The peripheral nerve stimulation is one of the current fundamental limitations of MRI for cardiac studies, since it limits the speed at which the gradients can be operated. In general this limitation is on the order of 20 Tesla/sec over 120 μsec (24). Currently, most manufacturers have gradient systems that can reach the peripheral stimulation threshold; further pushing of the envelope may not be worthwhile until this issue is overcome.

In addition to the inherent safety issues associated with MRI, the cardiac patient has other special concerns. Generally, the patient is monitored visually by eye or through a camera, the respiratory rate is monitored with a bellows, oxygenation with pulse oxymetry, and heart rate with ECG. Classically, the ECG is used to monitor rhythm and provide some information on acute ischemic events. However, in the magnet, the ECG is perturbed by the flowing blood and movement of the heart (27). The movement of the conductive material in a magnetic field sets up a Lorenz force that results in a voltage that is picked up in the ECG leads. Careful placement of the ECG leads on the chest in a much closer cluster than ordinarily used can reduce some of these effects (28). In general, this effect is not significant in determining the QRS complex for monitoring rate or arrythmias, but it does interfere with the weaker T wave. This makes the evaluation of S-T segments for ischemia difficult. To overcome this limitation, it is generally advised for stress test studies or for unstable patients, that the near real-time functional imaging of the heart be used to monitor the condition of the myocardium, much like what is used in cardiac ultrasound. Most state-of-the-art systems today have this type of monitoring available either as a product or in testing.

REFERENCES

1. Lauterbur P. Image formation by reduced local interactions: examples employing nuclear magnetic resonance. *Nature* 1973;242:190–195.
2. Mansfield P, Pykett IL. Biological and medical imaging by NMR. *J Magn Res* 1978;29:355–373.
3. Moon RB, Richard JH. Determination of intracellular pH by 31P magnetic resonance. *J Biol Chem* 1973;248:7276–7278.
4. Williams GD, Mosher TJ, Smith MB. Simultaneous determination of intracellular magnesium and pH from the three 31P NMR chemical shifts of ATP. *Anal Biochem* 1993;214:458–467.
5. Reeder SB, Faranesh AZ, Boxerman JL, et al. *In vivo* measurement of T2* and field inhomogeneity maps in the human heart at 1.5 T. *Magn Res Med* 1998;39:988–998.
6. Scholz TD, Martins JB, Skorton DJ. NMR relaxation times in acute myocardial infarction: relative influence of changes in tissue water and fat content. *Magn Reson Med* 1992;23:89–95.
7. Mathur-De VR, Lemort M. Invited review: biophysical properties and clinical applications of magnetic resonance imaging contrast agents. *Br J Radiol* 1995;68:225–247.
8. Hennig J, Nauerth A, Friedburg H. RARE imaging: a fast imaging method for clinical MR. *Magn Res Med* 1986;3:823–833.
9. Haase A, Frahm J, Matthaei D, et al. FLASH imaging: rapid NMR imaging using low flip-angle pulses. *Magn Reson Med* 1986;67:258–266.
10. Edelman RR, Manning WJ, Burstein D, et al. Coronary arteries: breath-hold MR angiography [comments]. *Radiology* 1991;181:641–643.
11. Feinstein JA, Epstein FH, Arai AE, et al. Using cardiac phase to order reconstruction (CAPTOR): a method to improve diastolic images. *J Magn Reson Imaging* 1997;7:794–798.
12. Kim RJ, Lima JA, Chen EL, et al. Fast 23Na magnetic resonance imaging of acute reperfused myocardial infarction. Potential to assess myocardial viability. *Circulation* 1997;95:1877–1885.
13. Schaefer S, Balaban RS. *Cardiovascular magnetic resonance spectroscopy.* Norwell: Kluwer Academic Publishers, 1993.
14. Brown TR, Kincaid BM, Ugurbil K. NMR chemical shift imaging in three dimensions. *Proc Natl Acad Sci* 1982;79:3523–3526.
15. Ordidge RJ, Connelly A, Lohman JAB. Image-selected *in vivo* spectroscopy (ISIS). A new technique for spatially selective NMR spectroscopy. *J Magn Res* 1986;66:283–294.
16. Bottomley PA. Spatial localization in NMR spectroscopy, *in vivo. Ann NY Acad Sci* 1987;508:333–348.
17. Shellock FG, Kanal E. *Magnetic resonance. Bioeffects, safety and patient management.* New York: Raven Press, 1994.
18. Budinger T. Nuclear magnetic resonance (NMR) *in vivo* studies: known thresholds for health effects. *J Comput Assist Tomogr* 1981;5:800–811.
19. Schenck J. Health and physiological effects of human exposure to whole body 4 teskal magnetic fields during MRI. In: Magin R, Liburdy R, Persson B, eds. *Biological effects and safety aspects of nuclear magnetic resonance imaging and spectroscopy.* New York: New York Academy of Sciences, 1991:285–301.
20. Food and Drug Administration. Magnetic resonance diagionstic device: panel recommendations and report on petitions for MR reclassification. *Federal Register* 1988;53:7575–7579.
21. Pavlicek W, Geisinger M, Castle L, et al. The effects of nuclear magnetic resonance on patients with cardiac pacemakers. *Radiology* 1983;147:149–153.
22. Persson BRR, Stahlberg F. *Health and safety of clinical NMR examinations.* Boca Raton, FL: CRC Press, 1989.
23. Bottomley PA, Edelstein W. Power deposition in whole body NMR imaging. *Med Phys* 1981;8:510–512.
24. Food and Drug Administration. Guidance for the submission of premarket notifications for magnetic resonance diagnostic devices. Washington, DC: FDA, 1998.
25. Reily J. *Electrical stimulation and electropathology.* Cambridge: Cambridge University Press, 1992.
26. Budinger T. Thresholds for physiological effects due to RF and magnetic fields used in NMR imaging. *IEEE Trans Nucl Sci* 1979;26:2821–2825.
27. Keltner J, Roos M, Brakeman P, et al. Magnetohydrodynamics of blood flow. *Magn Res Med* 1990;16:139–149.
28. Dimick RN, Hedlund L, Herfkens RJ, et al. Optimizing electrocardiograph electrode placement for cardiac-gated magnetic resonance imaging. *Invest Radiol* 1987;22:17–22.

CHAPTER 29

Magnetic Resonance Imaging of Cardiac Structure

Jens Bremerich, Gautham P. Reddy, and
Charles B. Higgins

The unique capability of magnetic resonance imaging (MRI) to provide images with high soft tissue contrast and spatial resolution in any plane makes it an excellent modality to define cardiac structure. The major clinical use of MRI for cardiac diagnosis during the first 15 years of its existence has been the depiction of pathoanatomy. Important indications for MRI for the demonstration of structural abnormalities have been in congenital heart disease, pericardial disease, cardiac and paracardiac masses, and some cardiomyopathies, especially arrhythmogenic right ventricular dysplasia and complications of myocardial infarction. This chapter describes current MRI techniques and applications for imaging of abnormalities of structure in specific cardiac diseases.

TECHNIQUE

MRI of the heart frequently requires ECG gating, because cardiac and blood motion during image acquisition degrade quality. In prospective gating, image acquisition is synchronized to the cardiac cycle, and the pulse sequence is initiated by the gating signal. Retrospective gating refers to image acquisition that is not synchronized to the cardiac cycle. The ECG signal is recorded simultaneously with MR image data and images are reconstructed later by assignment of the acquired data to various phases of the cardiac cycle as indicated by the recorded ECG signal.

J. Bremerich: Department of Radiology, University of Basel, CH-4031 Basel, Switzerland.

G. P. Reddy: Department of Radiology, University of California–San Francisco, San Francisco, California 94143.

C. B. Higgins: Department of Radiology, University of California–San Francisco Medical School, San Francisco, California 94143.

ECG-gated spin-echo MR images acquired in the coronal or sagittal plane give an overview of the thoracic anatomy. A TR of one cardiac cycle or approximately 0.7 to 1.0 s and TE of approximately 14 ms provide predominantly T1 weighting. Slice thicknesses of 3 to 5 mm in infants and children and 5 to 10 mm in adults are typically used. Additional images in the transverse plane or in oblique planes allow precise depiction of cardiac structure.

In traditional spin-echo MRI, acquisition of an image with a matrix of 256 × 256 requires 256 phase encoding steps over a period of 256 cardiac cycles. Because acquisition of a phase encoding step takes only a fraction of the cardiac cycle, imaging data is usually acquired from multiple slices at progressively greater delays after the ECG gating signal. Although this technique, known as multislice acquisition, is time efficient, one has to be aware that the images in different slice locations are acquired at different phases of the cardiac cycle. Multislice imaging can be extended to a multislice multiphase acquisition by repeating the sequence several times, each time cycling the order of acquisition at each anatomic level.

Respiratory motion artifacts can be reduced by acquiring an entire image during a single breath hold. The very short TR typically used in cine MRI permits regrouping of the data into segments each comprised of several phase encoding steps. This is known as segmented k-space, turbo, or breath hold cine imaging. For example, the 128 phase-encoding steps that are required for an image with a matrix of 128 × 128 could be acquired in 16 segments, each comprised of a segment of 8 phase-encoding steps. Thus, the acquisition can be completed within a breath-hold period of 16 cardiac cycles. In a different cine MRI-based approach, the acquisition time can be shortened substantially by using a coarse matrix and very short TR and TE. This approach produces images with low spatial resolution in approximately 600 to 2,000 ms. These images can be weighted to T1 or T2 contrast by applying preparatory pulses such as inversion recovery pulses. This technique has been used to monitor the passage of a bolus of paramagnetic contrast medium such as Gd-DTPA through the heart to detect hypoperfused myocardium (1,2). Another approach to shorten the image acquisition time is to produce multiple echoes with different phase encoding values after each excitation.

It is possible to acquire an entire image after a single excitation. This strategy is referred to as echo-planar imaging (EPI). Tomographic images can be acquired within 40 to 100 ms.

QUANTIFICATION OF VENTRICULAR VOLUME AND MASS

Ejection fraction and mass are important parameters in assessment of cardiovascular disease and in monitoring the effect of therapy. LV volume and mass can be estimated by echocardiography, gated or first-pass radionuclide imaging, and x-ray cineangiocardiography, but these methods rely on sampling of cardiac dimensions and calculations based on geometric assumptions. In contrast, cine MRI can provide three-dimensional data containing the entire heart, with sequential images throughout the cardiac cycle, which can be viewed as cine loops. Typical parameter settings for cine MRI are TR of 20 to 35 ms, TE of 4 to 20 ms, and flip angle of 35° to 60° to acquire 16 phases evenly spaced through the cardiac cycle (3). Cine MRI generates a blood pool signal that is white and produces high contrast between the blood pool and the myocardium (Fig. 1). Direct measurements of cardiac volumes and mass from contiguous cine MR images (Table 1) are accurate and reproducible and thus can be used for serial measurements and to monitor the effect of therapy (4). Because of the use of a 3D data set, MRI should be

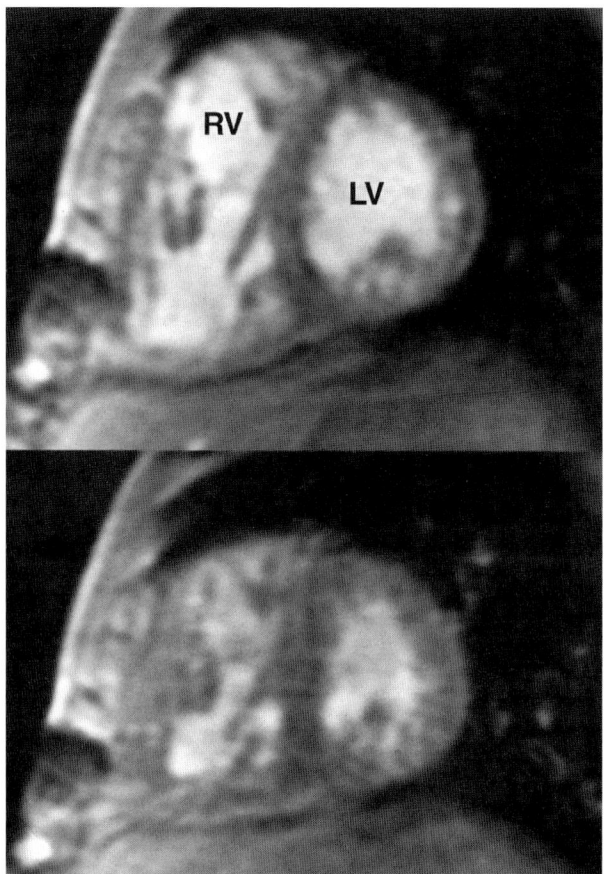

FIG. 1. Left and right ventricular mass can be measured from a stack of cine MR images acquired in the short axis. Images at the same location in end-diastole (**upper panel**) and end-systole (**lower panel**) are shown. Note that blood in the left (*LV*) and right (*RV*) ventricles has a bright appearance on cine MRI providing good distinction of myocardium and blood. End-diastolic volume can be calculated by adding the areas within the ventricle from each end-diastolic image from apex to base, and multiplying by slice thickness. Volume at end-systole can be computed in a similar fashion.

considered as the "gold standard" for the evaluation of left ventricular mass and volumes (4,5).

CONGENITAL HEART DISEASE

The major requirement for evaluation of congenital heart disease is the precise depiction of cardiovascular anatomy. ECG-gated MRI can be utilized with high diagnostic accuracy for assessment of morphologic features in simple and complex congenital heart disease (6).

MRI can demonstrate vascular anomalies such as coarctation of the aorta (Fig. 2) and abnormalities of the aortic arch such as double aortic arch, right aortic arch with retroesophageal left subclavian artery, and left aortic arch with aberrant right subclavian artery (7). Arch anomalies are best demonstrated on transverse images with 3-mm thickness. Coarctation is best visualized and measured on 3-mm thick oblique

TABLE 1. *Left ventricular dimensions, mass, and volumes on short axis images*

	Men	Women
End-diastolic wall thickness (cm)	0.95 ± 0.11*	
End-systolic wall thickness (cm)	1.64 ± 0.16*	
Wall thickening (%)	73.0 ± 18.1*	
LV mass (g)	158.3 ± 17.8	123.4 ± 8.3
LV end-diastolic volume (ml)	116.1 ± 15.9	108.4 ± 10.9
LV end-systolic volume (ml)	39.6 ± 7.9*	

* Includes both men and women.
LV, left ventricle.
(Adapted from ref. 66, with permission.)

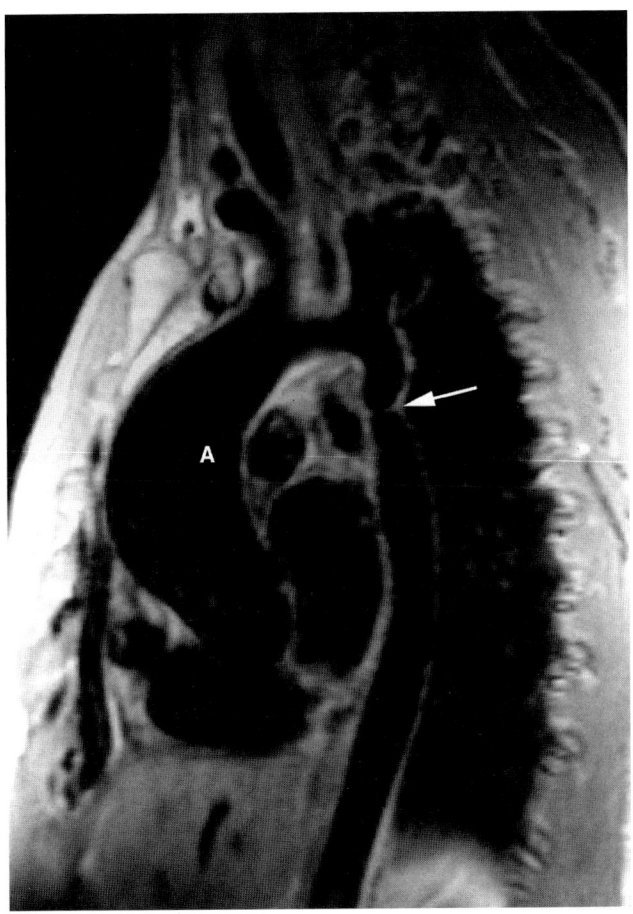

FIG. 2. Coarctation of the aorta. Oblique sagittal T1-weighted spin-echo (*SE*) image in the plane of the aortic arch. The juxtaductal coarctation is readily depicted (*arrow*). Note that blood appears black on T1-weighted SE images. *A,* ascending aorta.

artery. On transverse images the aorta can be identified by following the arch, and the pulmonary artery by its extension to the pulmonary arterial bifurcation. The origins of the aorta and pulmonary artery are revealed on sagittal or coronal images. In complete transposition, transverse images demonstrate the origin of the right-sided aorta from the normally positioned right ventricle and of the pulmonary artery from the left ventricle. In corrected transposition the aorta is on the left, arising from the abnormally positioned morphologic right ventricle, which is on the left of the anatomic left ventricle. The morphologic right ventricle can be identified by the following features: the right ventricular outflow tract separates the tricuspid from the pulmonary valve, and a muscular ring can be seen below the pulmonary valve on transverse MR images. The left ventricle is characterized by a lack of a complete muscular infundibulum. Other distinguishing features are a more ventrally positioned atrioventricular valve (tricuspid valve), a moderator band, and irregular apical ventricular septal surface for the right ventricle.

Congenital heart disease associated with right-sided outflow obstruction, such as tetralogy of Fallot, pulmonary atresia, and pulmonary artery stenosis, is assessed on consecutive transverse tomograms through the entire heart and pulmonary hila. These images demonstrate characteristic features of tetralogy of Fallot, such as narrowing of the right ventricular infundibulum, an enlarged anteriorly displaced overriding, a membranous ventricular septal defect (VSD), and hypertrophy of the right ventricle. The VSD can be readily detected on transverse MR images. The infundibulum and the pulmonary annulus are best depicted on sagittal to-

sagittal slices in the plane of the aortic arch. Velocity-encoded cine (VENC) MRI can be used to estimate the pressure gradient across the coarctation (8), as well as to quantify collateral flow (9). MRI can also be used for follow-up after surgical repair of coarctation.

Transverse or short axis MR images display the sinus venosum, secundum, and primum portions of the atrial septum (10). MRI has been found to be 90% sensitive and 90% specific for identifying defects at any level of the atrial septum (10). A potential pitfall is difficulty imaging the thin septum at the fossa ovalis that may produce little signal; thus, secundum atrial septal defects should be diagnosed with caution. Cine MRI can be helpful when atrial septal defects are suspected because small defects can be detected as a signal void at the site of the shunt.

The effectiveness of MRI for defining the pathoanatomy of abnormal ventriculoarterial connections such as transposition (Fig. 3), double outlet left ventricle, double outlet right ventricle (Fig. 4), and truncus arteriosus has been demonstrated (11). Transverse images at the base of the heart demonstrate the position of the aorta relative to the pulmonary

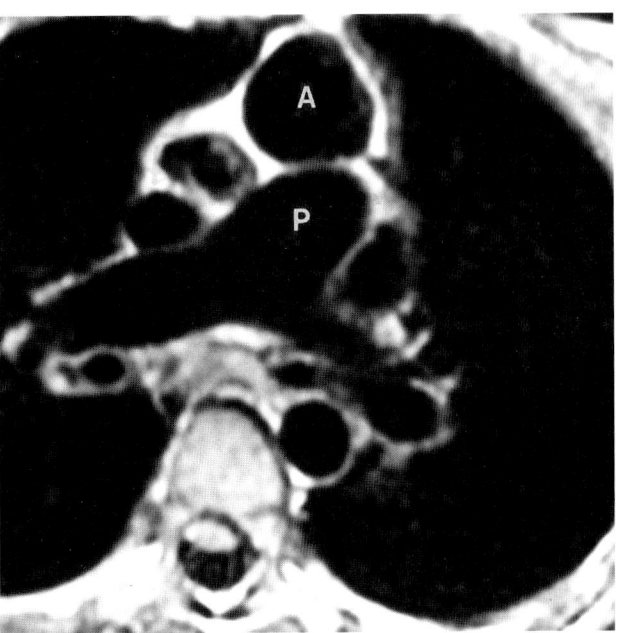

FIG. 3. Transposition of the great arteries. Axial T1-weighted SE MR image demonstrates the aorta (*A*) anterior to and to the left of the main pulmonary artery (*P*). (From ref. 11, with permission.)

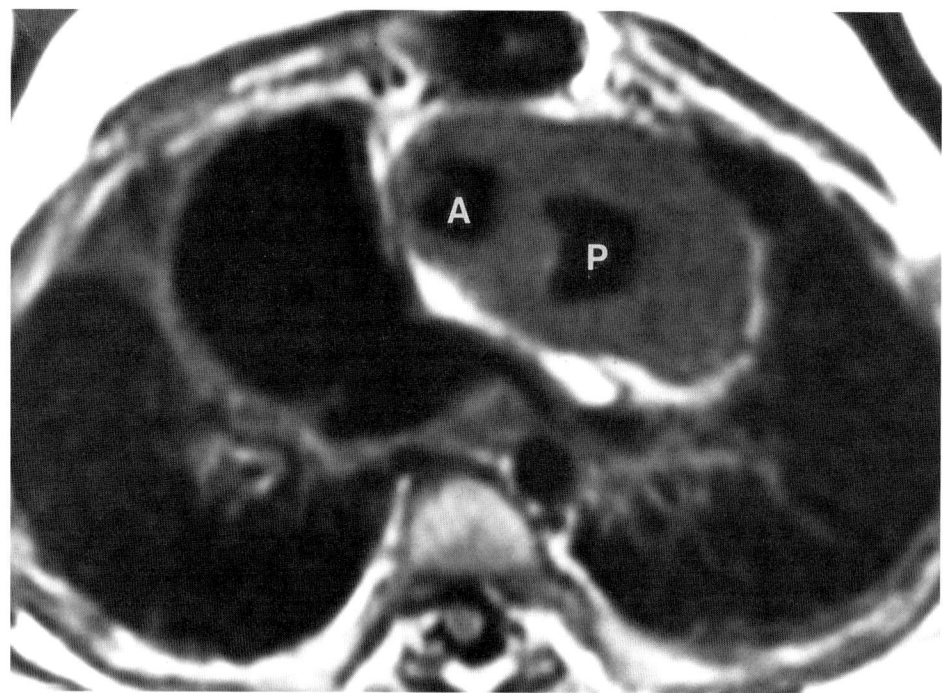

FIG. 4. Axial T1-weighted spin-echo MR image of a patient with double-outlet right ventricle. The image at the level just below the semilunar valves, demonstrates that both the aortic (*A*) and pulmonary (*P*) outflow tracts have a muscular wall, which is characteristic for the infundibulum of the right ventricle. (From ref. 67, with permission.)

mograms. Stenoses of the central pulmonary arteries are frequent in tetralogy of Fallot and can remain after surgical repair. These stenoses are best depicted on thin tomograms of 3-mm thickness acquired in the transverse plane for the main pulmonary artery or in oblique planes for left and right pulmonary arteries, such that the vessel of interest courses in the plane of imaging. The hemodynamic significance of pulmonary artery stenosis can be estimated by flow measurements with VENC-MRI in the main, right, and left pulmonary arteries (12). This method can be used to determine the blood flow to each lung. Because tetralogy of Fallot with severe pulmonary insufficiency after surgery can be associated with right ventricular failure, monitoring of right ventricular mass and function is important. Cine MRI is an excellent modality to monitor these parameters noninvasively and with high reproducibility (4), as discussed previously.

In complex ventricular anomalies such as single ventricle, transverse 5-mm thick slices are most useful to provide an overview of the complex ventricular anatomy and to define the atrioventricular and ventriculoarterial connections (13). MRI is used to identify a chamber as left or right ventricle, as discussed previously. A primitive type of single ventricle has morphologic features characteristic of neither a right nor a left ventricle.

In partial anomalous pulmonary venous return, transverse SE-MR imaging can clearly demonstrate abnormal connections to the superior vena cava, right atrium, or coronary sinus (14). A dilated coronary sinus may be a sign of anoma-

lous connection to this structure. MR images in transverse, sagittal, and coronal planes can demonstrate the anomalous pulmonary venous connection to the inferior vena cava in patients with the scimitar syndrome. Total anomalous pulmonary venous connection should be suspected, when no vessel can be identified entering the left atrium.

MRI has also been useful to depict anomalies of the systemic venous system such as a persistent left superior vena cava, atretic right superior vena cava with persistent left superior vena cava draining through an enlarged coronary sinus, or interruption of the inferior vena cava with azygos continuation.

The noninvasive nature, absence of ionizing radiation, and good reproducibility makes MRI an excellent method for monitoring cardiac morphology and ventricular volumes and mass after surgical correction of congenital heart disease. For example, MRI has demonstrated stenosis of pulmonary arteries after Jatene or arterial switch procedure employed for correction of transposition of the great arteries and for demonstrating stenoses of the right and left pulmonary arteries (Fig. 5) (15). Compared to echocardiography, MRI has the advantage of superior demonstration of conduits and anastomosis at the level of the great arteries (16,17). In the assessment of stenoses of conduits, anastomoses and baffles MRI provides information regarding (i) anatomic narrowing on SE-MRI, (ii) flow disturbances producing signal voids on cine MRI, and (iii) increased peak flow on VENC-MRI. MRI has been shown to be effective in demonstrating com-

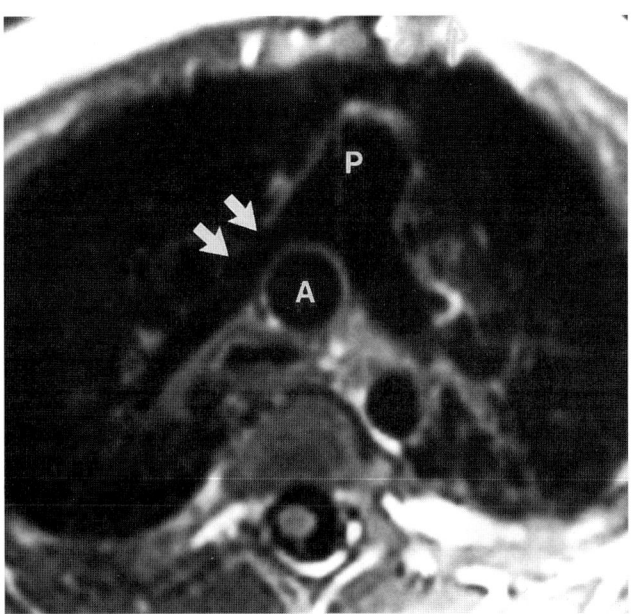

FIG. 5. Transposition of the great arteries after arterial switch (Jatene) procedure. The axial T1-weighted spin-echo MR image shows the main pulmonary artery (*P*) anterior to the ascending aorta (*A*). Note narrowing of the right pulmonary artery (*arrows*), which is a complication of this procedure. (From ref. 67, with permission.)

plications after surgical repair of Tetralogy of Fallot such as aneurysmal dilatation of the RV outflow and the consequences of pulmonary regurgitation on RV volumes, mass, and diastolic filling parameters (18–20).

PERICARDIAL DISEASE

The normal pericardium is identified on T1-weighted SE-MR images as a line of low signal intensity that is located between the high signal of pericardial fat on the outside and the epicardial fat on the inside. The thickness of normal pericardium is 1 to 2 mm, although values of up to 4 mm are not necessarily pathologic. The low signal intensity of the pericardium can be explained by its fibrous component in combination with the small quantity of pericardial fluid. On SE-MRI, some parts of the pericardium, particularly the region overlying the right atrium and the posterolateral wall of the left ventricle, may not be identifiable because of a paucity of epicardial fat. The pericardium is also not visible when it is contiguous with the lung (21,22). Small quantities of pericardial fluid posterior to the aorta in the superior pericardial recess of the transverse sinus or anterior to the aorta in the preaortic recess are considered normal. The posterior pericardial reflection about the pulmonary veins and inferior vena cava forms an inverted U-shaped pocket called the oblique pericardial sinus.

Pericardial effusion can be due to a variety of causes such as viral or idiopathic acute pericarditis, neoplasm, therapeutic doses of radiation, uremia, trauma, collagen vascular dis-

ease, and postpericardectomy and postinfarction (Dressler) syndromes. MRI is sensitive for the detection of small pericardial effusions. Small effusions are often noted along the right border or the posterolateral margin of the left ventricle. Larger effusions cause an asymmetric band around the heart and may distend the superior pericardial recess. When larger effusions occur, cine MRI is valuable in detecting compression or collapse of the right-sided heart chambers during ventricular diastole, which is a sign of cardiac tamponade. Pericardial fluid demonstrates high signal on cine MRI (23). Transudates usually produce low signal intensity on T1-weighted and high signal intensity on T2-weighted SE-MRI, whereas hemorrhagic or proteinaceous effusions demonstrate areas of medium or high signal intensity on T1-weighted SE-MRI and high intensity on T2-weighted images. Echocardiography affords excellent delineation of simple pericardial effusions, but it provides less optimal imaging of complex or loculated pericardial collections.

Constrictive pericarditis (Fig. 6) must be distinguished from restrictive cardiomyopathy because therapy for these two conditions is markedly different. Diagnostic difficulties arise because both constrictive pericarditis and restrictive cardiomyopathy can impair diastolic filling and thus can have similar clinical presentations and overlapping hemodynamic profiles at cardiac catheterization (24). Either CT or MRI can be used to demonstrate pericardial thickening, which is the most useful finding to diagnose constrictive pericarditis and exclude restrictive cardiomyopathy. In comparison with CT, MR has the advantages of obtaining images in multiple planes and assessing ventricular function. However, MRI lacks the ability to detect pericardial calcification. Pericardial thickening and calcification, however, must be interpreted with caution, because patients with prior cardiac surgery or the postpericardiotomy syndrome can have substantial pericardial thickening in the absence of constriction (25,26). In the appropriate clinical setting a pericardial thickness of >4 mm on SE-MR images is considered evidence of pericardial constriction (27). However, absence of pericardial thickening does not exclude constrictive pericarditis (27). Pericardial thickening can be localized and is most frequently demonstrated over the right ventricle (27).

Congenital absence of the pericardium may be complete or partial, and is most often left-sided. It is postulated that this defect is caused by premature obliteration of the embryonic duct of Cuvier, leading to incomplete formation of the parietal pericardium. In 3% of patients, the more common partial defect is associated with other congenital abnormalities, such as atrial septal defect, patent ductus arteriosus, or mitral valve abnormalities. Patients with partial absence of the left hemipericardium are at risk for herniation of the left atrial appendage, the entire left atrium, or both of the ventricles through the defect, which may lead to life-threatening cardiac strangulation or compression of the coronary arteries (28–30). MRI demonstrates the leftward protrusion of the left atrial appendage or the main pulmonary artery, as well as lung insinuates between the aorta and pulmonary

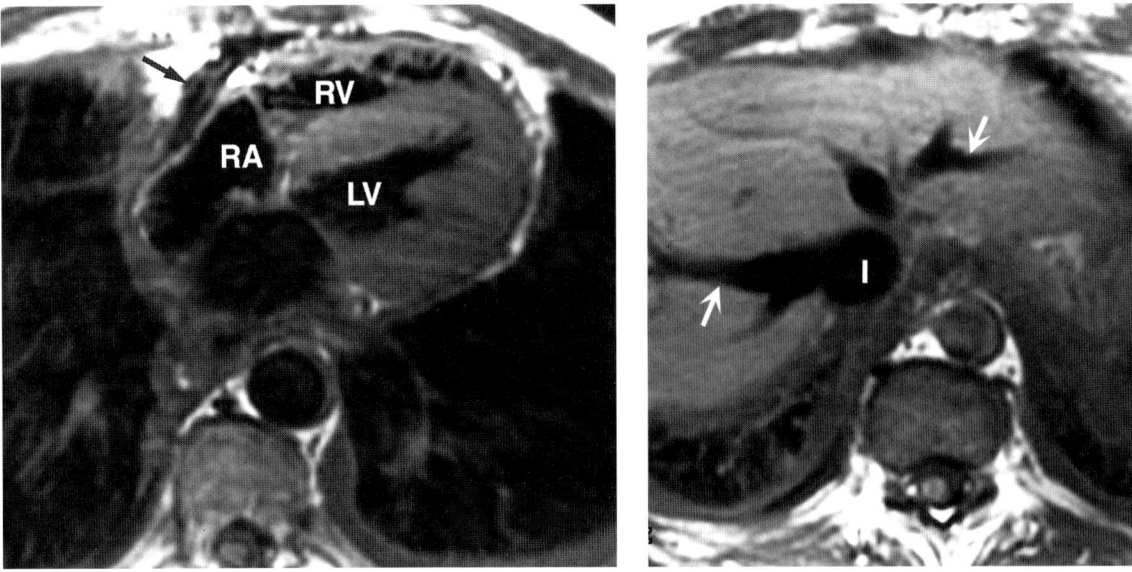

FIG. 6. Adult patient with constrictive pericarditis. **A:** Axial T1-weighted spin-echo MR image. Note tubular shape of the right ventricle (*RV*). In this case the right atrium (*RA*) in compressed, which is atypical. The pericardium is thickened, especially along the right side of the heart, where it is up to 10mm thick (*arrow*). *LV*, left ventricle. **B:** An axial image acquired through the liver reveals enlargement of the IVC (*I*) and hepatic veins (*arrows*).

artery and between the base of the heart and left hemidiaphragm (28,29).

CARDIAC AND PARACARDIAC MASSES

The most frequent intracardiac mass is thrombus, which is usually located within the left atrium or the left ventricle. Left atrial thrombus occurs in patients with mitral valve disease, and/or atrial fibrillation. Left ventricular thrombus occurs in patients with cardiomyopathy and after myocardial infarction. Thrombi can have a variable appearance on MR images, depending upon their age. Relatively fresh thrombi can produce high signal intensity, whereas older thrombi typically produce low signal intensity, particularly on T2-weighted images. The iron contained in thrombi can distort the regional magnetic field and decrease the signal intensity, referred to as magnetic susceptibility effect. This effect produces very low signal intensity on T2*-weighted cine images. Thus, the typical appearance of a thrombus is that of a mass with very low signal intensity on cine MR images. Unlike neoplastic masses, fresh thrombi are not vascularized; thus they do not enhance on T1-weighted SE-images after administration of MR contrast media.

Secondary cardiac neoplasms are 40 to 50 times more common than primary tumors of the heart (11). The most common secondary tumors are lung and breast cancer, lymphoma, and melanoma. Direct extension from adjacent mediastinal tumors or through vascular connections can also occur and are readily identified by MRI. The pulmonary vein can serve as a direct conduit for lung cancer and the inferior vena cava for cancer of the upper abdomen, such

as renal cell carcinoma. The definition of tumor extent is important, because involvement of atrial wall usually precludes removal of the entire tumor. Pericardium may also be invaded from adjacent lung and mediastinal tumor or by metastasis. The MRI features of tumor involvement of the pericardium are mass in the pericardial space, pericardial thickening, focal nodular lesions, and hemorrhagic effusion (31). Associated thickening of the myocardium may indicate myocardial invasion.

Primary tumors of the heart are rare, with an incidence of 0.0017 to 0.28% (32). Most primary tumors are benign. The most frequent benign tumors are myxoma and lipoma, typically located in the left and right atrium, respectively. Myxomas are typically attached by a stalk to the interatrial septum at the region of the fossa ovalis. Myxomas with a broad base of attachment to the atrial septum have also been described (11). A broad base, however, raises the suspicion of a malignant tumor (11). On T1-weighted SE-MRI, myxomas are of intermediate signal intensity, and they enhance after Gd-DTPA administration (33). On cine images, some myxomas produce low signal intensity due to their relatively high iron content.

Lipomas can be sessile, polypoid, or infiltrative. They are usually either subendocardial or subpericardial and occur most frequently in right atrium (32). Another associated abnormality is lipomatous hypertrophy. This tumorlike condition of the atrial septum is usually seen in obese elderly women and is characterized by fatty infiltration of the interatrial septum (34). Lipoma and lipomatous hypertrophy are recognized by signal intensities similar to subcutaneous fat, which is high signal intensity on T1-weighted SE-MR

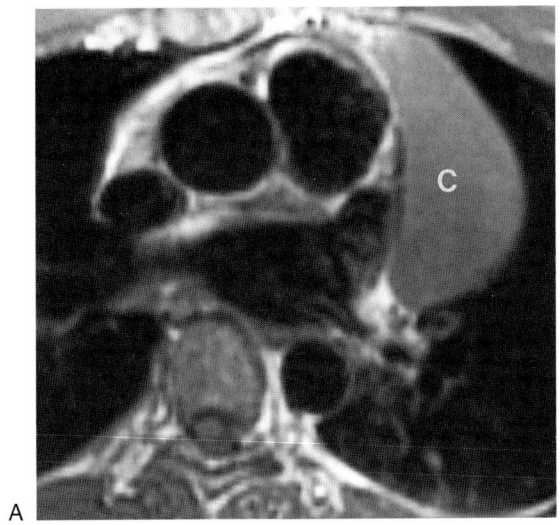
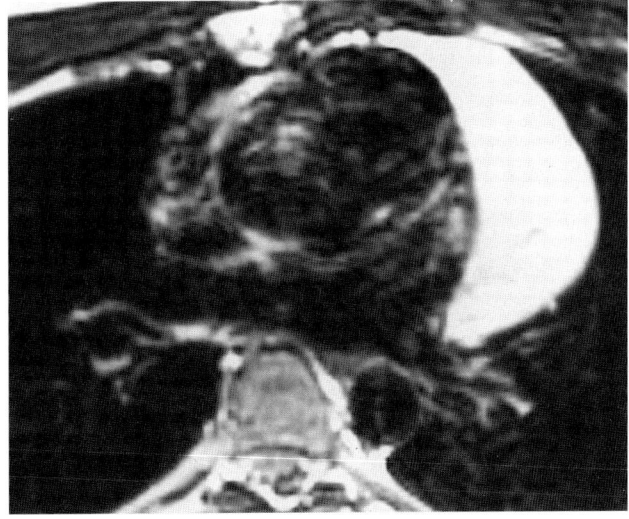

FIG. 7. Pericardial cyst (*C*) along left heart border. The cyst has intermediate signal intensity on spin echo T1-weighted image (**A**) and high signal intensity on fast spin-echo T2-weighted image (**B**).

images and low signal intensity when fat suppression techniques are applied.

Rhabdomyoma is the most frequent of all cardiac tumors in children. This tumor can vary in size and is frequently multiple, and it may be difficult to recognize because of its typically small size, intramural location, and signal characteristics similar to myocardium. Therefore, distortion of the myocardial wall may be the only evidence of rhabdomyoma.

Approximately 25% of all primary cardiac tumors are histologically malignant, and nearly all of these are sarcomas such as angiosarcoma, rhabdosarcoma, liposarcoma, fibrosarcoma, and malignant histiocytoma (32). The most frequent location is the right atrium. Primary cardiac lymphoma is rare and usually occurs in immunocompromised patients. MR features of malignant cardiac tumors are pericardial effusion, invasiveness and enhancement after Gd-DTPA administration. Because of the high spatial and contrast resolution, MRI can be used to evaluate size, shape, and extent of the tumor and to plan therapy (35,36).

Pericardial cysts are benign developmental lesions that are formed when a portion of the pericardium is pinched off during embryogenesis. Most pericardial cysts contain fluid and are well marginated. They are found most frequently in the right anterior cardiophrenic angle. On SE-MR images pericardial cysts are round or ovoid and are often contiguous with the normal pericardium. Uncomplicated cysts demonstrate low signal intensity on T1-weighted and high signal intensity on T2-weighted images (Fig. 7). Hemorrhagic or cysts filled with proteinaceous fluid show high signal intensity on T1-weighted images (37).

CARDIOMYOPATHY

Arrhythmogenic right ventricular dysplasia (ARVD) has been recognized as a cardiomyopathy of the right ventricular myocardium. Morphologic features of ARVD are partial or total replacement of the right ventricular myocardium with fat or fibrous tissue and/or thinning of the myocardium in the right ventricular free wall (Fig. 8). In adults, the normal right ventricular free wall is 3- to 4-mm thick. Fatty infiltration, wall thinning, and aneurysms of the right ventricular free wall can be seen on SE-images, and wall motion abnormalities on cine MRI (38,39). Intramyocardial fat must be carefully distinguished from normal epicardial fat and from

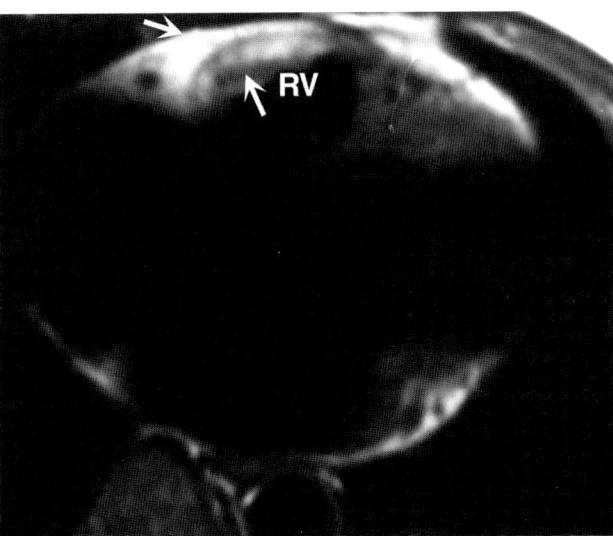

FIG. 8. Adult patient with arrhythmogenic right ventricular dysplasia. The T1-weighted spin-echo sequence employs a posterior saturation band (dark area posterior to the right ventricle) to reduce artifact from the blood in the left ventricle and atrium. The free wall of the right ventricle (*RV*) shows transmural fatty infiltration (*open arrow*) with bright signal intensity. Fatty infiltration of the myocardium should not be confused with subpericardial fat (*closed arrow*), which is a normal finding.

motion artifacts that propagate in the phase-encoding direction, producing spots of high signal intensity in the myocardium. MRI has been reported to be highly specific in the diagnosis of ARVD, although the sensitivity may be limited (40). The most convincing MR finding is transmural fat in the RV free wall. Rarely fat can also be detected in the septum of the left ventricle.

Congestive cardiomyopathy is characterized by systolic dysfunction, dilatation of the left ventricle, and in many cases dilatation of the right ventricle as well. Cine MRI demonstrates increase in LV end-diastolic and end-systolic volumes and decrease in stroke volume and ejection fraction. The thickness of the myocardium is usually normal, resulting in an overall increase in LV mass. Dilated cardiomyopathy can usually be distinguished from previous infarction, because the latter is typically characterized by focal wall thinning. MRI is useful for monitoring the effect of therapy in patients with congestive cardiomyopathy (41), because ventricular volumes and mass can be quantified with good reproducibility by cine MRI (4,42).

Hypertrophic cardiomyopathy is characterized by marked ventricular hypertrophy, small chamber volumes, systolic cavity obliteration, and diastolic dysfunction due to increased myocardial stiffness (Fig. 9). Hypertrophic cardiomyopathy is generally diagnosed and followed by echocardiography. The major role of MR imaging is documentation of unusual subtypes of this condition (43,44). The most common subtype is associated with asymmetric septal hypertrophy. In some patients, hypertrophy exists only in the outflow septum, whereas in others, the entire septum is hypertrophied. Other subtypes demonstrate homogeneous hypertrophy of the left ventricular myocardium or involvement of the apex only (45). Septal thickness of at least 15 mm and at least 1.3 to 1.5 times the thickness of the posterior wall

at end-diastole are considered diagnostic of hypertrophic cardiomyopathy. Measurements can be done on MR images in the four-chamber or the short-axis view (43,46–48). Left ventricular mass, volume, wall motion, and ejection fraction can be measured with cine MRI (44). Hypertrophic cardiomyopathy is frequently associated with abnormal systolic anterior motion of the anterior leaflet of the mitral valve, which can be detected by cine MRI.

The clinical and hemodynamic features of restrictive cardiomyopathy can overlap with those of constrictive pericarditis. MRI is helpful in distinguishing these two conditions. The major distinguishing feature is the thickness of the pericardium. In restrictive cardiomyopathy, pericardial thickness is usually normal. Less specific features of restrictive cardiomyopathy are enlargement of the atria, inferior vena cava, and hepatic veins, with normal volumes of the ventricles. Restrictive cardiomyopathy is frequently complicated by regurgitation of the atrioventricular valves, which can be demonstrated on cine MRI (49). In amyloid cardiomyopathy restriction can be associated with increased right atrial and ventricular wall thickness (50). Although the wall thickness of amyloid heart disease might be suggestive of hypertrophic cardiomyopathy, systolic function in the two diseases is different. As measured by ejection fraction and wall motion systolic function is normal or increased in hypertrophic cardiomyopathy, but it is decreased in amyloidosis.

Other infiltrative disease of the myocardium can cause typical signal changes. In cardiac sarcoidosis, intramyocardial nodules with high signal intensity on T2-weighted SE images have been described (51). Hemochromatosis has been found to produce low myocardial signal intensity on SE and particularly on gradient echo images (52). The low signal intensity on gradient images can be explained by the high sensitivity of this MR technique to regional distortions of the magnetic field induced by iron deposition in the myocardium. Cardiac hemochromatosis, however, is usually associated with congestive rather than with restrictive cardiomyopathy.

ISCHEMIC HEART DISEASE

In patients with suspected or known ischemic heart disease MR imaging can provide information about myocardial function, perfusion, and coronary anatomy as well as ventricular morphology.

Acute Myocardial Infarction

Acute myocardial infarction, particularly after reperfusion, produces a prolongation of the transverse relaxation time (T2), which is longer than the T2 of normal myocardium (~61 ms and ~41 ms, respectively, in canine myocardium [53]). This regional difference in T2 can be demonstrated on T2-weighted MR images as higher signal intensity of infarcted myocardium compared to normal myocardium. The T2 prolongation evolves within 24 h after onset of infarction and remains visible for 7 to 10 days (54,55).

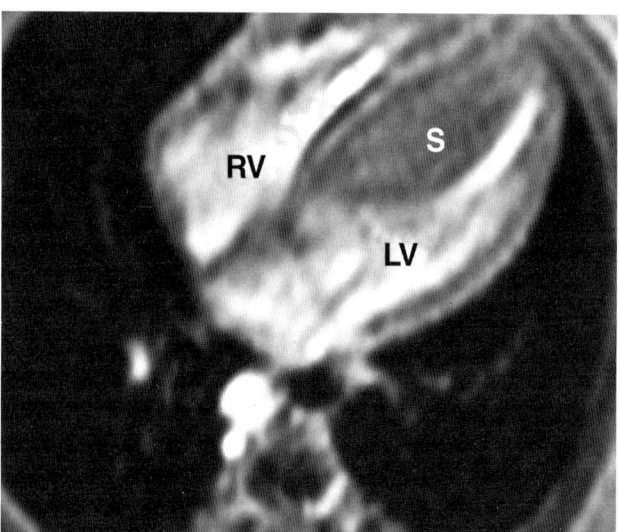

FIG. 9. Adult patient with hypertrophic cardiomyopathy. Blood in the left (LV) and right (RV) ventricle appears bright on this cine MR image. Note asymmetric hypertrophy of the septum (S).

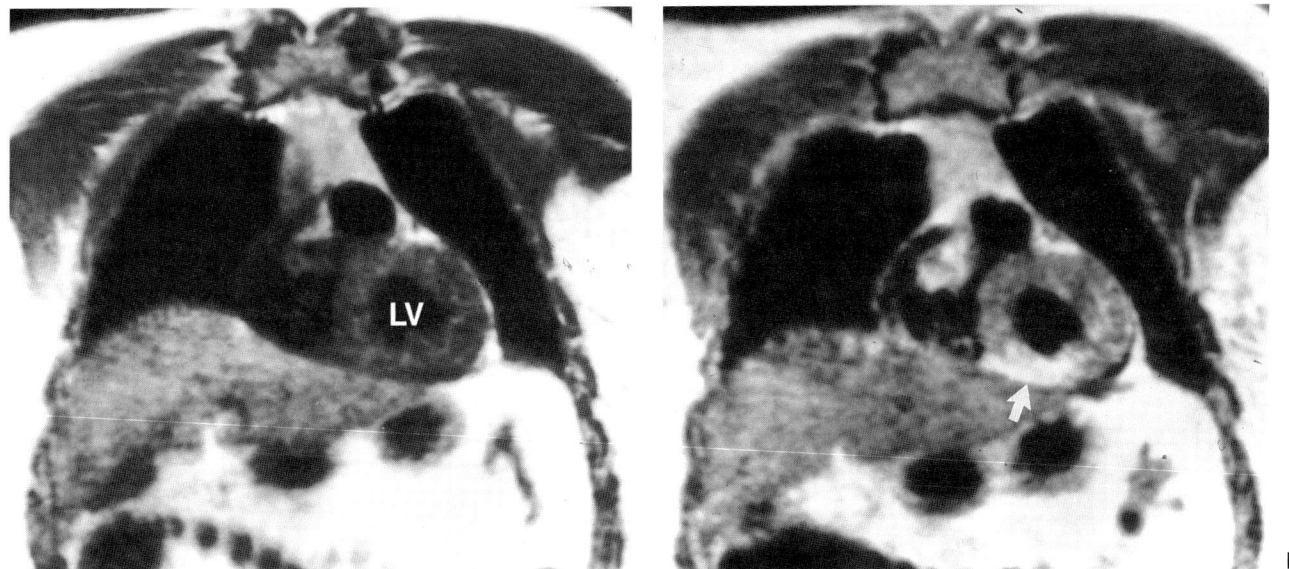

FIG. 10. T1-weighted spin-echo MRI in an adult patient with subacute myocardial infarction. **A:** Normal and infarcted myocardium are not distinguishable on the coronal precontrast image. **B:** After administration of the extracellular MR contrast media Gd-DTPA, however, infarction of the inferior wall can be clearly delineated as a hyperenhanced zone (*arrow*). Hyperenhancement can be attributed to distribution of Gd-DTPA in the expanded extracellular space in infarction. *LV*, left ventricle. (From ref. 11, with permission.)

Ischemic myocardial injury and infarction have also been demonstrated using extracellular MR contrast media such as gadolinium chelates (Fig. 10). On contrast-enhanced T1-weighted MR images, myocardial infarction enhances more intensely than normal myocardium. This hyperenhancement, can persist weeks to months after infarction, and is more intense in reperfused infarction than in occluded infarction (56). The spatial extent of hyperenhanced myocardium correlates well with the fixed scintigraphic defect in patients with acute myocardial infarction (56).

Complications of Myocardial Infarction

True left ventricular aneurysms can be recognized on MR images as severe wall thinning (less than 2 mm in thickness), bulging of the left ventricular wall with a wide ostium, and paradoxical motion. True aneurysms are typically located in the anterolateral wall or at the apex of the left ventricle (Fig. 11). False left ventricular aneurysms represent rupture of the myocardium with encapsulation by the fused pericardial layers. False aneurysms of the left ventricle usually have a

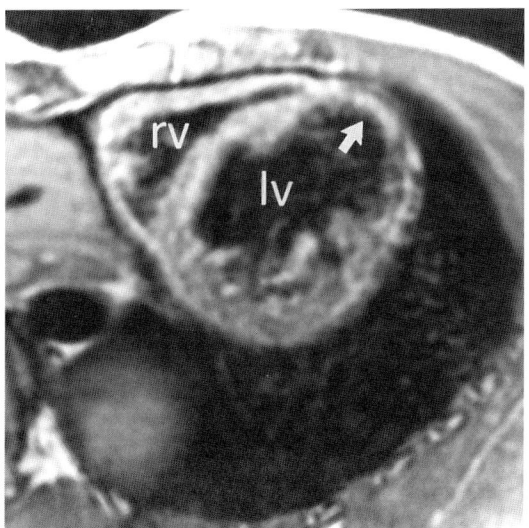
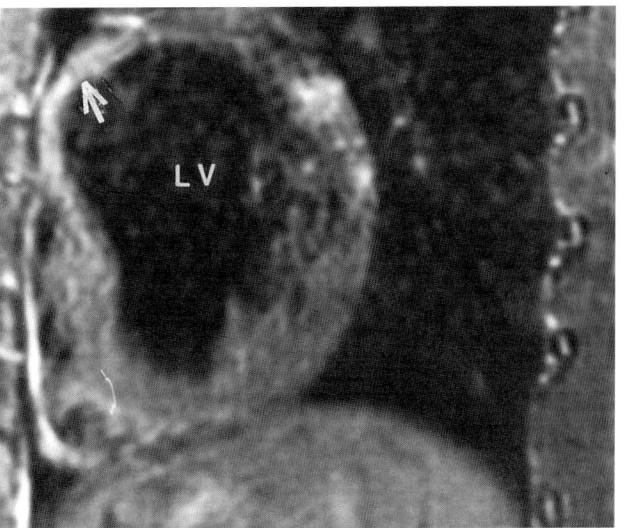

FIG. 11. Axial (**A**) and sagittal (**B**) T1-weighted spin-echo images of a boy who had a traumatic myocardial infarction that is now complicated by a true aneurysm of the left ventricle (*LV*). Note bulging and thinning of the LV wall at the aneurysm (*arrow*) with broad-based communication to the left ventricular chamber.

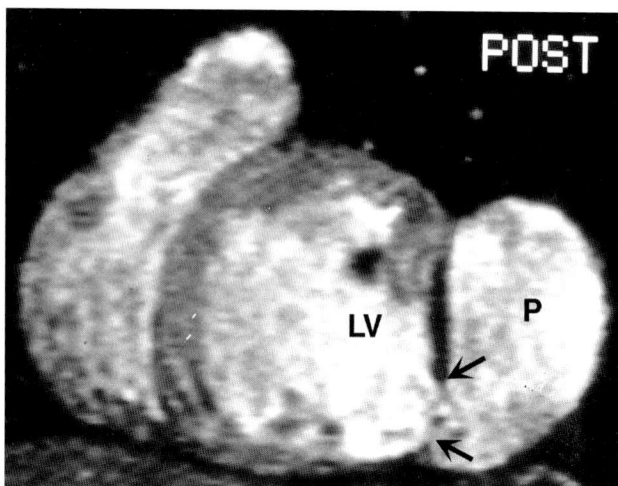

FIG. 12. Adult patient with false or pseudoaneurysm (*P*) of the left ventricle (*LV*). Oblique Gd-DTPA enhanced gradient echo image shows a narrow neck (*arrows*) between the left ventricle and the pseudoaneurysm. (From ref. 11, with permission.)

relatively small ostium (Fig. 12) and are typically located in the posterior or diaphragmatic wall. Both true and false aneurysms can be demonstrated with SE and cine MRI. Cine MRI can demonstrate wall motion through the cardiac cycle as well as the presence of thrombi within aneurysms (57).

Ventricular septal defect is another complication after myocardial infarction. Cine MRI can depict the location of the ventricular septal defect and permit clear distinction from valvular lesions. The pulmonary to systemic flow ratio (Q_p/Q_s) can be estimated by measuring pulmonary artery and aortic flow with VENC-MRI, thus quantifying the shunt volume.

Due to the unique ability of MRI to measure LV wall thickness reliably and with high reproducibility (4), the remodeling process of the left ventricle after acute myocardial infarction can be monitored and followed with sequential MRI examinations. After myocardial infarction, MRI usually demonstrates focal thinning of the left ventricular myocardium and enlargement of the left ventricle. In contrast, congestive (or dilated) cardiomyopathy is characterized by a uniform left ventricular wall thickness. The remodeling process can lead to left ventricular dilatation and progressive thinning of the myocardial wall adjacent to the infarcted region. Sequential MR imaging has been used experimentally to demonstrate the effectiveness of drugs in limiting detrimental morphologic changes (58).

VALVULAR HEART DISEASE

Valvular stenosis and regurgitation are readily identified on cine MR images because valvular dysfunction is usually associated with jet flow. Turbulent flow disturbs rephasing of the MRI signal. Therefore, stenosis or regurgitation typically produce a sharply demarcated area of diminished or

absent signal persisting for most of the systolic or diastolic period. This signal void must be distinguished from flow patterns in normal valves. Unlike signal voids caused by valve dysfunction, signal voids in normal individuals are characterized by their shorter duration of 50 to 100 ms (59). The length of the signal void on MR images correlates with the severity of aortic valve stenosis (60). Moreover, the total area of signal loss on cine MR images correlates significantly with severity of mitral regurgitation as determined by Doppler ultrasound or contrast ventriculography (61). However, the appearance of the signal void can be affected by variations acquisition parameters such as TE and in display settings such as window width and level. Consequently, quantitative assessment and sequential monitoring of the severity of valvular regurgitation by cine MRI requires strict standardization of both imaging and display parameters (62). The size of the signal void can also be affected by other factors, such as ventricular function, aortic pressure, ventricular pressure, and size of the regurgitant orifice.

Another approach to assess valvular heart disease is velocity-encoded cine MRI. This technique allows analysis of flow profiles in all cardiac valves and quantification of regurgitant volumes (63). The peak velocity across a stenotic valve can be measured, and the pressure gradient can be estimated using the modified Bernoulli equation. Pressure gradients estimated by velocity-encoded MRI and Doppler ultrasound are closely correlated (64). Highly reproducible quantification of both valvular dysfunction and ventricular function indicates the potential of MRI for monitoring valvular heart disease.

Valvular morphology can also be demonstrated with MRI. Echo-planar imaging time resolution is in the millisecond range and therefore can be used for examination of valve motion (65). Morphologic evaluation of mitral valve leaflets is superior on interleaved (multishot) echo-planar images, although temporal resolution is somewhat compromised in comparison to single-shot EPI (65).

REFERENCES

1. Schaefer S, van Tyen R, Saloner D. Evaluation of myocardial perfusion abnormalities with gadolinium-enhanced snapshot MR imaging in humans. *Radiology* 1992;185:795–801.
2. Bremerich J, Buser P, Bongartz G, et al. Noninvasive stress testing of myocardial ischemia: comparison of GRE-MRI perfusion and wall motion analysis to 99 mTc-MIBI-SPECT, relation to coronary angiography. *Eur Radiol* 1997;7:990–995.
3. Sechtem U, Pflugfelder PW, White RD, et al. Cine MR imaging: potential for the evaluation of cardiovascular function. *Am J Roentgenol* 1987;148:239–246.
4. Semelka RC, Tomei E, Wagner S, et al. Interstudy reproducibility of dimensional and functional measurements between cine magnetic resonance studies in the morphologically abnormal left ventricle. *Am Heart J* 1990;119:1367–1373.
5. Higgins CB. Which standard has the gold? *J Am Coll Cardiol* 1992; 19:1608–1609.
6. Kersting-Sommerhoff BA, Diethelm L, Teitel DF, et al. Magnetic resonance imaging of congenital heart disease: sensitivity and specificity using receiver operating characteristic curve analysis. *Am Heart J* 1989; 118:155–161.
7. Kersting-Sommerhoff BA, Sechtem UP, Fisher MR, et al. MR imaging

of congenital anomalies of the aortic arch. *Am J Roentgenol* 1987;149:
9–13.

8. Rees S, Somerville J, Ward C, et al. Coarctation of the aorta: MR imaging in late postoperative assessment. *Radiology* 1989;173:499–502.

9. Steffens JC, Bourne MW, Sakuma H, et al. Quantification of collateral blood flow in coarctation of the aorta by velocity encoded cine magnetic resonance imaging. *Circulation* 1994;90:937–943.

10. Diethelm L, Dery R, Lipton MJ, et al. Atrial-level shunts: sensitivity and specificity of MR in diagnosis. *Radiology* 1987;162:181–186.

11. Higgins CB, Hricak H, Helms CA. *Magnetic resonance imaging of the body*, 3rd ed. Philadelphia: Lippincot-Raven, 1996:409–518.

12. Caputo GR, Kondo C, Masui T, et al. Right and left lung perfusion: *in vitro* and *in vivo* validation with oblique-angle, velocity-encoded cine MR imaging. *Radiology* 1991;180:693–698.

13. Kersting-Sommerhoff BA, Diethelm L, Stanger P, et al. Evaluation of complex congenital ventricular anomalies with magnetic resonance imaging. *Am Heart J* 1990;120:133–142.

14. Masui T, Seelos KC, Kersting-Sommerhoff BA, et al. Abnormalities of the pulmonary veins: evaluation with MR imaging and comparison with cardiac angiography and echocardiography. *Radiology* 1991;181:645–649.

15. Blakenberg F, Rhee J, Hardy C, et al. MRI vs echocardiography in the evaluation of the Jatene procedure. *J Comput Assist Tomogr* 1994;18:749–754.

16. Duerinckx AJ, Wexler L, Banerjee A, et al. Postoperative evaluation of pulmonary arteries in congenital heart surgery by magnetic resonance imaging: comparison with echocardiography. *Am Heart J* 1994;128:1139–1146.

17. Martinez JE, Mohiaddin RH, Kilner PJ, et al. Obstruction in extracardiac ventriculopulmonary conduits: value of nuclear magnetic resonance imaging with velocity mapping and Doppler echocardiography. *J Am Coll Cardiol* 1992;20:338–344.

18. Rebergen SA, Chin JG, Ottenkamp J, et al. Pulmonary regurgitation in the late postoperative follow-up of tetralogy of Fallot. Volumetric quantitation by nuclear magnetic resonance velocity mapping. *Circulation* 1993;88:2257–2266.

19. Niezen RA, Helbing WA, van der Wall EE, et al. Biventricular systolic function and mass studied with MR imaging in children with pulmonary regurgitation after repair for tetralogy of Fallot. *Radiology* 1996;201:135–140.

20. Jacobstein MD, Fletcher BD, Nelson AD, et al. Magnetic resonance imaging: evaluation of palliative systemic-pulmonary artery shunts. *Circulation* 1984;70:650–656.

21. Stark DD, Higgins CB, Lanzer P, et al. Magnetic resonance imaging of the pericardium: normal and pathologic findings. *Radiology* 1984;150:469–474.

22. Sechtem U, Tscholakoff D, Higgins CB. MRI of the normal pericardium. *Am J Roentgenol* 1986;147:239–244.

23. Duerinckx AJ, Higgins CB. Valvular heart disease. *Radiol Clin North Am* 1994;32:613–630.

24. Vaitkus PT, Kussmaul WG. Constrictive pericarditis versus restrictive cardiomyopathy: a reappraisal and update of diagnostic criteria. *Am Heart J* 1991;122:1431–1441.

25. Olson MC, Posniak HV, McDonald V, et al. Computed tomography and magnetic resonance imaging of the pericardium. *Radiographics* 1989;9:633–649.

26. Randall PA, Trasolini NC, Kohman LJ, et al. MR imaging in the evaluation of the chest after uncomplicated median sternotomy. *Radiographics* 1993;13:329–340.

27. Masui T, Finck S, Higgins CB. Constrictive pericarditis and restrictive cardiomyopathy: evaluation with MR imaging. *Radiology* 1992;182:369–373.

28. Gutierrez FR, Shackelford GD, McKnight RC, et al. Diagnosis of congenital absence of left pericardium by MR imaging. *J Comput Assist Tomogr* 1985;9:551–553.

29. Altman CA, Ettedgui JA, Wozney P, et al. Noninvasive diagnostic features of partial absence of the pericardium. *Am J Cardiol* 1989;63:1536–1537.

30. Miller SW. Imaging pericardial disease. *Radiol Clin North Am* 1989;27:1113–1125.

31. Barakos JA, Brown JJ, Higgins CB. MR imaging of secondary cardiac and paracardiac lesions. *Am J Roentgenol* 1989;153:47–50.

32. Colucci W, Schoen F, Braunwald E. Primary tumors of the heart. In: Braunwald E, ed. *A textbook of cardiovascular medicine*. Philadelphia: WB Saunders, 1977:1465–1477.

33. Semelka RC, Shoenut JP, Wilson ME, et al. Cardiac masses: signal intensity features on spin-echo, gradient-echo, gadolinium-enhanced spin-echo, and TurboFLASH images. *J Magn Reson Imaging* 1992;2:415–420.

34. Applegate PM, Tajik AJ, Ehman RL, et al. Two-dimensional echocardiographic and magnetic resonance imaging observations in massive lipomatous hypertrophy of the atrial septum. *Am J Cardiol* 1987;59:489–491.

35. Freedberg RS, Kronzon I, Rumancik WM, et al. The contribution of magnetic resonance imaging to the evaluation of intracardiac tumors diagnosed by echocardiography. *Circulation* 1988;77:96–103.

36. Lund JT, Ehman RL, Julsrud PR, et al. Cardiac masses: assessment by MR imaging. *Am J Roentgenol* 1989;152:469–473.

37. Vinee P, Stover B, Sigmund G, et al. MR imaging of the pericardial cyst. *J Magn Reson Imaging* 1992;2:593–596.

38. Auffermann W, Wichter T, Breithardt G, et al. Arrhythmogenic right ventricular disease: MR imaging vs angiography. *Am J Roentgenol* 1993;161:549–555.

39. Blake LM, Scheinman MM, Higgins CB. MR features of arrhythmogenic right ventricular dysplasia. *Am J Roentgenol* 1994;162:809–812.

40. Menghetti L, Basso C, Nava A, et al. Spin-echo nuclear magnetic resonance for tissue characterization in arrhythmogenic right ventricular cardiomyopathy. *Heart* 1996;76:467–470.

41. Doherty NEd, Seelos KC, Suzuki J, et al. Application of cine nuclear magnetic resonance imaging for sequential evaluation of response to angiotensin-converting enzyme inhibitor therapy in dilated cardiomyopathy. *J Am Coll Cardiol* 1992;19:1294–2302.

42. Suzuki J, Caputo GR, Masui T, et al. Assessment of right ventricular diastolic and systolic function in patients with dilated cardiomyopathy using cine magnetic resonance imaging. *Am Heart J* 1991;122:1035–1040.

43. Higgins CB, Byrd BFd, Stark D, et al. Magnetic resonance imaging in hypertrophic cardiomyopathy. *Am J Cardiol* 1985;55:1121–1126.

44. Suzuki J, Chang JM, Caputo GR, et al. Evaluation of right ventricular early diastolic filling by cine nuclear magnetic resonance imaging in patients with hypertrophic cardiomyopathy. *J Am Coll Cardiol* 1991;18:120–126.

45. Webb JG, Sasson Z, Rakowski H, et al. Apical hypertrophic cardiomyopathy: clinical follow-up and diagnostic correlates. *J Am Coll Cardiol* 1990;15:83–90.

46. Arrive L, Assayag P, Russ G, et al. MRI and cine MRI of asymmetric septal hypertrophic cardiomyopathy. *J Comput Assist Tomogr* 1994;18:376–382.

47. Park JH, Kim YM, Chung JW, et al. MR imaging of hypertrophic cardiomyopathy. *Radiology* 1992;185:441–446.

48. Sardanelli F, Molinari G, Petillo A, et al. MRI in hypertrophic cardiomyopathy: a morphofunctional study. *J Comput Assist Tomogr* 1993;17:862–872.

49. Wagner S, Auffermann W, Buser P, et al. Diagnostic accuracy and estimation of the severity of valvular regurgitation from the signal void on cine magnetic resonance images. *Am Heart J* 1989;118:760–767.

50. Borer JS, Henry WL, Epstein SE. Echocardiographic observations in patients with systemic infiltrative disease involving the heart. *Am J Cardiol* 1977;39:184–188.

51. Riedy K, Fisher MR, Belic N, et al. MR imaging of myocardial sarcoidosis. *Am J Roentgenol* 1988;151:915–916.

52. Blankenberg F, Eisenberg S, Scheinman MN, et al. Use of cine gradient echo (GRE) MR in the imaging of cardiac hemochromatosis. *J Comput Assist Tomogr* 1994;18:136–138.

53. Tscholakoff D, Higgins CB, Sechtem U, et al. MRI of reperfused myocardial infarct in dogs. *Am J Roentgenol* 1986;146:925–930.

54. McNamara MT, Higgins CB, Schechtman N, et al. Detection and characterization of acute myocardial infarction in man with use of gated magnetic resonance. *Circulation* 1985;71:717–724.

55. Johnston DL, Mulvagh SL, Cashion RW, et al. Nuclear magnetic resonance imaging of acute myocardial infarction within 24 hours of chest pain onset. *Am J Cardiol* 1989;64:172–179.

56. Lima JA, Judd RM, Bazille A, et al. Regional heterogeneity of human myocardial infarcts demonstrated by contrast-enhanced MRI. Potential mechanisms. *Circulation* 1995;92:1117–1125.

57. Dooms GC, Higgins CB. MR imaging of cardiac thrombi. *J Comput Assist Tomogr* 1986;10:415–420.

58. Saeed M, Wendland MF, Seelos K, et al. Effect of cilazapril on regional left ventricular wall thickness and chamber dimension following acute myocardial infarction: *in vivo* assessment using MRI. *Am Heart J* 1992; 123:1472–1480.
59. Mirowitz SA, Lee JK, Gutierrez FR, et al. Normal signal-void patterns in cardiac cine MR images. *Radiology* 1990;176:49–55.
60. Mitchell L, Jenkins JP, Watson Y, et al. Diagnosis and assessment of mitral and aortic valve disease by cine-flow magnetic resonance imaging. *Magn Reson Med* 1989;12:181–197.
61. Pflugfelder PW, Sechtem UP, White RD, et al. Noninvasive evaluation of mitral regurgitation by analysis of left atrial signal loss in cine magnetic resonance. *Am Heart J* 1989;117:1113–1119.
62. Suzuki J, Caputo GR, Kondo C, et al. Cine MR imaging of valvular heart disease: display and imaging parameters affect the size of the signal void caused by valvular regurgitation. *Am J Roentgenol* 1990; 155:723–727.
63. Kilner PJ, Firmin DN, Rees RS, et al. Valve and great vessel stenosis: assessment with MR jet velocity mapping. *Radiology* 1991;178: 229–235.
64. Eichenberger AC, Jenni R, von Schulthess GK. Aortic valve pressure gradients in patients with aortic valve stenosis: quantification with velocity-encoded cine MR imaging. *Am J Roentgenol* 1993;160:971–977.
65. Davis CP, McKinnon GC, Debatin JF, et al. Single-shot versus interleaved echo-planar MR imaging: application to visualization of cardiac valve leaflets. *J Magn Reson Imaging* 1995;5:107–112.
66. Semelka RC, Tomei E, Wagner S, et al. Normal left ventricular dimensions and function: interstudy reproducibility of measurements with cine MR imaging. *Radiology* 1990;174:763–768.
67. Reddy GP, Higgins CB. MRI of congenital heart disease. In: Passariello R, ed. *Magnetic resonance in medicine multimedia virtual textbook*. Luxembourg: Euromultimedia S.A., 1997–98. Available at: [http://medic-online.net/mr/higgins/index.html].

CHAPTER 30

Imaging of Function

Christopher M. Kramer

Magnetic resonance imaging (MRI) is becoming increasingly applied to the cardiovascular system as clinicians and investigators bring to bear newer technologic advances in magnetic resonance (MR) hardware and software. The many advantages include its three-dimensional imaging capabilities that eliminate the constraints on other imaging modalities imposed by the position and orientation of the heart in the chest or by tissue attenuation. Imaging is possible in any desired plane. In addition, newer rapid imaging techniques allow evaluation of cardiac structure and function in one or a few breath holds. Wall thickening and ejection fraction are easily evaluated using cine MRI techniques. With automated analytic techniques, quantitation of left ventricular (LV) mass and volumes is becoming simplified. Newer methods for evaluation of intramyocardial function include myocardial tagging and phase velocity techniques. The response to pharmacologic stress in acute and chronic ischemic heart disease can be evaluated with these techniques. Function can be evaluated in many other disease states, including valvular heart disease and cardiomyopathies. MRI can evaluate the function of all of the cardiac valves, including prostheses. To evaluate intracardiac shunts, cine MRI can demonstrate flow between chambers, and phase velocity methods can measure ratios of pulmonary and systemic blood flows. In this chapter, all of the MRI methods for evaluating LV and valvular function will be reviewed.

VENTRICULAR SIZE AND FUNCTION

Global Left Ventricular Size and Function

Spin Echo Imaging

Several techniques exist for measuring LV volumes and ejection fraction. Historically, multislice, multiphase spin-echo imaging (Fig. 1) has been used to measure LV mass, stroke volume, and ejection fraction (EF) (1). This imaging

is a "black blood" technique that creates excellent contrast between blood and myocardium. Limitations with this technique include limited temporal resolution and long imaging times (from 20 to 40 minutes). These can be overcome by imaging only at end diastole and end systole (2); however, predicting end-systolic timing is fraught with potential error.

Gradient Echo Cine Imaging

Cine MRI can be used to provide multiple frames in a single slice with good contrast between myocardium and blood and can be displayed in a cine loop to evaluate function and blood flow. This white blood technique has been shown to be quite accurate for measuring LV volumes (3–5) (Figs. 2 and 3). Breath-holding techniques may be used to acquire multiple phase-encoding steps within each cardiac cycle, thus significantly decreasing the acquisition time for single slice and reducing respiratory artifacts (6). More recently, a conventional 1.5T MR scanner has been modified by an interactive workstation to allow real-time dynamic acquisition and display without cardiac gating or breath holding (7). When compared to echocardiographic imaging in patients with difficult acoustic windows, the real-time interactive MRI performed much better in visualization of all of the wall segments.

Echo Planar Imaging

The fastest method of acquiring structural information of the heart is echo-planar imaging, which requires one single pulse (8). Spatial resolution may be somewhat limited, however, and availability is not uniform among MRI centers as the hardware is quite expensive. Signal-to-noise ratio is poor and flow motion-induced artifacts can be a problem (9–11).

Imaging Strategies

The Simpson's rule multislice method and the biplane area-length method are the two most commonly used tech-

C. M. Kramer: Departments of Medicine and Radiology, University of Virginia, Charlottesville, Virginia 22908.

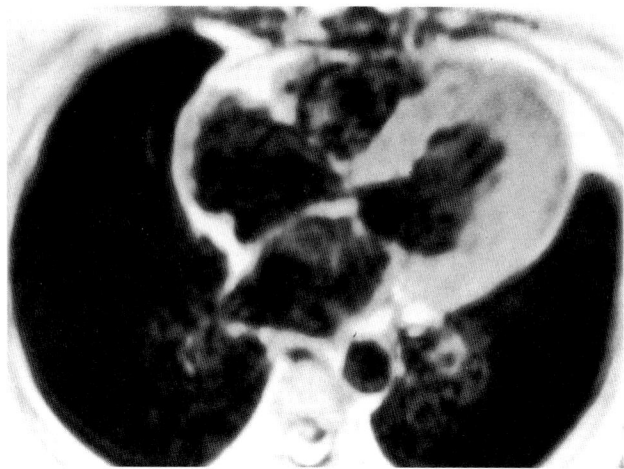

FIG. 1. An axial spin-echo "black blood" image, equivalent to an echocardiographic, four-chamber long-axis image. All four cardiac chambers and the descending thoracic aorta are seen.

niques to measure LV volumes. The former involves imaging multiple slices in the LV short-axis plane and summing the volumes generated by each slice based on the slice thickness. This can be performed with contiguous slices or with a gap between slices that requires multiplying the volumes by an interslice correction factor. Advantages of the Simpson's rule are the coverage of the entire heart and the elimi-

nation of any geometric assumptions, which is especially important in deformed left ventricles, such as those postinfarction. However, any obliquity of the acquisition may lead to errors in the measurement, and imaging at the base can create difficulties in differentiating basal LV from left atrium.

The area-length method can be performed using a single or biplane imaging strategy and uses the assumption that the LV is an ellipsoid. Two- and four-chamber long-axis planes can be used to define the radii of the ellipsoid in three dimensions, and the volume of the ellipsoid can be calculated using the formula as per Figure 4. The advantages of the area-length method are ease and speed of acquisition of the requisite imaging planes. The disadvantages include geometric assumptions made that will not hold true in deformed ventricles such as the postinfarction LV.

Requirements for Quantitation

Several potential pitfalls in the quantitation of LV parameters must be overcome. For one, the spatial resolution must be commensurate with the LV size with in-plane resolution of, at most, 1 to 2 mm. Reducing slice thickness to the minimum needed to cover the LV and optimizing slice orientation is important to minimize partial volume effects that occur at the edges of LV structures. In addition, careful electrocar-

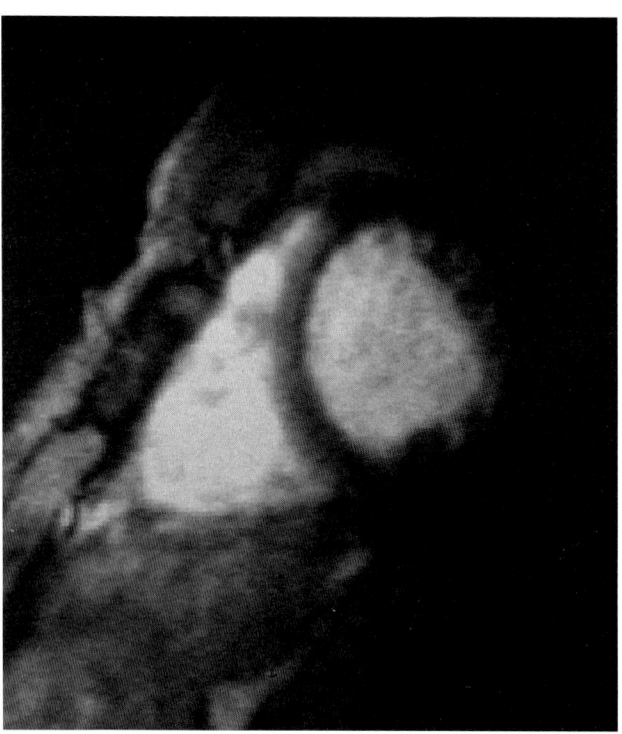

FIG. 2. End-diastolic, short-axis gradient echo cine "white blood" image in a double oblique plane in the basal left ventricle (LV). Note the excellent border definition between chamber and blood with visualization of LV trabeculae.

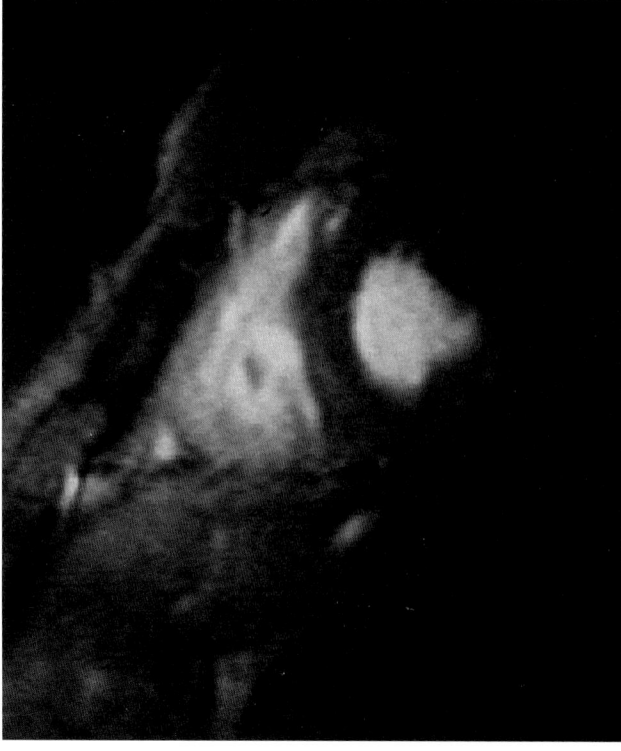

FIG. 3. End-systolic, short-axis gradient echo cine "white blood" image in the same plane and from the same image series as Figure 2. Wall thickening is uniform throughout the left ventricle short axis.

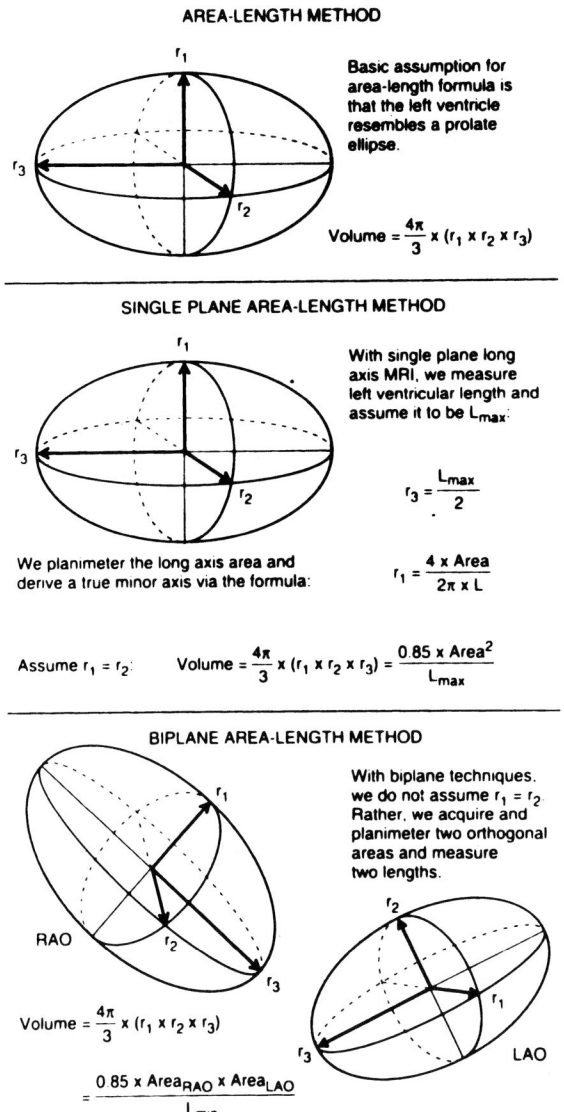

AREA-LENGTH METHOD

Basic assumption for area-length formula is that the left ventricle resembles a prolate ellipse.

$$\text{Volume} = \frac{4\pi}{3} \times (r_1 \times r_2 \times r_3)$$

SINGLE PLANE AREA-LENGTH METHOD

With single plane long axis MRI, we measure left ventricular length and assume it to be L_{max}.

$$r_3 = \frac{L_{max}}{2}$$

We planimeter the long axis area and derive a true minor axis via the formula:

$$r_1 = \frac{4 \times \text{Area}}{2\pi \times L}$$

Assume $r_1 = r_2$:

$$\text{Volume} = \frac{4\pi}{3} \times (r_1 \times r_2 \times r_3) = \frac{0.85 \times \text{Area}^2}{L_{max}}$$

BIPLANE AREA-LENGTH METHOD

With biplane techniques, we do not assume $r_1 = r_2$. Rather, we acquire and planimeter two orthogonal areas and measure two lengths.

RAO

LAO

$$\text{Volume} = \frac{4\pi}{3} \times (r_1 \times r_2 \times r_3)$$

$$= \frac{0.85 \times \text{Area}_{RAO} \times \text{Area}_{LAO}}{L_{min}}$$

FIG. 4. Three variants of the area-length method for estimating left ventricle volumes. At **top** is the basic area-length method that makes the assumption that the left ventricle resembles a prolate ellipse. With single-plane MRI (**middle panel**), left ventricle LV length is measured, long-axis area is measured, and volume is calculated by the formula shown. With the biplane method (**bottom panel**), two lengths and two areas are calculated, and the volume is calculated. (From ref. 152, with permission.)

diographic gating is essential to volumetric imaging with MRI. Respiratory gating or breath-hold imaging further improves image quality.

Left Ventricular Mass

Left ventricular mass is an important prognostic indicator, even in broad-based population studies (12). MRI requires no three-dimensional assumptions, ionizing radiation, or dependence on acoustic windows to obtain an accurate mea-

surement of LV mass. The volume of muscle is measured using the Simpson's rule from short-axis slices and multiplied by the specific gravity of myocardium (1.05 g/cm^2). Using an older 0.5T system that limited them to transaxial planes, Florentine et al. (13) found excellent correlation between MRI-derived measures of LV mass and that from postmortem LV mass in animals ($r = 0.95$). Keller et al. (14) found a better correlation ($r = 0.98$) when short-axis slices were used in a canine model. Due to partial volume effects and difficulties with border detection in these early studies, MRI slightly overestimated LV mass in comparison to actual LV mass. With improved hardware and reduced slice thickness during image acquisition, these limitations have been overcome. Maddahi et al. (15) confirmed the improved accuracy of the short-axis imaging acquisition over other planes in a canine model.

Accuracy of MRI for LV mass determination has been validated in animal models of valvular and ischemic heart disease. Manning and colleagues (16) studied both normal rats and rats with aortic regurgitation secondary to leaflet disruption, finding an excellent correlation with postmortem mass ($r = 0.98$) and an increase in LV mass as early as 5 days after the onset of aortic regurgitation. Shapiro et al. (17) demonstrated excellent correlation between LV mass postmortem in a canine infarction model that measured at either end diastole ($r = 0.94$) or end systole ($r = 0.98$) by MRI, establishing MRI as an accurate method of measuring mass in deformed left ventricles (Fig. 5). The accuracy of MRI has been recently demonstrated in hearts as small as that of the mouse (18). Franco et al. showed that in a transgenic mouse model of LV hypertrophy, the correlation between multislice, multiphase MRI and autopsy mass was excellent ($r^2 = 0.95$). Ruff et al. (19) demonstrated good agreement between MRI and autopsy and low intraobserver and interobserver variability in the measurements (5% for both) (Fig. 6).

MRI has been established as an accurate technique in man as well. Katz et al. (20) found a tight correlation between MR-derived measures of LV mass in cadaveric hearts with the actual mass ($r = 0.99$). In a group of 40 volunteers, they also found excellent intraobserver variability ($r = 0.96$, standard error of estimate, or SEE, 11.1g) and interobserver variability ($r = 0.91$, SEE 17.8g). Germain and associates (21) compared the reproducibility of MRI measurement of LV mass to that of M-mode echocardiography. They found that, when each study was repeated 4 days apart, MR was more reproducible ($r = 0.96$) when compared to M-mode echo ($r = 0.89$). Bottini et al. (22) demonstrated that in hypertensive patients the precision of LV mass measurement (11g) was much better than that of M-mode echo (26g). Yamaoka et al. (23) compared MRI with ultrafast computed tomography (CT) and contrast left ventriculography in 20 patients. Mass determined by left ventriculograpy was higher than that by MRI or CT, and the latter two methods correlated closely, especially when papillary muscles and trabeculae were included in the analysis.

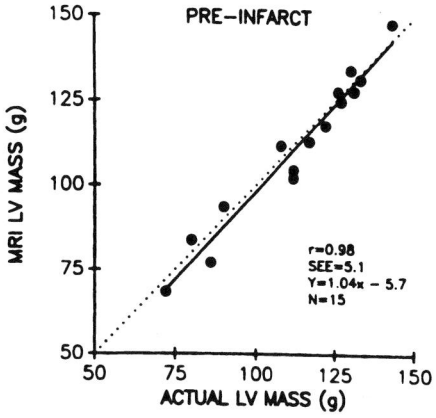
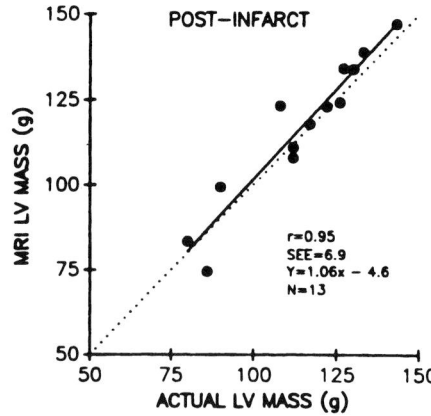

FIG. 5. Regression plots of left ventricular (*LV*) mass by actual weight versus multislice MRI-derived mass in a canine model before (**left panel**) and after myocardial infarct (**right panel**). The *dotted line* represents the line of identity. (From ref. 17, with permission.)

Methods have recently been developed to reduce the requisite imaging time to measure LV mass. Aurigemma and colleagues (24) found a single-phase method correlated closely to a method that acquired the end-diastolic phase on each short-axis slice in 20 normal volunteers (r = 0.99), with an underestimation by the single-phase method of 5 g on average. McDonald and associates (25) used a snapshot gradient echo technique to measure LV and RV (right ventricular) mass in a canine model with an overall acquisition time of 5 minutes or less. The measured difference between MRI-measured mass and autopsy was quite low at 4.4 ± 1.7 g.

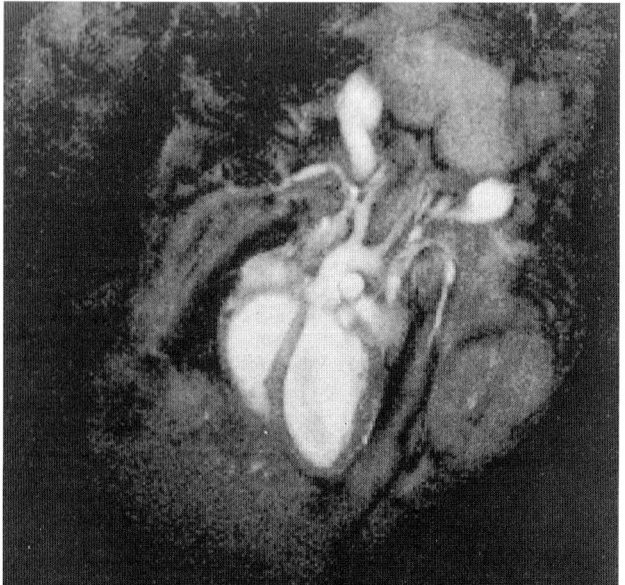

FIG. 6. Coronal end-diastolic cine magnetic resonance image from a mouse with a field of view of 35 mm × 35 mm and matrix 256 × 256. The left ventricle, right ventricle, and great vessels are well visualized. (From ref. 19, with permission.)

Clinical studies using MRI to evaluate LV mass have been increasing in number. In female endurance athletes, Riley-Hagan et al. (26) found increased LV mass in proportion to the increased LV end-diastolic volume compared to normal volunteers. Globits and associates (27) demonstrated increased LV mass in a cohort of 11 patients 2 months after orthotopic heart transplantation that correlated with cyclosporine levels. Using MRI, Kramer et al. (28) demonstrated a trend downward in LV mass during the first 8 weeks after first reperfused anterior MI. Others have used MRI to examine the effect of angiotensin converting enzyme inhibitors on LV mass in dilated cardiomyopathy (29) and in patients in the first 3 months after Q-wave myocardial infarction, in which LV mass fell significantly (30).

Left Ventricular Volumes and Ejection Fraction

The accurate quantitation of LV volumes and ejection fraction is important prognostic information in the setting of myocardial infarction (31) and valvular regurgitation (32). MR provides three-dimensional data, requiring no geometric assumptions to evaluate ventricular dimensions. The first validation study of MRI volumetrics was performed on ventricular casts by Rehr et al. (33) using spin echo techniques with an excellent correlation (r = 0.99) (Fig. 7). A similar study using silicone-rubber casts of canine left ventricles demonstrated an excellent correlation between water displacement and MR measured LV and RV volumes (r = 0.98 and 0.99, respectively) (34).

The lack of a gold standard has hindered correlative studies between MR and other techniques. The correlation with contrast ventriculography is quite good, although, in early studies, MRI tended to underestimate LV volume (35). Using a spin echo technique and Simpson's rule, Markiewicz et al. (34) demonstrated that MRI underestimated LV volume as measured by thermodilution techniques in the dog. Longmore et al. (36) showed that spin-echo MRI measures

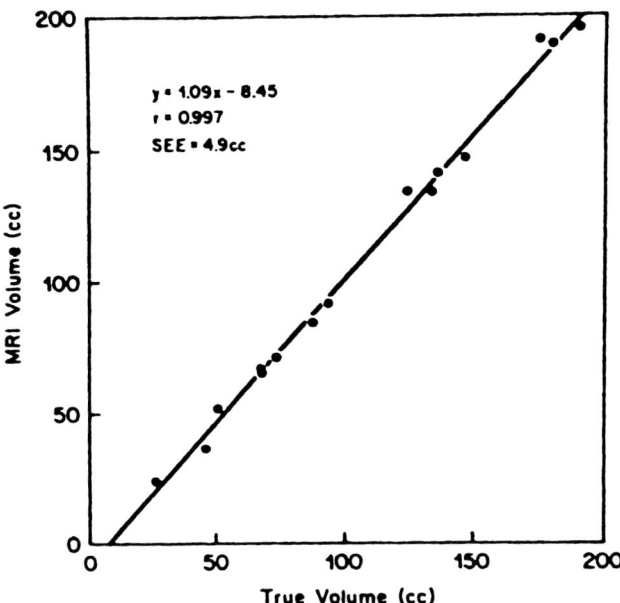

FIG. 7. Correlation between MRI and displacement volume for left ventricular casts with *r* = 0.997. (From ref. 33, with permission.)

of LV volumes in 40 patients, half of them normal volunteers and half with angina, correlated well with contrast ventriculography. Any individual volume measurement in the control population was associated with an error of approximately 2%. Other studies have documented *r* values between 0.84 and 0.98 for the correlation with contrast ventriculography (37,38).

Dilworth et al. (39) showed that volumes derived from a multislice MRI acquisition correlated better with catheterization-based volumes and EF than a single-plane axial MR image. Cranney et al. (4) studied 21 patients and compared biplane cine MRI, short-axis multislice spin-echo MRI, and contrast ventriculography (Fig. 8). Both MRI techniques tended to underestimate cath-derived end-diastolic volumes and EF. Potential explanations for the underestimation include: (i) interpretation of slowly moving blood near the endocardium at end diastole on the MRI as wall; (ii) inadequate analysis of the base from short-axis MR images, or (iii) overestimation on the ventriculogram due to dye filling the LV trabeculae. Lawson and colleagues (40) examined 77 patients with regional and 37 with global LV dysfunction, using techniques similar to those of Cranney (4), and found an *r* value greater than 0.91 relative to biplane ventriculography.

Studies of interstudy and interobserver variability have been performed with MRI techniques. Semelka et al. (41) used short-axis cine MRI in human volunteers and in patients with dilated cardiomyopathy and left ventricular hypertrophy (LVH) (42) to demonstrate excellent interstudy reproducibility. In the patients with deformed ventricles, they found interstudy variability of less than 5% for end-diastolic volumes and for end-systolic volumes, less than 5% for di-

lated cardiomyopathy and less than 8.5% for LVH. Pattynama (43) and colleagues studied variability in 2 subjects who underwent 20 repeated studies using spin-echo and cine MRI. They found no difference in reproducibility between techniques. Intra- and interobserver variability were low, and interexamination variance contributed more to total variance. Lorenz and colleagues (44) studied 75 healthy subjects with cine MRI and found interobserver and interstudy variability of 5 to 6%. This study established a normative data base to compare future studies (Table 1).

Most of the aforementioned studies measuring LV volumes also studied LV ejection fraction (EF). Several studies have examined the use of MRI for measuring EF only. Utz et al. (45) studied 11 patients with a Simpson's rule and found a good correlation (*r* = 0.88) with contrast ventriculography. A correlation of 0.79 was found when the area-length method was compared to contrast ventriculography (46). Van Rossum et al. (47) compared single-slice and multislice strategies against left ventriculography and found a strong correlation for the multislice method (*r* = 0.98) and

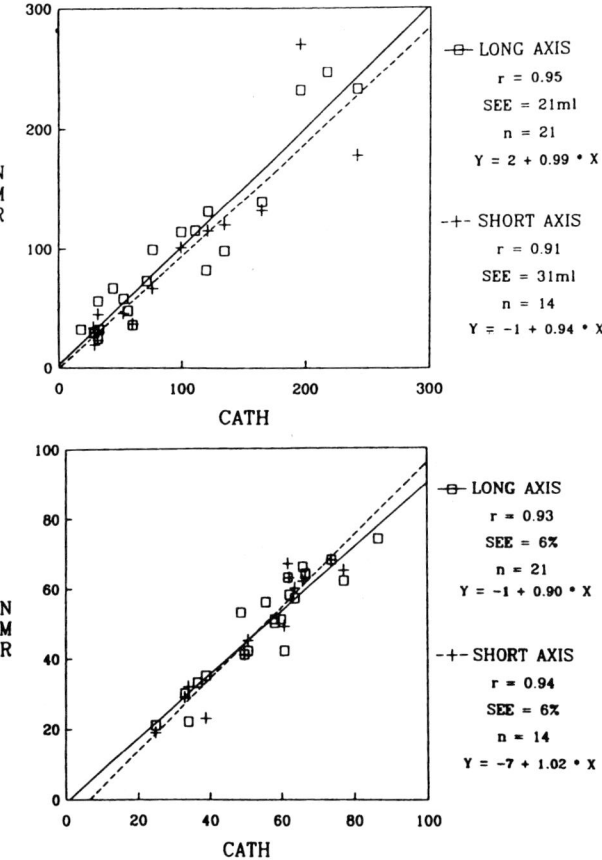

FIG. 8. Correlation of multislice, multiphase spin echo and long-axis cine MRI (NMR) and contrast ventriculography for assessment of left ventricle end-systolic volume (**top panel**). At **bottom** is the correlation of the same techniques for ejection fraction determination. *NMR*, nuclear magnetic resonance. (From ref. 4, with permission.)

TABLE 1. *Normal ventricular parameters derived from 47 normal males and 28 normal females using cine MRI and Simpson's method that may serve as normal reference values.[a]*

	All (n = 75)	Males (n = 47)	Females (n = 28)
LV ED volumes (mL)	121 ± 34 (55–187)	136 ± 30 (77–195)	96 ± 23 (52–141)
RV ED volumes (mL)	138 ± 40 (59–217)	157 ± 35 (88–227)	106 ± 24 (58–154)
LV ES (mL)	40 ± 14 (13–67)	45 ± 14 (19–72)	32 ± 9 (13–51)
RV ES (mL)	54 ± 21 (12–96)	63 ± 20 (23–103)	40 ± 14 (12–68)
IVSM (g)	54 ± 13 (28–80)	61 ± 11 (40–82)	42 ± 8 (26–58)
LVFWM (g)	104 ± 27 (44–150)	117 ± 22 (75–159)	82 ± 19 (46–119)
LVTM (g)	158 ± 39 (82–234)	178 ± 31 (118–238)	125 ± 26 (75–175)
RVFWM (g)	46 ± 11 (25–67)	50 ± 10 (30–70)	40 ± 8 (24–55)
LV EF (%)	67 ± 5 (57–78)	67 ± 5 (56–78)	67 ± 5 (56 –78)
RV EF (%)	61 ± 7 (47–76)	60 ± 7 (47–74)	63 ± 8 (47–80)
LVSV (mL)	82 ± 23 (36–127)	92 ± 21 (51–33)	65 ± 16 (33–97)
RVSV (mL)	84 ± 24 (37–131)	95 ± 22 (52–138)	66 ± 16 (35–98)
LVTM/LVEDV (g/mL)	1.33 ± 0.18 (0.98–1.68)	1.34 ± 0.19 (0.96–1.71)	1.31 ± 0.16 (0.99–1.63)
RVFWM/RVEDV (g/mL)	0.35 ± 0.06 (0.23–0.47)	0.33 ± 0.06 (0.21–0.44)	0.38 ± 0.05 (0.28–0.48)
LVTM/RVM	3.46 ± 0.66 (2.16–4.76)	3.64 ± 0.72 (2.23–5.04)	3.17 ± 0.43 (2.33–4.01)
CO (L/min)	5.2 ± 1.4 (2.42–8.05)	5.8 ± 3.0 (2.82 ± 8.82)	4.3 ± 0.9 (2.65–5.98)

[a] Ventricular parameters (mean ± 1 SD) with 95% confidence intervals (1.96 SD) in parentheses.
EF, ejection fraction; *CO*, cardiac output; *LVEDV, RVEDV*, left and right ventricular end diastolic volume; *LVES, RVES*, left and right ventricular end systolic volume; *IVSM*, interventricular septal mass; *LVFWM, RVFWM*, left and right ventricular free wall mass; *LVSV, RVSV*, left and right ventricular stroke volume: *LVTM*, left ventricular total mass; *RVM*, right ventricular mass.
(From ref. 44, with permission.)

a weak correlation with the single-slice technique. Gaudio et al. (48) compared MRI and radionuclide ventriculography in 32 patients with dilated cardiomyopathy and found a strong correlation ($r = 0.91$). These authors noted that MRI underestimated EF when compared to the nuclear method.

Cine MRI has been used to measure changes in LV volumes in congenital heart disease, both repaired and unrepaired. In 35 children with functional single ventricle, Fogel et al. (49) demonstrated that no changes in LV volume, mass, or ejection fraction occurred 6 to 9 months after the hemi-Fontan procedure, but that major decreases in all indices occurred 1 to 2 years after the Fontan procedure.

MRI has evolved into the reference method for evaluation of LV volumes and global function to compare new imaging modalities. Buck et al. (50) studied 23 patients with stable LV aneurysms and compared left ventricular end-diastolic volume (LVEDV), left ventricular end-systolic volume (LVESV), and left ventricular ejection fraction (LVEF) using three-dimensional echocardiography, two-dimensional echo, and biplane cineventriculography and using three-dimensional MRI as the gold standard. These investigators demonstrated that three-dimensional echo was quite accurate relative to the MR technique (Fig. 9).

Global Right Ventricular Size and Function

Right Ventricular Mass

The right ventricle is difficult to quantify in terms of mass and volumes because of its nongeometric shape. MR imaging can be used to measure RV mass, although precision is less than that for the LV. Doherty and associates (51) used

MRI in normal subjects and patients with dilated cardiomyopathy, demonstrating no difference in RV mass between groups, but showing excellent intra- and interobserver variability. Katz et al. (52) used spin-echo images of normals and patients with pulmonary hypertension and demonstrated good intra- and interobserver variability as well as a significant correlation between measured pulmonary artery pressure and RV mass ($r = 0.75$). Cine MRI was used by Lorenz et al. (53) to evaluate LV and RV mass and volumes in 22 patients after atrial repair of transposition of the great arteries (TGA). These investigators found markedly elevated RV mass in the patients late after repair.

Right Ventricular Volumes and Ejection Fraction

Because of the inability to model the right ventricle (RV), a multislice technique is optimal for measuring volumes and ejection fraction (EF). Boxt et al. (54) performed a study using a multislice spin-echo technique and Simpson's rule to measure RV volumes (Fig. 10). When compared to water displacement from RV casts, the correlation was excellent ($r = 0.98$). In patients with pulmonary hypertension, intra- and interobserver variability for measurement of RV end-diastolic volume index were good (10.3% and 5.8%, respectively). In a study by Pattynama et al. (55), the standard deviation for measurement of RV mass was 5.9 g and for RVEF 6.0%. Lorenz et al., in the study mentioned above (53), found normal RV cavity size and only mildly depressed RVEF in patients after atrial repair of TGA. Helbing et al. (56) studied gradient echo MR techniques as measurement of RV volumes and ejection fraction in 20 children with congenital heart disease and in 22 normal children and found

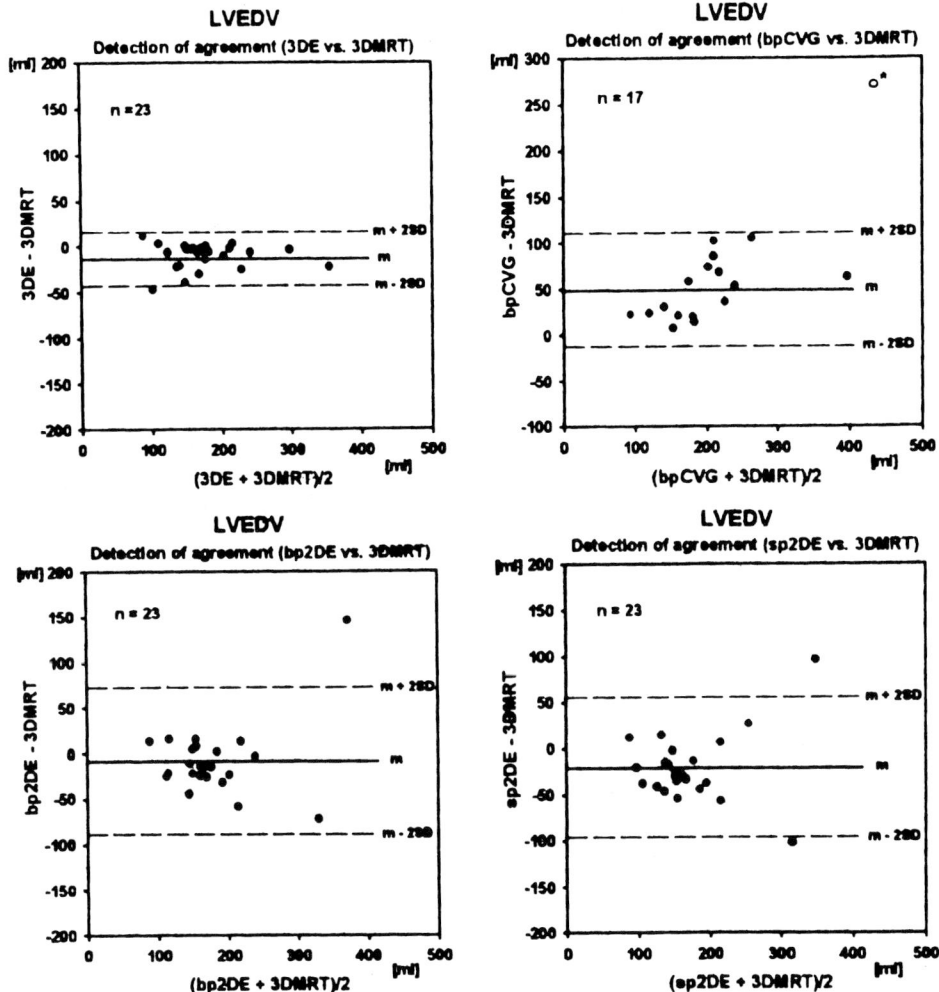

FIG. 9. Results of LV ejection fraction plotted as differences between methods and analysis of agreement. Note that the tightest agreement was for three dimensional echocardiography (*3DE*) versus three-dimensional MR tomography (*3D MRT*). *bp CVG*, biplane cineventriculography; *bp 2DE*, biplane two-dimensional echocardiography; *sp2DE*, single-plane, two-dimensional echocardiography; *outlier excluded from analysis. (From ref. 50, with permission.)

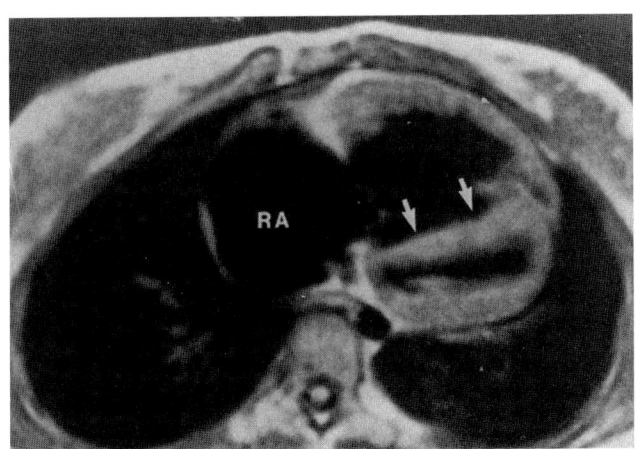

FIG. 10. Axial image at the level of the tricuspid valve in a patient with primary pulmonary hypertension. The right atrium (*RA*) is markedly enlarged. The right ventricle is markedly dilated and hypertrophied, and the interventricular septum (*arrows*) is flattened due to the volume and pressure overload. (From ref. 54, with permission.)

close correlation between RV and LV stroke volumes (r = 0.96).

Regional Left Venticular Function

The assessment of regional ventricular function is an integral part of the evaluation of patients with ischemic heart disease. A number of methods have been developed over recent years to accurately measure the function of the LV wall on a regional basis include cine MRI with the centerline approach, MR tagging, and phase velocity imaging.

Cine Magnetic Resonance Imaging

Cine magnetic resonance imaging (cine MRI) measures wall thickening, which is reduced early during ischemia. Wall thickening more accurately reflects the extent of myocardial dysfunction in ischemic heart disease than does wall motion (57). Limitations of other methods, such as echocardiography, include the problem of through-plane motion that can lead to imaging different regions of myocardium at end diastole and end systole. MRI can limit this problem because the imaging is defined in three-dimensional space. Peshock et al. (58) have measured regional wall thickening in normal subjects showing that the maximum systolic wall thickening is 60%. This group also studied patients with regional LV dysfunction in the setting of coronary artery disease. Compared to biplane ventriculography, MRI demonstrated re-

duced maximal percent systolic wall thickening with a sensitivity of 94% and specificity of 80%. Lotan et al. (59) studied 55 patients with cine MR and compared the results with biplane ventriculography. For 275 segments in the right anterior oblique view, absolute agreement was noted in 62% of segments and agreement within one wall-motion scoring grade was found in 96%. Similar results were found in the left anterior oblique view with complete agreement in 66% of segments and within one grade in 92% of segments.

Cine MRI has been studied in the setting of acute myocardial infarction to evaluate regional wall thickening. In 17 patients with wall-motion abnormalities identified by left ventriculography after Q-wave MI, Akins et al. (60) demonstrated abnormalities on MRI in 16 of the 17 patients. Wall thickness was reduced at the site of infarction, as was wall thickening. Meese and colleagues (61) studied 25 patients 1 week after thrombolytic therapy for acute MI. They showed good concordance between regional wall motion from MRI and left ventriculography.

More quantitative methods of assessing wall thickening have recently been developed. Holman et al. (62) used a centerline method initially developed for contrast ventriculography to measure wall thickening (Fig. 11). Endocardium and epicardium are contoured and 100 equidistant chords, each representing the wall thickness at that point, are placed perpendicular to the endocardial contour. The increase in length of each chord is calculated in order to calculate wall thickening. These investigators performed cine MRI in 25

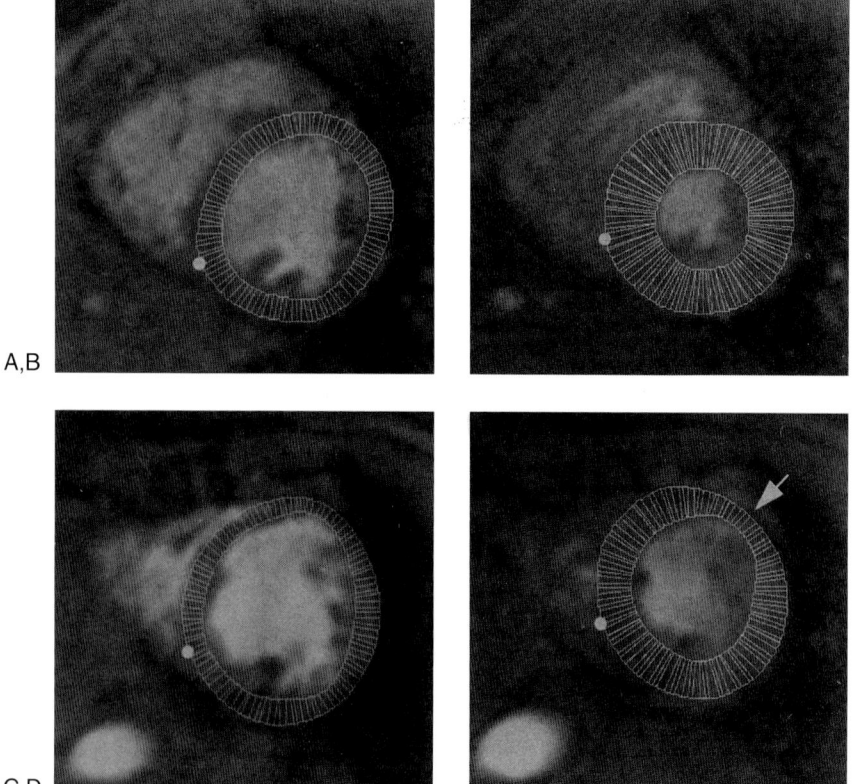

A,B

C,D

FIG. 11. These images demonstrate the quantitation of wall thickening from short-axis, gradient echo cine images at the mid-papillary level at end diastole (**A**) and end systole (**B**), using the centerline method (Holman). The endocardial and epicardial contours are shown as well as 100 equidistant chords, each representing the wall thickness at that point, that are placed perpendicular to the endocardial contour. The increase in length of each chord is calculated in order to calculate wall thickening. The starting points (*white dots*) on the end-diastolic and end-systolic images are used to correct for rotational motion. In a patient after anterior myocardial infarction, wall thinning is seen at end diastole (**C**) and lack of wall thickening at end-systole (**D**, *arrow*). (From ref. 62, with permission.)

patients on day 21 plus or minus 2 days following anterior MI and calculated the extent of dysfunctional myocardium as compared to a database of 48 normal volunteers. The enzymatically calculated infarct size correlated strongly with LV dysfunction as defined by the cine MRI ($r = 0.92$). Mean wall thickening in the distribution of the left anterior descending (LAD) artery was 46% plus or minus 8% compared to 87% plus or minus 3% in normals ($P < 0.001$), although wall thickness was not different at end-diastole.

Three-dimensional techniques for mapping wall thickening using cine MRI have been demonstrated to be superior to wall motion analysis for differentiating ischemic versus nonischemic regions in a dog model of acute ischemia (63).

Myocardial Tagging

In the past decade methods have been developed to track myocardial material points through the cardiac cycle to map regional ventricular function and quantify intramyocardial strains. Magnetic resonance tagging is a method in which magnetization is saturated within the imaging plane to "tag" the region of interest. This approach was initially reported by Zerhouni et al. (64) in 1988 and later adapted by Axel and colleagues (65) so that multiple parallel planes of saturation could be generated throughout the imaging plane. The tags or stripes remain embedded in myocardium and deform during systole, allowing the tracking of material points throughout the cardiac cycle. Different patterns of tags can be applied, including parallel one-dimensional lines, a two-dimensional grid (Fig. 12) (64), or radial stripes (66).

Validation of MR tagging for measuring myocardial wall thickening was performed initially by Beyar et al. (67) using a three-dimensional volume element approach, first in phantom studies and later in normal dogs and dogs with acute ischemia. Lima et al. (68) later validated this three-dimensional technique against sonomicrometers. One-, two-, and three-dimensional volume element approaches for calculating wall thickening were compared to sonomicrometers, and the best correlation was found with the three-dimensional method ($r = 0.95$). MRI overestimated the sonomicrometry values, an overestimation likely due to the effect of local dysfunction produced by the placement of sonomicrometry crystals in the myocardium.

Tag tracking was first performed on normal subjects using radial tags to measure myocardial torsion (69). Apical endocardial torsion was 19.1 ± 2.0 degrees in the counterclockwise direction (as viewed from the apex) and was 8 ± 1.9 degrees in the epicardium. Torsion increased with increasing distance from base to apex. Rogers et al. (70) used MR tagging to describe the systolic long-axis shortening of the LV, which is greatest at the base (moving 12.8 ± 3.8mm toward the apex). The mid-LV moved 6.9 ± 2.6mm, while the apex was nearly stationary, moving only 1.6 ± 2.2mm. Clark et al. (71) performed a one-dimensional analysis of intramyocardial shortening in normal volunteers. These investigators found a transmural and longitudinal gradient in intramyocar-

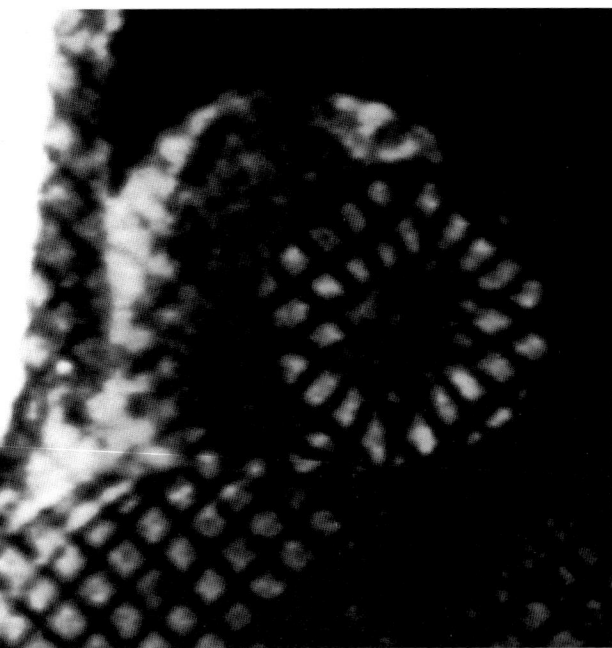

FIG. 12. Short-axis, gradient echo-tagged end-systolic image in a double oblique plane in the basal left ventricle in a normal subject. Note that the tag stripes deform greatest at the subendocardium and least within the subepicardium. No tag deformation is seen in stationary tissues such as the diapraghm in this breath-hold image.

dial shortening throughout the LV with the greatest shortening at the subendocardium (44% ± 6%) relative to the midwall (30% ± 6%) and subepicardium (22% ± 5%) and in the apex, relative to more basal regions.

Intramyocardial shortening has been examined in a variety of patient groups. In hypertensive patients with left ventricular hypertrophy and normal ejection fraction, Palmon et al. (72) demonstrated reduced circumferential and longitudinal shortening (Fig. 13). Mean subendocardial circumferential shortening was 29% ± 6% in hypertensive subjects compared to 44±6% in normal subjects ($P = 0.0001$). Therefore, hypertensive patients demonstrate contractile dysfunction despite the presence of normal overall pump function. In patients with hypertrophic cardiomyopathy, reduced percent circumferential shortening has been demonstrated in the anterior, septal, and inferior walls in regions characterized histologically by myofibrillar disarray and interstitial fibrosis (73) (Fig. 14). Longitudinal shortenening was likewise reduced relative to normals in the septum, most markedly in the base, but was normal in the lateral free wall.

The advent of k-space segmentation and breath-hold tagged imaging (74) has allowed imaging of patients with more acute heart disease. A study of 28 patients on day 5 after first anterior MI with single-vessel LAD disease demonstrated reduced circumferential shortening in basal lateral and midinferior regions, remote from the infarcted territory (75) (Fig. 15). Potential explanations for this dysfunction include abnormal coronary flow reserve in these regions,

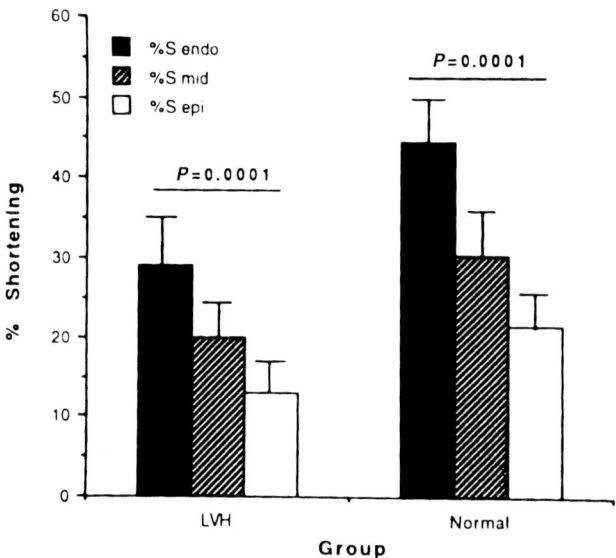

FIG. 13. Bar graph showing percent of circumferential shortening (*%S*) in endocardium (*endo*), midwall (*mid*), and epicardium (*epi*) in normal subjects (*n* = 10) and in subjects with left ventricular hypertrophy (*LVH, n* = 26). Note the gradient in *%S* from endocardium to epicardium in both groups and the reduced shortening in *LVH* at all levels compared to normals. (From ref. 72, with permission.)

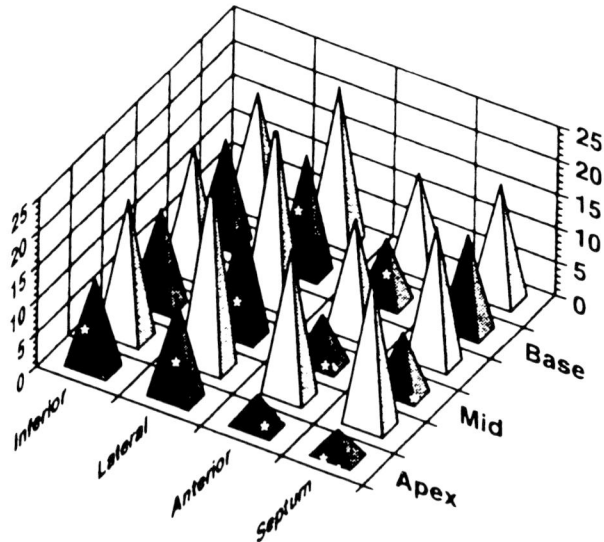

FIG. 15. Three-dimensional graph of intramyocardial circumferential shortening in 28 patients after first reperfused anterior myocardial infarction (*black pyramids*) and 10 human volunteers (*white pyramids*). *P < 0.05 versus normal subjects. Shortening is depressed as expected in the infarcted apex and midanterior, septal, and lateral walls, but was unexpectedly depressed in the basal lateral wall and trended lower in the midinferior wall, regions remote from the infarction. (From ref. 75, with permission.)

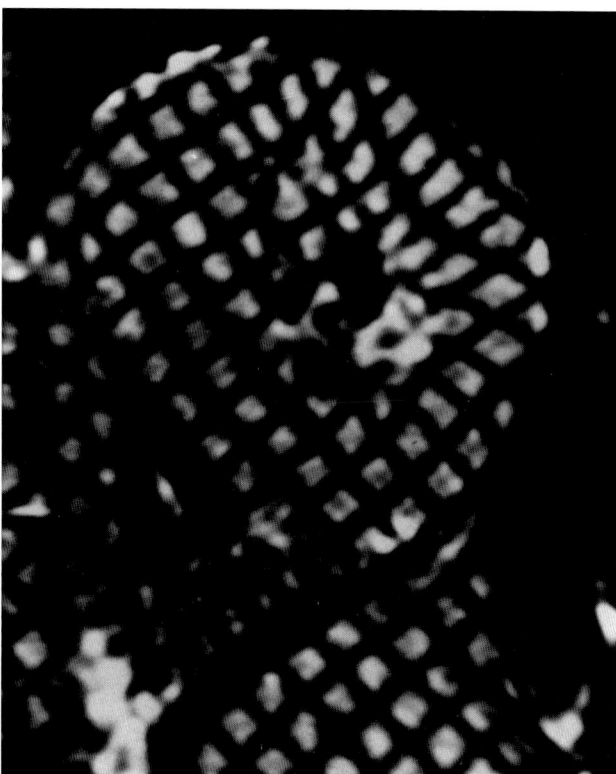

FIG. 14. Short-axis tagged double oblique image in the mid-left ventricle in a patient with hypertrophic cardiomyopathy. There is significant hypertrophy and reduced deformation of the anterior wall (*9 o'clock* to *12 o'clock* on the image), septum (*6 o'clock* to *9 o'clock*), and inferior wall (*3 o'clock* to *6 o'clock*).

altered local mechanical load, or tethering to infarcted regions. When 26 of these patients were imaged with breath-hold MR tagging 8 weeks later (28), remote region dysfunction had resolved, and circumferential shortening had improved in the infarcted apex and midanterior and midseptal regions. Despite the improvement in regional function and improved ejection fraction from 39% ± 12% to 45% ± 14%, LV end-diastolic volume index increased from 82 ± 24 mL/ m² to 96 ± 27 mL/m².

Regional myocardial strain or deformation in two and three dimensions can be analyzed using a finite element approach (76,77). This technique is based on the assumption that strain within a complex structure may be computed by subdividing it into small "elements" that have homogeneous properties. Using the tag intersections as trackable points, intramyocardial strain can be calculated without including bulk motion of the whole heart. The original position of each tag intersection is compared to the position at a deformed state and a tensor describing the magnitude and direction (vector) of displacement defined. By defining a tensor made up of two perpendicular tag segments, the magnitude and direction of maximal deformation may be computed. These values can be transformed to the "heart" coordinate system in which strain in the radial (wall thickening), and circumferential (i.e., circumferential shortening) may be determined.

Marcus et al. (78) used two-dimensional analysis techniques to demonstrate that the greatest abnormalities in strain parameters in 10 patients after anterior MI in comparison to normal subjects were within infarcted regions. These investigators found a decrease in systolic lengthening in the midanteroseptum from 1.27 ± 0.04 to 1.10 ± 0.06 and an increase in remote posterolateral regions (1.48 ± 0.11 compared to 1.36 ± 0.07 in normal volunteers). In patients with idiopathic dilated cardiomyopathy (IDC), MacGowan and colleagues (79) analyzed tagged images in a two-dimensional fashion. They then derived fiber direction from *ex vivo* hearts. These investigators demonstrated that endocardial and epicardial fiber strain was reduced in the patients with IDC compared to normal subjects and that cross-fiber strain was similarly reduced in the endocardium of patients. Shortening in the cross-fiber direction was relatively preserved in patients with IDC.

Three-dimensional analytic techniques have been applied in a variety of clinical populations. Young et al. (77) studied 7 patients with hypertrophic cardiomyopathy and compared their three-dimensional strain characteristics with 12 normal subjects. The principal strain associated with three-dimensional maximal contraction was slightly depressed throughout, especially in the basal septum (−0.18 ± 0.05 versus −0.22 ± 0.02 in normals) and anterior walls (−0.20 ± 0.05 versus −0.23 ± 0.02), whereas LV torsion was actually greater in hypertrophic cardiomyopathy (HCM) patients (19.9 ± 2.4 degrees versus 14.6 ± 2.7 degrees). Dong et al. (80) demonstrated that the reduced regional function demonstrated in such patients with MR tagging correlated with the extent of hypertrophy.

Patients with chronic right ventricular pressure overload have been studied with MR tagging. Dong et al. (81) used three-dimensional analysis in 9 patients with RV pressure overload and demonstrated reduced thickening and circumferential and longitudinal shortening in the septum. The flattening of the septum at end-systole also lead to reduced endocardial circumferential shortening in other LV regions. Fayad et al. (82) examined RV regional function using one-dimensional tags in 7 patients with chronic pulmonary hypertension and showed that regional short-axis shortening and long-axis shortening were reduced in patients. The greatest decrease in regional function was in the right ventricular outflow tract (RVOT) and basal septum.

Tagging has been used to evaluate regional ventricular function in repaired and unrepaired congenital heart disease. In 33 children with a single ventricle who underwent staged reconstruction leading to the Fontan procedure, Fogel et al. (83) demonstrated that patients before hemi-Fontan or after the Fontan had the highest compressive strains. Regional heterogeneity of strain was least in the Fontan group. In all patients, radial contraction was greatest in the superior walls and least in the inferior walls. Fogel et al. have also used tagging to study ventricular-ventricular interactions by comparing single right ventricle after Fontan to patients with transposition of the great arteries after atrial inversion procedure (84,85). These authors found that strain was greatest and heterogeneity of strain least in patients with the latter. They concluded that the pulmonary pumping LV interacted

with the systemic RV to allow for increased absolute strain but more homogenous strain than a systemic RV without an attached LV.

Phase Velocity Imaging

The MR velocity mapping technique encodes the velocity of moving structures quantitatively in the phase of the MR signal rather than the magnitude that is used for most MR images. The velocity of the myocardium can be measured throughout the cardiac cycle (Fig. 16) and can be derived for each point on the wall (86). A limitation of this technique is that wall velocity is the principal measurement. To derive displacement of a point, velocity must then be multiplied by time, and the accuracy becomes limited by the accuracy of the cumulative velocity measurements. In addition, velocity is usually measured in one plane while deriving two- or three-dimensional velocity requires multiple acquisitions, so that the clinical utility of the resultant long scanning time is decreased. Clinical applications of phase velocity mapping have been limited. Karwatowski et al. demonstrated regional differences in normal volunteers (87) and in patients with ischemic heart disease (88).

van Wedeen et al. (89) developed an MR method of depicting myocardial strain-rate or the incremental change in deformation per unit of time (the time between image phases). The strain-rate tensor (Fig. 17) at each tensor at each pixel is represented by a rhomboid that depicts the effect of the measured strain rate on a square at each locus. In this way, the myocardial state of motion at a particular point in time during the cardiac cycle can be displayed without cine images. Beache et al. (90) used this technique to

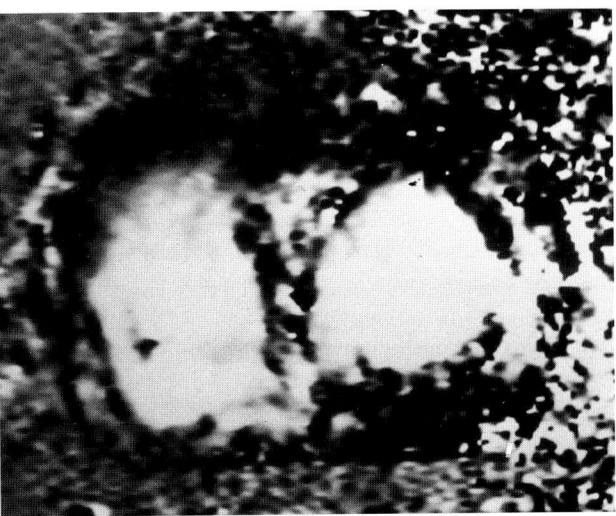

FIG. 16. Phase contrast image in the short-axis plane at mid-diastole in a normal subject. The velocity of the moving structures, i.e., intracavitary blood and myocardium is encoded and is directional (*white* is one direction and *black* the other). These signals can be processed to create a "velocity map" of the region of interest.

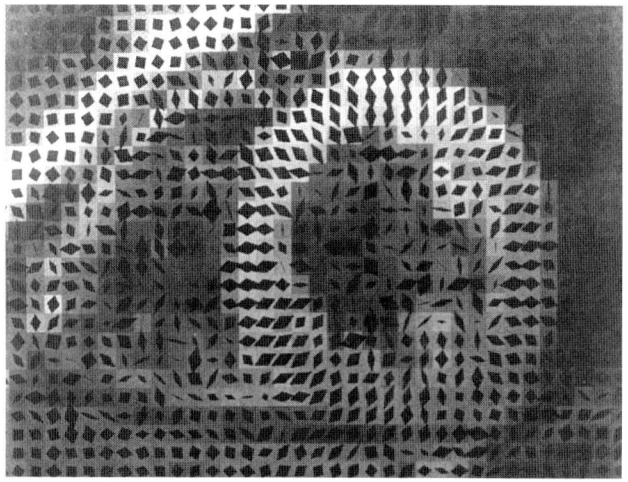

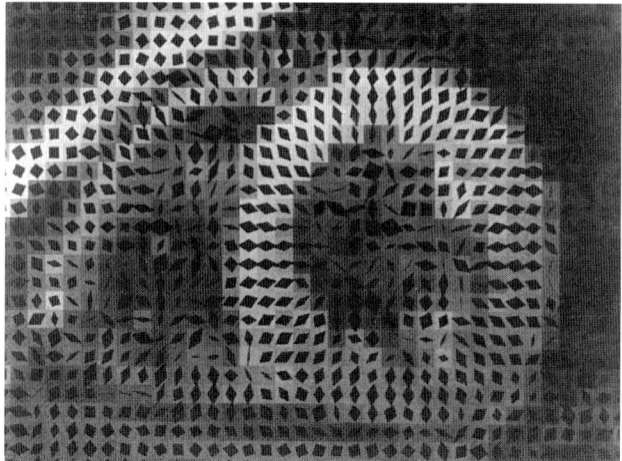

FIG. 17. Motionless movie of myocardial strain rate from echo planar short-axis images during systole. The strain-rate tensor at each tensor at each pixel is represented by a rhomboid that depicts the effect of the measured strain rate on a square at each locus. In this way the myocardial state of motion at a particular point in time during the cardiac cycle can be displayed without cine images. Strain rates are oriented in a radial direction in the myocardium, consistent with normal thickening and circumferential shortening. (From ref. 89, with permission.)

map systolic and diastolic intramural mechanics in 11 controls and 8 patients with hypertrophic cardiomyopathy, demonstrating an increase in the heterogeneity of strain-rate in diastole in patients with hypertrophic cardiomyopathy.

Diastolic Function

The evaluation of diastolic function is a newer application of MRI. Cine MRI has been performed at 32 phases of the cardiac cycle using semiautomatic analysis to define LV volumes at each time point (91). The ratio of early-to-late peak filling rates and the percentage of LV filling during early diastole distinguished patients with diastolic dysfunction from normal subjects. In another study of patients with in-

creased wall thickness and normal Doppler echocardiographic measures of diastolic function, cine MRI demonstrated abnormalities in diastolic function (92).

Functional Response to Pharmacologic Stress

Normal Subjects

Progressive adrenergic stress, using dobutamine, has become an important method for the detection of provocable myocardial ischemia. Cine magnetic resonance imaging has been used in conjunction with dobutamine stress to evaluate wall thickening in normal subjects (93). These investigators studied 23 patients, but they were limited by long image acquisition times to imaging only at rest and during peak dobutamine infusion (15 μg/kg/min). They evaluated wall thickening and changes in endocardial areas from 6 slices from apex to base. Power et al. (94) studied 13 normal subjects during dobutamine infusion to a peak dose of 20 μg/kg/min with tagged cine MRI. Mean percent circumferential shortening increased from 21% $\pm$ 4% to a maximum of 26% $\pm$ 3% at 10 μg/kg/min dobutamine before any increase in heart rate or blood pressure occurred (Fig. 18).

Ischemia

The clinical utility of dobutamine stress echocardiography for diagnosing ischemia in the presence of coronary artery disease is well documented (95). Several studies have been performed using dobutamine stress in an MRI environment to diagnose ischemia. Pennell et al. (96) studied 25 patients with angina and abnormal exercise electrocardiograms with dobutamine stress to a maximal dose of 20μg/kg/min. Dobutamine induced chest discomfort in 96% of the patients, and 11 of 25 completed the full protocol to 20μg/kg/min. The wall motion abnormalities noted by cine MRI during stress

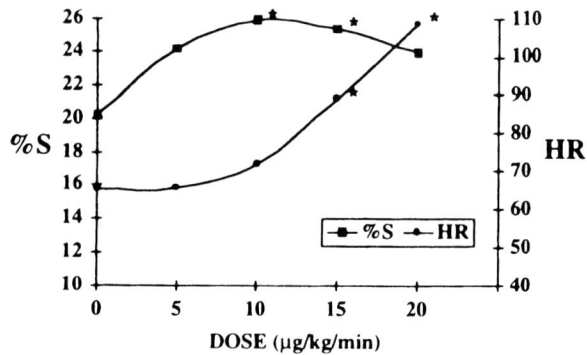

FIG. 18. Percent circumferential shortening (*squares*, on the left y axis) and heart rate (*circles*, on the right y axis) plotted against increasing doses of dobutamine (from 0 to 20 μg/kg/min). Percent shortening increases up to 10μg/kg/min dobutamine and then plateaus, whereas heart rate does not increase until the 15μg/kg/min dose. *$P < 0.01$ versus baseline. (From ref. 94, with permission.)

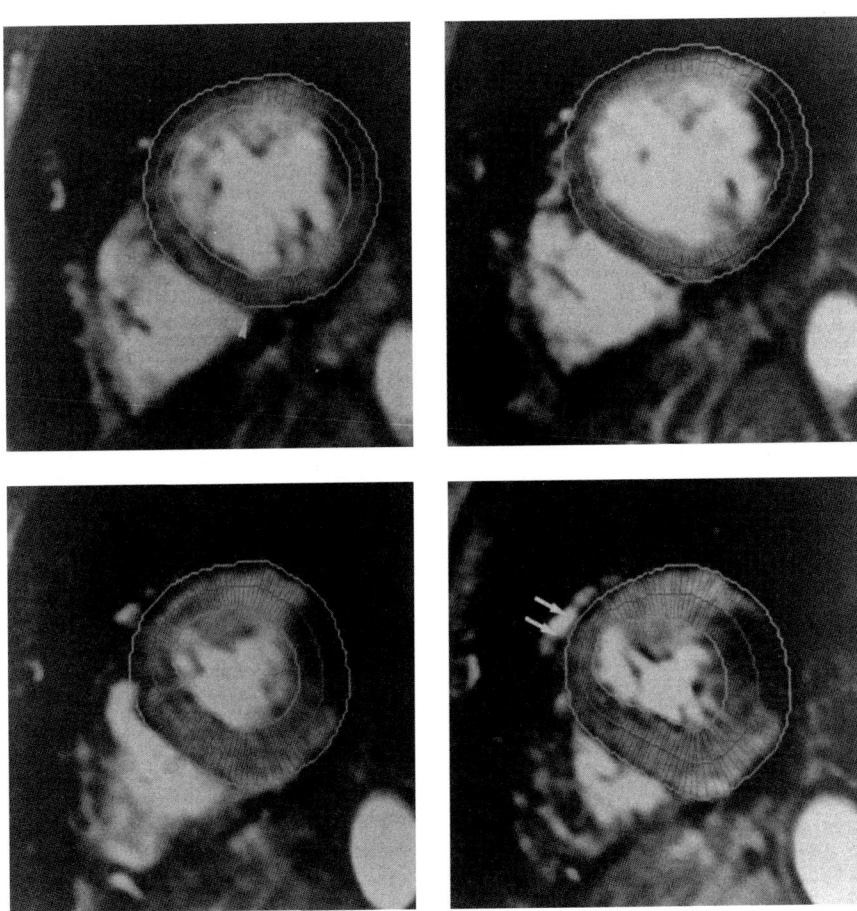

FIG. 19. Four short-axis images at the midpapillary level at end diastole (**top**) and end systole (**bottom**) at rest (**left**) and at peak dobutamine (**right**) in a patient with coronary artery disease in the left anterior descending coronary artery (**right**). Wall thickening is normal around the short axis at rest on the left and reduced in the anterior wall at peak dobutamine on the right (*arrows*). (From ref. 100, with permission.)

imaging corresponded to the location and extent of reversible ischemia on thallium scintigraphy in 95% of patients.

Van Rugge et al. (97) qualitatively analyzed wall motion with cine MRI and dobutamine infusion in patients with coronary disease and found a sensitivity of 81% and specificity of 100%. The same investigators employed a more quantitative approach using cine MRI and the centerline method in 39 patients with coronary artery disease and 10 normal subjects (98) (Fig. 19). This quantitative technique increased the sensitivity to 91% at the expense of a lower specificity (80%). In 32 patients with coronary artery disease, Baer et al. (99) showed an overall sensitivity of 84% for dobutamine stress MRI when compared with single-photon emission computed tomography MIBI scans. These results for dobutamine MRI compare quite favorably with dobutamine stress echocardiography and underscore the safety of the procedure in the MR environment.

Viability after Acute Myocardial Infarction

The evaluation of myocardial viability, defined as contractile reserve of dysfunctional myocardium, becomes important in the setting of the post-MI patient and the patient with chronic ischemic heart disease who is a candidate for revascularization. Imaging methods, such as dobutamine stress echocardiography (DSE), have been applied in these

situations (100). Cine MRI without tagging has been used recently to examine postinfarct viability. Dendale et al. (101) studied 37 patients early after acute MI with low-dose dobutamine cine MRI and echo using qualitative assessment of wall motion for both imaging modalities. Concordance between DSE and dobutamine cine MRI in identifying viable and nonviable segments was 81% in the 24 patients who had a follow-up study. The sensitivity and specificity of dobutamine MRI was 91% and 69%, respectively, and of DSE, 82% and 85%, respectively. Overall accuracy was not different (79% for MRI and 83% for echocardiography).

Dendale et al. (102) used follow-up MRI rather than follow-up echocardiography to validate the findings of early post-MI dobutamine cine MRI for predicting viability. These investigators studied 20 patients with a recent reperfused first MI, 14 of whom were subsequently revascularized by coronary artery bypass and angioplasty. A semiquantitative analysis of dobutamine response in short-axis MR images was used. Of these patients, 45% demonstrated viability with low-dose dobutamine infusion. On a per patient basis, the positive predictive and negative predictive values were 89% and 73%, respectively, with an overall accuracy of 80%. On a per-segment basis, accuracy was 74%. In akinetic segments compared to hypokinetic segments, the positive predictive value was higher but the negative predictive value lower.

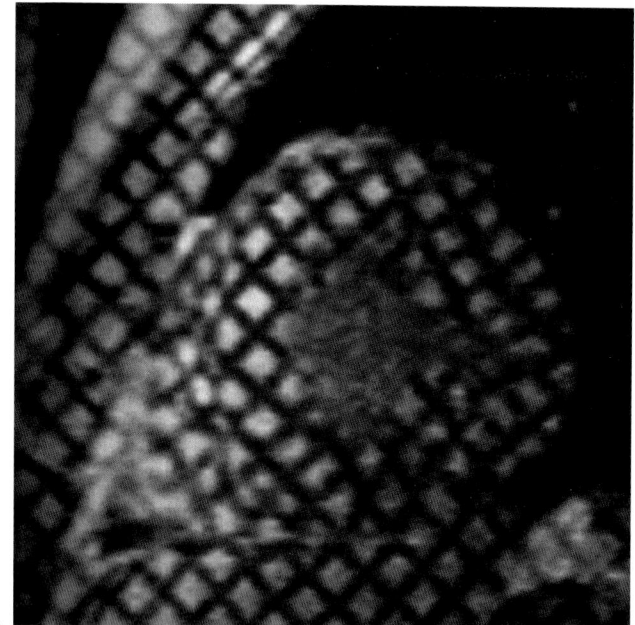

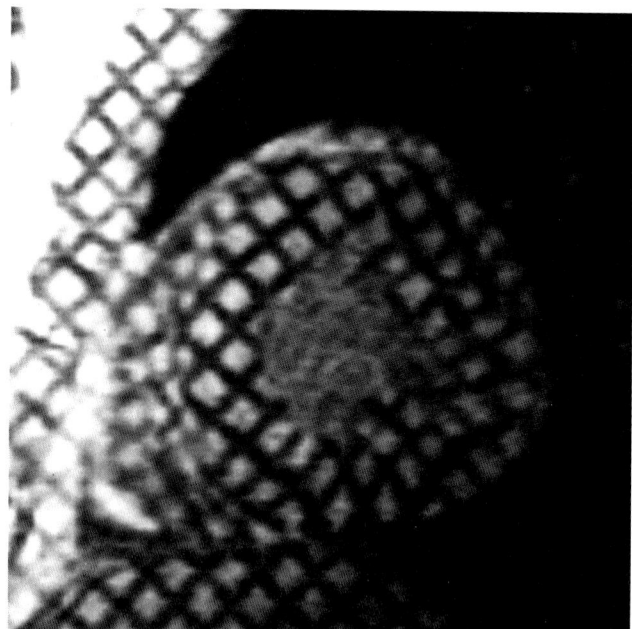

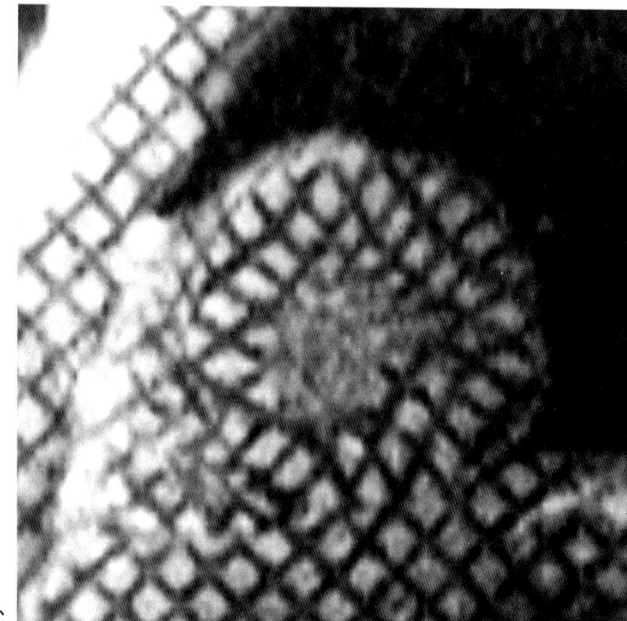

FIG. 20. A: End-systolic apical magnetic resonance tagged short-axis image in a patient on day 5 after anterior myocardial infarct (MI). The right ventricular apex and interventricular septum lie from *6 o'clock* to *9 o'clock* on the image, the anterior wall from *9 o'clock* to *12 o'clock,* the lateral wall from *12 o'clock* to *3 o'clock,* and the inferior wall from *3 o'clock* to *6 o'*clock. Percent intramyocardial circumferential shortening (%S) was −3% in the anterior wall denoting stretching rather than shortening, 3% in the septum (reduced compared to the normal data base), and 15% in the lateral wall (also reduced). **B:** End-systolic apical magnetic resonance tagged short-axis image in the same patient at the end of the 10 μg/kg/min dobutamine stage. Qualitatively, there is no longer stretching in the anterior wall, but otherwise it is difficult to discern significant changes within other regions. Quantitatively, %S increased normally (≥5% increase) in all walls. **C:** End-systolic apical magnetic resonance tagged short-axis image in the same patient at 8 weeks post-MI. Function has improved all around the short axis, and the end-systolic cavity area is reduced. Quantitatively, %S has increased to 24% in the anterior wall, 18% in the septum, and 27% in the lateral wall, all of which fall within the range of normal. (From ref. 103, with permission.)

Therefore, low-dose dobutamine MRI underestimated viability in akinetic segments.

Geskin et al. (103) studied 20 patients with a first reperfused MI on day 4 and week 8 post-MI with tagged MRI and low-dose dobutamine (5 and 10 g/kg/min) (Fig. 20). Mean %S was 15% ± 11% at baseline, increased to 16% ± 10% at 5 μg/kg/min dobutamine, 21% ± 10% at peak, and to 18% ± 10% at 8 weeks. The increase in %S with peak dobutamine was greater in dysfunctional myocardium (+ 9% ± 10%) than in normal tissue (+4% ± 12%). In dysfunctional regions that responded normally to peak dobutamine (greater than or equal to a 5% increase in %S), the increase in %S from baseline to 8 weeks post-MI (+9% ± 9%) was greater than in those regions that did not respond

normally (+5% ± 9%, *P* < 0.04). On a per-region basis, the sensitivity of the normal response to peak dobutamine (a greater than or equal to 5% increase in %S) for the return of function to normal was 87% with a specificity of 43%. The positive predictive accuracy was 56%, and the negative predictive accuracy 83%. Midmyocardial and subepicardial response to dobutamine were predictive of functional recovery, but the subendocardial response was not.

Viability in Chronic Myocardial Infarction

Dobutamine MRI has been studied as a predictor of viability after revascularization in patients with chronic LV dysfunction. Baer et al. (104) studied the predictive value of low-dose dobutamine MRI compared to the gold standard of flourine-18 fluorodeoxyglucose positron emission tomography (FDG PET) for viability in 35 patients with chronic infarction (more than 4 months old) (Fig. 21). They demonstrated that MRI findings of end-diastolic wall thickness of less than 6mm and wall thickening of less than 1mm were indicative of lack of viability. When these two findings were combined, the sensitivity was 88% and specificity was 87% with positive predictive accuracy of 92% for signs of viability on FDG-PET images. When dobutamine MRI was compared to dobutamine transesophageal echocardiography

(TEE) using the same definition of viability (105), the sensitivities were 77% and 81% and the specificities were 94% versus 100%, respectively.

In a subsequent study, the same group evaluated 43 patients with a chronic infarct with baseline MRI and a repeat study after revascularization to measure functional recovery (106). Recovery was noted in 63% of patients. The dobutamine-induced wall thickening was similarly as sensitive for functional recovery as for end-diastolic wall thickness (89% versus 92%) but much more specific (92% versus 56%).

VALVULAR HEART DISEASE

Techniques

Spin Echo

Multislice, multiphase spin-echo techniques give excellent border definition for measurement of chamber volumes, ejection fraction, and mass but are no longer used as frequently due to the poor temporal resolution and the long acquisition times required. The technique has been used for measurement of differences in right and left ventricular stroke volumes to measure regurgitant volumes in isolated valvular regurgitation (107,108).

Cine Gradient Echo

Cine gradient echo MRI is a ''white blood'' technique that has the advantage of providing multiple sequential images through the cardiac cycle in a single slice with excellent temporal resolution and border detection. Abnormal flow can cause dephasing of spins, which then results in a signal void (109,110) and can be used for identification of regurgitant or stenotic valvular lesions. Breath-hold cine MR techniques using a segmented k-space approach allows multiphase imaging of a single slice in a single breath hold.

Velocity-encoded Cine

The ability of MRI to measure the phase shifts of protons as they move through a magnetic field gradient is termed velocity-encoded (VEC) or phase-contrast cine MR imaging. The degree of phase shift can be measured to determine velocity of flow because phase shift is proportional to motion over time. A magnitude and a phase image are displayed, and the direction of velocity encoding can be selected in any three-dimensional orientation. The velocity map may be through-plane, with the jet perpendicular to the imaging plane, or in-plane, with the chosen plane including the jet. The Bernoulli equation ($\Delta P = 4V^2$) is used to relate velocity (V) to the pressure difference (ΔP) on either side of a stenotic orifice. Measures of velocity can be integrated over an area of interest, such as a blood vessel or cardiac chamber, and a flow volume calculated. This method has been validated with flow phantoms by Meier et al. (111) and on flow

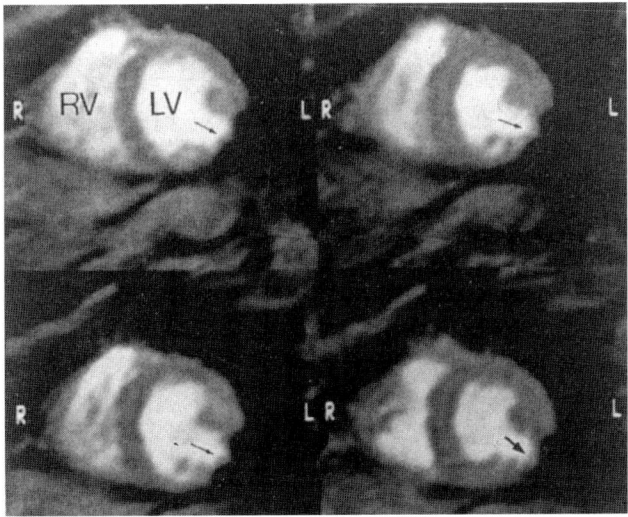

A

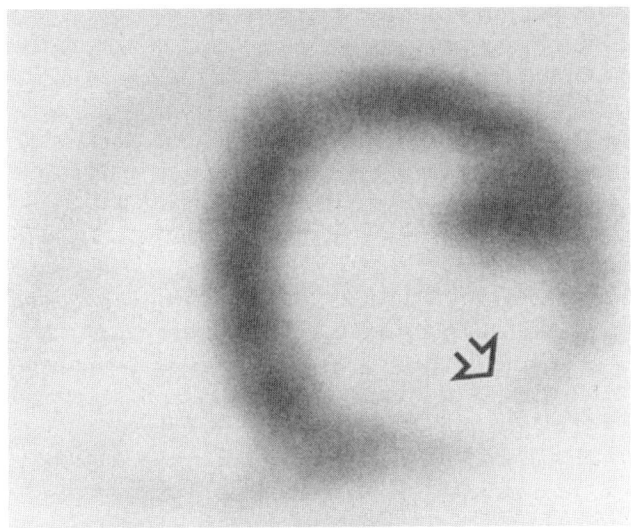

B

FIG. 21. Midventricular short-axis tomograms of a patient s/p inferolateral myocardial infarction. **A:** The magnetic resonance images are rest (**top set**) and dobutamine stress (**lower set**) at end diastole (**left**) and end systole (**right**). Wall thickness is reduced at end diastole and wall thickening is reduced in the inferolateral region both at rest and with dobutamine (*arrows*). This corresponds well with the [^{18}F]fluorodeoxyglucose (FDG) positron emission tomograph, (**B**) which demonstrates markedly reduced FDG uptake. *R*, right; *RV*, right ventricle; *L*, left; *LV*, left ventricle. (From ref. 104, with permission.)

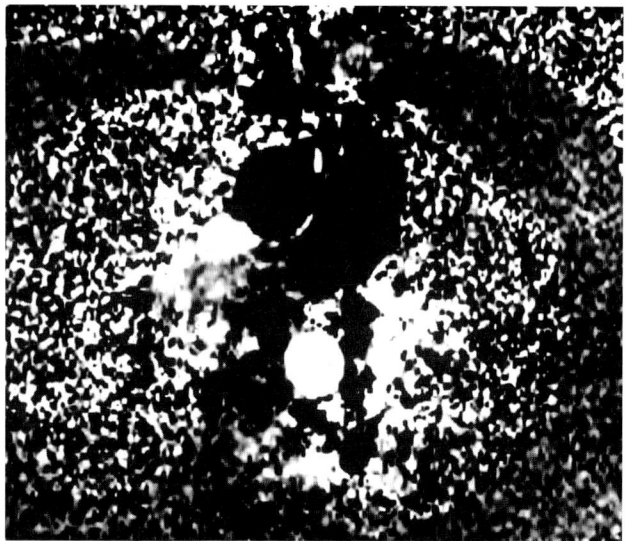

FIG. 22. Axial velocity-encoded cine image during early systole demonstrating flow in the ascending aorta toward the head (*white circle*) and flow toward the feet in the descending aorta (*black circle*).

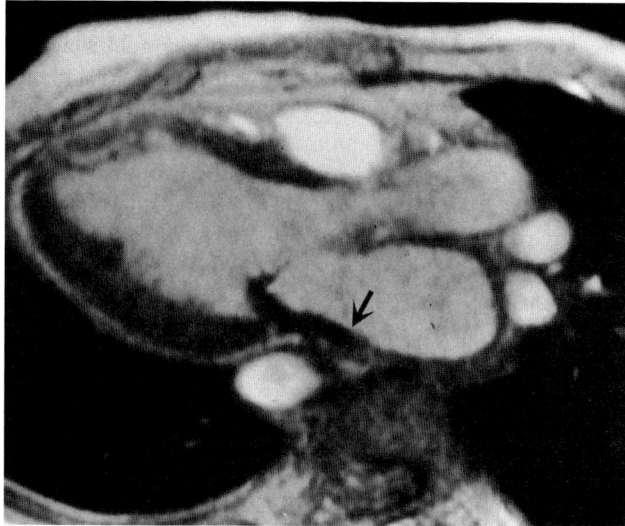

FIG. 23. Double oblique midsystolic gradient echo cine image through the left ventricle, mitral valve, left atrium, and aorta demonstrating an eccentric jet of mitral regurgitation represented by the signal void along the posterolateral left atrium (*arrow*).

in the aorta and pulmonary artery of normal subjects (112,113) (Fig. 22).

Potential limitations of the VEC MRI technique include the malalignment of the flow direction and the direction of flow encoding. The error is proportional to the cosine of the difference between the two angles and, therefore, the larger the angle, the greater the error. To counteract this limitation, a three-dimensional flow encoding method can be applied to improve the accuracy (114), although temporal resolution suffers and the true peak velocity may be missed. Another potential limitation is the presence of higher order motion, which can lead to nonlinearity of phase velocity. This problem can be conquered by using an ultrashort flow-encoding gradient (115). Finally, aliasing is a potential limitation. To prevent aliasing, the operator must choose a velocity to encode prior to the acquisition that is higher than the predicted maximal velocity.

Echo Planar Imaging

The fastest MR imaging technique available is echo planar imaging (EPI) in which acquisition times are in tens of milliseconds. However, this technique is not universally available due to the specialized hardware requirements. Nonetheless, single-shot EPI can be used to quantitate flow (114). Valve leaflet motion has also been studied with this technique (116).

Quantitation

Regurgitant Lesions

Using gradient echo cine techniques, regurgitation is recognized as signal voids, and their size correlates well with

color Doppler echocardiographic jet size (117) (Fig. 23). Many factors, however, can alter the size of signal void, reducing its effectiveness at quantitating the severity of regurgitation. These include hardware differences, complexities of regurgitant orifice size and volume, inclusion of nonregurgitant blood in jets, orientation of the imaging plane, changes in echo time (TE), etc. (118).

Other more quantitative techniques include the proximal convergence zone method, LV and RV stroke volume differences, and velocity-encoded cine MRI. The proximal convergence zone method is based on the continuity principle, such that the product of the hemispheric surface area of the proximal convergence zone and the velocity through the zone is an estimate of regurgitant flow rate. This method has been applied to aortic regurgitation (AR) and found to differentiate grades of AR (119,120).

In patients with single, isolated regurgitant lesions, the difference between RV and LV stroke volume can be calculated to estimate regurgitant volume (12,122). With more than one regurgitant lesion, this calculation is inaccurate. Two different methods are used to measure regurgitant flow by velocity-encoded MRI (VEC MRI). In one, regurgitant volume is calculated as the difference between LV and RV stroke volumes as measured from velocities in the aorta and pulmonary artery, respectively. This technique has been applied with excellent results in patients with AR (123,124).

Stenotic Lesions

Similar to Doppler echocardiography, the interrogation of stenotic valvular lesions makes use of the continuity equation to estimate functional valvular area. Velocity-encoded

MRI has theoretic advantages in that there are no limitations on maximum velocity measures, and it is a three-dimensional technique so the true direction of flow across the stenotic orifice can be examined. Potential limitations of these techniques include that alignment of the VEC slice truly perpendicular to the stenotic jet is problematic in eccentric jets and its distance from the stenotic valve may cause difficulties. If it is too far removed from the valve, signal loss can occur due to turbulence. If it is too close to the valve, the leaflets may interfere with the measurement of the jet velocity. In addition, image analysis can be a prohibitively long process. More recent work suggests that the use of short TE times (less than 4 msec) and using a plane parallel to the stenotic jet (in-plane velocity mapping) improves accuracy of velocity measures (125,126).

Individual Valvular Lesions

Mitral Regurgitation

Early work in the area of quantitation of mitral regurgitation was performed with the technique of measuring signal void from cine MRI. In a study of 26 patients with mitral regurgitation (MR), the extent and degree of signal loss correlated well with the severity of mitral regurgitation by either Doppler echocardiography or contrast ventriculography (127). Aurigemma and colleagues (128) measured the ratio of maximal flow void to left atrial and LV area in 40 patients with mitral regurgitation and found a good correlation with pulsed or color Doppler echocardiography.

Most of the recent work in measuring the volume of MR has been performed with VEC MRI. Fujita et al. (129) demonstrated in 19 patients with isolated mitral regurgitation, that by measuring regurgitant fraction using mitral inflow and aortic outflow velocities, the mitral regurgitation severity correlated well with color Doppler echocardiographic methods ($r = 0.87$). Hundley et al. (130) compared VEC MRI data with angiographic measures and found an excellent correlation for LVEDV ($r = 0.95$), LVESV ($r = 0.95$), and regurgitant fraction ($r = 0.96$) (Fig. 24).

Aortic Regurgitation

AR has been measured using cine MRI with evaluation of the created signal void (Fig. 25). Wagner et al. (117) used this technique in aortic regurgitation (AR) and mitral regurgitation (MR) to demonstrate high diagnostic accuracy (over 92%) for both techniques. Aurigemma and co-workers (131) used the same methods in AR as for MR and again demonstrated excellent correlation with Doppler. Sondergaard et al. (123) used the regurgitant volume approach in 10 patients with AR with an excellent correlation ($r = 0.97$) to aortic root angiography. They used VEC MRI to demonstrate close correlations of LV end-diastolic volume and regurgitant volume to the angiographic methods. Using VEC MRI, Dulce et al. (132) showed high accuracy ($r = 0.98$) and interstudy reproducibility ($r = 0.97$) of the tech-

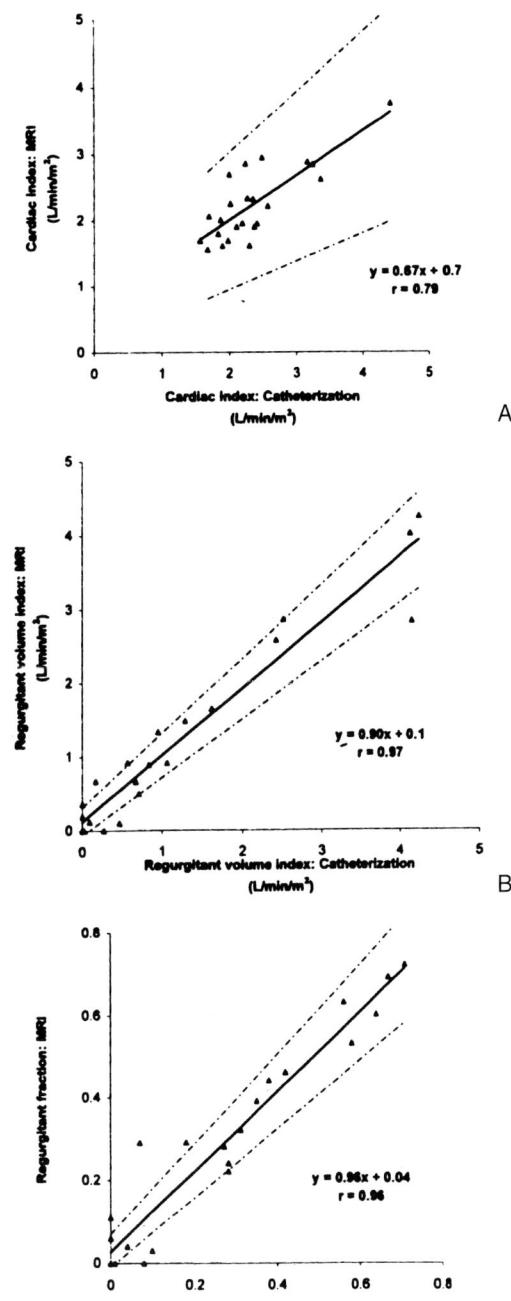

FIG. 24. Scatterplots demonstrating correlations between MRI and catheterization values for cardiac index (**A**), regurgitant volume index (**B**), and regurgitant fraction (**C**). *Dashed lines* represent the ± 95% confidence intervals for the regression equations. (From ref. 130, with permission.)

nique for measuring retrograde diastolic flow in the ascending aorta in chronic AR, which is equivalent to AR volume. Another method was developed by Ambrosi et al. (133) who applied a transverse saturation band above the aorta and measured its retrograde movement in the ascending and descending aorta. The presence of marked retrograde movement of the saturation band was 100% sensitive for angiographic grade III or IV AR in 24 patients.

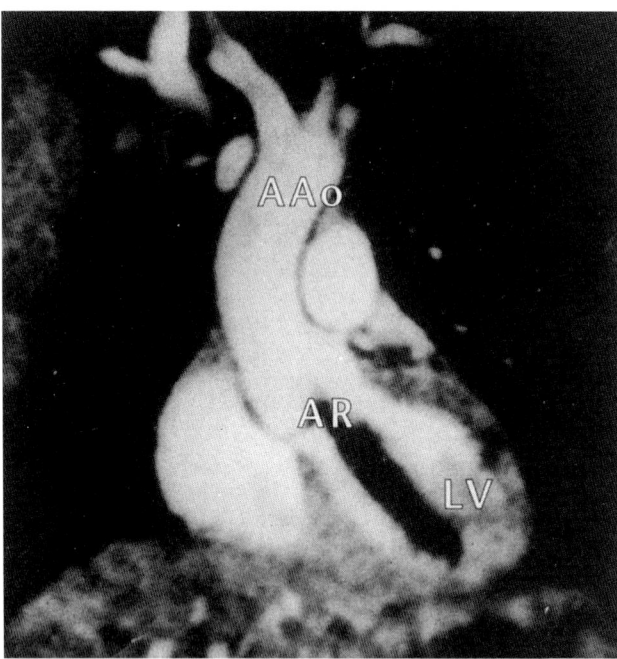

FIG. 25. Coronal middiastolic gradient echo cine image in a patient with severe aortic regurgitation (*AR*) shown as the signal void extending from the aortic valve into the left ventricle (*LV*). *AAo,* ascending aorta. (From ref. 153, with permission.)

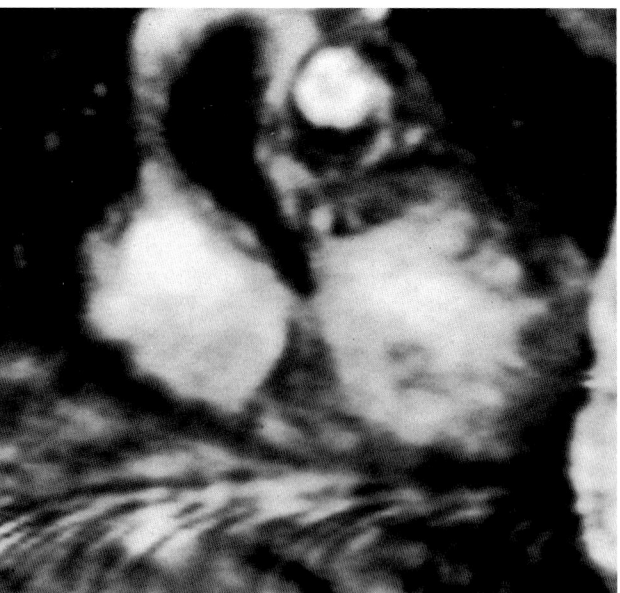

FIG. 26. Coronal gradient echo cine image in late systole in a patient with calcific aortic stenosis. The signal void from the high-velocity turbulent jet of flow distal to the aortic valve extending into the ascending aorta is demonstrated.

Mitral Stenosis

In mitral stenosis (MS), cine gradient echo imaging can demonstrate a signal void extending into the LV during diastole. Mitchell and colleagues (134) compared the size of signal loss relative to LV cross-sectional area and catheter-measured pressure gradients and found a good correlation ($r = 0.77$). Cosolo et al. (135) studied 20 patients with MS and found a significant correlation ($r = 0.81$) between the maximum mitral leaflet separation by cine MRI with mitral valve area measured by Doppler echocardiography. In 16 patients with MS, Heidenreich et al. (136) used VEC MRI to measure peak and mean mitral gradients and demonstrated significant correlation with Doppler echo with r values ranging form 0.82 to 0.95. Kilner et al. (137) used VEC MRI with short echo time (TE = 3.6 msec) to show excellent agreement in peak gradients in both mitral and aortic stenosis.

Aortic Stenosis

Both cine and VEC MRI have been used to assess the severity of aortic stenosis (AS). Mitchell et al. (134) used the length of signal loss distal to the aortic valve to grade the severity of AS with a good correlation with pressure gradients (Fig. 26). de Roos and colleagues (138) studied 17 patients with moderate or severe AS. They found that the properties of the imaging that correlated with more severe AS included narrow high-velocity jets that extended well

into the aorta distal to the valve and the presence of a prestenotic acceleration signal void proximal to the valve. Using VEC MRI, Eichenberger and associates (139) demonstrated excellent correlation for measurement of pressure gradient with Doppler echocardiography ($r = 0.96$) and cardiac catheterization ($r = 0.97$). Kilner et al. (125) showed excellent agreement between VEC MRI and Doppler echo in 11 patients with AS. Sondergaard et al. (140) used similar techniques to estimate valve area in AS and found a mean difference of 0.1 cm^2 from Doppler echo derived estimates.

Other Valvular Lesions

Velocity-encoded cine MRI has been used by investigators to interrogate the function of the tricuspid valve. Nakagawa et al. (141) described the velocity profile of normal tricuspid inflow, which was elliptical in nature. Rebergen et al. (142) compared tomographic tricuspid valve volume flow with VEC MRI in healthy children and patients after Mustard or Senning repair and found a close agreement in both groups ($r = 0.98$ in normal controls and 0.94 in patients). The same group found that measurements of pulmonary regurgitation volume in 18 patients after repair of tetrology of Fallot with VEC MRI closely correlated with tomographically determined volumes ($r = 0.93$) (143).

Prosthetic Valves

The safety of imaging prosthetic valves in high field MR scanners has been well documented (144,145) (Fig. 27). The lone exception is the Starr-Edwards ball cage prosthesis.

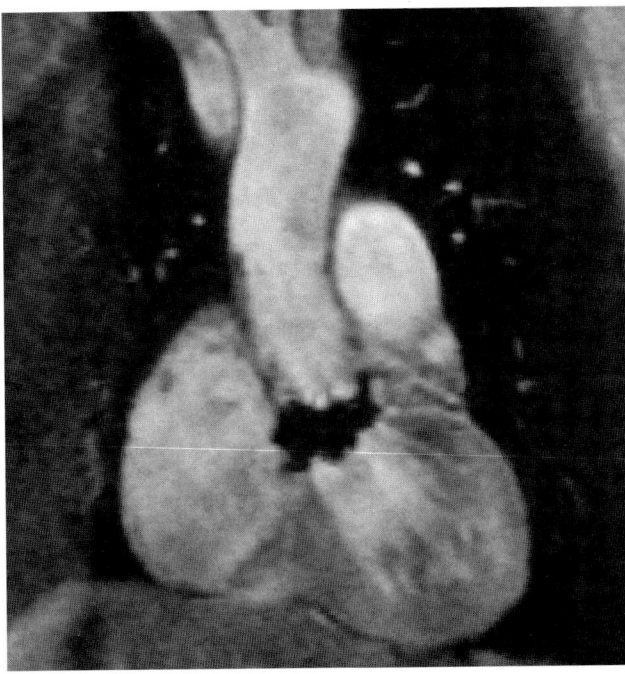

FIG. 27. Coronal gradient echo cine image in a patient after aortic valve replacement with a St Jude's mechanical prosthesis. Note the dark signal void due to the metallic prosthesis extending beyond the prosthesis into the basal left ventricle and aortic root.

Deutsch et al. (146) compared cine MRI with transesophageal color Doppler echocardiography to differentiate physiologic versus pathologic regurgitant flow in 47 patients. Grading of jet severity was identical in 75% of the prostheses and the quantification of jet length and area correlated well between methods.

INTRACARDIAC SHUNTS

Two major techniques are available to quantify intracardiac shunts and assess their severity: cine MRI (147) and VEC MRI (148). The cine method calculates stroke volume for the right and left ventricles using methods described earlier in this chapter, and the difference is the extent of the shunt. Two limitations of this technique are that the presence of aortic or pulmonary regurgitation complicates the stroke volume determination and that ventricular septal defect (VSD) shunting cannot be calculated in this manner. Using phase velocity techniques, the ratio of pulmonary to systemic blood flow (Q_p/Q_s) can be calculated by measuring peak flow and cross-sectional areas of the pulmonary artery and aorta in planes perpendicular to the proximal portions of the respective great vessels (149).

Atrial septal defects (ASD) are the most common intracardiac shunt lesion. Holmvang et al. (150) demonstrated that spin-echo imaging overestimated the major diameter and area of ASD due to septal thinning adjacent to a secundum ASD. However, (VEC) cine MRI measurements agreed

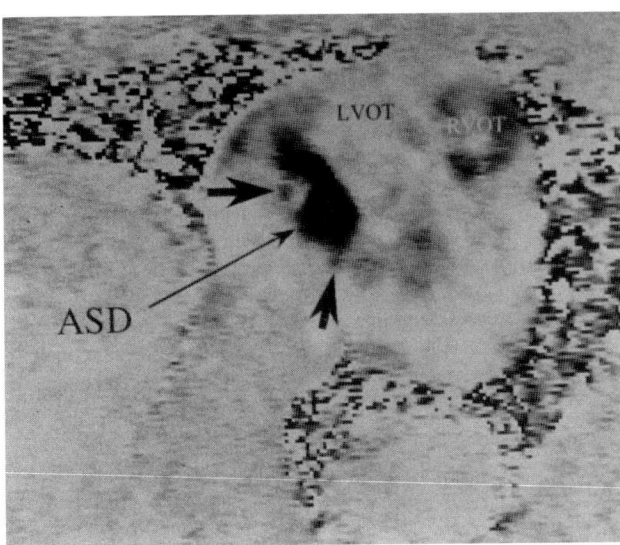

FIG. 28. Phase velocity map viewed from the right atrium in an oblique transaxial plane in a patient with a large atrial septal defect (*ASD*) (maximum diameter 3.5 cm). The *long arrow* points to the flow across the ASD and the *thick arrows* indicate fenestrations in the atrial septum. *LVOT*, left ventricular outflow tract; *RVOT*, right ventricular outflow tract. (From ref. 149, with permission.)

closely with catheterization measures of defect size ($r = 0.93$) (Fig. 28). Hundley et al. (151) compared VEC MRI and oximetric and indicator dilution methods for estimating shunt magnitude in a variety of intracardiac shunts. They found that the two methods correlated well with $r = 0.94$. MRI correctly identified the 12 patients with a Q_p/Q_s of less than 1.5 and the 9 patients with a Q_p/Q_s greater than or equal to 1.5.

REFERENCES

1. Fisher MR, von Schulthess GK, Higgins CB. Multiphasic cardiac magnetic resonance imaging: normal regional left ventricular wall thickening. *Am J Roentgenol* 1985;145:27–30.
2. Caputo GR, Suzuki JI, Kondo C, et al. Determination of left ventricular volume and mass using biphasic spin-echo MR imaging: comparison with cine MR. *Radiology* 1990;177:773–777.
3. Sechtem U, Pflugfelder PW, Gould RG, et al. Measurement of right and left ventricular volumes in healthy individuals with cine MR imaging. *Radiology* 1987;163:697–702.
4. Cranney GB, Lotan CS, Dean L, et al. Left ventricular volume measurement using cardiac axis NMR imaging-validation by calibrated ventricular angiography. *Circulation* 1990;82:154–163.
5. Buser PT, Aufferman W, Holt WW, et al. Noninvasive evaluation of global left ventricular function with use of cine nuclear agnetic resonance. *J Am Coll Cardiol* 1989;13:1294–1300.
6. Chien D, Atkinson DJ, Edelman RR. Strategies to improve contrast in turboFLASH imaging: reordered phase encoding and k-space segmentation. *J Magn Reson Imaging* 1991;1:63–70.
7. Yang PC, Kerr AB, Liu AC, et al. New real-time interactive cardiac magnetic resonance imaging system complements echocardiography. *J Am Coll Cardiol* 1998;32:2049–2056.
8. Pykett IL, Rzedzian RR. Instant images of the body by magnetic resonance. *Magn Res Med* 1987;5:563–571.
9. Lamb HJ, Doornbos J, van der Velde EA, et al. Echoplanar MRI of the heart on a standard system: validation of measurements of left

ventricular function and mass. *J Comp Assist Tomog* 1996;20: 942–949.

10. Nishimura D, Irarrazabal P, Meyer C. A velocity k-space analysis of flow effects in echo-planar and spiral imaging. *Magn Reson Med* 1995;33:549–556.

11. Unterweger M, Debatin JF, Leung DA, et al. Comparison of echoplanar and conventional cine-magnetic resonance data acqusition strategies. *Invest Radiol* 1994;29:994–1000.

12. Haider AW, Larson MG, Benjamin EJ, et al. Increased left ventricular mass and hypertrophy are associated with increased risk for sudden death. *J Am Coll Cardiol* 1998;32:1454–1459.

13. Florentine MS, Grosskreutz CL, Chang W, et al. Measurement of left ventricular mass *in vivo* using gated nuclear magnetic resonance imaging. *J Am Coll Cardiol* 1986;8:107–112.

14. Keller AM, Peshock RM, Malloy CR, et al. *In vivo* measurement of myocardial mass using nuclear magnetic resonance imaging. *J Am Coll Cardiol* 1986;8:113–117.

15. Maddahi J, Crues J, Berman DS, et al. Noninvasive quantification of left ventricular mass by gated proton magnetic resonance imaging. *J Am Coll Cardiol* 1987;10:682–692.

16. Manning WJ, Wei JY, Fossel ET, et al. Measurement of left ventricular mass in rats using electrocardiogram-gated magnetic resonance imaging. *Am J Physiol* 1990;258:H1181–H1186.

17. Shapiro EP, Rogers WJ, Beyar R, et al. Determination of left ventricular mass by magnetic resonance imaging in hearts deformed by acute infarction. *Circulation* 1989;79:706–711.

18. Franco F, Dubois SK, Peshock RM, et al. Magnetic resonance imaging accurately estimates LV mass in a transgenic mouse model of cardiac hypertrophy. *Am J Physiol* 1998;274:H679–H683.

19. Ruff J, Wiesmann F, Hiller K-H, et al. Magnetic resonance microimaging for noninvasive quantification of myocardial function and mass in the mouse. *Magn Reson Imag* 1998;40:43–48.

20. Katz J, Milliken M, Stray-Gunderson J, et al. Estimation of human myocardial mass with MR imaging. *Radiology* 1988;169:495–498.

21. Germain P, Roul G, Kastler B, et al. Inter-study variability in left ventricular mass measurement: comparison between M-mode echocardiography and MRI. *Eur Heart J* 1992;13:1011–1019.

22. Bottini PB, Carr AA, Prisant LM, et al. Magnetic resonance imaging compared to echocardiography to assess left ventricular mass in the hypertensive patient. *Am J Hypertens* 1995;8:221–228.

23. Yamaoka O, Yabe T, Okada M, et al. Evaluation of left ventricular mass: comparison of ultrafast computed tomography, magnetic resonance imaging, and contrast left ventriculography. *Am Heart J* 1993; 126:1372–1379.

24. Aurigemma G, Davidoff A, Silver K, et al. Left ventricular mass quantitation using single-phase cardiac magnetic resonance imaging. *Am J Cardiol* 1992;70:259–262.

25. McDonald KM, Parrish T, Wennberg P, et al. Rapid, accurate and simultaneous noninvasive assessment of right and left ventricular mass with magnetic resonance imaging using the snapshot gradient method. *J Am Coll Cardiol* 1992;19:1601–1607.

26. Riley-Hagan M, Peshock RM, Stray-Gundersen J, et al. Left ventricular dimensions and mass using magnetic resonance imaging in female endurance athletes. *Am J Cardiol* 1992;69:1067–1074.

27. Globits S, De Marco T, Schwitter J, et al. Assessment of early left ventricular remodeling in orthotopic heart transplant recipients with cine magnetic resonance imaging: potential mechanisms. *J Heart Lung Transplant* 1997;16:504–510.

28. Kramer CM, Rogers WJ, Theobald TM, et al. Dissociation between changes in intramyocardial function and left ventricular volumes in the 8 weeks after first anterior myocardial infarction. *J Am Coll Cardiol* 1997;30:1625–1632.

29. Doherty NE, Seelos KC, Suzuki J, et al. Application of cine nuclear magnetic resonance imaging for sequential evaluation of response to angiotensin-converting enzyme inhibitor therapy in dilated cardiomyopathy. *J Am Coll Cardiol* 1992;19:1294–1302.

30. Foster RE, Johnson DB, Barilla F, et al. Changes in left ventricular mass and volumes in patients receiving angiotensin-converting enzyme inhibitor therapy for left ventricular dysfunction after Q-wave myocardial infarction. *Am Heart J* 1998;136:269–275.

31. White HD, Norris RM, Brown MA, et al. Left ventricular end-systolic

volume as the major determinant of survival after recovery from myocardial infarction. *Circulation* 1987;76:44–51.

32. Borow KM, Green LH, Mann T, et al. End-systolic volume as a predictor of post operative left ventricular performance in volume overload from valvular regurgitation. *Am J Med* 1980;68:655–663.

33. Rehr RB, Malloy CR, Filipchuk NG, et al. Left ventricular volumes measured by MR imaging. *Radiology* 1985;156:717–719.

34. Markiewicz W, Sechtem U, Kirby R, et al. Measurement of ventricular volumes in the dog by nuclear magnetic resonance imaging. *J Am Coll Cardiol* 1987;10:170–177.

35. Edelman RR, Thompson R, Kantor H, et al. Cardiac function: evaluation with fast-echo MR imaging. *Radiology* 1987;162:611–615.

36. Longmore DB, Klipstein RH, Underwood SR, et al. Dimensional accuracy of magnetic resonance in studies of the heart. *Lancet* 1985;1: 1360–1362.

37. Just H, Holubarsch C, Friedburg H. Estimation of left ventricular volume and mass by magnetic resonance imaging: comparison with quantitative biplane angiography. *Cardiovas Intervent Radiol* 1987; 10:1–4.

38. MacMillan RM, Murphey JL, Kresh JY, et al. Left ventricular volumes using cine-MRI: validation with catheterization ventriculography. *Am J Cardiac Imaging* 1990;4:79.

39. Dilworth LR, Aisen AM, Mancini GB, et al. Determination of left ventricular volumes and ejection fraction by nuclear magnetic resonance imaging. *Am Heart J* 1987;113:24–32.

40. Lawson MA, Blackwell GG, Davis ND, et al. Accuracy of bi-plane long-axis left ventricular volume determined by cine magnetic resonance imaging in patients with regional and global dysfunction. *Am J Cardiol* 1996;77:1098–1104.

41. Semelka RC, Tomei E, Wagner S, et al. Normal left ventricular dimensions and function: interstudy reproducibility of measurements with cine MR imaging. *Radiology* 1990;174:763–768.

42. Semelka RC, Tomei E, Wagner S, et al. Interstudy reproducibility of dimensional and functional measurements between cine magnetic resonance studies in the morphologically abnormal left ventricle. *Am Heart J* 1990;119:1367–1373.

43. Pattynama PM, Lamb HJ, van der Velde EA, et al. Left ventricular measurements with cine and spin-echo MR imaging: a study of reproducibility with variance component analysis. *Radiology* 1993;187: 261–268.

44. Lorenz CH, Walker S, Morgan VL, et al. Normal human right and left ventricular mass, systolic function, and gender differences by cine magnetic resonance imaging. *J Cardiovasc Magn Reson* 1999;1:7–21.

45. Utz J, Herfkens RJ, Heinsimer JA, et al. Cine MR determination of left ventricular ejection fraction. *Am J Roentgenol* 1987;148:839–843.

46. Buckwalter KA, Aisen AM, Dilworth LR, et al. Gated cardiac MRI: ejection fraction determination using the right anterior oblique view. *Am J Roentgenol* 1986;147:33–37.

47. Van Rossum AC, Visser FC, Sprenger M, et al. Evaluation of magnetic resonance imaging for determination of left ventricular ejection fraction and comparison with angiography. *Am J Cardiol* 1988;62: 628–633.

48. Gaudio C, Tanzilli G, Mazzarotto P, et al. Comparison of left ventricular ejection fraction by magnetic resonance imaging and radionuclide ventriculography in idiopathic dilated cardiomyopathy. *Am J Cardiol* 1991;67:411–415.

49. Fogel MA, Weinberg PM, Chin AJ, et al. Late ventricular geometry and performance changes of functional single ventricle throughout staged Fontan reconstruction assessed by magnetic resonance imaging. *J Am Coll Cardiol* 1996;28:212–221.

50. Buck T, Hunold P, Wentz KU, et al. Tomographic three-dimensional echocardiographic determination of chamber size and systolic function in patients with left ventricular aneurysm. *Circulation* 1997;96: 4286–4297.

51. Doherty NE, Fujita N, Caputo GR, et al. Measurement of right ventricular mass in normal and dilated cardiomyopathic ventricles using cine magnetic resonance imaging. *Am J Cardiol* 1992;69:1223–1228.

52. Katz J, Whang J, Boxt LM, et al. Estimation of right ventricular mass in normal subjects and in patients with primary pulmonary hypertension by nuclear magnetic resonance imaging. *J Am Coll Cardiol* 1993; 21:1475–1481.

53. Lorenz CH, Walker ES, Graham TP Jr, et al. Right ventricular performance and mass by use of cine MRI late after atrial repair of transposition of the great arteries. *Circulation* 1995;92[Suppl II]:II233–II239.

54. Boxt LM, Katz J, Kolb T, et al. Direct quantitation of right and left ventricular volumes with nuclear magnetic resonance imaging in patients with primary pumonary hypertension. *J Am Coll Cardiol* 1992; 19:1508–1515.

55. Pattynama PM, Lamb HJ, Van der Velde EA, et al. Reproducibility of MRI-derived measurements of right ventricular volumes and myocardial mass. *Magn Reson Imaging* 1995;13:53–63.

56. Helbing WA, Rebergen SA, Maliepaard C, et al. Quantification of right ventricular function with magnetic resonance imaging in children with normal hearts and with congenital heart disease. *Am Heart J* 1995;130:828–837.

57. Lieberman AN, Weiss JL, Jugdutt BI, et al. Two-dimensional echocardiography and infarct size: relationship of regional wall motion and thinning to the extent of myocardial infarction in the dog. *Circulation* 1981;63:739–746.

58. Peshock RM, Rokey R, Malloy CM, et al. Assessment of myocardial systolic wall thickening using nuclear magnetic resonance imaging. *J Am Coll Cardiol* 1989,14:653–659.

59. Lotan CS, Cranney GB, Bouchard A, et al. The value of cine nuclear magnetic resonance imaging for assessing regional ventricular function. *J Am Coll Cardiol* 1989;14:1721–1729.

60. Akins EW, Hill JA, Sievers KW, et al. Assessment of left ventricular wall thickness in healed myocardial infarction by magnetic resonance imaging. *Am J Cardiol* 1987;59:24–28.

61. Meese RB, Spritzer CE, Negro-Vilar R, et al. Detection, characterization and functional assessment of reperfused Q-wave acute myocardial infarction by cine magnetic resonance imaging. *Am J Cardiol* 1990; 66:1–9.

62. Holman ER, Buller VGM, de Roos A, et al. Detection and quantification of dysfunctional myocardium by magnetic resonance imaging. *Circulation* 1997;95:924–931.

63. Azhari H, Sideman S, Weiss JL, et al. Three-dimensional mapping of acute ischemic regions using MRI: wall thickening versus motion analysis. *Am J Physiol* 1990;259:H1492–H1503.

64. Zerhouni E, Parrish D, Rogers WJ, et al. Human heart: tagging with MR imaging—a method for noninvasive measurement of myocardial motion. *Radiology* 1988;169:59–64.

65. Axel L, Dougherty L. MR imaging of motion with spatial modulation of magnetization. *Radiology* 1989;171:841–845.

66. Bolster BD Jr, McVeigh ER, Zerhouni EA. Myocardial tagging in polar coordinates with use of striped tags. *Radiology* 1990;177: 769–772.

67. Beyar R, Shapiro EP, Graves WL, et al. Quantification and validation of left ventricular wall thickening by a three-dimensional volume element magnetic resonance imaging approach. *Circulation* 1990;81: 297–307.

68. Lima JAC, Jeremy R, Guier W, et al. Accurate systolic wall thickening by nuclear magnetic resonance imaging with tissue tagging: correlation with sonomicrometers in normal and ischemic myocardium. *J Am Coll Cardiol* 1993;21:1741–1751.

69. Buchalter MB, Weiss JL, Rogers WJ, et al. Noninvasive quantification of left ventricular rotational deformation in normal humans using magnetic resonance imaging myocardial tagging. *Circulation* 1990;81: 1236–1244.

70. Rogers WJ, Shapiro EP, Weiss JL, et al. Quantification of and correction for left ventricular systolic long-axis shortening by magnetic resonance tissue tagging and slice isolation. *Circulation* 1991;84: 721–731.

71. Clark N, Reichek N, Bergey P, et al. Normal segmental myocardial function; assessment by magnetic resonance imaging using spatial modulation of magnetization. *Circulation* 1991;84:67–74.

72. Palmon LC, Reichek N, Yeon SB, et al. Intramural myocardial shortening in hypertensive left ventricular hypertrophy with normal pump function. *Circulation* 1994;89:122–131.

73. Kramer CM, Reichek NR, Ferrari VA, et al. Regional heterogeneity of function in hypertrophic cardiomyopathy. *Circulation* 1994;90: 186–194.

74. McVeigh ER, Atalar E. Cardiac tagging with breath-hold cine MRI. *Magn Reson Med* 1992;28:318–327.

75. Kramer CM, Rogers WJ, Theobald T, et al. Remote noninfarcted region dysfunction soon after first anterior myocardial infarction: a magnetic resonance tagging study. *Circulation* 1996;94:660–666.

76. Young AA, Imai H, Chang C-N, et al. Two-dimensional left ventricular deformation during systole using magnetic resonance imaging with spatial modulation of magnetization. *Circulation* 1994;89:740–752.

77. Young AA, Kramer CM, Ferrari VA, et al. Three-dimensional deformation in hypertrophic cardiomyopathy. *Circulation* 1994;90: 854–867.

78. Marcus JT, Gotte MJW, van Rossum AC, et al. Myocardial function in infarcted and remote regions early after infarction in man: assessment by magnetic resonance tagging and strain analysis. *Magn Res Med* 1997;38:803–810.

79. MacGowan GA, Shapiro EP, Azhari H, et al. Noninvasive measurement of shortening in the fiber and cross-fiber directions in the normal human left ventricle and in idiopathic dilated cardiomyopathy. *Circulation* 1997;96:535–541.

80. Dong SJ, MacGregor JH, Crawley AP, et al. Left ventricular wall thickness and regional systolic function in patients with hypertrophic cardiomyopathy: a three-dimensional tagged magnetic resonance imaging study. *Circulation* 1994;90:1200–1209.

81. Dong SJ, Crawley AP, MacGregor JH, et al. Regional left ventricular systolic function in relation to the cavity geometry in patients with chronic right ventricular pressure overload. *Circulation* 1995;91: 2359–2370.

82. Fayad ZA, Ferrari VA, Kraitchman DL, et al. Right ventricular regional function using MR tagging: normals versus chronic pulmonary hypertension. *Magn Res Med* 1998;39:116–123.

83. Fogel MA, Gupta KB, Weinberg PM, et al. Regional wall motion and strain analysis across stages of Fontan reconstruction by magnetic resonance tagging. *Am J Physiol* 1995;269:H1132–H1152.

84. Fogel MA, Weinberg PM, Fellows KE, et al. A study in ventricular-ventricular interaction. Single right ventricles compared with systemic right ventricles in a dual chamber circulation. *Circulation* 1995;92: 219–230.

85. Fogel MA, Weinberg PM, Gupta KB, et al. Mechanics of the single left ventricle. A study in ventricular-ventricular interaction II. *Circulation* 1998;98:330–338.

86. Pelc LR, Sayre J, Yun K, et al. Evaluation of myocardial motion tracking with cine-phase contrast magnetic resonance imaging. *Invest Radiol* 1994;29:1038–1042.

87. Karwatowski SP, Mohiaddin R, Yang GZ, et al. Assessment of regional left ventricular long-axis motion with MR velocity mapping in healthy subjects. *J Magn Reson Imaging* 1994;4:151–155.

88. Karwatowski SP, Mohiaddin RH, Yang GZ, et al. Regional myocardial velocity imaged by magnetic resonance in patients with ischaemic heart disease. *Br Heart J* 1994;72:332–338.

89. van Wedeen VJ, Weisskoff RM, Reese TG, et al. Motionless movies of myocardial strain-rates using stimulated echoes. *Magn Res Med* 1995;33:401–408.

90. Beache GM, Wedeen VJ, Weisskoff RM, et al. Intramural mechanics in hypertrophic cardiomyopathy: functional mapping with strain-rate MR imaging. *Radiology* 1995;197:117–124.

91. Hoff FL, Turner DA, Wang JZ, et al. Semiautomatic evaluation of left ventricular diastolic function with cine magnetic resonance imaging. *Acad Radiol* 1994;1:237–242.

92. Kudelka AM, Turner DA, Liebson PR, et al. Comparison of cine magnetic resonance imaging and Doppler echocardiography for evaluation of left ventricular diastolic function. *Am J Cardiol* 1997;80: 384–386.

93. van Rugge FP, Holman ER, van der Wall EE, et al. Quantitation of global and regional left ventricular function by cine magnetic resonance imaging during dobutamine stress in normal human subjects. *Eur Heart J* 1993;14:456–463.

94. Power T, Kramer CM, Shaffer AL, et al. Breathold dobutamine magnetic resonance tissue tagging: normal left ventricular response. *Am J Cardiol* 1997;80:1203–1207.

95. Sawada SG, Segar DS, Ryan T, et al. Echocardiographic detection of coronary artery disease during dobutamine infusion. *Circulation* 1991; 83:1605–1614.

96. Pennell DJ, Underwood SR, Manzara CC, et al. Magnetic resonance

imaging during dobutamine stress in coronary artery disease. *Am J Cardiol* 1992;70:34–40.

97. van Rugge FP, van der Wall EE, de Roos A, et al. Dobutamine stress magnetic resonance imaging for detection of coronary artery disease. *J Am Coll Cardiol* 1993;22:431–439.

98. van Rugge FP, van der Wall EE, Spanjersberg SJ, et al. Magnetic resonance imaging during dobutamine stress for detection and localization of coronary artery disease. *Circulation* 1994;90:127–138.

99. Baer FM, Voth E, Theissen P, et al. Gradient-echo magnetic resonance imaging during incremental dobutamine infusion for the localization of coronary artery stenoses. *Eur Heart J* 1994;15:218–225.

100. Smart SC, Sawada S, Ryan T, et al. Low-dose dobutamine echocardiography detects reversible dysfunction after thrombolytic therapy of acute myocardial infarction. *Circulation* 1993;88:405–415.

101. Dendale PAC, Franken PR, Waldman G-J, et al. Low-dosage dobutamine magnetic resonance imaging as an alternative to echocardiography in the detection of viable myocardium after acute infarction. *Am Heart J* 1995;130:134–140.

102. Dendale P, Franken PR, Holman E, et al. Validation of low-dose dobutamine magnetic resonance imaging for assessment of myocardial viability after infarction by serial imaging. *Am J Cardiol* 1998;82:375–377.

103. Geskin G, Kramer CM, Rogers WJ, et al. Quantitative assessment of myocardial viability post-infarction by dobutamine magnetic resonance tagging. *Circulation* 1998;98:217–223.

104. Baer FM, Voth E, Schneider CA, et al. Comparison of low-dose dobutamine gradient-echo magnetic resonance imaging and positron emission tomography with [^{18}F]-fluorodeoxyglucose in patients with chronic coronary artery disease. *Circulation* 1995;81:1006–1015.

105. Baer FM, Voth E, LaRosee K, et al. Comparison of dobutamine transesophageal echocardiography and dobutamine magnetic resonance imaging for detection of residual myocardial viability. *Am J Cardiol* 1996;78:415–419.

106. Baer FM, Thiessen P, Schneider CA, et al. Dobutamine magnetic resonance imaging predicts contractile recovery of chronically dysfunctional myocardium after successful revascularization. *J Am Coll Cardiol* 1998;31:1040–1048.

107. Glogar D, Globits S, Neuhold A, et al. Assessment of mitral regurgitation by magnetic resonance imaging. *Magn Reson Imaging* 1989;7:611–617.

108. Globits S, Frank H, Mayr H, et al. Quantitative assessment of aortic regurgitation by magnetic resonance imaging. *Eur Heart J* 1992;13:78–83.

109. Evans AJ, Blinder RA, Herfkens RJ, et al. Effects of turbulence on signal intensity in gradient echo images. *Invest Radiol* 1988;23:512–518.

110. Evans AJ, Hedlund LW, Herfkens RJ, et al. Evaluation of steady and pulsatile flow with dynamic MRI using limited flip angles and gradient refocused echoes. *Magn Reson Imaging* 1987;5:475–482.

111. Meier D, Maier S, Boesiger P. Quantitative flow measurements on phantoms and on blood vessels with MR. *Magn Reson Med* 1988;8:25–34.

112. Bogren HG, Klipstein RH, Firmin DN, et al. Quantitation of antegrade and retrograde blood flow in the human aorta by magnetic resonance velocity mapping. *Am Heart J* 1989;17:1214–1222.

113. Kondo C, Caputo GR, Semelka R, et al. Right and left ventricular stroke volume measurements with velocity encoded cine NMR imaging: *in vitro* and *in vivo* evaluation. *Am J Roentgenol* 1991;157:9–16.

114. Firmin DN, Klipstein RH, Hounsfield GL, et al. Echo-planar high-resolution flow velocity mapping. *Magn Reson Med* 1989;12:316–327.

115. Sondergaard L, Thomsen C, Stahlberg F, et al. Mitral and aortic valvular flow: quantification with MR phase mapping. *J Magn Reson Imaging* 1992;2:295–302.

116. Davis CP, McKinnon GC, Debatin JF, et al. Single-shot versus interleaved echo-planar MR imaging: application to visualization of cardiac valve leaflets. *J Magn Reson Imaging* 1995;5:107–112.

117. Wagner S, Auffermann W, Buser P, et al. Diagnostic accuracy and estimation of the severity of valvular regurgitation from signal void on cine MRI. *Am Heart J* 1989;118:760–767.

118. Suzuki J, Caputo GR, Kondo C, et al. Cine MR imaging of valvular heart disease: display and imaging parameters affect the size of the signal void caused by valvular regurgitation. *Am J Roentgenol* 1990;155:723–727.

119. Yoshida K, Yokoshikawa J, Hozumi T, et al. Assessment of aortic regurgitation by the acceleration flow signal void proximal to the leaking orifice in cine-magnetic resonance imaging. *Circulation* 1991;83:1951–1955.

120. Cranney GB, Benjelloun H, Perry GJ, et al. Rapid assessment of aortic regurgitation and left ventricular function using cine nuclear magnetic resonance imaging and the proximal convergence zone. *Am J Cardiol* 1993;71:1074–1081.

121. Underwood SR, Klipstei RH, Firmin DN, et al. Magnetic resonance assessment of aortic and mitral regurgitation. *Br Heart J* 1986;56:455–462.

122. Sechtem U, Plugfelder PW, Cassidy MM, et al. Mitral and aortic regurgitation: quantification of regurgitant volumes with cine MR imaging. *Radiology* 1988;167:425–430.

123. Sondergaard L, Lindvig K, Hildebrandt P, et al. Quantification of aortic regurgitation by magnetic resonance velocity mapping. *Am Heart J* 1993;125:1081–1090.

124. Honda N, Machida K, Hashimoto M, et al. Aortic regurgitation: quantitation with MR imaging velocity mapping. *Radiology* 1993;186:189–194.

125. Kilner PJ, Firmin DN, Rees RSO, et al. Valve and great vessel stenosis: assessment with MR jet velocity mapping. *Radiology* 1991;178:229–235.

126. Kilner PJ, Monzara CC, Mohiuddin RH, et al. Magnetic resonance jet velocity mapping in mitral and aortic valve stenosis. *Circulation* 1993;87:1239–1248.

127. Pflugfelder PW, Sechtem UP, White RD, et al. Non-invasive evaluation of mitral regurgitation by analysis of left atrial signal loss in cine magnetic resonance. *Am Heart J* 1989;117:1113–1119.

128. Aurigemma G, Reichek N, Schiebler M, et al. Evaluation of mitral regurgitation by cine MRI. *Am J Cardiol* 1990;66:621–625.

129. Fujita N, Chazouilleres AF, Hartiala MM, et al. Quantification of mitral regurgitation by velocity encoded cine nuclear magnetic resonance imaging. *J Am Coll Cardiol* 1994;23:951–958.

130. Hundley WG, Li HF, Willard JE, et al. Magnetic resonance imaging assessment of the severity of mitral regurgitation: comparison with invasive techniques. *Circulation* 1995;92:1151–1158.

131. Aurigemma G, Reichek N, Schiebler M, et al. Evaluation of aortic regurgitation by cardiac cine MRI, planar analysis and comparison to Doppler echocardiography. *Cardiology* 1991;78:430–439.

132. Dulce MC, Mostbeck GH, O'Sullivan M, et al. Severity of aortic regurgitation: interstudy reproducibility of measurements with velocity-encoded cine MR imaging. *Radiology* 1992;185:235–240.

133. Ambrosi P, Faugere G, Desfossez L, et al. Assessment of aortic regurgitation severity by magnetic resonance imaging of the thoracic aorta. *Eur Heart J* 1995;16:406–409.

134. Mitchell L, Jenkins JP, Watson Y, et al. Diagnosis and assessment of mitral and aortic disease by cine flow magnetic resonance imaging. *Magn Reson Med* 1989;12:181–197.

135. Cosolo GC, Zampa V, Rega L, et al. Evaluation of mitral stenosis by cine magnetic resonance imaging. *Am Heart J* 1992;123:1252–1260.

136. Heidenreich PA, Steffens J, Fujita N, et al. Evaluation of mitral stenosis with velocity-encoded cine-magnetic resonance imaging. *Am J Cardiol* 1995;75:365–369.

137. Kilner PJ, Wann LS, Firmin D, et al. Three directional magnetic resonance flow imaging of the human heart. *Dynam Cardiovasc Imaging* 1989;2:104–109.

138. de Roos A, Reichek N, Axel L, et al. Cine MR imaging in aortic stenosis. *J Comput Assist Tomogr* 1989;13:421–425.

139. Eichenberger AC, Jenni R, von Schultehess GK. Aortic valve pressure gradients in patients with aortic valve stenosis: quantification with velocity-encoded cine MR imaging. *Am J Roentgenol* 1993;160:971–977.

140. Sondergaard L, Hildebrandt P, Lindvig K. Valve area and cardiac output in aortic stenosis: quantification by magnetic resonance velocity mapping. *Am Heart J* 1993;126:1156–1164.

141. Nakagawa Y, Fujimoto S, Nakano H, et al. Magnetic resonance velocity mapping of normal transtricuspid velocity profiles. *Int J Card Imaging* 1997;13:433–436.

142. Rebergen SA, Helbing WA, van der Wall EE, et al. MR velocity

mapping of tricuspid flow in healthy children and in patients who have undergone Mustard or Senning repair. *Radiology* 1995;194:505–512.

143. Rebergen SA, Chin JGJ, Oeenkamp J, et al. Pulmonary regurgitation in the late postoperative follow-up of tetralogy of Fallot. *Circulation* 1993;88:2257–2266.

144. Soulen RL, Budinger TF, Higgins CB. Magnetic resonance imaging of prosthetic heart valves. *Radiology* 1985;154:705–707.

145. Randall PA, Kohman LJ, Scalzetti EM, et al. Magnetic resonance imaging of prosthetic cardiac valves *in vitro* and *in vivo*. *Am J Cardiol* 1988;62:973–976.

146. Deutsch HJ, Bachmann R, Sechtem U, et al. Regurgitant flow in cardiac valve prostheses: diagnostic value of gradient echo nuclar magnetic resonance imaging in reference to transesophageal two-dimensional color Doppler echocardiography. *J Am Coll Cardiol* 1992;19:1500–1507.

147. Sechtem U, Pflugfelder P, Cassidy MC, et al. Ventricular septal defect: visualization of shunt flow and determination of shunt size by cine magnetic resonance imaging. *Am J Roengenol* 1987;149:689–692.

148. Brenner LD, Caputo GR, Mostbeck G, et al. Quantification of left to right atrial shunts with velocity encoded cine nuclear magnetic resonance imaging. *J Am Coll Cardiol* 1992;20:1246–1250.

149. Taylor AM, Stables RH, Poole-Wilson PA, et al. Definitive clinical assessment of atrial septal defect by magnetic resonance imaging. *J Cardiovasc Magn Reson* 1999;1:43–49.

150. Holmvang G, Palacios IF, Vlahakes GJ, et al. Imaging and sizing of atrial septal defects by magnetic resonance. *Circulation* 1995;92:3473–3480.

151. Hundley WG, Li HF, Lange RA, et al. Assessment of left-to-right intracardiac shunting by velocity-encoded, phase-difference magnetic resonance imaging. *Circulation* 1995;91:2955–2960.

152. Martin ET, Fuisz AR, Pohost GM. Imaging cardiac structure and pump function. In: Reichek N, ed. *Cardiology clinics.* Philadelphia: WB Saunders, 1998;16(2):135–160.

153. Kramer CM. Magnetic resonance imaging of cardiac structures. In: Lee RT, Braunwald E, eds. *Atlas of cardiac imaging, current medicine.* Philadelphia: Current Medicine, 1998.

CHAPTER 31

Myocardial Perfusion and Magnetic Resonance Imaging

Anthon R. Fuisz and Gerald M. Pohost

Myocardial perfusion imaging has become one of the essential diagnostic components of clinical cardiology. Using radiopharmaceuticals, echogenic compounds, and radioopaque contrast agents or microspheres, myocardial perfusion can be measured and defects in perfusion detected. The optimal perfusion test would have a number of strengths. First, it would have a proven track record demonstrating its ability to detect ischemic heart disease with reasonable sensitivity and specificity. Second, it would be widely available and accepted by most clinicians. Third, it could assess myocardial viability. Fourth, it would have the potential to stratify risk. Finally, it should be able to provide additional accurate data about overall myocardial function that might assist the interpretation of the perfusion study.

Radionuclide techniques have accomplished most of these requirements. Unfortunately they do have certain disadvantages. The problem of attenuation is unavoidable, given the position of the heart within the chest, surrounded by substantial tissue thickness between myocardium and the gamma camera or positron emission tomography (PET) detector. Attenuation correction algorithms reduce this effect with PET imaging. With single photon emission computed tomography (SPECT) imaging, attenuation correction approaches have been disappointing, although they have not been fully exploited (Fig. 1).

Magnetic resonance imaging has developed into an important diagnostic tool. Its application to the evaluation of the cardiovascular system has been more recent. With its high resolution and its ability to track nontoxic paramagnetic con-

trast agents without ionizing radiation, magnetic resonance imaging (MRI) provides an alternative strategy for myocardial perfusion imaging. Already cardiovascular MRI (CMR) has been shown to provide accurate means to characterize myocardial structure and function (1), to assess valvular function (2), and to detect aortic disease (3). Magnetic resonance spectroscopy can be used to assess intracellular myocardial metabolism at rest and with stress in a variety of important disease processes (4,5).

MRI also has the potential to measure myocardial perfusion. First, perfusion can be measured through the tracking of a bolus of interstitial contrast agents like gadolinium chelates (e.g., Gd DTPA). The distribution of such agents can be used to evaluate the distribution of myocardial perfusion either using a qualitative approach by comparing differences in signal intensity (Fig. 1) or in a semiquantitative manner using specific algorithms that recognize other image characteristics (Fig. 2). Second, myocardial perfusion can be quantified by applying equations to the resultant time intensity curves, using a Fermi function model for constrained deconvolution (6-8). This technique places more rigid constraints on the delivery mode of the contrast compared with a qualitative perfusion evaluation, but allows the computation of blood flow to a given segment of myocardium with reasonable precision, and thus the detection of abnormal myocardial perfusion.

Myocardial perfusion can also be evaluated without the use of contrast agents through the technique of BOLD imaging. This technique uses differences in the MR properties of oxygenated blood compared with deoxygenated blood to calculate flow through the myocardium (9). While still in development, this technique has much to offer in perfusion, and in cardiac imaging in general.

A. R. Fuisz: Division of Cardiology, Department of Medicine, University of Alabama at Birmingham, Birmingham, Alabama 35294.

G. M. Pohost: Department of Medicine, University of Alabama at Birmingham, Birmingham, Alabama 35294.

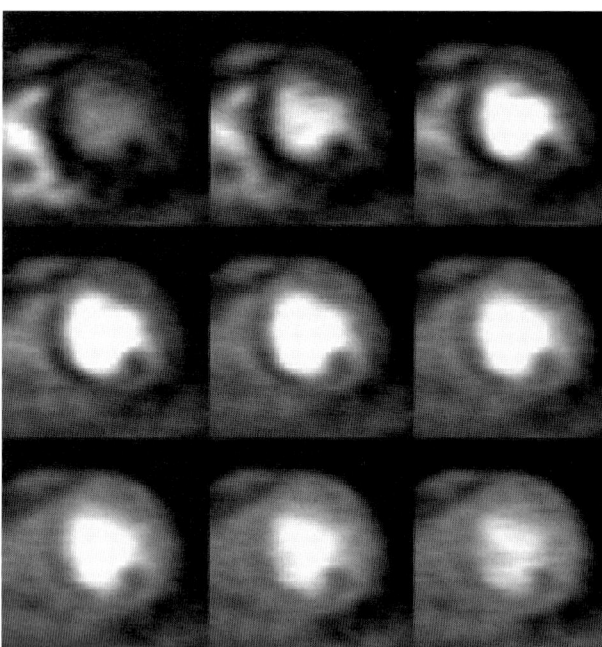

FIG. 1. Magnetic resonance (MR) perfusion images and radionuclide images in the same patient. The radionuclide images were read as having an anterior defect. The MR images were read as normal. Cath later confirmed the normal coronary anatomy. The presence of breast implants may have contributed to the false-positive radionuclide result.

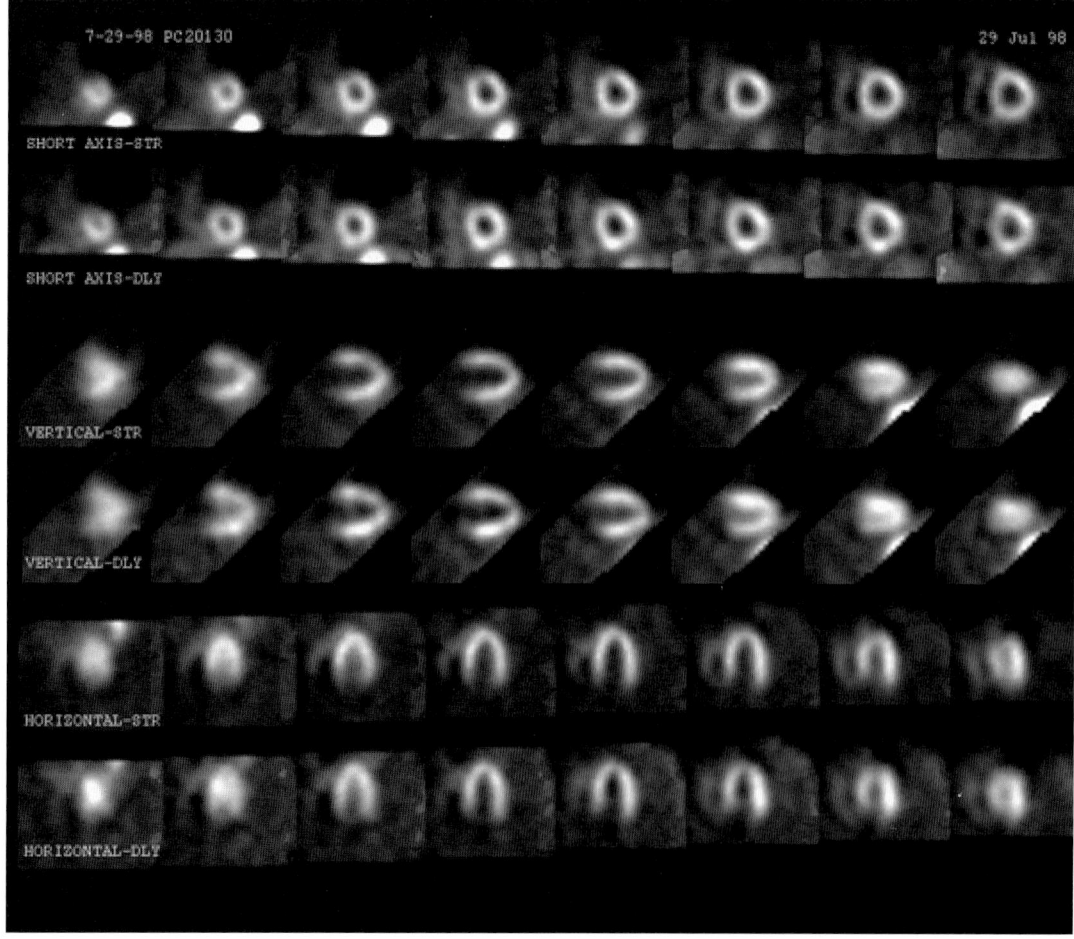

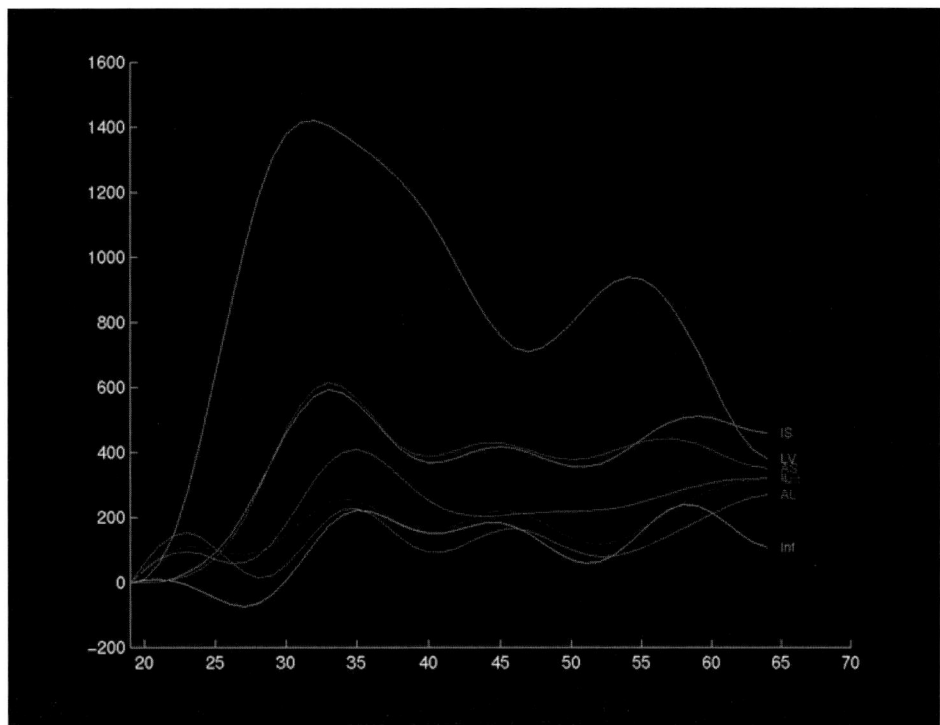

FIG. 2. Time intensity curves of the type used to do semiquantitative analysis of regional perfusion. The x axis is time in seconds, and the y axis represents intensity in arbitrary units. Slopes of the myocardial segments are normalized to the slope of the left ventricular cavity and compared to one another.

AGENTS USED FOR MR PERFUSION

The agents used for magnetic resonance perfusion imaging change local image parameters through their paramagnetic nature. A variety of these agents are used. The main agents used are chelates of gadolinium, which affect both T1 and T2, although the T1 effect is the most important in MR perfusion imaging. These agents are predominately excreted through the kidney, but unlike iodinated x-ray contrast medium have little risk of nephrotoxicity or anaphylaxis. One agent that has proven useful in our experience with MR perfusion is gadoteridol (Gd-HP-DO3A) (Bracco Diagnostics, Inc., Princeton, New Jersey). This agent has similar imaging characteristics to gadolinium DTPA, but has a much lower viscosity (at 20 degrees centigrade, Gd-DTPA has a viscosity of 4.9cP, while gadoteridol has a viscosity of 2.0cP), which facilitates the high flow rates needed for intravenous injection for perfusion imaging.

The principal weakness of the currently available agents is that they can readily diffuse out of the vascular compartment, complicating the analysis of time-intensity curves. This difficulty is currently the focus of substantial research activity. Newer MR contrast agents that remain within the blood pool (10-18) or are extracted by the myocardial cell provide alternative and more reliable approaches for quantification in MR perfusion imaging and are likely to be available clinically in the not distant future.

Superparamagnetic iron oxides particles have also been shown to be useful for evaluating MR perfusion since they

remain within the blood pool. This approach also requires further development and testing.

MAGNETIC RESONANCE PERFUSION IMAGING METHODS

Clinical magnetic resonance perfusion imaging is ideally carried out on a newer generation system with hardware that can support the high-speed imaging required for this type of examination (Fig. 3). Older hardware can be used but the resolution and the number of slices acquired are limited.

The first part of the MR perfusion protocol involves the initial acquisition of the standard cardiac examinations (transverse, two-chamber and four-chamber views). These images can identify abnormalities that might help explain a chest pain syndrome (and otherwise be missed by the perfusion study), including pericardial effusion, chest wall abnormalities, aortic dissection, and wall motion abnormalities suggesting previous myocardial infarction (MI). Studies have also shown the ability of MR techniques to assess bypass graft patency, which provides valuable additional information in the interpretation of a perfusion study (19,20). The images in the standard examination are also used to select the short-axis slices that will be imaged in the perfusion acquisition. Resting perfusion imaging is then performed. Ideally, a power injector is used to inject the gadolinium chelate through a peripheral intravenous (i.v.) line at the

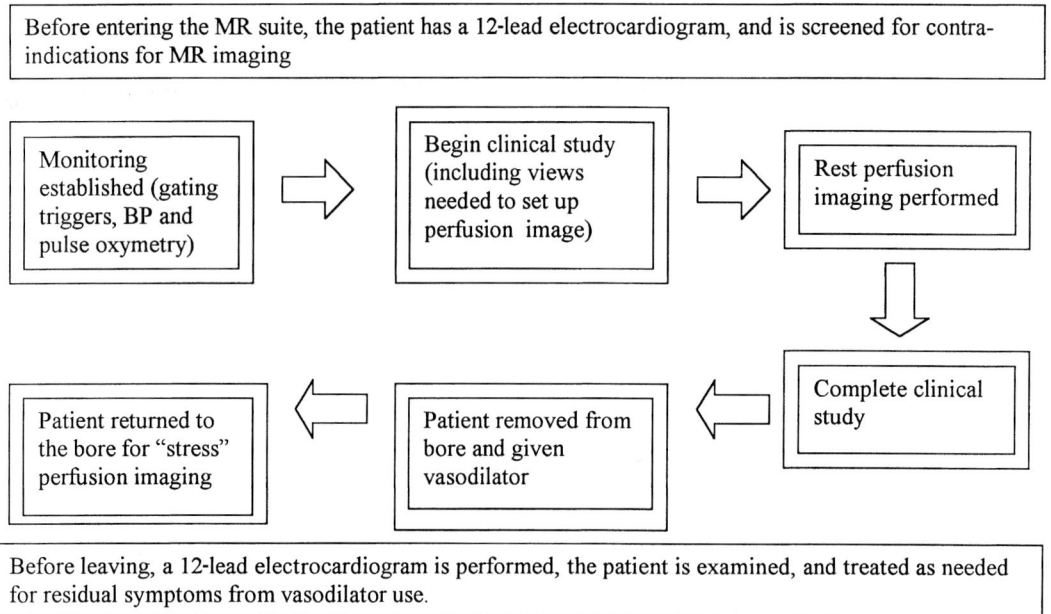

Before entering the MR suite, the patient has a 12-lead electrocardiogram, and is screened for contra-indications for MR imaging

Monitoring established (gating triggers, BP and pulse oxymetry)

Begin clinical study (including views needed to set up perfusion image)

Rest perfusion imaging performed

Complete clinical study

Patient returned to the bore for "stress" perfusion imaging

Patient removed from bore and given vasodilator

Before leaving, a 12-lead electrocardiogram is performed, the patient is examined, and treated as needed for residual symptoms from vasodilator use.

FIG. 3. Chart describing the organization of a magnetic resonance perfusion examination. *BP,* blood pressure.

rates of 5 to 10mL/sec. The use of a power injector allows bolus shapes to be more reproducible than those achievable with hand injections, and allows the bolus to be given while viewing the console of the MR system. Quantitative myocardial perfusion imaging generally requires the introduction of the paramagnetic contrast via a central venous line. The dose of paramagnetic contrast agent requires a compromise between the optimal signal-to-noise and avoiding the nonlinear nature of contrast enhancement, which can occur in the higher concentrations of the gadolinium-based agents. For the perfusion sequences, a time resolution, which allows slices to be acquired with every heart beat, is ideal. Within this time frame, the goal should be to acquire as many short-axis slices as is possible with the hardware being used. The injection of the contrast is triggered once a steady electrocardiogram (ECG)-gate is obtained, and usually at the seventh cardiac cycle in the sequence. About 60 seconds of cardiac cycles are then acquired. It is convenient at this time to perform short-axis multiphase images of the left ventricle to allow time for the contrast agent to diffuse out of the myocardium. The patient can then be withdrawn from the bore of the magnet and be given the vasodilator for the stress portion of the study. This agent can be dipyridamole or adenosine, generally given at the same doses and rates as used in radionuclide imaging. Adenosine may be potentially more useful, secondary to the sensitivity of the MR perfusion technique to inadequate vasodilatation. In contrast to radionuclide imaging, the patient is not usually monitored with a 12-lead ECG during this portion of the study. Though uncommon, ECG changes with dipyridamole will go undetected in MR perfusion imaging, mandating close supervision by a physician able to deal with the possible complications. In spite of this, hundreds of these studies have been performed safely. The stress imaging acquisition is then performed in the same manner as the resting study. The higher coronary flow rates achievable postvasodilatation make the time resolution even more important than in the resting images, with every heart beat resolution ideal.

The question of performing these studies in a breath hold is an important one. With a compliant and generally healthy patient, it is possible to perform these studies in a breath hold, as the majority of the important data is acquired in approximately 20 seconds. Strategies used elsewhere in cardiac MRI for respiratory gating are less applicable to this application, as the loss of even a small portion of the data can make a great difference in the interpretation. In the patient who is unable to be studied in a breath hold, the images can be acquired while the patient is freely breathing, and then registered in a postprocessing procedure (21). While this is somewhat dependent on image quality, it is still preferable in many patients, and a requirement if quantitative analysis of the perfusion images is to be performed. Another important feature of MR perfusion imaging, which is different from other cardiac MRI procedures, is the desirability of a specific gating algorithm, which is able to accurately gate with the available ECG. When acquiring clinical images, missing a few cardiac cycles may actually improve the final result, by excluding R-R intervals that are significantly different from the rest. In perfusion imaging, those lost R-R intervals may have contained the information that would have allowed ischemic myocardium to be distinguished from normal segments.

INTERPRETATION OF MAGNETIC RESONANCE PERFUSION IMAGES

The interpretation of cardiac perfusion images has brought some unexpected clinical challenges. With the expectation of high-resolution images unfettered by acoustical limitations, MRI perfusion images should be easier to accurately read than the corresponding images produced by radionuclide imaging or echocardiographic techniques. The higher resolution of MR perfusion imaging seems, however, to demonstrate regional flow heterogeneity even in patients with angiographically normal coronary arteries. Additionally, imaging artifacts can produce the appearance of defects to unfamiliar readers. Finally, it appears that the first-pass nature of MR perfusion imaging necessitates adequate vasodilatation to yield accurate results, which is not always achievable with the standard dose of dipyridamole (22).

The images are most easily read qualitatively in cine form, with a normal study demonstrating enhancement of the right ventricular cavity, followed by the left ventricular cavity, and finally enhancement of the myocardium, discernibly from epicardium to endocardium. Delay in enhancement in a segment with eventual normalization is the pattern seen in ischemia, with prolonged delay, the pattern seen in scar. Distinguishing scar from ischemia can also be assisted by the data present in the short-axis images (wall thickness and wall motion). Delayed hyperenhancement in segments may provide information about a segment's viability (23,24).

Semiquantitative analysis of perfusion images is done with two main goals. The first is to use image parameters to detect regional perfusion defects and to measure the effect of the vasodilatory agent used. The second is to allow semiquantification of blood flow and the derivation of flow indices in a particular region of interest (25). Algorithms are being developed that can detect ischemic territories once regions of interest are drawn in the appropriate myocardial segments. Parameters obtained from the time-intensity curves are compared as they vary within a segment from rest-to-stress and among the different myocardial segments analyzed. The ratio of the slope of the time-intensity curves in the rest-and-stress images can be used as a surrogate for perfusion index, which can be used to establish the adequacy of the vasodilatation and the normalcy of the myocardial segments in question. Adding the peak value achieved in the time-intensity curves to the ratios may be of value in distinguishing segments with rapid washin but poor overall increase in intensity (which may occur in infarction supplied by an open artery) from segments with rapid washin and normal peak values for intensity.

Unfortunately, these algorithms may not be applicable across different platforms, as signal characteristics inherent in images acquired with body coils are different from those acquired with surface coils. The development of useful semiquantitative ischemia algorithms will require the development of large databases of images with corresponding angiograms.

QUANTITATIVE PERFUSION

Like many other imaging techniques, the interpretation of magnetic resonance perfusion images requires practice and improves with experience. Minimizing this potential problem is possible in MR perfusion, through the adoption of a purely quantitative method for analyzing the images generated. Using the concept that the regional signal/time changes are proportional to the concentration of agent in the myocardium (which remains true at the lower doses of gadolinium agents) and an input function derived from the passage of contrast through the left ventricular cavity or the aorta, the blood flowing through a segment of myocardium can be modeled. In experimental systems, quantitative perfusion analysis based on these concepts has shown good agreement with perfusion measured by more traditional means.

APPLICATIONS OF MR PERFUSION

Table 1 summarizes the results of MR perfuson studies done to date. MR perfusion is currently in use as part of

TABLE 1. *Summary of MR perfusion studies performed to date*

Date	Authors	Topic studied	N	Vasodilator	Sensitivity	Specificity
1990	Wilke et al.	MR perfusion in CAD and normal volunteers	23	Not Determined	Good comparable data SPECT vs. MR	
1991	Manning et al.	First-pass MRI perfusion in patients with CAD	17	Not Determined	Excellent match with zones of infarction	
1992	Schaefer et al.	Imaging in 1- and 2-vessel CAD and normals	10	Dipyridamole	vs. angiography 65%	76%
1993	Klein	Perfusion in chronic CAD	5	Dipyridamole	Retrospective: 92%	75%
1994	Eichenberger et al.	Perfusion in ischemic heart disease	10	Dipyridamole	65%	76%
1994	Hartnell et al.	Perfusion in myocardial ischemia	18	Dipyridamole	vs. angiography 92% vs. thallium 92%	100% 100%
1994	Wilke et al.	Perfusion in stable CAD and normal volunteers	18	Dipyridamole	vs. SPECT 90%	

(continued)

CHAPTER 32

Magnetic Resonance Angiography of the Great Vessels and the Coronary Arteries

Peter G. Danias, Robert R. Edelman, and
Warren J. Manning

Magnetic resonance imaging (MRI) has many applications. One of the most important is MRI of the blood vessels, or magnetic resonance angiography (MRA). The ability to visualize the blood vessels using MRA is related to the fact that the signal that leads to the increased intensity within arteries and veins is related to blood motion. Accordingly, angiography can be performed without the need for contrast agents. Nevertheless, under certain conditions, particularly when imaging smaller vessels such as the coronary arteries, paramagnetic contrast agents can be helpful for improved visualization. This chapter focuses on the present and potential clinical applications of MRA.

PRESENT CLINICAL APPLICATIONS

Imaging of the Aorta

Over the last decade, MRA has been recognized as the premier technique for aortic imaging. MRA compares favorably to contrast x-ray aortography because it has no associ-

P. G. Danias: Department of Medicine, Harvard Medical School; Cardiovascular Division, Department of Medicine, Beth Israel Deaconess Medical Center, Boston, Massachusetts 02115.
R. R. Edelman: Department of Radiology, Harvard Medical School; Department of Radiology, Beth Israel Deaconess Medical Center, Boston, Massachusetts 02115.
W. J. Manning: Departments of Medicine and Radiology, Harvard Medical School, Boston, Massachusetts 02114; Cardiac Magnetic Resonance Center, Beth Israel Deaconess Medical Center, Boston, Massachusetts 02115.

ated procedural risks, iodinated contrast load, or ionizing radiation exposure. It has the advantage of being a three-dimensional technique. In addition, MR imaging of the aorta can provide information on wall composition, wall thickness, and intraluminal thrombus, whereas conventional aortography only depicts the lumen. Transthoracic and even transesophageal echocardiography (TTE and TEE, respectively) have limited ability to visualize the entire thoracic aorta. The superior border of the aortic arch and the origins of the great vessels often cannot be adequately assessed in adults using these ultrasound approaches. Furthermore, the somewhat invasive nature of TEE results in patient discomfort and risk, whereas the MR examination is very well tolerated by the majority of subjects. Finally, x-ray computerized tomography (CT) can only provide transverse sections, has associated x-ray exposure, and requires significant intravenous iodinated contrast load. The relatively large aortic diameter (20–35 mm), the rapid blood flow inside the lumen, and the relative immobility of the aortic arch and the descending thoracic aorta are additional characteristics favorable for MR imaging. Spin-echo (black-blood) techniques offer a "static" view of the vessel and are usually employed to visualize the aortic anatomy, because they offer high contrast between the lumen and the vessel wall. Aortic MRA per se, using gradient-echo (white-blood) techniques, with or without use of contrast enhancement, also can provide a comprehensive evaluation of aortic anatomy. For example, with the use of maximum intensity projections (MIP) to reconstruct the aorta and aortic arch vessels, one can obtain a 3D appreciation of the thoracic aortic anatomy (Fig. 1).

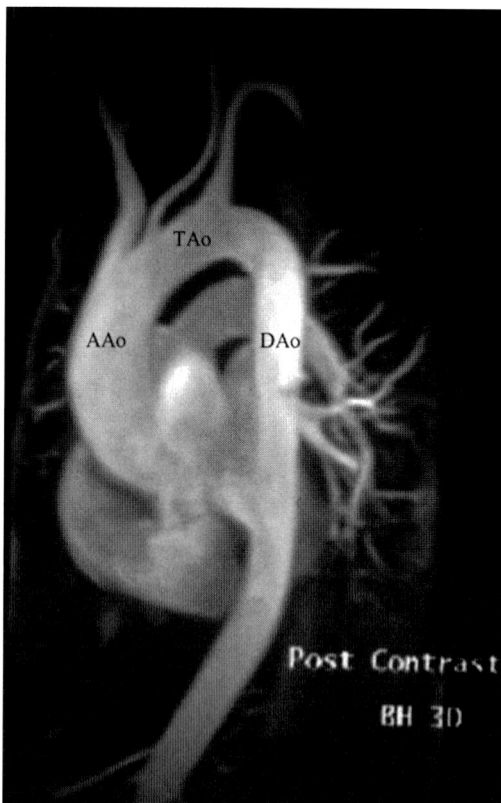

FIG. 1. Breath-hold (*BH*) Gd-DTPA-enhanced 3D imaging and reconstruction of the aorta, including the ascending aorta (*AAo*), transverse (*TAo*), and descending thoracic aorta (*DAo*) and the origins of the great vessels.

Flow

Gradient-echo MR sequences, including "time-of-flight" and "phase-contrast" approaches, have been used to measure aortic flow. The technical aspects, merits, and disadvantages of such techniques are beyond the scope of this chapter and have been discussed elsewhere (see Chapters 28–30). MRA can reliably measure the aortic flow and the elastic properties of the aorta. Several investigators (1,2) have shown that stroke volume and cardiac output MR measurements by direct flow measurement in the ascending thoracic aorta are in close agreement with measurements of the same parameters using the Simpson rule (disk-area method) from contiguous left ventricular short-axis images in systole and diastole. Additionally, aortic mean and instantaneous flow MR determinations are in close agreement with analogous Doppler echocardiographic data (2). Flow measurements of the ascending aorta may also be measured during bicycle ergometer exercise (up to 100 W) in healthy volunteers. Despite the exercise-induced thoracic motion, internally consistent measurements of flow and calculations of cardiac output are obtained (3).

Aortic MRA offers the potential to study the complex flow hemodynamics throughout the cardiac cycle. In both normal subjects and patients with coronary artery disease, flow in the aortic root is helical and reverses at the distal

ascending and transverse aorta (4). Vortices of clockwise and counterclockwise flow are generated in the left and right coronary sinuses, respectively, and are largely responsible for coronary artery filling. Although the study of the complex hemodynamics of the aortic flow is a field of active investigation, its role for clinical practice is uncertain at the present time.

Intravenous gadolinium (Gd-DTPA) is often used for aortic MRA to improve the contrast between the aorta and the surrounding structures. Contrast-enhanced MRA is widely used for the evaluation of patients with known or suspected aortic dissection, penetrating aortic ulcerations, and aortic aneurysms. These conditions are discussed in greater detail below.

Aortic Dissection

Aortic dissection is defined as the separation of a portion of the vascular intima from the media, and the generation of a second "false" lumen within the aortic wall. Thus an intimal dissection flap is formed, with distinct entry and exit points. Both therapy options and patient prognosis largely depend on the location and proximal extent of the dissection. Thus, the adequate visualization of the dissection flap is of highest clinical significance. Although the clinical presentation of this condition is usually dramatic, establishing the diagnosis is occasionally difficult and delay of appropriate therapy may be associated with an increased morbidity and mortality.

MR imaging is uniquely suited to assess aortic dissection, due to the ability to obtain tomographic images in virtually any plane. Aortic MRA is currently considered the "gold standard" for both establishing the diagnosis and identifying the entry and exit points (Fig. 2). Although spin-echo techniques are most commonly used and can readily identify the dissection flap, gradient-echo MRA, both without and with Gd-DTPA administration, offer high diagnostic yield. Flow

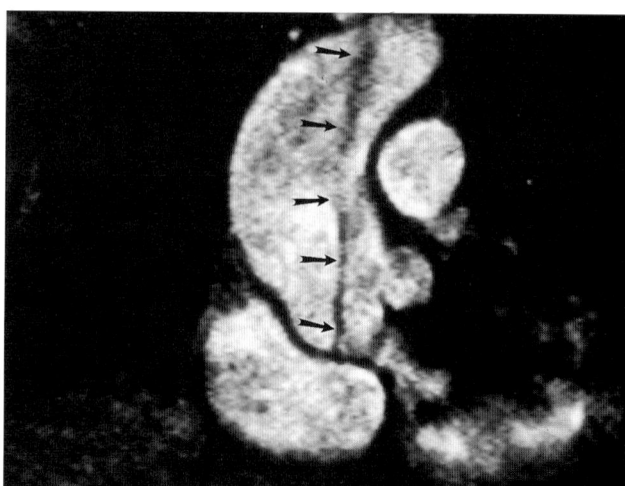

FIG. 2. Coronal slice of the ascending aorta using a breath-hold 2D gradient-echo sequence. Note the dissection flap (*arrows*) in the ascending aorta.

TABLE 1. *Detection and classification of thoracic aortic dissection, according to 4 noninvasive imaging modalities*

	Sensitivity (%)	Specificity (%)	Accuracy (%)	Positive predictive value (%)	Negative predictive value (%)
Type A dissection (ascending aorta)					
TTE	78.1	86.7	84.1	71.4	90.3
TEE	96.4	85.7	90	81.8	97.3
CT	82.6	100	94.9	100	93.3
MRI	100[a]	98.6[a,b]	99.0[a]	96.8[a]	100[a]
Type B dissection (descending aorta)					
TTE	10.0	100	80.4	100	80.0
TEE	100	96.4	97.1	88.2	100
CT	96.0	88.9	91.1	80.0	98.0
MRI	96.5[a]	100[c]	99.0[a]	100[c]	98.7[a]
All dissections					
TTE	59.3	83.0	69.8	81.4	61.9
TEE	97.7	76.9	90.0	87.7	95.2
CT	93.8	87.1	91.1	91.8	90.0
MRI	98.3[a]	97.8[a,b]	98.0[a]	98.3[a]	97.8

[a] $P < 0.05$ for TTE vs. MR.
[b] $P < 0.05$ for TEE vs. MR.
[c] $P < 0.05$ for CT vs. MR.
(From ref. 5, with permission.)

in the true and false aortic lumens can also be visualized and quantified.

In a large prospective study, Nienaber et al. (5) compared four noninvasive imaging tests for aortic dissection in clinically stable patients with suspected aortic dissection. One hundred and ten patients were evaluated by MRI, contrast-enhanced CT, TTE, and monoplane TEE. Test results were compared to contrast x-ray aortography, operative and autopsy findings. Aortic MRA was shown to have sensitivity and specificity both approaching 100% (Table 1). However, the MR examination was rather lengthy (39 ± 16 min), significantly longer compared to other noninvasive tests. Although the safety of MR aortography in very large series of unselected patients has not been reported, there is a concern that the lengthy examination may increase morbidity and mortality in unstable patients by delaying therapy. Aortic MRA has the advantage (relative to x-ray CT) that concomitant aortic valve involvement (presenting as aortic insufficiency) can be assessed in patients with suspected aortic dissection, though echocardiography is usually superior for quantitation of the severity of aortic regurgitation. With MRI the pericardium and involvement of great vessels are also readily appreciated, as well as the origin of the coronary arteries. However, MRA requires significant patient cooperation, and bulk motion during the examination results in motion artifacts, which considerably decrease the diagnostic yield of the examination. The interpretation of thoracic MR aortography should always be performed by qualified physicians, as the incidence of pitfalls that may lead to erroneous diagnosis is considerable (6).

Aortic Aneurysm

Aortic aneurysms have been reported in approximately 10% of autopsy series and the most common etiology is atherosclerosis. It is recognized that for the thoracic aorta, an aneurysm diameter that exceeds 6 cm (7 cm for patients at high operative risk) or one that is rapidly expanding, carries substantial risk for spontaneous rupture, and surgical repair is thus often indicated. The high spatial resolution of MR allows for precise measurements of the aortic diameter, which are of particular importance during the periodic follow-up of patients with known aortic aneurysms. Spin-echo techniques can reliably visualize the outer aortic diameter, whereas maximum intensity projections from gradient-echo sequences (with or without Gd-DTPA contrast enhancement) depict the internal lumen (Fig. 3). The interpretation of gradient-echo images should be performed with caution,

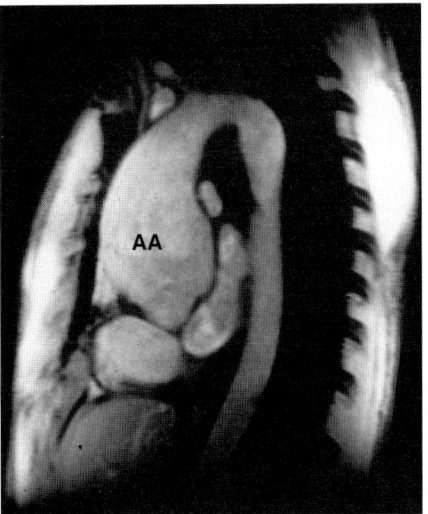

FIG. 3. Sagittal image obtained with a breath-hold 2D gradient-echo sequence with a large field-of-view, indicating a large aortic root aneurysm (*AA*).

as extensive thrombosis of the aneurysmal sac but without compromise of the luminal diameter may give the false impression of a normal vessel caliber. As compared with CT, MRA is unable to visualize focal aortic wall calcifications. However, MR has the significant advantage of not requiring iodinated x-ray contrast: an issue that is of particular significance, because of the incidence of co-existent renal disease and increased risk for contrast-induced nephropathy.

Congenital Diseases

The detailed description of MR imaging in simple and complex congenital heart disease is beyond the scope of this chapter and is discussed elsewhere (see Chapters 56–58), but there are certain congenital abnormalities that merit specific mention in reference to aortic MR imaging. These include the Marfan syndrome and coarctation of the aorta, disorders that are occasionally diagnosed in adolescents and young adults.

Marfan Syndrome

This genetic disorder is characterized by abnormal collagen synthesis, which results in abnormal elastic properties of a wide variety of tissues. Among these, the involvement of the media of the aortic wall results in weakening of the vessel wall and subsequent aneurysmal dilatation. Spontaneous aortic rupture is a common occurrence and cause of death in patients with Marfan syndrome. Surgical repair of ascending aorta aneurysms is recommended when the vessel diameter exceeds 5.5 cm, and in particular for those at high risk (women planning pregnancy, those with a family history of the Marfan syndrome with aortic dissection/rupture, and those with rapid aortic dilatation) surgery should be considered sooner.

MR imaging of the aorta is ideal both for initial assessment and for comparative follow-up studies of these individuals. Although standard TTE is most commonly used for assessment of the proximal ascending aorta, the improved accuracy and precision of MR imaging, coupled with the ability to obtain high-resolution images of the entire thoracic aorta in all compliant patients, place MR imaging as the new "gold standard" for the evaluation of this population.

Areas of research investigation include the MR assessment of the elastic properties of the aorta, with the evaluation of aortic distensibility, force of ejection, and pulse wave velocity. These parameters may be of benefit for the follow-up and evaluation of treatment adequacy in patients with Marfan syndrome that receive beta-blocker therapy to prevent aortic root dilatation.

Coarctation

This congenital vascular disease is characterized by the focal narrowing of the aortic lumen, most commonly immediately distal to the takeoff of the left subclavian artery, and is often seen in concert with congenital bicuspid aortic valve.

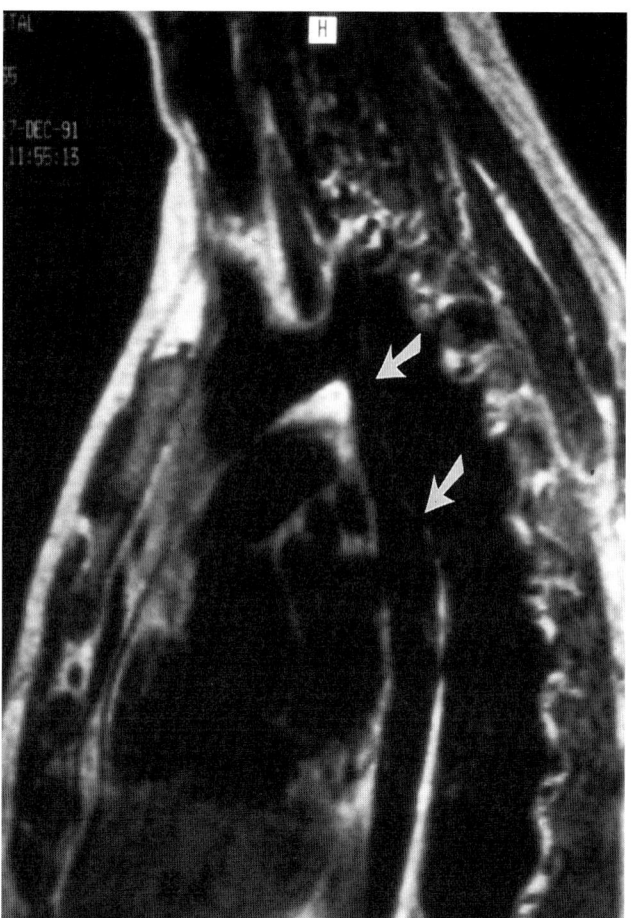

FIG. 4. Sagittal slice through the aortic arch and descending thoracic aorta, obtained using a spin-echo sequence during free breathing. The aortic diameter significantly narrows (*arrows*) distal to the left subclavian artery, establishing the diagnosis of aortic coarctation.

Though the pressure gradient across the stenosis can usually be evaluated by TTE with Doppler from the suprasternal approach, the anatomic location of this abnormality makes it difficult for other conventional noninvasive techniques to adequately visualize the length and precise location of the coarctation. Because of the ability to image with unrestricted angulations, aortic MRA is ideal for the delineation of this congenital abnormality (Fig. 4). At the same session flow velocity in the aorta can also be accurately measured. Thus, MR aortography, combining anatomic imaging and flow measurements, can be used to thoroughly assess the significance and evolution of this disorder.

MAGNETIC RESONANCE OF THE PULMONARY ARTERY

Compared to imaging of the aorta, MR imaging of the pulmonary artery is more challenging but is also becoming common. The pulmonary vasculature is particularly susceptible to artifacts related to motion, as the lungs expand and collapse during free breathing. Additionally, pulmonary ar-

TABLE 2. *Summary of pulmonary MRA studies for detection of pulmonary embolism (acute or chronic)*

Study	Technique	# Patients	Sensitivity (%)	Specificity (%)
	Spin-echo		31–84	25–100
Schiebler et al. 1993 (31)	SPAMM	18[a]	26–91	33–100
	TOF		25–88	33–100
Grist et al. 1993 (32)	GRE	20	96 (92–100)	62
Erdman 1994 (33)	Spin-echo (some + GRE)	64	90	77
	Spin-echo		50	44
Hatabu et al. 1994 (34)	SPAMM + spin-echo	12	88	100
	GRE cine + spin-echo		75	100
Loubeyre et al. 1994 (35)	Contrast-enhanced	23	70	100
Bergin et al. 1997 (36)	Contrast-enhanced	30	92 (90–93)	92 (87–96)
Meaney et al. 1997 (37)	Contrast-enhanced	30	100 (57–100)	95 (87–100)

[a] Segmental analysis.
GRE, gradient-echo; *SPAMM*, spatial modulation of magnetization; *TOF*, time-of-flight.

teries branch in a complex 3D fashion, and their diameter progressively decreases with each bifurcation. Finally, signal loss occurs at the vessel-lung interface, due to significant differences in magnetic susceptibility between blood/tissue and air. Although spin-echo approaches can be used to define the anatomy of the pulmonary trunk and the proximal portions of the right and left main pulmonary arteries, gradient-echo techniques (with or without contrast enhancement) are the mainstay of pulmonary MRA.

The evaluation and diagnosis of congenital abnormalities of the pulmonary trunk are discussed in Chapters 56–58. For clinical purposes in adult diagnostic imaging, the most significant application of pulmonary MRA is for the diagnosis of acute (and chronic) pulmonary thromboembolism. Thrombus embolization to segmental or subsegmental branches of the pulmonary artery is not infrequently encountered in chronically ill or debilitated patients with other medical problems or following major abdominal/pelvic surgery, and is associated with considerable morbidity and mortality. Because the signs and symptoms associated with pulmonary embolism are often nonspecific (tachycardia, dyspnea, cough, hemoptysis, chest pain, hypotension) and because the condition requires anticoagulation, occasionally thrombolysis, and rarely thrombectomy, therapies with considerable associated complications, it is important to promptly and reliably establish the diagnosis. The current "gold standard" for the diagnosis of pulmonary embolism is contrast x-ray pulmonary angiography, a procedure with considerable morbidity, cost, and associated risk for these compromised patients. Although radionuclide ventilation-perfusion scans are widely used and offer high sensitivity for the diagnosis of pulmonary embolism, the test specificity is low (~40% indeterminate scans), limiting the diagnostic yield of this test. Pulmonary MRA has been demonstrated to be an excellent noninvasive alternative: in several studies it has been shown to have an approximate overall sensitivity and specificity close to 90% (Table 2). Similar to conventional angiography, pulmonary emboli present as an abrupt discontinuation (signal void) of the arterial lumen (Fig. 5). Adjacent slices have

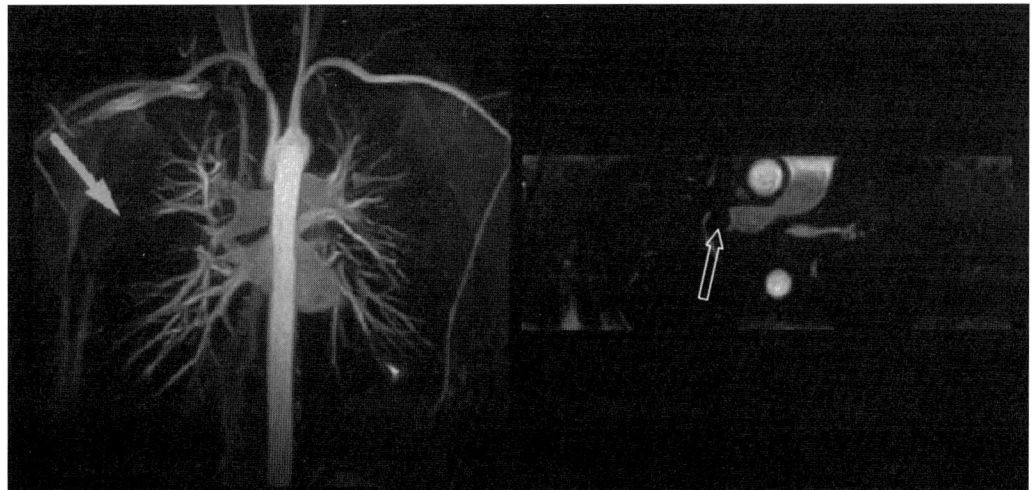

FIG. 5. MR pulmonary angiogram with Gd-DTPA contrast-enhancement acquired using a 3D breath-hold gradient-echo sequence. **Left panel:** The white *arrow* indicates an abrupt cutoff in a branch of the right pulmonary artery, suggesting a pulmonary artery embolism. The aorta and great vessels are also visualized. **Right panel:** A transverse slice at the level of the proximal right pulmonary artery demonstrates the filling defect (*open arrow*) in the vessel lumen.

to be carefully evaluated to exclude the out-of-plane course of the apparently occluded pulmonary artery.

MR imaging has also been shown to accurately detect pulmonary arteriovenous malformations (AVM). In a series of 11 patients, using spin-echo, gradient-echo, and phase contrast imaging, Silverman and colleagues (7) reported 100% accuracy in detecting lesions 1 to 6 cm in diameter. Although not a very common condition, the significant left-to-right shunt with larger AVM may result in high-output heart failure, and therefore establishing the diagnosis has clinical relevance.

MAGNETIC RESONANCE OF THE INFERIOR AND SUPERIOR VENAE CAVA

Both superior and inferior venae cava are vessels with large diameter and are relatively immobile. Therefore, they are not subject to significant motion artifacts and can be readily imaged by MR. Accurate flow measurements can also be obtained and their flow velocity pattern has been shown to be biphasic (8). Tricuspid regurgitation, constrictive/restrictive cardiac physiology, impaired systolic and diastolic right ventricular function, all result in impaired flow-velocity patterns within both venae cava and can be accurately determined by MR. However, the significant dependence of caval flow on the hemodynamic loading conditions, as well as the significant variability of these parameters within each subject, limit the clinical value of this information.

Another application of MRA of the great thoracic veins is for diagnosis of the superior vena cava (SVC) syndrome. This condition is characterized by engorgement of the SVC due to partial obstruction of drainage to the right atrium, commonly due to mediastinal neoplasm. Although contrast-enhanced CT imaging is commonly used for diagnosis of this disorder, MR imaging is superior, because it avoids the iodinated contrast osmotic load and decreases the likelihood for allergic reaction in patients who may already have laryngeal edema.

PULMONARY VEINS

The evaluation of pulmonary veins using MRA is most commonly performed to assess congenital abnormalities, and in particular anomalous pulmonary venous return to the right atrium. Although spin-echo MR imaging has been shown to be superior to both echocardiography and conventional angiography (9), gradient-echo approaches appear to have an even higher sensitivity in detecting partial anomalous pulmonary venous return (10) (Fig. 6). Anomalous pulmonary vein flow or pulmonary-to-systemic flow ratios can be quantified using phase-velocity methods. A more extensive discussion of the use of magnetic resonance to diagnose this and other congenital anomalies is presented elsewhere (see Chapters 56–58).

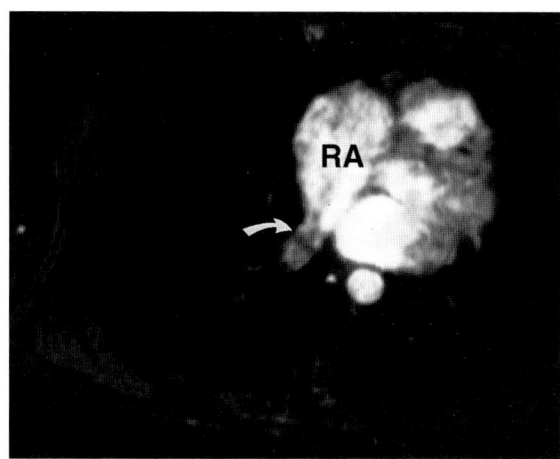

FIG. 6. Anomalous pulmonary venous return. Transverse slice acquired with a breath-hold 2D gradient-echo sequence, showing the right inferior pulmonary vein (*curved arrow*) draining into the right atrium (*RA*).

MAGNETIC RESONANCE OF THE CORONARY ARTERIES

Coronary contrast x-ray angiography (see Chapter 25) is the established "gold standard" for evaluation of the major epicardial coronaries. However, this invasive technique has associated morbidity, results in significant ionizing radiation exposure, and is rather costly. A noninvasive alternative approach that lacks these negative attributes is coronary MRA, which can assess both the anatomy and flow dynamics of the coronary circulation. However, even with rapid imaging MR sequences, cardiac motion and spatial resolution requirements necessitate that data are acquired over many successive heartbeats. Image blurring and motion artifacts occur during free-breathing coronary MRA. Additional impediments to high-resolution coronary MRA include the small diameter of the coronary arteries, their proximity to cardiac veins and to large blood pools (both atria and ventricles), the distance from the radiofrequency receiver coil (especially for the left circumflex coronary artery), and the strong signal from the surrounding epicardial fat.

Various approaches have been used to overcome these limitations and to allow submillimeter resolution coronary MRA. High-quality electrocardiographic (ECG) gating is an absolute necessity, usually in combination with k-space segmentation. Breath-holding, respiratory gating with diaphragmatic navigators or respiratory bellows, repetitive coached breathing, and correction of respiratory displacement based on navigator position data have all been used to compensate for respiratory bulk cardiac displacement and to attenuate motion artifacts. In combination with these motion suppression approaches, selective fat saturation with or without myocardial suppression prepulses, 3D imaging, ultrafast techniques, and intravascular contrast agents have all been used to improve the spatial resolution of coronary MRA.

Anatomy

Early studies using conventional ECG-gated MR spin-echo techniques demonstrated the feasibility of visualization of the coronary artery ostia in humans. With the introduction of gradient-echo imaging with k-space segmentation and breath-holding, imaging of extensive portions of the coronaries became possible. As first described in humans by Edelman et al. (11), the acquisition of multiple phase-encoding steps during each cardiac cycle can be used for acquisition of a 2D image in 15 to 20 sec. With this approach, breath-holding can be used to "freeze" respiratory motion, and a series of consecutively acquired 2D images spanning the proximal coronary tree are obtained. In most of the subsequent coronary MRA studies, the heart has been imaged during a 100-msec window in mid-diastole, a period of relative cardiac diastasis (so that cardiac motion would be minimized), but with rather high coronary blood flow. Typically, eight interleaved phase encoding steps are acquired during each cardiac cycle, necessitating 16 successive heart beats to complete a 128 (=8 × 16) ×256 matrix. Other typical imaging parameters include frequency selective pre-pulse for fat signal suppression, slice thickness of 3 to 4 mm and field-of-view of 240 mm. These parameters yield an in-plane spatial resolution of approximately 1.9 × 0.9 mm. However, repetitive breath-holding is fatiguing and greatly limits sequence development.

Although for the initial attempts for coronary MRA utilized breath-holding to minimize respiratory motion artifacts, the ability to compensate for respiratory motion using respiratory bellows or MR navigators now allows for free breathing coronary MRA. In conjunction with software and hardware advances (gradients, receiver coils), free-breathing 3D navigator methods for coronary MRA have become widely available. During a typical 3D study, a 30-mm thick slab can be imaged, with a 3-mm slice thickness and in-plane resolution of 0.5 × 0.5 mm (Fig. 7). With 3D approaches there is improved slice registration and enhanced signal-to-noise ratio, advantages that are of great importance for imaging of the tortuous coronary arteries. In addition, the introduction of intravascular contrast agents (which dramatically increase the T1 relaxation time of blood) improve the contrast-to-noise ratio and have provided encouraging initial results. Currently there is active investigation in this field to optimize free-breathing 3D coronary MRA, with and without contrast enhancement. The proximal portions of the major coronary arteries can be visualized in the vast majority of compliant subjects. In general, the right coronary artery, left main, and the left anterior descending coronary arteries are relatively easier to image, due to their less tortuous and more predictable course and their relatively anterior location. Consequently, the length of the right and left anterior descending coronary arteries that can be reliably visualized is typically longer than that for the left circumflex artery.

Coronary MRA has also been demonstrated to accurately measure the diameter of angiographically normal coronary vessels. The MR-measured average coronary vessel diameter (2.8–4.8 mm) is similar to previously reported anatomic (reference) values and correlates closely with the corresponding measurement from conventional angiography.

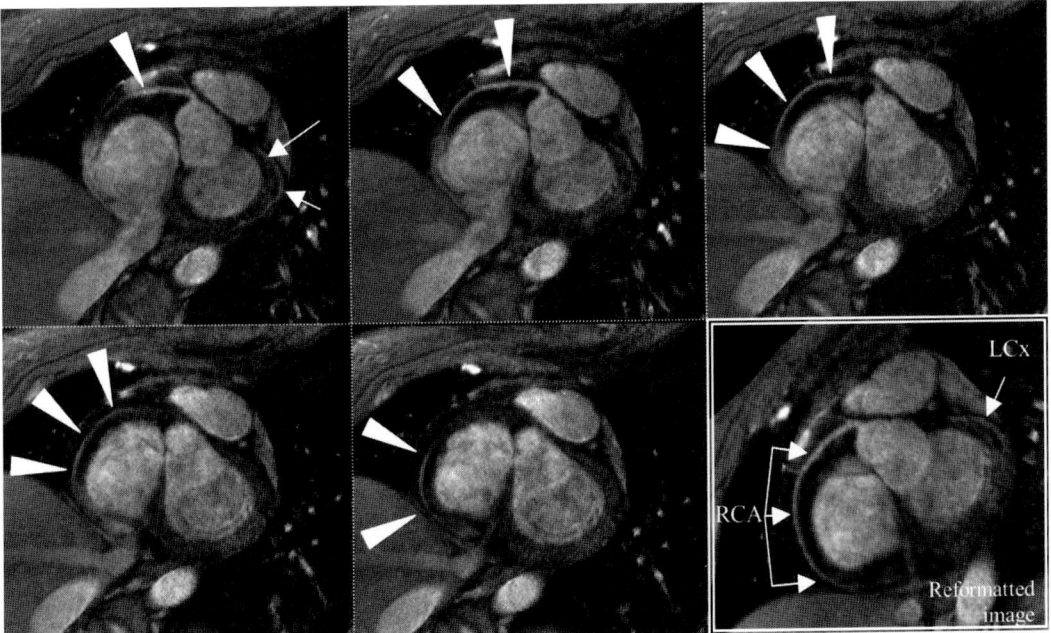

FIG. 7. Oblique coronary MRA from a free-breathing navigator-gated 3D image acquisition with prospective slice correction. In plane resolution is 0.5 × 0.5 mm. The entire right coronary artery (*RCA*) (*arrowheads*) and portion of the left circumflex coronary artery (*LCx*) (*arrows*) can be seen. (Courtesy of M. Stuber, Ph.D., and R. Botnar, Ph.D.)

Anomalous Coronaries

Coronary MRA is uniquely suited for the detection and course delineation of anomalous coronary arteries. Compared with conventional x-ray contrast angiography that is a projection method, coronary MRA can obtain images in any orientation and can thus reliably present the relationships of the various anatomic structures in any user-defined plane. Though rather uncommon, occurring in only 0.6–1.2% of adults, specific coronary anomalies have been associated with increased mortality. In particular, when an anomalous left anterior descending or right coronary artery courses between the ascending aorta and main pulmonary artery (Fig. 8), transient obstruction of flow in the coronary vessel may occur, resulting in extensive myocardial ischemia and sudden death. Therefore, the accurate identification and delineation of the course of the coronary arteries are of great clinical significance. This information is also of importance for preoperative evaluation, in cases referred for surgical revascularization.

At least three "blinded" comparative studies, collectively including 47 patients with coronary anomalies, have demonstrated that coronary MRA is as good as, if not superior to, conventional invasive angiographic imaging for this disorder (12–14). Many experienced laboratories now consider MR imaging as the "gold standard" for defining the anatomic course of these anomalous vessels.

Coronary Artery Disease

The assessment of native vessel coronary atherosclerosis using coronary MRA is a field of intense research activity. Although current techniques have a relatively limited spatial

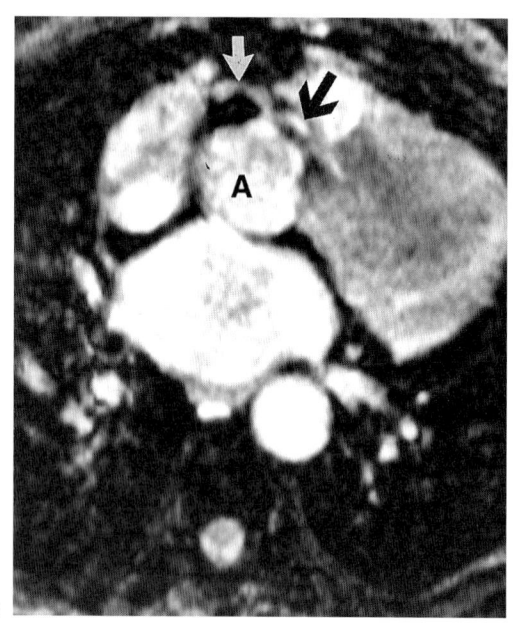

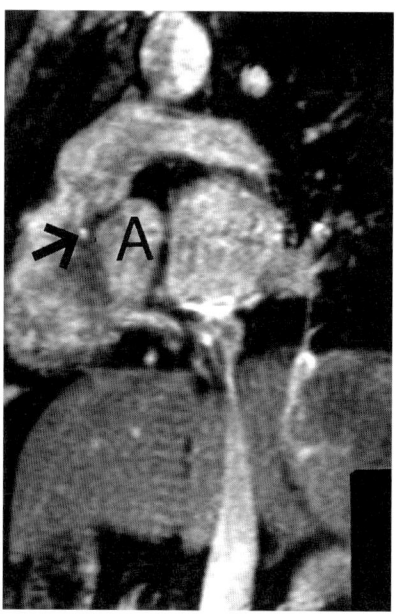

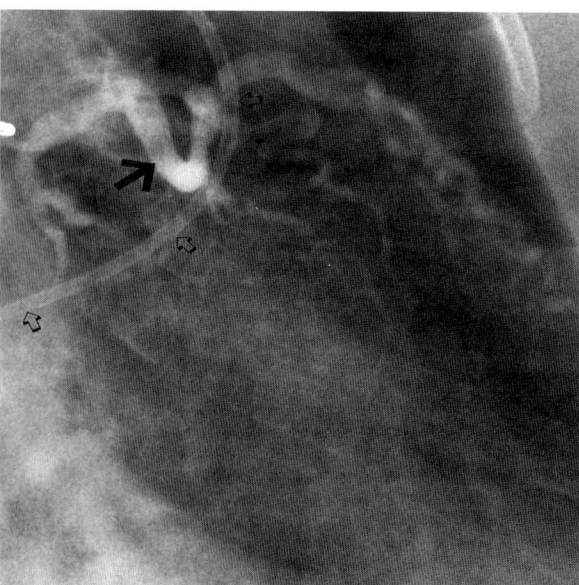

FIG. 8. A: Transverse coronary MRA image showing an anomalous common coronary artery arising from the right cusp and bifurcating to right coronary artery (*white arrow*) and left coronary artery (*black arrow*). The left coronary artery courses anterior to the aorta (*A*) and posterior to the right ventricular outflow tract. **B:** An oblique MRA image also demonstrates the course of the left coronary artery (*arrow*) between the aorta (*A*) and the right ventricular outflow tract. The conventional x-ray angiogram (right anterior oblique projection) from this patient (**C**) confirms the coronary anomaly. Note the anomalous left coronary artery (*arrow*) and its relation to the pulmonary artery catheter (*arrowheads*). (From ref. 14, with permission.)

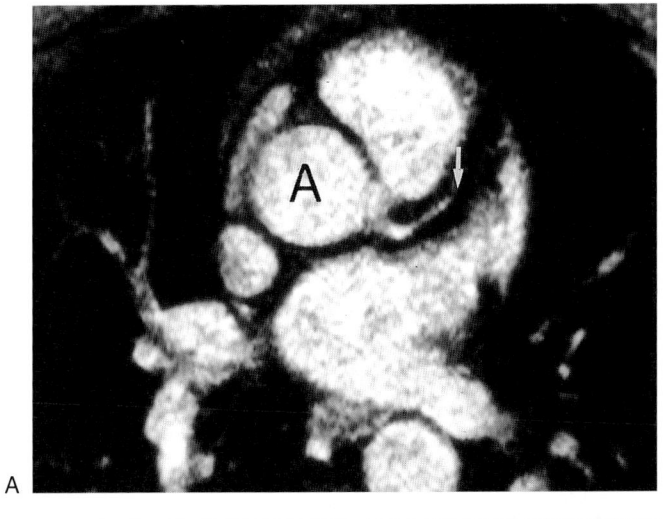

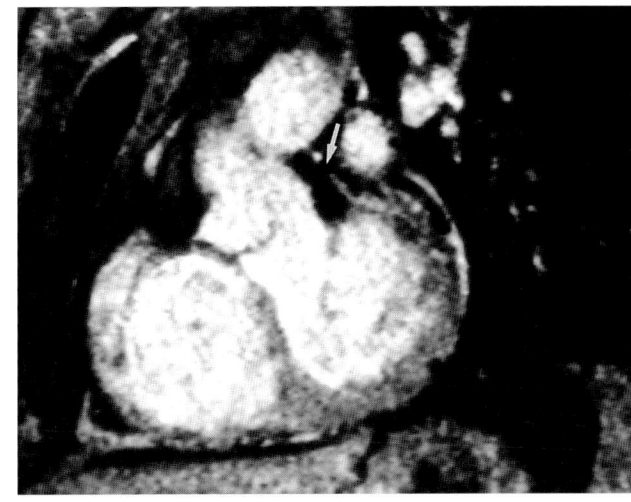

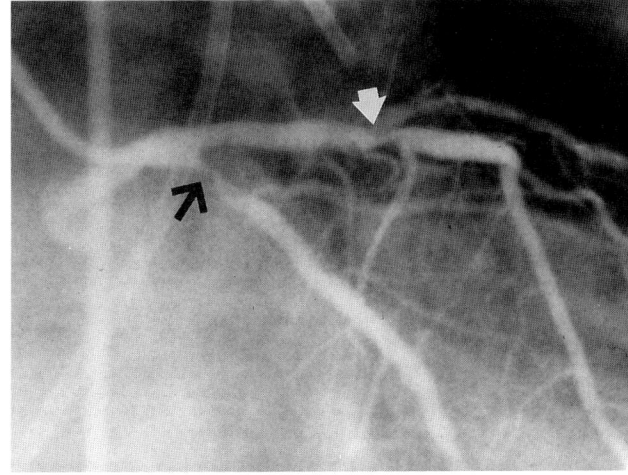

FIG. 9. Coronary MRA using a breath-hold 2D gradient-echo sequence, demonstrating a stenosis in the left anterior descending coronary artery. Both the transverse slice at the level of the aortic root (*A*) (**A**) and a coronal slice (**B**) show a signal void in the proximal vessel (*arrow*). Corresponding x-ray angiogram (**C**) confirms a stenosis at the same site (*white arrow*), and also a moderate stenosis at the proximal left circumflex coronary artery (*black arrow*). (From ref. 16, with permission.)

resolution, which precludes *quantitative* coronary MRA, the ability to qualitatively evaluate proximal and mid-coronary artery stenoses has been demonstrated in several clinical series. In most of the recent studies, segmented k-space gradient echo techniques with rectangular or spiral k-space trajectories are used to image flow inside the coronary arteries. With this approach, high signal intensity (bright blood) represents normal blood flow and low signal (signal void) either turbulent blood flow (high velocity at the site of stenosis) or total vessel occlusion (complete absence of flow) (Fig. 9).

Manning et al. (15) first reported on coronary MRA in comparison with conventional angiography in 39 patients with coronary disease confirmed by x-ray contrast angiography. Coronary MRA was performed using breath-hold 2D imaging. In this patient population, coronary MRA images of 98% of the major epicardial arteries were of adequate quality for evaluation. Overall sensitivity and specificity of coronary MRA for correctly classifying individual vessels as having or not having significant CAD (>50% diameter stenosis on conventional contrast angiography) was 90% and 92%, respectively. Subsequent studies (17–23) have reported variable sensitivity and specificity values for detect-

ing coronary disease (Table 3). Differences in patient selection, technique, and imaging parameters (including different spatial and temporal resolution) likely account for the wide variability. In the study by Pennell et al. (22), the severity of MR signal loss as a function of the degree of stenosis was also evaluated and was found to closely correlate with the percentage diameter stenosis. More recently, coronary MRA was also used to evaluate patients with coronary disease and balloon angioplasty, and was found to have high diagnostic yield for assessing restenosis (19).

In patients with recent myocardial infarction coronary MRA has been shown to accurately evaluate the presence of antegrade flow in the infarct-related artery (24–26). The noninvasive determination of patency influences therapy and prognosis in these patients, as it is believed that a patent coronary artery following myocardial infarction decreases the likelihood for remodeling and arrhythmogenesis.

Coronary Artery Bypass Grafts

MR imaging of coronary bypass grafts (both saphenous veins and internal mammary arteries) is facilitated by their relatively stationary anterior position, their relatively straight

TABLE 3. *Summary of coronary MRA studies for the detection of significant CAD (>50% stenoses)*

Investigators	Technique	Respiratory suppression	# Subjects	# Vessels with stenoses (%)	Sensitivity for <50% diameter stenosis	Specificity in detecting CAD
Manning et al. 1993 (15)	2D seg. GRE	BH	39	52 (35)	90 (71–100)	92 (78–100)
Duerinckx et al. 1994 (22)	2D seg. GRE	BH	21	27 (34)	63 (0–73)	(37–82)
Post et al. 1996 (21)	3D GRE	Retrospective nav. gating	20	21 (27)	38 (0–57)	95 (85–100)
Pennell et al. 1996 (22)	2D seg. GRE	BH	39	55 (35)	85 (75–100)	
Hu et al. 1996 (38)	2D interleaved spiral	BH	23	27	63	
Post et al. 1997 (20)	2D seg. GRE	BH	35	35 (28)	63 (0–100)	89 (73–96)
Müller et al. 1997 (19)	3D GRE	Retrospective nav. gating	35	54 (31)	83 (50–100)	94 (85–100)
Kessler et al. 1997 (18)	3D GRE	Retrospective nav. gating	73	43	65	88
Yoshino et al. 1997 (39)	2D seg. GRE	BH	31	31 (100–directed)	86	98
Woodard et al. 1998 (17)	3D GRE	Retrospective nav. gating	10	10 (25)	70	73

Sensitivity and specificity values are reported as mean (individual vessel range).
Seg., segmented k-space; *GRE*, gradient echo; *BH*, breath-hold; *nav.*, navigator.

and predictable course, and their larger diameter (compared to the native coronary vessels). Presence of flow is visualized as a signal void (spin-echo) and as bright signal (gradient-echo imaging) in the anatomic location corresponding to the expected graft position. Identification of flow in at least two slices obtained at different planes perpendicular to the expected bypass graft course suggests patency (Fig. 10). If, however, the presence of flow is suggested at only one level,

graft patency is considered "indeterminate," and if there is no evidence of flow in any portions of the graft, the graft is considered occluded. More recently, Gd-DTPA-enhanced 3D coronary MRA has been reported to have higher sensitivity (95–100%) for patency of both saphenous venous and internal mammary grafts. Data from several studies with and without use of MR contrast, comparing MR imaging data with contrast angiography, are summarized in Table 4.

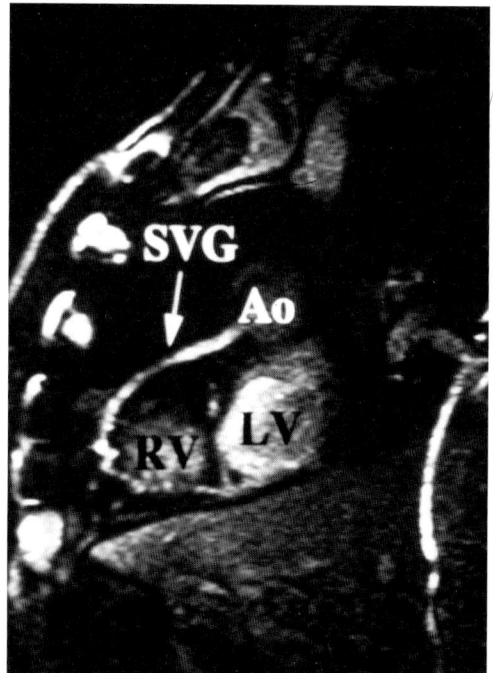
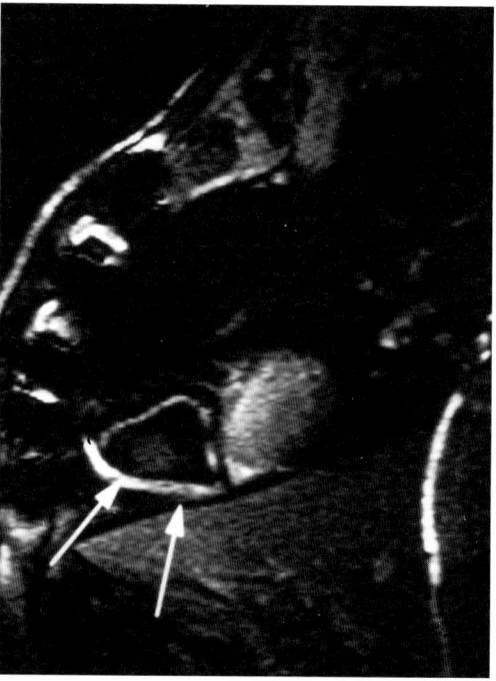

FIG. 10. Breath-hold MRA of a saphenous vein coronary artery bypass graft. Adjacent images show the graft (*SVG*) extending from the proximal aorta (*Ao*) to the posterior descending coronary artery. *LV*, left ventricle; *RV*, right ventricle. (From ref. 27, with permission.)

TABLE 4. *Summary of studies evaluating MRA for the assessment of coronary artery bypass graft patency*

	# Patients	# Grafts	% Patent	% Sensitivity	% Specificity
Spin Echo					
White et al. 1987 (40)	25	72	69	86	72
Rubinstein et al. 1987 (41)	20	47	62	90	72
Jenkins et al. 1988 (42)	16	41	63	89	73
Galjee et al. 1996 (43)	47	84	74	98	85
Gradient Echo					
White et al. 1988 (44)	28	28	52	93	86
Aurigemma et al. 1989 (45)	45	45	73	88	100
Galjee et al. 1996 (43)	47	84	74	98	88
Kessler et al. 1997 (18)	7	19	79	87	100
Flow Mapping					
Hoogendoorn et al. 1995 (46)	18	23	70	100/80 (PC/flow)	88/100 (PC/flow)
Contrast enhanced MRA					
Davies et al. 1997 (47)	8	54	39	100	24
Winterspreger et al. 1997 (48)	14	39	87	80/100 (SVG/IMA)	–
Vrachliotis et al. 1996 (49)	15	45	67	93	97
Winterspreger et al. 1998 (50)	27	76	79	94/96 (SVG/IMA)	85/67 (VSG/IMA)

pts, patients; *PC*, phase contrast; *SVG*, saphenous vein graft; *IMA*, internal mammary artery.

Although the patency or absence thereof can be usually confidently determined using MRA, the evaluation of adequacy of flow or the assessment of graft atherosclerotic disease is more challenging. Implanted metallic clips, markers, or intracoronary stents often create signal voids due to magnetic susceptibility. These artifacts, which are commonly located in very close proximity to the coronary arteries or grafts, preclude the assessment of these vessels.

Flow

MR phase velocity approaches have been used to quantify coronary artery blood flow. Although the extensive description of the principles of flow imaging are outside the scope of this chapter, in general, MR angiographic flow measurements are based on the modification of the MR blood signal as it crosses perpendicularly the imaging plane. Based either on net phase-change of the precessing flowing spins as they travel across a magnetic field gradient (phase-contrast technique), or on signal intensity changes due to inflow-effects (inflow or time-of-flight approach), blood velocity information can be obtained. By simultaneously measuring the coronary artery diameter, the instantaneous blood flow can be quantitatively assessed.

Coronary blood flow can be measured both during resting conditions and following pharmacologic vasodilatation. The relative change of flow velocity (and coronary flow rate) between the two states (rest-vasodilatation), represents the coronary flow reserve, a sensitive marker of epicardial and microvascular coronary artery disease. In patients with epicardial vessel atherosclerosis, the abnormal flow reserve can be used as an objective measurement to assess the need for revascularization. The accuracy of these measurements is limited by partial volume averaging effects (due to small vessel cross-sectional area), as well as by cardiac and respiratory motion and tortuous course of the coronary artery.

To overcome these limitations, several investigators measured global cardiac perfusion by assessing blood flow in the coronary sinus and/or the proximal aorta. Although these measurements are technically easier than direct coronary flow measurements, the global assessment of the coronary circulation is of little clinical value for evaluation of focal coronary stenoses. More recently, improvements in hardware and software have allowed for local coronary artery blood flow assessment. Edelman and colleagues (28) first reported on humans on direct measurement of right coronary and left anterior descending coronary artery flow using breath-holding with k-space segmentation. Various modifications of the phase contrast approach have been used to measure coronary flow in experimental animals, normal volunteers, patients with coronary disease, or patients with hypertrophic cardiomyopathy. Using coronary MRA, the biphasic pattern of flow in the right coronary artery and left anterior descending coronary artery, with the characteristic diastolic augmentation, have been demonstrated and shown to correlate well with intracoronary Doppler ultrasound measurements in humans (29,30). Relative changes of blood flow after intravenous administration of vasodilators (adenosine or dipyridamole) and after isometric exercise have also been used to measure coronary flow reserve in normal individuals and patients with heart disease. In normal human coronaries, a 3- to 5-fold increase of resting blood flow and velocity can be measured after pharmacologic vasodilatation, whereas a decreased (<2) ratio of flow reserve suggests impaired flow dynamics and is frequently encountered in epicardial or microvascular coronary artery disease.

REFERENCES

1. Bogren HG, Klipstein RH, Firmin DN, et al. Quantitation of antegrade and retrograde blood flow in the human aorta by magnetic resonance velocity mapping. *Am Heart J* 1989;117:1214–1222.
2. Kondo C, Caputo GR, Semelka R, et al. Right and left ventricular stroke volume measurements with velocity-encoded cine MR imaging: *in vitro* and *in vivo* validation. *Am J Roentgenol* 199;157:9–16.
3. Niezen RA, Doornbos J, van der Wall EE, et al. Measurement of aortic and pulmonary flow with MRI at rest and during physical exercise. *J Comput Assist Tomogr* 1998;22:194–201.
4. Bogren HG, Mohiaddin RH, Kilner PJ, et al. Blood flow patterns in the thoracic aorta studied with three-directional MR velocity mapping: the effects of age and coronary artery disease. *J Magn Reson Imaging* 1997;7:784–793.
5. Nienaber CA, von Kodolitsch Y, Nicolas V, et al. The diagnosis of thoracic aortic dissection by noninvasive imaging procedures [see comments]. *N Engl J Med* 1993;328:1–9.
6. Solomon SL, Brown JJ, Glazer HS, et al. Thoracic aortic dissection: pitfalls and artifacts in MR imaging. *Radiology* 1990;177:223–228.
7. Silverman JM, Julien PJ, Herfkens RJ, et al. Magnetic resonance imaging evaluation of pulmonary vascular malformations. *Chest* 1994;106:1333–1338.
8. Mohiaddin RH, Wann SL, Underwood R, et al. Vena caval flow: assessment with cine MR velocity mapping. *Radiology* 1990;177:537–541.
9. Masui T, Seelos KC, Kersting-Sommerhoff BA, et al. Abnormalities of the pulmonary veins: evaluation with MR imaging and comparison with cardiac angiography and echocardiography. *Radiology* 1991;181:645–649.
10. White CS, Baffa JM, Haney PJ, et al. Anomalies of pulmonary veins: usefulness of spin-echo and gradient-echo MR images. *Am J Roentgenol* 1998;170:1365–1368.
11. Edelman RR, Manning WJ, Burstein D, et al. Coronary arteries: breath-hold MR angiography. *Radiology* 199;181:641–643.
12. Vliegen HW, Doornbos J, de Roos A, et al. Value of fast gradient echo magnetic resonance angiography as an adjunct to coronary arteriography in detecting and confirming the course of clinically significant coronary artery anomalies. *Am J Cardiol* 1997;79:773–776.
13. Post JC, van Rossum AC, Bronzwaer JG, et al. Magnetic resonance angiography of anomalous coronary arteries. A new gold standard for delineating the proximal course? *Circulation* 1995;92:3163–3171.
14. McConnell MV, Ganz P, Selwyn AP, et al. Identification of anomalous coronary arteries and their anatomic course by magnetic resonance coronary angiography. *Circulation* 1995;92:3158–3162.
15. Manning WJ, Li W, Edelman RR. A preliminary report comparing magnetic resonance coronary angiography with conventional angiography. *N Engl J Med* 1993;328:828–832.
16. McConnell MV, Manning WJ, Edelman RR. MRA of coronary arteries. In: Higgins CB, HricaK H, Helms CA, eds. *Magnetic resonance imaging of the body*, 3rd ed. Philadelphia: Lippincott-Raven, 1996:1427.
17. Woodard PK, Li D, Haacke EM, et al. Detection of coronary stenoses on source and projection images using three-dimensional MR angiography with retrospective respiratory gating: preliminary experience. *Am J Roentgenol* 1998;170:883–888.
18. Kessler W, Achenbach S, Moshage W, et al. Usefulness of respiratory gated magnetic resonance coronary angiography in assessing narrowings > or = 50% in diameter in native coronary arteries and in aorto-coronary bypass conduits. *Am J Cardiol* 1997;80:989–993.
19. Müller MF, Fleisch M, Kroeker R, et al. Proximal coronary artery stenosis: three-dimensional MRI with fat saturation and navigator echo. *J Magn Reson Imaging* 1997;7:644–651.
20. Post JC, van Rossum AC, Hofman MB, et al. Clinical utility of two-dimensional magnetic resonance angiography in detecting coronary artery disease. *Eur Heart J.* 1997;18:426–433.
21. Post JC, van Rossum AC, Hofman MB, et al. Three-dimensional respiratory-gated MR angiography of coronary arteries: comparison with conventional coronary angiography. *Am J Roentgenol* 1996;166:1399–1404.
22. Pennell DJ, Bogren HG, Keegan J, et al. Assessment of coronary artery stenosis by magnetic resonance imaging. *Heart* 1996;75:127–133.
23. Duerinckx AJ, Urman MK. Two-dimensional coronary MR angiography: analysis of initial clinical results. *Radiology* 1994;193:731–738.

24. Hundley WG, Clarke GD, Landau C, et al. Noninvasive determination of infarct artery patency by cine magnetic resonance angiography. *Circulation* 1995;91:1347–1353.
25. Dendale P, Franken PR, Meusel M, et al. Distinction between open and occluded infarct-related arteries using contrast-enhanced magnetic resonance imaging. *Am J Cardiol* 1997;80:334–336.
26. Kramer CM, Rogers WJ, Geskin G, et al. Usefulness of magnetic resonance imaging early after acute myocardial infarction. *Am J Cardiol* 1997;80:690–695.
27. Manning WJ, Cheng D, Edelman RR. Functional cardiac imaging. In: Edelman RR, Hesselink JR, Zlatkin MB, eds. *Clinical magnetic resonance imaging*, vol. 2, 2nd ed. Philadelphia: WB Saunders, 1996:1788.
28. Edelman RR, Manning WJ, Gervino E, et al. Flow velocity quantitation in human coronary arteries with fast, breath-hold MR angiography. *J Magn Reson Imaging* 1993;3:699–703.
29. Hundley WG, Lange RA, Clarke GD, et al. Assessment of coronary arterial flow and flow reserve in humans with magnetic resonance imaging. *Circulation* 1996;93:1502–1508.
30. Globits S, Sakuma H, Shimakawa A, et al. Measurement of coronary blood flow velocity during handgrip exercise using breath-hold velocity encoded cine magnetic resonance imaging. *Am J Cardiol* 1997;79:234–237.
31. Schiebler ML, Holland GA, Hatabu H, et al. Suspected pulmonary embolism: prospective evaluation with pulmonary MR angiography. *Radiology* 1993;189:125–131.
32. Grist TM, Sostman HD, MacFall JR, et al. Pulmonary angiography with MR imaging: preliminary clinical experience. *Radiology* 1993;189:523–530.
33. Erdman WA, Peshock RM, Redman HC, et al. Pulmonary embolism: comparison of MR images with radionuclide and angiographic studies. *Radiology* 1994;190:499–508.
34. Hatabu H, Gefter WB, Axel L, et al. MR imaging with spatial modulation of magnetization in the evaluation of chronic central pulmonary thromboemboli. *Radiology* 1994;190:791–794.
35. Loubeyre P, Revel D, Douek P, et al. Dynamic contrast-enhanced MR angiography of pulmonary embolism: comparison with pulmonary angiography. *Am J Roentgenol* 1994;162:1035–1039.
36. Bergin CJ, Hauschildt J, Rios G, et al. Accuracy of MR angiography compared with radionuclide scanning in identifying the cause of pulmonary arterial hypertension. *Am J Roentgenol* 1997;168:1549–1555.
37. Meaney JF, Weg JG, Chenevert TL, et al. Diagnosis of pulmonary embolism with magnetic resonance angiography. *N Engl J Med* 1997;336:1422–1427.
38. Hu B, Meyer C, Macovski A, et al. Multi-spiral magnetic resonance coronary angiography [abstract]. *Proc Int Soc Magn Reson Med* 1996;1:176.
39. Yoshino H, Nitatori T, Kachi E, et al. Directed proximal magnetic resonance coronary angiography compared with conventional contrast coronary angiography. *Am J Cardiol* 1997;80:514–518.
40. White RD, Caputo GR, Mark AS, et al. Coronary artery bypass graft patency: noninvasive evaluation with MR imaging. *Radiology* 1987;164:681–686.
41. Rubinstein RI, Askenase AD, Thickman D, et al. Magnetic resonance imaging to evaluate patency of aortocoronary bypass grafts. *Circulation* 1987;76:786–791.
42. Jenkins JP, Love HG, Foster CJ, et al. Detection of coronary artery bypass graft patency as assessed by magnetic resonance imaging. *Br J Radiol* 1988;61:2–4.
43. Galjee MA, van Rossum AC, Doesburg T, et al. Value of magnetic resonance imaging in assessing patency and function of coronary artery bypass grafts. An angiographically controlled study. *Circulation* 1996;93:660–666.
44. White RD, Pflugfelder PW, Lipton MJ, et al. Coronary artery bypass grafts: evaluation of patency with cine MR imaging. *Am J Roentgenol* 1988;150:1271–1274.
45. Aurigemma GP, Reichek N, Axel L, et al. Noninvasive determination of coronary artery bypass graft patency by cine magnetic resonance imaging. *Circulation.* 1989;80:1595–1602.
46. Hoogendoorn LI, Pattynama PM, Buis B, et al. Noninvasive evaluation of aortocoronary bypass grafts with magnetic resonance flow mapping. *Am J Cardiol* 1995;75:845–848.
47. Davies C, Hany T, Kaufmann P, et al. Coronary artery bypass grafts: 3D MR angiography [abstract]. *Proc Int Soc Magn Reson Med* 1997;2:834.

48. Winterspreger B, von Smekal A, Engelmann M, et al. Determination of coronary artery bypass graft (CABG) patency using gadolinium enhanced 3D magnetic resonance angiography: correlation with coronary angiography [abstract]. *Proc Int Soc Magn Reson Med* 1997;1: 444.

49. Vrachliotis TG, Bis KG, Aliabadi D, et al. Contrast-enhanced breath-hold MR angiography for evaluating patency of coronary artery bypass grafts. *Am J Roentgenol* 1997;168:1073–1080.

50. Wintersperger B, Engelmann M, von Smekal A, et al. Patency of coronary bypass grafts: assessment with breath-hold contrast-enhanced MR angiography-value of a non-electrocardiographically triggered technique. *Radiology* 1998;208:345–351.

CHAPTER 33

Magnetic Resonance
Spectroscopy

Roberto Kalil-Filho, Gerald M. Pohost, and
Robert G. Weiss

Nuclear magnetic resonance (NMR) spectroscopy of the heart has been performed since the work of Jacobus et al. (1) and Garlick et al. (2) in 1977 before the development of magnetic resonance imaging. Early studies were performed using hearts isolated from small laboratory animal models, e.g., the rat. There are several nuclei that can be observed using NMR spectroscopic methods that have now, or have in the future, the potential to be of considerable clinical value in the study of the myocardium. These include: phosphorus-31 (^{31}P), hydrogen-1 (^{1}H), sodium-23 (^{23}Na), fluorine-19 (^{19}F), and carbon-13 (^{13}C). All but ^{13}C are the predominant forms of the given element in nature. ^{13}C represents 1.1% of naturally abundant carbon and is a stable, nonradioactive isotope. At the present time, the largest clinical experience is with ^{31}P NMR spectroscopy. Phosphorus-31 NMR spectra depict ATP, phosphocreatine (PCr), 2,3 diphosphoglycerol (DPG), and, sometimes, inorganic phosphate (Fig. 1). For the purposes of the present chapter, only ^{31}P will be discussed. The reader interested in NMR spectroscopy is referred to other monographs (2–4).

Cardiac ^{31}P NMR spectroscopy is the only method to noninvasively quantify cardiac high-energy phosphate metabolism in humans. It is a powerful tool that has the potential to directly detect myocardial ischemia and other types of myocardial injury. A variety of techniques, such as NMR spectroscopic imaging, have been described that can be used to acquire spatially localized ^{31}P NMR spectra from the myocardium and are summarized in prior reviews (3–8).

R. Kalil-Filho: Heart Institute, CEP-05409-010, São Paulo, Brazil.
G. M. Pohost: Department of Medicine, University of Alabama at Birmingham, Birmingham, Alabama 35294.
R. G. Weiss: Department of Medicine, Johns Hopkins University School of Medicine; Johns Hopkins Hospital, Baltimore, Maryland 21287.

However, the definite niche for cardiac ^{31}P NMR spectroscopic methods is still evolving, and this chapter will review the clinical studies of cardiac metabolism conducted with ^{31}P NMR spectroscopy.

MYOCARDIAL VIABILITY

In the past decade, myocardial viability has been intensely investigated because its identification can significantly impact patient treatment decisions. In patients with coronary artery disease (CAD), alterations in myocardial blood flow may result in regional or global left ventricular (LV) contractile dysfunction that may improve partially or completely after restoration of blood flow (9). This recovery implies that the dysfunctional or "hibernating" myocardium is ultimately viable.

Another dysfunctional, but viable, myocardial state is known as "stunning." Stunning dysfunction occurs transiently after an episode of severe ischemia despite restoration of myocardial blood flow (10,11). In general, the following three indices for myocardial viability have been described (12): (i) preserved coronary flow (adequate perfusion); (ii) preserved wall motion (systolic wall thickening); and (iii) preserved metabolism. The current magnetic resonance (MR) imaging and spectroscopy techniques provide a great potential to measure all three indices of viability. Adequate perfusion can be assessed by spin-echo, gradient-echo, and/or ultra-fast MR imaging, systolic wall thickening by cine MR imaging, and the presence of metabolic integrity can be determined by NMR spectroscopy. These noninvasive and versatile techniques have led to an increased clinical interest and research in recent years in the potential for *in vivo* measurement of myocardial metabolism by using MR spectroscopy.

Bottomley et al. (13) first studied the high-energy myocar-

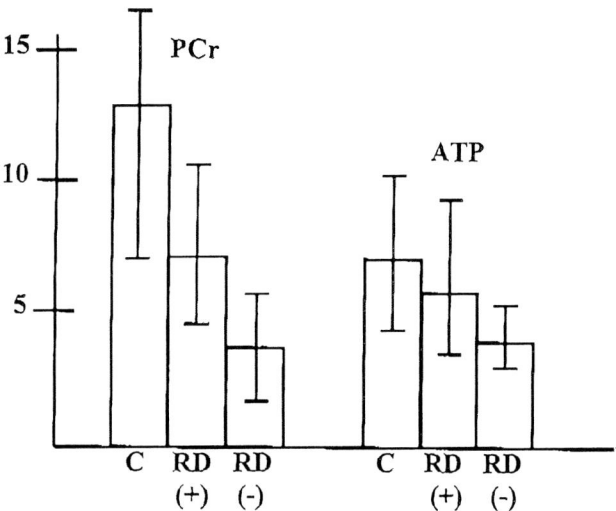

FIG. 1. Mean ± SD for phosphocreatine (*PCr*) and *ATP* in controls (*C*), in those patients who demonstrated defect that redistributed thallium scan (*RD*[+]) and in those patients with defect that showed no redistribution (*RD*[−]).

dial phosphate metabolism of patients with an acute anterior myocardial infarction. Cardiac-gated, ^{31}P magnetic resonance depth-resolved surface coil spectroscopy (DRESS) was performed 5 to 9 days after the onset of symptoms. Significant reductions in the phosphocreatine (PCr) to inorganic phosphate (Pi) ratio and elevations in the Pi to adenosine triphosphate (ATP) ratio were observed in endocardially or transmurally derived NMR spectra when compared with the values from epicardially displaced spectra and values from 7 healthy volunteers. However, contamination of the Pi resonances by other phosphate compounds, including blood 2,3-diphosphoglycerate, precluded precise spectral quantification of Pi and pH determination. The results indicated that localized ^{31}P NMR spectroscopy may be used to assess cellular energy reserve directly in clinical myocardial infarction and to evaluate the metabolic response to interventions. Mitsunami et al. (14) investigated 6 patients with previous Q-wave myocardial infarction (QMI), 6 with previous non-Q-wave myocardial infarction (NQMI), and 9 controls by the ECG-gated, DRESS technique. The infarct extent score of T1-201 scintigraphy was determined in 3 patients with QMI and in 4 patients with NQMI. Although no significant differences were found among the three groups in the relative phosphocreatine (PCr) to adenosine triphosphate (ATP) ratio (PCr/ATP), significant reductions were observed in the absolute amount of PCr normalized by the standard hexamethylphosphoric triamide (HMPT), (PCr/HMPT), or by both HMPT and LVW (PCr/HMPT/LVW) for QMI patients ($P < 0.05$), and in ATP/HMPT/LVW for QMI and NQMI patients ($P < 0.01$) as compared with controls. Their findings suggest that *in vivo* ^{31}P spectroscopy can detect reductions in high-energy phosphate levels in infarcted nonviable myocardium that may be useful in evaluating myocardial viability. Yabe et al. (15) also measured the

content of phosphocreatine (PCr) and ATP *in vivo* in the human heart. In that study, PCr and ATP contents were measured by ^{31}P NMR spectroscopy in myocardial segments defined as reversible ischemia or as scar by exercise T1-201 imaging. Forty-one subjects with stenosis of the left anterior descending coronary artery (greater than 50%) and 11 healthy control subjects (*C*) comprised the study group. Patients were divided into three groups on the basis of exercise T1-201 imaging: a reversible T1-201 defect group who demonstrated redistribution at late image (*RD* [+]), a fixed T1-201 defect group (*RD* [−]), and a control group(*C*). While the subjects lay supine in the magnet, ^{31}P NMR spectra were obtained from the anterior and apical regions of the left ventricle by slice-selected, one-dimensional chemical shift imaging. For metabolic quantification, a phosphate standard was placed at the center of the surface of the coil. An analysis of variance revealed significant differences among the three groups with respect to the mean PCr at rest (*C*, 12.14 ± 4/25; *RD*[+], 7.64 ± 3.00; *RD*[−], 3.94 ± 2.21 μmol/g wet heart tissue, mean ± SD, $P < 0.05$) as well as a significant decrease in ATP at rest (*C*, 7.72 ± 2.97; *RD* [+], 6.35 ± 3.17; *RD* [−] 4.35 ± 1.52 μmol/g wet wt heart tissue, $P < 0.05$) (Fig. 2). Compared with healthy control subjects, PCr content decreased significantly in patients with both exercise-related reversible and fixed T1-201 defects, and ATP content decreased significantly in subjects with fixed thallium defects. These results suggest that the clinical measurement of myocardial ATP by ^{31}P NMR spectroscopy may be useful for evaluating myocardial viability.

Moka et al. (16) clinically studied energy metabolism *in vivo* after nontransmural anterior myocardial infarction. ^{31}P NMR cardiac spectra in patients with stenosis of the left anterior descending coronary artery (LAD) and anterior wall hypokinesia on "optimal" antiischemic medications compared to those of healthy volunteers. The volume of interest was placed over the anterior myocardial wall identified by magnetic resonance imaging (MRI). To separate the influ-

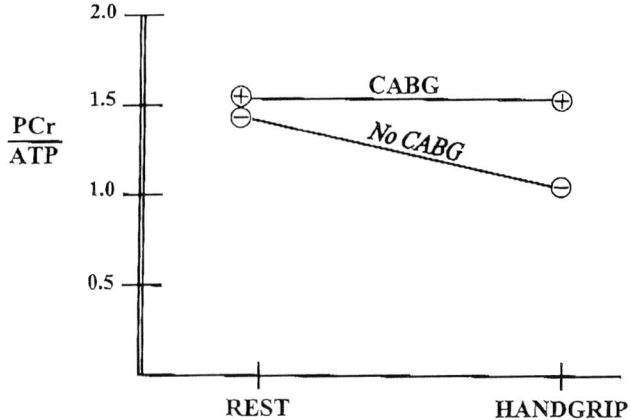

FIG. 2. Plot represents all patients with ≥70% stenosis of the left anterior descending corornary artery. One group underwent successful bypass surgery ([+] *CABG*); the other group had no intervention ([−] *CABG*).

ence of significant coronary stenosis but without hypo-kinesia, additional patients (group B) with LAD disease but without left ventricular dysfunction were examined. The effect of antiischemic medication on the phosphorus spectra was evaluated in patient group C, which had the same clinical features as group A. In these patients, NMR spectroscopic imaging was first performed without antiischemic medication (discontinued for less than 1 day) and then repeated during intravenous application of glyceroltrinite (GTNO). The mean PCr/ATP was significantly lower in patients after nontransmural myocardial infarction (MI) (group A) (1.24 ± 0.18) than in healthy volunteers (1.74 ± 0.23; $P < 0.01$, unpaired t-test). Patients with normal left ventricular function (group B) had a mean PCr/ATP (1.64 ± 0.22) similar to those of normal controls (1.74 ± 0.23). After GTNO infusion, the cardiac PCr/ATP of group C rose from 1.12 ± 0.08 to 1.32 ($P < 0.01$, paired t-test). Thus, hypokinetic myocardium after nontransmural infarction is characterized by lower PCr/ATP ratios. Their findings may reflect degenerative changes of myocytes due to disturbed microperfusion in viable areas of the infarct or to the remodeling process within viable myocytes in the infarct region.

Kalil-Filho et al. (17) investigated whether alterations in cardiac high-energy phosphates occurred in postischemic "stunned" human myocardium. Cardiac high-energy phosphates are reduced during experimental and clinical ischemia. Persistently abnormal myocardial high-energy phosphate metabolism has been hypothesized as a mechanism contributing to postischemic stunning, but not consistently observed in animal models of stunning. We studied 29 patients with a first anterior myocardial infarction (MI) who underwent successful reperfusion within 6 hours of the onset of chest pain. These patients underwent ^{31}P NMR spectroscopy a mean of 4 days after MI for measurement of left ventricular contractility and relative high-energy phosphate metabolites. Twenty-one patients underwent a second ^{31}P NMR spectroscopy study a mean of 39 days after MI. Eight volunteers served as control subjects. Global and infarct area wall motion scores improved significantly between the early and late studies. However, in regions that demonstrated spontaneous improvement in function ("stunned" myocardium), no difference was found between the early cardiac PCr/APT ratio of reperfused patients and that of control subjects ([mean ± SD] 1.51 ± 0.17 versus 1.61 ± 0.18, respectively, $P =$ NS), or between the early and late study that resulted in "stunned" patients (1.51 ± 0.17 versus 1.53 ± 0.17, respectively, $P =$ NS). For alpha of 0.05, the study had a 90% power to detect a 9% difference. These clinical observations are consistent with most earlier work in animal models of ischemia-reperfusion showing that stunned myocardium has normal high-energy phosphate ratios. It demonstrates for the first time in humans that relative cardiac high-energy phosphates are not altered or reduced in stunned human myocardium.

MYOCARDIAL ISCHEMIA

Weiss et al. (18) studied stress-induced, ischemia-related metabolic changes with spatially localized cardiac ^{31}P NMR spectroscopy before, during, and after continuous isometric handgrip exercise. The mean (± SD) PCr/ATP in the anterior left ventricular wall at rest was 1.72 ± 0.15 and 1.59 ± 0.31 in age-matched, normal subjects and in patients with nonischemic heart disease. These ratios did not change during the handgrip exercise in either group. However, in patients with left main coronary artery or LAD stenosis greater than or equal to 70%, the ratio decreased from 1.45 ± 0.3 at rest to 0.91 ± 0.24 during exercise ($P < 0.001$) and recovered to 1.27 ± 0.38 within after exercise. Repeat exercise testing in 5 patients after revascularization (balloon angioplasty or bypass surgery) yielded PCr/ATP values of 1.60 ± 0.20 at rest and 1.62? ± 0.18 during exercise, as compared to 1.51 ± 0.19 at rest and 1.02 ± 0.26 during exercise before revascularization ($P < 0.02$) (Fig. 2). The decrease in the PCr/ATP ratio during handgrip exercise in patients with coronary disease reflects a transient imbalance between oxygen supply and demand in myocardium with comprised blood flow or metabolic evidence of inducible ischemia. Exercise testing with ^{31}P NMR is a specific method for assessing the effect of ischemia on myocardial high-energy phosphate metabolism and for monitoring the response to ischemic therapies. Figure 3 illustrates a normal resting ^{31}P NMR study.

Yabe et al. (19) studied the relationship between cardiac ^{31}P NMR spectroscopy during handgrip stress in relation to exercise ^{201}Tl imaging. Twenty-seven patients with LAD coronary artery stenosis greater than or equal to 75% and 11 normal controls were studied. Patients were divided into two groups on the basis of exercise ^{201}Tl imaging: a redistribution ^{201}Tl defect group (RD [+]) on the delayed image, and a fixed ^{201}Tl defect group (RD [−]). While lying supine within the magnet, subjects performed handgrip exercise at 30% of maximal force once in every two cardiac cycles. ^{31}P MR spectra were collected before and during exercise. There were significant differences among the three groups (control (C), redistribution (RD[+]), and no redistribution (RD[−]) pattern) as follows: $C =$ 1.85 0.28; RD[+] 1.60 ± 0.19; and RD[−] = 1.24 ± 0.30, $P < 0.05$. PCr/ATP decreased significantly from 1.60 ± 0.19 at rest to 0.96 ± 0.28 during exercise ($P < 0.011$) in the RD [+] group, but did not change significantly from 1.24 ± 0.30 to 1.19 ± 0.28 during exercise in the RD[−] group. Similarly, the ratio did not change in the control group (1.85 ± 0.28 at rest versus 1.90 ± .23 during exercise). Contrary to normal subjects or patients with a fixed thallium defect, the PCr/ATP ratio was significantly reduced during exercise in patients with a reversible thallium defect. It appears that patients with fixed defects had reductions in total PCr and ATP (15) and that the PCr/ATP from some residual noninvolved myocardium is unchanged during stress. These results demonstrate and confirm that ^{31}P NMR spectroscopy with handgrip exercise testing is a sensitive method for detecting myocardial ischemia.

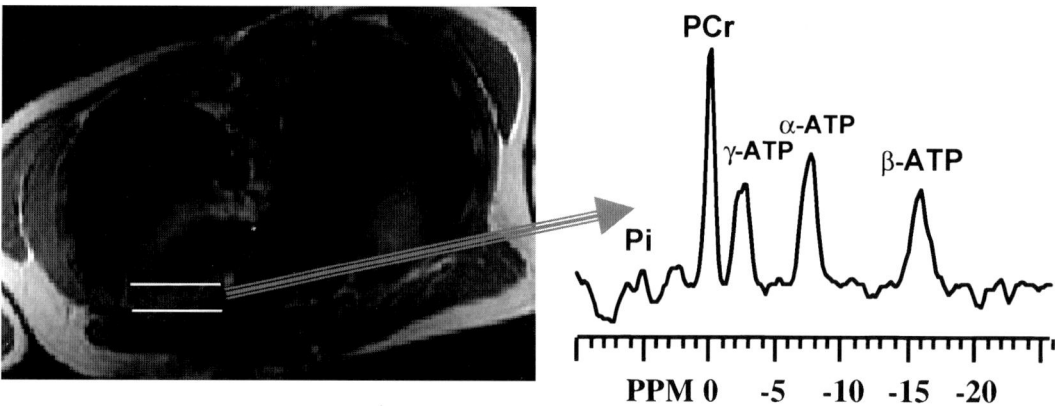

FIG. 3. Cardiac magnetic resonance (MR) image (**left**) and corresponding ^{31}P MR spectrum (**right**) from a normal human heart. The spin-echo MR image depicts the left venticle, and the portion of the left ventricle (between the *horizontal white lines*) from the ^{31}P MR spectrum was obtained with a one-dimensional chemical shift imaging sequence. The ^{31}P MR spectrum was acquired in about 10 minutes, and the peaks represent creatine phosphate (*PCr*), the three phosphate resonances of *ATP*, and inorganic phosphate (*Pi*).

DILATED CARDIOMYOPATHY AND HEART FAILURE

Abnormalities in high-energy phosphates and energy reserve have been identified in most experimental models of heart failure, and the energy reserve hypothesis of heart failure has been proposed by Ingwall (20) and others. Many clinical studies have been performed with magnetic resonance spectroscopy in order to determine whether abnormalities in cardiac high-energy phosphate metabolism can be detected in patients with dilated cardiomyopathy.

Schaefer et al. (21) found an increase in the phosphodiester/ATP in subjects with mild heart failure, while the PCr/ATP ratio was not statistically significantly reduced. They also later reported no changes in cardiac PCr/ATP during dobutamine stress in heart failure subjects (22). Hardy and collaborators, (23) who studied more severely affected individuals, were the first to report significant reductions in the myocardial PCr/ATP ratio at rest in adults with dilated cardiomyopathy and heart failure. These reductions were observed at rest in heart failure subjects with both ischemic and nonischemic etiologies. In 1992, Neubauer et al. (24) identified a significant correlation between the PCr/ATP ratio and NYHA class of heart failure for patients with dilated cardiomyopathy, the ratio being lower for more severe cases. There was no clear correlation though, between PCr/ATP and left ventricular ejection fraction or fractional shortening. They also reported that 6 patients with dilated cardiomyopathy, who were studied before and after 3 months of drug treatment, had an improvement of the NYHA status and a concomitant improvement in PCr/ATP.

In 1995, Neubauer et al. (25) studied the clinical and hemodynamic correlates of impaired cardiac high-energy phosphate metabolism in patients with heart failure due to dilated cardiomyopathy (DCM). They studied 14 volunteers and 23 patients with dilated cardiomyopathy. They observed that the PCr/ATP ratios were significantly reduced in DCM patients (1.54 ± 0.10) with mean ejection fraction of 34%, as compared to those of normal volunteers (2.02 ± 0.11; $P < 0.05$). The PCr/ATP ratios correlated with the clinical severity of heart failure as estimated by the NYHA class, and they also correlated with the left ventricular ejection fraction of the left ventricular end-diastolic wall thickness.

In 1997, Neubauer et al. (26) reported on survival and energetics in patients with dilated cardiomyopathy who were followed for 2.5 years. Patients were divided into two groups, one with a normal PCr/ATP and another with a reduced ratio. In the normal PCr/ATP group, the cardiovascular mortality was 5% as compared with 40% in the reduced PCr/ATP group. They also observed that the cardiac PCr/ATP was a better predictor of survival than left ventricular ejection fraction (EF) or NYHA class. They concluded that the myocardial PCr/ATP is a predictor of both total and cardiovascular mortality in patients with dilated cardiomyopathy.

Thus, abnormalities in ^{31}P NMR spectroscopy that determined high-energy phosphate metabolism have been noted at rest in subjects with moderate-to-severe heart failure, and such abnormalities predict outcomes and survival. Further work should be done to characterize the extent of metabolic abnormalities in heart failure and the role of reduced energy reserve in the pathogenesis of human heart failure.

HYPERTROPHIC CARDIOMYOPATHY

Several authors used NMR spectroscopy to evaluate cardiac energy metabolism in subjects with left ventricular hypertrophy and others with hypertrophic cardiomyopathy (HCM). Weiss et al. (18) observed no significant decrease in the myocardial PCr/ATP ratio at rest in patients with left ventricular hypertrophy. de Roos et al. (27) found a lower myocardial PCr/ATP ratio in 8 patients with HCM compared with 9 controls (1.32 ± 0.29 vs 1.65 ± 0.26). Likewise, Sakuma et al. (28) found abnormal phosphate cardiac metabolites in patients with HCM. They studied 19 patients with HCM and 6 normal volunteers. The PCr/ATP ratio in patients (1.07 ± 0.10, mean ± SE) was significantly lower than that in normal volunteers (1.71 ± 0.13, P < 0.01). The metabolic changes in HCM did not always correlate with perfusion abnormalities on T1-201 single-photon emission computed tomography imaging. Also, the ratio of PDE/PCr did not differ significantly between the two groups.

Jung et al. (29) used ^{31}P NMR spectroscopy to study HCM patients and normal volunteers. Patients with HCM had reduced cardiac PCr/ATP at rest as compared to normal subjects. In a subset with severe septal hypertrophy, they also observed increased Pi/PCr. The higher Pi/PCr may be caused by a relatively inadequate oxygen supply in severely hypertrophied myocardium. Many studies demonstrated a decrease in myocardial high-energy phosphate ratios at rest in HCM patients, but the pathophysiologic mechanism responsible for altered metabolism has not yet been elucidated, although a reduction in vasodilator reserve may be a contributing factor.

TRANSPLANTED HEARTS

Studies in laboratory animals have shown that a relationship between reductions in the myocardial PCr/ATP can even precede, by a few days, the development of histologic evidence of rejection (31). However, the mechanism for altered metabolism in experimental transplant rejection is unknown. Inspired by these experimental studies, one might expect that ^{31}P NMR spectroscopic methods could provide a noninvasive means of detecting early rejection in patients. Nonetheless, several human studies have failed to show a close relationship between the myocardial PCr/ATP and the degree or severity or rejection.

The first published work to evaluate cardiac high-energy phosphate metabolism in transplant patients and to compare cardiac PCr/ATP with histologic evidence of rejection was that of Bottomley et al. (32) in 14 patients on 19 occasions from 1 to 6 years after transplantation. On average, patients with mild rejection (detected with endomyocardial biopsy) have a reduced cardiac PCr/ATP ratio (1.57 ± 0.50, mean ± standard deviation) as compared to those of 17 healthy control subjects (1.93 ± 0.2; P < 0.01). Ratios of PCr to inorganic phosphate also appeared lower whenever detectable. However, ^{31}P NMR spectroscopy could not distinguish mild from moderate histologic rejection and, therefore, could not distinguish patients who required augmented therapy for rejection. This was true when comparing ^{31}P NMR spectra either with the current or future biopsy (sensitivity, 50%, and specificity, 73%, with the use of cardiac-averaged PCr/ATP values for each heart; sensitivity, 88%, and specificity, 55%, with the use of the lowest myocardial PCr/ATP measured in each heart). An explanation for the difference between human and animal studies might be the absence of immunosuppressive medication in the animal studies, leading to more severe, acute rejection in animal models. Another explanation is the problematic measurements derived from myocardial biopsies. A given focus might be biopsied many times and generate inadequate data.

Van Dobbenburgh et al. (33) studied the energy metabolism of 25 excised human donor hearts arrested with cardioplegic solution with ^{31}P NMR spectroscopic methods before implantation and correlated this cardiac output measured with the thermodilution in heart patients. No significant correlation was observed between the cardiac index of heart transplant patients during the first hours after transplantation and the PCr/ATP or the intracellular pH at the time of reperfusion. However, 1 week after transplantation, a significant correlation was observed between the cardiac index and the PCr/ATP, phosphomonoesterase/ATP, and the PCr/Pi at the time of reperfusion. In contrast, the pH at the time of reperfusion showed a poor correlation with the cardiac index 1 week after transplantation. It was concluded that functional recovery after human heart transplantation is related to the metabolic condition of the hypothermic donor heart.

Unfortunately, despite promising results in the laboratory, the available clinical evidence does not yet support the use of ^{31}P NMR spectroscopy as a diagnostic modality for grading the severity of transplant rejection. Although reductions in cardiac PCr/ATP have been observed in transplant rejection, metabolic abnormalities do not correlate with the severity of biopsy-determined histologic rejection. This, in part, may be related to the reliability of the myocardial biopsy. However, for the present, PCr/ATP should not be used to detect and manage allograft rejection. Future developments, such as the measurement of absolute concentrations of the ^{31}P metabolites, may improve this potential clinical application of NMR spectroscopy.

MICROVASCULAR DISEASE

Buchthal and colleagues (34) have used handgrip exercise ^{31}P NMR spectroscopy at 1.5T in women with no significant CAD as part of the Women's Ischemia Syndrome Evaluation (WISE) Study. These investigators found that approximately 20% of 35 women who underwent coronary angiography for chest pain had a significant decrease in PCr/ATP during exercise stress. It is likely that these changes may be related to microvascular disease with resultant ischemia in those patients with a positive PCr/ATP response. Further data are being acquired and studies are being performed at higher field (~ 4.0T) (35) to evaluate changes in Pi/ATP and pH in their patients.

SUMMARY

In conclusion, ^{31}P NMR spectroscopy is the only method to noninvasively assess human myocardial energy metabolism. Clinical studies using ^{31}P NMR spectroscopy have defined the ratios and levels of high-energy phosphates in normal human myocardium. Reductions in myocardial high-energy phosphate ratios have been observed at rest in subjects with dilated cardiomyopathy and heart failure, correlate with the severity of clinical heart failure, and predict outcomes and mortality. Exercise-induced reductions in cardiac high-energy phosphates are reproducibly observed in patients with significant coronary artery disease and inducible ischemia, but not in normal, age-matched subjects or patients with valvular regurgitation. Ultimately, ^{31}P NMR spectroscopy may be the magnetic resonance procedure of choice to assess myocardial viability.

The future of ^{31}P NMR spectroscopic methods will be enhanced by efforts to improve the sensitivity of the technique and, thus, the ability to detect metabolites throughout the entire heart and to do so with improved spatial resolution. In addition to ^{31}P spectroscopic methods, ^{1}H spectroscopic applications should ultimately provide a means of quantifying myocardial metabolism with improved spatial resolution. This has recently been shown to reliably quantify total creatine levels throughout both anterior and posterior myocardium and to detect significant creatine reductions in infarcted, nonviable myocardium (36). The eventual ability to perform metabolic imaging of high-energy phosphates (37–39) or creatine (40) would add another complementary dimension to cardiac MRI imaging.

REFERENCES

1. Jacobus WE, Taylor GJ IV, Hollis DP, et al. Phosphorus nuclear magnetic resonance of perfused working rat hearts. *Nature* 1977;265:756–758.
2. Garlick PB, Radda GK, Seeley PJ. Phosphorus NMR studies on perfused heart.
3. Schaefer S, Balaban R, eds. *Cardiovascular magnetic resonance spectroscopy.* Kluwer Academic Publishers, Amsterdam, The Netherlands, 1992.
4. Bottomley PA. MR spectroscopy of the human heart: the status and the challenges. *Radiology* 1994;191:593–612.
5. Ingwall JS, Weiss RG. ^{31}P NMR spectroscopy. The noninvasive tool for the study of the biochemistry of the cardiovascular system. *Trends Cardiovasc Med* 1993;2:29–37.
6. Bottomley PA, Hardy CJ, Roemer PB, et al. Problems and expediencies in human ^{31}P spectroscopy: the definition of localized volumes, dealing with saturation and the technique-dependence of quantification. *NMR Biomed* 1989;20:284–289.
7. Weiss RG, Bottomley PA. Cardiac magnetic resonance spectroscopy: principles and applications. In: *Marcus cardiac imaging: a companion to Braunwald's heart disease.* Philadelphia: WB Saunders, 1996.
8. Schaefer S. Clinical nuclear magnetic resonance spectroscopy: insight into metabolism. *Am J Cardiol* 1990;66:45F–50F.
9. Rahimtoola SH. A perspective on three large multicenter randomized clinical trials of coronary bypass surgery for chronic stable angina. *Circulation* 1985;72:V123–V135.
10. Diamond GA, Forrester JS, deLuz PL, et al. Post-extrastystolic potentiation of ischemic myocardium by atrial stimulation. *Am Heart J* 1978;95:204–209.
11. Braunwald E, Kloner RA. The stunned myocardium: prolonged, postischemic ventricular dysfunction. *Circulation* 1982;66:1146–1149.
12. Wijns W, Vatner SF, Camici PG. Hibernating myocardium. *N Engl J Med* 1998;339:173–181.
13. Bottomley PA, Herfkens RJ, Smith LS, et al. Altered phosphate metab-

olism in myocardial infarction: P-31 MR spectroscopy. *Radiology* 1987;165:703–707.
14. Mitsunami K, Okada M, Inoue T, et al. In vivo 31P nuclear magnetic resonance spectroscopy in patients with old myocardial infarction. *Jpn Circ J* 1992;56:614–619.
15. Yabe T, Mitsunami K, Inubushi T, et al. Quantitative measurements of cardiac phosphorus metabolites in coronary artery disease by ^{31}P magnetic resonance spectroscopy. *Circulation* 1995;92:15–23.
16. Moka D, Sechtem U, Theissen P, et al. [Non-transmural anterior wall infarct: changes in myocardial energy metabolism in remaining vital myocardium](German). *Z Kardiol* 1997;86:113–120.
17. Kalil-Filho R, de Albuquerque CP, Weiss RG, et al. Normal high energy phosphate ratios in "stunned" human myocardium. *J Am Coll Cardiol* 1997;30:1228–1232.
18. Weiss RG, Bottomley PA, Hardy CJ, et al. Regional myocardial metabolism of high-energy phosphates during isometric exercise in patients with coronary artery disease. *N Engl J Med* 1990;323:1593–1600.
19. Yabe T, Mitsunami K, Okada M, et al. Detection of myocardial ischemia by ^{31}P magnetic resonance spectroscopy during handgrip exercise. *Circulation* 1994;89:1709–1716.
20. Ingwall JS. Is cardiac failure a consequence of decreased energy reserve? *Circulation* 1993;87:VII-58–VII-62.
21. Schaefer S, Gober JR, Schwartz GG, et al. In vivo phosphorus-31 spectroscopic imaging in patients with global myocardial disease. *Am J Cardiol* 1990;65:1154–1161.
22. Schaefer S, Schwartz GG, Steinman SK, et al. Metabolic response of the human heart to inotropic stimulation: in vivo phosphorus-31 studies of normal and cardiomyopathic myocardium. *Magn Reson Med* 1992;25:260–272.
23. Hardy CJ, Weiss RG, Bottomley PA, et al. Altered myocardial high-energy phosphate metabolites in patients with dilated cardiomyopathy. *Am Heart J* 1991;122:795–801.
24. Neubauer S, Krahe T, Schindler R, et al. ^{31}P Magnetic resonance spectroscopy in dilated cardiomyopathy and coronary artery disease: altered cardiac high-energy phosphate metabolism in heart failure. *Circulation* 1992;86:1810–1818.
25. Neubauer S, Horn M, Pabst T, et al. Contributions of ^{31}P magnetic resonance spectroscopy to the understanding of dilated heart muscle disease. *Eur Heart J* 1995;16:115–118.
26. Neubauer S, Horn M, Cramer M, et al. Myocardial phosphocreatine-to-ATP ratio is a predictor of mortality in patients with dilated cardiomyopathy. *Circulation* 1997;96:2190–2196.
27. deRoos A, Doornbos J, Luten PR, et al. Cardiac metabolism in patients with dilated and hypertrophic cardiomyopathy: assessment with proton-decoupled ^{31}P MR spectroscopy. *J Magn Reson Imaging* 1992;2:711–719.
28. Sakuma H, Takeda K, Tagami T, et al. ^{31}P MR spectroscopy in hypertrophic cardiomyopathy: comparison with Tl-201 myocardial perfusion imaging. *Am Heart J* 1993;125:1323–1328.
29. Jung W, Sieverding L, Breuer J, et al. ^{31}P NMR spectroscopy detects metabolic abnormalities in asymptomatic patients with hypertrophic cardiomyopathy. *Circulation* 1998;97:2536–2542.
30. Canby RC, Evanochko WT, Bennett LV, et al. Monitoring the bioenergetics of cardiac allograft rejection using in vivo ^{31}P nuclear magnetic resonance spectroscopy. *J Am Coll Cardiol* 1987;9:1067–1074.
31. Fraser CD, Chacko VP, Jacobus WE, et al. Early phosphorus 31 nuclear magnetic bioenergetic changes potentially predict rejection in heterotopic cardiac allografts. *J Heart Transplant* 1990;9:197–204.
32. Bottomley PA, Weiss RG, Hardy CJ, et al. Myocardial high-energy phosphate metabolism and allograft rejection in patients with heart transplants. *Radiology* 1991;181:67–75.
33. Van Dobbenburgh JO, Lahpor JR, Wooley SR, et al. Functional recovery after human heart transplantation is related to the metabolic condition of the hypothermic donor heart. *Circulation* 1996;94:2831–2836.
34. Buchthal SD, den Hollander JA, Rogers WJ, Pohost GM for the WISE Investigators. Metabolic evidence of ischemia in women with chest pain but no or minimal coronary artery disease. Proceedings of the ISMRM, May 1999;1:149.
35. Den Hollender JA, Buchthal SD, Pohost GM. Fast low-angle ^{31}P MRSI of the human heart at 4.1 tesla. Proceedings of the ISMRM, May 1999.
36. Bottomley PA, Weiss RG. Creatine depletion in nonviable, infarcted myocardium measured by noninvasive MRS. *Lancet* 1998;351:714–718.

37. Hetherington HP, Luney DJ, Vaughan JT, et al. 3D ^{31}P spectroscopy imaging of the human heart at 4.1T. *Magn Reson Med* 1995;33: 427–431.

38. Twieg B, Myerhoff DJ, Hubesch B, et al. Phosphorus-31 magnetic resonance spectroscopy in humans by spectroscopic imaging: localized spectroscopy and metabolite imaging. *Magn Reson Med* 1989;12:291–305.

39. Hardy CJ, Bottomley PA, Rohling KW, et al. An NMR phased array for human cardiac ^{31}P spectroscopy. *Magn Reson Med* 1992;28: 54–64.

40. Bottomley PA, Lee Y, Weiss RG. Total creatine in muscle: imaging and quantification with proton MR spectroscopy. *Radiology* 1997;204: 403–410.

CHAPTER 34

Future Perspectives

Mark Doyle, Gerald M. Pohost, and
M. Eduardo Kortright

One must appreciate the role of other noninvasive imaging modalities to make a considered statement concerning the future of cardiovascular magnetic resonance (CMR). Naturally, as with other modalities, CMR has its proponents—i.e., those who have "hitched their wagon" to it— as well as its detractors—i.e., those who see no expanded role for CMR. Before discussing the future, it is instructive to define CMR. Thus, CMR is a set of diagnostic procedures based on the phenomenon of nuclear magnetic resonance (NMR). There are other types of magnetic resonance that take place in different atomic locations, e.g., electron spin (magnetic) resonance. Thus, strictly speaking, the term magnetic resonance is incomplete as we now use it, since, for medical diagnosis, we are in fact using NMR (as opposed to the more encompassing MR). For simplicity, the term CMR will be used for all magnetic resonance methods applied to the cardiovascular system. There are several CMR methods: magnetic resonance imaging (MRI), magnetic resonance angiography (MRA), and magnetic resonance spectroscopy (MRS). All these methods can potentially be performed in a single system, but commercially available systems usually do not perform MRS. The newest systems have been optimized for cardiovascular (CV) diagnosis and are able to perform high-speed, virtually "real time" imaging. Given these developments, proponents see a bright future in which CMR is the dominant cardiovascular imaging technology. However, it is possible to hold the opposite view, i.e., that CMR will play a relatively small role and that its use would be restricted to highly specialized centers or to use as a technique of last

resort. Currently, there is broad agreement among both groups that (from an informational perspective) MRI is the modality of choice for evaluating cardiac function and morphology in addition to visualizing the morphology of the aorta and its branches (1). However, the list of functions not *routinely* performed by MRI is substantial, and this list, in part, explains why there are two opposing views of CMR's future. At the present time, the functionality offered at a general MRI site does not permit routine visualization of the coronary arteries, valvular structures, and myocardial perfusion distribution. While these features are currently not available at the majority of MRI sites, they are being actively explored by a number of research groups (including ours). The belief among MR proponents is that these research and development areas will mature, and will form part of a comprehensive cardiovascular evaluation.

Currently, medical practice seeks to reduce costs by streamlining operations and automating interpretation using advanced computational methods. An effective diagnostic modality must balance the cost and the benefit (2). Thus, it is instructive to determine the minimum requirements for CMR to allow it to establish a position in the CV diagnostic armamentarium from which it can develop its full potential.

A recent cost analysis indicated that, currently, CMR is not economically viable as an independent diagnostic modality (3). Presently, for most cardiology practices, utilizing CMR requires sharing the resource with a number of other specialties, such as neurology and orthopedics. Otherwise, a scanner dedicated exclusively to CMR could remain idle for unacceptable periods of time. Thus, to capture a larger diagnostic market segment, it is necessary for the routine CMR examination to advance beyond providing basic ventricular function and cardiac morphology, albeit with more diagnostic information than other CV imaging modalities.

If CMR could replace other procedures of existing technologies, while providing excellent morphologic and functional assessment, then its economic benefits would increase

M. Doyle: Department of Medicine, University of Alabama at Birmingham, Birmingham, Alabama 35294.

G. M. Pohost: Department of Medicine, University of Alabama at Birmingham, Birmingham, Alabama 35294.

M. E. Kortright: Department of Computer Science, University of New Orleans, New Orleans, Louisiana 70148.

remarkably. The economic benefits of a scenario in which CMR could optimally assess morphology, function, perfusion, viability, and coronary arteries would make it quite cost-beneficial for the examination of patients with suspected ischemic heart disease. Then we must ask if CMR can mature sufficiently to either completely or partially replace the useful applications of existing diagnostic modalities. To answer this fundamental question, other key questions must be addressed:

- Most fundamentally, can MR adequately and rapidly image perfusion, viability, the coronary arteries, and intracoronary plaque?
- Can all such features be integrated into a single scanner?
- Can the large amount of data generated be processed rapidly to produce qualitative and quantitative diagnostic information?

FEASIBILITY

To address the question concerning the basic ability of CMR to image a wide variety of cardiac features and functions it would be useful to perform a limited review of the literature. A recent computer search of the medical literature yielded over 1,400 references to the cardiac applications of MRI, and over 2,400 dealing with vascular applications. Given the complexity of imaging the moving heart compared to the more stationary peripheral vasculature, it is easy to understand why vascular MRA research is more advanced than cardiac imaging and to appreciate that MRA will probably be even more successful in the future. This notwithstanding, there are numerous papers documenting the ability of MRI to image many important aspects of the heart structure and function. Present applications of MR in selected cardiovascular applications have been highlighted earlier, and while an extensive review of CMR is beyond the scope of this chapter, it is clear that high quality cardiovascular imaging is now possible. Let us focus on the direct imaging of the heart since peripheral vascular MRI is rapidly progressing, and, indeed, has already found substantial clinical applications.

Characteristics that favor the *clinical* feasibility of CMR are its low risk, moderate cost, diagnostic potential, and high patient acceptance. In a recent study comparing patient acceptance of MR angiography versus x-ray angiography, a number of different criteria were considered, including how much a person would pay to avoid either procedure and the effect that the procedure had on performance of daily activities. It was concluded that MRA was preferred by the vast majority of patients (4). Thus, the lack of need for catheterization with injection of frequently painful radioopaque media for MRI is seen as a major benefit by the patient. Additionally, since no prolonged recovery period is required for the patient and further diagnostic or interventional procedures can be knowledgeably performed after an MR examination, MR can reduce patient stay, the duration of the catheterization procedure, and the use of catheterization laboratory with the result that cost reduction can be anticipated.

INTEGRATION

The hundreds of published cardiac CMR papers mentioned only amount to about 2% of the medical MR literature. Considering the prevalence of cardiovascular disease in the population, this low percentage of CMR publications indicates that, as a modality, MR is grossly underutilized by the cardiovascular community. In practice, manuscripts reporting new approaches and new results are driven by clinical demand. The low utilization of cardiac MR is likely due to (i) lack of knowledge among physicians, (ii) inadequate technical capabilities of the majority of available scanners, and (iii) the paucity of expertise in CMR. By using existing knowledge of appropriate MR technology in today's scanners, it is possible to envisage scanners with very powerful capabilities for imaging the cardiovascular system. However, due to the complex nature of MR and the relatively large number of technical variations available, it becomes difficult for manufacturers to service and support all these variations. One possible solution would be for manufacturers to design highly modular systems, with well-defined interface protocols for each hardware and software component.

Additionally, many cardiovascular techniques require substantial data processing, both prior to and after image generation. Recently, a time-resolved, three-dimensional vascular imaging approach was successfully implemented, but required substantial off-line processing (5). Some acknowledgment of the growing requirement for computing capabilities is being made to accommodate, for example, the rapid cardiac imaging approach involving spirals, an approach that requires specialized processing prior to image generation; to that end, a separate computer is supplied by one manufacturer (6,7). However, rather than being regarded as the exception, advanced data processing capabilities should be factored into the design of a viable CMR unit.

RAPID SCAN TIME

Can the multiple CMR imaging functions be performed in a reasonable amount of time? It is now possible to assess ventricular function within several minutes using the "real-time" type of acquisition and display available on the newest cardiovascular "tailored" systems. When considering CMR scanner speed, it should be noted that every imaging function need not be applied to every patient. Nevertheless, to be most successful (especially with third-party carriers) CMR will need to replace the information acquired by one or more existing modalities. Given that at present a number of separate imaging procedures are typically performed on each cardiac patient, the functionality of a number of displaced modalities will have to be performed during the MR session. Ideally, these functions would be performed in a single session.

Regarding acquisition speed, consider the possible usage of an MR unit that would be used to perform perfusion imaging in addition to cardiac function and morphology. At our institution, approximately 30 cardiac perfusion examinations are performed daily by nuclear cardiology. These studies include patient preparation, exercise stress or adenosine/dipyridamole infusion, radiopharmacutical administration and single photon emission computed tomography (SPECT) imaging on at least two occasions requiring at least 2 hours of study time. However, the instrumentation and housing costs of MR are more expensive than those for nuclear cardiology, although the costs associated with radiation safety add cost to nuclear cardiology that are not present for CMR studies. For a CMR unit to match the costs of nuclear cardiology would require completing the function, morphology, and perfusion study within 30 minutes. Thus, to be cost competitive, it is necessary for the entire MRI procedure to be performed rapidly. One approach is to apply ''real-time'' scanning strategies. Next, patients should be prepared for scanning in a place remote from the scanner. This can be achieved by use of multiple detachable scanner tables on which ECG signal and possibly IV access are established prior to connecting to the scanner.

To date, advances in scan speed have followed advances in gradient technology. However, gradient speed is limited, since as speed increases, the possibility of stimulation of the peripheral nerves increases (8). Hence, the gains in scan speed associated with further advances in gradient technology are somewhat limited. A partial solution to this problem is provided by other scanning strategies to reduce the time of image acquisition. Recent advances have been achieved

by the simultaneous acquisition of spatial harmonics (SMASH) multiple surface coil approach (9). With SMASH, a limited portion of k-space is sampled with several surface coils, and, then, combining the data from all coils after acquisition, a high resolution imaging study is reconstructed from the lower resolution coil acquisitions. Another approach introduced by our group is called BRISK (10,11). BRISK uses the similarity that exists between multiple phases of typical cardiac cine scans. With BRISK, data are sampled in a sparse manner and interpolated after acquisition to allow the generation of high-resolution images. The common feature shared by both SMASH and BRISK is that substantial processing is necessary prior to image generation. Currently, such postprocessing is performed off-line, introducing delays between data acquisition and image display. The challenge to manufacturers is to incorporate adequate computing capacity to allow for the rapid postprocessing required for strategies such as BRISK and SMASH.

OPTIMIZING RESOLUTION

It is not sufficient to achieve rapid scan times only, since high resolution is essential for maintaining the high quality advantage of MR images. One problematic culprit that can compromise resolution is respiratory motion by the patient. A widely adopted solution is to have the subject briefly suspend breathing. Breath-hold approaches can virtually eliminate respiratory artifacts (12,13). Respiratory artifacts can be quite significant, as shown by the example in Figure 1 of a nonbreath-hold study compared to a breath-hold quantitative flow image obtained with turbo-BRISK. A disadvan-

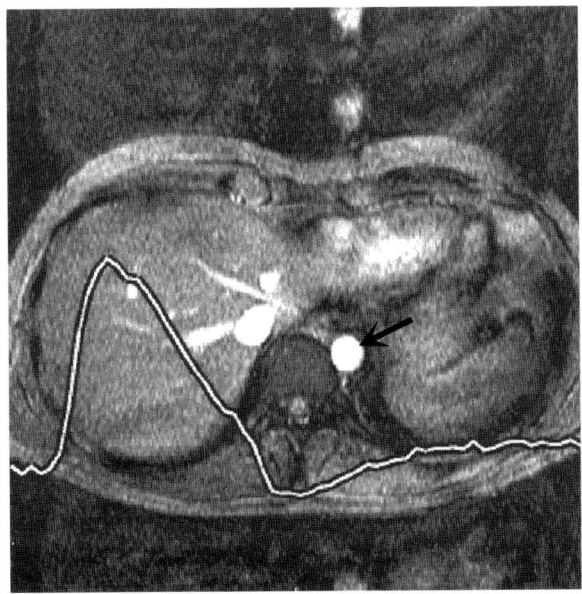
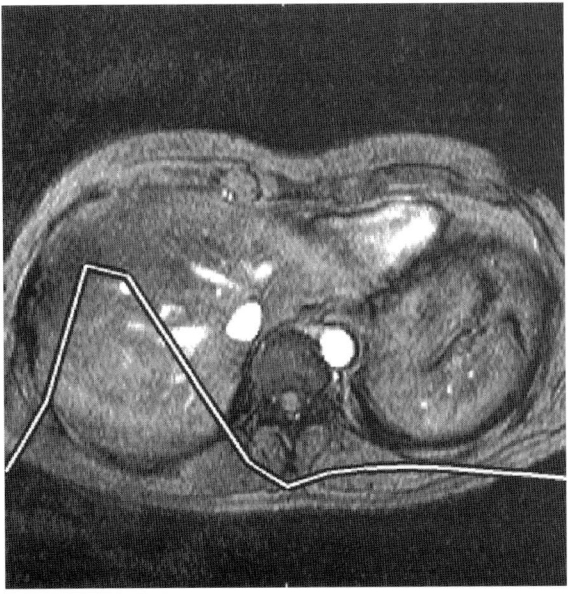

FIG. 1. Magnitude images with average velocity-time plots superimposed for flow in the descending aorta (*arrow*) for (**A**), a scan of several minutes duration, and (**B**), a turbo-BRISK acquisition acquired in a 20-sec breath hold. Notice in (**A**) the motion and flow artifacts are most visible outside of the body cavity, but are also present in the body section. In the breath-hold image (**B**), notice the absence of motion artifacts together with sharp edges.

tage of the breath-hold approach is that scan time is necessarily restricted to 20 to 30 seconds, which ultimately places restrictions on the resolution achievable. Another disadvantage is related to the ability of a given cardiovascular patient to continue a breath hold for 20 seconds or so. An additional disadvantage is that after each breath hold, a recovery time on the order of 30 to 40 seconds is required, making breath-hold approaches only about 25% efficient for multiple acquisitions. Recently, a specialized approach was introduced that uses a second imaging method applied during the CMR acquisitions to track diaphragm motion (13–15). Standard imaging is then synchronized to a particular diaphragmatic position and consequently is synchronized to the patient's breathing. This ''navigator'' approach avoids breath-holding. However, by operating the scanner in a respiratory gated mode, images are acquired only at (for example) end expiration, and the scan efficiency is again only 25 to 40%. The accuracy required of the respiratory compensation strategy depends on the imaging mode and the features being imaged. For instance, evaluation of cardiac function with two-dimensional imaging does not require fine resolution, and, in this case, other methods have proven useful to compensate for respiratory motion without prolonging the scan time (16). In contrast, coronary artery imaging requires very high resolution, and respiratory k-space reordering approaches are not as applicable (17,18). Thus, if prolonged acquisition times are to be avoided, either the intrinsic scan rate has to increase and/or alternative respiratory compensation strategies have to be developed.

Of course, if fewer scans per patient are in fact sufficient for diagnosis, then the need for rapid scanning is not as urgent as it first appears. Current clinical referral patterns are heavily biased by the widely disparate risks of each diagnostic modality, resulting in more scans than would be performed if risks were ignored or not present. For example, a person presenting with chest pain, but having a low pretest probability of coronary artery disease (CAD), might currently be referred for a radionuclide perfusion examination, given its low risk. Although a negative scan does not guarantee the absence of CAD, the sensitivity and specificity of radionuclide imaging for detection of CAD is in the mid-90s (19). Given the patient's low pretest probability in this example, a negative scan result might be enough to convince a physician that the patient does not warrant a (higher risk) catheterization procedure. If, on the other hand, CMR could image the coronary arteries directly, then the need for a diagnostic perfusion examination is reduced. Nevertheless, the need for perfusion scanning is not eliminated for all patient groups, in view of its ability to assess risk.

THE QUANTITATIVE REVOLUTION

The fourth condition is the ability to rapidly generate quantitative information. The medical literature is rich in comparisons of quantitative versus qualitative approaches for evaluation of diagnostic procedures. In such compari-

sons, the trend presented in the literature is that quantitative approaches are more reproducible than qualitative approaches. While reproducibility alone does not guarantee accuracy, it is nevertheless a necessary requirement for accurate clinical diagnosis. Currently, quantitative approaches have been applied to a wide variety of CV parameters including:

- cardiac function, via tagging and velocity mapping
- valvular function, via velocity imaging
- vascular evaluation, via velocity imaging and angiography
- cardiac metrics, such as mass, wall thickness, ventricular cavity dimensions, and shape, via cine imaging
- perfusion assessment, via contrast distribution

With CMR's ability to perform quantitative evaluation, it might be anticipated that its clinical benefits would be recognized and extensively used. Surprisingly, in most laboratories, quantitative approaches are infrequently used. One very practical reason for this is that quantitation typically requires higher levels of quality control, access to advanced processing technology, and additional personnel time to provide the necessary input. To quote Blase Carabello, ''In general, when accuracy and applicability compete in the clinical arena, applicability wins'' (20). In the absence of competition, qualitative evaluations are sufficient for a modality to flourish. However, in the context of competition among diagnostic modalities, the issue of quantitation gains added importance. When the same service is offered by competing technologies, improved accuracy warrants the extra effort required by quantitation.

Unfortunately, current quantitative approaches are not ideal. To enhance clinical applicability, a quantitative approach should be almost completely automatic, highly intuitive to the physician, and rapid to apply. Such an approach should allow the physician to make real-time decisions. Currently, a major impediment to quantitation is the high level of user input required. For example, to quantitate mass, volumes, and ejection fractions generally requires manually outlining cardiac borders in a number of slices and for a number of cardiac phases; to quantitate flow through a valve might involve defining a three-dimensional surface encompassing the valve. Some degree of automation is frequently attempted, but with varying degrees of success (21). Reducing the need for user-input must be addressed by improving image quality, faster computers, and enhanced processing approaches. At present, data processing is recognized as a requirement for any CMR package. However, the time involved for user input is currently disproportionate to the significance of the information obtainable. Thus, the requirement for rapid and extensive data processing capabilities to derive cardiac metrics presents another challenge to manufacturers.

One possible approach to limiting the time required for quantitative assessment is to target the region to be assessed. For example, tagged images allow an immediate visual estimation to be made of regional cardiac function, as can be

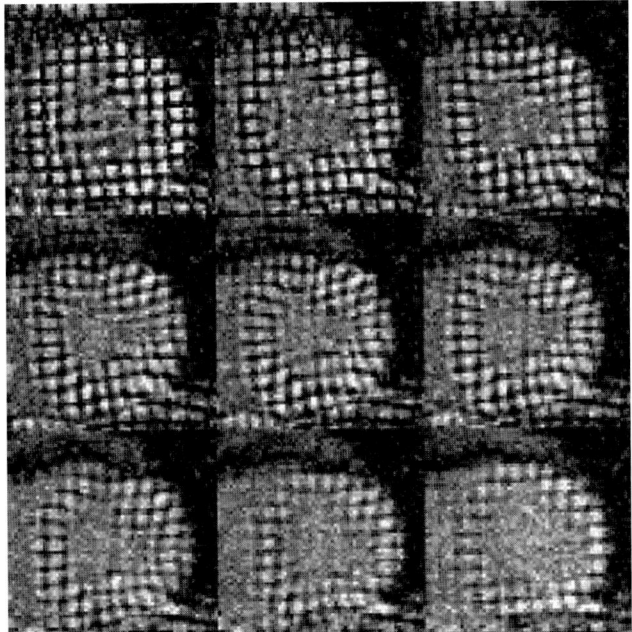

FIG. 2. Short-axis view of the left ventricle at the midlevel with tags applied as a regular grid at the ECG "R" wave. Nine consecutive views of the same plane are shown as the cardiac cycle advances (from **top left** to **bottom right**). Systolic and diastolic motion of the myocardium is observed as deformation of the grid tags.

seen in the example of a tagged data set given in Figure 2. Observation of cardiac tags provides an excellent signal for the diagnostician to focus on certain walls for quantitative analysis (22). This approach effectively minimizes the amount of data that must be processed. In contrast, three-dimensional tagged images or velocity images of three-dimensional flow fields are very difficult to visually interpret. In such complex cases, inadequate image display can limit the ability to focus quantitative efforts. In other words, if the physician does not realize that a certain analysis will improve clinical assessment, then that analysis will not be performed. Thus, improved visualization is another requirement for the optimal MR system.

THE VIRTUAL IMAGING SUITE

As MR technology advances and real-time imaging becomes routine, there will be an increased need for an easy-to-use interface for the physician or technician combining automatic display of images with quantitation. The image presentation modes of existing modalities have, to some extent, contributed to their success. Thus, if CMR is to provide the functionality of other modalities, it may be advantageous to assimilate their best aspects of data display. Additionally, CMR should be equipped with a number of different interface tools to better acquire data, each tool tailored to a partic-

ular imaging paradigm. Other modalities and areas from which CMR could benefit include:

- echocardiography for morphology, function, and valves
- x-ray angiography for vessels
- radionuclide medicine for perfusion
- virtual reality for blood flow

To assess cardiac function, morphology, and valve function, an on-screen echocardiography probe might be displayed and applied to a computer-generated heart model. Thus, imaging planes could be rapidly selected in an intuitive manner. Such an approach was recently featured in an article by Hardy et al. (23). On the computer screen, a generic model of a three-dimensional heart was displayed, and features from the patient-derived images, such as the apex, were mapped to the model. This allowed the orientation of each real-time view to be visualized relative to the three-dimensional computer model.

To assess vasculature patency, the display could simulate the x-ray angiography format. In this mode, projective views of the vasculature would be displayed, permitting physician-friendly assessment. When interrogating regions for stenoses assessment, CMR generated three-dimensional tomographic cross-sections would be used to calculate stenoses accurately. If quantitative velocity methods are available to determine vascular blood flow, contrast agent injection can be simulated (24). This would allow vessel-filling and vessel-emptying times to be determined as in x-ray angiography. In addition, regions of plaque could be located, and their size and extent evaluated. This could allow risk assessment.

Perfusion might best be analyzed in the manner familiar to radionuclide SPECT users. The conventional, multiple-slice, rest and stress stacked myocardial slices could be simulated. Given that MR contrast agents typically pass through the vascular system while radionuclide agents are taken up in the heart, then some reformatting of the dynamic MRI data would be necessary to simulate radionuclide images. An example of the contrast agent dynamics for a conventional first-pass MRI perfusion study is shown in Figure 3. On the other hand, agents that are efficiently extracted from the blood pool could be developed that would more closely simulate radionuclide myocardial perfusion scanning.

Recent advances in virtual reality make this visualization technique ideally suited to CMR's intrinsic three-dimensional nature. It can be envisaged that, with a suitable display, combined with motion sensitive gloves, the physician could "enter" the data set (25). For instance, to examine valve function, the physician would make his way to the appropriate chamber and visualize the stenotic jet. To assess the jet, he would hold his gloved hand in the flow field, and, using either pressure feedback or a digital readout, the highest velocity would be quickly identified. If this seems too futuristic, it might be instructive to invest approximately 50 cents in an amusement arcade to experience the level of virtual reality perceptions routinely achievable today.

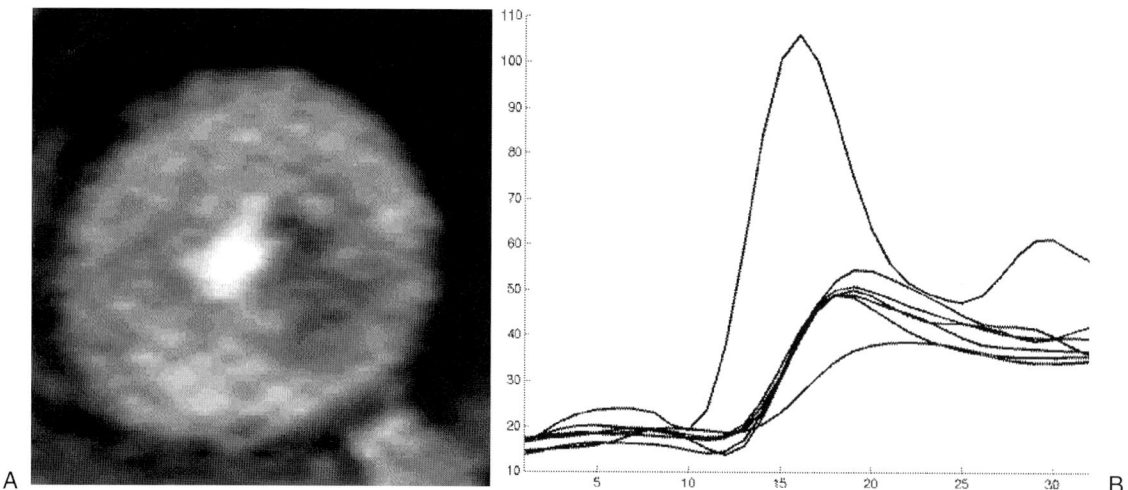

FIG. 3. One frame of a first-pass dynamic series is shown in (**A**). For the left ventricular blood pool and several myocardial regions, the average time-intensity curves are shown in (**B**), obtained with alternate heartbeat temporal resolution (the vertical axis represents intensity in arbitrary units, and the horizontal axis represents time in frames). A perfusion defect is indicated by the low-amplitude curve, corresponding to the region of low intensity in the image.

VIABILITY AND METABOLISM

Another one of CMR's unique features is the ability to evaluate the concentration of a number of metabolites, such as high-energy phosphates (using P-31), lipid (using H-1), cell membrane integrity (using Na-23), and others. While CMR imaging described earlier is based on the resonance of the hydrogen nucleus or proton, many other nuclei in nature manifest the phenomenon of nuclear magnetic resonance. Also, using spectroscopy approaches, it is possible to identify a clinical species. For example, the three ATP peaks on the P-31 spectrum are each located in different positions relative to the main P-31 peak. By placing a circular copper coil on the surface of the chest over the heart, spectra can be derived. In the

future, images displaying the distribution of ATP in the myocardium could be superimposed on a high-resolution hydrogen image. The severity of an ischemic insult could be assessed by the changes in myocardial energetics in patients with chest pain syndromes but without significant angiographically identifiable coronary disease (Fig. 4).

ATHEROSCLEROTIC PLAQUE DETECTION

The detection of intravascular plaques has traditionally been performed by x-ray catheterization. There are several disadvantages to this approach that CMR can potentially overcome: (i) X-ray views are projections of the vascular tree, which, while they provide excellent vessel "roadmaps," require that the degree of stenosis be inferred from the projective views. In contrast, CMR has the potential to provide tomographic views, which allow for examination of the vessel cross-section. (ii) X-ray angiograms only provide views of the vascular lumens; however, it is generally known that in the progression of vascular disease, the vascular lumen is the last physiologic feature to be compromised. CMR offers the possibility of being able to view the projective "road-maps" and also the tomographic views to examine vessel wall thickness. (iii) X-ray catheterization is an invasive procedure while CMR can be either noninvasive or minimally invasive.

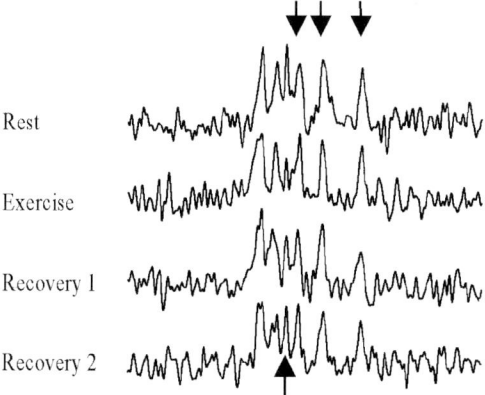

FIG. 4. ³¹P spectra from a patient with a greater than 90% mid- and distal left anterior descending coronary artery stenosis (PCr, *up arrow;* ATP peaks, *3 down arrows*). There is an approximately 45% drop in the PCr /ATP ratio during handgrip stress exercise that is not quite fully recovered even at 18 minutes after stress (*Recovery 1* at 9 minutes and *Recovery 2* at 18 minutes poststress).

The major disadvantage of CMR approaches at present is that the images generated are generally of lower resolution compared to x-ray images. Assuming that CMR image resolution increases in the future, then the full potential of CMR for vessel evaluation can be realized. In particular, the potential of CMR not just to determine the size and extent of plaques but to identify their constituents may make the diagnosis of "stable" or "vulnerable" plaques a part of the CMR vocabulary (26).

CONCLUSION

CMR has already declared itself as a viable diagnostic modality to assess cardiac structure and ventricular function. However, to be optimal and widely employed, CMR should exploit its ease of selection of slice orientation, its rapidity of data acquisition, and its versatility in data viewing and processing modes. Factors favoring the expansion of CMR are its low risk and noninvasive nature. Additionally, there are several advantageous imaging features of CMR: (i) its ability to visualize heart structures in three dimensions without contrast agents; (ii) the ability of MR to generate RF tag lines to most effectively assess regional wall motion dynamics; (iii) CMR spectroscopy's ability to look directly at myocardial metabolites, such as ATP, phosphocreatine, and lipids; and (iv) CMR's ability to characterize tissues, such as plaque, using relaxometry (i.e., T1 and T2 assessment). It has been estimated that over the 10-year period of 1980 to 1990, utilization of imaging procedures in the United States increased by 30 to 60% compared to the previous decade (27). Most of the increase occurred in high technology modalities such as echocardiography, computed tomography, and magnetic resonance imaging (which, in 1980, did not exist as a clinical option). Reasons cited for this dramatic growth included attempts to reduce the time required to make a diagnosis, to increase the certainty of diagnosis, and responsiveness to patient demands. Thus, global health-care trends, ongoing CMR research and development, and improvements in scanner hardware and software indicate that a bright future is guaranteed. The proverbial "one-stop-shop" will be a reality, i.e., using one modality, it will be possible to determine ventricular structure and function, myocardial perfusion, coronary artery (and graft) patency, and myocardial viability. In addition, the ability to assess valve function, to detect pericardial disease, to diagnose idiopathic right ventricular disease, to assess morphologies, function, and shunt size in congenital heart disease all provide ample justification for the conviction that CMR will be the most important diagnostic imagining modality for cardiovascular disease of the 21st century.

REFERENCES

1. Higgins CB, Sajuma H. Heart disease: functional evaluation with MR imaging. *Radiology* 1996;199:307–315.
2. Lipper MH, Hillman BJ, Pates RD, et al. Ownership and utilization of MR imagers in the commonwealth of Virginia. *Radiology* 1995:195:217–221.
3. Martin ET, Pohost GM. Magnetic resonance imaging of the cardiovascular system: can it be cost effective. In: Higgins CB, Ingwall JS, Pohost GM, eds. *Current and future applications of magnetic resonance in cardiovascular disease.* Armonk, NY: Futura Publishing, 1998.
4. Swan JS, Fryback DG, Lawrence WF, et al. MR and conventional angiography: work in progress toward assessing utility in radiology. *Acad Radiol* 1997;4(7):475–482.
5. Korsec FR, Frayne R, Grist TM, et al. Time-resolved contrast-enhanced 3D MR angiography. *Magn Reson Med* 1996;36:345–351.
6. Kerr AB, Pauly JM, Hu BS, et al. Real-time interactive MRI on a conventional scanner. *Magn Reson Med* 1997;38(3):355–367.
7. Liao JR, Pauly JM, Pelc NJ. MRI using piecewise-linear spiral trajectory. *Magn Reson Med* 1997;38(2):246–252.
8. Budinger TF, Fischer H, Hentschel D, et al. Physiological effects of fast oscillating magnetic field gradients. *J Comput Assist Tomogr* 1991;15(6):909–914.
9. Sodickson DK, Manning WJ. Simultaneous acquisition of spatial harmonics (SMASH): fast imaging with radiofrequency coil arrays. *Magn Reson Med* 1997;38(4):591–603.
10. Doyle M, Walsh EG, Blackwell GG, et al. Block regional interpolation scheme for k-space (BRISK): a rapid cardiac imaging technique. *Magn Reson Med* 1995;33:163–170.
11. Doyle M, Walsh EG, Foster RE, et al. Rapid cardiac imaging with turbo BRISK. *Magn Reson Med* 1997;37:410–417.
12. Davis CP, Liu PF, Hauser M, et al. Coronary flow and coronary flow reserve measurements in humans with breath-held magnetic resonance phase contrast velocity mapping. *Magn Reson Med* 1997;37:537–544.
13. Keegan J, Firmin D, Gatehouse P, et al. The application of breath hold phase velocity mapping techniques to the measurement of coronary artery blood flow velocity: phantom data and initial *in vivo* results. *Magn Reson Med* 1994;31:526–536.
14. Wang Y, Grimm RC, Felmlee JP, et al. Algorithms for extracting motion information from navigator echoes. *Magn Reson Med* 1996;36(1):117–123.
15. Felmlee JP, Ehman RL, Riederer SJ, et al. Adaptive motion compensation in MRI: accuracy of motion measurement. *Magn Reson Med* 1991;8(1):207–213.
16. Bailes DR, Gilderdale DJ, Bydder GM, et al. Respiratory ordered phase encoding (ROPE): a method for reducing respiratory motion artefacts in MR imaging. *J Comp Assist Tomogr* 1985;9(4):835–838.
17. Wang Y, Riederer SJ, Ehman RL. Respiratory motion of the heart: kinematics and the implications for the spatial resolution in coronary imaging. *Magn Reson Med* 1995;33(5):713–719.
18. Hofman MB, Wickline SA, Lorenz CH. Quantification of in-plane motion of the coronary arteries during the cardiac cycle: implications for acquisition window duration for MR flow quantification. *J Magn Reson Imaging* 1998;8(3):568–576.
19. McClellan JR, Dugan TM, Heller GV. Patterns of use and clinical utility of exercise thallium-201 single photon emission-computed tomography in a community hospital. *Cardiology* 1996;87(2):134–140.
20. Carabello BA. Mitral valve regurgitation. In: O'Rourke RA, McCall D, eds. *Current problems in cardiology*, St. Louis, MO: Mosby 1998; 23(4):197–244.
21. van der Geest RJ, Buller VG, Jansen E, et al. Comparison between manual and semiautomated analysis of left ventricular volume parameters from short-axis MR images. *J Comp Assist Tomogr* 1997;21(5):756–765.
22. McVeigh ER, Bolster BD Jr. Improved sampling of myocardial motion with variable separation tagging. *Magn Reson Med* 1998;39(4):657–661.
23. Hardy CJ, Darrow RD, Pauly JM, et al. Interactive coronary MRI. *Magn Reson Med* 1998;40:105–111.
24. Steinman DA, Eithier CR, Rutt BK. Combined analysis of spatial and velocity displacement artifacts in phase contrast measurements of complex flow. *J Magn Reson Imaging* 1997;7:339–346.
25. Trelease RB. The virtual anatomy practical: a stereoscopic 3D interactive multimedia computer examination program. *Clin Anat* 1998;11(2):89–94.
26. Gutstein DE, Fuster V. Pathophysiology and clinical significance of atherosclerotic plaque rupture. *Cardiovasc Res* 1999;41(2):323–333.
27. Mettler FA, Briggs JE, Carchman R, et al. Use of radiology in U.S. general short-term hospitals: 1980–1990. *Radiology* 1993;189:377–380.

CHAPTER 35

Current Evidence on Cost Effectiveness of Noninvasive Cardiac Testing

Leslee J. Shaw, Steven D. Culler, and
Edmund R. Becker

CURRENT HEALTH CARE ENVIRONMENT

Health care expenditures will have increased from 4% of the United States gross domestic product almost four decades ago to an estimated 14.5% by the end of this decade (1). In 1996, for the first time, the United States spent more than one trillion dollars on health care—13.6% of the gross domestic product or almost one seventh of all the output in the United States, more than twice what was spent in 1985 (1). By the year 2000, the United States Health Care Financing Administration predicted that unless the government initiates major health care reform, health spending will reach $1.7 trillion annually (18.1% of the gross domestic product) and $16 trillion (32% of the gross domestic product) by the year 2030 (2). Whereas in 1990, 15.4% of federal government expenditures went for health care, by the year 2000, it is estimated that 28.8% of government expenditures will go toward health care. The Social Security trust fund, from which Medicare draws for health care expenditures, is expected to be bankrupt by the turn of the decade requiring the government to either double payroll taxes or cut benefits by about one half.

A number of public and private efforts have been initiated in an attempt to constrain resource use and decrease the

L. J. Shaw: Department of Medicine, Health Policy and Management, Emory University, Atlanta, Georgia 30322.

S. D. Culler: Department of Health Policy and Management, Rollins School of Public Health at Emory University, Atlanta, Georgia 30322.

E. R. Becker: Department of Health Policy and Management, Rollins School of Public Health at Emory University, Atlanta, Georgia 30322.

overall costs of health care in the United States since the early 1980s. In general, regulatory efforts have attempted to reduce health care payment levels or place providers at risk for services rendered. Starting in 1983, revisions to the Medicare reimbursement system were instituted in the form of prospective payment systems, "lump sum" payments for hospitalizations by diagnosis. Part B of the Medicare system instituted resource-based relative value fee schedules for physician services in 1992. Recently, emphasis has shifted to decreasing reimbursement for outpatient services. In the next year, the introduction of Ambulatory Patient Classifications will bring a bundled payment for "like" services (e.g., computed tomography with and without contrast enhancement) to the hospital outpatient clinic setting. Furthermore, it is expected that, with revisions to the Medicare fee schedule in 1999, reductions in reimbursement for the practice expense portion of Medicare payments will range from 18 to 66%. For cardiac imaging, greater reductions are expected for rest echocardiograms, with lesser reductions for radionuclide imaging, and an increase in payments for stress echocardiography.

New provider systems, such as managed care, have instituted mechanisms to decrease health care costs based upon the premise that there is a substantial overutilization of medical services; see Chapter 68 (3,4). Due to their lower cost premiums, managed care organizations have had significant growth in the United States health care marketplace, with varying rates of penetration by state from 33 to 75%. By definition, managed care is the organization and integration of the delivery of medical services. A managed care organization establishes an arrangement between clinicians and institutions that typically includes financial incentives for lowering and limiting resource use by providing the care in the most effective setting.

Despite the growing penetration of managed care in the United States, most contractual agreements for noninvasive cardiac testing are still based on a reduced fee-for-service arrangement. Such a contractual arrangement reimburses on a cost-per-test basis that is usually below the standard charge for that facility. Legislative proposals for the Medicare program would require the lowest fee-for-service payment to guide all contractual agreements for that service, thus further decreasing the per-unit cost of care. Contractual reductions in charges are expected to continue.

Although managed care organizations vary considerably, most systems limit access to specialty care and put controls on resource utilization (i.e., preventing unnecessary test use or medical services). One method used to limit access to specialty care is case managers or physician gatekeepers that review and approve the use of specialty care and, in some cases, cardiac imaging services. The job of the gatekeeper is to review and evaluate the necessity of a medical procedure. The gatekeeper's role is to provide a mechanism to moderate overutilization by denying unnecessary referrals.

Managed care organizations have had a profound effect on health care expenditures. Recent evidence suggests that the growth in health care spending has attenuated in the past few years; in 1993, the percentage of gross domestic product was only 12.3 versus 9.3% in 1983 (4). Furthermore, higher rates of mammography and vaccinations as well as declines in premature births have been attributed to the focus on preventive services by managed health care plans (4). Despite the focus on limiting resource use, a recent report suggests that managed care has not resulted in worsening outcomes across an array of diseases (5), although long-term differences may be observed for chronic diseases as a result of deferment of care. Individual premium payments have also declined in the past few years. It is estimated that managed care organizations saved upward of $250 billion in 1997 alone (4). Despite reducing the rate of health care spending, a number of managed care organizations posted heavy financial losses in 1997 (including Kaiser Permanente and Oxford Health Plan), resulting in increases in premiums ranging from 8 to 20% in 1999 (4). Approximately two thirds of all managed health plans reported suboptimal financial performance in 1998. Although the reason for these losses is unclear, it may be argued that deferred or denied care may precipitate patient presentation with a worsening clinical status later on in the course of a disease process. Other reasons include caring for an aging population, the increase in long-term member longevity, and less patient selection bias. Many managed care organizations are also abandoning the gatekeeper concept, as care has been shown to be less efficient, in particular for certain types of specialty care (e.g., cardiac services). In addition, difficulties in accessing specialty care have prompted an outcry among many patients. Lawmakers have responded by proposing varying forms of the "Patient's Bill of Right" that could increase regulation of managed care services. As a consequence of a lack of continuity of care and declines in patient satisfaction, a number of managed care organizations have instituted open panel options (increased access to specialty care), as well as carve-out contracts for specialty services (6).

The accreditation of health care organizations has also undergone a reorganization in order to assess the quality of health care provided by a given institution. The Joint Commission of Accreditation of Health care Organizations, the accrediting body of more than 14,000 organizations, integrated outcomes and performance measures into the 1997 accreditation process. The focus of these efforts has been on continuous improvement of outcomes as a surrogate for the quality of care provided to patients. Cardiac services were one of the first services included in this new process and outcome evaluation process.

Overall, the environment for health care delivery is one of increasing efforts on controlling cost while, at the same time, providers find it necessary to show that they can provide effective, high quality health care with a minimum number of services.

COSTS OF ISCHEMIC HEART DISEASE

For cardiovascular disease, total costs approach $287 billion annually (7). This includes a direct cost of coronary disease of $124 billion for hospital, $27 billion for physician, $11 billion for home health services, and $16 billion for prescription drug costs. The indirect cost of ischemic heart disease may be defined as a measure of lost productivity due to morbidity and premature death as a result of atherosclerotic disease (e.g., travel time, out-of-pocket expenses, work productivity, lost wages, caretaker services, premature death). Lost productivity as a result of morbidity has been estimated to be $27 billion annually, while costs resulting from mortality equal $82 billion annually. The American College of Cardiology data bases documented that approximately half of all medical payments to cardiologists, including that for diagnostic testing, was related to the diagnosis of coronary disease. Diagnostic procedure use includes 12 to 15 million two-dimensional echocardiograms, 6 million exercise electrocardiograms, 5 million stress myocardial perfusion scans, 1.1 million cardiac catheterizations, and 1.5 million stress echocardiograms (Table 1). Despite efforts to

TABLE 1. *National estimates of noninvasive cardiac procedure use*

Test modality	National utilization estimates
Exercise treadmill	6 million
Rest echocardiography	12–15 million
Stress echocardiography	1.5 million
Stress perfusion imaging	5.2 million
Radionuclide angiography	100,000
Diagnostic catheterization	1.1 million

constrain health care resource use, annual growth rates for noninvasive testing since 1993 have approached 10%.

A major factor contributing to the rising cost of health care has been the development and growth of new technology (9–11). During the past two decades, the growth and development of cardiac imaging technology has been exponential, including tomographic nuclear imaging, technetium-99m-based radioisotopes, positron emission tomography, electron beam computed tomography, harmonic ultrasound imaging, as well as the development of new ultrasound contrast agents. Traditional methods to gain approval for use in this country include an important emphasis on safety and efficacy. Efficacy for an imaging modality may be defined as the ability of a new agent to be comparable to the "gold standard" for that imaging device.

Effectiveness, however, examines how well the new technique may be diagnostically or prognostically accurate in a variety of patient subsets as applied in daily clinical decision-making. Effectiveness includes the ability of the test to classify patients and the likelihood of false-positive and false-negative (cost waste) test results to evaluate extraneous resource use in the health care system. Many of the technological advances in cardiac imaging in the past two decades were introduced without undergoing scientific testing of the effectiveness of the procedure. Moreover, new technologies were often associated with higher charges even though there were few data to justify such increases. For payers, the rising costs of tests contributed to increase insurance premium costs, as well as to shrinking insurance benefits.

Cost containment efforts over the last 5 years have seen a paradigmatic shift in which payers, consumers, and the Health Care Financing Administration are requiring a more thorough evaluation of the effectiveness of any device prior to its use in every day clinical decision-making. The aim of requiring a higher threshold of evidence is to reduce test utilization, in particular, inappropriate use or the use of tests that provide little or marginal information. Evidence suggests that diagnostic procedures may be overused by 30 to 40% (3) and that the efficient use of noninvasive cardiac testing may be used to control higher inpatient, invasive procedure costs (11). In a recent report, control of precatheterization testing was proposed as a means of reducing more expensive, interventional cardiovascular procedures (11). The future of cardiac imaging, as proposed in this framework of economic changes, will depend on its ability to provide relevant clinical and economic information for enhanced diagnostic and therapeutic decision-making.

Accordingly, cardiac imaging techniques will play a critical role in enhancing cost savings, increasing efficiency, and streamlining the early detection and treatment of coronary disease. In the workup of suspected ischemia, the outpatient management of disease remains a viable method for controlling costs. On average, 35 to 40% of health care premiums are used for inpatient health care services, with only 8% being used for outpatient care. In general for primary and secondary prevention strategies, outpatient venues will become vital to orchestrating efficiency within health care.

FORMING A QUALITY FRAMEWORK WITHIN CARDIAC IMAGING

An outcome may be defined as the degree to which the process of care provides improvement in the health of the patient (12). The Institute of Medicine (12) defined health care quality as the degree to which health services both increase the likelihood of a desired health outcome and are consistent with current practice standards. Effectiveness assessment entails the evaluation of two components of health care: quality (outcome assessment) and value (cost). Reductions in health care cost will not be valued by society if they place a patient at undue risk. As such, reductions in health care cost have to be defined within a quality framework. In this framework, patient outcomes will be central to the assessment of health care quality. Outcome assessment allows for a safety net in preserving health care quality in an environment focusing on controlling health care spending.

In cardiac imaging, outcome assessment includes the ability of a test to define a patient's risk of significant (i.e., ≥75% coronary stenosis) coronary artery disease. For higher risk populations or those with established disease, the estimation of disease may be severe, multivessel coronary disease. Frequently, the diagnostic accuracy of a test is defined using the test sensitivity, i.e., true + /(true + + false −) and specificity, i.e., true − / (true − + false +). For prognosis, the ability of a test to form low-, intermediate-, and high-risk strata may simplistically define the ability of a test to predict near-term and long-term important cardiac outcomes. Cardiac outcomes may be defined as cardiac death, nonfatal myocardial infarction, as well as unstable angina or coronary revascularization. A complete evaluation of outcomes is beyond the scope of this chapter; however, we will attempt to highlight relevant outcome data and an evaluation of the current level of evidence for each of the commonly used modalities.

Among the commonly used noninvasive test modalities, those that have been in existence for a longer period of time generally have a greater body of outcomes evidence. Treadmill testing and nuclear cardiac imaging have been available testing modalities for two or more decades. The treadmill test has been incorporated into many large multicenter randomized trials, and its diagnostic and prognostic accuracy has been established across a wide array of patient subsets (13–16). For nuclear cardiology imaging, a number of recent multicenter, large observational series on risk stratification have been reported (17–19). By comparison, newer modalities, such as echocardiography, positron emission tomography (PET) imaging, or magnetic resonance imaging (MRI), have less extensive outcome data. In the area of echocardiography, a number of investigators are actively developing outcome databases and the American Society of Echocardiography currently supports grants in outcome research.

ECONOMIC PRINCIPLES

Societal Standards for an Economic Benefit

Increasing health care costs have placed a disproportionate burden on the individual health care consumer, resulting in higher out-of-pocket costs of care in addition to increasing premiums and declining coverage for beneficiaries and their dependents. Consumers have become frustrated with the limited choice of providers and with constrained access to services approved by their health insurance company. The result of these concerns has increased interest in evaluating the societal benefit for making informed economic choices in health care. The aim of economic analyses is to develop an understanding of the cost of alternative health care testing or therapies (ranging from the use of digoxin therapy as compared with the use of seat belts or disk brakes in automobiles). As the benefit of an economic decision to society is the focus of the analysis, societal standards are developed into a common metric in the form of a league table for the comparison of any economic analysis. Although there are limited cost data for cardiac imaging, we will formulate a synopsis of available data in a league table.

Cost Components to Health Care Diagnosis and Prognosis

Based on recent work in a number of large randomized trials (e.g., Emory Angioplasty-Surgery Trial [EAST] and Clinical Outcomes, Revascularization, and Aggressive Drug Evaluation [COURAGE]), a standard method for the estimation of direct medical care costs has evolved (20–24). Total cost of a hospital episode may be estimated by adjusting

charge information using hospital- or departmental-wide cost-to-charge ratios. Using this approach, the total cost of each hospitalization is calculated as the product between total billed charges during the hospital episode found in the claims data base by the hospital's overall cost-to-charge ratio available from the Medicare cost report (20–24). Physician professional costs may also be estimated using the resource-based relative value scale (RBRVS) methodology. From hospitals with centralized professional billing, all physician services (defined by current procedural terms [CPT] codes and modifiers) and physician charges over the entire episode of care can be collected. Using the relative value weights from the Medicare Fee Schedule, relative value units (RVUs) may be assigned to each CPT code and the total RVUs summarized (20–24). To convert the service RVUs into cost estimates, two different conversion factors are available, one from the Medicare national conversion factor and the other from the national conversion factor based on Blue Cross/Blue Shield (BCBS) or the Health Insurance Association of America (HIAA) data. Cost components include drug costs, testing procedural costs for the hospital or clinic, and indirect costs.

Technical Efficiency

An obvious benefit of the increasing technology in cardiac imaging has been the improved resolution and definition of cardiac structures that are currently available. Cardiac magnetic resonance imaging is an example of improved detection and identification of structures and physiology that may allow for a reduction in the need for duplicate testing. Additionally, improvements in radioisotope and tomo-

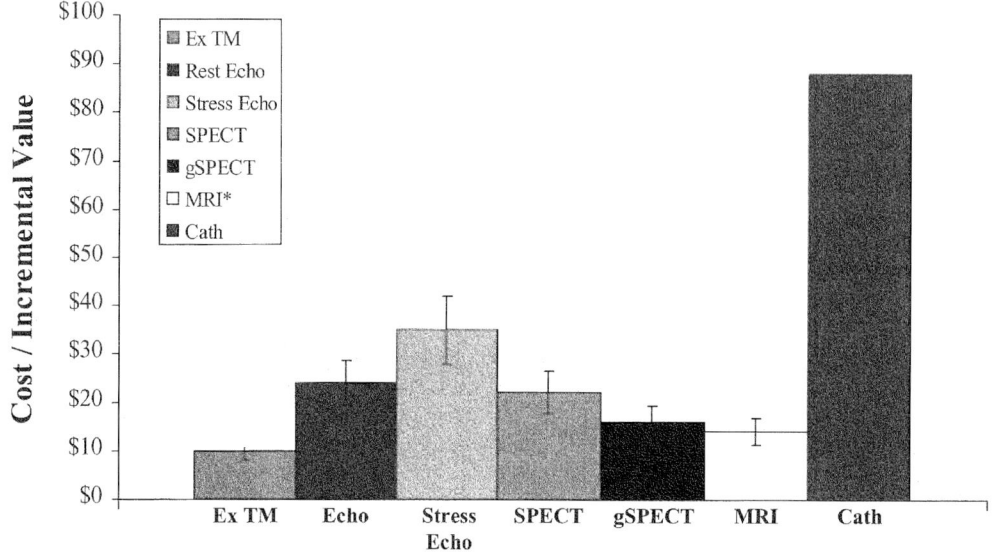

FIG. 1. Incremental cost by added value of test information. *Ex TM*, exercise treadmill; *Echo*, exercise echocardiogram; *SPECT*, stress myocardial perfusion imaging or single photon emission computed tomography; *gSPECT*, gated SPECT; *MRI**, estimates of cost per incremental value for cardiac magnetic resonance imaging; *Cath*, cardiac catheterization.

graphic techniques have resulted in a 20 to 30% improved diagnostic and prognostic accuracy. As imaging modalities have moved from qualitative two-dimensional images to three-dimensional images, from unenhanced to contrast enhanced images, from single head to multihead cameras, and so on, the improvements in temporal and spatial resolution result in enhanced technical efficiency. That is, by providing additional information for the diagnosis of coronary artery disease, early and efficient treatment is possible. In addition to technical improvements, the development of computerized databases to track the diagnosis and prognosis of coronary disease based upon noninvasive risk markers has also provided supportive information upon which to base individual patient management.

However, the development of new contrast agents, improved radioisotopes, camera or software systems, to name a few, have been associated with higher test charges (up to $2,500). In order to evaluate the economic value of these improvements, the incremental cost of new diagnostic information becomes the deciding factor for any new modality. An example of such an analysis is depicted in Figure 1. In this figure, the incremental value of noninvasive risk markers is compared to their added cost. For example, an additional 10% of new information from treadmill testing is obtained by incorporating ST depression, exertional chest pain, and exercise time into a patient's estimation of disease (13) at an added cost of less than $100 or an incremental cost of $10. By comparison, myocardial perfusion information adds approximately 30% new information above and beyond the treadmill test at an added cost of approximately $400 or at an incremental cost of $22. When ventricular function is added, for example, using gated single photon emission computed tomography (SPECT), the incremental cost decreases to $16. Although little data is available for cardiac magnetic resonance imaging, it is possible that the incremental value of the test could exceed other available modalities, thus yielding a greater technical efficiency (i.e., lower cost/incremental value).

Allocative Efficiency

Another form of efficiency that may be defined examines the classification of risk as determined by the noninvasive test. Using a 2 × 2 risk marker table (Table 2), of all the

TABLE 2. *Classification of expected costs by noninvasive test results*

Test result	Negative outcome	Positive outcome
Negative	Low cost (True −)	Cost waste (False +)
Positive	Cost waste (False −)	High cost (True +)

True −, posttest resource use is low; *True +*, posttest resource use is appropriately high including catheterization and intervention (if necessary); *False −*, after negative test, patient presents with documented coronary disease (e.g., acute myocardial infarction); *False +*, after positive test, patient is found to have no coronary disease (e.g., normal catheterization).

positive test results, results from catheterization, or from follow-up outcomes, reveal that these results are either true-positive or false-positive test results. Of all the negative test results, patients may be classified based on either true-negative or false-negative test results. A test that classifies the greatest number of patients as true positive or negative would achieve the greatest allocative efficiency. Although no test could be expected to achieve perfect classification, test cost waste may be determined from false-positive test results (e.g., a patient undergoing catheterization with normal coronaries) or false-negative test results (e.g., a patient being admitted for acute myocardial infarction after a normal test result). In perusing the literature, the goal for test classification would be to reduce the number of patients being misclassified to the range of 10 to 15%.

TYPES OF ECONOMIC ANALYSES

Cost Minimization Principles

Although the principle of cost minimization appears self-descriptive, it defines the lowest cost strategy *given* similar outcomes between the test comparison of interest. A number of examples of cost savings analyses have been published (25–37). In 1995, Berman and colleagues (26) compared incremental cost savings of alternative diagnostic testing strategies for patients with and without an abnormal rest electrocardiogram. The results of this analysis are depicted in Table 3. If a patient has a normal rest electrocardiogram, the lowest cost strategy was an initial exercise electrocardigram, followed by selective nuclear imaging and catheterization for patients with abnormal test results (i.e, 25% lower costs than that of direct catheterization). The lowest cost diagnostic strategy for patients with an abnormal rest electrocardiogram was initial nuclear imaging, followed by selective catheterization (i.e., 38% lower cost than direct catheterization). A similar analysis was published by Marwick et al. (28) in evaluating women at risk for coronary disease with exercise echocardiography. A stepwise diagnostic strategy, defined as referral to an echocardiogram for patients with an abnormal exercise tolerance test and catheterization limited to patients with an abnormal stress echocardiogram, was associated with the lowest evaluation costs (i.e., $663 per patient) as compared to other test strategies (Fig. 2). Recent analyses using outcome-based matching to form similar cohorts undergoing cardiac catheterization and nuclear imaging have compared the diagnostic and follow-up test costs for patients with stable chest pain symptoms (19). For low-to-high pretest risk patients, a 30 to 41% cost savings may be achieved by limiting cardiac catheterization to patients with provocative ischemia on their stress myocardial perfusion scan.

Resource Efficiency

The cost efficiency of noninvasive testing is based on several factors including the effectiveness of subsequent

TABLE 3. *Incremental testing strategies for cost savings*

Strategy	Cost/Patient		Cost/Patient	
	− ECG		+ ECG	
Direct catheterization	$2,800		$2,800	
ETT + selective nuc + cath	$2,089	25%	$2,013	
Nuclear + cath	$1,729		$2,240	
Nuclear + selective cath	$2,118		$1,726	38%

ECG, rest electrocardiogram; *ETT*, exercise tolerance test; selective nuc, selective nuclear testing in patients with an abnormal *ETT*; cath, cardiac catheterization; selective cath, catheterization in patients with an abnormal nuclear test.

treatment, accuracy of testing, the cost of testing, and the direct health benefits and resource use resulting from the testing procedure (31). A number of reports have examined the principle of selective resource use in high-risk patients (19,25,27). The principle of selectivity of resource use has been explored in a variety of patient subsets, including the acute evaluation of chest pain in the emergency department and in suspected coronary disease patients (30,37). This principle may be explained by optimizing the use of less expensive resources and limiting higher cost test use to the highest risk patients (Fig. 3). Resource efficiency, in addition to detailing the up-front cost of test(s), may also include consideration of the induced, downstream resource use patterns. We can illustrate this principle by evaluating the diagnostic workup of suspected coronary disease patients. In this setting, the patient presents to an outpatient visit where the clinical risk assessment is the first line and lowest cost portion of the evaluation strategy. By optimizing the clinical risk assessment, (stratifying patient-risk subsets), referrals should be limited to at-risk patients only. Conversely, lower risk patients receive a ''watchful waiting'' approach to care, with initiation of primary prevention strategies (i.e., risk factor control). In the emergency department, lower risk patients are shifted to the lower cost, outpatient setting. In the

evaluation of suspected coronary disease, only patients who have a positive exercise test are referred to cardiac imaging, thus controlling costs for all patients and limiting the use of coronary angiography to few patients with an abnormal test. The goal of selective resource use is to limit more expensive testing by identifying a large proportion of patients who are classified as low risk. Thus, cost efficiency within the diagnostic workup of patients with suspected or known coronary disease (including a variety of patient subsets) may be achieved by risk stratification at each juncture of the patient evaluation process.

The economic advantages of an outcomes-based strategy have been recently reported (25–37). In 1994, Christian and colleagues (29) demonstrated that myocardial perfusion tomography was cost-inefficient for identifying patients with left main or three vessel coronary artery disease (CAD) in a population of patients with a normal rest electrocardiogram. More recently, a similar analysis was performed using a prognostic endpoint (26). In this analysis of 5,083 patients, the cost of identifying patients at risk of cardiac death or myocardial infarction was $5,179 per event, or $3,652 if testing was limited to patients at intermediate to high likelihood of CAD (Fig. 4).

In most outcome data bases of suspected coronary disease,

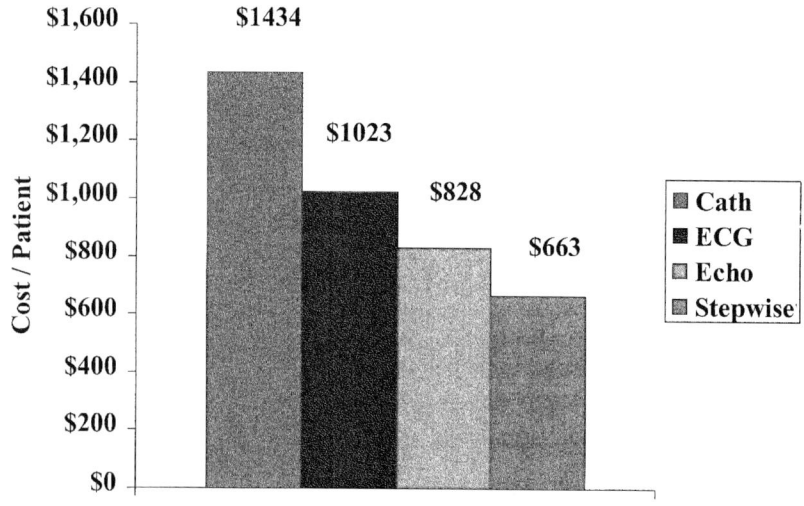

FIG. 2. Cost efficiency of stress echocardiography in 161 women. *Cath*, cardiac catheterization; *ECG*, exercise electrocardiogram; *Echo*, exercise echocardiogram; *Stepwise*, stress echocardiogram in ETT +, catheterization in echocardiogram +; *ETT*, exercise tolerance test.

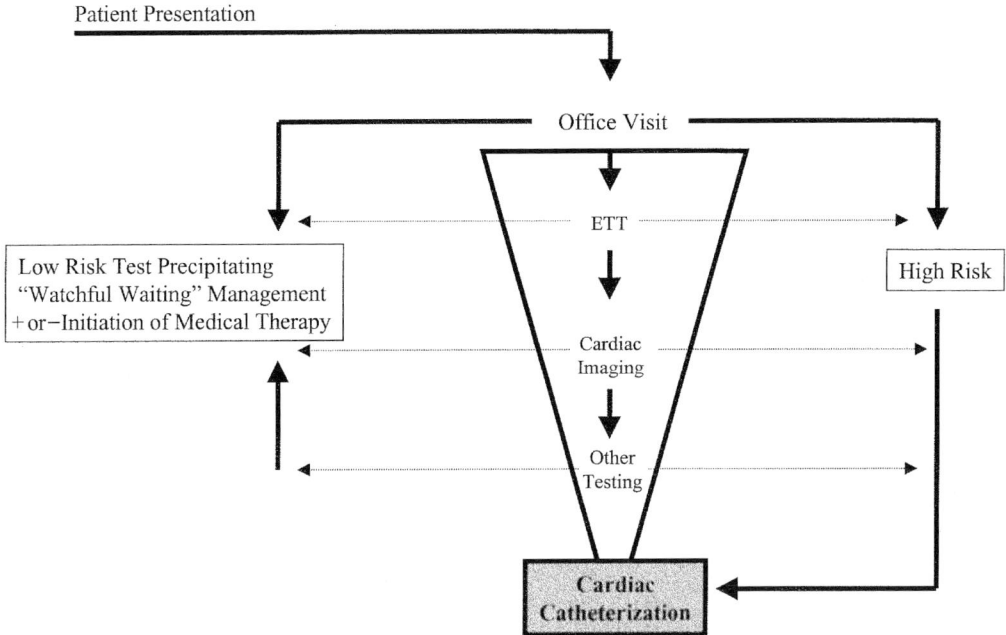

FIG. 3. Principle of selective resource use. *ETT*, exercise tolerance test.

60 to 80% of all patients are low risk. These patients use fewer resources during 3 years of posttesting (i.e, low-cost patients). In the acute setting, as many as 90% of patients have a negative scan, thus limiting admission to a small percentage of patients. In the acute setting, appropriately shifting patients to the lower cost outpatient setting provides a tremendous opportunity for cost savings. However, discharging patients should not result in an increase of out-of-hospital infarcts or cardiac arrests, events that are the number one reason for litigation in emergency departments, driving costs exponentially upward. A number of noninvasive-based diagnostic strategies in the emergency department using nuclear imaging (37,38), exercise testing (39), echocardiography (40), and electron beam computed tomography (41) with cost savings ranging from 10 to 40% for discharged patients have been reported (42,43).

Cost Effectiveness Analysis

Tests that identify risk and early treatment have been shown to have a benefit in terms of improved survival. Tests that effectively initiate early treatment provide a link to an economic benefit as a result of efficient and effective health care strategies decreasing admissions and overuse of health care services and improving patient outcomes. Tests that are highly accurate have a lower rate of false-positive tests (i.e, decreased cost waste due to overuse of cardiac catheterization) and lower rate of false-negative tests (i.e., decreased cost waste due to a reduction in hospitalization for unstable angina or myocardial infarction). These clinical principles form the basis for cost-effectiveness analysis.

Cost-effectiveness analysis techniques may be used when comparing varying test modalities (20–24). Cost-effective-

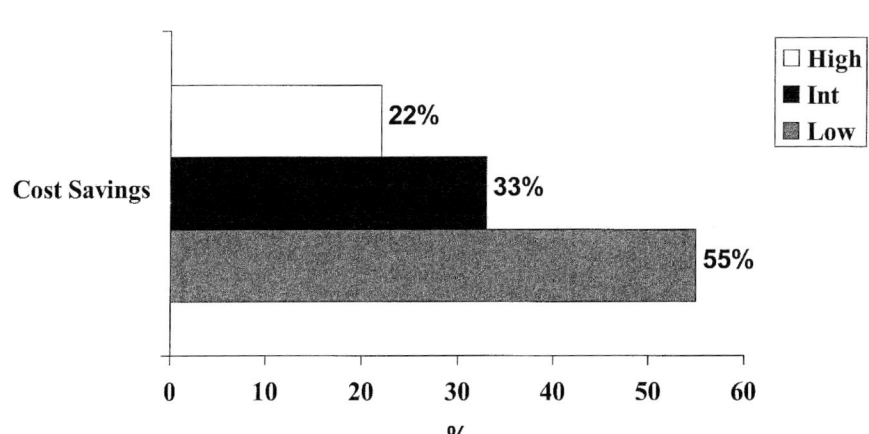

FIG. 4. Incremental cost savings with stress myocardial perfusion imaging: cost savings by implementing a selective cardiac catheterization strategy for patients with a high-risk perfusion scan (i.e., summed stress score greater than 8). *N* equals 5,083; 17% reduction in catherization rate. *Int*, intermediate.

TABLE 4. *League table of cost effectiveness data on noninvasive cardiac testing*

Test modality	Low	Int	High	List
Diagnostic catheterization		xx	$$	High pretest risk
Stress nuclear	$$	$$	$$	Low, Int, High: elderly with symptoms
				Intermediate: stable chest pain with suspected or known CAD, preoperative risk before vascular surgery
				Abnormal rest ECG
Exercise echo		$$		Intermediate: stable chest pain in women
Exercise treadmill	$	$$		Low: Asymptomatic ≥1 cardiac risk factor
				Intermediate: Known CAD or Intermediate Pretest Risk

CAD, coronary heart disease; ECG, electrocardiogram; Int, intermediate; *Echo*, echocardiogram; *xx*, cost ineffective, *$$* = cost effectiveness ratio <$50,000 per life year saved; *$*, moderately cost effectiveness ratio <$100,000 per life year saved; *List*, pretest clinical risk (low, intermediate, or high) with published cost-effectiveness data.

ness analysis may be defined as the incremental cost of one test or test-driven strategy over another divided by the incremental benefit of the same test or therapy. Such an analysis relates the economic resources consumed by the test in relation to the benefits attained by that test and is illustrated in the following equation:

$$Incremental\ CE = \frac{C_{Test\ \#1} - C_{Test\ \#2}}{O_{Test\ \#1} - O_{Test\ \#2}}$$

where *Incremental CE*$_{Test\ \#1}$ is the incremental cost-effectiveness of *Test #1* compared to *Test #2*, where *C* equals mean cost, and *O* equals mean outcome.

Using this equation, it is easy to see that in order to be more cost-effective, one needs to optimize either the numerator or denominator of the equation or both. A comparison that results in reduced cost and improved outcomes is termed a dominant strategy. By reducing costs and/or improving outcomes, we can improve the cost-effectiveness of a test. When outcomes are similar, the appropriate analysis is one of cost savings. General principles of cost-effectiveness include the fact that testing is (i) cost-effective in patient subsets for which the test is diagnostically and prognostically accurate, and (ii) cost-effectiveness ratios become more favorable with an increasing patient risk (i.e, secondary prevention or known coronary disease populations) in the population. For example, the cost-effectiveness of preoperative screening prior to vascular surgery is more advantageous for patients with an intermediate pretest probability of CAD who are symptomatic or have a prior CAD history as compared with lower risk, asymptomatic patients without any cardiac risk factors (36).

Improvements in survival are not directly related to a diagnostic test; instead, the results of the test are used to initiate therapy. Thus, a diagnostic test has only an indirect benefit on survival, rendering the calculation of cost-effectiveness ratios difficult (i.e., the denominator of Δ outcome). Much of our existing cardiac imaging outcomes data do not effectively link posttest decision-making in terms of the decision to initiate medical therapy posttest that may alter outcome in a patient. Despite the limitations, a number of investigators have reported the cost-effectiveness of a variety of diag-

nostic techniques and patient settings. Goldman et al. (32) presents a compendium of cost-effectiveness data in a league table that details a common metric for comparing the value to society of medical services and therapies. Table 4 reports on cost-effectiveness data from Goldman, as well as from several recent reports (31,35,37).

DEVELOPMENT OF COST-BASED DISEASE MANAGEMENT STRATEGIES

Using the available clinical and economic outcome data, it is now possible to define clinical guidelines for care of patients who may benefit from referral to cardiac testing. The purpose of a guideline is to reduce variability in resource use (i.e., cost of care) and outcomes by defining pathways of care. Disease management is a further refinement of the outcomes-based guideline that incorporates both the clinical and economic outcomes of care. The basis of disease management is that there is an optimal set of interventions that result in improved patient outcomes at lower health care costs. The theory for disease management is based on the reported significant variation in the diagnosis and treatment of different health care delivery systems. Major components of a disease management program include screening, procedures or interventions, and measurement of outcomes (clinical, economic, and humanistic—i.e., quality of life). The aim of a disease management strategy is to integrate cost-quality issues into clinical decision-making. An assessment of quality (i.e., outcomes) given the amount of resources that are expended on the cost of care may then ultimately be used to derive value in health care. A successful management strategy will result in an improvement in overall efficiency of the health care, a reduction in overall cost of care as a result of shifting care to lower cost venues, enhanced clinical decision-making, and improved short- and long-term outcomes of the patient.

Disease management strategies may be used to develop a rationale strategy to control costs in cardiology. Evidence exists that the use of a lower cost test that is effective at identifying coronary disease and cardiac event risk may serve as an initial screen, allowing for a more selective use of cardiac catheterization (19). The criteria of a quality test would be one that had a minimal false-positive rate (i.e., a low rate of diagnostic cost waste and a minimal false-negative rate or cost waste due to unstable angina or myocardial infarction admissions). The resulting disease management strategy would be conservative, limiting cardiac catheterization to patients with demonstrable ischemia or abnormal test findings (44). Cost savings would be accrued by identification of patients expected to have normal test results who receive a "watchful waiting" approach rather than additional resources for care (18,27,34,35).

Based on the guidelines of the American College of Cardiology/American Heart Association, indications for percutaneous interventions include patients with one-vessel disease with a moderate-large area of ischemic myocardium subtending a significant coronary stenosis (including class I or II angina). Despite these recommendations, there has been a 10- to 20-fold increase in the use of percutaneous interventions in this country, particularly for patients with Canadian Cardiovascular Society class I angina. Thus, implementing a selective use of cardiac catheterization for patients with a prior, demonstrable area of ischemia could have profound economic implications on the cost of care for cardiac patients. An estimated $3.5 million cost savings per 1,000 patients tested with a 40% reduction in the rate of cardiac catheterization could be attained (19). A similar estimation of cost savings was reported by Hachamovitch et al. (27). In this report on 5,083 patients, when catheterization was limited to patients with a high-risk nuclear scan, a 17% reduction in the rate of coronary angiography would be observed (26).

One example of a proposed disease management strategy using a cardiac imaging test will be used in the upcoming Clinical Outcomes, Revascularization, and Aggressive Drug Evaluation (COURAGE) trial and is detailed in Figure 5.

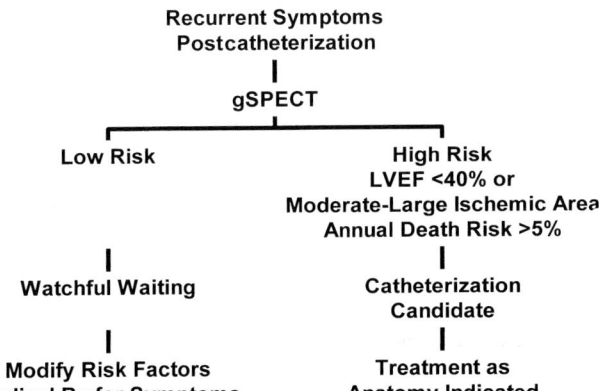

FIG. 5. Substudy using nuclear testing in the COURAGE trial of PTCA versus medical therapy. Retest as symptoms warrant or every 1–2 years. COURAGE, Clinical Outcomes, Revascularization, and Aggressive Drug Evaluation; *gSPECT*, gated single photon emission computed tomography; *LVEF*, left ventricle ejection fraction; *PTCA*, percutaneous transluminal coronary angioplasty; *Rx*, medical therapy.

The COURAGE trial is a 3,260 patient randomized, controlled trial of percutaneous transluminal coronary angioplasty (PTCA) plus medical therapy as compared with optimal medical therapy alone in reducing major cardiac events (including death or myocardial infarction). Patient inclusion is limited to those with catheterization-defined coronary disease without significant left ventricular dysfunction or three-vessel coronary disease (or its equivalent). The primary aim of this strategy is to define an optimal strategy for nuclear imaging for the assessment of recurrent symptoms for patients with known coronary disease.

COST FINDINGS RELATED TO NONINVASIVE TESTING TECHNIQUES

Standards for evaluation of economic analysis are listed in Table 5. For a cost savings model, outcomes should be equivalent between the comparative test groups so that any lowering of costs is not achieved at the expense of health care quality. Thresholds for economic efficiency in cost-effectiveness analysis are less than $50,000 per life-year saved with many health policy analysts recommending lowering that standard to somewhere in the range of $20,000 to $40,000 per life-year saved. For the remainder of this chapter, a synopsis of available economic data on noninvasive diagnostic testing will be provided.

Exercise Electrocardiography

In 1986, Chaitman reviewed the existing diagnostic accuracy data on exercise electrocardiography (ECG) testing with average sensitivity values in the range of 60 to 65% (16). Cardiac imaging modalities have uniformly higher accuracy values. Additional reviews on postmyocardial infarction testing have been published by Froelicher et al. (46) and Shaw et al. (47). A number of recent reports are available establishing the diagnostic and prognostic accuracy of treadmill testing in symptomatic patients with suspected coronary artery disease (47,13,14). In an analysis of 2,758 symptomatic patients, Shaw and colleagues (14) reported that the Duke treadmill score, a composite index of exercise time, exertional chest pain, and ST depression, was able to provide accurate estimates of patient's likelihood of significant and severe coronary disease as well as 5-year survival, regardless of gender (Fig. 6). These results have been similarly applied to a cohort of 976 women (14).

The routine workup of a patient with suspected coronary artery disease is depicted in Figure 7. This figure depicts patients proceeding from the outpatient clinic to the exercise treadmill laboratory, to a cardiac imaging laboratory, or to cardiac catheterization. Theoretically, the principle of selective resource use may be applied to the diagnostic workup of patients such that risk stratification is optimized for lower cost tests before referral to a more expensive scan. In the case of exercise electrocardiography, optimization of testing includes evaluation of more than ST segment changes but

TABLE 5. *Rules for cost analysis*

Economic models	Example	Rules
Cost savings = (cost$_A$ − cost$_B$) /equivalent outcome Cost benefit = (cost$_A$ − cost$_B$)	Compare cost (upfront + induced) of two tests given a similar test accuracy Compare costs of Test A management strategy as compared with Test B management strategy	Equal outcomes in order to assure quality All resource use and outcomes are converted into dollars (including outcomes) Cost difference <$0 is favored after dollar conversion of all inputs
Cost-effectiveness = (cost$_A$ − cost$_B$) (outcomes$_A$ − outcome$_B$)	Incremental cost-effectiveness of Test A versus Test B; comparing the induced resources used in relation to the accuracy of the test achieved to detect disease amenable to life saving treatment	

also includes consideration of hemodynamic, chronotropic, and functional capacity, as well as exertional symptoms. The Duke treadmill score is an example of the incorporation of several risk markers into a score for diagnostic and prognostic risk assessment (13). This score is being incorporated into the Marquette treadmill systems for individual patient risk estimation.

A number of studies have examined the diagnostic and prognostic accuracy as well as cost-efficiency of employing exercise echocardiography or stress myocardial perfusion scintigraphy following a routine exercise treadmill test. Use of cardiac imaging is cost-efficient when a stepped testing approach is used (26–28). Accordingly, cardiac imaging is employed only for patients with an abnormal or indeterminate exercise electrocardiogram. For both stress echocardiography and nuclear imaging, significant cost savings is achieved when postexercise test referral was limited to patients with an abnormal or indeterminate exercise treadmill test results.

Test use that is cost-effective (i.e., less than or equal to $40,000 per life year saved) includes the use of an exercise electrocardiogram for patients with known coronary disease, intermediate risk patients, or asymptomatic patients with one or more cardiac risk factors (31). Test use that is too costly (i.e., more than $100,000 per life year saved) includes the use of an exercise electrocardiogram in asymptomatic patients.

Exercise Echocardiography

The first publication on the diagnostic accuracy of exercise echocardiography was reported by Wann and colleagues in 1979 (49). Since that time, there have been a number of reports on the diagnostic accuracy of stress-induced ventricular dyssynergy. Two recent metaanalyses of the diagnostic accuracy of exercise echocardiography were reported (49,50) (Fig. 8). A synthesis of 49 reports revealed the sensitivity and specificity of new or worsening wall motion abnormality at 88% and 84%, respectively (49). Several recent

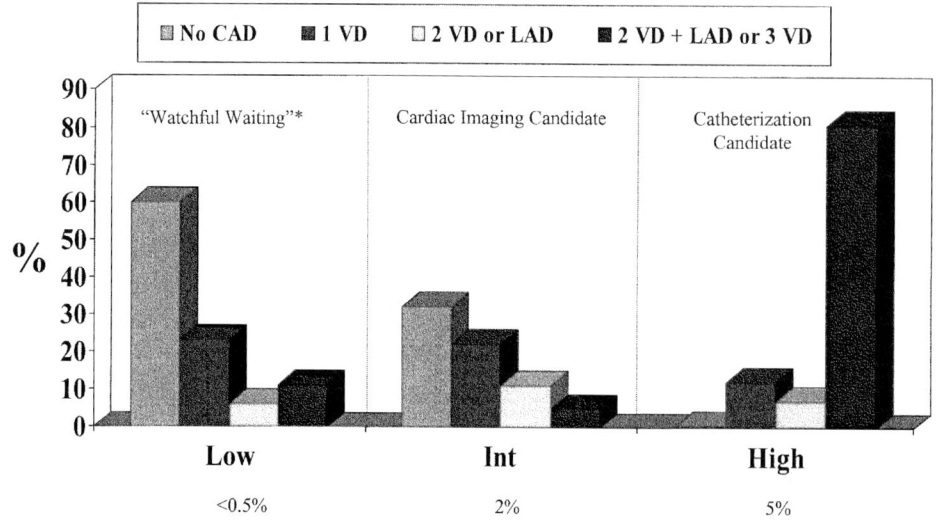

FIG. 6. Estimation of significant and severe coronary disease and annual cardiac mortality in 2,758 stable chest pain patients. *CAD*, coronary artery disease; *VD*, vessel disease; *LAD*, left anterior descending; "Watchful Waiting,"* modify risk factors and symptomatic medical therapy.

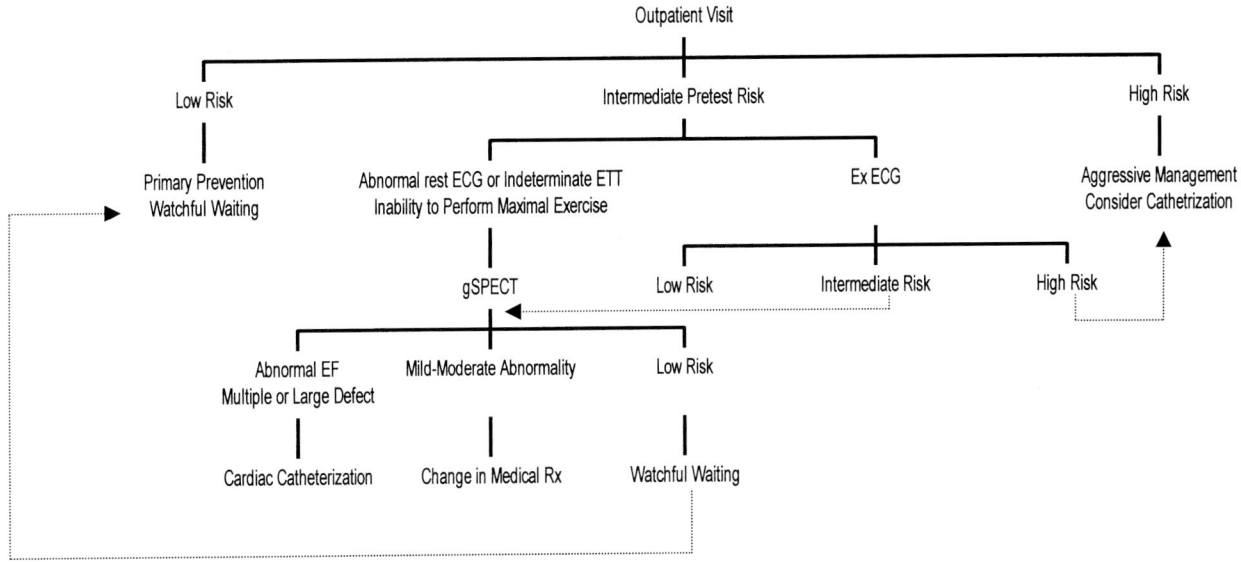

FIG. 7. Routine workup of suspected cardiac ischemia. *ECG*, electrocardiogram; *ETT*, exercise tolerance test; *ExECG*, exercise ECG; *EF*, ejection fraction; *gSPECT*, gated single photon emission computed tomography; *Rx*, medical therapy.

reports on the prognostic value of stress echocardiography have revealed incremental risk stratification for patients with stress-induced wall motion abnormalities (51–56). These results have been confirmed for varying patient subsets including post-myocardial infarction, women, and patients with suspected or known coronary disease (51–57). In the largest series reported to date, Poldermans et al. (54) reported 3-year, cardiac-event-free survival in 1,737 patients. In a multivariable Cox model, significant estimators of cardiac death or myocardial infarction included the presence of stress-induced ischemia (hazard ratio = 3.3) and extensive rest wall motion abnormalities (hazard ratio = 1.9). In a similar analysis from the Mayo Clinic on 860 patients with known or suspected coronary disease, 2-year outcomes were increased with the percentage of abnormal segments at peak stress and an abnormal left ventricular end-systolic volume response

to dobutamine stress echocardiography (56). Dobutamine stress echocardiography added 28.5% new information (i.e., incremental value) above clinical data in this Mayo series (56). For exercise echocardiography, McCully et al. (56) reported on survival in 1,325 patients with a normal, maximal exercise echocardiogram; ensuing, annual cardiac-event-free survival was 0.9%.

Currently, there are several reports on the costs of care associated with exercise echocardiography. One report by Marwick et al. (28) reported on the evaluation costs in 161 women with suspected coronary disease (Fig. 2). This report evaluated the diagnostic test cost for (i) exercise ECG followed by cardiac catheterization in women with an abnormal exercise ECG, (ii) exercise echocardiography in women with an abnormal exercise ECG, and (iii) direct cardiac catheterization. Total cost of care was $663 for a stepwise diagnostic

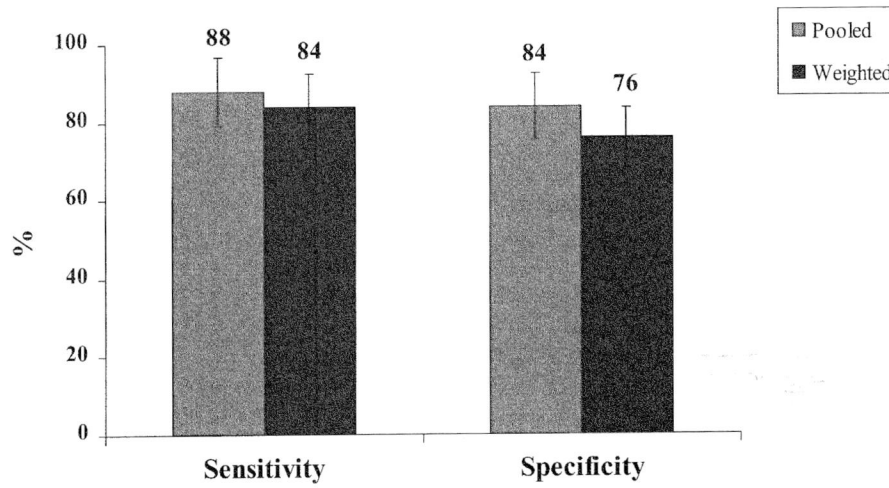

FIG. 8. Diagnostic accuracy of stress echocardiography from 49 published reports in 4,056 patients. *Pooled*, pooled data analysis; *Weighted*, weighted average by proportional sample size.

testing strategy (echocardiography in patients with an abnormal exercise ECG and catheterization for patients with an abnormal echocardiogram) as compared with costs ranging from 20 to 54% higher for testing including (i) stress echocardiography followed by catheterization, (ii) exercise ECG followed by catheterization, and (iii) direct coronary angiography. In another report by Rubin and colleagues (58), evaluation (or assessment) costs were compared for patients undergoing preoperative risk stratification prior to vascular surgery using dobutamine stress echocardiography. Using a simple selection algorithm, the preoperative test costs were compared for patients undergoing a selective testing approach, defined as preoperative testing with dobutamine stress echocardiography for patients with one or more clinical risk factors. Patients considered at high risk and requiring cardiac catheterization were those with a stress-induced wall motion abnormality. Low-risk patients without clinical risk markers did not undergo preoperative testing. These results reveal that, when preoperative testing is limited to a selected patient cohort with cardiac risk factors, the average testing costs could be lowered $214 for low-risk patients (58).

The cost-effectiveness of stress echocardiography has been recently explored in a decision model by Redberg (59). This analysis explored a variety of testing strategies for the evaluation of symptomatic women with suspected coronary artery disease (including stress Tl-201 imaging, exercise ECG, and no noninvasive testing. Table 6 details the results of this decision model using a marginal cost-effectiveness analysis comparing stress echocardiography with other techniques using a base case of a 55-year-old woman. The results reveal that for women with definite, probable, and nonspecific chest pain, echocardiography resulted in a dominant strategy (that is, both the outcomes and costs were lower with echocardiography, resulting in a negative cost-effectiveness ratio) when compared with Tl-201 imaging in women. Stress echocardiography was also cost-effective (i.e., less than $20,000 per quality-adjusted life years saved) when compared with exercise ECG testing. These results reveal an important concept: namely, that, for women, Tl-201 imaging

with a higher rate of breast artifact may be less accurate and lead to more costly care than would echocardiography.

Contrast-enhanced Echocardiography and Harmonic Imaging

Approximately 10 to 15% of routine two-dimensional echocardiograms are suboptimal (i.e., endocardial visualization in less than or equal to four of six myocardial segments in an apical four-chamber view). Recently, new intravenous ultrasound agents, including Albunex and Optison (Molecular Biosystems, Inc.), have been approved for left ventricular opacificition by the Food and Drug Administration (FDA). A number of other agents are currently in phase III studies for the evaluation of left ventricular opacification. Contrast-enhanced echocardiography has also been shown to define myocardial perfusion (currently in phase II clinical trials) and improve the Doppler signal (particularly helpful in low-flow states) in addition to aiding in endocardial border delineation. For echocardiography, there are several important patient subsets for whom visualization of the endocardial border is difficult (e.g., body habitus, obesity, and lung disease). For myocardial contrast echocardiography, the major advantages are the real-time interpretation of data allowing for enhanced laboratory throughput, fewer hours lost for employers (i.e., less lost productivity), and enhanced clinical decision-making.

A critical step in assimilation of new technology is whether the incremental benefit is worth the added cost. A compendium of literature and expert experiences on contrast echocardiography have been published in several review papers (60–62). A synthesis of reports reveals that myocardial contrast echocardiography provides clear definition of regional wall motion and thickening and enhances delineation of the left ventricular chamber for patients with technically difficult images (60–63). Myocardial contrast echocardiography also enhances diagnostic confidence in the clinical value of stress echocardiographic imaging with improvements in image quality in approximately 50% of patients (60–63). From a 203-patient, multicenter series, Optison imaging resulted in a higher percentage of studies (74%) converted to diagnostic echocardiograms as compared to the first generation agent, Albunex (26%, $P < 0.0001$), using a blinded core laboratory interpretation (63). Diagnostic yield may be defined as sufficient information in order to answer the principal diagnostic question (i.e., reason for referral), despite incomplete endocardial visualization. The results of a secondary analysis of 203 patients revealed that the diagnostic yield was enhanced with Optison (87%) as compared to a noncontrast (49%) echocardiogram ($P < 0.001$). Similar results have been reported with other unapproved agents revealing a 91 to 97% visualization of left ventricular segments with myocardial contrast echocardiography (64). Other agents, not yet FDA approved, have revealed modest concordance rates of contrast-enhanced wall motion to nuclear perfusion abnormalities (range, 54 to 61%) (64).

TABLE 6. *Cost-effectiveness of exercise echocardiography as compared with other noninvasive testing modalities in women with suspected coronary disease*[a]

	Marginal cost-effectiveness per QALY		
	T1-201	ECG ($)	No test ($)
Definite angina			
Echo	Dominated	16,305	21,215
Probable angina			
Echo	Dominated	15,510	12,088
Nonspecific CP			
Echo	Dominated	8,555	9,580

[a] Scenario designed for 55-year-old woman.

QALY, quality-adjusted life year; *Echo*, exercise echocardiogram; T1-201, exercise thallium-201; *ECG*, exercise electrocardiography; *CP*, chest pain.

Due to the recent approval of myocardial contrast echocardiography agents, few reports have documented the estimation of prognostic outcomes. A recent report has documented the value of myocardial contrast echocardiography in estimating improvement in regional ventricular function for patients undergoing coronary revascularization (65). From this report, myocardial contrast echocardiography had an excellent negative predictive value (>80%) for estimating attenuated regional function at 60 days postsurgery (66). A moderately strong correlation (0.5) was reported between contrast wall motion scores and nuclear perfusion defect severity ($P < 0.0001$) for the estimation of myocardial viability in 21 patients with chronic coronary disease (66). Using myocardial contrast echocardiography before and at 3 months postrevascularization, the negative and positive predictive value was 87 and 81% for improved regional function recovery ($n = 24$ with acute myocardial infarction) (67).

Incremental Value of Harmonic Imaging

Harmonic imaging has also been proposed as a new method to improve detection of echocardiographic abnormalities over fundamental echocardiography (64,68). Harmonic imaging differs from fundamental imaging by transmitting ultrasound at one frequency and receiving at twice the transmitted frequency. This technique has been used to enhance myocardial visualization. In order to evaluate the true incremental value of myocardial contrast echocardiography, it is imperative to discern the amount of independent information defined by harmonic imaging alone. In a recent report by Spencer and colleagues (68) in 20 patients, harmonic images had less clutter and better myocardial blood contrast. Furthermore, individual segments had enhanced visualization with harmonic imaging in 30 to 70% of apical four-chamber views. During dobutamine stress testing, the overall number of interpretable segments improved 20% with the use of harmonic imaging. Many segments traditionally difficult to image were improved with harmonic imaging with more segments being clinically interpretable during stress testing (68).

For patients with an initially suboptimal echocardiogram, diagnostic information sufficient in order to aid in patient management may still be gleaned in 25 to 30% of patients (63,68). Furthermore, using available literature, it is estimated that harmonic imaging provides a modest improvement in visualization (approximately 20%) with the greatest improvement being derived with myocardial contrast harmonic echocardiography (63–65,68).

Augmented image quality provides a means for improved patient management in the form of decreased echocardiographic-induced cost waste (i.e., false-positive tests) and a reduction in duplicate testing for patients at risk for a poor acoustic window (e.g., elderly, pulmonary disease). Shaw and colleagues (69) have published on the cost savings that may be achieved with Optison contrast echocardiography. The principle underlying these analyses is that improved technical efficiency with contrast enhancement results in a reduction in downstream resource use. For the patient who does not receive Optison, the principal diagnostic question still remains despite a suboptimal echocardiogram, and, as such, patient management may be misdirected or less efficient given inadequate information considered for patient management. This point is best illustrated with an example of a patient whose noncontrast study exhibited poor visualization. In this case, the noncontrast study revealed poor visualization of the apex. The echocardiographer interpreted the findings as myocardial thinning in that segment with akinesis of the apical wall. On injection of Optison, the entire apex filled with contrast revealing normal wall thickness as well as hypokinesis of the apical wall. Management of this patient would vary if the myocardial wall were considered akinetic and thinned as compared with being seen as only hypokinetic and of normal thickness.

Using this reasoning, improved diagnostic certainty lowers patient care costs and decreases extraneous resource use. In a secondary analysis (69) of 203 patients undergoing noncontrast and contrast (intravenous Optison, 3 mL) echocardiography, the results of this analysis revealed that the diagnostic yield was enhanced with the use of intravenous Optison (by approximately 40%) as compared to noncontrast echocardiogram ($P < 0.001$). Due to improved image quality in this difficult-to-image patient cohort, follow-up testing was recommended in 42% of noncontrast echocardiograms and in only 12% of Optison contrast echocardiograms ($P < 0.001$). The resultant costs were 18% lower with the use of intravenous Optison contrast agent ($P < 0.0001$). Use of Optison increased the initial diagnostic cost by $110 but resulted in a decrease (17 to 70%) in confirmatory transesophageal echocardiography, catheterization, or nuclear studies. Diagnostic accuracy was improved 2.7-fold for patients with a nondiagnostic echocardiogram receiving Optison with substantial cost savings of $319 per patient. The use of Optison could, then, result in a dominant strategy of improved effectiveness and cost savings (69). In addition to improved accuracy, recent reports have suggested that Optison is able to reduce the intraobserver and interobserver variability in the evaluation of regional wall motion abnormalities (70). Repeatability of any technique becomes a critical component for the identification of a true threshold of change for serial evaluation of worsening ventricular function (70). Prior reports in noncontrast echocardiography have suggested as much as 50% variability in repeated estimates of left ventricular ejection fraction may be observed (60–68).

Nuclear Cardiology

Over the past two decades, cardiovascular scintigraphic techniques have been established as an effective clinical tool for detecting CAD and estimating future risk of major cardiac outcomes (25,26,29,30,71–75). Nuclear techniques have been increasingly applied to the assessment of patient risk; a critical element in assessing cost-effectiveness (25,26, 29,30,71–75).

Stress Myocardial Perfusion Imaging

A growing body of evidence supports the fact that the extent and severity of perfusion abnormalities are strong and independent estimators of a patient's risk of cardiac death and myocardial infarction. Several recent reports have revealed a consistent pattern of low rates of major cardiac events for patients with a low-risk or normal perfusion scan—i.e., less than or equal to 1% annually [17,26,29,30]). The extent and severity of perfusion defects (26) are associated with incrementally higher outcome rates. From the Cedars-Sinai and Mid-America Heart Institute ($N = 20,340$), annual rates of cardiac death and myocardial infarction are depicted in Figure 9 for patients with a normal, mildly abnormal, moderately abnormal, and severely abnormal myocardial perfusion scan (75). Annual rates of cardiac death range from 0.1 to 1.3% ($P < 0.00001$); annual rates of cardiac death or myocardial infarction range from 0.3 to 2.3% ($P < 0.00001$). In addition to the results of the perfusion scan, other nuclear indices have also been found to yield significant prognostic information. Lung uptake of thallium on stress images has been found to be a powerful predictor of outcome by Cox proportional hazards analysis (30). Transient dilatation of the left ventricle during exercise or pharmacologic stress as measured by comparing the rest and stress images has been found to be an excellent predictor of future events (30).

Ventricular Function Imaging

Risk markers of stress-induced left ventricular dysfunction include a diagnostic threshold ejection fraction (EF) of 50%, prognostic threshold EF of less than or equal to 35%, a failure to augment ejection fraction with exertion, and segmental wall dysynergy (72,73). It has long been established that resting left ventricular function is a strong prognosticator of long-term mortality (76). Shaw and colleagues (77) (Fig. 10) published a metaanalysis of exercise-gated and first-pass ventricular function data. An inverse relationship may be observed between peak exercise left ventricular ejection fraction and event-free survival with increasing event rates as left ventricular ejection fraction decreases. These results have application to the newly developed software for determination of gated ejection fraction in the postexercise phase of testing. With little added cost to testing due to the automated gated acquisition methodologies, the need for additional testing, at least ventricular function testing, is minimized.

Cost Implications

From the clinical outcome data, risk increases proportionally with the extent and severity of perfusion and function abnormalities. Cost of care will also increase related to the risk on the nuclear scan and the underlying risk in the population. Total costs of care are higher in older and higher risk patients (29). For example, in a comparison of younger and older patients, higher rates of postnuclear referral to catheterization for younger men drive higher costs of care (Fig. 11). Thus, it is expected that nuclear testing will result in substantially greater resource needs for those patients with abnormal test results. Costs will be minimized through effective increases in survival. The greater body of outcome evidence and observational data on posttest resource use allow for precise determination of the induced costs associated with nuclear imaging.

With nuclear testing, a number of economic strategies

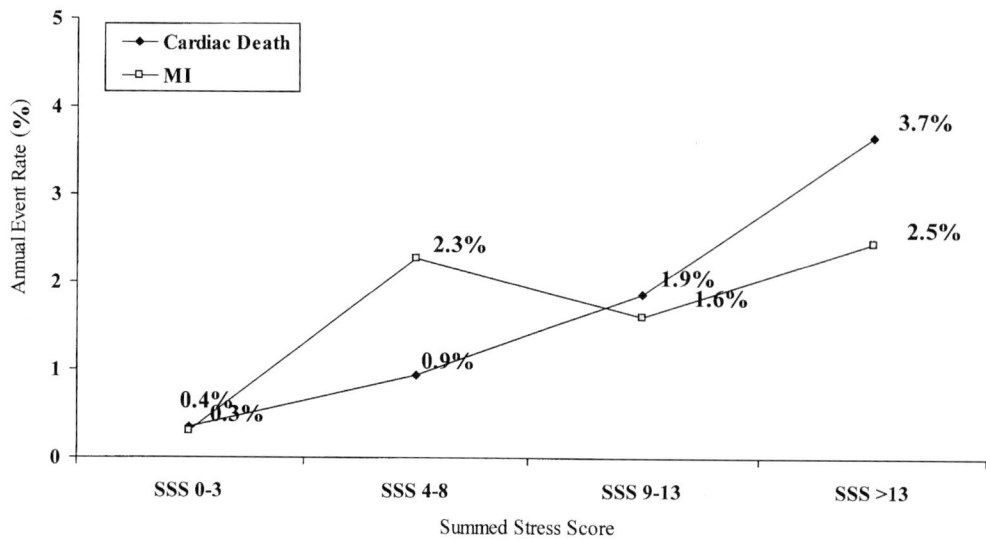

FIG. 9. Risk stratification by the extent and severity of nuclear perfusion abnormalities in 20,340 patients. *MI*, myocardial infarct.

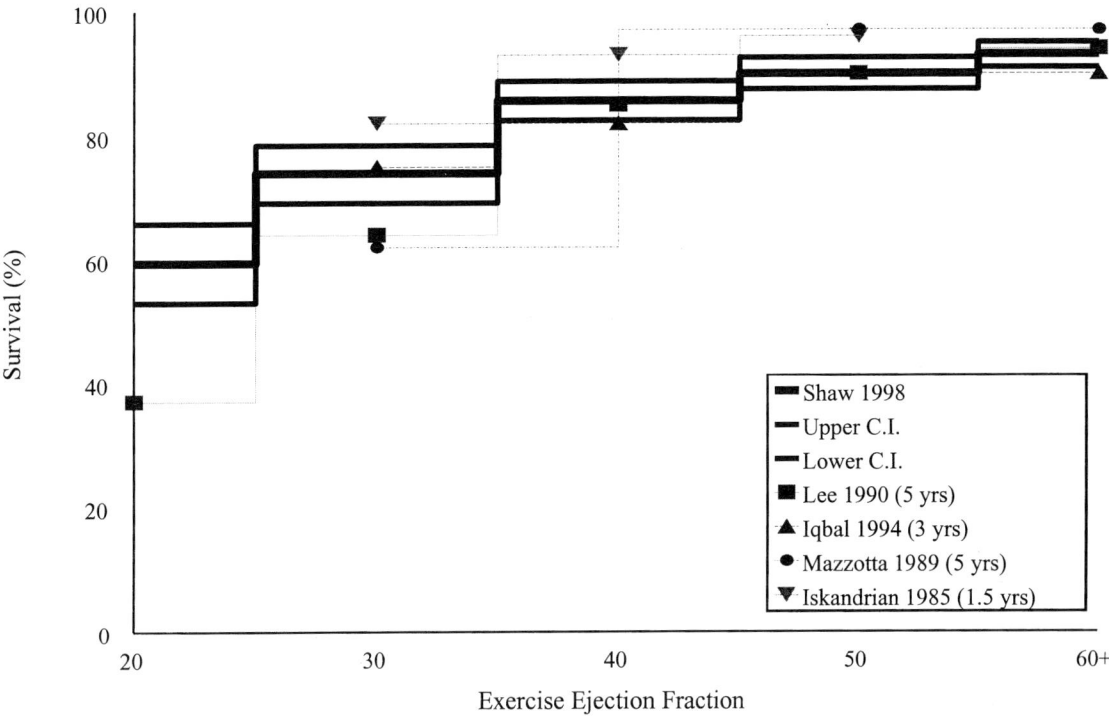

FIG. 10. Metaanalysis of gated and first-pass radionuclide imaging: prognosis by peak left ventricular ejection fraction. *C.I.*, confidence interval. (From ref. 77, with permission.)

may be optimized, including selectivity of resource use, test classification, technical efficiency by improved test accuracy, and cost-effectiveness as a result of early identification and treatment of risk. As a result of dramatic improvements in resolution and in software, nuclear imaging allows for a number of economic advantages. Improved resolution with nuclear imaging (e.g., multiheaded cameras, tomographic imaging) as well as software advances (e.g., gated SPECT, attenuation correction) have allowed for a more precise delineation of changes in myocardial perfusion and function.

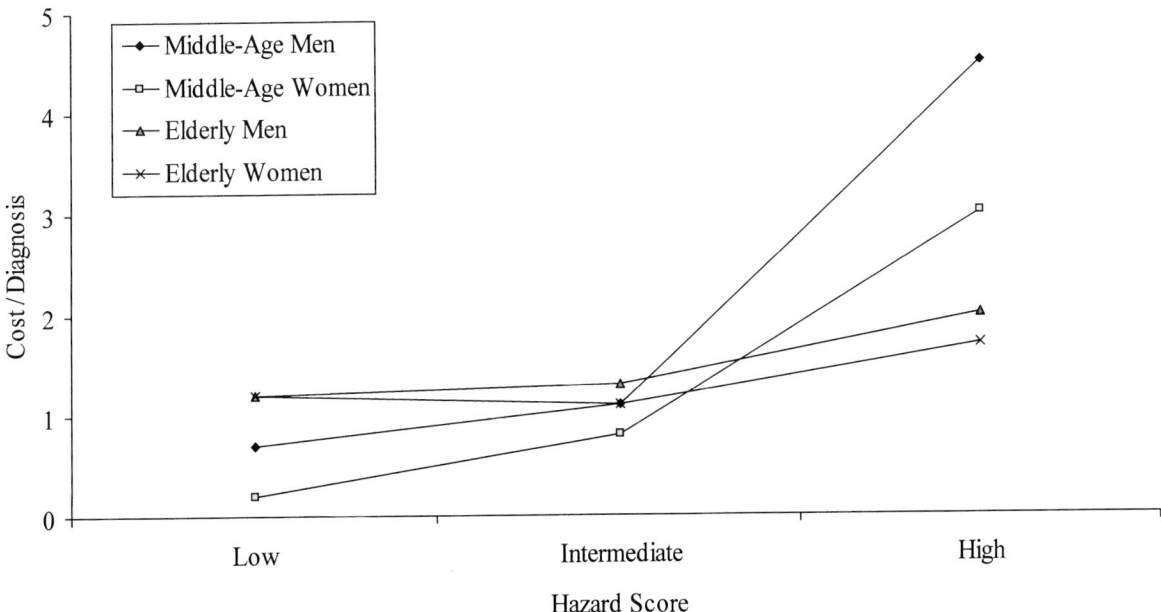

FIG. 11. Two-year costs of care by hazard risk for stress Tl-201 imaging. Middle age, age 65 or younger; Elderly, more than 65 years of age.

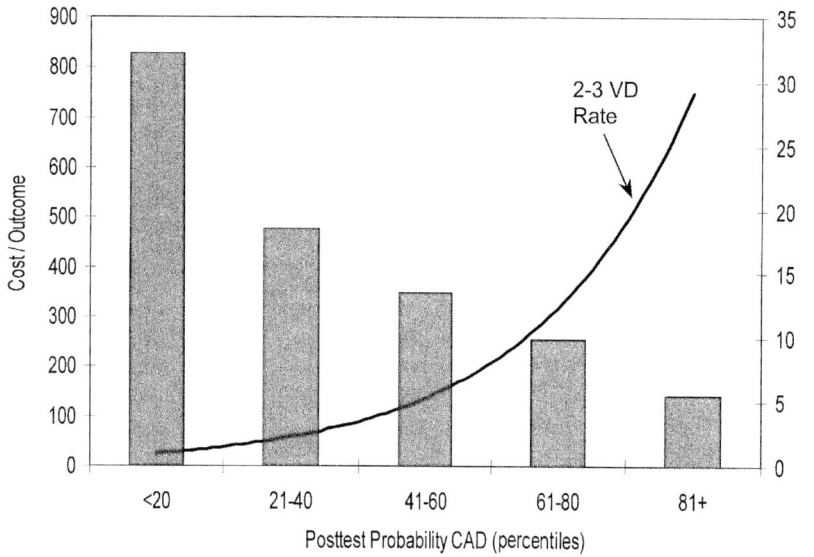

FIG. 12. Diagnostic cost to identify severe coronary artery disease. The point of reference is population costs and disease rates, approximately 25% of the catheterization rate. *CAD*, coronary artery disease; *VD*, vessel disease.

The ensuing patient care patterns become more efficient as a result of improved detection of physiologic abnormalities, that is, lower false-positive and false-negative test rates, resulting in nuclear-induced cost-efficiency of care.

The economic implications of an outcomes-based strategy were reported as early as 1994 when Christian and colleagues (29) demonstrated that myocardial perfusion scintigraphy was cost-inefficient for identifying patients with three-vessel or left main CAD in a population with a normal resting electrocardiogram. They illustrated the concept that testing is more cost-efficient for patient subsets for which the test is diagnostically more accurate. This relates to the cost per disease classification rate or the number of disease prevalence cases identified. From the Economic of Noninvasive Diagnosis study ($n = 8,411$), examples of the cost to identify severe coronary disease and cardiac death or myocardial infarction are depicted in Figures 12 and 13. More recently, in an analysis of 5,083 patients, the cost of identifying patients at risk of cardiac death or myocardial infarction was

$5,179 per event, $3,652 if testing was limited to patients at intermediate-to-high likelihood of coronary disease (26). This recent analysis from the Cedars-Sinai group also evaluates the incremental cost savings of two posttest catheterization strategies: (i) catheterization in all patients with any nuclear abnormality as compared with (ii) catheterization for patients with a high risk (i.e., summed stress score >8) (Fig. 4). The definition of a high-risk nuclear scan was based on the extent and severity of perfusion abnormalities and related to identification of a cohort of patients at highest risk of 2-year cardiac death or myocardial infarction. Patients with a high-risk scan (i.e., summed stress score greater than 8) have a higher prevalence of multivessel coronary disease or disease amenable to revascularization and would benefit, in terms of improved survival, from referral to angiography. The ensuing cost savings from such an approach ranged from 22 to 55% for high-to-low pretest risk patients with an overall reduction in coronary angiography of 17% (26).

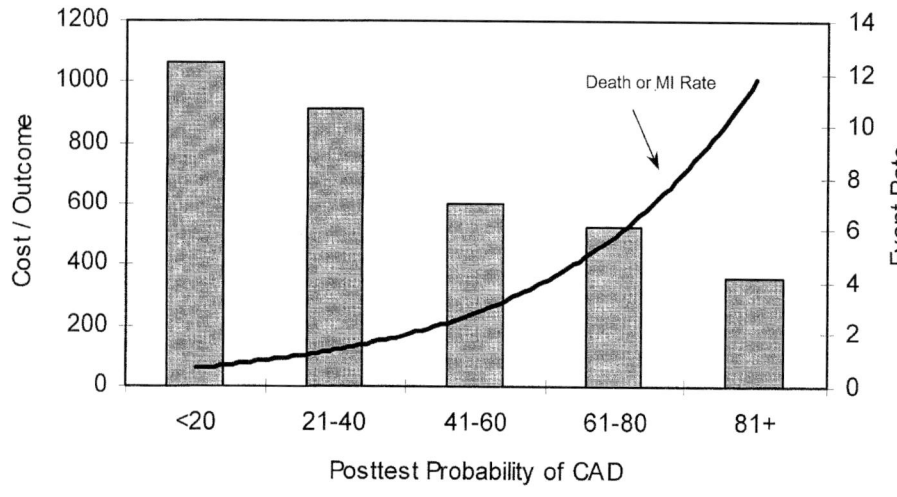

FIG. 13. Cost to identify death or myocardial infarction. The point of reference is population costs and event rates. *CAD*, coronary artery disease; *MI*, myocardial infarct.

TABLE 7. *Net cost savings of early rest Tc-99m tetrofosmin for acute chest pain evaluation*

Admission criteria: abnormal perfusion scan	Amount: % or $
Percent acute MI detected	90%
Percent reduction in hospital admissions	57%
Mean cost savings in dollars	$4,258

Selectivity of resource use has also been explored in the emergency department evaluation of acute chest pain imaging, in preoperative risk assessment, and in suspected or known coronary disease (Fig. 3) (26,28,33,34). The principle behind selective resource use may be explained by optimization of less expensive resources and limited referral of only those highest risk patients. In the emergency department, low-risk patients (i.e., no perfusion defects) are shifted to the lower cost, outpatient setting. In the evaluation of suspected coronary disease, only patients who have a positive exercise electrocardiogram are referred to nuclear imaging, thus controlling costs for all patients and limiting the use of expensive coronary angiography to a fraction of evaluated patients. On average, 60 to 80% of all patients have a low-risk test with few resources used during 3-year posttesting (i.e, low-cost patients) (17). In the emergency department setting, as many as 90% of patients have a negative perfusion scan, thus limiting admission to a small percentage of patients (37,42). When only patients with an abnormal rest perfusion scan are admitted to the hospital, a total of $4,258 cost savings may be achieved (Table 7)(42).

There has been a dramatic increase in the use of invasive cardiac procedures. A number of reports from the RAND Corporation have documented as high as 50% inappropriate use as judged by a review panel of medical experts (3,4). The routine pathway of care for a patient with coronary disease often starts from a noninvasive test, proceeding to coronary angiography, and then an interventional procedure. Thus, the effective limitation of catheterization use can lead to substantial cost savings; the rate-limiting step is if the deferment of angiography may achieve equivalent outcomes.

A recent example of the potential cost savings that may be accrued with a nuclear imaging-driven diagnostic strategy was recently reported from the Economics of Noninvasive Diagnosis multicenter study group (19). To determine observational differences in diagnostic and long-term costs of care by the initial choice of a coronary disease diagnostic testing modality (i.e., invasive versus noninvasive), 11,372 prospectively consecutive stable angina patients with predefined pretest clinical risk profiles (61% male, age 60 ± 12 years) who were referred for stress myocardial perfusion tomography or cardiac catheterization were enrolled in a 3-year outcome study. The composite 3-year costs of care were compared for two patient management strategies: (i) direct cardiac catheterization (aggressive) and (ii) initial stress myocardial perfusion imaging and selective catheterization

of high-risk patients (conservative). Observational comparisons of aggressive as compared with conservative testing strategies revealed that the average composite cost of care was higher for direct cardiac catheterization in all clinical risk subsets (range, $2,878 to $4,579), as compared with stress myocardial perfusion imaging plus selective catheterization (range, $2,387 to $3,010) (Fig. 14) for clinically low-risk, intermediate-risk, and high-risk patients with stable chest pain (P < 0.0001). Significant cost savings for stable chest pain patients were related to a decreased need for additional testing for patients with a low-risk nuclear scan and a higher use of PTCA for patients proceeding directly to cardiac catheterization. Importantly, the two cohorts had similar rates of cardiac death or myocardial infarction (P > 0.20). These data reveal that patients who undergo a more aggressive diagnostic strategy have higher diagnostic costs and greater rates of intervention and follow-up costs for lower risk, stable chest pain patients without a resultant improvement in outcome. The lack of improvement in 3-year outcomes decries the aggressive management approach and supports the cost savings yielded by using noninvasive testing for patients with stable chest pain symptoms.

Cost-effective care may be defined as patient management resulting in greater (or equivalent) improvement in outcome while minimizing the overall costs of care. For tests that identify risk and allow for early treatment with improved survival, cost-effective care is possible. Early treatment is linked to an economic benefit as a result of efficient and effective health care strategies that decrease admissions and overuse of health care services as well as those that result in improved survival. Tests that are highly accurate have a lower rate of false-positive tests (i.e., decreased cost waste due to overuse of cardiac catheterization) and lower rate of false-negative tests (i.e., decreased cost waste due to a reduction in hospitalization for unstable angina or myocardial infarction). Economic principles state that cost-effectiveness ratios become more favorable with increasing risk in the population. For example, the cost-effectiveness of preoperative screening prior to vascular surgery was more advantageous for patients with an intermediate pretest probability of CAD who are symptomatic or have a prior coronary disease history (36). Ziffer and colleagues (38) recently reported the cost-effectiveness of nuclear imaging in the emergency department. Using a threshold analysis (i.e., a likelihood of cardiac complications >0.25), recent evidence suggests that the use of SPECT imaging in the emergency department results in cost per event saved of $18,530 and cost per life-year saved of $71,257 (37).

An analysis of the cost-effectiveness of stress myocardial perfusion imaging in the END study population is presented in Figure 15 for patients by their pretest risk of coronary disease. Since $50,000 per life-year saved is the threshold for economic efficiency, the use of stress myocardial perfusion imaging for stable chest pain patients is cost-effective for intermediate-risk patients. An exception to this is elderly

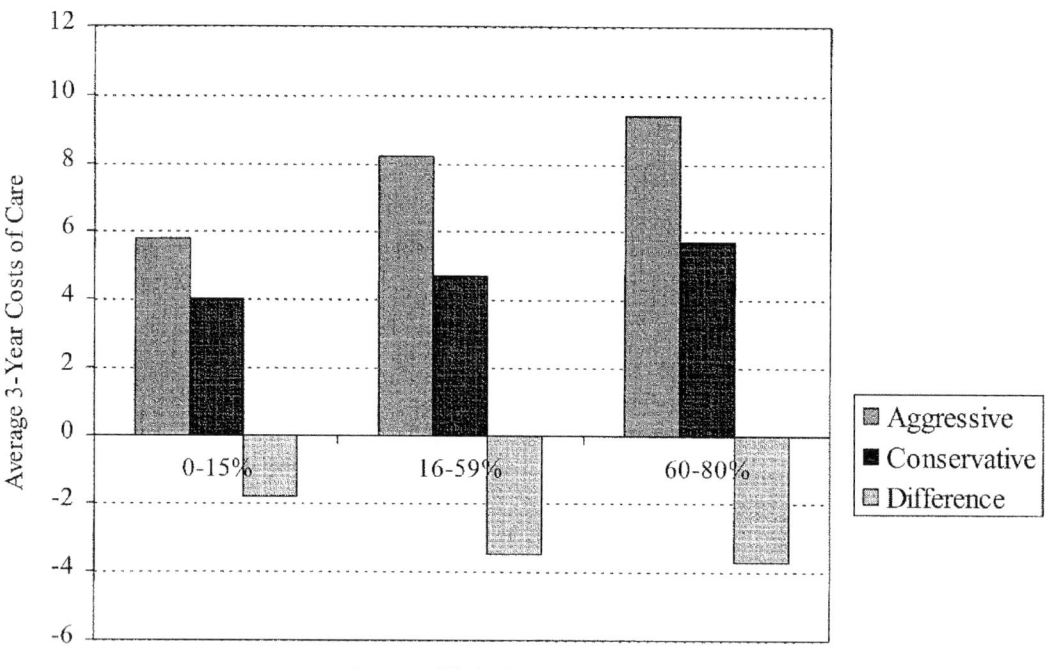

FIG. 14. Potential cost savings by requiring stress-induced nuclear ischemia prior to referral to cardiac catheterization in stable chest pain patients. *Aggressive management,* direct catheterization in patients with stable chest pain symptoms; *Conservative management,* a management strategy that includes initial stress myocardial perfusion imaging followed by selective catheterization in patients with documented stress-induced ischemia.

patients (i.e., age 65 years or older) where stress myocardial perfusion imaging in symptomatic patients was cost-effective for low-, intermediate-, and high-risk patients.

Electron-beam Computed Tomography

Theoretically, pathophysiologic measures detected within the coronary vasculature have distinct advantages in disease detection over conventional noninvasive imaging modalities. Electron-beam computed tomography (EBCT) provides

such measures in the determination of the amount of coronary artery calcium. Using an evidence-based approach to the evaluation of current published literature on EBCT, it appears that the evidence is preliminarily positive with published reports from small sample sizes (published reports on EBCT have a median sample size of 140) (78). The sensitivity and specificity for the detection of significant coronary disease is 76 to 91% and 45 to 59% in 3,581 patients (Table 8) (78).

Although EBCT is a relatively new technique, a prelimi-

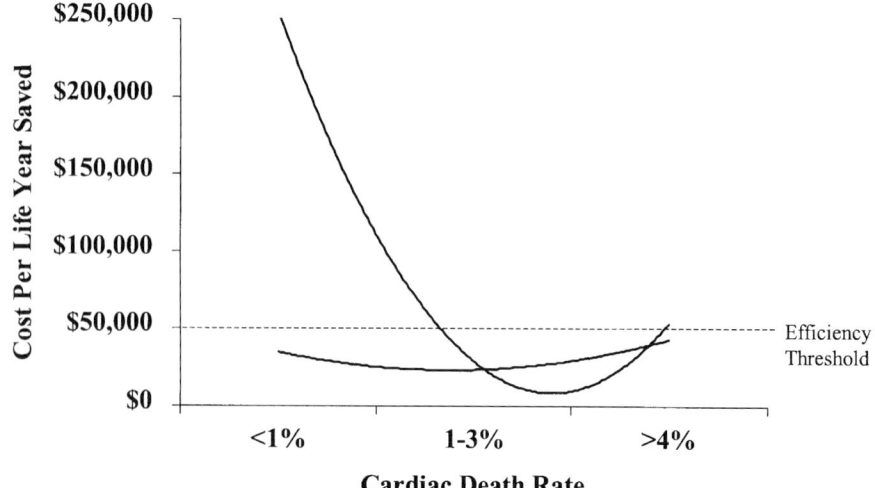

FIG. 15. Cost-effectiveness analysis in 8,411 stable chest pain patients undergoing stress nuclear imaging.

TABLE 8. *Review of published reports on the diagnostic accuracy of electron beam computed tomography*

Study	Year	Sensitivity (%)	Specificity (%)
Tanenbaum	1989	88.4	100.0
Agatston	1990	100.0	28.0
Breen	1992	100.0	47.2
Bielak	1994	82.5	85.0
Kaufmann	1995	92.8	66.7
Devries	1995	96.7	41.3
Kajimani	1995	77.0	86.0
Rumberger	1995	99.4	25.7
Braun	1996	92.5	72.7
Budoff	1996	94.6	43.8
Detrano	1996	70.0	71.0
Fallavollita	1996	87.5	58.6
Baumgart	1997	94.7	21.4
Schmermund	1997	99.1	58.3
Kennedy	1998	95.6	30.5
Schmermund	1998	67.9	66.7
Pooled Statistics		90.5	48.9
Median		93.7	58.5
Average		89.9	56.4
Weighted Average		76.2	45.2

nary cost analysis has been published using available data from the Mayo Clinic (79). Charges for EBCT are slightly higher than that of routine treadmill tests but less than for an echocardiogram or nuclear test; the average charge for EBCT is approximately $350 (limited CT of the chest). Using a 213-patient series, a calcium score of 168 had a 71% and 90% sensitivity and specificity, respectively (79). Using a cost simulation model, EBCT used to identify coronary disease achieved a cost that was least in intermediate-risk patients (79) (Fig. 16).

Magnetic Resonance Imaging

In recent years, clinical applications for cardiac magnetic resonance imaging (MRI) have increased dramatically. Technical advantages in MRI include enhanced spatial resolution, characterization of myocardial tissue, and highly accurate, three-dimensional imaging (80). Recent advancements in the field of cardiac MRI are numerous and include the assessment of ventricular function (tagging), myocardial perfusion (ultrafast imaging), and the evaluation of coronary anatomy (MR angiography) (80). Cardiac MRI allows for the accurate assessment of anatomy, left ventricular volume and mass, wall thickness, and cardiac metabolism (i.e., spectroscopy) and perfusion (contrast enhancement). Recent advances in software development for MRI perfusion analysis programs should allow for enhanced sensitivity and specificity for the detection of coronary disease (81). The possibility that any single type of test can provide information on multiple-risk parameters increases the attractiveness of MRI both as a tool for diagnosis and cost-efficiency (80).

Further developments in cardiac MRI include detection of coronary anatomy. The impact of a noninvasive test able to determine the extent of coronary disease (only previously defined with angiography) could have an enormous impact on the diagnostic costs of care (82). Improvements in accuracy would directly impact technical efficiency, with resultant improvements in diagnosis and patient management over other noninvasive tests and cost savings per patient diagnosis. Much lower rates of procedural complications are expected with MRI as compared to angiography; providing further cost savings to the health care system. Estimated diagnostic costs could be halved with the availability of cardiac MR angiography. Furthermore, the replacement of multiple tests within a diagnostic workup could result in substan-

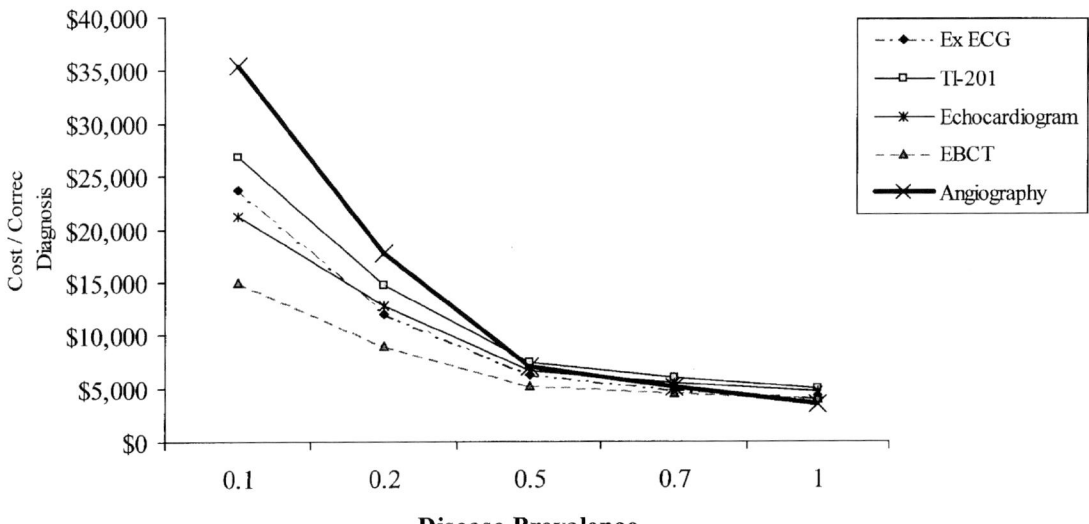

FIG. 16. Cost simulation model exploring costs to correctly diagnose coronary disease as a function of disease prevalence for EBCT as compared with other diagnostic test modalities. *Ex ECG*, exercise electrocardiography; *Tl-201*, exercise thallium-201 imaging; *EBCT*, electron beam computed tomography. (Adapted from ref. 79, with permission.)

tial cost savings. For example, the assessment of coronary stenosis combined with perfusion could aid substantially in reducing costs of care as well as providing enhanced information to guide patient management (83).

The rate-limiting step to cost-efficiency with cardiac MRI is the achievement of equivalent accuracy. Clinical studies of MR perfusion using visual and parametric analysis of signal intensity time curves have reported sensitivity and specificity values in the range of 60 to 90% when compared with coronary angiography and nuclear techniques (83). An 83% concordance with Tl-201 was recently reported by Ramani and colleagues (84) when assessing contrast MRI myocardial viability in 24 patients with stable coronary artery disease and left ventricular dysfunction.

In addition to diagnosis, the intensity of treatment is often based on the underlying risk of cardiac complications. The accuracy and reproducibility of MRI allows for its use when serially evaluating progressive or worsening disease or for medical therapy monitoring (85). The precise delineation of risk with MRI measures would allow for improved patient management. Although risk assessment data is limited due to the newness of cardiac MRI techniques, in a small series of 44 acute infarct patients, the presence and absence of microvascular obstruction (i.e., hypoenhancement) by contrast-enhanced MRI was associated with a 45 and 9% cardiac event rate over 16 months (86). Cardiac event rates also increased with infarct size (range, 30 to 71% for small to large infarcts).

Thus, the use of a highly accurate technique, such as MRI, could result in improved health care quality and economic value when compared to our current diagnostic workup of patients.

SUMMARY

A review of evidence warranting the use of a noninvasive test reveals that a substantial body of evidence is being developed on the economic implications of noninvasive test use. Economic implications define how improved accuracy and risk assessment affect the costs of resource utilization induced by a test. As outcome data is the key to defining expected resource use and rates of important adverse events, the body of evidence is more well developed in modalities that have been in existence for extended periods of time (e.g., nuclear imaging). However, new improvements in less expensive imaging modalities may provide potential cost savings in years to come. Despite the disparity in available outcome evidence, an increasing body of evidence suggests that substantial cost savings for most noninvasive tests is possible when cardiac imaging-driven diagnostic pathways are defined based on diagnostic and prognostic outcome data. In general, the savings are greatest in routine diagnostic evaluations and are achieved by limiting the use of expensive cardiac catheterization. For acute or in-hospital imaging, cost savings are also possible by shifting care to the outpatient setting. This may be accomplished, for example, by

early discharge of patients with normal imaging results. By appropriate referral of intermediate-risk patients with suspected coronary disease in the evaluation of suspected ischemia, including preoperative risk stratification, cost savings is also possible when compared to routine use of an imaging modality.

Cost-effectiveness is defined by a ratio of the incremental costs per life-year saved. For a noninvasive test, cost-effectiveness analyses define the marginal costs induced by a test in relation to the outcomes achieved by the test. An economic principle reveals that as test use becomes increasingly clinically effective, cost-effectiveness parallels this effectiveness. In this case, it is more clinically effective to use cardiac imaging modalities for intermediate pretest risk patients (as a result of a substantially greater incremental value when compared with lower and higher risk patients). The resulting care is also more cost-effective in use of cardiac imaging in intermediate-risk patients when compared with lower or higher pretest risk patients. Additional cost-effectiveness data are available for the use of cardiac imaging in the emergency department, preoperative risk stratification, as well as for testing in stable chest pain patients with suspected coronary disease.

As the data unfold on the economic advantages possible with cardiac imaging modalities, it is likely that comparative statements about the societal impact of test choices may be more clearly defined. Until then, we await additional data from well-controlled observational or randomized trials in order to define clearly the estimation of clinical and economic outcome with cardiac imaging techniques.

APPENDIX. MAJOR COST COMPONENTS OF AN ECONOMIC ANALYSIS

Type of resource	Data source
Hospital	Hospital billing systems (UB-92)
Physician	Resource base relative value scale
Outpatient	Patient self-reported office and clinic visits
	Patient self-reported prescription drug use
Patient indirect costs	Patient travel costs and lost work productivity

REFERENCES

1. Levit KR, Lazensby HC, Braden BR, et al. National health expenditures. *Health Affairs* 1996;17(1):35–51.
2. Burner ST, Waldo DR, McKusick DR. National health care expenditures. *Health Care Financing Review* 1996;14:1–30.
3. Kahn KL, Kosecoff J, Chassin MR, et al. Measuring the clinical appropriateness of the use of a procedure. Can we do it? *Med Care* 1988;26(4):415–422.
4. Chassin MR, Kosecoff J, Solomon DH, et al. How coronary angiography is used. Clinical determinants of appropriateness. *JAMA* 1987;258(18):2543–2547.
5. *Time* Internet site: *www.time.com/magazine/1998/dom/980713/cover1.html.* Accessed March 2000.

6. Luft HS. Medicare and managed care. *Ann Rev Pub Health* 1998;19: 459–475.

7. *Am J Managed Care* July 1998;4, Special Issue, Agency for Health Care Policy & Research Conference on Contracting for Specialty Services, SP11–SP100.

8. American Heart Association Internet site: *http:/www.amhrt.org/ stats/1997.*

9. Ginzberg E. *Health services research.* Cambridge, MA: Harvard University Press, 1991.

10. Fuchs VR. *The future of health policy.* Cambridge, MA: Harvard University Press, 1993.

11. Stevens R. *In sickness and in wealth.* New York: Basic Books, 1989.

12. Wennberg DE, Kellett MA, Dickens JD, et al. The association between local diagnostic testing intensity and invasive cardiac procedures. *JAMA* 1996;275:1161–1164.

13. Vibbert S, Reichard J. *The medical outcomes & guidelines sourcebook.* Washington, DC: Faulkner & Gray, 1992.

14. Shaw LJ, Peterson ED, Kesler K, et al. Use of a prognostic treadmill score in identifying diagnostic coronary disease subgroups and altering patient management. *Circulation* 1998;98(16):1622–1630.

15. Alexander KP, Shaw LJ, Shaw LK, et al. Diagnostic and prognostic value of the Duke treadmill score in women. *J Am Coll Cardiol* 1998; 32(6):1657–1664.

16. Chaitman BR. The changing role of the exercise electrocardiogram as a diagnostic and prognostic test for chronic ischemic heart disease. *J Am Coll Cardiol* 1986;8(5):1195–1210.

17. Chaitman BR, McMahon RP, Terrin M, et al. for the TIMI II Investigators. Impact of treatment strategy on predischarge exercise test in the thrombolysis in myocardial infarction (TIMI) II trial. *Am J Cardiol* 1993;71(2):131–138.

18. Brown KA. Prognostic value of myocardial perfusion imaging: state of the art and new developments. *J Nucl Cardiol* 1996;3(6)[Pt 1]: 516–537.

19. Shaw LJ, Hachamovitch R, Peterson ED, et al. Using an outcomes-based approach to identify candidates for risk stratification after exercise treadmill testing. *J Gen Int Med* 1999;14:1–9.

20. Shaw LJ, Hachamovitch R, Berman DS, et al. for the Economics of Noninvasive Diagnosis (END) Multicenter Study Group. The economic consequences of available diagnostic and prognostic strategies for the evaluation of stable angina patients: an observational assessment of the value of pre-catheterization ischemia. *J Am Coll Cardiol* 1999;33: 661–669.

21. Finkler SA. *Cost accounting for health care organizations: concepts and applications.* Gaithersburg, MD: Aspen Publishers, 1994.

22. Laupacis A, Feeny D, Detsky AS, et al. How attractive does a new technology have to be to warrant adoption and utilization? Tentative guidelines for using clinical and economic evaluations. *Can Med Assoc J* 1992;146:473–481.

23. Weinstein MC, Stason WB. Cost-effectiveness of coronary artery bypass surgery. *Circulation* 1982;66(5)[Pt 2]:III56–66.

24. Mark D. Medical economics and health policy issues for interventional cardiology. *Textbook of interventional cardiology,* 2nd ed. Philadelphia, PA: WB Saunders Co, 1993.

25. Weintraub WS, Mauldin PD, Becker ER, et al. A comparison of the costs and quality of life after coronary angioplasty or coronary surgery for multivessel coronary artery disease: results from the Emory Angioplasty versus Surgery Trial (EAST). *Circulation* 1995;92:2831–2840.

26. Berman DS, Hachamovitch R, Kiat H, et al. Incremental value of prognostic testing in patients with known or suspected ischemic heart disease: a basis for optimal utilization of exercise technetium-99m sestamibi myocardial perfusion single-photon emission computed tomography. *J Am Coll Cardiol* 1995;26:639–647.

27. Hachamovitch R, Berman DS, Shaw LJ, et al. Incremental prognostic value of myocardial perfusion single photon emission computed tomography for the prediction of cardiac death: differential stratification for risk of cardiac death and myocardial infarction. *Circulation* 1998;97: 535–543.

28. Marwick TH, Anderson T, Williams MJ, et al. Exercise echocardiography is an accurate and cost-efficient technique for detection of coronary artery disease in women. *J Am Coll Cardiol* 1995;26:335–341.

29. Christian TF, Miller TD, Bailey KR, et al. Exercise tomographic thal-

lium-201 imaging in patients with severe coronary artery disease and normal electrocardiograms. *Ann Int Med* 1994;121(11):825–832.

30. Shaw LJ, Miller DD, Romeis JC, et al. Prognostic value of noninvasive risk stratification and coronary revascularization in nonelderly and elderly patients referred for evaluation of clinically suspected coronary artery disease. *J Am Geriatr Soc* 1996;44:1190–1197.

31. Berman D, Hachamovitch R, Lewin H, et al. Risk stratification in coronary artery disease: implications for stabilization and prevention. *Am J Cardiol* 1997;79(12B):10–16.

32. Goldman L, Garber AM, Grover SA, et al. Task Force 6. Cost-effectiveness of assessment and management of risk factors. *J Am Coll Cardiol* 1996;27:1020–1030.

33. Shaw LJ, Eisenstein EL, Hachamovitch R, et al. for the Economics of Noninvasive Diagnosis Multicenter. A primer of biostatistic and economic methods for diagnostic and prognostic modeling in nuclear cardiology: part II. *J Nucl Cardiol* 1997;4:52–60.

34. Shaw LJ, Hachamovitch R, Marwick TH, et al. Cost-effectiveness analysis of stress myocardial perfusion imaging in stable angina patients: influence of age and pretest risk of coronary disease. *J Am Coll Cardiol* 1997;29:137A.

35. Shaw LJ, Hachamovitch R, Marwick TH, et al. Does the use of noninvasive testing reduce short- and long-term costs of care? *Circulation* 1996;94:I-168(abst).

36. Shaw LJ, Dittrich HC, West H, et al. Cost-effectiveness of myocardial contrast echocardiography as compared to nuclear perfusion imaging in the diagnosis of coronary disease. *J Am Soc Echo* 1998;11(5):512.

37. Shaw LJ, Hachamovitch R, Eisenstein E, et al. Cost implications of implementing a selective preoperative risk screening approach for peripheral vascular surgery patients. *Am J Managed Care* 1997;3: 1817–1827.

38. Ziffer J, Nateman DR, Janowitz WR, et al. Improved patient outcomes and cost-effectiveness of utilizing nuclear cardiology protocols in an emergency department chest pain center: two-year results in 6,548 patients. *J Nucl Med* 1998;39(5):139P.

39. Tatum JL, Jesse RL, Kontos MC, et al. Comprehensive strategy for the evaluation and triage of the chest pain patient. *Ann Emerg Med* 1996;29:116–125.

40. Hamm CW, Goldman BU, Heeschen C, et al. Emergency room triage of patients with acute chest pain by means of rapid testing for cardiac troponin T or troponin I. *New Engl J Med* 1997;337:1648–1653.

41. Laudon DA, Vukov LF, Breen JF, et al. Use of electron beam computed tomography in the evaluation of chest pain patients in the emergency department. *Ann Emerg Med* 1999;33:15–21.

42. Fleischman KE, Goldman L, Robiolio PA, et al. Echocardiographic correlates of survival in patients with chest pain. *J Am Coll Cardiol* 1994;23:1390–1396.

43. Radensky PW, Hilton TC, Fulmer H, et al. Potential cost-effectiveness of initial myocardial perfusion imaging for assessment of emergency department patients with chest pain. *Am J Cardiol* 1997;79:595–599.

44. Heller GV, Stowers SA, Hendel RC, et al. Clinical value of acute rest technetium-99m tetrofosmin tomographic myocardial perfusion imaging in patients with acute chest pain and nondiagnostic electrocardiograms. *J Am Coll Cardiol* 1998;31:1011–1017.

45. Ryan TJ, Bauman WB, Kennedy JW, et al. Guidelines for percutaneous transluminal coronary angioplasty. A report of the American Heart Association/American College of Cardiology Task Force on Assessment of Diagnostic and Therapeutic Cardiovascular Procedures (Committee on Percutaneous Transluminal Coronary Angioplasty). *Circulation* 1993;88(6):2987–3007.

46. Froelicher VF, Perdue S, Pewen W, et al. Application of meta-analysis using an electronic spreadsheet to exercise testing in patients with myocardial infarction. *Am J Med* 1987;83:1045–1054.

47. Shaw LJ, Peterson ED, Kesler K, et al. A meta-analysis of predischarge risk stratification after acute myocardial infarction with stress electrocardiographic, myocardial perfusion, and ventricular function imaging. *Am J Cardiol* 1996;78:1327–1337.

48. Froelicher VF, Lehmann KG, Thomas R, et al. The electrocardiographic exercise test in a population with reduced workup bias. *Ann Intern Med* 1998;128:965–974.

49. Wann LS, Faris JV, Childress RH, et al. Exercise cross-sectional echocardiography in ischemic heart disease. *Circulation* 1979;60: 1300–1308.

50. Kelsey AM, Shaw LJ, Ryan T. Fifteen years of exercise echocardiography: a meta-analysis. *Circulation* 1997;96(8):I-276(abst).

51. Heupler S, Mehta R, Lobo A, et al. Prognostic implications of exercise echocardiography in women. *J Am Coll Cardiol* 1997;30:414–420.

52. Picano E, Severi S, Michelassi C, et al. Prognostic importance of dipyridamole-echocardiography test in coronary artery disease. *Circulation* 1989;80:450–457.

53. Severi S, Picano E, Michelassi C, et al. Diagnostic and prognostic value of dipyridamole echocardiography in patients with suspected coronary artery disease. *Circulation* 1994;89:1160–1173.

54. Poldemans D, Fioretti PM, Boersma E, et al. Long-term prognostic value of dobutamine-atropine stress echocardiography in 1737 patients with known or suspected coronary artery disease. *Circulation* 1999; 99:757–762.

55. Chuah S, Pellikka PA, Roger VL, et al. Role of dobutamine stress echocardiography in predicting outcome in 860 patients with known or suspected coronary artery disease. *Circulation* 1998;97:1474–1480.

56. McCully RB, Roger VL, Mahoney DW, et al. Outcome after normal exercise echocardiography and predictors of subsequent cardiac events. *J Am Coll Cardiol* 1998;31:144–149.

57. Fleischman KE, Hunnink MGM, Kuntz KM, et al. Exercise echocardiography or exercise SPECT imaging? *JAMA* 1998;280:913–920.

58. Rubin DN, Ballal RS, Marwick TH. Outcomes and cost implications of a clinical-based algorithm to guide the discriminate use of stress imaging before noncardiac surgery. *Am Heart J* 1997;134:83–92.

59. Redberg RF. Diagnostic testing for coronary artery disease in women and gender differences in referral for revascularization. *Cardiol Clin* 1998;16:67–77.

60. Kaul S. Myocardial contrast echocardiography: 15 years of research and development. *Circulation* 1997;96:3745–3760.

61. Feinstein SB, Becher H, Macioch JE, et al. Rush-Presbyterian-St. Luke's clinical use of contrast echocardiography. *Amer J Cardiol: A Continuing Education Atlas* 1998:1–48.

62. Kaul S. Myocardial contrast echocardiography. *Curr Prob Cardiol* 1997;22:549–635.

63. Cohen JL, Cheirif J, Segar DS, et al. Improved left ventricular endocardial border delineation and opacification with Optison (FS069), a new echocardiographic contrast agent. *J Am Coll Cardiol* 1998;32:746–752.

64. Marwick TH, Brunken R, Meland N, et al. Accuracy and feasibility of contrast echocardiography for detection of perfusion defects in routine practice. *J Am Coll Cardiol* 1998;32:1260–1269.

65. Meza M, Ramee S, Collins T, et al. Knowledge of perfusion and contractile reserve improves the predictive value of recovery of regional myocardial function postrevascularization. *Circulation* 1997;96: 3459–3465.

66. Vernon S, Kaul S, Powers ER, et al. Myocardial viability in patients with chronic coronary artery disease and previous myocardial infarction. *Am Heart J* 1997;134:835–840.

67. Agati L, Voci P, Autore C, et al. Combined use of dobutamine echocardiography and myocardial contrast echocardiography in predicting functional recovery after coronary revascularization in patients with recent myocardial infarction. *Eur Heart J* 1997;18:771–779.

68. Spencer KT, Bednarz J, Rafter PG, et al. Use of harmonic imaging without echocardiographic contrast to improve two-dimensional image quality. *Am J Cardiol* 1998;82:794–799.

69. Shaw LJ, Gillam L, Feinstein S, et al. for the Optison Multicenter Study Group. Technology assessment in the managed care era: use of an intravenous contrast agent (FS069-Optison) to enhance cardiac diagnostic testing. *Am J Managed Care* 1998;4:SP169–SP176.

70. Crouse LJ, Cheirif J, Hanly DE, et al. Opacification and border delineation improvement in patients with suboptimal endocardial border delineation in routine echocardiography. *J Am Coll Cardiol* 1993;22: 1494–1500.

71. Iskandrian AS, Hakki AH, Kane-Marsh S. Prognostic implications of exercise thallium-201 scintigraphy in patients with suspected or known coronary artery disease. *Am Heart J* 1985;110:135–143.

72. Ladenheim ML, Kotler TS, Pollock BH, et al. Incremental prognostic power of clinical history, exercise electrocardiography and myocardial perfusion scintigraphy in suspected coronary artery disease. *Am J Cardiol* 1987;59(4):270–277.

73. Lee KL, Pryor DB, Pieper KS, et al. Prognostic value of radionuclide angiography in medically treated patients with coronary artery disease. A comparison with clinical and catheterization variables. *Circulation* 1990;82(5):1705–1717.

74. Jones RH, Johnson SH, Bigelow C, et al. Exercise radionuclide angiocardiography predicts cardiac death in patients with coronary artery disease. *Circulation* 1991;84(3)[Suppl]:I52–I58.

75. Berman DS, Hachamovitch R, Shaw LJ, et al. Prognostic risk stratification with SPECT imaging: results from a 20,340 patient multicenter registry. *J Am Coll Cardiol* 1998;31:410A.

76. Peterson ED, Shaw LJ, Califf RM for the American College of Physicians (ACP). Clinical guidelines for risk stratification after myocardial infarction. *Ann Intern Med* 1997;126:556–560.

77. Shaw LJ, Heinle SK, Borges-Neto S, et al. for the Duke Noninvasive Research Working Group. Prognosis in patients with coronary artery disease by equilibrium radionuclide measurements of left ventricular function during exercise. *J Nucl Med* 1998;39:140–146.

78. O'Rourke RA, Rumberger J, Brundage B, et al. Evaluation of electron beam computed tomography. *J Am Coll Cardiol* 2000 (in press).

79. Rumberger JA, Behrenbeck T, Breen JF, et al. Coronary calcification by electron beam computed tomography and obstructive coronary artery disease: a model for costs and effectiveness of diagnosis as compared with conventional cardiac testing methods. *J Am Coll Cardiol* 1999; 33:453–462.

80. van der Wall EE, van Rugge FP, Vliegen HW, et al. Ischemic heart disease: value of MR techniques. *Int J Cardiac Imaging* 1997;13: 179–189.

81. Kortright ME, Doyle M, Walsh EG, et al. Computer environment for qualitatitive/quantitative myocardial perfusion analysis in the women's ischemia syndrome evaluation study. *J Am Coll Cardiol* 1999;33:9A.

82. Post JC, van Rossum AC, Hofman MBM, et al. Three dimensional respiratory gated MR angiography of coronary arteries. *Am J Roentgenol* 1996;166:1399–1404.

83. Crnac J, Schmidt MC, Theissen P, et al. Assessment of myocardial perfusion by magnetic resonance imaging. *Herz* 1997;22:16–28.

84. Ramani K, Judd RM, Holly TA, et al. Contrast magnetic resonance imaging in the assessment of myocardial viability in patients with stable coronary artery disease and left ventricular dysfunction. *Circulation* 1998;98:2687–2694.

85. Johnson DB, Foster RE, Barilla F, et al. Angiotensin converting enzyme inhibitor therapy affects left ventricular mass in patients with ejection fraction >40% after acute myocardial infarction. *J Am Coll Cardiol* 1997;29:49–54.

86. Wu K, Elias Z, Judd RM, et al. Prognostic significance of microvascular obstruction by magnetic resonance imaging in patients with acute myocardial infarction. *Circulation* 1998;97:765–772.

SECTION II

Clinical Applications

CHAPTER 36

Chronic Stable Angina

Robert A. O'Rourke

Ischemic heart disease remains a major public health problem. Chronic stable angina is the first indication of ischemic heart disease in about 50% of patients (1,2). The reported annual incidence of angina is 213 per 100,000 population over the age of 30 (3).The incidence of angina can also be calculated by extrapolating from the number of myocardial infarctions (MIs) in the United States (4). Accordingly, the number of patients with stable angina can be calculated as 30 × 550,000 or 16.5 million (2). This approximation does not include patients who fail to seek medical attention for their chest pain or who are shown to have a noncardiac cause of chest discomfort (2).

Despite a recent reduction in cardiovascular deaths, ischemic heart disease is still the leading cause of mortality in the United States and causes one of every 4.8 deaths (5). Many patients are hospitalized for the assessment and treatment of stable chest pain syndromes, and many patients with chronic stable angina are unable to perform normal activities for varying periods of hours or days, and thus have a diminished quality of life. The economic costs of chronic coronary heart disease are enormous with direct costs of hospitalization greater than $15 billion a year (2).

The main objective of this chapter is to discuss the usefulness of noninvasive tests for the cost-effective diagnosis and risk stratification of patients with suspected or definite coronary heart disease, emphasizing the role of various imaging modalities for both diagnosis and risk stratification, the difference between the two often being arbitrary. The perioperative risk assessment of patients for noncardiac surgery is also discussed.

It must be emphasized that *not every patient needs every test* and that a markedly positive, low-level electrocardiogram (ECG) exercise test precludes the need for additional, more costly imaging studies prior to coronary angiography and, likely, myocardial revascularization. The use of addi-

tional noninvasive imaging tests in this situation is usually financially driven.

DIAGNOSIS

Definition of Angina

Angina is a clinical syndrome that consists of discomfort or pain in the chest, jaw, shoulder, back, or arm. It is typically precipitated or aggravated by exertion or emotional stress and relieved by nitroglycerin. Angina usually occurs in patients with coronary artery disease (CAD), affecting one or more large epicardial arteries. However, angina often is present in individuals with valvular heart disease, hypertrophic cardiomyopathy, and uncontrolled hypertension (2). It also occurs in patients with normal coronaries and myocardial ischemia due to coronary artery spasm or endothelial dysfunction. The symptom of angina is often observed in patients with noncardiac disorders affecting the esophagus, chest wall, or lungs.

Steps in Diagnosis Prior to Noninvasive Testing

History and Physical Examination

The first step is to obtain a detailed description of the symptom complex that is used by the clinician to characterize the chest pain or chest discomfort. Five descriptors are usually considered: (i) location, (ii) quality, (iii) duration of the discomfort, and the factors that (iv) induce and (v) relieve the pain.

After the description of the chest discomfort is obtained, the physician makes an integrated assessment of the symptom complex. The most commonly used classification scheme for chest pain divides patients into three groups: typical angina, atypical angina, or noncardiac chest pain (Table 1) (6).

Following a comprehensive interview concerning the chest pain, the presence of risk factors for coronary artery disease (CAD) should be determined. Smoking, hyperlipid-

R. A. O'Rourke: Department of Medicine, Division of Cardiology, University of Texas Health Science Center at San Antonio, San Antonio, Texas 78284.

504 SECTION II / CLINICAL APPLICATIONS

TABLE 1. *Clinical classification of chest pain*

Typical angina (definite)
  1. Substernal chest discomfort with a characteristic
    quality and duration that is:
      a. provoked by exertion or emotional stress, and
      b. relieved by rest or nitroglycerin
Atypical angina (probable)
  Meets two of the three characteristics above
Noncardiac chest pain
  Meets one or none of the typical anginal characteristics

(From ref. 6, with permission.)

emia, diabetes, hypertension, and a family history of premature CAD increase the likelihood of CAD. A past history of cerebrovascular or peripheral vascular disease also increases the probability of CAD.

The physical examination is often normal in patients with stable angina. However, an examination performed during an episode of pain can be beneficial. A third or fourth heart sound, a mitral regurgitant murmur, a paradoxically split S_2, bibasilar pulmonary rales, or palpable cardiac impulses that disappear when the pain subsides are all predictive of CAD. Evidence of noncoronary atherosclerotic disease—a carotid bruit, diminished pedal pulse, or abdominal aneurysm—increases the likelihood of CAD. An elevated blood pressure, xanthomas, and retinal exudates indicate the presence of CAD risk factors (2).

Clinical Assessment of the Likelihood of Coronary Artery Disease

The clinicopathologic study performed by Diamond and Forrester (7) demonstrated that it is possible to predict the probability of CAD after the history and the physical examination. By combining data from a series of angiography studies performed in the 1960s and the 1970s, they showed that simple clinical observations of pain type, age, and sex were powerful predictors of the probability of CAD.

The utility of the Diamond and Forrester approach was confirmed subsequently in prospective studies at Duke and Stanford (8–10). In both men and women referred to cardiology specialty clinics for cardiac catheterization or for cardiac stress testing, the initial clinical characteristics most helpful in predicting CAD were determined. In these studies, age, sex, and pain type were the most powerful predictors (7,11) (Tables 2 and 3). Smoking, Q-waves, or ST-T changes on

ECG, hyperlipidemia, and diabetes strengthened the predictive abilities of these models.

Electrocardiogram and Chest Roentgenogram

A resting 12-lead electrocardiogram (ECG) should be recorded in all patients with symptoms suggestive of angina; however, it will be normal in up to 50% of patients with chronic stable angina (2). ECG evidence of left ventricular hypertrophy (LVH) or ST-T wave changes consistent with myocardial ischemia favor the diagnosis of angina pectoris. Evidence of prior Q-wave MI on the ECG makes CAD very likely.

The presence of arrhythmias (e.g., as atrial fibrillation or ventricular tachyarrhythmias) on the ECG in patients with chest pain also increase the probability of underlying CAD (2); however, these arrhythmias are frequently caused by other types of cardiac disease. Various degrees of atrioventricular (AV) block occur in patients with chronic CAD, but have a very low specificity for the diagnosis. Left anterior fascicular block, right bundle-branch block, and left bundle-branch block often are present in patients with CAD and frequently indicate multivessel CAD. However, these findings also lack specificity for the diagnosis of chronic stable angina.

An ECG obtained during chest pain is abnormal in about 50% of patients with angina and a normal resting ECG. Sinus tachycardia occurs commonly; bradyarrhythmias are less common. ST-segment elevation or depression establishes a high likelihood of angina and indicates ischemia at a low work load, portending an unfavorable prognosis. Many high-risk patients with severe episodes of angina need *no* further noninvasive testing. Coronary arteriography usually defines the severity of coronary artery stenoses and defines the necessity and feasibility of myocardial revascularization. In patients with ST-T wave depression or inversion on the resting ECG, "pseudonormalization" of these abnormalities during pain is another indicator that CAD is likely (2). The occurrence of tachyarrhythmias, A-V block, left anterior fascicular block, or bundle-branch block during chest pain also increases the probability of coronary heart disease and often leads to coronary arteriography.

The chest roentgenogram is often normal in patients with

TABLE 2. *Pretest likelihood of CAD in symptomatic patients according to age and sex* (combined Diamond/Forrester and CASS data)*[a]

Age in years	Nonanginal chest pain		Atypical angina		Typical angina	
	Men	Women	Men	Women	Men	Women
30–39	4	2	34	12	76	26
40–49	13	3	51	22	87	55
50–59	20	7	65	31	93	73
60–69	27	14	72	51	94	86

[a] Each value represents the percent with significant CAD on catheterization.
CAD, coronary artery diseases; *CASS*, Coronary Artery Surgical Study.
(From refs. 7 and 11, with permission.)

TABLE 3. *Comparing pretest likelihoods of CAD in low-risk symptomatic patients with high-risk symptomatic patients—Duke database[a]*

| Age in years | Nonanginal chest pain | | | | Atypical angina | | | | Typical angina | | | |
| | Men | | Women | | Men | | Women | | Men | | Women | |
	Low	High	Low	High	Low	High	Low	High	Low	High	Low	High
35–44	3	35	1	19	8	59	2	39	30	88	10	78
45–54	9	47	2	22	21	70	5	43	51	92	20	79
55–64	23	59	4	25	45	79	10	47	80	95	38	82
65	49	69	9	29	71	86	20	51	93	97	56	84

[a] Each value represents the percent with significant CAD. The first is the percentage for a low-risk, middle-age patient without diabetes, smoking, or hyperlipidemia. The second is that of the same age patient with diabetes, smoking, and hyperlipidemia. Both high- and low-risk patients have normal resting ECGs. If ST-T wave changes or Q waves had been present, the likelihood of CAD would be higher in each entry of the table.
(From ref. 10, with permission.)

stable angina pectoris. Its usefulness as a routine test is *not* well established. It is more likely to be abnormal in patients with previous or acute MI, those with a noncoronary artery cause of chest pain, and those with noncardiac chest discomfort.

Coronary artery calcification increases the likelihood of symptomatic CAD. *Fluoroscopically detectable* coronary calcification is correlated with major vessel occlusion in 94% of patients with chest pain (2); however, the sensitivity of the test is only 40%.

Electron beam computed tomography (EBCT) (see Chapter 28) is being used with increased frequency for the detection and quantification of coronary artery calcification (12). In studies of *selected* patients, the sensitivity of a positive EBCT detection of calcium for the presence of CAD varied from 85 to 100%; the specificity ranged from only 41 to 76%; the positive predictive value varied considerably from 55 to 84% and the negative predictive value from 84 to 100% (13). The role of EBCT has been controversial. A recent report of an ACC/AHA expert consensus writing group does *not* recommend EBCT for screening of asymptomatic patients for CAD or for its use in most patients with chest pain (14). Its use in the assessment of asymptomatic patients frequently results in a large number of unnecessary and expensive further testing.

Exercise Electrocardiogram Stress Testing

Exercise (ECG) testing is a well-established procedure that has been in widespread clinical use for many decades (15). Although usually a safe procedure, both MI and death occur at a rate of up to 1 per 2,500 tests. Absolute contraindications to exercise testing include acute MI within 2 days, cardiac arrhythmias causing symptoms or hemodynamic compromise, symptomatic and severe aortic stenosis, symptomatic heart failure, acute pulmonary embolus or infarction, acute myocarditis or pericarditis, and acute aortic dissection. Relative contraindications include: left main coronary artery stenosis, moderate aortic stenosis, electrolyte abnormalities, systolic hypertension greater than 200 mg Hg, diastolic

blood pressure greater than 100 mm Hg, tachyarrhythmias or bradyarrhythmias, hypertrophic cardiomyopathy, and other forms of outflow tract obstruction, mental or physical impairment leading to an inability to exercise adequately, and high-degree A-V block.

For optimizing the information obtained, the protocol should be tailored to the individual patient with exercise lasting *at least 6 minutes*. Exercise capacity should be reported in estimated METs of exercise, (one MET is the standard basal oxygen uptake of 3.5 mL/kg/min) and also in minutes.

The ECG, heart rate, and blood pressure should be carefully monitored and recorded during each stage of exercise, as well as during ST-segment abnormalities and chest pain. The patient should be monitored continuously for transient rhythm disturbances, ST-segment changes, and other ECG manifestations of myocardial ischemia. Although exercise testing often is stopped when subjects reach a standard percentage of predicted maximum heart rate, there is *great variability* in maximum heart rates among individuals, and predicted values may be suboptimal for some patients. *Absolute indications* for termination of the test include: a decline in systolic blood pressure of greater than 10 mm Hg from baseline despite an increase in work load when accompanied by other evidence of ischemia; moderate-to-severe angina; increasing ataxia, dizziness, or near syncope; signs of poor perfusion such as cyanosis or pallor; technical difficulties in monitoring the ECG or systolic blood pressure; subject's desire to stop; sustained ventricular tachycardia; or ST elevation greater than 1.0 mm in leads without diagnostic Q waves.

The interpretation of the exercise test should include symptomatic response, exercise capacity, hemodynamic response, and ECG changes. The occurrence of ischemic chest pain consistent with angina is important, particularly if it necessitates termination of the test. Abnormalities in exercise capacity and the systolic blood pressure or the heart rate response to exercise are important findings. The most important ECG findings are ST depression and ST elevation. The most commonly used definition for a positive exercise test is greater than or equal to one millimeter of horizontal or downsloping ST-segment depression or elevation for at least 60 to 80 milliseconds after the end of the QRS complex (Fig. 1**A** and **B**).

A metaanalysis of 147 published reports describing 24,074 patients who underwent both coronary angiography and exercise testing found wide variation in sensitivity and specificity (15). The mean sensitivity was 68%, and the mean specificity was 77%. When the analysis considered only studies that excluded patients with a prior MI, the mean sensitivity was 67%, and the mean specificity was 72%. When the analysis was restricted to the few studies that avoided workup bias by including only patients who agreed in advance to have both exercise testing and coronary angiography, the sensitivity was 50% and the specificity was 90% (16). *Therefore, the true diagnostic value of the exercise ECG relates to its relatively high specificity.* The modest sensitivity of the exercise ECG is generally lower than that of imaging procedures (17,18).

Diagnostic testing is most valuable when the pretest probability of obstructive CAD is intermediate. In these conditions, the test result has the largest effect on the posttest probability of disease and, thus, on clinical decisions. Intermediate probability has been arbitrarily defined as between 10 and 90% (19); this definition has been utilized in several studies (20,21) including ACC/AHA exercise test guidelines (15).

Special Issues in Electrocardiogram Exercise Testing

Digoxin produces abnormal exercise-induced ST-depression in 25 to 40% of apparently healthy normals (22). Whenever possible, it is recommended that *beta blockers* (and other antiischemic drugs) be withheld for 48 to 72 hours prior to exercise stress testing for the diagnosis of patients with suspected CAD. When beta blockers cannot be stopped, ECG exercise testing usually will still be positive in patients at high risk.

Exercise-induced ST-depression usually occurs with *left bundle branch block* and often has no association with ischemia (23). In *right bundle branch block*, ST-depression in the left chest leads (V_{5-6}) or inferior leads (II, AVF), has the same significance as it does when the resting ECG is normal.

LVH with repolarization abnormalities on the resting ECG is associated with more false-positive test results due to decreased specificity. Even in hypertensive patients with LV hypertrophy on echo but not on ECG, false-positive ST-segment changes often occur with exercise (24).

Resting ST-segment depression is a marker for adverse cardiac events in patients with and without known CAD (15). Additional exercise-induced ST-segment depression in the patient with 1 mm resting ST-segment depression is a reasonably sensitive indicator of CAD.

The difficulties of using exercise testing for diagnosing obstructive CAD in *women* have led to speculation that stress imaging may be preferred instead of standard stress testing. However, there are insufficient data to justify replacing standard exercise testing with stress imaging *routinely* when evaluating women for CAD. In many women with a low pretest likelihood of disease, a negative exercise test will be sufficient, and imaging procedures will not be required (15).

Resting Echocardiography

Echocardiography can be useful for establishing a diagnosis of CAD and in defining the consequences of CAD in certain patients with chronic chest pain presumed to be chronic stable angina. However, most patients undergoing a *diagnostic* evaluation for angina *do not need* a resting echocardiogram.

Chronic ischemic heart disease, whether or not associated with angina, can result in impaired systolic left ventricular function. The extent and severity of regional and global abnormalities are important considerations in choosing appropriate medical or surgical therapy.

Echocardiographic findings that may help establish the diagnosis of chronic ischemic heart disease include regional systolic wall motion abnormalities, such as hypokinesis, akinesis, dyskinesis, and failure of a wall segment to thicken normally during systole (18) (Fig. 2). Care must be taken to distinguish chronic CAD as a cause of ventricular septal wall motion abnormalities from other conditions such as left bundle-branch block, presence of an intraventricular pacemaker, right ventricular volume overload, or prior cardiac surgery.

Mitral regurgitation demonstrated by Doppler echocardiography may result from global left ventricular systolic dysfunction, regional papillary muscle dysfunction, scarring and shortening of the chordae tendineae, papillary muscle rupture, or other causes (18).

Stress Imaging

Patients who are good candidates for cardiac stress testing *with imaging* for the diagnosis of CAD as opposed to exercise ECG alone include those in the following categories: (i) complete left bundle-branch block, electronically paced ventricular rhythm, preexcitation syndromes, and other similar ECG conduction abnormalities; (ii) patients who have greater than 1 millimeter of resting ST-segment depression—including those with LVH or taking drugs such as digitalis; (iii) patients who are unable to exercise to a level high enough to give meaningful results on routine stress ECG (these patients should be considered for pharmacologic stress imaging test); and (iv) patients with angina who have undergone prior revascularization, in whom localization of ischemia, establishing the functional significance of lesions, and demonstrating myocardial viability are important considerations (see Chapter 39).

Several methods can be used to induce stress: (i) exercise

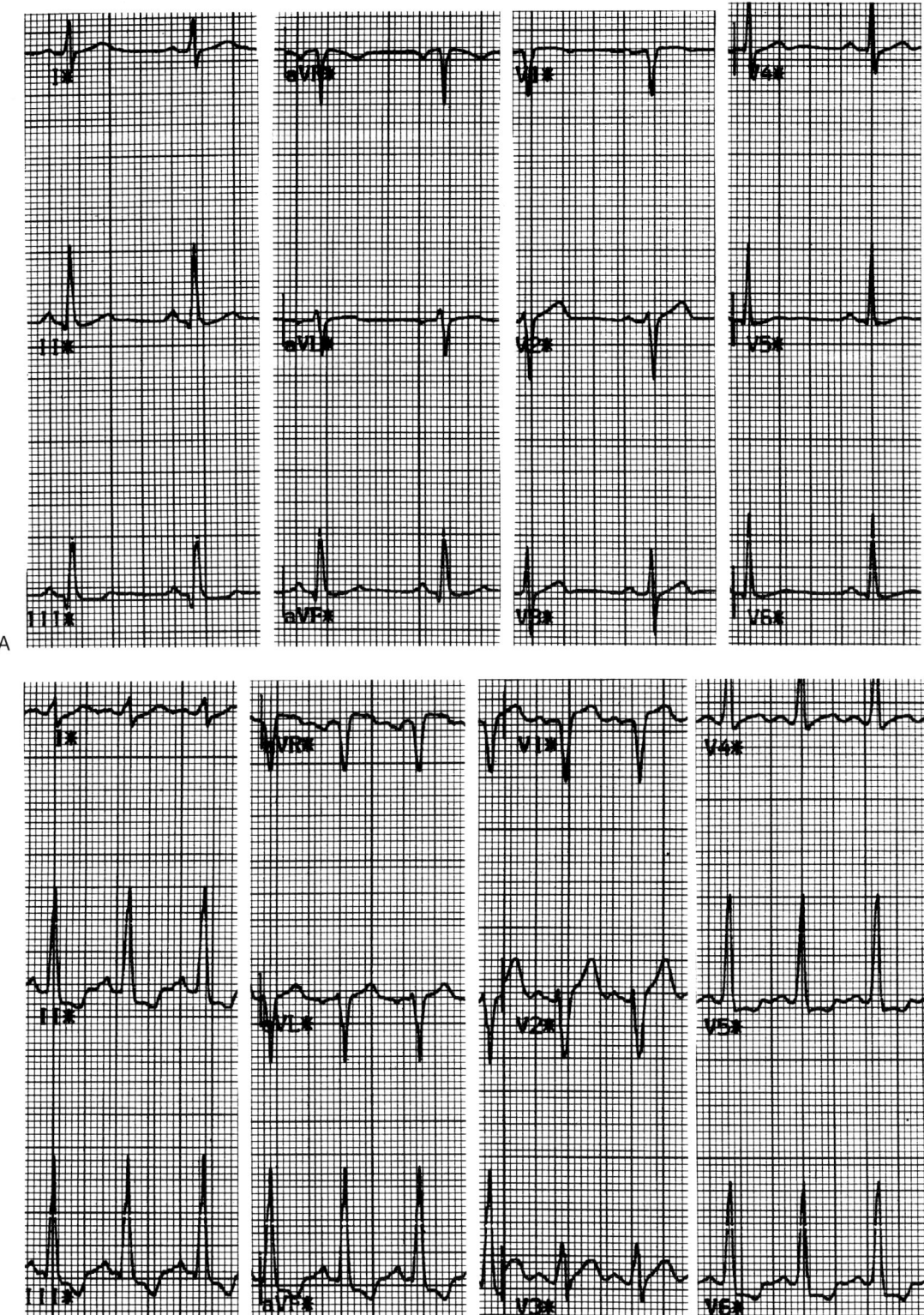

FIG. 1. A: Normal resting ECG at a heart rate of 75 beats/min in a 50-year-old man with exertional chest pain. **B:** Positive test with ≥2 mm ST-T wave downward sloping depression in leads II, III, AVF, V₅ and V₆ at a heart rate of 126 beats/min during stage 2 of a Bruce exercise test. Arteriography showed severe three-vessel coronary artery disease.

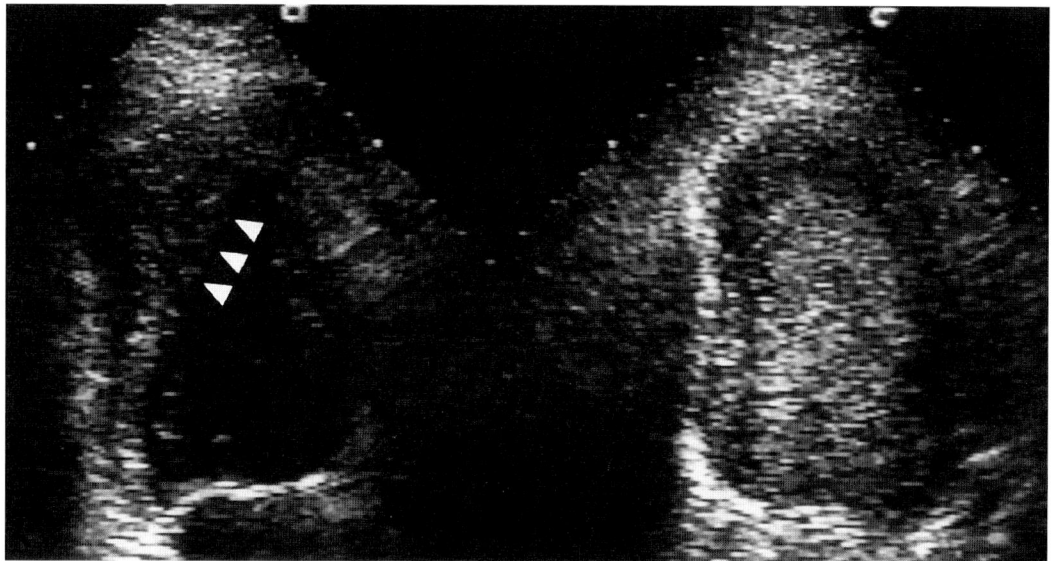

FIG. 2. Apical 2-chamber views from a 67-year-old man with apical segmental wall motion abnormalities. **Left panel** shows increased dense-echoes along the inferoapical region (*arrowheads*) suggestive of an apical thrombus. **Right panel** is a similar view after intravenous contrast injection of 0.5 mL of Optison. The apical region is completely filled with microbubbles, *excluding* the diagnosis of the previously suspected thrombus.

(treadmill or bicycle) and (ii) pharmacologic techniques (dobutamine or vasodilator drugs). When the patient can exercise to develop an appropriate level of cardiovascular stress for 6 to 12 minutes, exercise stress, (generally using a treadmill) is preferred to pharmacologic stress. However, when the patient cannot exercise to the appropriate level or in other specified circumstances (e.g., when stress echocardiography is being used in the assessment of myocardial viability), pharmacologic stress may be preferable. Three drugs are commonly used as substitutes for exercise stress testing: dipyridamole, adenosine, and dobutamine. Dipyridamole and adenosine are vasodilators that are commonly used in conjunction with myocardial perfusion scintigraphy, whereas dobutamine is a positive inotropic (and chronotropic) agent commonly used in conjunction with echocardiography (see Chapter 5).

Myocardial Perfusion Imaging

In patients with suspected or known chronic stable angina, the largest accumulated experience in myocardial perfusion imaging has been with the isotope thallium-201; however, the available evidence suggests that the newer isotopes technetium (Tc)-99m sestamibi and technetium-99m tetrofosmin provide similar diagnostic accuracy (25–33). Thus, for the most part, thallium-201, Tc-99m sestamibi, or Tc-99m tetrofosmin can be used interchangeably, with a similar diagnostic accuracy for CAD.

Myocardial perfusion imaging may use either planar or single photon emission computed tomographic (SPECT)

techniques and visual analyses (34) or quantitative techniques. Quantification using horizontal (35) or circumferential (36) profiles may improve the test's sensitivity, especially in patients with single-vessel disease. For thallium-201 planar scintigraphy, average reported values of sensitivity and specificity (not corrected for posttest referral bias) have been in the range of 83% and 88%, respectively, by visual analysis, and 90% and 80%, respectively, for quantitative analyses (2). Thallium-201 SPECT is generally more sensitive than planar imaging for diagnosing CAD, localizing hypoperfused vascular segments, identifying left anterior descending and left circumflex coronary artery stenoses, and correctly predicting multivessel CAD (2). The average sensitivity and specificity of exercise thallium-201 SPECT imaging (uncorrected for referral bias) are in the range of 89% and 76%, respectively, for qualitative analyses and 90% and 70%, respectively, for quantitative analysis (2).

Since the introduction of dipyridamole- or adenosine-induced coronary vasodilation as an adjunct to thallium-201 myocardial perfusion imaging (37), pharmacologic stress has become an alternative to exercise in the noninvasive diagnosis of CAD (38). Dipyridamole planar scintigraphy has a high sensitivity (90% average) and acceptable specificity (70% average) for detection of CAD (17). Dipyridamole SPECT imaging with thallium-201 or Tc-99m sestamibi appears to be at least as accurate as planar imaging (39). Results of myocardial perfusion imaging during adenosine infusion are similar to those obtained with dipyridamole and exercise imaging (17). Evidence of CAD is demonstrated by redistribution defects comparing stress and resting scintigrams (is-

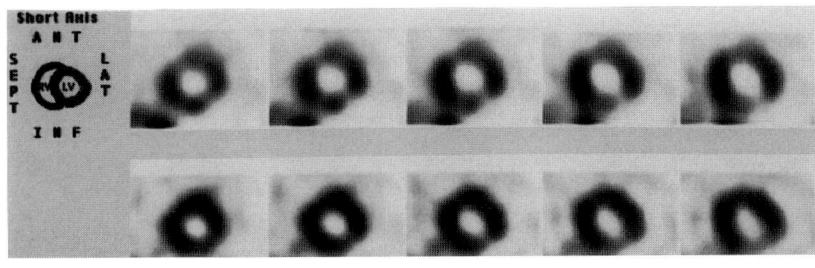

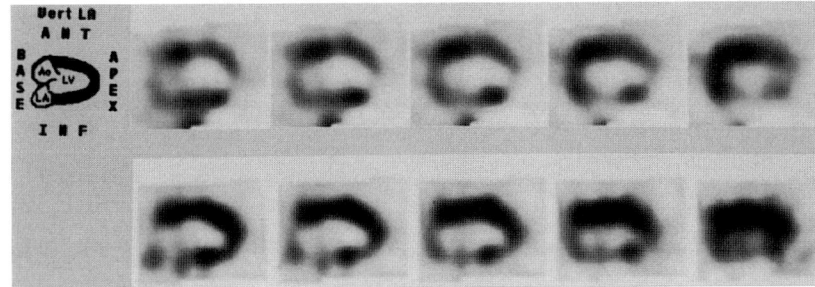

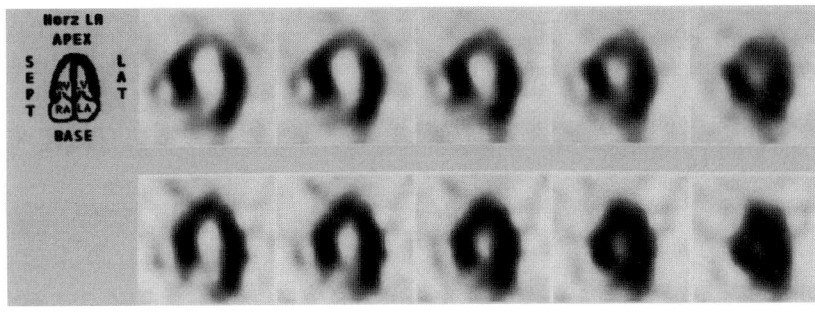

FIG. 3. SPECT Tl-201 scintigrams with exercise (1st horizontal column of each set) and 3 hours later. There is redistribution ischemia affecting anterior and anteroseptal areas and apex and partial reversal of the inferior wall defect. Coronary angiography showed a completely occluded right coronary artery and 80% stenosis of the mid-left anterior descending coronary artery.

chemia); fixed defects at rest (scar), and by LV dilation or lung uptake of isotope during stress (Figs. 3–5).

Stress Echocardiography

Stress echocardiography relies on imaging LV segmental wall motion and thickening during stress compared with baseline. Echocardiographic findings suggestive of myocardial ischemia include: (i) decease in wall motion in one or more LV segments with stress, (ii) decrease in wall thickening in one or more LV segments with stress, and (iii) compensatory hyperkinesis in complementary (nonischemic) wall segments (Figs. 5–9). The advent of digital acquisition and storage, as well as side-by-side (or quad screen) display of cine loops of LV images acquired at different levels of (rest or) stress, have facilitated efficiency and accuracy in interpretation of stress echocardiograms (17).

Stress echocardiography has been reported to have sensitivity and specificity for detecting CAD similar to stress myocardial imaging. In 36 studies reviewed, including 3,210 patients, the range of reported overall sensitivities (uncorrected for posttest referral bias) ranged from 70 to 97%. The average figure was 85% for overall sensitivity for exercise echocardiography and 82% for dobutamine stress echo-

cardiography (18). As expected, the reported sensitivity of exercise echocardiography for multivessel disease was higher (average: approximately 90%) than the sensitivity for single-vessel disease (average: approximately 79%) (18). In this series of studies, specificity ranged from 72 to 100%, with an average of approximately 86% for exercise echocardiography and 85% for dobutamine echocardiography.

Pharmacologic stress echocardiography is best accomplished using dobutamine since it enhances myocardial contractile performance and wall motion, which can be evaluated directly by echocardiography. Dobutamine stress echocardiography has substantially higher sensitivity than *vasodilator* (dipyridamole or adenosine) *stress echocardiography* for detecting coronary artery stenoses (40). In a recent review of 36 studies, average sensitivity and specificity (uncorrected for referral bias) of dobutamine stress echocardiography in the detection of CAD were in the range of 82% and 85%, respectively (2).

Special Issues in Stress Imaging

The sensitivity of the exercise imaging study for the diagnosis of CAD appears to be lower in patients taking *beta-blockers* (41). Nevertheless, in patients who exercise to a

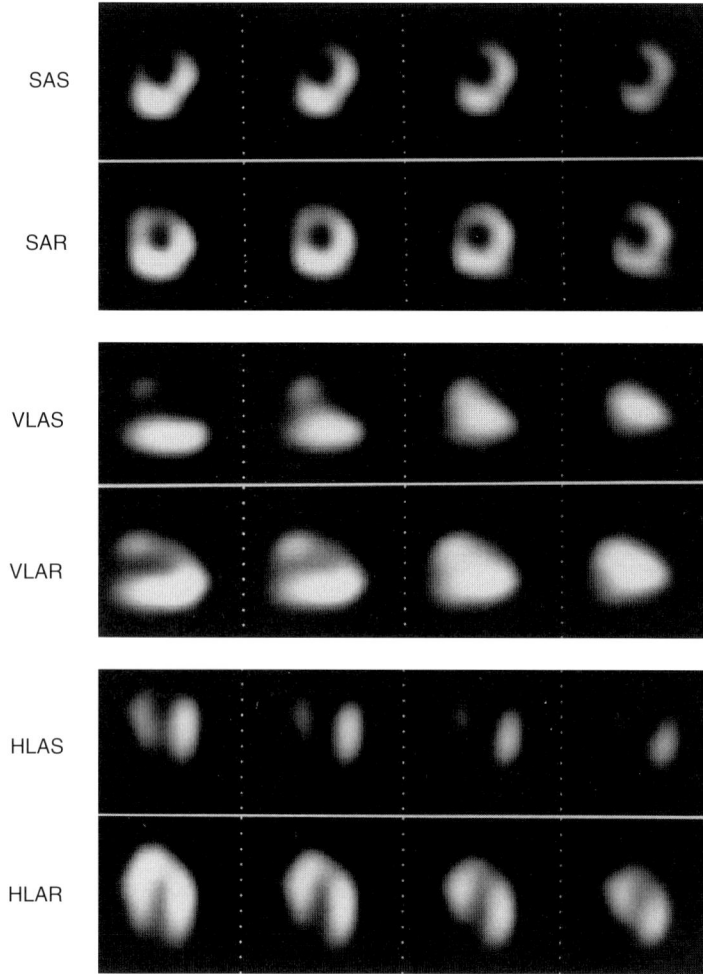

SAS

SAR

VLAS

VLAR

HLAS

HLAR

FIG. 4. SPECT Tl-201 scintigrams immediately following dipyridamole stress(s) (**top row**, each set) and 3 hours later (**bottom row**, each set) in short-axis, vertical long-axis, and horizontal long-axis tomographic views. There are severe anterior and anteroseptal reversible defects in this patient with a 90% stenosis of the proximal left anterior descending coronary artery. *SAS*, short axis—stress; *SAR*, short axis—rest; *VLAS*, vertical long axis—stress; *VLAR*, vertical long axis—rest; *HLAS*, horizontal long axis—stress; *HLAR*, horizontal long axis—rest.

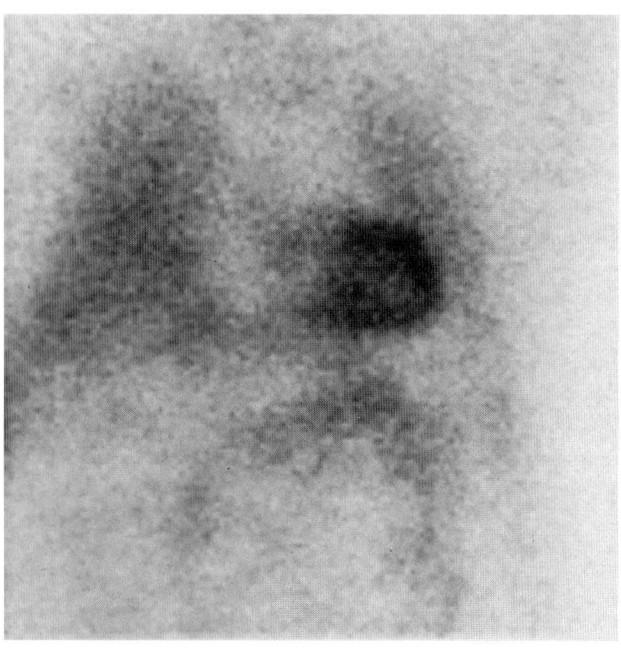

FIG. 5. Planar anterior-posterior view early after Tl-201 exercise test in a patient with severe three-vessel coronary artery disease. There is increased lung uptake of isotopes as compared to normal.

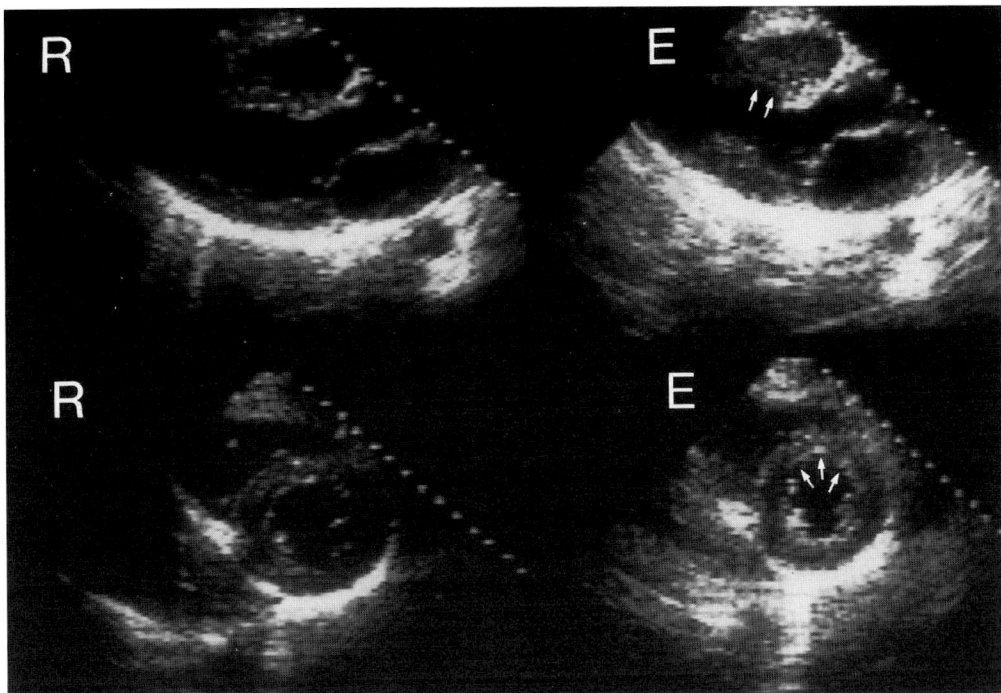

FIG. 6. Abnormal exercise stress echocardiography. Systolic frames from the parasternal long-axis (**upper panel**) and short-axis views of the left ventricle (**lower panel**) at rest (*R*) and immediately after exercise (*E*). Note the development of segmental wall motion abnormalities (*arrows*) along the anterior and septal segments. At angiography, single-vessel, 95% luminal stenosis of the proximal left anterior descending coronary artery was found.

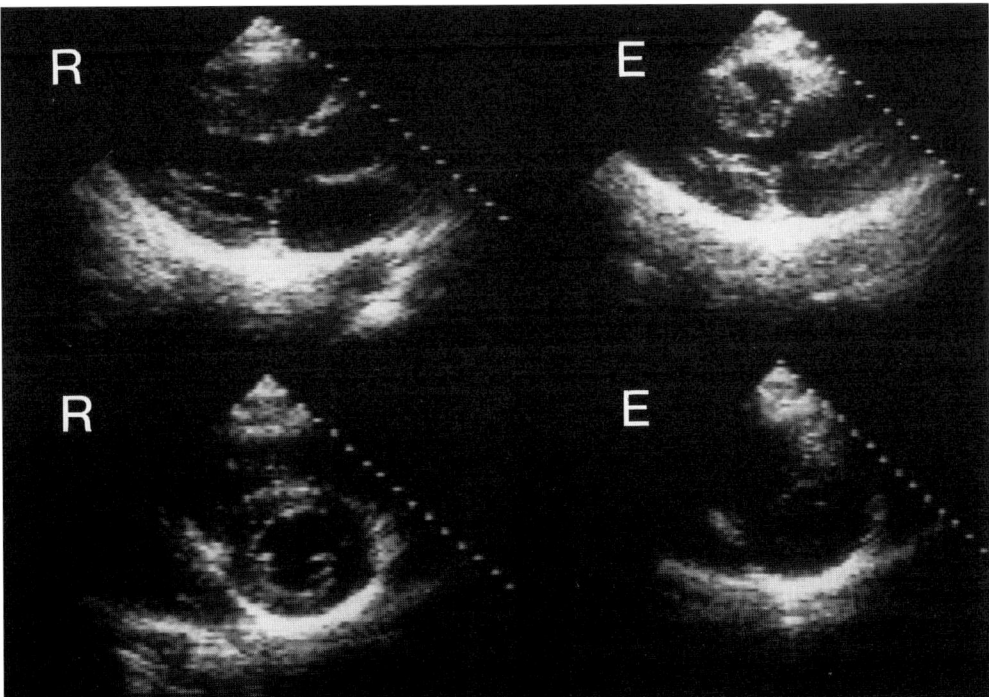

FIG. 7. Normalized exercise stress echocardiography. Same patient as in Figure 6 after successful coronary angioplasty and stent deployment at the proximal left anterior descending coronary artery. Systolic frames from the parasternal long-axis (**upper panel**) and short-axis (**lower panel**) at rest (*R*) and immediately after exercise (*E*). Compare to Figure 6 to appreciate the absence of the previously noted segmental wall motion abnormalities.

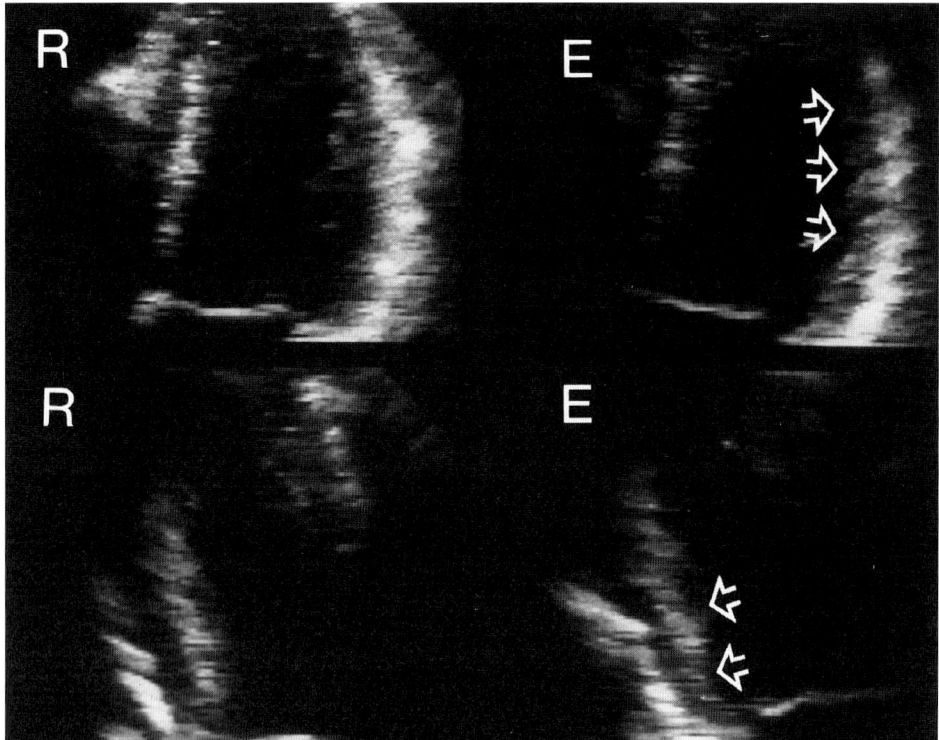

FIG. 8. Abnormal exercise stress echocardiography. Systolic frames from the apical four-chamber view (**upper panel**) and apical two-chamber view (**lower panel**) at rest (*R*) and immediately after exercise (*E*). Note the development of segmental wall motion abnormalities along the lateral segments on the four-chamber view (*arrows*) and the inferobasal segments from the two-chamber view (*arrows*). Development of multiple segmental wall motion abnormalities at stress suggests the presence of multivessel disease.

submaximal level, perfusion or echocardiographic imaging still affords higher sensitivity than the exercise ECG alone (18).

Several studies have observed an increased prevalence of myocardial perfusion defects in the interventricular septum during exercise imaging, in the absence of angiographic coronary disease, in patients with *left bundle-branch block* (42). Multiple studies have found that perfusion imaging with pharmacologic vasodilation is more accurate for identifying CAD in patients with left bundle-branch block (43). In contrast, only a single small study has reported on the diagnostic utility of stress echocardiography in the presence of left bundle-branch block (44).

The treadmill ECG test is less accurate for diagnosis in women, who have a generally lower pretest likelihood of CAD than men (15). Myocardial perfusion imaging or echocardiography could be a logical addition to treadmill testing in this circumstance. However, the sensitivity of thallium perfusion scans may be lower in women than in men (12). Photon attenuation artifacts due to breast attenuation, usually manifest in the anterior wall, can be an important consideration in the interpretation of women's perfusion scans, especially when thallium-201 is used as a tracer. Similar artifacts involving the inferior wall are common in very obese patients. This is a less common problem with ECG-gated technetium 99m sestamibi SPECT (45).

Comparison of Myocardial Perfusion Imaging and Echocardiography

In an analysis of 11 studies (46) involving 808 patients who had contemporaneous treadmill (or pharmacologic) stress echocardiography and myocardial perfusion scintigraphy, the overall sensitivity was 83% for stress perfusion imaging versus 78% for stress echocardiography ($P = $ NS). On the other hand, overall specificity tended to favor stress echocardiography (86% versus 77%, $P = $ NS).

More recently, Fleishmann et al. (47) performed a metaanalysis on 44 articles that examined the diagnostic accuracy of exercise tomographic myocardial perfusion imaging or exercise echocardiography. The overall sensitivity and specificity, respectively, were 85% and 77% for exercise echocardiography; 87% and 64% for exercise myocardial perfusion imaging; and 52% and 71% for exercise ECG. These results were not adjusted for referral bias.

SPECT has afforded diagnostic improvement over planar imaging for more precise localization of the vascular territo-

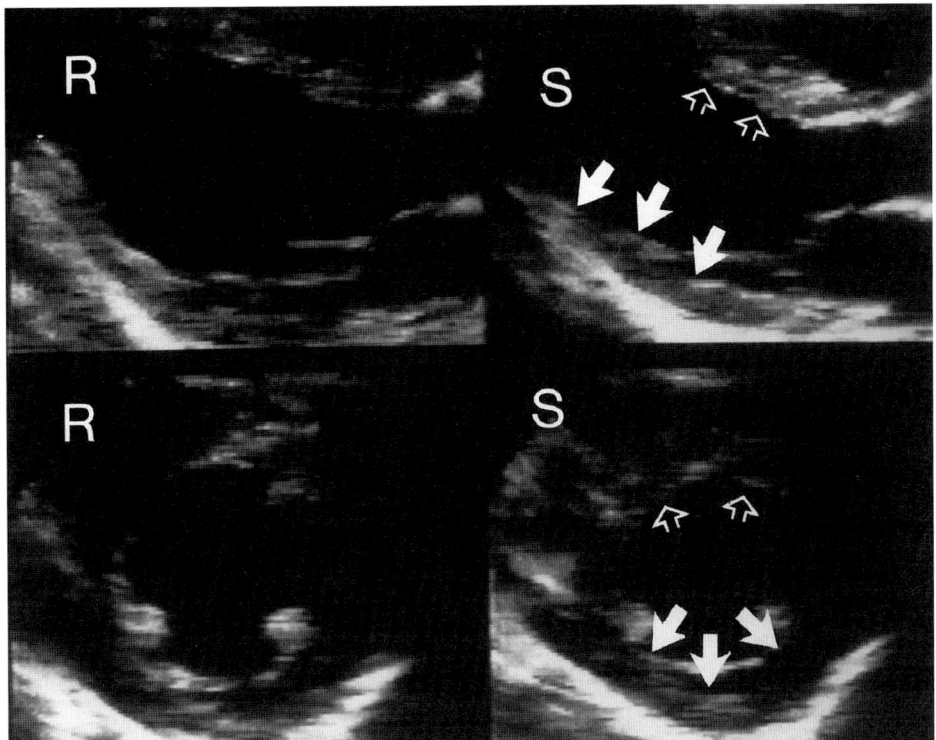

FIG. 9. Positive dobutamine stress echocardiography to identify myocardial viability. Systolic frames from the parasternal long-axis (**upper panel**) and short-axis views of the left ventricle (**lower panel**) in a 77-year-old man known to have multivessel disease and prior inferior wall myocardial infarction. Dobutamine stress echocardiography was performed to assess myocardial viability for possible revascularization. At rest (*R*), akinesis and thinning of the inferoseptal and inferolateral segments were noted consistent with prior transmural inferior wall myocardial infarction, whereas the anterior and septal segments showed moderate hypokinesis. During stress (*S*) induced by dobutamine infusion (20 μg/k/min), the inferior segments remained akinetic representing an old scar and, thus, no viability (*solid arrows*), whereas the anterior and septal segments showed increased systolic thickening and endocardial inward motion (*open arrows*) consistent with viable myocardium.

ries involved, particularly for identifying left circumflex coronary artery stenoses and predicting multivessel CAD (17). In data reported by O'Keefe et al. (46) from 10 published studies, there was a trend toward improved localization of coronary disease by stress myocardial perfusion imaging as compared to stress echocardiography (79 versus 65%). For localization of disease to the circumflex coronary artery, the radionuclide method conferred a significant advantage in sensitivity (72 versus 33%, $P < 0.001$).

Echocardiographic and radionuclide stress imaging have complementary roles and both add value to routine stress ECG under circumstances outlined above. The choice of which test to perform depends importantly on issues of local expertise, available facilities, and considerations of cost-effectiveness. A summary of the comparative advantages of stress myocardial perfusion imaging and stress echocardiography is provided in Table 4 (2).

Coronary Angiography

Recommendations for coronary angiography to establish a diagnosis of coronary heart disease are listed in Table 5

TABLE 4. *Comparative advantage of stress myocardial perfusion imaging and stress echocardiography in diagnosis of coronary artery disease*

Advantages of Stress Myocardial Perfusion Imaging
1. Higher technical success rate
2. Higher sensitivity, especially for single vessel coronary disease involving the left circumflex
3. Better accuracy in evaluating possible ischemia when multiple resting LV wall motion abnormalities are present
4. More extensive published data on evaluation of prognosis
Advantages of Stress Echocardiography
1. Higher specificity
2. Versatility—more extensive evaluation of cardiac anatomy and function
3. Greater convenience/efficacy/availability
4. Lower cost

(From ref. 15, with permission.)

TABLE 5. *Recommendations for coronary angiography to establish a diagnosis in patients with suspected angina, including patients with known CAD who have a significant change in anginal symptoms*

Class I
1. Patients with known or possible angina pectoris who have survived sudden cardiac death.

Class IIa
1. Patients with an uncertain diagnosis after noninvasive testing in whom the benefit of a more certain diagnosis outweighs the risk and cost of coronary angiography.
2. Patients who cannot undergo noninvasive testing due to disability, illness, or morbid obesity.
3. Patients with an occupational requirement for a definitive diagnosis.
4. Patients who by virtue of young age at onset of symptoms, noninvasive imaging, or other clinical parameters are suspected to have a nonatherosclerosis cause for myocardial ischemia (coronary artery anomaly, Kawasaki's disease, primary coronary artery dissection, radiation-induced vasculoplasty).
5. Patients in whom coronary artery spasm is suspected and provocative testing may be necessary.
6. Patients with a high pretest probability of left main or three-vessel CAD.

Class IIb
1. Patients with recurrent hospitalizations for chest pain in whom a definite diagnosis is judged necessary.
2. Patients with an overriding desire for a definitive diagnosis, and with a greater than low probability of CAD.

Class III
1. Patients with significant comorbidity in whom the risk of coronary arteriography outweighs the benefit of the procedure.
2. Patients with an overriding personal desire for a definitive diagnosis and with a low probability of CAD.

Class I: Conditions for which there is evidence and/or general agreement that a given procedure or treatment is useful and effective. Class II: Conditions for which there is conflicting evidence and/or a divergence of opinion about the usefulness/efficacy of a procedure or treatment. Class IIa: Weight of evidence/opinion is in favor of usefulness/efficacy. Class IIb: Usefulness/efficacy is less well established by evidence/opinion. Class III: Conditions for which there is evidence and/or general agreement that the procedure/treatment is not useful/effective and in some cases may be harmful.
CAD, coronary artery disease.

according to the ACC/AHA/ACP Guidelines on Chronic Stable Angina (2).

RISK STRATIFICATION

Introduction

The prognosis for the patient with chronic coronary artery disease is usually related to four patient factors. Left ventricular function is the strongest predictor of long-term survival in patients with CAD, and the ejection fraction is the most commonly used measure of the presence and the degree of LV dysfunction. The anatomic extent and severity of athero-sclerotic involvement of the coronary arteries is the second predictive factor. The number of stenosed coronary arteries is the most common measure of this characteristic. A third patient factor influencing prognosis is evidence of a recent coronary plaque rupture, indicating a substantially greater short-term risk for cardiac death or nonfatal MI. Worsening clinical symptoms with unstable features is the major clinical marker of a complicated plaque. The fourth prognostic factor is general health and noncoronary comorbidity.

Steps in Determining Prognosis Prior to Noninvasive Testing

History and Physical Examination

Very useful information relevant to prognosis can be obtained from the history. This includes demographics such as age and gender, as well as a medical history focusing on hypertension, diabetes, hypercholesterolemia, smoking, peripheral vascular or arterial disease, and previous MI (2). As discussed in the section on "Diagnosis," the description of the patient's chest discomfort can usually be readily assigned to one of three categories: (i) typical angina, (ii) atypical angina, and (iii) nonanginal chest pain.

The physical examination may be useful in risk stratification by defining the presence or absence of signs that might alter the probability of *severe* CAD. Useful findings include those suggesting: vascular disease (abnormal fundi, decreased peripheral pulses, bruits); long-standing hypertension (blood pressure, abnormal fundi); aortic valve stenosis or hypertrophic obstructive cardiomyopathy (systolic murmur, abnormal carotid pulse, abnormal apical pulse); left heart failure (third heart sound, displaced apical impulse, bibasilar rales), or right heart failure (jugular venous distension, hepatomegaly, ascites, pedal edema.)

Hubbard et al. (48) identified five clinical parameters that were independently predictive of severe three-vessel or left main CAD including age, typical angina, diabetes, gender, and prior MI and developed a 5-point cardiac risk score.

Electrocardiogram and Chest Roentgenogram

Patients with chronic stable angina who have resting ECG abnormalities are at greater risk than those with normal ECGs (2). Evidence of one or more prior MIs on ECG indicates an increased risk for cardiac events. In fact, the presence of Q-waves in multiple ECG leads, often accompanied by an R-wave in lead V_1 (posterior infarction), frequently is associated with a markedly reduced LV ejection fraction, an important determinant of the natural history of patients with CAD.

Califf et al. (49) demonstrated that the aggregation of certain historical and ECG variables in an "angina score," offers prognostic information that is independent of, and incremental to, that detected by catheterization. The angina score was comprised of three differentially weighted variables: (i) the "anginal course," (ii) anginal frequency, and (iii) resting ECG ST-T wave abnormalities.

On the chest roentgenogram, the presence of cardiomegaly, a left ventricular aneurysm, or pulmonary venous congestion are associated with a poorer long-term prognosis than occurs in patients with a normal chest x-ray.

The presence of calcium in the coronary arteries on chest x-ray or fluoroscopy in patients with symptomatic CAD suggests an increased risk of cardiac events (2). Although the presence and amount of coronary artery calcification by *electron beam computed tomography* correlate to some extent with the severity of CAD; there is considerable patient variation and many false positives (14).

Noninvasive Testing for Risk Stratification

Assessment of Left Ventricular Function

LV global systolic function and volumes are important predictors of prognosis in patients with cardiac disease. In patients with chronic ischemic heart disease, LV ejection fraction *measured* at rest by either echocardiography or radionuclide angiography is predictive of long-term prognosis; as LV ejection fraction declines, subsequent mortality increases. A resting ejection fraction of less than 35% is associated with an annual mortality rate of more than 3% per year (2).

Radionuclide LV ejection fraction may be measured at rest using a gamma camera, a technetium-99m tracer, and first-pass or gated equilibrium blood pool angiography (17) or by gated SPECT perfusion imaging using a technetium-based isotope (50). LV diastolic function can also be estimated by radionuclide ventriculography (17). LV systolic function can also be measured by quantitative two-dimensional echocardiography (17) and LV diastolic function assessed by transmitral valve Doppler recordings (18).

In patients with chronic stable angina and a history of previous MI, segmental wall motion abnormalities can be seen in both the zone(s) of prior infarction and in areas with ischemic "stunning" or "hibernation" of myocardium that are nonfunctional but still viable (2,51). In patients with chronic ischemic heart disease, the presence, severity, and mechanism of mitral regurgitation can be detected reliably using transthoracic two-dimensional imaging and Doppler echocardiographic techniques (18).

Echocardiography is the definitive test for detecting intracardiac thrombi (18). Left ventricular thrombi are most common in stable angina pectoris patients who have significant left ventricular wall motion abnormalities. In patients with anterior and apical infarctions, the presence of left ventricular thrombi denotes an increased risk of both embolism and death (52).

Electrocardiogram Exercise Testing

Unless cardiac catheterization is clearly indicated, symptomatic patients with suspected or known CAD should usually undergo exercise testing to assess the risk of future cardiac events, unless they have confounding features on their resting ECG or are unable to exercise. Also, documentation of exercise-induced ischemia is desirable for most patients who are being evaluated for revascularization (2).

Several studies have shown that risk assessment in patients with a normal ECG who are not taking digoxin and are physically capable *usually* should start with the exercise test (2,53–55). In contrast, a stress-imaging technique should be used for patients with ECG evidence of LVH, widespread resting ST-depression (greater than 1 mm), complete left bundle-branch block, ventricular paced rhythm, or preexcitation. The primary evidence that exercise testing can be used to estimate prognosis and assist in management decisions consists of seven observational studies (2,56,58). One of the strongest and most consistent prognostic markers is the maximum exercise capacity.

A second group of prognostic markers relates to exercise-induced ischemia. ST-segment depression and ST-segment elevation (in leads without pathologic Q waves and not in AVR) best summarize the prognostic information related to ischemia (56). Other variables are less powerful, including angina, the number of leads with ST-segment depression, the configuration of the ST-depression (downsloping, horizontal, or upsloping), and the duration of ST deviation into the recovery phase.

The Duke Treadmill Score combines this information and provides a way to calculate risk (15,56,57,59,60). The Duke Treadmill Score equals exercise time in minutes minus 5 times the ST-segment deviation in mm (during or after exercise) minus 4 times the angina index (which has a value of 0, if there is no angina; 1, if angina occurs; and 2, if angina is the reason for stopping the test). Among outpatients with suspected CAD, the two thirds of patients with scores indicating low risk had a 4-year survival of 99% (average annual mortality of 0.25%), and the 4% who had scores indicating high risk had a 4-year survival of 79% (average annual mortality rate of 5%) (see Table 6). Recent studies (59,60) indicate that this approach is equally applicable in men and women.

TABLE 6. *Survival according to risk groups based on DUKE treadmill scores*[a]

Risk group (score)	Percentage of total	Four-year survival	Annual mortality (%)
Low (≥ +5)	62	0.99	0.25
Moderate (−10 to +4)	34	0.95	1.25
High (< −10)	4	0.79	5.0

[a] Patients with a predicted average annual cardiac mortality of less than or equal to 1% per year (low-risk score) can be managed medically without need for cardiac catheterization. Patients with a predicted average annual cardiac mortality of greater than or equal to 3% per year (high-risk score) should be referred for cardiac catheterization.

(From ref. 72, with permission.)

Stress Imaging

Stress imaging studies using radionuclide myocardial perfusion imaging techniques or two-dimensional echocardiography at rest and during stress are useful for risk stratification and determining the most beneficial management strategy for patients with chronic stable angina (2). Whenever possible, treadmill or bicycle exercise should be used as the most appropriate form of stress since it provides the most information concerning patients' symptoms, cardiovascular function, and hemodynamic response during usual forms of activity (15). In fact, the inability to perform a bicycle or exercise treadmill test is in itself a negative prognostic factor for patients with chronic CAD.

In patients who cannot perform an adequate amount of bicycle or treadmill exercise, various types of pharmacologic stress are useful for risk stratification (17,18). The selection of the type of pharmacologic stress will depend on specific patient factors such as the patient's heart rate and blood pressure, the presence or absence of bronchospastic disease, the presence of left bundle-branch block or a pacemaker, and the likelihood of ventricular arrhythmias (see prior discussion).

Myocardial perfusion imaging has played a major role in the risk stratification of patients with CAD. Either planar or single photon emission computed tomography (SPECT) imaging utilizing thallium-201 or technetium-99m-perfusion tracers with images obtained at stress and during rest, provide important information concerning the severity of functionally significant CAD (2,17,61).

Stress echocardiography has been used more recently for assessing patients with chronic stable angina; thus, the amount of prognostic data obtained with this approach is somewhat limited. Nevertheless, the presence or absence of inducible myocardial wall motion abnormalities has useful predictive value in patients undergoing exercise or pharmacologic stress echocardiography. A negative stress echocardiography study denotes a low cardiovascular event rate during follow-up (2,18,62,63).

Myocardial Perfusion Imaging

Normal poststress thallium scan results are highly predictive of a benign prognosis even in patents with known coronary disease (17). A collation of 16 studies involving 3,594 patients followed for a mean of 29 months indicated a rate per year of cardiac death and MI of 0.9%, almost no different from that of the general population. In a recent prospective study of 5,183 consecutive patients who underwent myocardial perfusion studies during stress and later at rest, patients with normal scans were at low risk ($< 0.5\%$/year) for cardiac death and MI during 642 ± 226 days of mean follow up, and rates of both outcomes increased significantly with worsening scan abnormalities (64).

The number, extent, and site of abnormalities on stress myocardial perfusion scintigrams reflect the location and severity of functionally significant coronary artery stenoses. Lung uptake of thallium-201 on postexercise or pharmacologic stress images is an indicator of stress-induced global left ventricular dysfunction and is associated with pulmonary venous hypertension in the presence of multivessel CAD (65). Transient poststress ischemic left ventricular dilatation also correlates with severe two-or-three vessel CAD. Several studies have suggested that SPECT may be more accurate than planar imaging for determining the size of defects, for detecting coronary and, particularly, left circumflex CAD, and for localizing abnormalities in the distribution of individual coronary arteries (2,17). However, more false-positive results are likely to result from photon attenuation during SPECT imaging (17).

Information concerning both myocardial perfusion and ventricular function at rest may be helpful in determining the extent and severity of coronary disease (2,17). This combined information can be obtained by performing two separate exercise tests (e.g., stress perfusion scintigraphy and stress radionuclide ventriculography) or by combining the studies after a single exercise test (e.g., first-pass radionuclide angiography with technetium-99-based agents followed by perfusion imaging or perfusion imaging utilizing ECG gating). The use of ECG-gated technetium sestamibi SPECT imaging provides important prognostic information concerning LV ejection fraction and the extent of reversible ischemia.

The treadmill ECG test is less accurate for the diagnosis of coronary heart disease in women who have a lower pretest likelihood then men (15). However, the sensitivity of thallium perfusion scans may be lower in women then in men (2,17). Artifacts due to breast attenuation usually manifest in the anterior wall and can be an important consideration in the interpretation of women's scans, especially when thallium-201 is used as a tracer (17). As mentioned previously, Tc-99m sestamibi may be preferable to thallium-201 scintigraphy in women with large breasts and those with breast implants for determining prognosis as well for diagnosing CAD (17).

Pharmacologic stress perfusion imaging is preferable to exercise perfusion imaging in patients with left bundle-branch block. Recently, 245 patients with left bundle-branch block underwent SPECT imaging with thallium-201 ($n = 173$) or technetium 99m sestamibi ($n = 72$) during dipyridamole ($n = 153$) or adenosine ($n = 92$) stress (66). The 3-year survival was 57% in the high-risk group compared to 87% in the low-risk group ($P = 0.001$).

Stress Echocardiography

Stress echocardiography is both sensitive and specific for detecting inducible myocardial ischemia in patients with chronic stable angina (18). Compared with standard exercise treadmill testing, stress echocardiography provides an additional clinical value for detecting and localizing myocardial ischemia. The results of stress echocardiography may provide important prognostic value. Several studies indicate that patients at low, intermediate, and high risk for cardiac events can be stratified by the presence or absence of inducible wall motion abnormalities on stress echocardiography testing.

However, the value of a negative study compared to a negative thallium study needs to be further documented since there is less follow-up data as compared to radionuclide imaging. The presence of ischemia on the exercise echocardiogram is independent and incremental to clinical and exercise data in predicting cardiac events both in men and women (67,68).

The prognosis is not benign in patients with a positive stress echocardiographic study. In this subset, morbid or fatal cardiovascular events are more likely, but the overall event rates are rather variable. Hence, the cost-effectiveness of using routine stress echocardiographic testing to establish prognosis is uncertain.

Coronary Angiography

The availability of potent but expensive strategies to reduce the long-term morbidity and mortality of CAD mandate determination of patients most likely to benefit because of increased risk. This poses a major challenge to both the cardiovascular specialist and the primary care physician.

Assessment of cardiac risk and decisions regarding further testing usually begin with simple, repeatable, and inexpensive assessments of history and physical examination and extend to noninvasive or invasive testing depending on outcome. Clinical risk factors are in general additive, and a crude estimate of 1-year mortality can be obtained from these variables.

Risk stratification of patients with chronic stable angina by stress testing with exercise or pharmacologic agents has been shown to permit identification of groups of patients with low, intermediate, or high risk for subsequent cardiac events (5,17,19). Although one recent study (64) suggested that myocardial perfusion imaging can identify patients who are at low risk of death but increased risk of nonfatal MI, the major current focus of noninvasive risk stratification is on subsequent patient mortality. The objective is to identify patients in whom coronary angiography and subsequent revascularization might improve survival. Such an approach can only be effective if the patient's prognosis on medical therapy is sufficiently poor that it can be improved.

Previous experience in the randomized trials of coronary artery bypass grafting demonstrated that patients randomized to initial coronary artery bypass graft (CABG) had a lower mortality than those treated with medical therapy only if they were at substantial risk (69). Low-risk patients, who did not have a lower mortality with CABG, were those who had a 5-year survival of about 95% with medical therapy. This is equivalent to an annual mortality of 1%. As a result, coronary angiography to identify patients whose prognosis can be improved is inappropriate when the patient's esti-

mated annual mortality is less than or equal to 1%. In contrast, patients with a survival advantage with CABG, such as those with three-vessel disease, have an annual mortality of greater than or equal to 3%. Coronary angiography is appropriate for patients whose mortality risk is in this range.

Noninvasive test findings that identify high-risk patients are listed in Table 7. Patients identified as high risk are generally referred for coronary arteriography independent of their symptomatic status. Noninvasive tests, when appropriately utilized, are less costly than coronary angiography and have an acceptable predictive value for adverse events. This is most true when the pretest probability of severe CAD is low. When the pretest probability of severe CAD is high, direct referral for coronary angiography without noninvasive testing has been shown to be most cost-effective since the total number of tests is reduced (70).

TABLE 7. *Noninvasive risk stratification*

A. High-risk (> 3% annual mortality rate)
  1. Severe resting left ventricular dysfunction (LVEF < 35%)
  2. High-risk Duke treadmill score (score ≤ −11)
  3. Severe exercise left ventricular dysfunction (exercise LVEF < 35%)
  4. Stress-induced large perfusion defect (particularly if anterior)
  5. Stress-induced multiple perfusion defects of moderate size
  6. Large, fixed perfusion defect with LV dilatation or increased lung uptake (thallium-201)
  7. Stress-induced moderate perfusion defect with LV dilatation or increased lung uptake (thallium-201)
  8. Echocardiographic wall motion abnormality (involving > two segments) developing at low dose of dobutamine (≤10 mg/kg/min) or at a low heart rate (< 120 beats/min)
  9. Stress echocardiographic evidence of extensive ischemia
B. Intermediate-risk (1%–3% annual mortality rate)
  1. Mild/moderate resting left ventricular dysfunction (LVEF = 35% to 49%)
  2. Intermediate-risk Duke treadmill score (−11 < score < 5)
  3. Stress-induced moderate perfusion defect without LV dilatation or increased lung uptake (thallium-201)
  4. Limited stress echocardiographic ischemia with a wall motion abnormality only at higher doses of dobutamine involving ≤ two segments
C. Low-risk (< 1% annual mortality rate)
  1. Low-risk treadmill score (score ≥ 5)
  2. Normal or small myocardial perfusion defect at rest or with stress*
  3. Normal stress echocardiographic wall motion or no change of limited resting wall motion abnormalities during stress*

*Although the published data are limited, patients with these findings will probably not be at low risk in the presence of either a high-risk treadmill score or severe left ventricular dysfunction (LVEF 35%).
LV, left ventricle; *LVEF*, left ventricle ejection fraction.
(From ref. 7, with permission.)

OTHER NONINVASIVE TESTS

While ECG exercise testing, radionuclide ventriculography, resting two-dimensional and Doppler echocardiography, stress myocardial perfusion imaging, and stress echocardiography are the usual noninvasive tests employed in patients with chronic stable angina as indicated, certain other noninvasive tests have been utilized in some patients wtih chronic stable angina. These include ambulatory ECG recordings, magnetic resonance imaging, and positron emission tomography.

Ambulatory Electrocardiogram Recordings

Ambulatory ECG recordings have been utilized to detect symptomatic and asymptomatic episodes of myocardial ischemia in individuals during their normal activities. This is a relatively insensitive technique for detecting coronary artery disease even when there is 0.08 seconds of ST-segment depression for 60 seconds or greater, the usual definition for a positive test. It should be emphasized that this test is not a reliable diagnostic test for determining the presence of myocardial ischemia (15), and its role in monitoring therapy in patients with known ischemic heart disease is still under investigation. It was not recommended for screening for myocardial ischemia in a recent ACC/AHA Clinical Guidelines (71).

Magnetic Resonance Imaging

Magnetic resonance imaging is an excellent technique for defining left ventricular systolic and diastolic function, wall motion, and the presence of valvular regurgitation. Because it is a three-dimensional imaging modality, it is probably the most accurate methodology for determining ventricular volumes and function. When magnetic resonance is applied with dobutamine, it provides a mechanism for ischemia detection using induced wall motion abnormalities. Magnetic resonance has the potential to image perfusion and the coronary arteries, giving it great potential for comprehensive evaluation of the heart in patients with chronic stable angina (see Chapter 31).

Positron Emission Tomography

This technique is extremely useful for defining areas of myocardial tissue that are active metabolically in the presence of normal or markedly diminished myocardial perfusion. When available, this technique is applicable to many patients who have severely diminished left ventricular function and for whom a decision must be made as to whether or not improved coronary blood flow to these regions would result in the perfusion of contracting myocardium. This topic is reviewed in great detail in Chapter 14.

PERIOPERATIVE RISK STRATIFICATION PRIOR TO NONCARDIAC SURGERY

Introduction

Perioperative cardiac risk assessment of patients undergoing noncardiac surgery is a common clinical activity. The

TABLE 8. *Steps in evaluation of patients for noncardiac surgery*

1. Assessment of clinical markers
2. Assessment of functional capacity
3. Risk severity of surgical procedure
4. Noninvasive testing
5. Cardiac catheterization and coronary angiography

importance of this approach to patient management has increased markedly over the past two decades because an aging population and the need for cost containment are strong catalysts for the gradual yet dramatic changes in health care delivery. Undoubtedly, physicians will need objective data more frequently to justify decision-making; and "cost-effective" clinical pathways will be necessary to obtain full reimbursement for physician services.

In 1996, the American Heart Association/American College of Cardiology (AHA/ACC) published a set of step-wise guidelines for perioperative risk assessment (72). This is a methodical and systematic approach assessing predictors of intra- and postoperative morbidity and mortality. This evaluation relies on assessment of clinical history, ECG, functional capacity, left ventricular function, and prior history of MI. It is a safe and economical strategy that, combined with good clinical judgment on the part of the physician, results in an excellent clinical outcome.

The goal of preoperative risk stratification is to reduce overall perioperative morbidity and mortality in patients wtih CAD. Steps in the risk evaluation of patients for noncardiac surgery are listed in Tables 8 to 11 and Figure 10.

TABLE 9. *ACC/AHA clinical markers for perioperative risk assessment*

Major
Unstable coronary syndromes
Recent myocardial infarction
Unstable or severe angina
Uncompensated congestive heart failure
Significant arrhythmias
High-grade atrioventricular block
Symptomatic ventricular arrhythmias
Supraventricular tachycardia with uncontrolled ventricular rate
Severe valvular disease

Intermediate
Mild angina
Prior myocardial infarction by history or pathological QRS
Compensated or prior congestive heart failure
Diabetes mellitus

Minor
Advanced age
Abnormal electrocardiogram (LBBB, LVH, ST-T abnormalities)
Rhythm other than sinus
Low functional capacity
History of stroke
Uncontrolled systemic hypertension

LBBB, left bundle-branch block; *LVH*, left ventricular hypertrophy.

TABLE 10. *Estimated energy requirements for various activities*

1 MET	Can you take care of yourself?
	Eat, dress, or use the toilet?
	Walk indoors around the house?
	Walk a block or two on level ground at 2–3 mph or 3.2–4.8 km/h?
4 METs	Do light work around the house like dusting or washing dishes?
	Climb a flight of stairs or walk up a hill?
	Walk on level ground at 4 mph or 6.4 km/h?
	Run a short distance?
	Do heavy work around the house like scrubbing floors or lifting or moving heavy furniture?
	Participate in moderate recreational activities like golf, bowling, dancing, double tennis, or throwning a baseball or football?
>10 METs	Participate in strenuous sports like swimming, singles tennis, football, basketball, or skiing?

MET, metabolic equivalent.
(From the Duke Activity Status Index and AHA Exercise Standards, with permission.)

TABLE 11. *Cardiac risk* stratification for noncardiac surgical procedures*

High risk
Emergent major operations, particularly in the elderly
Aortic and other major vascular
Peripheral vascular
Anticipated prolonged surgical procedures associated with large fluid shifts and/or blood loss
Intermediate risk
Carotid endarterectomy
Head and neck
Intraperitoneal and intrathoracic
Orthopedic
Prostate
Low risk†
Endoscopic procedures
Superficial procedure
Cataract
Breast

*Combined incidence of cardiac death and nonfatal myocardial infarction.
† Do not generally require further preoperative cardiac testing.

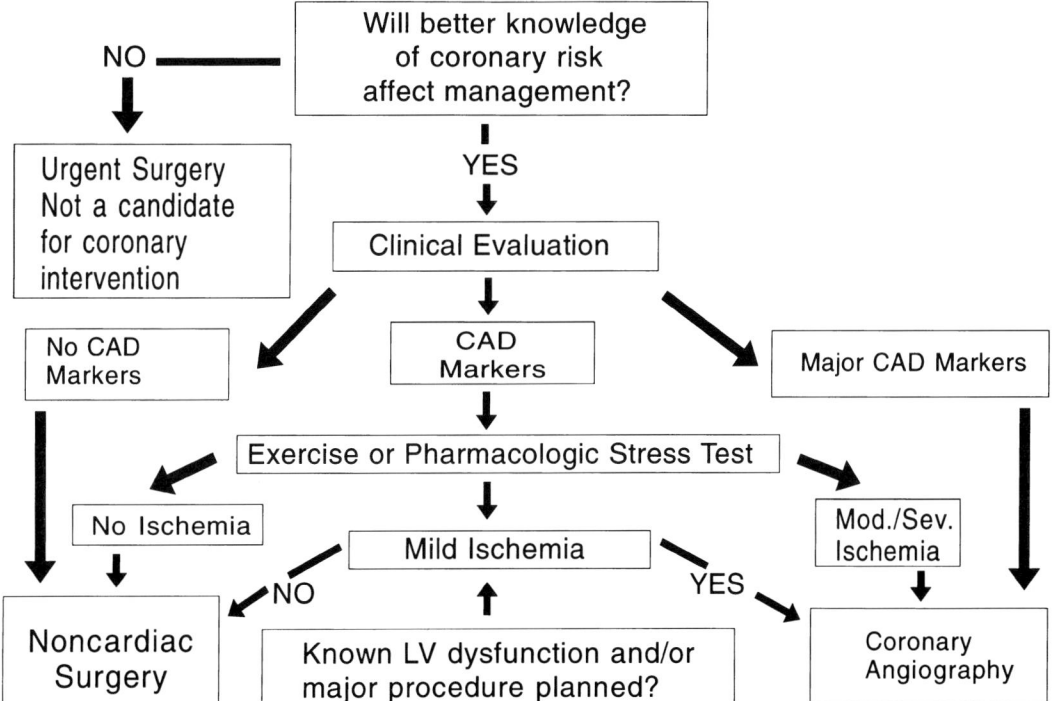

FIG. 10. Algorithm for assessment and management of coronary artery disease (CAD). CAD markers: age, 70 years or older; prior angina; prior myocardial infarction; previous congestive heart failure and/or ventricular arrhythmias; diabetes mellitus; and Q waves on the resting electrocardiogram. Major CAD markers: recent myocardial infarction (MI) complicated by angina, congestive heart failure, or positive stress test; unstable or new onset angina; recent non-Q-wave anterior MI; more than two CAD markers in selected patients. Exercise testing: preferred when possible because functional capacity is more correlated with adverse outcomes than is ischemia. The combination of major ischemia at low functional capacity is especially worrisome. Moderate-to-severe ischemia: ischemia in multiple coronary territories in association with transient left ventricular dysfunction and/or low workload, e.g., less than 4 to 6 METS. *LV*, left ventricular; *METS*, metabolic equivalents.

The purpose of preoperative evaluation is not to "give medical clearance" per se but rather to evaluate the patient's current medical status, detect stress-induced ischemia using noninvasive methods when necessary, and to make recommendations about patient management during the entire perioperative period.

Clinical Evaluation

The primary care physician or the physician most familiar with the patient is responsible for the pivotal act of performing the initial clinical examination, an assessment the physician will use in the attempt to accurately categorize low-, intermediate-, and high-risk patient profiles. A decision must then be made, either individually or in concert with a consultant, regarding future discourse.

The cornerstone of the risk assessment requires a very thorough physical examination, a meticulous clinical history, a chest radiograph, and an ECG. The clinical history must include a reliable and valid assessment of the patient's functional capacity and quality of life, an estimation that can be difficult to gauge accurately during routine office visits.

Exercise capacity should be reported in estimated metabolic equivalents (METs) of exercise. The definition of the term MET consists of the resting VO_2 for a 70 kg, 40-year-old male, with 1 MET equivalent to 3.5 mL/min/kg of body weight. Work activities are thus calculated in multiples of METs (Table 10).

Patient Stratification Using Noninvasive Testing

Successful perioperative cardiac testing should achieve both short- and long-term risk assessment. The major difficulty with stratification is the use of potentially unnecessary preoperative testing and the consequent possibility of requisite additional testing (if initial results are equivocal).

Important factors to consider when determining CAD clinical markers include the existence of known CAD, a history of myocardial revascularization procedures within the past 5 years or normal coronary angiography within the past 2 years.

Further testing following clinical assessment is necessary only when the additional information may alter patient treatment and perioperative outcome (73). In general, indications for further cardiac testing and treatments do not differ from those in the nonoperative setting, but their timing is dependent on such factors as the urgency of surgery, patient risk factors, and special surgical considerations (72).

Because of the suboptimal sensitivity of tests such as exercise ECG monitoring and exercise or pharmacologic stress testing using myocardial perfusion imaging or two-dimensional echo, the negative predictive value may not be sufficient when evaluating patients at high pretest probability of serious events on clinical grounds. It is especially important in the low-risk group to avoid costly and unnecessary tests that may lead to false-positive results.

When there is intermediate risk as due to either a preponderance of disease markers or due to few disease markers but high-risk surgery, further testing is indicated; this is the group most likely to benefit from additional noninvasive testing.

Assessment of Functional Capacity

One of the most important indicators of risk in the patient with known or suspected coronary artery disease is functional status. Several studies have shown that patients able to meet a high functional (physiologic) demand on testing have a low cardiac event rate.

If the patient's functional level is unclear by the clinical assessment or likely is low (less than 4 METS), an objective functional (stress) test should be performed for more accurate measurement. Pharmacologic stress testing offers an excellent alternative in cases where patients are unable to exercise adequately due to deconditioning, obesity, age, or where they are to undergo orthopedic, peripheral vascular, or neurosurgical procedures (73).

Assessment of Left Ventricular Function

The assessment of LV function also starts with the initial clinical assessment. Reduced LV function often results in symptoms of congestive heart failure (CHF), including dyspnea on exertion, orthopnea, and paroxysmal nocturnal dyspnea. On physical examination, a third heart sound is often present, and there may be jugular venous distention, pulmonary rales, and tachycardia. The most frequently used diagnostic modalities for the assessment of LV include echocardiography and MUGA (multiple gate acquistion) scanning; the latter widely considered the gold standard among noninvasive studies for *quantitative* measurements of left ventricular ejection fraction (LVEF). An alternative is gated technetium sestamibi SPECT, which provides information about ischemia and LV function.

There are conflicting data regarding the relationship between depressed LV and postoperative adverse cardiac events. The data from both radionuclide scintigraphy and echocardiographic studies suggest that resting LVEF is a relatively insensitive and nonspecific independent marker for postoperative myocardial infarction and cardiac death. However, LV systolic or diastolic dysfunction may predict the occurrence of postoperative CHF.

Specific Testing Modalities

Exercise Treadmill Test

Exercise testing is widely available, relatively inexpensive, and is preferred over pharmacologic imaging when possible; functional capacity is better correlated with adverse outcomes than ischemia. The exercise treadmill test is able to provide an estimate of functional capacity, hemodynamic response to exercise, potential for catecholamine-induced cardiac arrhythmias, and exercise myocardial ischemic threshold.

Multiple studies using ST segment depression of greater than or equal to 1 mm or horizontal downsloping depression as a positive test for ischemia indicate a 2-to-3-fold increased risk of perioperative events in patients with ST-segment depression on preoperative stress testing.

Exercise Stress Myocardial Perfusion Imaging

The addition of myocardial perfusion imaging, either thallium-201 or technetium sestamibi to exercise stress testing, increases the sensitivity for the identification of patients with coronary artery stenosis.

The joint ACC/AHA Perioperative Guidelines summarized current data regarding preoperative myocardial perfusion imaging methods. The positive predictive value of thallium redistribution following stress testing for MI or death ranged from 4 to 20% in selected reports. The negative predictive value is very high (approximately 99%); thus, the prognosis associated with a normal scan is excellent. In the nonoperative ambulatory setting among patients with chest pain, exercise thallium scintigraphy data are additive to those from coronary angiography in identifying those at high risk for subsequent late events.

Certain radionuclide findings indicating higher risk include: the severity of perfusion defect, number of reversible defects, uptake of isotope by the lung (indicating pulmonary venous hypertension), LV dilatation (depressed LV systolic function with stress), presence of fixed perfusion abnormalities (prior MI), and marked ST segment changes associated with angina during pharmacologic stress imaging (74).

Dipyridamole Myocardial Perfusion Imaging

Dipyridamole thallium scintigraphy (DTS) is the most widely used pharmacologic stress test before noncardiac surgery in patients unable to exercise. In many studies, the dipyridamole thallium scintigraphy result has been the single most important factor for determining cardiac risk. DTS has been accepted as an extremely sensitive, noninvasive diagnostic test with an excellent negative predictive value but *low positive predictive value.* A normal dipyridamole thallium scintigraphy has an excellent negative predictive value for an uncomplicated perioperative course, regardless of clinical risk factors. Patients with fixed defects have had an increased perioperative cardiac event compared with patients who had normal scans. Risk stratification is improved when the results of DTS are integrated with clinical markers referred for testing for vascular surgery.

Patients with multiple thallium defects are much more likely to have multivessel CAD, and, within this subgroup, the positive predictive value of postoperative cardiac death or MI approaches 30%. Other radionuclide markers of LV dysfunction, such as LV dilatation or lung uptake, indicate patients at very high risk of perioperative events.

Dobutamine Stress Echo

In myocardial ischemia, regional wall motion abnormalities occur before ECG changes and angina. When stress images are compared with resting images, ischemia is made evident by worsening wall motion.

Doubtamine stress echo (DSE) is a feasible, safe, and useful modality for cardiac risk stratification before surgical procedures; its accuracy appears comparable to myocardial perfusion imaging, and it has the additional advantages of having a relatively lower cost and providing additional information regarding LV function and valvular abnormalities.

In six studies published between 1991 and 1993 (75), the same methodologic limitations as seen in the evaluations using other noninvasive techniques, chiefly, referral and detection bias, were also present with DSE. Unfortunately, there was not a uniform criterion for a positive test. In these six studies, only 2 of 317 patients with a negative result had either an MI or cardiac death postoperatively (negative predictive value greater than 99%). However, the positive predictive value for these serious events is low (pooled estimate, 15%; range, 7 to 23%).

In 1996, Shaw et al. (76) published the results of a meta-analysis of 15 nonrandomized trial reports on preoperative risk stratification using both dipyridamole-thallium imaging (10 reports with 1,994 total patients) and dobutamine stress echocardiography (5 reports with 445 total patients). Meta-analysis of the 15 studies suggest that the prognostic value for perioperative ischemic events is comparable between available techniques but that the accuracy varies with coronary artery disease prevalence.

Dobutamine Stress MRI

Ambulatory (Holter) Electrocardiogram Recording

Mangano et al. compared the relative sensitivity of preoperative versus intraoperative and postoperative ECG monitoring in consecutive men with known or suspected CAD before noncardiac surgery. Ischemia on preoperative ambulatory ECG recording was found to be less than 30% sensitive for all perioperative cardiac events, whereas ischemia in the early postoperative period was much more sensitive. Intraoperative ischemia, although not uncommon, was less sensitive and specific compared with abnormalities observed in the early postoperative period.

Coronary Angiography

Coronary angiography is a testing modality that is used when previously conducted noninvasive tests have indicated that there is a strong change of moderate-to-severe myocardial ischemia. It is neither cost-effective nor clinically appropriate to perform cardiac catheterization in all vascular surgery candidates. Indications for coronary angiography are

TABLE 12. *Indications for coronary angiography in perioperative evaluation before (or after) noncardiac surgery*

Patients with suspected or proven CAD

Class I
High-risk results during noninvasive testing
Angina pectoris unresponsive to adequate medical therapy
Most patients with unstable angina pectoris
Nondiagnostic or equivocal noninvasive test in a high-risk patient undergoing a high-risk noncardiac procedure
Class II
Intermediate-risk results during noninvasive testing
Nondiagnostic or equivocal noninvasive test in a lower-risk patient undergoing a high-risk noncardiac surgical procedure
Urgent noncardiac surgery in a patient convalescing from acute perioperative MI
Class III
Low-risk noncardiac surgery in a patient with known CAD and low-risk results on noninvasive testing
Screening for CAD without appropriate noninvasive testing
Asymptomatic after coronary revascularization, with excellent exercise capacity ($\leq$7 METs)
Mild stable angina in patients with good LV function, low-risk noninvasive test results
Patient is not a candidate for coronary revascularization because of concomitant medical illness
Prior technically adequate normal coronary angiogram within 5 years
Severe LV dysfunction (e.g., ejection fraction <20%) and patient not considered candidate for revascularization procedure
Patient unwilling to consider coronary revascularization procedure results will affect management

designated as class I, II, or III by the ACC/AHA Task Force on Clinical Practice Guidelines (Table 12).

REFERENCES

1. Kannel WB, Feinleib M. Natural history of angina pectoris in the Framingham study. Prognosis and survival. *Am J Cardiol* 1972;29:154–163.
2. Gibbons RJ, Chatterjee K, Daley J, et al. ACC/AHA/ACP guidelines for the management of chronic stable angina: a report of the American College of Cardiology/American Heart Association/American College of Physicians Task Force on Practice Guidelines (Committee on the Management of Patients with Chronic Stable Angina). *J Am Coll Cardiol* 1999 (in press).
3. Elveback LR, Connolly DC, Melton LJ III. Coronary heart disease in residents of Rochester, Minnesota. VII. Incidence, 1950 through 1982. *Mayo Clin Proc* 1986;61:896–900.
4. Ryan TJ, Anderson JL, Antman EM, et al. ACC/AHA guidelines for the management of patients with acute myocardial infarction. A report of the American College of Cardiology/American Heart Association Task Force on Practice Guidelines (Committee on Management of Acute Myocardial Infarction). *J Am Coll Card* 1996;28:1328–1428.
5. The American Heart Association. *Biostatistical fact sheets*. Dallas, TX: American Heart Association, 1997.
6. Diamond GA, Staniloff HM, Forrester JS, et al. Computer-assisted diagnosis in the noninvasive evaluation of patients with suspected coronary disease. *J Am Coll Cardiol* 1983;1:444–455.
7. Diamond GA, Forrester JS. Analysis of probability as an aid in the clinical diagnosis of coronary-artery disease. *N Engl J Med* 1979;300:1350–1358.
8. Pryor DB, Harrell FE, Lee KL, et al. Estimating the likelihood of significant coronary artery disease. *Am J Med* 1983;75:771–780.
9. Sox HC, Hickam DH, Marton KI, et al. Using the patient's history to estimate the probability of coronary artery disease: a comparison of primary care and referral practices [published erratum appears in *Am J Med* 1990;89(4):550]. *Am J Med* 1990;89:7–14.
10. Pryor DB, Shaw L, McCants CB, et al. Value of the history and physical in identifying patients at increased risk for coronary artery disease. *Ann Intern Med* 1993;118:81–90.
11. Chaitman BR, Bourassa MG, Davis K, et al. Angiographic prevalence of high-risk coronary artery disease in patient subsets (CASS). *Circulation* 1981;64:360–367.
12. Wexler L, Brundage B, Crouse J, et al. Coronary artery calcification: pathophysiology, epidemiology, imaging methods, and clinical implications. A statement for health professionals from the American Heart Association Writing Group. *Circulation* 1996;94:1175–1192.
13. Mautner SL, Mautner GC, Froehlich J, et al. Coronary artery disease: predication with *in vitro* electron beam CT. *Radiology*1994;192:625–630.
14. O'Rourke RA, Brundage BH, Froelicher VF, et al. ACC/AHA consensus document on electron beam computed tomography for the diagnosis of coronary artery disease. *J Amer Coll Cardiol* 2000 (in press).
15. Gibbons RJ, Balady GJ, Beasley JW, et al. ACC/AHA guidelines for exercise testing: executive summary. A report of the American College of Cardiology/American Heart Association Task Force on Practice Guidelines (Committee on Exercise Testing). *J Am Coll Cardiol* 1998.
16. Froelicher VF, Lehmann KG, Thomas R, et al. The electrocardiographic exercise test in a population with reduced workup bias: diagnostic performance, computerized interpretation, and multivariable prediction. Veterans Affairs Cooperative Study in Health Services #016 Quantitative Exercise Testing and Angiography (QUEXTA) Study Group. *Ann Intern Med* 1998;128:965–974.
17. Ritchie JL, Bateman TM, Bonow RO, et al. Guidelines for clinical use of cardiac radionuclide imaging. Report of the American College of Cardiology/American Heart Association Task Force on Assessment of Diagnostic and Therapeutic Cardiovascular Procedures (Committee on Radionuclide Imaging), developed in collaboration with the American Society of Nuclear Cardiology. *J Am Coll Cardiol* 1995;25:521–547.
18. Cheitlin MD, Alpert JS, Armstrong WF, et al. ACC/AHA Guidelines for the clinical application of echocardiography. A report of the American College of Cardiology/American Heart Association Task Force on Practice Guidelines (Committee on Clinical Application of Echocardiography). Developed in collaboration with the American Society of Echocardiography. *Circulation* 1997;95:1686–1744.
19. Diamond GA, Forrester JS, Hirsch M, et al. Application of conditional probability analysis to the clinical diagnosis of coronary artery disease. *J Clin Invest* 1980;65:1210–1221.
20. Goldman L, Cook EF, Mitchell N, et al. Incremental value of the exercise test for diagnosing the presence or absence of coronary artery disease. *Circulation* 1982;66:945–953.
21. Melin JA, Wijns W, Vanbutsele RJ, et al. Alternative diagnostic strategies for coronary artery disease in women: demonstration of the usefulness and efficiency of probability analysis. *Circulation* 1985;71:535–542.
22. LeWinter MM, Crawford MH, O'Rourke RA, et al. The effects of oral propranolol, digoxin, and combination therapy on the resting and exercise electrocardiogram. *Am Heart J* 1977;93:202–209.
23. Whinnery JE, Froelicher VF, Stuart AJ. The electrocardiographic response to maximal treadmill exercise in asymptomatic men with left bundle branch block. *Am Heart J* 1977;94:316–324.
24. Mercado M, O'Rourke RA. Unpublished data.
25. Kiat H, Berman DS, Maddahi J. Comparison of planar and tomographic exercise thallium-201 imaging methods for the evaluation of coronary artery disease. *J Am Coll Cardiol* 1989;13:613–616.
26. Iskandrian AS, Heo J, Kong B, et al. Use of technetium-99m isonitrile (RP-30A) in assessing left ventricular perfusion and function at rest and during exercise in coronary artery disease, and comparison with coronary arteriography and exercise thallium-201 SPECT imaging. *Am J Cardiol* 1989;64:270–275.
27. Taillefer R, Laflamme L, Dupras G, et al. Myocardial perfusion imaging with Tc-99m-methoxy-isobutyl-isonitrile (MIBI): comparison of short and long time intervals between rest and stress injections. Preliminary results. *Eur J Nucl Med* 1988;13:515–522.

28. Maddahi J, Kiat H, Van Train FK, et al. Myocardial perfusion imaging with technetium-99m sestamibi SPECT in the evaluation of coronary artery disease. *Am J Cardiol* 1990;66:55E–62E.

29. Kahn JK, McGhie I, Akers MS, et al. Quantitative rotational tomography with 201T and Tc-99m 2-methoxy-isobutyl-isonitrile. A direct comparison in normal individuals and patients with coronary artery disease. *Circulation* 1989;79:1282–1293.

30. Wackers FJ, Berman DS, Maddahi J, et al. Technetium-99m hexakis 2-methoxyisobutyl isonitrile: human biodistribution, dosimetry, safety, and preliminary comparison to thallium-201 for myocardial perfusion imaging. *J Nucl Med* 1989;30:301–311.

31. Maisey MN, Mistry R, Sowton E. Planar imaging techniques used with technetium-99m sestamibi to evaluate chronic myocardial ischemia. *Am J Cardiol* 1990;66:47E–54E.

32. Maddahi J, Kiat H, Friedman JD, et al. Technetium-99m-sestamibi myocardial perfusion imaging for evaluation of coronary artery disease. In: Zaret BL, Beller GA, eds. *Nuclear cardiology: state of the art and future directions.* St. Louis: Mosby, 1993:191–200.

33. Zaret BL, Rigo P, Wackers FJ, et al. Myocardial perfusion imaging with 99m TC-tetrofosmin. Comparison to Tl-201 imaging and coronary angiography in a phase III multicenter trial. *Circulation* 1995;91:313–319.

34. Detrano R, Janosi A, Lyons KP, et al. Factors affecting sensitivity and specificity of a diagnostic test: the exercise thallium scintigram. *Am J Med* 1988;84:699–710.

35. Watson DD, Campbell NP, Read EK, et al. Spatial and temporal quantitation of plane thallium myocardial images. *J Nucl Med* 1981;22:577–584.

36. Garcia E, Maddahi J, Berman D, et al. Space/time quantitation of thallium-201 myocardial scintigraphy. *J Nucl Med* 1981;22:309–317.

37. Gould KL. Noninvasive assessment of coronary stenoses by myocardial perfusion imaging during pharmacologic coronary vasodilatation. I. Physiologic basis and experimental validation. *Am J Cardiol* 1978;41:267–278.

38. Verani MS. Pharmacologic stress myocardial perfusion imaging. *Curr Probl Cardiol* 1993;18:481–525.

39. Parodi O, Marcassa C, Casucci R, et al. Accuracy and safety of technetium-99m hexakis 2-methoxy-2-isobutylisonitrile (Sestamibi) myocardial scintigraphy with high dose dipyridamole test in patients with effort angina pectoris: a multicenter study. Italian Group of Nuclear Cardiology. *J Am Coll Cardiol* 1991;18:1439–1444.

40. Dagianti A, Penco M, Agati L, et al. Stress echocardiography: comparison of exercise, dipyridamole and dobutamine in detecting and predicting the extent of coronary artery disease [published erratum appears in *J Am Coll Cardiol* 1995;26(4):1114]. *J Am Coll Cardiol* 1995;26:18–25.

41. Hockings B, Saltissi S, Croft DN, et al. Effect of beta adrenergic blockade on thallium-201 myocardial perfusion imaging. *Br Heart J* 1983;49:83–89.

42. DePuey EG, Guertler-Krawczynska E, Robbins WL. Thallium-201 SPECT in coronary artery disease patients with left bundle branch block. *J Nucl Med* 1988;29:1479–1485.

43. O'Keefe JH Jr, Bateman TM, Barnhart CS. Adenosine thallium-201 is superior to exercise thallium-201 for detecting coronary artery disease in patients with left bundle branch block. *J Am Coll Cardiol* 1993;21:1332–1338.

44. Mairesse GH, Marwick TH, Arnese M, et al. Improved identification of coronary artery disease in patients with left bundle branch block by use of dobutamine stress echocardiography in comparison with myocardial perfusion tomography. *Am J Cardiol* 1995;76:321–325.

45. Smanio PE, Watson DD, Segalla DL, et al. Value of gating of technetium-99m sestamibi single-photon emission computed tomographic imaging. *J Am Coll Cardiol* 1997;30:1687–1692.

46. O'Keefe JH, Barnhart CS, Bateman TM. Comparison of stress echocardiography and stress myocardial perfusion scintigraphy for diagnosing coronary artery disease and assessing its severity. *Am J Cardiol* 1995;75:25D–34D.

47. Fleischmann KE, Hunink MGM, Kuntz KM, et al. Exercise echocardiography or exercise SPECT imaging? A meta-analysis of diagnostic test performance. *JAMA* 1998;280(10):913–920.

48. Hubbard BL, Gibbons RJ, Lapeyre AC, et al. Prospective evaluation of a clinical and exercise-test model for the prediction of left main coronary artery disease. *Ann Intern Med* 1993;118:81–90.

49. Califf RM, Mark DB, Harrell FE, et al. Importance of clinical measures

50. of ischemia in the prognosis of patients with documented coronary artery disease. *J Am Coll Cardiol* 1998;11:20–26.

50. Germano G, Erel J, Lewin H, et al. Automatic quantitation of regional myocardial wall motion and thickening from gated technetium-99m sestamibi myocardial perfusion single-photon emission computed tomography. *Circulation* 1996;93:463–473.

51. Oh JK, Gibbons RJ, Christina TF, et al. Correlation of regional wall motion abnormalities detected by two-dimensional echocardiography with perfusion defect determined by technetium 99m sestamibi imaging in patients treated with reperfusion therapy during acute myocardial infarction. *Am Heart J* 1996;131:32–37.

52. Spirito P, Bellotti P, Chiarella F, et al. Prognostic significance and natural history of left ventricular thrombi in patients with acute anterior myocardial infarction: a two-dimensional echocardiographic study. *Circulation* 1985;72:774–780.

53. Gibbons RJ, Zinsmeister AR, Miller TD, et al. Supine exercise electrocardiography compared with exercise radionuclide angiography in noninvasive identification of severe coronary artery disease. *Ann Intern Med* 1990;112:743–749.

54. Ladenheim ML, Kotler TS, Pollock BH, et al. Incremental prognostic power of clinical history, exercise electrocardiography and myocardial perfusion scintigraphy in suspected coronary artery disease. *Am J Cardiol* 1987;59:270–277.

55. Mattera JA, Arain SA, Sinusas AJ, et al. Exercise testing with myocardial perfusion imaging in patients with normal baseline electrocardiograms: cost savings with a stepwise diagnostic strategy. *J Nucl Cardiol* 1998;5:498–506.

56. Mark DB, Hlatky MA, Harrell FE, et al. Exercise treadmill score for predicting prognosis in coronary artery disease. *Ann Intern Med* 1987;106:793–800.

57. Morrow K, Morris CK, Froelicher VF, et al. Prediction of cardiovascular death in men undergoing noninvasive evaluation for coronary artery disease. *Ann Intern Med* 1993;118:689–695.

58. Brunelli C, Cristofani R, L'Abbate A. Long-term survival in medically treated patients with ischaemic heart disease and prognostic importance of clinical and electrocardiographic data (the Italian CNR Multicentre Prospective Study OD1). *Eur Heart J* 1989;10:292–303.

59. Shaw LS, Peterson ED, Shaw LK, et al. Use of prognostic treadmill score in identifying diagnostic coronary disease subgroups. *Circulation* 1998;98:1622–1630.

60. Alexander KP, Shaw LJ, Delong ER, et al. Value of exercise treadmill testing in women. *J Am Coll Cardiol* 1998;32:1657–1664.

61. Boyne TS, Koplan BA, Parsons WJ, et al. Predicting adverse outcome with exercise SPECT technetium-99m sestamibi imaging in patients with suspected or known coronary artery disease. *Am J Cardiol* 1997;79:270–274.

62. Williams MJ, Odabashian J, Lauer MS, et al. Prognostic value of dobutamine echocardiography in patients with left ventricular dysfunction. *J Am Coll Cardiol* 1996;27:132–139.

63. Afridi I, Quinones MA, Zoghbi WA, et al. Dobutamine stress echocardiography: sensitivity, specificity, and predictive value for future cardiac events. *Am Heart J* 1994;127:1510–1515.

64. Hachamaovitch R, Berman DS, Shaw LJ, et al. Incremental prognostic value of myocardial perfusion SPECT for the prediction of cardiac death: differential stratification for risk of cardiac death and myocardial infarction. *Circulation* 1998;97:533–543.

65. Cox JL, Wright LM, Burns RJ. Prognostic significance of increased thallium-201 lung uptake during dipyridamole myocardial scintigraphy: comparison with exercise scintigraphy. *Can J Cardiol* 1995;11:689–694.

66. Wagdy HM, Hodge D, Christian TF, et al. Prognostic value of vasodilator myocardial perfusion imaging in patients with left bundle branch block. *Circulation* 1998;97:1563–1570.

67. Marwick T, D'Hondt AM, Baudhuin T, et al. Optimal use of dobutamine stress for the detection and evaluation of coronary artery disease: combination with echocardiography or scintigraphy, or both? *J Am Coll Cardiol* 1993;22:159–167.

68. Marwick TH. Use of stress echocardiography for the prognostic assessment of patients wtih stable chronic coronary artery disease. *Eur Heart J* 1997;18[Suppl D]:D97–101.

69. Califf RM, Armstrong PW, Carver JR, et al. Stratification of patients into high, medium and low risk subgroups for purposes of risk factor management. *J Am Coll Cardiol* 1996;27:1007–1019.

70. Patterson RE, Eisner RL, Horowitz SF. Comparison of cost-effective-

ness and utility of exercise ECG, single photon emission tomography, positron tomography and coronary angiography for diagnosis of coronary artery disease. *Circulation* 1995;91:51–68.

71. Crawford MH, Bernstein SJ, Deedwania PC, et al. ACC/AHA guidelines for ambulatory electrocardiography: a report of the American College of Cardiology/American Heart Association Task Force on Practice Guidelines (Committee to Revise the Guidelines for Ambulatory Electrocardiography). *J Am Coll Cardiol* 1999;34(3):912–948.

72. Guidelines for perioperative cardiovascular evaluation for noncardiac surgery: a report of the American College of Cardiology/American Heart Association Task Force on Practice Guidelines (Committee on Perioperative Cardiovascular Evaluation for Noncardiac Surgery). *J Am Coll Cardiol* 1996;27:910–948.

73. Chaitman BR, Miller DD. Perioperative cardiac evaluation for noncardiac surgery. Noninvasive cardiac testing. *Prog Cardiovasc Dis* 1998; 40:405–418.

74. Hendel RC, Whitfield SS, Villegas BJ, et al. Prediction of late cardiac events by dipyridamole thallium imaging undergoing elective vascular surgery. *Am J Cardiol* 1992;70:1243–1249.

75. Kloehn GC, O'Rourke RA. Perioperative risk stratification in patients undergoing noncardiac surgery. *S Int Care Med* 1999 (in press).

76. Shaw LJ, Eagle KA, Gersh BJ, et al. Meta analysis of intravenous dipyridamole thallium 201 imaging (1985 to 1994) and dobutamine echocardiography (1991 to 1994) for risk stratification before vascular surgery. *J Amer Coll Cardiol* 1996;27:787–798.

77. Mark DB, Hlatky MD, Harrell FE, et al. Exercise treadmill score for predicting prognosis for coronary artery disease. *Ann Int Med* 1993: 118:689–690.

Imaging in Cardiovascular Disease, edited by Gerald M. Pohost et al., Lippincott Williams & Wilkins, Philadelphia © 2000

CHAPTER 37

Imaging in Acute Coronary Syndromes

Maria G. Sciammarella, Elias H. Botvinick, and Robert A. O'Rourke

Acute coronary syndromes (ACS), unstable angina, non-Q (or non-ST segment elevation) and Q wave myocardial infarction are dynamic processes that have common pathophysiologic mechanisms. A coronary atherosclerotic plaque ruptures and a mural or occlusive thrombus forms, impairing or totally interrupting the perfusion of the myocardium. Consequently, the clinical spectrum of patients arriving in the emergency department with ischemic chest pain at rest ranges from unstable angina, due to partial coronary occlusion, to acute myocardial infarction, due to complete coronary occlusion. The recognition, interruption, and reversal of this dynamic process are the main therapeutic objectives in the acute setting. This chapter will review the application of perfusion imaging and associated or alternative methods in three specific clinical conditions: unstable angina, non-Q wave myocardial infarction, and patients with low-to-intermediate risk of acute myocardial ischemia presenting to the emergency department with chest pain.

UNSTABLE ANGINA AND NON-Q INFARCTION

Background

For many years we have assumed that those with unstable angina have a dynamic syndrome requiring active and early intervention, angiography, and revascularization. However, evidence has been accumulating that many of these patients

M. G. Sciammarella: Division of Cardiology and Nuclear Medicine, University of California–San Francisco, San Francisco, California 94143.

E. H. Botvinick: Division of Cardiology, University of California–San Francisco Medical Center, San Francisco, California 94143.

R. A. O'Rourke: Department of Medicine, Division of Cardiology, University of Texas Health Science Center at San Antonio, San Antonio, Texas 78284.

may respond well to conservative medical management. This relates to the nature of the associated pathophysiology where the condition is generally related to a nonocclusive yet unstable atheromatous process. Several clinical trials (1–4) in patients with both unstable angina and non-Q wave infarction as well as a reported late follow-up study (5) have demonstrated a lack of significant differences in the rate of death or nonfatal myocardial infarction among those treated medically or with revascularization. Since most patients with unstable angina and non-Q infarction can be symptomatically controlled with medical therapy, a sufficient, noninvasive method may permit reduced risk and cost of revascularization in all but those with refractory treatment or with high risk of future events in spite of symptomatic control. Myocardial perfusion imaging may serve this purpose (Fig. 1).

Unstable Angina

See discussion below: Triage of Patients Presenting to the Emergency Department with Chest Pain.

Exercise Testing

Although exercise testing with electrocardiographic recordings can be performed in unstable angina patients who have been stabilized with medical therapy (6–8), it often provides inadequate prognostic value. In these studies, exercise induced ST depression was related to subsequent events, but the lack of induced ischemic ST changes did not indicate a reduced risk and could not differentiate between high- and low-risk groups (6,7). In fact, in the study by Wilcox and co-workers (6), patients without induced ST changes had a 21% event rate.

Mark and co-workers developed and validated the Duke Treadmill Score, which combined elements of exercise test performance, including treadmill time or METS achieved,

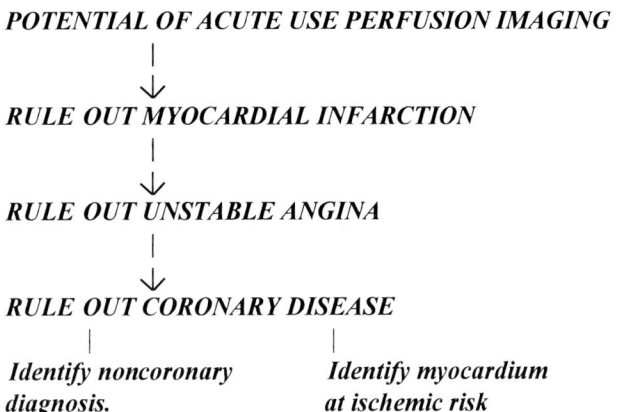

FIG. 1. Potential of acute use of myocardial perfusion imaging.

amount of induced ST segment depression, and severity of the angina to derive a single value related to the likelihood, risk, and outcome of coronary disease. The Duke Treadmill Score has been found to be a reliable method for risk stratification in coronary artery disease (CAD) and was applied for this purpose in the *Unstable Angina: Diagnosis in Management. Clinical Practice Guideline No. 10* (9).

Echocardiography

The utility of echocardiography in identifying patients with unstable angina has now been evaluated in a limited number of studies involving a relatively small number of subjects. Generally, rest echocardiography has been applied. Nixon and co-workers (10) evaluated 19 patients with chest pain and with no prior myocardial infarct (MI) with a rest echocardiogram at admission and before discharge. The authors found that the absence of improvement in wall-motion score between admission and discharge was associated with a more complicated postdischarge course. Stein and co-workers (11) studied 63 patients with unstable angina with an echocardiogram at admission. They reported a sensitivity of 92% and a specificity of 69% for predicting major in-hospital complications.

Studies are generally subjective and qualitative with few studies of risk stratification and outcomes. Risk stratification generally relates to the left ventricular ejection fraction, which is not measured at stress echocardiography, either with exercise or with pharmacologic stress. Regional wall motion abnormalities may persist with prolonged ischemia due to myocardial "stunning" or hibernation and may relate to the size of the "risk zone." However, these postischemic defects are generally short-lived and, unlike perfusion scintigraphy, there is no good evidence of echocardiography sensitivity hours after chest pain resolution. Wall motion abnormalities have been found to resolve rapidly if imaged serially after chest pain presentation with ST abnormalities but no infarction. Such imaging must be done during chest pain or sensitivity falls to unacceptable levels. This is documented

in the studies of Gibler and Jeroudi and co-workers (12,13). In these studies the sensitivity of wall motion abnormalities by echocardiography was reduced in the absence of chest pain, and echocardiography was of little value when done late, at approximately 5 hours after presentation.

Most important is the ability to stratify patients by risk with known or suspected unstable angina. In general, as in unstable angina, the diagnostic and risk stratification abilities of perfusion scintigraphic methods exceed those of echocardiography methods (14,15). Lin and co-workers (16) evaluated the "incremental prognostic value" of 226 consecutive patients with medically treated unstable angina who underwent exercise echocardiography. The stress echocardiogram was not used for decision-making, and 38 patients who were not studied went to revascularization. A positive stress echocardiogram was related to a 9% event rate, but the event rate in those with a normal stress echo study was still 3% per year. This compares to the hard event rate of approximately 1% in patients with coronary disease and negative stress perfusion images (15).

Perfusion Scintigraphy

Among 1,187 patients classified by Shaw et al. (17) with the Duke Treadmill Score to an intermediate coronary risk group (34 to 70%), 84% could be reclassified to low- or high-risk subgroups, 70.3% to low-risk, and 14.2% to high-risk, respectively, when myocardial perfusion scintigraphy was added. So even with the Duke treadmill score, many patients are classified as intermediate risk with ambiguous prognosis and related management decisions.

Several studies present evidence that myocardial perfusion imaging may provide prognostic data that can assess risk in patients with unstable angina and thus guide medical therapy (18) (Fig. 2; see also Color Plate 15 following page 294). Hillert and co-workers (19) found that 15 of 19 patients with reversible Tl-201 perfusion defects developed infarction or recurrent unstable angina as compared to 2 of 18 (P < 0.001) without evidence of redistribution during a 12-week follow-up. Madsen and co-workers (20) used planar thallium imaging in a group of patients with unstable angina who were then followed for 15 months. Of those with a reversible defect on symptom-limited, stress perfusion imaging performed after admission for a noninfarction chest pain syndrome, 21% suffered a nonfatal myocardial infarction or death as opposed to only 3% of patients without reversible perfusion defect during a 14-month follow-up.

Marmur and co-workers (21) evaluated the predictive value of a positive stress electrocardiogram (ECG), stress myocardial perfusion images, ambulatory ECG, and coronary angiogram in 54 patients presenting with unstable angina and found that the only predictor of events was the presence of reversible perfusion defects. Among 52 unstable angina patients studied by Brown and co-workers (22), the only significant predictor of death or myocardial infarction, was the presence of a reversible exercise perfusion defect (22). Those with reversible defects had a hard event rate of 26%, while those with none had a 3% (< 1% per year) rate

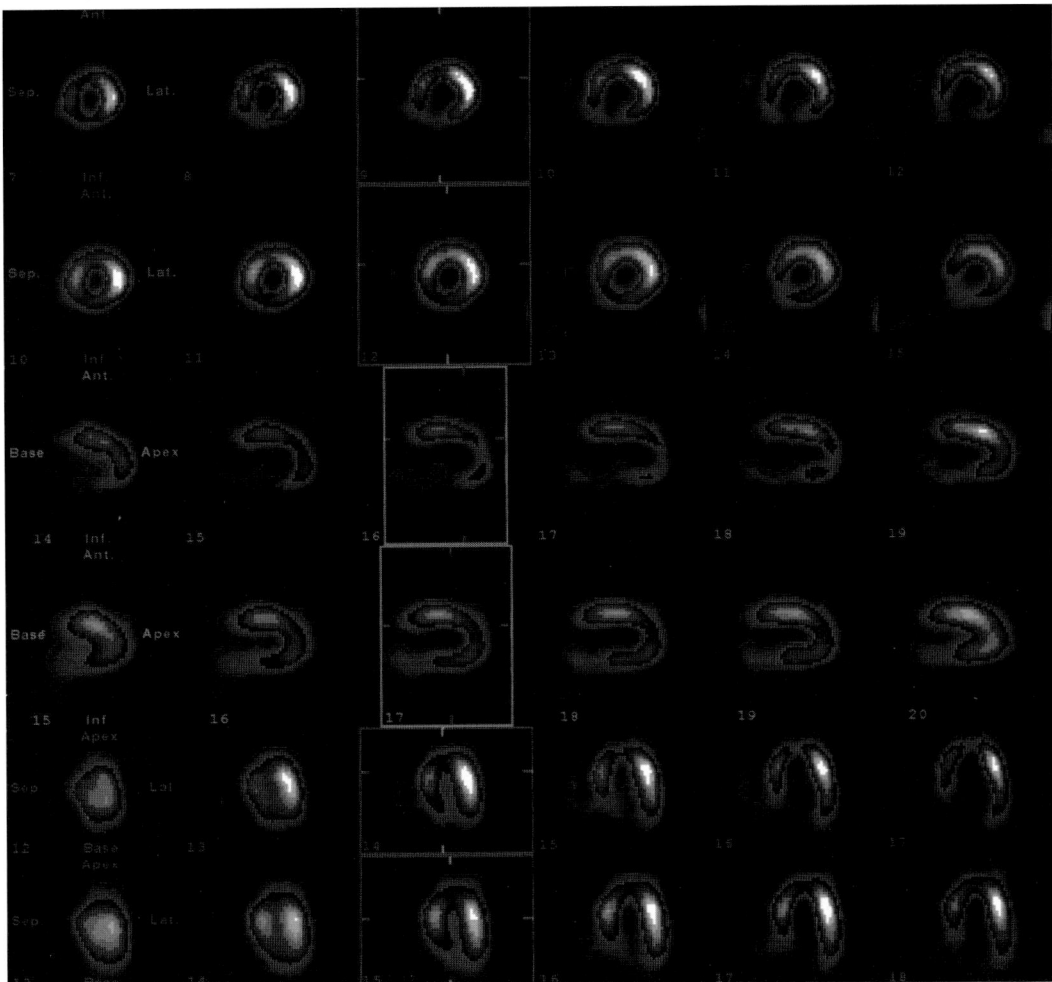

FIG. 2. Unstable angina with extensive myocardium at ischemic risk. Shown are the stress Tl-201 single-photon emission computed tomography myocardial perfusion images in a 74-year-old male with unstable angina and severe coronary artery disease. Short-axis slices **(top)**, vertical long-axis slices **(middle)**, and horizontal long-axis slices **(bottom)**. In each view, the postexercise images are shown above, while those acquired after Tl-201 at rest are displayed below. A severe reversible perfusion defect is evident in the apical, inferior, and posterior-septal left ventricular walls. Coronary angiography demonstrated severe coronary artery disease in the right coronary artery and left circumflex artery vessels. (See also Color Plate 15 following page 294.)

over the 39 months of the study. The stress ECG had no prognostic value in these patients. Stratmann and co-workers (23) found similar results in 126 medically stabilized unstable angina patients. Of 40 patients, 10 patients (25%) with reversible defects suffered hard events, compared to only 1 of 86 (1%) without reversible defects ($P < 0.001$). Again, neither fixed defects nor the stress ECG were predictive of events. These and other workers (24) performed dipyridamole myocardial perfusion imaging with Tc-99m sestamibi prior to discharge in 128 medically treated patients with unstable angina who were at intermediate pretest clinical risk. They were then followed for 16 months plus or minus 11 months. Events, both ''hard'' and ''soft'' were noted in 10% with normal studies and 69% with defects ($P < 0.01$). The perfusion scan was the only independent predictor of outcome. A noninvasive strategy of risk stratification based on

stress perfusion imaging can well separate high- from low-risk subgroups and serve as a basis for selecting those most likely to benefit from aggressive management (Fig. 2). A major advantage of perfusion scintigraphy is its ability to identify abnormalities in the setting of unstable angina even after pain resolution. (See discussion below.)

Guidelines developed under the sponsorship of the Agency of Health Care Policy Research (AHCPR) have indicated a clear role for the use of nuclear testing in patients admitted with unstable angina (9). These guidelines suggest that many such patients can be treated medically after appropriate risk stratification. This strategy is widely supported by the published data and is applied daily in the many patients presenting to the stress testing laboratory for stress test evaluation in the setting of atypical or rest pain (25). Here, although ambiguous at presentation, many of these patients demonstrate scintigraphic evidence of ischemia. Given the nature of their presenting symptoms, the diagnosis of unstable angina must be applied to their syndrome.

The management approach developed under the current AHCPR *Guidelines* recommends referral to catheterization with hemodynamic instability or the failure of medical treatment to control ischemia. Hemodynamically stabilized patients with medically controlled ischemia are candidates for a noninvasive management approach. Within this approach, those patients classified as low risk by clinical factors, patients who probably did not have unstable angina initially, can be managed as outpatients and referred to stress testing within 72 hours of initial admission. Patients at intermediate to high risk who have been stabilized and are free of recurrent angina, evidence of pump dysfunction, or significant ventricular arrthymias are also candidates for this approach. The initial test in these patients would be exercise testing in those patients with a normal resting ECG. Patients with abnormal or uninterpretable rest ECGs or who are on digoxin would undergo exercise stress perfusion imaging.

A table included in the AHCPR *Guidelines* demonstrates the far greater difference in event rate between normal and abnormal stress perfusion scintigrams than between normal and abnormal stress ECGs, attesting to the greater ability of the scintigraphic method to risk stratify these patients. Again, given the lesser accuracy of the exercise ECG and the superior prognostic ability of the scintigraphic method, proceeding directly to stress scintigraphy is a common approach. Those patients unable to exercise would undergo pharmacologic stress perfusion imaging. Certainly dobutamine stress is not well advised in patients with ongoing or recently symptomatic unstable angina who are also potential candidates for stress echocardiographic studies.

The AHCPR *Guidelines* recommend that the decision to apply stress echocardiography or stress perfusion imaging should be guided by local availability and expertise, but present no data regarding the value of stress echocardiography in patients with unstable angina. (See above: Echocardiography in Unstable Angina and below: Triage of Patients Presenting to the Emergency Department with Chest Pain). Data documenting the value of myocardial perfusion imaging to risk stratify and guide management in patients with unstable angina is strong and growing increasingly compelling.

NON-Q WAVE (NON-ST ELEVATION) MYOCARDIAL INFARCTION

See below: Triage of Patients Presenting to the Emergency Department with Chest Pain.

Overview

Non-Q wave myocardial infarctions are generally partial or "incomplete" infarctions. With the expectation that many patients with this condition are at high risk and will experi-

ence a subsequent event, they are generally managed with an invasive strategy.

Stress Echocardiography

Wang and co-workers (26) studied 168 patients with a Q wave and 105 patients with a non-Q wave MI with dobutamine echocardiography. Although patients with both Q and non-Q MI and a negative study had a higher event-free survival than those with a negative test, the event rate was nonetheless substantial: 14.8% in patients with Q-wave MI and 23.8% in patients with non-Q MIs.

Stress Perfusion Scintigraphy

Several clinical trials noted earlier (1–5) in patients with unstable angina or non-Q wave infarction have demonstrated no significant differences in the rate of death or nonfatal myocardial infarction among those treated medically or with revascularization. A noninvasive method may identify a population well treated conservatively without angiography or revascularization. Here, as with unstable angina, myocardial perfusion imaging may well serve as an able "gatekeeper" to angiography.

The TIMI IIIB Trial (5) randomized 1,473 patients with unstable angina or non-Q infarction to an invasive approach with angiography within 48 hours and revascularization as the primary treatment option, or conservative management where medical therapy was primary and angiography with cross-over to the aggressive-invasive management group reserved only for refractory angina and recurrent or significant ischemia on stress ECG or perfusion imaging. The mortality and infarction rate and overall event rate over the first year was 6% and did not differ between those treated with aggressive and conservative management strategies.

The VANQWISH Study (Veterans Affairs Non-Q Wave Infarction Strategies in Hospital) (27) randomized 920 patients with non-Q wave infarction to either an invasive strategy, where patients underwent angiography within 72 hours after diagnosis and were managed based on the findings, or to a conservative, ischemia-guided strategy, where medical therapy was instituted and noninvasive testing with perfusion imaging was applied early to determine if an indication for coronary angiography was present. The number of hard end-points as well as the number of revascularization procedures was significantly higher in the invasive strategy group at hospital discharge, at 1 month and at 1 year. Overall mortality did not differ between groups. This and other studies suggest that most patients with non-Q-wave infarction do not benefit from routine, early invasive management and revascularization. There is no convincing data supporting routine angiography after uncomplicated infarction, non-Q wave infarction, or unstable angina. A noninvasive assessment is particularly applicable in patients who have minimal risk factors or in patients with clear cut unstable angina or non-Q infarction, who are stable with an uncomplicated

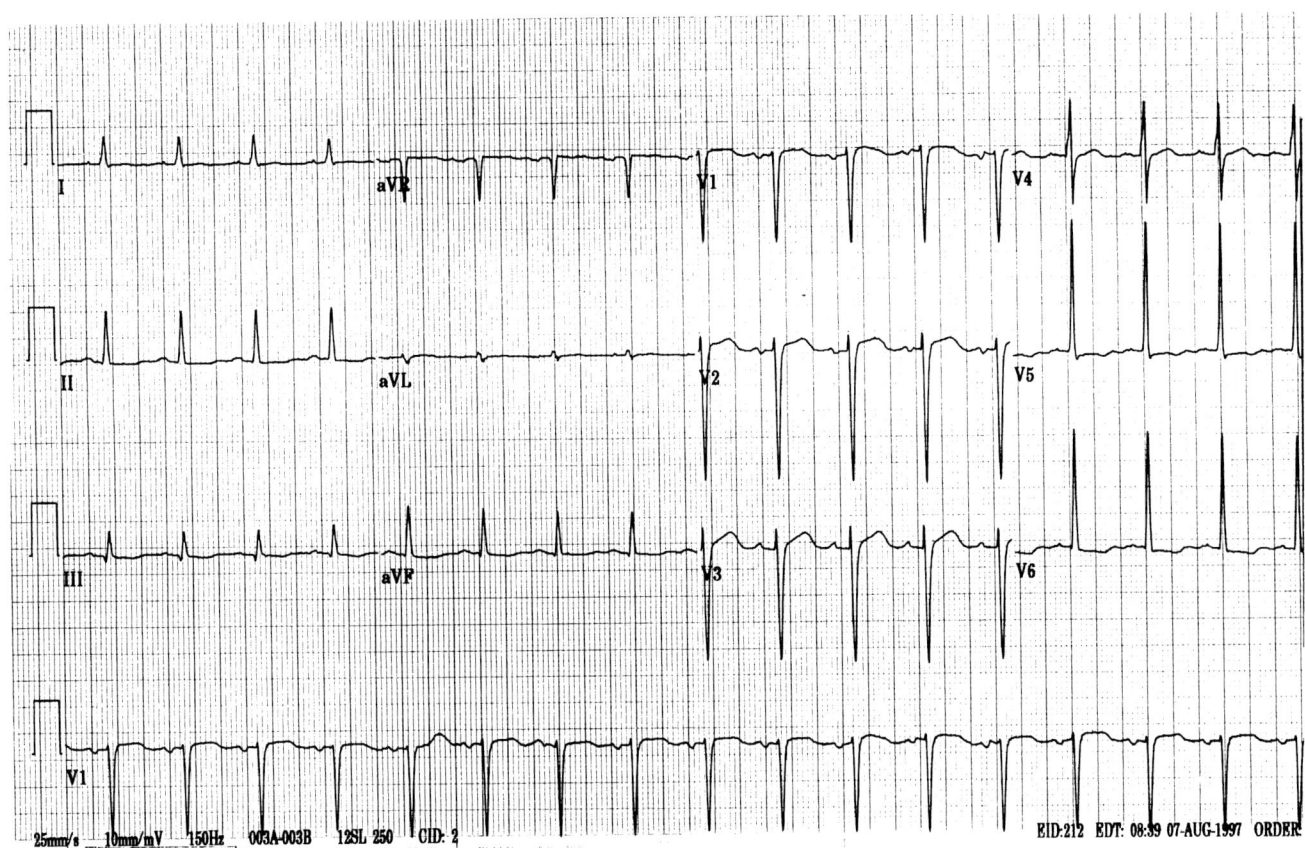

FIG. 3. Non-Q wave myocardial infarction with extensive myocardium at ischemic risk: electrocardiogram. Shown is the electrocardiogram of a 72-year-old man, admitted with non-Q wave myocardial infarction. The patient presented with nocturnal breathlessness that awakened him from sleep and progressed to respiratory failure.

course and respond quickly to medical therapy. In these medically stabilized patients, either exercise or pharmacologic stress testing with perfusion imaging could effectively stratify patients into low- and high-risk subsets (Figs. 3–6; see also Color Plates 16–18 following page 294).

TRIAGE OF PATIENTS PRESENTING TO THE EMERGENCY DEPARTMENT WITH CHEST PAIN

The Problem

Every year nearly 6 million people present to the emergency department in the United States with chest pain or other symptom suggesting the possibility of acute myocardial infarction (AMI). More than half of these, over 3 million people, are admitted to acute care units or to monitored beds with the diagnosis of ROMI (rule out myocardial infarction). However, less than one third of these patients are eventually shown to have had an acute coronary event.

Patients with noncardiac chest pain and a normal or nonspecifically abnormal ECG are generally sent home and those with classic pain and acute ST segment elevation are admitted and treated aggressively. However, patients with suggestive chest pain and normal or nonspecific ECG findings are generally admitted with a low documented event rate, in the range of 10 to 20%. This is the largest patient group admitted with the diagnosis of ROMI (rule out MI)! While these patients have an excellent short-term prognosis, they absorb most of the costs. Thus, providing routine hospital care to patients with low risk of having an acute coronary ischemic syndrome may not be time- or cost-effective (28).

Yet as many as 5 to 10% of patients with an AMI are misdiagnosed and released from the emergency department (29). Patients with a missed diagnosis of AMI have a high mortality rate, and the failure to diagnose and treat AMI patients in the emergency department has a poor outcome (29), accounting for the largest settlements of malpractice lawsuits (30). For these reasons, most physicians treat such patients conservatively and so admit too many patients to the hospital with what eventually proves to be noncardiac chest pain.

The problem and the remaining challenge are the prompt identification of the few high-risk patients not evident within an otherwise relatively low-risk population presenting to the emergency department. The goal is to admit to the hospital only patients with high probability of an ACS and not to admit patients with a low likelihood of an ACS.

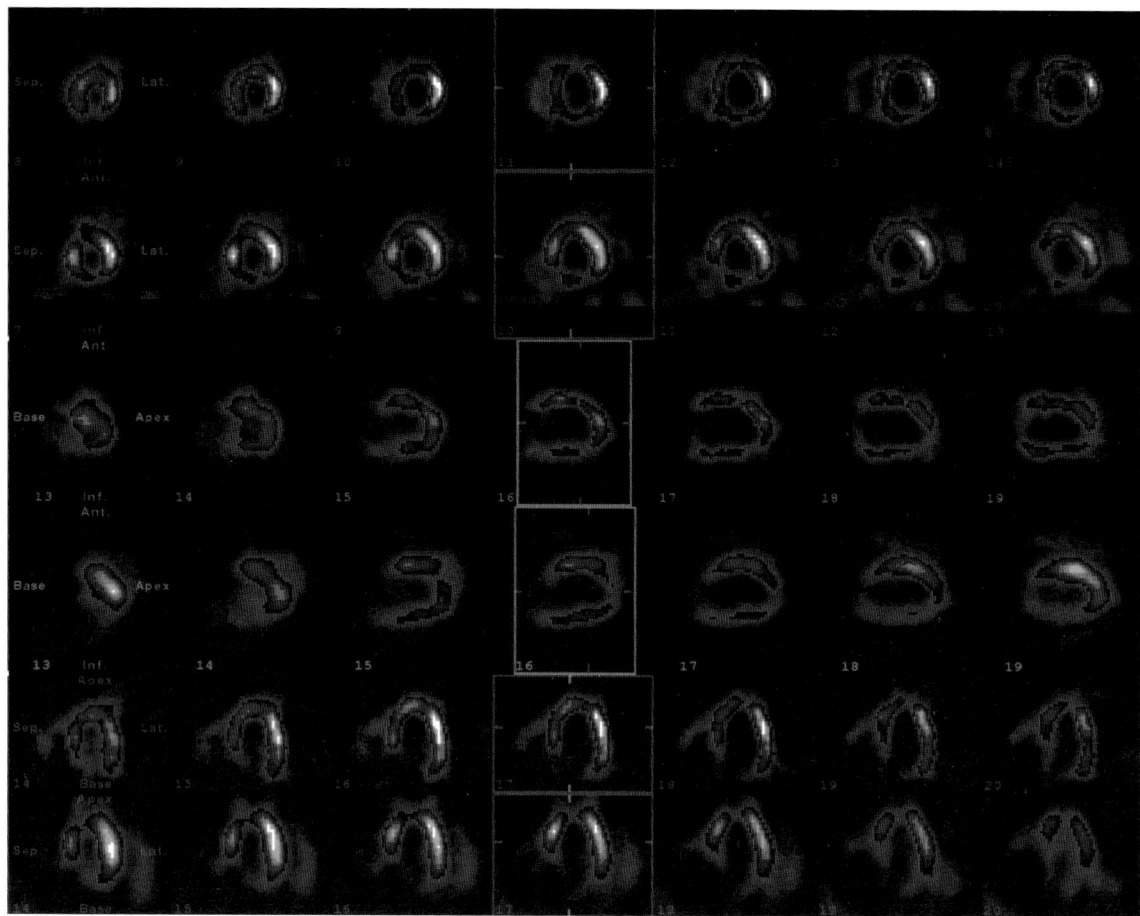

FIG. 4. Non-Q wave myocardial infarction with extensive myocardium at ischemic risk: electrocardiogram (ECG). Shown in the same format as Figure 2 are the dual isotope stress gated single-photon emission computed tomography myocardial perfusion images that belong to the 72-year-old man whose ECG is shown in Figure 3. In each view, the postdipyridamole images are shown **above**, while those acquired earlier, after Tl-201 at rest, are displayed **below**. Evident are left ventricular dilatation associated with inferior, anterior, and septal perfusion defects that show partial reversibility. Concomitant gated images reveal a dilated left ventricle with global left ventricular dysfunction and an ejection fraction of 28%. (See also Color Plate 16 following page 294.) (From Pharmacologic stress in nuclear medicine self-study III: cardiology, with permission.)

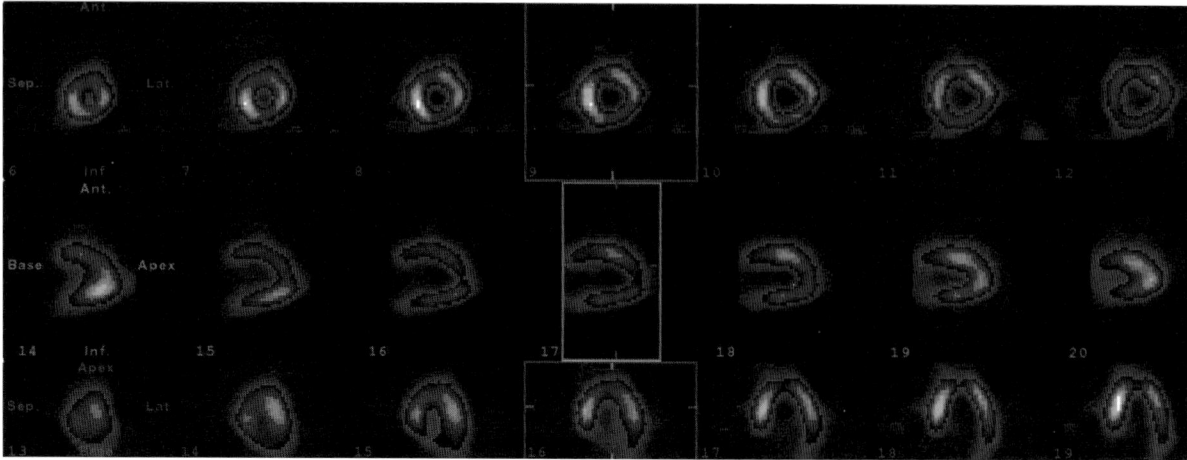

FIG. 5. Non-Q wave myocardial infarction with extensive myocardium at ischemic risk. Shown are the 24-hour delayed 201-TL images performed in the patient presented in Figure 4. The myocardial perfusion is completely normal. The evidence of complete redistribution, viability, and widespread left ventricular dysfunction brought aggressive evaluation and management, with a strong likelihood of functional improvement after revascularization. (See also Color Plate 17 following page 294.) (From Pharmacologic stress in nuclear medicine self-study III: cardiology, with permission.)

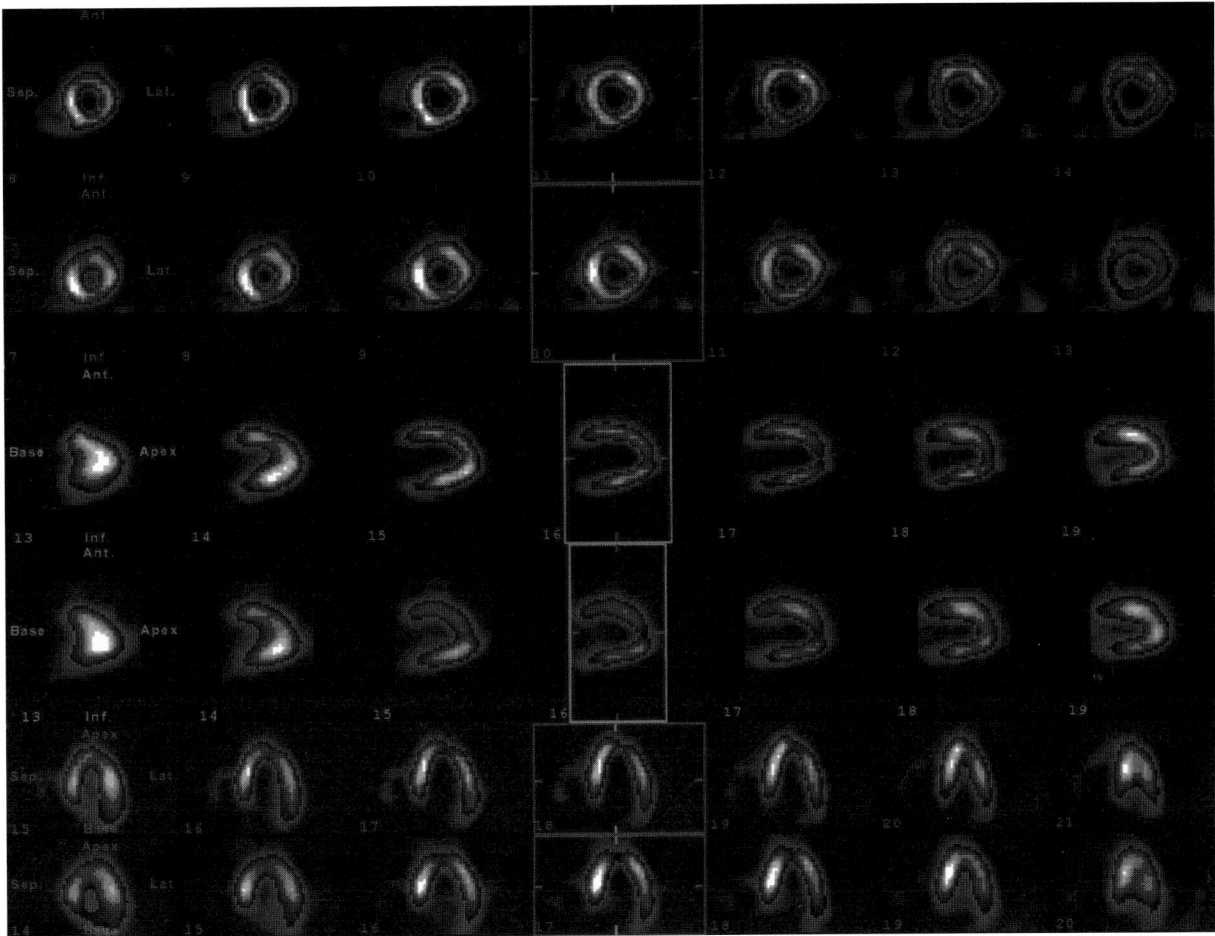

FIG. 6. Non-Q wave myocardial infarction with extensive myocardium at ischemic risk after revascularization procedure. Shown in the same format as Figure 2 are the dual isotope stress gated single-photon emission computed tomography (SPECT) myocardial perfusion images obtained 8 weeks after surgery in the same 72-year-old man presented in Figures 4 and 5. The left ventricle is reduced in size, myocardial perfusion is normal, and the calculated ejection fraction by gated SPECT is 50%. The images were acquired at Stage IV of the Bruce protocol. (See also Color Plate 18 following page 294.) (From Pharmacologic stress in nuclear medicine self-study III: cardiology, with permission.)

The Cost

The overall cost of such management, a long-standing source of income to hospitals, is in the range of $3 to $5 billion annually! With continued reforms and the wider application of managed care, it will be the "providers" who will be paying this bill. It is important then to develop a more efficient and cost-effective triage procedure for patients presenting with ROMI.

The efficient management of this population requires that we reduce delays in therapy, inappropriate admissions, dispositions, and costs. The strategy to achieve the goal is based on appropriate clinical evaluation with an appropriate selection of laboratory and noninvasive tests. From a clinical perspective, it is important to recognize that patients with unstable angina as well as those with acute myocardial infarction have a pathophysiology in common as well as a spectrum of presentation; this must be recognized and then optimally differentiated and risk stratified in patients pre-

senting to the emergency department. Thus, strategies for triage, diagnosis, and treatment of the acute chest pain patient should identify all ACS.

What is really needed is a fast and inexpensive method to determine the presence, site, extent, and severity of ongoing acute myocardial ischemia, evidence of the presence, site, and extent of AMI, and the state of left and right left ventricular function. This evaluation permits identification of myocardium at ischemic risk, likely the most important factor in coronary disease risk stratification. Can a single method provide all this information? Is there any method with a high enough predictive value of a negative test that permits safe patient discharge from the emergency department?

Alternative Diagnostic Approaches

Several diagnostic approaches have been evaluated to improve emergency department triage and to aid management in these patients. These approaches include the application of clinical algorithms and acute testing to telescope diagnosis/evaluation. Among the latter, serum cardiac enzymes analysis, exercise testing, echocardiography, and myocardial perfusion scintigraphy, have been applied alone or in combination.

Clinical Algorithms

Based on population studies relating the resting ECG and available clinical parameters to the likelihood of infarction, this is the simplest approach to estimate the risk of AMI in patients presenting to the emergency department with possible ACS (31). Early during the evaluation it may be difficult to separate unstable angina from non-ST segment elevation MI. Some investigators have demonstrated a correlation between ACS and the character of chest pain and other presenting factors. However, this chest pain is ambiguous and coronary risk factors do not differentiate between individual episodes. Also, many presenting with these characteristic symptoms or signs have no coronary disease (32).

Only 50 to 60% of patients presenting with AMI have diagnostic changes on the ECG. As many as 44% of patients with AMI have a normal ECG or no changes from a previous tracing (33). Although the presence of ST-segment elevation greater than 1 mm on the initial resting ECG, identifies patients with chest pain having a very high likelihood of AMI, its absence does not exclude AMI or significant coronary risk (31). Most patients who present to the emergency department for evaluation of chest pain have symptoms and ECG findings that fall between the extremes of classic high likelihood and very low likelihood groups.

Lee and co-workers (34) designed a multivariate algorithm to identify patients presenting to the emergency department with chest pain and a low risk of having an acute MI. The algorithm was prospectively validated in 2,684 patients for predicting the risk of acute MI based on both clinical and ECG data acquired in the emergency department. Among the 1,727 patients at high risk based on the algorithm, 1,230 (61%) had an AMI or unstable angina. However, of the 957 (36%) patients who were classified as low risk by the algorithm, 771 (81%) did not have abnormal cardiac enzymes or recurrent chest pain during 12 hours of observation and were eligible for discharge from the emergency department. Yet among these 771 patients, 17 (2.1%) had a nonfatal MI, a coronary death, or underwent coronary revascularization soon after triage. One hundred eighty-six patients initially identified as "low-risk" patients were identified later (while still in the emergency department) as requiring hospital admission, and at least 145 of 771 (19%) patients who were identified for early discharge from the emergency department had an ACS as the final diagnosis. Overall, 331 (35%) of those patients assigned to the low-risk group with normal or nondiagnostic ECG had a final diagnosis of either acute myocardial infarction or unstable angina. More recently, Goldman and co-workers (35) have expanded on earlier

work, applying a patient-profile clinical algorithm to predict those needing intensive care among all who present to the emergency department with acute chest pain.

Although, these algorithms separate patients into high- and low-risk patients and identify well patients belonging to clearly high-risk and clearly very low-risk subgroups, there are major omissions. Many with intermediate categorization are indeterminate in diagnosis, risk, and management plan. Algorithms alone are not enough.

Acute Testing to Telescope Diagnosis and Evaluation

Serum Cardiac Enzyme Analysis

Biochemical markers, enzymes that appear in the serum after myocardial cell death, have been considered the "gold standard" for the diagnosis of AMI. They are a particularly important part of the assessment of patients presenting to the emergency department with chest pain and a nondiagnostic ECG. Such a method, if sensitive and timely enough, allows ruling out AMI if the results are negative. Unlike prior methods that provided a retrospective diagnosis without time to act, currently available assays provide adequate and immediate information that could help guide patient management.

Cardiac enzymes including CK isoforms, troponins T and I, and myoglobin offer considerable promise for speeding the diagnosis of AMI and increasing its specificity (36). Although generally not thought to be released with unstable angina, this is, in fact, a clinical diagnosis and can be related to a small enzyme rise. The diagnostic accuracy of these enzymes depends on their individual kinetics and on the time after the onset of the event (chest pain) at which the sample is drawn. For all cardiac enzymes, however, the negative predictive value of the initial sample often is inadequate to rule out AMI, and the method overall may not be optimal in excluding ACSs.

Long experience reveals the gross lack of specificity of total CK values and less so of CK-MB. However, CK-MB requires 8 to 12 hours to evolve after symptoms for its highest sensitivity, and tissue specificity is an issue. Again, CK-MB mass and troponin T do not achieve their maximum negative predictive value to ROMI until 12 hours after the onset of chest pain.

Both troponins T and I represent a new generation of cardiac biochemical markers that may provide an important additional clinical tool for the assessment of the ACS. Cardiac levels of troponin T and I seem to be highly sensitive and specific for myocardial necrosis, to increase quickly, and to remain elevated for prolonged periods. Each of these may improve the ability to detect myocardial infarction, but the earlier peak of troponin I makes it more optimal for application in emergency department triage. A sensitivity of 100% has been reported for troponin T in the diagnosis of AMI, but with a low specificity of 78%, compared with 92% for creatine kinase. However, when unstable angina was excluded, the specificity improved to 97%. Several studies have demonstrated that patients who have acute chest pain, a nondiagnostic ECG, and serum elevation of either troponin I or troponin T have a worse outcome compared to those with no enzyme elevation. Patients with an elevated troponin level but normal MBCK levels are generally considered to have a non-Q wave MI.

Myoglobin is a relatively small protein that is abundant in muscle cytosol, both skeletal and myocardial. It is released early after tissue injury and may be elevated as early as 1 hour after myocardial injury and often peaks within 3 to 5 hours. It is cleared rapidly by the kidneys, and levels may return to baseline in 6 to 12 hours. Myoglobin has an 89% negative predictive value for ruling out AMI after 6 hours of chest pain onset, but its accuracy as a marker of necrosis decreases rapidly after 7 hours; it may not be diagnostic in AMI patients who present late. However, myoglobin is not a cardiac specific marker and has a relatively low specificity especially in patients with renal insufficiency.

Blood samples taken earlier than 8 hours from the onset of chest pain have a reduced likelihood of enzyme elevation. Patients presenting early with AMI or unstable angina and a nondiagnostic ECG must be identified and differentiated from those whose chest pain is of noncardiac origin, as must those with unstable angina who never release enzymes.

Even when considered together, clinical evaluation, the ECG, and serum enzymes have limitations and restricted accuracy for determining those patients with ACS among the many patients who present to the emergency department with chest pain.

Exercise Testing

The group to be targeted by this and other diagnostic approaches includes patients in whom the suspicion of CAD is high enough to consider admission to the hospital but low enough so the decision is questionable. Exercise testing in the emergency department has been used to triage ROMI patients with the diagnosis of ACS by identification of exercise-induced ischemia (37,38).

Lewis and co-workers (37) performed early treadmill testing in 93 nonconsecutive low-risk patients admitted to the hospital from the emergency department to ROMI with interpretable rest ECG. A modified Bruce protocol was performed immediately on admission, with a median time of less than 1 hour. Of 12 patients, 6 with a positive, ischemic exercise ECG had significant coronary artery disease by angiography. Among 81 patients with negative ($n = 59$) or nondiagnostic ($n = 22$) exercise ECGs, 44 were discharged immediately; while 37 of these 81 patients, (26 with a negative test) were observed for 24 or more hours. There were 2 noncardiac deaths, and 1 patient had a late and unsuspected AMI after negative testing in this initial study group. The exercise test identified most patients with events, as well as a low-risk subgroup, which could be discharged or admitted.

However, this study had no control subjects, and a select population was studied with a very low infarct rate.

The same group (38) conducted a prospective study in 212 heterogeneous low-risk emergency department chest pain patients, as indicated by clinical and ECG criteria. Immediate exercise testing was performed before serum cardiac enzymes were measured. Twenty-eight (13%) patients had positive exercise ECGs, of whom 23 had further evaluation that revealed evidence of CAD in 13 (57%). One hundred twenty-five (59%) patients had negative exercise test results and 59 (28%) had nondiagnostic tests. All patients with negative stress tests and 93% with nondiagnostic exercise tests were discharged directly from the emergency department. Thirty-day follow-up was done in 201 (95%) patients and revealed no mortality in any patient. Stress testing was said to be related to early discharge of many with negative tests and was, therefore, highly cost-effective as a triage measure in this population.

What is the value of acute exercise testing in such a low likelihood population with not a single diagnosed infarction? In this group, the simple decision to exercise the patient acutely, without waiting for enzyme results, was likely enough to exclude AMI and permit an out-patient evaluation.

In another study, Gibler and co-workers (39) performed exercise testing in 791 patients presenting to the emergency department with chest pain. Negative enzymes ruled out AMI. Among 52 patients with coronary artery disease, 14 were abnormal for a sensitivity of 29%, a specificity of 99%, and a negative predictive value of 98%, and a poor positive predictive value. Here, the method missed many with acute coronary syndromes.

Krasuski and co-workers (40) recently demonstrated the cost-effectiveness of weekend and holiday treadmill testing to triage 135 emergency department chest pain patients who were of high enough likelihood that they would generally need admission if stress testing were unavailable. They were compared with a "low or very low" likelihood group of 182 patients as defined by Goldman and co-workers (35) and managed with outpatient elective stress testing within 48 hours of their emergency department visit. Eighty-eight of 90 (98%) with negative tests and 28 of 39 (72%) with equivocal tests were discharged on the same day as testing. Six patients, 2 among 28 (4%) with "consistent but not diagnostic" stress ECGs and 4 of 6 (66%) with frankly abnormal tests, went on to angiography and revascularization. No patient died in the 6-month follow-up, and outcomes were otherwise similar in this higher risk compared to the parallel low-risk group followed.

In a diverse and ambiguous group of chest pain patients presenting for ROMI, would a negative exercise test be enough to exclude disease? In some studies, the answer is an emphatic affirmative, in others, it is not. Clearly, the implications of Bayes theorem have as much or more to do with the outcome of studies as does related test accuracy.

However, we have more experience with stress testing and stress imaging than that simply presented in reference to patients presenting for emergency department triage. We

TABLE 1. *Ideal triage method*

Analytic characteristics	Biologic characteristics
Simple assay	High myocardial "concentration"
Rapid turnaround	Not present in other tissues
High precision	Not detected in normal
Quantitative	Released rapidly in response to injury
	Persists for a reasonable duration
	Released in proportion to injury
	Little to no population variation
	Clinical characteristics
	Very sensitive and specific
	Optimal for diagnosis, prognosis
	Can influence therapy and outcomes

know that in many clinical settings, imaging has been shown to be superior to stress testing alone for diagnosis, and, generally, for prognosis in coronary disease.

Either exercise or pharmacologic stress associated with echocardiography or myocardial perfusion scintigraphy may be more appropriate in some cases for patient's triage and management. Also, rest imaging may be helpful in some patients (Table 1).

Rest Echocardiography

See above: Echocardiography in Unstable Angina.

Several studies have documented a high sensitivity and specificity of rest echocardiography in detecting AMI (41)). When rest echocardiography was applied in patients with known ACS in a series of studies (40), it demonstrated wall motion abnormalities in 89 to 100% of patients with transmural MI and in approximately 79 to 86% of patients with a non-Q MI. However, overall, there was difficulty recognizing wall motion abnormalities with small transmural or non-Q MIs, diffuse wall motion abnormalities were nonspecific for CAD. It may be of value for rapid discrimination to assess the cause of ambiguous ST abnormalities in patients presenting without prior infarction and prior normal ECG or in patients with a high likelihood of AMI and ongoing pain. However, in the larger population that we evaluate in our emergency department, the findings are not supportive of its wide application. Studies have applied echocardiography to the evaluation of patients presenting with possible ACS with varying criteria.

Sasaki and co-workers (42) performed rest echocardiography in 46 emergency department patients who were admitted for chest pain with normal ECG and CK. Patients with prior MI, significant valvular disease, cardiomyopathy, prior cardiac surgery, and left bundle-branch block (LBBB) were excluded. Eight of the 18 patients undergoing echocardiography during chest pain had wall motion abnormalities. Six of the 8 patients with positive echocardiographic findings actually had AMIs. One of the 10 patients without wall mo-

tion abnormalities also had an AMI. Of the 28 patients who had undergone echocardiography after chest pain relief, 10 had abnormal studies and 18 had normal studies. Eight of the 10 with abnormal studies had AMIs, and none of the 18 with normal studies had AMIs. Thus, in this *small selective* series, sensitivity of echocardiography for detecting myocardial infarction was 86%, and the specificity was 82% during chest pain but 100% and 90%, respectively, in the absence of ongoing chest pain. A positive study during pain or after pain relief correlated with the development of AMI, but a negative study finding after pain relief did not detect underlying CAD in a significant percentage; a negative study even during pain did not eliminate the possibility of AMI.

Peels and co-workers (43) studied 43 patients with ongoing pain and nondiagnostic ECGs in the emergency department. Again, patients with prior MI, with known CAD, or who had revascularization procedures were excluded as well as patients whose ultrasound window was technically inadequate. Sensitivity for ACS was 88% (22 of 25) with a specificity of 78% (14 of 18), and, for AMI, it was 92% (12 of 13) and 53% (16 of 30), respectively. Regional asynergy could not distinguish ischemia from infarction. Although these results are encouraging, the fraction of emergency department patients to which these results are applicable is likely small, since they best apply to those without technical limitations or to those with a positive coronary history who have ongoing chest pain when studied.

Sabia and co-workers (44) applied two-dimensional echocardiography in 180 high-risk chest pain patients within 4 hours of presentation to the emergency department. Three observers blinded to the clinical data, ECG, and enzymes read the studies. Adequate studies were achieved in 94%. Diagnostic criteria included only segmental wall motion abnormalities, in a coronary distribution. Among 30 patients with AMI, 29 had adequate studies, and 27 (93%) of these had segmental wall motion abnormalities, and only 9 with diagnostic ECG changes. Of the 60 patients without regional or global left ventricular dysfunction, 2 patients (4%) had AMI. Fortuitously, none of the 22 (13%) patients with global dysfunction and without regional abnormalities had AMI. Of the 87 patients with regional wall motion abnormalities, 31% experienced AMIs. If global left ventricular systolic dysfunction was excluded, the sensitivity of segmental wall motion abnormalities was 93%, with a limited specificity, 49%, in part because of the 31 patients with previous MI, and negative and positive predictive values of 100%, and 31%, respectively. Among patients not admitted, 2 had AMI. The study demonstrates the nonspecificity and problematic reproducibility of the method for evaluation of the presence and etiology of wall motion abnormalities, well demonstrated in other settings (45).

Kontos and co-workers (46) studied 140 patients with possible ACS by rest echocardiography in the emergency department. Wall motion abnormalities were evident in 20 of 21 (95%) of those patients with AMI. There were no wall motion abnormalities in 43, 1 with an AMI, and 5 with sig-

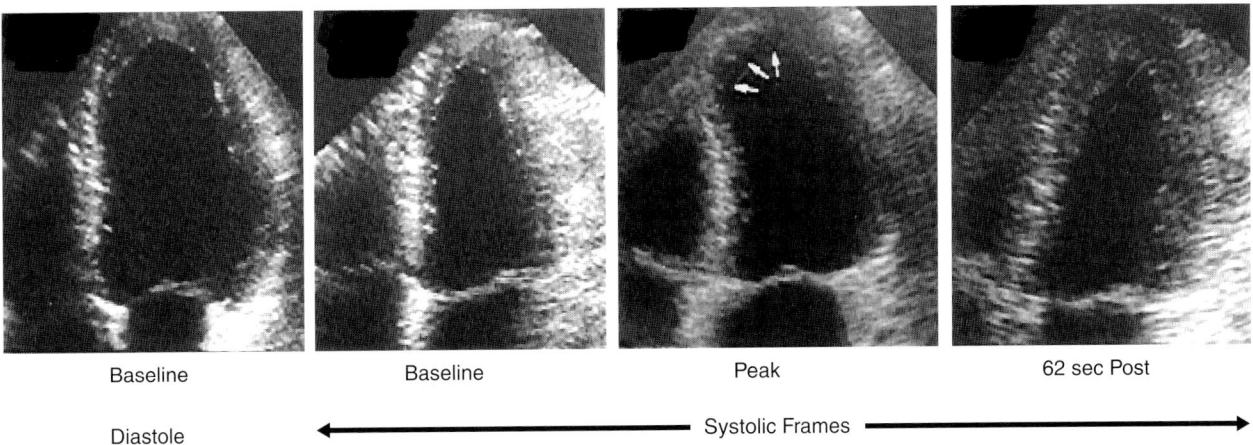

Baseline   Baseline   Peak   62 sec Post

Diastole   ←————————— Systolic Frames —————————→

FIG. 7. Stress echocardiography. Serial apical four-chamber views in a 51-year-old man who underwent supine bicycle exercise. Discrete regional asynergy is noted in the distal septum and apex consistent with ischemia in the left anterior descending coronary artery distribution. The regional systolic wall motion abnormality disappeared at 62 seconds postexercise. Patient had a 75% stenosis on the proximal left anterior descending artery; no other significant disease was noted. (Courtesy of Dr. Miguel Zabalgoitia and Dr. Robert O'Rourke, Universtiy of Texas, Health Science Center, San Antonio, Texas.)

nificant coronary stenoses or abnormal stress myocardial perfusion images. The sensitivity for predicting AMI or significant coronary artery disease was 84% with a negative predictive value of 82%. Several patients with AMI and unstable angina were missed.

In the emergency department, the criteria of echocardiographic wall motion abnormalities must be applied to a range of diagnostic categories and will be less useful, although rest echocardiography in the emergency department showed initial promise, it is insensitive for distinguishing ischemia in the absence of gross wall motion abnormalities and nonspecific for the diagnosis of AMI. When seeking ACS among ambiguous patients in the emergency department setting, echocardiography has a false-negative rate that precludes discharging all patients with negative findings. In addition, abnormal studies remain nonspecific due to prior infarction or noncoronary causes of ventricular dysfunction.

Stress Echocardiography

See above: Echocardiography in Unstable Angina.

Trippi and co-workers (47) reported the results of dobutamine stress echocardiography applied by the on-call ultrasonographer and emergency department staff to triage patients presenting to the emergency department with chest pain and a low MI and coronary likelihood, with normal rest wall motion, a normal ECG and initial CK-MB mass. The study was then transmitted to the on-call cardiologist who read the study on a laptop computer. The discharge of 41 patients after a normal dobutamine stress echocardiogram brought a decrease in costs from $1,580 to $665 without adverse events at 30 days. Colon and co-workers (48) studied 75 emergency department patients with nondiagnostic electrocardiograms by exercise (64%) or dobutamine stress

echocardiography (36%) after a 4-hour observation period. All 5 patients with coronary disease were identified with abnormal stress wall motion.

While limited reports indicate some efficacy, the poor reproducibility of the method (45), the frequent insufficiency of the dobutamine effect (50) and the problematic nature of dobutamine stress in the setting of ACS make this the less desirable method of pharmacologic stress. Beyond this, several studies demonstrate the poor ability of the method to risk stratify coronary patients and differentiate risk between those with positive and negative echocardiographic findings. The prognostic information obtained with treadmill or bicycle exercise is better, particularly the latter, which images segmental motion at peak exercise (Fig. 7).

MYOCARDIAL PERFUSION SCINTIGRAPHY

Overview

Rest myocardial perfusion imaging is now being included in the algorithm for the emergency department triage and management of ACS (Fig. 1). Myocardial perfusion scintigraphy is a valuable and appealing tool for evaluating patients presenting to the emergency department with chest pain because it allows assessment of the full dynamic process of ACS, early in the cascade of ischemic events, enabling detection of ischemia prior to evolving myocardial infarction, and providing key data for early risk assessment and therapeutic decisions.

Tl-201 Rest Imaging

Several studies documented the usefulness of myocardial perfusion imaging with thallium-201 (Tl-201) at rest to evaluate myocardial perfusion and viability in patients with acute ischemic coronary syndromes. Several other studies have demonstrated myocardial defects on rest ^{201}Tl images acquired with injection during the postpain state, without evidence of acute ST-segment changes, or old or recent MI in patients with unstable angina pectoris. The Tl-201 method was successfully applied to evaluate the extent of myocardium at ischemic risk and the prognosis of patients with unstable angina, and it has been used in variant angina and to determine the cause of rest ECG abnormalities as well.

Wackers and co-workers were the first to demonstrate the ability of myocardial perfusion imaging to risk stratify in the acute setting. From 1976 to 1979, the authors published several studies demonstrating that planar imaging with thallium-201 can be a sensitive predictor of myocardial infarction (50,51) and unstable angina (52). Wackers et al. (50) imaged 200 MI patients with planar Tl- 201 within the first 24 hours of symptom onset. Sensitivity was 82% (165/200), but this value decreased over time. Sensitivity was 100% (44 of 44) within the first 6 hours, but decreased to 79% when imaging was performed later than 48 hours. Early sensitivity was in part related to early postinfarction ischemia. The same group (52) imaged 98 unstable angina patients with planar Tl-201 imaging during a pain-free period within 18 hours of chest pain resolution. Tl-201 planar sensitivity was 76% for identifying patients with a complicated hospital course. But when image findings were combined with electrocardiographic findings, a poor outcome was predicted with 94% sensitivity. Again, the incidence of abnormal perfusion studies decreased as the time after resolution of pain increased. These same authors (51) subsequently evaluated the risk stratification capability of Tl-201 planar imaging in patients with no evidence of prior MI and normal or nondiagnostic ECG who were admitted to rule out MI. Two hundred and three patients were studied within 10 hours after their last chest pain episode. All 34 patients with infarction and 27 (58%) of those with unstable angina had abnormal myocardial perfusion studies, whereas none of the 98 patients with stable angina or atypical chest pain had abnormal myocardial perfusion studies. Of the 47 patients with diagnosis of unstable angina, 27 had an abnormal myocardial perfusion study; however, in the subset of patients presenting with unstable angina that progressed to myocardial infarction, the sensitivity was 100%.

In a prospective study at one institution, Van der Wieken and co-workers (53) studied 149 patients with acute chest pain and nondiagnostic ECGs to evaluate acute Tl-201 planar imaging as a decision tool. Patients were injected as soon as possible after presentation, and no patient was injected longer than 12 hours after resolution of pain. Myocardial perfusion defects were present in 57 patients and acute MI developed in 35. Among the 149 patients with normal or equivocal ECG, only 1 of the 79 with normal myocardial perfusion study developed AMI. When equivocal and normal scans were reported together, the sensitivity was very high (97% with a relatively high specificity of 79% and positive predictive value of 54% for the detection of AMI).

Also, for the detection of coronary artery disease, they reported a sensitivity of 96%, with a specificity of 79%, and negative and positive predictive values of 97% and 71%, respectively.

Other workers reported that the rest Tl-201 study could be used to distinguish between an AMI and unstable angina in patients admitted with prolonged chest pain. The patients were injected with Tl-201 in the emergency department, and imaging was acquired shortly thereafter. Patients in whom AMI was ruled out demonstrated resting defects that had shown delayed redistribution. Patients who fulfilled the criteria for myocardial infarction had persistent perfusion defects on serial scans. Freeman and co-workers (54) performed quantitative planar Tl-201 studies in 66 patients with unstable angina. Injection of the tracer was performed at a mean of 5.6 hours after chest pain. Perfusion abnormalities were seen in 83% of patients with coronary stenoses of more than or equal to 50% or greater but in only half of patients with less severe disease. The sensitivity of Tl-201 defects or washout abnormalities for detection of significant coronary stenosis was 67% with specificity of 59%. Likewise, 11 of 18 patients (61%) who had in-hospital cardiac events had resting Tl-201 defects, whereas only 8 of 25 (32%) without cardiac events had resting perfusion defects.

Hakki and co-workers (55) also demonstrated a correlation between the degree of stenosis and the presence of perfusion defects on rest Tl-201 imaging when patients were injected while pain free.

Brown and co-workers (56) performed rest/redistribution planar Tl-201 scintigrams in 65 patients with anginal syndromes and demonstrated reversible perfusion defects in all patients with rapidly progressive angina.

Even though Tl-201 is an excellent perfusion tracer, the available data indicate a relatively poor diagnostic accuracy in the setting of AMI, or unstable angina, with a particularly low specificity.

Rest Myocardial Perfusion Imaging with Tc-99m Based Agents

The properties of generator production, linear uptake with coronary blood flow, and myocardial uptake with minimal redistribution have made Tc-99m labeled perfusion tracers (sestamibi and tetrosfosmin) very attractive diagnostic tools for the assessment of AMI and ACSs (Table 3). An accurate reflection of coronary blood flow coupled with favorable physical imaging properties permits using these compounds to measure the acute area at risk and, subsequently, the index event infarct size in patients with AMI. The accuracy of these measurements has been validated in both animal and clinical studies (57–60). These studies (61,62) reveal that when Tc-99m-sestamibi is injected during coronary occlusion, perfusion imaging accurately defines the risk area for several hours after the initial injection, even when reperfusion occurs. The limited redistribution of Tc-99m sestamibi allows the immediate injection of the radiotracer during or

TABLE 2. *Echocardiography for the triage of patients presenting to the Emergency Department with chest pain*

Advantages	Disadvantages
Real time	WMA nonspecific for AMI or
Valvular, hemodynamics	CAD
Cost?	Insensitive to small MI
	WMA does not correlate with
	MI or ischemia size
	Cannot differentiate MI from
	ischemia
	Depends on short-lived
	"stunning"
	Technical inadequate studies
	Qualitative analysis
	Reproducibility
	Limited, difficult, and possibly
	dangerous, pharmacologic
	stress method
	Availability/logistics

AMI, acute myocardial infarct; *CAD*, coronary artery disease; *MI*, myocardial infarct; *WMA*, wall motion abnormality.

soon after symptom resolution, with accurate imaging still possible late after chest pain subsides or on patient stabilization, without interfering with immediate treatment. This forms the physiologic rationale for the use of Tc-99m sestamibi in ACSs, from unstable angina to AMI. Tc-99m sestamibi can be administered intravenously in the emergency department during the episode of chest pain and imaged later. Thus, Tc-99m sestamibi imaging at rest is suitable for distinguishing patients with ACSs from those with atypical rest chest pain of noncardiac origin. Therefore, acute myocardial perfusion imaging is now being included more frequently in the algorithm for the triage and management of ACS with very promising results. The study by Christian and co-workers (59) demonstrates the value of the method

TABLE 3. *Perfusion scintigraphy for the triage of patients presenting to the Emergency Department with chest pain*

Advantages	Disadvantages
Perfusion + Function − Single rest study	Costs?
Perfusion more sensitive than wall motion	Availability/ Logistics
	Differentiate acute and remote MI
Reproducibility	Not real time
Defects persist long after clinical ischemia	"Radiation"
Quantitative (normal data base)	
Quantitative relation to MI, ischemia and prognosis, as continuous variables	
Choice of pharmacologic stress method—dilator stress sensitive	
Rare inadequate study	

MI, myocardial infarct.

in identifying patients with acute coronary occlusion not recognized by ECG changes; the study by Gibbons and co-workers (60) demonstrates the value of the method when applied serially to assess the effect of intervention with reperfusion therapy.

Two studies (61,62) focused on the diagnostic capability of resting Tc-99m sestamibi single-photon emission computed tomography (SPECT) myocardial perfusion imaging to detect significant coronary artery disease in patients with unstable angina. Gregoire and co-workers (61) studied 45 patients with clinical suspicion of unstable angina. Tc-99m sestamibi was injected during chest pain and imaged 6 hours later. Those patients with an abnormal scan had a repeat study at rest 24 to 48 hours later while pain free. The sensitivity and specificity of studies performed during pain was 96% and 79%, respectively. Injection while asymptomatic was associated with a lower sensitivity of 35% and slightly higher specificity of 84%.

Bilodeau and co-workers (62) compared the results of Tc-99m sestamibi SPECT imaging with injection during active chest pain and when pain free with ECG data and coronary anatomy in a selected group of 45 patients with acute chest pain and suspected unstable angina. The sensitivity for coronary artery disease detection with Tc-99m sestamibi SPECT imaging was 96% when injected during chest pain, with a specificity of 79%. This was significantly higher than the 65% sensitivity of ECG done during chest pain. Even when patients were pain free at the time of Tc-99m sestamibi injection, myocardial perfusion imaging demonstrated improved sensitivity compared with the rest ECG. Additionally, Tc-99m sestamibi SPECT imaging was able to localize coronary disease, and the location of the perfusion defect correlated with the most severe coronary lesion in 88% of cases.

This study was confirmed by Varetto and co-workers (63) who used Tc-99m sestamibi SPECT imaging to assess 64 emergency department patients at low-to-moderate risk with a normal ECG. Tc-99m sestamibi SPECT imaging provided a sensitivity of 100%, with a specificity of 92%. None of the patients with normal perfusion imaging subsequently was shown to have evidence of coronary artery disease or had a cardiac event over an 18-month follow-up. Among the 30 patients with abnormal Tc-99m sestamibi SPECT studies, 13 had AMI and 14 unstable angina, and 6 cardiac events occurred during the follow-up. The negative predictive value for both short-term and long-term events was 100%. Another important finding in this study is that among the 14 patients with unstable angina and abnormal Tc-99m sestamibi SPECT studies, 12 had complete normalization on follow-up imaging 24 hours after the acute event. This specific finding demonstrated that acute sestamibi myocardial imaging is a useful tool for the identification of the ACS without AMI in this population. Also, the study reported that 11 of 14 patients with unstable angina were injected with the radionuclide a mean of 4.7 hours after chest pain remission, suggesting the existence of a period of time after an ischemic event during which diagnostic accuracy is not jeopardized.

Hilton and co-workers (64) assessed the risk stratification and prognostic potential of acute sestamibi myocardial perfusion imaging in 102 patients presenting to the emergency department with typical angina, and normal or nondiagnostic ECGs. Those with a history of MI were excluded. All patients were injected during chest pain. Image findings were interpreted as normal, equivocal, or clearly abnormal. Those patients with coronary events could not be separated from those with any coronary events on the basis of age, gender, and type of pain, coronary risk factors, the physical examination, or rest ECG. Overall, only 1 patient (1.5%) among 70 with a normal scan had a cardiac event, bypass surgery. Thus, the predictive value of a negative test was 98%. Among 17 patients with a positive scan, 12 had cardiac events, and the positive predictive value was 71%. However, among 34 patients with normal images and subsequent stress testing and/or coronary angiography, none had coronary disease and all were event free after 18 months. Multivariate regression analysis demonstrated that an abnormal sestamibi study was the only predictor of an adverse cardiac event ($P = 0.009$). An abnormal myocardial perfusion study had a sensitivity of 94% and specificity of 83%, with overall accuracy of 88% for the prediction of all cardiac events, and the study had sensitivity of 100% with specificity of 78% for AMI. The emergency department imaging study separated 85% of the population into a low (1 to 2%) and high (70%) risk group. Furthermore, its high specificity permitted reduction of admission based on image findings. In these two studies (63,64), a normal rest emergency department sestamibi myocardial perfusion study had a benign long-term outcome with no events in 166 patients followed for 3 to 18 months (65).

Kjoller and co-workers (66) studied the risk stratification potential of acute myocardial perfusion imaging in patients within 2 hours of chest pain resolution; they concluded that the technique was not useful. However, this study differs from the studies discussed above because the study was performed in a high-risk population with a high incidence of a prior MI (40%) or acute MI (54%), with a portable planar imaging camera in the coronary unit. AMI was the only end point considered; thus the sensitivity was high (96%), and the specificity extremely low (8%). Among 62 patients without AMI, 57 had an abnormal imaging study. Thus, the low specificity is clearly associated with the end point, AMI, because many perfusion defects seemed to be related to acute myocardial ischemia in the absence of AMI. Overall, the data in these studies (61–66) demonstrated that acute rest when positive Tc-99m sestamibi has a high sensitivity for detecting AMI and an excellent negative predictive value when normal.

Recently, the risk stratification of acute myocardial perfusion imaging has been evaluated with Tc-99m tetrosfosmin. In a multicenter study, Wackers and co-workers (67) demonstrated the benefits of a normal rest tetrofosmin SPECT perfusion image in 357 patients presenting to the emergency department with chest pain and a normal or nondiagnostic ECG. Patients were injected during or within 6 hours of symptom cessation. Follow-up evaluation was performed for an additional 30 days after hospital discharge. SPECT, as well as cardiac events, were reviewed in a blinded manner and were not available to the admitting physician. Two hundred and four studies (57%) were normal, and 153 (43%) were abnormal. Of the 20 (6%) patients with AMI, 18 had abnormal images, and a sensitivity of 90%, whereas only 2 had normal images, with a negative predictive value of 99%. Multiple logistic regression analysis demonstrated abnormal SPECT imaging to be the best predictor of AMI and significantly better than clinical data. Although the incidence of AMI with negative perfusion study was higher than that reported in nonblinded studies, a negative study indicated a small infarction and was associated with good prognosis (68).

The risk stratification and prognostic value of AMI with the addition of simultaneous functional evaluation from rest gated Tc-99m sestamibi SPECT has been assessed (69). Nicholson and co-workers (70) reported the data from 12 studies performed in the acute setting with gated rest Tc-99m sestamibi SPECT and provided a substantial improvement in specificity (69 to 97%) and positive predictive value (38 to 97%).

Investigators at the Medical College of Virginia developed a risk-based systematic strategy for rapid triage and evaluation of patients presenting to the emergency department with chest pain (71). It serves as an early model in the application of this method. Risk assessment was assigned within 30 minutes of presentation and was based on the initial emergency department presentation, chest pain, and presenting ECG. A critical pathway that suggests a subsequent evaluation and intervention defines each of five risk levels. level 1: AMI-acute thrombolysis or percutaneous transluminal coronary angioplasty; level 2: AMI or unstable angina—admitted to CCU; level 3: probable unstable angina; level 4: possible unstable angina; level 5: noncardiac chest pain—appropriate outpatient referral. Level 3 and 4 patients presented ambiguities of diagnosis and management and were evaluated by gated acute myocardial perfusion imaging. Patients with equivocal or abnormal studies were admitted to the hospital and assigned to level 2 or 3, as appropriate. Patients with normal perfusion and function were discharged and scheduled to return within 72 hours for a follow-up stress test with perfusion imaging. The results of the subsequent stress perfusion imaging were combined with those of the normal resting study to form one perfusion study. Using this template, these investigators conducted an observational study (72) to assess the safety and efficacy of a systematic evaluation and triage strategy, including immediate resting gated myocardial perfusion imaging in patients presenting to the emergency department with chest pain of possible cardiac origin. Studied were 1,187 patients consecutive patients. Within 60 minutes of presentation, each patient was assigned to one of the five levels on the basis of risk. Levels

3 and 4 registered 438 patients triaged into these moderate- and low-risk levels; they underwent acute resting myocardial perfusion imaging with injection of sestamibi in the emergency department. Patients were followed for 1 year to determine the incidence of cardiac events. Among the 338 with normal studies, no AMI or deaths occurred, and only 10 revascularizations (3%) were performed. Among the 100 patients with abnormal or equivocal studies, there were 11 AMIs, 32 revascularizations, and 9 cardiac deaths. The sensitivity of immediate resting myocardial perfusion imaging for AMI was 100% with a specificity of 78%. During 1-year follow-up, patients with normal findings had a revascularization event rate of 3% with no AMI or death. Patients with abnormal imaging findings had a 42% event rate, with 11% experiencing MI and 8% cardiac death. Multivariate analysis revealed that an abnormal rest myocardial perfusion imaging

study was the only independent predictor of AMI. In patients with abnormal imaging, the risk for AMI and for myocardial revascularization was significantly higher than in patients with normal findings (7% versus 0%, and 32% versus 2%, respectively). This data supports the safety and value of this strategy, employing gated rest sestamibi SPECT imaging that appears to be an effective method for the rapid triage of relatively low-risk emergency department chest pain patients. The method permits discrimination of unsuspected high-risk patients who require prompt admission and adequate treatment from those who really are at low risk and who may be evaluated as outpatients. An additional potential logistic advantage is that emergency department injection can be used as the first part of an exercise Tc-99m sestamibi evaluation if the resting study is negative and the patient is stable (Fig. 8; see also Color Plate 19 following page

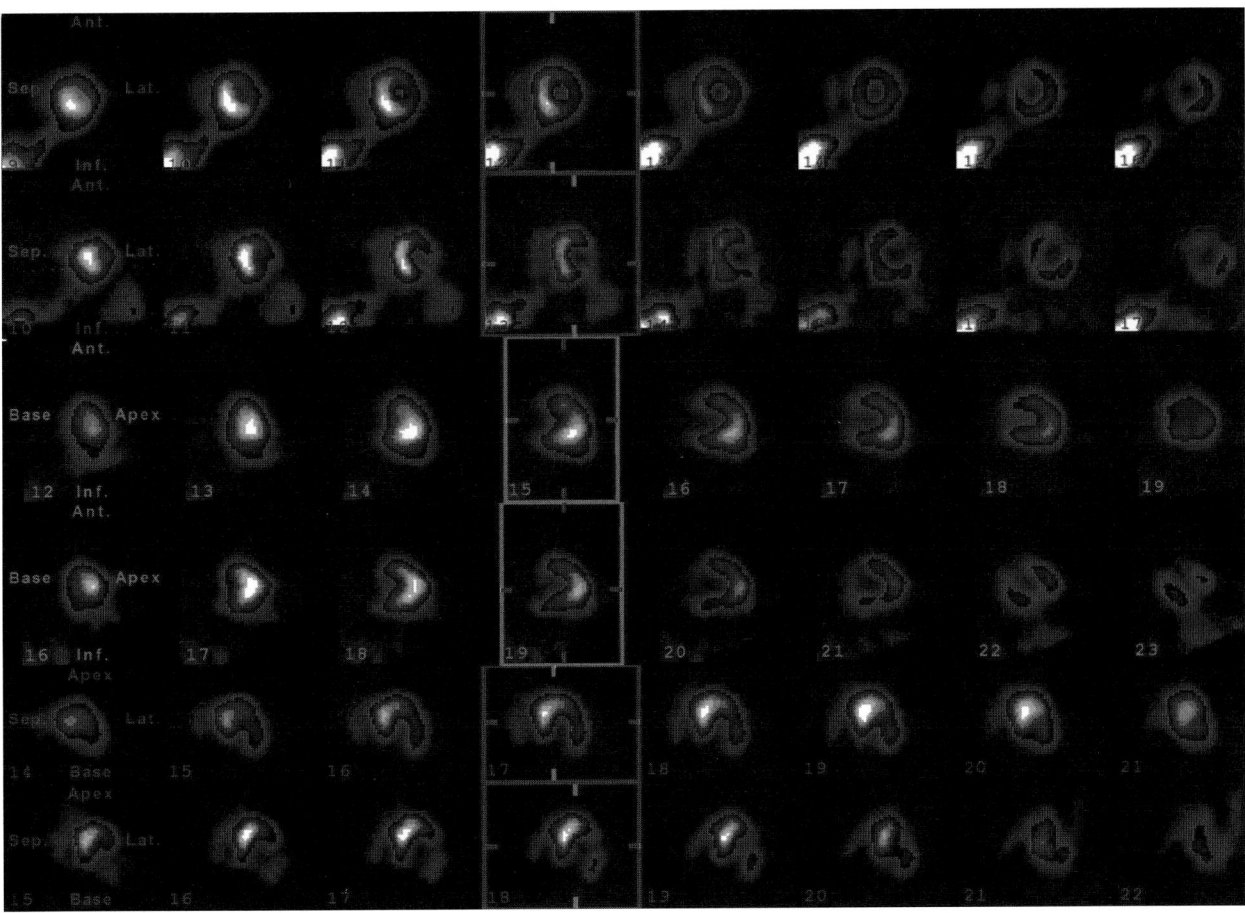

FIG. 8. End-diastolic (ED) chest pain. Shown in the same display as Figure 2 are rest and dipyridamole gated Tc-99m MIBI myocardial perfusion images in an obese 84-year-old woman with chest pressure. Her electrocardiogram shows right bundle-branch block. In each view, rest Tc-99m MIBI images at presentation to the emergency department are shown above while those acquired after dipyridamole are shown below. There is evidence of subtle decreased uptake of the tracer in the lateral wall on rest ED images. Gated single-photon emission computed tomography images showed normal global and regional wall motion. These findings suggest myocardial ischemia as the cause of the perfusion defect. The dipyridamole images show a dense and extensive myocardial perfusion defect in the same lateral wall region. These findings demonstrate the presence of myocardium at ischemic risk, likely in the distribution of the left circumflex coronary artery. Coronary angiography showed a tight proximal lesion of the left circumflex coronary artery. (See also Color Plate 19 following page 294.) (From Pharmacologic stress in nuclear medicine self study III: cardiology, with permission.)

294). This would permit the most complete and expeditious evaluation with early discharge of normal patients.

Even with these encouraging results, it is important to note that the technique is imperfect, and its implementation in the emergency department setting requires a multidisciplinary effort. Some small infarcts could be missed, and a small, but significant, portion of the population will have suboptimal studies due to technical factors. Another crucial aspect is information transfer, necessary if the information from acute imaging is to be inappropriately applied in clinical decision-making.

STRESS Tc-99m SESTAMIBI MYOCARDIAL PERFUSION SCINTIGRAPHY

What is the best time to stress patients who present to the emergency department with low-to-intermediate likelihood of ACS? The value of gated rest SPECT Tc-99m sestamibi, followed by a stress study was evaluated in 135 emergency department patients with chest pain and a low probability for AMI. Abnormal gated perfusion scans were noted in 47 (35%), and, among the 22 who subsequently underwent cardiac catheterization, 96% had evidence of coronary artery disease. Of the 88 patients with a normal rest perfusion study, 55 had stress Tc-99m sestamibi and 7 had coronary angiography. Forty-five of the 55 (82%) had normal stress images and were without events on follow-up, while 6 of 7 (86%) with angiography had normal coronary vessels. These data support the use of acute rest sestamibi imaging as an effective method for risk stratification, complemented, where appropriate, by stress imaging to guide management (71).

COMPARISON OF ECHOCARDIOGRAPHY AND MYOCARDIAL PERFUSION IMAGING

While both two-dimensional echocardiography and myocardial perfusion imaging with sestamibi can identify patients at low and high risk, the scintigraphic studies appear to present the possibility of superior diagnosis and risk stratification in this as in other clinical settings. However, comparative studies are few. In their earlier study, Varetto and co-workers (63) demonstrated both superior sensitivity and specificity of the scintigraphic method.

Kontos and co-workers (72) conducted a study in 185 patients presenting to the emergency department with chest pain and low-to-moderate risk for myocardial ischemia on the basis of the presenting history, physical examination, and ECG. The patients underwent both echocardiography and myocardial perfusion imaging within 4 hours of emergency department presentation. Positive echocardiography was defined as the presence of segmental wall motion abnormalities or moderate-to-severe global systolic dysfunction; a positive perfusion imaging was defined as a perfusion defect in association with abnormal wall motion or wall thickening, or both. Overall agreement between the two techniques was high (concordance, 89%; κcoefficient, 0.74) in the 27 patients who had MI or underwent coronary angiography. For all patients, concordance was 89%, with a κ of 0.66.

COST-EFFECTIVENESS

Two published studies (73,74) have addressed the cost-effectiveness of myocardial perfusion imaging with Tc-99m sestamibi for emergency department triage. Radensky and co-workers (73) evaluated the impact of acute imaging on the disposition of patients. The authors demonstrated that, due to the results of acute sestamibi imaging in 50 consecutive patients presenting to the emergency department, 68% were triaged to a less acute unit and 58% were sent home. A total of 69.37 hospital days were saved at an absolute cost savings of $786 per patient. During a subsequent 10-month follow-up included in this cost-effective analysis, no AMIs or deaths occurred in 30 patients with a normal imaging study. Similar results were reported by other investigators (74), who noted that prior to the use of acute Tc-99m sestamibi imaging in the emergency department, patients with suspicious chest pain and nondiagnostic ECG had a 96% hospital admission rate. After perfusion imaging was introduced, the admission rate fell to approximately 60%. In addition, a 17% reduction in hospital costs, with a $923 saving per patient was realized in the group undergoing imaging versus the group undergoing clinical and ECG evaluation alone. During the follow-up of 180 patients from 3 to 12 months, no events were seen in those with a negative scan.

Recently, one study has addressed the cost-effectiveness of using myocardial perfusion imaging with Tc-99m tetrofosmin in emergency department patients. A normal SPECT study as a criterion not to admit patients would result in a 57% reduction in hospital admissions, with a mean cost saving per patient of $4,258 (69). These data support acute emergency department Tc-99m SPECT imaging as being cost-effective and clinically valuable in ambiguous patients presenting to the emergency department with chest pain of suspected cardiac origin.

SUMMARY

Jesse and co-workers present an in depth review of the subject (75). The evaluation of chest pain in the emergency department setting should be systematic, risk based, and goal driven. The initial evaluation is based on the patient history, a focused physical examination, and the ECG. This information is enough to categorize patients into groups as high, moderate, and low risk. However, the data from many studies suggests that such an initial evaluation will fail to identify a limited but important number of patients who harbor significant coronary risk, but appear otherwise to be low risk. Further, these patients need early identification in order to permit appropriate intervention and event reduction. It is very important to improve the sensitivity of the evaluation process to identify these patients. Success has been reported with a number of strategies including emergency imaging. Particularly promising is emergency department-related stress testing and imaging with Tc-99m based perfusion agents. Early provocative testing, either exercise or pharmacologic stress testing may also be effective. The added value of each of these tests lies only in their application as a part of a systematic protocol to evaluate all patients with acute chest pain presenting to the emergency department. These tests must be done efficiently, cost-effectively, and in a manner that will aid recognition and reduce the time required to treat ACSs.

REFERENCES

1. National Cooperative Study Group. Unstable angina. National Cooperative Study group to compare surgical and medical therapy. In-hospital experience and initial follow-up results in patients with one, two and three vessel disease. *Am J Cardiol* 1978;42:839–848.
2. Scott SM, Deupree RH, Sharma GVRK, et al. VA study of unstable angina: 10-year results show duration of surgical advantage for patients with impaired ejection fraction. *Circulation* 1994;90[Suppl]:120–123.
3. Luchi RJ, Scott SM, Deupree RH. Comparison of medical and surgical treatment for unstable angina. *N Engl J Med* 1987;316:977–984.
4. The TIMI IIIB Investigators. Effects of tissue plasminogen activator and a comparison of early invasive and conservative strategies in unstable angina and non-Q-wave myocardial infarction. *Circulation* 1994; 89:545–1556.
5. Anderson HV, Cannon CP, Stone PH, et al. One year results of the thrombolysis in myocardial infarction TIMI Phase IIIB clinical trial. A randomized comparison of tissue type plasminogen activator versus placebo and early invasive versus early conservative strategies in unstable anginal and non-Q wave myocardial infarction. *J Am Coll Cardiol* 1995;26:1643–1650.
6. Wilcox I, Freedman SB, Allman KC, et al. Prognostic significance of a predischarge exercise test in patients with suspected unstable coronary artery disease. *Am J Cardiol* 1991;18:677–683.
7. Butman SM, Olsen HG, Gardin JM, et al. Submaximal exercise testing after stabilization of unstable angina pectoris. *J Am Coll Cardiol* 1984; 4:667–673.
8. Swahn E, Areskog M, Berglund U, et al. Predictive importance of clinical findings and a predischarge exercise test in patients with suspected unstable coronary artery disease. *Am J Cardiol* 1987;59(4): 208–214.
9. Department of Health and Human Services. *Unstable angina: diagnosis in management. Clinical practice guideline No. 10.* Washington D.C.: Department of Health and Human Services, Public Health Service, Agency for Healthcare Policy and Research. National Heart, Lung and Blood Institute, AHCPR publication number 94-0602, March 1994.
10. Nixon JV, Brown CN, Smitherman TC. Identification of transient and persistent segmental wall motion abnormalities in patients with unstable angina by two dimensional echocardiography. *Circulation* 1982; 65:1497–1503.
11. Stein JH, Neumann A, Preston LM, et al. Admission echocardiography predicts in hospital cardiac events in patients with unstable angina. *J Am Coll Card* 1996;27:377A.
12. Gibler WB, Runyon JP, Levr RG, et al. A rapid diagnostic and treatment center for patients with chest pain in the emergency department. *Ann Emerg Med* 1995;25;18.
13. Jeroudi Mo, Cherif J, Habib GB, et al. Prolonged wall motion abnormalities after chest pain at rest in patients with unstable angina: a possible manifestation of myocardial stunning. *Am Heart J* 1994;127: 1241–1250.
14. Botvinick EH. Stress imaging: current clinical options for the diagnosis, localization, and evaluation of coronary artery disease. *Med Clin North Am* 1995;79(5):1025–1061.
15. Brown KA. Do stress echocardiography and myocardial perfusion imaging have the same ability to identify the low-risk patient with known or suspected coronary artery disease? *Am J Cardiol* 1998;81: 1050–1053.
16. Lin SS, Lauer MS, Marwick T. Risk stratification of patients with medically treated unstable angina using exercise echocardiography. *Am J Cardiol* 1998;82:720–724.
17. Shaw LH, Hachamovitch R, Isjandrian AE. Treadmill test scores: attributes and limitations [editorial]. *J Nucl Cardiol* 1997;4:74.
18. Brown KA. Management of unstable angina: the role of noninvasive risk stratification in nuclear cardiology and managed care: from challenge to opportunity. *J Nucl Cardiol* 1997;4[Suppl]:S164–S168.
19. Hillert MC, Narahara KA, Smitherman TC, et al. Thallium-201 perfusion imaging after the treatment of unstable angina pectoris: relationship to clinical outcome. *West J Med* 1996;145:335–340.
20. Madsen JK, Stubgaard M, Utne HE, et al. Prognosis and thallium-201 scintigraphy in patients admitted with chest pain without confirmed acute myocardial infarction. *Br Heart J* 1998;59:184–189.
21. Marmur JD, Freeman MR, Langer A, et al. Prognosis in medically stabilized unstable angina: early Holter ST monitoring compared with predischarge exercise thallium tomography. *Ann Int Med* 1990;113: 575–581.
22. Brown KA. Prognostic value of thallium-201 myocardial perfusion imaging in patients with unstable angina who respond to medical treatment. *J Am Coll Cardiol* 1991;17:1053–1057.
23. Stratmann HG, Younis LT, Wittry MD, et al. Exercise technetium-99m myocardial tomography for the risk stratification of men with medically treated unstable angina pectoris. *Am J Cardiol* 1995;76: 236–240.
24. Stratmann HG, Tamesis BR, Younis LT, et al. Prognostic value of predischarge dipyridamole technetium-99m sestamibi myocardial tomography in medically treated patients with unstable angina. *Am Heart J* 1995;130:734–740.
25. Zhu YY, Botvinick EH, Dae MW, et. al. Dipyridamole perfusion scintigraphy: the experience with its application in 170 patients with known or suspected unstable angina. *Am Heart J* 1991;121:33–40.
26. Wang CH, Cherng WJ, Hua CC, et al. Prognostic value of dobutamine echocardiography in patients after Q-wave or non-Q-wave myocardial infarction. *Am J Cardiol* 1998;82:38–42.
27. Boden WE, O'Rourke RA, Crawford MH, et al. for the Veterans Affairs Non-Q Wave Infarction Strategies in Hospital (VANQWISH) Trial Investigators. Outcomes in patients with acute non-Q wave myocardial infarction randomly assigned to an invasive as compared with a conservative management strategy. *N Engl J Med* 1998;338:1785–1792.
28. Finenberg RA, Scadden D, Goldman L. Care of patients with low probabiltiy of acute myocardial infarction: cost effectiveness of alternatives to coronary-care unit admissions. *N Engl J Med* 1984;310: 1301–1307.
29. Lee TH, Rouan GW, Weisberg MC, et al. Clinical characteristics and natural history of patients with acute myocardial infarction sent home from the emergency room. *Am J Cardiol* 1987;60:219–224.
30. Rusnak RA, Stair TO, Hansen K, et al. Litigation against the emergency physician: common features in cases of missed myocardial infarction. *Ann Emerg Med* 1989;18:1029–1034.
31. Goldman L, Cook EF, Brand DA, et al. A computer protocol to predict myocardial infarction in emergency department patients with chest pain. *N Engl J Med* 1988;318:797–803.
32. Lee TH, Cook EP, Weisberg M, et al. Acute chest pain in the emergency room. Identification and examination in low risk patients. *Arch Intern Med* 1985;145:65–69.
33. Young GP, Green TR. The role of single ECG, creatine kinase, and CKMB in diagnosing patients with acute chest pain. *Am J Emerg Med* 1993;11:444–449.
34. Lee TH, Jarez G, Cook EF, et al. Ruling out acute myocardial infarction: a prospective multicenter validation of a 12-hour strategy for patients at low risk. *N Engl J Med* 1991;324:1239.
35. Goldman L, Cook EF, Johnson PA, et al. Prediction of the need for intensive care in patients who present to emergency departments with acute chest pain. *N Engl J Med* 1996;334:1498–1504.
36. Adams JE, Bodor GS, Davila Roman VG, et al. Cardiac troponin I. A marker with high specificity for cardiac injury. *Circulation* 1993;88: 101–106.
37. Lewis WR, Amsterdam EA. Utility and safety of immediate exercise testing of low-risk patients admitted to the hospital for suspected acute myocardial infarction. *Am J Cardiol* 1994;74:987–990.
38. Kirp JD, Turnispseed S, Lewis WR, et al. Evaluation of chest pain in low-risk patients presenting to the emergency department: the role of the immediate exercise testing. *Ann Emerg Med* 1998;32:1–7.

39. Gibler WB, Runyon JP, Levr RG, et al. A rapid diagnostic and treatment center for patients with chest pain in the emergency department. *Ann Emerg Med* 1995;25:1–8.
40. Krasuski RA, Hartley LH, Lee TH, et al. Weekend and holiday exercise testing in patients with chest pain: clinical outcomes and cost savings. *J Gen Intern Med* 1999;14(1):10–14.
41. Horowitz RS, Morganroth J, Parrotto C, et al. Inmediate diagnosis of acute myocardial infarction by two dimensional echocardiography. *Circulation* 1982;65:323–329.
42. Sasaki H, Charuzi Y, Beeder C, et al. Utility of echocardiography for the early detection of assessment of patients with nondiagnostic chest pain. *Am Heart J* 1986;112:494–497.
43. Peels CH, Visser CA, Funke-Kupper AJ, et al. Usefulness of two-dimensional echocardiography for inmediate detection of myocardial ischemia in the emergency room. *Am J Cardiol* 1990;65:687–691.
44. Sabia P, Afrookteh A, Touchstone DA, et al. Value of regional wall motion abnormality in the emergency room diagnosis of acute myocardial infarction: a prospective study using two-dimensional echocardiography. *Circulation* 1991;84[Suppl I]:I-85–I-92.
45. Hoffmann R, Lethen H, Marwick T, et al. Analysis of interinstitutional observer agreement in interpretation of dobutamine stress echocardiograms. *J Am Coll Cardiol* 1996;27:330–336.
46. Kontos MC, Arrowood JA, Paulson WH, et al. Ability of echocardiography in the emergency department to detect myocardial ischemia in patients presenting with chest pain. *J Am Soc Echocardiol* 1995;8:346A.
47. Trippi JA, Kopp G, Lee KS, et al. The feasibility of dobutamine stress echocardiography in the emergency department with telemedicine interpretation. *J Am Soc Echocardiol* 1996;9:113–118.
48. Colon PJ, Cheirif J, Guarisco J, et al. Rapid triage of patients presenting to the emergency department with chest pain using stress echocardiography. *J Am Soc Echocardiol* 1995;8:29F.
49. Ballal RS, Secknus MA, Mehta R, et al. Cardiac outcomes in coronary patients with submaximal dobutamine stress echocardiography. *Am J Cardiol* 1997;80:725–729.
50. Wackers FJ, Busemann-Sokole E, Samson G, et al. Value and limitations of thallium-201 scintigraphy in the acute phase of myocardial infarction. *N Engl J Med* 1976;295:1–5.
51. Wackers FJTh, Lie KI, Liem KL, et al. Thallium-201 scintigraphy in unstable angina pectoris. *Circulation* 1978;57:738–742.
52. Wackers FJTh, Lie KI, Liem KL, et al. Potential value of thallium-201 scintigraphy as a means of selecting patients for the coronary care unit. *Br Heart J* 1979;41:111–117.
53. van der Wieken LR, Kan G, Belfer AJ, et al. Thallium scanning to decide CCU admission in patients with non diagnostic electrocardiograms. *Int J Cardiol* 1983;4:285–295.
54. Freeman MR, Williams AE, Chisholm RJ, et al. Role of resting thallium 201 perfusion in predicting coronary anatomy, left ventricular wall motion, and hospital outcome in unstable angina patients. *Am Heart J* 1989;117:306–314.
55. Hakki A-H, Iskandrian AS, Kane SA, et al. Thallium-201 myocardial perfusion scintigraphy and left ventricular function at rest in patients with rest angina pectoris. *Am Heart J* 1984;108:326–332.
56. Brown K, Okada RD, Boucher CA, et al. Serial thallium-201 at rest with unstable and stable angina. Relationship of myocardial perfusion at rest to presenting clinical syndrome. *Am Heart J* 1983;106:70–77.
57. Verani MS, Jeroudi MO, Mahmarian JJ, et al. Quantification of myocardial infarction during coronary occlusion and myocardial salvage after reperfusion using cardiac imaging with technetium-99 hexakis 2 methoxyisobutyl isonitrile. *J Am Coll Cardiol* 1988;12(6):1573–1581.
58. Sinusas AJ, Trauman KA, Bergin JD, et al. Quantification of area at risk during coronary occlusion and degree of myocardial salvage after reperfusion with technetium-99-m- methoxyisobutyl-isonitrile. *Circulation* 1990;82:1424–1437.

59. Christian TF, Clements IP, Gibbons RJ. Noninvasive identification of myocardium at risk in patients with acute myocardial infarction and nondiagnostic electrocardiograms with technetium-99m sestamibi. *Circulation* 1991;83:1615–1620.
60. Gibbons RJ, Verani MS, Behrenbeck T, et al. Feasibility of tomographic Tc-99m hexakis-2-methoxyl-2-methylpropyl-isonitrile imaging for the assessment of myocardial area at risk and the effect of acute treatment in myocardial infarction. *Circulation* 1989;980:1277–1286.
61. Gregoire J, Theroux P. Detection and assessment of unstable angina using myocardial perfusion imaging: comparison between technetium-99m sestamibi SPECT and 12 lead electrocardiogram. *Am J Cardiol* 1990;66:42E–46E.
62. Bilodeau L, Theroux P, Gregoire J, et al. Technetium-99m sestamibi tomography in patients with spontaneous chest pain: correlations with clinical, electrocardiographic and angiographic findings. *J Am Coll Cardiol* 1991;18:1684–1691.
63. Varetto T, Cantalupi D, Altieri A, et al. Emergency room technetium-99m sestamibi imaging to rule out acute myocardial ischemic events in patients with nondiagnostic electrocardiograms. *J Am Coll Cardiol* 1993;22:1804–1808.
64. Hilton TC, Thompson RC, Williams HJ, et al. Technetium-99m sestamibi myocardial perfusion imaging in the emergency room evaluation of chest pain. *J Am Coll Cardiol* 1994;23:1016–1022.
65. Hilton TC, Stowers SA, Fulmer H. Ninety-day follow-up of ED patients with chest pain and normal or non-diagnostic ECG who undergo acute cardiac imaging with Tc-99m sestamibi. *J Am Coll Cardiol* 1995;25:192A.
66. Kjoller E, Nielsen SL, Carlsen J, et al. Impact of inmediate and delayed myocardial scintigraphy on therapeutic decisions in suspected acute myocardial infarction. *Eur Heart J* 1995;16:909–913.
67. Wackers FJ, Heller GV, Stowers SA, et al. Normal rest tetrofosmin SPECT imaging in patients with chest pain and normal or nondiagnostic ECG in the emergency department is associated with lower need for subsequent cardiac catheterization and revascularization. *J Am Coll Cardiol* 1997;29:196A.
68. Heller GV, Stowers SA, Hendel RC, et al. Clinical value of acute rest techneteium-99m tetrosfosmin tomographic myocardial perfusion imaging in patients with acute chest pain and nondiagnostic electrocardiograms. *J Am Coll Cardiol* 1998;31:1011–1017.
69. Tatum JL, Jesse RL, Kontos MC, et al. A comprehensive strategy for the evaluation and triage of the chest pain patient. *Ann Emerg Med* 1997;29:116–125.
70. Nicholson CS, Tatum JL, Jesse RL, et al. The value of gated Tc-99m sestamibi perfusion imaging in acute ischemic syndromes. *J Nucl Cardiol* 1995;22:S57.
71. Tatum JL, Ornato JP, Jesse RL, et al. A diagnostic strategy using Tc-99m sestamibi for evaluation of patients with chest pain in the emergency department. *Circulation* 1994;90:I-367A.
72. Kontos MC, Arrowood JA, Jesse RL, et al. Comparison between 2-dimensional echocardiography and myocardial perfusion imaging in the emergency department in patients with possible ischemia. *Am Heart J* 1998;136:724–733.
73. Radensky PW, Hilton TC, Fulmer H, et al. Potential cost effectiveness of initial myocardial perfusion imaging for assessment of emergency department patients with chest pain. *Am J Cardiol* 1997;79:595–599.
74. Weissman I, Dickinson CZ, Dworkin HJ, et al. Cost-effectiveness of myocardial perfusion imaging with SPECT in the emergency department evaluation of patients with unexplained chest pain. *Radiology* 1996;199:353–357.
75. Jesse RL, Kontos MC. Evaluation of chest pain in the emergency department. *Curr Prob Cardiol* 1997;22:149–236.

CHAPTER 38

Evaluation of Patients after Intervention

Daniel S. Berman, Michael J. Zellweger,
Leslee J. Shaw, Howard C. Lewin,
Eric A. Dubois, John D. Friedman,
and Guido Germano

Coronary artery revascularization and aggressive medical intervention have become powerful therapies in the management of ischemic heart disease. Although coronary angiography provides a clinically valuable measure of the severity of ischemic heart disease and is the principal method to which noninvasive methods have been compared, its invasive nature precludes its routine use in the evaluation of patients after intervention. Furthermore, angiography provides predominantly anatomic assessments and does not standardly assess physiologic significance of an individual coronary stenosis. Noninvasive stress testing with its ability to provide information about physiologic significance of stenoses and risk stratification of coronary artery disease (CAD) patients is ideally suited to assess patients after intervention (1–5).

D. S. Berman: University of California–Los Angeles School of Medicine, Los Angeles, California 90025; Department of Imaging/Nuclear Medicine, Cedars-Sinai Medical Center, Los Angeles, California 90048.

M. J. Zellweger: Department of Cardiology, University Hospital Basel, CH-4031 Basel, Switzerland.

L. J. Shaw: Department of Medicine, Health Policy and Management, Emory University, Atlanta, Georgia 30322.

H. C. Lewin: Department of Medicine, University of California–Los Angeles School of Medicine, Los Angeles, California 90024; Department of Imaging/Cardiology, Cedars-Sinai Medical Center, Los Angeles, California 90048.

E. A. Dubois: Department of Cardiology, Academic Medical Center, University of Amsterdam, 1105 AZ Amsterdam, The Netherlands.

J. D. Friedman: Department of Cardiology/Nuclear Medicine, Cedars-Sinai Medical Center, Los Angeles, California 90048.

G. Germano: Department of Radiological Sciences, University of California–Los Angeles School of Medicine, Los Angeles, California 90024; Department of Medicine, Cedars-Sinai Medical Center, Los Angeles, California 90048.

Risk stratification has been shown to have the greatest incremental value and cost-effectiveness in patients for whom the diagnosis of coronary artery disease is already established or for whom the probability of coronary artery disease is high (2,3,5). The extent and severity of coronary disease is a strong prognosticator but its direct assessment currently requires use of an invasive procedure. The extent and severity of disease may also be estimated using less expensive, noninvasive techniques that may provide equivalent information with respect to prediction of subsequent cardiac events (3,4,6).

When devising a risk assessment tool, detection of the amount of ischemic burden and the extent of left ventricular dysfunction are valuable tools for outcomes assessment. From noninvasive imaging, recent evidence suggests that varying outcomes may be estimated by combining measures of myocardial ischemia with ventricular function data (7). Measures of the amount of myocardial ischemia (i.e., ST depression, stress-induced perfusion defects) are proposed estimators of ischemic events, including acute ischemic syndromes (unstable angina or myocardial infarction). Conversely, the extent of left ventricular dysfunction has been shown to be strongly related to the frequency of cardiac death. Thus, using empiric risk stratification and linking noninvasive measures to effective therapeutic interventions could provide an optimal approach to patient management, which could lead to enhanced event-free survival for patients with known coronary disease.

Noninvasive testing can also play an important complementary role in patients who have undergone catheterization. In those patients for whom uncertainty exists regarding therapeutic options after cardiac catheterization, noninvasive testing may be used for risk stratification, while patients at high risk may be referred to revascularization. Evidence in the literature suggests, however, that this is not common practice. Topol and colleagues (8) recently reported that, in a cohort of 2,000 patients with private medical insurance, only 29% had exercise testing of any type performed prior to single-vessel angioplasty. It is possible that a significant proportion of these patients had no inducible ischemia; indeed, many patients with single-vessel coronary artery disease do not have inducible ischemia by cardiac imaging and are clearly at low risk of subsequent adverse outcomes (2). The implications of these considerations with respect to health-care policy and the costs of medical care are significant, since many of these patients might have been spared the risk of this procedure (and the health-care system spared the cost of the procedure) if noninvasive testing had been performed.

There have been several reports suggesting an overuse of cardiac catheterization (9,10). In a recent analysis of 305 metropolitan areas, the use of cardiac catheterization had a direct influence on the rate of coronary revascularization that was unrelated to the rate of coronary disease in the population but was strongly correlated to an increasingly aggressive approach to coronary disease treatment (10). For noninvasive testing, if referral to cardiac catheterization is limited to those with a high posttest risk, the subsequent diagnostic yield of catheterization for significant coronary disease, as well as for survival estimates, could be enhanced. The use of coronary revascularization could then be more selectively applied to patients who receive the greatest risk benefit.

In very practical terms, the posttest care of patients may be guided by information derived from the cardiac noninvasive test. That is, ventricular function and myocardial perfusion information may be integrated into a clinical pathway. An obvious benefit of directed posttest management is that it allows for selectivity of an expensive resource use (i.e., cardiac catheterization and revascularization). Another direct benefit of this approach is that only those patients at high posttest risk are referred to cardiac catheterization, resulting in an enhanced diagnostic yield from cardiac catheterization. The enhanced diagnostic yield will result in catheterization of a greater number of patients with a significant coronary stenosis and a lower number of patients with nonobstructive disease being referred to catheterization (i.e., a commonly used quality indicator of appropriateness of referral to catheterization). Since the benefit of treatment is directly related to the risk in the population, referral of patients to cardiac catheterization should be recommended for patients who have a high risk noninvasive test (e.g., left ventricular ejection fraction $\leq 35\%$, extensive perfusion abnormalities, or possibly left ventricular dilatation). This is based on the principle that the prevalence of severe disease and risk of major cardiac outcomes is high in each of the aforementioned categories (7,11). These patients warrant an aggressive management approach that includes referral to coronary angiography.

With respect to patients who have undergone revascularization, if severe symptoms recur after myocardial revascularization, coronary angiography is usually directly indicated to determine if repeat revascularization is needed to reduce symptoms. However, in less symptomatic or asymptomatic patients with extensive silent ischemia before revascularization, consideration of repeat revascularization should deal with the prediction of patients at increased risk for cardiac death, who may warrant repeat revascularization for purposes of improving survival. In this regard, noninvasive stress testing is of particular importance, as the direct referral to angiography may prompt unnecessary repeat revascularization. Since the evaluation of patients with coronary artery disease is extensively discussed in Chapter 37 this chapter will focus only on the postintervention assessment.

FOLLOW-UP OF PATIENTS AFTER PERCUTANEOUS TRANSLUMINAL ANGIOPLASTY

Introduction

Percutaneous transluminal angioplasty (PTCA) was introduced in 1977 by Gruentzig (12,13). More than 400,000 PTCA procedures are carried out each year in the United States alone by balloon angioplasty or related technologies (14). This figure now exceeds the number of coronary bypass surgeries. Interventional cardiovascular procedure costs approach $10 billion annually, approximately 1% of all U.S. health-care expenditures (14). The technique remains limited by two persistent difficulties: acute vessel closure during intervention and restenosis during the first 6 months of follow-up (15–17). PTCA restenosis rates without stenting range between 20 and 65%, depending on the method of follow-up and the criteria used to define restenosis (12,15–18). Successfully dilated total coronary occlusions have a higher rate of angiographic restenosis at 6 months than dilated stenoses (19).

Intracoronary stenting has shown clinical efficacy in reducing rates of reocclusion and restenosis (20). By early 1999, more than 1 million stents had been implanted in patients worldwide. Patients with stents show a lower restenosis or reocclusion rate than patients undergoing PTCA without stenting; however, an average restenosis rate of 20% (15 to 32%) (11,21) in native vessels has been reported and long-term results of stenting in saphenous-vein graft lesions show average restenosis rates of 36% (18 to 59%) (15,21).

Fourteen to 33% of patients with restenosis have silent restenosis without recurrent symptoms (22,23). The positive predictive value of symptoms for the occurrence of angiographic restenosis is approximately 60%, whereas the likelihood that asymptomatic patients are free from angiographic restenosis (negative predictive value) has been reported to be about 85%. Patients with silent ischemia documented by exercise electrocardiography, thallium-201 scintigraphy, or radionuclide angiography have been shown to have a prognosis similar to patients with angina (23).

Clinical Follow-up and Exercise Testing

Ischemic symptoms due to restenosis generally develop within 3 to 6 months after the coronary angioplasty, with a peak incidence between the second and third month. Patients presenting with recurrent angina greater than 6 months after PTCA are more likely to have progression of coronary artery disease at other sites than restenosis (24). For patients with clear angina prior to PTCA and in whom symptoms are ameliorated by PTCA, clinical monitoring for the development of new symptoms is probably an appropriate post-PTCA approach. However, for patients with less clear symptoms prior to PTCA, stress testing with or without imaging should be considered. In a study of 78 patients with single-vessel coronary artery disease undergoing single-vessel PTCA, Roth et al. (25) have reported sensitivity and specificity rates of angina for detecting restenosis of 50% and 68%, respectively, with a positive and negative predictive value of 38% and 78%.

The development of chest pain during the exercise stress test is also a poor marker for restenosis, with a sensitivity of only 24 to 63% (23,26–32). Furthermore, electrocardiographic changes are not highly accurate for detecting restenosis, with sensitivities ranging between 15 and 79% and specificity ranging between 33 and 88%. The mean value for sensitivity and specificity from these studies is 56% and 73%, respectively (23,26–32). Despite these less than impressive overall results in general PTCA populations, for patients with single-vessel disease, a normal resting electrocardiogram (ECG) and a positive stress-ECG before angioplasty, exercise testing without imaging may be useful in the prediction of restenosis (33). In a single study, reported by el-Tamimi et al., 31 patients with single-vessel disease and positive stress ECG before intervention were assessed after PTCA for restenosis. Fourteen of 31 patients had an angiographically significant restenosis. The sensitivity and specificity of testing was 79 and 82% at 3 days after angioplasty and increased to 93 and 100% at 1 to 6 months post-PTCA ($N = 14$). In this highly selected population, only 1 of 17 patients without restenosis had a false-positive treadmill test (34).

Follow-up by Nuclear Methods

Although nuclear cardiology testing before PTCA could be useful to define the presence and extent of ischemia, it has been noted that only a minority of patients undergo stress testing prior to PTCA (35). The American College of Cardiology (ACC) database reported that approximately 45% of all patients undergoing percutaneous interventions had provocative testing prior to PTCA. When both pre- and post-PTCA studies have been available, several have shown that there is an improvement in myocardial perfusion after successful PTCA. This improvement has been noted with both reversible and nonreversible defects (as illustrated in the example in Fig. 1) (36,37). Current American College of Cardiology/American Heart Association (ACC/AHA) guidelines for PTCA note that documentation of stress-induced ischemia is desirable for most patients undergoing evaluation for revascularization, particularly for patients with mild-moderate angina (CCSC I-II, i.e., Canadian Cardiovascular Society Class I or II) (38). The 1993 ACC/AHA guidelines for percutaneous interventions include a criterion based on an assessment of provocative ischemia (38). According to this guideline for patients with only CCSC I-II angina, PTCA is indicated only when there are moderate to large areas of ischemia on noninvasive testing.

There is a physiologic basis for using cardiac imaging modalities in this setting based on data revealing that patients with significant coronary lesions exhibit reductions in coronary flow reserve. Scintigraphic variables and measured flow reserve show a strong correlation. Miller and colleagues (39) studied a cohort of patients with intermediate coronary stenoses, comparing the results of quantitative coronary angiography, sestamibi single-photon emission computed tomography (SPECT) imaging, and Doppler flow probe, measured coronary reserve. The results of this study demonstrated the best correlation to be between flow reserve measurements and sestamibi uptake (89% agreement, κ statistic = 0.78). The results of these studies suggest that in those patients with equivocal catheterization results, perfusion imaging can identify those lesions that are physiologically significant and, thus, those patients who are at greater risk. Subsequently, decisions regarding revascularization in these cases, particularly with PTCA, can be based on both physiologic and anatomic data. From a clinical standpoint, myocardial perfusion scintigraphy is more commonly used to assess patients following PTCA. A number of reports have indicated that nuclear imaging has been shown to be accurate for the detection of restenosis. Using thallium-201 SPECT, Hecht et al. (40) demonstrated that nuclear testing is accurate in defining the presence of restenosis, whether or not complete revascularization was achieved with PTCA. They compared the sensitivity and specificity for detecting restenosis by exercise electrocardiography and Tl-201 SPECT in 116 patients. The sensitivity was 93 versus 52%, and the specificity was 77 versus 64% for SPECT and exercise electrocardiography, respectively (40). Subsequent work by Hecht et al. (41) demonstrated that Tl-201 SPECT is accurate for detection of restenosis in symptomatic as well as asymptomatic patients.

Pfisterer et al. (23) described ischemia on thallium scintigraphy in 28% of 405 patients who underwent PTCA 6 months before the nuclear testing. Of these 112 patients, follow-up angiography revealed significant stenosis in the artery supplying the ischemic zone in 101 (97%) of the cases. Of these, 80 (77%) represented restenosis in the angioplastied vessel, 21 (23%) represented *de novo* lesions. In contrast, results of exercise electrocardiography were negative

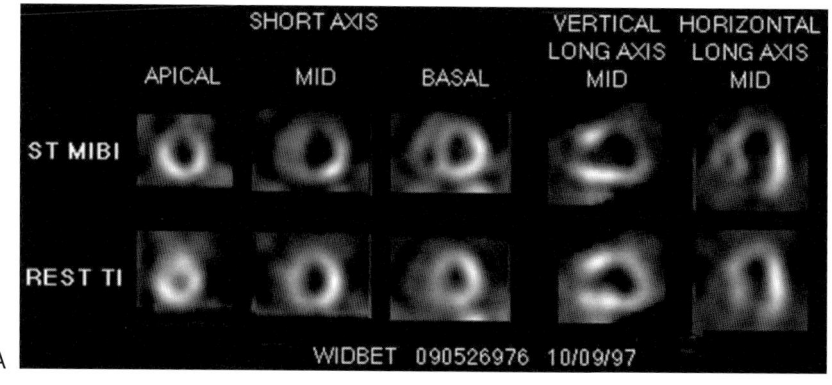

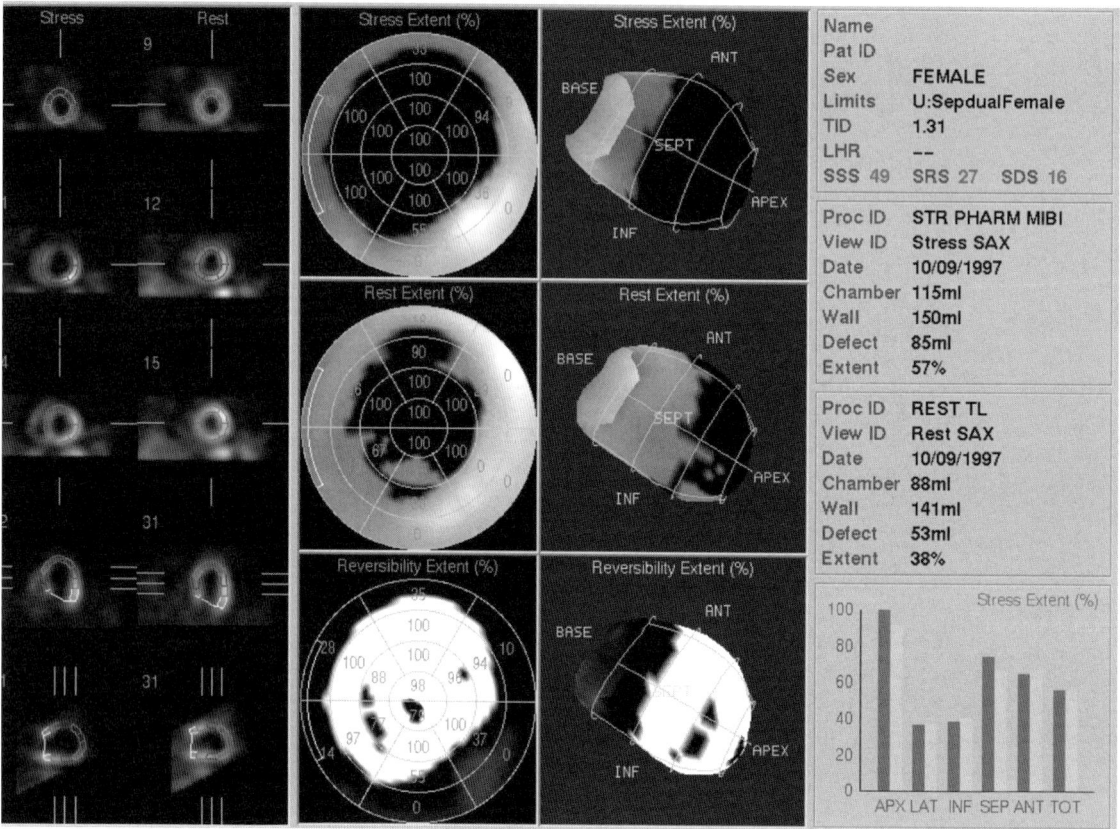

FIG. 1. A: Adenosine stress sestamibi/rest thallium-201 myocardial perfusion SPECT images in an 83-year-old female with typical angina. The summed stress score is extremely high at 49. The transient ischemic dilatation ratio is elevated at 1.31. The findings demonstrate evidence of severe ischemia throughout the left anterior descending coronary artery (LAD) territory. The poststress ejection fraction is severely reduced at 29%. Coronary angiography performed 5 days after testing revealed a 95% proximal LAD stenosis. **B:** Quantitative perfusion SPECT (QPS) analysis of the patient shown in **A**. Extensive, largely reversible defect is noted throughout the LAD territory. The quantitative stress defect extent is 57% in this patient. *(continued)*

in 74% of patients with scintigraphic ischemia and angiographic stenosis. Angiographic degree of restenosis was similarly high in patients with symptomatic and silent ischemia (23). A similar report on the detection of restenosis by Tc-99m sestamibi after successful percutaneous coronary angioplasty in 37 patients was published by Milan et al. (42). They reported a sensitivity of 87.5% and a specificity of

78% for the detection of restenosis. Overall sensitivity rates between 76 and 94% (mean value 89%) and specificity rates between 46 and 84% (mean value 75%) have been published (23,28,33,42–44).

Although the restenosis rate following coronary stenting is lower than that following balloon angioplasty, restenosis remains an important clinical problem with stenting. Prelim-

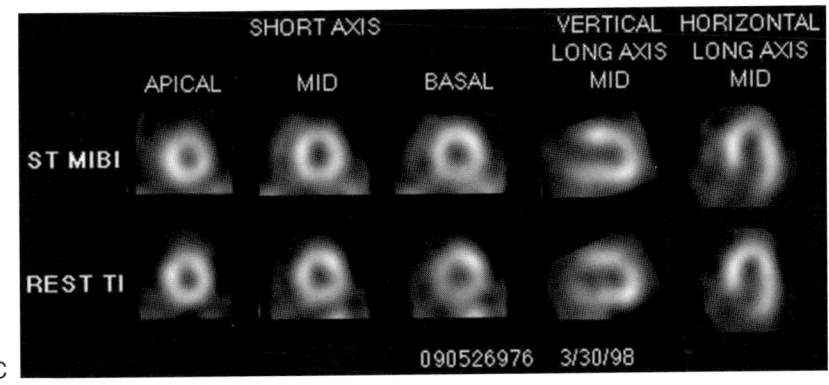

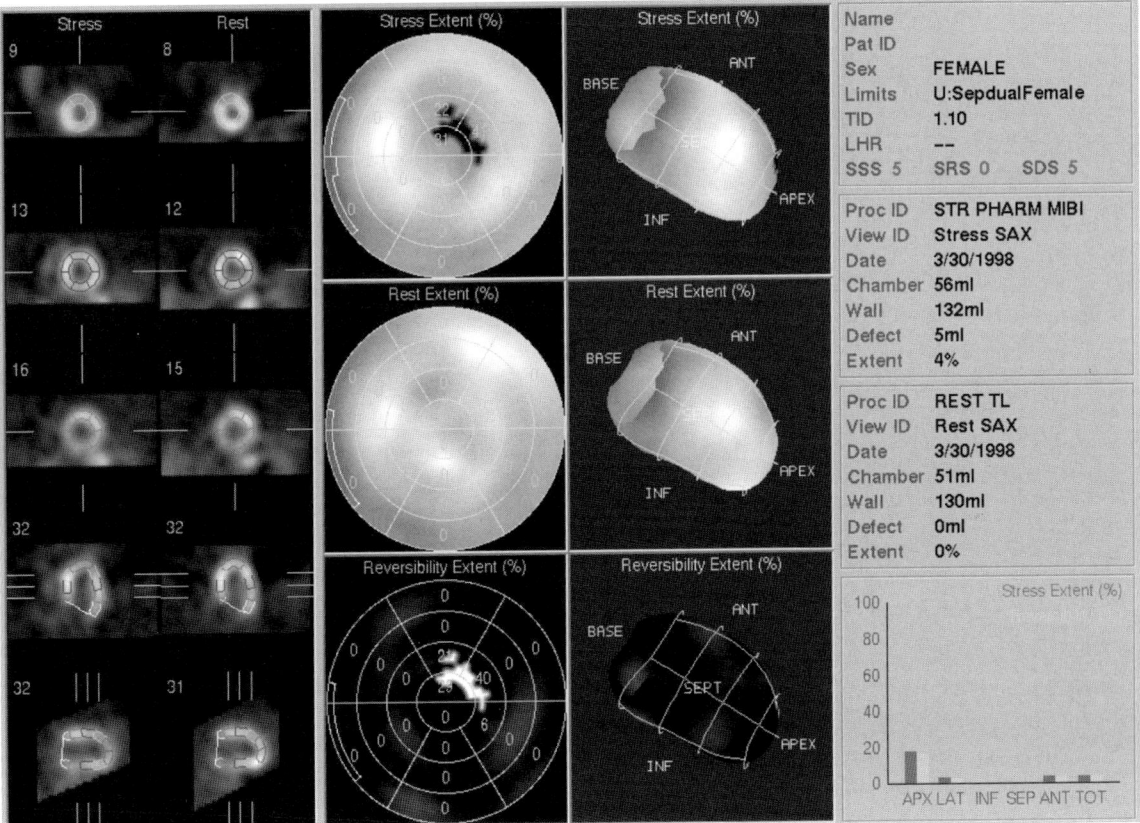

FIG. 1. *Continued.* **C:** Adenosine stress myocardial perfusion SPECT of the same patient illustrated in **A** at 5 months following rotational atherectomy and balloon angioplasty with stenting of the proximal LAD. At this time, the patient was asymptomatic. The myocardial perfusion SPECT study is essentially normal, demonstrating dramatic improvement in myocardial perfusion. **D:** Quantitative perfusion SPECT (QPS) analysis of the post-PTCA SPECT shown in **C**. The QPS study is nearly normal, confirming the visual findings and demonstrating marked improvement compared with pre-PTCA (**B**). The poststress left ventricular ejection fraction was 57%, with normal left ventricular wall motion. *PTCA*, percutaneous transluminal coronary angioplasty; *SPECT*, single-photon emission computed tomography.

inary data have suggested myocardial perfusion imaging sensitivities between 85 and 94% and specificities between 83 and 86% for detecting restenosis after coronary stenting (45,46).

The use of nuclear testing very early after angioplasty is controversial. Early data suggest that improved myocardial perfusion could be documented very early after PTCA.

Stress thallium scintigraphy may predict late restenosis even if it is performed within 24 hours after angioplasty (sensitivity 77%, specificity 67%) (47). Other early reports, however, showed that the nuclear test may be falsely positive early following PTCA, causing some to conclude that early testing post-PTCA is not useful (26,48). It has been reported that partially reversible or persistent defects might be noted shortly after PTCA (48,49), with no angiographic evidence of abnormality in the vessels. Resolution of these early reversible defects is often observed on subsequent tests (48,50).

Several explanations for the higher false-positive rate of stress myocardial perfusion SPECT early following PTCA have been proposed, including stunned vasa vasorum in the coronary artery undergoing angioplasty affecting vasodilator reserve, distal embolization of atheromatous material, and local vascular trauma, to name a few. In a recent review, nuclear imaging had a high positive and negative predictive value for restenosis when imaging was delayed approximately 2 to 4 weeks following the index procedure (51). From this review, there was a steady decline in the rate of false-positive scans as time from the index procedure elapsed, although median sample size was small (n = 63 patients).

Despite the observation of an early increased false-positive rate, recent experience has suggested that the frequency of the early post-PTCA false-positive myocardial perfusion study is much lower than previously observed. Miller et al. (51) proposed that post-PTCA false-positive rates may be less of a concern today due to improved resolution with Tc-99m agents as well as improved restoration of blood flow with new interventional techniques. Therefore, for practical purposes, when there is a significant question as to the adequacy of a high-risk angioplasty procedure, early performance of stress nuclear testing is considered to be clinically useful.

Prognostic Impact by Nuclear Follow-up

Although simply knowing whether restenosis is present can be of clinical importance for some patients, from a practical standpoint, the most important question in asymptomatic or minimally symptomatic patients following angioplasty is related to risk assessment. To date, there have been no published manuscripts dealing specifically with risk assessment of the post-PTCA patient. In a preliminary report from our institution assessing the cardiac event rate and referral to catheterization in patients undergoing stress sestamibi myocardial perfusion SPECT 1 month to 1 year following PTCA, we showed the results in 539 patients studied with rest thallium-201/stress 99m-technetium sestamibi dual isotope myocardial perfusion SPECT. The hard event rate (cardiac death or myocardial infarction) and total event rate (hard events and late bypass surgery occurring >60 days following testing) increase significantly as a function of SPECT abnormality. In a Cox proportional hazards model, the summed stress score (SSS), derived from the stress perfusion scores of 20 SPECT segments (see Chapter 13), as well as the type of stress (adenosine versus treadmill exercise test) performed, were the only significant predictors of hard events. Furthermore, the referral rates to early catheterization following SPECT were directly proportional to the

degree of scan abnormality (52). For patients without angina, the total event rate was comparable to those with angina. The relationship between scan findings and event rates was similar for patients with and without angina. From these preliminary results, we conclude that stress myocardial perfusion SPECT plays an important role in the clinical management of the post-PTCA patient. There appears to be an appropriate use of nuclear scan results in guiding decisions after catheterization, with low catheterization rates following nuclear scanning in patients with little evidence of ischemia.

In addition to assessing the ability of nuclear scanning to detect restenosis, the previously mentioned work of Pfisterer et al. (23) also evaluated the prognostic implications of silent ischemia by myocardial perfusion imaging. These investigators demonstrated that prognosis in patients with silent ischemia was remarkably similar to that of symptomatic patients. These observations suggest that silent ischemia due to restenosis after angioplasty has significant prognostic importance that may be improved by repeat angioplasty (23). Considerations should be given to routine stress testing for this entity.

In addition to providing perfusion information, gated myocardial perfusion SPECT can be used to assess regional and global ventricular function after PTCA. As discussed in Chapters 13 and 19, this technique provides accurate quantitative measurements of left ventricular ejection fraction and left ventricular volumes as well as semiquantitative assessment of regional wall motion. To date, there have been no reports of the use of gated SPECT in the post-PTCA patient. However, due to its improved ability to detect severe and extensive coronary artery disease over perfusion imaging alone, it is reasonable to assume that this method will provide increased sensitivity (with probably slightly decreased specificity) for detecting significant restenosis. Given the powerful prognostic content of gated perfusion SPECT information, the techniques of gated SPECT may also prove superior to perfusion SPECT alone in risk stratification of the post-PTCA patient. Thus, on the basis of the available evidence, myocardial perfusion imaging after PTCA is useful in identifying restenosis in risk stratifying patients, and appears to have a significant impact on the clinical management of post-PTCA patients.

Follow-up by Echocardiography

Stress echocardiography, using exercise, pharmacologic, or pacing stress, is also widely used clinically and can help assess patients following PTCA. Stress echocardiographic techniques have been used to detect restenosis in patients after PTCA with diagnostic accuracies comparable to nuclear imaging (53,54). Specifically, a high concordance has been observed between exercise stress echocardiography and exercise thallium-201 SPECT (54). Takeuchi et al. (55) compared dobutamine stress echocardiography and Tl-201 SPECT for detecting restenosis after PTCA. In 53 patients, they describe sensitivities of 78% and 74% and specificities of 93% and 93% for stress echocardiography and SPECT, respectively. For detecting restenosis following PTCA by echocardiography, sensitivity has been reported between 78 to 90% and specificity between 76% and 93%, depending on stress modalities and on whether the patient achieved the target heart rate at peak exercise (53–57). To date there have been no prognostic or risk stratification manuscripts reporting the results of stress echocardiography following PTCA.

Recommendations for Follow-up Patients Who Undergo Percutaneous Transluminal Angioplasty

Due to the high incidence of restenosis and its prognostic implications, as well as because of the progressive nature of coronary artery disease, it is clear that follow-up is essential for patients undergoing PTCA. The previous discussion demonstrates that clinical information, stress electrocardiography, stress myocardial perfusion SPECT, and stress echocardiography have a potential role in the assessment of the post-PTCA patient. Figures 2–4 summarize our recommendations for the assessment of the post-PTCA patient based on the patient's symptoms and angiographic findings before PTCA.

For patients with single-vessel disease (Fig. 2), who had typical angina prior to PTCA and whose symptoms were relieved by the revascularization procedure, it would be reasonable to follow symptoms in the assessment of potential restenosis. If typical angina recurs within the first 6 months following PTCA, restenosis would be likely and repeat coronary angiography indicated. In patients with single-vessel disease who develop nonanginal or atypical anginal symptoms in the first 6 months following PTCA, noninvasive

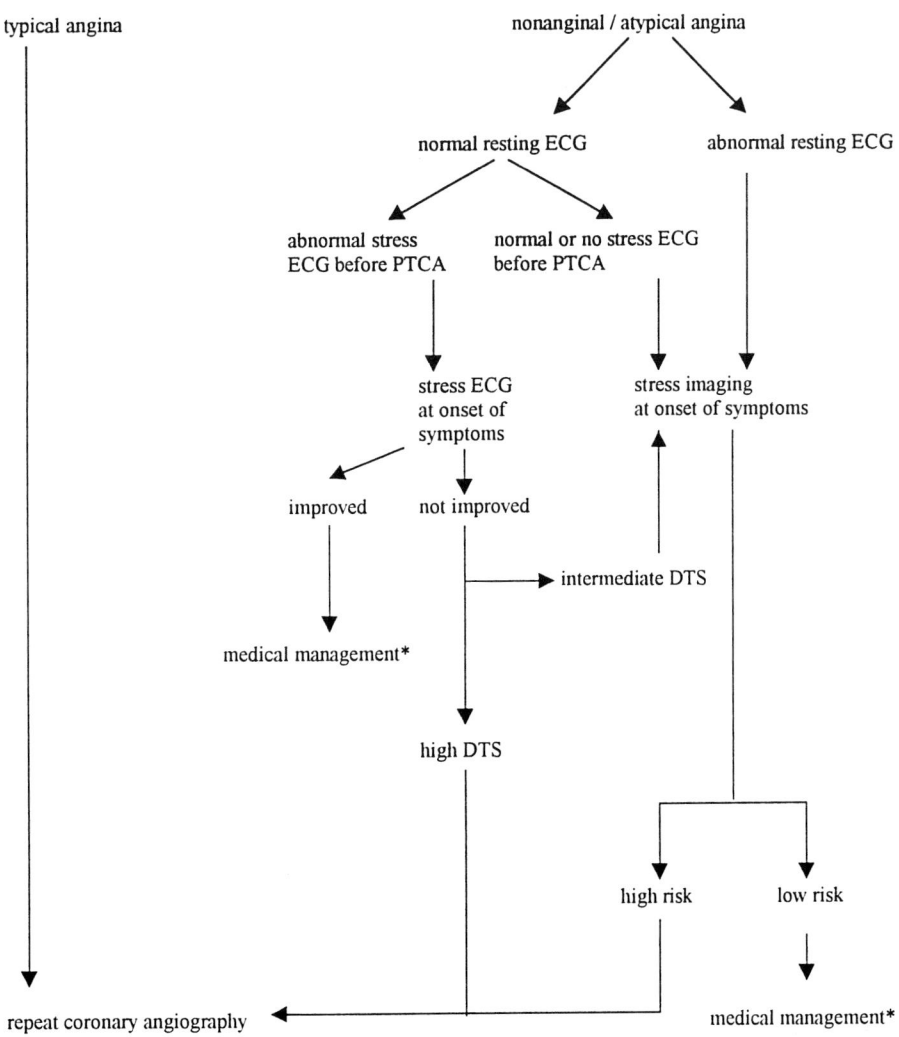

FIG. 2. Algorithm for the post-PTCA follow-up of symptomatic patients with single-vessel disease. *If time of testing <3 months, repeat test at 3–6 months. *ECG*, electrocardiogram; *DTS*, Duke Treadmill Score; *PTCA*, percutaneous transluminal coronary angioplasty.

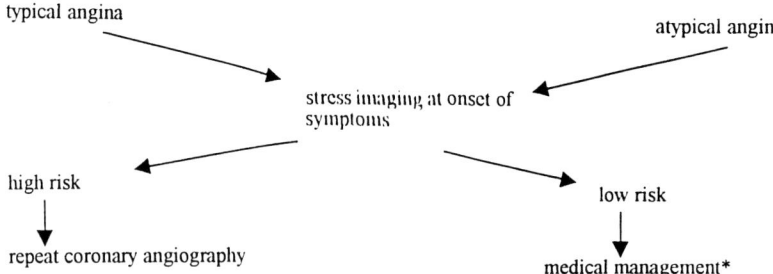

FIG. 3. Algorithm for the post-PTCA follow-up of symptomatic patients with multivessel disease. *If time of testing <3 months, repeat test at 3–6 months. *PTCA*, percutaneous transluminal coronary angioplasty.

testing becomes useful, since catheterizing all patients with atypical symptoms would not be cost-effective and could result in an overuse of repeat revascularization.

Further subdivision of these patients with single-vessel disease is based on the resting ECG findings. Those with an abnormal resting ECG (left bundle-branch block, left ventricular hypertrophy, etc.) are excellent candidates for nuclear or echocardiographic testing. For single-vessel disease patients with a normal resting ECG, standard ECG stress testing without imaging may be useful. For all of the exercise procedures (with or without imaging), we consider it critically important that the patients be able to achieve a maximal level of stress or develop an ischemic response to exercise. Patients who do not have an adequate treadmill stress test should be referred for pharmacologic stress imaging. In

order to maximize the likelihood of achieving a high level of stress, we recommend that patients be taken off beta blockers and negative chronotropic calcium channel antagonists, when clinically appropriate, for 48 hours prior to exercise testing. Thus, nonnuclear stress testing is particularly effective for patients who have had stress testing prior to PTCA.

We generally recommend a comprehensive evaluation of the treadmill test using an approach that takes into account both clinical and electrocardiographic responses to stress. The most widely validated approach in this regard is the Duke treadmill score, which is based on exercise duration, the degree of ST-segment depression, and the presence and degree of chest pain observed during exercise (58). A recent report using the Duke treadmill score has shown an enhanced

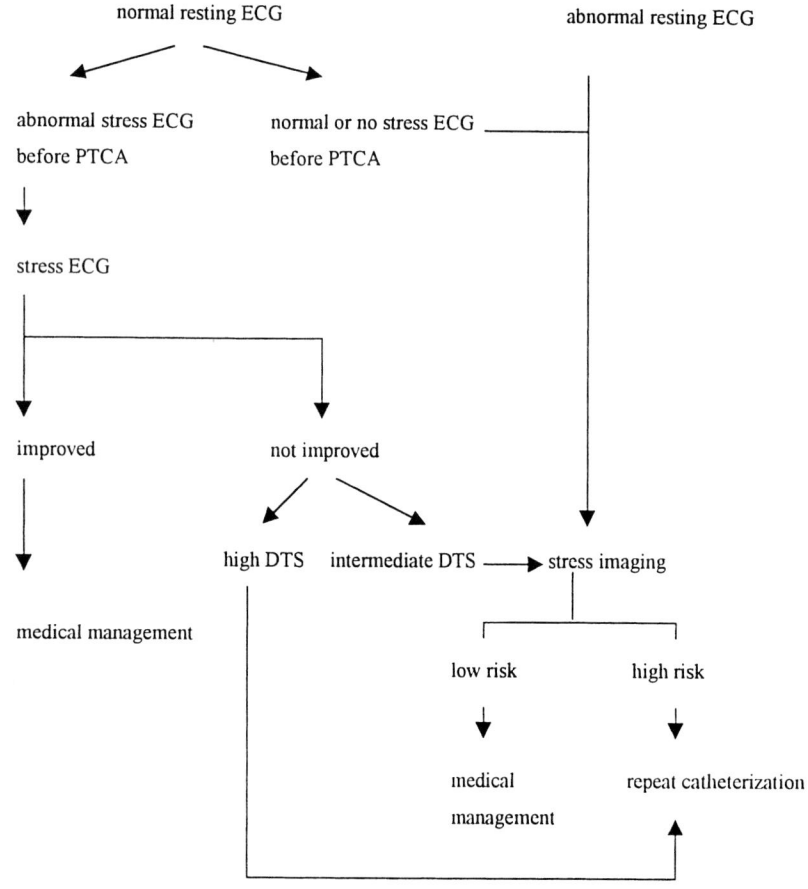

FIG. 4. Algorithm for follow-up of asymptomatic patients (3 to 6 months after PTCA). *DTS*, Duke Treadmill Score; *PTCA*, percutaneous transluminal coronary angioplasty.

ability to identify a significant coronary stenosis or severe coronary disease using this index, as compared to electrocardiographic or symptomatic parameters documented during stress testing (58). If the results of the stress ECG show improvement compared to the pre-PTCA study and reveal a low to intermediate risk Duke treadmill score, the patients could be classified as being at low risk and could be followed with continued medical therapy. If a high-risk Duke treadmill score (≤ 10) were observed (an uncommon but important observation) patients would be appropriately referred directly for repeat coronary angiography. If an intermediate Duke treadmill score were observed, stress imaging would be useful in further defining the patients who are most likely to benefit from angiography (2,59).

If single-vessel disease patients had a normal resting ECG and normal or no stress ECG prior to PTCA, when atypical symptoms recur, stress imaging should be considered. Patients at high risk after stress imaging would be excellent candidates for repeat coronary angiography. Patients at low risk could be followed with continued medical therapy.

Figure 3 illustrates our suggested approach to patients with multivessel disease before PTCA who develop symptoms in the post-PTCA period. Unless the patients are unstable, patients with multivessel disease who develop typical angina would be candidates for stress-imaging procedures before repeat coronary angiography to better determine the culprit lesion and to be best prepared for appropriate intervention. Since coronary stenting has become common, and since single-vessel stenting is frequently performed (often with staged procedures in multivessel disease), identification of the culprit lesion would appear to be even more important in the poststenting era than it was previously. Since stress-imaging procedures have highest sensitivity for detecting the most critically stenosed areas, these modalities are particularly effective in identifying the culprit lesion (42,60). Following stress imaging, low-risk patients could then be treated with medical management, whereas those found to be at high risk would be excellent candidates for repeat angiography (1,6).

Standard nonimaging stress testing could be applied in patients with multivessel disease prior to PTCA, as shown for patients with single-vessel disease in Figure 2. However, since the stress electrocardiogram does not provide information regarding the culprit vessel (location of ischemia by ECG is not predictive of location of ischemia by coronary angiography or myocardial perfusion SPECT [61,62]), this approach frequently provides inadequate clinical information for appropriate clinical management (i.e., selection of the appropriate lesion for PTCA).

Our approach to patients without symptoms is illustrated in Figure 4. If patients had angina prior to PTCA, which was relieved by PTCA, the approach would be the same as that applied to any chronic coronary artery disease patient. If, however, the patients had minimal or no symptoms prior to PTCA, then noninvasive stress testing would be indicated to evaluate the likelihood of restenosis and, if present, to

risk stratify the patient. In general, we would suggest that such patients be followed up between 3 to 6 months following PTCA, since this is the period in which restenosis is most likely to occur. The approach is the same as that shown in Figure 2 for the patients with nonanginal or atypical chest pain.

FOLLOW-UP OF PATIENTS AFTER CORONARY ARTERY BYPASS GRAFTING

Introduction

Following its introduction by Favaloro in 1969 (63), coronary artery bypass grafting (CABG) has become widely utilized for treatment of CAD. In 1996, CABG was performed on 367,000 patients in the United States (14). Over time, the results have continued to improve (64–67). With more widespread use of PTCA, CABG is now performed on higher risk patients with more advanced age, impaired left ventricular systolic function, extensive coronary artery disease, and history of myocardial infarction. The long-term efficacy of CABG is ultimately limited by graft stenosis and by progression of disease in native vessels. Saphenous vein graft occlusion rates have recently been reported to be 8% early, 13% at 1 year, 20% at 5 years, 41% at 7.5 years, 41% at 10 years, and 45% after 11.5 years (66,67). FitzGibbon et al. (67) observed that the greatest incidence of graft occlusions and of severe graft atherosclerosis occurred at 7.5 years after surgery. The time interval between 5 and 10 years corresponds to the period in which severe symptoms often recur after CABG. They reported an annual graft occlusion rate of approximately 2.1%. More than 48% of patients had significant graft disease at 5 years after CABG, 81% after 15 years. In contrast to the saphenous vein, arterial conduits, such as the internal mammary artery, more often remain free of atherosclerosis until late after surgery. Internal mammary patency rates of over 80% have been reported at 10 years after surgery (68).

In follow-up of patients after CABG, cardiovascular imaging can be used to document intraoperative cardiac injury or improved perfusion or function after revascularization, to demonstrate or predict graft disease or stenosis, and to predict subsequent cardiac events. The high frequency of occlusion or stenosis in bypass grafts, added to the known tendency of coronary artery disease to progress, makes the late post-CABG risk assessment of particular clinical importance.

Various studies have concluded that symptoms are not reliable predictors of graft patency or stenosis (69). Silent ischemia detected by exercise testing and ambulatory electrocardiography is present in 15 to 33% of the patients 1 year after CABG (70). New development or recurrence of chest pain provides a sensitivity of only 60% and a specificity of 20% for graft occlusion (69). Routine nonimaging stress testing has also been reported to have a low sensitivity

(60%), despite a high specificity (86%) for detecting a graft occlusion or stenosis (70).

Nuclear Methods

Nuclear methods can be used for evaluation of both left ventricular function and perfusion in patients after CABG. Although improvement of ventricular function may be noted as early as the first days after revascularization (71–73), the timing of the assessment of left ventricular ejection fraction is important because an early evaluation may underestimate the degree of recovery. An improvement in ejection fraction has been reported by Ghods et al. (73) up to 2 months after surgery.

A common finding after CABG, which was first described with radionuclide angiography but has been noticed also with gated SPECT and echocardiography, is abnormal septal motion postoperatively (74,75). It has been demonstrated that abnormal postoperative septal motion is usually associated with normal septal perfusion and viability (76).

In the absence of perioperative injury or abrupt graft closure, myocardial perfusion imaging after CABG surgery will usually show improvement of coronary perfusion in the revascularized territories (77,78). The degree of stress-induced perfusion abnormality preoperatively is related to the likelihood of extensive improvement in the postoperative state (78).

Cardiac radionuclide imaging has been shown to be able to identify graft stenosis or occlusion. Pfisterer et al. (79) described sensitivity, specificity, and accuracy of 80%, 88%, and 86%, respectively, using planar thallium imaging in patients who had undergone CABG 1 year prior to the nuclear testing. Lakkis et al. (80) described an 80% overall-sensitivity and 87% overall-specificity (with sensitivity 82%, 92%, and 75% and specificity 90%, 91%, 75% for left anterior descending artery, right coronary artery, and left circumflex artery, respectively) for exercise thallium-201 SPECT evaluation in 50 patients. They compared the nuclear results to the results of exercise electrocardiography, which showed a sensitivity of 31% and a specificity of 93%. The same group published a study assessing graft stenosis late after CABG by adenosine thallium-201 SPECT in 109 patients. They reported a sensitivity of 96% and a specificity of 61%. The observed sensitivity for detecting graft stenosis is comparable to the sensitivity for detecting stenosis in native vessels. The authors explained the relatively low specificity by the fact that bypasses were frequently supplying myocardium partly scarred from a previous myocardial infarction and unbypassed native disease proximal to the grafts, or progression of native disease distal to the grafts (81).

The available evidence suggests that nuclear tests provide excellent information about graft patency in patients who have undergone CABG surgery, for both vein grafts (79–83), as well as for internal mammary artery (84) and gastroepiploic artery grafts (85). Despite the ability to detect graft stenosis or occlusion, nuclear testing is seldom used

for this purpose alone on a clinical basis, since the finding of graft stenosis does not necessarily imply the need to consider repeat revascularization. Thus, the primary clinical application of nuclear testing in patients following CABG is risk stratification.

Prognostic Impact of Nuclear Stress Testing

Risk stratification of the post-CABG patient is an important clinical consideration in patient management. Although exercise testing alone (without imaging) has been evaluated (86–88), in general, these studies have shown little or no prognostic value for isolated exercise testing in this patient cohort. A study by Weiner et al. (88), the single study showing prognostic value of exercise testing, reported only modest differences in survival based on stress testing results.

In contrast, several studies have shown that after evaluation of treadmill and exercise data, myocardial perfusion SPECT (Tl-201 as well as Tc-99m sestamibi) provides incremental prognostic information for patients after bypass surgery (72,83). In a study of 294 patients undergoing exercise Tl-201 SPECT ≥ 5 years after CABG and followed for 31 ± 11 months, Palmas et. al. (89) demonstrated that shortness of breath and peak exercise heart rate were significant clinical predictors of cardiac death or nonfatal myocardial infarction. Two scintigraphic variables added significant prognostic information to the clinical model: the Tl-201 summed reversibility score (a measure of the extent and severity of reversible defects) and the presence of increased lung uptake of Tl-201. The nuclear data doubled the amount of information of a multivariate model as measured by the global chi-square. Nallamothu et al. (90) reported similar incremental information for stress Tl-201 SPECT, even when coronary angiographic variables were taken into account. In 250 patients undergoing stress Tl-201 SPECT and coronary angiography, 58 ± 50 months after CABG, no significant prognostic value was provided by clinical, stress, or angiographic variables. In contrast, the extent of the Tl-201 perfusion abnormality, multivessel perfusion defects, and increased lung thallium uptake were significant independent predictors of events.

Lauer et al. (83) have demonstrated that even in asymptomatic patients after CABG, thallium perfusion defects and impaired exercise capacity are strong and independent predictors of subsequent death or nonfatal myocardial perfusion (83). In a study of 873 asymptomatic patients undergoing exercise Tl-201 SPECT a mean of 7 years after CABG and followed-up for 3 years, exercise capacity (≤6 metabolic equivalent tests [METs]) and Tl-201 perfusion defects were independently predictive of cardiac death and nonfatal myocardial infarction. Nine percent of asymptomatic patients with perfusion defects died over the 3-year follow-up versus 3% ($P = 0.0004$) for those without perfusion defects.

To date, Miller et al. (91) have published the only prognostic study with respect to risk stratification early after

CABG. They included 405 patients, who had exercise thallium-201 testing two years after CABG and were followed-up for a median duration of 5.8 years after nuclear testing. Of these patients, 34% were asymptomatic. Increasing age, shorter exercise duration, and the number of abnormal thallium-201 segments after exercise have been shown to be significant independent predictors for total mortality. A *post hoc* analysis revealed that SSS was the strongest independent predictor for total mortality. The 5-year survival free of coronary death or myocardial infarction was 93% for patients without angina and a normal image or small postexercise defect versus 71% for patients with angina and a medium or large defect.

With stress Tc-99m sestamibi SPECT, our group has published preliminary data reporting annual cardiac death rates of 0.8%, 1.3%, and 3.2% in 865 patients undergoing SPECT more than 5 years after surgery for normal, mildly abnormal, and moderately to severely abnormal scans, respectively (92), as judged by the summed stress score (5). Further preliminary data from our group compared the prognostic value of dual isotope myocardial SPECT, in 628 patients who underwent CABG less than 5 years before nuclear testing to that observed in 916 patients whose nuclear tests were performed more than 5 years after CABG. The patients studied less than 5 years post-CABG had significantly fewer cardiac deaths or nonfatal myocardial infarctions (hard events) than patients who had CABG more than 5 years before nuclear testing. Also, patients without symptoms and CABG less than 5 years before nuclear testing had a significantly lower hard event rate than patients with symptoms. The annual cardiac death rate in the group tested less than 5 years after CABG was low at 0.9% (93).

With respect to exercise radionuclide angiography (RNA), Borges-Neto et al. (94) have reported the long-term follow-up of 182 patients undergoing exercise RNA and coronary angiography less than 3 years after CABG. The exercise ejection fraction was the strongest predictor of cardiac death, contributing beyond clinical and catheterization data. Since the summed stress score on myocardial perfusion SPECT is the perfusion correlate of peak exercise ejection fraction, reflecting the extent of ischemia and infarction, similar results would be expected from assessment of this more widely available variable.

Follow-up of Coronary Artery Bypass Graft Patients by Echocardiography

As with nuclear testing, stress echocardiography can also be utilized in follow-up of patients following bypass surgery. Kafka et al. (95) performed exercise echocardiography in 182 patients after CABG, patients in whom coronary angiography was also performed. In 93 of the 118 cases with vascular compromise on angiography (greater than or equal to 50% stenosis), exercise echocardiography was abnormal (sensitivity 79%). In 78 of the 95 cases without evidence of vascular compromise on angiography, exercise echocardiog-

raphy was normal (specificity 82%). Importantly, the greater the number of regions with vascular compromise on angiography, the more likely was an abnormal finding on exercise echocardiography.

With dobutamine, transesophageal echo has been reported to be superior to transthoracic echo for the detection of ischemia after CABG surgery. Sensitivity increased from 78 to 93%; the specificity of transesophageal echocardiography was 93% (96). Pezzano et al. (97,98) documented graft patency of internal mammary graft artery to left anterior descending coronary artery in 49 of 58 patients by dipyridamole Doppler echocardiography. Goto et al. published results on left internal thoracic artery graft patency using the left supraclavicular echocardiographic view (no stress) in 25 patients and found a sensitivity of 71.4% and a specificity of 100% for graft patency.

On the basis of the available evidence, therefore, it would appear that stress echocardiography and stress nuclear techniques have similar efficacy in assessing bypass graft patency. However, it is generally acknowledged that abnormal septal motion that occurs normally postoperatively makes interpretation of echocardiography in the postoperative patient somewhat difficult. In contrast, interpretation of myocardial perfusion studies in the postoperative patient provides no reported additional difficulty. Possibly of even greater importance, to date, there has been very limited information available with respect to risk stratification of the postoperative patient using stress echocardiographic techniques.

Computed Tomography

Several studies have demonstrated the feasibility of assessing graft patency using electron beam computed tomography (EBCT) with intravenous contrast injection at rest. Sensitivities of 94%–100% and specificities of 97%–100% have been reported for detecting coronary bypass graft patency (99–101). The accuracy appears to be independent of the vessel that was bypassed and has not been statistically significantly different for saphenous veins compared with internal mammary grafts (99–101). EBCT is a promising noninvasive screening method for evaluation of graft patency following CABG. The limitation of this method is that it does not provide information about graft stenosis but only shows graft patency. In addition, the method is not widely available at this time. Less explored is this method's potential to provide information about the progression of coronary artery disease following CABG by serial assessment of coronary calcification. In the future, it is likely that multislice mechanical CT scanners will play an important role in assessment of graft patency.

Magnetic Resonance Imaging

The feasibility of magnetic resonance imaging for assessing bypass graft patency has also been assessed. Magnetic resonance imaging (MRI) reached sensitivities of up to 93% and specificities of up to 97% for the documentation of graft patency (102–104), with a κ-value comparing MRI and coronary angiography of 0.9 (102). By combining standard MRI techniques with MR phase velocity mapping, the flow rate in the graft can be measured, potentially allowing assessment of graft stenosis as well as simple patency (103). This method can also be used with adenosine stress to evaluate myocardial perfusion at rest and stress in regions supplied by bypass grafts. Some difficulty is encountered with MRI due to artifacts caused by metallic structures left in place following bypass surgery. For example, Okamura et al. (104) described the interference of sternal wires (stainless steel) and hemoclips with the interpretation of MRI and the consequent reduction in sensitivity for assessing graft patency. Higher sensitivity could be expected if the type of metal used in the sternal wires and hemoclips at CABG did not distort the MRI signal. Although highly promising, this method is limited in its clinical application due to the lack of standardized protocols for routine clinical assessments. Although MRI scanners are abundant, relatively few centers have established experience in assessment of graft patency or rest and stress perfusion or function studies.

RECOMMENDATIONS

The management of the post-CABG patient depends on multiple factors, probably the most important being the patient's symptoms. In patients who become severely symptomatic after CABG, direct catheterization is frequently indicated. In some of these patients, however, the imaging techniques can be of help in defining the culprit lesion. Stress nuclear methods or MRI/CT assessments of graft patency could be useful in these circumstances. Although stress echocardiography could be considered, the difficulty in assessing wall motion abnormalities in the postoperative patient may limit the general effectiveness of this procedure in this setting.

In the less symptomatic patient or in asymptomatic patients following late bypass, noninvasive risk stratification plays an important clinical role.

Our recommendations for assessment of the post-CABG patient are illustrated in Figure 5. When typical or atypical symptoms reoccur following bypass surgery, nuclear stress imaging should be considered. Patients with a benign prognosis, on the basis of the imaging finding, would be candidates for intensive medical therapy while those with a predicted high event rate would be candidates for coronary angiography, with consideration for possible repeat revascularization. Since silent ischemia can be both severe and extensive, even patients without symptoms should be considered for testing.

In the first several years following bypass surgery, routine stress imaging is not recommended, since, in general, the risk of cardiac events is low for asymptomatic patients in this period. Of course, patients who are at particularly high risk early postoperatively, despite their asymptomatic state, would be candidates for early stress testing. Such patients might include those with extensive coronary disease and incomplete revascularization, as well as younger patients with accelerated atherosclerosis. Approximately 5 years after bypass surgery, since the frequency of multiple-vessel graft stenosis or occlusion as well as progression of disease in native coronary arteries is expected to be relatively high, consideration should be given to performing a stress nuclear procedure even in asymptomatic patients. If the test results are indicative of a high likelihood of subsequent cardiac events, strong consideration would then be given to referral to coronary angiography.

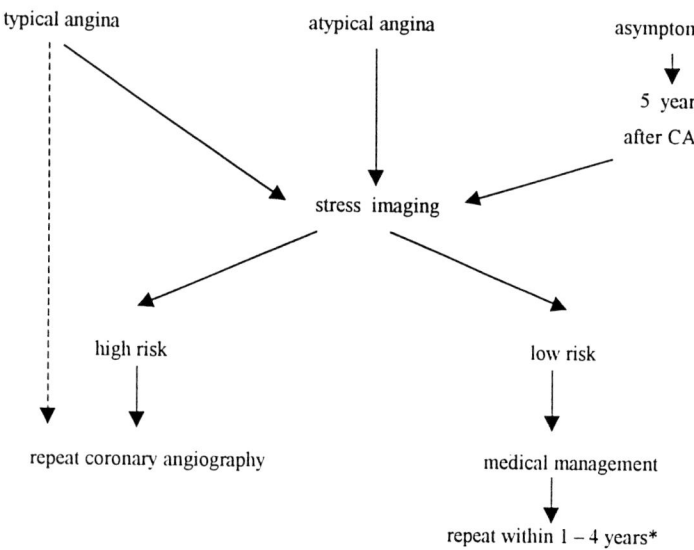

FIG. 5. Algorithm for patients after CABG. *Depending on symptoms, risk factors (control of hypertension, lipids), coronary anatomy, and surgical procedure. *CABG,* coronary artery bypass graft surgery.

MEDICAL INTERVENTION

Introduction

Plaque rupture is now widely accepted as the inciting factor in acute coronary ischemic syndromes. Furthermore, impaired vasomotion accompanying atherosclerotic plaque rupture in the setting of a subcritical stenosis has been advocated as a major factor contributing to progressive disease and myocardial necrosis. Atherosclerosis is now considered to be a complex physiology of inflammation within the coronary artery wall often resulting in acute plaque rupture and reduced blood flow to the myocardium. This insight into the atherosclerotic process has been used to develop an array of medical therapies aimed at reducing lipids available for deposition in the vessel wall and attenuating the level of detrimental circulating neurohumoral substances (as occurs with ACE inhibitors [105–107], in addition to other factors that affect a reduction in ensuing cardiac risk). HMG-CoA-reductase inhibitors, for example, exhibit a beneficial effect by modifying endothelial function, inflammatory responses, plaque stability, and thrombus formation (108–110).

Perfusion defect size and severity have been shown in large multicenter observational series to be strongly correlated with the presence and extent of high-grade coronary stenoses and, most importantly for medical therapy, to document flow to the coronary bed (1,2,5). To the extent that coronary flow reserve is effected by the atherosclerotic process, coronary disease progression and the response of therapeutic interventions may be monitored with cardiac imaging techniques. There are limited data on the use of cardiac imaging techniques to document effective medical management. However, effective cholesterol lowering has been shown to improve myocardial perfusion reserve by nuclear imaging in hypercholesterolemic patients (111–113), indicating that impairment of reactive hyperemia may play a more central role in identifying cardiac outcomes and for targeting medical therapy. This is due to the fact that alterations in coronary flow reserve may result not only from fixed stenosis but also from intrinsic wall elasticity, integrity of the endothelium, and vasodilator responsiveness within the arterial wall. Just as improvements in perfusion may document therapeutic success, worsening of defect size and severity may identify patients for whom additional lipid lowering therapy or invasive intervention may be indicated.

For cardiac imaging, the central noninvasive risk marker to assess flow is myocardial perfusion imaging. Although efforts are underway to develop an estimation of intravascular volume with myocardial contrast echocardiography, the current gold standard for the assessment of perfusion is nuclear imaging with SPECT or PET (positron emission tomography). Myocardial perfusion imaging may prove useful in assessing agents that alter vasomotor tone and coronary endothelial function, such as lipid-lowering drugs. This notion is supported by the improved clinical outcome without evidence of angiographic lesion regression in virtually all of the lipid trials.

Sequential perfusion imaging may be useful in assessing the efficacy of antiischemic therapy and cardiac interventions. Preliminary data suggest that perfusion imaging may be useful to assess the antiischemic effects of various medical therapies for patients with coronary artery spasm as well as in the setting of fixed obstructive lesions. Nitrates, calcium antagonists, and beta-blocker therapy, used alone or in combination, have been shown to effectively reduce the extent of stress-induced scintigraphic ischemia in small patient samples, and the use of risk-based empiric treatment will result in improved patient outcome. For example, after acute myocardial infarction, Dakik et al. (114) recently showed in a prospective, randomized pilot study of patients with extensive ischemia after acute myocardial infarction that intensive medical therapy prevents myocardial ischemia to a degree comparable to that achieved by a combination of PTCA and medical therapy. The sequential SPECT results suggested that patients showing an early reduction of ischemia on medical therapy have as favorable event-free survival at 1 year as patients undergoing revascularization. These early observations suggest that by providing an objective means for assessment of the early response to a trial of medical therapy, serial imaging studies may expand the indications for medical as opposed to revascularization therapies in a variety of clinical settings.

In patients with coronary artery disease, medical therapy is a cornerstone of patient management. A large number of studies document the benefit of medical therapy in patients with chronic stable angina. In considering the methods for follow-up and monitoring of patients who undergo medical therapy, a number of factors should be considered. They should be followed by reproducible methods. If exercise treadmill tests are used for assessment of therapy, common endpoints include exercise duration, maximal ST-segment depression, and the time of onset of angina. The use of nuclear testing in assessing response to medical therapy poses interesting additional considerations. If maximal exercise or pharmacologic stress is used before and after therapy, a potential beneficial effect of medical therapy could be obscured; i.e., if the patient exercises to a much greater workload after therapy before injection of a perfusion tracer, the observed perfusion defects may be the same as before therapy, even if myocardial perfusion was improved at the same workload as achieved before treatment. A stress imaging protocol that avoids this pitfall is to ensure that the heart rate or the double product achieved (blood pressure × heart rate at peak exercise) is the same in both baseline and follow-up tests. We would propose a protocol that allows the conventional exercise endpoints of maximal exercise duration, etc., to be obtained while deriving scintigraphic information from exercise to the same workload as baseline. This protocol involves the exercise injection of Tc-99m sestamibi or tetrofosmin at the same workload as during the baseline study, providing a directly comparable perfusion measurement on follow-up imaging, with continuation of the exercise until the standard clinical endpoints of maximal exercise are achieved.

Reproducibility of Nuclear Testing Results

There are several studies that show excellent reproducibility for myocardial perfusion SPECT. Mahmarian et al. (115) published data that showed that quantitative exercise Tl-201 tomography is highly reproducible and can be used to accurately interpret temporal changes in myocardial perfusion in individual patients. A greater than or equal to 10% change in total perfusion defect size defined the 95% confidence interval for exceeding the intrinsic variability of the tomographic technique.

Previous results from our group showed a high intraobserver agreement in 80 patients with a κ value of 0.82 for stress studies and a κ value of 0.73 for resting studies. We have also demonstrated the defect extent and severity, as measured by automatic quantitative analysis of exercise dual isotope myocardial perfusion SPECT (116) evaluated in 30 patients who had two exercise dual-isotope studies 31 days plus or minus 16 days apart, are highly stable measurements and can reliably detect changes of greater than or equal to 10% from baseline (117). When gated SPECT is employed, in addition to providing reproducible assessment of various indices of myocardial perfusion, the method provides highly reproducible measurements of left ventricular ejection fraction and left ventricular volumes, as discussed in Chapter 19. Figure 6 illustrates the application of serial myocardial perfusion SPECT to monitor medical therapy in a patient with chronic coronary artery disease.

Reproducibility of Echocardiographic Methods

To date, there is only one report on the reproducibility of stress echocardiography. In this study of 15 patients undergoing dobutamine stress, there was excellent reproducibility in assessment of segmental wall motion on repeated studies and excellent interobserver agreement ($\kappa = 0.86$ for each) (55). In contrast, in a large, multicenter study of interobserver agreement in interpretation of dobutamine stress echocardiograms, Hoffmann et al. (118) reported excellent interobserver agreement only when studies were graded as good to excellent in quality. However, this subgroup represented only 40% of the cohort; in the remaining 60% of the patients, the agreement ranged from only 43 to 74%. With exercise echocardiography, with the inherent greater amount of patient motion and respiratory variation, even poorer reproducibility would be expected. These considerations, as well as the absence of a widely accepted, objective quantitative method for interpretation, limit the effectiveness of stress echocardiography in the serial assessment of the effects of medical interventions.

Reproducibility of Electron-beam Computed Tomography Methods

Electron-beam computed tomography is a promising new tool for the evaluation of coronary artery disease. Callister et al. (119) showed a better reproducibility for the volumetric calcium score than for the traditional coronary calcium score. Fifty-two patients underwent two studies carried out a few minutes apart. The medium percentage change was 9% for the volumetric and 15% for the traditional score. As with the graft patency application, the widespread use of this approach for serial assessment of medical therapy awaits the broader dissemination of the technology.

Reproducibility of Magnetic Resonance Imaging Methods

MRI has great promise for serial assessment of medical therapy. The ability to provide reproducible quantitation of ventricular volumes and mass is already being used in clinical trials. The more widespread use of this approach for assessment of medical therapy for the guiding of patient management on a practical, clinical basis awaits further dissemination of expertise and clinical availability of the measurements. With respect to evaluation of the effects of medical therapy on myocardial perfusion, MRI is not yet widely used clinically, due to the lack of standardized, objective approaches to the assessment of rest and stress perfusion.

Myocardial Perfusion and Antiischemic Drugs

Mahmarian et al. (120) tested transdermal nitroglycerin in a randomized, double blind, placebo controlled trial using quantitative thallium-201 tomography. Patients in the active group had a significant reduction in their total perfusion defect size (average 8.9%), which was most apparent in those with the largest ($\geq$20%) baseline defects (average reduction = 11.4%).

Similar results have been reported with isosorbide dinitrate when administered to patients with coronary disease. Lewin et al. (121) collected data that showed a decrease in defect extent in patients treated once daily with extended-release isosorbide mononitrate (120 mg/day) for 30 to 35 days. Total defect extent was decreased by 13% and total defect severity was reduced by 14% from baseline to the last study. This study employed rest thallium-201/exercise Tc-99m sestamibi separate acquisition dual-isotope myocardial perfusion SPECT protocol (121).

Combination antiischemic medications including calcium antagonists, beta blockers, and nitrate therapy are commonly used in patients with chronic coronary artery disease. A number of studies have also documented the effects of medical therapy on stress-induced ischemia (122–124). Cid et al. (122) demonstrated that patients taking one or more antiischemic medications during dobutamine SPECT had a significant reduction in the likelihood of an abnormal scan.

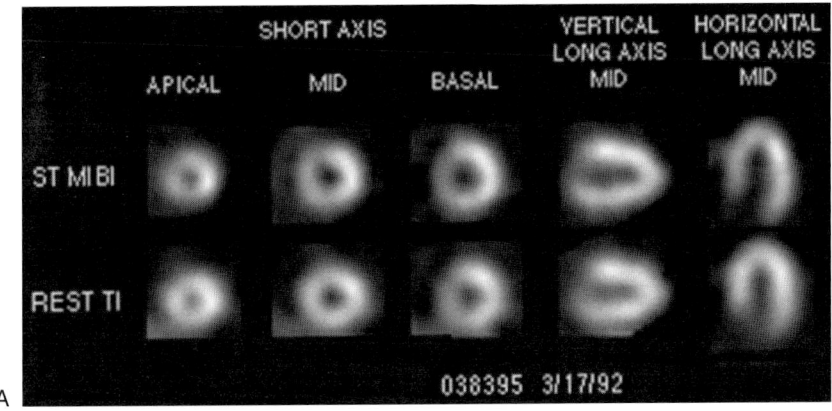

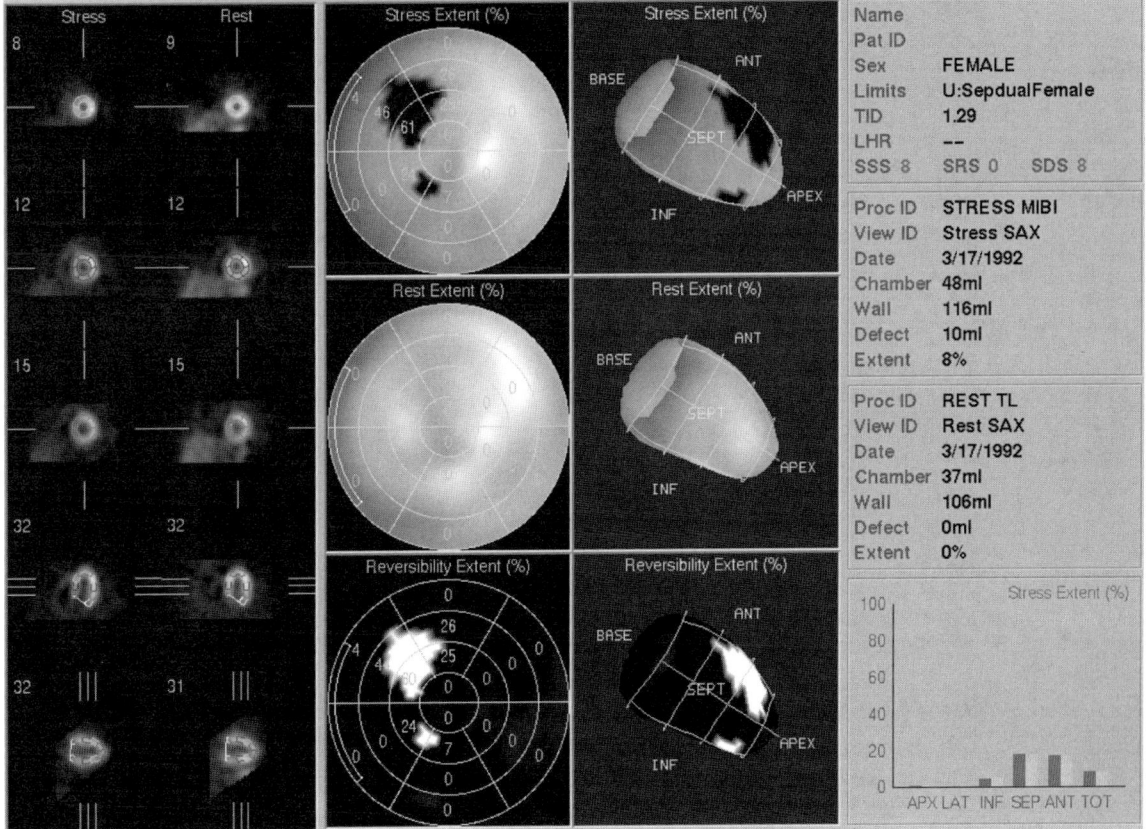

FIG. 6. A: Exercise sestamibi/rest TI-201 myocardial perfusion SPECT in a 69-year-old female with atypical angina following an acute myocardial infarction showing a small reversible defect in the left anterior descending artery (LAD) territory. **B:** Quantitative perfusion SPECT (QPS) analysis of the patient shown in **A**. The quantitative stress defect extent was 8%, and the computer derived summed stress score was 8. Subsequent coronary angiography revealed a 70% proximal LAD stenosis and a 40% right coronary artery (RCA) narrowing. The patient subsequently underwent medical management. Compare **A** and **B** with **C** and **D**. *(continued)*

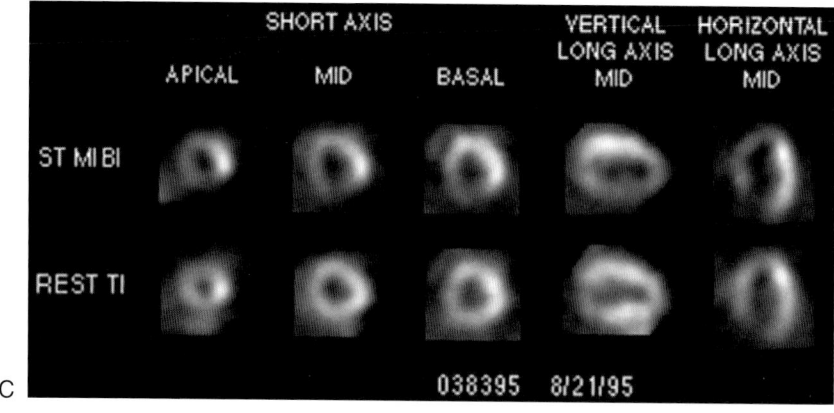

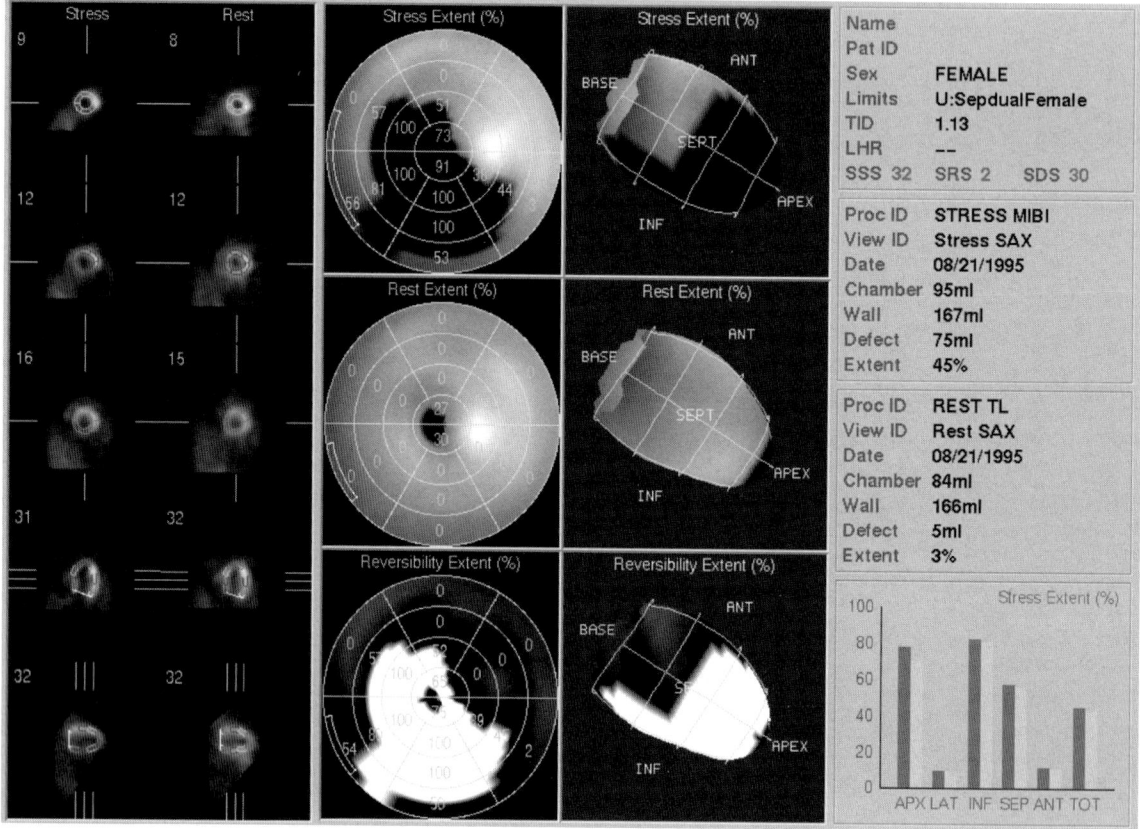

FIG. 6. *Continued.* **C:** Exercise stress sestamibi/rest thallium-201 myocardial perfusion SPECT in the same patient as shown in **A**, three years later. The patient still had only atypical angina. The SPECT findings now demonstrate evidence of extensive reversible ischemia in the LAD and RCA territories. Based on the severity of the perfusion defects, critical stenoses of these two vessels can be predicted. Coronary angiography the day following testing revealed a subtotal mid-LAD stenosis and a 95% proximal RCA stenosis. The minimal abnormality on the resting thallium study indicated that the area of prior myocardial infarction was small. **D:** Quantitative perfusion SPECT (QPS) analysis of the SPECT study shown in **C**. The QPS study demonstrated a stress perfusion defect extent of 45%, with large abnormalities in the LAD and RCA territories. The summed stress score was markedly elevated at 32. Objective documentation of worsening of stress myocardial perfusion is provided by the study. *SPECT*, single-photon emission computed tomography.

Furthermore, Shehata et al. (123) reported the acute effects of propranolol administration on dobutamine-induced perfusion defects in patients with coronary artery disease. In this latter series, dobutamine SPECT was performed on separate days with and without pretreatment of intravenous propranolol. The results indicated that total and ischemic perfusion defect size was reduced 22% and 32%, respectively, following propranolol administration.

When using pharmacologic vasodilator stress, Dakik and colleagues (114) reported the results of sequential adenosine SPECT to compare the efficacy of medical therapy versus coronary angioplasty for suppressing ischemia in 44 postmyocardial infarction patients whose initial perfusion scan exhibited a large area of ischemia (114). Approximately 30 days after the initiation of therapy, a 37 and 23% reduction in total and ischemic perfusion defect size was observed with antiischemic therapy. The reduction in total (12 to 15%) and ischemic (12%) perfusion defect size was similar for patients randomized to intensive medical therapy versus coronary angioplasty. Sharir et al. (124) studied the effects of combination antiischemic medications on perfusion defect size in 21 patients with chronic coronary disease who had dipyridamole SPECT. Baseline SPECT was performed off antiischemic medications and then repeated following administration of either calcium antagonists, nitrates, and/or beta blockers. The results indicated a 24 to 33% reduction in defect size with antiischemic medications.

Despite the reported benefit of medical therapies on reducing stress-induced defect patterns, it is important to determine how reductions in the extent of abnormalities affect event-free survival. In the ACME (Angioplasty Compared to Medicine) study, 270 patients were randomized to receive antiischemic therapy or coronary angioplasty (125). Thallium-201 planar scintigraphy was performed at baseline and after 6 months of therapy. Survival was significantly improved for patients who had normalized perfusion with either therapy as compared to those with persistent ischemia (92 versus 82%, $P = 0.02$) (125). In the more recent study in acute myocardial infarction patients by Dakik et al. (114) described above, it was reported that event-free survival was 96% for patients who had a significant reduction in perfusion defect size compared to 65% for those who exhibited no major reduction in nuclear perfusion defects.

A synopsis of these results indicates that preliminary evidence in small patient samples shows that perfusion imaging may be used to assess the efficacy of antiischemic therapy as well as to provide a measure for tracking future risk of cardiac outcomes.

Lipid Lowering Drugs

Improvement of myocardial perfusion by short-term fluvastatin therapy was shown by Eichstädt et al. (126) They presented 17 males that were treated for 12 weeks and then followed-up by thallium-201 scintigraphy. In ischemic segments, myocardial perfusion increased by 30%. In normal segments, perfusion increased by only 5%. The change in perfusion rate between ischemic and normal segments was statistically significant (126). The authors concluded that LDL (low-density lipoprotein) lowering by HMG-CoA reductase inhibitors improved myocardial perfusion, especially in areas of ischemia (126,127).

Siebelink et al. (128) have reported the use of PET scanning to assess fluvastatin therapy in 15 asymptomatic subjects with elevated cholesterol levels. Fluvastatin treatment significantly increased coronary flow reserve, documented by serial 13N-ammonia PET imaging at rest and during pharmacologic stress. Reduction of cholesterol levels may have a direct beneficial cardiac effect in primary prevention that can be assessed with imaging techniques. Using SPECT in 10 patients with known coronary artery disease and proven hypercholesterolemia who were treated with diet and cholesterol-lowering medication, serial quantitative SPECT examination showed that a 42% reduction of mean LDL cholesterol was associated with a 53% reduction of mean stress perfusion score (129).

EBCT may also be of use in documenting the impact of cholesterol lowering on coronary artery disease. As noted above, in a recent study evaluating serial changes in calcified coronary volume as assessed by EBCT, Callister et al. (119) showed that measurement of the calcified coronary volume is highly reproducible. In a subsequent study (130), the authors evaluated the serial change for this measurement in a group of patients. They postulated that aging plaques may become smaller in volume while becoming denser. In patients not undergoing HMG-CoA reductase therapy or not achieving an LDL less than 120 mg percent on therapy, all had an increase in the calcified coronary volume over a 1-year period. In contrast, of patients receiving HMG-CoA reductase inhibitors and whose LDL on treatment was less than 120 mls percent, more than 60% demonstrated a reduction of the calcified coronary volume over the same time. Since the measurement of calcified coronary volume is nearly automatic with EBCT, this technique may provide a useful tool in evaluating the effects of medical therapy.

RECOMMENDATIONS FOR SERIAL CLINICAL ASSESSMENT OF PATIENTS UNDERGOING MEDICAL THERAPY

Of the various imaging methods, at the present time SPECT or PET techniques are the most well-validated for purposes of serial quantitative assessment of myocardial perfusion. These methods are likely to be useful for the care of individual patients in documenting the response to standard medical therapies in a variety of clinical settings, as well as in assessing the efficacy of new medical therapies in clinical trials. For other cardiac assessments, such as serial assessment of myocardial mass in patients with left ventricular hypertrophy (LVH) or in assessing serial changes in left ventricular volumes, several of the imaging methods are effective. Particularly noteworthy in this regard are the high reproducibilities of gated SPECT and MRI measurements.

REFERENCES

1. Hachamovitch R, Berman DS, Kiat H, et al. Effective risk stratification using exercise myocardial perfusion SPECT in women: gender-related differences in prognostic nuclear testing. *J Am Coll Cardiol* 1996;28(1):34–44.
2. Hachamovitch R, Berman DS, Shaw LJ, et al. Incremental prognostic value of myocardial perfusion single photon emission computed tomography for the prediction of cardiac death: differential stratification for risk of cardiac death and myocardial infarction. *Circulation* 1998; 97(6):535–543.
3. Ladenheim ML, Kotler TS, Pollock BH, et al. Incremental prognostic power of clinical history, exercise electrocardiography and myocardial perfusion scintigraphy in suspected coronary artery disease. *Am J Cardiol* 1987;59(4):270–277.
4. Brown KA. Prognostic value of thallium-201 myocardial perfusion imaging. A diagnostic tool comes of age. *Circulation* 1991;83(2): 363–381.
5. Berman DS, Hachamovitch R, Kiat H, et al. Incremental value of prognostic testing in patients with known or suspected ischemic heart disease: a basis for optimal utilization of exercise technetium-99m sestamibi myocardial perfusion single-photon emission computed tomography. *J Am Coll Cardiol* 1995;26(3):639–647.
6. Hachamovitch R, Berman DS, Kiat H, et al. Exercise myocardial perfusion SPECT in patients without known coronary artery disease: incremental prognostic value and use in risk stratification. *Circulation* 1996;93(5):905–994.
7. Sharir T, Germano G, Lewin HC, et al. Prognostic value of myocardial perfusion and function by gated SPECT in the prediction of non-fatal myocardial infarction and cardiac death. *Circulation* 1999;100:I-383.
8. Topol EJ, Ellis SG, Cosgrove DM, et al. Analysis of coronary angioplasty practice in the United States with an insurance-claims data base. *Circulation* 1993;87(5):1489–1497.
9. Wennberg DE, Kellett MA, Dickens JD, et al. The association between local diagnostic testing intensity and invasive cardiac procedures. *JAMA* 1996;275(15):1161–1164.
10. Kuhn EM, Hartz AJ, Baras M. Correlation of rates of coronary artery bypass surgery, angioplasty, and cardiac catheterization in 305 large communities for persons age 65 and older. *Health Serv Res* 1995; 30(3):425–436.
11. Sharir T, Germano G, Kavanagh PB, et al. Incremental prognostic value of post-stress left ventricular ejection fraction and volume by gated myocardial perfusion single photon emission computed tomography. *Circulation* 1999;100:1035–1042.
12. Gruentzig AR, King SB III, Schlumpf M, et al. Long-term follow-up after percutaneous transluminal coronary angioplasty. The early Zurich experience. *N Engl J Med* 1987;316(18):1127–1132.
13. Gruentzig AR, Senning A, Siegenthaler WE. Nonoperative dilatation of coronary-artery stenosis: percutaneous transluminal coronary angioplasty. *N Engl J Med* 1979;301(2):61–68.
14. American Heart Association: *http://www.amhrt.org*.
15. Goy JJ, Eeckhout E. Intracoronary stenting. *Lancet* 1998;351: 1943–1949.
16. Braunwald E. *Heart disease: a textbook of cardiovascular medicine*, 5th ed. Philadelphia: WB Saunders, 1997.
17. Kuntz RE, Baim DS. Defining coronary restenosis. Newer clinical and angiographic paradigms. *Circulation* 1993;88(3):1310–1323.
18. Nobuyoshi MK, Kimura T, Nosaka H, et al. Restenosis after successful percutaneous transluminal coronary angioplasty: serial angiographic follow-up of 229 patients. *J Am Coll Cardiol* 1988;12(3): 616–623.
19. Violaris AG, Melkert R, Serruys PW. Long-term luminal renarrowing after successful elective coronary angioplasty of total occlusions. A quantitative angiographic analysis. *Circulation* 1995;91(8): 2140–2150.
20. De Jaegere EF, Popma JJ, Serruys PW. Clinical trials on intracoronary stenting. *Semin Intervent Cardiol* 1996;43(1):233–245.
21. Fischman DL, Leon MB, Baim DS, et al. A randomized comparison of coronary-stent placement and balloon angioplasty in the treatment of coronary artery disease. Stent Restenosis Study Investigators. *N Engl J Med* 1994;331(8):496–501.
22. Popma JJ, van den Berg EK, Dehmer GJ. Long-term outcome of patients with asymptomatic restenosis after percutaneous transluminal coronary angioplasty. *Am J Cardiol* 1988;62(17):1298–1299.
23. Pfisterer M, Rickenbacher P, Kiowski W, et al. Silent ischemia after percutaneous transluminal coronary angioplasty: incidence and prognostic significance. *J Am Coll Cardiol* 1993;22(5):1446–1454.
24. Joelson JM, Most AS, Williams DO. Angiographic findings when chest pain recurs after successful percutaneous transluminal coronary angioplasty. *Am J Cardiol* 1987;60(10):792–795.
25. Roth A, Miller HI, Keren G, et al. Detection of restenosis following percutaneous coronary angioplasty in single-vessel coronary artery disease: the value of clinical assessment and exercise tolerance testing. *Cardiology* 1994;84(2):106–113.
26. Breisblatt WM, Barnes JV, Weiland F, et al. Incomplete revascularization in multivessel percutaneous transluminal coronary angioplasty: the role for stress thallium-201 imaging. *J Am Coll Cardiol* 1988; 11(6):1183–1190.
27. Bengston JR, Honan MB, et al. Detection of restenosis after elective percutaneous transluminal coronary angioplasty using the exercise treadmill test. *Am J Cardiol* 1990;65:28–34.
28. Marie PY, Danchin N, Karcher G, et al. Usefulness of exercise SPECT-thallium to detect asymptomatic restenosis in patients who had angina before coronary angioplasty. *Am Heart J* 1993;126(30)[Pt 1]:571–577.
29. Scholl JM, Chaitman BR, David PR, et al. Exercise electrocardiography and myocardial scintigraphy in the serial evaluation of the results of percutaneous transluminal coronary angioplasty. *Circulation* 1982; 66(2):380–390.
30. Rosing DR, Van Raden MJ, Mincemoyer RM, et al. Exercise, electrocardiographic and functional responses after percutaneous transluminal coronary angioplasty. *Am J Cardiol* 1984;53(12):36C–41C.
31. Wijns WSP, Reiber JHC, et al. Early detection of restenosis after successful percutaneous transluminal coronary angioplasty by exercise-redistribution thallium scintigraphy. *Am J Cardiol* 1984;53: 36C–41C.
32. O'Keefe JH Jr, Lapeyre AC, Holmes DR Jr, et al. Usefulness of early radionuclide angiography for identifying low-risk patients for late restenosis after percutaneous transluminal coronary angioplasty. *Am J Cardiol* 1988;61(1):51–54.
33. Ernst SM, Hillebrand FA, Klein B, et al. The value of exercise tests in the follow-up of patients who underwent transluminal coronary angioplasty. *Int J Cardiology* 1985;7(3):267–279.
34. el-Tamimi H, Davies GJ, Hackett D, et al. Very early prediction of restenosis after successful coronary angioplasty: anatomic and functional assessment. *J Am Coll Cardiol* 1990;15(2):259–264.
35. Legrand V, Mancini GB, Bates ER, et al. Comparative study of coronary flow reserve, coronary anatomy and results of radionuclide exercise tests in patients with coronary artery disease. *J Am Coll Cardiol* 1986;8(5):1022–1032.
36. Eichhorn EJ, Konstam MA, Salem DN, et al. Dipyridamole thallium-201 imaging pre- and post-coronary angioplasty for assessment of regional myocardial ischemia in humans. *Am Heart J* 1989;117(6): 1203–1209.
37. Liu P, Kiess MC, Okada RD, et al. The persistent defect on exercise thallium imaging and its fate after myocardial revascularization: does it represent scar or ischemia? *Am Heart J* 1985;110(5):996–1001.
38. Ryan TJ, Kennedy JW, Keriakes DJ, et al. Guidelines for percutaneous transluminal coronary angioplasty. A report of the American Heart Association/American College of Cardiology Task Force on assessment of diagnostic and therapeutic cardiovascular procedures. *Circulation* 1993;88:2987–3007.
39. Miller DD, Younis LT, Bach RG, et al. Correlation of pharmacological Tc-99m-sestamibi myocardial perfusion imaging with poststenotic coronary flow reserve in patients with angiographically intermediate coronary artery stenoses. *Circulation* 1994;89(5):2150–2160.
40. Hecht HS, Shaw RE, Bruce TR, et al. Usefulness of tomographic thallium-201 imaging for detection of restenosis after percutaneous

transluminal coronary angioplasty. *Am J Cardiol* 1990;66(19): 1314–1318.

41. Hecht HS, Shaw RE, Chin HL, et al. Silent ischemia after coronary angioplasty: evaluation of restenosis and extent of ischemia in asymptomatic patients by tomographic thallium-201 exercise imaging and comparison with symptomatic patients. *J Am Coll Cardiol* 1991;17(3): 670–677.

42. Milan E, Zoccarato O, Terzi A, et al. Technetium-99m-sestamibi SPECT to detect restenosis after successful percutaneous coronary angioplasty. *J Nucl Med* 1996;37(8):1300–1305.

43. Pirelli S, Danzi GB, Massa D, et al. Exercise thallium scintigraphy versus high-dose dipyridamole echocardiography testing for detection of asymptomatic restenosis in patients with positive exercise tests after coronary angioplasty. *Am J Cardiol* 1993;71(12):1052–1056.

44. Pfisterer ME, Gradel C. Assessment after myocardial revascularization. In: Underwood R, ed. *Nuclear medicine in clinical diagnosis and treatment P.D.* London: Churchill Livingstone, 1429–1438.

45. Milavertz JTM, Hodge D, et al. SPECT myocardial perfusion imaging in patients who have undergone coronary artery stenting. *J Am Coll Cardiol* 1997;29:228A(abst).

46. Petrakian A, Ahmad A, Badruddin S, et al. Value of myocardial perfusion tomography in the assessment of post-stent coronary restenosis. *J Am Coll Cardiol* 1997;29:228A(abst).

47. Hardoff R, Shefer A, Gips S, et al. Predicting late restenosis after coronary angioplasty by very early (12 to 24 h) thallium-201 scintigraphy: implications with regard to mechanisms of late coronary restenosis. *J Am Coll Cardiol* 1990;15(7):1486–1492.

48. Manyari DE, Knudtson M, Kloiber R, et al. Sequential thallium-201 myocardial perfusion studies after successful percutaneous transluminal coronary artery angioplasty: delayed resolution of exercise-induced scintigraphic abnormalities. *Circulation* 1988;77(1):86–95.

49. Iskandrian AS, Lemlek J, Ogilby JD, et al. Early thallium imaging after percutaneous transluminal coronary angioplasty: tomographic evaluation during adenosine-induced coronary hyperemia. *J Nucl Med* 1992;33(12):2086–2089.

50. Hirzel HO, Nuesch K, Gruentzig AR, et al. Short- and long-term changes in myocardial perfusion after percutaneous transluminal coronary angioplasty assessed by thallium-201 exercise scintigraphy. *Circulation* 1981;63(5):1001–1007.

51. Miller DD, Verani MS. Current status of myocardial perfusion imaging after percutaneous transluminal coronary angioplasty. *J Am Coll Cardiol* 1994;24(1):260–266.

52. Lewin HC, Hachamovitch R, Cohen I, et al. Stress SPECT in patients following recent PTCA: prognostic value and risk stratification. *J Nucl Med* 1997;38:130P(abst).

53. Flachskampf FA, Hoffmann R, von Dahl J, et al. Functional assessment of PTCA results by stress echocardiography: when and how to test. *Eur Heart J* 1995;16[Suppl J]:31–34.

54. Fioretti PM, Pozzoli MM, Ilmer B, et al. Exercise echocardiography versus thallium-201 SPECT for assessing patients before and after PTCA. *Eur Heart J* 1992;13(2):213–219.

55. Takeuchi M, Sonoda S, Miura Y, et al. Reproducibility of dobutamine digital stress echocardiography. *J Am Soc Echocardiogr* 1997;10(4): 344–351.

56. Hoffmann R, Lethen H, Flachskampf FA, et al. Exercise echocardiography performed early and late after percutaneous transluminal coronary angioplasty for prediction of restenosis. *Eur Heart J* 1995;16(12): 1872–1879.

57. Merthes H, Nixdorf U, Mohr-Kahaly S, et al. Exercise echocardiography for the evaluation of patients after nonsurgical coronary artery revascularization. *J Am Coll Cardiol* 1993;21:1087–1093.

58. Shaw LJ, Peterson ED, Shaw LK, et al. Use of a prognostic treadmill score in identifying diagnostic coronary disease subgroups. *Circulation* 1998;98(16):1622–1630.

59. Shaw LJ, Peterson ED, Lewin HC, et al. Using an outcomes-based approach to identify candidates for risk stratification after exercise treadmill testing. *J Gen Int Med* 1999;14:10–14.

60. Breisblatt WM, Weiland FL, Spaccavento LJ. Stress thallium-201 imaging after coronary angioplasty predicts restenosis and recurrent symptoms. *J Am Coll Cardiol* 1988;12(5):1199–1204.

61. Mark DB, Hlatky MA, Lee KL, et al. Localizing coronary artery obstructions with the exercise treadmill test. *Ann Intern Med* 1987; 106:53–55.

62. Kang X, Berman DS, Kimchi EY, et al. Maximal ST depression during exercise dose not localize myocardial ischemia. *Am Coll Cardiol* 1998;31:267A(abst).

63. Favaloro RG. Saphenous vein graft in the surgical treatment of coronary artery disease. Operative technique. *J Thorac Cardiovasc Surg* 1969;58(2):178–185.

64. Yusuf S, Zucker D, Peduzzi P, et al. Effect of coronary artery bypass graft surgery on survival: overview of 10-year results from randomised trials by the Coronary Artery Bypass Graft Surgery Trialists Collaboration. *Lancet* 1994;344(8922):563–570.

65. Christakis GT, Ivanov J, Weisel RD, et al. The changing pattern of coronary artery bypass surgery. *Circulation* 1989;80(3)[Pt 1]: 1151–1161.

66. Bourassa MG. Fate of venous grafts: the past, the present and the future. *J Am Coll Cardiol* 1991;17(5):1081–1083.

67. FitzGibbon GM, Leach AJ, Kafka HP, et al. Coronary bypass graft fate: long-term angiographic study. *J Am Coll Cardiol* 1991;17(5): 1075–1080.

68. Grondin CM, Campeau L, Lesperance J, et al. Comparison of late changes in internal mammary artery and saphenous vein grafts in two consecutive series of patients 10 years after operation. *Circulation* 1984;70(3)[Pt 2]:1208–1212.

69. Di Luzio V, Sowton E. Angina in patients with occluded aorto-coronary vein grafts. *Br Heart J* 1980;43:426–435.

70. Kennedy HL, Seiler SM, Sprague MK, et al. Relation of silent myocardial ischemia after coronary artery bypass grafting to angiographic completeness of revascularization and long-term prognosis. *Am J Cardiol* 1990;65(1):14–22.

71. Greenberg BH, Hart R, Botvinick EH, et al. Thallium-201 myocardial perfusion scintigraphy to evaluate patients after coronary bypass surgery. *Am J Cardiol* 1978;42(2):167–176.

72. Iskandrian AE, Tecce MA, et al. Simultaneous assessment of left ventricular perfusion and function with technetium-99m-sestamibi after coronary artery bypass grafting. *Am Heart J* 1993;126: 1199–1203.

73. Ghods M, Pancholy S, Cave V, et al. Serial changes in left ventricular function after coronary artery bypass: implications in viability assessment. *Am Heart J* 1995;129(1):20–23.

74. Gray R, Maddahi J, Berman D, et al. Scintigraphic and hemodynamic demonstration of transient left ventricular dysfunction immediately after uncomplicated coronary artery bypass grafting. *J Thorac Cardiovasc Surg* 1979;77(4):504–510.

75. Righetti A, Crawford MH, O'Rourke RA, et al. Interventricular septal motion and left ventricular function after coronary bypass surgery: evaluation with echocardiography and radionuclide angiography. *Am J Cardiol* 1977;39(3):372–377.

76. Okada RD, Murphy JH, Boucher CA, et al. Relationship between septal perfusion, viability, and motion before and after coronary artery bypass surgery. *Am Heart J* 1992;124(5):1190–1195.

77. Verani MS, Marcus ML, Spoto G, et al. Thallium-201 myocardial perfusion scintigrams in the evaluation of aorto-coronary saphenous bypass surgery. *J Nucl Med* 1978;19(7):765–772.

78. Lurie AJ, Salel AF, Berman DS, et al. Determination of improved myocardial perfusion after aortocoronary bypass surgery by exercise rubidium-81 scintigraphy. *Circulation* 1976;54(6)[Suppl]:III20.

79. Pfisterer M, Emmenegger H, Schmitt HE, et al. Accuracy of serial myocardial perfusion scintigraphy with thallium-201 for prediction of graft patency early and late after coronary artery bypass surgery. A controlled prospective study. *Circulation* 1982;66(5):1017–1024.

80. Lakkis NM, Mahmarian JJ, Verani MS. Exercise thallium-201 single photon emission computed tomography for evaluation of coronary artery bypass graft patency. *Am J Cardiol* 1995;76(3):107–111.

81. Khoury AF, Rivera JM, Mahmarian JJ, et al. Adenosine thallium-201 tomography in evaluation of graft patency late after coronary artery bypass graft surgery. *J Am Coll Cardiol* 1997;29(6):1290–1295.

82. Zimmerman R, Tillmanns H, Knapp WH. Noninvasive assessment of coronary artery bypass patency: determination of myocardial thallium-201 washout rates. *Eur Heart J* 1988;9:319–327.

83. Lauer MS, Lytle B, Pashkow F, et al. Prediction of death and myocar-

dial infarction by screening with exercise-thallium testing after coronary-artery-bypass grafting. *Lancet* 1998;351(9103):615–622.

84. Johnson AM, Kron IL, Watson DD, et al. Evaluation of postoperative flow reserve in internal mammary artery bypass grafts. *J Thorac Cardiovasc Surg* 1986;92(5):822–826.

85. Kusukawa J, Hiroto Y, Kawamura K, et al. Efficacy of coronary artery bypass surgery with gastroepiploic artery. Assessment with thallium 201 myocardial scintigraphy. *Circulation* 1989;80(3)[Pt 1]:I135–140.

86. Dubach P, Froelicher V, Klein J, et al. Use of the exercise test to predict prognosis after coronary artery bypass grafting. *Am J Cardiol* 1989;63:530–533.

87. Yli-Mäyry S, Huikuri HV, Airaksinen J, et al. Usefulness of a postoperative exercise test for predicting cardiac events after coronary artery bypass grafting. *Am J Cardiol* 1992;70:56–59.

88. Weiner DA, Ryan RJ, Parsons L, et al. Prevalence and prognostic significance of silent and symptomatic ischemia after coronary artery bypass surgery: a report from the coronary artery surgery study (CASS) randomized population. *J Am Coll Cardiol* 1991;18:343–348.

89. Palmas W, Bingham S, Diamond GA, et al. Incremental prognostic value of exercise thallium-201 myocardial single-photon emission computed tomography late after coronary artery bypass surgery. *J Am Coll Cardiol* 1995;25(2):403–409.

90. Nallamothu N, Hohnson JH, Bagheri B, et al. Utility of stress single-photon emission computed tomography (SPECT) perfusion imaging in predicting outcome after coronary artery bypass grafting. *Am J Cardiol* 1997;80:1515–1521.

91. Miller TD, Christian TF, Hodge DO, et al. Prognostic value of exercise thallium-201 imaging performed within 2 years of coronary artery bypass graft surgery. *J Am Coll Cardiol* 1998;31:848–854.

92. Lewin HC, Hachamovitch R, Cohen I, et al. Stress SPECT in patients more than five years following bypass surgery: incremental prognostic value and risk stratification. *J Nucl Med* 1997;38,[Suppl]40P–41P(abst).

93. Zellweger MJ, Dubois EA, Lai S, et al. Risk of cardiac death in patients early and late after CABG using stress myocardial perfusion SPECT: implications for appropriate clinical strategies. *J Nucl Med* 1999;40:7P.

94. Borges-Neto S, Shaw LJ, Kesler K, et al. Usefulness of serial radionuclide angiography in predicting cardiac death after coronary artery bypass grafting and comparison with clinical and cardiac catheterization data. *Am J Cardiol* 1997;79:851–855.

95. Kafka H, Leach AJ, Fitzgibbon GM. Exercise echocardiography after coronary artery bypass surgery: correlation with coronary angiography. *J Am Coll Cardiol* 1995;25(5):1019–1023.

96. Hoffmann R, Lethen H, Falter F, et al. Dobutamine stress echocardiography after coronary artery bypass grafting. Transthoracic vs biplane transoesophageal imaging. *Eur Heart J* 1996;17(2):222–229.

97. Pezzano A, Cali G, Milazzo A, et al. Transthoracic 2D echo color Doppler assessment of internal mammary artery to left anterior descending coronary artery graft. *Int J Cardiac Imaging* 1995;11(3):177–184.

98. Goto Y, Kadowaki K, Sato T, et al. Noninvasive assessment of left internal thoracic artery graft patency using transthoracic echocardiography. *Nippon Kyobu Geka Gakkai Zasshi—J Jap Assoc Thoracic Surg* 1993;41:2013–2018.

99. Bateman TM, Gray RJ, Whiting JS, et al. Prospective evaluation of ultrafast cardiac computed tomography for determination of coronary bypass graft patency. *Circulation* 1987;75(5):1018–1024.

100. Stanford W, Rooholamini M, Rumberger J, et al. Evaluation of coronary bypass graft patency by ultrafast computed tomography. *J Thorac Imaging* 1988;3(2):52–55.

101. Achenbach S, Moshage W, Ropers D, et al. Noninvasive, three-dimensional visualization of coronary artery bypass grafts by electron beam tomography. *Am J Cardiol* 1997;79(7):856–861.

102. Vrachliotis TG, Bis KG, Aliabadi D, et al. Contrast-enhanced breath-hold MR angiography for evaluating patency of coronary artery bypass grafts. *Am J Roentgenol* 1997;168(4):1073–1080.

103. van Rossum AC, Galjee MA, Doesburg T, et al. The role of magnetic resonance in the evaluation of functional results after CABG/PTCA. *Int J Cardiac Imaging* 1993;9[Suppl 1]:59–69.

104. Okamura Y, Mochizuki Y, Iida H, et al. Evaluation of coronary artery

bypass grafts with magnetic resonance imaging. *Nippon Kyobu Geka Gakkai Zasshi—J Jap Assoc Thoracic Surg* 1997;45(6):874–877.

105. Packer M. Do angiotensin-converting enzyme inhibitors prolong live in patients with heart failure, treated in clinical practice? *J Am Coll Cardiol* 1996;28:1323–1327.

106. Swedberg K, Eneroth P, et al. Hormones regulating cardiovascular function in patients with severe congestive heart failure and in their relation to mortality. CONSENSUS Trial Study Group. *Circulation* 1990;82:1730–1736.

107. Packer M. The neurohumoral hypothesis: a theory to explain the mechanism of disease progression in heart failure. *J Am Coll Cardiol* 1992;20:248–254.

108. Russel R. Atherosclerosis, an inflammatory disease. *N Engl J Med* 1999;340:115–126.

109. Bellosta S, Bernini F, Ferri N, et al. Direct vascular effects of HMG-CoA reductase inhibitors. *Atherosclerosis* 1998;137[Suppl]:101–109.

110. Laufs U, La Fata V, et al. Upregulation of endothelial nitric oxide synthase by HMG-CoA reductase inhibitors. *Circulation* 1998;97:1129–1135.

111. Gould KL. Reversal of coronary atherosclerosis. Clinical promise as the basis for noninvasive management of coronary artery disease. *Circulation* 1994;90(3):1558–1571.

112. Gould KL, Ornish D, Scherwitz L, et al. Changes in myocardial perfusion abnormalities by positron emission tomography after long-term, intense risk factor modification. *JAMA* 1995;274(11):894–901.

113. Yokoyama I, Ohtake T, Momomura S, et al. Reduced coronary flow reserve in hypercholesterolemic patients without overt coronary stenosis. *Circulation* 1996;94(12):3232–3238.

114. Dakik HA, Farmer J, Kleiman NS. Images in cardiovascular medicine. Fistula between left main, left anterior descending, and pulmonary arteries. *Circulation* 1998;97(20):2091–2092.

115. Mahmarian JJ, Moye LA, Verani MS, et al. High reproducibility of myocardial perfusion defects in patients undergoing serial exercise thallium-201 tomography. *Am J Cardiol* 1995;75(16):1116–1119.

116. Sharir T, Berman DS. A novel approach for myocardial SPECT quantitation: validation of an automatic segmental scoring method. *Circulation* 1998;98[Suppl 1]:1588(abst 3099).

117. Lewin HC, Sharir T, Germano G, et al. Reproducibility of dual isotope myocardial perfusion SPECT using a new quantitative perfusion SPECT (QPS) approach. *J Am Coll Cardiol* 1999;33:483A(abst).

118. Hoffmann R, Lethen H, Marwick T, et al. Analysis of interinstitutional observer agreement in interpretation of dobutamine stress echocardiograms. *J Am Coll Cardiol* 1996;27:330–336.

119. Callister TQ, Cooil B, Raya SP, et al. Coronary artery disease: improved reproducibility of calcium scoring with an electron-beam CT volumetric method. *Radiology* 1998;208(3):807–814.

120. Mahmarian JJ, Fenimore NL, Marks GF, et al. Transdermal nitroglycerin patch therapy reduces the extent of exercise-induced myocardial ischemia: results of a double-blind, placebo-controlled trial using quantitative thallium-201 tomography. *J Am Coll Cardiol* 1994;24(1):25–32.

121. Lewin HC, Berman DS. Achieving sustained improvement in myocardial perfusion: role of isosorbide mononitrate. *Am J Cardiol* 1997;79(12B):31–35.

122. Cid E, Verani MS, Mahmarian JJ. Factors affecting the diagnostic accuracy of quantitative single photon tomography combined with dobutamine stress. *J Nucl Med* 1996;37:58P.

123. Shehata AR, Gillam LD, Mascitelli VA, et al. Impact of acute propranolol administration on dobutamine-induced myocardial ischemia as evaluated by myocardial perfusion imaging and echocardiography. *Am J Cardiol* 1997;80:268–272.

124. Sharir T, Livschitz S, Rabinowitz B, et al. Anti-ischemic drugs reduce size of reversible defects in dipyridamole/submaximal exercise Tl-201 SPECT imaging. *J Nucl Cardiol* 1997;4:S71.

125. Parisi AF, Hartigan PM, Folland ED. Evaluation of exercise thallium scintigraphy versus exercise electrocardiography in predicting survival outcomes and morbid cardiac events in patients with single- and double-vessel disease. Findings from the Angioplasty Compared to Medicine (ACME) Study. *J Am Coll Cardiol* 1997;30(5):1256–1263.

126. Eichstadt HW, Eskotter H, Hoffman I, et al. Improvement of myocardial perfusion by short-term fluvastatin therapy in coronary artery disease. *Am J Cardiol* 1995;76(2):122A–125A.

127. Mostaza JM, del Valle Gornez, Martinez M, et al. Incremento de la perfusion miocardica durante el tratamiento hipolipemiante en pacientes con cardiopatia isquemica. *Revis Esp Cardiol* 1996;49(9):669–674.

128. Siebelink HMJ, Van Boven AJ, et al. Cholesterol lowering in primary prevention improves coronary flow reserve and coronary vascular resistance. *Circulation* 1998;98[Suppl]:195(abst 480).

129. Schwartz RG, et al. Serial quantitative single photon emission computed tomography monitors improved myocardial perfusion accompanying cholesterol reduction therapy. *Circulation* 1998;98[Suppl]:195(abst 478).

130. Callister TQ, Raggi P, Dooil B, et al. Effect of HMG-CoA reductase inhibitors on coronary artery disease as assessed by electron-beam computed tomography. *N Engl J Med* 1998;339:1972–1978.

CHAPTER 39

Myocardial Viability

Clinical Applications

Robert O. Bonow

The incidence and clinical significance of left ventricular dysfunction have increased dramatically in the past several decades. The number of deaths annually from heart failure has increased steadily during the last quarter century, and heart failure is now the leading cause of hospital admission in patients covered by Medicare. Coronary artery disease (CAD) is in large part responsible for this rise in heart failure morbidity and mortality, and coronary artery disease is now the major cause of heart failure in the developed countries of the world (1), having surpassed valvular heart disease and hypertension as the leading etiology of left ventricular (LV) dysfunction and heart failure. Coronary artery disease is responsible for over two thirds of cases of heart failure in the United States (Fig. 1). Moreover, the mortality rate of patients with heart failure caused by CAD is significantly greater than that of patients with heart failure caused by nonischemic etiologies (2).

Conversely, patients with CAD and LV dysfunction have a significantly reduced survival rate compared to patients with preserved LV function (Fig. 2); LV function has been established as among the most important determinants of long-term prognosis in patients with ischemic heart disease (3–7). Thus, among patients with LV dysfunction, those with CAD have the worst outcome, and, among patients with CAD, those with LV dysfunction have the worse outcome.

This has important diagnostic and therapeutic implications. First, it is critically important to identify those patients with symptomatic heart failure (as well as those with asymptomatic LV dysfunction) who have CAD, because these patients require aggressive secondary prevention strategies (8). In addition, a large subset of patients with CAD and LV

dysfunction should be considered candidates for myocardial revascularization.

A number of surgical series have demonstrated that the survival of patients with CAD and LV dysfunction is improved significantly by myocardial revascularization compared to medical therapy (9–14), with the magnitude of survival benefit with surgery ranging from 10 to 54%. The incremental survival benefit with surgery compared to medical treatment is also greater in patients with LV dysfunction compared to those with normal LV function (Fig. 3). Although all of these surgical series were retrospective and nonrandomized, the consistent finding of enhanced survival with coronary artery bypass graft (CABG) surgery suggests that the possibility of revascularization should at least be considered in every patient. However, even with surgery, patients with LV dysfunction have a greater mortality compared to patients with normal LV function, whether treated medically or surgically (Fig. 3), and the immediate operative risk may be 10% or greater in patients with significant LV dysfunction. Thus, the patients who may ultimately benefit the most from revascularization are also those in whom revascularization poses the greatest risk.

Proper identification of patients for revascularization includes selection of those with the potential for clinical improvement or survival benefit in whom the risks of revascularization procedures are justified. Thus, diagnostic testing has a role in determining those patients with LV dysfunction who have underlying CAD, and also in identifying those with established CAD who are suitable candidates for myocardial revascularization.

During the past decade, noninvasive imaging to determine the presence and magnitude of dysfunctional but viable myocardium has also become an important component in the evaluation of patients with depressed LV function. It is now apparent that LV dysfunction resulting from CAD is not

R. O. Bonow: Division of Cardiology, Northwestern University Medical School; Division of Cardiology, Northwestern Memorial Hospital, Chicago, Illinois 60611.

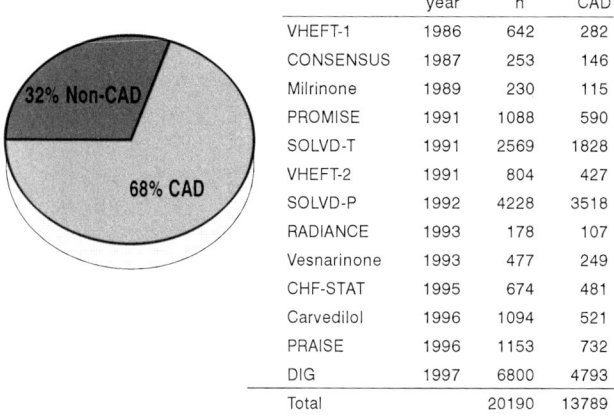

	year	n	CAD
VHEFT-1	1986	642	282
CONSENSUS	1987	253	146
Milrinone	1989	230	115
PROMISE	1991	1088	590
SOLVD-T	1991	2569	1828
VHEFT-2	1991	804	427
SOLVD-P	1992	4228	3518
RADIANCE	1993	178	107
Vesnarinone	1993	477	249
CHF-STAT	1995	674	481
Carvedilol	1996	1094	521
PRAISE	1996	1153	732
DIG	1997	6800	4793
Total		20190	13789

FIG. 1. Prevalence of coronary artery disease (CAD) in 13 randomized multicenter heart failure treatment trials reported in the *New England Journal of Medicine* from 1986 to 1997. The number of patients (n) is indicated for each trial, as is the number with CAD. Underlying CAD was present in 68% of patients. (From ref. 1, with permission.)

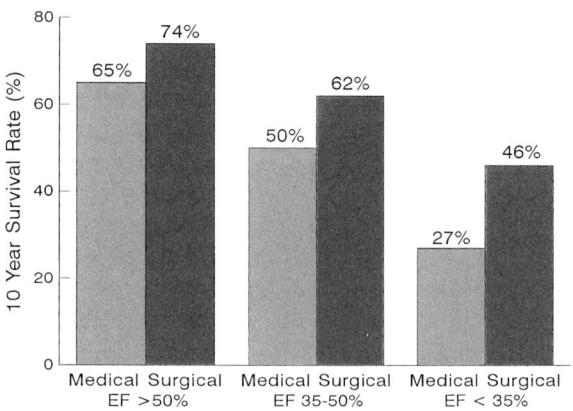

FIG. 3. Survival in patients with coronary artery disease from the Duke database. Data are shown for patients with normal LV function (**left panel**), mild-moderate LV dysfunction (**middle panel**), and severe LV dysfunction (**right panel**). Survival rates in patients undergoing coronary artery bypass surgery are compared to those treated medically for each subgroup. Although survival rates are higher with surgery compared to medical therapy across the spectrum on left ventricular function, the incremental benefit of surgery is greatest in patients with the most severe LV dysfunction. (From ref. 13, with permission.)

always an irreversible process related to previous myocardial infarction, because LV function improves substantially in many patients, and may even normalize, after myocardial revascularization (15–20). The percentage of patients with LV dysfunction undergoing myocardial revascularization who subsequently demonstrate a substantial improvement in LV function varies among reported series, related in part to patient selection factors and adequacy of the myocardial revascularization procedures. This percentage, however, is not inconsequential as it has been estimated that 25 to 40% of patients with chronic CAD and LV dysfunction have the potential for significant improvement in ventricular function after revascularization (20–25), as shown in Figure 4.

The current and evolving noninvasive methods for identi-

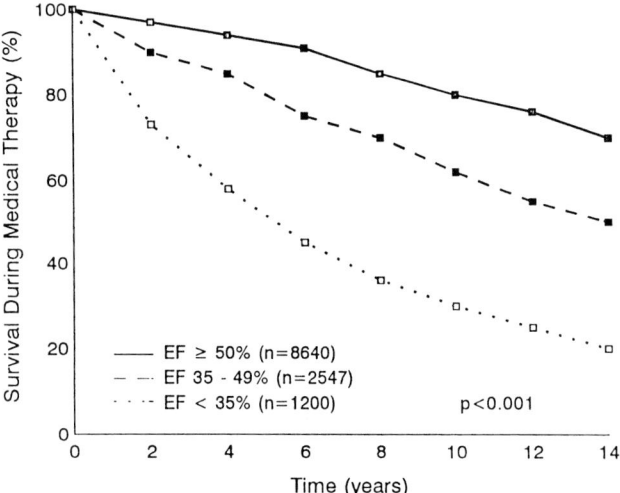

FIG. 2. Influence of resting LV ejection fraction (*EF*) on survival during medical therapy in patients in the Coronary Artery Surgery Study Registry. (From ref. 7, with permission.)

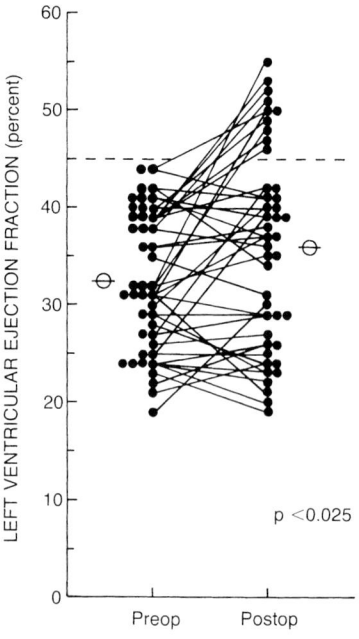

FIG. 4. Left ventricular ejection fraction at rest by radionuclide ventriculography before (*Preop*) and 6 months after (*Postop*) coronary artery bypass surgery in 43 patients with preoperative left ventricular dysfunction. The *dashed line* at 45% indicates the lower limit of normal resting ejection fraction. Although operation resulted in only a small increase in mean ejection fraction, substantial increases in ejection fraction were observed in 15 patients (35%), and postoperative ejection fraction was normal in 10 patients (23%). (From ref. 24, with permission.)

fying myocardial ischemia and/or myocardial viability have been discussed at length in previous chapters of this book. This chapter will focus on the applications of these methods to improve selection of patients with LV dysfunction for myocardial revascularization and on the impact of revascularization on LV function, symptoms, and prognosis.

IDENTIFICATION OF VIABLE MYOCARDIUM

A number of clinically reliable physiologic markers can be employed for determining the presence and extent of viable myocardium in patients with coronary artery disease and LV dysfunction, using standard noninvasive imaging techniques. These include indexes of regional myocardial blood flow using perfusion tracers and assessment of regional wall motion and regional systolic wall thickening, which may be assessed by echocardiography, cine magnetic resonance imaging (MRI), or gated single-photon emission tomography (SPECT) imaging. Measures of regional blood flow and/ or function are helpful in identifying viable tissue if they are normal or near-normal. However, in patients with underperfused but viable myocardium, blood flow, wall motion, and wall thickening may be severely reduced or absent (16–19). For this reason, radionuclide tracers that reflect intact cellular metabolic processes or cell membrane integrity, as well as methods to assess regional LV function during inotropic stimulation to elicit contractile reserve, have intrinsic advantages over indexes of blood flow and function at rest. In keeping with these concepts, positron emission tomography (PET) to evaluate myocardial metabolism using ^{18}F-fluorodeoxyglucose (FDG), SPECT imaging with thallium-201 or technetium-99m perfusion tracers to evaluate membrane integrity, and low-dose dobutamine echocardiography to evaluate myocardial inotropic reserve have evolved over the past two decades with excellent clinical results and are now in widespread practice.

Predicting Recovery of Left Ventricular Function

The overall accuracies of PET, SPECT, and dobutamine echocardiography (echo) for predicting recovery of regional LV function after myocardial revascularization are similar, based on the results of multiple published studies (Fig. 5), although dobutamine echo and PET imaging with metabolic tracers appear to have greater specificity compared to SPECT imaging, while SPECT has greater sensitivity (20,26). This translates into higher positive predictive values (in the range of 83%) for PET and dobutamine echo compared to thallium SPECT (in the range of 68%), but higher negative predictive values for SPECT (90%) compared to both PET and dobutamine echo (83%), as indicated in Figure 5. Several studies have also demonstrated the ability to predict improvement in global as well as regional LV function, in that ejection fraction (EF) increases after revascularization in patients in whom large regions of dysfunctional myocar-

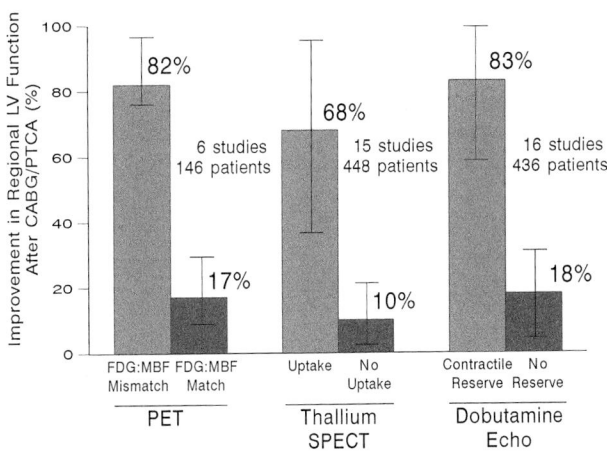

FIG. 5. Likelihood of improved regional left ventricular (*LV*) function after revascularization based on noninvasive methods to detect viable myocardium from 6 studies using positron emission tomography (*PET*), in which enhanced ^{18}F-fluorodeoxyglucose (*FDG*) uptake relative to myocardial blood flow (*MBF*) was used as a marker of viability; 15 studies using single-photon emission computed tomography (*SPECT*), in which thallium uptake was used as a marker of viability; and 16 studies using dobutamine echocardiography, in which contractile reserve was used as a marker of viability. The range of values reported by the individual studies is indicated by the horizontal bars connected by vertical lines. The light shaded bars indicate the positive predictive value and the dark bars the inverse of the negative predictive value. *CABG*, coronary artery bypass graft; *PTCA*, percutaneous transluminal angioplasty. (From ref. 20, with permission.)

dium are identified as viable by these noninvasive techniques (27–30).

Myocardial Viability versus Myocardial Ischemia

The diagnostic accuracy for predicting improvement in function after revascularization with both dobutamine echo and thallium SPECT imaging is enhanced when these studies demonstrate evidence of both myocardial viability and inducible ischemia. For example, an increase in regional contraction with dobutamine administration is a very specific marker of viable tissue, as necrotic or fibrotic myocardium does not manifest contractile reserve. However, the important clinical question is usually not merely whether viable tissue is present in dysfunctional myocardium, but whether that viable tissue has the potential to improve in function after revascularization. In this context, contractile reserve may be observed in regions in which recovery of function is not likely after revascularization, such as cardiomyopathic tissue in patients with dilated cardiomyopathy and myocardium remote from a large myocardial infarction that has undergone remodeling. Regional function would be expected to improve after revascularization in neither of these latter situations despite the presence of contractile reserve. Several studies indicate that a more specific finding for predicting recovery of function after revascularization is a biphasic response during dobutamine echo (31,32), that is, an initial increase in regional function at low doses of dobutamine followed by deterioration of regional function at higher doses. The finding of contractile reserve at low-dose administration of dobutamine is evidence of viability, and the subsequent decline in function with higher doses of dobutamine is evidence of superimposed inducible ischemia. It is the finding of ischemia in this setting that provides specific evidence that the contractile dysfunction at rest is closely linked to a critical coronary artery stenosis and that restoration of myocardial blood supply is likely to result in improved systolic function.

Similar observations regarding the distinction between viable tissue in dysfunctional myocardial regions and viable tissue with the potential for functional recovery have been made with perfusion imaging using thallium and technetium-99m tracers. The regional uptake and retention of thallium and sestamibi are dependent on the active, energy-dependent cation exchange mechanisms of sarcolemmal and mitochondrial membranes of viable myocytes, and, hence, the regional tracer activity measured in dysfunctional myocardial segments is directly proportional to the relative amount of viable myocytes and inversely proportional to the extent of fibrosis (33,34). Thus, the level of regional thallium or sestamibi activity at rest, a marker of the extent of viable tissue, should have predictive value regarding recovery of function after revascularization. This has been shown to be the case, as a continuum exists between regional thallium-201 activity and the likelihood of functional recovery after revascularization (35,36) (Fig. 6). Similar data have been reported with technetium-99m sestamibi (36). This continual relationship also indicates that the accuracy of this prediction is greatest

at either extreme of the activity spectrum, with high levels of thallium or sestamibi activity indicating a high probability of recovery of function and very low levels a low probability of functional recovery. However, in regions with intermediate levels of thallium or sestamibi activity, the certainty with which recovery of function can be predicted is much lower, and in dysfunctional segments with activity levels in the range of 50 to 60% compared to normal segments, the prediction of functional recovery is reduced to a 50/50 proposition. It is noteworthy that SPECT imaging cannot differentiate between a 50% transmural reduction in perfusion and subendocardial scar with a normally perfused epicardial layer, both of which may result in the appearance of a similar perfusion defect at rest. This poor predictive accuracy in regions with borderline tracer activity at rest can be improved significantly by determining whether there is also evidence of reversible ischemia. For the same level of thallium activity at rest, myocardium that demonstrates reversible ischemia (that is, lower relative thallium activity during exercise) has a significantly greater likelihood of improving function after revascularization than does myocardium in which there is a fixed reduction in thallium activity during exercise and at rest (37).

Thus, both myocardial perfusion imaging and dobutamine echo are concordant in that the demonstration of inducible ischemia is a more specific finding regarding the potential for recovery of function after revascularization than is the mere demonstration that the underlying myocardium contains viable tissue. The biphasic response to dobutamine and the finding of a reversible or partially reversible perfusion defect appear to have similar diagnostic implications. Nonetheless, it is also important to note that, in terms of patient outcome, there may be other advantages resulting from revascularization of viable tissue beyond the recovery of systolic function. Hence, there may be advantages to identifying the relative extent of underperfused but viable myocardium in regions with contractile dysfunction, even if there is no reversal of systolic dysfunction after revascularization. Restoration of blood flow to viable tissue may have important effects to attenuate LV remodeling after myocardial injury, lessen the potential for serious ventricular arrhythmias, and reduce the risk of future fatal acute ischemic events (20). In this regard, the detection of viable myocardium, especially viable myocardium that is ischemic, is a means to unmask jeopardized myocardium that identifies patients with CAD and LV dysfunction who are at particularly high risk.

Evolving Diagnostic Methods

The ability of metabolic PET imaging, SPECT perfusion imaging, and dobutamine echo to detect viable myocardium are well established, as are the limitations of these techniques. Exciting new methods for assessing viability are also undergoing clinical evaluation. PET imaging is not widely available, but it is possible to image the high energy photons from positron-emitting tracers by modifying standard

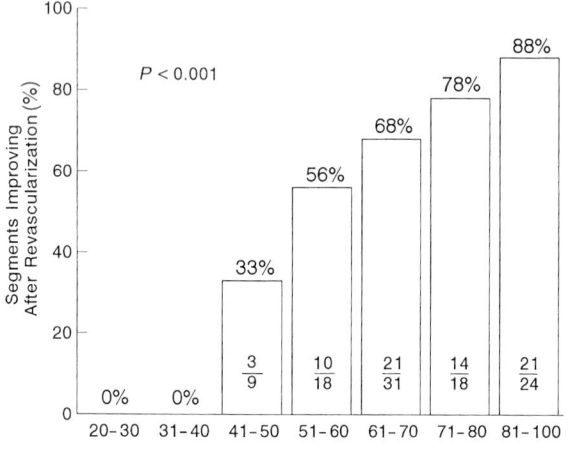

FIG. 6. Demonstration of the nearly linear relationship between the percent of peak thallium activity on rest-redistribution imaging and the likelihood of segmental improvement after revascularization. Although various cutoff values have been proposed as "thresholds" for viability, this figure indicates the continuous nature of this relationship. (From ref. 35, with permission.)

SPECT equipment with high-energy collimators and/or coincidence detection. The preliminary data from several laboratories (38,39) suggests that SPECT imaging of FDG yields diagnostic information comparable to PET imaging (although the spatial resolution is considerably lower with SPECT). Contrast echocardiography to assess microvascular integrity has been demonstrated to predict myocardial viability in patients with acute myocardial infarction using intracoronary injection of ultrasonic contrast agents (40,41). Noninvasive viability assessment using intravenous administration of these agents is forthcoming soon (42). Magnetic resonance imaging (MRI) methods have also emerged recently, using dobutamine stress to assess contractile reserve (43) or contrast enhancement techniques with gadolinium DTPA to assess extent of necrotic and/or fibrotic myocardium (44), with very promising early results. Contrast echocardiography and contrast MRI have enormous potential because of the ability to evaluate transmural perfusion and infarction patterns, thereby differentiating patients with transmural ischemia and/or infarction from those in whom the process is localized only to the subendocardial regions. In particular, the enhanced spatial resolution of MRI improves its usefulness for more accurate differentiation of viable from nonviable myocardium than the current noninvasive standards.

PREDICTING IMPROVED PATIENT OUTCOME

Medical Therapy versus Revascularization in Patients with Viable Myocardium

The demonstration of viable myocardium in patients with CAD and LV dysfunction appears to identify patients with particularly poor prognosis with medical therapy; the available data indicate that these patients have improved survival with revascularization. These observations, initially made with PET imaging, have now been extended to SPECT imaging and dobutamine echocardiography.

Several investigators using PET have reported that myocardial revascularization in patients with underperfused but metabolically active myocardium significantly improves survival results compared with medical therapy. Two separate studies (Fig. 7), reported results in a total of 87 patients with LV dysfunction (mean ejection fraction, 31%). Eitzman et al. (45) reported a 1-year mortality rate of 33% in patients treated medically, compared to a mortality rate of only 4% in patients undergoing coronary artery bypass surgery or angioplasty. Similarly, the mortality rates with medical therapy versus revascularization were 50% and 12%, respectively, in the data reported by Di Carli et al. (46). Many of the patients studied by Di Carli et al. were referred for PET evaluation from the heart failure program at their institution. In addition to improved survival, patients with myocardial viability by PET who underwent revascularization also manifested a significant improvement in heart failure symptoms

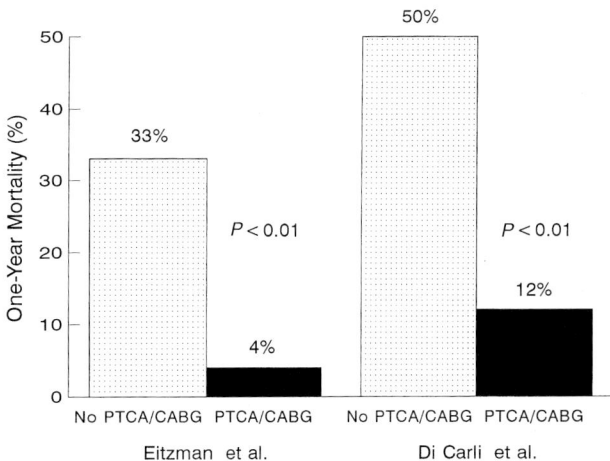

FIG. 7. One-year mortality in patients with left ventricular dysfunction and evidence of viable myocardium, as determined by FDG:blood flow mismatch on PET imaging by Eitzman et al. (45) and Di Carli et al. (46). In both studies, patients treated medically had a greater 1-year mortality rate compared to patients undergoing myocardial revascularization. *CABG*, coronary artery bypass graft; *FDG*, ^{18}F-fluorodeoxyglucose; *PET*, positron emission tomography; *PTCA*, percutaneous transluminal angioplasty. (From refs. 45 and 46, with permission.)

(46) and objective exercise tolerance (47) compared to patients who were treated medically.

Parallel findings have been reported in studies using SPECT imaging with thallium-201. In a small series of 85 patients with evidence of myocardial viability by thallium imaging, Gioia et al. (48) assessed outcome of those treated medically compared to those undergoing myocardial revascularization. Survival and survival without myocardial infarction tended to be significantly higher in those treated with revascularization (Fig. 8). Preliminary data from an Italian multicenter study support these observations. Among 85 patients with LV dysfunction (mean ejection fraction,

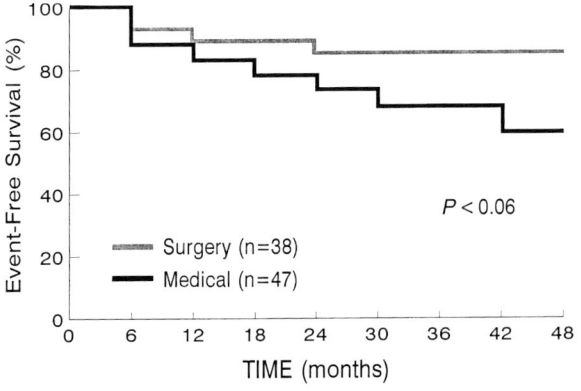

FIG. 8. Survival in patients with LV dysfunction and viable myocardium as assessed by thallium-201 SPECT imaging. Survival is greater in patients undergoing myocardial revascularization compared to patients treated medically. (From ref. 48, with permission.)

35%) and evidence of myocardial viability by thallium imaging, survival and survival without myocardial infarction were enhanced in those treated with myocardial revascularization, compared to those patients treated medically (49).

Similar to the experience gained with PET and thallium SPECT as well as the earlier experience assessing inotropic reserve with epinephrine infusions and postextrasystolic potentiation during left ventriculography (50), the identification of viable myocardium with dobutamine echocardiography also appears to provide important prognostic information in patients with LV dysfunction (51–53). Patients with inotropic reserve appear to have an initial survival advantage compared to those patients without inotropic reserve (which cannot be explained by differences in baseline left ventricular function, symptoms, or coronary anatomy), but this initial advantage is lost over a 12-to-24 month period (53). Two recent studies (52,53) have reported concordant findings indicating that survival is enhanced by myocardial revascularization among patients with LV dysfunction who manifest inotropic reserve with dobutamine. Afridi et al. (52) reported the outcome of 318 patients with chronic CAD and LV ejection fraction less than 35% who underwent dobutamine echocardiography and who were followed for a mean of 1.5 years. The mortality rate was 6% in the group manifesting contractile reserve who underwent revascularization, but 20% in those with contractile reserve who were treated medically. Similarly, Chaudhry et al. (53) followed 80 patients with CAD disease and LV ejection fraction of less than 40% (mean 28%) after dobutamine echo and observed a survival rate of 93% at 3 years in patients with contractile reserve who underwent revascularization, compared to 49% in those treated medically (Fig. 9).

Thus, data from clinical studies employing PET, thallium SPECT, and dobutamine echocardiography provide concor-

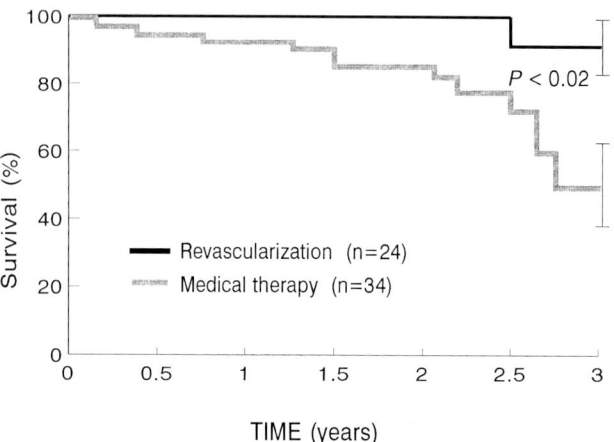

FIG. 9. Survival in patients with left ventricular dysfunction and viable myocardium as assessed by contractile reserve on low-dose dobutamine echocardiography. Survival was significantly greater in patients undergoing myocardial revascularization compared to patients treated medically. (From ref. 53, with permission.)

dant information suggesting that patients with CAD and LV dysfunction, who have evidence of viable myocardium within dysfunctional regions, represent a group at particularly high risk during the course of medical therapy. This risk appears to be reduced significantly by a strategy of myocardial revascularization. There are major limitations in these studies that should be addressed, and, because of these limitations, definitive conclusions cannot be reached at this time. These studies all represent retrospective, nonrandomized series involving relatively small numbers of patients. In addition, patient selection biases likely were present, and the factors used for selecting some patients for revascularization and others for medical therapy are unspecified. It is unclear if other predictors of outcome, such as severity of angina or inducible myocardial ischemia, were used to guide the selection toward revascularization. Clearly, prospectively designed, randomized trials involving large numbers of patients would be required to resolve these issues. However, the overall concordance of the available results thus far, obtained using three independent imaging methods from multiple centers, supports the concept that patients with LV dysfunction and evidence of myocardial viability represent a high-risk group with a high cardiac event rate; this poor prognosis may be reduced considerably by revascularization of the viable but underperfused myocardium. These observations support the concept that methods to detect myocardial viability and ischemia have important clinical relevance in patients after myocardial infarction and/or patients with heart failure.

Selection of Patients for Revascularization

The issue of survival in patients with viable myocardium treated medically or surgically is one of the important determinants of the prognostic importance of viability assessment in patients with LV dysfunction. Another equally important question is whether viability assessments are necessary in making the decision for revascularization. Considering the survival advantage of coronary artery bypass surgery noted in large registries of patients in which the results of surgery have been compared to medical therapy in patients with LV dysfunction (Fig. 3), coupled with the apparent improved outcome with revascularization of patients who have evidence of viable myocardium (noted above), one might argue that a preoperative viability assessment is not necessary and adds little, except cost. The controversy is whether revascularization should be considered in all patients with CAD and LV dysfunction with or without evidence of viable myocardium. Such an aggressive strategy must be balanced by the high operative risk of 10% or greater in patients with severe LV dysfunction; even with surgery, patients with severe left ventricular dysfunction have a relatively poor long-term outcome (Fig. 3).

Several series have provided important data that address this particular question. Pagley et al. (54) reported the outcome of patients with LV dysfunction (mean ejection frac-

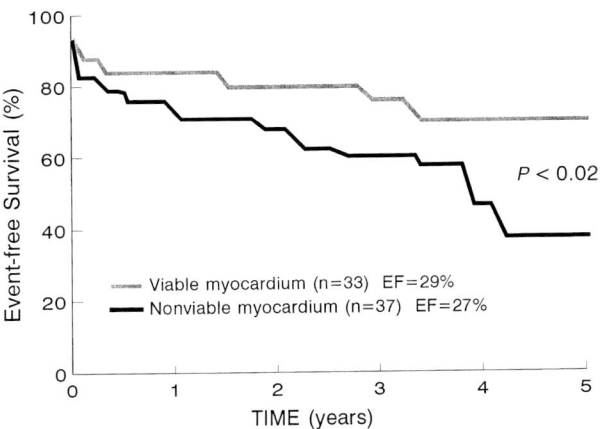

FIG. 10. Survival in patients with left ventricular dysfunction undergoing coronary artery bypass surgery, all of whom underwent preoperative perfusion imaging with thallium-201. Perioperative and long-term postoperative survival was significantly greater in patients with evidence of substantial myocardial viability than in patients with less evidence of viable myocardium. (From ref. 54, with permission.)

tion, 28%) after coronary artery bypass surgery, all of whom underwent preoperative thallium imaging. Patients with evidence of myocardial viability had a significantly lower perioperative and long-term postoperative mortality rate than did patients without myocardial viability (Fig. 10). Similar findings were reported by Haas et al. (55) with metabolic PET imaging. In this latter study, 34 patients with LV dysfunction (mean ejection fraction, 28%) who underwent a preoperative PET study and were referred for bypass surgery on the basis of myocardial viability had significantly better perioperative and long-term survival than did 35 patients (mean ejection fraction, 29%) who did not undergo imaging preoperatively and were referred for surgery on the basis of clinical and angiographic findings. The perioperative mortality in the latter group was 11%, whereas there were no early deaths in the group with preoperative viability assessment.

These data from the nuclear cardiology literature are supported by the results of the prognostic studies of dobutamine echocardiography noted previously. Afridi et al. (52) reported mortality rates of 6% in patients who demonstrated contractile reserve on preoperative dobutamine echocardiograms, compared to 17% in patients without contractile reserve, at a mean follow-up interval of 1.5 years after revascularization. Chaudhry et al. (53) reported similar findings, with very poor survival in patients who underwent myocardial revascularization in the absence of contractile reserve.

The same caveats noted earlier apply to the interpretation of these data regarding the application of viability measures for selecting patients with left ventricular dysfunction for myocardial revascularization. The available data all represent retrospective analyses of clinical data bases, with important potential patient selection biases. To date, there have been no large-scale, randomized, prospectively designed trials to address this issue. However, in the absence of such

definitive trial data, it is noteworthy that the current data do demonstrate remarkable consistency.

CLINICAL IMPLICATIONS

The identification of myocardial viability in patients with LV dysfunction has several important clinical implications. Recovery of LV function after revascularization appears to result in an improved prognosis and an amelioration of symptoms. Although it is important to interpret the results of the studies reported to date with some degree of caution, the overall concordance of the results supports the concept that patients with viable but dysfunctional myocardium represent a high-risk group with a high cardiac event rate, and that this poor prognosis may be reduced considerably by revascularization of the viable but underperfused myocardium.

The data with both PET and SPECT methods are more fully developed than the more recent data with dobutamine echocardiography, but the assessment of contractile reserve with dobutamine has shown enormous promise. It is now clear that a number of dysfunctional myocardial regions will manifest metabolic evidence of viability, with either FDG or thallium uptake, but lack inotropic reserve during dobutamine administration (56–58). It is conceivable that some hibernating regions are so delicately balanced between the reductions in flow and function, that any catecholamine stimulation to increase oxygen demands will merely result in ischemia and inability to elicit contractile reserve. Whether the PET or SPECT information is more accurate than the dobutamine echocardiographic data regarding the potential for such regions to improve in function after revascularization awaits further study. MRI and contrast echocardiography have recently emerged as additional diagnostic tools for the assessment of myocardial viability. Their precise role in the diagnostic assessment of myocardial viability is currently under intense investigation.

Above all, the clinical relevance of viability assessment by these and other imaging modalities requires extensive study. Over 80% of dysfunctional myocardial regions identified as viable by these various imaging techniques may improve after revascularization, but the specific patients likely to benefit clinically from this information are not fully delineated. At present, the identification of viable myocardium is only one factor that enters into the equation to recommend or not recommend revascularization in the patient with impaired LV function. As in any other patient with CAD, this decision should also be based on clinical presentation, coronary anatomy, LV function, and evidence of inducible ischemia. Increasingly, however, determination of the viability of myocardial territories to be revascularized plays a pivotal role in this decision-making process. Definitive, accurate, and cost-effective methods are essential to make this determination, and noninvasive techniques to assess myocardial function will be called on with increasing frequency in the future for this purpose.

REFERENCES

1. Gheorghiade M, Bonow RO. Heart failure in the United States: a manifestation of coronary artery disease. *Circulation* 1998;97:282–289.
2. Bart BA, Shaw LK, McCants CB Jr, et al. Clinical determinants of mortality in patients with angiographically diagnosed ischemic or non-ischemic cardiomyopathy. *J Am Coll Cardiol* 1997;30;1002–1008.
3. Bruschke AVG, Proudfit WL, Sones FM. Progress study of 590 consecutive nonsurgical cases of coronary artery disease followed 5–9 years. II. Ventriculographic and other correlations. *Circulation* 1973;47: 1154–1163.
4. Hammermeister KE, DeRouen TA, Dodge HT. Variables predictive of survival in patients with coronary disease: selection by univariate and multivariate analysis from the clinical, electrocardiographic, exercise, arteriographic, and quantitative angiographic evaluations. *Circulation* 1979;59:421–430.
5. Harris PJ, Harrel FE, Lee KL, et al. Survival in medically treated coronary artery disease. *Circulation* 1979;60:1259–1269.
6. Mock MB, Ringqvist I, Fisher LD, et al. Survival of medically treated patients in the Coronary Artery Surgery Study (CASS) registry. *Circulation* 1982;66:562–568.
7. Emond M, Mock MB, Davis KB, et al. Long-term survival of medically treated patients in the Coronary Artery Surgery Study (CASS) Registry. *Circulation* 1994;90:2645–2657.
8. Smith SC, Blair SN, Criqui MH, et al. Consensus Panel statement: preventing heart attack and death in patients with coronary artery disease. *Circulation* 1995;92:3–4.
9. Faulkner SL, Stoney WS, Alford WC. Ischemic cardiomyopathy: medical versus surgical treatment. *J Thorac Cardiovasc Surg* 1977;74: 77–82.
10. Alderman EL, Fischer P, Litwin GC, et al. Results of coronary artery surgery in patients with poor left ventricular function (CASS). *Circulation* 1983;68:785–795.
11. Pigott J, Kouchoukous N, Oberman A, et al. Late results of surgical and medical therapy for patients with coronary artery disease and depressed left ventricular function. *J Am Coll Cardiol* 1985;5:1036–1045.
12. Bounous EP, Mark DB, Pollock BG, et al. Surgical survival benefits for coronary disease patients with left ventricular dysfunction. *Circulation* 1988;78[Suppl I]:I-151–I-157.
13. Muhlbaier LH, Pryor DB, Rankin JS, et al. Observational comparison of event-free survival with medical and surgical therapy in patients with coronary artery disease: 20 years of follow-up. *Circulation* 1992; 86[Suppl II]:II-198–II-204.
14. Baker DW, Jones R, Hodges J, et al. Management of heart failure. III. The role of revascularization in the treatment of patients with moderate or severe left ventricular dysfunction. *JAMA* 1994;272:1528–1534.
15. Rahimtoola SH. Coronary bypass surgery for chronic angina-1981: a perspective. *Circulation* 1982;65:225–241.
16. Braunwald E, Rutherford JD. Reversible ischemic left ventricular dysfunction: evidence for "hibernating" myocardium. *J Am Coll Cardiol* 1986;8:1467–1470.
17. Rahimtoola SH. The hibernating myocardium. *Am Heart J* 1989;117: 211–213.
18. Ross J Jr. Myocardial perfusion-contraction matching: implications for coronary artery disease and hibernation. *Circulation* 1991;83: 1076–1083.
19. Dilsizian V, Bonow RO. Current diagnostic techniques of assessing myocardial viability in hibernating and stunned myocardium. *Circulation* 1993;87:1–20.
20. Bonow RO. Identification of viable myocardium. *Circulation* 1996;94: 2674–2680.
21. Rozanski A, Bernard D, Gray R, et al. Preoperative prediction of reversible myocardial asynergy by postexercise radionuclide ventriculography. *N Engl J Med* 1982;307:212–213.
22. Brundage BH, Massie BM, Botvinick EH. Improved regional ventricular function after successful surgical revascularization. *J Am Coll Cardiol* 1984;3:902–908.
23. Dilsizian V, Bonow RO, Cannon RO, et al. The effect of coronary artery bypass grafting on left ventricular systolic function at rest: evidence for preoperative subclinical myocardial ischemia. *Am J Cardiol* 1988;61: 1248–1254.
24. Bonow RO, Dilsizian V. Thallium-201 for assessing myocardial viability. *Semin Nucl Med* 1991;21:230–241.
25. Elefteriades JA, Tolis G Jr, Levi E, et al. Coronary artery bypass grafting in severe left ventricular dysfunction: excellent survival with improved ejection fraction and functional state. *J Am Coll Cardiol* 1993; 22:1411–1417.
26. Bax JJ, Wijns W, Cornel JH, et al. Accuracy of currently available techniques for predicting functional recovery after revascularization in patients with left ventricular dysfunction due to chronic coronary artery disease: comparison of pooled data. *J Am Coll Cardiol* 1997;30: 1451–1460.
27. Tillisch JH, Brunken R, Marshall R, et al. Reversibility of cardiac wall-motion abnormalities predicted by positron tomography. *N Engl J Med* 1986;314:884–888.
28. Lucignani G, Paolini G, Landoni C, et al. Presurgical identification of hibernating myocardium by combined use of technetium-99m hexakis 2-methoxyisobutylisonitrile single photon emission tomography and fluorine-18 fluoro-2-deoxy-D-glucose positron emission tomography in patients with coronary artery disease. *Eur J Nucl Med* 1992;19: 874–881.
29. Carrel T, Jenni R, Haubold-Reuter S, et al. Improvement in severely reduced left ventricular function after surgical revascularization in patients with preoperative myocardial infarction. *Eur J Cardiothorac Surg* 1992;6:479–484.
30. Ragosta M, Beller GA, Watson DD, et al. Quantitative planar rest-redistribution 201Tl imaging in detection of myocardial viability and prediction of improvement in left ventricular function after coronary bypass surgery in patients with severely depressed left ventricular function. *Circulation* 1993;87:1630–1641.
31. Chen C, Li L, Chen LL, et al. Incremental doses of dobutamine induce a biphasic response in dysfunctional left ventricular regions subtending coronary stenoses. *Circulation* 1995;92:756–766.
32. Afridi I, Kleiman NS, Raizner AE, et al. Dobutamine echocardiography in myocardial hibernation: optimal dose and accuracy in predicting recovery of ventricular function after coronary revascularization. *Circulation* 1995;91:663–670.
33. Zimmerman R, Mall G, Rauch B, et al. Residual ^{201}Tl activity in irreversible defects as a marker of myocardial viability: clinicopathological study. *Circulation* 1995;91:1016–1021.
34. Medrano R, Lowry RW, Young JB, et al. Assessment of myocardial viability with Tc-99m sestamibi in patients undergoing cardiac transplantation: a scintigraphic/pathological study. *Circulation* 1996;94: 1010–1017.
35. Perrone-Filardi P, Pace L, Prastaro M, et al. Dobutamine echocardiography predicts improvement of hypoperfused dysfunctional myocardium after revascularization in patients with coronary artery disease. *Circulation* 1995;91:2556–2565.
36. Udelson JE, Coleman PS, Matherall JA, et al. Predicting recovery of severe regional ventricular dysfunction: comparison of resting scintigraphy with thallium-201 and technetium-99m sestamibi. *Circulation* 1994;89:2552–2561.
37. Kitsou AN, Srinivasan G, Quyyumi AA, et al. Stress-induced reversible and mild-to-moderate irreversible thallium defects: are they equally accurate for predicting recovery of regional left ventricular function after revascularization? *Circulation* 1998;98:501–508.
38. Bax JJ, Cornel JH, Visser FC, et al. Prediction of recovery of regional ventricular dysfunction following revascularization: comparison of F18-fluorodeoxyglucose SPECT, thallium stress-reinjection SPECT and dobutamine echocardiography. *J Am Coll Cardiol* 1996;28: 558–564.
39. Srinivasan G, Kitsiou AN, Bacharach SL, et al. [^{18}F]Fluorodeoxyglucose single photon emission computed tomography: can it replace PET and thallium SPECT for the assessment of myocardial viability? *Circulation* 1998;97:843–850.
40. Ragosta M, Camarano G, Kaul S, et al. Microvascular integrity indicates myocellular viability in patients with recent myocardial infarction: new insights using myocardial contrast echocardiography. *Circulation* 1994;89:2562–2569.
41. deFillipe CR, Willet DR, Irani WN, et al. Comparison of myocardial contrast echocardiography and low-dose dobutamine stress echocardiography in predicting recovery of left ventricular function after coronary revascularization in chronic ischemic heart disease. *Circulation* 1995;91:990–998.
42. Kaul S. Myocardial contrast echocardiography: 15 years of research and development. *Circulation* 1997;96:3745–3760.
43. Baer FM, Theissen P, Schneider CA, et al. Dobutamine magnetic resonance imaging predicts contractile recovery of chronically dysfunction

myocardium after successful revascularization. *J Am Coll Cardiol* 1998;31:1040–1048.

44. Ramani K, Judd RM, Holy TA, et al. Contrast magnetic resonance imaging in the assessment of myocardial viability in patients with stable coronary artery disease and left ventricular dysfunction. *Circulation* 1998;98:2687–2694.

45. Eitzman D, Al-Aouar Z, Kanter HL, et al. Clinical outcome of patients with advanced coronary artery disease after viability studies with positron emission tomography. *J Am Coll Cardiol* 1992;20:559–565.

46. Di Carli MF, Davidson M, Little R, et al. Value of metabolic imaging with positron emission tomography for evaluating prognosis in patients with coronary artery disease and left ventricular dysfunction. *Am J Cardiol* 1994;73:527–533.

47. Di Carli MF, Asgarzadie F, Schelbert HR, et al. Quantitative relation between myocardial viability and improvement in heart failure symptoms after revascularization in patients with ischemic cardiomyopathy. *Circulation* 1995;92:3436–3444.

48. Gioia G, Powers J, Heo J, et al. Prognostic value of rest-redistribution tomographic thallium-201 imaging in ischemic cardiomyopathy. *Am J Cardiol* 1995;75:759–762.

49. Gimelli A, Marzullo P, Landi P, et al. Value of thallium-201 viability imaging for evaluating prognosis in patients with ischemic left ventricular dysfunction. *J Am Coll Cardiol* 1996;27:90A(abst).

50. Nesto RW, Cohn LH, Collins JJ, et al. Inotropic reserve: a useful predictor of increased 5 year survival and improved postoperative left ventricular function in patients with coronary artery disease and reduced ejection fraction. *Am J Cardiol* 1982;50:39–44.

51. Williams MJ, Olabshian J, Lauer MS, et al. Prognostic value of dobu-tamine echocardiography in patients with left ventricular dysfunction. *J Am Coll Cardiol* 1996;27:132–139.

52. Afridi I, Grayburn P, Panza J, et al. Myocardial viability during dobutamine echocardiography predicts survival in patients with coronary artery disease and severe left ventricular systolic dysfunction. *J Am Coll Cardiol* 1998;32:921–926.

53. Chaudhry FA, Tauke JT, Alessandrini RS, et al. Prognostic implications of contractile reserve in patients with coronary artery disease and severe left ventricular dysfunction. *J Am Coll Cardiol* 1999;34:730–738.

54. Pagley PR, Beller GA, Watson DD, et al. Improved outcome after coronary artery bypass surgery in patients with ischemic cardiomyopathy and residual myocardial viability. *Circulation* 1997;95:793–800.

55. Haas F, Haehnel CJ, Picker W, et al. Preoperative positron emission tomographic viability assessment and perioperative and postoperative risk in patients with advance ischemic heart disease. *J Am Coll Cardiol* 1997;30:1693–1700.

56. Panza JA, Dilsizian V, Laurienzo JM, et al. Relation between thallium uptake and contractile response to dobutamine: implications regarding myocardial viability in patients with chronic coronary artery diseases and left ventricular dysfunction. *Circulation* 1995;91:990–998.

57. Perrone-Filardi P, Pace L, Prastaro M, et al. Assessment of myocardial viability in patients with chronic coronary artery disease: rest-4 hour-24 hour thallium-201 tomography versus dobutamine echocardiography. *Circulation* 1996;94:2712–2719.

58. Sawada, S, Elsner G, Segar DS, et al. Evaluation of patterns of perfusion and metabolism in dobutamine-responsive myocardium. *J Am Coll Cardiol* 1997;29:55–61.

CHAPTER 40

Mitral Valve Disease

Blase A. Carabello

The mitral valve allows free flow of blood from the left atrium to the left ventricle (LV) in diastole and forces undirectional forward flow into the aorta during systole by preventing regurgitation into the left atrium. Either stenosis or regurgitation may produce the picture of left heart failure (pulmonary congestion and diminished forward output), even if left ventricular function remains normal. Additionally, both conditions may lead to left ventricular pump or muscle dysfunction. Imaging of the mitral valve and blood flow through the LV is extremely useful in assessing valve function and its role as a cause of heart failure. Echocardiography provides excellent views of the mitral valve. Magnetic resonance allows quantification of regurgitation using phase velocity mapping and optimal assessment of LV function, including ventricular volumes, mass, and wall stress.

MITRAL REGURGITATION

Overview

In assessing the patient with mitral regurgitation (MR), four questions should be addressed. These are as follows:

1. What is the etiology of the mitral valve disease?
2. How severe is the MR and is it severe enough to cause clinically important pathophysiology?
3. If the disease is severe, what is the optimum time for correcting the MR?
4. Can the valve be repaired or must it be replaced?

Cardiac imaging, especially with echocardiography, forms the mainstay in answering these questions.

Question 1: What Is the Etiology of Mitral Regurgitation?

Primary Mitral Regurgitation

The mitral valve consists of its annulus, the mitral valve leaflets, the chorda tendineae, and the papillary muscles.

B. A. Carabello: Department of Medicine, Baylor College of Medicine; Department of Medicine, Veterans Administration Medical Center, Houston, Texas 77030.

When it is an abnormality of one of these components of the mitral valve that is responsible for regurgitation, the term primary MR is used. Common causes of primary MR include mitral valve prolapse, spontaneous chordal rupture, coronary artery disease with attendant ischemia and papillary muscle dysfunction, infective endocarditis, and rheumatic heart disease (1).

When left ventricular dilatation due to myocardial dysfunction has led to papillary muscle malalignment and annular enlargement, mitral regurgitation occurring under these circumstances is termed secondary MR.

Identifying the etiology of mitral regurgitation is important in assessing prognosis and in predicting whether or not the valve can be repaired or must be replaced if surgical correction is eventually necessary. For instance, when posterior leaflet prolapse of a myxomatous valve is the cause of mitral regurgitation, there is a high likelihood of repair. On the other hand, when there is severe rheumatic deformity of the valve, repair might be impossible even when the best surgical expertise is available. Because the issue of repair versus replacement is usually crucial, transesophageal echocardiography (TEE) with its excellent imaging of the mitral valve is used to help resolve the likely course of surgical management. Shown in Figure 1 are echocardiographic images of two of the typical etiologies of primary MR. Figure 1A demonstrates the echocardiographic image of the typically thickened and redundant leaflets of a patient with mitral valve prolapse. Figure 1B demonstrates a patient with a flail leaflet due to ruptured chordae tendineae.

Question 2: How Severe Is the MR and What Are the Pathophysiologic Consequences?

The pathophysiologic changes that accompany the development of acute mitral regurgitation are important (2). The acute volume overload produced by the sum of regurgitant and forward flows increases LV sarcomere length, thereby increasing end diastolic volume. The new pathway for ejection (into the left atrium) unloads the LV, allowing

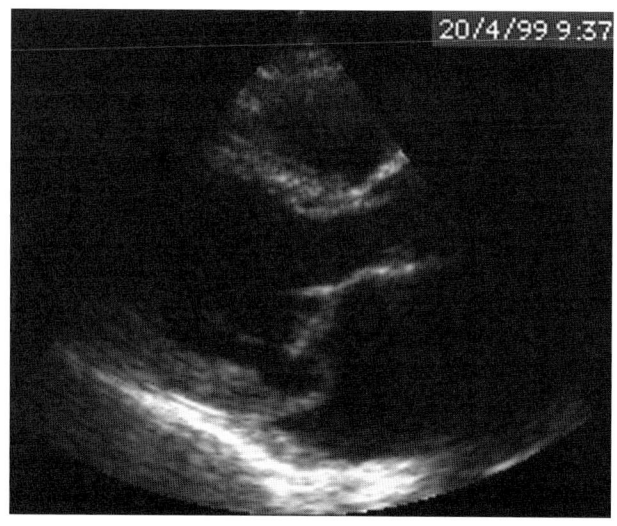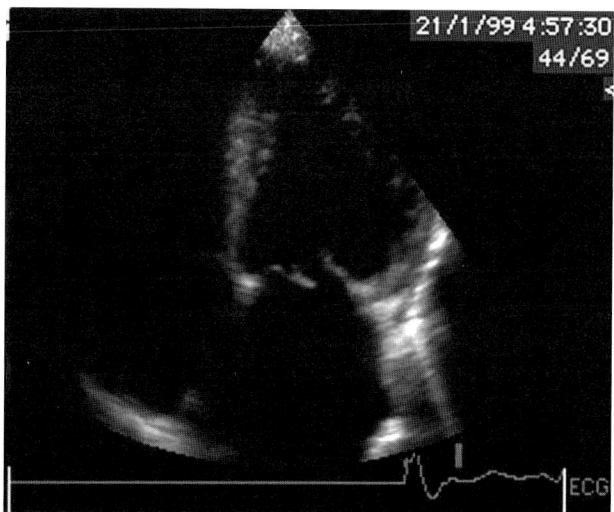

FIG. 1. Echocardiographic images of mitral valve prolapse due to a flail leaflet obtained from parasternal view (**A**) and apical four-chamber view (**B**).

more complete emptying and thereby reducing end systolic volume. The result of these changes is an increase in total stroke volume. However, because a substantial portion of the total stroke volume is regurgitated into the left atrium (LA), forward stroke volume decreases. At the same time, volume overload on the small unprepared LA and LV increases LV, LA, and pulmonary venous pressure in turn, leading to pulmonary congestion.

Clinical Presentation

Almost all patients with acute severe MR are symptomatic with dyspnea and orthopnea. During physical examination, palpation finds the apical impulse in its normal position. S_1 is reduced in intensity and is followed by a systolic murmur, which usually radiates to the axilla. The murmur is usually associated with a third heart sound. Although the murmur of MR is typically described as a holosystolic murmur, in acute MR, the high left atrial pressure during ventricular systole (V wave) diminishes the driving gradient between the LV and left atrium, and the murmur may be foreshortened. Examination of the lungs detects pulmonary rales as evidence of pulmonary congestion.

TABLE 1. *Angiographic grades of mitral regurgitation*

+1	Whiff of contrast enters the left atrium but does not opacify it completely
+2	Complete opacification of the left atrium but less densely than the left ventricle
+3	Equal opacification of left atrium and left ventricle
+4	Opacification of the left atrium, its appendage, and pulmonary veins Atrial opacification exceeds ventricular opacification

Diagnostic Studies

Echocardiography and Magnetic Resonance

In acute severe MR, the left atrium and LV are not enlarged. However, the favorable loading conditions of MR augment ejection performance producing hyperdynamic LV systolic performance. Frequently, the etiology of the MR can be demonstrated on transthoracic echocardiography (TTE). However, in many cases, color flow study during TTE underestimates the severity of the MR. If severe MR is suspected on clinical grounds but not demonstrated by TTE, TEE, or magnetic resonance imaging are often helpful in resolving the issue as well as in establishing the anatomic cause of the MR (3).

Cardiac Catheterization

Right heart catheterization usually demonstrates pulmonary hypertension and elevated pulmonary capillary wedge pressure. Although unreliable in chronic MR (4), in acute MR, a large V wave is usually present, because the LA is still small and unable to accommodate the volume overload. The left ventriculogram demonstrates regurgitation of contrast from the LV into the LA and its appearance is used to semiquantitatively assess the severity of the mitral regurgitation present (Table 1). If there is a suspicion that the etiology of MR might be ischemic in nature, coronary arteriography should be performed.

CHRONIC MITRAL REGURGITATION

The transition from acute to chronic compensated MR is accomplished by the development of eccentric cardiac hypertrophy. As sarcomeres are laid down in series and the myocytes elongate, chamber volume increases. Because of the still favorable loading conditions present in compensated MR, ejection performance is enhanced, permitting return of forward stroke volume toward normal. At the same time, LA enlargement allows for accommodation of the regurgitant volume, allowing left atrial pressure to return toward normal. In this situation, the patient may be remarkably well compensated without symptoms, even during fairly strenuous activity.

During physical examination, palpation of the precordium finds the apical impulse displaced downward and to the left. An apical thrill may be noted. There is a holosystolic murmur that radiates toward the axilla. If the mitral regurgitation is due to incompetence of the anterior leaflet, murmur radiation may be to the back or to the top of the head. A third heart sound in the case of severe MR does not necessarily indicate congestive heart failure but rather reflects the rapid filling of the LV from a large LA filling volume. The chest is clear to auscultation and the neck veins are not elevated.

Diagnostic Studies

Electrocardiogram

The electrocardiogram usually shows LA abnormality and LV hypertrophy. The chest x-ray shows an enlarged heart with normal lung fields.

Echocardiography and Magnetic Resonance

The echocardiogram remains the primary tool used to gauge the severity of MR. Phase velocity magnetic resonance methods provide an alternative to the echocardiogram to evaluate severity. Neither imaging approach is perfect and continues to evolve. In severe chronic MR, both two-dimensional echocardiography and magnetic resonance imaging should demonstrate enlargement of both the LA and LV. The absence of chamber enlargement suggests that either the MR is not severe or has not been chronic. Severity assessment is aided by imaging using color flow Doppler studies or phase velocity magnetic resonance. Even in severe MR, the regurgitant orifice is relatively small, on the order of 0.3 cm². As blood is driven into the orifice, it accelerates, and it is this acceleration of red blood cells that is detected by color flow Doppler and phase velocity mapping.

Visual Estimation and Color Flow Mapping

In this technique, the severity of the amount of MR is based upon the appearance of the depth and breadth of the mitral regurgitant jet (5,6). This technique is highly subjective but usually is adequate in assessing whether regurgitant flow is severe versus absent or trivial. However, more precise evaluation of MR severity is not afforded easily by this subjective method. Color flow mapping was an attempt to improve on this technique. Here, mapping of the area of the regurgitant jet on the LA side of the valve is used either as

an absolute area or normalized to the LA area to assess severity of MR. Greater relative areas indicate more severe MR. Although this technique was initially greeted with enthusiasm, several limitations have subsequently been defined, limiting its use (7). If flow is directed toward one of the walls of the LA, the jet size is confined and MR severity may be underestimated (8). Machine gain setting can also affect the breadth of the jet, independent of regurgitant volume (9). These limitations have reduced the use of color flow mapping because the extra time it requires is not justified by increased accuracy. On the other hand, the Doppler jet still gives important information regarding the pathology involved. In single leaflet regurgitation, the jet is usually directed away from the affected leaflet—i.e., in posterior leaflet prolapse, the jet is directly anterior. Conversely, incomplete mitral valve closure is usually associated with a central jet.

Proximal Isovelocity Surface Area Method

As shown in Figure 2 (see also Color Plate 20 following page 294), as the regurgitant jet approaches the ventricular side of the mitral regurgitant orifice, it assumes a hemispherical shape (10,11). This observation can be used to calculate regurgitant flow if jet area and velocity are known (flow = area × velocity). At the outside of the convergence zone, the hemispherical area (area = $2\Pi r^2$) is large, and the velocity is low. As the jet moves toward the orifice, the area decreases while the velocity increases. By establishing the hemispherical area at the point of aliasing where velocity is known from the machine settings, regurgitant flow can be calculated. The

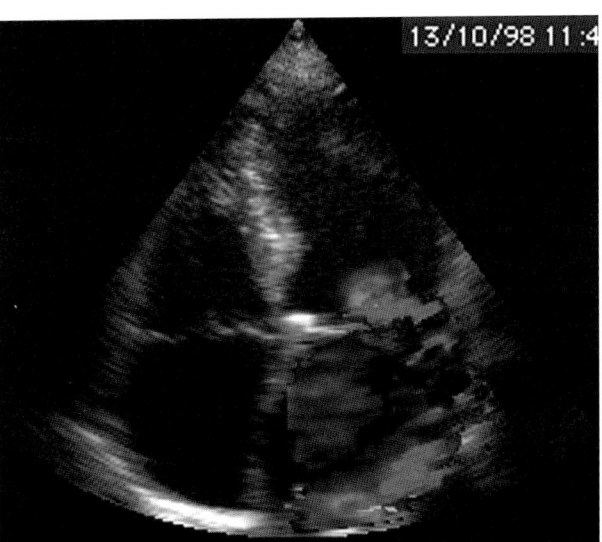

FIG. 2. Proximal convergence of the mitral regurgitation jet on the left ventricular side of the mitral valve is shown. A schematic is presented for determining the area of the jet at the site of aliasing. When this area is multiplied by the aliasing velocity, flow can be obtained. (See also Color Plate 20 following page 294.)

radius term for the area calculation is the length of a line from the edge of the convergence zone to the mitral valve plane.

While the proximal isovelocity surface area (PISA) method increases the ability to quantify MR, numerous limitations have prevented it from developing widespread acceptance in clinical practice. In some cases, the convergence zone is difficult to discern, making the method impractical. In cases where the convergence zone can be detected, the method is still operator dependent (12). By choosing a convergence zone that is too far distant from the actual regurgitant orifice, the contour may be oblong rather than hemispheric, causing overestimation of the radius term and, therefore, overestimation of true flow. If a convergence zone too close to the orifice is chosen, flattening of the zone may cause underestimation of radius and, therefore, underestimation of regurgitant flow. Further, to calculate radius, the exact position of the mitral plane must be known but can be difficult to pinpoint. Lastly, this method gives only instantaneous flow. Because regurgitant flow varies throughout the systolic cycle, instantaneous flow may or may not reflect the magnitude of overall regurgitant flow.

The PISA method can be extended to calculate regurgitant orifice area (13,14). By interrogating the regurgitant orifice, the maximum regurgitant velocity can be determined. By dividing maximum flow from the PISA method by maximum velocity, the peak regurgitant orifice area can be calculated. Larger orifice areas are consistent with more severe MR and areas above 0.3 cm^2 usually indicate severe MR.

Quantitative Doppler Echocardiography

In MR, the flow crossing the mitral valve in diastole represents the total mitral flow (regurgitant plus forward flow). On the other hand, the flow leaving the aortic valve in systole represents forward flow. By subtracting forward flow from total flow, regurgitant flow is obtained (15). By dividing regurgitant flow by total flow, regurgitant fraction is obtained. Total flow is calculated by multiplying the diastolic mitral time-velocity integral times the diastolic mitral valve area. Then, by multiplying the systolic aortic time velocity integral times aortic outflow tract area, forward flow is obtained. In this way, regurgitant flow and regurgitant fraction can be calculated. This method is probably the most accurate for determining the quantity of MR. However, it is time intensive and has not gained widespread clinical usage.

The Vena Contracta Method

The width of the jet as it leaves the regurgitant orifice or vena contracta should represent an approximation of the size of the regurgitant orifice. Using quantitative Doppler flow as a gold standard, this method has been shown to be superior to visual estimation and color flow mapping in assessing MR (16). However, the method also has its limitations. The size of the vena contracta is load dependent and changes unpredictably with changes in afterload (17).

Cardiac Catheterization

When surgery is contemplated, cardiac catheterization is employed to help establish the severity of MR if severity remains unclear following clinical and echocardiographic assessment. Because coronary disease can be the etiology of MR, coronary arteriography is usually performed at this time. During cardiac catheterization, right heart pressures are recorded. In the symptomatic patient with MR, the pulmonary capillary wedge pressure should be elevated reflecting the hemodynamic cause of symptoms. There may or may not be a large V wave depending on the ability of the left atrium to accommodate the volume overload. If hemodynamics are normal at rest, exercise should be performed to confirm that there is a hemodynamic cause for the patient's symptoms. Cardiac output is measured using the thermodilution or Fick techniques. A left ventriculogram is then performed using a large volume (60 cc's) of contrast. The intensity to which the LA is opacified during this procedure helps gauge the severity of the MR. Contrast ventriculography has the potential to add additional data to Doppler echocardiography because, during contrast injection, actual flow, rather than the velocity of flow, is visualized. However, this method is only semiquantitative and has its own limitations in assessing MR severity (10,18,19). A common error in performing ventriculography is injection of too little contrast to adequately opacify both the enlarged LV and enlarged LA. The result is under opacification and an underestimation of the severity of MR.

As with quantitative Doppler techniques, quantitative cine angiography can also be performed. By calculating the end-diastolic and end-systolic volumes angiographically, using the area-length method or Simpson's rule, total left ventricular stroke volume is obtained (19). By subtracting forward stroke volume (that obtained by dividing Fick or thermodilution cardiac output by heart rate) regurgitant flow is obtained. As with quantitative echocardiography, regurgitant fraction equals regurgitant flow divided by total flow. This technique can provide an excellent means for quantitating the severity of MR. Unfortunately, in many laboratories, the lack of attention to detail in calculating ventricular volumes detracts from the accuracy of the method. Thus, today *quantitative* angiography is not widely employed in most centers.

Apart from the vagaries noted above in using both echocardiography and invasive techniques to assess the severity of MR, day-to-day changes in hemodynamics and loading conditions also affect severity. Small changes in blood pressure can greatly affect the orifice area and the gradient for systolic retrograde flow and worsen or diminish MR. It is not at all uncommon for different methods applied at different times to derive entirely different assessments of the severity of MR in a given patient. Frequently, these differences are attributed to the method of severity assessment when in fact they should be attributed to changes in the patient's physiologic state from one evaluation to the next.

Question 3: If Mitral Regurgitation Is Severe, When Should Surgical Correction Be Undertaken?

Until very recently, the outcome of surgery for nonischemic MR was poor. Age-corrected survivorship was only 50 to 60% at 10 years compared to 90% for patients undergoing aortic valve replacement for aortic stenosis (20). Operative mortality was also higher for MR compared to that for other valvular heart diseases. The reasons for poor outcome in MR stemmed from lack of recognition of the proper timing of surgery and also from surgery that damaged or removed the mitral valve apparatus, causing, in turn, ventricular dysfunction. In the transition from compensated to decompensated MR (2), the myocardium, injured from prolonged volume overload has decreased contractility. Thus, the ventricle remains larger at end systole because of its inability to expel blood, resulting in an increase in end-systolic volume. At the same time, LA pressure becomes elevated causing the symptoms of pulmonary congestion. Enlargement of the LV increases the radius term of the Laplace relationship, increasing systolic wall stress (afterload) despite the LA ejection pathway, which tends to unload the ventricle. Nonetheless, augmented preload still enhances ejection fraction. In the case shown (Fig. 3), despite the presence of significant LV dysfunction, ejection fraction is normal, 60%. In the past, physicians relying on ejection fraction to help time surgery delayed too long before referring patients for mitral valve replacement. Several lines of evidence suggest that left ventricular dysfunction is often present when ejection fraction falls below 60%. Figure 4 demonstrates that when ejection fraction falls below 60%, whether mitral valve repair or replacement is performed, survival is reduced (21). Other studies have found a similar cut-point for preoperative ejection fraction leading to reduced postoperative ejection fraction (22) and decreased contractility (23). Alternatively, end-systolic volume or dimension, which is less affected by the preload that augments ejection fraction in MR, has been used to help time surgery. As shown in Figure 5, when end systolic dimension approaches 45 mm, the probability of a bad outcome following surgery increases (24). This benchmark was virtually the same as that found by Zile and colleagues (25). Crawford et al., (26) who examined end systolic volume, found a cutoff of 50 cc/m², which translates to an end-systolic dimension of approximately 45 mm. Thus, even asymptomatic patients should usually be referred for mitral valve surgery when ejection fraction approaches 60% or when end-systolic dimension approaches 45 mm. However, if symptoms have developed, surgery should be performed even if LV function has not deteriorated to the levels noted above. The presence of symptoms alone,

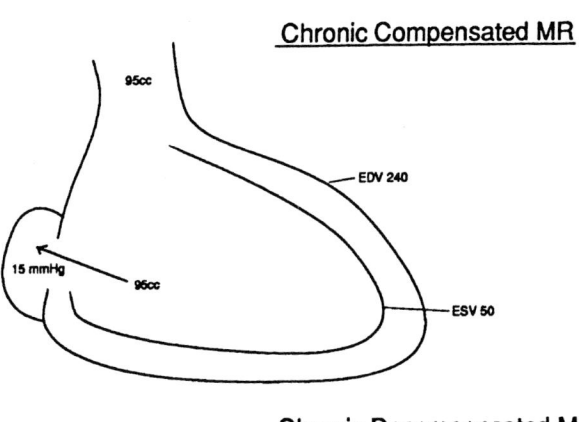

Chronic Compensated MR

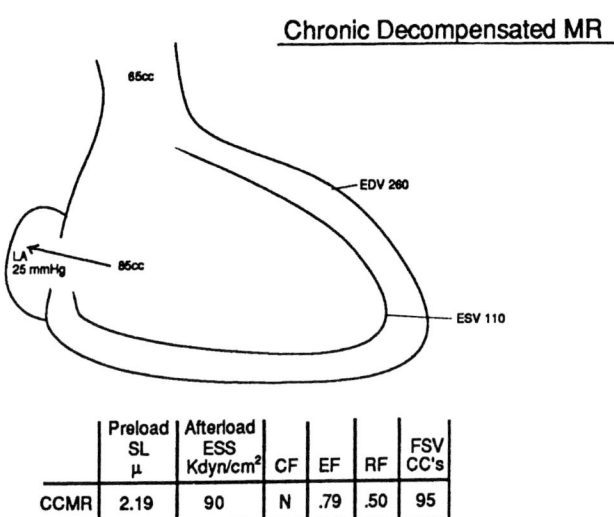

Chronic Decompensated MR

	Preload SL μ	Afterload ESS Kdyn/cm²	CF	EF	RF	FSV CC's
CCMR	2.19	90	N	.79	.50	95
CDMR	2.19	120	↓	.58	.57	65

FIG. 3. The transition from compensated to decompensated mitral regurgitation (MR) is shown. The ventricle is now impaired by contractile dysfunction, in turn reducing its ability to shorten so that end-systolic volume (*ESV*) increases. Although MR often was thought of as a lesion that reduces afterload, afterload actually increases in the decompensated phase, further impairing ejection and acting in concert with contractile dysfunction to increase ESV. Impaired contraction leads to further left ventricle dilatation, which produces yet more MR. Regurgitant fraction (*RF*) increases and forward stroke volume (*FSV*) is diminished. However, high preload still augments ejection fraction (*EF*), which may remain in the "normal" range. *CF*, contractile function; *CCMR*, chronic compensated MR; *CDMR*, chronic decompensated MR; *EDV*, end-diastolic volume; *ESS*, end-systolic stress; *LA*, left atrium; *SL*, sarcomere length.

in the face of normal left ventricular function, has been found to worsen prognosis (27).

Thus, in the timing of mitral valve surgery for MR, serial echocardiography is indispensable. Patients with moderate-to-severe symptoms should undergo echocardiography at least yearly to provide surveillance of possible development of occult LV dysfunction. When there is evidence that LV dysfunction is developing, cardiac catheterization should be performed for the purposes of coronary arteriography and,

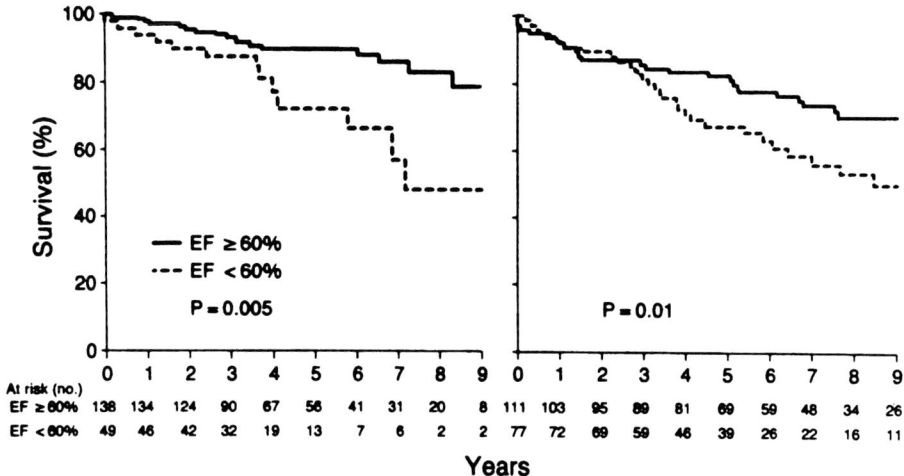

FIG. 4. Postoperative survival for patients with mitral regurgitation undergoing mitral valve surgery is demonstrated. Whether mitral valve repair (**left**) or mitral valve replacement (**right**) was employed, survivorship was similar to that of an aged-matched well comparison group as long as ejection fraction (*EF*) exceeded 60% prior to surgery. (From ref. 21, with permission.)

if necessary, to confirm the severity of the hemodynamic abnormalities associated with MR.

Question 4: Will Mitral Valve Repair or Mitral Valve Replacement Be Performed?

Three types of mitral valve surgery can be performed for MR. These include: (i) the previously standard operation in which the native mitral valve and the subvalvular apparatus

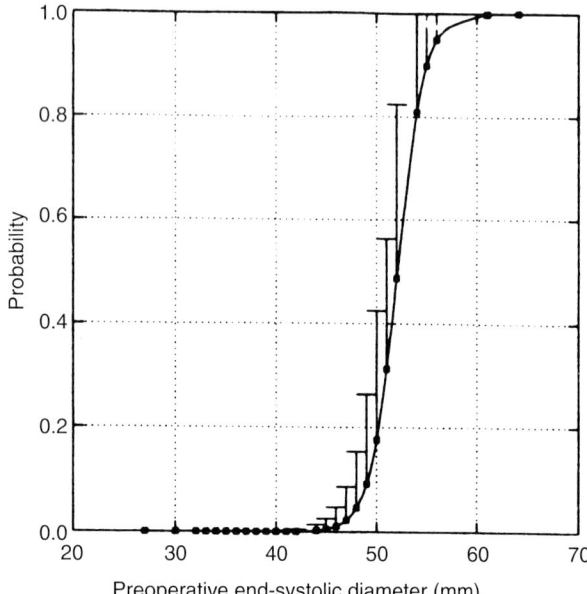

FIG. 5. The probability of a bad postsurgical outcome is plotted against preoperative end-systolic dimension for patients with mitral regurgitation. The probability of a poor outcome increases rapidly as end-systolic dimension exceeds 45 mm. (From ref. 24, with permission.)

were removed and a prosthesis installed; (ii) a mitral valve repair in which the native valve is conserved; and (iii) a mitral valve replacement retaining part or all of the native valve by which the normal continuity between the leaflets and the apparatus is preserved. Because of the physiologic importance of the mitral valve apparatus, outcome depends on which operation is performed. It is now clear that the mitral valve apparatus not only maintains mitral valve competence, but is also an integral working part of the LV. The mitral apparatus helps maintain the ellipsoid shape of the LV and coordinates LV contraction. Isolated removal of the mitral valve apparatus in a normal ventricle, by itself, causes substantial LV dysfunction (28–33). Thus, during mitral valve surgery, the integrity of the mitral valve and its apparatus should be maintained whenever possible.

When a mitral valve repair can be performed, the benefits of apparatus-continuity are coupled with the benefits of avoiding a prosthetic valve and its potential complications of valve failure, thromboembolism, or the need for anticoagulation. Preoperative echocardiography, usually employing the transesophageal approach, is crucial in assessing repairability. When just the posterior leaflet or chorda tendineae are involved, repair usually can be performed. When both leaflets are involved, repair is still possible, but its likelihood diminishes. Currently, with the use of TEE, the prediction of which procedure eventually will be performed is approximately 80% accurate (34). This is a crucial area for preoperative imaging because it affects the timing of surgery. The most controversial issue surrounds the asymptomatic patient with normal LV function. While the standard policy now is to delay surgery until either symptoms or early objective signs of LV dysfunction develop, elective repair prior to these benchmarks could be entertained if repair were certain. In this case, no prosthesis would be employed, and, thus, the patient would be spared the risks of prosthetic valves and anticoagulation. The situation would then be similar to that of an atrial-septal defect repair in which surgery is routinely performed in asymptomatic patients because repair can be performed at a low operative risk, without the use of a prosthetic device, reliably preventing late-term complications.

At the other end of the spectrum, patients with severe LV dysfunction who would not be candidates for mitral valve replacement with chordal disruption (which would cause a prohibitive worsening in ventricular function), may still survive surgery and improve postoperatively if the mitral valve apparatus can be spared. In this group, preoperative imaging with accurate prediction of outcome is paramount in determining whether or not surgery should be performed.

Other Issues in the Timing of Surgery

It should be noted that age-corrected surgical mortality is increased for mitral valve surgery in patients over the age of 70 (35). Mortality is greatest in those patients with coronary disease and in those patients requiring mitral valve replacement. While symptomatic elderly patients should not be denied surgery because of age, there is no compelling reason to pursue surgery in asymptomatic aged patients.

Advanced Left Ventricular Dysfunction

The question often arises as to the point at which LV function has so deteriorated that mitral surgery is impossible. In view of recent success in operating on patients with dilated cardiomyopathy and secondary MR with ejection fractions as low as 0.15, this question is hard to answer (36). As long as the mitral apparatus is left intact, patients with very low ejection fractions may benefit from surgery. However, if the apparatus cannot be conserved, surgery in patients with an ejection fraction of less than 0.50 and certainly less than 0.40 have a high risk and reduced benefit.

ISCHEMIC MITRAL REGURGITATION

Ischemic MR occurs when papillary muscle dysfunction, alone or in concert with wall motion abnormalities, prevents valve coaptation. It must be distinguished from mitral regurgitation originating from other causes (rheumatic disease, etc.) in patients who happen to have coexistent coronary disease. Despite improved outcome for nonischemic MR, prognosis for ischemic disease remains poor. Survival is only 50% at 5 years (37–39). This poor outcome stems from the inherent LV dysfunction responsible for the MR and from the progressive nature of the underlying coronary disease.

Unlike nonischemic MR, where mitral valve repair is clearly the operation of choice, there is no consensus regarding the best operation for ischemic MR. Because the valve itself is usually normal in ischemic MR, it leaves little for the surgeon to repair. Indeed, Cohn et al. (37) has recommended

mitral valve replacement as the treatment of choice because long-term outcome was superior to repair. Alternatively, Bolling and colleagues (40) have noted successful repair with an excellent result even in elderly patients with ischemic MR.

MEDICAL THERAPY OF MITRAL REGURGITATION

Acute severe MR nearly always results in symptoms due to pulmonary congestion and decreased forward output. Arterial vasodilators are the treatment of choice in the absence of hypotension (41). Vasodilators such as nitroprusside reduce aortic impedance and preferentially increase aortic (forward) output while simultaneously decreasing regurgitant flow and left atrial pressure. In the case of hypotension, vasodilators cannot be used; instead aortic balloon counterpulsation is used to increase forward output while supporting blood pressure. Once stable, MR is surgically corrected.

Because vasodilators are effective in treating acute MR, their use in chronic MR seems intuitive. This notion is further bolstered by the successful use of vasodilators in aortic regurgitation (42). However, afterload in chronic MR is usually normal. Vasodilators lower afterload to potentially subnormal levels, resulting in loss of LV mass. While reversal of hypertrophy is often taken to be beneficial, it must be remembered that the ventricle in MR is a thin-walled dilated spheroid with a lower than normal mass-to-volume ratio (43). Reduction in mass could conceivably impair ventricular performance when mitral valve competency is regained. While this concept is speculative, there are currently no large trials supporting the use of vasodilators in asymptomatic patients and, currently, available data do not support the use of vasodilators in asymptomatic patients (44,45). Conversely, improvement has been demonstrated in symptomatic patients treated with ACE inhibitors (46), but surgery may be the preferred treatment in this group.

MITRAL STENOSIS

Etiology

Rheumatic heart disease is the cause of almost all cases of acquired mitral stenosis (MS). The disease is three to four times more common in women than in men, even though rheumatic fever attacks slightly more men. The reason for female predominance is unknown. Because of the difficulties in establishing the diagnosis of a previous episode of rheumatic fever, a rheumatic origin is often difficult to prove.

Occasionally, severe mitral annular calcification can restrict orifice area in the absence of a rheumatic involvement, constituting a second etiology for MS.

Symptomatic patients with mitral stenosis complain of dyspnea on exertion, orthopnea, and paroxysmal nocturnal dyspnea. Because it is the right ventricle (RV) that must develop the pressure needed to drive blood across the stenotic mitral valve, MS eventually leads to a pressure over-load on the RV. Secondary reversible pulmonary vasocon-striction often complicates the disease, eventually causing RV failure by worsening the RV pressure overload. In such cases, patients also complain of ascites and edema.

The symptoms above are typical for any patient with heart failure. Other but rarer symptoms, which are more specific for MS, include hoarseness as the enlarged left atrium impinges on the left recurrent laryngeal nerve (Ortner's syndrome) and dysphagia. Angina with normal coronaries may occur in patients with pulmonary hypertension, presumably due to right ventricular hypertrophy and ischemia. Hemoptysis is more common and is thought to occur when left atrial hypertension ruptures small, thin-walled bronchial veins.

Diagnostic Studies

Electrocardiogram

In patients in sinus rhythm, there is left atrial abnormality, right axis deviation, and signs of RV hypertrophy that may be present. As the disease progresses, atrial fibrillation becomes common. However, the onset of atrial fibrillation corresponds more to advancing age than to various hemodynamic parameters of stenosis severity.

Chest X-ray

Figure 6 is a chest x-ray showing many classic features of mitral stenosis. As the LA enlarges, it causes straightening

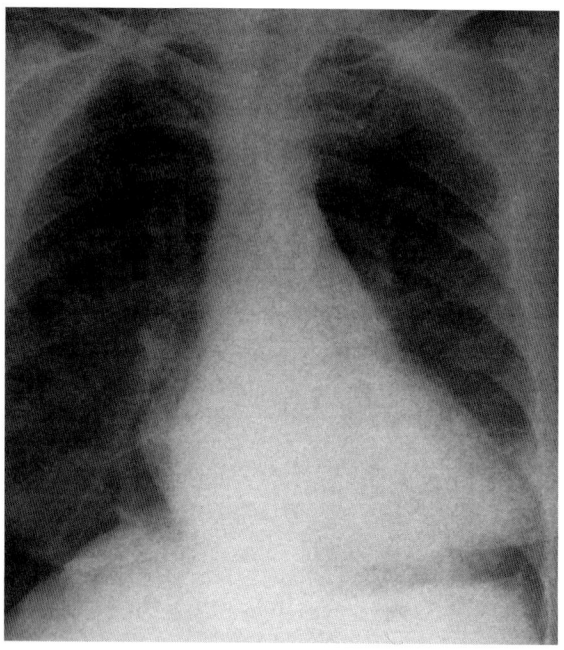

FIG. 6. A chest x-ray of a patient with mitral stenosis is demonstrated. Enlargement of the left atrium causes straightening of the left heart border. The left atrium is seen as a double density inside the shadow of the right atrium at the right heart border. Chronic pulmonary venous hypertension has led to the development of Kerley B lines.

of the left heart border. The enlarged LA is also seen as a double density at the right heart border, where the LA is seen just inside the right atrium (RA). Chronic pulmonary venous hypertension leads to edema and thickening of pulmonary septae (Kerley B lines). In the lateral view, RV enlargement causes obliteration of the retrosternal air space.

Echocardiography

Echocardiography is the key to confirming the diagnosis of mitral stenosis and in assessing its severity. The echocardiogram in MS demonstrates doming and thickening of the valve leaflets, which are restricted in motion. The technique also images pathology of the subvalvular apparatus and detects concomitant MR and LA enlargement, and it can estimate left ventricular function. Surprisingly, LV ejection performance is decreased in approximately one third of patients with MS (47–49). Decreased ejection performance in MS accrues in part from increased afterload due to reflex vasoconstriction secondary to reduced forward output. Additionally, restricted LV inflow diminishes preload reserve that normally compensates for afterload mismatch (50).

How Severe Is the Mitral Stenosis?

The normal mitral valve area is 4 to 5 cm^2. Little hemodynamic disturbance, even during exercise, occurs until the valve area is reduced to 2.0 cm^2 (Table 2). When valve area decreases to 1.5 to 2.0 cm^2, mild symptoms may develop, although in some cases more severe exercise limitation may be noted. When valve area is reduced to 1.0 to 1.5 cm^2 (moderately severe disease), symptoms intensify and limit lifestyle. When valve area narrows to less than 1.0 cm^2 (severe disease), pulmonary hypertension develops, severely limiting activity and worsening prognosis. Symptoms have been a key to the prognosis of the disease and the benefit to surgery. For patients with New York Heart Association class IV symptoms, the survival benefit to surgery compared to medical therapy is quite large (Fig. 7) (51). For class II and class III, there is still a survival benefit, mostly to class III patients, but the benefit is less marked. Thus, mechanical intervention should probably be planned at the onset of mild-to-moderate symptoms. However, because pulmonary hypertension also worsens prognosis, mechanical intervention should be undertaken even in the asymptomatic patient if pulmonary hypertension is present (52).

During echocardiography, the mitral valve orifice can be planimetered accurately in the short-axis view (Fig. 8). Although this technique may overestimate valve area, if there is additional subvalvular obstruction, many consider this to be the most accurate way of assessing mitral valve area (53). A complementary method of valve area assessment is the use of the pressure half-time technique (54). Using continuous wave Doppler, the mitral inflow velocity can be imaged. In more severe disease, the gradient across the valve persists throughout diastole, and the decay in velocity is slow. In

TABLE 2. *Severity of mitral stenosis*

Severity	MVA	Gradient	PAP	Symptoms
Mild	>2.0 cm²	Only with exercise	nl	NYHA I
Moderate	1.5–2.0 cm²	5–10 mm Hg	nl	NYHA I or II
Moderately severe	1.0–1.5 cm²	5–15 mm Hg	nl	NYHA I, II, or III
Severe	<1.0 cm²	≥15 mm Hg	↑	NYHA I–IV

MVA, mitral valve area; *NYHA*, New York Heart Association class; *PAP*, pulmonary artery pressure.

less severe disease, the decay in velocity is more rapid. By dividing the empiric constant of 220 by the time it takes for inflow velocity to fall from its peak to the peak divided by the square root of 2 (pressure half-time method) (Fig. 8), the mitral valve area can be estimated. In general, these techniques have fairly good agreement between each other and with calculations obtained from catheterization data. However, in a given subject, substantial discrepancies may exist. Thus, valve area by itself should not be the only factor used to determine the severity of mitral stenosis. This parameter must be taken in context with the overall clinical and hemodynamic picture.

Because the presence of pulmonary hypertension adversely affects outcome, pulmonary pressure should be estimated during echocardiography when tricuspid regurgitation is present. In this technique, the reverse systolic gradient between RV and RA is used to estimate RV pressure. Doppler interrogation of the tricuspid valve regurgitant jet determines its maximum velocity and, in turn, allows one to calculate peak RV pressure. For instance, a peak velocity (V)

of the regurgitant jet across the tricuspid valve of 3 m/sec indicates a peak gradient of 36 mm Hg between RV and RA as calculated by the modified Bernoulli equation (gradient = $4V^2$). If right atrial pressure were 10 mm Hg (either assumed or measured by neck vein elevation), a peak RV pressure of 46 mm Hg (36 + 10) is calculated. In the absence of pulmonic stenosis, this is the same pressure as peak pulmonary artery pressure.

Cardiac Catheterization

In most cases, all the hemodynamic information needed to assess the severity of mitral stenosis can be determined echocardiographically. However, when discrepancies between clinical and echocardiographic data make stenosis severity uncertain, hemodynamic measurements made during cardiac catheterization can be used to assess mitral valve area using the Gorlin formula (55), which relies upon the transmitral gradient (*h*) and cardiac output (*CO*) to calculate mitral valve area (*MVA*).

$$MVA = \frac{CO/DFP \times HR}{0.85 \times \sqrt{2\,gh}}$$

where *DFP* is the diastolic filling period (in seconds), *HR* is the heart rate, *h* is the gradient, and *g* is acceleration due to gravity. It should be pointed out that it was for the mitral valve that the Gorlins developed the empiric correction factor (0.85) needed to match their hemodynamic calculations of valve area with actual valve areas. Probably because of this validation, there has been good agreement between invasive and noninvasive estimations of mitral valve area. In using the Gorlin formula to calculate area, the two pieces of data used in the calculation, cardiac output and pressure gradient, must be obtained properly. The gold standard for cardiac output determination is the Fick method (56).

The wedge pressure has been a reliable surrogate for true left atrial pressure, provided it is properly measured (57,58). However, if a damped pulmonary artery pressure rather than true wedge pressure is obtained, overestimation of LA pressure and transmitral gradient will occur. In order to be certain that a wedge pressure rather than a damped pulmonary artery pressure is being recorded, highly oxygenated LA blood should be withdrawn from the catheter in the wedge position. If poorly oxygenated pulmonary artery blood is withdrawn instead, the catheter must be repositioned.

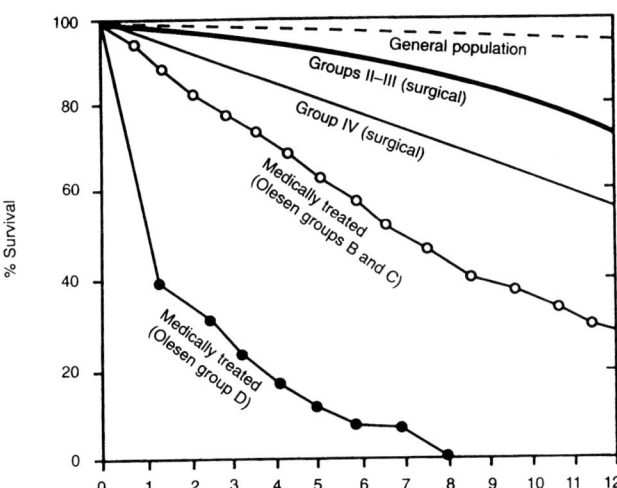

FIG. 7. Outcome for patients with mitral stenosis according to symptom class is demonstrated. Severely symptomatic patients (Olesen group D) had substantially worse survival when treated medically than did similarly severely symptomatic patients (Group 4) treated surgically. Moderately symptomatic patients (Olesen groups B and C) also fared worse than their surgically treated counterparts, but the difference was less. As patients become less symptomatic, the differences between medical versus surgical therapy also lessens. (From ref. 51, with permission.)

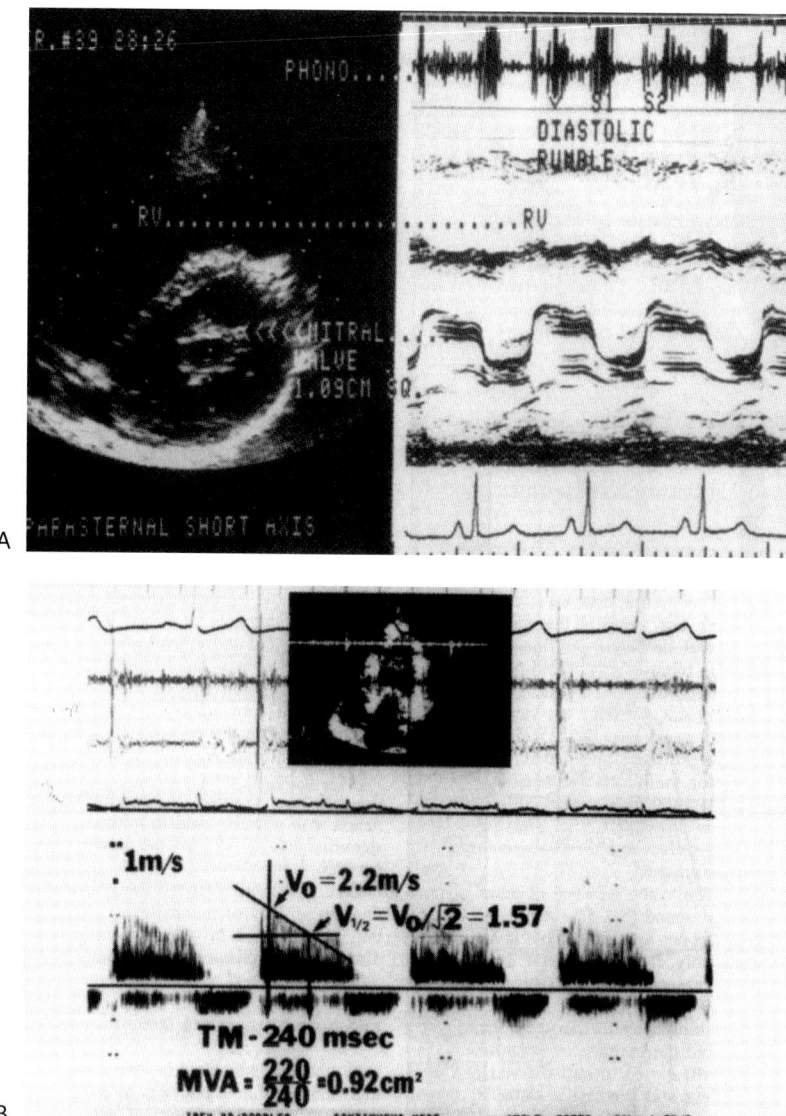

FIG. 8. A: Cross-sectional image of the mitral valve used to planimeter its area. M-mode echocardiogram is at the right. This very stenotic valve has an orifice area of 1.09 cm². *RV*, right ventricle. **B:** The Doppler flow pattern for a patient with mitral stenosis. It demonstrates delay in decay of low velocity that is maintained by the transmitral gradient. This principle, in turn, is used to calculate the pressure half-time that is divided into the empirical constant of 220 to calculate a mitral valve area (*MVA*). V_o, velocity at valve opening; *TM*, time from T_o to $T_{1/2}$. (From ref. 76, with permission.)

During cardiac catheterization, coronary arteriography should also be performed in patients with risk factors for coronary disease and in those patients with a history of angina.

The Timing of Intervention

Intervention should be performed when the patient develops more than mild symptoms or if there is asymptomatic pulmonary hypertension (52–59). Mitral stenosis can be corrected by balloon valvotomy, by surgical repair of the valve, or by valve replacement. In appropriately chosen valves, balloon valvotomy has been shown to be as effective as open

commissurotomy at both early and mid-term results (60). While there are occasionally cases where open repair can affect a better result than valvulotomy, this is impossible to predict preoperatively. Therefore, for most patients, expected correction entails either a percutaneous balloon valvotomy or mitral valve replacement.

Echocardiographic valve score has been used as the primary preprocedural predictor of the success of balloon valvotomy (61). Valves are graded on leaflet mobility, calcification, leaflet thickness, and disease of the subvalvular apparatus. Each category is given a score of zero to 4, where zero is normal and 4 is severely diseased. Since MS exists in all cases being evaluated, the minimum score is usually

4. In general, valvotomy has been successful for scores of 8 or less. However, some patients with worse scores still benefit from valvotomy. Thus, while surgery usually should be recommended in patients with high valve scores, valvotomy may still be employed if the patient is at a high surgical risk. It has become standard practice to perform a TEE to look carefully for left atrial thrombus prior to the valvotomy. Valve scoring is usually performed during this echocardiogram. If the valve score is low and there is no evidence of left atrial clot, the patient proceeds to balloon valvotomy. If a clot is present, a 3-month trial of warfarin anticoagulation is undertaken and is followed by repeat transesophageal echocardiography. If the clot has disappeared, valvotomy is then performed. If clot is still present, open surgical commissurotomy is performed instead.

Valvotomy carries a less than 1% risk while surgery in the absence of pulmonary hypertension carries a risk of less than or equal to 3%. Although pulmonary hypertension increases surgical risk substantially, it is not clear that it also increases the risk of balloon commissurotomy. Thus, in cases of advanced pulmonary hypertension, commissurotomy is probably the procedure of choice unless the valve is so severely deformed and heavily calcified that success is unlikely. Following balloon valvotomy, the risk of restenosis is low for at least 5 years. While it can be anticipated that restenosis will occur with longer follow-up, it is likely that recurrence will not occur for about 10 years on average, based on previous results of closed surgical commissurotomy.

A more problematic group is that group of patients that is entirely asymptomatic except for the presence of atrial fibrillation. Because atrial fibrillation becomes more permanent the longer it exists, early conversion to normal sinus rhythm is advisable whenever possible. It is likely, but not proven, that commissurotomy will help in controlling atrial arrhythmias by allowing for a reduction in left atrial size. While still controversial, many physicians provide mechanical relief of MS, if, at the onset of atrial fibrillation, the arrhythmia cannot be easily controlled and converted to sinus rhythm. This is especially true if it is obvious that a balloon commissurotomy can be performed, sparing the patient the risks inherent in prosthetic valves.

MITRAL VALVE PROLAPSE

The term "mitral valve prolapse" (MVP) encompasses a wide clinical spectrum, ranging from a variant of normal physiology to severely abnormal, anatomically deformed mitral valves. At the normal end of the spectrum, physiologic changes that reduce LV volume can result in MVP when diminished volume decreases tension on the chorda tendinea, allowing more travel of the mitral valve so that it becomes superior to the mitral annulus during systole. Such conditions include tachycardia, thyrotoxicosis, and volume depletion. Patients in this category are probably at no risk, or at very little risk, for the complications of MVP (infective

endocarditis, etc.). On the other end of the spectrum are deformed redundant mitral valves undergoing myxomatous proliferation. It is these patients who are susceptible to the complications of MVP syndrome, including endocarditis, valvular incompetence, arrhythmias, and stroke (62–65).

Definition

Classically, mitral valve prolapse has been diagnosed during physical examination by the findings of a midsystolic click followed by a late systolic murmur. However, not all prolapsing mitral valves produce these findings. In defining MVP, echocardiography is the best technique for demonstrating the mitral valve superior to the mitral annular plane during systole. Approximately a decade ago, it was realized that the mitral annulus has the shape of a hyperbolic paraboloid (saddleback) and does not form a straight plane (Fig. 9). For this reason, mitral valve prolapse seen in the four-chamber echocardiographic view must be confirmed in the parasternal long-axis view (66). That is, in the four-chamber view, the humps of the saddle may be mistaken for MVP,

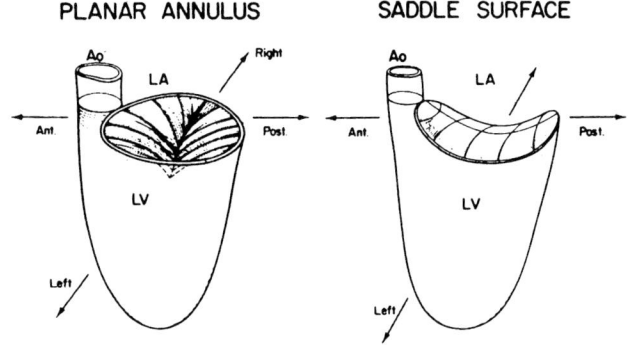

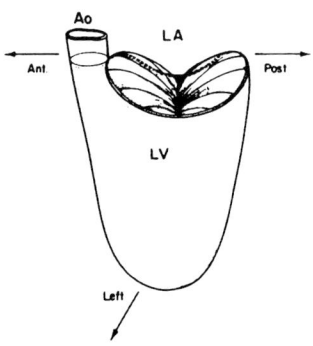

FIG. 9. A schematic of the saddleback shape of the mitral valve annulus is demonstrated. It is important to keep this shape in mind when diagnosing that the mitral valve leaflets have become superior to the "plane" (mitral valve prolapse) during systole. *Ao*, aorta; *Ant*, anterior; *LA*, left atrium; *LV*, left ventricle; *Post*, posterior. (From ref. 77, with permission.)

thereby overestimating the prevalence of the condition and overdiagnosing the disease.

Mitral Valve Prolapse Syndrome

The majority of patients with MVP are asymptomatic. However, some complain of chest pain atypical for myocardial ischemia, palpitation, and presyncope or syncope. Panic disorder has often been associated with mitral valve prolapse (67). However, it remains to be proven whether prolapse is the cause of the symptoms noted above. Rather than MVP causing the symptoms, it is more likely that autonomic dysfunction that leads to volume depletion and tachycardia causes a small LV, allowing the mitral valve to prolapse (68). The origin of chest pain is also unclear. It has been suggested that mitral valve prolapse causes excessive tension on the papillary muscles producing papillary muscle ischemia and chest pain. In fact, patients with MVP may have abnormal thallium perfusion scans (69), reduced ejection performance (70), and ECG abnormalities, especially in the inferior leads (71). However, it still remains to be proven that the prolapse is the cause of these abnormalities rather than an associated phenomenon.

Diagnosis

Physical Examination

Mitral valve prolapse is normally diagnosed during physical examination when the classic midsystolic click and end systolic murmur are heard. In any given case, one or both findings may be heard or both may be absent even in echocardiographically proven mitral valve prolapse. The click occurs when the elongated chorda tendineae and mitral valve leaflets are stretched taut in midsystole. The murmur develops when the elongated chorda tendineae allow extension of the valve leaflets beyond coaptation allowing MR. As the disease progresses, the MR intensifies, and the murmur becomes more holosystolic in nature. Various maneuvers during physical examination may be useful in making the diagnosis. Maneuvers that decrease LV volume (change in posture from recumbent to standing, Valsalva maneuver, or amyl nitrate inhalation) produce greater prolapse and, therefore, an earlier appearance of the click in systole and a louder and more holosystolic murmur. Maneuvers that increase LV volume (leg raising or squatting) reduce the effective length of the chorda tendineae and cause the click to occur later in systole or even to disappear while the murmur decreases in intensity and occurs later in systole.

Electrocardiogram

The electrocardiogram in MVP is usually normal. However, it may show nonspecific ST and T wave abnormalities, especially in the inferior leads (71).

Echocardiography

Echocardiography is the primary means for confirming the diagnosis of MVP. The diagnosis is made when one or both mitral valve leaflets is demonstrated superior to the mitral annulus. As noted, this should be confirmed in both the four-chamber and long-axis views. Even in patients in whom the diagnosis is clear from physical examination, echocardiography still should be performed at least once because it adds significant prognostic information regarding valve morphology. It is those patients with MVP who have thickened, redundant, and clearly abnormal valves who suffer the vast majority of complications from the disease (72). Apart from the diagnosis of the prolapse itself, echocardiography adds information regarding the severity of MR and its progression on follow-up examinations.

Cardiac Catheterization

Except for its usefulness in assessing the hemodynamics and severity of MR, cardiac catheterization has little role to play in the diagnosis of mitral valve prolapse.

Natural History

Progression to MR

The progression to severe MR is slow and unpredictable. In one study, there was a 25-year span between when the murmur was first heard and when the disease had progressed to the point of requiring mitral valve surgery (65). In general, older patients are more likely to progress than other patients. However, this probably simply represents the presence of the disease for a longer period of time. Men are more likely to develop severe MR than are women.

Endocarditis

Mitral valve prolapse may be the most common predisposing cause of endocarditis in the nondrug abusing population, constituting a major need for diagnosing the disease so that endocarditis prophylaxis may be employed in appropriate situations (73). It is the patients with a murmur and thickened redundant valve leaflets who are especially susceptible to endocarditis, and it is clearly these patients who require antibiotics prior to bacteremic procedures (64). For the patients with prolapse diagnosed echocardiographically but who have otherwise normal valves and no murmur, prophylaxis is controversial.

Arrhythmias

Atrial arrhythmias are common in patients with mitral valve prolapse. As noted above, cause and effect is usually difficult to ascertain. It may be that it is those patients with autonomic dysfunction, who are prone to atrial tachyarrhythmias, that have MVP because of reduced chamber volume. However, serious arrhythmias have been diagnosed in patients with mitral valve prolapse who seem to have no other cause (74). Sudden death has been occasionally reported (75). However, the incidence of severe arrhythmias has never been established but is probably quite low.

Stroke

Patients with mitral valve prolapse have an increased risk of stroke. It is thought that the prolapsing valve, or possibly the mitral regurgitant jet, causes an area of endothelial denudation, producing a site for platelet aggregation and thrombus formation. While the overall risk is low, some patients with embolic stroke have no other explanation other than MVP.

Therapy

Endocarditis Prophylaxis

The most important therapy in the patient with MVP is protection against infective endocarditis. It remains debatable exactly which patients require prophylaxis. However, the patient with a misshapened thickened valve, especially in the presence of the murmur of MR, is at high risk and requires prophylaxis. At the other end of the spectrum, the patient with an otherwise normal valve and no murmur is *probably* at very low risk, and prophylaxis often is not employed.

Other Therapies

For patients with unexplained chest pain with mitral valve prolapse, beta-blockade has been advocated. No large randomized trials exist to prove efficacy; thus, this therapy has been used empirically. It seems helpful in some cases.

Because of the potential for stroke, those patients with clearly redundant valves may receive daily aspirin therapy, although there is no proof that this therapy is effective.

REFERENCES

1. Waller BF, Howard J, Fess S. Pathology of mitral valve stenosis and pure mitral regurgitation: part II. *Clin Cardiol* 1994;17(7):395–402.
2. Carabello BA. Mitral regurgitation: basic pathophysiologic principles. Part 1. *Mod Concepts Cardiovasc Dis* 1988;57(10):53–58.
3. Castello R, Fagan L Jr, Lenzen P, et al. Comparison of transthoracic and transesophageal echocardiography for assessment of left-sided valvular regurgitation. *Am J Cardiol* 1991;68:1677–1680.
4. Fuchs RM, Heuser RR, Yin FC, et al. Limitations of pulmonary wedge V waves in diagnosing mitral regurgitation. *Am J Cardiol* 1982;49(4):849–854.
5. Miyatake K, Izumi S, Okamoto M, et al. Semiquantitative grading of severity of mitral regurgitation by real-time two-dimensional Doppler flow imaging technique. *J Am Coll Cardiol* 1986;7(1):82–88.

6. Spain MG, Smith MD, Grayburn PA, et al. Quantitative assessment of mitral regurgitation by Doppler color flow imaging: angiographic and hemodynamic correlations. *J Am Coll Cardiol* 1989;13(3):585–590.
7. Shah PM. Quantitative assessment of mitral regurgitation. *J Am Coll Cardiol* 1989;13(3):591–593.
8. Chen CG, Thomas JD, Anconina J, et al. Impact of impinging wall jet on color Doppler quantification of mitral regurgitation. *Circulation* 1991;84(2):712–720.
9. Sahn DJ. Instrumentation and physical factors related to visualization of stenotic and regurgitant jets by Doppler color flow mapping. *J Am Coll Cardiol* 1988;12(5):1354–1365.
10. Recusani F, Bargiggia GS, Yoganathan AP, et al. A new method of quantification of regurgitant flow rate using color Doppler flow imaging of the flow convergence region proximal to a discrete orifice. An *in vitro* study. *Circulation* 1991;83(2):594–604.
11. Bargiggia GS, Tronconi L, Sahn DJ, et al. A new method for quantification of mitral regurgitation based on color flow Doppler imaging of flow convergence proximal to regurgitant orifice. *Circulation* 1991;84(4):1481–1489.
12. Simpson IA, Shiota T, Gharib M, et al. Current status of flow convergence for clinical applications: is it a leaning tower of PISA? *J Am Coll Cardiol* 1996;27(2):504–509.
13. Vandervoort PM, Rivera JM, Mele D, et al. Application of color Doppler flow mapping to calculate effective regurgitant orifice area. An *in vitro* study and initial clinical observations. *Circulation* 1993;88(3):1150–1156.
14. Enriquez-Sarano EM, Seward JB, Bailey KR, et al. Effective regurgitant orifice area: a noninvasive Doppler development of an old hemodynamic concept. *J Am Coll Cardiol* 1994;23(2):443–451.
15. Enriquez-Sarano EM, Bailey KR, Seward JB, et al. Quantitative Doppler assessment of valvular regurgitation. *Circulation* 1993;87(3):841–848.
16. Hall SA, Brickner ME, Willett DL, et al. Assessment of mitral regurgitation severity by Doppler color flow mapping of the vena contracta. *Circulation* 1997;95(3):636–642.
17. Kizilbash AM, Willett DL, Brickner ME, et al. Effects of afterload reduction on vena contracta width in mitral regurgitation. *J Am Coll Cardiol* 1998;32(2):427–431.
18. Carabello BA. What exactly is 2 – 3 + mitral regurgitation [editorial]? *J Am Coll Cardiol* 1992;19(2):339–340.
19. Croft CH, Lipscomb K, Mathis K, et al. Limitations of qualitative angiographic grading in aortic or mitral regurgitation. *Am J Cardiol* 1984;53(11):1593–1598.
20. Lindblom D, Lindblom U, Qvist J, et al. Long-term relative survival rates after heart valve replacement. *J Am Coll Cardiol* 1990;15(3):566–573.
21. Enriquez-Sarano M, Tajik AJ, Schaff HV, et al. Echocardiographic prediction of survival after surgical correction of organic mitral regurgitation. *Circulation* 1994;90(2):830–837.
22. Schuler G, Peterson KL, Johnson A, et al. Temporal response of left ventricular performance to mitral valve surgery. *Circulation* 1979;59:1218–1231.
23. Wisenbaugh T. Does normal pump function belie muscle dysfunction in patients with chronic severe mitral regurgitation? *Circulation* 1988;77:515–525.
24. Wisenbaugh T, Skudicky D, Sareli P. Prediction of outcome after valve replacement for rheumatic mitral regurgitation in the era of chordal preservation. *Circulation* 1994;89:191–197.
25. Zile MR, Gaasch WH, Carroll JD, et al. Chronic mitral regurgitation: predictive value of preoperative echocardiographic indexes of left ventricular function and wall stress. *J Am Coll Cardiol* 1984;3:235–242.
26. Crawford MH, Souchek J, Oprian CA, et al. Determinants of survival and left ventricular performance after mitral valve replacement. Department of Veterans Affairs Cooperative Study on Valvular Heart Disease. *Circulation* 1990;81(4):1173–1181.
27. Ling LH, Enriquez-Sarano M, Seward JB, et al. Clinical outcome of mitral regurgitation due to flail leaflet. *N Engl J Med* 1996;335:1417–1423.
28. Rushmer RF. Initial phase of ventricular systole: asynchronous contraction. *Am J Physiol* 1956;184:188–194.

29. Hansen DE, Sarri GE, Niczyporuk MA, et al. Physiologic role of the mitral apparatus in left ventricular regional mechanics, contraction synergy and global systolic performance. *J Thorac Cardiovasc Surg* 1989; 97:521–533.

30. Goldman ME, Mora F, Guarino T, et al. Mitral valvuloplasty is superior to valve replacement for preservation of left ventricular function: an intraoperative two-dimensional echocardiographic study. *J Am Coll Cardiol* 1987;10:568–575.

31. Carabello BA. The mitral valve apparatus: is there still room to doubt the importance of its preservation [Editorial]? *J Heart Valve Dis* 1993; 2:250–252.

32. David TE, Burns RJ, Bacchus CM, et al. Mitral valve replacement for mitral regurgitation with and without preservation of chordae tendineae. *J Thorac Cardiovasc Surg* 1984;88:718–725.

33. Rozich JD, Carabello BA, Usher BW, et al. Mitral valve replacement with and without chordal preservation in patients with chronic mitral regurgitation: mechanism for differences in postoperative ejection performance. *Circulation* 1992;86:1718–1727.

34. Hellemans IM, Pieper EG, Ravelli AC, et al. Prediction of surgical strategy in mitral valve regurgitation based on echocardiography. The ESMIR Research Group of the Interuniversity Cardiology Institute of The Netherlands. *Am J Cardiol* 1997;79:334–338.

35. Enriquez-Sarano M, Schaff HV, Orszulak TA, et al. Valve repair improves the outcome of surgery for mitral regurgitation. A multivariate analysis. *Circulation* 1995;91(4):1022–1028.

36. Bach DS, Bolling SF. Improvement following correction of secondary mitral regurgitation in end-stage cardiomyopathy with mitral annuloplasty. *Am J Cardiol* 1996;78(8):966–969.

37. Cohn LH, Rizzo RJ, Adams DH, et al. The effect of pathophysiology on the surgical treatment of ischemic mitral regurgitation: operative and late risks of repair versus replacement. *Eur J Cardiothorac Surg* 1995;9(10):568–574.

38. Lamas GA, Mitchell GF, Flaker GC, et al. Clinical significance of mitral regurgitation after acute myocardial infarction. Survival and Ventricular Enlargement Investigators. *Circulation* 1997;96(3): 827–833.

39. Tcheng JE, Jackman JD Jr, Nelson CL, et al. Outcome of patients sustaining acute ischemic mitral regurgitation during myocardial infarction. *Ann Intern Med* 1992;117(1):18–24.

40. Bolling SF, Deeb GM, Bach DS. Mitral valve reconstruction in elderly, ischemic patients. *Chest* 1996;109(1):35–40.

41. Horstkotte D, Schulte HD, Niehues R, et al. Diagnostic and therapeutic considerations in acute, severe mitral regurgitation: experience in 42 consecutive patients entering the intensive care unit with pulmonary edema. *J Heart Valve Dis* 1993;2(5):512–522.

42. Scognamiglio R, Rahimtoola SH, Fasoli G, et al. Nifedipine in asymptomatic patients with severe aortic regurgitation and normal left ventricular function. *N Engl J Med* 1994;331(11):689–694.

43. Carabello BA. The relationship of left ventricular geometry and hypertrophy to left ventricular function in valvular heart disease. *J Heart Valve Dis* 1995;4[Suppl II]:S132–S139.

44. Wisenbaugh T, Sinovich V, Dullabh A, et al. Six-month pilot study of captopril for mildly symptomatic, severe isolated mitral and isolated aortic regurgitation. *J Heart Valve Dis* 1994;3(2):197–204.

45. Marcotte F, Honos GN, Walling AD, et al. Effect of angiotensin-converting enzyme inhibitor therapy in mitral regurgitation with normal left ventricular function. *Can J Cardiol* 1997;13(5):479–485.

46. Schön JR. Hemodynamic and morphologic changes after long-term angiotensin converting enzyme inhibition in patients with chronic valvular regurgitation. *J Hypertens* 1994;12[Suppl 4]:S95–104.

47. Gash AK, Carabello BA, Cepin D, et al. Left ventricular ejection performance and systolic muscle function in patients with mitral stenosis. *Circulation* 1983;67:148–154.

48. Hildner FJ, Javier RP, Cohen LS, et al. Myocardial dysfunction associated with valvular heart disease. *Am J Cardiol* 1972;30(4):319–326.

49. Heller SJ, Carleton RA. Abnormal left ventricular contraction in patients with mitral stenosis. *Circulation* 1970;42:1099–1110.

50. Ross J Jr. Afterload mismatch and preload reserve: a conceptual framework for analysis of ventricular function. *Prog Cardiovasc Dis* 1976; 18:255–264.

51. Roy SB, Gopinath N. Mitral stenosis. *Circulation* 1968;38[Suppl V]: 68–76.

52. Vincens JJ, Temizer D, Post JR, et al. Long-term outcome of cardiac surgery in patients with mitral stenosis and severe pulmonary hypertension. *Circulation* 1995;92[Suppl II]:137–142.

53. Martin RP, Rakowski H, Kleiman JH, et al. Reliability and reproducibility of two dimensional echocardiograph measurement of the stenotic mitral valve orifice area. *Am J Cardiol* 1979;43:560–568.

54. Hatle L, Brubakk A, Tromsdal A, et al. Noninvasive assessment of pressure drop in mitral stenosis by Doppler ultrasound. *Br Heart J* 1978;40:131–140.

55. Gorlin R, Gorlin SG. Hydraulic formula for calculation of the area of the stenotic mitral valve, other cardiac valves, and central circulatory shunts. I. *Am Heart J* 1951;41:1–29.

56. Dehmer GJ, Firth BG, Hills LD. Oxygen consumption in adult patients during cardiac catheterization. *Clin Cardiol* 1982;5:436.

57. Lange RA, Moore DM, Cigarroa RG, et al. Use of pulmonary capillary wedge pressure to assess severity of mitral stenosis: is true left atrial pressure needed in this condition? *J Am Coll Cardiol* 1989;13:825.

58. Alpert JS. The lessons of history as reflected in the pulmonary capillary wedge pressure. *J Am Coll Cardiol* 1989;13:830.

59. American College of Cardiology/American Heart Association. ACC/AHA guidelines for the management of patients with valvular heart disease. A report of the American College of Cardiology/American Heart Association Task Force on practice guidelines (Committee on Management of Patients with Valvular Heart Disease). Committee Members: Bonow RO, Carabello B, DeLeon AC, Edmunds LH, Fedderly BJ, Freed MD, Gaasch WH, McKay CR, Nishimura RA, O'Gara PT, O'Rourke, RA, Rahimtoola SH.

60. Reyes VP, Raju BS, Wynne J, et al. Percutaneous balloon valvuloplasty compared with open surgical commissurotomy for mitral stenosis. *N Engl J Med* 1994;331(15):961–967.

61. Wilkins GT, Weyman AE, Abascal VM, et al. Percutaneous balloon dilatation of the mitral valve: an analysis of echocardiographic variables related to outcome and the mechanism of dilatation. *Br Heart J* 1988; 60:299–308.

62. Duren DR, Becker AE, Dunning AJ. Long-term follow-up of idiopathic mitral valve prolapse in 300 patients: a prospective study. *J Am Coll Cardiol* 1988;11(1):42–47.

63. Wilcken DE, Hickey AJ. Lifetime risk for patients with mitral valve prolapse of developing severe mitral regurgitation requiring surgery. *Circulation* 1988;78(1):10–14.

64. Mills P, Rose J, Hollingsworth J, et al. Long-term prognosis of mitral-valve prolapse. *N. Engl J Med* 1977;297(1):13–18.

65. Kolibash AJ Jr, Kilman JW, Bush CA, et al. Evidence for progression from mild to severe mitral regurgitation in mitral valve prolapse. *Am J Cardiol* 1986;58(9):762–767.

66. Levine RA, Stathogiannis E, Newell JB, et al. Reconsideration of echocardiographic standards for mitral valve prolapse: lack of association between leaflet displacement isolated to the apical four chamber view and independent echocardiographic evidence of abnormality. *J Am Coll Cardiol* 1988;11(5):1010–1019.

67. Mavissakalian M, Salerni R, Thompson ME, et al. Mitral valve prolapse and agoraphobia. *Am J Psychiatry* 1983;140(12):1612–1614.

68. Gaffney FA, Karlsson ES, Campbell W, et al. Autonomic dysfunction in women with mitral valve prolapse syndrome. *Circulation* 1979; 59(5):894–901.

69. Butman S, Chandraratna PA, Milne N, et al. Stress myocardial imaging in patients with mitral valve prolapse: evidence of a perfusion abnormality. *Cathet Cardiovasc Diagn* 1982;8(3):243–252.

70. Gottdiener JS, Borer JS, Bacharach SL, et al. Left ventricular function in mitral valve prolapse: assessment with radionuclide cineangiography. *Am J Cardiol* 1981;47(1):7–13.

71. Lobstein HP, Horwitz LD, Curry GC, et al. Electrocardiographic abnormalities and coronary arteriograms in the mitral click-murmur syndrome. *N Engl J Med* 1973;289:127–131.

72. Marks AR, Choong CY, Sanfilippo AJ, et al. Identification of high-risk and low-risk subgroups of patients with mitral-valve prolapse. *N Engl J Med* 1989;320(16):1031–1036.

73. McKinsey DS, Ratts TE, Bisno AL. Underlying cardiac lesions in adults with infective endocarditis. The changing spectrum. *Am J Med* 1987;82(4):681–688.

74. DeMaria AN, Amsterdam EA, Vismara LA, et al. Arrhythmias in the

mitral valve prolapse syndrome. Prevalence, nature and frequency. *Ann Intern Med* 1976;84(6):656–660.

75. Savage DD, Levy D, Garrison RJ, et al. Mitral valve prolapse in the general population. 3. Dysrhythmias: The Framingham Study. *Am Heart J* 1983;106(3):582–586.

76. Assey ME, Usher BW, Carabello BA. The patient with valvular heart disease. In: Pepine CJ, Hill JA, Lambert CR, eds. *Diagnostic and therapeutic cardiac catheterization,* 2nd ed. Baltimore: Williams & Wilkins, 1994.

77. Levine RA, Triulze MO, Harrigan P, et al. The relationship of mitral annular shape to the diagnosis of mitral valve prolapse. *Circulation* 1987;75(4):756–767.

CHAPTER 41

Aortic Valve Disease

Alex Durairaj and P. Anthony N. Chandraratna

Echocardiography of the aortic valve along with Doppler assessment of flow across the valve has become essential in the evaluation of aortic valve disease. There has been good correlation with catheterization data such that catheterization-based hemodynamic data may not be necessary to guide medical or surgical treatment in some patients (1). Echocardiography has also proved useful in the serial follow-up of these patients.

ANATOMY OF THE AORTIC VALVE

The aortic root is delineated by the bases of the semilunar leaflets proximally, and the sino-tubular ridge distally; it consists of a fibrous annulus, three leaflets, fibrous interleaflet triangles, and three dilated segments of the aortic wall called the *sinuses of Valsalva*. The long axis of the outflow tract is directed rightward and anteriorly. The *annulus fibrosus* forms a three-pronged coronet; the three triangular portions below the annulus are composed of fibrous and muscular tissue that extends from the outflow tract. The lower border of each crescent-shaped leaflet adheres to the annulus, forming a cusp (2). The free edge is thin with a thickening at the tip called the *node of Arantius*. Fine collagenous bundles radiate from the node to the attached border, forming a ridge that serves as the surface where the cusps abut when the valve is closed. This ridge is 25% thicker than the free edge of the leaflet (3). The *lunula* is the portion above this closing line. There is adequate leaflet tissue to allow a few millimeters of overlap during valve closure (4). Each sinus is named after the coronary artery that arises within the sinus. The right coronary sinus is to the right and anterior; the left coronary sinus is to the left and posterior; the noncoronary sinus is to the right and posterior. These *sinuses of Valsalva*

are dilatations of the arterial wall that extend from the base of the cusps to the supraaortic ridge. During systole, the fibroelastic wall of the root dilates and the open valve orifice appears triangular; blood enters the sinuses forming vortices that keep the leaflets in their midposition, preventing occlusion of the coronary ostia, as well as initiating approximation of the leaflets as systole ends.

The normal trileaflet valve is ideally suited to perform its function; competent enough to prevent significant diastolic regurgitation, while opening adequately so as not to interfere with systolic ejection. Bileaflet valves are adequate to prevent significant regurgitation, but will obstruct outflow to some extent without considerable elastic stretch. Quadricuspid valves pose no obstruction, but lack adequate support to prevent regurgitation (5).

Focal thickening of the aortic valve commonly occurs as part of the normal aging process; there has been no correlation between valve thickness and sex, height, weight, or body surface area. Within each leaflet, the thickest structure is the node, which is more than twice as thick as the free edge. The closing ridge is the next thickest part (3). The node and the closing ridge thicken with age especially after the fifth decade; Lorz et al. (6) found the incidence of excessive aortic valve thickening to be 28% in patients over the age of 70. The free edges thin and Lambl's excrescences develop. Among the individual leaflets, the noncoronary leaflet is thicker than either right or left leaflet. It has been postulated that this may be due to the higher diastolic pressure this cusp endures because it does not have a coronary ostia to relive some of the pressure (3,7).

Imaging Planes

The aortic valve is imaged primarily from the parasternal long- and short-axis views. The parasternal views are orthogonal to each other and often provide information with regard to the etiology of aortic pathology. The valve can also be viewed from the apical five-chamber, apical long-axis, and subcostal views. These positions, along with the suprasternal

A. Durairaj: Division of Cardiology, Keck School of Medicine, Southern California Medical Center, Division of Cardiology, Los Angeles County and University of Southern California, Los Angeles, California 90033.

P. A. N. Chandraratna: University of California–Irvine, Orange, California 92868; Cardiology Section, Long Beach Veterans Administration Medical Center, Long Beach, California 90822.

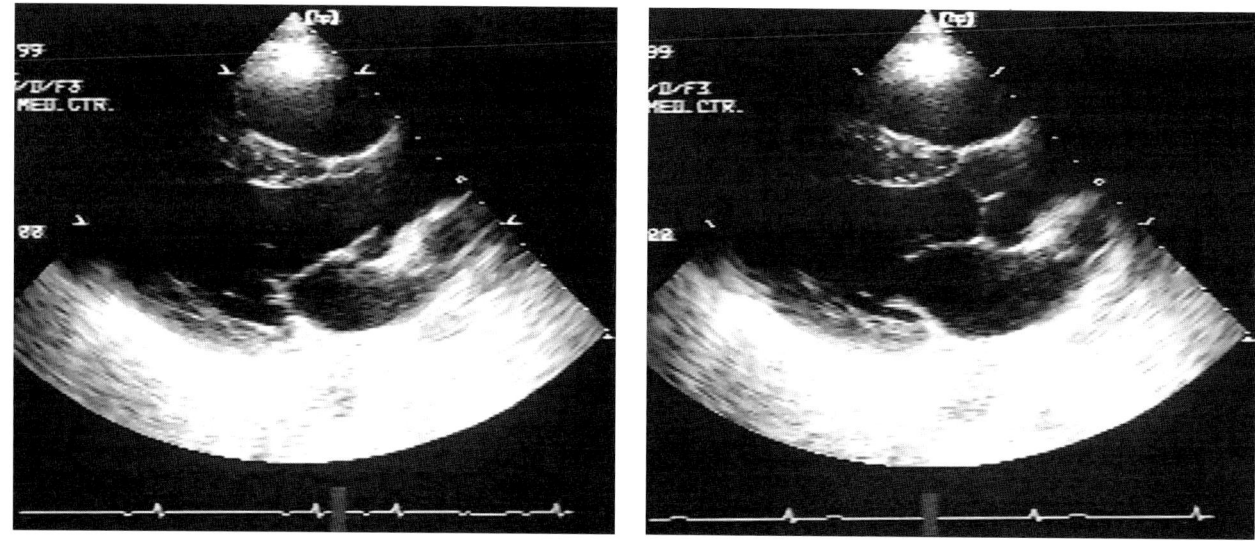

FIG. 1. Normal aortic valve in systole and diastole. **A:** In systole, the right and noncoronary leaflets form thin lines parallel to the aorta. The bulge behind each valve are the sinuses. **B:** In diastole, the coapted edges of the leaflets produce a linear echo in the middle of the left ventricular outflow tract. The body of the leaflets are oriented parallel to the echo beam and are often not visualized.

notch and the right parasternal area, direct the ultrasound beam in parallel with aortic flow and are suitable for Doppler interrogation.

The parasternal long-axis view cuts the aortic valve in an anteroposterior direction. By convention, the ventricle is to the left and the image plane is oriented such that it passes through the right and noncoronary leaflets. In diastole, only the coapted free edges of the aortic cusps are seen. They are oriented perpendicular to the imaging plane and form a thin linear echo in the midportion of the aortic root. The bodies of the leaflets are parallel to the imaging plane and are not well visualized. At peak systole, the bodies of the cusps are forced open; they are now oriented perpendicular to the imaging plane and form thin linear echoes that parallel the aortic root (Fig. 1). The parasternal view is useful in differentiating valvular stenosis from outflow obstruction caused by subvalvular or supravalvular disease. It can also demonstrate valve thickening and calcification and reduced leaflet excursion, prompting further in-depth studies to evaluate the severity of stenosis.

The parasternal short axis cuts the aorta in cross-section at the level of the aortic annulus. In diastole, the commissures of the valves should be visualized in a configuration likened to an upside-down Mercedes Benz logo. In systole, the free edges of the cusps produce an orifice that appears as a triangle with curved sides. The parasternal short-axis view enables characterization of valve leaflet morphology. In both of the parasternal views, aortic flow is oriented perpendicular to the imaging plane. These views provide poor Doppler signals to assess flow velocity. The parasternal long-axis view, however, is useful for color-flow mapping of the turbulent aortic regurgitant jet. Likewise, the parasternal short-axis view can assist in measuring the area of the regur-

gitant jet and in distinguishing valvular from paravalvular leaks.

The apical five-chamber view places the imaging plane parallel to the left ventricular outflow tract. This vantage point is useful for visualizing doming of the body of the leaflets as well as thin subvalvular membranes. These structures would be perpendicular to the apical imaging plane and hence produce better echoes. This is also the ideal orientation for Doppler interrogation of the aortic flow velocity and aortic regurgitant signal.

AORTIC STENOSIS

Etiology

Congenital malformations, calcific (degenerative), and rheumatic fusion of the commissures comprise the vast majority of the causes of aortic stenosis (8). Other rarer causes include a large, obstructive infective vegetation (usually fungal), homozygous type II hyperlipoproteinemia, Paget disease of bone, systemic lupus erythematosus, rheumatoid involvement, ochronosis, and irradiation (9,10). It also may result from an autoimmune process.

Within the last decade, degenerative calcification has become the most common cause of aortic stenosis in Western countries, accounting for 51% of all causes of isolated aortic stenosis in one series (11,12). Lipid deposits accumulate at the site of degeneration of the collagenous stroma. These deposits act as a nidus for calcification. This process affects the base and extends to the free margins, leaving the commissures free of fusion in most cases (Fig. 2). This process limits the mobility of the cusps and is found typically in the late eight and ninth decades. The prevalence of aortic leaflet

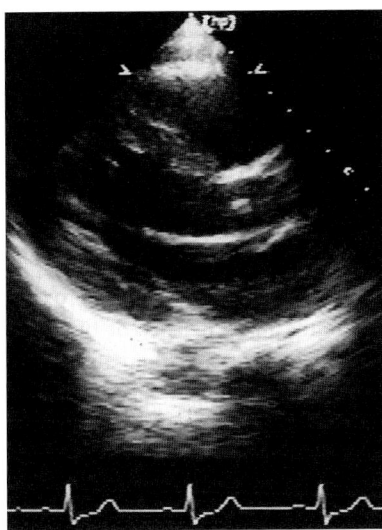

FIG. 2. Calcified aortic valve. The valve produces a larger echo-dense image.

thickening and aortic stenosis is 26% and 2%, respectively, in patients over age 65 (13). A similar process occurs in bicuspid valves, but much sooner, most frequently in the sixth and seventh decades (Fig. 3). Unicuspid valves produce severe obstruction and are the most common cause of symptomatic aortic stenosis in infants. In patients aged 15–65 years with aortic stenosis, 60% are bicuspid, 25–30% are tricuspid, and 10% are unicuspid (9). Besides age and a congenitally deformed valve, clinical factors associated with aortic valve calcification include hypertension and lower body mass index; predictors of aortic stenosis are age and serum ionized calcium (13,14).

Rheumatic valvulitis results from an altered immune response to infection with group A streptococcus. An antigenic response to streptococcus cross-reacts against the host tissue. This inflammatory response causes adhesions and fusion of the commissures. It is often accompanied by retraction and stiffening of the cusps causing combined stenosis and insufficiency. Rheumatic disease typically affects the mitral valve, followed by a combination of both mitral and aortic valves. Less commonly, the aortic valve is the only valve affected. Prior to this decade, rheumatic involvement was the most common cause of aortic stenosis, decreasing from 48% of cases in 1965 to 11% in 1990 in a series from the Mayo Clinic (11). The pathophysiology, natural history, clinical findings, and management of aortic stenosis is discussed in detail elsewhere (9,15).

Qualitative Assessment

Attempts to quantify the severity of aortic stenosis using 2-D echocardiography have been disappointing. It does, however, provide a qualitative assessment of the severity of aortic stenosis, which may be used to screen patients who need more detailed investigation. Observation of the normal excursion of at least one of the leaflets is highly indicative of noncritical aortic stenosis. The absence of any observed movement suggests severe stenosis is likely. The severity of calcification of the aortic valve is not a reliable predictor of the degree of stenosis. In young patients with aortic stenosis secondary to congenital or rheumatic disease, calcification may be absent. Systolic doming of the aortic valve leaflets is often observed in these patients in association with significant stenosis (16,17).

Maximal aortic cusp separation has been studied as a more objective means of assessing the severity of aortic valve stenosis. The parasternal long-axis view is used to measure the maximal separation of the right and noncoronary cusps. Qualitative assessment of the valves accurately distinguishes normal valves from abnormal aortic valve leaflets, although this single-plane slice of the aortic valve cannot accurately predict aortic valve area. In one series, all patients with normal valves had a maximal separation of >15mm, while those with critical aortic stenosis had a maximal separation of ≤11mm. Difficulty arose in separating noncritical aortic stenosis from critical stenosis (16). Accurate image acquisition is crucial; if the 2D plane is directed toward the outer area of the commissures, maximal separation will be underestimated. Another source of error arises in patients with decreased cusp motion secondary to impaired left ventricular function.

Although planimetry of the mitral valve has been useful in grading mitral stenosis, the same success has not been reported with aortic stenosis. Several factors contribute to this shortcoming. First, the aortic valve moves in an inferior-superior direction during the cardiac cycle, thus moving into and out of the plane of the parasternal short-axis view. Second, the aortic valve is smaller, the same margin of error afforded the mitral valve would misclassify the severity of

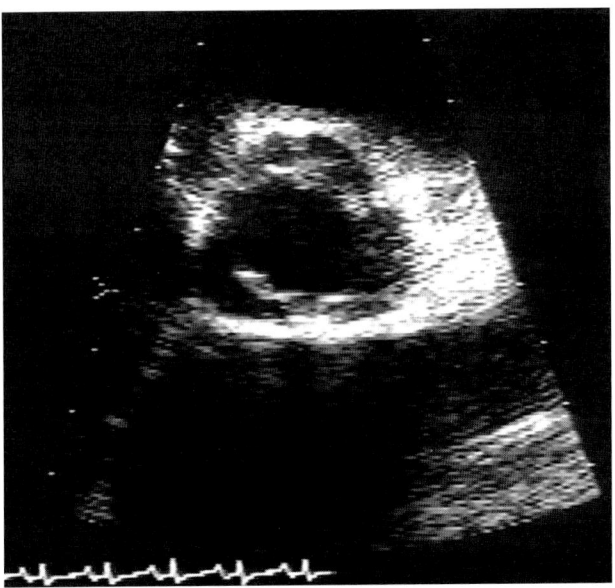

FIG. 3. Bicuspid aortic valve. The opening is more elliptical in contrast to the triangular shape of a tricuspid valve.

TABLE 1. *Suggested criteria for grading the degree of aortic stenosis*

Degree of stenosis	AVA (cm^2)	AVA index (cm^2/m^2)	Peak velocity (m/s)	Peak gradient (mm Hg)	Mean gradient (mm Hg)
Probably mild					<20
Uncertain			<4.0	<60	20–50
Mild	>1.5	>0.9			
Moderate	>1.0–1.5	>0.6–0.9			
Likely severe			4.0–4.5	60–79	50–69
Severe	<0.8–1.0	<0.4–0.6	>4.5	>80	>70

$$AVA = \frac{SV}{44.5(SEP)\sqrt{MPG}}$$

where SV is the stroke volume, SEP is the systolic ejection period, and MPG is the mean pressure gradient. All variables listed above can be derived via Doppler measurements. The calculated aortic valve area using the Gorlin equation has correlated well with catheter-derived data (21,35–37). The Gorlin equation has an empiric constant in its calculation, which may be a source of error. The calculated aortic valve is flow dependent, particularly when the cardiac output is less than 4.5 l/min. In such patients, when the cardiac output is low, dobutamine infusion increases forward output substantially (38). This may help differentiate patients with severe aortic stenosis from patients with a decreased effective orifice area caused by a low cardiac output.

Continuity Equation

The continuity equation exploits the principle that the flow through the left ventricular outflow tract is equal to the flow through the stenotic aortic orifice. Blood flow equals cross-sectional area times the mean velocity. Thus, we derive the continuity equation:

$$A_{LVOT} \times v_{LVOT} = AVA \times v_{AV}$$

where A_{LVOT} is the area of the left ventricular outflow tract at which v_{LVOT}, the mean velocity, is measured and v_{AV} is the mean velocity at the vena contracta. The diameter of the left ventricular outflow tract is routinely measured in the parasternal long-axis view. In the optimal imaging plane, the anterior and posterior walls of the aorta should be parallel, the sinuses of Valsalva should be symmetric, and the base of the aortic valve leaflets should be clearly visualized. The left ventricular outflow tract measurement should then be taken at the inside edges of the annulus at the base of both the right and noncoronary cusps of the aortic valve. The area of the left ventricular outflow tract is calculated by:

$$A_{LVOT} = \pi \left(\frac{D_{LVOT}}{2} \right)^2$$

where D_{LVOT} is the measured diameter. The Doppler echocardiographic equivalent of the mean velocity is the velocity-

time integral. The velocity of the left ventricular outflow tract is obtained from pulsed-wave Doppler interrogation from the apical five-chamber view. Theoretically, the signal should be recorded at the same location that was used to measure the outflow tract diameter. Logistically, this can be difficult as the diameter is measured from the parasternal view. Also, the outflow tract moves during systole further complicating this measurement.

Solving the continuity equation for the aortic valve area yields:

$$AVA = \pi \left(\frac{D_{LVOT}}{2} \right)^2 \frac{VTI_{LVOT}}{VTI_{AV}}$$

The velocity time integral is tedious to trace; a much simpler measurement would be the peak velocity. Studies have shown that the ratio of the peak velocities at the left ventricular outflow tract and the aortic valve are an adequate substitute for the velocity time integral (36,39,40).

Theoretically, the aortic valve area calculated by continuity equation should not be dependent on flow, however, clinical studies show that there is some change with flow (41). The continuity equation assumes that the left ventricular outflow tract is circular, when it is actually more elliptical. It also assumes that the outflow tract has a constant shape. Given these shortcomings, the aortic valve area derived from the continuity equation still correlates well with catheter-based data. It consistently underestimates the aortic valve area obtained using the Gorlin equation. This is felt to be secondary to an underestimation of the left ventricular outflow tract area (39).

Clinical Applications of Echocardiography in Aortic Stenosis

Echocardiography has proved useful in the diagnosis of aortic stenosis. Otto et al. (42) were able to develop a prediction rule for patients with symptomatic aortic stenosis. If the maximal aortic jet velocity was greater than 4.0 m/s, aortic valve replacement was recommended, conversely, if the peak velocity was less than 3.0 m/s, aortic valve replacement was not needed. When the peak velocity was between 3 to 4 m/s, a Doppler-derived aortic valve area was calculated. For those patients with an aortic valve area less than or equal to 1 cm^2 an aortic valve replacement was recommended; for those with a valve area greater than or equal to 1.7 cm², aortic valve replacement was not recommended. In the intermediate group with an aortic valve area between 1.0 to 1.7 cm², the degree of aortic insufficiency was the determining factor. The rule has a total error rate of 3.9% in their prospective study of 77 patients.

Studies by Otto et al. (43) have also documented the reproducibility of repeat echocardiographic readings for serial observation of asymptomatic patients with aortic stenosis. Serial echocardiographic studies have shown an average increase in aortic jet velocity by 0.32 ± 0.34 m/s, an average increase in the mean gradient by 7 ± 7mm Hg, and an average decrease in the valve area by 0.12 ± 0.19 cm² annually (44). It should be noted that these are average changes over a mean of 2.5 years. There was marked individual variability in the rate of hemodynamic progression of aortic stenosis. The initial echocardiographic severity of aortic stenosis was the strongest predictor of outcome. Additionally, the rate of increase of the peak aortic jet velocity and functional status score was predictive of outcome. At 2 years, 84 ± 16% of patients with a peak aortic jet velocity less than 3 m/s were free of death or aortic valve replacement, compared to 21 ± 18% and 66 ± 13% for patients with a peak velocity >4.0 m/s and between 3–4 m/s, respectively. This argues for an individualized approach to the follow-up of patients with asymptomatic aortic stenosis.

Progression of severity of aortic stenosis has been assessed by changes in pressure gradients and aortic valve area. The pressure gradient is said to increase by 10–15 mm Hg per year (43–51), however, in some patients it increases by as much as 15–19 mmHg per year while others show little or no change or even an actual decrease. Aortic valve areas are said to decrease by 0.1 to 0.3 cm² per year (44,51–54) and the average rate of change has ranged from 0.10 to 0.15 cm² per year. The 95% confidence limit of echocardiographic Doppler-derived aortic valve area to that obtained by cardiac catheterization ranges from ±0.4 to 0.8 cm² (55,56). Moreover, Otto and co-workers (43) have documented that although stenosis severity progresses more rapidly in patients who develop symptoms requiring aortic valve replacement, these patients cannot be identified at the initial study. Progression of aortic stenosis does not necessarily occur in linear manner but usually in a step-wise manner. Furthermore, depending on the time interval used to obtain the linearized rate, the rate of change can vary over a wide range, for example, from 0.004 cm²/year to 1.3 cm²/year (27).

Other Techniques

Cardiac catheterization and 2D with Doppler echocardiography are the two techniques for adequately assessing the severity of stenosis. Nuclear medicine techniques and computed MRI provide information on left ventricle wall stress and ejection fraction.

AORTIC REGURGITATION

Etiology

Aortic regurgitation may result from diseases of either the aortic valve or the ascending aorta, or both. The primary processes include retraction, prolapse, trauma, or perforations of the cusps, widening or prolapse of the commissures, dilatation of the annulus, and dilatation or dissection of the ascending aorta (57). The vast majority of cases, accounting for more that 96% of the Mayo Clinic series of cases of aortic regurgitation were secondary to postinflammatory disease, aortic root dilatation, incomplete closure of a congenitally bicuspid valve, and infective endocarditis.

Postinflammatory changes of the aortic valve can be seen with ankylosing spondylitis, rheumatoid arthritis, psoriatic arthritis, Reiter syndrome, systemic lupus erythematosus, and rheumatic heart disease. Rheumatic valvulitis stands apart as the most frequent cause of postinflammatory involvement of the aortic valve. In the Mayo Clinic series, postinflammatory aortic valve disease accounted for the majority (51%) of the cases of aortic regurgitation prior to 1980. This decreased to 29% in 1980, most likely because of the decreasing incidence of acute rheumatic fever (10,11,57).

Aortic root dilatation has become an increasingly more common cause of aortic regurgitation. In the same Mayo Clinic series, the incidence of aortic root dilatation increased from 17% before 1980 to 37% in 1980, surpassing postinflammatory aortic valve disease as the predominant cause of aortic regurgitation (11). In 90% of these cases, the etiology of aortic root dilatation was idiopathic, however, myxomatous changes affecting the aortic valve was noted in the majority of these valves. Degeneration has been implicated as the most common cause of pure aortic regurgitation requiring aortic valve replacement (58). Other identified causes of aortic root dilatation include aortitis, from syphilis, giant-cell arteritis, or Takayasu disease, the Marfan syndrome, aortic dissection, hypertension, Ehlers-Danlos syndrome, osteogenesis imperfecta, and pseudoxanthoma elasticum (9,10).

Although the most common sequelae of congenital bicuspid aortic valves is dystrophic calcification causing aortic stenosis, roughly one third of excised bicuspid valves suffer from some degree of aortic regurgitation. Cusp prolapse is the most frequent structural cause of aortic regurgitation in these valves (Fig. 5). Aortic root dilatation and aortic dissection are other factors causing aortic regurgitation and may be related to the abnormal structural integrity of the ascending aorta. Lastly, congenitally bicuspid valves are more prone to infective endocarditis (59).

Infective endocarditis is the most common cause of acute aortic regurgitation (60). Infective endocarditis affecting a previously stenotic valve may cause a combination of aortic stenosis and regurgitation. Rarely, a massive vegetation may produce pure aortic stenosis. Other potential causes of aortic regurgitation include cusp prolapse from a supra cristo ventricular septal defect or subaortic stenosis, quadricuspid aor-

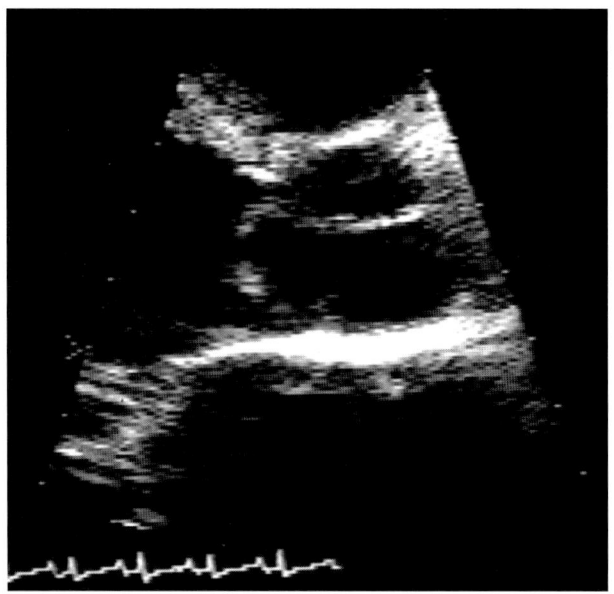

FIG. 5. Aortic valve prolapse. The body and tips of the leaflets are seen proximal to the plane of the aortic root.

tic valves, trauma to the aortic cusps, "Fen-Phen" valvulopathy, and hypertensive episodes. Lastly, a trivial degree of aortic regurgitation may be a normal variant. The incidence of this finding increases with age (5).

Two-dimensional and M-mode echocardiography can aid in revealing the etiology of aortic regurgitation. Due to the limitations of these modalities, incomplete or eccentric closure of the aortic cusps are nonspecific signs of aortic regurgitation.

Effect of the regurgitant jet on intracardiac structures can be demonstrated with 2D and M-mode echocardiography. High-frequency diastolic fluttering of the anterior mitral leaflet is a specific observation in aortic regurgitation. Depending on the direction of the regurgitant jet, fluttering may also be seen in other neighboring structures including the posterior mitral leaflet, ventricular septum, and posterior wall. In severe cases of aortic regurgitation, left ventricular end-diastolic pressure rises rapidly and may exceed left atrial pressure, causing premature closure of the mitral valve and premature aortic cusp opening. These findings are dependent on the RR interval and disappear with a tachycardia (61). M-mode echocardiography is especially helpful in demonstrating these features, as cardiac events can be easily timed to the electrocardiogram.

The effects of aortic regurgitation on the left ventricle can be used to differentiate acute from chronic aortic regurgitation. In acute aortic regurgitation, the ability of the left ventricle to dilate is limited. Thus, end diastolic pressure is markedly increased, hence premature mitral valve closure and premature aortic cusp opening are more common in acute aortic regurgitation (33,61). In chronic aortic regurgitation, increased end diastolic volume results in an enhanced stroke volume via Frank-Starling mechanisms. This elevates

the systolic blood pressure and increases myocardial wall stress and in response the ventricle hypertrophies. The regurgitant volume results in chronic volume overload of the left ventricle and causes a gradual dilatation of the chamber. The net effect is a tremendous increase in left ventricular mass. It should be noted that as the left ventricle dilates in chronic aortic regurgitation, it becomes more globular; consequently, echocardiographically based left ventricular mass calculations are not as accurate. As the compensatory mechanisms of the ventricle are exhausted, left ventricular dysfunction ensues, initially during exercise, eventually at rest. Other signs of progressive deterioration of the heart's ability to compensate include left atrial enlargement and right ventricular dilatation. The clinical findings, natural history, and management of acute and chronic aortic regurgitation are described elsewhere (9,15,60).

Doppler Assessment

Doppler interrogation of the aortic valve is the primary noninvasive modality to detect aortic regurgitation. All Doppler techniques are sensitive and especially specific in the qualitative diagnosis of aortic regurgitation. The following echocardiographic characteristics of the regurgitant jet have been studied: color flow mapping, pressure half-time, signal intensity, reversal of flow in the abdominal aorta, and regurgitant fraction. However, an accurate method to quantitatively assess aortic regurgitation has been elusive. This is due both to a lack of an accurate gold standard, namely angiography (62), and the influence of changes in hemodynamics (63,64), anatomical factors (65), and machine settings (66) on Doppler measurements. Use of multiple parameters in conjunction with the clinical presentation should be incorporated when making an assessment regarding the severity of aortic regurgitation; any one particular method may be limited.

With aortic regurgitation, reversal of blood flow occurs through an incompetent aortic valve back into the left ventricle. The velocity of this blood is high, correlating with the high pressure differential between the aorta and left ventricle throughout diastole. This can be detected by pulsed-wave and continuous-wave Doppler. The pulsed wave signals can be plotted by software into a two-dimensional color map of the extent of the regurgitant jet through the aortic valve and into the left ventricle (Fig. 6; see also Color Plate 21 following page 294). Quantification of the severity of aortic regurgitation has been attempted by measurement of various parts of this regurgitant jet map. Two such measurements are jet length and jet area. Unfortunately, these measures have correlated poorly with the angiographic grade of regurgitation (63,67,68). The regurgitant jet is a complex three-dimensional structure. It can be difficult to adequately represent it in a two-dimensional image. The jet can also be distorted by hitting structures within the left ventricle (69) and by incoming mitral flow. Lastly, the jet is influenced by hemo-

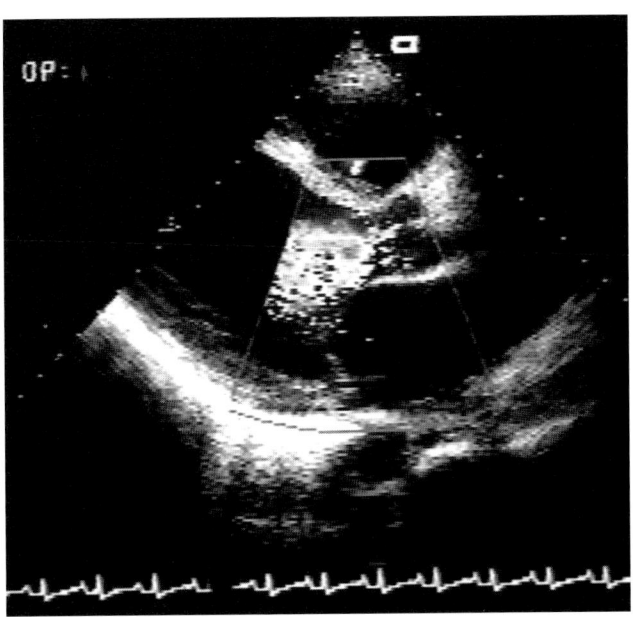

FIG. 6. Color flow Doppler with severe aortic regurgitation. The color flow signal occupies the majority of the left ventricular outflow tract and has a lot of turbulence as witnessed by mosaicism. (See also Color Plate 21 following page 294.)

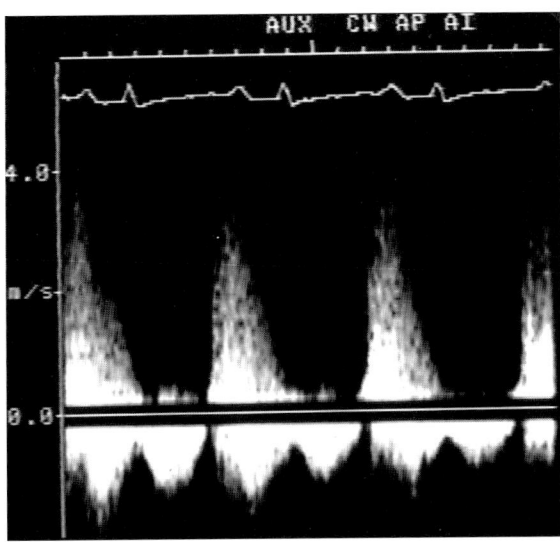

FIG. 7. Continuous-wave Doppler with severe aortic regurgitation. The slope of the continuous-wave signal is greater than 3 m/s^2.

dynamic factors such as left ventricular compliance and systemic vascular resistance.

Color flow mapping shows the turbulence of the regurgitant jet as it crosses the aortic valve. The dimensions of this jet at the level of the aortic valve show a relationship to the regurgitant orifice area. In the parasternal long-axis view, the jet height at the aortic valve is used and in the parasternal short-axis view, the jet area at the level of the valve is used. These values are often indexed to the diameter of the left ventricular outflow tract and the left ventricular outflow area, respectively. Both sets of measurements have shown better correlation to the angiographic grade of aortic regurgitation. A jet height-to-left ventricular outflow tract diameter ratio less than 25% reliably separates mild from moderate aortic regurgitation. Similarly, a ratio greater than 65% separates severe from moderate aortic regurgitation (5,33,61,67). Color flow mapping has serious limitations in assessing the severity of eccentric regurgitant jets (Table 2).

Continuous-wave Doppler examination of the left ventricular outflow tract records the instantaneous velocity of the regurgitant blood across an incompetent aortic valve. The velocity in turn is proportional to the pressure gradient across the aortic valve. In severe aortic regurgitation, the aortic end-systolic pressure is increased since the left ventricle ejects both forward stroke volume as well as the regurgitant volume. As blood flows backward across the incompetent aortic valve during diastole, the left ventricular pressure rises rapidly while the aortic diastolic pressure drops. Consequently, the continuous-wave Doppler tracing will show a high initial instantaneous velocity, which rapidly declines as the aortic diastolic pressure approaches left ventricular pressures. In milder forms of aortic regurgitation, the initial velocity will be lower and the velocity decay will be slower. The characteristics of this decay are represented by both the slope of the decay and the pressure half-time. Generally, a slope of greater than 3 m/sec^2 suggests severe aortic regurgitation as does a pressure half-time of less than 250 msec (Fig. 7). A pressure half-time greater than 400 msec more commonly implies mild aortic regurgitation (5,33,68,70). Unfortu-

TABLE 2. *Suggested criteria for grading the degree of aortic regurgitation*

Degree of regurgitation	JH/LVOH	JSAA/LVOA	Deceleration slope (m/sec^2)	Pressure half-time (ms)	Retrograde abdominal flow
1+	<24%	<4%		>400	
2+	25–46%	4–24%			
3+	47–64%	25–59%			Holodiastolic
4+	>65%	>60%	>3	<250	Holodiastolic
Correlation with angiography	R = 0.91	R = 0.86	R = 0.70	R = 0.62	
Sensitivity for 3–4+ AR	94%	92%		100%	
Specificity for 3–4+ AR	97%	97%	97%		
Accuracy	96%	93%	86%		

JH, jet height; *LVOH,* LV outflow height; *JSA,* jet surface area; *LVOA,* LV outflow area.

nately, there are also inherent limitations to this technique. The diastolic pressure gradient is influenced by systemic vascular resistance, left ventricular compliance, and the heart rate. An increase in systemic vascular resistance, a reduction in left ventricular compliance, and an increase in the heart rate all increase the slope of the diastolic velocity decay (61). As a result, these measures are used only to differentiate severe regurgitation.

Normally in the abdominal aorta, there is only forward systolic flow. There may be a minimal amount of early diastolic flow reversal, reflecting distal runoff in the coronary and carotid arteries. This early diastolic flow reversal may be accentuated by mild aortic regurgitation. Holodiastolic flow reversal in the abdominal aorta has been proposed as a means of distinguishing mild from severe aortic regurgitation. In a small study by Takenaka et al. (71), holodiastolic flow reversal in the abdominal aorta was 100% sensitive. The only misclassification in this study was in a patient with a patent ductus arteriosus.

The regurgitant fraction is the regurgitant volume expressed as a percentage of total stroke volume:

$$RF = \frac{TSV - SV}{TSV}$$

where TSW is the total flow across the aortic valve in systole, and SV is the effective forward stroke volume. As mentioned previously, the flow across a valve can be calculated by echocardiography by multiplying the mean velocity by the outflow area. TSV can be calculated using this method across the aortic valve; SV can be calculated using any other nonregurgitant valve, typically the pulmonic or mitral valve. The main limitation of this method is the difficulty involved in accurately making the numerous measurements needed. When successful, however, echocardiographically derived regurgitant fraction has correlated well with catheterization based data (72–74). A regurgitant fraction greater than 55% is regarded as severe aortic regurgitation; a regurgitant fraction less than 30% implies mild aortic regurgitation (5).

Clinical Applications of Echocardiography in Aortic Regurgitation

Patients with mild-to-moderate aortic regurgitation that does not progress should have a normal life expectancy. Patients with severe aortic regurgitation are known to have a long asymptomatic period; after symptoms develop, their five-year mortality is about 25% (9). The best predictor of the development of symptoms is left ventricular systolic dysfunction at rest; the best predictors of left ventricular systolic dysfunction are increased left ventricular size (end-diastolic size >70 mm or end-systolic size >50 mm) and left ventricular systolic dysfunction during exercise (9). Two-dimensional and M-mode echocardiography are useful in the follow-up of asymptomatic patients with aortic regurgitation

by providing serial measurements of left ventricular size and function (75). This data could be helpful in deciding the optimal timing for valve replacement. Valve replacement has been shown to decrease left ventricular volume and hypertrophy to some degree, and to increase left ventricular systolic function. This is more likely to occur if left ventricular dysfunction has been present for less than 12 months (76). Based on this data, a reasonable approach to surveillance of severe aortic regurgitation would be routine echocardiographic assessment every 6 to 12 months.

Other Techniques

In some centers with expertise in nuclear cardiology, serial radionuclide ventriculograms to assess LV volume and function at rest may be an accurate and cost-effective alternative to serial echocardiograms. However, there is no justification for routine serial testing with both an echocardiogram and a radionuclide ventriculogram. Serial radionuclide ventriculograms are also recommended in patients with suboptimal echocardiograms, patients with suggestive but not definite echocardiographic evidence of LV systolic dysfunction, and patients for whom there is discordance between clinical assessment and echographic data. In centers with specific expertise in cardiac magnetic resonance imaging, serial magnetic resonance imaging may be performed in place of radionuclide angiography for the indications listed above. In addition to accurate assessment of LV volume, mass, wall thickness, and systolic function, cardiac magnetic resonance imaging may also be used to quantify the severity of valvular regurgitation (15).

Serial exercise testing is also not recommended routinely in asymptomatic patients with preserved systolic function. However, exercise testing may be invaluable to assess functional capacity and symptomatic responses in patients with equivocal changes in symptomatic status.

REFERENCES

1. Slater J, Gindea AJ, Freedberg RS, et al. Comparison of cardiac catheterization and Doppler echocardiography in the decision to operate in aortic and mitral valve disease. *J Am Coll Cardiol* 1991;17:1026–1036.
2. Williams PL, Warwick R, Dyson M, et al., eds. *Gray's anatomy*, 37th ed. New York: Churchill Livingstone, 1989:711–712.
3. Sahasakul Y, Edwards WD, Naessens JM, et al. Age-related changes in aortic and mitral valve thickness: implications for two-dimensional echocardiography based on an autopsy study of 200 normal human hearts. *Am J Cardiol* 1988;62:424–430.
4. Sutton JP III, Ho SY, Anderson RH. The forgotten interleaflet triangles: a review of the surgical anatomy of the aortic valve. *Ann Thoracic Surg* 1995;59:419–427.
5. Weyman A, Griffin BP. Left ventricular outflow tract: the aortic valve, aorta, and subvalvular outflow tract. In: Weyman A, ed. *Principles and practice of echocardiography*. Philadelphia: Lea & Febiger, 1994: 498–574.
6. Lorz W, Cottier C, Gyr N. The prevalence of aortic stenosis in an elderly population: an echocardiographic study in a small Swiss community. *Cardiol Elderly* 1993;1:511–515.
7. Chiang HT, Lin M. Echocardiographic evaluation of thickened aortic valve and its relation to aortic stenosis and regurgitation. *Chung Hua i Hsueh Tsa Chih Chinese Med J* 1992;50:443–447.

8. Selzer A. Changing aspects of the natural history of valvular aortic stenosis. *New Engl J Med* 1987;317:91.
9. Rahimtoola, SH. Aortic valve disease. In: Schlant R, Alexander RW, eds. *Hurst's the heart,* 9th ed. New York: McGraw-Hill, 1988: 1759–1787.
10. Rose AG. Etiology of valvular heart disease. *Curr Opinion Cardiol* 1996;11:98–113.
11. Dare AJ, Veinot JP, Edwards WD, et al. New observations on the etiology of aortic valve disease: a surgical pathologic study of 236 cases from 1990. *Human Pathology* 1993;24:1330–1338.
12. Passik CS, Ackermann DM, Pluth JR, et al. Temporal changes in the causes of aortic stenosis: a surgical pathologic study of 646 cases. *Mayo Clinic Proc* 1987;62:119–123.
13. Stewart BF, Siscovick D, Lind BK, et al. Clinical factors associated with calcific aortic valve disease. Cardiovascular Health Study. *J Am Coll Cardiol* 1997;29:630–634.
14. Mautner GC, Mautner SL, Cannon R, et al. Clinical factors useful in predicting aortic valve structure in patients > 40 years of age with isolated valvular aortic stenosis. *Am J Cardiol* 1993;72:194–198.
15. Bonow RO, Carabello B, Leon AC, et al. ACC/AHA Guidelines for the management of patients with valvular disease. *J Am Coll Cardiol* 1998;32:1486–1588.
16. DeMaria AN, Bommer W, Joye J, et al. Value and limitations of cross-sectional echocardiography of the aortic valve in the diagnosis and quantification of valvular aortic stenosis. *Circulation* 1980;62: 304–312.
17. Weyman AE, Feigenbaum H, Dillon JC, et al. Cross-sectional echocardiography in assessing the severity of valvular aortic stenosis. *Circulation* 1975;52:828.
18. Hoffmann R, Flachskampf FA, Hanrath R. Planimetry of orifice area in aortic stenosis using multiplane transesophageal echocardiography. *J Am Coll Cardiol* 1993;22:529–534.
19. Kim CJ, Berglund H, Nishioka T, et al. Correspondence of aortic valve area determination from transesophageal echocardiography, transthoracic echocardiography, and cardiac catheterization. *Am Heart J* 1996; 132:1163–1172.
20. Cormier B, Iung B, Porte JM, et al. Value of multiplane transesophageal echocardiography in determining aortic valve area in aortic stenosis. *Am J Cardiol* 1996;77:882–885.
21. Oh JK, Taliercio CP, Holmes DR Jr, et al. Prediction of the severity of aortic stenosis by Doppler aortic valve area determination: prospective Doppler-catheterization correlation in 100 patients. *J Am Coll Cardiol* 1988;11:1227–1234.
22. Harrison MR, Gurley JC, Smith MD, et al. A practical application of Doppler echocardiography for the assessment of severity of aortic stenosis. *Am Heart J* 1988;115:622–628.
23. Currie PJ, Seward JB, Reeder, GS, et al. Continuous-wave Doppler echocardiographic assessment of severity of calcific aortic stenosis: a simultaneous Doppler-catheter correlative study in 100 adult patients. *Circulation* 1985;71:1162.
24. Callahan MJ, Tajik A.J, Su-Fan Q, et al. Validation of instantaneous pressure gradients measured by continuous-wave Doppler in experimentally induced aortic stenosis. *Am J Cardiol* 1985;56:989.
25. Smith MD, Dawson PL, Elion JL, et al. Correlation of continuous wave Doppler velocities with cardiac catheterization gradients: an experimental model of aortic stenosis. *J Am Coll Cardiol* 1985;6:1306.
26. Currie PJ, Hagler DJ, Seward JB, et al. Instantaneous pressure gradient: a simultaneous Doppler and dual-catheter correlative study. *J Am Coll Cardiol* 1986;7:800.
27. Rahimtoola SH. ''Prophylactic'' valve replacement for mild aortic valve disease at the time of surgery for other cardiovascular disease? . . . NO. *J Am Coll Cardiol* 1999;33:2009–2015.
28. Feigenbaum H. *Echocardiography,* 5th ed. Philadelphia: Lea & Febiger, 1993:195–196.
29. Niederberger J, Schima H, Maurer G, et al. Importance of pressure recovery for the assessment of aortic stenosis by Doppler ultrasound. Role of aortic size, aortic valve area, and the direction of the stenotic jet *in vitro. Circulation* 1996;94:1934–1940.
30. Williams GA, Labovitz AJ, Nelson JG, et al. Value of multiple echocardiographic views in the evaluation of aortic stenosis in adults by continuous wave Doppler. *Am J Cardiol* 1985;55:445.
31. Teirstein P, Yeager M, Yock PG, et al. Doppler echocardiographic measurement of aortic valve area in aortic stenosis: a noninvasive application of the Gorlin Formula. *J Am Coll Cardiol* 1986;8:1059–1065.
32. Yeager M, Yock PG, Popp RL. Comparison of Doppler-derived pressure gradient to that determined at cardiac catheterization in adults with aortic valve stenosis: implications for management. *Am J Cardiol* 1986; 57:644–648.
33. Oh JK, Seward JB, Tajik AJ. *The echo manual* 2nd ed. Philadelphia: Lippincott-Raven, 1999.
34. Rahimtoola SH. Valvular heart disease: a perspective. *J Am Coll Cardiol* 1983;1:199–215.
35. Otto CM, Pearlman AS, Comess KA, et al. Determination of the stenotic aortic valve area in adults using Doppler echocardiography. *J Am Coll Cardiol* 1986;7:509–517.
36. Skjaerpe T, Hegrenaes L, Hatle L. Noninvasive estimation of valve area in patients with aortic stenosis by Doppler ultrasound and two-dimensional echocardiography. *Circulation* 1985;72:810–818.
37. Zoghbi WA, Farmer KL, Soto JG, et al. Accurate noninvasive quantification of stenotic aortic valve area by Doppler echocardiography. *Circulation* 1986;73:452–459.
38. Bermejo J, Garcia-Fernandez MA, Torrecilla EG, et al. Effects of dobutamine on Doppler echocardiographic indexes of aortic stenosis. *J Am Coll Cardiol* 1996;28:1206–1213.
39. Baumgartner H, Kratzer H, Helmreich G, et al. Determination of aortic valve area by Doppler echocardiography using the continuity equation: a critical evaluation. *Cardiology* 1990;77:101–111.
40. Otto CM, Pearlman AS, Gardner CL, et al. Simplification of the Doppler continuity equation for calculating stenotic aortic valve area. *J Am Soc Echocardiography* 1988;1:155–157.
41. Burwash IG, Pearlman AS, Kraft CD, et al. Flow dependence of measures of aortic stenosis severity during exercise. *J Am Coll Cardiol* 1994;24:1342–1350.
42. Otto CM, Pearlman AS. Doppler echocardiography in adults with symptomatic aortic stenosis. Diagnostic utility and cost-effectiveness. *Arch Int Med* 1988;148:2553–2560.
43. Otto CM, Pearlman AS, Gardner CL. Hemodynamic progression of aortic stenosis in adults assessed by Doppler echocardiography. *J Am Coll Cardiol* 1989;13:545–550.
44. Otto CM, Burwash IG, Legget ME, et al. Prospective study of asymptomatic valvular aortic stenosis: clinical, echocardiographic, and exercise predictors of outcome. *Circulation* 1997:95:2262–2270.
45. Chetlin MD, Gertz EW, Brundage BH, et al. Rate of progression of severity of valvular aortic stenosis. *Am Heart J* 1979;96:689–700.
46. Nestico PF, De Pace NL, Kimbris D, et al. Progression of isolated aortic stenosis: analysis of 29 patients having more than 1 cardiac catheterization. *Am J Cardiol* 1983;52:1054–1058.
47. Roger VL, Tajik AJ, Bailey KR, et al. Progression of aortic stenosis in adults: new appraisal using Doppler echocardiography. *Am Heart J* 1990;119:331–338.
48. Davies SW, Gershlick A, Balcon R. Progression of valvular stenosis: a long-term retrospective study. *Eur Heart J* 1991;12:10–14.
49. Faggiano P, Ghizzoni G, Sorgato A, et al. Rate of progression of valvular aortic stenosis in adults. *Am J Cardiol* 1992;70;229–233.
50. Peter M, Hoffman A, Parker C, et al. Progression of aortic stenosis: role of age and concomitant coronary artery disease. *Chest* 1993;103: 1715–1719.
51. Brener SJ, Duffy CI, Thomas JD, et al. Progression of aortic stenosis in 394 patients: relation to changes in myocardial and mitral valve dysfunction. *J Am Coll Cardiol* 1995;25:305–310.
52. Bogart DB, Murphy BL, Wong BY, et al. Progression of aortic stenosis. *Chest* 1979;76:391–396.
53. Jonasson R, Jonasson B, Nordlander R, et al. Rate of progression of severity of valvular aortic stenosis. *Acta Med Scand* 1983;213:51–54.
54. Wagner S, Selzer A. Patterns of progression of aortic stenosis: a longitudinal hemodynamic study. *Circulation* 1982;65:709–712.
55. Rahimtoola SH. Perspective on valvular heart disease: an update. In the ACC 40th Anniversary Seminar. *J Am Coll Cardiol* 1989;14:1–23.
56. Rahimtoola SH. Perspective on valvular heart disease: update II. In: Knoebel S, ed. *Era in cardiovascular medicine.* New York: Elsevier, 1991:45–70.
57. Olson LJ, Subramanian R, Edwards WD. Surgical pathology of pure aortic insufficiency: a study of 225 cases. *Mayo Clin Proc* 1984;59: 835–841.
58. Tonnemacher D, Reid C, Kawanishi D, et al. Frequency of myxomatous degeneration of the aortic valve as a cause of isolated aortic regurgitation severe enough to warrant aortic valve replacement. *Am J Cardiol* 1987;60:1194–1196.

59. Subramanian R, Olson LJ, Edwards WD. Surgical pathology of combined aortic stenosis and insufficiency: a study of 213 cases. *Mayo Clin Proc* 1985;60:247–254.
60. Rahimtoola SH. Recognition and management of acute aortic regurgitation. *Heart Dis Stroke* 1993;2:217–221.
61. Meyer T, Sareli P, Pocock WA, et al. Echocardiographic and hemodynamic correlates of diastolic closure of mitral valve and diastolic opening of aortic valve in severe aortic regurgitation. *Am J Cardiol* 1987;59:1144–1148.
62. Croft CH, Lipscomb K, Mathis K, et al. Limitations of qualitative angiographic grading in aortic or mitral regurgitation. *Am J Cardiol* 1984;53:1593–1598.
63. Switzer DF, Yoganathan AP, Nanda NC, et al. Calibration of color Doppler flow mapping during extreme hemodynamic conditions *in vitro*: a foundation for a reliable quantitative grading system for aortic incompetence. *Circulation* 1987;75:837–846.
64. Reimold SC, Maier SE, Fleischmann KE, et al. Dynamic nature of the aortic regurgitant orifice area during diastole in patients with chronic aortic regurgitation. *Circulation* 1994;89:2085–2092.
65. Thomas JD, O'Shea JP, Rodriguez L, et al. Impact of orifice geometry on the shape of jets: an *in vitro* Doppler color flow study. *J Am Coll Cardiol* 1991;17:901–908.
66. Stevenson JG. Critical importance of gain, pulse repetition frequency, and carrier frequency on apparent 2D color Doppler jet size. *Circulation* 1988;78:II-12.
67. Perry GJ, Helmcke F, Nanda NC, et al. Evaluation of aortic insufficiency by Doppler color flow mapping. *J Am Coll Cardiol* 1987;9:952.
68. Dolan MS, Castello R, St Vrain JA, et al. Quantitation of aortic regurgitation by Doppler echocardiography: a practical approach. *Am Heart J* 1995;129:1014–1020.
69. Stevenson JG. Lessons provided by color flow imagery: disturbed flow jets tend to adhere to adjacent walls. *J Am Coll Cardiol* 1987;9:3A.
70. Grayburn PA, Handshoe R, Smith MD, et al. Quantitative assessment of the hemodynamic consequences of aortic regurgitation by means of continuous wave Doppler recordings. *J Am Coll Cardiol* 1987;10:135–141.
71. Takenaka K, Daestani A, Gardin JM, et al. A simple Doppler echocardiographic method for estimating severity of aortic regurgitation. *Am J Cardiol* 1986;57:1340–1343.
72. Rokey R, Sterling LL, Zoghbi WA, et al. Determination of regurgitant fraction in isolated mitral or aortic regurgitation by pulsed Doppler two-dimensional echocardiography. *J Am Coll Cardiol* 1986;7:1273–1278.
73. Kitabatake A, Ito H, Inoue M, et al. A new approach to noninvasive evaluation of aortic regurgitant fraction by two-dimensional Doppler echocardiography. *Circulation* 1985;72:523–529.
74. Kandath D, Nanda NC. Assessment of aortic regurgitation by noninvasive techniques. *Current Prob Cardiol* 1990;15:45–58.
75. McDonald IG, Jelinek M. Serial M-mode echocardiography in severe chronic aortic regurgitation. *Circulation* 1980;62:1291.
76. Bonow RO, Dodd JT, Maron BJ, et al. Long-term serial changes in left ventricular function and reversal of ventricular dilatation after valve replacement for chronic aortic regurgitation. *Circulation* 1988:78(5,Pt 1):1108–1120.

CHAPTER 42

Tricuspid and Pulmonary Valve Disease

Paulo A. Ribeiro and Muayed Al-Zaibag

DIAGNOSIS OF TRICUSPID VALVE DISEASE

The diagnosis of tricuspid valve disease is challenging since the symptoms and physical signs can be masked by concomitant mitral valve disease. Currently, the state of the art in imaging and diagnosis of the tricuspid valve is two-dimensional echocardiography (2-DE), complemented with Doppler hemodynamic assessment. These combined noninvasive techniques, that are widely available, achieve a precise and cost-effective anatomic and physiologic assessment of the tricuspid valve. We will discuss specific echocardiographic features that may pinpoint an accurate etiological diagnosis of tricuspid disease.

Pathology of the Normal Tricuspid Valve and Echocardiographic Correlations

The histologic composition of the tricuspid valve consists of three different layers; the atrial surface consisting of collagen and elastin fibers, the middle layer composed of myxomatous connective tissue, and the collagen fibers that constitute the bulk of the ventricular side of the valve (1). The normal tricuspid valve has a complex anatomic structure that can be readily evaluated by 2-DE. The annular circumference of the valve in men is 11.4 ± 1.1 cm and in females is 10.8 ± 1.3 cm (2). The anterior leaflet is almost always the largest, while the posterior leaflet may have between one and four scallops (2). Two-dimensional echocardiography is the best imaging technique to assess the tricuspid leaflets (Figs. 1 and 2). The anterior leaflet is seen in the four-chamber and right ventricular inflow view. The posterior leaflet

is assessed from the lower parasternal right ventricular inflow. The single septal leaflet is the smallest, and can be imaged from the two-dimensional echocardiographic (2-DE) apical four-chamber view; leaflets are avascular and thin in normal valves. Bright echoes indicate that the leaflets are thick or calcified, such as is found in rheumatic tricuspid disease. The anatomic features are readily detected by 2-DE that can differentiate between the normal tricuspid leaflet insertion and displaced leaflets, such as in Ebstein's anomaly; the tricuspid leaflets attach toward the right ventricular apex, and part of the right ventricular (RV) cavity becomes atrialized.

The subvalvular tricuspid apparatus is composed of three papillary muscles; the anterior has a moderator band attached to it, usually readily detected by 2-DE. The medial tricuspid papillary muscles may be rudimentary in adults. On average, 25 chordae tendineae insert into the tricuspid valve, 7 to the anterior leaflet, 6 to the posterior leaflet, 9 into the septal leaflet, and 3 into the commissural areas (2). The chordae tendineae commonly arise from the papillary muscle or from the muscle of the posterior or septal walls of the RV. Two-dimensional echocardiography images the papillary muscles and chordae attachments and can differentiate between normal, thin chordae and fused and matted chordae that exhibit abnormal bright echoes, such as in rheumatic tricuspid heart disease and endomyocardial fibrosis. There are five types of chordae tendineae: fan-shaped, free-edge, rough, deep, and basal chordae (2). The basal chordae are the shortest and measure an average of 0.6 cm; the deep and rough chordae can be as long as 2.2 cm (2). The fan-shaped chordae form precise landmarks for the commissures and distinguish clefts from the genuine commissures of the leaflets. The deep chordae, not present in the mitral valve, appear to provide a second arcade for leaflet attachment to the larger tricuspid valve annulus and leaflets. The free-edge chordae are characteristic of the tricuspid valve. They are single and may originate in the apex of the papillary muscle from its base and

P. A. Ribeiro: Department of Cardiology, Loma Linda University Hospital, Loma Linda, California 92354.

M. Al-Zaibag: Department of Cardiology, Loma Linda University Medical Center, Loma Linda, California 92354; Cardiac Sciences Department, King Fahad National Guard Hospital, Riyadh, Saudi Arabia.

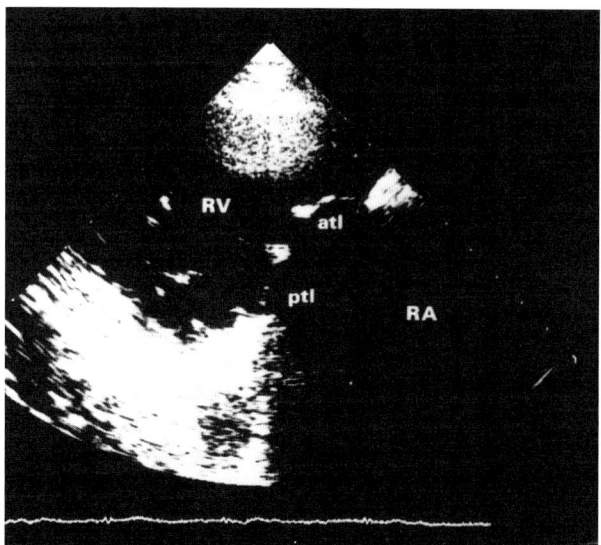
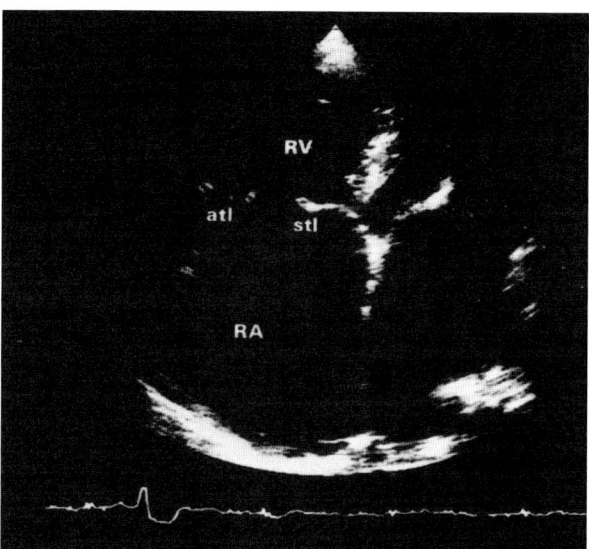

FIG. 1. Two-dimensional echo study: right ventricular inflow view (**left panel**) and apical four-chamber view (**right panel**), showing thickened tricuspid leaflets with restricted motion and diastolic doming. These are the echocardiographic features of rheumatic tricuspid stenosis. *RA,* right atrium; *RV,* right ventricle; *atl,* anterior leaflet of tricuspid valve; *ptl,* posterior leaflet of tricuspid valve; *stl,* septal leaflet of tricuspid valve.

insert into the leaflets' free edge. In males, the length of the anteroposterior commissure measures an average of 1.1 cm, the posterior septal, 0.8 cm, and the anteroseptal, 0.6 (2). Although the tricuspid commissures are not readily seen on 2-DE, the normal motion of the edges of the leaflets indicate that they are anatomically free.

Pathologic Findings in Tricuspid Stenosis: Echocardiographic Correlations

From the series of 363 surgically excised tricuspid valves at the Mayo Clinic (3) reported in 1988, the etiology of

the tricuspid valve disease was rheumatic in 53% of cases, congenital heart disease in 26%, pulmonary venous hypertension in 15%, infective endocarditis in 3%, and trauma or carcinoid in 1% (Table 1). More recently, the Mayo Clinic has reported cases of tricuspid stenosis due to use of ergot alkaloids and Fen/Phen drugs (4,5).

Pathologic findings show that rheumatic tricuspid stenosis (TS) exhibits leaflet fibrosis and retraction, commissural fusion, and, in some cases, chordae matting (1,2). The commissures are not well distinguishable, as they are covered by a continuous curtain of valve tissue. Calcification of tricuspid valve is distinctively rare. Pathologically, the tricuspid leaf-

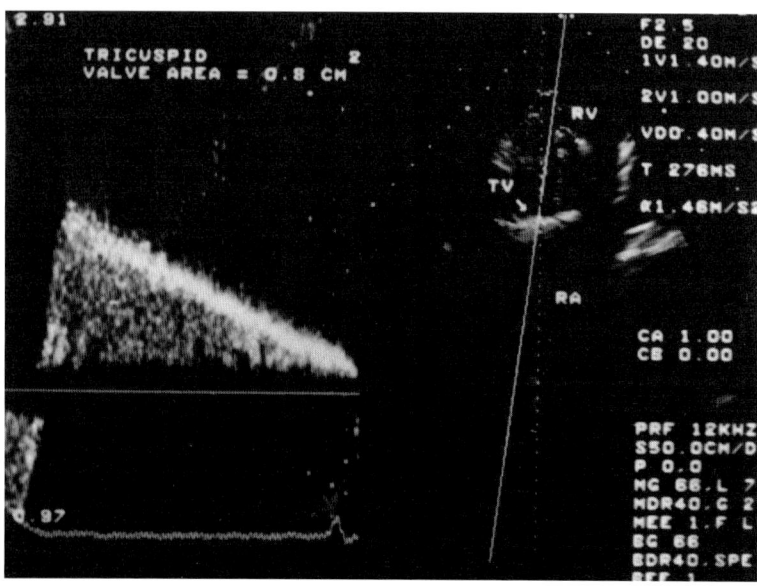

FIG. 2. Continuous-wave Doppler flow signal across the tricuspid valve, showing increased diastolic flow velocity. The velocity deceleration is slow, and the pressure half-time is prolonged, indicative of tricuspid stenosis. Using 220/pressure half-time, the TVA equals 0.8 cm². *TVA,* tricuspid valve area.

TABLE 1. *Etiology of tricuspid valve stenosis*

Rheumatic heart disease
Congenital heart disease
Carcinoid heart disease
Endomyocardial fibrosis
Tumor involving tricuspid valve
Localized constrictive pericarditis
Lupus erythematosus
Use of ergot alkaloids
Fen/Phen valvulopathy

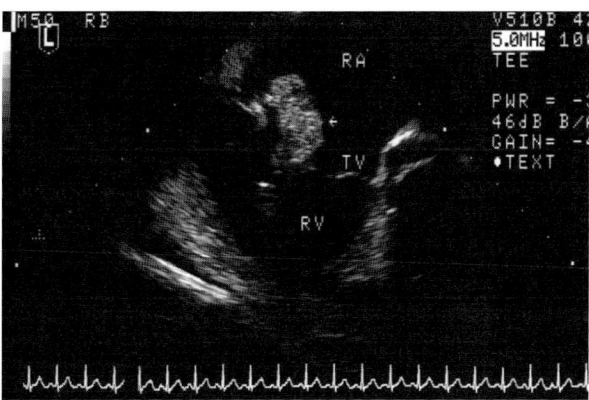

FIG. 4. Transesophageal echocardiographic echo study of the right ventricular inflow showing a large vegetation (*arrow*) attached to the tricuspid valve. (Courtesy of Ramesh Bansal, M.D.)

lets are less thickened compared to the mitral valve. The subvalvular chordae are uncommonly fused and matted. The 2-DE diagnosis of rheumatic tricuspid stenosis occurs in 3 to 4% of patients with rheumatic heart disease (6). The echocardiographic features include leaflet thickening, diastolic doming as a result of the commissural fusion, and decreased mobility (Fig. 1) (1,2,7,8). These findings are characteristic of rheumatic heart disease (6).

Carcinoid heart disease can distort the tricuspid leaflets, and the chordae tendineae can be thickened (9–12). Deposits of dense plaques of carcinoid tumor cells in the leaflets cause decreased motion and immobility in extreme cases with tricuspid stenosis. Two-dimensional echocardiographic features of tricuspid stenosis in carcinoid disease include leaflet thickening, with leaflets that are immobile in the semiopen position and with bright echoes from the deposits of tumor cells in chordae tendineae (9). Two-dimensional echocardiography and Doppler flow signal may be characteristic for carcinoid heart disease (13). Lupus erythematosus can lead to tricuspid stenosis in rare cases. Pathologic findings would also include pericardial effusion and mitral valve Libman-Sacks vegetations, readily detected by 2-DE (Figs. 3 and 4).

Endomyocardial fibrosis may involve the tricuspid valve

and subvalvular apparatus and cause tricuspid stenosis (10). Tricuspid regurgitation (TR) with an enormous right atrium are usual findings on 2-DE, together with the distinctive features of this disease, include bright echoes obliterating the RV apex, best seen in the apical four-chamber view and (right ventricular) inflow tract view.

Congenital tricuspid stenosis is rare and few cases of Ebstein's anomaly have been described (11). This abnormality presents with varying degrees of TR and is usually associated with atrial septal defect or a patent foramen ovale. The pathologic findings consist of displacement and attachment of the tricuspid valve into the body of the RV. The four-chamber apical view is the best view to establish the extent of tricuspid valve displacement and reduction of the functional size of the RV (14–16). These echocardiographic features are characteristic of Ebstein's anomaly (Fig. 5; see also Color Plate 22 following page 294).

Pathophysiology of Tricuspid Valve Stenosis

The tricuspid valve is a large orifice compared to the mitral valve, and it measures at least 7 cm^2 (1,2). With such large area, tricuspid valve stenosis (TS) must be severe to be physiologically important. The tricuspid pressure gradient assessed by hemodynamic studies or Doppler echocardiography is the hemodynamic hallmark used routinely to assess to significance of TS (Fig. 2) (13,17–21). There are inherent limitations in calculating the Gorlin tricuspid valve area during cardiac catheterization, particularly in patients with significant TR (12). Doppler-derived tricuspid valve area can be evaluated using the pressure half-time of tricuspid valve inflow Doppler signal, using the equation described by Hatle (Fig. 2) (13). A good correlation has been demonstrated between the Gorlin and Doppler tricuspid valve area.

A low cardiac output is the major hemodynamic disturbance secondary to tricuspid obstruction (12). A mean diastolic gradient of 2 mm Hg across the valve is considered to be indicative of severe tricuspid stenosis. With a low cardiac

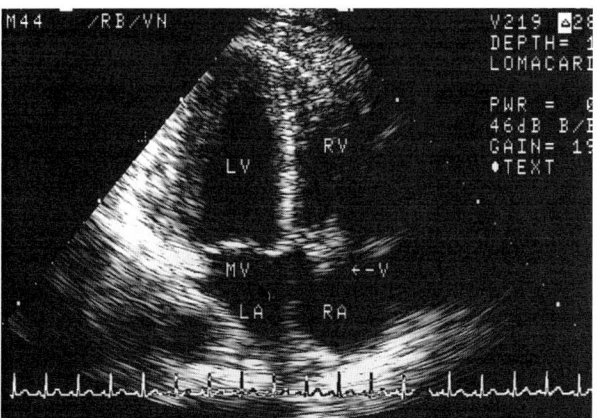

FIG. 3. Two-dimensional echo study: apical four-chamber view with left ventricle showing abnormal bright echoes attached to the tricuspid valve (*v*, vegetation) in a patient with infective endocarditis. *LA,* left atrium; *LV,* left ventricle; *MV,* mitral valve; *RA,* right atrium; *RV,* right ventricle. (Courtesy of Ramesh Bansal, M.D.)

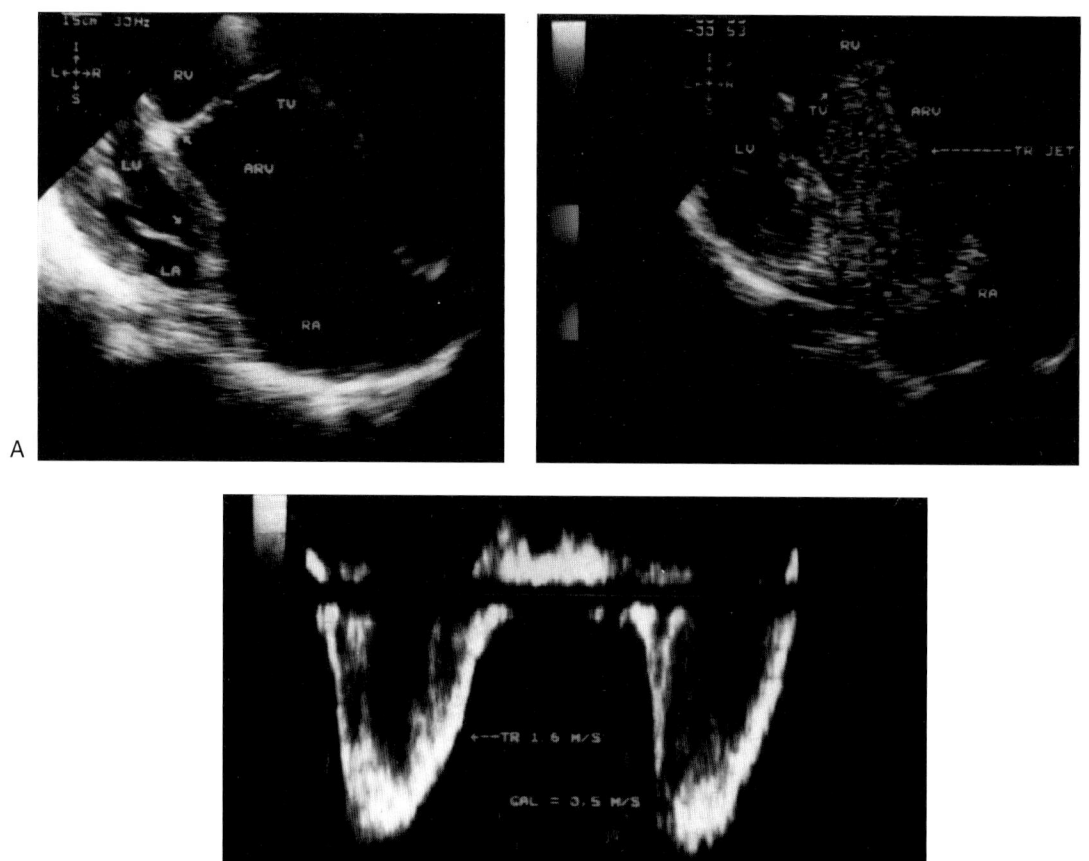

FIG. 5. Two-dimensional echocardiograph of the right ventricular inflow view without color (**A**) and with color flow (**B**), showing marked inferior displacement of the tricuspid valve diagnostic of Ebstein's anomaly. Color-flow imaging shows severe tricuspid regurgitation (TR). **C:** Image shows color-wave Doppler signal of the TR jet, showing feature of high "V" wave pressure in the right atrium. *RA,* right atrium; *RV,* right ventricle; *TV,* tricuspid valve. (See also Color Plate 22 following page 294.) (Courtesy of Ramesh Bansal, M.D.)

output and slow heart rate, there may be no gradient across the valve despite the presence of severe TS. Atropine or fluid challenge may be necessary to expose occult tricuspid valve gradients (22). With exercise, the decrease in RV diastolic filling period, secondary to increase in heart rate, causes an increase in mean atrial pressure and tricuspid gradient, with a concomitant decrease in RV diastolic pressure (22). The associated rise in right atrial pressure is presumably due to the reduced time period for RV filling. Cardiac output usually can only increase twofold at peak exercise in patients with TS. This accounts for the patients' symptoms of tiredness, fatigue, and shortness of breath with exercise.

The mean right atrial pressure is normal in the majority of patients with severe TS. The high right atrial pressures observed in patients with severe TS usually indicates concomitant tricuspid valve regurgitation (22), or, alternatively, a failing RV (23–29). Right atrial pressure tracing exhibits a prominent A wave in the majority of patients with sinus rhythm and a slow Y descent, indicative of the loss of the

rapid filling phase of the RV (12). Similar findings can be extrapolated noninvasively from the Doppler flow signal (Fig. 2). In a few patients, the A wave may be similar to the V wave; this may indicate that the right atrium is failing, and, in our opinion, heralds the development of atrial fibrillation.

History and Clinical Examination in Tricuspid Valve Stenosis

In developing nations, the great majority of patients with TS are due to rheumatic heart disease. In the Western world, rheumatic TS is dwindling, and other, more unusual etiological and new causes of stenosis are emerging, such as tricuspid carcinoid heart disease and use of ergot alkaloids (4).

The time interval between the episode of rheumatic fever and onset of symptoms varies from a few months to four decades. Tricuspid stenosis is nearly always associated with concomitant mitral stenosis, the latter usually dominating

TABLE 2. *Physical signs of tricuspid stenosis*

Slow Y descend (jugular venous pulse)
Prominent A wave (jugular venous pulse)
Diastolic rumble (tricuspid focus)
Increased murmur intensity (inspiration)
Tricuspid opening snap (prior mitral opening snap)
Diastolic thrill (rare)

TABLE 3. *Echocardiographic and Doppler diagnosis of tricuspid stenosis*

Two-dimensional echocardiography (2-DE)
Pulsed-wave Doppler (PWD)
Continuous-wave Doppler (CWD)
Color flow imaging (CFI)

the clinical picture. Shortness of breath with exertion is present in all cases of isolated TS, reflecting the low cardiac output in these patients. Hemoptysis and pulmonary infarction may occur as a result of emboli from thrombus in the right atrium. Hepatomegaly, ascites, and ankle edema may prevail in those patients with concomitant severe tricuspid regurgitation who have elevated mean right atrial pressures and RV dysfunction. Orthopnea and paroxysmal nocturnal dyspnea is experienced in patients with TS and usually is associated with significant mitral valve stenosis.

The clinical detection of TS may be difficult, since the physical features can be masked by an associated mitral stenosis; isolated tricuspid valve stenosis is a rare clinical entity. In patients with sinus rhythm, the large A wave in the jugular venous pulse is prominent and increases with inspiration (Table 2). The Y descent is slow, due to the absence of the rapid RV filling phase. Astute clinical cardiologists may be able to diagnose TS from the neck veins' characteristic wave forms. The diastolic murmur is mainly presystolic and terminates well before the first heart sound. A left-sided sternal diastolic rumble is not pathognomonic for TS, as patients with severe pure TR may exhibit diastolic flow murmurs (14). The tricuspid opening snap may be present, and it occurs prior to the mitral valve opening snap in severe tricuspid valve stenosis. The tricuspid rumble usually increases with inspiration and decreases or even disappears with expiration (12). The diastolic thrill may be palpable, but this is very uncommon (12). For those patients who initially present with atrial fibrillation, the tricuspid murmur occurs mainly in the early diastolic period. With a low heart rate or hypovolemia, the murmur may vanish, as there is a longer period for RV filling and the tricuspid diastolic valve gradient is abolished.

Electrocardiographic and Radiologic Findings in Tricuspid Stenosis

In pure tricuspid stenosis, the patients are usually in sinus rhythm (12). The significant electrocardiographic (ECG) findings are the tented P waves, greater than 3 mm, best seen in the inferior leads. A normal QRS access in the absence of ECG criteria for RV hypertrophy may be the clue for the diagnosis. Interestingly, the PR interval is prolonged in half of the patients with tricuspid stenosis. A prominent right heart border on chest x-ray indicates right atrial dilatation or hypertrophy secondary to tricuspid obstruction. Despite severe TS, some patients exhibit a normal chest x-ray, since

the right atrium dilates mildly. Other concomitant radiologic abnormalities, such as an enlarged left atria or pulmonary trunk, indicate concomitant mitral valve disease.

Echocardiographic and Doppler Assessment in Tricuspid Stenosis

Historically, the M-mode decrease in the E to F slope was a useful echocardiographic feature of TS (15). Several authors showed that this feature lacked specificity (15). With the advent of 2-DE, the tricuspid leaflets and subvalvular apparatus can be assessed from the apical four-chamber view, RV inflow, short-axis view, and the subcostal views (Fig. 1). The classic echocardiographic features of TS include leaflet thickening with restricted motion and diastolic doming of all three leaflets (30). The sensitivity and specificity of these 2-DE characteristics of TS have been variable. Daniels et al. (16) showed that only 4 of 9 patients who exhibited the echocardiographic features of TS had hemodynamic significant obstruction. In contrast, other studies demonstrated 100% sensitivity of the echo features of TS (30). We showed that only 57% of patients with diastolic doming of all three leaflets and restricted motion exhibited hemodynamic significant TS (6). In a minority of patients with occult TS, the diastolic gradient can be exposed with atropine or fluid challenge. These studies clearly indicate that restricted motion and diastolic doming are very sensitive markers of commissural fusion and some decrease in tricuspid valve area, but they are not a precise marker of hemodynamically significant TS.

Doppler studies are ideally suited noninvasive techniques to assess the significance of tricuspid valve gradients (Table 3) (13,15). There is a difference between the catheter fluid filled hemodynamic and Doppler gradients, since the latter measure an instantaneous gradient. The right ventricular inflow view and four-chamber view should be used for Doppler studies of the tricuspid valve (Fig. 2).

The pulsed Doppler sample is placed in the RV close to the tricuspid valve, giving a signal with a profile similar to that seen in mitral stenosis (Table 4). The right-sided cham-

TABLE 4. *Doppler characteristics of tricuspid valve stenosis*

Flame-shape jet (CFI)
Increased pressure-half time (CWD + PWD)
Increased early diastolic velocity (PWD + CWD)
Increased peak and mean diastolic gradients (PWD + CWD)
Reduced tricuspid valve area (PWD + CWD)

CFI, color flow imaging; *CWD,* continuous-wave Doppler; *PWD,* pulsed wave Doppler.

ber blood velocities are lower compared to those of the left side. The initial diastolic tricuspid velocity is increased, and there is a decrease in its decline, with a longer pressure half-time. Diastolic velocities correlate well with the severity of TS. With the modified Bernoulli equation, peak and mean diastolic gradients can be derived from the tricuspid flow velocities. There is a good correlation between the Doppler and cardiac catheterization tricuspid diastolic gradients (Table 4). In severe TS, the velocity may exceed the pulsed Doppler resolution and exhibit aliasing. Continuous-wave Doppler studies will provide similar information in these cases (Table 4) (Fig. 2).

Hatle et al. (13) described the use of the pressure half-time tricuspid inflow signal, together with the empirical constants of 220 to calculate Doppler tricuspid valve area (Fig. 2). The Doppler tricuspid valve area results correlate well with the Gorlin tricuspid valve area. The color flow Doppler does not define the severity of TS. A diastolic color flame-shaped jet across the tricuspid valve indicates flow disturbance, and the images are useful to enable ideal parallel alignment of the continuous wave Doppler, particularly in eccentric jets. This will enable accurate diastolic gradient and tricuspid valve area calculations.

Hemodynamic and Angiographic Findings in Tricuspid Stenosis

The classic hemodynamic findings in TS are a markedly reduced resting cardiac output and a diastolic gradient greater than or equal to 2 mm Hg (Table 5) (12). This fails to increase normally in response to exercise. A large A wave exceeding the V wave by more than 5 mm Hg indicates severe TS (12). We have observed a few patients with severe TS who exhibited similar A- and V-wave amplitude, indicating that the RV is failing, or, alternatively, that the TR is hemodynamically important (Table 5). Interestingly, the mean right atrial pressure may be normal in many of the patients with severe TS.

The tricuspid diastolic gradient of 2 mm Hg is considered to be diagnostic for severe tricuspid valve stenosis, and can be similarly detected by Doppler echocardiography. The gradient may be absent in the early stages of TS, since advanced stenosis is required to be physiologically significant (22). The tricuspid valve gradient increases with volume overload and an increase in heart rate. The decrease in RV filling

TABLE 5. *Hemodynamic features of tricuspid stenosis*

Tricuspid diastolic gradient ≥2 mm Hg
Slow Y descent (RA)
Large A wave (RA)
Decreased cardiac output (CO)
Failure of CO to increase with exercise
Reduced Gorlin tricuspid valve area

RA, right atrium; *CO,* cardiac output.

period, secondary to tachycardia, causes an increase in mean right atrial pressure and tricuspid valve gradient. There are inherent limitations in calculating the tricuspid valve area using the Gorlin formula. The major source of inaccuracies occur with concomitant TR that is present in nearly all patients, which results in the underestimation of tricuspid valve area calculation. Two identical right atrium and right ventricular catheters are required to measure the tricuspid gradient simultaneously, since the gradient may be very small as a result of the high degree of compliance of the right atrium and systemic venous system. Not surprisingly, the original study results between anatomic and tricuspid Gorlin valve area showed a poor correlation, in the absence of a gold standard method of calculating tricuspid valve area (12). The Doppler-estimated tricuspid valve area appears to correlate fairly well with the Gorlin calculation tricuspid valve area. Doppler is the most accurate technique to measure instantaneous gradient of the tricuspid valve, without some of the pitfalls of fluid-filled catheters. Doppler is the gold standard technique for assessing the gradient across the tricuspid valve.

Pitfalls in Clinical Diagnosis of Tricuspid Stenosis

Since the clinical features of TS may be overshadowed by concomitant mitral stenosis, the diagnosis should be suspected in all patients with rheumatic valve stenosis, particularly in those with atrial fibrillation.

The two-dimensional echocardiographic features of TS are leaflet thickening and diastolic doming of all three leaflets, indicating some degree of commissural fusion, but these are not precise indicators of TS (Fig. 1). Many patients who exhibit the echocardiographic features of TS have valve areas of around 3 cm². Hemodynamic studies were indicated for diagnostic purposes. At the present time, the gold standard is Doppler, with the Doppler studies taken across the tricuspid valve that will accurately measure instantaneous gradient and tricuspid valve area.

The classic hemodynamic hallmark of TS is the 2 mm Hg tricuspid valve gradient, measured after two identical fluid-filled catheters placed in the right atrium and right ventricle, respectively (12). Provocative measures are necessary to expose occult gradients in a minority of patients with severe TS. The gradient could be measured in the echocardiography laboratory by Doppler at rest, and after provocative measures with fluid challenge, atropine, or dopamine.

In patients with concomitant severe TR, the mean tricuspid gradient may measure more than 2 mm by Doppler as a result of the large V wave in the absence of organic TS (Table 5). This can be detected on the Doppler envelope with an early and rapid descending of the gradient across the tricuspid valve, secondary to the large V wave (Fig. 5). The color Doppler will be complementary to the pulsed- and continuous-wave Doppler studies in these cases (Table 3).

Pathologic Findings in Tricuspid Regurgitation

Pathologic findings in many cases of pure TR exhibit a dilated tricuspid valve annulus and otherwise an anatomically normal valve (17,18). The annulus measurement is significantly larger in patients with the so-called functional TR, secondary to pulmonary hypertension (18). The pathologic features of purely TR may include fibrosis, leaflet retraction, and chordae fusion. Some patients with rheumatic heart disease may exhibit commissural fusion (1,2). As we discussed in the tricuspid valve section, the different pathologic causes of TS may cause a wide spectrum of degree of TR (Table 6).

Pathologic Findings in Tricuspid Regurgitation: Echocardiographic Correlations

As described in the tricuspid stenosis section of this chapter, the majority of patients with the described pathologic findings of rheumatic TS have concomitant regurgitation (Table 6). Therefore, the typical echocardiographic features of TS, i.e., diastolic doming and restricted leaflet motion, are a marker for the rheumatic etiology of tricuspid disease (1,2,17). Congenital malformation of the tricuspid valve leads to a wide spectrum of degrees of regurgitation. Ebstein's tricuspid valve displacement is readily detected by 2-DE and establishes the cause for the regurgitation (Fig. 5).

The pathophysiologic findings in carcinoid heart disease and endomyocardial fibrosis of the tricuspid were described in the tricuspid stenosis section (11). The 2-DE features are characteristic for the underlying cause for the TR. Trauma may rupture the anterior papillary muscle and cause severe tricuspid regurgitation. Transesophageal echocardiography (TEE) is ideally suited to establish the diagnosis. Myocardial infarction secondary to a proximal right coronary artery occlusion may be the underlying etiology for TR; pathologically, the papillary muscle of the tricuspid valve is necrotic or scarred (19). Two-dimensional echocardiography will show areas of right ventricular wall motion abnormalities, together with abnormal, dense echo signals from the papillary muscle.

In infective endocarditis, the tricuspid leaflets may exhibit vegetations or perforation and the chordae tendineae can be ruptured (3). Two-dimensional echocardiography will demonstrate the above features to establish the etiology of the tricuspid regurgitation (Fig. 5). A floppy prolapsed tricuspid valve has an annulus that can measure more than 14 cm, with a larger leaflet area compared to other etiologies of tricuspid pathology (3). The apical four-chamber view with the leaflet hammocking into the right atrium is usually demonstrated in tricuspid prolapse and Marfan's disease (20).

Frequently, pure TR pathologically exhibits only a dilated valve annulus. This finding is common in patients with pulmonary hypertension, i.e., functional tricuspid regurgitation. Two-dimensional echocardiographic measurement of the tricuspid annulus in the apical four-chamber view and parasternal right ventricular inflow aids in the etiological diagnosis of functional TR.

Pathophysiology of Tricuspid Regurgitation

The symptoms of patients with TR are a result of the severity of the cardiovascular hemodynamic disturbance, particularly the increase in mean right atrial pressure and decrease in cardiac output. Conceivably, the decreased renal perfusion leads to sodium and fluid retention and may be responsible for many of the right-sided heart failure symptoms.

The pathophysiology of certain types of TR is well understood; these types include leaflet cusp perforation as a result of endocarditis; tricuspid papillary muscle necrosis following right ventricular infarction; severe tricuspid valve chordae involvement in endomyocardial fibrosis, chordae fusion, and failure of the tricuspid coaptation in rheumatic heart disease; and marked tricuspid valve prolapse in Marfan's disease. Echocardiography can usually differentiate readily between these different types of tricuspid valve regurgitation.

The mechanism underlying the pathophysiology of functional tricuspid regurgitation with normal anatomic tricuspid valve leaflets and subvalvular apparatus appears to be annular dilatation (17,18). This has been documented in functional tricuspid regurgitation by echocardiographic, angiographic, and pathologic studies (3,21,29). The severity of tricuspid valve regurgitation correlates significantly with the size of the tricuspid valve annulus, both in systole and diastole (17,18). The annulus dilatation is thought to be secondary to RV dilatation in patients with increased RV afterload.

The pathophysiologic mechanism behind the annular dilatation in functional TR has important clinical implications. The annular dilatation may reflect anatomic and geometrical changes of the RV; in this case, surgical treatment with annulus size reduction is indicated. Alternatively, functional tricuspid regurgitation may simply reflect primary RV failure.

TABLE 6. *Etiology of tricuspid valve regurgitation*

Rheumatic heart disease
Myxomatous tricuspid valve
Tricuspid prolapse/Marfan's
Infective endocarditis
Congenital heart disease
Carcinoid heart disease
Endomyocardial fibrosis
Trauma
Myocardial infarction
Use of ergot alkaloids
Fen/Phen drugs
Rheumatoid arthritis
Radiation therapy
Functional

The diagnosis and annulus measurements are readily done by 2-DE (21).

There are inherent limitations in evaluating RV ejection fraction as an index of RV systolic function. Tricuspid regurgitation reduces RV afterload and leads to falsely high RV ejection fraction calculation. Abnormally high levels of pulmonary pressure and resistance may increase the degree of TR (18). There is an inverse relation between RV ejection fraction and pulmonary artery pressure. Thus, the objective evaluation of RV function is complex, particularly in the context of TR and increased pulmonary vascular resistance. The evaluation of RV ejection fraction is hampered by methodological problems and, in normal subjects, has a large variability between 35 to 75% (31).

Symptoms and Physical Signs in Patients with Tricuspid Regurgitation

Most commonly, patients with TR present with symptoms of shortness of breath with exercise (23). That is a consequence of decreased cardiac output. A high right atrial pressure may also lead to symptoms of right heart failure, such as distended neck veins, ascites, and ankle swelling (32). Clinically, this can be detected with jugular venous pressure that will be increased with a prominent V wave. The classic signs of TR are present in about one third of patients with significant TR (14). Patients may have a systolic murmur in the tricuspid area. This may be difficult to detect in patients with fast atrial fibrillation or concomitant severe mitral regurgitation. The murmur is pansystolic, rough, high pitched, and loudest in the tricuspid area, but it can also be heard at the apex (14). The murmur increases with inspiration in a minority of patients.

The majority of patients with TR are in atrial fibrillation and may exhibit features of RV failure. The liver is frequently palpable and ankle edema will be present in 50%. One quarter of the patients will show distended neck veins, ascites, and wasting. A pulsating liver and cyanosis are detected in 10% of patients (14). There is a wide variability of the character of the tricuspid valve murmur. According to some authors the murmur is detected in all patients.

Ninety percent of those patients who have severe TR will have the Carvallo sign with a pulsatile liver and prominent V waves on the neck veins. Uncommonly, patients may be jaundiced and cyanosed due to low cardiac output and liver congestion. Splenomegaly is rare and probably related to portal hypertension in those patients who develop liver cirrhosis. Since isolated severe TR is distinctively rare, the clinical features are often masked by those associated with mitral valve disease (25). In two cases of isolated organic TR, the patients presented with classic features of TR.

The natural history of severe TR is difficult to determine, as mitral valve disease nearly always dominates the clinical picture. The clinical diagnosis and its severity are at times difficult to assess.

Electrocardiography and Radiologic Features in Tricuspid Valve Regurgitation

The great majority of patients with TR present with atrial fibrillation as a result of right atrium dilation and increased wall thickness. For the minority who are in sinus rhythm, the P wave is typically broad and notched in standard leads, with associated P mitrale (14). The QRS axis is vertical or right, and complete right bundle-branch block is observed in 51% of patients. QRS complex is seen in lead V1 in 44% of patients. An intrinsic deflection in leads V1 and V2 is also found in the majority of patients.

Patients that present with significant TR nearly always exhibit cardiomegaly. The enlargement of the pulmonary artery shadow is commonly seen and indicates pulmonary hypertension. The lung fields are oligemic in half of the patients. Hemosiderosis of the lungs and pleural effusion may be part of the clinical picture of patients with longstanding severe TR.

Two-dimensional Echocardiography and Doppler Studies in Tricuspid Regurgitation

Doppler techniques are the gold standard for the detection and quantification of the severe TR (Table 3). Continuous, pulsed, and color flow Doppler are each important imaging modalities for these patients (Fig. 5). Four different echo Doppler approaches have been studied: contrast echocardiography, continuous-wave Doppler; pulse Doppler; and color flow Doppler.

1. The 2-DE characteristics of TR show a dilated right atrium and ventricle, and a paradoxical motion of the interventricular septum (26). The M-mode or 2-DE recording of the inferior vena cava, after contrast injection in the arm vein, will show contrast visualization in the inferior vena cava during ventricular systole (27). The 2-DE measurement of the tricuspid annulus from the four-chamber view may help in differentiating between functional and structural TR.

2. *Continuous wave Doppler* is useful in assessing the presence and severity of TR. It is most commonly used to assess pulmonary artery systolic pressure using the modified Bernouilli equation. There is a good correlation between pulmonary artery pressure assessed during right heart cardiac catheterization and TR velocity Doppler-derived pulmonary artery pressure. In patients with severe tricuspid regurgitation, a large V wave will be present in the right atrium. The Doppler envelope will exhibit early peaking and a midsystolic rapid deceleration as a result of a large V wave. In contrast, in mild TR, these features will not be present (Fig. 5) (26). A typical round midsystolic signal of flow velocity across the tricuspid valve can be acquired when the flow is parallel to the Doppler probe. The signal intensity correlates with the degree of TR (24). The inability to obtain a complete envelope usually indicates that the

degree of TR is mild. In contrast, an intense signal is a marker of moderate to severe TR (Fig. 5) (26).

3. The degree of TR can be assessed by *pulsed Doppler* by mapping the length and width of the tricuspid jet into the right atrium (27). Great care must be taken in mapping the right atrium, in order to enable the detection of eccentric tricuspid jets. A ratio of forward versus reverse flow in the hepatic veins further contributes to the quantification of TR (28).

4. *Color flow Doppler* is a simple and reliable technique to quantify the severity of tricuspid regurgitation (29). A systolic color mosaic jet is demonstrated in the right atrium, arising close to the tricuspid valve, by measuring the regurgitant flow area, the jet length, and the ratio of regurgitation area to that of the right atrium from the apical four-chamber and parasternal RV inflow views. Systolic flow reversal by pulse wave or color flow Doppler in the hepatic veins indicates a severe degree of TR. An IVC and hepatic veins 2-DE and Doppler signals aid in an indirect calculation of right atrial pressure (28).

The etiology of TR can, in the majority of cases, be determined by a detailed 2-DE study of the tricuspid valve, right atrium, and RV, combined with Doppler pulmonary artery systolic pressure evaluation and indirect IVC or hepatic two-dimensional echo assessment of right pressure (Table 6) (28). In rheumatic heart disease, the tricuspid valve may exhibit features of TS, i.e., doming and thickening of all three leaflets, or, alternatively, 2-DE features of thickness of the leaflets with concomitant rheumatic mitral valve disease.

Carcinoid heart disease exhibits a Doppler flow signal that is very suggestive for the diagnosis. Tricuspid leaflets are held open and immobile in the semiopen position with free TR on color flow Doppler (9). The chordae tendineae may exhibit echocardiographic features of thickening and fusion secondary to invasion by the carcinoid tumor. The 2-DE features of endomyocardial fibrosis (10) are distinct from those of carcinoid heart disease (9), although both can invade the subvalvular tricuspid apparatus.

Echocardiographic studies of the tricuspid valve in endomyocardial fibrosis usually do not exhibit features of stenosis with immobile leaflets. Bright echoes obliterate the apical portion of the RV and the right atrium that is invariably dilated. The four-chamber view and RV inflow tract usually show best the bright echoes on the RV apex, representing thrombus and fibrosis obliterating this portion of the RV, and extending to the tricuspid subvalvular apparatus. The echocardiographic characteristics of Ebstein's anomaly are classic with displacement of tricuspid leaflet insertion, and atrialized portion of the RV.

Tricuspid valve prolapse can account for another etiology of TR and is demonstrated by 2-DE, particularly in the apical four-chamber view. Rarely, the 2-DE findings may demonstrate a flail tricuspid chordae as a cause of TR. Trauma to the tricuspid valve or rupture of the papillary muscle follow-

ing an RV infarct may be the underlying etiology (19). Flail leaflet or chordae are ideally detected by transesophageal echocardiography (TEE) examination. Masses may be seen with 2-DE studies of the tricuspid valve, that may represent a benign tumor, such as fibroelastoma or myxoma. These echocardiographic features may be difficult to differentiate from vegetations due to infective endocarditis. TEE is ideally suited to detect perforation in the tricuspid leaflets, either secondary to trauma or endocarditis. The visualization of pacemaker lead through the tricuspid valve detected by echocardiography may be the underlying etiology of TR.

The hemodynamic disturbances observed in TR are increased right atrial pressure and decreased cardiac output. Cardiac output fails to increase with exercise. The decrease in renal blood flow may lead to sodium and fluid retention and contribute to right heart failure (14). The mean right atrial pressure is abnormally high with large V waves. The rapid, wide descent appears with inspiration. There is a wide hemodynamic spectrum of severity of TR.

In mild TR, the mean right atrial pressure may be normal with prominent V-waves. The ventricularization of the pattern of the right atrial pressure may be total in patients with severe TR and right atrial and ventricle pressure may be equal.

Right ventricular angiography is a valid method for the diagnosis of tricuspid insufficiency using the Ubago technique (29). Using special catheters, TR is not detected in normal subjects using this technique. The technique is invasive and not cost-effective; the gold standard is 2-DE with Doppler techniques. Furthermore, the catheter can at times artificially increase the degree of TR.

Pitfalls in the Diagnosis of Tricuspid Regurgitation

The clinician should be aware that the classic clinical features of TR are present in only a minority of patients who have severe valve regurgitation. The majority of patients may exhibit a systolic murmur that increases with inspiration and could be confused with mitral regurgitation murmur. There is a marked variability of tricuspid valve murmur, depending on preload and heart rate. Contrary to general belief, the failure of this systolic murmur to increase with inspiration does not exclude TR. The presence and severity of TR is influenced by preload and afterload, and, therefore, the character of the murmur may vary (33). The results of the echo Doppler studies should take this observation into consideration, and this may explain the variability in the degree of TR observed in longitudinal serial studies.

The noninvasive cardiologist should also realize that detection of TR is common in normal subjects (34). Doppler studies are very sensitive in their detection of TR. Since physiologic TR occurs in the majority of patients, a TR signal can commonly be detected. Characterization of the regurgitation Doppler jet is important in differentiating between physiologic and pathologic TR.

Angiography has constituted the gold standard technique for evaluation of severe TR, although it is mandatory to use special techniques to avoid increasing the degree of regurgitation with malposition of the catheter across the tricuspid valve (35). There may be a discrepancy between the angiographic and hemodynamic degree of severity of TR. In our experience, the echo/Doppler or angiographic degree of TR can be severe, while the hemodynamic data may exhibit only mild-to-moderate hemodynamic disturbance. Discrepancy between the hemodynamic and the angiographic Doppler assessment of TR may at times constitute a challenge and create difficulties in clinical decision-making for the clinician. Integration of the results of invasive and noninvasive diagnostic techniques with a thorough clinical assessment are of paramount importance in achieving the correct management decision in each patient's case. These patients, who have been at bed rest before cardiac catheterization, may have had a large dose of diuretics with prolonged periods of fasting and may be volume depleted. The gold standard technique for evaluation of TR is, at present, the pulsed and color Doppler.

PULMONARY VALVE

Congenital heart disease accounts for the great majority of abnormalities of the pulmonary valve. Rheumatic heart disease virtually never involves the pulmonary valve. Since patients with severe pulmonary stenosis may be asymptomatic, the diagnosis is established by physical examination and confirmed by imaging techniques, i.e., 2-DE and Doppler studies, or angiography with hemodynamic studies.

Pathologic Findings in Pulmonary Valve Disease

Congenital pulmonic stenosis is the most common valvular lesion in children and may be associated with other cardiac defects. Pathologically, the valve exhibits the characteristic features with a dome-shaped stenosis with commissural fusion and a minute central opening. Dysplastic pulmonary valve occurs in 10% of cases of congenital pulmonary stenosis and may be associated with Noonan syndrome (36). Commonly associated with a small pulmonary valve annulus, in pulmonary atresia (37) associated with Fallot's tetralogy, the commissures may be completely fused with no opening. A pulmonary valve with four equal cusps is not uncommon and is usually of no clinical significance. The pulmonary valve can be involved in carcinoid (8), as the tumor cells may lead to thickening and to restricted leaflet motion with concomitant stenosis. Functional pulmonic valve regurgitation may occur in the context of pulmonary hypertension with dilatation of the annulus and structural leaflet abnormalities.

Clinical Features in Pulmonary Valve Disease

The symptoms of pulmonic stenosis (PS) are related to the associated cardiac defects and severity of the obstruction.

Patients with a mild-to-moderate degree of PS are asymptomatic and lead a normal active life. Patients with severe PS may be asymptomatic until late adulthood. Symptoms may develop in patients with PS particularly when the RV fails. Infants born with severe PS present with heart failure and cyanosis as a result of shunting via a patent foramen ovale.

Pulmonic stenosis presents with an ejection systolic murmur at the left sternal border and a systolic thrill when the obstruction is severe. The length of the murmur is related to the severity of the stenosis. With severe stenosis, the murmur is louder, longer, and harsher. The pulmonic component of the second heart sound is soft. A characteristic early systolic ejection click is detected at the pulmonary focus. The click helps establish the differential diagnosis between pulmonary valve stenosis, subpulmonary obstruction, and ventricular septal defect. Patients with pulmonary hypertension may develop a Graham Steell early diastolic murmur of pulmonic regurgitation.

Electrocardiographic and Radiologic Findings in Pulmonary Valve Disease

The electrocardiogram may be normal in mild PS. The ECG will exhibit right axis deviation and features of RV hypertrophy in moderate-to-severe cases of PS. The P pulmonale may also develop in the inferior ECG leads. The chest x-ray shows a dilated main pulmonary trunk without cardiomegaly. The lung fields are usually normal but, in severe pulmonic stenosis, may exhibit oligemia.

Echocardiographic and Doppler Studies in Pulmonary Valve Disease

Echo Doppler is the technique of choice for imaging the pulmonary valve and evaluating the physiology of the obstruction and the degree of pulmonary regurgitation (Fig. 6; see also Color Plate 23 following page 294). To assess the pulmonary valve morphology, two-dimensional echocardiography is done in the parasternal short-axis and subcostal views. Patients with pulmonic valve stenosis will exhibit a thick and domed valve with restriction of cusp motion. The main pulmonary artery is frequently dilated as a consequence of the poststenotic jet. From the parasternal long-axis view, the pulmonary artery bifurcation is usually well visualized. Bright echoes in adult patients indicate calcium deposits in the leaflets. In severe cases, the RV exhibits concentric hypertrophy. Normally, the RV wall thickness measures 3 to 4 mm. The measurement of the annulus together with the valve echocardiographic appearance helps establish the diagnosis of dysplastic valve (36).

Continuous-wave Doppler, using the modified Bernoulli equation, enables the calculation of peak and mean pulmonic transvalvular gradients (37). Studies have shown an excellent correlation between the Doppler and cardiac catheterization gradients (38). Traditionally, the pressure gradient cal-

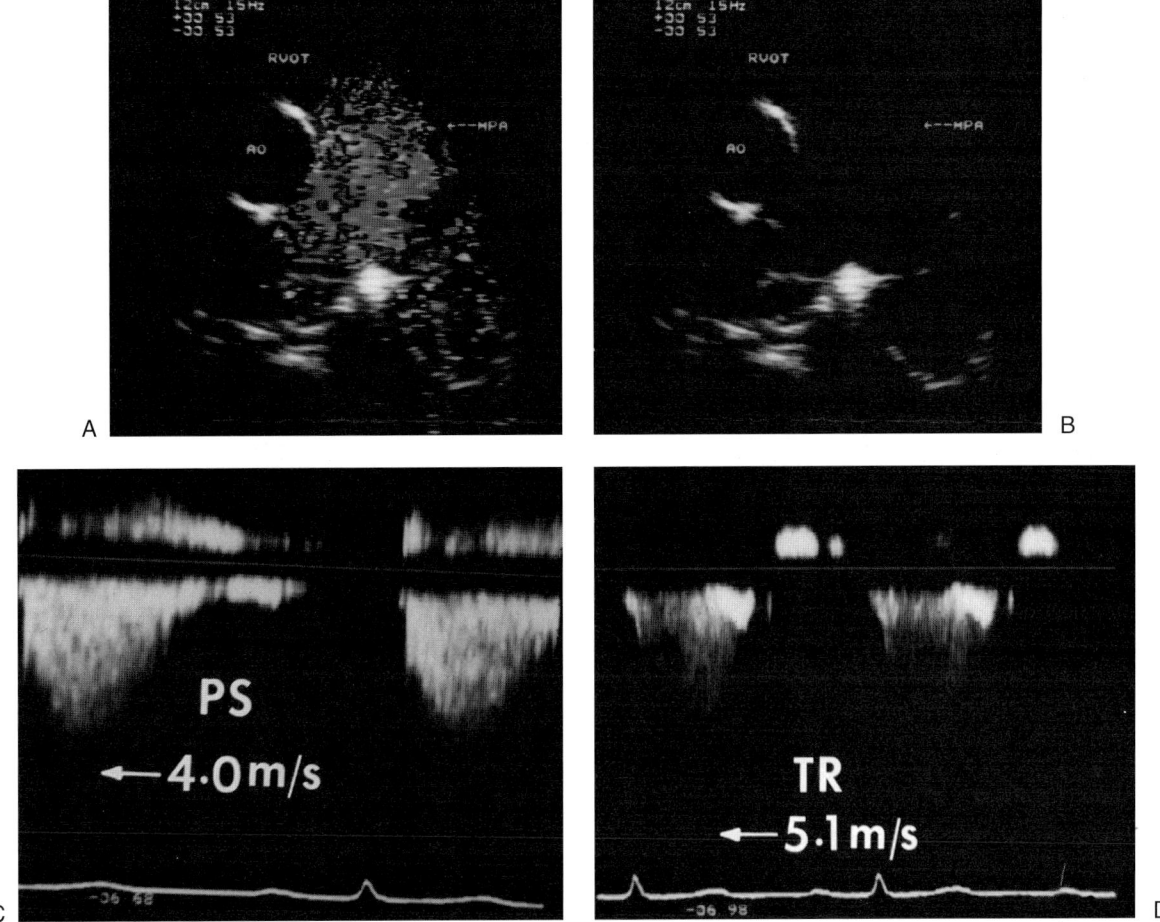

FIG. 6. Parasternal two-dimensional echocardiographic study from a patient with severe valvular pulmonic stenosis (*PS*): **A:** Panel shows the mosaic-like color flow jet of PS during systole in the main pulmonary artery (MPA). **B:** Panel of the same image without color, showing dilated MPA. **C:** Panel of continuous-wave Doppler (CWD) study of the PS jet showing velocity of 4 m/sec, consistent with a peak gradient of 64 mm Hg. **D:** Image shows trace of *TR*, using CWD. The TR velocity is 5.1 m/sec, consistent with right ventricular systolic pressure of 110 mm Hg. *TR,* tricuspid regurgitation. (See also Color Plate 23 following page 294.) (Courtesy of Ramesh Bansal, M.D.)

culation by continuous wave Doppler is the method of choice to assess the severity of the PS as well as the results of balloon valvotomy and surgical repair (39). Theoretically, one can calculate pulmonary valve area using the continuity equation.

Some patients may present with concomitant RV infundibular stenosis. Doppler flow signal pattern in these patients exhibits the dagger-shaped late systolic envelope typical of dynamic obstruction. Sampling from the apical or subcostal approach may in some cases be more accurate than from the short-axis view. Color flow mapping typically demonstrates the level of the pulmonary obstruction and aids in the diagnosis. It is also valuable in allowing optimal continuous wave Doppler alignment with the jet for accurate assessment of velocity. Pulsed wave Doppler sampling from the RV outflow tract and pulmonic valve also is of value in localizing the level of obstruction (38). In patients with more than one level of pulmonary obstruction or pulmonic valve regurgita-

tion, continuous wave Doppler may overestimate the pressure gradient. In contrast, in patients with severe pulmonary valve stenosis and RV failure, the Doppler signal that reflects velocity may underestimate the degree of stenosis.

The degree of concomitant pulmonary incompetence and the derangement of RV filling can be accurately assessed by Doppler studies (40). Color Doppler is a very sensitive and accurate means of assessing the degree of pulmonic valve regurgitation (40). Since this is a very sensitive technique, the differentiation between physiologic and genuine pathologic pulmonic incompetence may at times be difficult (41–44). Color flow jets that extend less than 1 cm into the RV outflow tract are usually classified as physiologic. Echocardiographic studies in which the degree of regurgitation on color flow image (CFI) extend more than 1 cm indicates pathology. There is no validation of the criteria that differentiates between mild, moderate, and severe pulmonary valve regurgitation. This is due, in part, to the fact that no gold standard technique is available to enable a correlative study.

Pulmonary angiography is plagued with limitation of passing a catheter through the pulmonary valve and injecting into the pulmonary artery. Pulsed-wave Doppler can define the area of pulmonary incompetence (43). The signal pattern does not quantify the severity of the TR. In contrast, the intensity of the velocity signal and the shape of the continuous-wave Doppler correlates with the severity of the pulmonary regurgitation. There is a maximal early diastolic peak velocity similar to that observed in aortic regurgitation with a gradual diastolic decrease. Continuous-wave Doppler signal also can be used for measuring pulmonary artery pressure accurately (44). Severe pulmonary incompetence exhibits a Doppler signal with a rapid velocity deceleration that virtually disappears in late diastole, as the right ventricular and right atrial pressures equalize (45). In patients with concomitant PS and regurgitation, the increased flow across the pulmonary valve increases the velocity across it, and this may overestimate the true gradient.

Echocardiography is the best imaging technique to detect vegetation or tumor attached to the pulmonary valve. Endocarditis is uncommon in the pulmonary valve, unless the patients also have a concomitant ventricular septal defect. The most common benign tumor attached to the pulmonary valve is fibroelastoma. Rare cases of thickening of the pulmonary valve with concomitant pulmonary incompetence may be secondary to carcinoid heart disease or ergot alkaloid deposits.

Angiography and Hemodynamic Studies in Pulmonary Valve Disease

Angiography of the right ventricle in the lateral or anteroposterior view is an established method in diagnosing pulmonic stenosis. The negative contrast jet shows the classic doming of the pulmonary valve together with the jet across the tight opening of the pulmonary valve. The main pulmonary artery usually exhibits poststenotic dilation. For measurement of the gradient, a pull-back is usually done from the pulmonary artery to the RV, and a gradient of 50 mm Hg is usually indicative of moderate to severe PS.

CONCLUSIONS

The clinical diagnosis of tricuspid and pulmonary valve disease is made after a detailed clinical history and cardiovascular physical examination. Two-dimensional echocardiography and Doppler are the best techniques to confirm the diagnosis and assess severity of the tricuspid and pulmonary valve lesions and establish the etiology of the disease.

ACKNOWLEDGMENTS

We are grateful to Sally Angell for the superb secretarial work in typing the manuscript. Our thanks to Dr. Ramesh Bansal for his personal prints used in this chapter.

REFERENCES

1. Virmani R. The tricuspid valve. *Mayo Clinic Proc* 1988;63:943–946.
2. Silver MD, Lam JHC, Rangathan N, et al. Morphology of the human tricuspid valve. *Circulation* 1971:43;333–348.
3. Hauck AJ, Freeman DP, Ackerman DM, et al. Surgical pathology of the tricuspid valve: a study of 363 cases spanning 25 years. *Mayo Clinic Proc* 1988;63:851–863.
4. Redfield MM, Holmes DR, Edwards WD, et al. Valve disease associates with ergot alkaloid use: echocardiographic and pathologic correlations. *Ann Intern Med* 1992;117:50–52.
5. Connolly HM, Crary JL, McGoon MD, et al. Valvular heart disease associated with fenfluramine-phentermine. *New Engl J Med* 1997;9: 581–588.
6. Ribeiro PA, Zaibag MA, Sawyer W. A prospective study comparing the hemodynamic with the cross-sectional echocardiographic diagnosis of rheumatic tricuspid stenosis. *Eur Heart J* 1989;10:120–126.
7. Cook WT, White PD. Tricuspid stenosis with particular reference to diagnosis and prognosis. *Br Heart J* 1941;3:147–152.
8. Carpena C, Kay JH, Mendex AM, et al. Carcinoid heart disease: surgery for tricuspid and pulmonary lesions. *Am J Cardiol* 1973;32:229–233.
9. Callahan JA, Wroblewski EM, Reeder GS, et al. Echocardiographic features of carcinoid heart disease. *Am J Cardiol* 1982;50:762–768.
10. Davies J, Ball JD. The pathology of endomyocardial fibrosis in Uganda. *Br Heart J* 1955;17:337–342.
11. Shiina A, Seward JB, Edwards WD, et al. Two-dimensional echocardiographic spectrum of Ebstein's anomaly: detailed anatomic assessment. *J Am Coll Cardiol* 1984;3:356–370.
12. Kitchen A, Turner R. Diagnosis and treatment of tricuspid stenosis. *Br Heart J* 1964;26:354–359.
13. Hatle L, Angelsen B. *Doppler ultrasound in cardiology: physical principles and clinical application*, 2nd ed. Philadelphia: Lea & Febiger, 1985:170–176.
14. Salazar E, Levine HD. Rheumatic tricuspid regurgitation. The clinical spectrum. *Am J Med* 1962;33:111–129.
15. Feigenbaum H. *Echocardiography*, 3rd ed. Philadelphia: Lea & Febiger, 1981:239–327.
16. Daniels SJ, Mintz GS, Kotler MN. Rheumatic tricuspid valve disease: two-dimensional echocardiographic, haemodynamic, and angiographic correlations. *Am J Cardiol* 1983;51:492–496.
17. Tei C, Pilgrim JP, Shah PM, et al. The tricuspid valve annulus study of size and motion in normal subjects and in patients with tricuspid regurgitation. *Circulation* 1982;66:665–771.
18. Morrison DA, Ouitt T, Hammermeister KE. Functional tricuspid regurgitation and right ventricular dysfunction in pulmonary hypertension. *Am J Cardiol* 1988;62:108–112.
19. Zone DD, Botti RE. Right ventricular infarction with tricuspid insufficiency and chronic heart failure. *Am J Cardiol* 1976;37:445–448.
20. Arbulu A, Asfaw I. Tricuspid valvulectomy without prosthetic replacement. Ten years of clinical experience. *J Thorac Cardiovasc Surg* 1981; 82:684–691.
21. Mikami T, Kudo T, Sakurai N, et al. Mechanisms for development of functional tricuspid regurgitation determined by pulsed Doppler and two-dimensional echocardiography. *Am J Cardiol* 1984;53:160–164.
22. Xavier de Brito AH, Seuff JA, Toledo AN, et al. Early stages of tricuspid stenosis. *Am J Cardiol* 1966;18:57–63.
23. Cha SD, Desai RS, Gooch AS, et al. Diagnosis of severe tricuspid regurgitation. *Chest* 1982;82:726–731.
24. Glancy DL, Marcus FI, Cuadra M, et al. Isolated organic tricuspid regurgitation. *Am J Med* 1969;46:989–995.
25. Miyatake K, Okamoto M, Konishata N, et al. Evaluation of tricuspid regurgitation by pulsed Doppler and two-dimensional echocardiography. *Circulation* 1982;66:777–784.
26. Nimura Y, Miyatake K, Okamoto M, et al. Pulsed Doppler echocardiography in the assessment of tricuspid regurgitation. *Ultrasound Med Biol* 1984;10:239–247.
27. Pennestri F, Loperfido F, Salvatori MP, et al. Assessment of tricuspid regurgitation by pulsed Doppler ultrasonography of the hepatic veins. *Am J Cardiol* 1984;54:363–368.
28. Ubago JL, Figueiroa A, Ochoteco A, et al. Analysis of the amount of tricuspid valve annular dilatation required to produce functional tricuspid regurgitation. *Am J Cardiol* 1983;52:155–158.

29. Coelho E. Physiopathologic study (clinical and experimental) of the tricuspid valve. *Am J Cardiol* 1959;3:517–523.

30. Nanna M, Chandrepapna A, Reid C, et al. Value of two-dimensional echocardiography in detecting tricuspid stenosis. *Circulation* 1977;67: 221–224.

31. Maddahi J, Berman DS, Matsouka DT, et al. A new technique for assessing right ventricular ejection fraction using rapid multiple gated equilibrium cardiac pool scintigraphy. *Circulation* 1979;60:581–589.

32. Muller O, Schillingford J. Tricuspid incompetence. *Br Heart J* 1954; 16:195–198.

33. Yoshid K, Yoshikawa J, Shakudo M, et al. Colour Doppler evaluation of valvular regurgitation in normal subjects. *Circulation* 1988;78: 840–847.

34. Ubago JL, Figueroa A, Colman T, et al. Right ventriculography as a valid method for the diagnosis of tricuspid insufficiency. *Cathet Cardiov Diagn* 1981;7:433–451.

35. Emmanouilides GC, Baylen BG. Pulmonary stenosis. In: Adams FH, Emmanouilides GC, eds. *Heart disease in infants, children, and adolescents*, 3rd ed. Baltimore: Williams & Wilkins, 1983.

36. Freed MD, et al. Critical pulmonary stenosis with dimunitve right ventricle in neonates. *Circulation* 1973;48:875–881.

37. Kosturakis D, Allen HD, Goldberg SJ, et al. Noninvasive quantification of stenotic semilunar valve areas by Doppler echocardiography. *J Am Coll Cardiol* 1984;3:1256–1262.

38. Johnson GL, Kwan OL, Handshoe S, et al. Accuracy of combined two-dimensional echocardiography and continuous-wave Doppler recordings in the estimation of pressure gradient in right ventricular outlet obstruction. *J Am Coll Cardiol* 1984;3:1013–1018.

39. Mullins CE, Ludomirsky A, O'Laughlin MP, et al. Balloon valvuloplasty for pulmonic valve stenosis: two-year follow-up: hemodynamic and Doppler evaluation. *Cathet Cardiovasc Diagn* 1988;14: 76–81.

40. Berger M, Hecht SR, van Tosh A, et al. Pulsed and continuous wave Doppler echocardiographic assessment of valvular regurgitation in normal subjects. *J Am Coll Cardiol* 1989;13:1540–1545.

41. Nimura Y, Miyatake K, Izumi S. Physiological regurgitation identified by Doppler techniques. *Echocardiography* 1989;6:385–392.

42. Yoshida K, Yoshikawa J, Shakudo M, et al. Color Doppler evaluation of valvular regurgitation in normal subjects. *Circulation* 1988;78: 840–847.

43. Kostuchi W, Vandenbossche J, Friart A, et al. Pulsed Doppler regurgitant flow patterns of normal valves. *Am J Cardiol* 1986;58:309–313.

44. Masuyama T, Kodama K, Kitabatake A, et al. Continuous-wave Doppler echocardiographic detection of pulmonary regurgitation and its application to noninvasive estimation of pulmonary artery pressure. *Circulation* 1986;74:484–492.

45. Miyatake K, Okamoto M, Konoshita N, et al. Pulmonary regurgitation studied with the ultrasonic pulsed Doppler technique. *Circulation* 1982; 65:969–976.

46. Noonan JA. Hypertelorism with Turner phenotype: a new syndrome with associated congenital heart disease. *Am J Dis Child* 1968;116: 373.

CHAPTER 43

Evaluation of Prosthetic Heart Valves

Miguel Zabalgoitia and Mohammed A. Oraby

The optimal management of patients with prosthetic heart valves requires serial assessment of valve function and left ventricular (LV) performance. Symptoms of fatigue, dyspnea, and exercise intolerance in patients with prosthetic heart valves may be due to valve dysfunction or to a variety of comorbid conditions. Doppler echocardiography is the imaging modality of choice in evaluating patients with known or suspected prosthetic valve dysfunction because it provides reliable information regarding native and prosthetic valve structure and function, reproducible hemodynamic data for serial examinations, and accurate assessment of regional and global systolic LV contractility (1). Since its clinical introduction a decade ago, transesophageal echocardiography (TEE) has been widely accepted as a test that allows superior anatomic and functional assessment of native and prosthetic valves, and, thus, it has changed the diagnostic ability of ultrasound from a predominantly ''stage of limitations'' into a more accurate recognition of prosthetic malfunction.

This chapter presents a practical approach to the use of Doppler echocardiography in prosthetic heart valves in a frame of cost containment. Evaluation of cost and effectiveness of diagnostic testing tends to be complex, because it involves not only the test itself, but also the treatment strategies that follow (2). In assessing the cost analysis of a diagnostic test, one must answer the following questions: (i) Is the test involved in the clinical decision-making process?, (ii) Does the test lead toward the treatment of choice?, (iii) What is the accuracy of the test?, (iv) What is the cost of the test, and (v) What is the morbidity of the test? Although a formal cost analysis of echocardiography for assessing prosthetic heart valves is lacking, the answer to each of the preceding questions is clearly favorable. Thus, the clinician's perception of echocardiography in evaluating these patients is not only that it is a widely accepted test but also a highly cost-effective tool.

FUNDAMENTAL PRINCIPLES PERTAINING TO PROSTHESES

Before describing normal and abnormal prosthetic valve characteristics, it is important to review briefly several fundamental ultrasound principles as they relate to cardiac valve prostheses.

Modified Bernoulli Equation

The blood flow velocity through a narrow orifice is related to the pressure difference between the two chambers as described by the Bernoulli principle, which is used to convert flow velocity (m/sec) to pressure gradient (mm Hg). The modified Bernoulli equation used in prosthetic valves is the same as that used in native valves:

$$Pressure\ gradient\ =\ 4 \cdot V_{MAX}^{2}$$

where V_{MAX} is the maximal (peak) velocity across the valve orifice. It is important to recognize that the modified Bernoulli equation neglects the effects of acceleration and viscous losses, and yet it is quite accurate when compared to simultaneous obtained catheter-derived pressure gradients (3). Whenever the outflow tract velocity is greater than 1 m/sec, such as in patients with concomitant aortic regurgitation, this velocity should be subtracted from V_{MAX}. For aortic valves, both maximal instantaneous and mean gradients are calculated, whereas for mitral valves only the mean gradient is calculated.

M. Zabalgoitia: Department of Medicine; Department of Echocardiography, University of Texas Health Science Center at San Antonio, San Antonio, Texas 78229.

M. A. Oraby: Department of Medicine/Cardiology, University of Texas Health Science Center at San Antonio; Department of Medicine/Cardiology, University Hospital, San Antonio, Texas 78229.

Pressure Recovery

Recording valve gradients that appear to be an "overestimation," when compared with those at catheterization, may result from distal pressure recovery, which refers to the conversion of *kinetic* energy present at the valve level to *pressure* energy distal to the valve (4). When flow passes through the prosthesis, components of velocity and momentum are directed inward, causing the flow to continue to contract distally for a short distance. This point of maximal constriction is called *vena contracta* and occurs downstream distally from the anatomic location of the prosthesis. As the jet expands and decelerates beyond the vena contracta, the associated turbulence results in an increase in aortic pressure ("pressure recovery"), such that, when aortic pressure is measured in the distal ascending aorta, the LV/aortic *pressure difference* is less than if the aortic pressure was measured at the vena contracta. The degree of pressure recovery may be as high as a mean of 10 mm Hg in small St. Jude valves challenged under physiologic flow rates. The magnitude of pressure recovery is greater with larger valve areas and with smaller aortic roots. Thus patients with severe prosthetic stenosis and poststenotic aortic root dilation may show *less* pressure recovery than patients with mild to moderate stenosis and normal aortic root dimensions.

Pressure recovery and vena contracta are important concepts to consider when Doppler- and catheter-derived pressure gradients are compared. *Since continuous-wave Doppler measures velocity at the level of the vena contracta (physiologic variable), and catheterization measures the difference between LV and the fully recovered static pressure in the aorta, it is the catheter-derived data that must be interpreted with caution.* Failure of the invasive technique to record the gradient at the vena contracta may explain some of the reported discrepancies (5).

Continuity Equation

An important limitation of Doppler velocities (and derived pressure gradients) is that they are volume and rate dependent. When transvalvular flow is decreased, such as in patients with significant systolic LV dysfunction, Doppler velocities may only be moderately elevated despite severe obstruction. Thus, comparisons may be confounded by interval changes in flow volume and rate. For these reasons, calculation of valve areas, in addition to mean pressure gradients, should be routinely calculated.

The equation of continuity can be used to estimate aortic as well as mitral valve areas. For the aortic valve area (*AVA*), one can use either velocity time integrals or peak velocities (*V*):

$$AVA = A_{LVOT} \cdot V_{LVOT} / V_{TRANSPROSTHESIS}$$

where A_{LVOT} is the cross-sectional area of the outflow tract measured from the two-dimensional parasternal long-axis view, V_{LVOT} is the velocity proximal to the valve from an apical view using pulse-wave Doppler, and $V_{TRANSPROSTHESIS}$

is the velocity through the prosthesis from an apical view using continuous-wave Doppler. Since the direction of the aortic jet across a prosthetic valve is unpredictable and often eccentric, all three acoustic aortic windows (apical, suprasternal, and right parasternal) need to be interrogated to detect the highest velocity signal. Continuity equation areas correlate well with the various valve sizes (6). The largest source of variability in calculating the area from this equation is the accurate and reliable measurement of the LV outflow tract. When this diameter is difficult to obtain from the precordial window, TEE offers an excellent alternative, as has previously been reported from our laboratory (7).

For the mitral valve area (*MVA*) the continuity equation is:

$$MVA = (AVA \cdot VTI_{AORTIC}) / VTI_{TRANSPROSTHESIS}$$

where *AVA* is the cross-sectional aortic valve area as measured from the parasternal long-axis view, VTI_{AORTIC} is the velocity time integral across the native aortic valve, and $VTI_{TRANSPROSTHESIS}$ is that across the mitral prosthesis (8). The continuity equation, based on the principle of *conservation of mass*, assumes that flow across the mitral prosthesis and the second valve are equal. Thus, in patients with more than mild mitral regurgitation, the preferred method to estimate the valve area is the pressure half-time. In the presence of aortic regurgitation, the pulmonic valve area and flow can be used in lieu of the aortic valve. However, the limiting step in using the pulmonic valve is the accurate and reproducible measurement of the right ventricular outflow tract from the precordial approach. An important advantage of the continuity equation is its relative independence from valvular gradient and chamber compliance. However, the measurements for the continuity equation are more cumbersome to obtain than those for the pressure half-time formula.

The aortic and mitral valve areas calculated from invasive data using the Gorlin formula have been useful for making clinical decisions over many years. However, the Gorlin formula and continuity equation have different governing principles with a similar goal. The continuity equation relates the physiologic flow area of the vena contracta, whereas the Gorlin formula assumes a laminar flow passing through a flat orifice. Neither of these two conditions—laminar flow nor a flat orifice—occur physiologically in either native or prosthetic valve stenosis (9). Thus, it should not be expected that the two valve areas be identical to each other. The accuracy, reproducibility, and ability to predict the patient's outcome are certainly more important than the degree of agreement between the two measurements.

Doppler Velocity Index

Doppler velocity index (*DVI*) is a dimensionless ratio of the LV outflow tract velocity to that through the prosthesis:

$$DVI = V_{LVOT} / V_{TRANSPROSTHESIS}$$

Since it is *independent* of valve size, this index is particularly useful when the cross-sectional area of the LV outflow tract cannot be obtained. Since the velocity proximal to the valve is subtracted from that across the prosthesis, the patient serves as his/her own control, with flow being the main dependent factor: the higher the index, the larger the area and, in contrast, the lower the index, the smaller the area. The index values calculated from 25 normally functioning St. Jude Medical aortic valves were 0.39 ± 0.07 (range, 0.28 to 0.55). In a small group of patients with severe stenosis of St. Jude Medical aortic valves requiring reoperation, the Doppler velocity index was 0.19 ± 0.05 (range, 0.12 to 0.27), which was significantly different from normal values at the $p < 0.05$ level (10).

Valve Resistance

Resistance is the quotient of gradient and flow: $R = \Delta P/Q$. This hemodynamic parameter was suggested by Ford et al. (11) as an alternative method to the Gorlin formula for assessing severity of *native* aortic stenosis. Valve resistance can be calculated from echo-Doppler data as:

$$Resistance = \Delta P \cdot ET / SV \cdot 1.33$$

where ΔP is the mean pressure gradient in mm Hg, *ET* is ejection time in seconds, and *SV* is stroke volume in mL/min. The ratio of mm Hg to mL/min is converted to dynes $\cdot$ sec $\cdot$ cm^{-5} when multiplied by 1.33. In conditions characterized by variation of flow, valve resistance remains more constant than the area calculated by the Gorlin formula. However, in considering valve resistance, one must recognize that: (i) most data have been derived from *native* valve stenosis, not from prostheses; (ii) no information is available during changing flow conditions, such as exercise; and (iii) there is virtually no clinical data on prosthetic *mitral* valves. Saad et al. (10) studied two groups of patients with prosthetic aortic malfunction (predominant stenosis versus predominant regurgitation) and compared them with a control group. Effective orifice area (continuity equation), Doppler velocity index, and valve resistance are all effective in separating the groups. However, it is unclear whether valve resistance *per se* adds clinically significant information beyond that derived by valve area and Doppler velocity index. Valve resistance in patients with small aortic valve areas, relatively low flow velocities, and severe LV systolic dysfunction may be helpful to differentiate severe prosthetic valve stenosis from a low cardiac output state, as it does in patients with native aortic stenosis (12).

Leakage Backflow

This is a *normal* regurgitant flow that occurs when the occluder has already been seated in its closed position and flow leaks between and around the occluder assembly. Leakage backflow is characteristic of mechanical devices. This ''built-in'' regurgitation has the theoretical advantage to prevent stasis and thrombus formation through a ''washing''

mechanism. Leakage backflow are low-velocity, non-aliasing jets encoded in a homogenous color, red or blue, depending on the location of the transducer. In contrast, abnormal regurgitant jets are wide, large, and frequently eccentric, extending far into the proximal chamber, displaying a mosaic pattern indicative of turbulent flow (13).

ECHOCARDIOGRAPHY OF NORMAL PROSTHETIC HEART VALVES

There are two types of prosthetic heart valves: mechanical and biological. Table 1 depicts the currently FDA-approved prosthetic heart devices for use in this country. Since no prosthetic valve has an effective orifice area as large as a native valve, normally functioning prostheses are thus *inherently* stenotic. In general, the smaller the device size is, the higher the velocities are, and the smaller is the area. Flow velocities and gradients vary depending on the type, size, and position of the prosthesis. Other factors that affect pressure gradients include LV function, heart rate, and duration of systolic ejection or diastolic filling times, depending on the anatomic valve in question. Table 2 describes the normal range of Doppler values for prosthetic valves in the aortic and mitral positions derived from published series (14–17).

For practical purposes, the same systematic approach used in native valves apply to artificial valves. Doppler examination is the cornerstone in assessing prosthetic valve stenosis or regurgitation. Increased flow through a prosthesis increases the transvalvular velocity, just as decreased flow decreases it as well. Thus, *a relatively high gradient in the setting of a hyperkinetic state (such as anemia or sepsis) does not necessarily indicate stenosis. Conversely, a slightly elevated gradient in the setting of severe LV dysfunction may be indicative of significant stenosis.*

Echocardiography has some limitations primarily related to the interface between the ultrasound and the foreign material composing the devices. The intense reverberations projected behind the prosthesis can mask normal structures

TABLE 1. *Prosthetic heart valves currently approved in the United States*

Type	Model	First year
Ball-in-cage	Starr-Edwards	1965
Single-tilting disc	Medtronic-Hall	1977
	OmniScience	1978
Double-tilting disc	St. Jude Medical	1977
	Duromedics	1982
	Carbomedics	1986
Porcine	Hancock Standard	1970
	Hancock MO	1978
	CE Standard	1971
	CE Supra Annular	1982
Pericardial	Carpentier-Edwards	1982
Homograft	Non-commercial	1962
	Commercial	1984
Autologous	Non-commercial	1967

CE, Carpentier-Edwards; *MO*, modified orifice.

TABLE 2. *Normal Doppler values for aortic and mitral prostheses*

Aortic prostheses	Peak velocity (m/s)	Mean gradient (mm Hg)	Area mean (cm²)	Area range (cm²)
Starr-Edwards	3.1 ± 0.5	24 ± 4	*	*
Bjork-Shiley	2.5 ± 0.6	14 ± 5	2.2	1.6–2.9
St. Jude Medical	3.0 ± 0.8	11 ± 6	2.4	1.8–3.4
CarboMedics	2.5 ± 0.5	14 ± 5	2.3	1.8–3.2
Medtronic Hall	2.6 ± 0.3	12 ± 3	*	*
OmniScience	2.8 ± 0.4	14 ± 3	*	*
Aortic Homograft	0.8 ± 0.4	7.1 ± 3	2.2	1.7–3.1
Hancock	2.4 ± 0.4	12 ± 2	1.8	1.4–2.3
Carpentier-Edwards	2.4 ± 0.5	14 ± 6	1.8	1.2–3.1
Mitral prostheses	Peak velocity (m/s)	Mean gradient (mm Hg)	Area mean (cm²)	Area range (cm²)
Starr-Edwards	1.8 ± 0.4	4.6 ± 2.4	2.1	1.2–2.5
Bjork-Shiley	1.6 ± 0.3	5.0 ± 2.0	2.4	1.6–3.7
St. Jude Medical	1.6 ± 0.3	5.0 + 2.0	2.9	1.8–3.9
Medtronic Hall	1.7 ± 0.3	3.1 ± 0.9	2.4	1.5–3.9
OmniScience	1.8 ± 0.3	3.3 ± 0.9	1.9	1.6–3.1
Hancock	1.5 ± 0.3	4.3 ± 2.1	1.7	1.3–2.7
Carpentier-Edwards	1.8 ± 0.2	6.5 ± 2.1	2.5	1.6–3.5

* Insufficient data available.
(Data from refs. 14–17, with permission.)

or create artifacts leading to a misdiagnosis (i.e., thrombus). To utilize echocardiography at its maximal capacity, one should be aware of the most common technical errors or "pitfalls" (18) and aware of some practical suggestions on how to minimize them (Table 3). A very helpful and frequently overlooked practice in evaluating prosthetic valves is the comparison with prior studies. The importance of a timely postoperative study cannot be overemphasized. This initial study establishes the baseline gradient and area for that particular valve, in that patient, at that time. This "hemodynamic fingerprint" profile can then be used in the future if prosthetic valve malfunction becomes a concern. The frequency with which Doppler echocardiographic studies should be performed routinely in uncomplicated patients is uncertain. In general bioprostheses need to be followed more closely than mechanical valves because of the unavoidable risk of structural deterioration after 5 years in the mitral position and after 8 years in the aortic position. A practical schedule is recommended in Table 4.

The importance of the technical aspects in recording a complete and thorough Doppler echocardiographic examination should be obvious. The quality of the echocardiographic recording is an essential ingredient for an accurate interpretation of data and for patient management. The premise that *the real value of echocardiography is bearing in the hand of the beholder* has been successfully tested over time; the more complex and difficult the condition, the stronger the premise holds.

Mechanical Valves

These include the ball-in-cage, the single tilting-disk, and the double tilting-disk mechanisms. Of the ball-in-cage design, only the Starr-Edwards valve has endured. When the

TABLE 3. *Echocardiography of prosthetic heart valves: limitations and pitfalls*

Technical limitations/ pitfalls	Suggestions
Reverberations and acoustic shadowing	Optimize gain settings Use alternative view where area of interest is not "obscured" by the device Consider TEE (i.e., mitral position)
Failure to obtain maximal velocity	Guide with color-flow in case of mitral valve Use suprasternal, right supraclavicular, and right parasternal in case of aortic valve
Under or over estimation of valve gradient or effective orifice area	Include proximal velocity in continuity equation if $V_1 > 1$m/sec (i.e., aortic regurgitation) Consider *pressure recovery* Use *mean* gradient rather than peak gradient
Unexpectedly high valve gradient or abnormally small orifice area	Consider clinical setting (tachycardia, anemia, high cardiac output state) and repeat study under more "steady" conditions Calculate Doppler velocity index Calculate valve resistance Consider *prosthesis-patient* mismatch Remeasure LVOT diameter or consider TEE for this purpose Consider stress echocardiography to exclude valve dysfunction

LVOT, left ventricular outflow tract; *TEE,* transesophageal echocardiography.

TABLE 4. *Recommendations for Doppler echocardiography follow-up in patients with prosthetic heart valves*

Patient category	Recommendation*
A. Early follow-up	
Biological or mechanical	Baseline in all patients < 6 weeks post-op
B. Late follow-up	
Bioprosthetic valves	Every 2–3 years for the first 6 years, then every year
Mechanical valves	Every 3–5 years
C. Clinical suspicion of valve dysfunction	
Mitral position	TEE
Aortic position	Precordial study first, it suboptimal or clinically inconsistent, proceed with TEE

* Implies transthoracic studies unless otherwise specified. *TEE,* transesophageal echocardiography.

silicone rubber ball retracts toward the apex of the cobalt-chromium cage, blood passes through the valve orifice and flows between the ball and the stents.

In single-tilting valves, when the pyrolytic carbon disk opens, blood flows through two unequal (major and minor) orifices, and the disk remains open with an angle of less than 80 degrees, which favors closure by a backflow mechanism. Color in normal single-tilting disk valves includes leakage backflow around the central strut and between the disk and the sewing ring. The Medtronic-Hall valve has a characteristic large central backflow jet that can extend far into the proximal chamber with aliasing, whereas the peripheral jets are nonaliased, low-velocity flows (13).

The double-tilting disk prostheses, like St. Jude Medical and CarboMedics, have an opening angle greater than 80 degrees, resulting in little deviation of flow through the valve orifice. The two-dimensional imaging of a normally functioning bileaflet valve includes the sewing ring and two distinct linear echoes during valve opening. Identification of the two hemidiscs may be problematic with the standard precordial approach, particularly in the aortic position. As illustrated in Figure 1, TEE visualizes the hemidiscs quite well in the mitral position. Doppler gradients through the side orifices closely approximate the transvalvular and net pressure gradients (4). Color flow demonstrates leakage backflow at the disk periphery, at the central closure line, and at the hinge points. The CarboMedics valve is a newer version of the bileaflet mechanism with recessed pivots that result in larger regurgitant backflow jets, which may extend far back into the receiving chamber, but are nonaliased, low-velocity jets.

Biological Valves

These include *autografts* harvested from the same patient, *homografts* harvested from cadaveric human hearts, and *heterografts* harvested or tailored from another species, particularly porcine. An important advantage of all biological valves is the absence of need for chronic anticoagulation. The Ross procedure is an autotransplant of the pulmonic valve into his or her aortic position, with a bioprosthesis replacing the pulmonic valve. This operation is in itself a double valve replacement to solve a single problem, and, as such, it has the attendant early and late risks. The aortic homograft is the preferred substitute in young patients. The major advantages of autografts and homografts are their relative resistance to infection and the excellent hemodynamic profile, most notably in smaller sizes. Pre- or intraoperative TEE measurement of the aortic annulus is frequently used to select the correct valve size (19). The Carpentier-Edwards pericardial valve represents a new generation of bioprosthesis with a different manufacturing design to improve longevity (20).

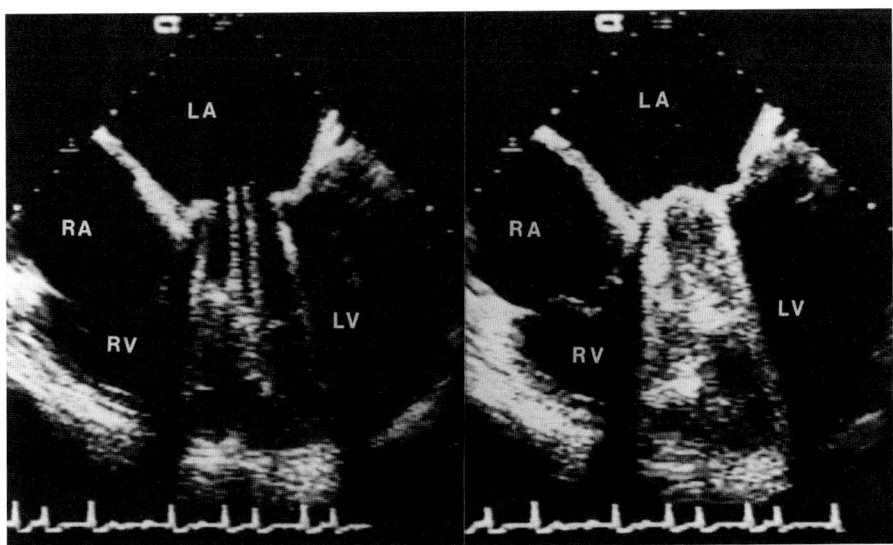

FIG. 1. Transesophageal imaging of a normally functioning St. Jude Medical mitral prosthesis in its opening (**A**) and closing (**B**) positions. *LA,* left atrium; *LV,* left ventricle; *RA,* right atrium; *RV,* right ventricle.

A,B

ECHOCARDIOGRAPHY OF PROSTHETIC VALVE DYSFUNCTION

In addition to a careful clinical examination, transthoracic Doppler echocardiography should be part of the initial assessment. As it overcomes the problem of left atrial shadowing seen when mitral mechanical prostheses are imaged from the apical precordial window, TEE has significantly improved the diagnostic ability of ultrasound to detect common and uncommon valve abnormalities (7). Table 5 depicts several clinical conditions where TEE is frequently indicated. However, because of its increased sensitivity, the operator requires experience and clinical judgment. Cardiac catheterization and angiography may provide definitive confirmation; however, based on clinical and economical grounds, their use should be restricted to patients in whom echocardiography, including TEE, has not provided a definitive diagnosis. Description of prosthetic valve dysfunction should follow recommended guidelines (21).

Structural Deterioration

This is a dysfunction resulting from an *intrinsic* valve problem causing stenosis or regurgitation, and includes stress fracture, poppet or disk escape, calcification, degeneration, and torn leaflet.

Mechanical Valves

Primary malfunction is rarely encountered in the currently available mechanical prostheses (22). Old versions of the Starr-Edwards valve had a rare failure called *ball variance*, which refers to conformational changes in the ball, presum-

ably due to lipid absorption. Ball variance could result in emboli from thrombus formed on the irregular cracked ball surface, in stenosis due to thrombosis, or in regurgitation due to sticking of the ball within the cage. The Convexo-Concave version of the Bjork-Shiley valve had several cases of strut fracture resulting in disk embolization and its subsequent removal from the United States market. However, this valve was implanted in thousands of patients in this country who continue to need clinical and echocardiographic follow-up.

Biological Valves

For most recipients of bioprosthetic valves, structural deterioration is probably inevitable if he or she lives long enough. Findings of leaflet thickening in the absence of endocarditis most likely represent calcific degeneration. However, a thickened and often irregular cusp(s) appearance can also be seen in endocarditis. Thus, the echocardiographic interpretation of "fibrocalcific changes" on bioprosthetic cusps should be based on the overall clinical context. Calcific degeneration may lead to stenosis due to restricted cusp motion or to regurgitation due to flail cusp(s). Figure 2 illus-

TABLE 5. *Prosthetic valve conditions where TEE is indicated*

Stenotic valves
  Suspected acute valve thrombosis
  Follow-up of thrombolytic therapy for valve thrombosis
  Abnormal precordial Doppler velocities without an obvious cause
Regurgitation
  All mitral prosthesis if suspected moderately severe (3+) or severe (4+)
  Aortic prostheses with clinical and precordial echo discrepancies
  Aortic valve conduits for evaluation of proximal aorta
Thromboembolic event
  Stroke, transient ischemic attacks, or other peripheral embolism
  Nondiagnostic precordial echocardiogram
Endocarditis
  Could be the initial study with a high clinical suspicion
  Spiking fevers despite appropriate antibiotic therapy
  Unexplained development of congestive heart failure
  Suspicion of sepsis-related complications i.e., abscess, dehiscence, mycotic aneurysm
  Pre- or intraoperative assessment

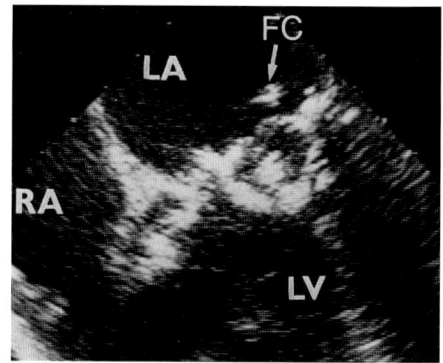

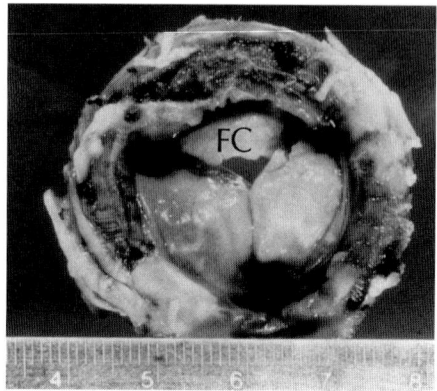

FIG. 2. A: Upper panel illustrates the transesophageal imaging of a degenerated bioprostheses in the mitral position associated with severe regurgitation. The patient presented with classic symptoms of severe congestive heart failure. *Arrow* indicates the flail cusp (*FC*). **B**: Lower panel depicts the excised bioprosthesis. *LA,* left atrium; *LV,* left ventricle; *RA,* right atrium.

trates a classic flail bioprosthetic cusp in the mitral position as seen from the transesophageal approach, which was later documented at surgery. *Echocardiographic detection of a flail cusp is important since almost always it is associated with severe prosthesis regurgitation.* The rate of bioprosthetic failure increases slowly until the 6th year, and then progresses rapidly due to tissue degeneration, erosion, and calcification. The incidence of porcine bioprosthesis failure is 25% at 10 years and more than 60% at 15 years (23). Although the single most attractive advantage of bioprosthetic valves is that anticoagulation usually is not needed, *the increased risk of reoperation is a serious alternative consideration compared to the reduced risk of bleeding due to no anticoagulation.* Significant improvement has been achieved with the last generation of Carpentier-Edwards pericardial aortic valves with a 94% actuarial rate of freedom from valve-related death, 84% freedom from complications, and 97% freedom from reoperation (20).

Nonstructural Dysfunction

Nonstructural dysfunction includes abnormalities leading to prosthetic valve stenosis or regurgitation, such as entrapment by pannus or suture, and inappropriate sizing (also called *patient-prosthesis mismatch*), in which the prosthesis is structurally normal, but the hemodynamics are consistent with a greater degree of stenosis than would be expected for that type of valve and size (24). The mismatch results because the valve area is inadequate for the patient's body surface area. A valve perfectly acceptable for a small, sedentary patient may be inadequate for a larger, physically active individual. This problem is typically seen in patients with small aortic annulus size as well as in those in whom the primary native valve lesion was stenosis. Clinically, the patient fails to improve or may even be symptomatically worse. Not only is their persistent hemodynamically significant aortic stenosis unlikely to regress under these loading conditions, but also LV hypertrophy. In some patients, the inadequate hemodynamics may only be apparent at higher cardiac output. Therefore, in patients with exertional dyspnea suggesting valve obstruction without evidence of a primary valve dysfunction at rest, stress echocardiography may be helpful. The diagnosis of patient-prosthesis mismatch requires exclusion of intrinsic valve dysfunction. This further emphasizes the need for a baseline study before hospital discharge or soon afterward.

Thrombosis

Mechanical prostheses are inherently thrombogenic, and, thus, the most common malfunction is due to thrombotic obstruction, a major cause of morbidity and mortality, despite the routine use of anticoagulants. Thrombosis most often results in stenosis; however, some degree of regurgitation is common since the thrombus may preclude a complete valve sealing. Bileaflet valves may present a unique problem

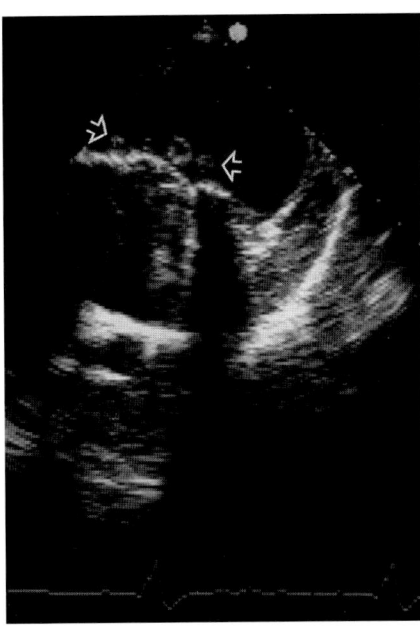

FIG. 3. Tranesophageal imaging of a St. Jude Medical mitral prosthesis demonstrating thrombi. The patient presented with right hemiparesis. Multiple thrombi are noted (*arrows*) on the atrial aspect of the prosthesis. On the actual recording, the thrombi were highly mobile as they were on the flow path. Compare with the normal characteristics of the St. Jude Medical on Figure 1.

as thrombosis can "freeze" only one hemidisc. Figure 3 depicts the transesophageal imaging of a patient who presented with right hemiparesis. Multiple small thrombi are noted on the atrial aspect of the St. Jude Medical mitral valve. All patients with mechanical valves must receive warfarin therapy and have the international normalized ratio (INR) maintained between 2.5 and 3.5. In patients with a higher risk for thromboembolism, such as those in atrial fibrillation, prior thromboembolism, severe LV dysfunction, or a hypercoagulable state, the INR should be maintained between 3.5 and 4.5. The incidence of thrombosis on warfarin is around 0.5% per year, but the risk is considerably higher without anticoagulation (25). The risk of thrombosis is slightly higher in the mitral, as opposed to the aortic position, and the risk of mechanical valve thrombosis in the tricuspid position is unacceptably high (annual rate of 4%) due to the relatively lower flow rate through the right-sided chambers (26). No data are available for valves in the pulmonic position.

TEE is a cost-effective tool ideally suited for the rapid diagnosis of suspected valve thrombosis and in evaluating the efficacy of thrombolytic therapy (27,28). Since TEE can be performed at the bedside in the emergency room or the intensive care unit, it may be a life-saving procedure. Although reoperation is frequently recommended, thrombolytic therapy can be used in critically ill patients who are inadequate candidates for reoperation. Mortality associated with emergent surgery in acute valve thrombosis may be as high as 30 to 40%, depending on preoperative functional

TABLE 6. *Clinical efficacy and complications of thrombolytic therapy in prosthetic valve thrombosis*

				Complications			
Position	No. of valves	Clinical success (%)	Reobstruction (%)	Embolism (%)	Stroke (%)	Bleed* (%)	Deaths (%)
Mitral	122	81	18	10	4	11	7
Aortic	51	86	16	10	2	8	6
Tricuspid	28	86	19	4	0	32	0
Pulmonary	6	100	17	0	0	0	0
Total	207	84	18	9	3	14	6

* Nondisabling bleed.
(From ref. 31, with permission.)

class, urgency of the operation, and concomitant coronary artery disease (29). Table 6 presents a summary of a comprehensive review of the English literature by Hurrel et al. (30), beginning in 1971 when thrombolytic therapy for prosthetic valve obstruction was first reported (31). These data revealed an 84% success rate in restoring normal valve function, an 18% recurrence of thrombosis, a 9% embolism rate, a 3% stroke rate, a 14% nondisabling bleed rate, and a 6% mortality rate. Patients who have a large clot, those with evidence of valve obstruction, and those who are in New York Heart Association functional class III or IV because of prosthetic thrombosis should undergo immediate reoperation. However, *thrombolytic therapy should be considered as a lifesaving procedure for those patients who have an unacceptable high-risk for a reoperation* (32).

Streptokinase has been the most frequently used lytic agent for this purpose; it has enjoyed a higher success rate (84%) over urokinase (57%) and tissue plasminogen activator (67%). Duration of lysis depends on resolution of pressure gradients and valve areas to near-normal by serial Doppler examinations. Lysis should be stopped at 24 hours if there is no hemodynamic improvement, or after 72 hours even if hemodynamic recovery is incomplete. If thrombolytic therapy is successful, it should be followed by intravenous heparin until warfarin achieves an INR between 2.5 and 3.5. If partially successful, thrombolytic therapy may be followed by a combination of subcutaneous heparin twice daily (activated partial thromboplastin time of 55 to 80 sec) plus warfarin (INR 2.5 to 3.5) for a 3-month period (32).

During a TEE examination, a group of thin filamentous structures of a few millimeters long moving independently of the valve may be seen on the atrial side of mitral prostheses or on the ventricular side of aortic prostheses. These filamentous structures or *fibrin strands* can be distinguished from vegetations or thrombi by their chaotic movement in and out of the imaging plane. Fibrin strands are more commonly seen on mechanical valves, and they have been associated with a higher incidence of embolic events (33); however, they can also be seen in normally functioning prostheses (34). Thus, further studies are needed to determine the significance of fibrin strands before clinical decisions are made based solely on their presence. In the meantime, identification of fibrin strands in otherwise normally

functioning valves should be considered an incidental finding.

Endocarditis

Based on large series, the incidence of endocarditis is similar in mechanical and bioprosthetic valves, occurring at an annual rate of 1.2% per year (35,36). When compared to native valves, prosthetic valve endocarditis is more likely to be associated with abscesses and conduction abnormalities. Vegetations typically appeared as irregular echoes attached to valvular or perivalvular components commonly moving with the flow path. Infected bioprostheses usually result in leaflet destruction, whereas, in mechanical valves, the vegetations may interfere with the occluding mechanism, resulting in either stenosis or regurgitation. Large (>10 mm) vegetations are associated with an increased incidence of embolic complications (37). When thrombosis or perivalvular leak occurs during an active prosthetic valve endocarditis, they should be reported within this latter category (21).

The early and accurate identification of septic complications has a significant impact on clinical decisions. A perivalvular abscess or a fistulous tract is associated with a worse prognosis and indicate the need for aggressive medical and surgical therapies. *Findings suggestive of a perivalvular abscess in a patient with prosthetic valve endocarditis include persistent sepsis despite appropriate antibiotics, new or worsening congestive heart failure, and new first-degree AV block or incomplete right bundle-branch block.* Echocardiographic findings include valve rocking, mycotic aneurysm, and an echo-lucent space within the adjacent structures. As indicated in Table 7, identification of an abscess may be very difficult from the transthoracic approach. However, TEE has dramatically improved the ability to detect vegetations and abscesses in both native and prosthetic valves (7,38,39). Figure 4 illustrates the typical findings of an abscess on the posterior aspect of a St. Jude Medical valve in the aortic position creating a fistulous tract between the aorta and the LV outflow tract with severe aortic regurgitation. Although the routine use of TEE in all patients with suspected endocarditis is controversial, *in high-risk patients, such as those with prosthetic heart valves, TEE should be regularly performed if there is a reasonable level of suspicion, even if the trans-*

TABLE 7. *Sensitivity and specificity of transthoracic vs. TEE in detecting vegetations and abscesses complicating prosthetic valve endocarditis*

				TTE		TEE	
Author	Year	Reference	No. of patients	Sens (%)	Spec (%)	Sens (%)	Spec (%)
Mugge*	1989	37	105	58	ID	90	ID
Taams*	1990	38	33	36	100	100	100
Daniel**	1991	39	118	28	99	87	95

* Detection of vegetations; ** detection of abscesses; ID, insufficient data to calculate specificity; *Sens,* sensitivity; *Spec,* specificity; *TEE,* transesophageal echocardiography; *TTE,* transthoracic echocardiography.

thoracic echocardiogram is normal. This is a practical and cost-effective approach particularly in patients who have failed to improve on medical therapy. Fistulous tracts connecting the abscess with adjacent structures, such as the left atrium, right atrium, or right ventricle, can be tracked during the TEE color flow examination.

Prosthetic Stenosis

Aortic Position

A careful echo-Doppler examination may provide essential hemodynamic and etiologic information in prosthetic

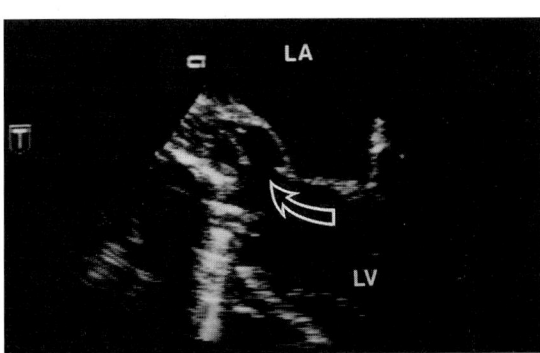

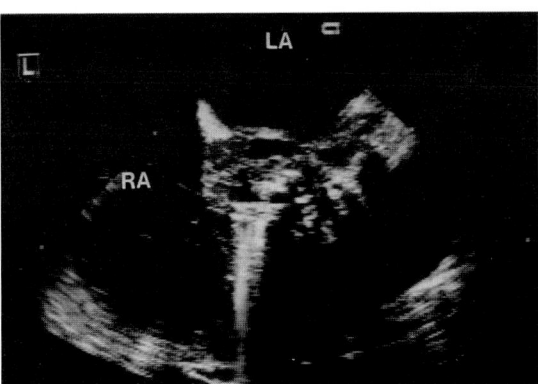

FIG. 4. Transesophageal imaging of a Medtronic-Hall aortic valve demonstrating a perivalvular abscess. The **upper panel** depicts an echo-lucent cavity (*arrow*) on the posterior aspect of the prosthesis corresponding to a fistulous tract communicating the aorta with the LV outflow tract creating prosthesis dehiscence and severe regurgitation. The **lower panel** is the cross-sectional view of the perivalvular abscess in the same patient. *LA,* left atrium; *LV,* left ventricle; *RA,* right atrium.

aortic stenosis. Frequently, the initial suspicion of valve stenosis is the incidental finding of high flow velocities during a routine Doppler examination. Significant overestimation of the continuous-wave Doppler signals may occur in the presence of concomitant regurgitation and in the presence of small orifices (40). When catheter-derived gradients are available, the comparison should be made between the two *mean* gradients. The catheter *peak-to-peak* gradient should not be compared with the Doppler gradients since the former is not an instantaneous event (3). TEE is the ideal means by which to determine the *cause* of the obstruction, such as thrombus, vegetation, pannus formation, or calcific degeneration. Common indications for TEE in patients with prosthetic stenosis are listed in Table 5. In an asymptomatic patient with elevated transvalvular velocities but otherwise unremarkable TEE examination, obstruction due to fibrous tissue ingrowth (pannus formation) is the most likely explanation. In these cases, a close Doppler follow-up examination is recommended; if symptoms develop, reoperation should be considered.

Mitral Position

Assessment of prosthetic mitral stenosis severity includes estimation of the mean pressure gradient and valve area (41). In changing hemodynamic conditions, such as exercise, the valve area remains more constant than the pressure gradients. Mitral valve area should be calculated using the pressure half-time and the continuity equation. Color flow may help in aligning the Doppler beam parallel to the main flow stream. The valve gradient should be combined with the pressure half-time to differentiate prosthetic stenosis from increased transvalvular volume. Increased E-wave velocity in the absence of a prolonged deceleration time may be due to mitral regurgitation; on the other hand, an E-wave velocity greater than 2.5 m/sec and a pressure half-time greater than 200 msec is highly suspicious for prosthetic mitral stenosis. A TEE examination should be considered if the *cause* is unclear. Also, TEE may permit the selective sample of velocities through the central and the side orifices in cases of bileaflet mechanical prostheses. This is important because pressure recovery is less when the velocities are recorded through the side orifices (4).

Prosthetic Regurgitation

Prosthetic valve regurgitation can be transvalvular or peri-valvular in origin, and it should be differentiated from the normal backflow leakage frequently found in mechanical valves. Pathologic regurgitation is characterized by large, wide, frequently eccentric jets commonly colored with a mosaic pattern indicative of turbulent flow. In general, assessment of prosthetic valve regurgitation follows similar principles as those with native valves, but quantitation is often more difficult.

Aortic Position

Potential sources of regurgitation, such as primary failure, ring dehiscence, or vegetations, should be sought. Assess-

ment includes several echo Doppler indices, such as the height of the regurgitant jet relative to the outflow tract. Eccentric jets may overestimate the severity of regurgitation. The pressure half-time may be useful in differentiating chronic from acute regurgitation. In general, acute (and often severe) regurgitation shows a rapid slope decay indicative of markedly elevated LV end-diastolic pressure. Although highly specific, this finding is not sensitive for the diagnosis of severe regurgitation as the slope decay may be altered by changes in LV compliance, stiffness, heart rate, and cardiac rhythm. Thus, a patient with severe *chronic* aortic regurgitation and a compliant LV may have an aortic-LV diastolic pressure slope similar to that seen in patients with mild or moderate regurgitation. The amount of flow reversal in the descending aorta also correlates with severity. Normal flow

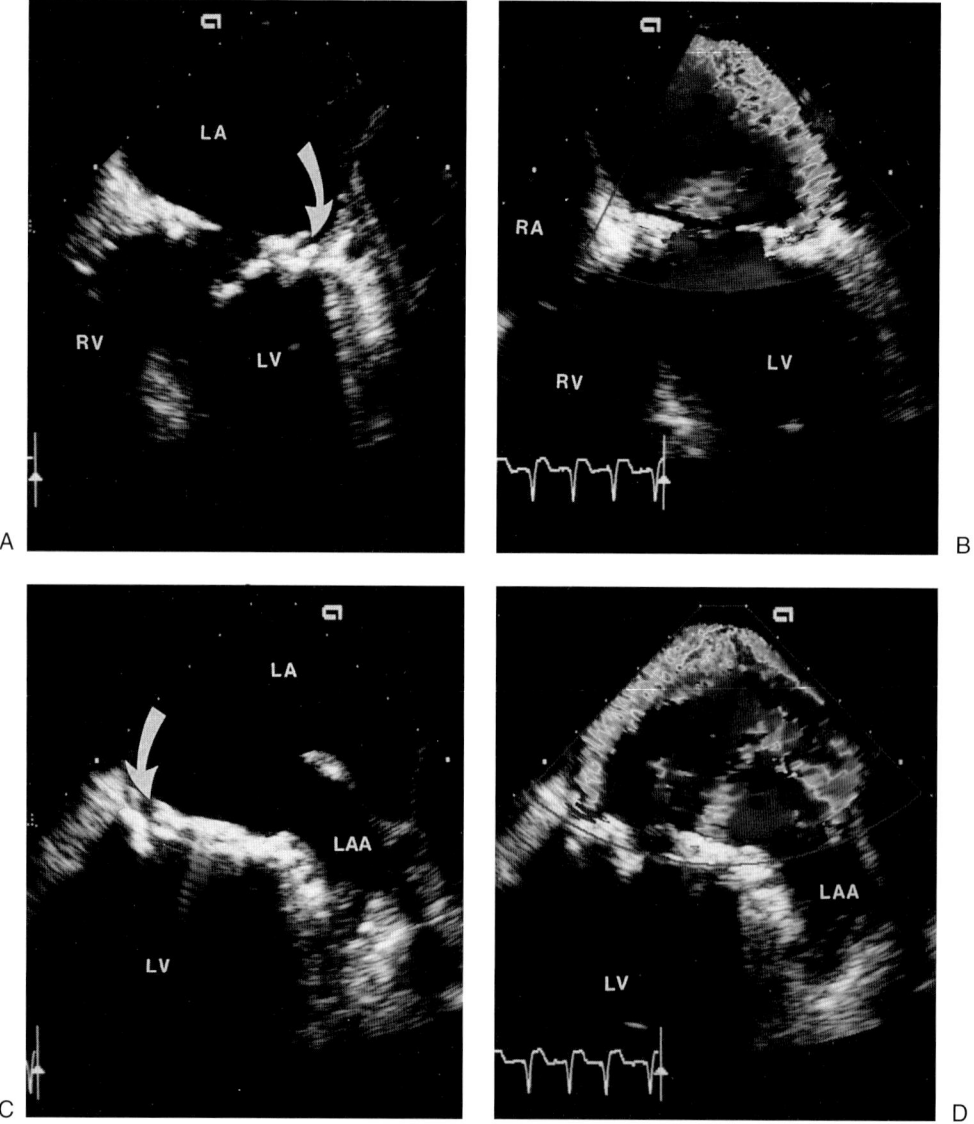

FIG. 5. Transesophageal imaging in a patient with a dehiscent mitral bioprosthesis. **A** and **C:** Both panels depict a drop-out of echoes (*arrows*) between the sewing ring and the mitral annulus from the transverse and longitudinal views. **B** and **D:** The panels show a large eccentric jet of severe regurgitation that "hugs" the atrial wall. *LA,* left atrium; *LAA,* left atrial appendage; *LV,* left ventricle; *RA,* right atrium; *RV,* right ventricle. (See also Color Plate 24 following page 758.)

reversal is confined to early diastole, whereas persistence throughout diastole is consistent with severe regurgitation. TEE can be very useful in detecting the cause of regurgitation and in differentiating its origin (valvular versus perivalvular).

Mitral Position

In the presence of severe mitral regurgitation, the E-wave velocity is increased, but the pressure half-time is short. The direction of the jet may provide important information. Very eccentric jets, "hugging" the atrial wall, are commonly indicative of severe regurgitation despite their narrow width and relatively small percent area within an enlarged left atrium. Figure 5 (see also Color Plate 24 following page 758) illustrates the TEE imaging of a patient with a dehiscent Hancock (porcine graft) prosthesis in the mitral position with a very eccentric regurgitant jet directed toward the posterolateral aspect of the left atrium and eventually entering into the left superior pulmonary vein. An eccentric jet of severe mitral regurgitation loses momentum and velocity as it contacts the atrial wall despite a large volume, a phenomenon known as the *coanda* effect (42).

Color Doppler demonstration of flow conversion, also known as PISA (proximal isovelocity surface area), on the ventricular side of the valve has been used to assess severity (43). When fluids enter the regurgitant orifice, they tend to accelerate to reach a peak velocity at the neck of the orifice. Concentric hemispheres, defined by their velocity magnitude, are successively smaller in radius as the velocity increases. A recent evaluation of transthoracic methods for evaluating prosthetic mitral regurgitation compared the proximal zone of acceleration, the intensity of the Doppler signal, and the size of the color Doppler jet within the left atrium (44). The proximal zone of acceleration or flow conversion was more sensitive but less specific for predicting significant regurgitation; it was the only precordial sign of severe mitral regurgitation in 40% of the patients studied.

Despite the benefits of the precordial approach, evaluation of prosthetic regurgitation continues to be a problem because the left atrium is obscured by the reverberations from the metallic material of the device. Evaluation of prosthetic mitral regurgitation from the apical views is commonly suboptimal. However, because of the anatomical relationship between the esophagus and the left atrium, TEE overcomes this important technical limitation (18). *Thus, assessment of prosthetic mitral regurgitation is not only a solid indication for TEE, but also the standard of diagnostic approach for these patients.*

The morphology of the pulmonary vein Doppler waveform is dependent on both volume of regurgitation and left atrial properties. Pulmonary vein flow characteristics have been useful in assessing severity in native valve regurgitation. The typical pattern seen with increasing severity is loss of the systolic wave amplitude with eventual "reversal" of this wave flow. These changes, however, should not be interpreted as an absolute measure of regurgitant severity. Pulmonary venous flow reversal is more likely to occur in acute than in chronic regurgitation because, in the former condition, the left atrium is less compliant. In addition, characterization of pulmonary vein flows in prosthetic mitral regurgitation is lacking, and, thus, extrapolation of data acquired in the native mitral valve should be carefully done.

Stress Echocardiography in Assessing Prosthetic Valve Function

In assessing prosthetic valves, one may encounter patients with symptoms that suggest valve dysfunction in whom the two-dimensional and Doppler flow pattern appear normal. Under these circumstances, stress echocardiography may elicit abnormal hemodynamics suggesting early valve dysfunction or a patient-prosthesis mismatch. Conversely, a normal hemodynamic stress response can be reassuring. Valve gradients, areas, changes in regurgitation severity, and estimation of the systolic pulmonary artery pressure can all be calculated at rest and at different levels of stress. Table 8 summarizes the most recent data (45–49).

TABLE 8. *Exercise Doppler hemodynamics in prosthetic valves[a]*

Aortic position	Patients	Valve sizes (mm)	Mean gradient (mm Hg)		
			Rest	Exercise	Increase (%)
Carpentier-Edwards	4	21	15 ± 3	21 ± 3	70
Medtronic-Hall	14	21	15 ± 4	24 ± 6	80
Medtronic-Hall	14	21–27	9 ± 4	15 ± 6	83
St. Jude Medical	17	21–27	11 ± 4	18 ± 7	81

Mitral position	Patients	Valve sizes	Mean gradient (mm Hg)		
			Rest	Exercise	Increase (%)
Bjork-Shiley	11	25–31	4.9 ± 1.8	10.3 ± 2.9	100
Starr-Edwards	6	28–32	4.6 ± 1.2	12.6 ± 4.1	130
St. Jude Medical	17	26–32	2.5 ± 1.4	5.1 ± 3.5	102
Medtronic-Hall	15	26–32	3.0 ± 1.1	7.0 ± 2.9	116

[a] Exercise protocols utilized were symptom-limited treadmill, upright, or supine bicycle protocols.
(Data from refs. 45–49, with permission.)

Dobutamine echocardiography provides an alternative means for patients unable or unwilling to undergo an exercise protocol. In 25 patients with normally functioning mechanical aortic prostheses, dobutamine echocardiography reached more often an arbitrary target heart rate (>85%) as compared with bicycle ergometry. A normal hemodynamic response consisted in an increase of near 100% from baseline on peak flow velocity, mean, and maximal instantaneous gradients (50). For the patient with decreased LV function and prosthetic aortic stenosis of undetermined severity, dobutamine echocardiography may be useful in determining its severity. However, the use of dobutamine echocardiography in aortic stenosis has not been fully investigated.

SUMMARY

Other imaging techniques, such as radionuclide ventriculography, myocardial perfusion imaging, positron emission tomography, and magnetic resonance imaging have little if any role compared to echocardiography in the assessment of prosthetic heart valves.

Although the clinical examination is an essential component in assessing patients with suspected prosthetic valve malfunction, the fact is that these patients are almost never referred to surgery on the basis of clinical information alone. When the echocardiographic data does not suggest prosthetic valve dysfunction, other comorbid diseases should be considered, including *native* valve malfunction, LV systolic and/or diastolic dysfunction, coronary artery disease, and pericardial disease. Stress echocardiography should be considered whenever symptoms appear on exertion and when the two-dimensional images, including those from TEE, have not detected an apparent abnormality. Nowadays, prosthetic valve dysfunction has emerged as a solid indication for TEE.

Finally, one must remember that valve replacement is not "curative" in itself. By replacing an abnormal native valve for an artificial device, we have replaced one disease state by another that will require clinical follow-up, antithrombotic medication, antibiotic prophylaxis, and prompt recognition of potentially disastrous complications unique to this "new" condition. Any patient with a prosthetic heart valve who does not improve after surgery or who later shows deterioration of functional capacity should undergo Doppler echocardiography and, if necessary, a TEE examination to determine the cause. Despite the fact that clinical models for cost analysis of echocardiography in prosthetic heart valves are lacking, the "clinical wisdom" from clinical practice in this area has led us to recognize echocardiography in the critical pathway of patients with prosthetic heart valves.

REFERENCES

1. Zabalgoitia M. Echocardiographic assessment of prosthetic heart valves. *Curr Probl Cardiol* 1992;17:267–325.
2. Kuppersmith J, Holmes-Rovner M, Hogan A, et al. Cost-effectiveness analysis in heart disease, I: general principles. *Prog Cardiovasc Dis* 1994;37:161–184.
3. Burstow DJ, Nishimura RA, Bailey KR, et al. Continuous wave Doppler echocardiographic measurement of prosthetic valve gradients. A simultaneous Doppler-catheter correlative study. *Circulation* 1989;80:504–514.
4. Vandervoort PM, Greenberg NL, Pu M, et al. Pressure recovery in bileaflet heart valve prostheses. *Circulation* 1995;92:3464–3472.
5. Chambers JB. Is pressure recovery an important cause of "Doppler aortic stenosis" with no gradient at cardiac catheterization? *Heart* 1996;76:381–383.
6. Chafizadeh ER, Zoghbi WA. Doppler echocardiographic assessment of the St. Jude Medical prosthetic valve in the aortic position using the continuity equation. *Circulation* 1991;83:213–223.
7. Zabalgoitia M, Herrera CJ, Chaudry FA, et al. Improvement in the diagnosis of bioprosthetic valve dysfunction by transesophageal echocardiography. *J Heart Valve Dis* 1993;2:595–603.
8. Dumesnil JG, Honos GN, Lemieux M, et al. Validation and applications of mitral prosthetic valvular areas by Doppler echocardiography. *Am J Cardiol* 1990;65:1443–1448.
9. Burwash IG, Thomas DD, Sadahiro M, et al. Dependence of Gorlin formula and continuity equation valve areas on transvalvular volume flow rate in valvular aortic stenosis. *Circulation* 1994;89:827–835.
10. Saad RM, Barbetseas J, Olmos L, et al. Application of the continuity equation and valve resistance to the evaluation of St. Jude medical prosthetic aortic valve dysfunction. *Am J Cardiol* 1997;80:1239–1242.
11. Ford LE, Feldman T, Chiu YC, et al. Hemodynamic resistance as a measure of functional impairment in aortic valvular stenosis. *Circ Res* 1990;66:1–7.
12. Cannon JD, Zile MR, Crawford FA, et al. Aortic valve resistance as an adjunct to the Gorlin formula in assessing the severity of aortic stenosis in symptomatic patients. *J Am Coll Cardiol* 1992;20:1517–1523.
13. Hixson CS, Smith MD, Mattson MD, et al. Comparison of transesophageal color flow Doppler imaging of normal mitral regurgitant jets in St. Jude Medical and Medtronic-Hall cardiac prostheses. *J Am Soc Echocardiogr* 1992;5:57–62.
14. Alam M, Rosman HS, Lakier JB, et al. Doppler and echocardiographic features of normal and dysfunctioning bioprosthetic valves. *J Am Coll Cardiol* 1987;10:851–888.
15. Reisner SA, Melter RS. Normal values of prosthetic valve Doppler echocardiographic parameters: a review. *J Am Soc Echocardiogr* 1988;1:201–210.
16. Laske A, Jenni R, Maloigne M, et al. Pressure gradients across bileaflet aortic valves by direct measurement and echocardiography. *Ann Thorac Surg* 1996;61:48–57.
17. Chakraborty B, Quek S, Pin DZ, et al. Doppler echocardiographic assessment of normally functioning Starr-Edwards, CarboMedics and Carpentier-Edwards valves in aortic position. *Angiology* 1996;47:481–489.
18. Zabalgoitia M, Garcia M. Pitfalls in the echo-Doppler diagnosis of prosthetic valve disorders. *Echocardiography* 1993;10:203–212.
19. Jaffe WM, Coverdale A, Roche AH, et al. Doppler echocardiography in the assessment of the homograft aortic valve. *Am J Cardiol* 1989;63:1466–1470.
20. Aupart MR, Sirinelli AL, Diemont FF, et al. The last generation of pericardial valves in the aortic position: ten-year follow-up in 589 patients. *Ann Thorac Surg* 1996;61:615–620.
21. Edmunds LH Jr, Clark RE, Cohn LH, et al. Guidelines for reporting morbidity and mortality after cardiac valvular operations. *J Thorac Cardiovasc Surg* 1996;112:708–711.
22. Grunkemeier GL, Starr A, Rahimtoola SH. Prosthetic heart valve performance: long-term follow-up. *Curr Probl Cardiol* 1992;17:329–406.
23. Rahimtoola SH. Perspective on valvular heart disease: an update. *J Am Coll Cardiol* 1989;14:1–23.
24. Rahimtoola SH. The problem of valve prosthesis-patient mismatch. *Circulation* 1978;58:20–24.
25. Cannegieter SC, Rosendaal FR, Briet E. Thromboembolic and bleeding complications in patients with mechanical heart valve prostheses. *Circulation* 1994;89:635–641.
26. Thornburn CW, Morgan JJ, Shananhan MX, et al. Long-term results of tricuspid valve replacement and the problem of prosthetic valve thrombosis. *Am J Cardiol* 1983;51:1128–1132.
27. Dzavik V, Cohen G, Chan KL. Role of transesophageal echocardiography in the diagnosis and management of prosthetic valve thrombosis. *J Am Coll Cardiol* 1991;18:1829–1833.

28. Young E, Shapiro SM, French WJ, et al. Use of transesophageal echocardiography during thrombolysis with tissue plasminogen activator of a thrombosed prosthetic mitral valve. *J Am Soc Echocardiogr* 1992;5:153–158.

29. Husebye DG, Pluth JR, Schaff HV, et al. Reoperation on prosthetic heart valves: an analysis of risk factors in 552 patients. *J Thorac Cardiovasc Surg* 1983;86:543–552.

30. Hurrel DG, Schaff HV, Tajik AJ. Thrombolytic therapy for obstruction of mechanical prosthetic valves. *Mayo Clin Proc* 1996;71:605–613.

31. Luluaga IT, Carrera D, D'Oliveira J, et al. Successful thrombolytic therapy after acute tricuspid-valve obstruction. *Lancet* 1971;1:1067–1068.

32. Lengyel M, Fuster V, Keltai M, et al. Guidelines for management of left-sided prosthetic valve thrombosis: a role for thrombolytic therapy. *J Am Coll Cardiol* 1997;30:1521–1526.

33. Orsinelli DA, Pearson AG. Detection of prosthetic valve strands by transesophageal echocardiography: clinical significance in patients with suspected cardiac source of embolism. *J Am Coll Cardiol* 1995;26:1713–1718.

34. Stoddard MF, Dawkins PR, Longaker RA. Mobile strands are frequently attached to the St. Jude Medical mitral valve prosthesis as assessed by two-dimensional transesophageal echocardiography. *Am Heart J* 1992;124:671–674.

35. Bloomfield P, Wheatley DJ, Prescott RJ, et al. Twelve-year comparison of a Bjork-Shiley mechanical heart with a porcine bioprosthesis. *N Engl J Med* 1991;324:573–579.

36. Hammermeister KE, Henderson WG, Burchfiel CM, et al. Comparison of outcome after valve replacement with a bioprosthesis versus a mechanical prosthesis: initial 5 year results of a randomized trial. *J Am Coll Cardiol* 1987;10:719–732.

37. Mugge A, Daniel WG, Frank G, et al. Echocardiography in infective endocarditis: reassessment of prognostic implications of vegetation size determined by the transthoracic and the transesophageal approach. *J Am Coll Cardiol* 1989;14:631–638.

38. Taams MA, Gussenhoven EJ, Boss E, et al. Enhanced morphological diagnosis in endocarditis by transesophageal echocardiography. *Br Heart J* 1990;63:109–113.

39. Daniel WG, Mugge A, Martin RP, et al. Improvement in the diagnosis of abscesses associated with endocarditis by transesophageal echocardiography. *N Engl J Med* 1991;324:795–800.

40. Flachskampf FA, Kohler J, Ask P, et al. Overestimation of flow velocity through leaks in mechanical valve prostheses and through small orifices by continuous-wave Doppler. *J Am Soc Echocardiogr* 1997;10:904–914.

41. Chalmers JB. How should we describe forward flow through replacement mitral valves using echocardiography? *J Heart Valve Dis* 1995;4[Suppl I]:S55–S58.

42. Chao K, Moises VA, Shandas R, et al. Influence of the Coanda effect on color Doppler jet area and color encoding. *In vitro* studies using color Doppler flow mapping. *Circulation* 1992;85:333–341.

43. Yoshida K, Yoshikawa J, Akasaka T, et al. Value of acceleration flow signals proximal to the leaking orifice in assessing the severity of prosthetic mitral valve regurgitation. *J Am Coll Cardiol* 1992;19:333–338.

44. Cohen GI, Davison MB, Klein AL, et al. A comparison of flow convergence with other transthoracic echocardiographic indexes of prosthetic mitral regurgitation. *J Am Soc Echocardiogr* 1992;5:620–627.

45. Tatineni S, Barner HB, Pearson AC. Rest and exercise evaluation of St. Jude Medical and Medtronic-Hall prostheses. *Circulation* 1989;80[Suppl I]:16–23.

46. Wiseth R, Levang OW, Tangen G. Exercise hemodynamics in small (<21mm) aortic valve prostheses assessed by Doppler echocardiography. *Am Heart J* 1993;125:138–146.

47. Reisner SA, Lichtenberg GS, Shapiro JR, et al. Exercise Doppler echocardiography in patients with mitral prosthetic valves. *Am Heart J* 1989;118:755–759.

48. Halbe DW, Woodruff RC, Ojile MC, et al. Non-invasive exercise-evaluation of St. Jude and Medtronic-Hall prosthetic heart valves. *Circulation* 1988;78[Suppl II]:16–23.

49. van den Brink RB, Verheul HA, Visser CA, et al. Value of exercise Doppler echocardiography in patients with prosthetic or bioprosthetic cardiac valves. *Am J Cardiol* 1992;69:367–372.

50. Zabalgoitia M, Kopec K, Oneschuk L, et al. Use of dobutamine echocardiography in assessing mechanical aortic prostheses: comparison with exercise echocardiography. *J Heart Valve Dis* 1997;6:253–257.

CHAPTER 44

Infective Endocarditis

Marcus F. Stoddard

Infective endocarditis encompasses all infections of any endocardial site of the heart or intracardiac prosthetic material by a myriad of microorganisms, but more typically is characterized by a bacterial infection of cardiac valvular endocardium. The disease may result in serious sequelae and is often life threatening with a mortality ranging from 10 to 40% (1–3). The impact of this disease on health-care cost has been substantial, and cumulative incremental costs have been estimated at $46,132 per case in the United States (4). The clinical diagnosis of infective endocarditis in the modern era is challenging because the ''classic findings'' of infective endocarditis as described by Sir William Osler are seldom present (5). Although an irrefutable diagnosis of infective endocarditis can only be made by histologic confirmation, this is not feasible or necessary in the vast majority of patients with infective endocarditis. A vegetation or excrescence, particularly involving cardiac valves, is the classic pathologic lesion associated with infective endocarditis. Transthoracic two-dimensional echocardiography (TTE), first shown to be useful in the assessment of infective endocarditis over 25 years ago (6), remains the most widely employed imaging technique for the diagnosis of vegetations due to endocarditis. The finding of vegetation by TTE coupled with clinical criteria strengthens the diagnosis of endocarditis and allows expeditious and appropriate medical therapy. However, the sensitivity of TTE for vegetation may be significantly limited in several situations, such as technically inadequate acoustic windows, small vegetations (i.e., less than 5 mm in size) and the presence of prosthetic material (see Chapter 2). Transesophageal echocardiography (TEE) circumvents many of the limitations of TTE for the detection of pathologic lesions due to infective endocarditis by imaging from transesophageal and transgastric acoustic windows. As such, echocardiography continues to play an ever-expanding role in the evaluation of patients with possible infec-

tive endocarditis. Newer echocardiographic techniques, such as three-dimensional echocardiography, promise to further broaden and refine the role of echocardiography in the diagnosis and management of this protean and often devastating disease.

This chapter discusses the role of echocardiography, particularly TEE in the evaluation and management of adult patients with suspected and/or proven infective endocarditis. The limitations of echocardiography, in select circumstances, are duly noted. Recommendations on the first-line use of TTE versus TEE are offered. Lastly, the potential impact of echocardiography on health-care cost in the diagnosis of endocarditis is discussed.

DIAGNOSTIC CRITERIA FOR INFECTIVE ENDOCARDITIS

Patients with infective endocarditis may present with nonspecific constitutional symptoms such as intermittent fever and chills, malaise, myalgias, or weight loss. Splinter hemorrhages or Roth spots may be present on examination but are more frequently absent. In subjects experiencing severe valve injury, the presentation may be fulminant with symptoms and signs of heart failure, sepsis, or cardiogenic shock. Suspicion of infective endocarditis should be entertained in patients with persistent bacteremia and a new or changed murmur and/or systemic embolism. The nonspecific and protean clinical manifestations of infective endocarditis makes it abundantly clear that misdiagnoses of infective endocarditis are common. Importantly, incorrect diagnosis in patients with or without infective endocarditis may have grave consequences, which lead to life-threatening sequelae from the disease or inappropriately prolonged hospitalization with concomitant unnecessary expenses, respectively.

Standardized clinical criteria for the diagnosis of infective endocarditis have been proposed and found to be of some use (7). However, such criteria are overly strict and insensitive,

M. F. Stoddard: Department of Medicine, University of Louisville; Department of Medicine, Division of Cardiology, University Hospital, Louisville, Kentucky 40292.

TABLE 1. *Duke criteria for infective endocarditis (see Table 2 for definitions)*

I. Definite infective endocarditis
   A. Pathologic criteria
      1. Microorganisms: demonstrated by culture or histology in a
         a. Vegetation in-situ, or
         b. Vegetation that embolized, or
         c. Intracardiac abscess, or
      2. Pathologic lesions (vegetation or intracardiac abscess: confirmed by histology showing active endocarditis
   B. Clinical criteria using definitions in Table 2
      1. Two major criteria, or
      2. One major and three minor criteria, or
      3. Five minor criteria
II. Possible infective endocarditis
   A. Findings consistent with but fall short for definite endocarditis (I.) but
   B. Findings do not meet criteria for rejected infective endocarditis (III.)
III. Rejected infective endocarditis
   A. Firm alternative diagnosis for manifestations of endocarditis, or
   B. Resolution of symptoms of endocarditis without antibiotics or with antibiotic therapy of ≤ 4 days, or
   C. No pathologic evidence of infective endocarditis at surgery or autopsy after antibiotic therapy of ≤ 4 days.

(Adapted from ref. 8, with permission.)

TABLE 2. *Definitions of Duke major and minor criteria for infective endocarditis*

I. Major criteria
   A. Positive blood culture for infective endocarditis
      1. Typical microorganism for infective endocarditis from two separate blood cultures:
         a. Streptococcus viridans, streptococcus bovis, HACEK group, or
         b. Community-acquired staphylococcus auresis or enterococcus, in the absence of a primary focus, or
      2. Persistently positive blood culture, defined as recovery of a microorganism consistent with infective endocarditis from:
         a. Blood cultures drawn more than 12 hours apart, or
         b. Three of three, or a majority of four or more blood cultures drawn over a span of > 1 hour.
   B. Evidence of endocardial involvement
      1. Echocardiogram consistent with endocarditis
         a. Oscillating intracardiac mass on valve or supporting structures, or in path of regurgitant jets, or on prosthetic material in the absence of alternative explanation, or
         b. Abscess, or
         c. New dehiscence of prosthetic valve, or
      2. New valvular regurgitation (increase or change in preexisting murmur not sufficient)
II. Minor criteria
   A. Predisposition
      1. Predisposing heart condition, or
      2. Intravenous drug use, or
   B. Fever (≥ 100.4°F)
   C. Vascular phenomena
      1. Major arterial emboli, septic pulmonary infarcts, mycotic aneurysm, intracranial hemorrhage, or Janeway lesions, or
   D. Immunologic phenomena
      1. Glomerulonephritis, Osler nodes, Roth spots or rheumatoid factor, or
   E. Microbiologic evidence
      1. Positive blood culture but not meeting major criterion for serologic evidence of active infection with organism consistent with infective endocarditis
   F. Echocardiogram: findings consistent with infective endocarditis but not meeting major criterion such as
      1. Nodular valvular thickening, nonoscillating masses or valvular fenestrations.

(Adapted from ref. 8, with permission.)

requiring histologic confirmation of infective endocarditis (7). Noting the limitations of schemas based on mere clinical criteria, investigators from Duke (8) proposed criteria for infective endocarditis that incorporate echocardiographic findings (Tables 1 and 2). In this retrospective study, it was shown that the sensitivity of the clinical diagnosis of pathologically proven infective endocarditis was considerably enhanced by coupling echocardiographic results with clinical, blood culture, and pathologic findings (i.e., sensitivity increased from 51 to 80%). Importantly, recent studies further suggest that the more sensitive Duke criteria are highly specific (9).

Echocardiography, particularly TEE, is very sensitive and specific for detecting vegetations and the structural complications of endocarditis, such as abscess, mycotic aneurysm, fistula, and flail leaflets. In addition, the prognostic value of echocardiography for predicting morbid events and individuals at higher risk of death from endocarditis has been determined (10). The sensitivity, specificity, and predictive value of echocardiography has made it essential in the evaluation of patients with suspected or proven endocarditis. Accordingly, this chapter will focus primarily on the various echocardiographic methods for detecting vegetations and structural complications from infective endocarditis, and their prognostic value.

NATIVE VALVE INFECTIVE ENDOCARDITIS: SENSITIVITY AND SPECIFICITY OF ECHOCARDIOGRAPHY

The echocardiographic detection of a vegetation is influenced by multiple factors that include echogenicity, mobility, size and location of the vegetation, presence of prosthetic material, transducer frequency and equipment sensitivity, technical skills of the sonographer, interpretative expertise of the echocardiographer, and pretest probability of endocarditis.

In addition, the specificity of echocardiography for native valve infective endocarditis may be lowered by erroneous diagnoses attributable to lesions that mimic vegetations, such as Lambl's excrescences, valvular fibrin strands, ruptured or redundant chordae, nonspecific valvular thickening, or calcification, etc.

Impact of Vegetation Properties and Location

Although a vegetation is an excrescence visualized as a mass on two-dimensional echocardiography, distinguishing a vegetation from the many other types of masses seen by echocardiography is not always straightforward and requires knowledge of its most and least characteristic properties and locations. Features most characteristic of a vegetation include a mass with an echogenicity similar to that of myocardium, attached on the site of a valve leaflet in the path of a turbulent jet, lobulated or pedunculated in shape and displaying unrestricted mobility, particularly if prolapsing (Table 3; Figs. 1 and 2). In contrast, an immobile, sessile, highly reflectile or calcified intracardiac mass, particularly if not associated with valvular apparatus, is less likely to be a vegetation from active infective endocarditis. Echocardiographic masses with some but not all of the characteristic features of a vegetation are likely to have an intermediate probability of being a vegetation and may be due to nonspecific valvular thickening from degeneration, myxomatous valves, ruptured chordae, calcification, fibrin strands, etc. (see Chapters 2 and 40–42).

The size and, potentially, the location of a vegetation also impacts the sensitivity of echocardiography, particularly TTE, in infective endocarditis. For example, Erbel et al. (11) showed a sensitivity of only 25% for vegetations less than

TABLE 3. *Characteristics of an echogenic mass most or least likely to be representative of a vegetation*

| | Vegetation features | |
Characteristic	Most characteristic	Least characteristic
Echogenicity	Myocardial gray scale	Highly reflectile (Gray scale of calcium)
Shape	Lobulated/pedunculated	Sessile or stringlike
Location	Valve/side of valve exposed to turbulent jet	Mural or side of valve not exposed to turbulent jet
Mobility	Unrestricted motion	Immobile

5 mm and 69% for vegetations of 5 to 10 mm, but 100% for vegetations greater than 10 mm by two-dimensional TTE. Gilbert et al. (12) noted that TTE was completely insensitive for detection of vegetations less than 3 mm. Although technological improvements, since the report of Gilbert et al. (12), in two-dimensional resolution may have enhanced the sensitivity of TTE for detection of small vegetations, this has yet to be shown. Alternatively, the sensitivity of TEE appears little affected by vegetation size and remains in excess of 90% despite vegetations less than 5 mm (11).

Although unproven, it is likely that echocardiography in particular is less sensitive for detection of pulmonic and tricuspid valve and nonvalvular vegetations as compared to aortic and mitral valve vegetations. Complete visualization of the aortic or mitral valve is often more technically feasible by TTE or TEE as compared to the pulmonic or tricuspid valve.

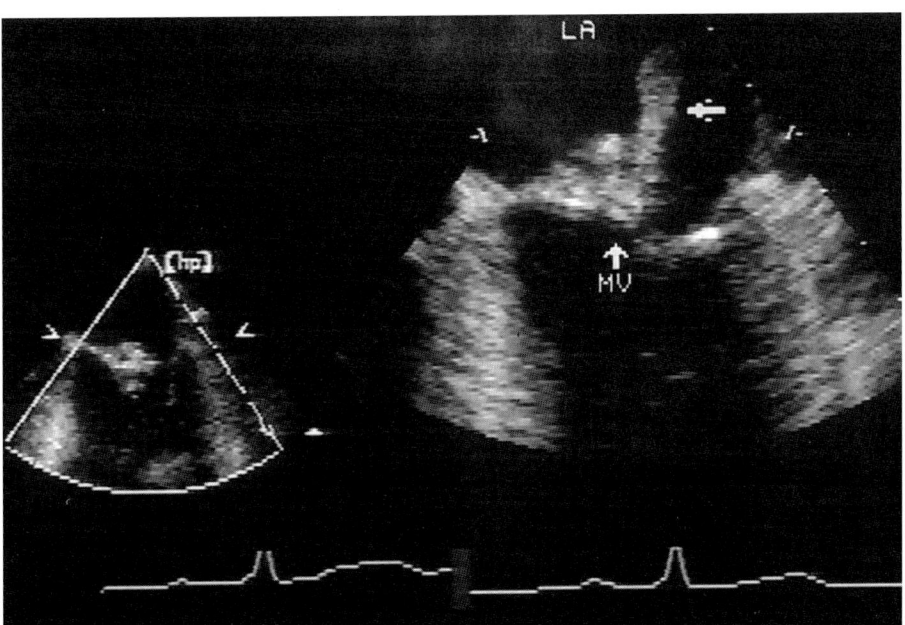

FIG. 1. Transesophageal echocardiography horizontal view showing large vegetation (*arrow*) attached to mitral valve (*MV*) and extending into the left atrium (*LA*). This mass was highly mobile in real-time and showed many of the typical features of a vegetation (see text for details).

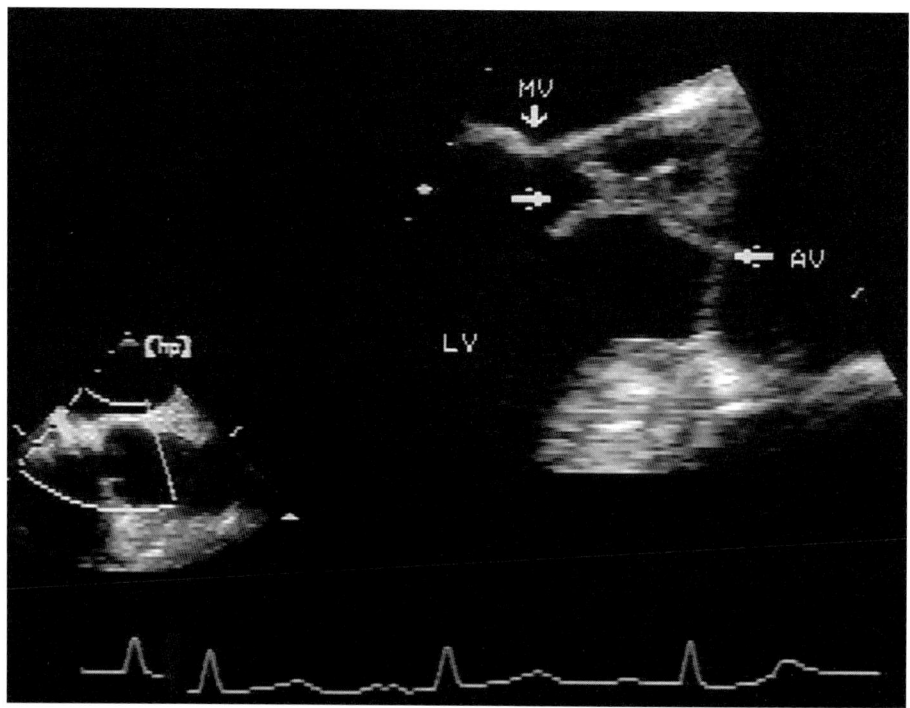

FIG. 2. Transesophageal echocardiography long-axis view showing large vegetation (*arrow*) attached to aortic valve (*AV*) that was highly mobile and prolapsed into the left-ventricular outflow tract. This density showed characteristic features of a vegetation (see text for details). *LV,* left ventricle; *MV,* mitral valve.

Sensitivity of Echocardiography for Vegetations

From the earlier discussion, it is apparent that some variance in the reported sensitivity and specificity of echocardiography for endocarditis would be expected on the basis of the echocardiographic criteria chosen, vegetation sizes, and location unique to the population being studied, as well as the quality of the technical performance and interpretative expertise of examiners. The results of earlier studies summarized by O'Brien and Geiser (13) reported sensitivities that varied from 43 to 100%, with an overall sensitivity of 79%

for the detection of vegetations by two-dimensional TTE in infective endocarditis.

More recent echocardiographic studies (11,14–20) comparing the sensitivities of TTE and TEE for native valve vegetations suggest that earlier reported values (13) are likely inflated (Table 4). All studies comparing the two techniques have consistently shown that TEE is substantially more sensitive than TTE for detecting vegetations, with an overall sensitivity in excess of 90% for TEE and approximately 60% for TTE (Table 4). Although these recent studies have definitively confirmed that TEE is more sensitive than

TABLE 4. *Comparative studies of sensitivity and specificity of transthoracic (TTE) versus transesophageal (TEE) echocardiography for vegetations in native valve infective endocarditis*

Study	Sensitivity*		Specificity**	
	TTE%	TEE%	TTE%	TEE%
Erbel et al. (11)	55 (11/20)	100 (20/20)	98 (70/71)	98 (70/71)
Daniel et al. (14)	60 (53/88)	99 (83/88)	—	—
Mügge et al. (15)	68 (47/69)	94 (65/69)	—	—
Taams et al. (16)	71 (15/21)	86 (18/21)	—	—
Shively et al. (17)	69 (11/16)	94 (15/16)	92 (46/50)	98 (49/50)
Pedersen et al. (18)	33 (2/6)	100 (6/6)	89 (8/9)	100 (9/9)
Birmingham et al. (19)	30 (10/33)	88 (29/33)	100 (30/30)	97 (29/30)
Shapiro et al. (20)	68 (23/34)	97 (33/34)	91 (31/34)	91 (31/34)
Total	60 (172/287)	94 (269/287)	95 (185/194)	97 (188/194)

* Data represent number of vegetations; ** data represent number of patients without vegetations, correctly identified by TTE or TEE.

TABLE 5. *Comparative studies of transthoracic (TTE) versus transesophageal (TEE) echocardiography in detection of native tricuspid and pulmonic valve vegetations*

Study	No of pts	TV vegetation*		PV vegetation*	
		TTE	TEE	TTE	TEE
San Roman et al. (21)	48	21/21	21/21	—	—
Herrera et al. (22)	7	3/4	4/4	2/3	3/3
Mügge et al. (15)	2	2/2	2/2	—	—
Pedersen et al. (18)	5	1/2	2/2	—	—
Birmingham et al. (19)	31	0/1	1/1	—	—
Shapiro et al. (20)	30	5/8	8/8	0/3	3/3
Total	121	32/38 (84%)	38/38 (100%)	2/6 (33%)	6/6 (100%)

No. of Pts, number of patients with suspected infective endocarditis; *PV*, pulmonic valve; *TV*, tricuspid valve; *data presented as number of TV or PV vegetations detected by TTE or TEE/number of TV or PV vegetations.

TTE for left-sided (e.g., aortic or mitral valve) vegetations, the same cannot be unequivocally stated for their comparative sensitivities for right-sided (e.g., pulmonic or tricuspid valve) vegetations. A compilation of six studies (15,18–22) suggests that TEE, as compared to TTE, detects only slightly more tricuspid valve vegetations in patients with suspected endocarditis (Table 5). However, the delineation of the tricuspid valve with a monoplane TEE probe, as was used in these studies, may often prove difficult. It is unclear if the advent of multiplane TEE will further widen the yield of TEE compared to TTE (23). Although not ideally imaged by TEE, the pulmonic valve is more fully delineated by TEE as compared to TTE. As such, anecdotal reports (20,22–24) suggesting a better detection of pulmonic valve vegetations by TEE versus TTE are probably correct (Table 5).

Specificity of Echocardiography for Vegetations

A high specificity of TTE for native valve vegetations, typically in excess of 95%, has been consistently shown (Table 4). Despite the better sensitivity of TEE, comparative studies (11,14,16–20) confirm that the high specificity of TTE is maintained by TEE (Table 4). These impressive results are partly attributable to the experience of investigators conducting such studies who are abundantly aware of the many entities which may mimic or simulate a vegetation by TEE (25). The advent of multiplane TEE, providing an enhanced ability to define intracardiac structures, should maintain the reported high specificity of TEE for native valve vegetations when applied in clinical practice by less experienced examiners (23).

Sensitivity and Specificity of Echocardiography for Structural Complications of Native Valve Infective Endocarditis

Equally as important as the detection of vegetations is the determination of potential structural complications from infective endocarditis. Formation of myocardial abscess, fistula, mycotic aneurysm, valvular aneurysm or perforation, or a flail leaflet are serious complications of infective endocarditis and harbingers of morbid events and higher mortality. Either one of these entities may warrant surgical intervention. Unquestionably, echocardiography, particularly TEE, has been crucially important in the diagnosis of these complications from endocarditis.

Prior to the advent of echocardiography, the diagnosis of myocardial abscess was primarily made postmortem (26). Two-dimensional TTE quickly proved to be a major advance in the clinical diagnosis of this potentially life-threatening complication of infective endocarditis (27–29). Myocardial abscesses from endocarditis are more frequently in the periaortic valvular region as compared to other perivalvular areas (30,31). Although Ellis et al. (29), in a retrospective study, reported a sensitivity of 86% (19 of 22) and specificity of 88% (21 of 24) for TTE in the detection of myocardial abscesses, subsequent studies have shown significant limitations of this technique when compared to TEE (31,32). Employing the "classic" echocardiographic criterion for myocardial abscess, namely echolucent areas within the myocardium or fibrosa, Daniel et al. (31) showed that TEE was considerably more sensitive than TTE for detecting abscesses associated with native valve endocarditis (i.e., 87 versus 27%). Specificities for both techniques were excellent (i.e., <95%).

TEE also is superior to TTE in the precise delineation of the anatomic extent of subaortic complications in aortic valve endocarditis (32). The mitral-aortic intervalvular fibrosa is a complex interannular junctional zone between portions of the anterior mitral leaflet and the aortic valve. Complications from infective endocarditis in this zone are schematically depicted in Figure 3 and include abscess, aneurysm, fistula, and rupture. Precise characterization of these complications aided by TEE is often critical in determining the appropriate surgical intervention. Two-dimensional and color flow Doppler TTE is a useful technique for detecting mitral valvular perforation. However, it appears limited for the diagnosis of aortic valve perforation (33). Transesophageal echocardiography more accurately defines this serious complication of the mitral or aortic valve (33). Although not

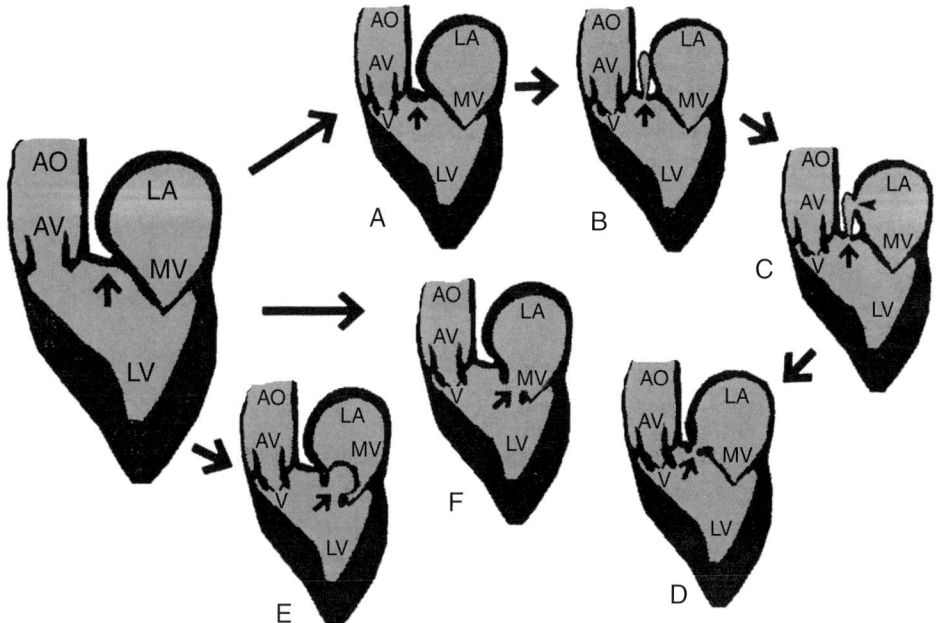

FIG. 3. Schematic of the long-axis view of the heart and subaortic structures with primary endocarditis of the aortic valve. **A–D:** The panels represent complications of secondary infection of the mitral-aortic intervalvular fibrosa (*arrow*). **A** shows mitral-aortic intervalvular fibrosa abscess; **B** shows aneurysm; **C** shows rupture of the aneurysm into the left atrium (*arrowhead*); and **D** shows rupture of the mitral-aortic intervalvular fibrosa into the left atrium without formation of an aneurysm. **E** and **F** show complications resulting from secondary infection of the anterior mitral leaflet. **E** demonstrates formation of an aneurysm, and **F** shows perforation of the anterior mitral leaflet. *AO,* aorta; *AV,* aortic valve; *LA,* left atrium; *LV,* left ventricle; *MV,* mitral valve. (From ref. 32, with permission.)

unanticipated, TEE appears superior to TTE in the detection and characterization of valvular aneurysms from infective endocarditis (34). Color flow Doppler monoplane TEE, on occasion, may underestimate the severity of tricuspid valve regurgitation relative to TTE. Thus, TTE assumes an important role when significant tricuspid regurgitation is felt to complicate endocarditis, but unconfirmed by monoplane TEE. However, in my experience multiplane TEE has eliminated this potentially important limitation of monoplane TEE.

Why Is TEE Superior to TTE?

The explanation for TEE's unequivocal superiority over TTE for left-sided vegetations and structural complications from infective endocarditis is straightforward in most respects, but enlightening in others (Table 6). Current TEE probes image at frequencies greater than or equal to 5.0 mHz as compared to the 2.5 to 3.5 mHz range commonly used for TTE in adults. The esophageal window for TEE affords a closer proximity of the transducer to the aortic and mitral valves. Thus, it is understandable that the resolution of TEE would be superior to TTE. In addition, multiplane TEE offers a better intuitive three-dimensional assessment of the extent of disease and lessens false positives as compared to monoplane TEE by displaying anatomy more fully. Equally

important is the capability to interrogate the entire aortic and, especially, mitral valve apparatus by TEE. For example, with multiplane TEE, the tomographic plane can be swept through the entire surface of the mitral valve leaflets, chordae tendineae, annulus, and papillary muscles in search for endocarditic lesions. Standard transthoracic echocardiographic views (e.g., parasternal long- and short-axis, and apical four-, two- and three-chamber planes) as commonly performed do not completely image the entire mitral or aortic valve apparatus. A nonstandard approach, coupled with standard views, of sweeping through the valvular apparatus in intermediate and "oblique" planes, much in the manner of

TABLE 6. *Factors promoting the superiority of transesophageal echocardiography (TEE) over transthoracic echocardiography for left-sided lesions due to endocarditis*

Higher ultrasound frequency
  ≥5.0 vs. 2.5 MHz—enhances TEE resolution
More proximity to valves
  Enhances TEE resolution
Multiplane views
  More three-dimensional, allowing better assessment of extent of disease and fewer false positives
Complete visualization of entire valvular apparatus
  Enhances sensitivity of TEE

TEE, is necessary to fully visualize valve anatomy (35). We have adopted this broader approach in our laboratory when confronted with the potential diagnosis of endocarditis.

PROSTHETIC VALVE INFECTIVE ENDOCARDITIS SENSITIVITY AND SPECIFICITY OF ECHOCARDIOGRAPHY

Factors that influence the sensitivity and specificity of echocardiography for native valve endocarditis, as discussed earlier, also impact the echocardiographic detection of prosthetic valve vegetations or complications. In addition, acoustic shadowing from prosthetic valve material obstructs passage of ultrasound, possibly obscuring lesions distal to the valve, which potentially lowers the sensitivity of echocardiography. Thus, it is not unexpected that the sensitivities for prosthetic versus native valve endocarditis are less with two-dimensional TTE (approximately 35 versus 60%) or TEE (approximately 85 versus 95%). Conversely, the specificity of echocardiography for prosthetic versus native valve endocarditis appears similar. However, false positives for prosthetic valve endocarditis may occur from an erroneous interpretation of artifactual phantoms, sewing ring suture, fibrin strands (36), surgically severed or retained chordae tendineae (37), or periprosthetic material—entities associated with prosthetic valves.

Compilation of the results from six studies (15,17–19,38,39) shows a better sensitivity of TEE (85%) for vegetations from prosthetic valve endocarditis as compared to that of TTE (36%) (Table 7). Daniel et al. (31) have shown that TEE as compared to TTE is more sensitive for abscess complicating prosthetic valve endocarditis (88 versus 31%), but equally specific (94 versus 100%). Perivalvular abscess occurs more commonly with prosthetic compared to native valve endocarditis and may be detected by TEE more frequently than vegetations in prosthetic valve endocarditis (e.g., 50 versus 33%) (16). As such, the role of TEE for recognition of abscess may be crucial in the diagnosis

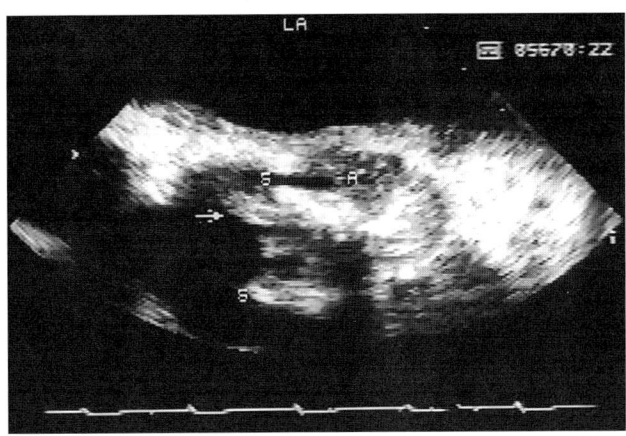

FIG. 4. Transesophageal echocardiography oblique short-axis view of bioprosthetic aortic valve with paravalvular abscess (*A*) and vegetation (*arrow*). Two of the struts (*S*) of the valve are seen. *LA,* left atrium.

of prosthetic valve endocarditis (Fig. 4). However, anterior aortic root abscesses identified in 3 patients by TTE but missed by TEE in the study of Taams et al. (16) emphasizes the complementary role of these two echocardiographic modalities. Prosthetic valve dehiscence may be the only abnormality present in infective endocarditis and is more easily detected and fully delineated by TEE. Although a diagnosis of endocarditis should not be made on the basis of valvular dehiscence alone, when coupled with appropriate clinical signs, this isolated echocardiographic finding would strongly support that diagnosis. Small periprosthetic valvular regurgitant jets are recognized immediately after valve replacement by TEE and should not be misdiagnosed as due to endocarditis. However, an expanding area of dehiscence is more specific and supports the notion that serial TEE may be necessary in evaluating patients with possible prosthetic valve endocarditis but a finding of ''minor'' valvular dehiscence on initial TEE. Echocardiography, particularly TEE, plays an important role in the detection of additional complications of prosthetic valve endocarditis, such as fistula, mycotic aneurysm, etc. (Fig. 5).

Impact of Valve Type and Position and Type of TEE Probe on Sensitivity of TEE for Prosthetic Valve Endocarditis

The completeness of a TEE examination for prosthetic valve endocarditis is significantly influenced by the type and position of the prosthetic valve being evaluated and the type of TEE probe. These factors are likely to impact the sensitivity of TEE for prosthetic valve endocarditis in individual patients. In general, mechanical valves are more difficult to fully image than bioprosthetic or tissue valves (e.g., homografts). One noticeable exception to this rule are the mechanical bileaflet tilting disk valves when in the mitral position, which can be as completely imaged, if not more so, as that

TABLE 7. *Sensitivity of transthoracic (TTE) and transesophageal (TEE) echocardiography for prosthetic valve infective endocarditis vegetations*

Study	Sensitivity*	
	TTE %	TEE %
Mügge et al. (15)	27 (6/22)	77 (17/22)
Shively et al. (17)	0 (0/3)	100 (3/3)
Pedersen et al. (18)	43 (3/7)	100 (7/7)
Birmingham et al. (19)	0 (0/2)	100 (2/2)
Daniel et al. (38)	36 (12/33)	82 (27/33)
Zabalgoitia et al. (39)	44 (19/44)	86 (38/44)
Total	36 (40/111)	85 (94/111)

*Data represent number of vegetations.

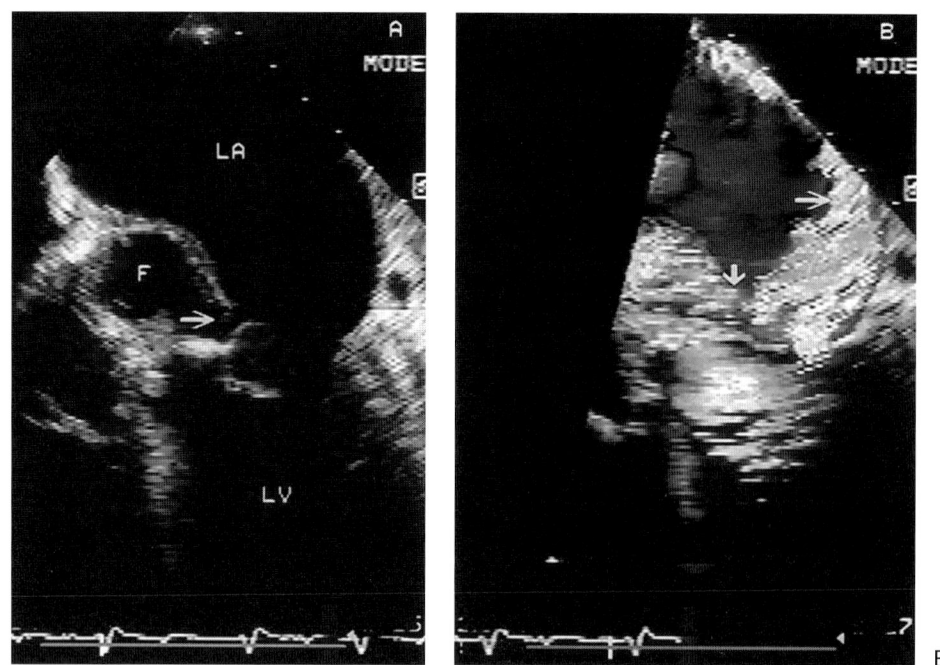

FIG. 5. Transesophageal echocardiography five-chamber plane of false aneurysm (*F*) that ruptured (*arrow*) into the left atrium (*LA*) complicating prosthetic valve endocarditis (**A**). Continuous flow from the site of rupture (*down arrow*) into the left atrium and along the lateral left atrial wall (*rightward arrow*) was well seen with color Doppler (**B**). *LV,* left ventricle.

of bioprostheses with TEE. The thoroughness by which mechanical valves can be examined is heterogeneous and depends on the specific valve design. Ball-in-cage valves are typically more demanding to fully image compared to single leaflet or bileaflet tilting disk valves. A specific prosthetic valve type is more easily imaged in the mitral compared to the aortic position. For example, a bileaflet tilting disk valve in the mitral position is very easily imaged completely, but when placed in the aortic position this valve is the most challenging valve to fully examine and often only partially seen despite transgastric long-axis planes. A multiplane probe allows for a more thorough interrogation of prosthetic valves as compared to a biplane and, certainly, a monoplane TEE probe—particularly for valves in the aortic position.

CLINICAL IMPACT OF ECHOCARDIOGRAPHY IN NATIVE AND PROSTHETIC VALVE INFECTIVE ENDOCARDITIS

Prognostic Value of Echocardiography for Morbidity and Death from Endocarditis

Numerous studies (10,11,15,30,40–46) have reported specific TTE findings associated with a higher risk of death and complications from endocarditis (Table 8). Complications include cerebral, peripheral, and pulmonary embolism, heart failure, and sepsis. Death may occur from any of these entities and is more frequent in patients with virulent organisms, protracted illness prior to therapy, and prosthetic valves, or in the elderly.

Sanfilippo et al. (42), in a retrospective study of 204 patients with infective endocarditis, reported that increasing vegetation length was associated with more frequent complications. An echocardiographic score based on vegetation size, extent, echogenicity, and mobility had a 70% sensitivity and 92% specificity for complications in mitral valve endocarditis and a 76% sensitivity and 62% specificity in aortic valve endocarditis. Predicting specific complications from infective endocarditis and the need for prophylactic surgical intervention on the basis of echocardiographic findings remains controversial. Left-sided vegetations in excess of 10 mm have been associated with more frequent systemic embolism by some investigators (15,16,46), but not by others (11,40,42,47,48). Mügge et al. (15), in a study of 105 patients with infective endocarditis, reported that subjects with a vegetation greater than 10 mm had a higher incidence of embolism (47%) than did those with a vegetation less than or

TABLE 8. *Potentially useful echocardiographic predictors of morbidity and mortality from infective endocarditis*

Vegetation size > 10 mm
Mobile vegetation
Mitral vs. aortic vegetation
Vegetation echogenicity similar to myocardium
Enlarging vegetation in serial studies
Valve damage (e.g., flail/perforation)
Complication abscess/aneurysm/fistula
Left ventricular dysfunction

equal to 10 mm (19%), particularly when involving the mitral valve. Similarly, Jaffe et al. (10) noted embolism in 26% (8 of 32) of patients with vegetations greater than 10 mm, compared to 11% (2 of 18) of subjects with smaller or no vegetations. However, recent studies using TTE (47) or TEE (48) have shown no significant relationship between vegetation size and embolism. The variance in the results of these studies is unknown but may relate to differences in observation periods between patients with and without large vegetations or to differences in antecedent antibiotic treatment and its duration prior to echocardiography. Valvular vegetations may increase, decrease, or not change in size during therapy for endocarditis (47,50). Rohmann et al. (51) using serial TEE in 83 patients with endocarditis showed that subjects in which vegetations increased or were unchanged compared to those with vegetations that decreased had more embolic events (45 versus 17%), valve replacement (45 versus 2%) and death (10 versus 0%). Although the divergence in results of existing studies suggests that vegetation size cannot be used as an independent indicator to perform prophylactic surgery, clinicians are often confronted with "gigantic" vegetations that create a sense of unease and appear to justify a more aggressive surgical approach (Fig. 6). A metaanalysis by Tischler et al. (52) further supports the notion that echocardiographically detected left-sided vegetations greater than 10 mm predispose to an increased risk of systemic embolism and need for valve surgery.

The leading cause of death in infective endocarditis is congestive heart failure. Destruction of cardiac valves by this process causes valvular regurgitation. TTE using color-flow and spectral Doppler is a major advance in the noninvasive evaluation of valvular regurgitation. TEE is a useful adjunct to TTE for this same purpose, particularly in the assessment of prosthetic valves (see Chapter 43). Although the decision to intervene surgically in the treatment of patients with infective endocarditis is largely based on clinical considerations, several echocardiographic findings demand that surgical therapy be considered. These findings include: (i) ring abscess or fistula, which bestow an ominous prognosis and may worsen in the face of antibiotic therapy; (ii) severe valvular regurgitation, particularly if the mitral valve is involved and can be repaired; and (iii) mechanical prosthetic valve endocarditis, which makes eradication of infection with antibiotics alone difficult.

Does Echocardiography Impact Clinical Outcome in Infective Endocarditis?

The outcome of infective endocarditis depends critically on its early recognition and the initiation of appropriate medical and/or surgical therapy. Echocardiography expedites the diagnosis of endocarditis and helps guide the appropriate medical approach. Although blinded, randomized large-scale trials are lacking, several studies support the idea that echocardiography has an indispensable role in improving outcome in endocarditis (53,54). Schulz et al. (53) compared the clinical outcome in patients with native valve or prosthetic valve infective endocarditis. The in-hospital mortality (21 versus 17%) and mortality during a follow-up of 22 plus or minus 10 months (28 versus 25%) did not significantly differ between native and prosthetic valve endocarditis. In this study (53), prosthetic valve endocarditis did not have a worse prognosis than native valve endocarditis, results attributed to an improved diagnostic accuracy achieved by TEE, leading to comparable diagnostic latency periods in both groups. In a similar study, Werner et al. (54) found that infective endocarditis in elderly patients had a clinical outcome similar to that of younger patients. These results were attributed to the ability to diagnose endocarditis as early in the elderly as compared to younger patients because of TEE. This enabled a timely initiation of appropriate medical and surgical therapy.

ROLE OF ECHOCARDIOGRAPHY IN EVALUATION OF SUSPECTED NATIVE VALVE ENDOCARDITIS

When to Perform TTE versus TEE

Presentations prompting a clinical suspicion of infective endocarditis vary widely depending on the individual patient risk. Subjects presenting with fever, bacteremia, and new cardiac murmur are readily considered as having endocarditis. However, a high index of suspicion is needed for other patient subsets. For example, confusion or stroke is not an infrequent presentation of endocarditis in the elderly. Unex-

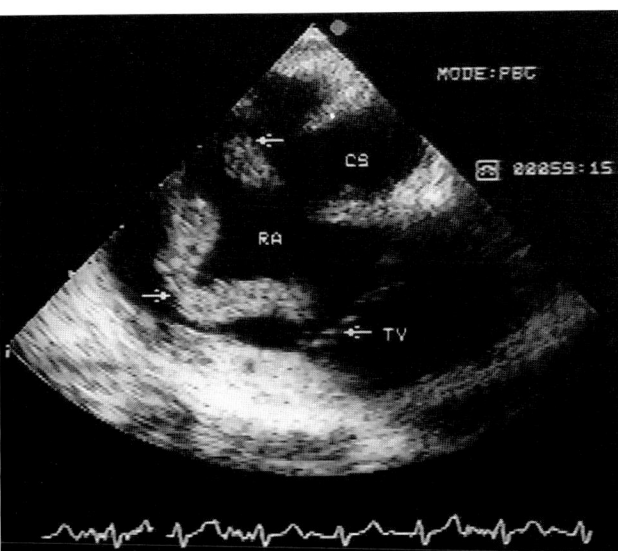

FIG. 6. Transesophageal echocardiography from a four-chamber plane demonstrating a "gigantic" sepentine vegetation (*arrows*) attached to the tricuspid valve (*TV*). This vegetation prolapsed into the coronary sinus (*CS*), inferior vena cava, and right ventricle. This patient expired 24 hours later of sepsis, pulmonary edema, and, presumably, pulmonary embolus. *RA*, right atrium.

TABLE 9. *When to perform transthoracic (TTE) and transesophageal (TEE) echocardiography for suspected native valve infective endocarditis?*

A. TTE performed as primary imaging test in all cases
B. TEE performed for following circumstances after TTE
   1. Nondiagnostic, equivocal, or technically inadequate TTE
   2. Normal TTE but clinical suspicion for endocarditis intermediate to high
   3. TTE negative for abscess or structural complication but clinical course suggestive
   4. Positive blood cultures without obvious noncardiac source and negative TTE

TABLE 10. *When to perform transthoracic (TTE) and transesophageal (TEE) echocardiography for suspected prosthetic valve infective endocarditis?*

A. TEE performed as primary imaging test in almost all cases
B. If TTE performed before TEE, when to do TEE?
   1. Negative, nondiagnostic, or inadequate TTE
   2. TTE positive for vegetation but structural complications (e.g., abscess, fistula) suspected on clinical grounds
   3. TTE positive for vegetations and nonsurgical treatment approach planned

plained fever or pulmonary infection in intravenous drug abusers should raise suspicion for infective endocarditis. Immunocompromised patients may present with unexplained deterioration in overall health. Chronic renal failure predisposes to native valve infective endocarditis because of degenerative valvular disease. A high index of suspicion must be reserved for such patients. TTE is reasonably sensitive for native valve endocarditis compared to TEE and justifies its use as the primary diagnostic imaging procedure of choice when this condition is suspected. Although TEE is superior to TTE for left-sided endocarditis, the potential risk of complications from this semiinvasive technique warrants some caution as a screening modality for native valve infective endocarditis. If TTE is inadequate for technical reasons or equivocal, most authorities would agree that TEE is then needed (18,19,55–57). However, disagreement remains whether TEE is (18,19) or is not (55–57) justified in the case of technically adequate and normal TTE. Some investigators (55–57) have reported that a negative TTE virtually excludes native valve infective endocarditis. Ultimately, the clinical suspicion for endocarditis should weigh heavily in the decision to proceed with TEE in the face of a normal TTE. In the opinion of this author, TEE should be considered despite a normal TTE if clinical suspicion is *intermediate* to *high* for endocarditis. These and other conditions that warrant consideration of TEE are shown in Table 9. A negative TEE, particularly with multiplane technology (23), makes the probability of native valve infective endocarditis very low (17,58). However, echocardiography cannot exclude endocarditis and repeat TEE should be considered when clinical suspicion warrants.

ROLE OF ECHOCARDIOGRAPHY IN EVALUATION OF SUSPECTED PROSTHETIC VALVE INFECTIVE ENDOCARDITIS

When to Perform TTE versus TEE

Unlike native valve infective endocarditis, in the opinion of this author, TEE should be used as a primary diagnostic imaging modality when prosthetic valve infective endocarditis is suspected. The sensitivity of TTE in this circumstance

is low, making it a problematic screening test. Practicing clinicians are often inappropriately reassured when a TTE fails to demonstrate vegetations or abscess, which is often the case,. Transesophageal echocardiography is a very safe and widely available test with considerably better sensitivity for prosthetic valve endocarditis. These features justify its role as a primary imaging test in this clinical condition. TTE may be needed in select circumstances as an adjunct to TEE. In cases in which TTE has been performed before TEE, a negative or nondiagnostic test warrants TEE. A TTE demonstrating prosthetic valve vegetations may not obviate the need for TEE in certain circumstances, such as clinical suspicion of endocarditis complications (e.g., abscess, fistula) or in individuals with planned nonsurgical treatment (Table 10) (59).

UNUSUAL SITES OF VEGETATIONS AND COMPLICATIONS OF INFECTIVE ENDOCARDITIS: VALUE OF TEE

Transesophageal echocardiography has virtually unlimited ability to interrogate nonvalvular intracardiac structures beyond valves in search of lesions attributable to infective endocarditis. Thus, TEE has a unique capability of diagnosing unusual sites of infective endocarditis that would be otherwise difficult to diagnose. Unusual sites of vegetations potentially diagnosable using TEE include the eustachian valve (60,61), thebesian valve, patent ductus (62), mural endocardium (63), pacer leads (64), central lines, and indwelling catheters. Rare complications of endocarditis may also be readily detected by TEE, such as descending thoracic aortic mycotic aneurysm (65) and ruptured membranous interventricular septum (66).

COST-EFFECTIVENESS OF ECHOCARDIOGRAPHY IN INFECTIVE ENDOCARDITIS

Medical decisions are increasingly shaped by financial considerations. Demonstrating the potential cost-effectiveness of echocardiography in the management of patients with suspected or proven infective endocarditis is necessarily a complex and daunting task, which as of yet has not been done. Compared to other cardiac imaging modalities (e.g., single-photon emission computed tomography imaging, positron emission tomography imaging, magnetic resonance imaging, or computed tomography), echocardiography, particularly TTE, is less expensive, making it a favorable option. Echocardiography may ultimately prove to be cost-effective in several ways. A major cost in the treatment of infective endocarditis is the protracted hospitalization required for intravenous antibiotics. Echocardiography may be useful in identifying patients at low risk for complications and expedite their management to an outpatient setting. Potential cost savings could accrue by identifying patients at high risk for complications (e.g., abscess) and low likelihood of nonsurgical cure, thereby shortening time to surgery and circumventing cumulative, incremental cost from management of preventable complications (e.g., embolism, heart failure, etc.) (67). Definitive echocardiographic findings confirming infective endocarditis may lessen cost by curtailing planned extensive evaluations for noncardiac sources of bacteremia. However, TTE, because of its widespread availability, lack of risk, and relatively inexpensive cost is often inappropriately employed without consideration of patient pretest probability of infective endocarditis. Practicing clinicians must use sound judgment in the construction of a medically appropriate framework for clinical decision-making in the usage of echocardiography in patients with suspected or proven endocarditis.

ECHOCARDIOGRAPHY IN CULTURE-NEGATIVE ENDOCARDITIS

Culture-negative endocarditis (defined as infective endocarditis despite persistently negative blood cultures) is a clinical dilemma for which echocardiography may play an important role. Mortality may be high, attributable to a delay in diagnosis and initiation of treatment (68). Echocardiography may be useful to delineate the vegetations and structural complications of endocarditis (69). It is probable that the emergence of echocardiography has shortened the time to diagnosis of culture-negative endocarditis, hastened initiation of antimicrobial therapy, and, thereby, potentially reduced morbidity and mortality (70).

ALTERNATIVE IMAGING MODALITIES TO ECHOCARDIOGRAPHY AND NEWLY EMERGING ECHOCARDIOGRAPHIC TECHNIQUES IN ENDOCARDITIS

Echocardiography is the undisputed imaging technique of choice in the evaluation of endocarditis. However, other imaging modalities have been reported in the assessment of endocarditis that include nuclear single-photon emission computed tomography, magnetic resonance imaging, and computed tomography. The advantages of echocardiography, particularly with the advent of TEE over these techniques for this clinical situation will make echocardiography

the procedure of choice in the assessment of endocarditis in the foreseeable future. These advantages include safety (TTE), flexibility, widespread availability, excellent sensitivity and specificity, and the ability to assess ventricular, native valve and prosthetic valve function, and competitive cost. In addition, newly emerging echocardiographic techniques and applications further solidify the role of echocardiography in the assessment of infective endocarditis. Three-dimensional echocardiography promises to allow a more comprehensive analysis of cardiac structure in the setting of endocarditis (71). Transesophageal echocardiography guided vegetation biopsy by a transvenous method may usher in a new era in the diagnosis of infective endocarditis, especially in culture-negative endocarditis (72). Nevertheless, magnetic resonance methods provide a safe alternative when TTE methods are unsuccessful and TEE is undesirable.

SUMMARY

In summary, echocardiography has an important and often pivotal role in the diagnosis and management of patients with infective endocarditis. TTE and TEE are complementary, but TEE is superior in sensitivity for vegetations, abscess, and other endocarditic complications. TTE should remain the first-line diagnostic imaging test in most patients with suspected native valve infective endocarditis by virtue of its safety, reasonable sensitivity, and unsurpassed specificity. However, TEE is essential in most patients with suspected prosthetic valve infective endocarditis. A negative TEE, particularly with multiplane imaging, makes endocarditis very unlikely. Repeat echocardiographic studies in patients with proven endocarditis may be of use in monitoring response to antibiotic therapy; failure of a vegetation to become smaller would denote a worse prognosis. Although cost-effectiveness data supporting a favorable cost-benefit ratio for echocardiography in infective endocarditis have not been reported, echocardiography has the potential to improve outcome by promoting an earlier diagnosis of endocarditis and expediting initiation of antimicrobial treatment. Lastly, technological developments (e.g., three-dimensional echocardiography) promise to further enhance the role of echocardiography in infective endocarditis.

REFERENCES

1. Bayliss R, Clarke C, Oakley C, et al. The microbiology and pathogenesis of infective endocarditis. *Br Heart J* 1983;50:513–519.
2. Malquarti V, Saradarian W, Etienne J, et al. Prognosis of native valve infective endocarditis: a review of 253 cases. *Eur Heart J* 1984;5:11–20.
3. Erbel R, Liu F, Ge J, et al. Identification of high-risk subgroups in infective endocarditis and the role of echocardiography. *Eur Heart J* 1995;16:588–602.
4. Frary CJ, Devereux RB, Kramer-Fox R, et al. Clinical and health care cost consequences of infective endocarditis in mitral valve prolapse. *Am J Cardiol* 1994;73:263–267.
5. Osler W. The Gulstonian Lectures on malignant endocarditis. *Br Med J* 1885;1:467–470;522–526;577–579.

6. Dillon JC, Feigenbaum H, Konecke LL, et al. Echocardiographic manifestations of valvular vegetations. *Am Heart J* 1973;86:698–704.

7. von Reyn CF, Levy BS, Arbeit RD, et al. Infective endocarditis: an analysis based on strict case definitions. *Ann Intern Med* 1981;94(Pt 1):505–518.

8. Durack DT, Lukes AS, Bright DK. New criteria for diagnosis of infective endocarditis: utilization of specific echocardiographic findings. Duke endocarditis service. *Am J Med* 1994;96(3):200–209.

9. Hoen B, Beguinot I, Rabaud C, et al. The Duke criteria for diagnosing infective endocarditis are specific: analysis of 100 patients with acute fever or fever of unknown origin. *Clin Infect Dis* 1996;23(2):298–302.

10. Jaffe WM, Morgan DE, Pearlman AS, et al. Infective endocarditis, 1983–1988: echocardiographic findings and factors influencing morbidity and mortality. *J Am Coll Cardiol* 1990;15:1227–1233.

11. Erbel R, Rohmann S, Drexler M, et al. Improved diagnostic value of echocardiography in patients with infective endocarditis by transesophageal approach. A prospective study. *Eur Heart J* 1988;9:43–53.

12. Gilbert BW, Haney RS, Crawford F, et al. Two-dimensional echocardiographic assessment of vegetative endocarditis. *Circulation* 1977;55:346–353.

13. O'Brien JT, Geiser EA. Infective endocarditis and echocardiography. *Am Heart J* 1984;108:386–394.

14. Daniel WG, Schröder E, Mügge A, et al. Transesophageal echocardiography in infective endocarditis. *Am J Cardiac Imag* 1998;2:78–85.

15. Mügge A, Daniel WG, Frank G, et al. Echocardiography in infective endocarditis: reassessment of prognostic implications of vegetation size determined by the transthoracic and the transesophageal approach. *J Am Coll Cardiol* 1989;14:631–638.

16. Taams MA, Gussenhoven EJ, Bos E, et al. Enhanced morphological diagnosis in infective endocarditis by transesophageal echocardiography. *Br Heart J* 1990;63:102–113.

17. Shively BK, Gurule T, Roldan C, et al. Diagnostic value of transesophageal compared with transthoracic echocardiography in infective endocarditis. *J Am Coll Cardiol* 1991;18:391–397.

18. Pedersen WR, Walker M, Olson JD, et al. Value of transesophageal echocardiography as an adjunct to transthoracic echocardiography in evaluation of native and prosthetic valve endocarditis. *Chest* 1991;100:351–356.

19. Birmingham GD, Rahko PS, Ballantyne F. Improved detection of infective endocarditis with transesophageal echocardiography. *Am Heart J* 1992;123:774–781.

20. Shapiro SM, Young E, De Guzman S, et al. Transesophageal echocardiography in diagnosis of infective endocarditis. *Chest* 1994;105:377–382.

21. San Roman JA, Vilacosta I, Zamorano JL, et al. Transesophageal echocardiography in right-sided endocarditis. *J Am Coll Cardiol* 1993;21:1226–1230.

22. Herrera CJ, Mehlman DJ, Hartz RS, et al. Comparison of transesophageal and transthoracic echocardiography for diagnosis of right-sided cardiac lesions. *Am Heart J* 1992;70:964–966.

23. Job FP, Franke S, Lethen H, et al. Incremental value of biplane and multiplane transesophageal echocardiography for the assessment of active infective endocarditis. *Am J Cardiol* 1995;75:1033–1037.

24. Shapiro SM, Young E, Ginzton LE, et al. Pulmonic valve endocarditis as an under diagnosed disease: role of transesophageal echocardiography. *J Am Soc Echocardiogr* 1992;5:48–51.

25. Stoddard MF, Liddell NE, Longaker RA, et al. Transesophageal echocardiography: normal variants and mimickers. *Am Heart J* 1992;6(24):1597–1598.

26. Ryon DS, Pastor BH, Myerson RM. Abscess of the myocardium. *Am J Med Sci* 1996;251:698–705.

27. Fox S, Cotler MN, Segal Bl, et al. Echocardiographic diagnosis of acute aortic valve endocarditis and its complications. *Arch Intern Med* 1977;137:85–89.

28. Mardelli TJ, Ogawa S, Hubbard FE, et al. Cross-sectional echocardiographic detection of aortic ring abscess in bacterial endocarditis. *Chest* 1978;74:576–578.

29. Ellis SG, Goldstein J, Popp RL. Detection of endocarditis-associated perivalvular abscesses by two-dimensional echocardiography. *J Am Coll Cardiol* 1985;5:647–653.

30. Aguado JM, Gonzalez-Vilchez F, Martin-Duran R, et al. Perivalvular abscesses associated with endocarditis: clinical features and diagnostic accuracy of two-dimensional echocardiography. *Chest* 1993;104:88–93.

31. Daniel WG, Mügge A, Martin RP, et al. Improvement in the diagnosis of abscesses associated with endocarditis by transesophageal echocardiography. *N Engl J Med* 1991;324:795–800.

32. Karalis DG, Bansal RC, Hauck AJ, et al. Transesophageal echocardiographic recognition of subaortic complications in aortic valve endocarditis: clinical and surgical implications. *Circulation* 1992;86:353–362.

33. De Castro S, d'Amati G, Cartoni D, et al. Valvular perforation in left-sided infective endocarditis: a prospective echocardiographic evaluation and clinical outcome. *Am Heart J* 1997;134(4):656–664.

34. Mollod M, Felner KJ, Felner JM. Mitral and tricuspid valve aneurysms evaluated by transesophageal echocardiography. *Am J Cardiol* 1997;79(9):1269–1272.

35. Gleason CB, Stoddard MF, Wagner SG, et al. A comparison of cardiac valvular involvement in the primary antiphospholipid syndrome versus anticardiolipin-negative systemic lupus erythematosus. *Am Heart J* 1993;125:1123–1129.

36. Stoddard MF, Dawkins PR, Longaker RA. Mobile strands are frequently attached to the St. Jude medical mitral valve prosthesis as assessed by two-dimensional transesophageal echocardiography. *Am Heart J* 1992;124:671–674.

37. Malaterre HR, Sunda M. Chordae tendineae mimicking vegetation after mitral valve replacement. *Ann Thorac Surg* 1996;62(3):944–945.

38. Daniel WG, Mügge A, Grote J, et al. Comparison of transthoracic and transesophageal echocardiography for detection of abnormalities of prosthetic and bioprosthetic valves in the mitral and aortic positions. *Am J Cardiol* 1993;71:210–215.

39. Zabalgoitia M, Herrera CJ, Chaudhry FA, et al. Improvement in the diagnosis of bioprosthetic valve dysfunction by transesophageal echocardiography. *J Heart Valve Dis* 1993;3:595–603.

40. Lutas EM, Roberts RB, Devereux RB, et al. Relation between the presence of echocardographic vegetations and the complication rate in infective endocarditis. *Am Heart J* 1986;112:107–113.

41. Buda AJ, Zotz R, LeMire MS, et al. Prognostic significance of vegetations detected by two-dimensional echocardiography in infective endocarditis. *Am Heart J* 1986;112:1291–1296.

42. Sanfilippo AJ, Picard MH, Newell JB, et al. Echocardiographic assessment of patients with infectious endocarditis: prediction of risk for complications. *J Am Coll Cardiol* 1991;18:1191–1199.

43. Rohmann S, Seifert T, Erbel R, et al. Identification of abscess formation in native valve infective endocarditis using transesophageal echocardiography: implications for surgical treatment. *Thorac Cardiovasc Surg* 1991;39:273–280.

44. Rohmann S, Erbel R, Darius H, et al. Prediction of rapid versus prolonged healing of infective endocarditis by monitoring vegetation size. *J Am Soc Echocardiogr* 1991;4:465–474.

45. Rohmann S, Erbel R, George G, et al. Clinical relevance of vegetation localization by transesophageal echocardiography in infective endocarditis. *Eur Heart J* 1992;12:446–452.

46. Lancelloti P, Galiuto L, Albert A, et al. Relative value of clinical and transesophageal echocardiographic variables for risk stratification in patients with infective endocarditis. *Clin Cardiol* 1998;21:572–578.

47. Heinle S, Wilderman N, Harrison K, et al. Value of transthoracic echocardiography in predicting embolic events in active infective endocarditis. *Am J Cardiol* 1994;74:799–801.

48. Castro SD, Magni G, Beni S, et al. Role of transthoracic and transesophageal echocardiography in predicting embolic events in patients with active infective endocarditis involving native cardiac valves. *Am J Cardiol* 1997;80:1030–1034.

49. Vuille C, Nidorf M, Weyman AE, et al. Natural history of vegetations during successful medical treatment of endocarditis. *Am Heart J* 1994;128(1):1200–1209.

50. Rohmann S, Erbel R, Darius H, et al. Effect of antibiotic treatment on vegetation size and complication rate in infective endocarditis. *Clin Cardiol* 1997;20(2):132–140.

51. Rohmann S, Erbel R, Darius H, et al. Prediction of rapid versus prolonged healing of infective endocarditis by monitoring vegetation size. *J Am Soc Echocardiogr* 1991;4:465–474.

52. Tischler MD, Vaitkus PT. The ability of vegetation size on echocardiography to predict clinical complications: a meta-analysis. *J Am Soc Echocardiogr* 1997;10(5):562–568.

53. Schulz R, Werner GS, Fuchs JB, et al. Clinical outcome and echocardiographic findings of native and prosthetic valve endocarditis in the 1990's. *Eur Heart J* 1996;17(2):281–288.

54. Werner GS, Schulz R, Fuchs JB, et al. Infective endocarditis in the

elderly in the era of transesophageal echocardiography: clinical features and prognosis compared with younger patients. *Am J Med* 1996;100: 90–97.

55. Lowry RW, Zoghbi WA, Baker WB, et al. Clinical impact of transesophageal echocardiography in the diagnosis and management of infective endocarditis. *Am J Cardiol* 1994;73:1089–1091.

56. Lindner JR, Case RA, Dent JM, et al. Diagnostic value of echocardiography in suspected endocarditis. *Circulation* 1996;93:730–736.

57. Irani WN, Grayburn PA, Afridi I. A negative transthoracic echocardiogram obviates the need for transesophageal echocardiography in patients with suspected native valve active infective endocarditis. *Am J Cardiol* 1996;78:101–103.

58. Sochowski RA, Chan KL. Implication of negative results on a monoplane transesophageal echocardiographic study in patients with suspected infective endocarditis. *J Am Coll Cardiol* 1993;21:216–221.

59. Bruss J, Jacobs LE, Kotler MN, et al. Utility of transesophageal echocardiography in the conservative management of prosthetic valve endocarditis. *Chest* 1992;102:1886–1888.

60. Georgeson R, Liu M, Bansal RC. Transesophageal echocardiographic diagnosis of eustachian valve endocarditis. *J Am Soc Echocardiogr* 1996;9(2):206–208.

61. Palakodeti V, Keen WD Jr, Rickman LS, et al. Eustachian valve endocarditis: detection with multiplane transesophageal echocardiography. *Clin Cardiol* 1997;20(6):579–580.

62. Mandel KE, Ginsburg CM. Staphylococcal endocarditis complicating a patent ductus arteriosus. *Pediatr Infect Dis J* 1994;13(9):833–834.

63. Shirani J, Keffler K, Gerszten E, et al. Primary LV mural endocarditis diagnosed by TEE. *J Am Soc Echocardiogr* 1995;8(4):554–556.

64. Federmann M, Dirsch OR, Jenni R. Pacemaker endocarditis. *Heart* 1996;75:446.

65. Jofe II, Emmi RP, Oline J, et al. Mycotic aneurysm of the descending thoracic aorta: the role of transesophageal echocardiography. *J Am Soc Echocardiogr* 1996;9:663–667.

66. Winslow TM, Friar DA, Larson AW, et al. A rare complication of aortic valve endocarditis: diagnosis with transesophageal echocardiography. *J Am Soc Echocardiogr* 1995;8:546–550.

67. Goldman ME, Fisher EA, Winters S, et al. Early identification of patients with native valve infectious endocarditis at risk for major complications by initial clinical presentation and baseline echocardiography. *Int J Cardiol* 1995;52:257–264.

68. Persanti EL, Smith IM. Infective endocarditis with negative blood cultures: an analysis of 52 cases. *Am J Med* 1979;66:43–50.

69. Rubenson DS, Tucker CR, Stinson EB, et al. The use of echocardiography in diagnosing culture-negative endocarditis. *Circulation* 1981;64: 641–646.

70. Ali AS, Trivedi V, Lesch M. Culture-negative endocarditis: a historical review and 1990s update. *Prog Cardiovasc Dis* 1994;37:149–160.

71. Kasprzak JD, Salustri A, Roelandt JR, et al. Comprehensive analysis of aortic valve vegetation with anyplane, paraplane, and three-dimensional echocardiography. *Eur Heart J* 1996;17:318–320.

72. Colvin EV, Lau YR, Samdarshi TE. Vegetation biopsy using transesophageal echocardiography guidance: a technique to aid in diagnosis of culture-negative endocarditis. *Cathet Cardiovasc Diagn* 1996;37: 215–217.

CHAPTER 45

Clinical and Pathological Features of Cardiomyopathy

Robert W. W. Biederman and
Gerald M. Pohost

The term "cardiomyopathy" is relatively recent in its appearance in the medical literature. Brigden is given the credit for coining the word "cardiomyopathy" in 1957 and a decade later it was defined by Goodwin (1) and later refined by the World Health Organization (2) as myocardial disease exclusive of coronary artery disease (3,4). Later the term was expanded to include primary and secondary cardiomyopathy, the latter to relate the myocardial derangement as dependent upon another initiating process. The term primary (or idiopathic) cardiomyopathy has become slandered in today's literature to mean left ventricular (LV) dysfunction of any unknown cause. For the purpose of this chapter, primary cardiomyopathy will denote nondefinable whereas secondary cardiomyopathy will describe definable causes. It should be noted that the World Health Organization/Scientific Council on Cardiomyopathies, and the task force on cardiomyopathies has proposed that the nomenclature of cardiomyopathy be made less ambiguous (2) (Table 1). Accordingly, the term "cardiomyopathy" should be used to describe the group previously known as "primary cardiomyopathy." Secondary cardiomyopathy should be replaced with the term *specific* heart muscle disease, substituting the known cause (Table 2). For instance, it should be ischemic *heart muscle disease*, not ischemic cardiomyopathy. Chapters 45 and 46 will adhere to this classification.

R. W. W. Biederman: Department of Cardiovascular Disease, Center for Nuclear Magnetic Resonance Research and Development; Department of Medicine, University of Alabama at Birmingham, Birmingham, Alabama 35223.
G. M. Pohost: Department of Medicine, University of Alabama at Birmingham, Birmingham, Alabama 35294.

The epidemiology of congestive heart failure in the U.S. attests to the increasing importance cardiomyopathies are occupying in health care. In 1990 there were 1 million hospitalizations with an adjusted cost of $7 billion, and it was the most common diagnosis-related group (DRG). Moreover, more than 75% of all CHF admissions occurred in the Medicare population. The trend for CHF as a product of cardiomyopathy shows no sign of stabilizing either. The annual incidence in 1970 was 250,000 cases, in 1988 there were 400,000 cases diagnosed, and in 1992 there were nearly 700,000 new cases seen. Thus, the current prevalence is estimated to be 5 million cases in the United States alone representing 1.5% of the population (5) and an extraordinary burden to our gross national product. When one considers the total costs to include lost productivity, the annual cost exceeds $40 billion. The mortality for cardiomyopathy that progresses to CHF despite the improvements in detection and treatment, as well as emerging nonmedical therapies, has barely made a dent in the overall mortality. It remains at 25% in 3 years for NYHA IV symptoms. Thus, it is incumbent upon clinicians and scientist to have better techniques for detection and treatment of a nationwide and certainly global problem.

This chapter will deal with an introduction to the class of cardiomyopathies (primary, secondary, and the dilated cardiomyopathies), and describe the pathology unique to each followed by current treatment strategies. The following chapter (Chapter 46) will deal more directly with specific imaging strategies relevant to each cardiomyopathic condition.

645

TABLE 1. *WHO/ISFC classification of CMX**

Dilated CMX	Restrictive CMX	Hypertrophic CMX
Dilation of LV, RV, or both	May exist without obliteration	Disproportionate hypertrophy of LV;
Dilation often severe accompanied by hypertrophy	Includes endocardial fibrosis and Loeffler cardiomyopathy	occasionally the RV
Impaired systolic function	Scarring effects either LV, RV, or both	Involves the septum more than the free wall; occasionally diffuse
CHF may/may not supervene	Involvement of AV valves is common but outflow tracts are spared	LV volume (typically normal or reduced)
May present with ventricular/atrial arrhythmias	Cavity obliteration characteristic in advanced disease	Systolic pressure gradient commonInheritance by autosomal dominance with incomplete penetrance
Death may occur at any stage		Morphologic changes usually more severe in the septum

*Heart muscle disease of unknown cause or associated with disorders of other symptoms. Disorders of the myocardium caused by systemic or pulmonary hypertension, coronary artery disease, valvular heart disease, or congenital heart disease has been excluded.

CMX, heart muscle disease; LV, left ventricle; RV, right ventricle; CHF, congestive heart failue; AV, atrioventricular.

TABLE 2. *Etiology of specific heart muscle disease*

A

Infections
  Bacterial
    Diphtheria
    Tuberculosis
    Typhoid fever
    Rheumatic fever
    Scarlet fever
    Meningococcal
    Pneumococcal
    Gonococcal
    Brucellosis
    Tetanus
    Meliodosis
    Tularemia
    Pertussis
  Spirochetal
    Syphilis
    Leptospirosis
    Lyme disease
  Rickettsial
    Typhus
    Rocky mountain spotted fever
  Viral
    Poliomyelitis
    Influenza
    Mumps
    Rubella
    Rubeola
    Variola
    Varicella
    Epstein-Barr
    Coxsackie B
    Echovirus
    Cytomegalovirus
    Hepatitis
    Rabies
    Mycoplasma
    Psittiacosis
    Herpes
    Encephalitis
    Arboviruses
  Mycoses
    Actinomycosis
    Blastomycosis
    Monoiliasis
    Aspergilliosis
    Histoplasmosis
    Coccidiomycosis

Cryptococcosis
    Candidiasis
  Protozoal
    Trypanosomiasis cruzi
    Toxoplasmosis
    Malaria
    Amebiasis
    Leishmaniasis
    Balantine coli
  Helminthic
    Trichinosis
    Echinococcosis
    Schistosomiasis
    Ascariasis
    Filariasis
    Paragonimiasis
    Strongyloides
    Cysticercoisis
    Visceral larval migrans

B
Granulomatous disease
    Sarcoid
    Wegener
Other inflammatory diseases
    Giant cell myocarditis
    Hypersentivity myocarditis
    Loeffler eosinophilia

C
Metabolic
  Endocrine
    Thiamine
    Acromegaly
    Thyrotoxicosis
    Hypothyroidism
    Pheochromcytoma
  Diabetes mellitus
  Familial storage disease
    Gylcogen storage disease
    Refsum disease
    Niemann-Pick
    Hand-Schüller-Christian disease
    Fabry
    Gangliosiderosis
    Sphingolipidoses
    Gaucher
    Sandhoff
    Mucopolysaccharide

Hunter-Hurler
    Whipple
  Nutritional
    Beriberi
    Kwashliorkor
    Scurvy
    Peliagra
    Selenium-Keshan disease
    Obesity
  Other
    Hypokalemia
    Carnitine
    Uremia
    Gout
    Oxalosis
    Porphyria

D
Deposits
    Hemochromatosis
    Oxalosis
    Ochronosis
    Amyloid
    Neoplasm
Connective tissue
    Rheumatoid heart disease
    Ankyloid spondylitis
    Systemic lupus erythematosus
    Scleroderma
    Dermatomyositus
    Periarteritis nodusum
Hematologic
    Polycythemia vera
    Leukemia
    Multiple myeloma
    Sickle cell anemia
    Anemia
    Henoch-Schönlein purpura
    TTP
Neoplastic diseases
    Primary neoplasm
    Metastatic neoplasm

E
Hereditary-Familial-Neuromuscular
    Progressive muscular dystrophy
    Duchenne
    Limb-Girdle of Erb

Fascio-scapular-humeral (Landozy-Dejerine)
    Humero-peronial ataxia
    Friedreich ataxia
    Myotonia atrophica-Steinart
    Myasthenia gravis
    Familial centronuclear myopathy
    Juvenile progressive spinal atrophy (Kugul-Berg-Welander)
    Neurofibromotisis

F
Endomyocardial disease
    Endomyocardial fibrosis
    Hypereosinophilic heart disease-Loeffler's
    Endocardial fibroelastosis
    Carcinoid (RV)

G
Toxins and drugs
    Adriamycin
    Amphetamines
    Antimony
    Arsenic
    Carbon monoxide
    Carbon tetrachloride
    Catecholamines
    Cobalt
    Cocaine
    Cyclophosphamides
    Emetine
    Ethyl alcohol
    Lithium
    Lead
    Methysergide
    Phenothiazines
    Phosphorus
    Tricyclics
    Zidovudine
    Radiation

H
Physiologic agents
    Heat strokes
    Hypothermia
    Tachycardia

I
Miscellaneous
    Peripartum

DILATED CARDIOMYOPATHY

The dilated cardiomyopathies are a group of diseases of unknown etiology that comprise the vast majority of this classification (Fig. 1; see also Color Plate 25 following page 758). Typically, this class of cardiomyopathies is determined by echocardiography, radionuclide gated blood pool imaging, or MRI.

Peripartum Cardiomyopathy

An unfortunate manifestation of cardiomyopathy either during or in the ensuing 3 months after pregnancy is peripartum cardiomyopathy. This entity presents with CHF symptoms. The incidence is not well known: approximately 1,000 U.S women will have peripartum cardiomyopathy each year, and for many, it will be fatal. The typical outcome of the disease is that one third fully recover, another third die in an acute phase or require transplantation, and the other third develop residual but stable LV systolic dysfunction.

The incidence of peripartum cardiomyopathies (PCM) represents almost 5% of all cardiomyopathies and 10–13%

of cardiomyopathies in women. The etiology and pathogenesis of PCM are still unknown. Infectious diseases, nutritional disorders, and immunologic processes have been reported but they do not account for the majority of the cases. Most interesting, immune responses to the foreign tissue of the placenta and fetus may explain the derangement of the immune function that triggers myocardial involvement. Occult myocardial dysfunction may be the most common pathogenic mechanism (7).

The pathology is similar to that of dilated cardiomyopathy. The etiology of this disease remains uncertain, but current evidence suggests that it is related to myocarditis of viral, autoimmune, or idiopathic mechanism (8). Also, nutrition appears to play a role in the etiology of this disease. The utility of immunosuppressive therapy remains uncertain. However, other advances in medical therapy with dilated cardiomyopathy and cardiac transplantation have significantly improved quality of life and survival in these patients (9). Peripartum cardiomyopathy may be another cardiac presentation of the antiphospholipid syndrome, in addition to the well-described valvular involvement as Airoldi and co-workers (10) have described.

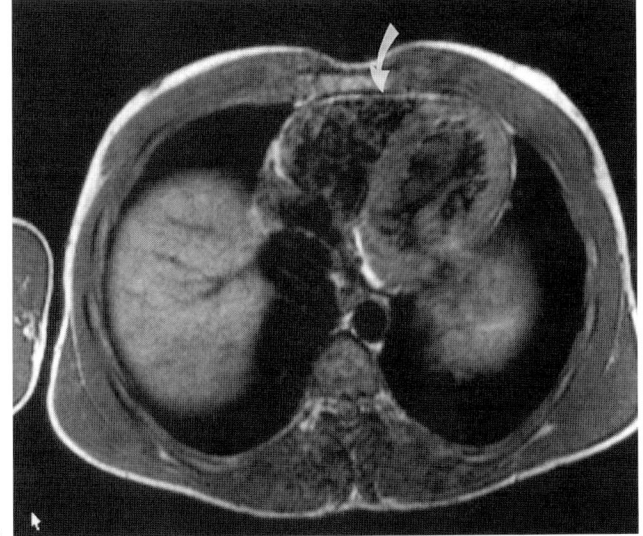

A

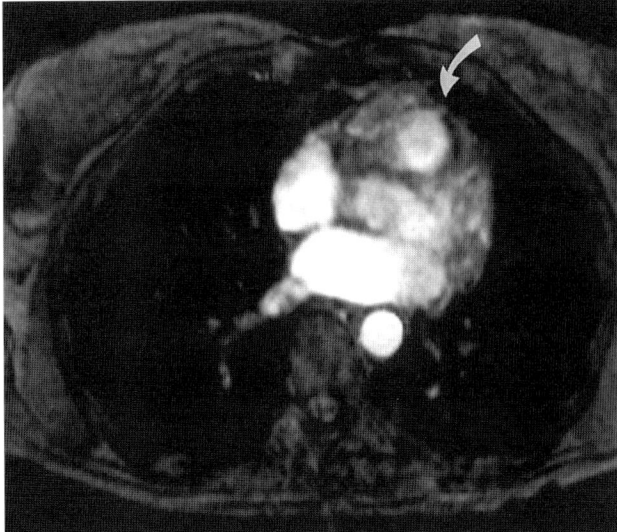

B

FIG. 1. A: Pathologic specimen of a patient with a dilated cardiomyopathy revealing biventricular chamber enlargement (the LV is on the right-hand side). (From ref. 6, with permission.) B: MRI of a 17-year-old male with electrophysiologic (EPS) confirmation of arrthymogenic right ventricular dysplasia (ARVD). Note the thinned RV free wall, which, on gradient echo images, revealed focal RV dyskinesia in the area of the thinned myocardium. C: MRI of a right ventricular outflow tachycardia located in the conus/ right ventricular outflow tract (RVOT) showing focal thinning 1.5 cm below the pulmonic valve. Interrogation of this area by EPS confirmed the diagnosis of a rapid inducible narrow complex tachycardia, which was subsequently radiofrequency ablated. (C is from ref. 6, with permission.) (See also Color Plate 25 following page 758.)

C

In a related area, controversy continues that women appear to be at increased risk for rejection after heart transplantation. Recent data suggest that it is the previous pregnancy, and not gender per se, that is associated with an increased frequency of rejection in females after heart transplantation in those patients with a peripartum cardiomyopathy (11). It continues to be unclear if childbirth or pregnancy trigger the onset of a latent cardiomyopathy syndrome.

Alcoholic Cardiomyopathy

As the name indicates, the incessant use of alcohol can lead in some patients to a form of cardiomyopathy. This is the major form of dilated cardiomyopathy in the Western world and may account for nearly one third of the adult population with cardiomyopathies (12). The clinical manifestations are similar to those of idiopathic cardiomyopathy yet the pathologic features are different. Alcoholic cardiomyopathy is seen to have an increase in intracellular lipid with swelling of the sarcolemma reticulum. Traditionally, nutritional deficiencies were thought to provide a major explanation for the induced LV dysfunction but it is now apparent that alcoholic cardiomyopathy can occur in absentia. Occasionally, cobalt may play a contributing role as a toxic metabolite (13) (see section on Toxic Cardiomyopathy).

Treatment for this cardiomyopathy must include abstinence, which can frequently lead to normalization of LV dysfunction. However, such normalization is, seen infrequently (due to compliance issues) but can occur in up to 30% of patients who are *truly* abstinent (14).

HIV Cardiomyopathy

Heretofore the incidence of cardiac involvement in human immunodeficiency virus (HIV) was felt to be low. However, the incidence of myocardial involvement in such patients is increasing. There appears to be a direct correlation between CD4 count and the level of myocardial dysfunction. The mechanism remains unclear at this time but a cellular response to myofibrils appears likely resulting in a myocarditis.

Recently, Lipshultz reported in a prospective, long-term clinical and echocardiographic follow-up study of 952 asymptomatic HIV-positive patients and a follow-up period of 60 ± 5.3 months. A diagnosis of dilated cardiomyopathy was made in 76 patients (8%). The annual incidence was estimated at an average rate of 15.9% per 1,000 patients. Interestingly, the incidence of dilated cardiomyopathy was higher in patients with a CD4 count. Additionally, all patients underwent endomyocardial biopsy for histologic, immunohistologic, and virologic assessment. A histologic diagnosis of myocarditis was made in 63 (83%) of the patients with dilated cardiomyopathy. Inflammatory infiltrates were analyzed and were predominantly composed of CD3 and CD8 lymphocytes. With staining for major histocompatibility complex class I antigens were positive in 71% of the patients. In the myocytes of 58 patients, HIV nucleic acid sequences were detected by in situ hybridization. An active myocarditis was documented in 36 of the 58 patients. Among these 36 patients, 6 were also infected with Coxsackievirus group B (17%), 2 with cytomegalovirus (6%), and 1 with Epstein-Barr virus (3%). This strongly supports a direct link in the pathogenesis of inducible myocarditis from HIV, probably due to an autoimmune process (15).

Even more important, subclinical cardiac abnormalities in HIV-infected children appear to be quite common and often progressive. Dilated cardiomyopathy and inappropriate LV hypertrophy have been seen. Lipshultz and colleagues (16) noted that LV function correlated with immune dysfunction at baseline but not longitudinally, suggesting that the CD4 cell count may not be a useful surrogate marker of HIV-associated LV dysfunction as opposed to the work of Barbaro and coworkers (15). More concerning was the recent report from Italy regarding their first cardiac transplant recipient who died of fulminant complications of AIDS. Neither the patient nor the organ donor belonged to any of the known risk groups for HIV infection. It was determined that he had contracted HIV from an earlier blood transfusion (17).

Approximately 14 million persons worldwide are estimated to be infected with HIV-1. More effective therapies have produced longer survival times for HIV-infected patients. Along with the decreased mortality comes a penalty in the emergence of previously unencountered HIV complications including HIV-related heart disease. The most common and life-threatening cardiovascular complication of HIV infection is the development of primary heart muscle disease associated with severe global left ventricular. Other less common forms of symptomatic heart disease in HIV-1-infected patients are pericardial effusion with cardiac tamponade, high-grade arrhythmia with sudden cardiac death, and systemic embolization caused by nonbacterial thrombotic endocarditis or endocarditis (18).

Obesity-associated Cardiomyopathy

With the recent addition of obesity as a cardiac risk factor it is remarkable that more has not been written on the subject of cardiomyopathy associated with obesity. Little is known on this subject. One might speculate that fatty infiltration, analogous to steatosis in the hepatic system, may be responsible. Periodically case reports appear indicating that, aside from obesity, no other explanation can be identified for the observed LV impairment (19). Obesity as a causal role is supported by the rapid improvement in LV dysfunction once the obesity is corrected. Hydrogen magnetic resonance spectroscopy could provide a means to track the amount and change in mobile fats present in such a cardiomyopathic state.

Arrythmogenic Right Ventricular Dysplasia

This unique and increasing in frequency, right-sided cardiomyopathy is described as partial or total replacement of the right ventricular (RV) wall by adipose or fibrous tissue. RV wall thinning and focal dyskinesias are the pathognomonic features. As well, the initiating clinical event is usually right ventricular reentry ventricular tachycardia (Fig. 1B and C). There is an autosomal dominant inheritance to this cardiomyopathy that maps to chromosome 14q23-q24 (20). The diagnosis is predicated on the constellation of electrocardiographic findings of Uhl sign in leads V1 and V2 and findings on the MRI, consistent with arrythmogenic right ventricular dysplasia (ARVD) including RV dysfunction and thinning (21) (see Chapter 46).

SECONDARY DILATED CARDIOMYOPATHY (SPECIFIC HEART MUSCLE DISEASE)

This refers to all cardiomyopathies associated with a known etiology. In general, specific heart muscle disease can be assessed with echocardiographic radionuclide gated blood pool imaging or MRI. In specific instances, Gallium-67 can be used.

Diabetic Cardiomyopathy

Diabetes is a strong cardiac risk factor for atherosclerotic heart disease. Accordingly, it has been difficult to define a cardiomyopathic syndrome in patients with diabetes that is not related to ischemic heart disease. Nevertheless, there may be some association between noncoronary diabetes and a cardiomyopathy independent of coronary artery disease. Rubler and co-workers (22) first described this association in 1972. Retrospective analysis from the Framingham Heart Study demonstrated a 2.5-fold higher incidence of CHF symptoms in patients with diabetes (and insulin) (23). A link has been suggested between diabetes and idiopathic cardiomyopathy. Potential mechanisms to explain myocardial dysfunction with dilation and the lack of coronary artery lesions include increased vascular permeability and increased glycosylation of collagen analogous to the glycosylation of hemoglobin. However, in this state, the collagen fibrils lose distensibility and resultant diastolic dysfunction ensues (24).

Disturbances of coronary circulation have been reported in diabetic patients with microvascular dysfunction without obstructive coronary atherosclerosis. Coronary blood flow reserve has been shown to be lower in diabetic patients than in controls. Similarly, total coronary resistance during hyperemia appears to be higher in diabetic patients compared with the control subjects. Surprisingly, no association was found between the coronary flow reserve and serum lipid or HbA1c values as compared to euglycemic controls (25).

Finally, contractile protein regulation may be altered in patients with diabetic cardiomyopathy. Recently Malhotra and Sanghi (26) showed diminished calcium sensitivity in the regulation of the cardiac actomyosin from diabetic hearts. It has been postulated that diminished calcium sensitivity along with shifts in cardiac myosin heavy chain (V1→V3) could contribute to the impaired cardiac function in the hearts of chronic diabetic rats. It has also been reported that sarcomeric proteins such as myosin light chain-2 (MLC-2) and troponin I (TnI) may be involved in regulating muscle contraction and in calcium sensitivity because phosphorylation of cardiac TnI is associated with altered maximum enzymatic activity (and calcium force relationship) in muscle preparations of diabetics (27). These results imply early impairment of coronary vascular reactivity and diminished contractile response in insulin-dependent diabetes mellitus patients, which may represent an early precursor of future coronary heart disease or may contribute to the pathogenesis of LV dysfunction and subsequent cardiomyopathy. Thus, it is likely that imaging of metabolic function would provide a means for early detection of a diabetic cardiomyopathic syndrome. PET (2,3 DPG) and MR (^{31}P) approaches might be useful in such evaluation.

Ischemic Cardiomyopathy

This topic has been covered extensively in Chapters 36–39, which provide the basis for the pathology of ischemic heart disease. However, several important concepts shall be elaborated with respect to the transition of ischemic heart with preserved LV function to the heart with LV dysfunction, i.e., "ischemic" cardiomyopathy. Once myocardial injury occurs (ischemic, stunned, hibernating, or infarcted myocardium), myocardial dysfunction may be indistinguishable from an idiopathic cardiomyopathy. Thus, identification of these manifestations of ischemic disease permit inclusion of treatment strategies that have an immense impact on myocardial function resulting in improved symptoms. Ideally, this translates into improved survival. Unstated is the concept that the distinction of ischemic cardiomyopathy versus nonischemic cardiomyopathy is the critical diagnosis to be made. Clearly, noninvasive imaging will play a major role in this evaluation (radionuclide perfusion imaging, stress echo, and MRI studies). Treatment strategies for the ischemic cardiomyopathy have become quite sophisticated, including balloon angioplasty with endovascular stents, coronary artery bypass grafting, percutaneous/transmural myocardial laser revascularization and, more recently, surgical reconstruction therapies (for patients with dilated ischemic cardiomyopathies). This markedly contrasts with the vast number of nonischemic cardiomyopathies in which supportive therapy is the mainstay in treatment modalities.

Bacterial Myocarditis

As compared to idiopathic cardiomyopathy or viral myocarditis, bacterial myocarditis is considered rare. As noted in a previous study from the Armed Forces Institute of Pathology, virtually any infectious agent can be associated with myocarditis.

Protozoal Myocarditis

The most common cause of myocarditis is *Trypanosoma cruzi*, which leads to Chagas disease. It is endemic in areas of South America where up to 50% of the population is thought to be infected. Up to 20% die in the acute phase. There can be a latent phase for up to 20 years and a chronic phase demonstrating dilated cardiomyopathy. *Toxoplasma gondii* is seen in immunosuppressed patients, especially in association with cardiac transplantation. It has also been observed in patients with the acquired immunodeficiency disorder (HIV) (see below). Typically, there are encysted organisms within the myocardium causing an inflammatory response. *Trichinella spiralis*, however, never encyst in the myocardium but cause nonspecific inflammatory manifestations in response to the death of the parasite (28).

Viral Myocarditis

Viral myocarditis is ubiquitous. Definitive cause and effect have been proven in cytomegalovirus. Other implicated agents include the enteroviruses, such as Coxsackie B. The latter is more commonly seen in younger males. Other viral vectors include adenoviruses and viruses that cause systemic disease: measles, rubella, mononucleosis, psittacosis, and giant cell myocarditis. The latter can be proven definitively by biopsy.

Hypersensitivity Cardiac Disease

Rarely, myocarditis has been associated with a number of drugs with toxic manifestations. Typically, the drugs cause either a hypersensitivity reaction or toxic myocarditis.

The most noteworthy is that of anthracycline toxicity. Usually, there is only a chronic phase after high-dose anthracycline administration for solid tumors. The myocardial manifestations correlate with the dose of drug. As doses exceed 450 mg/m^2 the risks increase. In the course of 6 months to 5 years indolent myocardial dysfunction can occur manifesting as dyspnea with exercise intolerance. An exceedingly rare form of hyperacute myocarditis can occur with anthracycline use. Death can occur within 48 h of an intravenous bolus of the drug.

Two types of myocyte damage are seen, those with myofibrillar loss and those with dilated sarcolemma reticulum. There is a grading scale to quantitate extent of myocardial involvement. The prior use or concomitant exposure to mediastinal irradiation is thought to be additive to the risk (29).

Transplant Rejection

The increasing utilization of cardiac transplantation for refractory CHF will lead to an increase in the incidence of cardiac rejection, another form of cardiomyopathy. This form of iatrogenic cardiomyopathy is characterized by several presentations:

Immediate heart failure can occur without an immune reaction. Most commonly, early heart failure is related to delay in organ reanastomosis with prolonged ischemic time or to trauma to the heart during procurement. A more recognized

but easily preventable form is right ventricular failure secondary to unrecognized pulmonary hypertension in a heart that is not prepared for the elevated residual pulmonary pressures. This can cause an acute fall in preload leading to hypotension and failure to wean from the heart-lung machine requiring a right ventricular assist device (30).

Hyperacute rejection is almost unheard of in the present era of accurate cross-matching of blood and major histocompatibility antigens. When present, clinical manifestations are immediate and pronounced. The heart quickly dilates, darkens from ischemia, and fails to contract. The histopathologic markers are consistent with severe hemorrhage into the interstitium. This is untreatable short of immediate retransplantation with another heart, usually not an option.

Acute rejection is typified by a high rate in the first 3 months of a perivascular infiltrate with or without endocardial lymphocyte infiltration. The offending T cells, as the agent of the cellular immune arm, are typically suppressed to a baseline state by Cyclosporine, Azathioprine, and prednisone. If such a perturbation of the immune system goes untreated, rejection can progress to involve the interstitium with or without myocyte death. This is termed moderate rejection. Myocyte necrosis is typically not enough in the early stage to cause CHF, but if progression to frank myocyte damage with hemorrhage remains, this is often the case. The immune response consists of a mixture of neutrophils, lymphocytes, and eosinophils. This presentation is typically treated with OKT3, a murine monoclonal antibody against the cytotoxic suppressor T cells. The rejection is formally graded by an International Society for Heart Transplantation working group classification (Chapter 50).

A recently recognized noncellular form of rejection is termed vascular rejection. This is a humoral immune response characterized by deposition of immunoglobulins IgM or IgG, compliment or fibrinogen into the vasculature. The hallmark is inflammation and infiltration into the vessels by lymphocytes. A concern is that, despite no real treatment (except retransplantation if in a hyperacute response) it may promote the emergence of an accelerated form of atherosclerosis (31). In view of its portability and rapid applicability, echocardiography would be the imaging approach of choice for the early stages of rejection. MRI might be added in the later phases.

RESTRICTIVE HEART MUSCLE DISEASE

Primary Restrictive

The histopathology finding in patients with primary (or idiopathic) cardiomyopathy are nonspecific and generally include cellular hypertrophy with marked increase in interstitial fibrosis. This translates clinically into an inability for myocardial relaxation during the active and passive portions of diastole. Typically, echocardiographic techniques are employed first to characterize restrictive disease. Measurements of relaxation such as $-dp/dt$, tau (T), depressed E:A ratios, and increased isovolumic relaxation time consistently confirm that systolic function may remain intact but diastolic dysfunction is the hallmark (32). Echocardiography, radionuclide cineangiography, and MRI can effectively assess diastolic dysfunction.

Clinical symptoms do not allow discrimination between diastolic and systolic dysfunction in a reproducible fashion. In fact, chest pain appears to be one of the most frequent complaints (second only to dyspnea) leading clinicians astray in their initial differential diagnosis. Hemodynamic studies reveal elevated central venous pressure with typically normal cardiac output and systolic function. LV end-diastolic volumes (LVEDV) are frequently small secondary to the restrictive process. LV mass tends to be increased while the atria are dilated secondary to increased filling pressures.

In sharp distinction from patients with primary dilated cardiomyopathy, mortality for restrictive disease is better (10–15%/year). Yet, this is of little solace as the mortality is inexorable with 10-year survival being 10–15%.

Sarcoidosis

Sarcoidosis involves the heart and circulation in several ways. It can cause cor pulmonale without any involvement of the heart. It can cause restrictive disease by virtue of deposition of the noncaseating granulomas within the myocardium. Often, however, in addition to diastolic involvement, there is increased arrhythmogenic potential either via conduction system infiltration or by direct myocardial infiltration in up to 20% of patients. The latter is due to myocardial fibrosis, which has become a recognized source for arrhythmogenesis (33). As compared to idiopathic dilated cardiomyopathy, sarcoidosis has very different clinical features, including female predominance, a high incidence of grave conduction disturbances and abnormal wall thickness, asymmetric wall motion abnormalities, and radionuclide perfusion defects preferentially affecting the anteroseptal and apical regions (34) (Fig. 2). Treatment for sarcoidosis is problematic since the etiology is not known. Reynolds and colleagues have determined it to be an alteration in CD4/CD8 ratio that responds well to immune modulating drugs. In addition to echo, MRI, and radionuclide cineangiography that assess ventricular function, Gallium-67 radionuclide imaging can localize myocardial involvement.

Hemochromatosis

Excessive amounts of iron pigment in the heart from hemolysis, hemosiderosis, or hemochromatosis can result in a cardiomyopathy. Pathology reveals characteristic hemosiderin deposits on a Prussian blue stain within the interstitium and sarcolemma. The transferrin saturation and the serum ferritin provide a combined sensitivity and specificity of >90% in the genetic form. As well, there is a gradation of deposition within the myocardium transmurally (Fig. 3) (35). Classically, this disorder is treated with phlebotomy. Chela-

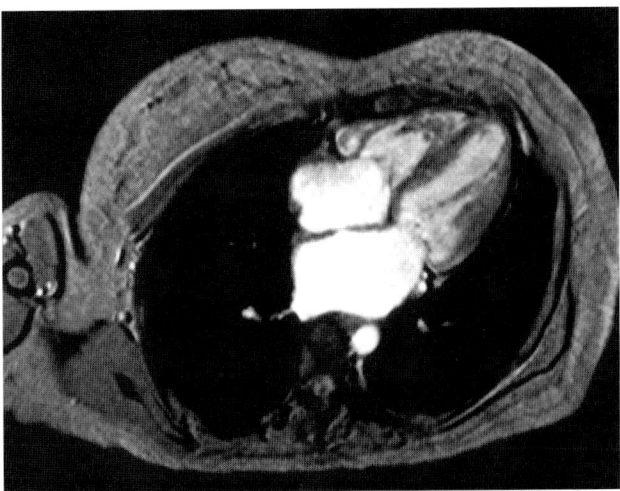

FIG. 2. Sarcoid heart disease is frequently associated with marked bi-atrial enlargement (right atrium measured 51 mm and the left atrium measured 56 mm) along with dilated inferior vena cava and normal LV/RV size MRI findings for restrictive cardiomyopathy (with or without an increase in left ventricular wall thickness).

tion therapy is used if the response to phlebotomy is inadequate. More recently, liver transplantation has been utilized with variable benefit on the myocardium.

Scleroderma

Myocardial involvement in scleroderma consists of fibrosis and can be found in up to 80% of the patients on autopsy.

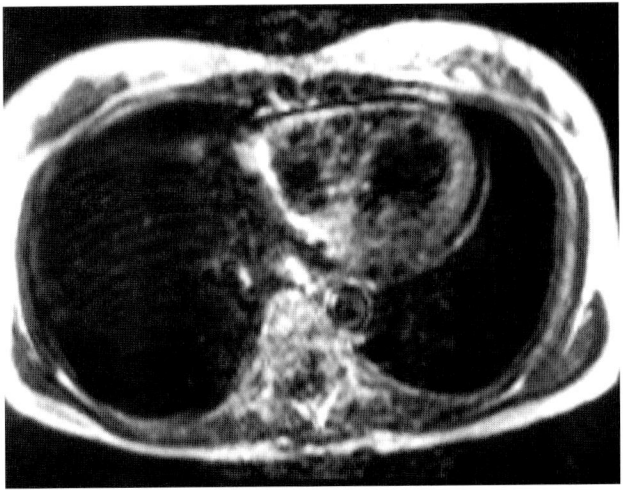

FIG. 3. A spin-echo image is shown from a 44-year-old female who initially presented in 3rd degree heart block. MRI was performed to evaluate for the possibility of structural heart disease, LVH on her EKG, and for quantitation of LV function. The abnormally low signal intensity from the MRI suggested a metallic substance within her liver. Hemochromatosis was suspected and confirmed by laboratory analysis. The patient had mild restrictive disease secondary to the cardiac infiltrative process.

The fibrosis may be patchy, be in both ventricles, or cause extensive myocardial scarring. Contraction band necrosis (similar to that observed with cocaine) can be seen. Patients with scleroderma typically present with RV systolic dysfunction but LV diastolic dysfunction is often a complicating factor especially in the presence of severe hypertension. Evidence of LV dysfunction can be seen in up to 75% of patients (36).

Treatment for scleroderma heart disease is mainly supportive with the addition of immune modifying agents in advanced cases. There is concern that overuse of such agents can provoke renal crisis that can be irreversible. ACE inhibitors are particularly helpful in addition to the overall beneficial effect they have on LV dysfunction.

Glycogen Storage Diseases

Fabry disease is an X-linked recessive disorder of glycosphingolipid metabolism due to a deficiency of the lysosomal enzyme α-galactosidase A as a consequence of many mutations. Interestingly, the cardiac manifestations are angina and myocardial infarctions despite angiographically normal coronaries. Accumulation of glycogen within the myocytes with resultant LV dysfunction and failure is the hallmark (37). Gaucher disease and Pompe disease may cause a pseudohypertrophic cardiomyopathy characterized by deposition of the glycogen in the myocardium. These diseases are observed only in children.

Endomyocardial Fibrosis

Loeffler (38) first described endomyocardial fibrosis (EMF) in 1930, and this entity is regularly included in the differential for restrictive cardiomyopathy but is rarely seen in the Western world. Nevertheless, it remains an entity of some intrigue. More than 100 cases have been reported, mostly on autopsy. The distinguishing pathological features are an eosinophilic infiltration and damage to the myocardium, typically, the endocardium. Fibrosis is a constant feature secondary to the toxic effects of the secretory protein released by the eosinophils as a granule basic protein (39). The restrictive process is similar to other processes that result in diastolic dysfunction with two distinct exceptions. There appears to be a hyperthrombotic response with deposition of thrombus onto the trabeculae, possibly due to the destruction of the most superficial layer of the endocardium. On occasion this thrombotic process can progress to gross limitation of cardiac stroke volume secondary to clot mass. As expected, systemic manifestations such as stroke often occur. The hallmark of EMF is a thick endocardial rind that subsequently forms around the endocardium. This rind is noncompliant and, despite essentially normal midwall and epicardial myocardial systolic function, both are restricted during diastole.

Biventricular dysfunction is often present, however, the presentations can be quite variable, ranging from no symptoms to severe CHF. Interestingly, EMF should be included in the differential of unexplained hypereosinophilia as it often serves as a harbinger long before the diagnosis is made (40).

ENDOCARDIAL FIBROELASTOSIS

Endocardial fibroelastosis (EFE) is primarily observed in infancy. There are several forms, which include endocardial sclerosis, fetal endocarditis, fetal endocardial fibroelastosis, and elastic tissue hyperplasia. The fetal forms are increasingly recognized with genotyping. The pathologic condition involves the LV and the mitral and aortic valves. The secondary form appears more frequently in aortic stenosis, hypoplastic left heart syndrome, and coarctation. The clinical features usually occur by 1 year of age and the presentation is similar to an idiopathic dilated cardiomyopathy with LV dysfunction and congestive heart failure. The particular features involve LV dilation with dense fibrosis along the endocardium that is the pathognomonic feature. Biopsy usually shows a fibrous invasion into the endocardium with elastic stains being positive. Almost always there is cardiac dilation; however, on occasion a contracted form of EFE can occur with elevated LA pressures and markedly elevated pulmonary pressures. Digoxin is the treatment of choice. This therapy appears to be more than supportive as reports exist that withdrawal of the drug can precipitate rapid CHF symptoms even after LV dilation has returned to normal, as is frequently observed (41).

SECONDARY RESTRICTIVE DISEASE

Amyloid

Amyloidosis is the most frequently reported restrictive cardiomyopathy. There are multiple entities of amyloid including primary, secondary, familial, and senile. All have in common the deposition of light chain amino acids into the myofibrils. These proteins are immunoglobulins deposited in the form of beta-pleated sheets that impart a strong tensile strength to the myocardium and inhibit deformation leading to impaired relaxation. Cardiac amyloid can exist as a sole entity but in 60% of the cases there is concomitant systemic involvement, primarily within the hepatic system. The large percentage of amyloid presentations have an underlying plasma-cell dyscrasia such as multiple myeloma, plasmacytoma, or monoclonal gammopathy of unknown significance (MGUS). A novel mutation in the transthyretin gene encoding 59 Thr-Lys associated with autosomal dominant hereditary systemic amyloidosis in an Italian kindred in whom cardiac involvement was a major feature identified recently. This illustrates the difficulty in diagnosis of cardiac amyloid, and the variable clinical phenotype in hereditary amyloidosis (42).

The average age of presentation is in the fifth decade and the hallmark is dyspnea at rest and on exertion. Occasionally, amyloidosis can present as high-degree heart block without prodromal CHF symptoms. Cardiac glycosides should be used with caution, if at all, because of an increased binding to the amyloid fibrils and consequent arrhythmias (43).

Regardless of its presentation, the prognosis is uniformly poor with very little survival by 24 months (<10%). In fact, many studies report no significant improvement in survival despite aggressive therapy (e.g., vincristine, adriamycin, and dexamethasone). Emerging therapies such as bone marrow replacement initially met with high expectations. But, with the findings that a systemic derangement in several cytokines, many of which are not located within the bone marrow, the likelihood for prolonged survival appears dismal (44).

Cardiomyopathy Associated with Neuromuscular Disease

Myocardial fibrosis, as well as fibrointimal proliferation, is the trademark of the cardiomyopathies associated with neuromuscular disease. For example, Friedrich ataxia, a form of progressive muscular dystrophy, and myotonic muscular dystrophy may present with a cardiomyopathy. It is a progressive and unrelenting process that, in addition to the muscular weakness, encumbers its victims with symptoms of CHF. Other disorders include Duchenne muscular dystrophy, limb-girdle of Erb, and Kearne-Sayre syndrome.

Cases of Becker muscular dystrophy (BMD) have been reported, which show only mild or subclinical skeletal muscle involvement with an overt dilated cardiomyopathy. Severe left ventricular dilation with reduced ejection fraction, which could be complicated by life-threatening arrhythmias, may occur in this disorder. Contrary to previous reports that indicated the involvement of 5'-end mutations in cardiomyopathies as a result of dystrophin gene alterations, a recent study showed that, despite the apparent concentration of deletions in two regions (5'-end and exons 47 through 49), there was no involvement of specific gene mutations in the development of this cardiomyopathy (45).

MELAS (myopathy, encephalopathy lactic acid stroke syndrome) is a rare but fascinating disorder characterized by red ragged fibers on muscle biopsy and involves the coronary arteries and mitochondrial enzymes causing a dilated cardiomyopathy (46).

NONDILATED HEART MUSCLE DISEASE

Hypertrophic Cardiomyopathy

Hypertrophic cardiomyopathy (HCM) presents as diastolic dysfunction. Until a few years ago the classic description for the pathologic derangement of hypertrophic cardiomyopathy was a disordered myofibrillar process typically localized to the interventricular septum. This has been confirmed by a clear genetic basis, but it remains unclear as to how alteration of tropomyosin, myosin, and other proteins leads to localization of the myofibrillar disarray to the septum (47). It is now clear that it is a heterogeneous process involving the sarcomere with at least 40 missence mutations ascribed to the β-myosin heavy chain 9 chromosome (14q11-q12) with others relegated to troponin-T. Recently, the genetic abnormalities for the entity has been seen in asymptomatic and elderly patients raising suspicion that the foundation for the disease may be more occult than previously expected (48).

The most common feature of HCM is asymmetric septal hypertrophy (ASH), which can be associated with subaortic obstruction and mitral regurgitation (Fig. 4A; see also Color Plate 26 following page 758). The narrowed LV outflow tract (LVOT) caused by the septal protrusion and the consequent anterior displacement of the anterior mitral leaflet and papillary muscles appears essential to the development of the gradient between the LVOT and the LV (subaortic stenosis). The protruding septum creates a Venturi effect resulting in systolic anterior motion of the mitral valve (SAM), which causes the subaortic obstruction (Fig. 4B and C). The mitral regurgitation occurs secondary to the failure of the leaflets to coapt and a funnel-like gap is formed such that regurgitant volume is directed eccentrically into the posterior portion of the left atrium. Importantly, the pressure gradient has been recognized to be a variable process in which, depending on loading condition, time of day, and heart rate, the gradient (and probably symptoms) will be temporarily dynamic (49).

Clinically, patients present with chest pain with or without ischemia, dyspnea, presyncope, and/or syncope. Unlike the restrictive cardiomyopathies, HCM can be frequently suggested from a physical examination. In addition to a loud murmur, dynamic auscultation can raise a high suspicion of HCM with simple bedside maneuvers (50).

The clinical course of HCM is also quite variable, even unpredictable. It is now becoming clear that the subaortic gradient is a poor predictor of events and clinical outcomes. Another potential predictive modality may be the underlying molecular genetic defect. Currently, risk factors for sudden death include young age, myocardial ischemia, syncope, a family history of sudden death, and sustained ventricular tachycardia. Myomectomy with relief of symptoms does not appear to be an important risk factor. All told, the risk of death ranges from 1 to 6% yearly. HCM is the most common cause of unexplained sudden death in an otherwise apparently healthy competitive athlete (51). Diastolic dysfunction is manifested as dyspnea on exertion likely secondary to decreased compliance, but also to the alterations in preload that occur with increased sympathetic tone that further increases gradient. Techniques to treat HCM have ranged from myomectomy, septal ablation therapy with alcohol, embolization of the first septal perforator, dual chamber pacing, and negative inotropic drugs. Each modality has its own enthusiasts, but the predominant data supports the concept of not using the gradient as the sole indicator of clinical success. Chief among the drawbacks in gradient measure-

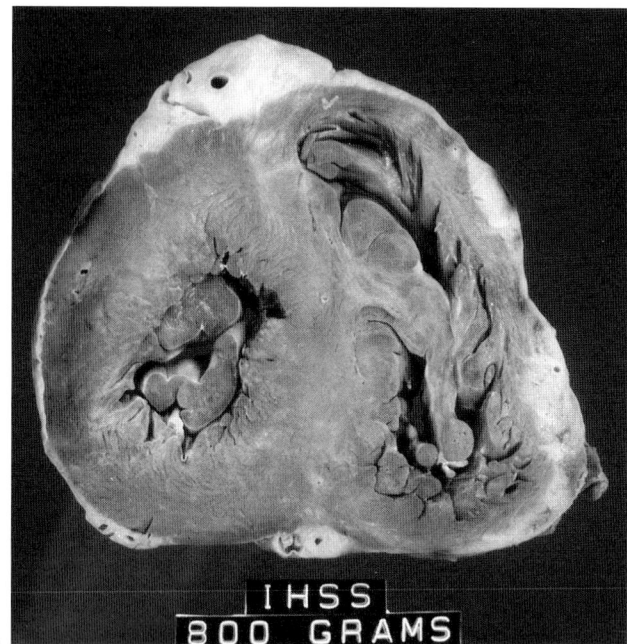

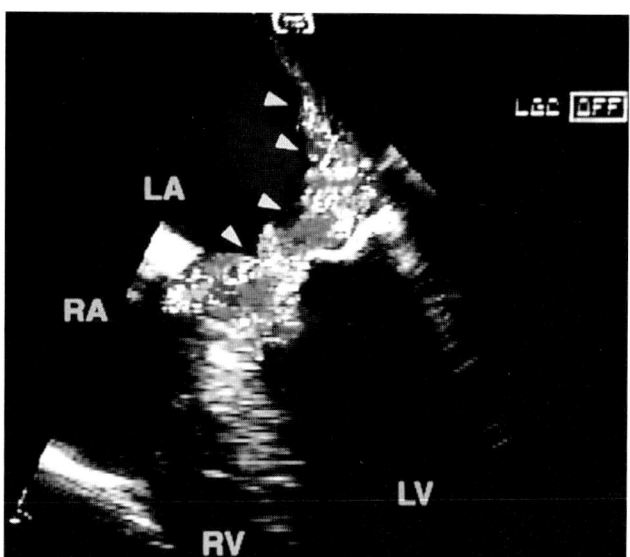

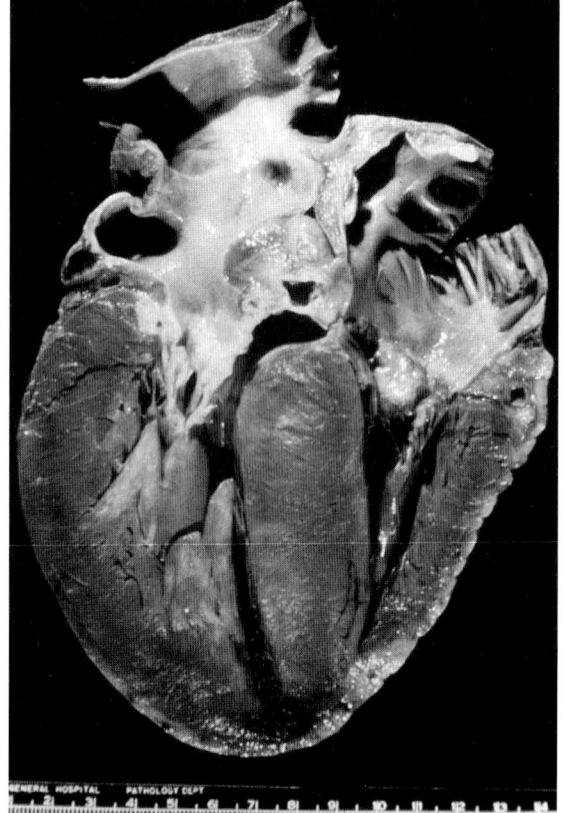

FIG. 4. A: Pathologic specimen of a patient with hypertrophic cardiomyopathy. The LV body weight ratio (g/kg) was in excess of 8:1 (normal 2.5:1). **B:** Systolic anterior motion (SAM) of the mitral valve is depicted in this patient with a variant of hypertrophic cardiomyopathy, hypertrophic obstructive cardiomyopathy. This was formerly known as idiopathic hypertrophic subaortic stenosis (IHSS). Note, SAM is present in both anterior and posterior mitral leaflets with non-coaptation. The resulting eccentric mitral jet (arrowheads) is demonstrated. M-mode (not shown) echocardiography demonstrated midsystolic preclosure of the aortic valve and course systolic fluttering. **C:** Pathologic specimen of a hypertrophic cardiomyopathic ventricle (without obstruction) revealing marked concentric hypertrophy. (See also Color Plate 26 following page 758.) (From ref. 6, with permission.)

ment is that it is dynamic, does not correlate with exercise capacity, and the reduction in syncopal events does not always correlate with reduction in the LVOT obstruction (52–54). Moreover, ventricular tachyarrhythmias may not always be the primary mechanism of sudden death in patients with HCM.

A less common form of HCM is localized to the LV apex most commonly seen in Japan, although more recent Western appearances have been reported. It is associated with striking T-wave inversion. Unlike the classic ASH, there does not appear to be a familial basis thus far described. There is usually only apical hypertrophy with no outflow tract obstruction. Generally, this form of HCM is associated with a favorable prognosis.

CONCLUSION

The cardiomyopathies are a heterogeneous collection of diseases with a multitude of pathological features and clinical manifestations. The sequelae are variable. There are, however, many clinical similarities. It is these similarities that generate the need for robust imaging strategies to allow noninvasive differentiation between the classes and subgroups of cardiomyopathies.

REFERENCES

1. Goodwin JF. Prospects and predictions for the cardiomyopathies. *Circulation* 1974;50:210–216.
2. Brandenburg RO, Chazov E, Cherian G. Report of the WHO/ISFC task force on the definition and classification of cardiomyopathies. *Br Heart J* 1980;44;672–673.
3. Brigden W. Uncommon myocardial diseases. The non coronary cardiomyopathies. *Lancet* 1957;2:1243–1249.
4. Fejfar Z. Accounts of international meetings: idiopathic cardiomegaly. *Bull WHO* 1968;28:979–992.
5. Abraham WT, Havranek EP. The economics of heart failure. *Heart Failure* 1998;14:8–9.
6. Nanda NC, Domansky MJ, eds. *Atlas of transesophageal echocardiography.* Baltimore: Williams & Wilkins, 1998.
7. Bertrand E. Post-partum cardiomyopathy: medical aspects, role of heart transplantation. *Arch Malad Coeur Vaiss* 1995;88:1635–1640.
8. Witlin AG, Mabie WC, Sibai BM. Peripartum cardiomyopathy: an ominous diagnosis. *Am J Obstet Gynecol* 1997;176(1 Pt 1):182–188.
9. Brown CS, Bertolet BD. Peripartum cardiomyopathy: a comprehensive review. *Am J Obstet Gynecol* 1998;178:409–413.
10. Airoldi ML, Eid O, Tosetto C, et al. Post-partum dilated cardiomyopathy in anti-phospholipid positive woman. *Lupus* 1996;5:247–250.
11. Johnson MR, Naftel DC, Hobbs RE, et al. The incremental risk of female sex in heart transplantation: a multiinstitutional study of peripartum cardiomyopathy and pregnancy. Cardiac Transplant Research Database Group. *J Heart Lung Transplant* 1997;16:801–812.
12. Piano MR, Schwertz DW. Alcoholic heart disease: a review. *Heart Lung* 1994;23:3–5.
13. Jarvis JQ, Hammond E, Meier R, et al. Cobalt cardiomyopathy. A report of two cases from mineral assay laboratories and a review of the literature. *J Occup Med* 1992;34:620–625.
14. Kouvaras G, Coikkincz D. Effects of alcohol on the heart: current views. *Angiology* 1986;37:592.
15. Barbaro G, Di Lorenzo G, Grisorio B, et al. Incidence of dilated cardiomyopathy and detection of HIV in myocardial cells of HIV-positive patients. (Gruppo Italiano per lo Studio Cardiologico dei Pazienti Affetti da AIDS). *N Engl J Med* 1998;339:1093–1099.
16. Lipshultz SE, Easley KA, Orav EJ, et al. Left ventricular structure and function in children infected with human immunodeficiency virus: the prospective P2C2 HIV Multicenter Study. Pediatric Pulmonary and Cardiac Complications of Vertically Transmitted Infection (P2C2 HIV) Study Group. *Circulation* 1998;97:1246–1256.
17. Calabrese F, Angelini A, Cecchetto A, et al. HIV infection in the first heart transplantation in Italy: fatal outcome. Case report. *APMIS* 1998;106:470–74.
18. Herskowitz A. Cardiomyopathy and other symptomatic heart diseases associated with HIV infection. *Curr Opin Cardiol* 1996;11:325–331.
19. Itoh H, Yamamoto M, Tanimoto N, et al. Simple obesity with cardiomyopathy of obesity. *Int Med* 996;35:876–879.
20. Rampazzo, A, Nava A, Danieli GA, et al. The gene for arrhythmogenic right ventricular cardiomyopathy maps to chromosome 14q23-q24. *Hum Mol Genet* 1994;3:959–964.
21. Blake LM, Scheinman MM, Higgins CB. MR features of arrhythmogenic right ventricular dysplasia. *Am J Roentgenol* 1994;152:809–813.
22. Rubler S, Dglugash J, Yuceoglu YZ, et al. New type of cardiomyopathy associated with diabetic glomerulerosclerosis. *Am J Cardiol* 1972;30:595–602.
23. Kannel WB, Hjortland M, Castelli WP. Role of diabetes in congestive heart failure: the Framingham study. *Am J Cardiol* 1974;34:29–34.
24. Brownlee M, Carami A, Viassara H. Advanced glycosylation end products in tissue and the biochemical basis of diabetic complications. *N Engl J Med.* 1988;318:1315–1321.
25. Pitkanen OP, Nuutila P, Raitakari OT, et al. Coronary flow reserve is reduced in young men with IDDM. *Diabetes* 1998;47:248–254.
26. Malhotra A. Sanghi V. Regulation of contractile proteins in diabetic heart. *Cardiovasc Res* 1997;34:34–40 and Rodrigues B, Cam MC, McNeill JH. Metabolic disturbances in diabetic cardiomyopathy. *Mol Cell Biochem* 1998;180:53–57.
27. Ziegelhoffer A, Ravingerova T, Styk J, et al. Mechanisms that may be involved in calcium tolerance of the diabetic heart. *Mol Cell Biochem* 1997;176:191–198.
28. Silver MM, Silver MD. Cardiomyopathies. In: Silver MD, ed. *Cardiovascular path,* 2nd ed. New York: Churchill Livingstone, 1991.
29. Billingham ME, Bristow M. Evaluation of anthracycline cardiotoxicity: predictive ability and functional correlation of endocardial biopsy. *Cancer Treat Symp* 1980;3:71–76.
30. Snoddy BS , Nanda, NC, Holman WL, et al. *Echo J: CV Ultra Tech* 1996;12:159–163.
31. Hammond EH, Yowell RL, Nunda S, et al. Vascular (humoral) rejection in heart transplantation: pathologic observations and clinical implications. *J Heart Transplant* 1989;8:430–443.
32. Wilmhurst PT, Katritsis D. Restrictive cardiomyopathy. *Br Heart J* 1990;63:323–329.
33. Peters NS, Wit AL. Myocardial architecture and ventricular arrhythmogenesis. *Circulation* 1998;97:1746–1754.
34. Yazaki Y, Isobe M, Hiramitsu S, et al. Comparison of clinical features and prognosis of cardiac sarcoidosis and idiopathic dilated cardiomyopathy. *Am J Cardiol* 1998;82:537–540.
35. Buja LM, Roberts WC. Iron in the heart: etiology and clinical significance. *Am J Med* 1971;51:209.
36. Anuari A, Graninger W, Scheider B, et al. Cardiac involvement in systemic sclerosis. *Arthritis Rheum* 1992;35:1356.
37. Eng CM, Desnick RJ. Molecular basis of Fabry disease: mutations and polymorphisms in the human alpha-galactosidase A gene. *Human Mutat* 1994;3:103.
38. Loeffler W. Endocarditis parietalis fibroplastica MI Bluteosinophiline. *Schweiz Med Wchnscr* 1930;66:817–820.
39. Spry CJ, Tai P, Davies J. The cardiotoxicity of eosinophils. *Post Grad Med J.* 1983;59:147–151.
40. Solley GO, Maldonado JE, Gleich GJ, et al. Endomyocardiopathy with eosinophilia. *Mayo Clin Proc* 1976;51:697–708.
41. Carcellar AM, Maroto E, Fouron JC. Dilated and contracted forms of primary endocardial fibroelastosis. *Br Heart J* 1990;63:311–315.
42. Booth DR, Tan SY, Hawkins PN, et al. A novel variant of transthyretin, 59 Thr—Lys associated with autosomal dominant cardiac amyloidosis in an Italian family. *Circulation* 1995;91:962–967.
43. Spyrou N Foale R. Restrictive cardiomyopathies. *Curr Opin Cardiol* 1994;9:344–349.
44. Gillmore JD, Davies J, Iqbal A, et al. Allogeneic bone marrow transplantation for systemic AL amyloidosis. *Br J Haem* 1998;100:226–228.
45. Melacini P, Fanin M, Danieli GA, et al. Myocardial involvement is very frequent among patients affected with subclinical Becker's muscular dystrophy. *Circulation* 1996;94:3168–3175.
46. Anan R, Nagagawa M, Miyata M, et al. Cardiac involvement in mitochondrial diseases. A study of 17 patients with documented motochondrial DNA defects. *Circulation* 1995;91:955–961.
47. Wigle DE, Rakowski H, Kimball BP, et al. Hypertrophic cardiomyopathy. *Circulation* 1995;92:1680–1692.
48. Niimura H, Bachinski LL, Sanswatanaroj S, et al. Mutations in the gene for cardiac myosin-binding protein C and late onset familial hypertrophic cardiomyopathy. *N Engl J Med* 1998;338:1248–1257.
49. Nishimura RA, Trusty JM, Hayes DL, et al. Dual-chamber pacing for hypertrophic cardiomyopathy: a randomized, double-blind, crossover trial. *J Am Coll Cardiol* 1997;29:435–441
50. Maron BJ, Bonow RO, Cannon RO, et al. Hypertrophic cardiomyopathy: interrelations of clinical manifestations, pathophysiology, and therapy. *N Engl J Med* 1987;316:780–789.

51. Maron BJ, Epstein SE, Roberts WC. Causes of sudden death in competitive athletes. *J Am Coll Cardiol* 1993;72:939–943.
52. Maron BJ. Appraisal of dual-chamber pacing therapy in hypertrophic cardiomyopathy: too soon for a rush to judgment? *J Am Coll Cardiol* 1996;27:431–432.
53. Nishimura RA, Hayes DL, Ilstrup DM, et al. Effect of dual-chamber pacing on systolic and diastolic function in patients with hypertrophic cardiomyopathy. Acute Doppler echocardiographic and catheterization hemodynamic study. *J Am Coll Cardiol* 1996;27:421–430.
54. Fananapazir L, McAreavey D. Therapeutic options in patients with obstructive hypertrophic cardiomyopathy and severe drug-refractory symptoms. *J Am Coll of Cardiol* 1998;1:259–264.

CHAPTER 46

Subsection C:

CARDIOMYOPATHIES AND OTHER SYNDROMES ASSOCIATED WITH CONGESTIVE HEART FAILURE

Evaluation of the Cardiomyopathies Using Imaging Techniques

Robert W. W. Biederman and
Gerald M. Pohost

This chapter examines the imaging modalities used to detect and characterize features of the cardiomyopathies. The clinical and pathologic features of the cardiomyopathies were addressed in the preceding chapter (Chapter 45). Both chapters are integrally related and together will provide an appreciation of the disease state and the appropriate imaging approach.

More traditional approaches, such as two-dimensional and Doppler echocardiography, as well as emerging techniques that include three-dimensional echocardiography, magnetic resonance imaging (MRI), including spectroscopy, single photon radionuclide and positron emission tomography (PET) will be discussed. The introduction to the chapter is devoted to the important and essential features that are to be imaged for each cardiomyopathic syndrome. Additionally, important imaging derived information, such as cardiac morphology, ventricular volumes and mass, and chamber function will be described. Myocardial perfusion and metabolism are also discussed. All of these technologies and approaches are discussed in depth throughout this book.

EVALUATION OF LEFT VENTRICLE VOLUME, EJECTION FRACTION, AND MASS

The measurement of ventricular volumes and mass provides important insights into the nature of the cardiomyo-

pathic syndrome. The advent of high resolution and three-dimensional techniques has provided the accuracy and resolution relevant for appropriate characterization. While cardiac catherization has remained the standard for imaging, it had suffered from the fact that it is two-dimensional and that its risk is higher than the noninvasive imaging methods. With the advent of two-dimensional echocardiography and radionuclide angiography in the mid-1970s and magnetic resonance in the early 1980s, the clinicians armamentarium was substantially widened. However, the techniques do not offer the same ability to quantitate and assess left ventricular (LV) volumes, morphology, and mass with high spatial and temporal resolution. Similarly, reproducibility was markedly different among the various imaging techniques.

Techniques

The first technique in the current imaging era to approximate ejection fraction (EF), LV end diastolic volume (EDV) and LV end systolic volume (ESV) with cardiomyopathy was echocardiography (M-mode and two-dimensional). Several adaptations of the idealized prolate ellipse were incorporated into volumetric computations including the "bullet" formula. However, it should be noted that, in pathologic hearts such volumetric calculations tend to be less accurate than those in healthy hearts. Subsequently, "Simpson's rule" was incorporated into volume measurements using stacked short-axis acquisitions with interslice interpolation to arrive at an estimated volume. This served a two-fold purpose: in addition to quantifying volume, echocardiography could interrogate LV wall thickness with higher fidelity than x-ray angiography using radioopaque contrast medium.

R. W. W. Biederman: Department of Cardiovascular Disease, Center for Nuclear Magnetic Resonance Research and Development; Department of Medicine, University of Alabama at Birmingham, Birmingham, Alabama 35223.

G. M. Pohost: Department of Medicine, University of Alabama at Birmingham, Birmingham, Alabama 35294.

Thus, a one-and then two-dimensional approach became the standard for estimating ventricular volumes and mass (1,2).

Nevertheless, the computation of volumes using Simpson's rule suffered from the inadequacy of the acoustic window and the variability in orientation of the standard views. Transesophageal echocardiography (TEE) overcame the problem of attenuation by the lungs (3). With Lauterbur's invention in 1972 that allowed nuclear magnetic resonance to image morphology and the subsequent initial application to the heart by Pohost and colleagues (4), cardiovascular MRI (CMR) was initiated as a clinical cardiovascular imaging modality. The ability of CMR to image in any plane orientation and in three dimensions remains a principle advantage over other imaging modalities. Thus, with high spatial resolution and lack of attenuation, MRI has become the gold standard for measuring volumes and mass.

The complex motion and geometry of the heart in many cardiomyopathies and in ischemic heart disease can be problematic for traditional imaging modalities. Though many studies have been performed to compare MRI with other techniques *in vivo*, there continues to be a conspicuous paucity of intramodality comparisons. Autopsy specimens have been used and have shown fair correlation between 0.85 and 0.90 (5). Due to limitations of autopsy-derived hearts, phantoms or casts filled or impregnated with methylmethacrylate have been used more successfully for such comparisons. Rehr and co-workers, using cast volume water displacement and MRI spin-echo volume determination, showed an excellent correlation ($r = 0.99$) with a SEE of 5.0 cm^2 (6). Markiewitz and colleagues correlated ventricular volumes with silicon casts from 19 excised dog hearts and found very good correlations for both ventricles. (LV, $r = 0.99$ and RV, $r = 0.98$) (7). *In vivo* work followed, showing high degrees of correlation, generally greater than $r = 0.91$, with many studies using *in vivo* models. The majority of these were in nonpathologic states where uniform application of certain geometric assumptions could be employed reliably (8–10).

The cardiomyopathic heart frequently assumes a globular shape and can significantly deviate from standard mathematical assumptions. Recognizing the need for validation of MRI techniques in nonidealized states, Semelkka and co-workers compared normals and patients with left ventricular hypertrophy and dilated cardiomyopathies in two separate imaging sessions. They showed that the interobserver variability for measuring end-diastolic volume (EDV) was 3.6% and 3.8%, while for the end-systolic volume (ESV) variability was 9.7% and 9.0% in the normal group. Interobserver variabilities were less than 5.0% for both EDV and ESV for patients with dilated cardiomyopathies and less than 8.5% for both EDV and ESV in left ventricular hypertrophy (11).

Ejection fraction (EF) is the mainstay for the evaluation of ventricular function, not because it is independent of loading conditions (it is not), but because it is easily determined and not dependent on absolute volumes. In the dilated cardiomyopathies where prognosis is a function of EF, measurement requires special attention. Although EF is frequently determined clinically, Rich and co-workers have demonstrated that the measurement has a SEE of $\pm 10\%$ ($r = 0.73$) (12). However, using Simpson's rule or radionuclide cineangiography, good correlations can be generated (0.78 to 0.93) (13,14).

By extrapolation, to achieve a correct EF, optimally calculated with accurate and reproducible volumetric determinations, it should follow that three dimensional imaging methods such as MRI would provide more accurate measurements. Thus, the majority of studies that evaluate LV volumes, also include EF as a standard calculation. In general, correlation in normals can be high ($r = 0.93$ to 0.97) (15,16). However, in dilated cardiomyopathy where LVEF is depressed, correlations are suboptimal. Thus, for EF evaluation, two-dimensional echo is not recommended and multiple gated equilibrium radionuclide cineangiography (MUGA) would be anticipated to provide less accurate data than three-dimensional methods like MRI.

The calculation of LV mass (LVM) has been well established and uses similar assumptions. As expected, higher resolution leads to improved accuracy and reproducibility. The Penn convention and the American Society of Echocardiography techniques use echocardiographic techniques to estimate mass with a high degree of accuracy and reproducibility. Furthermore, some of the original studies that demonstrated adverse effect of abnormal LV mass on morbidity and mortality used echocardiography (17). However, because of its geometric assumptions and two-dimensional nature, the variability in groups of patients may be too large for reliable use in the individual patient. This notion is demonstrated by Bottini and colleagues. The accuracy, precision, and reliability of LVM estimates by MRI were compared to data obtained by two-dimensional echo in hypertensive patients. MRI LV mass estimates were within 17.5 g (95% confidence interval) of the autopsy LV mass. The precision of LVM by MRI was over twice that observed with ECHO (SEE = ± 11 g versus ± 23 g). The reliability of MRI LV mass estimates were more consistent than that for two-dimensional-echo (SEE = ± 8 g versus ± 49 g). Furthermore, the number of patients needed to achieve a predetermined power level was a log-fold less—i.e; by echo, 550 patients were required to achieve a 95% confidence interval for detecting a difference of 10 grams, while only 17 patients were required with MRI. The authors concluded that MRI appeared to be a more precise and reliable method for measurement of LV mass, and would be more suitable than two-dimensional-echo for the clinical evaluation of the individual patient (18).

Dilated Cardiomyopathy

The term *dilated cardiomyopathy* (DCM) denotes a primary myocardial disorder of unknown cause. Classically, the finding of regional dysfunction in a dilated ventricle her-

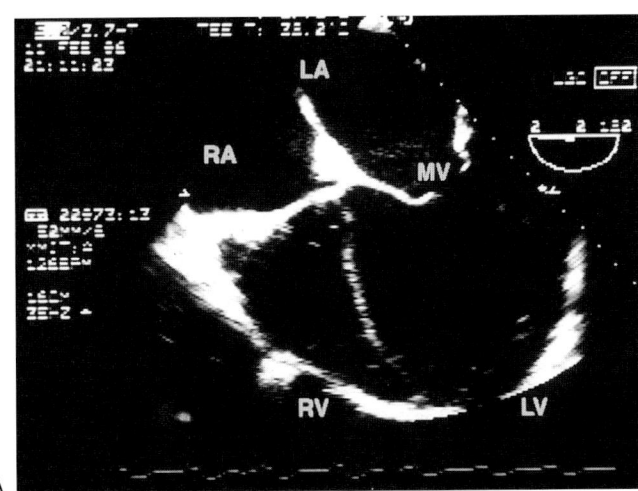
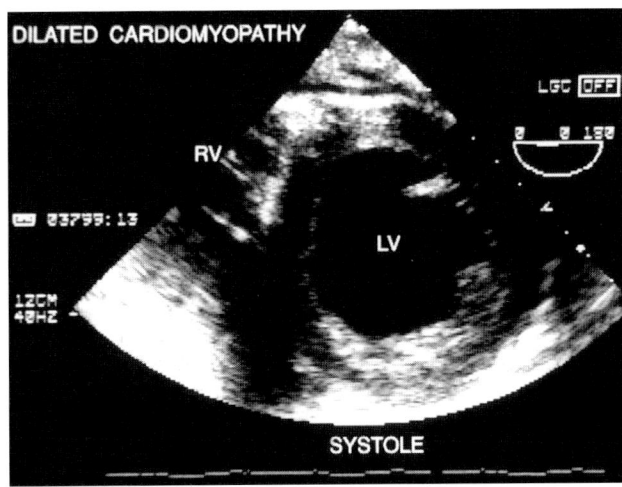

FIG. 1. A: Two-dimensional echocardiographic demonstration of a patient with an idiopathic dilated cardiomyopathy showing the four-chamber view as labeled: right ventricle (*RV*), left ventricle (*LV*), right atrium (*RA*), left atrium (*LA*), and mitral valve (*MV*). Note the biatrial and biventricular enlargement. (From ref. 95, with permission.) **B:** two-chamber view by magnetic resonance imaging of the same patient.

alds the presence of an ischemic origin. Echocardiographic evaluation of systolic function was the first technique to recognize consistently that this paradigm was incorrect (19,20). However, both two-dimensional and M-mode echocardiograms reveal characteristic signs of LV dilation including reduced shortening fraction (SF), presence or absence of biventricular involvement, the association of atrial enlargement, E-point separation on the parasternal view, and the presence of valvular disturbances (Fig. 1A). The finding of mitral annular dilation with failure of the mitral leaflets to coapt can readily be determined with high fidelity by transthoracic echocardiography (TTE) or TEE. This issue is of importance if mitral valve repair is an option vs. mitral valve replacement.

Incorporation of Doppler velocity analysis to estimate pulmonary artery pressure, LV outflow tract (LVOT) velocities as an indicator of cardiac output, and the acceleration slope (analogous to dp/dt) are clinically useful tools and can be readily performed by echocardiography. Likewise, diastolic indices of LV function can readily be obtained with a high degree of precision by echocardiography. These indices include diastolic flow, isovolumic relaxation time, and reversal of "s" and "d" waves for pulmonary venous flow. Commonly seen is a psuedonormalization pattern indicating increased filling pressure secondary to elevated EDP and left atrial (LA) pressure with a depressed early filling velocity (21). LA filling wave forms are helpful in evaluating the presence of concomitant restrictive disease, which is rapidly being recognized as one of the distinguishing features of dilated cardiomyopathy (21). Interestingly, the presence of concomitant diastolic dysfunction is reported in 50% to 60% of patients with dilated cardiomyopathy (22,23).

Physiology and Ventricular Function

Using echocardiography, Belardinelli and co-workers evaluated exercise training in patients with dilated cardiomyopathy and showed that there was improvement in diastolic indices of LV function. Fifty-five patients underwent a pulsed-Doppler echocardiographic study, a radionuclide angiographic study, and a cardiopulmonary exercise test before and after a 2-month exercise training program. In the trained subgroups there was a significant increase in rapid filling fraction, peak filling rate, peak early filling velocity, and E:A ratio. Stepwise logistic regression showed that Doppler LV diastolic filling patterns were independent predictors of overall cardiac events ($P = 0.02$), and a restrictive pattern had a worse prognosis compared with a normal filling pattern ($P = 0.007$). However, exercise training itself did not reach statistical significance as a predictor of cardiac events ($P = 0.54$). Thus, Doppler echocardiography may be a valuable tool in the prognostic assessment of patients with DCM who will benefit from exercise training (24).

There is considerable evidence that 17-1231-iodohexadecanoic acid (IHPA) and 15-(p-[1231]-iodophenyl)-pentadecanoic acid (IPPA), tracers of myocardial fatty acid metabolism, show that the clearance half-times in patients with dilated cardiomyopathy are markedly prolonged. More interestingly, there was significant heterogeneity between the clearance times from the interventricular septum and the inferior and posterolateral walls (25). In general, the delayed clearance was a hallmark of dilated cardiomyopathy and was not found in ischemic cardiomyopathy with equivalent LV dysfunction (26).

This pattern is also reflected in positron emission tomography (PET). Again, myocardial clearance has striking variability. Thus, the predictive power for the radionuclide tracers and their use in LV dysfunction is not convincing. The putative mechanisms for tracer behavior are only now becoming understood.

There is considerable diversity in the potential mechanisms for radionuclide-labeled fatty acid clearance in cardiomyopathy, particularly for the dilated form (see Table 2, Chapter 45). Nevertheless, metabolic insults can be observed with PET. Early studies employed ^{11}C-palmitate as an indicator of β-oxidation with multislice PET distribution to define the spatial distribution of myocardial fatty acids. Tomographic acquisitions in patients with dilated cardiomyopathy revealed heterogeneous distribution of ^{11}C-palmitate without a definable pattern to suggest a predictable decrease (or increase) in fatty acid metabolism. In addition, there was no predictable relationship between systolic thickening and the change in metabolism. This relationship held true when independently correlated to ^{201}Tl imaging (27) and with glucose loading. While there may have been more heterogeneity present than in the normal population, there was a trend toward lower EF in patients with abnormal metabolism in response to glucose administration as shown by Schelbert and associates (28). The switch from fatty acid metabolism to ketone bodies as a source of energy has been suggested as a way to account for such observations, (after glucose load, the citric acid cycle would be down regulated). Retrospectively, it is possible that fibrosis, microvascular disease, or even alterations in β-oxidation may explain some of the observed inconsistencies.

Additionally, ^{11}C-acetate as a tracer to follow the fate of Krebs cycle intermediates can be assessed. These studies compared favorably with the earlier ^{11}C-palmitate investigations. When an inotropic agent was added, the clearance of ^{11}C-acetate and myocardial efficiency increased, since the heart was operating on a more beneficial portion of the Frank-Starling curve. Furthermore, dobutamine augmented vasodilator properties and increased cardiac inotropy. MVO_2 and Laplacian analysis revealed wall tension to be favorably improved (29). Recent studies using ^{13}N-ammonia and ^{15}O-water have been performed to quantitate perfusion in dilated cardiomyopathy. In contrast, the investigators showed that perfusion was homogeneous at rest, yet perfusion reserve was dramatically reduced (30). Explanations for this characteristic include occult microvascular disease or reduction in coronary perfusion pressure secondary to the increase in EDP.

The evaluation of dilated cardiomyopathies has been aided tremendously through the use of MRI. The ability to evaluate dimensions, wall thickness, tissue characteristics, and certain anatomic considerations enables MRI to play a critical role (Fig. 1**B**). As previously mentioned, the primary role in the imaging of a dilated cardiomyopathy must be the exclusion of an ischemic etiology. In general, the role of MRI can fulfill four purposes: (i) exclusion of other disease entities, (ii) evaluation of ventricular wall thickness and

chamber dimensions, (iii) physiological evaluation of the cardiomyopathy, and (iv) tissue characterization.

The exclusion of other disease entities can be performed rapidly and accurately by spin-echo (dark blood) and gradient-echo (cine or bright blood) techniques to evaluate regional wall motion, myocardial wall thinning, or aneurysmal dilation suggestive of a previous myocardial infarction. Morphologic evaluations typically use multislice/multiphase acquisitions where the measurements of LV chamber dimensions and wall thickness are performed with respiratory and ECG gating. ECG gating is used to obtain different phases of the cardiac cycle and insure that each tomographic image obtained at the appropriate phase of the cardiac cycle. Transverse axial views are also gated, usually in the spin-echo mode, and are used to detect atrial enlargement. The views important to the cardiologist are the four-chamber (perpendicular to the intraventricular septum) and the two-chamber (parallel to the intraventricular septum and depicting the LA and LV). In addition, the standard short-axis slices are obtained using the gradient-echo approach so that radial shortening can be evaluated. In particular, the gradient-echo sequences (bright blood), normal blood motion appears white while the slower moving myocardium appears dark. Thus, intrinsic contrast is manufactured endogenously. This is in distinction to the exogenously supplied contrast used for x-ray angiography. The ''bright blood'' or cine sequence is most important for evaluating LV function and regional wall motion.

As described previously, estimation of volumes and mass is accurate and reproducible, and MRI should be considered as the ''gold standard'' for these measurements. Such measurements are particularly useful for following progression of disease and/or response to medications or interventions. As such, MRI arms the clinician with an unparalleled tool (31). However, it should be noted that this technique requires considerable attention to detail. An increased number of slices is necessary to increase the accuracy of mass determination. However, acquisition times will be longer.

Recently, it has been recognized that volumetric analyses may underestimate EDV because of failure to take into consideration the longitudinal shortening of the LV during systole. This results from failure to include the basal plane in the short axis view at the end of diastole. Clinically, it results in underestimation of stroke volume (SV), ejection fraction (EF), and cardiac output (CO). Recognition of this problem will improve the accuracy and reproducibility of such calculations. Marcus and colleagues have recommended inclusion of the most basal slice in EDV calculations and also correction, as needed, for computation of ESV (32).

The assessment of a particular cardiomyopathy utilizes cine MRI to examine wall thickening and ventricular function. If end-systolic pressure is known (or estimated), Laplacian stress analysis can be performed (33). Stroke volume may be calculated by either cine or multiple-gated spin-echo acquisitions. Additionally, the presence of valvular regurgitation can be assessed using gradient-echo techniques. In normal patients there is a marked base to apex gradient of wall thickening that MRI studies have shown to be markedly diminished in those with dilated cardiomyopathy (34).

Finally, a unique aspect of MRI is its ability to examine tissue character. Since the relaxation rates are frequently different in different organs and in different disease startes, knowledge of such relaxation rates can be exploited to offer diagnostic insight.

Specific Cardiomyopathies

Myocarditis—Viral, Protozoal, and Inflammatory

The first clue to a myocarditis is frequently enlargement of the cardiac silhouette on the chest x-ray. Two-dimensional echo is helpful in demonstrating the presence of global dysfunction of either or both ventricles (35). The utility of non-invasive imaging techniques frequently depends on the demonstration of an inflammatory pattern in conjunction with chamber dysfunction. Therefore, several methods have been employed to elucidate this pattern (Fig. 2**A**). Both antimyosin ^{111}In-labeled antibody and gallium-67 scanning have been used and myocardial uptake of these radiopharmaceuticals is helpful in establishing the diagnosis of myocarditis (36,37).

Friedrich and colleagues recently reported a novel application of MRI utilizing the principle of inflammation as a marker for imaging patients with biopsy-proven myocarditis. After meeting the inclusion criteria of ECG changes, reduced myocardial function, elevated creatine kinase, positive troponin T, serologic evidence for acute viral infection, exclusion of coronary heart disease, and positive antimyosin imaging, 19 patients were imaged by MRI. After intravenous administration of 0.1 mmol/kg gadolinium-DPTA, global signal enhancement of the left ventricular myocardium as compared to skeletal muscle with T1-weighted images were made. Measurements in 18 volunteers on days 2, 7, 14, 28, 72, and 84 after the onset of symptoms were compared. The investigators confirmed what had been suspected; acute myocarditis evolves from a focal to a more disseminated process during the first 2 weeks after onset of symptoms. In addition, the authors noted that the extent of increased signal distribution at day two was predictive of the LVEF at day 72 (38) (Fig. 2**B**).

Until recently, antimyosin antibody imaging was relegated to research interest only. However, in addition to adding sensitivity to the evaluation of the syndrome of myocardial infarction, it has been used as a means of detecting myocarditis. Recently Indium-111 antimyosin antibody imaging and thallium-201 were compared in patients with myocarditis and dilated cardiomyopathy. The distribution of each tracer and antimyosin/thallium-201 overlap were evaluated with single-photon emission computed tomography (SPECT). Comparisons between antimyosin and thallium-201 SPECT images were useful for evaluating the activity

of myocarditis and ongoing myocardial damage, particularly, in areas with no perfusion in patients with dilated cardiomyopathy, thus helping to differentiate between the cardiomyopathy and the myocarditis, even in the chronic stage (39).

The two most common causes of myocarditis is Epstein-Barr virus (EBV) and cytomegalovirus (CMV). Laroche-Traineau and co-workers reported that a patient with Glanzmann's thrombasthenia secreted an monoclonal antibody of EBV (B7) that reacted with the myosin heavy chain of human platelets. B7 specifically labeled myosin, but there was no labeling of aortic smooth muscle cells. Purified Fab fragments retained their affinity to myosin, suggesting that B7 may be useful in the imaging of myocardial necrosis after myocardial infarction, myocarditis, cardiac drug toxicosis, or allograft rejection (40). Unstated by the authors was the extrapolation that B7, if labeled with a radionuclide agent, may be a novel epitope to employ for myocardial necrosis analogous to antimyosin antibody.

In Brazil, where *Trypanosoma cruzi* is endemic and responsible for Chagas disease, the heart is the most commonly affected organ. The search for an improved method to detect and differentiate it from other cardiomyopathies is ongoing. Recently, eight patients underwent MRI with gadolinium enhancement to guide endomyocardial and surgical biopsies to sites with more intense inflammatory processes. The presence of the *T. cruzi* antigen correlated with the severity of myocardial inflammation as provided by the MRI-guided biopsy specimens and provided strong supportive evidence for the role of *T. cruzi* even in the chronic forms of Chagas heart disease (41). This imaging enhancement technique improved the sensitivity and specificity of the biopsy and will likely lead to reduced need for repeat biopsies, as well as a reduced number of incorrect medical regimens.

Other forms of hypersensitivity or drug induced myocarditis/cardiomyopathy have been investigated, albeit to a lesser extent. In 59 patients with a hematologic malignancy undergoing adriamycin chemotherapy, myocardial imaging was performed by SPECT with ^{123}I-metaiodobenzylguanidine (MIBG), an agent to determine the sympathetic nerve traffic in the heart. The relationship of the washout rate of MIBG to the total dose of adriamycin, the left ventricular ejection fraction, and the frequency of arrhythmias was evaluated. The MIBG washout rate was related to the total dose of adriamycin, suggesting that it is useful for evaluaing the extent of cardiac sympathetic nerve damage (42). Patients requiring adriamycin are at a particular disadvantage, as they need an effective antineoplastic agent, yet may be hindered from treatment by cardiotoxicity. Thus, this technique may provide insight as to when cardiotoxic doses are being approached, and avoid empirically limiting the effective dose.

Peripartum Cardiomyopathy

There are no large series of peripartum cardiomyopathy studied with modern imaging techniques. Anecdotal reports

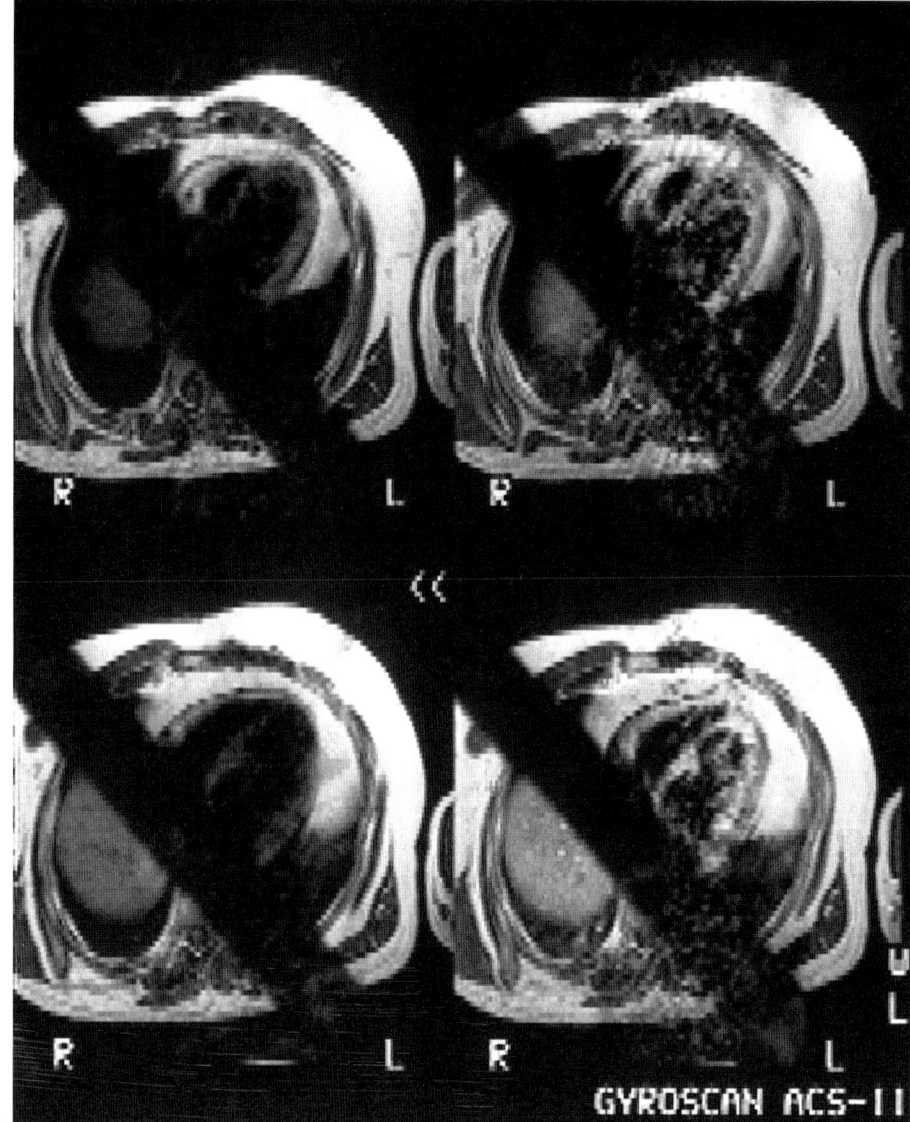

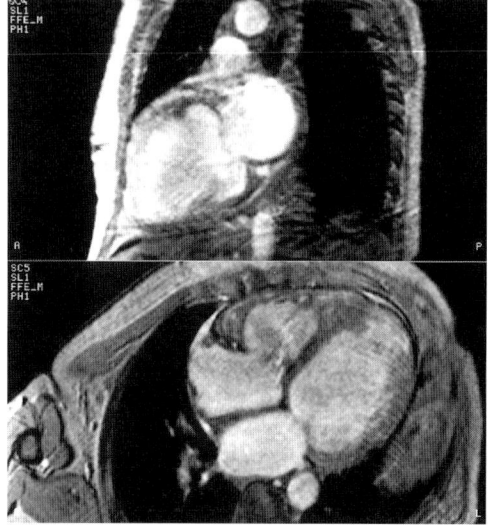

FIG. 2. **A:** Magnetic resonance imaging of a 56-year-old man with viral induced cardiomyopathy. His end-diastolic volume measured 680 mL (upper end of normal is 120 mL), his end-diastolic dimension measured 78 mL (upper limit of normal is 54 mm), and his ejection fraction measured 11%. The right anterior oblique and four-chamber views are displayed (left and right). The patient was referred for cardiac transplantation. **B:** Myocarditis diagnosed by Gadolinium DTPA in a 45-year-old man referred for chest pain and positive cardiac necrosis enzymes. Myocardial enhancement can be seen in the left ventricle pre- and postGadolinium in two representative slices (top and bottom). This technique utilizes a slab to suppress flow signal that would enter into the respective ventricles from the atrium thus increasing myocardial/chamber contrast. The patient had no coronary artery disease.

are scattered throughout the literature. An unusual presentation with hypertrophic cardiomyopathy (HCM) was recently reported in which two-dimensional and Doppler echocardiography was used to guide labor and delivery of a 35-year-old woman. There are no known associations of HCM and peripartum cardiomyopathy. As described in Chapter 45, the peripartum cardiomyopathy typically manifests as a dilated cardiomyopathy (43). Since myocarditis or other inflammatory processes have been one suspected etiology, it is tempting to speculate that an agent that can characterize inflammation may be of use—such as gadolinium-DPTA with MRI.

Alcoholic Cardiomyopathy

The cardiomyopathy associated with alcoholism is characteristically dilated, although the precise etiology is unknown. Improvement in LV dysfunction is commonly observed. While improvement is often not seen clinically (likely a social commentary on the disease rather than the pathophysiology), in controlled studies, marked improvements of even severe derangement in left and right ventricular function have been reported. Such clinical improvement is not typically observed in other cardiomyopathies. In peripartum cardiomyopathy and myocarditis is much less common.

Illustrating this point, Guillo and colleagues prospectively evaluated the long-term prognosis of 14 patients with alcoholic cardiomyopathy with severe congestive heart failure (CHF) after total abstinence. They noted significant improvement after 6 months (44).

Nineteen male patients with alcoholic cardiomyopathy and symptomatic left ventricular dysfunction with EFs 15% below baseline by echocardiography were followed. Improvement in cardiac performance and functional class was detected in about one-half of patients with alcoholic cardiomyopathy who abstained from alcohol, even in cases presenting with severe LVD (45).

A very interesting observation was made by Prazak and co-workers using echocardiography in which they showed that the mortality of patients with severe congestive heart failure and left ventricular dysfunction associated with alcoholic cardiomyopathy was significantly lower than that in patients with other idiopathic cardiomyopathies despite similar degrees of LV dysfunction and dilation. Overall survival at 1, 5, and 10 years was 100%, 81%, and 81% for the group with alcoholic cardiomyopathy and 89%, 48%, and 30% for the group with other idiopathic cardiomyopathies, respectively ($P = 0.041$). The differences were even more striking for transplant-free survival ($P = 0.005$). Thus, despite similar degrees of left ventricular dilatation, disease progression in alcoholic cardiomyopathy is markedly different from that of other idiopathic cardiomyopathies (46).

Further work has been done to elaborate the increased role of arrythmias in patients with alcoholic cardiomyopathy, though this is likely a function of the ventricular dilation per se and not critically dependent on the mechanism of the disease process (47). The process of hypertrophy and fibrosis is increasingly recognized as the substrate for arrhythmogenesis. In particular, at the membrane level, there are abnormal calcium handling and alterations in outward repolarizing potassium channels. The end result appears to be a delay in repolarization (48,49).

Human Immunodeficiency Virus Cardiomyopathy

Human immunodeficiency virus (HIV) cardiomyopathy is a recent addition to the long list of cardiomyopathies. The explosion in knowledge about HIV has had its influence in the cardiovascular field. The previously unexpected association between HIV and dilated cardiomyopathy is now more frequently being recognized and reported. The cardiovascular abnormalities in pediatric HIV, as well, are incompletely understood. Lipshultz and associates performed baseline echocardiograms as part of a prospective study on 196 vertically HIV-infected children. While 88% had symptomatic HIV infection only 2 patients had CHF at enrollment. Nevertheless, cardiac measurements were abnormal at baseline (decreased left ventricular fractional shortening, heart rate, LV dimension, mass, and wall stress). After 2 years of follow-up, most of the abnormal baseline cardiac measurements correlated with depressed CD4 cell count Z scores and the presence of HIV. While the LV chamber was dilated, LV hypertrophy also was noted in the setting of decreased height and weight (50,51).

In addition to the development of severe global left ventricular dysfunction, other less common forms of symptomatic heart disease in HIV-1-infected patients have been observed by echocardiography. These include pericardial effusion with cardiac tamponade and systemic embolization related to nonbacterial thrombotic endocarditis or bacterial endocarditis (52,53). Detection of myocardial dysfunction and other cardiac abnormalities was performed in a prospective cross-sectional echocardiographic study of 157 patients who were HIV-seropositive and acutely ill. Eighty men and 77 women were studied (mean age, 34 years). They were all heterosexual and none was a hemophiliac or an intravenous drug user. A high prevalence of echocardiographically detected myocardial and pericardial disease was found in this group of acutely ill HIV-infected patients with abnormalities seen in 79 (50%) patients: 14 of 151 (9%) had dilated cardiomyopathy; 33 of 151 (22%) had left ventricular dysfunction; and 9 of 151 (6%) had isolated right ventricular dilatation. This study was one of the first to demonstrate the high prevalence of cardiac involvement in advanced HIV (54).

Arrthymogenic Right Ventricular Dysplasia

As described in Chapter 47, arrythmogenic right ventricular dysplasia (ARVD) is a heart disease characterized by total or partial fat replacement of the myocardium that has recently been described as a cardiomyopathy but does not neatly fit into either the Goodwin or World Health Orga-

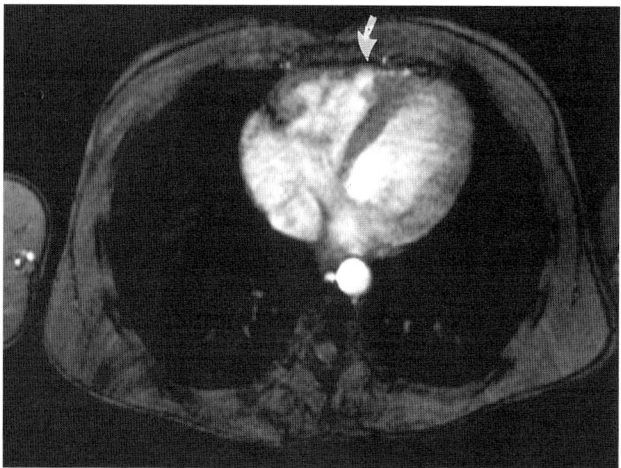

FIG. 3. Arrthymogenic right ventricular dysplasia. Note the thinned right ventricle (RV) free wall by gradient echo imaging revealed focal RV dyskinesia in the area of the thinned myocardium (*arrow*). This defect was confirmed by electrophysiologic testing, as well as an RV angiogram by x-ray angiography.

nization/International Society and Federation of Cardiology classifications. However, it is a heterogeneous pathologic disturbance within the right ventricle (RV) and, occasionally, the LV. The clinical criteria that have been agreed upon to describe ARVD are: (i) ventricular arrhythmias with a left bundle-branch block configuration; (ii) T-wave inversion in the anterior precordial leads; (iii) wall motion abnormalities observed using echocardiography and angiography; and (iv) cardiac failure not attributable to other heart diseases. In addition, other more nebulous morphologic characteristics have been observed. This has been most rigorously done with MRI imaging (Fig. 3). These additional criteria include: (i) high-intensity areas indicating fatty substitution of the myocardium, (ii) ectasia of the right ventricular outflow tract, (iii) dyskinetic bulges, (iv) dilation of the right ventricle, and (v) enlargement of the right atrium (55). Others, including the authors of this chapter, add the presence of RV wall thinning as another criterion for ARVD.

Other imaging techniques have been used to help detect ARVD, including ^{123}I-MIBG, [201]TlCl, ultrafast computed tomography (UFCT), and echocardiography for the detection of left or right ventricular involvement. In 15 patients with (ARVD), Takahashi utilized radionuclide ventriculography (RNV) and myocardial imaging with ^{123}I-MIBG, [201]TlCl, MRI, and UFCT in 15 patients with ARVD and in 10 normal volunteers to attempt to detect early myocardial involvement in patients with ARVD. Interestingly, 14 patients (93%) showed regional ^{123}I-MIBG defects, while 12 patients (80%) showed regional [201]TlCl defects. Abnormal UFCT or MRI findings suggested fatty involvement in the LV myocardium were demonstrated in 7 patients while 7 other patients showed regional ^{123}I-MIBG defects without abnormal UFCT and MRI findings. ^{123}I-MIBG was signifi-

cantly more sensitive than UFCT and MRI ($P < 0.05$). These findings indicate that myocardial imaging with ^{123}I-MIBG may be a more sensitive detector for early myocardial damage when ventricular involvement is not yet present (56).

Recently, ARVD has been found to have a genetic predisposition. Linkage analysis has revealed that autosomal dominant ARVD can be mapped to 14q23-q24 (ARVD1) and to 1q42-q43 (ARVD2). A third possible locus was assigned to 14q12-q22. Rampazzo and co-workers have reported the possibility of a fourth locus (ARVD4), mapping to 2q32 (57). In the future, the hallmark of morphologic ARVD will likely include chromosomal mapping for confirmation of the disease process.

Secondary Cardiomyopathy

Diabetic Cardiomyopathy

Imaging methods have done little to establish the presence of a diabetic dilated cardiomyopathy. To establish the existence of such a cardiomyopathy, one must exclude the presence of epicardial coronary artery disease. Recent experimental work supports a role for endothelial dysfunction as the basis of microvascular disease. Experimental evidence using ^{125}I-BMIPP autoradiography supports an aberration in fatty acid metabolism. Less myocardial activity was found in the dilated diabetic heart than in the control group indicating that myocardial fatty acid metabolism was less than in the former group (58). This concept is further supported by a report of simultaneous imaging ^{201}Tl and [^{123}I] betamethyliodophenylpentadecanoic acid (BMIPP), a fatty acid tracer. Regional wall motion abnormalities were seen by contrast angiography. In a patient with diabetic cardiomyopathy ^{201}Tl demonstrated transient perfusion defects in the inferoposterior wall of the left ventricle that correlated with reduced [^{123}I]BMIPP uptake. These results suggested that the impairment of myocardial free fatty acid metabolism may be a contributory factor for regional wall motion abnormalities, in addition to small-vessel coronary artery disease (59).

Collagen Vascular Disease

Systemic Lupus Erythematosis

Systemic lupus erythematosis (SLE) is rarely associated with a cardiomyopathy. However, reports using Indium-111-antimyosin Fab imaging demonstrate myocardial injury in SLE. Morguet and associates used antimyosin imaging in 2 patients with documented SLE with subsequent improvement with immunosuppressant therapy. Although the incidence specificity of Indium-111-antimyosin Fab uptake is unknown, this report suggests that it may be useful to screen for myocardial involvement in patients with SLE (60).

Systemic Sclerosis

Systemic sclerosis (SS) can involve the myocardium. Detection of this involvement, however, is difficult. Gallium-67 citrate has been proposed to delineate such involvement. Using MRI, echocardiography, and myocardial gallium-67 citrate imaging, Gaal and associates found increased myocardial gallium uptake in 5 of 16 patients. While both echocardiography and MRI revealed depressed LV function, only the gallium scans indicated the possibility of myocardial interstitial inflammation (61).

Symptomatic cardiac involvement in patients with SS indicates a very poor prognosis. Ferri and colleagues emphasized this in a recent study when they noted a vast discrepancy between the frequency of myocardial disease (25%) and myocardial fibrosis found at autopsy (81%). Using ultrasonic videodensitometric analysis, 35 patients with systemic sclerosis (age range, 22 to 65) and normal ventricular function by echo were studied along with 25 healthy controls matched for age and gender. All patients had a negative maximal exercise stress test. Patients with evidence of arterial hypertension, renal involvement, and diabetes were excluded. Echocardiographic images were digitized by a real-time videodigitizer (Tomtec Imaging Systems) and texture analysis was performed on the septum and the posterior wall. They found changes in the cyclic echo amplitude probably related to myocardial fibrosis in a large proportion of systemic sclerosis patients (88%). The presence of fibrosis and microcirculatory abnormalities potentially explains the link with LV dysfunction, electrical abnormalities, and sudden death that occur during the evolution of the disease (62). Cardiac MRI has been added to the armamentarium of imaging techniques for SS because of its ability to provide high-resolution anatomic and functional images in three dimensions (63). Also, thallium-201 has been used to demonstrate defects that may represent areas of myocardial infiltration. Thallium-201 in SS is variably accurate with 30% of patients showing scintigraphic but not always clinical evidence of cardiac involvement (64). Similarly, gallium-67 scanning may be helpful both prognostically and clinically in demonstrating the clinical improvements with corticosteroids (65) (Fig. 4).

Phosphorus-31 NMR Spectroscopy

Nuclear magnetic resonance (NMR) spectroscopy has been used to probe the biologic and chemical properties of the myocardium. Phosphorus-31 (^{31}P) in particular is used routinely for spectroscopic imaging. Reductions in the myocardial phosphocreatine (PCr)-to-ATP ratio measured noninvasively by ^{31}P-NMR spectroscopy in patients with heart failure due to dilated cardiomyopathy have indicated that cardiac energy metabolism is impaired. Neubauer and associates followed 39 patients with dilated cardiomyopathy for 2.5 years. The investigators tested whether the PCr/ATP ratio offered prognostic information. In addition, they compared LVEF and New York Heart Association (NYHA) class with PCr/ATP. At study entry, LVEF and NYHA class were determined, and cardiac PCr/ATP was measured by localized ^{31}P-NMR spectroscopy of the anterior myocardium. The total mortality was 26% during the study period. Patients were divided into two groups, one with normal PCr/ATP (>1.60, [1.98 ± 0.07]) in 19 healthy volunteers and one group with reduced PCr/ATP (<1.60, [1.30 ± 0.05]) in 20 patients. After 2.5 years, 8 of 20 (40%) patients with reduced PCr/ATP had died, all from cardiovascular causes. Of the 19 patients with normal PCr/ATP, only 2 had died (11%), only 1 of whom from cardiovascular causes. Importantly, Kaplan-Meier analysis showed significantly reduced cardiovascular mortality ($P = 1.016$) for patients with normal versus low PCr/ATP. Correspondingly, a Cox model for multivariate analysis showed that the PCr/ATP and NYHA class offered significant independent prognostic information on cardiovascular mortality. In addition to being predictive,

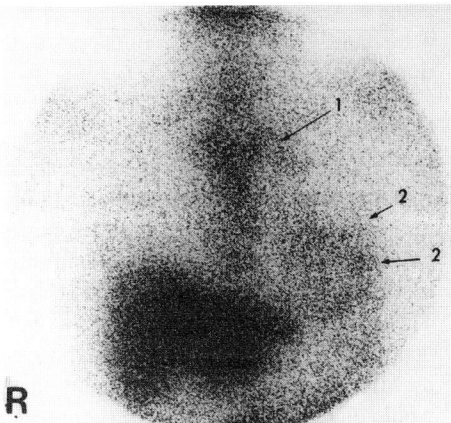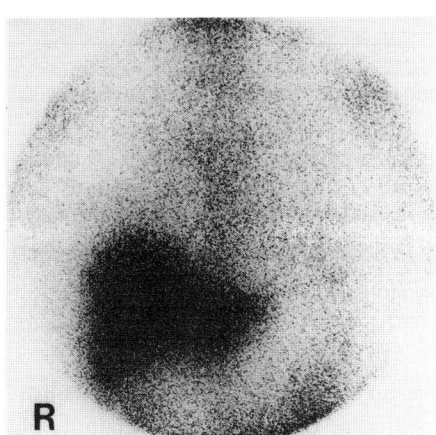

FIG. 4. Initial Galium-67 imaging of the chest (**left**) shows areas of increased activity in the mediastinal lymph nodes (*1*) and the heart (*2*) in the anterior projections. Biopsy specimen of a mediastinal node at exploratory thoracotomy disclosed noncaseating granuloma indicative of sarcoidosis. The patient was treated with corticosteroids. On repeat galium-67 imaging 3 months later (**right**), the areas of involvement previously seen are now less prominent. (From ref. 96, with permission.)

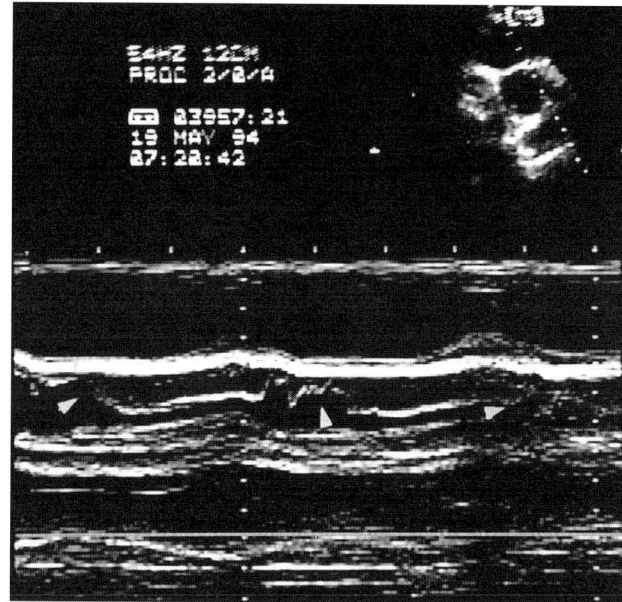

D

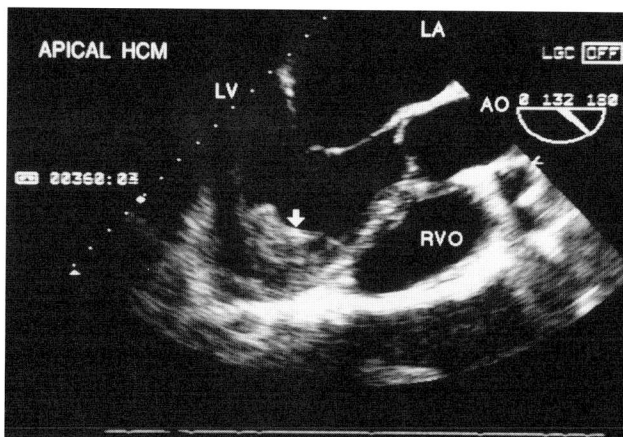

E

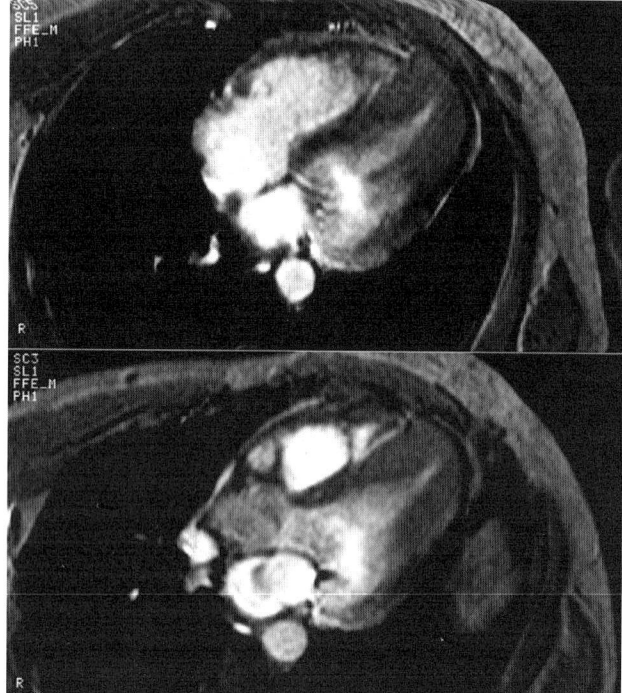

F

FIG. 5. *continued* **D:** Apical hypertrophy: five-chamber, two-dimensional echocardiography view with course aortic valve fluttering (arrows). **E:** Apical hypertrophy in a 49-year-old female. The **top** view is an MRI (magnetic resonance image) in the four-chamber projection, while the **bottom** view is in the more traditional outflow tract view. Both are in end diastole. As opposed to the LVOT obstructive variant, this Japanese variety predominantly effects the apex. In this case, the more basal wall thickness measures 11 mm each (posterior and anterior septal) while the apical myocardium had a maximum thickness of 21 mm each. *Ao,* aorta; *AV,* aortic valve; *LA,* left atrium; *LVOF,* left ventricular outflow tract; *RVO,* right ventricular outflow. (From ref. 95, with permission.)

niques. The mechanism for this observation is generally thought to be a Venturi effect created by the thickened septum, or an abnormal mitral valve and/or an anteriorly displaced anterior papillary muscle (77). During early systole the distal anterior mitral leaflet, and occasionally the posterior leaflet, move towards the apex. The remainder of the anterior leaflet moves towards the septum in the initial portion of LV contraction. At the end of LV contraction the distal mitral leaflet assumes its normal position just prior to ventricular relaxation. The amount of SAM appears to correlate with the magnitude of the intraventricular pressure gradient between the LV outflow tract and the LV. (Fig.

5C and **D**; see also Color Plate following page 000) These observations can be easily made in the parasternal view, but often the differentiation between leaflet and chordal SAM is not possible. The apical view facilitates this differentiation.

Continuous and pulsed-wave Doppler allow the interrogation of the LVOT, as well as the evaluation of the severity of induced mitral regurgitation. It is essential to differentiate the higher velocity LV outflow jet from the aortic flow and the jet of mitral regurgitation. Continuous-wave Doppler allows estimation of the pressure gradient by the Bernoulli formula. The peak gradient is obtained in mid- to late systole and can be estimated by $4V^2$ where V is the maximum instantaneous velocity. Recognizing that the aortic outflow velocity is not uniform and occurs at a time delayed from the onset of systole ensures that the interrogation of the jet of mitral regurgitation, frequently a higher velocity, is not confused with the LV outflow velocity (78). Cine MRI has been found to be sensitive and specific to the complexities of the dynamic mitral regurgitation associated with HCM (79).

Recently, Hada and colleagues used a newly emerged technique to interrogate diastolic properties in asymmetric septal hypertrophy (ASH). In 21 patients with ASH and in 24 age-matched normals, the E:A ratios measured by mitral inflow Doppler were not different between the groups (1.0 versus 1.1 m/sec). However, apical pulsed-Doppler tissue imaging revealed 'E' wave velocities of the septum that were significantly decreased in the hypertrophic group compared to the control group (4.0 ± 1.5 versus 8.1 ± 2.2 cm/sec). 'A' wave velocities were increased in the hypertrophic septum as well, resulting in a significantly lower E:A ratio (0.5 ± 0.3) compared to the E:A ratio (0.9 ± 0.3) of the normal septum. Furthermore, deceleration time of the 'E' wave and isovolumic relaxation time were markedly prolonged in the thickened septum compared to the normal septum (136 ± 51 versus 107 ± 28 m/sec and 91 ± 36 versus 63 ± 19 m/sec, respectively). Thus, despite the significantly hypertrophied septum, traditional diastolic indices were not abnormal at the time of measurement in this group of patients; yet, intramyocardial pulsed-Doppler echocardiography could detect regional diastolic myocardial dysfunction (80). This points to an earlier manifestation of the pathologic derangements in the hypertrophied septum than had heretofore been appreciated.

Two-dimensional echocardiography or MRI can easily assess traditional hypertrophic cardiomyopathy; however, the apical variant of hypertrophic cardiomyopathy may be difficult to diagnose using transthoracic echocardiography because of inconsistent imaging of the apical segment. Furthermore, the distribution of hypertrophy may be inaccurate and abnormalities in wall thickening underestimated. Multiplane transesophageal echocardiography allows high resolution imaging of all segments of the left ventricle, particularly the apex and can characterize this otherwise difficult pathology (81). This lesion in particular is well assessed noninvasively by MRI, which probably should be the imaging technique of choice (Fig. 5E and F).

Ventricular Function in Hypertrophic Cardiomyopathy

One important feature of MRI is its ability to evaluate ventricular function. Because of a combination of high spatial and temporal resolution, low signal-to-noise ratios and three-dimensional acquisitions, regional myocardial function can be readily, accurately, and reproducibly determined. Illustrating this concept, Sato and associates examined systolic wall thickening (%WT) and percent change of segmental wall area (%AR) by cine magnetic resonance imaging in 40 patients with HCM and 23 volunteers. Short-axis images of the left ventricle in normals were recorded at the base and the apex and were divided into five segments. While apical %WT and %AR segments in the control group were markedly increased as compared to the basal segments, the majority of the patients with HCM had reduced %WT and %AR in proportion to the degree of hypertrophy. Interestingly, the areas of least hypertrophy in the HCM patients had normal or even supernormal function. This led to the concept of a possible compensatory mechanism for the dysfunctional myocardium to preserve an otherwise remote depressed regional contractile function (82).

In one of the earliest clinical applications for MRI tissue tagging, Young and associates investigated three-dimensional myocardial strain in patients with HCM. Using finite element analysis, three-dimensional reconstruction was performed to measure circumferential, radial, and meriodonal strain. They noted that radial strain was mildly depressed, whereas meriodonal strain was markedly depressed in these patients. Circumferential strains were reduced primarily in the septum. Interestingly, torsion was enhanced in HCM patients, likely as a compensatory mechanism to augment ventricular function (76).

NMR spectroscopy, as stated earlier, has been used to probe the biochemical and energetic properties of the myocardium. In particular, phosphorus-31 (^{31}P) has been extensively used for spectroscopic imaging by NMR. As shown earlier, disturbed myocardial energy metabolism may occur in patients with primary hypertrophic cardiomyopathy. In order to obtain insight into cardiac energy metabolism 13 patients with HCM underwent chemical-shift imaging with a double resonant surface coil. A two-dimensional sequence in combination with slice selective excitation was used to acquire spectra of the anteroseptal region of the left ventricle. The chemical shifts of the phosphorus metabolites, intracellular pHi, and coupling constants J (alphabeta) and J (gammabeta) were calculated. Peak areas of 2,3-diphosphoglycerol (DPG), inorganic phosphate (Pi), and adenosine triphosphate (ATP) were determined and corrected for blood contamination, saturation, and differences in nuclear Overhauser enhancements. With respect to phosphocreatine/gamma-ATP ratio, pHi, or the coupling constants, no differences were found between patients with severe HCM and those with moderate HCM or a control group of healthy volunteers ($n = 16$). However, the PCr/Pi ratio of those with HCM differed significantly from controls probably mediated by an ischemically driven decreased oxygen supply in the severely hypertrophied myocardium (83). Using a variation of this technique decreased PCr/Pi has been suggested in patients with advanced hypertrophic cardiomyopathy (84).

The concept of an ischemic basis to the septal dysfunction in patients with HCM is not a new one. Using gated radionuclide cardiac blood pool scan (GCS), Pohost and colleagues interrogated the ventricular septum and correlated it with left ventricular function in 22 patients with HCM, 9 with valvular aortic stenosis, and 6 normals. Using echocardiography all patients with HCM had asymmetric septal hypertrophy, and 14 of 22 had systolic anterior motion of the anterior leaflet of the mitral valve. Only 2 of 8 patients with aortic stenosis and adequate echocardiograms had asymmetric septal hypertrophy. None had systolic anterior motion. The GCS demonstrated disproportionate upper septal thickening in 11, septal flattening in 16, and apical cavity obliteration in 17 patients. Importantly, a filling defect consistent with an ischemic basis was present in the region of the left ventricular outflow tract in 16 of the 22 patients with HCM. In the 9 patients with valvular aortic stenosis, 2 demonstrated septal flattening, 2 had cavity obliteration, and 2 had an outflow tract defect. Both patients with cavity obliteration demonstrated asymmetric septal hypertrophy (DVST) on echocardiogram. As opposed to the high predominance of ^{201}Tl defects in patients with HCM, only 2 aortic stenosis patients had a similar pattern. This finding helped to stimulate an intense area of investigation that is still ongoing today (85).

Septal Interventions

As discussed in Chapter 45, mortality and morbidity associated with hypertrophic obstructive cardiomyopathy (HOCM) is considerable. Various surgical and nonsurgical techniques have been undertaken to reduce the septal hypertrophy that invariably bulges into the LVOT. The expectation is that reduction of the septal protrusion will reduce the LV outflow tract gradient and, consequently, reduce clinical sequelae. This concept was recently tested by Nagueh and associates evaluating the ability of myocardial contrast echocardiography (MCE) to guide the targeted delivery of ethanol during nonsurgical septal reduction therapy (NSRT) and to assess the relation between the MCE risk area and infarct size determined by radionuclide methods. The investigators hypothesized that MCE could provide accurate delineation of the vascular territory of the coronary arteries enabling injection of ethanol into the correct coronary artery. Twenty-nine patients with HOCM and maximal medical therapy underwent NSRT. The left ventricular outflow tract (LVOT) gradient by Doppler echocardiography at baseline was 53 ± 16 mm Hg (mean ± SD). Diluted sonicated albumin (Albunex) was selectively injected into the septal perforator arteries during simultaneous transthoracic imaging. Immediately after MCE, ethanol was injected into the same vessel after NSRT. Accurate mapping of the vascular beds of the septal perforators was successfully attained in all patients by MCE. The LVOT gradient decreased to 12 ± 6 mm Hg (P < 0.001). The second phase of this study was performed 6 weeks after NSRT. Twenty-three patients underwent myocardial perfusion studies performed with single-photon emission computed tomography (SPECT). Mean SPECT septal perfusion defect size involved 9.5% ± 6% of the left ventricle and correlated well with MCE area (r = 0.7), with no statistically significant difference between the risk area estimated by MCE and that by SPECT. Thus, it appears that estimation of the size of the septal vascular

territory with MCE is accurate, safe, and feasible in essentially all patients undergoing NSRT. MCE may be able to delineate the perfusion bed of the septal perforators and predict the infarct size that follows ethanol injection (86). A comparable technique has recently been described by Faber and colleagues using percutaneous transluminal septal myocardial ablation (PTSMA) as an alternative technique for reducing the LV outflow tract gradient. Utilizing this technique, 91 patients underwent balloon occlusion using either coronary angiography or myocardial contrast echocardiography to identify the first septal artery. After 3 months of follow-up, the NYHA class was reduced (2.8 ± 0.6 to 1.1 ± 1.0, P = <0.0001), the mitral regurgitation grade was reduced and the SAM grade improved. More striking was the reduction in the LV outflow gradient. At rest, the gradient was reduced from 73.8 ± 35.4 to 14.6 ± 25.5, while after postextrasystolic beats the gradient was reduced from 149.3 ± 42.5 to 49.1 ± 48.7 (P = <0.0001 for both). Either of the aforementioned nonsurgical techniques would be of tremendous clinical benefit if it could be definitively shown that reducing the gradient has a favorable impact on morbidity and mortality (87).

FUTURE APPLICATIONS OF IMAGING TECHNIQUES

Imaging in the Surgical Correction of Nonischemic Cardiomyopathy

In 1999, there were more than 40,000 patients that were be possible candidates for cardiac transplantation. Unfortunately, less than 10% (approximately 2,300 to 2,400) patients received cardiac transplants. This disparity is chiefly driven by the finite supply of donor organs, a supply that appears to have reached a plateau. Emblematic of this dilemma has been the emergence of alternative surgical options not only to preserve or even forestall the need for transplantation, but also to potentially eliminate the need altogether. Along with emerging surgical techniques has come the development of imaging strategies which examine their mechanisms of function. Several modalities are described below.

Left ventricular partial ventriculectomy (LVPV), formerly referred to as the Batista procedure, involves surgical resection of the myocardium to reduce LV chamber volume in order to improve wall stress and thus ventricular performance. Twenty-four patients (age 46 ± 9 years) referred for heart transplantation underwent isolated LVPV or LVPV and mitral valve annuloplasty. All patients were in NYHA class III or IV due to dilated cardiomyopathy. Functional class, left and right ventricular ejection fraction (radionuclide), left ventricular end-diastolic and end-systolic diameter, and fractional shortening (by echocardiography), as well as hemodynamic variables were determined. The mean follow-up was 474 ± 174 days. Survival at 30, 180, and 365 days was 92 ± 6%, 67 ± 10%, and 63 ± 10%, respectively.

There were 9 deaths. Reporting on the surviving group of patients, the left ventricular end-diastolic diameters at baseline were 188 ± 27 and, at 1 year, 70 ± 5.3 mm, while the left ventricular end-systolic diameters were 73.5 ± 7.4 and 55 ± 5.5 mm, respectively. Fractional shortenings were 13 ± 3% and 22 ± 2%, respectively. The left ventricular ejection fractions were 18 ± 14 and 23.7 ± 6.1%, respectively. There was an improvement in the cardiac index from a baseline of 2.11 ± 0.52 to 2.53 ± 0.64 L/min at 1-year follow-up, suggesting that the systemic pattern of CHF had improved. Norepinephrine blood levels were reduced from 702 ± 258 to 439 ± 307 pg/mL. Despite the improvement, the mortality rate in this study was 37.5% (88).

Performing the same left ventricular partial ventriculectomy, McCarthy and associates reported the results of 57 patients who were alive at 3 months. The etiology of heart failure was dilated cardiomyopathy in 95% of the patients, and all had a left ventricular end diastolic dimension of greater than 7 cm. While all of the patients in NYHA functional classes III and IV, 54 patients (95%) were awaiting heart transplantation. Fifty-five patients had simultaneous mitral valve repair (the other 2 had mitral valve replacement) and over half the patients had tricuspid valve repair. At 3 months, the investigators noted improvement in left ventricular ejection fraction as measured by echocardiography at baseline of 14.4 ± 7.7 to 23.2 ± 10.7%, left ventricular end-diastolic volume decreased from 254 ± 85 to 179 ± 73 mL, and left ventricular end-diastolic diameter decreased from 8.4 ± 1.1 to 6.3 ± 0.9 cm, (all, $P < 0.001$). In addition, peak oxygen consumption (MVO_2) increased from 10.6 ± 3.9 to 15. ± 4.5 mL/kg per min. However, the cardiac index did not change (2.2 l/min per m²). Although the authors note that 40% of the patients had been on inotropic pharmaceuticals preoperatively, none were at 3 months. NYHA functional class improved from 3.6 ± 0.5 preoperatively to 2.2 ± 0.9 at 3 months ($P < 0.001$). Left ventricle assist device (LVAD) support was required as rescue therapy in 11 patients (17%). Actuarial freedom from procedure failure, defined as death or relisting for transplant, was 58% at 1 year. In-hospital mortality was 3.5% ($n = 2$). On follow-up, there were 7 late deaths (including 3 sudden deaths), giving an extrapolated actuarial patient survival of 82% at 1 year (89).

Criticisms of this technique include an unacceptable mortality, as high as 37.5%, and the deficiency of this technique as a pure approach since the majority of the patients underwent simultaneous mitral valve replacement. However, the technique is still in evolution. More importantly, this procedure pioneered the way for more plastic approaches to caring for a very complex group of patients in whom, short of transplantation, little could be done. And, importantly, in both investigations of LVPV, the echocardiogram and radionuclear imaging were critical for the evaluation of ventricular volumes. However, little emphasis was placed on the potential mechanisms of any improvement in ventricular contractility.

Most recently, Biederman and co-workers used MRI tissue tagging to analyze a novel method of surgical LV reduction for nonischemic cardiomyopathy, the Dor procedure. Particular attention was devoted to the myocardial performance pre- and postsurgical correction. As stated above, the results of the Batista procedure have been generally disappointing. Explanations include a failure to account for *a priori* regional wall function and disregard for cardiac fiber orientation. The Dor LV reconstruction approach (endoventricular circular patch plasty) attempts to address these issues by surgically restoring the typically spherical heart to a prolate-ellipse utilizing a single apical cut and a Dacron patch insertion. MRI analysis of the first Dor procedure on nonischemic dilated cardiomyopathy in the United States was performed on a 68-year-old white male with NYHA-IV symptoms. The patient underwent MRI examination with respiratory compensation (ROPE) and cardiac gating to obtain conventional and orthogonal-tissue tagged images in standard views. While baseline echocardiography found global LV dysfunction, qualitative MRI radiofrequency (RF) tagging analysis revealed segmental abnormalities which were confirmed at surgery. EDV at baseline and at 1 month were 303 and 242 mL, respectively. At 3 months, the EDV had decreased even more to 215 mL. Similarly, ESV was initially 238 and dropped to 189 mL at 1 month; however, at 3 months, ESV had further fallen to 166 mL. Likewise, indices of sphericity and qualitative strain patterns showed improvement. MRI analysis of a condition difficult to image in any other fashion, revealed that the excluded apical wrap was initially akinetic, and that it became paradoxical at 1 month. By 3 months, however, it was only tardykinetic. Importantly, volumetric indices and strain revealed beneficial remodeling, which occurred at a time remote from the surgery. This correlated well with marked clinical improvement despite reduced SV and a stable EF. Thus, in this one patient restoration of a favorable LV geometry suggested that reconfiguration to a prolate-ellipse may be superior to simple removal of myocardium (as in the Batista procedure) (Fig. 6). Although only in 1 patient, MRI analysis suggests that the Dor reconstruction technique for *non*ischemic dilated cardiomyopathy may be another option for patients under consideration for cardiac transplantation (90).

It should be noted that imaging investigations are currently underway in patients with ischemic cardiomyopathy in several centers throughout the world. More than 750 patients with ischemic cardiomyopathy worldwide have undergone the Dor procedure with operative mortality between 1% and 3%, which is clearly better than the natural evolution of the disease. Ejection fraction, only a marginal mathematical indicator of true contractile function, is increased an average of 10% for the group postoperatively.

Another alternative to transplantation in patients with nonischemic cardiomyopathy is dynamic cardiomyoplasty (DC) using the latissimus dorsi muscle as a wrap to "girdle" the ventricle during diastole and using pacing of that muscle to augment systolic function. This technique has been variably used for approximately 10 years. A cumulative database of

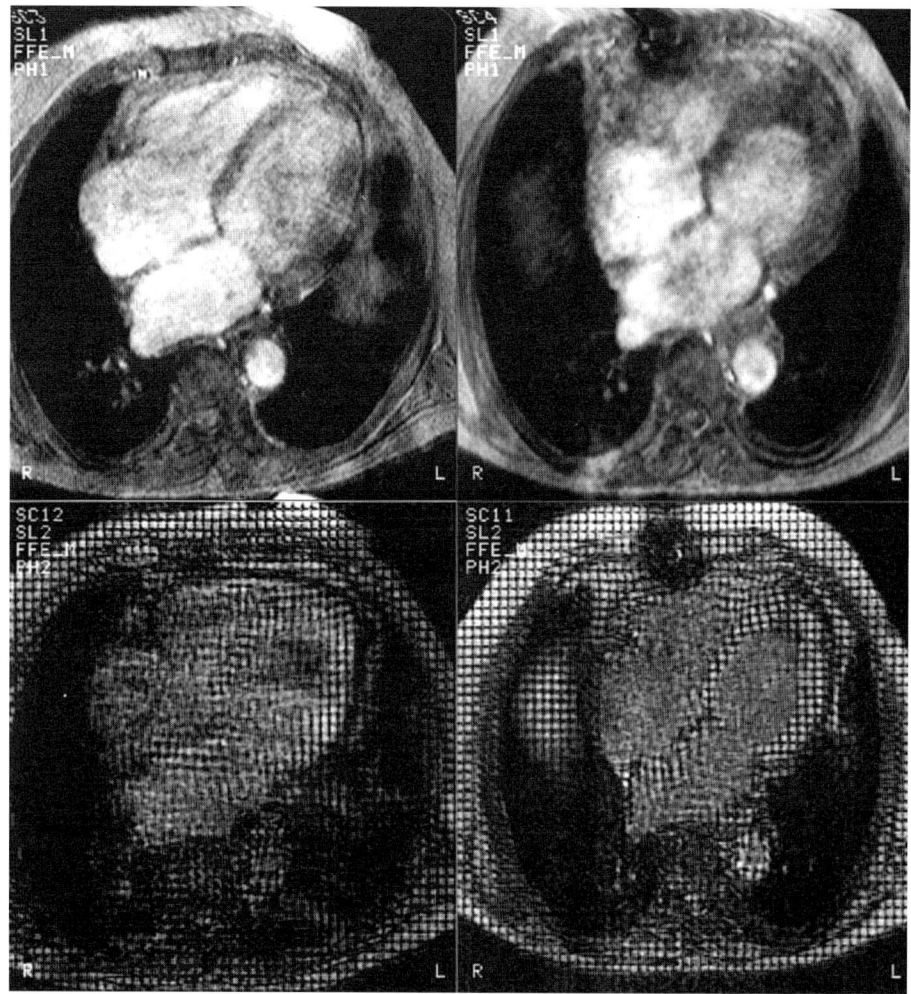

FIG. 6. A 68-year-old male with an idiopathic dilated cardiomyopathy with an end-diastolic volume (EDV) measuring 303 mL prior to the Dor procedure. Note the marked reduction in size presurgery (**A**) at 3-months postsurgery (**B**), measuring 215 mL. **C** and **D**: The two panels represent the same slice levels as **A** and **B**; however, radio-frequency tissue tagging has been employed to place a saturation grid across the myocardium in diastole. This RF pattern remains through systole, providing a definitive region of myocardium to be interrogated throughout the cardiac cycle. In this method, local intramyocardial strain (ε) can be quantitated.

preoperative patient characteristics and mortality after cardiomyoplasty has been recorded, consisting of 5-year follow-up and representing the worldwide experience of 42 medical centers. Actuarial survival ($n = 261$) was 88%, 80%, and 76% at 1, 3, and 6 months after cardiomyoplasty, respectively. Lower ejection fraction, increased number of major coronary arteries with greater than or equal to 70% stenotic lesions, and a lower chronotropic response to exercise were independent risk factors for early cardiovascular mortality. Notably, early risk of cardiovascular mortality was significantly reduced as centers gained experience with more than 3 patients (91).

More recently, sophisticated techniques have been applied to attempt to understand the mechanics of DC. Tissue imaging using Doppler ultrasound was used to assess the stimulated skeletal muscle contraction in 7 patients after left latis-

simus dorsi DC. Beat-to-beat variation in inferior wall motion was assessed by examining peak myograft velocities during 10 muscle-assisted and 10 nonassisted cardiac cycles. The temporal relationship between electrostimulation and myograft contraction, changes in cardiac geometry, and the effect of alterations in stimulation voltage and muscle synchronization were assessed. Augmentation of inferoposterior wall motion was present in 5 patients (mean peak systolic wall velocity: nonassisted, 2.5 cm/sec $\pm$ 0.5); assisted, 7.8 cm/sec $\pm$ 6.3) (92). Cardiac geometry probably maintains a more favorable chamber dimension that is thought to be due to the girdling effects of the muscle wrap (93).

In DC, the latissimus dorsi muscle is harvested on a vascular pedicle, manipulated through the rib cage, and fastened to the LV and RV. Following this manipulation, a pacemaker is connected and is stimulated. This surgical process causes an obligatory ischemic muscle with subsequent necrosis and degeneration. Harvesting the latissimus dorsi and simultaneously minimizing the ischemia is a subject of intense research and the concept of a vascular delay has emerged where the muscle is gradually harvested and slowly entrained with a pacemaker allowing for suitable vascular support to develop. In this role, MRI has been helpful in delineating the observed degeneration. Kalil Filho and associates performed MRI investigating the signal intensity of the *L. dorsi.*, compared it with the thoracic skeletal muscle, and found it to be increased. The signal intensity was similar to that of subcutaneous fat in those images outlining a noninvasive strategy to enable improved strategies for vascular harvesting (94).

Similar to the early years of cardiac transplantation, all of the alternative surgical approaches are rapidly evolving and will undoubtedly become an important strategy in the vast majority of patients who otherwise would be candidates for cardiac transplantation. Noninvasive imaging techniques will be essential to the success and clinical dissemination of these new surgical approaches.

REFERENCES

1. Devereux RB, Reichek N. Echocardiographic determination of LV mass in man: anatomic validation of the method. *Circulation* 1977;55: 613–618.
2. Liebsen PR, Devereux RB, Horan MJ. Hypertension research: echocardiography in the measurements of LV wall mass. *Hypertension* 1987; 9[Suppl II]:2.
3. Seward JB, Khandheria BK, Oh JK. Transesophageal echocardiography: technique, anatomic correlations, implementations and clinical applications. *Mayo Clin Proc* 1988;63:649–662.
4. Goldman MR, Pohost GM, Ingwall JS, et al. Nuclear magnetic resonance imaging: potential cardiac applications. *Am J Cardiol* 1980; 46(7):1278–1283.
5. Florintine MS, Grosskreutz, Chang W, et al. Measurement of left ventricular mass *in vivo* using gated nuclear magnetic resonance imaging. *J Am Coll Cardiol* 1986;8:107–109.
6. Rehr RB, Malloy CR, Filipchuk NG, et al. Left ventricular volumes measure by MR imaging. *Radiology* 1985;156:717–719.
7. Markiewitz W, Sechtem U, Kirby R, et al. Measurement of ventricular volumes in the dog by nuclear magnetic resonance imaging. *J Am Coll Cardiol* 1987;10:170–177.
8. Edelman RR, Thompson R, Kantor H. Cardiac function: evaluation with fast-echo MR imaging. *Radiology* 1987;162:611–615.
9. Cranney GB, Lotan CS, Dean L, et al. Left ventricular volume measurements using cardiac axis nuclear magnetic imaging: validation by calibrated ventricular angiography. *Circulation* 1990;82:154–163.
10. Dell'Italia LJ, Blackwell GC, Pearce WJ, et al. Assessment of ventricular volumes using cine magnetic resonance in the intact dog. A comparison of measurement methods. *Invest Radiol* 1994;2:162–166.
11. Semelka RC, Tomei E, Wagner S, et al. Interstudy reproducibility of dimension and functional measurements between cine magnetic resonance studies in the morphologically abnormal left ventricle. *Am Heart J* 1990;119:1367–1371.
12. Rich S, Sheikh A, Gallastengui J, et al. Determination of left ventricular ejection fraction by visual estimation during real-time two-dimensional echocardiography. *Am Heart J* 1982;104:603–607.
13. Folland ED, Parisi AF, Moynihan PF, et al. Assessment of left ventricular ejection fractions and volumes by real-time, two dimensional echocardiography and radionucleotides. *Circulation* 1979;60:760–765.
14. Carr KW, Engler RL, Forsythe JR, et al. Measurements of left ventricular ejection fraction by mechanical cross sectional echocardiography. *Circulation* 1979;59:1196–1199.
15. Benjelloun H, Cranney GB, Kirk KA, et al. Interstudy reproducibility

16. Dulce MC, Mostbeck GH, Friese KK. Quantification of left ventricular volumes and function with cine MR imaging: comparisons of geometric models with three-dimensional data. *Radiology* 1993;188(2):371.
17. Koren MJ, Devereux RB, Casale PN, et al. Relation of left ventricular mass and geometry to morbidity and mortality in uncomplicated essential hypertension. *Ann Int Med* 1991;114:345–352.
18. Bottini PB, Carr AA, Prisant LM, et al. Magnetic resonance imaging compared to echocardiography to assess left ventricular mass in the hypertensive patient. *Am J Hypertens* 1995;8(3):221–228.
19. Wallis DE, O'Connell JB, Henkin RE, et al. The value of echocardiographic regional wall motion abnormalities in dilated cardiomyopathies: a common finding and good prognostic sign. *J Am Coll Cardiol* 1984;4:674–670.
20. Medina R, Panidis IP, Morganroth J, et al. The value of echocardiographic regional wall motion abnormalities in detecting coronary artery disease in patients with or without a dilated left ventricle. *Circulation* 1985;109:799–803.
21. Xie GY, Berk MR, Smith MD, et al. Prognostic value of Doppler transmital flow patterns in patients with congestive heart failure. *J Am Coll Cardiol* 1994;24:132–138.
22. Werner GS, Schaefer C, Dirks R, et al. Doppler echocardiography assessment of left ventricular filling in idiopathic dilated cardiomyopathy during a one-year follow-up: relation to disease. *Am Heart J* 1993; 126:1408–1414.
23. Zile MR. Diastolic dysfunction and heart failure in hypertrophied hearts. *Congest Heart Fail* 1998;4(6):32–43.
24. Belardinelli R, Georgiou D, Cianci G, et al. Exercise training improves left ventricular diastolic filling in patients with dilated cardiomyopathy. Clinical and prognostic implications. *Circulation* 1995;91(11): 2775–2784.
25. Hock A, Freundlieb D, Vyska K. Myocardial imaging and metabolic studies with 17-123I-iodohexadecanoic acid in patients with congestive cardiomyopathy. *J Nucl Med* 1983;24:22–25.
26. Ugolini V, Hansen C, Kulkarni P. Abnormal myocardial fatty acid metabolism in dilated cardiomyopathy detected by 15-(p-[123I]-iodophenyl)-pentadecanoic acid and tomographic imaging. *Am J Cardiol* 1988;62:923–926.
27. Geltman EM, Smith JL, Beecher D, et al. Altered regional myocardial metabolism in congestive cardiomyopathy detected by positron emission tomography. *Am J Med* 1983;74:773–780.
28. Schelbert HR, Henze E, Sochor H, et al. Effects of substrate availability on myocardial C-11 palatate kinetics by positron emission tomography in normal subjects and patients with ventricular dysfunction. *Am Heart J* 1986;111:1055–1063.
29. Beanlands RS, Bach DS, Raylman R, et al. Acute effects of dobutamine on myocardial oxygen consumption and cardiac efficiency measured using carbon 11 acetate in patients with dilated cardiomyopathy. *J Am Coll Cardiol* 1993;22:1389–1394.
30. Abraham S, Fischman A, Alpert N. Regional heterogeneity of myocardial blood flow in humans with dilated cardiomyopathy. *J Nucl Med* 1994;35:23P.
31. Fujita N, Hartiala J, O'Sullivan, et al. Assessment of left ventricular diastolic function in dilated cardiomyopathy with cine magnetic resonance imaging: effect of angiotensin converting inhibitor, Benazapril. *Am Heart J* 1993;125:171–176.
32. Marcus JT, Gotte JW, DeWaal LK, et al. The influence of through-plane motion on left ventricular volumes measured by magnetic resonance imaging: implications for image acquisition and analysis. *J Cardiovasc Mag Res* 1999;(1):1–6.
33. Fujita N, Duerinex AJ, Higgins CB. Variation in left ventricular wall stress with cine magnetic resonance imaging: normal subjects versus dilated cardiomyopathy. *Am Heart J* 1993;125(5)[Pt 1]:1337–1344.
34. Buse PT, Aufferman W, Holt WW, et al. Noninvasive evaluation of global left ventricular function with the use of cine magnetic resonance. *J Am Coll Cardiol* 1989;13:1294–1298.
35. Pinamonti B, Alberti E, Cigagalotto A, et al. Echocardiographic findings in myocarditis. *Am J Cardiol* 1988;62:285–290.
36. Lambert K, Isaac D, Hendel, R. Myocarditis masquerading as ischemic heart disease: the diagnostic utility of antimyosin imaging. *Cardiology* 1993;82:415–417.
37. O'Connel, JB, Henkin RE, Robinson JA, et al. Gallium-67 imaging in

patients with dilated cardiomyopathy and biopsy proven myocarditis. *Circulation* 1984;70:58–62.

38. Friedrich MG, Strohm O, Schulz-Menger J, et al. Contrast media-enhanced magnetic resonance imaging visualizes myocardial changes in the course of viral myocarditis. *Circulation* 1998;97(18):1802–1809.

39. Yamada T, Matsumori A, Tamaki N, et al. Indium-111 antimyosin antibody imaging and thallium-201 imaging—a comparative myocardial scintigraphic study using single-photon emission computed tomography in patients with myocarditis and dilated cardiomyopathy. *Jap Circulation J* 1997;61(10):827–835.

40. Laroche-Traineau J, Clofent-Sanchez G, Daret D, et al. A human monoclonal antibody obtained from EBV-transformed B cells with specificity for myosin. *Brit J Haematol* 1995;91(4):951–962.

41. Bellotti G, Bocchi EA, de Moraes AV, et al. *In vivo* detection of Trypanosoma cruzi antigens in hearts of patients with chronic Chagas' heart disease. *Am Heart J* 1996;131(2):301–307.

42. Niitsu N, Yamazaki J, Nakayama M, et al. Usefulness of 123I-MIBG myocardial SPECT in patients with hematologic malignancies with chemotherapeutic agent-induced cardiomyopathy. *Gan To Kagaku Ryoho* [*Japanese Journal of Cancer & Chemotherapy*] 1995;22(13):1941–1945.

43. Wilansky S, Belcik T, Osborn R, et al. Hypertrophic cardiomyopathy in pregnancy. The use of two-dimensional and Doppler echocardiography during labor and delivery: a case report. *J Heart Valve Dis* 1998;7(3):355–357.

44. Guillo P, Mansourati J, Maheu B, et al. Long-term prognosis in patients with alcoholic cardiomyopathy and severe heart failure after total abstinence. *Am J Cardiol* 1997;79(9):1276–1278.

45. La Vecchia LL, Bedogni F, Bozzola L, et al. Prediction of recovery after abstinence in alcoholic cardiomyopathy: role of hemodynamic and morphometric parameters. *Clin Cardiol* 1996;19(1):45–50.

46. Prazak P, Pfisterer M, Osswald S, et al. Differences of disease progression in congestive heart failure due to alcoholic as compared to idiopathic dilated cardiomyopathy. *Eur Heart J* 1996;17(2):251–257.

47. Doni F, Kheir A, Manfredi M, et al. Alcoholic cardiomyopathy in the initial phase: the earliness of an arrhythmic substrate in relation to Doppler echocardiographic changes. *Cardiologia* 1996;41(1):69–70.

48. John RM. Is cardiac hypertrophy arrhythmogenic? *Congest Heart Fail* 1998;4(6):43–48.

49. Peters. *Circulation* 1998.

50. Lipshultz SE, Easley KA, Orav EJ, et al. Left ventricular structure and function in children infected with human immunodeficiency virus: the prospective P2C2 HIV Multicenter Study. Pediatric Pulmonary and Cardiac Complications of Vertically Transmitted HIV Infection (P2C2 HIV) Study Group. *Circulation* 1998;97(13):1246–1256.

51. Lipshultz SE. Dilated cardiomyopathy in HIV-infected patients [editorial]. *New Eng J Med* 1998;339(16):1153–1155.

52. Herskowitz A. Cardiomyopathy and other symptomatic heart diseases associated with HIV infection. *Curr Opin Cardiol* 1996;11(3):325–331.

53. Epstein JE, Eichbaum QG, Lipshultz SE. Cardiovascular manifestations of HIV infection. *Comp Ther* 1996;22(8):485–491.

54. Hakim JG, Matenga JA, Siziya S. Myocardial dysfunction in human immunodeficiency virus infection: an echocardiographic study of 157 patients in hospital in Zimbabwe. *Heart* 1996;76(2):161–165.

55. Midiri M, Finazzo M, Brancato M, et al. Arrhythmogenic right ventricular dysplasia: MR. *Eur Radiol* 1997;7(3):307–312.

56. Takahashi N, Ishida Y, Maeno M, et al. Noninvasive identification of left ventricular involvements in right ventricular dysplasia: comparison of 123I-MIBG, 201TlCl, resonance imaging and ultrafast computed tomography. *Ann Nucl Med* 1997;11(3):233–241.

57. Rampazzo A, Nava A, Miorin M, et al. ARVD4, a new locus for arrhythmogenic right ventricular cardiomyopathy, maps to chromosome 2 long arm. *Genomics* 1997;45(2):259–263.

58. Oshima M, Higashi S, Kikuchi Y, et al. Autoradiographic study of myocardial fatty acid metabolism in diabetic mouse using 125I-BMIPP. *Nippon Igaku Hoshasen Gakkai Zasshi* [*Nippon Acta Radiologica*] 1996;56(3):137–138.

59. Shimonagata T, Nanto S, Hori M, et al. A case of hypertensive-diabetic cardiomyopathy demonstrating left ventricular wall motion abnormality. *Diabet Care* 1996;19(8):887–891.

60. Morguet AJ, Sandrock D, Stille-Siegener M, et al. *J Nucl Med* 1995;36(8):1432–1435.

61. Gaal J, Hegedus I, Devenyi K, et al. Myocardial gallium-67 citrate

scintigraphy in patients with systemic sclerosis. *Ann Rheum Dis* 1995;54(10):856–858.

62. Ferri C, Di Bello V, Martini A, et al. Heart involvement in systemic sclerosis: an ultrasonic tissue characterisation study. *Ann Rheum Dis* 1998;57(5):296–302.

63. Chandra M, Silverman ME, Oshinski J, et al. Diagnosis of cardiac sarcoid aided by MRI. *Chest* 1996;110:562–565.

64. Kinney EL, Jackson GL, Reeves WC. Thallium-scan myocardial defects and echocardiographic abnormalities in patients without clinical cardiac dysfunction. *Am J Med* 1980;68:497–503.

65. Okayama K, Kurata C, Tuwarahara K. Diagnostic and prognostic value of myocardial scintigraphy with thallium-201 and gallium-67 in cardiac sarcoidosis. *Chest* 1995;107:330–334.

66. Neubauer S, Horn M, Cramer M, et al. Myocardial phosphocreatine-to-ATP ratio is a predictor of mortality in patients with dilated cardiomyopathy. *Circulation* 1997;96(7):2190–2196.

67. Narita M, Kurihara T. Evaluation of long-term prognosis in patients with heart failure: is cardiac imaging with iodine-123 metaiodobenzylguanidine useful? *J Cardiol* 1998;31(6):343–349.

68. Melacini P, Fanin M, Danieli GA, et al. Myocardial involvement is very frequent among patients affected with subclinical Becker's muscular dystrophy. *Circulation* 1996;94(12):3168–3175.

69. Miyoshi K, Fujikawa K. Comparison of thaliu-201 myocardial single-photon emission computed tomography and cine magnetic resonance imaging in Duschenne's muscular dystrophy. *Am J Cardiol* 1995;75(17):1284–1286.

70. Fabrizi GM, Lodi R, D'Ettorre M, et al. Autosomal dominant limb girdle myopathy with ragged-red fibers and cardiomyopathy. A pedigree study by *in vivo* 31P-MR spectroscopy indicating a multisystem mitochondrial defect. *J Neuro Science* 1996;137(1):20–27.

71. Oki T, Tabata T, Yamada H, et al. Difference in systolic motion velocity of the left ventricular posterior wall in patients with asymmetric septal hypertrophy and prior anteroseptal myocardial infarction. Evaluation by pulsed tissue Doppler imaging. *Jap Heart J* 1998;39(2):163–172.

72. Wigle ED, Sasson Z, Henderson MA. Hypertrophic cardiomyopathy. The importance of site and the extent of hypertrophy. *Prog Cardiovasc Dis* 1985;28:1–5.

73. Pons-Llado G, Carreras F, Borras X, et al. Comparison of morphological assessment of hypertrophic cardiomyopathy by magnetic resonance versus echocardiography imaging. *Am J Cardiol* 1997;79(12):1651–1656.

74. Kaul S, Tei C, Shah PM. Interventricular and free wall dynamics in hypertrophic cardiomyopathy. *J Am Coll Cardiol* 1983;1:1024–1029.

75. Nakatami S, White RD, Powell K, et al. Dynamic magnetic resonance imaging assessment of the effect of ventricular wall curvature on regional function in hypertrophic cardiomyopathy. *Am J Cardiol* 1996;77(8):618–622.

76. Young AA, Kramer CM, Ferrari VA, et al. Three-dimensional left ventricular deformation in hypertrophic cardiomyopathy. *Circulation* 1994;90:854–867.

77. Pollick C, Rakowoski H, Wigle ED. Muscular subaortic stenosis: the quantitative relationship between anterior systolic motion and the pressure gradient. *Circulation* 1984;69:43–48.

78. Nishimura R, Tajik AJ, Reeder GS. Evaluation of hypertrophic cardiomyopathy by Doppler color flow imaging: initial observations. *Mayo Clin Proc* 1986;61:631–635.

79. Fujita N, Chazouillers AF, Hartialla JJ. Quantification of mitral regurgitation by velocity encoding cine nuclear magnetic resonance imaging. *J Am Coll Cardiol* 1994;23:951–952.

80. Hada Y, Itoh N, Asakawa M, et al. Left ventricular wall motion dynamics of asymmetric septal hypertrophy: assessment by intramyocardial pulsed Doppler echocardiography. *J Cardiol* 1998;31(6):351–360.

81. Crowley JJ, Dardas PS, Shapiro LM. Assessment of apical hypertrophic cardiomyopathy using transoesophageal echocardiography. *Cardiology* 1997;88(2):189–196.

82. Sato T, Yamanari H, Ohe T, et al. Regional left ventricular contractile dynamics in hypertrophic cardiomyopathy evaluated by magnetic resonance imaging. *Heart Vessels* 1996;11(5):248–254.

83. Sieverding L, Jung WI, Breuer J, et al. Proton-decoupled myocardial 31P NMR spectroscopy reveals decreased PCr/Pi in patients with severe hypertrophic cardiomyopathy. *Am J Cardiol* 1997;80(3A):34A–40A.

84. Sieverding L, Jung WI, Breuer J, et al. Proton-decoupled myocardial 31P NMR spectroscopy reveals decreased PCr/Pi in patients with se-

vere hypertrophic cardiomyopathy. *Am J Cardiol* 1997;80(3A): 34A–40A.
85. Pohost GM, Vignola PA, McKusick KE, et al. Hypertrophic cardiomyopathy. Evaluation by gated cardiac blood pool scanning. *Circulation* 1977;55(1):92–99.
86. Nagueh SF, Lakkis NM, He ZX, et al. Role of myocardial contrast echocardiography during nonsurgical septal reduction therapy for hypertrophic obstructive cardiomyopathy. *J Am Coll Cardiol* 1998;32(1): 225–229.
87. Faber L, Seggewiss H, Gleichmanm U. Percutaneous transluminal septal myocardial ablation in hypertrophic obstructive cardiomyopathy. Results with respect to intraprocedural myocardial contrast echocardiography. *Circulation* 1998;98:2415–2421.
88. Bocchi EA, Bellotti G, Vilella de Moraes A, et al. Clinical outcome after left ventricular surgical remodeling in patients with idiopathic dilated cardiomyopathy referred for heart transplantation: short-term results. *Circulation* 1997;96[Suppl 9]:II-165–167.
89. McCarthy JF, McCarthy PM, Starling RC, et al. Partial left ventriculectomy and mitral valve repair for end-stage congestive heart failure. *Eur J Card-Thor, Surg* 1998;13(4):337–343.
90. Biederman RWW, Doyle M, Fuisz AR, et al. MRI analysis of the Dor left ventricular surgical reconstruction for non-ischemic dilated cardiomyopathy. *J Cardiovasc Mag Res* 1999;(1)[Suppl]:A27.
91. Rector TS, Benditt D, Chachques JC, et al. Retrospective risk analysis for early heart-related death after cardiomyoplasty. The Worldwide Cardiomyoplasty Group. *J Heart Lung Transplant* 1997;16(10): 1018–1025.
92. Grubb NR, Sutherland GR, Campanella C, et al. Latissimus dorsi muscle: assessment of stimulation after cardiomyoplasty with Doppler US tissue imaging. *Radiololgy* 1996;199(1):59–64.
93. Thornton BS, Hung WT. Dynamic stiffness and implications for assisting the operation of the left ventricle. *IMA J Math Appl Med Biol* 1996; 13(4):275–295.
94. Kalil Filho R, Bocchi E, Rosemberg L, et al. Evaluation of chronic morphological changes in the latissimus dorsi, after cardiomyoplasty, with magnetic resonance. *Arquiv Brasild Cardiol* 1995;65(3):221–225.
95. Nanda NC, Domansky MJ, eds. *Atlas of transesophageal echocardiography*. Baltimore: Williams & Wilkins, 1998.
96. Dubosovsy. Ga-67 and TI-201 imaging in sarcoidosis involving the myocardium. *Clin Nucl Med* 1981;6(3):120–121.

CHAPTER 47

Hypertrophic Cardiomyopathy

Pravin M. Shah and Robert W. W. Biederman

DEFINITION OF HYPERTROPHIC CARDIOMYOPATHY

Hypertrophic cardiomyopathy has been defined as cardiac hypertrophy of unknown etiology. This may be further characterized as inappropriate, often asymmetric hypertrophy with hyperdynamic systolic function and impaired diastolic function. It may co-exist with conditions known to be associated with ventricular hypertrophy such as hypertension and aortic stenosis; however, its extent and distribution are inappropriate to the underlying cause. The condition is commonly heredofamilial, although sporadic cases are not rare (1–3).

CLASSIFICATION

One classification scheme is based on the distribution of hypertrophy, namely, concentric and asymmetric. Asymmetric includes the following: (i) Septal: the interventricular septum is the more common site of pronounced asymmetric hypertrophy. (ii) Free wall: some patients with a more pronounced free wall hypertrophy have been described. (iii) Apical: the apical asymmetric hypertrophy is less common, but is often mistaken for coronary artery disease due to deeply inverted T-waves across the precordium.

A second classification scheme is based on the hemodynamics of intraventricular obstruction and includes the following: (i) obstructive: resting state and on provocation and (ii) nonobstructive.

Obstructive cases commonly involve the left ventricular

outflow tract. Infrequently, midventricular obstruction or right ventricular infundibular obstruction may be present with or without left ventricular outflow gradient.

It may be stressed that the original term idiopathic hypertrophic subaortic stenosis or IHSS (1) may apply only to cases with left ventricular obstruction. It is more appropriate to use the more generic term *hypertrophic cardiomyopathy*.

DIAGNOSTIC IMAGING

Echocardiography

Echocardiography is ideally suited to assess the structural and functional changes associated with hypertrophic cardiomyopathy (4–7).

Left Ventricle

The distribution of hypertrophy, whether concentric or asymmetric, can be evaluated by multiple cross sections. The asymmetric variety exhibits more advanced hypertrophy in one segment than others. The most common site of pronounced hypertrophy involves the upper one third to one half of the interventricular septum. Less commonly, free wall segments show the more pronounced hypertrophy. Generally, the posterobasal segment adjacent to the posterior mitral annulus maintains normal thickness or is least affected in hypertrophy. An uncommon form consists of predominant involvement of the apex, also termed apical asymmetric hypertrophy (AAH). This is often associated with deeply inverted T waves (8–9). The apical asymmetric hypertrophy (AAH) seen in Japan (so-called Japanese variety) is associated with normal thickness of the basal segments, whereas that seen in North America and Europe is generally associated with some basal wall hypertrophy. The ventricular walls often have a sparkling appearance. The left ventricular cavity dimensions are normal or small. There is endocardial thickening often seen in the upper interventricular septum and is

P. M. Shah: Loma Linda University School of Medicine, Loma Linda, California 92350; Noninvasive Cardiac Imaging and Academic Programs, Hoag Memorial Hospital Presbyterian, Newport Beach, California 92663.

R. W. W. Biederman: Department of Cardiovascular Disease, Center for Nuclear Magnetic Resonance Research and Development; Department of Medicine, University of Alabama at Birmingham, Birmingham, Alabama 35223.

thought to result from repeated contacts with the anterior mitral leaflet.

Right Ventricle

Although some degree of right ventricular hypertrophy is commonly seen in most cases, its distribution in the right ventricular infundibulum may be more pronounced in some, which provides an anatomic basis for infundibular obstruction.

Left Atrium

Dilatation of the left atrium is frequently noted and is generally mild. More severe dilatation may be present in long-standing cases with diastolic dysfunction and in the obstructive type with mitral regurgitation. Similarly, those with an independent mechanism of mitral regurgitation may have disproportionately dilated atrium.

The Valves

Characteristically, the anterior mitral leaflet is often thickened. It is shown to be elongated in many cases. Occasionally, the posterior leaflet may also be elongated. The systolic anterior motion of the mitral valve commonly involves the anterior mitral leaflet, occasionally the posterior mitral leaflet, and sometimes both participate together. The extent of systolic anterior motion (SAM) is variable, and, in more severe obstructive cases, it contacts the interventricular septum at or near the site of echo dense area of endocardial thickening (4). Occasionally, mitral valve prolapse may co-exist. Calcification of the mitral annulus is commonly observed in middle-aged and elderly subjects.

FUNCTIONAL OR HEMODYNAMIC CHANGES

Concerning systolic function, left ventricular ejection fraction is almost always increased, often resulting in near cavity obliteration. The rate of ejection is rapid, giving rise to the characteristic jerky upstroke to the carotid arterial pulse (10). In late stages, deterioration of function with depression of left ventricular (LV) ejection fraction may develop in rare cases and may resemble dilated cardiomyopathy or end-stage hypertensive heart disease.

With regard to diastolic function, nearly all cases exhibit some diastolic dysfunction, which in early cases consist of impaired relaxation with reversal of mitral inflow E/A ratio. The mitral inflow velocity E-wave deceleration time is characteristically prolonged, although hyperadrenergic type state of the myocardium may result in a shorter deceleration time. Similarly, mitral regurgitation may also influence the mitral Doppler wave form, resulting in a shorter deceleration time in presence of significant mitral regurgitation.

Pulmonary venous Doppler flow wave form typically shows a prominent prolonged A_r (atrial reversal) wave.

When A_r is longer in duration than mitral inflow A wave, the LV end diastolic pressure is nearly always elevated. This phenomenon reflects resistance to filling during atrial contraction in late diastole, resulting in longer reversal of flow in pulmonary veins.

With regard to intraventricular gradients, systolic intraventricular gradients are often observed and may be present at one of four sites (11): (i) LV outflow tract: This results in left ventricular outflow tract (LVOT) obstruction or muscular subaortic stenosis. (ii) Cavity obliteration: This results from rapid emptying of the left ventricular cavity responsible for transient intracavity high pressures and late systolic pressure gradients. Cavity obliteration may co-exist with outflow obstruction. (iii) Midventricle: Hypertrophy at a midpapillary muscle site results in midsystolic apposition of the ventricular walls separating an apical cavity from basal portion. The midventricular obstruction is uncommon and is generally not associated with evidence of outflow obstruction. (iv) Right ventricular infundibulum: The infundibular obstruction is purely muscular and dynamic, resembling congenital infundibular pulmonic stenosis. This is, however, associated with left ventricular hypertrophy in addition to right ventricular hypertrophy.

LVOT Obstruction or Muscular Subaortic Stenosis

Most obstructive cases have gradients across the LVOT, resulting in dynamic and variable outflow obstruction. This functional characteristic was responsible for the earlier name of the disease, idiopathic hypertrophic subaortic stenosis, or IHSS. The echo Doppler features are characteristic and consist of most if not all of the following features:

1. SAM or systolic anterior motion of the mitral valve
2. Narrowed LV outflow tract
3. Aortic valve preclosure
4. Pulsed-wave Doppler: high velocity aliased signal in LVOT
5. Color flow imaging: turbulence in LV outflow tract and mitral regurgitation
6. Continuous-wave Doppler: a dagger-shaped high velocity signal in LV outflow tract associated with outflow obstruction
7. Holosystolic signal of mitral regurgitation, which peaks in late systole

Systolic Anterior Motion

The systolic anterior motion (SAM) commonly involves the anterior mitral leaflet, or it may involve both leaflets but only rarely the posterior mitral leaflet. The conditions required for development of SAM include elongation of anterior and/or posterior leaflets, early systolic coaptation occurring at the midportion of the leaflet, leaving a residual portion of one or both leaflets in the left ventricle, hyperdynamic left ventricle, and a narrow outflow tract (12). There

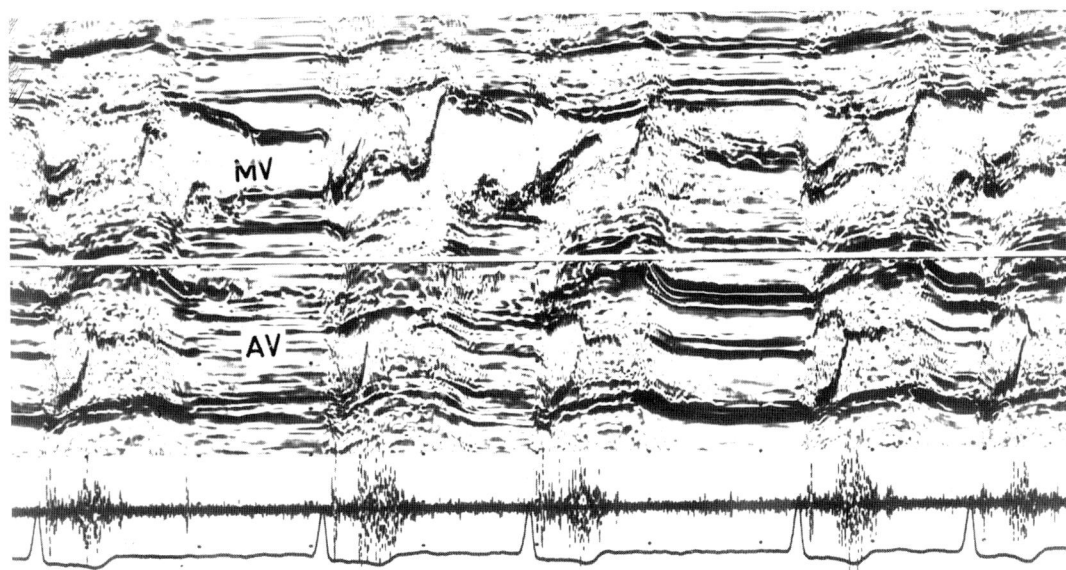

FIG. 1. Dual M-mode echocardiogram from the mitral valve (*MV*) and the aortic valve (*AV*) are shown along with phonocardiogram tracing and electrocardiogram showing atrial fibrillation lead. Note the varying extent of systolic anterior motion (SAM) in different beats along with varying intensity of the systolic murmur with changing cycle lengths. The aortic valve shows midsystolic preclosure. Note that the second and the fourth beats show more prominent SAM with earlier aortic valve preclosure and earlier onset and more intense murmurs.

is some suggestion that anterior displacement of the mitral apparatus may be a factor in some cases. The residual mitral leaflet appears to be sucked into the LV outflow tract by venturi-like forces following early rapid ejection. Thus, the SAM is initiated after onset of ejection and results in contact with the LV outflow tract and retreats at end of ejection. This progressive malcoaptation resulting from SAM results in increasing mitral incompetence in mid- and late systole. The leaflet-septal contact area marks the location of outflow obstruction (Fig. 1).

Narrowed Left Ventricular Outflow Tract

Narrowed left ventricular outflow tract occurs as a result of massive hypertrophy of interventricular septum. The distribution of septal hypertrophy is variable, but is often maximal at about 2 cm below the aortic annulus, where the thickness may exceed 20 mm. Some patients, however, exhibit marked thickness in the upper septum at the level of the aortic annulus.

Aortic Valve Preclosure

Aortic valve preclosure was described in the early M-mode literature and consists of midsystolic closing motion of one or more cusps followed by reopening in late systole. The cusp motion may reflect changes in flow rate across the outflow tract and/or the venturi forces playing a significant role.

Pulsed-wave Doppler

Pulsed-wave Doppler helps to localize the site of obstruction. On moving the sample volume from the left ventricular apex gradually toward and into the LV outflow tract, a sudden increase in peak systolic velocity is observed at the site of the SAM-septal contact and complex aliasing is observed into the outflow tract. This clearly localizes the site of increased velocity (i.e., increased gradient) and hence obstruction.

Color Flow Imaging

Color flow imaging provides a visual assessment of the increase in velocity by color reversal as flow approaches the site of SAM-septal contact and turbulence in the outflow tract timed after development of SAM. The mitral regurgitation is seen as progressive jet increasing after onset of SAM (Fig. 2). The extent of mitral regurgitation is dependent on the presence and severity of outflow obstruction. An independent etiology of mitral regurgitation may co-exist in a small minority of patients.

Continuous-wave Doppler

Continuous-wave Doppler provides two distinct jet profiles, one originating in the LV outflow and one across the mitral valve (Fig. 3). The LV outflow profile has a characteristic dagger shape, with early rapid increase in velocity after onset of ejection, reaching up to 2 m/sec. The velocity profile

Rapid, complete emptying is demonstrated by two-dimensional echo with near opposition of all the ventricular walls including the apex in midsystole. This translates into ejection fraction being 85 to 90%.

Pulsed Doppler in LV outflow tract may show higher velocity of rapid ejection, but without complex aliasing.

Color flow Doppler does not show turbulence in the outflow tract, but may show simple aliasing due to higher velocity.

Continuous-wave Doppler has a characteristic profile, consisting of a dagger shape with its "blade," or portion of increased velocity, being narrow. Thus, an initial increase in outflow velocity representing increased flow rate may reach up to 2.0 m/sec; and the subsequent increase representing intraventricular gradient occurs in late systole. Typically, the late peak occupies less than 40% of the ejection time. This is in striking contrast to the LV outflow obstruction, in which the gradient occupies a larger portion of ejection. Despite these criteria, a distinction may be difficult in presence of tachycardia, and other features of outflow obstruction such as leaflet SAM should be sought.

The phenomenon of cavity obliteration may co-exist with LV outflow obstruction, and in these patients all the features including continuous-wave Doppler profile of outflow obstruction will predominate.

Midventricular Obstruction

A small subset of patients exhibits midventricular obstruction, which should be differentiated from cavity obliteration. The following echo Doppler features permit accurate evaluation.

Two-dimensional echo shows opposition of the left ventricular walls at the level of papillary muscles noted in midsystole. This results in a distinct and separate apical cavity, and the apex is often thin and akinetic. The basal left ventricular cavity is of normal dimension and no SAM is observed.

Pulsed Doppler shows an early systolic velocity peak and a second late systolic or early diastolic flow peak from apex to the base.

Continuous-wave Doppler profile obtained from the apex may resemble a dagger shape similar to that described for the LV outflow obstruction. However, the midsystolic portion of the Doppler signal is often interrupted due to left ventricular wall opposition interfering with the continuous-wave Doppler signal from the apex.

Right Ventricular Outflow Obstruction

The right ventricular (RV) outflow composed of the infundibulum is surrounded circumferentially by muscle fibers. Thus, the RV outflow obstruction resembles congenital infundibular pulmonary stenosis, albeit associated with generalized hypertrophy of both ventricles. The echo Doppler features of RV outflow obstruction consist of the following.

1. RV infundibulum is hypertrophied and empties in midsystole from hypercontraction of the muscle fibers. This is best appreciated by transthoracic echo in parasternal short-axis view or by transesophageal echo in the vertical- (90 degrees) or long-axis planes (approximately 135 degrees).
2. Pulsed-wave Doppler shows complex aliasing in pulmonary outflow tract.
3. Color flow imaging demonstrates systolic turbulence in the pulmonary artery.
4. Continuous-wave Doppler exhibits a dagger-shaped profile that resembles that observed with the LVOT obstruction described above. This is best obtained from second or third left interspace aligning the Doppler signal to pulmonary outflow. The peak velocity accurately reflects the magnitude of RV outflow obstruction and may be estimated using the simplified Bernoulli equation (pressure gradient $= 4V^2$).
5. Tricuspid regurgitation (TR) signal when present shows increased velocity consistent with elevation in right ventricular systolic pressure. This should not be misinterpreted to indicate pulmonary hypertension. The TR velocity in concert with the right ventricular outtract velocity could help determine pulmonary arterial systolic pressure. Thus,

$$RV\ Systolic\ Pressure = 4V^2_{TR} + RA\ pressure$$
$$= 4V^2_{TR}$$
$$+ 10\ mm\ Hg\ (assumed\ RA\ pressure)$$

$$PA\ Systolic\ Pressure = RV\ Systolic\ Pressure$$
$$- RV\ outflow\ gradient$$
$$= [4V^2_{TR} + 10] - 4V^2R_{VO}$$

where V_{TR} is the tricuspid regurgitation velocity and V_{RVO} is the peak right ventricular outflow velocity.

ROLE IN INTRAOPERATIVE ASSESSMENT

Transesophageal echo (TEE) plays a key role in assisting an adequate surgical myectomy, while avoiding complication of iatrogenic ventricular septal defect. The results of myectomy may be immediately assessed intraoperatively as the patient is weaned off cardiopulmonary bypass. See Chapter 4.

ROLE IN CHEMICAL MYECTOMY

It has been proposed that chemical myectomy performed by injection of ethanol in the septal branch of the left anterior descending coronary artery results in a focal infarction of the upper LV septum, enlarging the LV outflow tract and thus providing a relief of outflow obstruction. This is at present an experimental procedure with significant morbidity and only about an 80% chance of success. In addition to providing accurate measurements of the outflow gradients, injection of ultrasonic contrast in the septal branch prior to injection of ethanol defines the specific segment to become infarcted (15). The septal distribution is variable among individuals, and, in some patients, the first septal may be the appropriate vessel, and in others, it may be the second septal branch. The immediate results can be confirmed; however, in some patients, a further drop in gradients is to be expected as progressive thinning of the LV septum takes place.

MAGNETIC RESONANCE IMAGING IN HYPERTROPHIC CARDIOMYOPATHY

The intrinsically three-dimensional imaging and spatial resolution provided by cardiac magnetic resonance imaging (MRI) affords a novel and robust means to interrogate the structure, physiology, and metabolism of hypertrophic cardiomyopathy.

While most aspects of hypertrophic cardiomyopathy are well delineated by two-dimensional and M-mode echocardiography, its limitations are related to the partial volume errors that are associated with an intrinsically one- or two-dimensional approach. Such errors tend to overestimate wall thickness due to nonperpendicular interrogation. MRI minimizes such partial volume errors and should provide a more reliable wall thickness estimate. Image acquisition is not dependant on finding a proper ''window'' nor is it limited by body habitus. These concepts were strengthened by Pons-Llado (16) and associates in a simultaneous evaluation of echocardiography and MRI in 30 patients with hypertrophic cardiomyopathy. Measuring wall thickness in predesignated LV segments, in addition to assessing the number of segments where LV wall thickness was greater than 15mm, these investigators found that echocardiography detected 221 of 330 total segments (67%), whereas MRI detected 320 (97%) segments. Interestingly, the authors noted that the degree of hypertrophy did not correlate with presence of an obstructive pattern or with the presence of diastolic dysfunction by Doppler.

The imaging of the left ventricular regional wall motion has generated some controversy concerning patients with hypertrophic cardiomyopathy. Several echocardiographic studies have indicated that the interventricular septum is usually severely hypokinetic as compared to the LV posterior and free walls. However, MRI reveals that septal motion is more complex. Nakatami and colleagues (17) evaluated the radius of curvature and the circumferential strain in the interventricular septum of patients with hypertrophic cardiomyopathy using MRI tissue tagging. Understanding that Laplacian analysis would indicate that a flattened septum would likely predict an overestimate of myocardial stress, the authors were able to show that the flattened septum corre-

lated with reduced circumferential shortening. In a further analysis, using multiple step-wise linear regression(s), these investigators found that both short- and long-axis curvatures significantly contributed to total endocardium circumferential shortening ($r = 0.87$, $P < 0.0001$). They hypothesized that the decreased septal deformation, as compared to the posterior wall, may be partly explained by the short- and long-axis curvatures being significantly flatter (in some instances a catenoid shape) (17). The author recognized that Laplacian stress analysis is imprecise for a thick-walled sphere with a uniform radius. Nevertheless, these assumptions appear geometrically valid and have been reproduced by other investigators.

MRI can easily assess traditional hypertrophic cardiomyopathy; however, the apical variant of hypertrophic cardiomyopathy found most frequently in Japanese literature may be difficult to diagnose using standard transthoracic echocardiography because of inconsistent imaging of the apical segment. Furthermore, the distribution of hypertrophy may be inappropriately assigned and abnormalities in wall thickening underestimated. Additionally, cine MRI has been found to be sensitive and specific to the location and pattern of mitral regurgitation with HCM (18). Finally, this lesion, in particular, is well assessed noninvasively by MRI and probably should be the imaging technique of choice (Fig. 5).

One of the more attractive features of MRI is its specific ability to evaluate LV function. In view of its increased spatial and temporal resolution with low signal-to-noise ratios, regional myocardial function can be easily, accurately, and reproducibly accomplished. As an example of this concept, Sato and associates examined systolic wall thickening (%WT) and percent change of segmental wall area (%SAR) by cine magnetic resonance imaging in 40 patients with hypertrophic cardiomyopathy (HCM) and 23 volunteers. The short-axis images of the LV in the normals were recorded at both base and apex and were divided into five segments. While apical %WT and %SAR segments in the control group were markedly increased as compared to the basal segments, the majority of the patients with HCM had reduced %WT and %SAR in proportion to the degree of hypertrophy. Importantly, the areas of least hypertrophy in the HCM patients had normal or even supernormal function. This has led to the concept of a possible compensatory mechanism for the dysfunctional myocardium to preserve otherwise remotely depressed regional contractile function (19).

In one of the earliest clinical uses for MRI tissue tagging, Young and co-workers (20) used finite element analysis in patients with HCM. Three-dimensional reconstruction was performed to measure circumferential, radial, and meriodonal strain. Young noted that radial strain was only mildly depressed, whereas meriodonal shortening was markedly depressed in these patients. Circumferential strains were reduced chiefly in the septum. Interestingly, torsion was enhanced in HCM patient hearts, which were, again, the most likely to compensate for the regions of reduced contractile dysfunction.

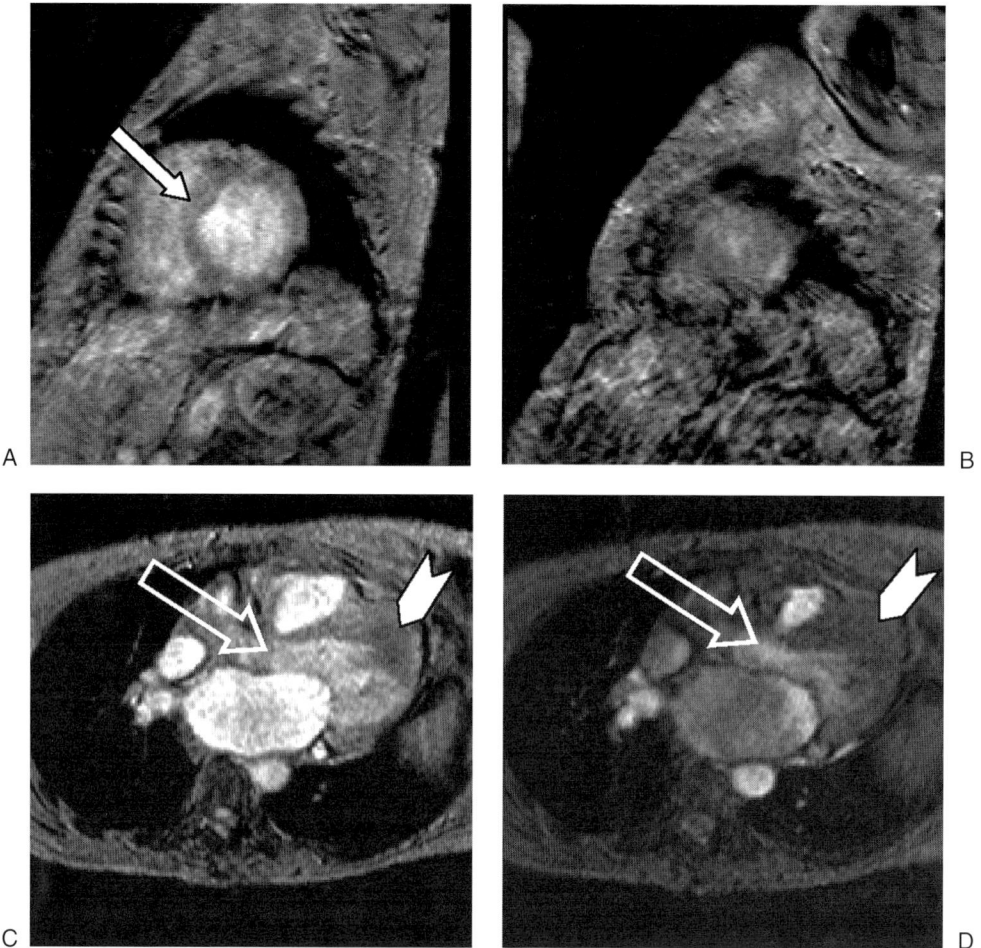

FIG. 5. Cardiac MRI depicting a 64-year-old white female North American patient with the apical variant of hypertrophic cardiomyopathy (HCM) presenting with dyspnea and chronic atrial fibrillation. The images were obtained using a gradient echo (bright blood) sequence. The top two panels represent a short-axis acquisition at the mid-left ventricle (LV) (**A**) and apex (**B**). Careful inspection reveals the miniscule apical cavity (**B**). The bottom two panels represent axial LV views with the outflow tract and apical myocardium seen in diastole (**C**) and systole (**D**). There is no outflow tract narrowing seen to initiate further investigation for possible HCM (*open arrows*). The apical LV chamber is almost entirely occupied by myocardium (*chevrons*). Note the absence of significant basal or midseptal hypertrophy (*solid arrows*) leading to the mischaracterization of this patient on earlier echocardiographic evaluations.

Nuclear magnetic resonance spectroscopy (NMR) has been used to probe the metabolic properties of the left ventricular myocardium. Phosphorus-31 (P^{31}) has been extensively used for NMR spectroscopy. Disturbed myocardial energy metabolism may occur in patients with hypertrophic cardiomyopathy. To obtain a noninvasive window into cardiac energy metabolism, 13 patients with HCM underwent spectroscopic imaging using a 1.5 T system with a double-resonant surface coil. A two-dimensional sequence in combination with slice selective excitation was used to acquire spectra of the anteroseptal region of the left ventricle. Peak areas of 2,3-diphosphoglycerol (DPG), inorganic phosphate (Pi), and adenosine triphosphate (ATP) were determined. Determining phosphocreatine (PCR)/gamma-ATP ratio or pHi yielded no difference between patients with severe HCM and those with moderate HCM. However, the PCR/Pi ratio of those with HCM differed significantly from control (n = 16). The underlying metabolic abnormality was probably mediated by ischemia related to the decreased oxygen supply in the severely hypertrophied myocardium (21). Using a variation of this technique, decreased PCR/Pi has been shown in patients with advanced hypertrophic cardiomyopathy (21). However, the ability to identify inorganic phosphate at 1.5 T (the highest field available for clinical practice) is limited. Accordingly, PCr/ATP is a more readily refined parameter at 1.5T. At higher fields, PCr/pH is more easily evaluated and appears more precise for identifying abnormal energy metabolism.

Radiofrequency tagging techniques and spectroscopy are currently in their investigative phase. It is likely that they will further enhance our ability to understand this pathological state and more appropriately intervene on its natural history.

CONCLUSION

Echocardiography has emerged as a noninvasive technique that provides an accurate diagnosis as well as hemodynamic profile in a patient suspected with hypertrophic cardiomyopathy. Indeed, the echocardiographic characterizations of left ventricular outflow obstruction and of left ventricular cavity obliteration have settled the disputes among experts about relevance of intraventricular gradients based on cardiac catheterization and angiographic studies. In subjects with suboptimal echo images by transthoracic echo, transesophageal approach is useful to provide evidence of hypertrophy and its distribution, of left ventricular outflow tract dimensions and flow dynamics, as well as function of the mitral valve. Magnetic resonance methods are a promising addition to echocardiography for diagnostic and post-therapeutic evaluation. Specifically, MR methods should be considered when there is uncertainty as to the extent of the hypertrophic process and when the apical variant is suspected.

REFERENCES

1. Braunwald E, Morrow AG, Cornell WP, et al. Idiopathic hypertrophic subaortic stenosis. *Am J Med* 1960;29:924–945.
2. Goodwin JF, Hollman A, Cleland WP, et al. Obstructive cardiomyopathy simulating aortic stenosis. *Br Heart J* 1960;22:403–414.
3. Wigle ED, Heimbecker RO, Gunton RW. Idiopathic ventricular septal hypertrophy causing muscular subaortic stenosis. *Circulation* 1962;26:325–340.
4. Shah P, Gramiak R, Kramer D. Ultrasound localization of left ventricular outflow obstruction in hypertrophic obstructive cardiomyopathy. *Circulation* 1969;40:3–11.
5. Popp R, Harrison D. Ultrasound in the diagnosis and evaluation of therapy of idiopathic hypertrophic subaortic stenosis. *Circulation* 1969;40:905–914.
6. Shah PM, Gramiak R, Adelman AG, et al. Role of echocardiography in diagnostic and hemodynamic assessment of hypertrophic subaortic stenosis. *Circulation* 1971;44:891–898.
7. Shah P, Gramiak R, Adelman A, et al. Echocardiographic assessment of the effects of surgery and propranolol on the dynamics of outflow obstruction in hypertrophic subaortic stenosis. *Circulation* 1972;45:516–521.
8. Sakamoto T, Tei C, Murayama M, et al. Giant negative T-wave inversion as a manifestation of asymmetric apical hypertrophy (AAH) of the left ventricle. Echocardiographic and ultrasonocardiotomographic study. *Jpn Heart J* 1976;7:611–629.
9. Tei C. Asymmetric apical hypertrophy-relationship to the giant T-wave inversion. *J Cardiol* 1978:121–141.
10. Murgo JP, Alter BR, Dorethy JF, et al. Dynamics of left ventricular ejection in obstructive and nonobstructive hypertrophic cardiomyopathy. *J Clin Invest* 1980;6:1369–1382.
11. Shah PM. Controversies in hypertrophic cardiomyopathy. *Curr Probl Cardiol* 1986;10:561–613.
12. Shah P, Taylor RD, Wong M. Abnormal mitral valve coaptation in hypertrophic obstructive cardiomyopathy: proposed role in systolic anterior motion of mitral valve. *Am J Cardiol* 1981;8:258–262.
13. Sasson G, Yock PG, Hatle LK, et al. Doppler determination of pressure gradient in hypertrophic cardiomyopathy. *J Am Coll Cardiol* 1988;11:752–756.
14. Murgo JP, Alter BR, Dorethy JD, et al. Dynamics of left ventricular ejection in obstructive and nonobstructive hypertrophic cardiomyopathy. *J Clin Invest* 1980;66:1369–1382.
15. Nagueh SF, Lakkis NM, He Z, et al. Role of myocardial contrast echocardiography during nonsurgical septal reduction therapy for hypertrophic obstructive cardiomyopathy. *J Am Coll Cardiol* 1998;32:225–229.
16. Pons-Llado G, Carreras F, Borras X, et al. Comparison of morphological assessment of hypertrophic cardiomyopathy by magnetic resonance versus echocardiography imaging. *Am J Cardiol* 1997;79(12):1651–1656.
17. Nakatami S, White RD, Powell K, et al. Dynamic magnetic resonance imaging assessment of the effect of ventricular wall curvature on regional function in hypertrophic cardiomyopathy. *Am J Cardiol* 1996;77(8):618–622.
18. Fujita N, Chazouillers AF, Hartialla JJ. Quantification of mitral regurgitation by velocity encoding cine nuclear magnetic resonance imaging. *J Am Coll Cardiol* 1994;23:951–952.
19. Sato T, Yamanari H, Ohe T, et al. Regional left ventricular contractile dynamics in hypertrophic cardiomyopathy evaluated by magnetic resonance imaging. *Heart Vessels* 1996;11(5):248–254.
20. Young AA, Kramer CM, Ferrari VA, et al. Three-dimensional left ventricular deformation in hypertrophic cardiomyopathy. *Circulation* 1994;90:854–867.
21. Sieverding L, Jung WI, Breuer J, et al. Proton-decoupled myocardial 31P NMR spectroscopy reveals decreased PCr/Pi in patients with severe hypertrophic cardiomyopathy. *Am J Cardiol* 1997;80(3A):34A–40A.

Restrictive Cardiomyopathy

Brian D. Hoit

According to the World Health Organization and International Society and Federation of Cardiology (WHO/ISFC), cardiomyopathies are heart muscle diseases of unknown etiology (1). While this definition acknowledges our ignorance, it has utility in that it differentiates the primary cardiomyopathies from known pathologic processes that disturb myocardial function such as ischemic, hypertensive, valvular, and congenital heart diseases. A generally accepted clinicopathologic classification scheme initially proposed by Goodwin includes dilated or congestive, hypertrophic, and restrictive/infiltrative cardiomyopathies (2). This chapter will focus on the least common cardiomyopathic class, i.e., the restrictive/infiltrative cardiomyopathies (heretofore to be referred to as restrictive).

Despite its relative rarity, restrictive cardiomyopathy has assumed importance in clinical cardiology for several reasons. First, restrictive cardiomyopathies exemplify the concept of diastolic heart failure (3); these diseases have as their central pathophysiologic component, abnormal ventricular diastolic compliance and impaired ventricular filling, with relatively preserved ventricular systolic function. Second, the hemodynamic and clinical manifestations of restrictive cardiomyopathy may mimic those produced by constrictive pericarditis, which, in contrast to restrictive cardiomyopathy, is a surgically curable disorder. Third, restrictive cardiomyopathy may present with interventricular conduction delays, heart block, or skeletal muscle disease and, therefore, be difficult to diagnose. Fourth, diagnostic criteria for restriction are not universally accepted, and the morphologic spectrum with hypertrophic cardiomyopathy and the presence of overlap syndromes (4) challenge our concepts of classification. Finally, echo Doppler assessment has become an important, noninvasive means of detecting the pathophysiol-

ogy, morphology, and, in some instances, the prognosis of the restrictive cardiomyopathies (5–7).

Restrictive cardiomyopathy may involve primarily either the myocardium or the endomyocardium and cause ventricular obliteration, either in isolation or in the setting of either systemic or iatrogenic disease. Irrespective of the etiology and nature of the myocardial pathophysiologic charaterics of the ventricles is that they have a small-to-normal size, that the myocardial walls are stiff, and that there are signs of restriction to inflow. Thus, despite normal (or near normal) systolic function, ventricular diastolic and atrial pressures are increased. Equalization of the diastolic pressures and a ''square root'' dip and plateau of early diastolic pressures of the right and left ventricles may be seen if the compliances of these chambers are similarly affected; thus, the hemodynamics of constrictive pericarditis may be simulated. Elevated atrial pressures produce systemic and pulmonary venous congestion, and relatively underfilled ventricles lead to reduced cardiac output and fatigue.

The chest x-ray usually reveals normal-sized ventricles, although enlargement of the atria and pericardial effusion may produce an enlarged cardiac silhouette. Pleural effusions and signs of pulmonary congestion may also be present.

DIAGNOSTIC FINDINGS

Both the echocardiogram and the cine magnetic resonance imaging studies infrequently identify the cause of restriction, but in many cases are useful to exculpate other causes of the syndrome. The Doppler technique has assumed an important role in characterizing the nature of transvalvular filling and in helping make the clinically crucial distinction between constrictive pericarditis and restrictive cardiomyopathy; most recently Doppler tissue velocities and coronary flow characteristics have been shown to be of value (6,8,9). These Doppler flow patterns and their respiratory changes are illus-

B. D. Hoit: Department of Medicine, Case Western Reserve University; Department of Cardiology, University Hospitals of Cleveland, Cleveland, Ohio 44106.

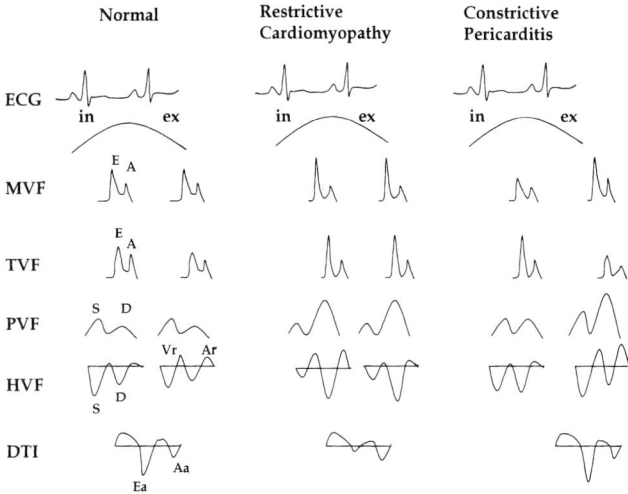

FIG. 1. Schematic of Doppler flows during inspiration (*in*) and expiration (*ex*) in normals, restrictive cardiomyopathy, and constrictive pericarditis. See text for details. *E,* early diastolic filling; *A,* atrial systolic filling; *S,* systolic flow; *D,* diastolic flow; *Vr,* V wave reversals; *Ar,* atrial systolic reversals; *Ea ,*early diastolic tissue velocites; *Aa,* late diastolic tissue velocities; *MVF,* mitral valve flow; *TVF,* tricuspid valve flow; *PVF,* pulmonary venous flow; *HVF,* hepatic venous flow; *DTI,* Doppler tissue imaging.

TABLE 1. *Mitral and tricuspid inflow and hepatic vein flow in normals, pericardial constriction, and restrictive cardiomyopathy*

Normal
  Mitral inflow
    a. No (~10%) respiratory variation in E velocity
    b. DT of 160 m/sec or more
  Tricuspid inflow
    a. Mild (~15%) respiratory variation in E velocity
    b. DT of 160 m/sec or more
  Hepatic vein
    a. Systolic forward (S) flow greater than diastolic forward (D) flow (in sinus—rhythm)
    b. Systolic forward less than diastolic forward flow (in atrial fibrillation)
    c. Slight increase in systolic (SR) and diastolic reversals (DR) with expiration
Constriction
  Mitral inflow
    a. Inspiratory E less than expiratory E (~25% change)
    b. DT, not always, but usually shortened (~160 m/sec)
  Tricuspid inflow
    a. Inspiratory E greater than expiratory E (~40% change)
    b. DT usually shortened (~160 m/sec)
  Hepatic vein
    a. Decreased diastolic forward flow with expiration
    b. Marked decrease in diastolic forward flow and increase in diastolic flow reversals with expiration
Restriction
  Mitral inflow
    a. No respiratory variation of E velocity
    b. Increased E velocity (usually ~1.0 m/sec)
    c. Decreased A velocity (usually ~0.5 m/sec)
    d. Increased E/A ratio (~2.0)
    e. Shortened DT of E (~160 m/sec)
  Tricuspid inflow
    a. Mild respiratory variation (~15%) in E velocity
    b. Increased E/A ratio (~2.0)
    c. Shortened DT of E (~160 m/sec)
  Hepatic vein
    a. Systolic forward flow (S) less than diastolic forward flow (D)
    b. Increase in systolic and diastolic flow reversals with inspiration

trated in Figure 1 and Table 1. In the normal subject, the early filling wave (E) of mitral flow is greater than the late, atrial systolic wave (A), and neither change significantly with respiration. In contrast, the E and A velocities of tricuspid valve flow increase slightly with inspiration. Pulmonary venous flow is generally biphasic, with a dominant wave during systole (S) and a smaller wave during diastole (D); respiratory changes are minimal and atrial systolic reversals are generally small. Hepatic vein flow consists of a larger S and smaller D wave with small reversals (V_r and A_r) after each wave, respectively. With expiration, S and D waves decrease and V_r and A_r increase. Doppler tissue imaging (DTI) shows a prominent longitudinal axis velocity in early diastole (E_a) and a smaller velocity after atrial contraction (A_a). In the patient with restrictive cardiomyopathy, the mitral valve flow shows an increased E/A ratio (≥ 2) with a short (<150 msec) deceleration time, a short isovolumic relaxation time (<70 msec), and no respiratory variation. The tricuspid valve flow shows an increased E/A ratio without respiratory variation and a shortened deceleration time and isovolumic relaxation time that shortens further with inspiration. The S/D ratio of pulmonary venous flow is less than 1, atrial reversals are increased (not shown in Fig. 1), and there is little respiratory variation. The S/D ratio of hepatic venous flow is less than 1, and prominent reversals are seen during inspiration. Doppler tissue imaging shows a striking decrease in E_a and a reversal of the E_a/A_a ratio. In patients with constrictive pericarditis, mitral valve, and tricuspid valve flows display a "restrictive" filling pattern, but exhibit marked respiratory variation. The isovolumic re-

laxation time shortens during expiration. The S/D of pulmonary venous flow is less than 1 with increased velocities (especially diastolic) in expiration, resulting in a further decrease in the S/D ratio. In contradistinction to restrictive cardiomyopathy, hepatic venous flow reversals occur in expiration. Early diastolic tissue velocities (E_a) are normal on DTI.

Despite the considerable interest in the reported ability to discriminate restrictive cardiomyopathy from constrictive pericarditis, there is not uniform agreement regarding the characteristic features of the Doppler indices, especially those of venous flows. Moreover, rigorous studies of the sensitivity and specificity of these Doppler findings are lacking, and relatively few patients have been examined. Thus, the diagnostic certainty is related to the number of "pathognomonic" findings in concert with clinical information and additional imaging studies.

In this regard, magnetic resonance imaging is useful because pericardial thickness can be accurately assessed in a pericardium greater than 4.0 mm thick, MRI can distinguish between constrictive and restrictive syndromes (10). Invasive hemodynamics may be helpful, and, occasionally, a histologic diagnosis is necessary.

Other magnetic resonance findings include reduced ventricular function and thickening of the diseased myocardium. The three-dimensional nature of magnetic resonance imaging (MRI) provides a means of accurately determining myocardial mass, which is increased in the restrictrive syndromes. Also, an approach known as phase velocity mapping provides means for evaluating flow patterns across the atrioventricular (AV) and the outflow valves. Although this approach is not yet widely used, it is available; and a number of investigations have described the abnormal patterns in restrictive syndromes (11).

One report suggested that radionuclide ventriculography could provide indices of left ventricular (LV) diastolic function that could differentiate constrictive from disease states (12). However, measurements of LV filling, such as the peak filling rate, time-to-peak filling, and various filling fractions require careful attention to technical detail. The need for stable heart rates, the lack of venous flows, and the inability to observe the influence of respiration on cardiac blood flows are important limitations to such applications of radionuclide ventriculography to the assessment of restrictive cardiomyopathy.

Myocardial Disease

Noninfiltrative Cardiomyopathies

Recent data suggest that idiopathic restrictive cardiomyopathy may be an autosomal dominant disorder involving myocardium, conduction tissue, and skeletal muscle, with resultant restrictive ventricular filling and heart failure, atrioventricular (AV) block, and distal skeletal myopathy, respectively (13). Deposition of the intermediate filament desmin has been linked to this syndrome and may represent a distinct pathologic entity; accumulation of desmin immunoreactive material on heart biopsy may be confirmed ultrastructurally (14,15).

Myocyte hypertrophy and fibrosis on endomyocardial biopsy is reported in restrictive cardiomyopathy, and the absence of myocyte disarray is an important pathologic distinction because hypertrophic cardiomyopathy may create diagnostic confusion. Overlap syndromes, characterized by physiologic evidence of restriction and myocyte hypertrophy but without disarray or echocardiographic left ventricular hypertrophy, may occur (16). A feature of both echocardiography and of cine MRI that can assist in distinguishing primary restrictive cardiomyopathy from cardiac amyloidosis (in addition to the associated clinical features) is the presence of a more dramatic increase in wall thickness and in mass, respectively, in the latter. In both disorders (and in restrictive

cardiomyopathies in general), ventricular dimensions are normal or reduced, systolic function is variable, and atrial dimensions are enlarged.

Two-dimensional and Doppler echocardiography provide a reliable and noninvasive measure of diagnosing primary restrictive cardiomyopathy in children (17). A dominant mitral E velocity, an increased pulmonary venous A reversal velocity and duration, and shortened mitral deceleration time are present in both children and adults with primary restrictive cardiomyopathy. On computed tomographic or magnetic resonance imaging scans, evidence of restrictive filling (e.g., right atrial and caval enlargement) are common in both restrictive cardiomyopathy and constrictive pericarditis. Again, MRI can be used to accurately assess pericardial thickness, which often provides the diagnosis. Pyrophosphate scans are no longer recommended since they are frequently falsely positive in primary restrictive cardiomyopathy.

Although endocardial fibroelastosis is not often associated with a restrictive cardiomyopathic syndrome, coronary artery disease with premature death is a major problem in these patients (18). Myocardial fibrosis, which may have a patchy distribution and can be present in both ventricles, is found in the majority of patients with scleroderma at autopsy. On echocardiography and on cine MRI, left ventricular wall thickening in the absence of hypertension may be seen. However, heart failure owing to either restrictive or dilated cardiomyopathy is rare (19).

Infiltrative Cardiomyopathies

Although there are several types of amyloidosis, cardiac involvement is most common in primary amyloidosis (AL type), which is caused by plasma cell production of immunoglobulin light chains (often in association with multiple myeloma). However, cardiac deposition of amyloid protein may occur in secondary amyloidosis due to chronic inflammation (AA type), familial, or senile amyloidosis (20,21). Mutations of the protein transthyretin (formerly prealbumin) are usually inherited as an autosomal dominant and produce peripheral and autonomic neuropathy in addition to cardiac disease (21). Amyloid deposits may be interstitial and widespread, resulting in restrictive cardiomyopathy, or they may be localized to (i) conduction tissue, resulting in heart block and ventricular arrhythmias, (ii) the cardiac valves, resulting in valvular regurgitation, (iii) the pericardium, resulting in constriction, and (iv) the coronary arteries, resulting in ischemia. Moreover, amyloid may be isolated to the subendocardium in senile amyloid and in amyloid secondary to chronic disease (22); deposition of amyloid and atrial natriuretic factor (ANF) in the atria are frequent in aged hearts (23). In some cases, the clinical picture is dominated by neuropathy and nephropathy, and cardiac involvement is not recognized.

The cardiac silhouette on the chest radiogram may be normal to moderately enlarged. The echocardiogram and cine MRI may reveal symmetrical wall thickness involving the right and left ventricles, a small or normal LV cavity and variable (but often depressed) systolic function, and left

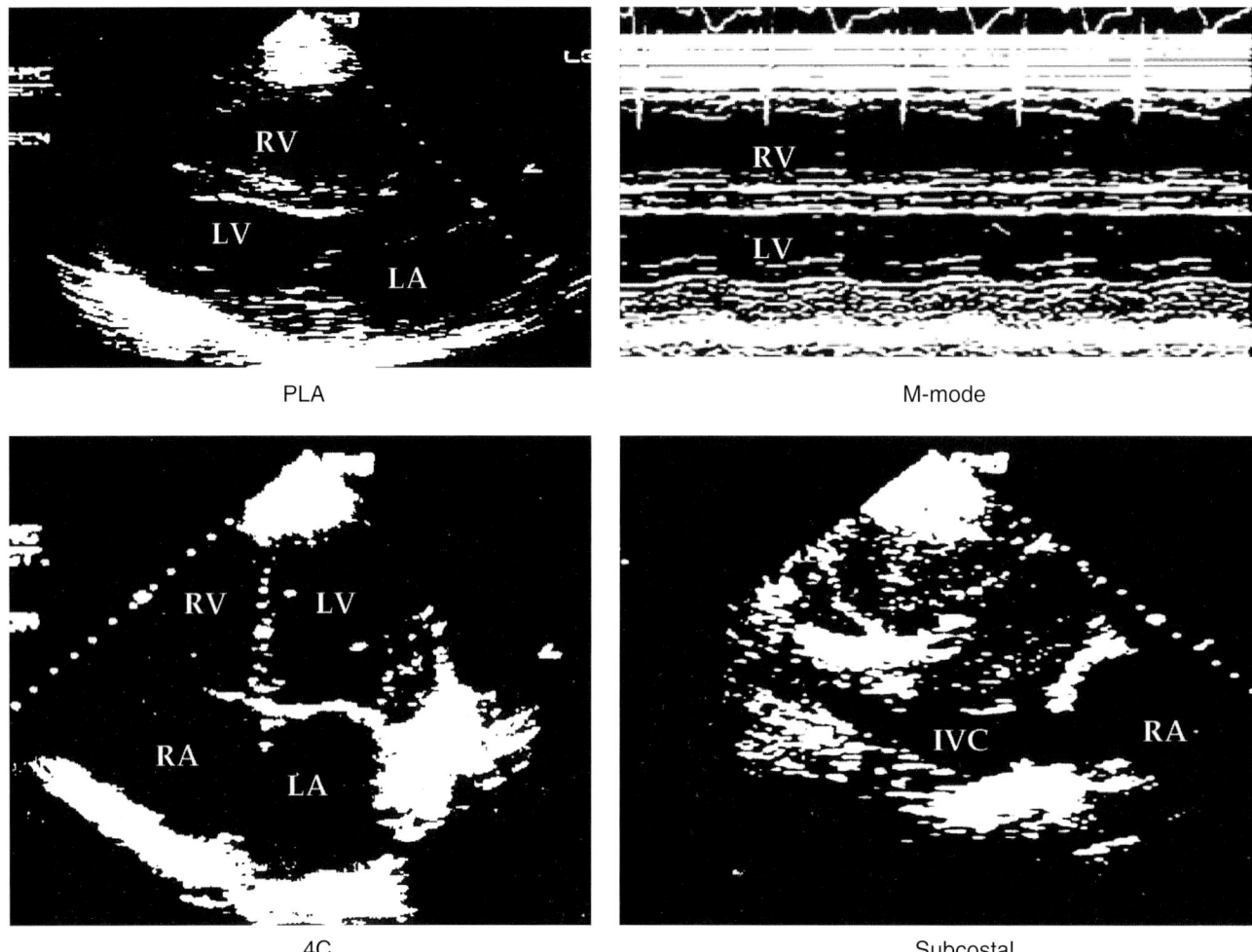

FIG. 2. M-Mode and two-dimensional echocardiogram from a patient with biopsy proven amyloidosis causing hemodynamic restriction. The left ventricular systolic function is mildly impaired, and there is biatrial enlargement and vena cava plethora. Left ventricular hypertrophy is best seen in the M-mode study. *PLA,* parasternal long axis; *4C,* four chamber view; *RV,* right ventricle; *LV,* left ventricle; *LA,* left atrium; *RA,* right atrium; *IVC,* inferior vena cava.

atrial enlargement and a small pericardial effusion (Fig. 2). The LV wall thickness may be an important prognostic variable (7). Digitized M-mode tracings reveal decreased rates of both systolic wall thickening and diastolic wall thinning and increased isovolumic relaxation time (24). Highly reflective echoes producing a granular or sparkling appearance and occurring in a patchy distribution are characteristic two-dimensional echo findings (25), but they are neither sensitive nor specific. Concentric hypertrophy, as occurs in hypertension or aortic stenosis, may produce a uniformly speckled or echo lucent appearance of the myocardium, and idiopathic hypertrophic cardiomyopathy may display a patchy, granular sparkling (26). Although they correlate with wall thickness, granular echoes may not be seen and, importantly, their recognition is subjective and is affected by ultrasound instrument settings. Thus, granular sparkling alone is an unreliable

finding. Two-dimensional echo also reveals thickening of the interatrial septum and valves (especially the AV valves), enlarged papillary muscles, and dilated atria and inferior vena cava (Fig. 2).

Doppler studies may show the restrictive pattern of left ventricular filling—i.e., a transmitral E/A ratio greater than or equal to 2 without respiratory variation, transmitral diastolic deceleration time less than 150 msec, and an isovolumic relaxation time less than or equal to 70 msec. The systolic-to-diastolic pulmonary venous flow ratio is less than 1 and atrial reversals increase with inspiration in the pulmonary and hepatic veins.

Abnormalities of left ventricular filling are also demonstrated with the LV time-activity curve from radionuclide ventriculography (27). Moreover, radionuclide imaging using technetium-99m pyrophosphate (or indium-111 antimyosin, which is no longer available for clinical studies) may be useful in diagnosis (28,29). The variable clinical, diagnostic, and prognostic features reflect the location, nature, and extent of amyloid deposition and the temporal course of the disease (30). Although both ventricles are generally involved, an endomyocardial biopsy of the right ventricle (most helpful if an abdominal fat aspirate is negative) may be falsely negative.

Other Infiltrative Diseases

Sarcoid granulomas involve the heart, but are frequently subclinical (31). Interstitial granulomatous inflammation initially produces diastolic dysfunction, but later and with more extensive involvement, it may produce systolic (at times focal) abnormalities (32). Localized thinning and dilatation of the basilar left ventricle resembling ischemic heart disease is characteristic (33). Pericardial effusions are common. Sarcoid pulmonary involvement is frequent and produces echo and Doppler findings of pulmonary hypertension and right heart failure. High-grade AV block, usually owing to the involvement of the conduction system, and ventricular arrhythmias may result in sudden cardiac death (34). Thallium-201 and gallium-67 have been used to indicate areas of myocardial involvement and have been used to predict the response to corticosteroids (35).

Even more dramatic are the regions of increased intensity on T2-weighted MRI associated with myocardial sarcoidosis. Gaucher's disease is due to an inherited deficiency of the enzyme β-glucocerebroside, which results in accumulation of cerebroside in the reticuloendothelial system, brain, and heart. Diffuse interstitial infiltration of the left ventricle occurs, but it is not often associated with symptoms of LV failure; LV wall and valvular thickening and pericardial effusion are seen on echo (36).

Storage Diseases

Myocardial iron deposition in hemochromatosis, either primary or secondary, usually produces dilated cardiomyopathy, but occasionally restrictive cardiomyopathy may be seen. One report suggests that cardiac involvement progresses temporally from a small, concentrically hypertrophied ("restrictive") LV with diastolic dysfunction to a dilated LV with systolic dysfunction (37). However, this progression is not universally accepted, and systolic abnormalities may require provocation (38). Granular sparkling and atrial enlargement may be seen on echocardiogram, but are nonspecific (39). Quantitative ultrasonic analysis (integrated backscatter) has been used experimentally to detect changes in the echo reflectivity of the myocardium owing to iron deposition in thalassemia major (40). Magnetic resonance images (T1-weighted) demonstrate reduced myocardial signal intensity. The liver in hemochromatosis is frequently not visible on MR images, a striking and diagnostic finding.

Fabry's disease, an X-linked, genetically heterogeneous disorder of glycosphingolipid metabolism caused by lysosomal ceramide deficiency, leads to the accumulation of glycolipid and may present with either a restrictive, hypertrophic or dilated cardiomyopathy, mitral regurgitation, ischemic heart disease, and aortic degeneration. Echocardiographic findings and magnetic resonance in restrictive cardiomyopathy mimic those seen in amyloid, and LV mass correlates with the severity of disease (41). Hypertension, mitral valve prolapse, and heart failure are common clinical presentations.

Pompe's disease (Glycogen Storage Type II) is due to an abnormality of glycogen storage that may produce restrictive cardiomyopathy. A hypertrophied, hypokinetic left ventricle in an infant with muscle hypotonia are characteristic findings; the echocardiographic manifestations may be indistinguishable from hypertrophic obstructive cardiomyopathy. Adults with glycogen storage type III (debranching enzyme deficiency) may have marked left ventricular hypertrophy on echocardiography (42).

Endomyocardial Disease

Endomyocardial Fibrosis and Hypereosinophilic Syndrome

Endomyocardial diseases that cause restrictive obliterative cardiomyopathies include endomyocardial fibrosis (EMF) and hypereosinophilic (Loeffler's) syndrome. The former accounts for 10 to 20% of deaths due to heart disease in equatorial Africa, but the disease is seen throughout the world. In contrast, Loeffler's endocarditis is seen mainly in countries with a temperate climate, and, although it shares similar pathologic features with EMF, it affects mainly men, is usually related to parasitic infections, and is characterized by intense eosinophila (greater than 1,500/mm) and thromboembolic phenomena (43,44).

Although their clinical presentations differ (EMF has a more insidious onset), the pathology and, therefore, cardiac imaging studies, are generally similar in the endomyocardial diseases. M-mode echo findings are nonspecific and digitized M-mode studies reveal a decreased peak filling rate and a decreased duration of the peak filling (45). On two-dimensional echo, apical obliteration of the right and/or left ventricle, apical thrombus, preservation of ventricular systolic function with thickening of the posterior atrioventricular valve apparatus and posterobasilar LV wall, echo densities in the endocardium, and small ventricular and large atrial cavities are noted (Fig. 3) (46). Involvement of the posterior mitral and tricuspid valve leaflets result in mitral and tricuspid regurgitation; less commonly, restricted motion may produce stenosis. Sparing of the outflow tracts are characteristic (47). Doppler interrogation yields typical patterns of restriction (increased E/A, decreased isovolumic relaxation time, decreased deceleration time), mitral and tricuspid regurgita-

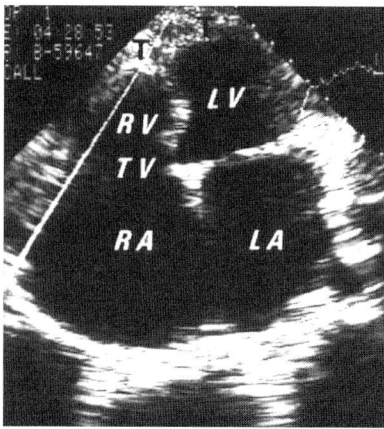 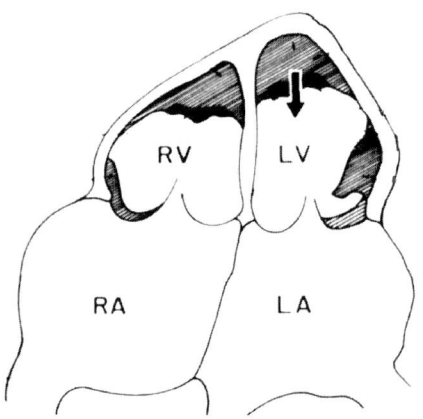

FIG. 3. Left panel: Echocardiogram from a patient with biventricular endomyocardial disease and advanced heart failure. Note the small ventricles, large atria, and obliterative thrombus (*T*) in the apices. *LA*, left atrium; *LV*, left ventricle; *RA*, right atrium; *RV*, right ventricle; *TV*, tricuspid valve. **Right panel:** Schematic of a four-chamber view illustrating potential pathologies in endomyocardial disease. *Arrow* denotes a potential inward motion of the obliterative process. (From ref. 47, with permission.)

tion and, less often, stenosis. Not surprisingly, the location, extent, and severity of involvement determine the clinical picture.

Carcinoid Syndrome

Involvement of the heart occurs as a late complication of carcinoid syndrome in approximately 50% of patients. Fibrous endocardial plaques comprised of smooth muscle cells in a stroma of collagen and acid mucopolysacharide on the tricuspid and pulmonic valves and right heart endocardium are characteristic; LV involvement is distinctly uncommon (48). Although tricuspid and pulmonic stenosis and regurgitation dominate the clinical picture, restrictive cardiomyopathy may occur. The chest x-ray is often normal, but cardiomegaly, and pleural effusions and nodules may be evident; unlike congenital pulmonic stenosis, there is no poststenotic dilatation of the pulmonary artery trunk (49). Two-dimensional echocardiography reveals thickened, retracted tricuspid and pulmonic valves and right atrial and ventricular enlargement; right atrial wall thickening may be seen on transesophageal echo. Low-velocity tricuspid and pulmonic regurgitation on Doppler indicate normal pulmonary arterial pressures, which is typical of carcinoid heart disease. Gradients across stenotic tricuspid and pulmonic valves are readily determined using Bernoulli gradient calculations.

Malignant Infiltration

Infiltrating tumors of the heart are generally metastatic (lung, breast, melanoma, lymphoma, leukemia), and they rarely produce restriction to ventricular filling unless the pericardium is involved. Infiltration is suggested by a localized increase in wall thickness, often associated with abnormal wall motion and pericardial effusion.

Iatrogenic Disease

Pericardial disease frequently complicates radiation therapy to the chest and may produce constrictive pericarditis;

however, endo- and myocardial involvement may produce restrictive cardiomyopathy, at times presenting years after radiation therapy has been completed (50). Anthracyclines (51) and methysergide (52) can cause endomyocardial fibrosis.

REFERENCES

1. WHO/ISFC Task Force. Definition and classification of cardiomyopathies. *Br Heart J* 1980;44:672–673.
2. Goodwin J, Oakley C. The cardiomyopathies. *Br Heart J* 1972;44: 672–673.
3. Shabetai R. Controversial issues in restrictive cardiomyopathy. *Postgrad Med J* 1992;68:S47–S51.
4. Wilmshurst P, Katritsis D. Restrictive and hypertrophic cardiomyopathies in Noonan syndrome: the overlap syndromes. *Heart* 1996;75: 94–97.
5. Appleton C, Hatle L, Popp R. Demonstration of restrictive ventricular physiology by Doppler echocardiography. *J Am Coll Cardiol* 1988;11: 757–768.
6. Klein A, Cohen G, Pietrolungo J, et al. Differentiation of constrictive pericarditis from restrictive cardiomyopathy by Doppler transesophageal echocardiographic measurements of respiratory variations in pulmonary venous flow. *J Am Coll Cardiol* 1993;22:1935–1943.
7. Cueto-Garcia L, Tajik A, Kyle R, et al. Serial echocardiographic observations in patients with primary systemic amyloidosis: an introduction to the concept of early (asymptomatic) amyloid infiltration of the heart. *Mayo Clin Proc* 1984;59:589–597.
8. Garcia M, Rodriguez L, Ares M, et al. Differentiation of constrictive pericarditis from restrictive cardiomyopathy: assessment of left ventricular diastolic velocities in longitudinal axis by Doppler tissue imaging. *J Am Coll Cardiol* 1996;27:108–114.
9. Akasaka T, Yoshida K, Yamamuro A, et al. Phasic coronary flow characteristics in patients with constrictive pericarditis. Comparison with restrictive cardiomyopathy. *Circulation* 1997;96:1874–1881.
10. Masui T, Finck S, Higgins C. Constrictive pericarditis and restrictive cardiomyopathy: evaluation with MR imaging. *Radiology* 1992;182: 369–373.
11. Mohiaddin RH, Pennell DJ. MR blood flow measurement. Clinical application in the heart and circulation. *Cardiol Clin* 1998;16(2): 161–187.
12. Gerson M, Fowler N. Differentiation of constrictive pericarditis and restrictive cardiomyopathy by radionuclide ventriculography. *Am Heart J* 1989;118:114–120.
13. Katristsis D, Wilmshurst P, Wendon J, et al. Primary restrictive cardiomyopathy: clinical and pathologic characteristics. *J Am Coll Cardiol* 1991;18:1230–1235.
14. Arbustini E, Morbini P, Grasso M, et al. Restrictive cardiomyopathy, atrioventricular block and mild to subclinical myopathy in patients with desmin-immunoreactive material deposits. *J Am Coll Cardiol* 1998; 31:645–653.

15. Zachara E, Bertini E, Lioy E, et al. Restrictive cardiomyopathy due to desmin accumulation in a family with evidence of autosomal dominant inheritance. *G Ital Cardiol* 1997;27:436–442.
16. Cooke R, Chambers J, Curry P. Noonan's cardiomyopathy: a non-hypertrophic variant. *Br Heart J* 1994;71:561–565.
17. Cetta F, O'Leary P, Seward J, et al. Idiopathic restrictive cardiomyopathy in childhood: diagnostic features and clinic course. *Mayo Clin Proc* 1995;70:634–640.
18. Navarro-Lopez F, Llorian A, Ferrer-Roca O, et al. Restrictive cardiomyopathy in psuedoxanthoma elasticum. *Chest* 1980;78:113–115.
19. Botstein G, LeRoy E. Primary heart disease in systemic sclerosis (scleroderma): advances in clinical and pathologic features, pathogenesis, and new therapeutic approaches. *Am Heart J* 1981;102:913–919.
20. Olson L, Gertz M, Edwards W, et al. Senile cardiac amyloidosis with myocardial dysfunction: diagnosis by endomyocardial biopsy and immunohistochemistry. *N Engl J Med* 1987;317:738–742.
21. Hesse A, Altland K, Linke R, et al. Cardiac amyloidosis: a review and report of a new transthyretin (prealbumin) variant. *Br Heart J* 1993; 70:111–115.
22. Looi L. Isolated atrial amyloidosis: a clinicopathologic study indicating increased prevalence in chronic heart disease. *Hum Pathol* 1993;24: 602–607.
23. Kawamura S, Takahashi M, Ishihara T, et al. Incidence and distribution of isolated atrial amyloid: histologic and immunohistochemical studies of 100 aging hearts. *Pathol Int* 1995;45:335–342.
24. Sutton MSJ, Reichek N, Kastor J, et al. Computerized M-mode echocardiographic analysis of left ventricular dysfunction in cardiac amyloid. *Circulation* 1982;66:790–799.
25. Nicolosi G, Pavan D, Lestuzzi C, et al. Prospective identification of patients with amyloid heart disease by two-dimensional echocardiography. *Circulation* 1984;70:432–437.
26. Bhandari AK, Nanda NC. Myocardial texture characterization by two-dimensional echocardiography. *Am J Cardiol* 1983;51:817–825.
27. Lenihan DJ, Gerson MC, Hoit BD, et al. Mechanisms, diagnosis, and treatment of diastolic heart failure. *Am Heart J* 1995;130:153–166.
28. Lekakis J, Nanas J, Moustafellou C, et al. Cardiac amyloidosis detected by Indium-111 antimyosin imaging. *Am Heart J* 1992;124:1630–1631.
29. Wizenberg T, Muz J, Sohn Y, et al. Value of myocardial Technetium-99m pyrophosphate scintigraphy in the non-invasive diagnosis of cardiac amyloidosis. *Am Heart J* 1982;103:468–479.
30. Cueto-Garcia L, Reeder G, Kyle R, et al. Echocardiographic findings in systemic amyloidosis: spectrum of cardiac involvement and relation to survival. *J Am Coll Cardiol* 1985;6:737–743.
31. Gibbons W, Levy R, Nava S, et al. Subclinical cardiac dysfunction in sarcoidosis. *Chest* 1991;100:44–50.
32. Valantine H, McKenna W, Nihoyannopoulos P, et al. Sarcoidosis: a pattern of clinical and morphological presentation. *Br Heart J* 1987; 57:256–263.
33. Burstow DJ, Tajik AJ, Bailey KR, et al. Two-dimensional echocardiographic findings in systemic sarcoidosis. *Am J Cardiol* 1989;63: 478–482.
34. Perry A, Vuitch F. Causes of death in patients with sarcoidosis: a morphologic study of 38 autopsies with clinicopathologic correlations. *Arch Pathol Lab Med* 1995;119:167–172.
35. Okayama K, Kurata C, Tawarchara K, et al. Diagnostic and prognostic value of myocardial scintigraphy with thallium-201 and gallium-67 in cardiac sarcoidosis. *Chest* 1995;107:330–334.
36. Saraclar M, Atalay S, Kocak N, et al. Gaucher's disease with mitral and aortic involvement: echocardiographic findings. *Pediatr Cardiol* 1991;13:56–58.
37. Arnett E, Nienhius A, Henry W, et al. Massive myocardial hemochromatosis: a structure-function conference at the National Heart and Lung Institute. *Am Heart J* 1975;90:777–787.
38. Dabestani A, Child J, Henze E, et al. Primary hemochromatosis: anatomic and physiologic characteristics of the cardiac ventricles and their response to phlebotomy. *Am J Cardiol* 1984;54:153–159.
39. Candell-Riera J, Lu L, Seres L, et al. Cardiac hemochromatosis: beneficial effects of iron and removal therapy. An echocardiographic study. *Am J Cardiol* 1983;52:824–829.
40. Lattanzi F, Bellotti P, Picano E, et al. Quantitative ultrasonic analysis of myocardium in patients with thalassemia major and iron overload. *Circulation* 1993;87:748–754.
41. Goldman M, Cantor R, Schwartz M, et al. Echocardiographic abnormalities and disease severity in Fabry's disease. *J Am Coll Cardiol* 1986;7:1157–1161.
42. Coleman R, Winter H, Wolf B, et al. Glycogen storage disease type III (glycogen debranching enzyme deficiency): correlation of biochemical defects with myopathy and cardiomyopathy. *Ann Int Med* 1992;116: 896–900.
43. Olsen E, Spry C. Relation between eosinophilia and endomyocardial disease. *Prog Cardiovasc Dis* 1985;27:241–254.
44. Shaper A. What's new in endomyocardial fibrosis? *Lancet* 1993;342: 255–256.
45. Davies J, Gibson D, Foale R, et al. Echocardiographic features of eosinophilic endomyocardial disease. *Br Heart J* 1982;48:434–440.
46. Gottdiener J, Maron B, Schooley R, et al. Two-dimensional echocardiographic assessment of the idiopathic hypereosinophilic syndrome: anatomic basis of mitral regurgitation and peripheral embolization. *Circulation* 1983;67:572–578.
47. Acquatella H, Schiller N, Puigbo J, et al. Value of two-dimensional disease with and without eosinophilia. A clinical and pathologic study. *Circulation* 1983;67:1219–1226.
48. Lundin L, Norheim I, Landelius J, et al. Carcinoid heart disease: relationship of circulating vasoactive substances to ultrasound-detectable cardiac abnormalities. *Circulation* 1988;77:264–269.
49. Pellikka P, Tajik A, Khandheria B, et al. Carcinoid heart disease: clinical and echocardiographic spectrum in 74 patients. *Circulation* 1993; 87:1188–1196.
50. Brosius FC, Waller BF, Roberts WC. Radiation heart disease: analysis of 16 young (aged 15 to 33 years) necropsy patients who received over 3,500 rads to the heart. *Am J Med* 1981;70:519–530.
51. Mortensen S, Olsen H, Baandrup U. Chronic anthracycline cardiotoxicity: haemodynamic and histopathological manifestations suggesting a restrictive endomyocardial disease. *Br Heart J* 1986;55:272–282.
52. Mason J, Billingham M, Friedman J. Methysergide-induced heart disease: a case of multivalvular and myocardial fibrosis. *Circulation* 1977; 56:889–890.

CHAPTER 49

Cardiac Imaging for Myocarditis

Igor F. Palacios

Inflammation of the cardiac muscle, or myocarditis can be produced by a large number of infectious organisms. The enteroviruses, especially Coxsackie B virus, are the more common cause of epidemic myocarditis (1,2). The clinical presentation of myocarditis varies from asymptomatic patients with normal left ventricular systolic function and electrocardiographic abnormalities during outbreaks of Coxsackie B virus to those with severe compromise of left ventricular systolic function, fulminant heart failure, and cardiogenic shock (1–5). Although chest pain due to myopericarditis can occur often, we have reported a group of patients with myocarditis who presented with manifestations mimicking acute myocardial infarction (6). These patients presented with typical coronary pain, electrocardiographic changes consistent with acute myocardial infarction, and elevation of serum levels of creatine kinase (MB fraction). Some of these patients presented with cardiogenic shock requiring temporary intraaortic balloon support. The finding of normal coronary arteries in such patients should lead to a high index of suspicion of myocarditis and prompt right ventricular biopsy and/or cardiac imaging (radionuclide or magnetic resonance) should be performed to determine the diagnosis. Myocarditis can also present as recurrent episodes of ventricular tachycardia and sudden death with or without ventricular dysfunction (1–5).

The incidence and clinical course of myocarditis are not well defined. Dilated cardiomyopathy is an important cause of congestive heart failure resulting in 50% mortality within 2 years of the diagnosis (1,4–5). Active myocarditis has been postulated to be the cause of acute onset of dilated cardiomyopathy and perhaps of a subset of patients with chronic dilated cardiomyopathy (3–5). Although the true incidence of antecedent myocarditis in patients with symp-

tomatic dilated cardiomyopathy remains uncertain, heart failure of recent onset due to acute dilated cardiomyopathy is one form of presentation of acute myocarditis (3–5). Some of the patients with the acute form could evolve to chronic dilated cardiomyopathy. It is possible that an adverse immunological response produced by the viral infection leads to progressive myocyte damage culminating in dilated cardiomyopathy. There is some evidence that supports this hypothesis (2,7–11). In selected murine strains, injection of Coxsackie B3 virus or encephalomyocarditis virus results in a self-limited infection of the myocardium (7). During the initial infective phase myocyte viral replication occurs, and it results within 7 to 10 days in interferon, macrophages, natural killer cells, and humoral antibody production. During this acute phase, minimal myocyte necrosis with sparse inflammatory infiltrate occur. As the virus is eliminated, lympho-mononuclear infiltrate intensifies. Chronic myocardial damage is produced by both autodirected T lymphocytes and humoral antibodies (2,7–11). In a murine model, dilated cardiomyopathy occurs by 1 year after the acute infection (11). Such a viral infection results in an autoimmune response that leads to progressive myocyte damage and dilated cardiomyopathy. It is possible that a similar pathological mechanism exists in humans.

MYOCARDIAL BIOPSY

A variety of studies have documented the difficulty that exists in establishing a precise diagnosis of myocarditis based on clinical, electrocardiographic, and serological findings (1–5). The definitive diagnosis of myocarditis can be made only by examination of myocardial tissue. Because myocardial biopsy provides histologic confirmation of clinically suspected myocarditis, it is currently the procedure of choice or ''gold standard'' for diagnosis. Before the use of endomyocardial biopsy in the assessment of patients with dilated cardiomyopathy and suspected myocarditis, the diag-

I. F. Palacios: Department of Medicine, Harvard Medical School; Cardiac Catheterization Laboratory, Department of Medicine, Massachusetts General Hospital, Boston, Massachusetts 02114.

nosis of acute myocarditis was dependent on clinical criteria. The presence of congestive heart failure of unknown cause preceded by a febrile viral illness with an associated four-fold increase in antibody titer to cardiotropic virus was a presumptive evidence of myocarditis, particularly if pericarditis or heart block were present. The technique of endomyocardial biopsy has been used in patients with dilated cardiomyopathy of unknown etiology to identify patients with myocarditis (3,12–20). The incidence of biopsy-documented myocarditis in patients with unexplained dilated cardiomyopathy varies widely (30,12–20). These controversial results are largely due to a difference in pathological interpretation of biopsy specimen. Furthermore, endomyocardial biopsy is subject to sampling error and the frequency with which this technique fails to detect myocarditis is unknown. This lack of correlation could be explained by a biopsy sampling error in a disease that is frequently focal or multifocal.

A major advance in the diagnosis of myocarditis was achieved in 1987 when a panel of cardiac pathologists, highly skilled in the interpretation of myocardial biopsy, met in Dallas, Texas, to establish a pathological definition of myocarditis to be used in a large, multicenter study designed to determine the efficacy of immunosuppressive therapy in patients with myocarditis (21). Myocarditis was defined as the presence of an inflammatory infiltrate associated with injury (necrosis or degeneration) to adjacent myocytes. This criteria allows that data from different studies could be compared accurately. With this classification *first or initial biopsies* are classified into three major histologic groups: (i) myocarditis—specimens showing an interstitial infiltrate and associated necrosis or degeneration of adjacent myocytes; (ii) borderline myocarditis—biopsies containing an interstitial inflammatory infiltrate but lacking myocyte necrosis and/or degeneration, repeat biopsy is recommended in these patients; and (iii) no myocarditis—specimen showing no interstitial inflammatory infiltrate. These specimens contain either normal myocardium, or nonspecific findings such as interstitial and/or replacement fibrosis and myocyte hypertrophy. *Repeat or successive biopsies* are classified as: (i) ongoing myocarditis—specimens that continue to show evidence of a persistent inflammatory infiltrate and ongoing degeneration or necrosis of adjacent myocytes; (ii) resolving myocarditis—specimens showing continued cellular inflammation but no evidence of myocyte necrosis; and (iii) resolved myocarditis—these biopsy specimens show resolution of both infiltrate and myocyte necrosis. Within each diagnostic category the following are evaluated: (i) the type of inflammatory infiltrate (lymphocytic, eosinophilic, neutrophilic, mixed, giant cell, granulomatous, etc); (ii) the distribution of inflammation (focal, confluent, or diffuse); (iii) the extent of inflammation (absent, mild, moderate, severe); (iv) the extent of acute injury; (v) the location of fibrosis (endocardial, interstitial, or both); (vi) the extent of fibrosis (scored separately for both endocardium and interstitium from 0–3); and (vii) the extent of hypertrophy (21). The type of inflammatory infiltrate is an important determinant of the

prognosis in patients with acute myocarditis. Davidoff et al. (22) reported that patients with "giant cell" myocarditis have a worse prognosis than those with "lymphocytic" myocarditis. Giant cell myocarditis was highly associated with ventricular tachycardia, heart block, and ultimately the requirement of a permanent pacemaker. Furthermore, an adverse event, either cardiac mortality or cardiac transplantation, was significantly greater in patients with giant cell myocarditis than those with lymphocytic myocarditis. In the Myocarditis Treatment Trial (23) patients with unexplained left ventricular dysfunction of less than 2-year duration, with a left ventricular ejection fraction of less than 45% and histological evidence of myocarditis on right ventricular endomyocardial biopsy were candidates for randomization in the study. In this study 2,305 patients with congestive heart failure less than 2-years' duration and of unknown etiology underwent right ventricular biopsy to determine eligibility for the trial. The diagnosis of myocarditis was made in only 209 patients (9.4%).

Even though the specificity of endomyocardial biopsy for diagnosing myocarditis is good, its sensitivity is questionable. Because sampling error must certainly occur, the frequency with which myocarditis exists but is not detected by myocardial biopsy is not known. In a selected group of 27 patients with acute dilated cardiomyopathy of recent onset (<6 months' duration) we demonstrated a lack of correlation between histological evidence of myocarditis in the biopsy and clinical signs suggestive of active myocarditis (a febrile virus-like illness preceding the onset of acute dilated cardiomyopathy), clinical evidence of pericarditis and laboratory abnormalities of inflammation such as elevation of the erythrocyte sedimentation rate, leucocytosis, and elevation in the serum concentration of creatinine kinase; scored with a number from 1 to 3 (3).

Because myocardial necrosis and cell infiltration are integral components of myocarditis, imaging techniques, previously shown to localize areas of myocardial necrosis and those used to identify areas of cell infiltration and inflammation, have been tested in patients with suspected myocarditis. Radionuclide techniques using either gallium-67 (Ga-67; an inflammation-avid radioisotope) or antimyosin antibody-labeled with indium-111 (a necrosis-avid radiotracer) and MRI using the distribution of gadolinium-DTPA have been used with promising results in patients with new onset of dilated cardiomyopathy and suspected myocarditis (24–29). Compared with the "gold standard" of myocardial biopsy these techniques are sensitive but nonspecific. Albeit, endomyocardial biopsy remains the gold standard for the diagnosis of myocarditis, it is possible that the lack of specificity of these radionuclide and MR techniques may be due to sampling error of the endomyocardial biopsy. The ideal technique for diagnosing myocarditis should have high sensitivity, low morbidity and low cost. Myocardial biopsy is safe when performed by experienced operators. However its morbidity, cost, and potential for sampling error due to the focal nature of myocarditis make the biopsy technique suboptimal. In contrast, inflammation (Ga-67) and necrosis (antimyosin) sensitive radionuclide imaging techniques are more suitable for this role.

GALLIUM-67 MYOCARDIAL SCINTIGRAPHY

Ga-67 myocardial scintigraphy has been used as noninvasive technique for detecting myocardial inflammatory lesions (24–27). This agent is routinely used to identify chronic inflammation with a reported sensitivity of 90%. Because inflammation is an obligatory component of myocarditis, the Ga-67 technique demonstrates increased radioactivity in patients with myocarditis.

Gamma camera imaging (now usually using a SPECT camera) is performed 72 hours after the intravenous administration of 8 mCi of Ga-67. Ga-67 is a gamma emitter with an energy for its main rays of 93 keV (42%) ($=$I), 184 keV (20%) ($=$II), and 300 keV (17%) ($=$III). Images are obtained using a gamma camera equipped with a parallel hole collimator adapted to medium energy (200–400 keV). There are several techniques-dependent sources of error that could decrease the sensitivity of this technique. Three to five views are obtained for each patient: anterior, 45° left anterior oblique (LAO), left lateral supplemented when necessary by 30°, and 60° LAO to allow better differentiation of the myocardial region from the sternal region and the vertebral column. Scans should be performed at 72 h after the intravenous injection of the radiopharmaceutical. If imaging is performed at 24 h after the injection, the Ga-67 may not clear the blood pool and result in a false positive scan. If scanning is performed at 48 h, the heart may be imaged but increased background activity may decrease the sensitivity. Most of the liver should be excluded from the field of view because it reduces counts detected from the myocardium. Finally, in lactating or premenstrual women, breast uptake may obscure myocardium. Myocardial uptake is measure in digitized images and a ratio computed between the mean uptake per pixel in the precordial region and the sternum is determined. The examination is considered as positive when this ratio is ≥1, doubtful if the ratio is <1, but with visible myocardial uptake, and negative if the precordial region is not different from the background.

The mechanism of Ga-67 accumulation in inflammatory zones requires plasma transport, with binding of the radioisotope to transferrin, especially to reach the zone. Local uptake depends on an increase in capillary permeability and the importance of the exudate. Intracellular accumulation occurs on the membranes of the polymorphonuclear leukocytes and, to a lesser extent, on the membranes of the lymphocytes and monocytes. Analysis of inflammatory exudates shows that the greatest part of Ga-67 accumulates in a transferrin and lactoferrin-bound form. Ga-67 imaging is useful clinically in the detection of noncardiac chronic inflammatory states. It has also been shown to be useful in the detection of inflammation in bacterial endocarditis, myocardial abscess, myocardial sarcoidosis, and pericardial disease.

An increase in myocardial Ga-67 uptake has been demonstrated in an experimental model of rabbit adrenergic myocarditis (30). O'Connell et al. (24,25) reported an excellent sensitivity in patients with biopsy documented myocarditis. Five of 6 (87%) biopsy samples with myocarditis showed dense Ga-67 uptake, whereas only 9 of 65 (14%) with negative biopsy samples were interrelated with equivocal positive Ga-67 scans (p < 0.001). Gallium uptake in these 9 patients was not as dense as those with biopsy proven myocarditis. Furthermore, although 5 of the 14 patients (36%) with positive Ga-67 scans had biopsy proven myocarditis, only 1 of 57 (1.8%) with a negative scan had a biopsy positive for myocarditis. In addition, changes in myocardium Ga-67 activity paralleled the clinical course of patients treated with immunosuppressive therapy for biopsy proven myocarditis. From 3 patients treated with immunosuppressive therapy, follow-up Ga-67 imaging showed that the scan became negative in 2 and changed from a diffuse pattern to a more localized pattern in the other one. They concluded that Ga-67 scanning may be a useful screening test for identifying patients with a high yield of biopsy proven myocarditis, and serial scans may eliminate the need for frequent biopsies in patients with proven myocarditis. The results from this study are in agreement with those of Camargo et al. (26) who compared endomyocardial biopsy and myocardial imaging with Ga-67 in 44 children with dilated cardiomyopathy. Evidence of myocarditis was demonstrated by endomyocardial biopsy in 32 (72.7%) patients; 21 (65.6%) of these had a positive Ga-67 scan and 11 (34.4%) had a negative scan. From the 12 patients that had a negative endomyocardial biopsy for myocarditis, 9 (75%) had a negative Ga-67 scan. Furthermore, the severity of inflammation in the biopsy was only mild in 9 of the 11 patients with positive biopsy and negative Gallium scans. Similarly, the authors concluded that the Ga-67 is a noninvasive diagnostic method with good sensitivity to establish the diagnosis of acute myocarditis in children with dilated cardiomyopathy. On the contrary, Bouhour et al. (27) found no correlation between Ga-67 imaging and endomyocardial biopsy findings in 91 patients with dilated cardiomyopathy and LVEF < 55%. Myocarditis defined as ≥5 mononuclear cells in the myocardial interstitium as counted in 20 fields at a magnification of ×400 was found in only four cases (4.4%). Ga-67 scans were negative in these four cases. Ga-67 scanning was positive in only 13 patients, none of which had a positive biopsy for myocarditis.

ANTIMYOSIN ANTIBODY CARDIAC IMAGING

Because myocyte necrosis is an obligatory component of myocarditis, monoclonal antimyosin Fab fragments labeled with Indium-111 have been used in patients suspected of having acute myocarditis (28,29,31–35). The technique is useful for detecting myocarditis in patients with both depressed and normal left ventricular function.

With this technique 500 μg of monoclonal antimyosin Fab fragments labeled with 1.5 mCi of Indium-111 are ad-

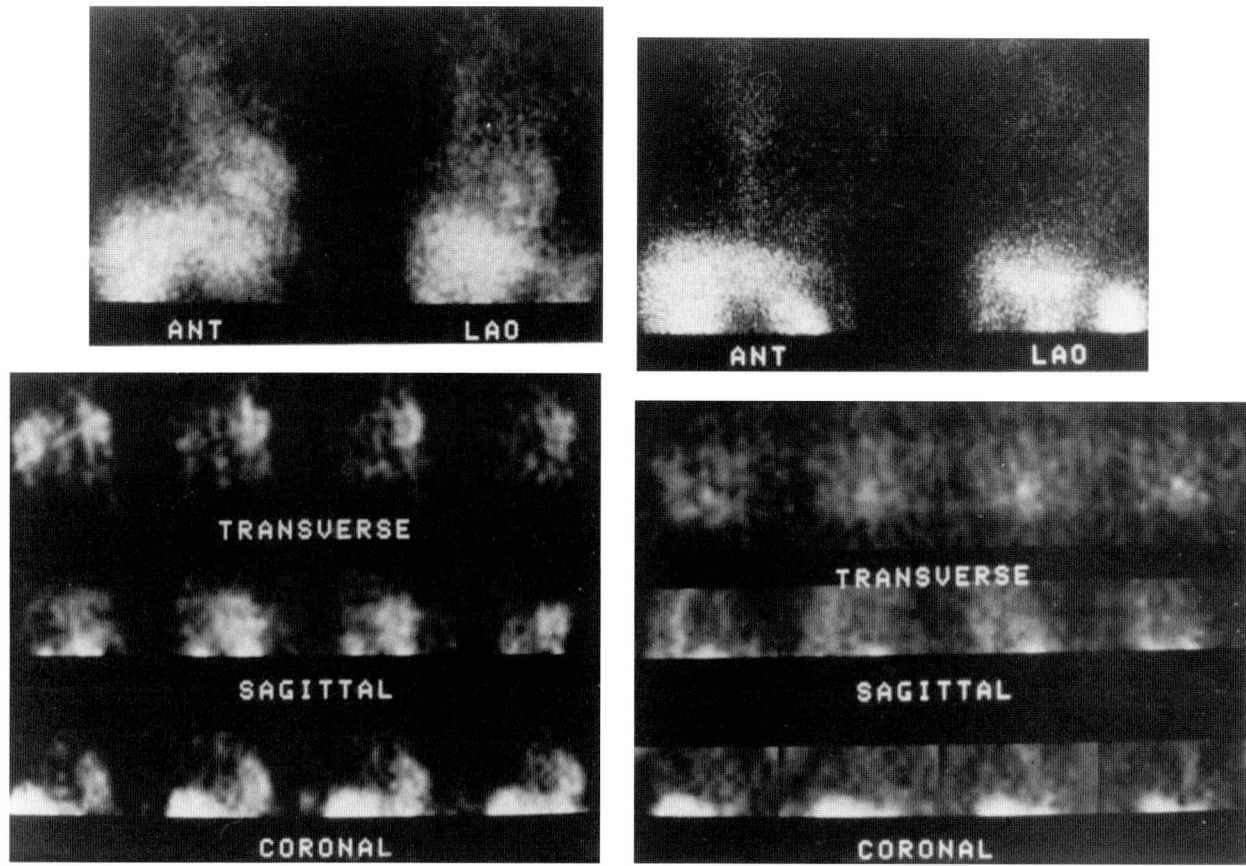

FIG. 1. Initial (**left panels**) and 6-month follow-up (**right panels**) antimyosin antibody imagines of a patient presenting with acute onset of dilated cardiomyopathy and biopsy proved acute myocarditis. Planar (**upper panels**) and tomographic reconstructions (**lower panels**) are shown. Intense diffuse tracer uptake is seen in the cardiac region in both the anterior (*ANT*) and the left anterior oblique (*LAO*) planar images and in the transverse, sagital and coronal tomographic reconstructions at the time of presentation (**left panels**). Her biopsy demonstrated acute myocarditis and her left ventricular ejection fraction (LVEF) was 34%. At 6-months follow-up (**right panels**) she had a normal antimyosin imaging. Nonspecific uptake is seen within the liver, spleen, and spine, but no activity is evident in the cardiac region in either the planar or the tomographic images. Her biopsy at follow-up showed healed myocarditis and her LVEF increased to 55%.

ministered through a peripheral vein and both planar and single-photon emission computed tomographic (SPECT) images are obtained at 48 h after administration of the agent. At 48 h the highest uptake is seen in the kidneys and then the hepatic regions. Some activities are present in the spleen and in the bone marrow. At 24 h the blood pool activity is too high for imaging of the myocardium. The plasma half-life of indium-111 labeled antimyosin antibody Fab is 5 hours. The plasma activity of the radiolabeled antibody decreases to 20% and to less than 10% at 24 and 48 h after the isotope injection. A scan is positive when focal or diffuse uptake of the tracer is present in the planar image and in at least two of the three tomographic reconstructions (Fig. 1). A scan is negative when no tracer is demonstrated in either planar or SPECT images or when faint activity is present in the planar image but not confirmed in the SPECT images. Antimyosin uptake can be analyzed quantitatively by the uptake ratio between the cardiac and the right lung regions.

When results of the scan and the biopsy were negative, the uptake ratio was less than 1.3. Positive results on antimyosin scan showed a much higher uptake of 1.69 ($p < 0.001$). There were no significant differences in this uptake ratio when the patients with positive scans were further divided into biopsies positive and negative (1.69 vs. 1.69). Carrio et al. (34) determined a heart to lung ratio and a visual score (0–3) in 16 antimyosin studies in 13 patients with suspected myocarditis. Eight normal controls had a ratio of 1.46 ± 0.04 and a score of 0. Patients with suspected myocarditis had an average ratio of 2.0 ± 0.5 and 11 of the 16 studies were visually positive with a score of 2 or 3. Evidence of myocarditis was demonstrated in the biopsy in only 4 of these patients showing ratios between 1.76 and 3.03 and a score of 2.

Radiolabeled Fab fragments of monoclonal antimyosin antibodies have been shown to bind to cardiac myocytes that have lost the integrity of their sarcolemmal membranes and exposed intracellular myosin to the extracellular fluid space (36–38). This image technique has been shown to localize areas of necrosis in patients with acute myocardial infarction (36–38). The general biodistribution of indium-111-labeled antimyosin antibody was studied in C3H/He mice with encephalomyocarditis virus infection by Kishimoto et al. (39). Significant myocardial uptake was demonstrated in 6 of 6 mice 10 days after viral infection and then subsided in 5 of 6 mice by 1 month. Pathological examination showed active and ongoing myocardial necrosis with dilated ventricles on day 10, less active necrosis and healing on day 20, and healing with increasing myocardial fibrosis in days 30 and 150. In the chronic stage, 2 of 5 mice on day 30 and 2 of 6 mice on day 150 had positive uptake. These findings support the role of antimyosin antibody imaging as a noninvasive method for the detection of the necrotic processes present in the acute and chronic stages of myocarditis.

Obrador et al. (35) compared antimyosin antibody uptake in 21 patients with dilated cardiomyopathy awaiting heart transplantation with the histological analyses of the explanted hearts. Antimyosin uptake was present in 15 patients (71%), but myocarditis in the explanted hearts was detected in only 7. In 11 patients there was an abnormal antimyosin scan and no histopathological evidence of myocarditis. These findings suggest ongoing myocyte damage in the absence of histological evidence of active myocarditis in patients with dilated cardiomyopathy.

Antimyosin imaging has been shown to be a useful technique for the diagnosis of myocarditis. The sensitivity, specificity, positive predictive value, and negative predictive value of antimyosin scintigraphy in patients suspected of having acute myocarditis were previously reported (28,29,31). The sensitivity is approximately 90–100%, specificity 50%, and negative predictive value 90%. Thus, the antimyosin scan can detect myocarditis and exclude myocarditis when compared with the myocarditis Dallas criteria.

In our first publication, with the use of this imaging technique, we compared the results of antimyosin antibody imaging with those of the myocardial biopsy in 28 patients clinically suspected of having myocarditis, 25 of whom had left ventricular ejection fractions less than 45% (28). Myocardial biopsy was positive for myocarditis in 9 (32%) patients, showed nonspecific findings in 13 patients (47%), and was normal in 6 patients (21%). Seventeen patients (61%) had positive scans. The scan was positive in the 9 patients who had evidence of myocarditis by biopsy and negative in the 11 who had no evidence of myocarditis by biopsy. The remaining 8 patients had positive antimyosin scans but no evidence of myocarditis by biopsy. Although this incongruity may be due to nonspecific antimyosin uptake, a lower sensitivity of myocardial biopsy due to sampling error is the more likely explanation for this discrepancy.

In a later publication we compared the results of antimyosin antibody imaging with those of right ventricular biopsy in 82 patients presenting with clinically suspected myocarditis, 74 of which had dilated cardiomyopathy of recent onset (<1-year duration) (29). Antimyosin antibody imaging was performed within 48 h of the right ventricular biopsy. Myocarditis was diagnosed by right ventricular biopsy in 18 patients (22%), a normal biopsy was present in 22 patients (27%), and nonspecific histopathological changes were present in the biopsy of the remaining 42 patients (51%). The antimyosin scan was positive in 45 patients (55%) and negative in 37 (45%). Fifteen of the 18 patients (83%) with biopsy-proved myocarditis had a positive scan. Three of the 37 patients (8.1%) with negative scans had evidence of myocarditis by biopsy. Thirty patients had a positive antimyosin scan and no evidence of myocarditis by myocardial biopsy. Using the right ventricular biopsy as a "gold standard" for diagnosing myocarditis, the following results were obtained: antimyosin scan sensitivity, 83%; antimyosin scan specificity, 53%; predictive value of a positive scan, 33%, and predictive value of a negative scan, 92%.

All but 2 of the 30 patients with positive scans and negative biopsies had dilated cardiomyopathy and presented with symptomatic heart failure. At 6-month follow-up, 16 of these 28 patients with dilated cardiomyopathy who had a positive scan and negative biopsy for myocarditis underwent a repeat evaluation of left ventricular ejection fraction by gated blood pool scan. Spontaneous improvement with a substantial increase in left ventricular ejection fraction occurred in 7 of them (Fig. 2). Because spontaneous improvement in ventricular function is a well-recognized feature of acute myocarditis, this data suggests that acute myocarditis was the cause of acute dilated cardiomyopathy and that myocardial biopsy failed to demonstrate the disease because of sampling error. Furthermore, improvement was demonstrated in 54% of the patients with positive scans (7 of the 10 patients with biopsy proved myocarditis and 7 of 16 with biopsy negative). In contrast, improvement occurred in only 18% of patients with

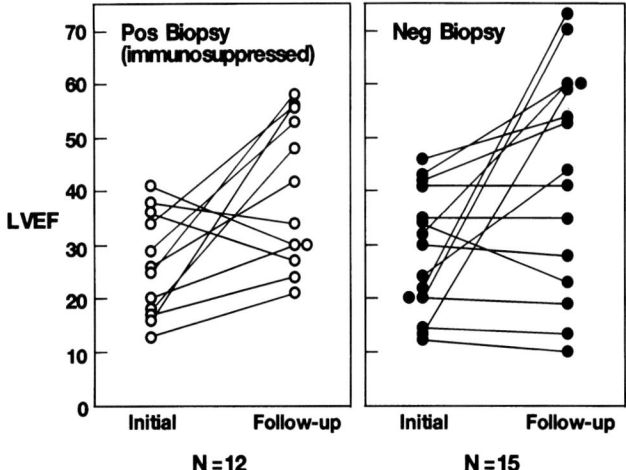

FIG. 2. Changes in left ventricular ejection fraction over time in patients with positive antimyosin antibody scans. Patients are divided into two groups, 12 with biopsy proved myocarditis treated with immunosuppression (**left panel**) and 15 without histological evidence of myocarditis (**right panel**).

negative scans ($p < 0.01$). Thus, antimyosin scan is useful as a screening method in the initial evaluation of patients with clinically suspected myocarditis. Furthermore, patients with positive scans are more likely to exhibit an increase in left ventricular ejection fraction within 6 months of follow-up, either spontaneously or during immunosuppressive therapy, than those with negative scans.

Narula et al. (31) compared the results of antimyosin antibody imaging with those of endomyocardial biopsy. They reported a 100% sensitivity, a 44% specificity, a positive predictive value of 48%, and a negative predictive value of 100%. Compared with myocardial biopsy, antimyosin scintigraphy has a higher sensitivity and higher negative predictive value for diagnosing myocarditis. However, a large number of patients suspected of myocarditis have negative biopsy and positive antimyosin scans. The more likely explanation for this finding is that the lack of sensitivity of endomyocardial biopsy is due to the focal nature of the disease.

Since spontaneous improvement is a frequent clinical manifestation of acute myocarditis, Narula et al. (31,32) examined the diagnostic accuracy of both antimyosin antibody imaging and endomyocardial biopsy using a significant improvement in left ventricular ejection fraction at follow-up as clinical evidence of myocarditis. They demonstrated that endomyocardial biopsy had a poor sensitivity (35%) but a high specificity (79%) for predicting a favorable outcome. Although, a positive biopsy predicted an improvement in ejection fraction, it failed to diagnose a large proportion of patients who subsequently improved. The predictive values of a positive and a negative endomyocardial biopsy were 55% and 63%, respectively. In contrast, antimyosin scan demonstrated a very high sensitivity (82 to 94%) in predicting improvement. The predictive values of a positive and a negative scan were 45 to 52% and 75 to 90%, respectively. The specificity was not as impressive (25 to 42%). Thus, a positive antimyosin scan has a significantly greater ability than myocardial biopsy to identify patients with acute onset of dilated cardiomyopathy likely to have an improvement in the ejection fraction over time.

Werner et al. (40) assessed the role of antimyosin antibody imaging in 36 patients with idiopathic dilated cardiomyopathy. All patients had a negative left ventricular endomyocardial biopsy for myocarditis. Thirteen of the 36 patients (36%) had positive scans and 23 (64%) had a negative scan. At 21 ± 12 months' follow-up there were two and ten cardiac deaths in the former and latter groups respectively ($p = 0.12$). The corresponding 2-year survival rates were 81 and 59%, respectively. This study suggests that ongoing cardiac myocyte damage occurs in a subgroup of patients with idiopathic dilated cardiomyopathy. The trend toward a more favorable clinical outcome in this group of patients with positive scans is in agreement with the results of Dec et al. (29) showing a greater incidence of improvement in ventricular function at follow-up in patients with positive antimyosin scans.

Lekakis et al. (33) examined the natural evolution of a positive antimyosin scan in 10 patients with acute myocarditis. These patients had evidence of myocarditis by positive endomyocardial biopsy and antimyosin scans. They underwent repeat assessment of left ventricular function and antimyosin scans at 1, 2, and 6 months. During follow-up 2.2 repeat antimyosin scans per patient were performed. Heart-to-lung ratio normalized (<1.6) within 1 month in 4 patients, within 2 months in 1 patient, and within 6 months in 2 patients; 3 patients continued to have positive antimyosin scan at 6 months, suggesting ongoing myocardial necrosis. Improvement in ventricular function was demonstrated at the end of follow-up in only 4 patients. Normalization or persistence of tracer uptake could not predict an improvement in left ventricular ejection fraction. These findings are in agreement with our previous study demonstrating a lack of correlation between the histological findings on repeat endomyocardial biopsy and changes in left ventricular ejection fraction early during immunosuppressive therapy in 20 patients with biopsy proved myocarditis (41). Improvement of LVEF occurred in patients with evidence of ongoing, healing, or healed myocarditis at follow-up myocardial biopsy. These 20 patients presented with heart failure due to dilated cardiomyopathy of recent onset (<6 months, LVEF ≤ 0.40). At repeat biopsy, 8 patients had evidence of ongoing myocarditis and 12 showed resolved myocarditis. Left ventricular ejection fraction improved in 8 of the 12 patients with resolved myocarditis. Left ventricular ejection fraction also improved in 4 of the 8 patients despite evidence of ongoing myocarditis in the biopsy. However, regardless of the histological findings on repeat biopsy, early improvement in ejection fraction was associated with an excellent long-term prognosis.

Thus, although antimyosin scintigraphy is useful for diagnosing myocarditis, an improvement in LVEF cannot be predicted on the basis of persistence or not of tracer uptake of repeat scans at follow-up.

Narula et al. (42) used antimyosin antibody imaging in 8 patients presenting with acute myocarditis masquerading as acute myocardial infarction. These 8 patients presented with chest pain and electrocardiographic changes similar to that of an acute myocardial infarction. These patients underwent coronary arteriography, endomyocardial biopsy, and antimyosin cardiac imaging. All 8 patients had normal coronary arteries. The antimyosin scan revealed diffuse, heterogeneous, and global left ventricular uptake in 7 patients. Myocardial biopsy was positive for myocarditis in 4 of the 7 patients with positive scans. Two more of the 7 patients had evidence of borderline myocarditis in the biopsy.

OTHER RADIOISOTOPE IMAGING MODALITIES

Thallium-201 (Tl-201) imaging has been found to be of value in differentiating patients with ischemic dilated cardiomyopathy from those with idiopathic dilated cardiomyopathy (43). Although in patients with idiopathic dilated cardiomyopathy, thallium uptake is relatively uniform, in patients with dilated cardiomyopathy owed to coronary artery disease a large defect in tracer uptake of greater than 40% of the image circumference can be detected reflecting massive myocardial replacement by fibrosis. Although small scattered defects in tracer uptake may be found in patients with dilated cardiomyopathy, the magnitude of these defects is usually less than 20% of the circumference and does not account for the extent of left ventricular dysfunction. Tl-201 imaging is valuable in the evaluation of patients with sarcoidosis (44). Myocardial involvement with sarcoid may produce multifocal regions of reduced tracer activity corresponding to regions of granuloma or scar. Tl-201 has also been used in patients with myocarditis but its results has not been very impressive. With this technique focal areas of reduced thallium uptake were documented by Tamaki et al. (45) in 3 of 6 patients with clinically documented myocarditis and by Bulkley et al. (43) in 3 of 8 patients with dilated cardiomyopathy. However, the imaging findings are nonspecific, resembling those of coronary artery disease.

Finally, indium-111 oxine-labeled granulocytes imaging was used by Becker et al. (46) in 17 patients with exudative perimyocardial disease. However, the technique yielded positive results in only 6 of the 17 patients, indicating a low sensitivity of this imaging modality.

MAGNETIC RESONANCE IMAGING

Myocardial edema has been demonstrated by magnetic resonance imaging using T2-weighted images in several case reports of patients with myopericarditis due to Lyme disease, acute viral myocarditis, systemic lupus erythematosus, and rheumatic myocarditis (47–49). However, T2-weighted images are susceptible to motion, and the image quality of the myocardium is poor. More recently, contrast media-enhanced MRI has been used to visualize the localization, activity, and extent of inflammation in patients with myocarditis. Friedrich et al. (50) recently reported their experience with the use ECG triggered, T1-weighted images before and after the application of 0.1 mmol/kg gadolinium in 19 patients with suspected myocarditis. These patients had clinical and laboratory data suggestive of acute myocarditis including electrocardiographic changes, reduced systolic function, elevated creatine kinase, positive troponin T, serological evidence for acute viral infection, exclusion of coronary artery disease, and positive antimyosin scintigraphy. Global relative signal enhancement of the left ventricular myocardium related to skeletal muscle were measured in these patients on days 2, 7, 14, 28, and 84 after the onset of symptoms and compared it with measurements of 18 volunteers. The global relative enhancement was higher in patients on days 2 (4.6 ± 0.3 vs. 2.5 ± 0.2; $p < 0.0001$); 7 (4.7 ± 0.5; $p < 0.0001$); 14 (4.6 ± 0.5; $p < 0.0002$); and 28 (3.9 ± 0.4; $p = 0.009$) but not on day 84 (3.1 ± 0.3; $p =$ NS). On day 2 the enhancement was focal, whereas at later points, the enhancement was diffuse suggesting that acute myocarditis evolves from a focal to a disseminated process during the first 2 weeks after the onset of symptoms. In patients with

evidence of ongoing disease, the values remained elevated. Belloti et al. (51) used magnetic resonance imaging with gadolinium enhancement to guide endomyocardial biopsy and surgical biopsies to sites with more intense inflammatory processes in 8 patients with Chagas heart disease. They found evidence of myocarditis in at least one myocardial fragment in all patients. Furthermore, *Trypanosoma cruzi* antigen was detected in 71% of the segments with histopathologic evidence of myocarditis while *T. cruzi* antigens were detected in only 16% of regions with only mild or absent myocarditis.

These preliminary results are encouraging and suggest that contrast-enhanced MRI may serve as a powerful noninvasive diagnostic tool in acute myocarditis.

REFERENCES

1. Fuster V, Gersh BJ, Giuliani ER, et al. The natural history of idiopathic dilated cardiomyopathy. *Am J Cardiol* 1981;47:525–531.
2. Woodruff JF. Viral myocarditis—a review. *Am J Pathol* 1980;101: 427–479.
3. Dec GW Jr, Palacios IF, Fallon JT, et al. Active myocarditis in the spectrum of acute dilated cardiomyopathies: clinical features, histologic correlates, and clinical outcome. *N Engl J Med* 1985;312:887.
4. Johnson RA, Palacios IF. Dilated cardiomyopathies of the adult (first part). *N Engl J Med* 1982;307:1051.
5. Johnson RA, Palacios IF. Dilated cardiomyopathies of the adult (second part). *N Engl J Med* 1982;307:1119.
6. Dec GW Jr, Waldman HW, Southern JF, et al. Viral myocarditis mimicking acute myocardial infarction. *J Am Coll Cardiol* 1992;20:85–89.
7. Huber SA, Lodge PA. Coxsackievirus B-3 myocarditis—Identification of different pathogenic mechanisms in DBA/2 and BALB/c mice. *Am J Pathol* 1986;122:284–291.
8. Huber SA, Lodge PA. Coxsackie virus B3 myocarditis in BALB/mice: evidence of autoimmunity to myocyte antigens. *Am J Pathol* 1984;116: 21–29.
9. Wilson FM, Miranda QR, Chason Jl, et al. Residual pathologic changes following murine Coxackie A and B myocarditis. *Am J Pathol* 1969; 55:253–265.
10. Paque RE, Gaunti CJ, Nealon TJ, et al. Assessment of cell-mediated hypersensitivity against Coxsackie B3 viral induced myocarditis utilizing hypertonic salt extracts of cardiac tissue. *J Immunol* 1978;120: 1672–1678.
11. Reyes MP, Ho KL, Smith E, et al. A mouse model of dilated-type cardiomyopathy due to Coxsackie virus B3. *J Infect Dis* 1981;155: 232–236.
12. Parrillo JE, Aretz HT, Palacios IF, et al. The results of transvenous endomyocardial biopsy can frequently be used to diagnose myocardial diseases in patients with idiopathic heart failure: endomyocardial biopsies in 100 consecutive patients revealed a substantial incidence of myocarditis. *Circulation* 1984;69:93.
13. Mason JW, Billingham ME, Ricci DR. Treatment of acute inflammatory myocarditis assisted by endomyocardial biopsy. *Am J Cardiol* 1980;45:1037.
14. Nippoldi TB, Edwards WD, Holmes DR Jr, et al. Right ventricular endomyocardial biopsy: Clinicopathologic correlates in 100 consecutive patients. *Mayo Clin Proc* 1982;57:407–481.
15. Fenoglio JJ Jr, Ursell PC, Kellogg CF, et al. Diagnosis and classification of myocarditis by endomyocardial biopsy. *N Engl J Med* 1983; 308:12–18.
16. Zee-Cheng CS, Tsai CC, Palmer DC et al. High incidence of myocarditis by endomyocardial biopsy in patients with idiopathic congestive cardiomyopathy and biopsy proven myocarditis. *J Am Coll Cardiol* 1984;3:63–70.
17. Unverferth DV, Fetters JK, Unverferth BJ, et al. Human myocardial histologic characteristics in congestive heart failure. *Circulation* 1983; 68:1194–1200.
18. Hosepud JD, McAnulty JH, Miles NR. Lack of objective improvement in ventricular systolic function in patients with myocarditis treated with azathioprine and prednisone. *J Am Colll Cardiol* 1985;6:797–801.

19. French WJ, Siegel RJ, Cohen AH, et al. Yield of endomyocardial biopsy in patients with biventricular failure: comparison of patients with normal versus reduced left ventricular ejection fraction. *Chest* 1986;90:181–184.
20. Cassling RS, Linder J, Sears TD, et al. Quantitation of inflammation in biopsy specimens from idiopathically failing or irritable hearts: Experience in 80 pediatric and adult patients. *Am Heart J* 1985;110:713–720.
21. Aretz HT, Billingham ME, Edwards WD, et al. Myocarditis, a histopathologic definition and classification. *Am J Cardiovasc Pathol* 1986;1:3.
22. Davidoff R, Palacios I, Southern J, et al. Giant cell versus lymphocytic myocarditis. A comparison of their clinical features and long-term outcomes. *Circulation* 1991;83:953–961.
23. Mason JW, O'Connell JB, Herskowitz A, et al. A clinical trial of immunosuppressive therapy for myocarditis: The Myocarditis Treatment Trial Investigators. *N Engl J Med* 1995;333:269–275.
24. O'Connell JB, Robinson JA, Henkin RE, et al. Immunosuppressive therapy in patients with congestive cardiomyopathy and uptake of gallium-67. *Circulation* 1981;64:780–786.
25. O'Connell JB, Henkin RE, Robinson JA, et al. Gallium-67 imaging in patients with dilated cardiomyopathy and biopsy proven myocarditis. *Circulation* 1984;70:58–62.
26. Camargo PR, Mazzieri R, Snitcowsky R, et al. Endomyocardial biopsy and myocardial imaging with 67-gallium in the diagnosis of active myocarditis in children with dilated cardiomyopathy. *Arquivos Brasileiros de Cardiologia* 1990;54:27–31.
27. Bouhour JB, Helias J, de Lajartre AY, et al. Detection of myocarditis during the first year after discovery of a dilated cardiomyopathy by endomyocardial biopsy and gallium-67 myocardial scintigraphy: prospective multicenter French study of 91 patients. *Eur Heart J* 1988;9:520–528.
28. Yasuda T, Palacios IF, Dec GW, et al. Indium-111 monoclonal antibody imaging in the diagnosis of acute myocarditis. *Circulation* 1987;76:306.
29. Dec GW, Palacios I, Yasuda T, et al. Antimyosin antibody cardiac imaging: its role in the diagnosis of myocarditis. *J Am Coll Cardiol* 1990;16:97–104.
30. Reeves WC, Jackson GL, Flickinger FW, et al. Radionuclide imaging of experimental myocarditis. *Circulation* 1981;63:640–644.
31. Narula J, Khaw BA, Dec GW, et al. Diagnostic accuracy of antimyosin scintigraphy in suspected myocarditis. *J Nucl Cardiol* 1996;3:371–381.
32. Narula J, Southern JF, Dec GW, et al. Antimyosin uptake and myofibrillar lysis in dilated cardiomyopathy. *J Nucl Cardiol* 1995;2:470–477.
33. Lekakis J, Nanas J, Prassopoulos V, et al. Natural evolution of antimyosin scan and cardiac function in patients with acute myocarditis. *Int J Cardiol* 1995;52:53–58.
34. Carrio I, Berna L, Ballester M, et al. Indium-111 antimyosin scintigraphy to assess myocardial damage in patients with suspected myocarditis and cardiac rejection. *J Nucl Med* 1988;29:1893–1900.
35. Obrador D, Ballester M, Carrio I, et al. Active myocardial damage

without attending inflammatory response in dilated cardiomyopathy. *J Am Coll Cardiol* 1993;21:1667–1671.
36. Khaw BA, Fallon JT, Strauss HW, et al. Myocardial infarct imaging of antibodies to canine cardiac myosin with indium-111-diethylenetriamine pentaacetic acid. *Science* 1980;209:295–297.
37. Khaw BA, Fallon JT, Beller GA, et al. Specificity of localization of myosin specific antibody fragments in experimental myocardial infarction: histologic, histochemical, autoradiographic and scintigraphic studies. *Circulation* 1979;60:1527–1531.
38. Khaw BA, Beller GA, Haber E, et al. Localization of cardiac myosin-specific antibody in myocardial infarction. *J Clin Invest* 1976;58:439–446.
39. Kishimoto C, Hung GL, Ishibashi M, et al. Natural evolution of cardiac function, cardiac pathology and antimyosin scan in a murine myocardial model. *J Am Coll Cardiol* 1991;17:821–827.
40. Werner GS, Figula HR, Muntz DL, et al. Myocardial Indium-111 antimyosin uptake in patients with idiopathic dilated cardiomyopathy: relation to hemodynamics, histomorphometry, myocardial enteroviral infection, and clinical course. *Eur Heart J* 1993;14:175–184.
41. Dec GW, Fallon JT, Southern JF, et al. Relation between histological findings on early repeat right ventricular biopsy and ventricular function in patients with myocarditis. *Br Heart J* 1988;60:332.
42. Narula J, Khaw BA, Dec GW Jr, et al. Brief report: Recognition of acute myocarditis masquerading as acute myocardial infarction. *N Engl J Med* 1993;328:100–104.
43. Bulkley BH, Hutchins GM, Bailey I, et al. Thallium-201 imaging and gated cardiac pool scans in patients with ischemic and idiopathic congestive cardiomyopathy. *Circulation* 1977;55:753–760.
44. Bulkley BH, Rouleau J, Strauss HW, et al. Sarcoid heart disease: diagnosis by thallium-201 myocardial perfusion imaging. *Am J Cardiol* 1976;37:125.
45. Tamaki N, Yonekura Y, Kadota K, et al. Thallium-201 myocardial perfusion imaging in myocarditis. *Clin Nucl Med* 1985;10:562–566.
46. Becker W, Borst V, Maisch B, et al. In-111-labeled granulocytes in inflammatory heart diseases. *Eur Heart J* 1987;8(suppl J):307–310.
47. Gagliardi MG, Bevilacqua M, Di Renzi P, et al. Usefulness of magnetic resonance imaging for diagnosis of acute myocarditis in infant and children, and comparison with endomyocardial biopsy. *Am J Cardiol* 1991;68:1089–1091.
48. Been M, Thompson BJ, Smith MA, et al. Myocardial involvement in systemic lupus erythematosus detected by magnetic resonance imaging. *Eur Heart J* 1988;9:1250–1256.
49. Chandraratna PA, Bradley WG, Kortman KE, et al. Detection of acute myocarditis using nuclear magnetic resonance imaging. *Am J Med* 1987;83:1144–1146.
50. Friedrich MG, Strohm O, Schultz-Menger J, et al. Contrast media-enhanced magnetic resonance imaging visualizes myocardial changes in the course of viral myocarditis. *Circulation* 1998;97:1802–1809.
51. Belloti G, Bocchi EA, de Moraes AV, et al. *In vivo* detection of trypanosoma cruzi antigens in hearts of patients with chronic Chagas' heart disease. *Am Heart J* 1996;131:301–307.

CHAPTER 50

Noninvasive Methods of Evaluating Cardiac Allograft Rejection

Brian A. Foley

The endomyocardial biopsy has been the mainstay in evaluating cardiac allografts for episodes of rejection since the beginnings of cardiac transplantation (1). Although effective, it is expensive, invasive, and not without a small but inherent risk to the patient. It must be performed frequently in the initial posttransplant period due to the increased incidence of rejection in the first 6 months after transplantation. The goal of frequent biopsies is to diagnose allograft rejection in its early stages to allow enhanced medical immunosuppression before the onset of hemodynamic compromise.

The rejection grading system is based on the number of white blood cells (WBCs) per high power field observed as determined subjectively by the pathologist (2). They are graded from 0 to 4 with grade 0 being the number of WBCs expected in nontransplanted myocardium (Fig. 1; see Color Plate 28 following page 758). Grade I rejection is a mildly elevated number of WBCs and is further subdivided into Ia and Ib based on the pattern of WBC clustering being focal or diffuse, respectively. Grade II is a more severe elevation in WBCs in a single isolated focus within otherwise grade 0 or 1 myocardium, and has no subdivisions. Grade III is a moderately severe elevation and is again subdivided into IIIa and IIIb as with grade I. Myocyte damage and hemodynamic compromise are sometimes associated with grade IIIa rejections, but less often in the current era of newer immunosuppressive medications. Grade IIIb is very severe rejection and is associated with myocyte necrosis and typically with hemodynamic compromise. Grade IV is very severe, and very rare in the current era, and is always associated with myocyte necrosis and hemodynamic compromise.

B. A. Foley: Department of Medicine, Division of Cardiology, University of Alabama at Birmingham, Birmingham, Alabama 35294.

Grades 0 to Ia rejections are the goal posttransplant. Grades Ib and II are typically treated initially with minor adjustments to the immunosuppressive regimen and heightened frequency of surveillance biopsies. They often resolve spontaneously back to grades 0 or Ia, but if persistent may require more aggressive enhancement of the immunosuppressive regimen. Grades III and higher always warrant aggressive treatment since they have a much higher incidence of continuing to progress to higher grades (3) and ultimately to hemodynamic compromise, with the potential of permanent damage to the organ or death.

The goal of any noninvasive monitoring method, therefore, is to mimic the grading scale of the endomyocardial biopsy, allowing the detection and treatment of rejection in its early stages before the morbidity and mortality begin to rise. Multiple imaging modalities have been investigated and can be subdivided into the following categories: quantification of WBC presence and/or myocyte necrosis within the myocardium; monitoring changes in various tissue characteristics; evaluation of hemodynamic changes including both systolic and diastolic changes; and monitoring of changes in electrical characteristics as rejection progresses.

QUANTIFICATION OF WBC PRESENCE AND MYOCARDIAL NECROSIS

In 1987 Eisen et al. (4) demonstrated in a canine model that labeling WBCs with indium-111 (^{111}In) could be used to quantify rejection in heterotopically transplanted hearts. Because the hearts were transplanted heterotopically the survival of the test animal was not dependent upon the transplanted organ. This allowed a group of 11 animals to be studied throughout the complete natural history of cardiac rejection, until the donor organ ceased to function. Another group of 5 animals was initially treated with cyclosporin and

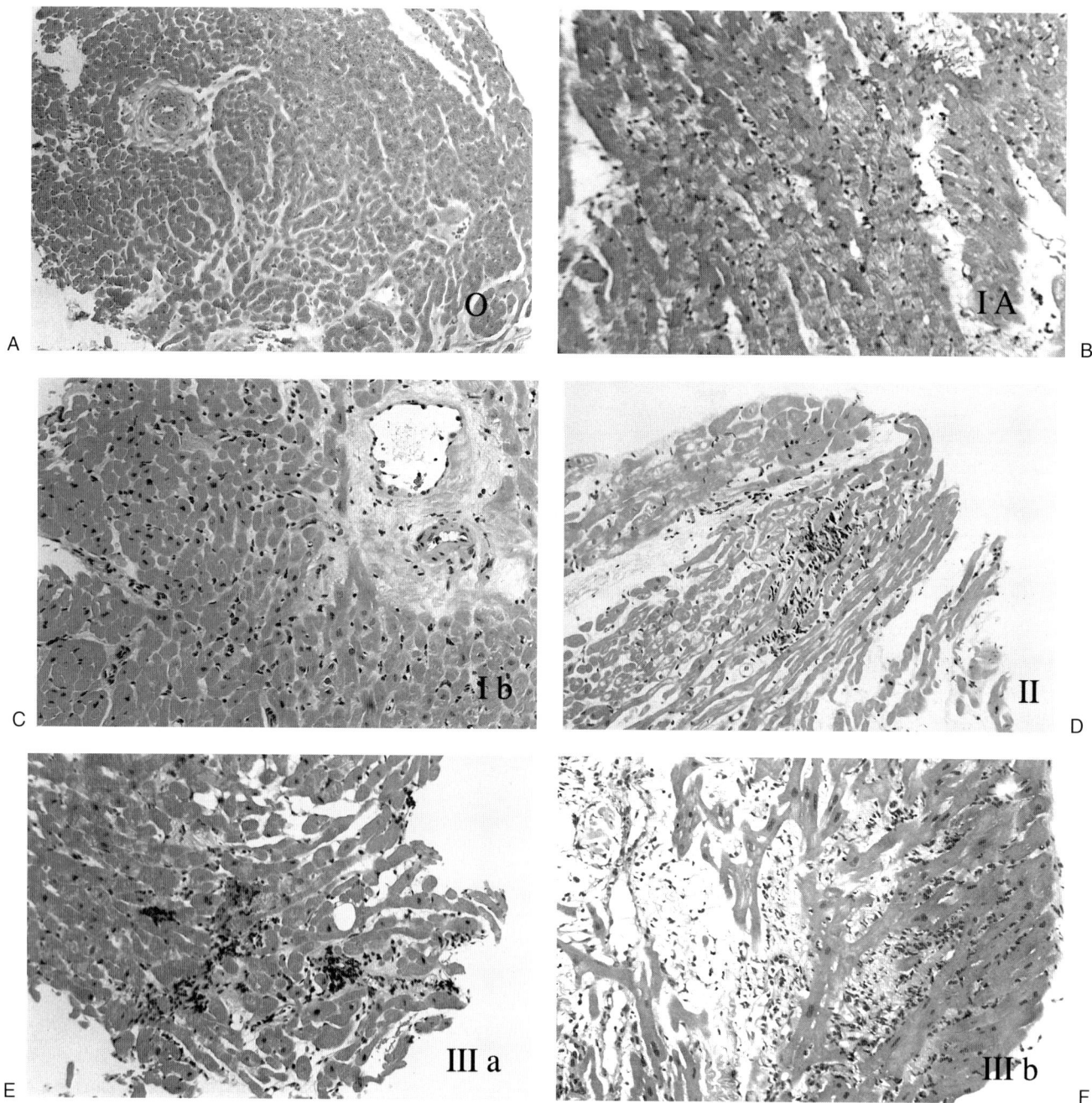

FIG. 1. Pathology of endomyocardial biopsy. **A:** Grade 0 is normal myocardium. **B:** Grade Ia is mild focal rejection. **C:** Grade Ib is mild diffuse rejection. **D:** Grade II is a single focus of high-grade rejection in an otherwise grade 0 or 1 biopsy. **E:** Grade IIIa is moderately severe focal rejection. **F:** Grade IIIb is severe diffuse rejection, note the myocyte necrosis. Grade IV is not shown due to its rarity, but has further infiltration than IIIb with more extensive myocyte necrosis diffusely. (See Color Plate 28 following page 758.)

prednisone to determine if the presence of these immunosuppressive medications altered the correlation of radionuclide imaging to rejection as determined by right ventricular (RV) biopsy. In addition, each animal served as its own control by comparing the scintigrams of the native heart to that of the transplanted organ. To correct for radioactivity of labeled lymphocytes circulating in the blood pool, the investigators

labeled red blood cells (RBCs) with technetium-99m (Tc-99m) and subtracted this image from the ^{111}In image. All episodes of moderate to severe rejection were detected by increases in ^{111}In image intensity greater than four standard deviations from the norm. All grade 0 or Ia rejections were read as normal. Unfortunately, only 75% (3 of 4) of the mild episodes (grades Ib or II) were detected, providing inadequate sensitivity in this critical range necessitating confirmation with biopsies. Other drawbacks of the technique included: exposure to levels of radiation allowing only 5 to 6 exams per year, lengthy image acquisition times, and confusion by co-morbidities such as ischemia-induced reperfusion injury, and concomitant infections.

A variation of this technique was used in a human trial in which a monoclonal Fab fragment, antimyosin, was labeled with ^{111}In. Developed originally to diagnose acute myocardial infarction, this antibody binds to the myosin that has leaked into the interstitial spaces from damaged myocardium, but not to myosin in undamaged cells (5). This trial was performed in a prospective manner on 38 patients undergoing orthotopic heart transplantation. After the first 70 scintigraphies the investigators determined that the heart to lung (H/L) ratio could not discriminate between rejection and nonrejection, but that a decrease in this ratio from the prior measurement was never associated with biopsy proven rejection. They completed the study with this as a prospective criterion. The negative predictive value of scintigraphy was 98% (95% confidence limits 90–100%). They predicted that 50% of the biopsies could be avoided using negative scintigraphy criterion. Unfortunately, the 2% incidence of grade IIIa rejections missed by this technique could have perilous consequences for those patients. Also, the dose of radiation delivered to the patient after repeated exams is equivalent to a ventriculogram. Although not observed in this study, antimyosin is murine in origin and the development of murine antibodies is possible. Finally, the incidence of rejection episodes in this study was very low at 10, thus necessitating a much larger controlled trial before conclusions are drawn.

One very interesting variation performed in a limited murine model involves simultaneous administration of ^{123}Iodine-labeled antimyosin and ^{111}In-labeled MHC class II antibodies (6). The use of the second isotope allowed the detection of upregulation of MHC class II antigens on cardiac myocytes correlating to earlier stages of rejection, before cell damage had occurred. This has the potential to increase the sensitivity and specificity of radionuclide techniques, but is still limited by the dose of radiation administered and the lack of human trials.

TISSUE CHARACTERIZATION IN CARDIAC REJECTION

Tissue characterization techniques allow the monitoring of changes in specific parameters of the allograft myocardium over time. Modalities that allow noninvasive detection include echocardiography, magnetic resonance cardiac imaging, and magnetic resonance spectroscopy of myocardial high-energy phosphate metabolism.

Echocardiographic Methods

As early as 1981 an increase in LV mass was noted to be associated with high-grade rejection. Sagar et al. (7) con-

ducted a study in 15 patients who were at least 3 months posttransplant, using M-mode echocardiography to determine the LV mass of the allograft. Echos were performed at the times of their routine 3-month surveillance biopsies and whenever a biopsy was performed due to suspicion of rejection. Technically optimal studies could be obtained in only 13 of the patients. There were 12 episodes of rejection in 7 patients. A 139% average increase in LV mass was noted, rising from 129.8 ± 11.8 g to 310 ± 130 g. LV mass subsequently returned to baseline with resolution of the rejection episode in 6 patients. The 7th patient did not show a reduction in LV mass and ultimately died of refractory rejection 6 months after transplant. This rather striking observation unfortunately only correlated well with high-grade rejection episodes of level 3A and higher, and was insensitive to the intermediate grades. In addition, this study was performed in the precyclosporin era of immunosuppression. The enhanced immunosuppression achieved with cyclosporin today has reduced the inflammation and edema associated with grade 3A level rejections significantly (8,9). Subsequent studies confirmed increase in LV mass with severe rejection, but to a much less extensive degree than in the precyclosporin era (10), and with correspondingly less sensitivity to intermediate grade rejections. This is of particular interest in the pediatric transplant population where increased technical difficulty and risk are associated with the performance of endomyocardial biopsies, and so echocardiographic assessment is often used as a substitute (11). Although increased LV mass is noted in this population as well, significant interobserver and intraobserver variability exists, thus limiting the utility of this technique (12).

In a more recent study Gill et al. (13) failed to demonstrate statistically significant increase in LV mass during cellular rejection. They did, however, note significantly increased LV mass in the setting of humoral, or "vascular," allograft rejection. This form of rejection is not associated with the histologic change of increased cellularity, and is not predicted by routine endomyocardial biopsy. It is much less common and, in general, tends to appear earlier after transplantation than cellular rejection, and tends to be associated with a worse prognosis (14,15). Immunofluorescent staining of endomyocardial biopsy specimens may reveal deposition of complement and immunoglobulin in the perivascular space as well as capillary leakage of fibrin (16). Immunofluorescent staining is not routinely performed in most transplant centers, however, due to the requirements of additional tissue extraction at the time of biopsy, increased cost, and relative infrequency of this form of rejection. For now echocardiographic detection of increased LV mass and decreased LV function remain the mainstay of detection of this form of allograft rejection.

Newer echocardiographic techniques include the use of ultrasonographic tissue characterization (UTC) techniques (17). UTC is the evaluation of the variability of the myocardial "texture" based on its acoustic properties. Variations in the microscopic structure of myocardium will influence its acoustic characteristics. Nonrejecting myocardium has a fairly consistent, even texture. Rejecting myocardium displays a much greater variability through a sample volume element. Using these techniques, indices of tissue homogeneity and heterogeneity have been defined. In one study, Gotteiner et al. (18) examined 22 pediatric patients ranging in age from 8 days to 17.5 years. There were 13 boys and 9 girls. Four different parameters were measured and combined to form a mathematical prediction. The sensitivity was 96% of first rejection episodes, 93% of moderate and severe rejection episodes, and 69% of all episodes. Unfortunately, chronic changes in tissue after an initial rejection episode limit the utility in subsequent episodes. In addition, the sample volumes are small, and can be deceived by the "patchy" character of cardiac rejection. Overall this technique has potential to evolve into a useful method as technology progresses, but for now is complex with inadequate sensitivity and specificity. Another variant of this technique involves the use of end-diastolic 2-dimensional integrated backscatter (2D-IB). This involves mathematical evaluation of the raw, unprocessed RF signal derived from the ultrasonic transducer. It again derives an index of tissue density variability. It also suffers from the same limitations, and is most sensitive only for tissue that is becoming edematous, implying severe rejection.

Magnetic Resonance Imaging Methods

Magnetic resonance imaging provides a sensitive measure of LV thickness and mass. As previously discussed, increased LV thickness and mass have been correlated with worsening grades of cardiac rejection. In this setting the MRI criteria for assessing myocardial rejection are similar to those used in echocardiography. Similar arguments apply to the limitations of these parameters, particularly in the cyclosporin era, because significant LV mass increase now tends to be limited to severe rejection episodes only.

Attempts have also been made to correlate the T1- and T2-weighted relaxation times with rejection. These parameters are unique to MRI and tend to reflect the quantity of tissue water within edematous myocardium. The greater the degree of inflammation, the more prolonged the T1 and T2 relaxation times. Aherne et al. (19) applied this technology to the tissue characterization of endomyocardial biopsy samples in heterotopic canine cardiac transplants in 1986. This study demonstrated a clear increase in the T2-weighted relaxation times in rejecting hearts as the rejection proceeded from mild to moderate by histologic examination. There was, however, no further prolongation as the rejection proceeded from moderate to severe. There was considerable overlap in the T1 relaxation times between nonrejecting and rejecting hearts, although this may have been distorted by variations in heart rate. There were no significant differences in the T2 or T1 relaxation times in animals treated with cyclosporin with the exception of two animals that showed simultaneous histologic evidence of rejection despite therapy. Wisenberg

et al. (20) performed a human trial in 1987. In this trial myocardium was imaged *in vivo* in 25 transplant patients, using 10 normal volunteers and 4 patients status post-nontransplant cardiac surgery as controls. Interestingly, in this trial, imaging during the first 25 days after transplantation revealed significant elevations in both the T1 and T2 relaxation times as well as increased wall thickness in all transplant patients, whereas nontransplant surgical patients had no evidence of elevation of any of the parameters. These abnormalities in the transplant population seemed to resolve after the initial 25-day time frame. In late images (after 25 days) prolongation of the T1 time, T2 time, or increase in wall thickness greater than 2 standard deviations from normal correctly identified 14 out of 15 rejection episodes, and 1 of 28 images was falsely labeled as rejecting when significant rejection was absent. The highly abnormal parameters during the initial 25-day period in this study were attributed to the prolonged ischemic time involved in transplantation as opposed to other cardiac surgeries. In this study the average ischemic time was 4 to 5 hours. In contradiction to the results of Wisenberg et al. a European trial in 29 heart transplant patients by Revel et al. (21), demonstrated no reliable prolongation of either the T1 or T2 relaxation times. They did, however, confirm the increase in LV wall thickness. There were, however, only 33 examinations in 29 patients, so little sequential data was available to correlate nonrejecting states with active rejection within the same patient. Additionally the grades of rejection did not exceed grades 1 to 2, thus only mild to moderate rejection was observed, which could possibly account for the absence of the changes characteristic in the Wisenberg trial. A subsequent trial by Doornbos et al. (22), in 7 transplant patients and 7 controls acquired 42 exams and again captured no biopsy grade greater than grade 2. This trial did show a trend toward prolongation of the T2 times in the grade 2 biopsy patients, but this trend was much too small to achieve statistical significance.

In an attempt to increase the sensitivity of MRI for the detection of rejection, Mousseaux et al. studied MRI data in 39 patients and 7 healthy volunteers with the addition of the myocardial contrast agent gadolinium tetraazacyclododecane (Gd-DTPA) during the study. This is a paramagnetic contrast agent that improves visualization and characterization, particularly of myocardial injury in ischemic heart disease (23). Although the authors found a significant increase in myocardial enhancement (ME) in rejecting patients, they were unable to accurately separate patients who needed enhanced immunosuppression from those not requiring intervention. They also noted significant difficulty with acquiring adequate image quality to perform T2 imaging analysis consistently. Most recently Marie et al. (24) used the "black blood" imaging sequence technique using combined spin-echo and inversion recovery MRI sequences. This allowed enhanced determination of the T2-weighted relaxation time. In 122 examinations performed in 75 patients, 52 were performed within 1 week of biopsy with no therapeutic changes made. ISHLT grade 2 or higher rejection was noted in 9 cases (5 grade 2 and 4 grade 3A). Using T2 prolongation greater than or equal to 2 standard deviations they achieved a sensitivity of 89% (8/9) and specificity of 91% (39/43).

Magnetic Resonance Spectroscopy Methods

One of the unique features of magnetic resonance technology is the ability to evaluate the energy metabolism of living tissue, *in vivo*, via analysis of the magnetic resonance spectrum of high-energy phosphates. Changes to these spectra parallel, and may precede, histologic changes of rejection. Canby et al. (25) initially applied this technology to a rat model of heterotopically transplanted hearts in 1987. Brown Norway rat hearts were transplanted heterotopically into the necks of Lewis rat recipients. Isografts between Lewis rat donors and recipients were used as controls. Measurements obtained on post-op day 2 were used as a baseline. Phosphocreatine (PCr) to inorganic phosphate (Pi) ratios were unchanged or increased in the isograft controls, but decreased progressively in the allografts, becoming statistically significant by day 4 compared to day 2. The PCr to adenosine triphosphate beta (ATP_B) ratios did not change in isografts, but were significantly decreased by day 4 in the allografts. In addition, intracellular pH increased in the allograft group initially followed by a shift to acidosis later. Bottomley et al. (26) later documented results in an *in vivo* MRS human trial of 14 patients. Spectroscopy was performed using a 1.5 Tesla MRI/MRS device with MRS surface coils. Again lower ratios of PCr/ATP_B were documented, and lower ratios of PCr/Pi were observed when they were detectable, but reliable differentiation of rejecting versus nonrejecting patients could not be achieved. Two attempts have been made by Walpoth et al. (27,28) to combine the MRI and MRS technologies, first in rats then in pigs, in an effort to improve the sensitivity and specificity of the technique. Unfortunately while confirming the changes in the aforementioned ratios, they were unable to reliably differentiate between non- and mildly rejecting myocardium. Only moderate and severe rejection was reliably detected.

Benvenuti et al. studied human endomyocardial biopsy tissue specimens in 46 biopsies performed 6 to 455 days after transplantation in 19 heart transplant recipients (29). All were on triple drug therapy including cyclosporin, Imuran, and steroids. Tissue ATP levels were measured by high-performance liquid chromatography. This confirmed by a traditional ''wet'' approach that tissue ATP levels were significantly reduced in hearts suffering moderate, but not mild rejection. There was also a trend, though not highly significant, for lower ATP levels in nonrejecting myocardium when compared to nontransplanted hearts. This observation led Evanochko et al. to consider if ongoing cardiac allograft vasculopathy (CAV) could be causing transient ischemic events in the transplanted myocardium, leading to the reduced ATP levels. CAV is a competing process of rejection that is as yet poorly understood. It typically does not present angiographically until after the first year post-

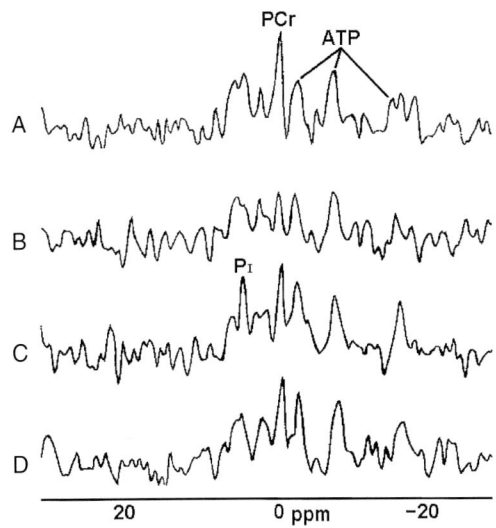

FIG. 2. Example of a positive ^{31}P MRS stress test. **A:** Baseline spectrum at rest. **B:** Positive response to handgrip, with decreased PCr peak. **C:** Initial recovery period with return of the PCr peak and increased P_I, suggesting ischemia during recovery. **D:** Late recovery with return to baseline values.

transplant, but is associated with microvascular hemodynamic abnormalities as well (30). To determine if an early ischemic component was involved, Evanochko et al. (31,32) performed a ^{31}P MRS stress test in 27 patients who had been transplanted from 4 to 159 months prior. Eight patients demonstrated a positive stress test with PCr/ATP ratios outside of two standard deviations from the mean, yet all of these patients had normal coronary arteriograms. Figure 2 is a representative example of a positive ^{31}P MRS stress test. Figure 2**A** is the baseline cardiac spectrum at rest. Figure 2**B** shows the positive response to a hand grip exercise with a decrease in the PCr peak demonstrated. In Figure 2**C** an initial recovery spectrum is shown with the PCr peak returning, but a significant increase in the Pi peak appears, suggestive of an ischemic event. Finally, in Figure 2**D** a late recovery spectrum is shown demonstrating return to baseline levels. Based on these findings the authors hypothesized that although CAV does not manifest angiographically until greater than 1 year after transplantation, it probably begins to develop at the microvascular level immediately after transplant. If so, then cardiac ^{31}P MRS might prove a very sensitive screening tool to discover this population early. This could potentially lead to significant reduction in the number of left heart catheterizations required for posttransplant monitoring of CAV.

EVALUATION OF HEMODYNAMIC CHANGES

A decrease in left ventricular systolic function in a cardiac transplant patient is considered hemodynamically compromising rejection until proven otherwise. Although advancing CAV with myocardial infarction, or CMV myocarditis can also cause depression of LV function, the patient must be treated presumptively and rapidly for rejection until another etiology is clearly documented. Even with treatment, each episode of hemodynamically compromising rejection statistically worsens the patient's long-term survival, and without treatment is uniformly fatal. In the absence of another well-proven etiology, even with an endomyocardial biopsy with no or only low-grade rejection, new onset of systolic LV dysfunction diagnosed by *any* method must *always* be treated as rejection as rapidly and aggressively as possible. Even though endomyocardial biopsy is considered the "gold standard" by which other modalities are measured, there are still episodes of "biopsy-negative" rejection that are very real, and often respond to therapy with enhanced immunosuppression. These events are usually referred to as "vascular" or "humoral" rejection, and immunofluorescent staining of endomyocardial biopsies often reveals evidence of antibody and/or complement deposition, as well as fibrin deposition (30) although the correlation is not absolute. Due to its speed and portability, the 2D echocardiogram has become the mainstay of diagnosis of these life-threatening events. Due to the worsening prognosis with these events, the goal of endomyocardial biopsy, or any noninvasive surrogate, is to diagnose cardiac rejection in its early stages while treatment with enhanced immunosuppression can prevent progression to hemodynamic compromise. The measurement of systolic function is therefore, by definition, inadequate for this task. Most studies of functional assessment have therefore concentrated on measurements of diastolic function in the hopes of finding a parameter that could be reliably measured, that adequately predates systolic compromise, and yet can be readily reversed with treatment to maintain a good prognosis.

Echocardiography has again predominated in the evaluation of diastolic functional parameters. As early as 1984, Dawkins et al. (33) explored the use of M-mode echocardiograms with simultaneous phonocardiograms to measure the isovolumic relaxation time (IVR). They postulated that acute rejection was associated with impairment of LV diastolic filling, giving rise to elevations in pulmonary arterial wedge pressures and thus earlier mitral valve opening with a resultant decrease in IVR. Their (pre-ISHLT) grading system of endomyocardial biopsies graded on a scale of 0 to 2 with 0 having no WBC infiltrate, 1 having increased WBC infiltrate but no cell necrosis, and 2 having more WBC infiltrate and myocyte cell necrosis. Normal subjects and transplant patients with grade 0 rejection had similar IVR times of 78 $\pm$ 12 msec in normal subjects and 72 $\pm$ 9 msec in transplant patients. With grade 1 rejection, there was no significant difference in IVR from grade 0, but with grade 2 rejection (approximately correlating to ISHLT grade 3b or 4) the IVR dropped by approximately 26% (range 5% to 86%) to 57 $\pm$ 12 msec. This provided a diagnostic sensitivity of 87% and specificity of 90%. Paulsen et al. (34) used a computer-assisted M-mode echo technique to evaluate diastolic parameters. They studied 9 patients with biopsy proven rejection compared with 10 normal controls, and found that the rapid

ventricular filling period prolonged from 155 $\pm$ 14 msec to 183 $\pm$ 16 msec, normalized peak filling rates decreased from 5.3 $\pm$ 0.8 sec^{-1} to 3.9 $\pm$ 0.4 sec^{-1}, and rates of posterior wall thinning decreased from 7.4 $\pm$ 1.0 sec^{-1} to 3.8 $\pm$ 0.6 sec^{-1}. Unfortunately no biopsy histologic grades were specified for correlation in this paper. With the advent of Doppler echocardiography Valantine et al. (36) documented that IVRT, peak early mitral flow velocity (M1), mitral flow velocity with atrial systole (M2), and the rate of decrease of M1 by the pressure half time (PHT) method all changed significantly consistent with advancing diastolic dysfunction as the histologic grade progressed from mild to moderate rejection. There were differences noted between no and mild rejection, but the overlap in values was high. All of the above studies suffered from small numbers of patients in the study group and lack of follow-up studies in the rejecting patients after treatment.

A confounding variable to the evaluation of diastolic dysfunction in the cardiac transplant patient is well-documented evolution of constrictive-restrictive physiology early postoperatively in most transplant patients, and its occult persistence on a long-term basis. Young et al. (35) in 15 cardiac transplant patients and 5 heart-lung transplant patients, documented a hemodynamic pattern of early (within the first month) systemic hypertension, elevations of the mean right atrial pressure, right ventricular end-diastolic pressure, mean pulmonary artery pressure, and mean pulmonary capillary wedge pressure with normal heart rates and cardiac outputs. These changes tended to resolve after the first month post-op, but even after normalization of these parameters the use of rapid volume infusion uncovered occult restrictive right atrial pressure patterns and appearance of a Kussmaul response not present prior to volume infusion. Valantine et al. (36) later performed a Doppler echocardiographic study with full hemodynamic correlation and documented a 15% persistence of frank restrictive-constrictive hemodynamics beyond 1 year posttransplant. They did not perform volume loading, and so occult persistence may have been even higher. The Doppler echocardiographic parameters of LV dysfunction (IVR, M1, M2, PHT), and the corresponding parameters of RV dysfunction (T1, T2, PHT), were all consistent and sensitive measures of diastolic function, correlating well with the invasive hemodynamic measurements. Of important note is that the degree of diastolic dysfunction had a correlation with the documented incidence of rejection, suggesting that recurrent rejection and fibrosis has a role in the development of diastolic dysfunction. Some of the patients with restrictive-constrictive physiology also developed clinically significant ventricular systolic dysfunction as well. Skowronski et al. (37) in a similar study with invasive hemodynamic correlation, showed that both the LV and RV diastolic parameters rose during rejection, but that the RV diastolic and minimum pressures remained elevated despite histological resolution of rejection confirmed by endomyocardial biopsy, again implying persistent negative effects of rejection episodes even with systolic and histologic resolution. These persistent effects make it more difficult to correctly diagnose rejection episodes based solely on diastolic functional data when comparing inter-individual data. Holzmann et al. (38) showed that establishing baseline data for each patient, then performing only intra-patient comparisons improved sensitivity and specificity, but unfortunately this was still insufficient to make consistent accurate predictions of rejection vs. nonrejection. Additional confounding variables in this study were the degree of inter- and intraobserver variability. Pellicelli et al. (39) also documented that the lack of AV synchrony between the recipient atria and the donor atria and ventricles also made the measurement of diastolic inflow properties less accurate.

Newer computer enhancements are improving the accuracy of measurement of diastolic parameters by echocardiogram, and helping to reduce the inter- and intraobserver variability. Hausmann et al. (40) has used acoustic quantification (AQ) to provide instantaneous calculation of cavity areas and has verified the initial restrictive pattern posttransplant typically resolves within the first 8 weeks, but lacks long-term follow-up data to date. Kimball et al. (41) applied automatic border detection algorithms to enhance the evaluation of diastolic function. This technique allowed good delineation of the rapid filling, diastasis, and atrial contraction phases of diastole. Interestingly, their data implied that the mechanism of diastolic dysfunction during rejection in their pediatric population subtly differed from that seen in the adult population. They noted predominantly impaired relaxation in children with decreased early diastolic filling and the maintenance of normal filling during atrial contraction. This contrasted with predominant compliance problems in adults, with increased early diastolic filling and left atrial hypertension. Both of these studies show promise for the early detection of ISHLT grade greater than 2 rejection, but will need larger, prospective trials for confirmation.

A unique study of LV diastolic function was performed by Yun et al. (42). These investigators implanted tantalum markers into the LV midwall of 15 transplant recipients at the time of transplantation. Using computer-assisted analysis of biplane cinefluoroscopic images they were able to perform detailed evaluation of the three-dimensional, time-varying LV chamber twist and untwist mechanisms. Although this would not be practical for routine screenings of rejection, it did provide elegant data showing that initial LV rapid recoil was markedly diminished during rejection. The maximum overall untwist rate (dT/dt$_{max}$) did not change during rejection, but the first 15% of diastolic filling was significantly lower. With resolution of rejection, these parameters reverted back toward baseline, but never returned to baseline completely, consistent with previous studies that have confirmed persistent diastolic abnormalities postrejection. This data could potentially be applied to newer MRI radiofrequency tagging methods to noninvasively measure the LV twist dynamics.

CHANGES IN ELECTRICAL CHARACTERISTICS

Attempts have been made to diagnose cardiac rejection by monitoring the electrical properties of the myocardium since the early days of cardiac transplantation. Decreases in QRS voltage as rejection progresses were originally described in 1966 by Lower et al. (43) in the canine model, and subsequently documented in humans as well. Hess et al. (44) described the Medical College of Virginia (MCV) protocol in humans, in which the sum of the QRS voltages in leads I, II, III, and V$_5$ are recorded. A decrease by 20% over 24 h was considered diagnostic of rejection. This was, however, during the precyclosporin era of cardiac transplantation. Much as with the correlation between LV mass and rejection, as the use of cyclosporin became more prevalent, the correlation between QRS voltage and rejection became less and less useful. In only the most advanced rejection cases is this classic finding apparent today. Other parameters retain some utility, however. Richartz et al. (44a) describe a correlation between the QTc interval and rejection. This group correlated the QTc by simple ECG monitoring on 65 adult cardiac transplant recipients between January of 1994 and April of 1997. There were 212 paired biopsy specimens and QTc intervals. Of these 177 were ISHLT histologic grade 0 to 3A (Texas Heart Institute (THI) grade 0–5), and 35 were ISHLT 3A to 4 (THI 6–10). The mean QTc in the former group was 449 ± 2 msec and in the latter was 517 ± 11 msec. Using an increase of 10% or more in the QTc as an indication of rejection yielded a sensitivity of 86% with a specificity of 88%. These are similar to values quoted for most of the other diagnostic modalities, but by a considerably cheaper and simpler modality. Still, 14% of rejections requiring therapy will be missed.

In a recent study, Bourge et al. (45) performed a multicenter study using an implanted pacemaker with epicardial leads having high-resolution telemetry capabilities in 30 patients at five transplant centers in the United States. During follow-up visits, intramyocardial electrograms (IEGMs) were recorded during intrinsic and paced activity. These were digitized in a laptop-based computer and transmitted via the Internet to the central data acquisition center. After processing, a rejection sensitive parameter (RSP) was calculated by fitting a normal distribution curve to the terminal part of the repolarization phase of the IEGM as in Figure 3**A**. This RSP is then mapped as a function of time as in Figure 3**B**. This figure demonstrates an individual patient who experienced two separate grade 3A rejections as marked. Using these parameters yielded a sensitivity of 83% and specificity of 58% for detecting significant rejection, but also yielded an impressive negative predictive value of 98%. The application of this modality as a screening tool would have allowed the elimination of 55% of the unnecessary EMBs. In a companion paper Grasser et al. (46) describe the variability of the measurement of the RSP with the time of day, posture, activity, and pacing. By applying these parameters to a next generation of devices the investigators hope to create an

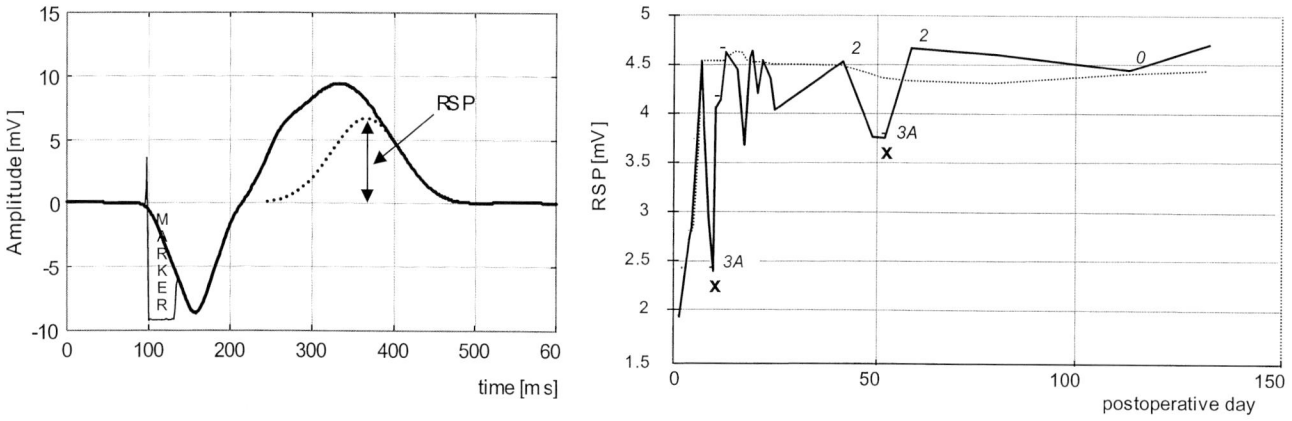

FIG. 3. The rejection sensitive parameter (*RSP*). **A** shows how a normal distribution is fitted to the terminal portion of the repolarization phase of the IEGM. **B:** An individual patient who had two episodes of grade 3a rejection, marked by the Xs.

automatic recording sequence that will monitor the patient at home during sleep. This should allow greater precision in detecting changes from the patient's baseline, earlier in the course of rejection.

DISCUSSION

The fundamental paradox faced by any noninvasive modality applied to the monitoring of cardiac transplant rejection is to attempt to make the diagnosis of rejection *before* adverse changes begin to occur in the tissue. In the age of cyclosporin, and soon even newer immunosuppressants, the inflammation resulting from WBC infiltration of the myocardium is significantly suppressed. The WBCs seem to be attracted into the myocardium, but are not activated as they were in the absence of cyclosporin. Unfortunately, virtually all of the modalities discussed are reliant upon some adverse effect, some *change* in the myocardium that effects either its function, tissue density, metabolic parameters or electrical characteristics. Many of these modalities now boast on the order of 90% sensitivity and specificity, but unfortunately that leaves 10% of the potentially life threatening episodes of rejection undiagnosed. When each episode of significant rejection causes lasting detrimental effects to the myocardium, this is clearly not an acceptable alternative. Although these newer technologies are now becoming capable of detecting exceedingly subtle changes to these parameters, the fundamental question remains, what can we use to detect WBC infiltration *before* any changes occur, and before any damage is done to the graft, or at least before any *permanent* damage is done. It is not unreasonable to consider that if the changes are caught at the very earliest onset, many of these effects might still be completely reversible, without worsening of the overall prognosis. The answer to this question will require further prospective studies, on a larger scale, with an eye toward outcome based on intention to treat. In the meantime, the endomyocardial biopsy remains the most reliable way of detecting early cardiac allograft rejection.

REFERENCES

1. Billingham ME. Diagnosis of cardiac rejection by endomyocardial biopsy. *Heart Transplantation* 1982;1:25–30.
2. Billingham ME, Cary NRB, Hammond ME, et al. A working formulation for the standardization of nomenclature in the diagnosis of heart and lung rejection: Heart Rejection Study Group. *J Heart Transplant* 1990;9:587–593.
3. Milano A, Caforio AL, Livi U, et al. Evolution of focal moderate (International Society for Heart and Lung Transplantation grade 2) rejection of the cardiac allograft. *J Heart Lung Transplantation* 1996; 15:456–460.
4. Eisen HJ, Eisenberg SB, Saffitz JE, et al. Noninvasive detection of rejection of transplanted hearts with indium-111-labeled lymphocytes. *Circulation* 1987;75:868–876.
5. Hesse B, Mortensen SA, Folke M, et al. Ability of antimyosin scintigraphy monitoring to exclude acute rejection during the first year after heart transplantation. *J Heart Lung Transplantation* 1995;14(pt 1): 23–31.
6. Isobe M, Sekiguchi M. Staging of cardiac rejection by simultaneous administration of ^{123}I-antimyosin and ^{111}In-anti MHC class II antibodies. *Acta Cardiologica* 1996;51:515–520.
7. Sagar KB, Hastillo A, Wolfgang TC, et al. Left ventricular mass by M-mode echocardiography in cardiac transplant patients with acute rejection. *Circulation* 1981;64(2 pt 2):II217–220.
8. Oyer PE, Stinson EB, Jamieson SW, et al. Cyclosporin-A in cardiac allografting: a preliminary experience. *Transplantation Proc* 1983;25: 1247–1252.
9. Oyer PE, Stinson EB, Jamieson SW, et al. Cyclosporine in cardiac transplantation: a 2½ year follow-up. *Transplantation Proc* 1983; 25(suppl 1):2546–2552.
10. Gill EA, Borrego C, Bray BE, et al. Left ventricular mass increases during cardiac allograft vascular rejection. *J Am Coll Cardiol* 1995; 25:922–926.
11. Kimball TR, Witt SA, Daniels SR, et al. Frequency and significance of left ventricular thickening in transplanted hearts in children. *Am J Cardiol* 1996;77:77–80.
12. Santos-Ocampo SD, Sekarski TJ, Saffitz JE, et al. Echocardiographic characteristics of biopsy-proven cellular rejection in infant heart transplant recipients. *J Heart Lung Transplantation* 1996;15(1 pt 1):25–34.
13. Gill EA, Borrego C, Bray BE, et al. Left ventricular mass increases during cardiac allograft vascular rejection. *Heart Transplantation* 1995; 25: 922–925.
14. Ensley RD, Hammond EH, Renlund DG, et al. Clinical manifestations of vascular rejection in cardiac transplantation. *J Transplant Proc* 1991; 23:1130–1132.
15. Herskowitz A, Soule LM, Ueda K, et al. Arteriolar vasculitis on endomyocardial biopsy: a histologic predictor of poor outcome and cyclosporine treated heart transplant recipients. *J Heart Transplantation* 1987;6(3):127–136.

16. Hammond EH, Yowell RL, Nunoda S, et al. Vascular (humoral) rejection in heart transplantation: pathologic observations and clinical implications. *J Heart Transplantation* 1989;8:430–443.
17. Gotteiner NL, Vonesh MJ, Crawford SE, et al. Myocardial acoustics in pediatric allograft rejection. *J Heart Lung Transplantation* 1996;15:596–604.
18. Angermann CE, Nassau K, Stempfle HU, et al. Recognition of acute cardiac allograft rejection from serial integrated backscatter analyses in human orthotopic heart transplant recipients. Comparison with conventional echocardiography. *Circulation* 1997;95:140–150.
19. Aherne T, Tscholakoff D, Finkbeiner W, et al. Magnetic resonance imaging of cardiac transplants: the evaluation of rejection of cardiac allografts with and without immunosuppression. *Circulation* 1986;74:145–146.
20. Wisenberg G, Pflugfelder PW, Kostuk WJ, et al. Diagnostic applicability of magnetic resonance imaging in assessing human cardiac allograft rejection. *Am J Cardiology* 1987;60:130–136.
21. Revel D, Chapelon C, Mathieu D, et al. Magnetic resonance imaging of human orthotopic heart transplantation: correlation with endomyocardial biopsy. *J Heart Transplantation* 1989;8:139–146.
22. Doornbos J, Verwey H, Essed CE, et al. MR imaging in assessment of cardiac transplant rejection in humans. *J Comput Assisted Tomogr* 1990;14:77–81.
23. Mousseaux E, Farge D, Guillemain R, et al. Assessing human cardiac allograft rejection using MRI with Gd-DOTA. *J Comput Assist Tomogr* 1993;17:237.
24. Marie PY, Cardeaux JP, Angioi M, et al. Detection and prediction of acute heart transplant rejection: preliminary results on the clinical use of a "black blood" magnetic resonance imaging sequence. *Transplantation Proc* 1998;30:1933–1935.
25. Canby RC, Evanochko WT, Barrett LV, et al. Monitoring the bioenergetics of cardiac allograft rejection using *in vivo* P-31 nuclear magnetic resonance spectroscopy. *J Am Coll Cardiol* 1987;9:1067–1074.
26. Bottomly PA, Weiss RG, Hardy CJ, et al. Myocardial high-energy phospate metabolism and allograft rejection in patients with heart transplants. *Radiology* 1991;181:67–75.
27. Walpoth BH, Lazeyras F, Tschopp A, et al. Assessment of cardiac rejection and immunosuppression by magnetic resonance imaging and spectroscopy. *Transplantation Proc* 1995;27:2088–2091.
28. Walpoth BH, Muller MF, Celik B, et al. Assessment of cardiac rejection by MR-imaging and MR-spectroscopy. *Eur J Cardio-Thoracic Surg* 1998;14:426–430.
29. Benvenuti C, Aptecar E, Deleuze P, et al. Myocardial high-energy phosphate depletion in allograft rejection after orthotopic human heart transplantation. *J Heart Lung Transplantation* 1994;13:857–861.
30. Lones MA. Clinical-pathologic features of humoral rejection in cardiac allografts: a study in 81 consecutive patients. *J Heart Lung Transplantation* 1995;14:151–162.
31. Evanochko WT, Buchthal S, den Hollander J, et al. Cardiac transplant patients assessed by the P-31 MRS stress-test. Abstract presented at:

First Annual Meeting of The Society of Cardiovascular Magnetic Resonance; Atlanta, January 31, 1998.
32. Evanochko WT, Buchthal SD, den Hollander JA, et al. Cardiac transplant patients respond to the ^{31}P MRS stress-test. *J Cardiovasc Magn Res* (in press).
33. Dawkins KD, Oldershaw PJ, Billingham ME, et al. Changes in diastolic function as a noninvasive marker of cardiac allograft rejection. *Heart Transplantation* 1983;3:286–294.
34. Paulsen W, Magid N, Sagar K, et al. Left ventricular function of heart allografts during acute rejection: an echocardiographic assessment. *Heart Transplantation* 1985;4:525–529.
35. Young JB, Leon CA, Short D, et al. Evolution of hemodynamics after orthotopic heart and heart-lung transplantation: early restrictive patterns persisting in occult fashion. *J Heart Transplantation* 1987;6:34–43.
36. Valantine HA, Appleton CP, Hatle LK, et al. A hemodynamic and Doppler echocardiographic study of ventricular function in long-term cardiac allograft recipients. *Circulation* 1989;79:66–75.
37. Skowronski EW, Epstein M, Ota D, et al. Right and left ventricular function after cardiac transplantation: changes during and after rejection. *Circulation* 1991;84:2409–2417.
38. Holzmann G, Gidding SS, Crawford SE, et al. Usefulness of left ventricular inflow Doppler in predicting rejection in pediatric cardiac transplant recipients. *Am J Cardiol* 1994;73:205–207.
39. Pellicelli AM, Cosial JB, Ferranti E, et al. Alteration of left ventricular filling evaluated by Doppler echocardiography as a potential marker of acute rejection in orthotopic heart transplant. *Angiology* 1996;47:35–41.
40. Hausmann B, Muurling S, Stauch C, et al. Detection of diastolic dysfunction: acoustic quantification (AQ) in comparison to Doppler echocardiography. *Int J Cardiac Imaging* 1997;13:301–310.
41. Kimball TR, Semler DC, Witt SA, et al. Noninvasive markers for acute heart transplant rejection in children with the use of automatic border detection. *J Am Soc Echocardiography* 1997;10:964–972.
42. Yun, KL, Niczyporuk MA, Daughters GT, et al. Alterations in left ventricular diastolic twist mechanics during acute human cardiac allograft rejection. *Circulation* 1991;83:962–973.
43. Lower RR, Dong E, Glasener FS. Electrocardiograms of dogs with heart homografts. *Circulation* 1966;33:455–460.
44. Hess ML, Hastillo A, Wolfgang TC, et al. The noninvasive diagnosis of acute and chronic cardiac allograft rejection. *Heart Transplantation* 1982;1:31–38.
44a. Richartz BM, Radovancevic B, Bologna MT, et al. Usefulness of the QTc interval in predicting acute allograft rejection. *Thorac Cardiovasc Surg* 1998;46:217.
45. Bourge R, Eisen H, Hershberger R, et al. Noninvasive rejection monitoring of cardiac transplants using high resolution intramyocardial electrograms: initial US multicenter experience. *Pace* 1998;21(Pt II):2338–2344.
46. Grasser B, Iberer F, Schreier G, et al. Intramyocardial electrogram variability in the monitoring of graft rejection after heart transplantation. *Pace* 1998;21(Pt II):2345–2349.

Imaging in Cardiovascular Disease, edited by Gerald M. Pohost et al., Lippincott Williams & Wilkins, Philadelphia © 2000

CHAPTER 51

Systolic Etiologies

Mark R. Starling

The quantification of left ventricular (LV) size and systolic performance has emerged as an important factor in the evaluation of patients with cardiovascular disease. It is essential for defining the severity of cardiac disease processes, for predicting the outcome of cardiac disease processes, for establishing the need for therapy, for guiding the selection of therapy, and for assessing the efficacy of a chosen therapy. Irrespective of the technology used to quantify LV size and systolic performance, the ability of invasive or noninvasive technologies to accomplish this important clinical objective depends upon whether the chosen technology is accurate, precise, and reproducible. The implication of an accurate test is that it is without error; thus, if we had an object of known size, the technology employed to determine the size of the object would do so within exact limits. Clinically, we may be able to use a technology that lacks accuracy, if all we wish to know is whether the size of an object is grossly normal or abnormal. This degree of inaccuracy would, however, not be useful if we wish to know the size of an object within specific limits upon which we would base a judgment for therapy. Further, the precision of a particular technology is dependent upon its ability to repeat successfully a measurement of object size within close specified limits. This is particularly applicable when we are attempting to determine the efficacy of a particular intervention or therapeutic strategy in managing a cardiovascular disease process. Whether a beneficial or detrimental effect occurs can be determined only if the measurement of the object exceeds or falls outside certain specified limits. Finally, the ability to reproduce measures of an object from a technology on the same images will, in part, introduce the range within which the technology can be deemed accurate. Thus, depending upon the specific clinical intent, the limits of the technology that is chosen to accomplish the task must be known.

We, therefore, examined the ability of invasive and noninvasive technologies to quantify LV size and systolic performance with the expectation of examining data that would allow recommendations for the type of technology, the approach to utilizing the technology, and the specified clinical condition or question to which the technology should be applied for quantifying LV size and systolic performance.

CINEVENTRICULOGRAPHY

The use of contrast cineventriculography (CVG) for quantifying LV size and systolic performance has had a long and storied history. This particular technology depends upon the accuracy, precision, and reproducibility of LV volumes, because LV systolic performance is directly related to LV size at end-diastole and end-systole, as it is with most, if not all, noninvasive technologies. The technical approaches to attaining high-quality CVG images and the methods of quantitating LV volumes determine the accuracy of this particular invasive technology.

In Vitro Cast Comparisons

Since the early approaches of Dodge and Baxley (1) and Kasser and Kennedy (2) for quantitating LV volumes from CVG images, further refinements, including: the development of new biplane CVG equipment and complex computer algorithms for quantifying LV size, have been compared to a single plane approach (3–13). Two methods have been employed. First, a comparison of biplane and single plane CVG volume calculations to true volumes (3–7); and, second, a comparison of these two methods in patients with and without LV wall motion abnormalities (8–13). Three studies have performed excellent comparisons of biplane and single plane CVG volumes with human heart cast volumes in multiple projections employing several processing techniques. In a comparison of orthogonal and nonorthogonal axial oblique and standard orthogonal oblique CVG images of 14 human heart specimens, Starling and Walsh (4) calculated

M. R. Starling: Division of Cardiology, Veterans Administration Medical Center, Ann Arbor, Michigan 48105.

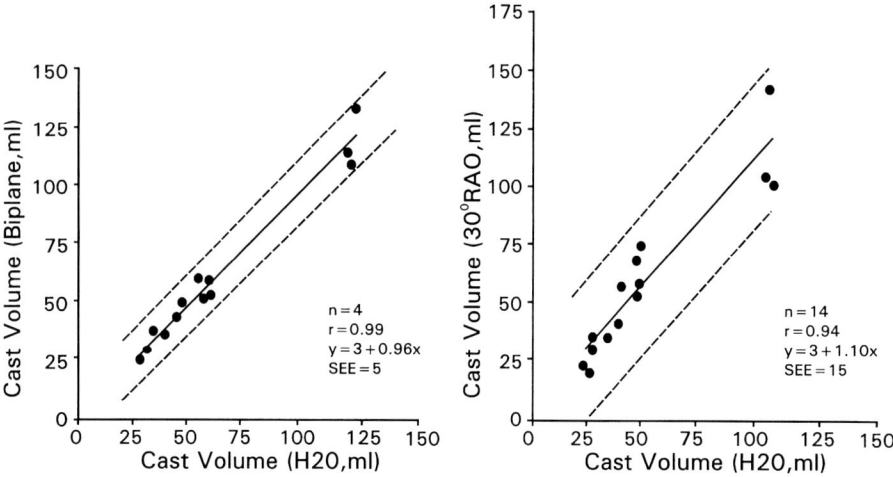

FIG. 1. Left panel: The standard biplane orthogonal oblique cine-ventriculographic volumes, on the ordinate, are compared to true volumes by water displacement, on the abscissa. **Right panel:** The single plane right anterior oblique cineventriculographic volumes, on the ordinate, are compared to true volumes by water displacement, on the abscissa. The true volumes are overestimated by the single plane right anterior oblique cineventriculographic approach, and the 95% confidence intervals are increased 300% in comparison to the standard biplane orthogonal oblique cineventriculographic approach. (From ref. 4, with permission.)

LV volumes using a Simpson's rule algorithm and demonstrated correlations with true volumes ($r = 0.99$ for all comparisons; SEE = 5–7 mL, Fig. 1). However, the mean biplane CVG orthogonal axial oblique views significantly overestimated true volumes (69 ± 43 ml vs. 60 ± 35 mL, $p < 0.01$). The nonorthogonal axial oblique and standard orthogonal oblique views did not differ significantly from true volumes (63 ± 35 and 60 ± 34 mL, respectively). Thus, it would appear that standard orthogonal oblique CVG images have a high correlation, low standard error, and little deviation from true volumes. When single plane right anterior oblique CVG images of the human heart casts were used to calculate LV volumes with an area-length formulation, there continued to be a correlation ($r = 0.94$); but there was a greater standard error of the estimate in comparison to any of the biplane CVG calculations ($p < 0.05$ to < 0.01). The single plane CVG area-length method overestimated true volumes by as much as 40% (Fig. 1), while the biplane CVG Simpson's rule method did not. Thus, even in comparison to true volumes from human heart casts without distortions in LV shape, biplane CVG can quantify LV volumes more accurately than a single plane area-length approach when Simpson's rule algorithm is employed.

Simpson's rule algorithm is a unique mathematical application to calculating volumes by dividing the long-axis into a series of perpendicular planes of infinite number (4,5). These thin planes are summed to calculate a ventricular volume. This concept provides an opportunity to incorporate distortions in LV shape without assuming a particular geometric form, which cannot be done with an area-length formulation. Thus, a Simpson's rule algorithm has the theoretic potential of providing more accurate quantification of LV volumes.

This concept was examined more specifically by Pietras and co-workers (6), who calculated biplane CVG volumes of 17 heart casts from orthogonal and nonorthogonal oblique views using an area-length formulation and a Simpson's rule algorithm. The cast volumes calculated from biplane CVG

images using the area-length formulation overestimated true volumes ($p < 0.002$), but the Simpson's rule algorithm did not differ significantly from true volumes. Thus, the Simpson's rule algorithm resulted in a more accurate quantification of true volumes.

Ino and co-workers (7) examined the impact of right ventricular (RV) hemodynamics on LV volume calculations from biplane CVG images using an area-length calculation from 30 postmortem human heart casts in two groups of patients: Group I had abnormal and Group II had normal RV hemodynamics. Although the correlations between the biplane CVG LV volumes were comparable ($r = 0.92$ and 0.99), there was substantial overestimation of the volumes ($p < 0.025$ and 0.05). Thus, this supports the contention that an assumption of LV shape may not account for alterations in LV geometry, such as those that may occur with abnormal RV hemodynamics. Subsequently, Ino et al. (8) employed a Simpson's rule algorithm to address this issue and calculated LV volumes from biplane CVG images and compared them to true volumes of postmortem human heart casts from patients with congenital heart disease in the presence and absence of abnormal RV hemodynamics. The correlations between calculated LV volumes from conventional and nonconventional biplane CVG views and true volumes ranged from 0.96 to 0.99. The regression equations obtained from conventional views and from the nonconventional views using the Simpson's rule algorithm did not differ, confirming that they were not affected by the hemodynamic state of the RV. Thus, their data support the contention that a more complex mathematical approach to calculating LV volumes, particularly in the presence of abnormal LV geometry, may be able to quantify more accurately LV volumes than when simplified assumptions of LV shape inherent to standard area-length formulations are applied.

In Vivo Patient Comparisons

The argument concerning whether biplane or single plane CVG of the LV is adequate for quantifying LV volumes and systolic performance is well known. These studies have focused on whether biplane or single plane CVG imaging should be performed in patients with ischemic heart disease and regional LV wall motion abnormalities. Walsh and colleagues (10) examined 59 patients with ischemic heart disease and performed frontal, lateral, and biplane CVG imaging for the calculation of LV volumes and ejection fractions. In those patients with segmental LV wall motion abnormalities secondary to a previous anterior transmural myocardial infarction, the single plane lateral LV ejection fractions exceeded the single plane frontal LV ejection fractions because of anterior contraction abnormalities. Nevertheless, both single plane LV ejection fractions differed from the biplane LV ejection fractions. Thus, they concluded that in the presence of segmental LV wall motion abnormalities secondary to ischemic heart disease, LV size calculated from biplane CVG images resulted in more accurate quantification of LV systolic performance.

Tate and coworkers (13) performed a retrospective analysis of 91 consecutive biplane CVG images to determine practical guidelines for identifying a need to perform biplane CVG imaging, particularly in laboratories where sequential injections may be required because of single plane equipment. By multivariate analysis, the only predictor of a higher LV ejection fraction calculated from biplane CVG was an anterior wall motion abnormality. When these data were tested prospectively in a separate group of 60 patients, the biplane CVG LV ejection fractions were systematically larger than the corresponding single plane CVG LV ejection fractions in patients with anterior wall motion abnormalities by an average of 0.05 ± 0.04 ejection fraction units. This was not so when anterior LV wall motion abnormalities were absent (Fig. 2). It is reasonable to conclude that accurate quantification of LV size and systolic performance can be best determined, particularly in the presence of regional LV wall motion abnormalities, using biplane CVG images and a Simpson's rule algorithm to account for alterations in LV shape.

Left Ventricular Wall Motion

There have been several studies performed examining the complexities of segmental LV wall motion (15–17). LeWinter and colleagues (15) analyzed whether significant regional differences in shortening existed and whether shortening characteristics in circumferentially oriented hoop axis fibers differed from the more longitudinally oriented fibers near the epicardium using ultrasound crystals placed at three levels of the LV free wall in animals. The mean shortening of the circumferential fibers at the apex averaged approximately 20% of their end-diastolic length, while the midventricular and basal segments averaged 13% and 14%, respectively. The epicardial fibers shortened only 5 to 6% of their end-diastolic length at all three sites. Thus, heterogeneity in regional LV systolic performance was clearly evident in this animal study.

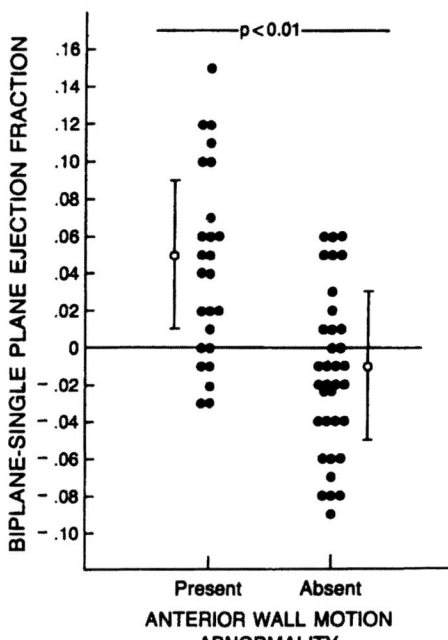

FIG. 2. The difference between biplane and single plane left ventricular ejection fractions for patients in whom an anterior wall motion was present or absent is illustrated. In those patients with an anterior wall motion abnormality, the biplane cineventriculographic left ventricular ejection fractions exceeded the single plane values by −0.03 to +0.15 ejection fraction units. Thus, in the presence of an anterior wall motion abnormality a single plane oblique cineventriculographic view underestimates left ventricular ejection fraction. (From ref. 13, with permission.)

Subsequent studies have been performed to document the complexities of segmental LV wall motion in humans using myocardial markers (16,17). These studies are based on data previously reported by Streeter and co-workers (18). This elegant pathologic study described the complex fiber orientation across the LV and concluded that models based on uniform myocardial fiber structure and function should have significant limitations. Hansen and co-workers (17) demonstrated several important aspects of segmental LV wall motion. First, segmental LV wall motion is not operational in a single plane; but, rather, it is operational in three-dimensional space where twist and torsional deformation are important contributors to the extent of LV regional contraction. Second, there is a lack of homogeneity in this motion throughout the LV. Third, torsional deformation is not sensitive to alterations in loading conditions; but it is sensitive to heart rate. Ingels and co-workers (16) have also used radiopaque markers implanted in the myocardial midwall of 58 patients and studied their motion with computer-aided fluoroscopy. They used the marker motion as the standard for segmental LV wall motion to determine the accuracy of five methods of measuring segmental LV wall motion. They observed that one method using radial measurements and fixed eternal polar coordinates showed significantly less error (26%) in measuring mid-wall marker motion than the other four methods (range 43–48%, $p < 0.000001$). Thus, although all methods of measuring segmental LV wall motion in humans assume homogeneity of motion, as well as linearity of wall motion, this is probably not true, since significant errors related to the complexity of LV wall motion in three-dimension space remain and are not incorporated into our present methodologies.

Accordingly, it must be appreciated that wall motion may be substantially more complex than simple long- and short-axis changes and that normal wall motion may vary throughout the LV and, thereby, require individual regional standards for comparison. Several approaches have been proposed for quantitating normal wall motion in different regions of the LV (19). These include the area, cord, and radial approaches with or without external references. Gelberg and colleagues (19) examined 17 control subjects and 17 subjects with abnormal regional LV systolic performance using three different quantitative methods of regional analysis of biplane CVG images. In their hands, the area method had the lowest failure rate and the best separation of normal from abnormal regional LV systolic performance; also, it seemed to best reflect the symmetry and uniformity of motion of the LV. Bhargava and coworkers (20) used a computer-assisted analysis of the percent change in the square root of the area in each of 12 consecutive 30-degree, pie-shaped LV segments from 40 normal subjects. They concluded that the square root of the area change permitted the establishment of objective confidence limits for normal wall motion, and it was useful as an index of regional LV systolic performance compared to the existing radius, area, hemicord, or cordal methods. However, objective evidence to support this contention was not forthcoming. Clayton and colleagues (21) attempted to answer the question whether a fixed external reference system would more accurately describe regional LV wall motion; and they observed, in contrast to other investigators (16), that an external reference system was not apparently superior to other systems for quantifying regional LV systolic performance.

Although several approaches have been used, Sheehan and co-authors (22) reported on the potential theoretic advantages to the application of the centerline method for quantitating regional LV systolic performance. Wall motion was measured along 100 cords constructed perpendicular to a center line drawn midway between the end-diastolic and end-systolic contours normalized for heart size. An abnormality in regional LV systolic performance was, thus, expressed in units of standard deviations from the mean motion from a reference sample population to indicate both the severity and significance of the segmental LV wall motion abnormality (Fig. 3). They demonstrated that the mean abnormality averaged over 100 cords correlated highly with the area LV ejection fraction ($r = 0.97$), and the full extent of regional LV wall motion abnormalities could be determined as the percent of the complete contour of the LV. The

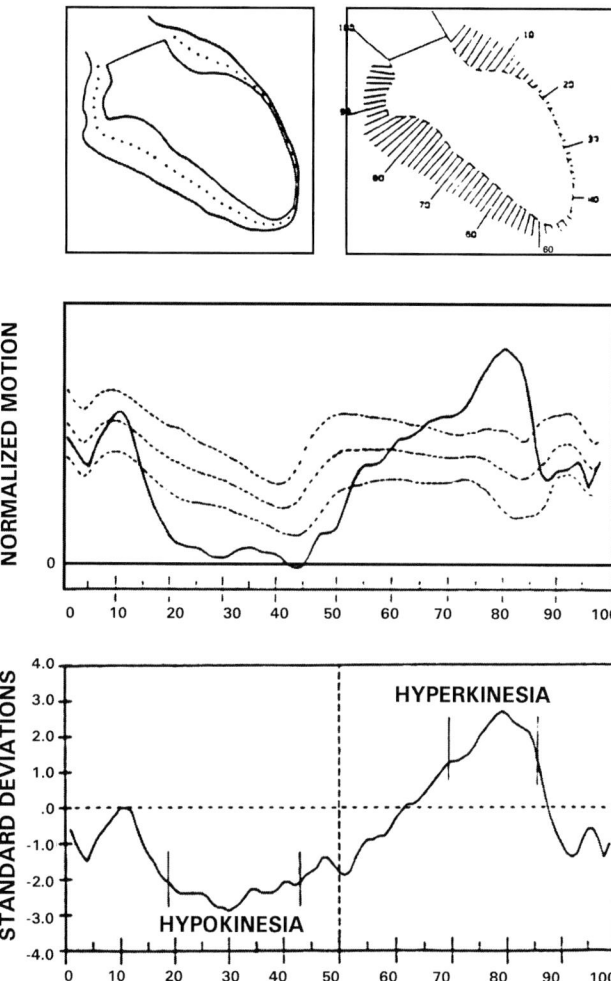

FIG. 3. The centerline method of regional left ventricular wall motion analysis is illustrated by superimposition of the end-diastolic and end-systolic left ventricular endocardial contours with a center line constructed by the computer midway between the two contours. Also illustrated is the location of hypokinetic segments in a patient with anterior infarction over the anterior and apical sectors. It is confined to the inferior sectors in most patients with an inferior myocardial infarction. (From ref. 22, with permission.)

severity of hypokinesis at the site of an acute myocardial infarction also correlated better with infarct size estimated from creatinine kinase release ($r = -0.78$) than did the area LV ejection fraction or the circumferential extent of hypokinesis. Thus, because the centerline method required no apex, origin, coordinate system, or LV geometric reference, it could be applied to all regions, irrespective of their orientations or dissimilarity of contour. Nevertheless, the argument over the optimal method for quantitating regional LV systolic performance highlights the complexity of regional LV wall motion and the difficulties of determining accurate, precise, and reproducible limits of normality. Although the centerline method may have advantages, any regional analysis of LV systolic performance is only a simplified approximation.

Error Analysis

There are several potential errors that must be considered when performing CVG to quantify LV volumes and systolic performance. These may include technical considerations, errors due to magnification and pincushion distortion, and the precision and reproducibility of the measurements. The effect of contrast medium on LV volumes and systolic performance was evaluated early by Vine and colleagues (23) on postoperative biplane CVG images in 10 patients in whom epicardial markers had been placed at the time of coronary artery bypass surgery. There was no significant effect on LV end-diastolic volumes; but an effect on LV end-systolic volumes occurred on the seventh beat after injection. There was a small but significant increase in LV systolic performance by the seventh beat after injection. Thus, injections of contrast do not have a significant impact on LV size or systolic performance through the sixth postinjection beat.

Although the effects of contrast may be minimal for the first few beats following injection, the effects of technique on the adequacy of delineating the LV cavity may have more wide-ranging consequences. It appears that the only determinant of CVG image quality is the location of the catheter at the LV apex at the time of injection.

Another technical aspect is the ability to correct for magnification and pincushion distortion that occurs with the utilization of x-ray equipment. Magnification correction, including the position of the geometric center of the LV, is important, since the absence of this kind of correction introduces up to a 28% error in the LV volume calculation (24). In a study by Baylen and colleagues (25), an external reference grid or an intracardiac radiopaque catheter balloon was used for quantifying LV volumes, which then were compared to true volumes from animals and infants with congenital heart disease. Both comparisons to true volumes were excellent ($r = 0.99$ for both, $p < 0.001$). Thus, to obtain accurate LV volumes, careful attention to the technical aspects of performing CVG and to correcting for magnification and pincushion distortion are required.

Similarly, reproducibility and observer variability need to be taken into account, particularly as they apply to quantifying LV size and systolic performance from sequential studies that may be required in certain kinds of investigations. Several studies have investigated the variability of LV size and systolic performance from biplane CVG images. An early study by Wexler and co-workers (26) examined CVG images from 14 medical centers participating in the coronary artery surgery study (CASS), which were systematically re-read at four designated control centers. The data were then compared to those calculated at the clinical site. The correlations for LV end-diastolic and end-systolic volumes and ejection fractions were 0.71, 0.84, and 0.79, respectively. A qualitative assessment of regional LV wall motion from both right

anterior and left anterior oblique images provided correlation scores of 0.83. When the precision of LV size and systolic performance was assessed by Rigaud and co-workers (27) on two sequential CVG acquisitions approximately 15 minutes apart at comparable heart rates and LV systolic and end-diastolic pressures in 19 patients undergoing coronary arteriography, there was a high degree of intra-observer consistency in the LV volume and systolic performance measures (<5%). Segmental LV wall motion had intra-observer variabilities ranging from 4 to 9% and inter-observer variabilities ranged from 7 to 14%. Thus, if CVG images are acquired with appropriate attention to detail and quantitative techniques are used, reasonably precise and reproducible determinations of LV size and systolic performance, particularly with biplane CVG imaging, can be obtained.

Chaitman and co-workers (28) found a high degree of precision and reproducibility for quantitative measures of LV size, systolic performance, and regional LV wall motion. A wide degree of variability was introduced when an objective analysis was compared to two observers' subjective analyses of LV size, systolic performance, and segmental wall motion. Thus, they concluded that a subjective analysis had a significant error rate and that the accuracy and reproducibility of this kind of analysis was poor. Thus, these data suggest that a subjective analysis of LV size, systolic performance, and regional LV wall motion from CVG images is probably neither accurate nor reproducible.

DIGITAL SUBTRACTION ANGIOGRAPHY

Because of the requirements for LV opacification, attention to technique details, accurate edge definition, and geometric assumptions, computerized densitometric analysis of digital subtraction angiograms using low-dose contrast injections was offered as an alternative method of quantifying LV size and systolic performance. A comparison of brightness in regions-of-interest at end-diastole and end-systole, which takes into account the third dimension independent of LV shape, a precondition of biplane CVG imaging (4), accomplished this task with a single plane view. Nissen and colleagues (29) used two mechanical heart models of differing geometry and demonstrated a correlation between the calculated and measured LV ejection fractions. Subsequently, they performed computer densitometric analysis of digital subtraction angiograms and compared the LV ejection fraction data with that from single plane and biplane area-length calculations in 72 patients, of whom half had had a prior myocardial infarction. There was a close correlation between the computer densitometric analysis, whether it was performed with a direct LV or intravenous injection and the single plane and biplane LV ejection fractions ($r = 0.91$ and 0.93, respectively) in those patients without a prior myocardial infarction. However, in the patients who had had a prior myocardial infarction, there was a substantial deterioration in the correlation of the computer densitometric analysis of the digital subtraction angiograms with single plane CVG

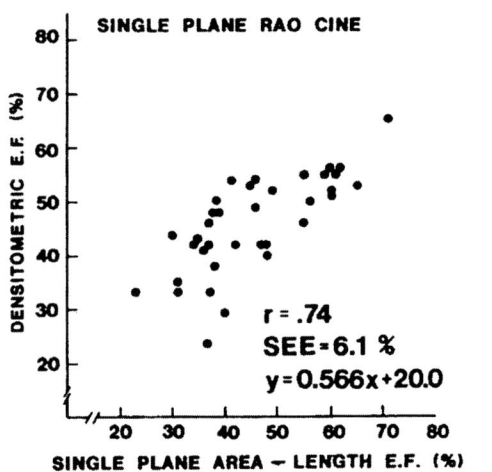

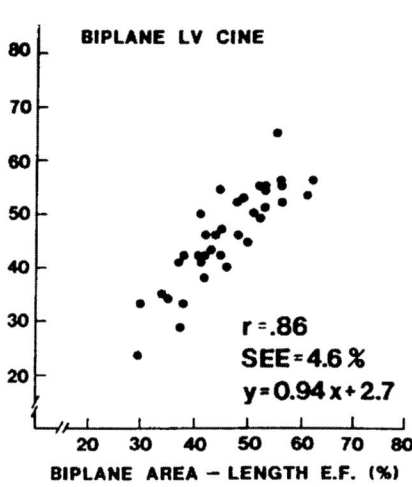

FIG. 4. The results of linear regression analyses comparing computer densitometric left ventricular ejection fractions to those from single plane right anterior oblique (**left panel**) and biplane (**right panel**) cineventriculography in patients with a previous myocardial infarction are illustrated. The deterioration in the correlation between the densitometric approach and single plane cineventriculography is clear, whereas the correlation with biplane cineventriculography is maintained. (From ref. 29, with permission.)

($r = 0.74$), while that with the biplane CVG was maintained ($r = 0.86$) (Fig. 4). Thus, it was concluded that LV ejection fractions from computer densitometric analysis of digital subtraction angiograms accurately quantified LV ejection fractions, irrespective of LV shape.

Realizing that the area-length method might lead to erroneous data, Lehmkuhl and co-workers (30) compared the densitometric approach with the area-length method from a single plane right anterior oblique digital subtraction angiogram for quantifying LV size and systolic performance and compared these data to that from contrast images of heart casts and CVG images from 54 patients that were analyzed by two independent observers. The phantom study demonstrated that the densitometric approach yielded estimation errors that were substantially less than those that occur when the area-length formulation was used ($p < 0.01$). Although comparable errors of the estimate for LV size and systolic performance were recorded for both methods in the patient study, the reliability of the densitometric approach significantly improved upon the area-length method ($p < 0.01$). Thus, the more complex densitometric approach to analyzing single plane digital subtraction angiograms accurately quantitated LV size and systolic performance, similar to the kinds of data obtained from biplane CVG.

RADIONUCLIDE VENTRICULOGRAPHY

LV Ejection Fraction

Multiple-gated acquisition (MUGA) scans of the distribution of a radioisotope in the cardiac blood pool were originally used as a means for quantifying LV systolic performance. The early studies of Strauss and co-workers (31) and others demonstrated the utility of this technique for quantifying LV systolic performance. Although the initial intent of developing MUGA scan technology was to quantify LV ejection fraction, the assumption was made that the time-activity curve reflected an LV volume curve, which was only proven later with the development of techniques for quantifying LV volumes (32).

There have been excellent studies comparing LV ejection fractions from MUGA scans with those from biplane CVG. Schelbert and co-workers (33) studied 20 patients, who had a diagnostic cardiac catheterization and a MUGA scan to calculate LV ejection fractions. There was a correlation between the MUGA LV ejection fractions and those from the biplane CVG ($r = 0.94$), suggesting that this nuclear approach was an accurate method of quantifying LV systolic performance. Similar correlations between LV ejection fractions by MUGA and those from biplane CVG were reported by Starling and co-investigators (34).

The accuracy and reproducibility of LV ejection fractions from MUGA scans have been examined by Wackers and co-authors (35), and they were excellent (1.4 ± 1.2 and 1.7 ± 1.5%, respectively). This error did not differ in patients with normal or reduced LV ejection fractions. When the precision of the MUGA LV ejection fractions was examined by obtaining studies on two separate occasions in 70 patients in two different formats: one on the same day approximately 1 to 2 hours apart and another on two separate days; the precision of the MUGA LV ejection fractions for all repeat studies performed on the same day and on separate days did not differ (3.3 ± 3.1 and 4.3 ± 3.1%, respectively). However, the precision of the LV ejection fractions by MUGA demonstrated a higher variability in patients with normal LV ejection fractions (5.4 ± 4.4%) compared to that in patients with reduced LV ejection fractions (2.1 ± 2.0%, $p < 0.01$). It can be concluded from these data that not only the accuracy, but also the precision and reproducibility of LV ejection fractions from MUGA scans in patients with normal and abnormal LV ejection fractions are highly acceptable. Thus, this technique represents a valuable, non-invasive alternative to biplane CVG for quantifying LV systolic performance.

Left Ventricular Volumes

Several different methods have been proposed for calculating LV volumes from MUGA scans including: geometric approaches (36), nongeometric or count-based approaches (37), and those that use an iterative build-up factor (38). To examine the utility of a geometric approach, Palacios and co-investigators (36) used an area-length calculation of LV volumes from MUGA scans and biplane CVG images and compared them to true volumes of 10 postmortem human hearts. The data obtained would suggest that both a geometric and a nongeometric approach to calculating LV volumes from MUGA scans is reasonable.

There have been several highly sophisticated approaches to calculating nongeometric, count-based LV volumes from MUGA scans. Initially, Dehmer and co-workers (37) studied a scintigraphic, nongeometric technique for quantitating LV volumes and compared them to single plane CVG LV volumes. The correlations were strong for LV end-diastolic ($r = 0.985$, SEE $= 16.2$ mL) and end-systolic volumes ($r = 0.988$, SEE $= 14.7$ mL). Subsequently, studies (37) compared LV volumes calculated from MUGA scans to those from biplane CVG. Although the count-based approach for calculating LV volumes from MUGA scans demonstrated correlations with those from biplane CVG ($r = 0.95$ and 0.98), this approach underestimated the LV end-diastolic volumes, while there was no difference in the LV end-systolic volumes. In a subsequent study (34), this group demonstrated that the time-activity curve represented LV volumes throughout the cardiac cycle (Fig. 5). Therefore, it can be concluded that accurate LV volumes can be calculated using nongeometric, count-based methodology.

The complexities of calculating LV volumes from MUGA scans is dependent upon several technical aspects, including: calculation of absorption factors (38), calculation of attenuation correction factors (39), obtaining appropriate blood samples (34,39), the edge detection algorithms and region-of-interest selection methods (37), and the potential for respiratory variation. Because of these considerations, the accuracy and reproducibility of LV volume determinations using a nongeometric approach has been examined. Although the reproducibility of the measurements by the same observer or different observers was found to be quite high by Verani and co-investigators (41), there were significant variations in individual studies, particularly between observers. Thus, in contrast to the high degree of reproducibility from case-to-case and precision between studies for MUGA LV ejection fractions, the LV volume calculations are more subject to technical considerations and observer variability, which may limit the routine clinical applicability of this approach for quantifying LV volumes.

Left Ventricular Wall Motion

Few studies have examined the value of MUGA scans for assessing regional LV systolic performance. Maddox and colleagues (42) evaluated regional LV ejection fractions using MUGA scans and compared them to those from CVG. The MUGA and CVG approaches were in agreement as to the presence or absence of segmental LV wall motion abnormalities in 84% of the regions examined. A comparison of regional LV ejection fractions demonstrated significant differences between regions with CVG determined normal [75 $\pm$ 3% (SEM)], hypokinetic ($44 \pm 3\%$, $p < 0.0005$), and akinetic ($24 \pm 5\%$, $p < 0.005$) wall motion. Thus, although the assessment of whether regional LV wall motion was normal or abnormal was useful from the MUGA scan and the analysis of regional LV systolic performance showed differences, there was overlap in the quantification of segmental LV wall motion compared to that determined by CVG.

Because of this limitation, Holman and co-workers (43) examined the utility of a paradoxic image by subtracting the background-corrected LV end-diastolic frame from the correspondingly adjusted end-systolic frame. This approach allowed for an assessment of whether regional LV wall mo-

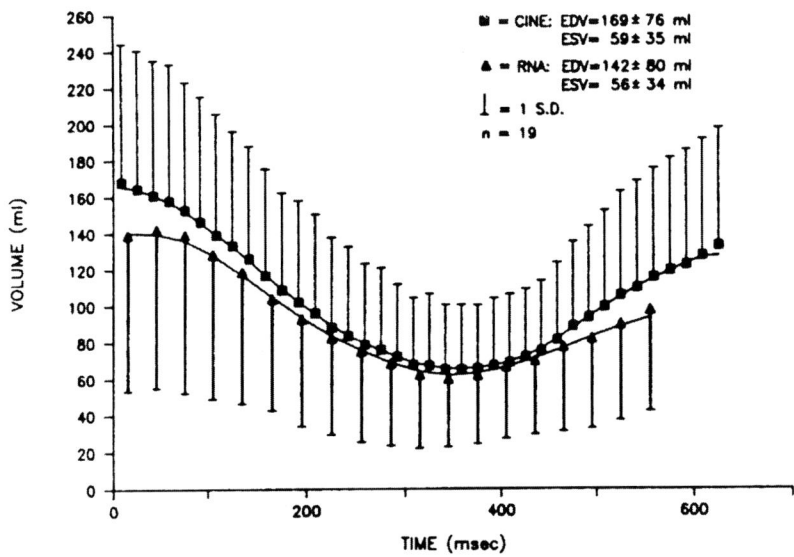

FIG. 5. The frame-by-frame mean left ventricular volume data are shown for biplane contrast cineventriculography (*CINE*) and MUGA (*RNA*) through a single cardiac cycle. Note the slight underestimation of the mean left ventricular end-diastolic volumes and the close correspondence of the end-systolic volumes confirming that the time-activity curve represents an LV volume curve. (From ref. 34, with permission.)

tion was either normal or mildly hypokinetic compared to akinetic or frankly dyskinetic. However, there was only excellent agreement for locating dyskinetic LV regions.

Phase analysis, either in animals or humans has been employed to examine whether there is a homogeneous pattern of contraction across the LV and to quantitate the uniformity of wall motion. In one animal study (44), MUGA scans were acquired both prior to and following ligation of the left circumflex coronary artery. There was correlation between the phase angle shift and phase amplitude and the extent of regional LV dyssynergy determined by regional crystal analysis, but the standard errors of the estimate and 95% confidence intervals were wide. In patients with normal LV wall motion and those with segmental LV wall motion abnormalities studied by Frais and co-investigators (45), there was uniformly a delay in the phase angle that corresponded to the site of abnormality. The mean phase angle (23.6 ± 15.7 degrees) differed from that in the patients with normal LV wall motion (7.6 ± 11.1 degrees, $p < 0.001$). In patients with more generalized segmental LV wall motion abnormalities, the LV phase image revealed multiple regions of inhomogeneous phase angles, and the mean phase angle averaged 56.4 ± 23.9 degrees. This value differed from that in patients with normal and isolated segmental abnormalities in LV wall motion ($p < 0.001$). The ability to quantitate discrete differences in LV wall motion in individual regions using phase analysis of MUGA scans remains difficult.

Tomography

Two forms of tomography have been evaluated: one using the MUGA scan and another using the myocardial perfusion image to quantify LV volumes, ejection fractions, and segmental wall motion. In an elegant study by Gill and co-investigators (46), MUGA cardiac blood pool tomograms were initially studied in a series of phantoms filled with 99m-technetium. They demonstrated a correlation of $r = 0.99$ between the tomographic volumes and true volumes. Subsequently, patient studies were recorded at 16 frames per cardiac cycle at each of 60 angles over 360 degrees of rotation; and the data were reconstructed and presented in an endless loop cine format of a set of sequentially beating tomographic slices in the apical four-chamber, short-axis, and long-axis oblique views. The LV volumes were compared to single plane CVG data and demonstrated correlations for both LV end-diastolic ($r = 0.94, p < 0.0001$, SEE = 20 mL) and end-systolic volumes ($r = 0.93, p < 0.001$, SEE = 24 mL) and ejection fractions ($r = 0.92, p < 0.001$, SEE = 0.08). However, despite the significant correlations, there were substantial underestimations of LV volumes as LV size increased. A visual assessment of regional LV wall motion using the 16-frame tomographic slices was reported as having an advantage over a similar interpretation of the planar images and, as expected, the single plane CVG images.

Recently, there have been several studies examining

whether gated 99m-technetium sestamibi myocardial perfusion images can quantify LV size and systolic performance simultaneously with an assessment of myocardial perfusion and viability. Williams and Taillon (47) evaluated the ability of sestamibi images processed by digital inversion to provide a semiautomated evaluation of the LV cavity and applied commonly available edge-detection software to quantify LV systolic performance. Left ventricular ejection fractions using this technique were compared to myocardial perfusion phantoms and single plane CVG data. The in vitro validation demonstrated that the myocardial perfusion LV ejection fractions correlated with those from the double-chamber phantom ($r = 1.00$). The in vivo relationships also demonstrated a correlation with the single plane CVG data ($r = 0.85$). Intra- and interobserver variability for the tomographic LV ejection fractions ranged between zero and 3 ejection fraction units.

There are also two studies that compared LV ejection fractions from gated 99m-technetium sestamibi myocardial perfusion images to MUGA scans (48,49). Although one study (48) demonstrated a correlation between these two techniques of only $r = 0.71$ ($p < 0.001$); the second study (49) demonstrated a more striking correlation between the LV ejection fractions of $r = 0.91$, a slope that was near unity, and little or no intra- or interoperator variability. Thus, there still remains variability in the strength of the relationships between the sestamibi and MUGA LV ejection fractions.

ECHOCARDIOGRAPHY

Two-dimensional Echocardiography

Two-dimensional echocardiographic images of the LV have been widely used to assess LV volumes, ejection fractions, and segmental LV wall motion. Although the most common approach to interpreting these images for LV volumes and systolic performance is subjective during visual examinations of the dynamic images, this may not be the optimal approach, despite its practicality.

Several in vivo studies have used two-dimensional echocardiographic images to calculate LV volumes and ejection fractions in patients, who had CVG or MUGA scan data for comparison (34,50). Two excellent early studies undertook to compare two-dimensional echocardiographic LV volumes and ejection fractions to those from biplane CVG (34,50). Both of these studies used optimal two-dimensional image pairs and a modified Simpson's rule algorithm to calculate LV end-diastolic and end-systolic volumes to compare to the corresponding biplane CVG data. Although both studies found a significant underestimation of LV volumes by this quantitative two-dimensional echocardiographic approach, the LV ejection fractions appeared accurate (Fig. 6). These data confirmed that LV volumes and systolic performance could be quantified from high-quality, two-dimensional echocardiographic images.

Subsequent studies compared two-dimensional echocar-

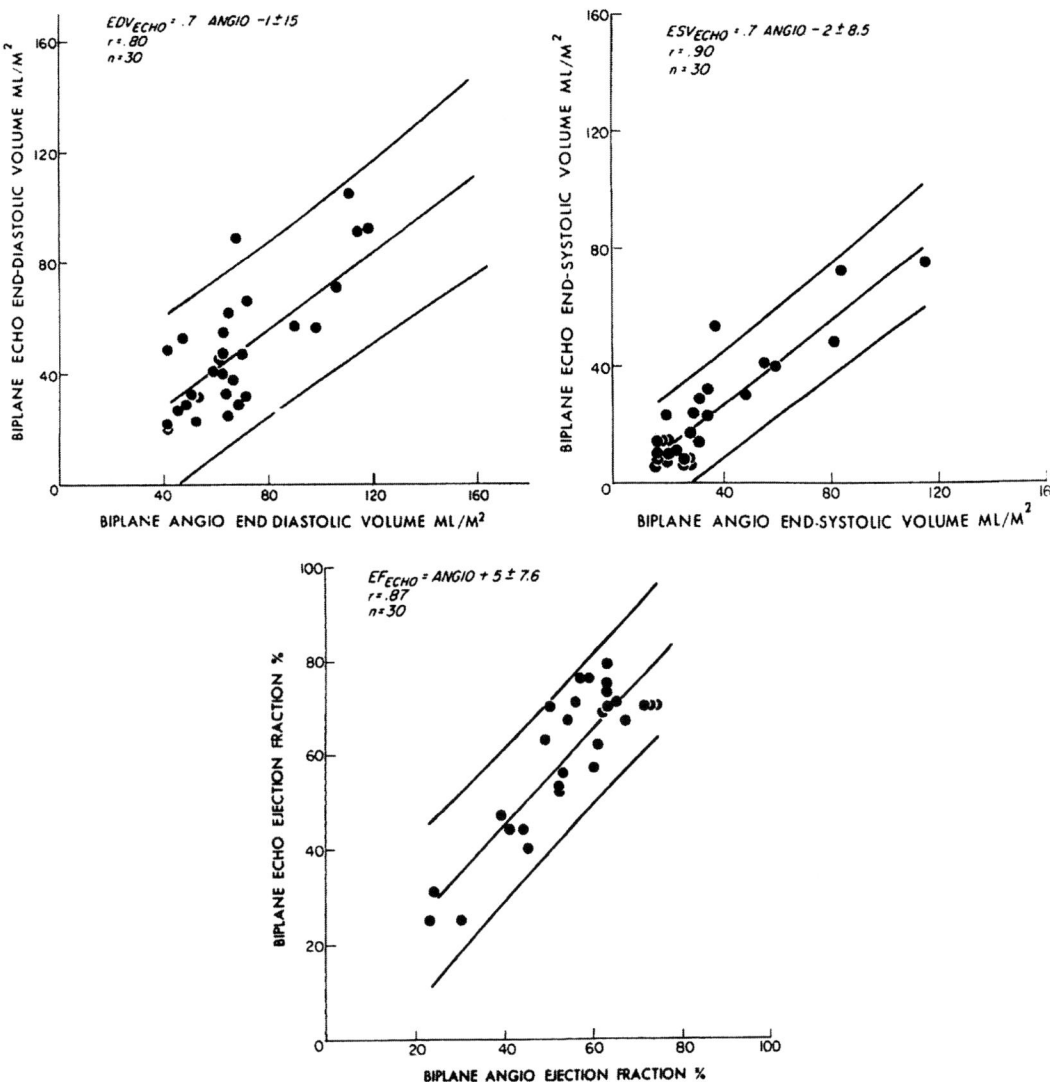

FIG. 6. Top left panel: The relationship between biplane two-dimensional echocardiographic left ventricular end-diastolic volumes indexed to body surface area, on the ordinate, and to biplane cineventriculographic end-diastolic volumes indexed to body surface area, on the abscissa, are shown. **Top right panel:** A similar comparison is shown for left ventricular end-systolic volumes. **Bottom panel:** A similar comparison is shown for left ventricular ejection fractions. The outer limit lines represent the 95% confidence intervals for the data. (From ref. 50, with permission.)

diographic LV volumes and ejection fractions to those from single plane CVG (51–56). In all instances, there were significant correlations but substantial underestimations of CVG LV volumes by echocardiography.

In addition, there have been comparisons of two-dimensional echocardiographic LV ejection fractions to those from MUGA scans. Folland and colleagues (51) compared two-dimensional echocardiographic LV ejection fractions to those calculated from CVG and MUGA scans and demonstrated correlations between the LV ejection fractions ($r = 0.75$; SEE $= 0.09$ and $r = 0.78$; SEE $= 0.10$, respectively). They concluded that this was a reasonable enough correlation to make useful clinical estimations of LV ejection fraction when they were calculated using quantitative echocardiographic methods.

There are also studies, that have compared two-dimensional echocardiographic determinations of segmental LV wall motion to those obtained from MUGA scans and CVG (56). The data obtained would suggest that there is better agreement between the degree of LV segmental dyssynergy identified by two-dimensional echocardiography and CVG than by MUGA scans.

Otterstad and co-investigators (53) studied serial two-dimensional echocardiograms in a core laboratory to address the precision and the reproducibility of the LV ejection fraction calculations. The deviations of LV ejection fractions between investigators on repeat echocardiograms was ± 5 ejection fraction units, but a systematic difference between investigators was noted. The co-efficients of variation ranged from 3 to 9% for different investigators, 3 to 6% for repeated measurements, and 7 to 19% for repeat echocardiographic examinations. When a 10% error in classification was accepted, the total variability ranged from 16 to 28%. Thus, what they established, in a short period of time, was that the echocardiographic image acquisition technique was the dominant component of variation, suggesting that standards need to be put in place for acquiring images and that the reproducibility of an individual evaluation is best served by a single investigator examining a sequence of high-quality images. Thus, even with careful quantitative echocardiographic approaches, there can be a substantial error introduced into the quantification of LV systolic performance.

Whether quantitative two-dimensional echocardiographic methods are required has been questioned. Several investigations have proposed that semiquantitative or visual analyses of two-dimensional echocardiographic images are sufficient, in and of themselves, for providing accurate estimates of LV systolic performance. Mueller and co-authors (54) reported that, in 40 patients undergoing biplane CVG, the best correlation for a visual estimate of LV ejection fractions came from a group of three blinded observers and ranged from $r = 0.75$ to 0.84. They noted, however, that all correlations improved when the quality of the studies improved, particularly when the definition of the endocardial surface exceeding 75% of the circumference of the LV. Nevertheless, differences persisted and one observer had systematically higher values than the other two, suggesting that interobserver variability may be substantial. Berning and co-authors (55) compared visual estimates of LV ejection fractions from two-dimensional echocardiographic images with those from MUGA scans and single plane CVG in patients with an acute myocardial infarction. Using one or the other of these standards, the correlation was good ($r = 0.93$), but the 95% confidence intervals for a single, visual two-dimensional echocardiographic estimate of LV ejection fraction was 17 ejection fraction units. Although these data suggested that a wide variation could occur on a visual estimate of LV ejection fraction, they commented that there was reasonable separation of patients into those who had LV ejection fractions that exceeded or were less than 40 ejection fraction units.

A more recent study (56) compared visual estimates of LV ejection fractions from two-dimensional echocardiographic images in 339 consecutive patients to those from MUGA scans and CVG. When the MUGA LV ejection fractions were divided into those that were normal, slightly reduced, moderately reduced, and severely reduced; there was substantial overlap among these groups when visual estimates of the two-dimensional echocardiographic images were used to estimate LV ejection fraction. The standard deviations in individual groups ranged from 12 to 13 ejection fraction units. In fact, the visual two-dimensional echocardiographic estimates of moderate and severe LV systolic dysfunction were not dissimilar, suggesting an important limitation of visual estimates of LV systolic performance. Van Royen and co-investigators (57) examined the accuracy and reproducibility of visual two-dimensional echocardiographic estimates of LV systolic performance by multiple echocardiog-raphers and compared them to quantitative MUGA LV ejection fractions processed by multiple nuclear technologists. They also examined the precision of these assessments after a 1-week interval. The relationship between the LV ejection fractions determined by both methods was good ($r = 0.81$, SEE $= 3.5$ ejection fraction units), but there were substantial differences in individual patients (limits of agreement, 24%). Intra- and interobserver reproducibility was reasonable for both methods, but they were substantially better for the MUGA than for the visual two-dimensional echocardiographic data (Fig. 7). Also, the limits of agreement were substantially better for the quantitative MUGA than the visual two-dimensional echocardiographic LV ejection fractions (2 to 4% vs. 13 to 17 %, respectively). Thus, the LV ejection fractions by these two techniques showed reasonably good agreement, but when a precise and reproducible LV ejection fraction was required for making patient management decisions, a quantitative MUGA scan was clearly superior to a visual analysis of two-dimensional echocardiographic images. Similarly, when a visual analysis of regional LV wall motion abnormalities on the two-dimensional echocardiographic images was performed in patients with ischemic heart disease by Peart and co-authors (58), there was substantial within and between interpreter variability. Upon repeat analysis of the same segment, one evaluator's agreement was 92%, whereas the other's was only 80%. Similarly, between evaluator agreement was 89% for some segments, but it was only 63% for other segments. Thus, within and between evaluator disagreement on regional LV wall motion abnormalities using a subjective assessment of two-dimensional echocardiographic images introduces a potential limitation for the general application of this noninvasive technique to analyzing sequential studies.

Transesophageal Echocardiography

Smith and co-authors (59) calculated LV volumes and ejection fractions from transesophageal echocardiograms using Simpson's rule, area-length, and diameter-length methods. Although reasonable correlations were obtained for LV end-diastolic ($r = 0.85$ to 0.88) and end-systolic volumes ($r = 0.93$ to 0.94) in comparison to single plane CVG data, there was a substantial underestimation of both volumes ($p < 0.003$). The LV ejection fractions were best predicted using the Simpson's rule algorithm ($r = 0.85$). These data suggest that, as with standard transthoracic echocardiography, transesophageal echocardiography underestimates LV volumes; but it may provide quantitatively accurate LV ejection fractions.

The reproducibility of assessments of LV ejection fraction by transesophageal echocardiography has been examined in quantitative and qualitative terms (60,61). Qualitative assessments of LV systolic performance between observers, the precision between studies, and the interstudy reproducibility were assessed by Deutsch and co-workers (61). Comparing the results of quantitative (60) and qualitative studies (61) suggests, once again, that, even using the transesopha-

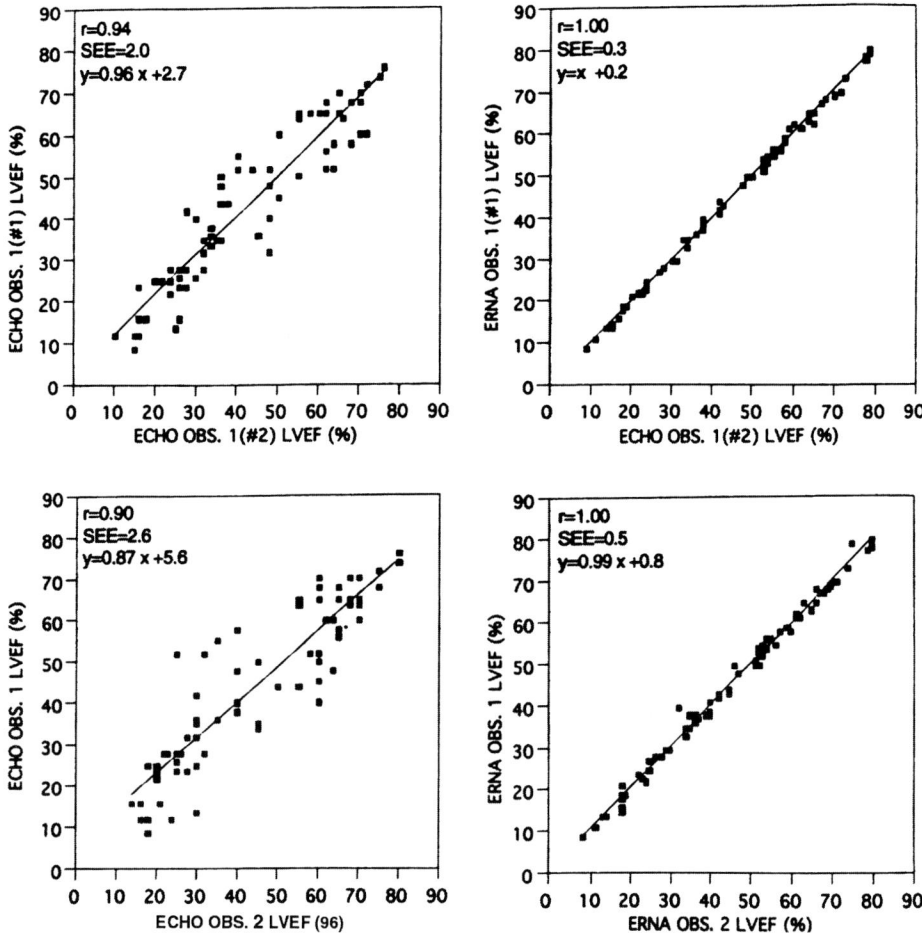

FIG. 7. Top panel: The correlation between the first and second visual estimates of left ventricular ejection fraction by echocardiographer 1 and between the first and second quantitative left ventricular ejection fraction by nuclear technologist 1 are shown. **Bottom panel:** The correlation between the visual estimates of left ventricular ejection fraction by two different echocardiographers and the correlation between the quantitative left ventricular ejection fractions by two nuclear technologists are shown. Note that the mean intraobserver variability is 2% for MUGA left ventricular ejection fractions and 15.3% for the two-dimensional echocardiographic visual estimates. Note also that the mean interobserver variability was 3.8% for the MUGA left ventricular ejection fractions and 18.1% for the two-dimensional echocardiographic visual estimates. (From ref. 57, with permission.)

geal approach, a quantitative assessment of LV systolic performance is more accurate, precise, and reproducible than subjective, visual estimations.

Three-dimensional Echocardiography

Because of difficulties with image quality and technical considerations regarding the quantification of LV systolic performance, the potential of three-dimensional echocardiography to provide a more complete assessment of LV size and systolic performance and, thereby, eliminate some of the difficulties with the two-dimensional approach is attractive. There have been excellent studies of three-dimensional reconstruction of *in vitro* simulations, heart models, or phantoms. Fazzalari and co-investigators (62) described the rela-

tionship between three-dimensional echocardiographic volumes of a phantom of known volume and found a linear regression equation that was near unity, a correlation coefficient of 1.0, and a standard error of the estimate of 3 mL. Thus, it can be concluded from these phantom studies that three-dimensional echocardiographic data can be acquired and analyzed to provide accurate quantification of volumes. These determinations of volume may be more accurate, at least in these phantom studies, than two-dimensional echocardiographic volume calculations.

Subsequently, there have been several studies that have attempted to compare three-dimensional echocardiographic determinations of LV size to those of single plane CVG (62–65). An early study by Nixon and colleagues (64) showed that three-dimensional echocardiographic LV end-diastolic and end-systolic volumes correlated with those from single plane CVG (0.95 and 0.94, respectively). The standard errors of the estimate were also small (9 mL and 7 mL, respectively).

Two subsequent studies by Sapin and co-investigators (65) and Kupferwasser and co-authors (63) also compared two- and three-dimensional echocardiographic LV volumes to those from single plane CVG. These studies suggested superiority of the three-dimensional echocardiographic approach to quantifying LV size compared to two-dimensional echocardiography.

There have also been studies to examine the value of three-dimensional echocardiography for quantifying LV systolic performance. Nosier and co-investigators (66) calculated three-dimensional echocardiographic LV ejection fractions and compared them to those from MUGA scans in patients with normal and abnormal LV shapes. The three-dimensional echocardiographic LV volume data was calculated using a Simpson's rule algorithm or an apical biplane modified Simpson's method. There was an excellent correlation, close limits of agreement, and nonsignificant differences between the three-dimensional echocardiographic and MUGA LV ejection fractions ($r = 0.99$), when Simpson's rule algorithm was used to calculate the echocardiographic LV volumes. Thus, these data demonstrated that three-dimensional echocardiography that used a Simpson's rule algorithm to calculate LV volumes could accurately quantify LV systolic performance.

Acoustic Quantification and Color Kinesis

Because of the potential difficulties of detecting endocardial borders, acoustic quantification has been developed as a technique for on-line detection of endocardial boundaries to provide a continuous display of LV area or volume changes and, therefore, LV systolic performance. The LV ejection fractions determined by two-dimensional echocardiographic acoustic quantification calculated from LV volumes obtained by both the area-length or Simpson's rule algorithm demonstrated a relationship with those from MUGA scans ($r = 0.92$, SEE = 4, $p < 0.05$) (67). Unfortunately, the acoustic quantification approach overestimated the MUGA LV ejection fractions with relatively wide limits of agreement $4 \pm 16\%$.

The ability to detect endocardial borders is also sometimes a limitation to quantitating regional LV systolic performance. The advent of color kinesis, a method for color encoding LV wall motion, as a tool to aid in the interpretation of regional LV wall motion in patients with regional dyssynergy has shown potential. Lang and co-investigators (68) investigated the feasibility and accuracy of quantitating segmental LV wall motion using a novel color kinesis analysis to provide an objective evaluation of regional LV systolic performance. They examined two-dimensional echocardiographic images from the short-axis and apical four-chamber views in 20 normal subjects and 40 patients with regional LV wall motion abnormalities. The LV end-systolic color

overlays were used to color encode LV endocardial motion throughout systole on a frame-by-frame basis. By developing histograms in the normal subjects that were highly consistent and reproducible, the patterns of contraction in the normal subjects could be used for an objective and automated interpretation of LV wall motion abnormalities. Thus, the advent of color kinesis to color encode regional LV wall motion and the potential for quantifying segmental LV systolic performance for objective interpretations of two-dimensional echocardiographic images is a new technique, that may have great promise.

CINE COMPUTED TOMOGRAPHY AND MAGNETIC RESONANCE IMAGING

There are two additional technologies that have been applied to quantifying LV size and systolic performance. These include cine computed tomography and magnetic resonance imaging. Although they are more widely used for other purposes, they have shown promise for quantifying LV size and systolic performance. Both of these approaches have the advantages of being gated to the electrocardiogram and of acquiring multiple slices of the LV whose areas can then be summed to obtain a volume. This process is similar to the Simpson's rule algorithm applied to biplane CVG and two-dimensional or three-dimensional echocardiography, which is probably the most accurate and precise mathematical approach to quantifying LV volumes. Thus, there is some data, although preliminary, to support the use of cine computed tomography for quantifying LV size and systolic performance (69).

There is much better data to support the use of magnetic resonance imaging for quantifying LV size and systolic performance. In contrast to the limited comparisons with cine computed tomography, studies with magnetic resonance imaging have been far more sophisticated and have used biplane CVG as the standard for comparing calculations of LV volumes, ejection fractions, segmental wall motion, and mass (see Chapters 29 and 30). Cranney et al. (70) systematically calculated magnetic resonance LV volumes and masses and compared them to biplane CVG data. In their initial study of 21 patients undergoing cardiac catheterization and magnetic resonance imaging within 3 days, they demonstrated that LV end-diastolic volumes were systematically underestimated by magnetic resonance imaging compared to biplane CVG ($p < 0.05$), while the LV end-systolic volumes were similar. They also reported that the intra- and interobserver variabilities in the volumetric determinations by magnetic resonance were only 11%. A subsequent study from this group systematically examined the precision and reproducibility of the magnetic resonance LV ejection fractions. These studies were rigorous and demonstrated the ability of magnetic resonance imaging to assess not only cardiac structure, but also quantify LV size, systolic performance, regional wall motion and mass.

Because of the ability of magnetic resonance imaging to so accurately quantitate LV mass, Holman and co-workers (71) evaluated regional LV wall thickening in 25 patients, who had had a prior myocardial infarction, and compared these data with that in 48 control subjects. The total extent of LV dysfunction defined as abnormalities in LV wall thickening by magnetic resonance imaging correlated with myocardial infarct size ($y = 0.90\ x + 0.92$, $p < 0.0001$). This study by Holman and co-workers suggests that an analysis of global LV mass and regional LV wall thickening may be a unique capability of magnetic resonance imaging for quantifying both global and, in this case, regional LV systolic performance (see also Chapters 29 and 30).

CLINICAL APPLICATIONS

Data from this discussion provide clear evidence that we have several imaging technologies available to us that accurately quantitate LV size, ejection fraction, segmental LV wall motion, and mass. It is appropriate to examine the clinical utility of these technologies and to scrutinize each in regard to whether they are accurate; precise, that is, can on two separate occasions provide the same data; and reproducible, that is, the same observer or a different observer can reexamine the same study and come up with a comparable result within narrow specified limits. The most extensive evaluation of this kind has been done for CVG. The conclusions that can be drawn from those investigations are that biplane CVG in normal and abnormal ventricles that use a Simpson's rule algorithm to calculate LV size provides accurate, precise, and reproducible quantitative LV volumes and systolic performance data. Geometric assumptions of area-length in normal or diseased ventricles, particularly when single plane CVG images are used, can lead to clinically spurious data as can visual analysis of these kinds of images.

Noninvasive imaging technologies each have their own usefulness and clinical place. It would appear that MUGA scans and magnetic resonance imaging most accurately, precisely, and reproducibly quantify LV systolic performance. More sophisticated comparisons will be required to confirm the abilities of 99m-technetium sestamibi myocardial perfusion imaging and cine computed tomography to quantify LV size and systolic performance. Two-dimensional echocardiography, particularly if a subjective, visual analysis is applied to the images, is fraught with error; but a quantitative approach for analyzing these images certainly improves upon a subjective estimate of LV size and systolic performance and is probably clinically valuable. The newer processing modalities, including: three-dimensional echocardiography as well as acoustic quantification and color kinesis of two-dimensional echocardiographic images, may enhance the quality of the echocardiographic images and, thereby, provide more accurate quantification of LV size, systolic performance and segmental wall motion.

If we examine the clinical question that is being asked, the invasive or noninvasive imaging technology that should be chosen to quantify LV systolic performance may vary. For example, if we wish to know whether the LV is normal or abnormal in its most crude sense, any noninvasive imaging modality may be satisfactory as long as a quantitative assessment is employed. However, if we are asking the question of whether or not there has been some incremental change in LV size, systolic performance, or regional LV wall motion, which is a far more complex question requiring far more accurate determinations of LV size and systolic performance, then the selection of noninvasive imaging technology becomes more difficult. The data suggest that whatever noninvasive imaging technology is chosen, its validity should be established in comparison to *in vitro* phantoms or hearts and to *in vivo* biplane CVG to clearly delineate its accuracy, precision, and reproducibility for quantifying LV size and systolic performance. It is also clear that a subjective analysis of any noninvasive imaging technology, particularly the widely applied two-dimensional echocardiographic approach, is so fraught with inaccuracy and variation in interpretation that it is probably not appropriate.

REFERENCES

1. Dodge HT, Baxley WA. Left ventricular volume and mass and their significance in heart disease. *Am J Cardiol* 1969;23:528–537.
2. Kasser IS, Kennedy JW. Measure of left ventricular volumes in man by single-plane cineangiocardiography. *Invest Radiol* 1969;4:83–90.
3. Dubel HP, Tschapek A. Axial oblique projections—volumetric studies into left ventricular cast specimens of man. *Eur J Radiol* 1984;4(2): 85–88.
4. Starling MR, Walsh RA. Accuracy of biplane axial oblique and oblique cineangiographic left ventricular cast volume determinations using a modification of Simpson's rule algorithm. *Am Heart J* 1985;110: 1219–1225.
5. Chapman CB, Baker O, Reynolds J, et al. Use of biplane cinefluorography for measurement of ventricular volume. *Circulation* 1958;18:1105.
6. Pietras RJ, Kondos GT, Juska J. Quantitative validation of cineangiographic axial oblique biplane left ventricular volume measurement. *Cathet Cardiovasc Diagn* 1987;13:157–161.
7. Ino T, Benson LN, Mikalian H, et al. Correlation of left ventricular angiographic casts and biplane left ventricular volumetry in infants and children. *Am J Cardiol* 1988;61:441–445.
8. Ino T, Benson LN, Mikalian H, et al. Determination of left ventricular volumes by Simpson's rule in infants and children with congenital heart disease. *Br Heart J* 1989;61:182–185.
9. Vogel, JH, Cornish D, McFadden RB. Underestimation of ejection fraction with single plane angiography in coronary artery disease: role of biplane angiography. *Chest* 1973;64:217–221.
10. Walsh W, Falicov RE, Pai AL. Comparison of single and biplane ejection fractions in patients with ischaemic heart disease. *Br Heart J* 1976; 38:388–395.
11. Rogers WJ, Smith LR, Bream PR, et al. Quantitative axial oblique contrast left ventricular: validation of the method by demonstrating improved visualization of regional wall motion and mitral valve function with accurate volume determinations. *Am Heart J* 1982;103: 185–194.
12. Hillis LD, Winniford MD, Dehmer GJ, et al. Left ventricular volumes by single plane cineangiography: *in vivo* validation of the Kennedy regression equation. *Am J Cardiol* 1984;53:1159–1163.
13. Tate DA, Weaver D, Dehmer GJ. Effect of an anterior wall motion abnormality on the results of single plane and biplane left ventriculography. *Am J Cardiol* 1992;70:791–796.
14. Brogan WC III, Glamann B, Lange RA, et al. Comparison of single and biplane ventriculography for determination of left ventricular volume and ejection fraction. *Am J Cardiol* 1992;69:1079–1082.

15. LeWinter MM, Kent RS, Kroener JM, et al. Regional differences in myocardial performance in the left ventricle of the dog. *Circ Res* 1975; 37:191–199.

16. Ingels NB Jr, Daughters GT II, Stinson EB, et al. Evaluation of methods for quantitating left ventricular segmental wall motion in man using myocardial markers as a standard. *Circulation* 1980;61:966–972.

17. Hansen DE, Daughters GT II, Alderman EL, et al. Torsional deformation of the left ventricular midwall in human hearts with intramyocardial markers: regional heterogeneity and sensitivity to the inotropic effects of abrupt rate changes. *Circ Res* 1988;62:941–952.

18. Streeter DD, Spotnitz HM, Patel DP, et al. Fiber orientation in the canine left ventricle during diastole and systole. *Circ Res* 1969;24: 339–347.

19. Gelberg HJ, Brundage BH, Glantz S, et al. Quantitative left ventricular wall motion analysis: a comparison of area, chord and radial methods. *Circulation* 1979;59:99–100.

20. Bhargava V, Warren S, Vieweg WV, et al. Quantitation of left ventricular wall motion in normal subjects: comparison of various methods. *Cathet Cardiovasc Diagn* 1980;6:7–16.

21. Clayton PD, Jeppson GM, Klausner SC. Should a fixed external reference system be used to analyze left ventricular wall motion? *Circulation* 1982;65:1518–1521.

22. Sheehan FH, Bolson EL, Dodge HT, et al. Advantages and applications of the centerline method for characterizing regional ventricular function. *Circulation* 1986;74:293–305.

23. Vine DL, Hegg TD, Dodge HT, et al. Immediate effect of contrast medium injection on left ventricular volumes and ejection fraction. A study using metallic epicardial markers. *Circulation* 1977;56:379–384.

24. Cascade PN, Wajszczuk WJ, Kerin NZ, et al. Determination and importance of the magnification factor in the calculation of ventricular volume: development of a simple, accurate method. *Cathet Cardiovasc Diagn* 1978;4:391–398.

25. Baylen B, Ogata H, French WJ, et al. Accurate internal correction for the magnification of cineangiocardiography in infants with congenital heart disease. *Am Heart J* 1984;107:113–118.

26. Wexler LF, Lesperance J, Ryan TJ, et al. Interobserver variability in interpreting contrast left ventriculograms (CASS). *Cathet Cardiovasc Diagn* 1982;8:341–355.

27. Rigaud M, Hardy A, Castadot M, et al. Variability and reproducibility of quantitative left ventricular angiography. *Cathet Cardiovasc Diagn* 1989;16:8–15.

28. Chaitman BR, DeMots H, Bristow D, et al. Objective and subjective analysis of left ventricular angiograms. *Circulation* 1975;52:420–425.

29. Nissen SE, Elion JL, Grayburn P, et al. Determination of left ventricular ejection fraction by computer densitometric analysis of digital subtraction angiography: experimental validation and correlation with area–length methods. *Am J Cardiol* 1987;59:675–680.

30. Lehmkuhl H, Altstidl R, Machnig T, et al. On-line evaluation of systolic performance by densitometry in digital left ventriculography. *Clin Cardiol* 1996;19:729–736.

31. Strauss HW, Zaret BL, Hurley PJ, et al. A scintiphotographic method for measuring left ventricular ejection fraction in man without cardiac catheterization. *Am J Cardiol* 1971;28:575–580.

32. Starling MR, Gross MD, Walsh RA, et al. Assessment of the radionuclide angiographic left ventricular maximum time-varying elastance calculation in man. *J Nucl Med* 1988;29:1368–1381.

33. Schelbert HR, Verba JW, Johnson AD, et al. Nontraumatic determination of left ventricular ejection fraction by radionuclide angiocardiography. *Circulation* 1975;51:902–909.

34. Starling MR, Crawford MH, Sorensen SG, et al. Comparative accuracy of apical biplane cross-sectional echocardiography and gated equilibrium radionuclide angiography for estimating left ventricular size and performance. *Circulation* 1981;63:1075–1084.

35. Wackers FJ, Berger HJ, Johnstone DE, et al. Multiple gated blood pool imaging for left ventricular ejection fraction: validation of the technique and assessment of variability. *Am J Cardiol* 1979;43:1159–1166.

36. Palacios I, Goldman M, Aretz T, et al. Comparison of contrast x-ray biplane cineangiography and technetium-99m radionuclide scans for measurement of ventricular volumes in human autopsy hearts. *Am Heart J* 1986;112:1032–1038.

37. Dehmer GJ, Lewis SE, Hillis LD, et al. Nongeometric determination of left ventricular volumes from equilibrium blood pool scans. *Am J Cardiol* 1980;45:293–300.

38. Starling MR, Dell'Italia LJ, Walsh RA, et al. Accurate estimates of absolute left ventricular volumes from equilibrium radionuclide angiographic count data using a simple geometric attenuation correction. *J Am Coll Cardiol* 1984;3:789–798.

39. Siegel JA, Maurer AH, Wu RK, et al. Absolute left ventricular volume by an iterative build-up factor analysis of gated radionuclide images. *Radiology* 1984;151:477–481.

40. Starling MR, Dell'Italia LJ, Nusynowitz ML, et al. Estimates of left ventricular volumes by equilibrium radionuclide angiography: importance of attenuation correction. *J Nuc Med* 1984;25:14–20.

41. Verani MS, Gaeta J, LeBlanc AD, et al. Validation of left ventricular volume measurements by radionuclide angiography. *J Nuc Med* 1987; 28:401–402.

42. Maddox DE, Wynne J, Uren R, et al. Regional ejection fraction: a quantitative radionuclide index of regional left ventricular performance. *Circulation* 1979;59:1001–1009.

43. Holman BL, Wynne J, Idoine J, et al. The paradox image: a noninvasive index of regional left ventricular dyskinesis. *J Nuc Med* 1979;20: 1237–1242.

44. Starling MR, Walsh RA, Lasher JC, et al. Quantification of left ventricular regional dyssynergy by radionuclide angiography. *J Nucl Med* 1987;28:1725–1735.

45. Frais M, Botvinick E, Shosa D, et al. Phase image characterization of localized and generalized left ventricular contraction abnormalities. *J Am Coll Cardiol* 1984;4:987–998.

46. Gill JB, Moore RH, Tamaki N, et al. Multigated blood-pool tomography: new method for the assessment of left ventricular function. *J Nuc Med* 1986;27:1916–1924.

47. Williams KA, Taillon LA. Gated planar technetium 99m-labeled sestamibi myocardial image inversion for quantitative scintigraphic assessment of left ventricular function. *J Nuc Med* 1995;2:285–295.

48. Boonyaprapa S, Ekmahachai M, Thanachaikun N, et al. Measurement of left ventricular ejection fraction from gated technetium-99m sestamibi myocardial images. *Eur J Nuc Med* 1995;22:528–531.

49. Calnon DA, Kastner RJ, Smith WH, et al. Validation of new counts-based gated single photon emission computed tomography method for quantifying left ventricular systolic function: comparison with equilibrium radionuclide angiography. *J Nucl Cardiol* 1997;4:464–471.

50. Schiller NB, Acquatella H, Ports TA, et al. Left ventricular volume from paired biplane two-dimensional echocardiography. *Circulation* 1979;60:547–555.

51. Folland ED, Parisi AF, Moynihan PF, et al. Assessment of left ventricular ejection fraction and volumes by real-time, two-dimensional echocardiography. A comparison of cineangiographic and radionuclide techniques. *Circulation* 1979;60:760–766.

52. Hecht HS, Taylor R, Wong M, Shah PM. Comparative evaluation of segmental asynergy in remote myocardial infarction by radionuclide angiography, two-dimensional echocardiography, and contrast cineventriculography. *Am Heart J* 1981;101:740–749.

53. Otterstad JE, Froeland G, St. John Sutton M, et al. Accuracy and reproducibility of biplane two-dimensional echocardiographic measurements of left ventricular dimensions and function. *Eur Heart J* 1997; 18:507–513.

54. Mueller X, Stauffer JC, Jaussi A, et al. Subjective visual echocardiographic estimate of left ventricular ejection fraction as an alternative to conventional echocardiographic methods: comparison with contrast angiography. *Clin Cardiol* 1991;14:898–902.

55. Berning J, Rokkedal Nielsen J, et al. Rapid estimation of left ventricular ejection fraction in acute myocardial infarction by echocardiographic wall motion analysis. *Cardiology* 1992;80:257–266.

56. Gottsauner-Wolf M, Schedlmayer-Duit J, Porenta G, et al. Assessment of left ventricular function: comparison between radionuclide angiography and semiquantitative two-dimensional echocardiographic analysis. *Eur J Nucl Med* 1996;23:1613–1618.

57. Van Royen N, Jaffe C, Krumholz H, et al. Comparison and reproducibility of visual echocardiographic and quantitative radionuclide left ventricular ejection fractions. *Am J Cardiol* 1996;77:843–850.

58. Peart I, Austin A, Hall R. Subjective analysis of cross-sectional echocardiograms: reproducibility and sources of variability. *Eur Heart J* 1987;8:171–178.

59. Smith MD, MacPhail B, Harrison MR, et al. Value and limitations of transesophageal echocardiography in determination of left ventricular volumes and ejection fraction. *J Am Coll Cardiol* 1992;19:1213–1222.

60. Ryan T, Burwash I, Lu J, et al. The agreement between ventricular

volumes and ejection fraction by transesophageal echocardiography or a combined radionuclear and thermodilution technique in patients after coronary artery surgery. *J Cardiothor Vasc Anest* 1996;10:323–328.

61. Deutsch HJ, Curtins JM, Leischik R, et al. Reproducibility of assessment of left ventricular function using intraoperative transesophageal echocardiography. *Thorac Cardiovasc Surg* 1993;41:54–58.

62. Fazzalari NL, Davidson JA, Mazumdar J, et al. Three-dimensional reconstruction of the left ventricle from four anatomically defined apical two-dimensional echocardiographic views. *Acta Cardiol* 1984;39:409–435.

63. Kupferwasser I, Mohr-Kahaly S, Stahr P, et al. Transthoracic three-dimensional echocardiographic volumetry of distorted left ventricles using rotational scanning. *J Am Soc Echo* 1997;10:840–852.

64. Nixon JV, Saffer SI, Lipscomb K, et al. Three-dimensional echoventriculography. *Am Heart J* 1983;106:435–443.

65. Sapin P, Schroeder K, Gopal A, et al. Comparison of two-dimensional and three-dimensional echocardiography with cineventriculography for measurement of left ventricular volume in patients. *J Am Coll Cardiol* 1994;24:1054–1063.

66. Nosier YF, Salustri A, Kasprzak JD, et al. Left ventricular ejection fraction in patients with normal and distorted left ventricular shape by three-dimensional echocardiographic methods: a comparison with radionuclide angiography. *J Am Soc Echo* 1995;11:620–630.

67. Chandra S, Bahl VK, Reddy SC, et al. Comparison of echocardiographic acoustic quantification system and radionuclide ventriculography for estimating left ventricular ejection fraction: validation in patients without regional wall motion abnormalities. *Am Heart J* 1997;133:359–363.

68. Lang R, Vignon P, Weinert L, et al. Echocardiographic quantification of regional left ventricular wall motion with color kinesis. *Circulation* 1996;93:1877–1885,

69. Bouchard A, Lipton MJ, Farner DW, et al. Evaluation of regional ventricular wall motion by ECG-gated CT. *J Comput Assisted Tomogr* 1987;11:969–974.

70. Cranney GB, Lotan CS, Baxley DL, et al. Left ventricular volume measurement using cardiac axis nuclear magnetic resonance imaging. Validation by calibrated ventricular angiography. *Circulation* 1990;82:154–163.

71. Holman ER, Buller VG, de Roos A, et al. Detection and quantification of dysfunctional myocardium by magnetic resonance imaging. A new three-dimensional method for quantitative wall-thickening analysis. *Circulation* 1997;95:924–931.

CHAPTER 52

Diastolic Etiologies

César Coello and Martin M. LeWinter

Recognition of the syndrome of clinical heart failure with elevated filling pressures and pulmonary congestion in the presence of preserved left ventricular contraction (normal systolic function) has led to the concept of diastolic heart failure. Early epidemiological data suggested that this condition was present in a substantial proportion of the patients evaluated for heart failure (1). Recognition of the high prevalence of this condition has motivated research over the last two decades. These efforts have been instrumental in the development of a better understanding of pathophysiology at both the cellular and organ level. The function of the heart during diastole is a complex process in which ventricular relaxation, the passive properties of the ventricle, and the characteristics of ventricular filling are closely interrelated. Accordingly, in conjunction with a consideration of imaging in relation to diastolic heart failure, it is useful to begin with an overview of the physiology and pathophysiology of diastole.

PHYSIOLOGY AND PATHOPHYSIOLOGY OF DIASTOLE

Phases of Diastole

The definition of diastole in itself has been an object of debate. For the purposes of this chapter, we shall consider ventricular diastole to be the period between closure of the aortic valve and closure of the mitral valve. (An alternative is to consider all of contraction-relaxation systole and events following completion of relaxation diastole.) The relation between ventricular pressure and volume during diastole is determined by three main factors, deactivation or active relaxation of the myofilaments, restoring forces, which are responsible for elastic recoil and diastolic suction, and the passive filling properties of the ventricular chamber. The

C. Coello: Department of Medicine, University of Vermont, Burlington, Vermont 05401.
M. M. LeWinter: Department of Medicine, University of Vermont; Cardiology Unit, Fletcher Allen Health Care, Burlington, Vermont 05401.

phases of diastole include isovolumic relaxation, early filling, diastasis, and atrial systole.

Isovolumic relaxation is the time between closure of the aortic valve and opening of the mitral valve. During this period inactivation of the myocytes (relaxation) is translated into decay of the intraventricular pressure to levels below atrial pressure, at which point the mitral valve opens and the phase of *rapid ventricular filling* ensues. It is important to keep in mind that myocyte relaxation continues after the isovolumic phase is complete and thus contributes to generation of both the intraventricular pressure and the atrioventricular pressure gradient responsible for the rapid filling phase. At the same time, a portion of the energy generated during systole may be converted to potential energy (in the form of a restoring force) and then to kinetic energy during rapid filling in the form of elastic recoil, or filling by suction. Suction in effect allows the ventricle to fill at lower pressures than would otherwise be the case. As discussed below, generation of restoring forces is complex; their magnitude is inversely related to the end-systolic volume.

The resulting early filling pattern and instantaneous relation between ventricular pressure and volume reflect a dynamic interaction between the time course of relaxation, conversion of restoring forces (when present) into elastic recoil, and the passive filling properties of the ventricle. As the pressures in the atrium and ventricle almost equilibrate, relaxation is completed, recoil forces are dissipated, and the velocity and volume of left ventricular filling drops markedly, corresponding to the phase of *diastasis*. During this phase and subsequently, the relation between ventricular pressure and volume is dominated by the fully relaxed, or passive filling properties of the ventricle. As described below, the passive relation between pressure and volume is curvilinear, and determined by chamber geometry, stiffness of the myocardial tissue, and external constraints such as the pericardium and the contralateral ventricle.

The *atrial filling phase* occurs when the left atrium contracts, resulting in additional filling of the ventricle, and ends when ventricular contraction closes the mitral valve. Although the portion of the stroke volume accounted for by atrial contraction has great variability, during this phase the relation between ventricular pressure and volume continues to be dominated by the passive relation.

Cellular Determinants of Myocyte Relaxation

Contraction of the mammalian cardiomyocyte begins with opening of L-type sarcolemmal calcium channels triggered by the propagation of an action potential. A relatively small amount of calcium enters the cytosol and activates the release of large amounts of calcium through opening of ryanodine receptor channels located in adjacent portions of the sarcoplasmic reticulum (SR) (calcium-induced calcium release). The resulting marked transient elevation of intracellular calcium allows calcium ions to occupy sites on the troponin C subunit of troponin, a regulatory protein complex decorating the actin molecule. This induces conformational changes in the troponin complex and another regulatory protein, tropomyosin, that ultimately releases the inhibition of actin-myosin crossbridge formation normally present at low levels of cytosolic calcium. Deactivation of this process (relaxation) requires removal of calcium ions from troponin C. The two primary mechanisms are an energy-requiring calcium transporting enzyme in the SR (the SR calcium ATPase, abbreviated SERCA-2) and Na-Ca exchange by a protein complex located in the sarcolemma. SERCA-2 reuptake of cytosolic calcium is ordinarily responsible for the largest proportion of calcium cycled per beat whereas the Na-Ca exchanger extrudes the relatively small amount of calcium that enters the cell through the L-type channels back into the extracellular space. In disease states, the balance between these two major processes of calcium disposition can vary considerably. The process of SERCA-2 reuptake of calcium is modulated by an adjacent SR protein, phospholamban, which ordinarily has an inhibitory effect on SERCA-2. This inhibition is relieved by cyclic AMP-mediated phosphorylation, resulting in more rapid reuptake of calcium ions and faster relaxation. Catecholamines increase contraction rate by virtue of cyclic AMP phosphorylation of L-type channels, augmenting calcium-induced calcium release, and relaxation rate by phosphorylation of phospholamban.

Failure of the normal mechanisms of reuptake and extrusion of calcium ions results in slowing of relaxation and/or an inability to restore calcium to normal diastolic levels, i.e., incomplete relaxation with excessive diastolic tension. Other determinants of relaxation rate are the affinity of calcium for the myofilaments and the kinetics of crossbridge dissociation. Alterations in calcium affinity appear to often play a role in modulation of relaxation by paracrine and autocrine substances.

Extracellular and Organ Level Control

Extracellular and organ level factors modulate the timing and rate of relaxation. As described by Brutsaert and co-

workers (3) and others (2,4) these include afterload, regional and temporal inhomogeneities, and paracrine factors.

Load has a complex and as yet incompletely understood interaction with relaxation (2,4–8). A direct influence of load on the length-dependency of calcium sensitivity of the myofilaments and crossbridge detachment rate may be operative. Additionally load may influence stretch-activated channels that modify trans-sarcolemmal calcium flux (9). Loads may have different effects depending on their timing. Increases in contraction loads delay the onset and modestly slow relaxation. In contrast, an increase in load that is timed during relaxation can have the opposite effect, resulting in earlier onset and more rapid relaxation. Relaxation loads may be pertinent to arterial wave reflection from the periphery back to the heart. Reduced arterial compliance, for instance due to aging, results in more rapid wave reflection and potentially may convert a relaxation load into a contraction load.

Increases in regional or temporal inhomogeneities of contraction or relengthening slow relaxation and filling rates. Examples include regional ischemia, hypertrophic cardiomyopathy, conduction abnormalities, and ventricular pacing. The mechanisms have not been fully elucidated, but likely are related to regional load variations.

An important and relatively recent development in the physiology of myocardial relaxation is the discovery of endocardial and vascular endothelial modulators (3,9,10). (Detailed consideration of this complex topic is beyond the scope of this chapter. The reader is referred to recent reviews for a more complete treatment.) This concept was first proposed by Brutsaert and co-workers (12), who noted that denudation of the endocardium of papillary muscle preparations resulted in an earlier onset and more rapid relaxation in conjunction with a very modest reduction of developed force, i.e., a disproportionate effect on relaxation. Subsequently, it became apparent that *vascular* endothelium also plays an important role in these responses. As is the case with vascular tissue in general, a key signaling molecule for these effects on myocardial function appears to be nitric oxide (NO). In isolated cardiac muscle and in the intact ventricle, NO surrogates and donors (e.g., nitroprusside) cause similar effects as described above, while inhibition of NO synthase (NOS) has opposite effects. Finally, cardiac myocytes themselves are capable of producing NO (an autocrine effect). Most effects of NO on myocardial function are thought to be mediated by cyclic GMP, although noncyclic GMP mediated effects have also been proposed. The effect of NO on relaxation appears to involve a decrease in myofilament calcium responsiveness rather than a direct effect on calcium reuptake and disposition. Although the physiologic significance of NO in control of myocardial relaxation has not yet been fully elucidated, it is likely important since so many vasoactive substances (e.g., bradykinin, substance P) ultimately modulate NO production. The short half-life of NO and responsiveness of vascular endothelium to changes in flow and shear stress suggest a role in short-time course responses. There is also some experimental evidence of NO involvement in the modulation of beta-adrenergic responses.

Other paracrine factors influence myocardial relaxation (10). Angiotensin II (AT II) produced in the myocardium has complex effects on myocardial function, although there is disagreement about their magnitude and significance. In hypertrophied hearts AT II increases contractility and slows relaxation. Effects in the normal heart are less clear. The mechanisms may involve calcium reuptake and increased myofilament sensitivity to calcium; however, they have not been fully elucidated. Additionally, activation of angiotensin-converting enzyme increases kininase activity; therefore, increased AT II levels are associated with reduced bradykinin activity, one result of which may be decreased NO mediated relaxation effects. The vascular endothelium also releases endothelin-1 (ET-1), a potent vasoconstrictor that also appears to delay and slow relaxation. Elevated ET-1 concentrations in congestive heart failure may implicate a role for this substance in slowed relaxation in patients with failing myocardium. Other locally released substances that may influence myocardial relaxation include natriuretic peptides, prostaglandins and adenylpurines. The physiologic and pathophysiologic significance of paracrine and autocrine modulators and their complex interactions are objects of current investigational interest.

Restoring Forces

Restoring forces are generated when the ventricle contracts to an end-systolic volume (ESV) below its equilibrium volume (Vo) (9,11), the volume in the fully relaxed state when transmural pressure is zero. Their magnitude is inversely proportional to the ESV. When ESV is below Vo, the chamber can be considered under compression due to storage of potential energy generated during contraction in functional springs in the myocardium. This energy is converted to kinetic energy in the form of elastic recoil, with resultant suction of blood from the atrium into the ventricle early during diastole, i.e., during the rapid filling phase (13). Suction is operative as a mechanism of filling whenever ESV is less than Vo, whether or not the left ventricular transmural pressure actually becomes negative. Because the normal early diastolic transmitral gradient is ordinarily only on the order of several mmHg, an ESV corresponding to even a slightly negative transmural pressure can have an important influence on filling. The fact that filling occurs simultaneously by other mechanisms that ordinarily prevent the left ventricular pressure from becoming negative obscures the presence of suction when it is present. Suction allows the ventricle to fill at lower pressures than would otherwise be the case. Its contribution to filling is dependent on ventricular loading conditions and contractility (14). Suction is likely most important under conditions of stress, when contractility is high and ESV small, for example during exercise. Correspondingly, in situations in which contractility is impaired

such that the ESV is increased, suction will tend to be reduced or lost as a mechanism of filling.

At the level of the cardiac myocyte, the potential energy of elastic recoil is stored by compression of titin, a giant protein that binds myosin to the Z line. Additionally, several aspects of the deformation of the ventricular chamber also have been proposed to contribute to restoring forces and diastolic suction (15,16). These include deformation of connective tissue, transmural variation in timing of contraction and relengthening, and torsional rotation of the ventricle (twist). Restoring forces and filling by suction have been extremely difficult to study experimentally in the intact circulation because of difficulties in measuring both Vo and the volume of mitral inflow accounted for by suction. New techniques employing nonfilling diastoles in the intact heart that allow measurement of fully relaxed pressure at small volumes have been developed to investigate this problem (11,14). Studies using these techniques indicate that restoring forces and suction are probably normally present over at least the lower portion of the physiologic range of filling and are increased by adrenergic stimulation.

The Pressure-volume Relationship of the Passive Ventricle

The intracavitary pressure-volume relationship (PVR) of the fully relaxed or passive ventricle is determined by the geometry of the chamber, the nature of the tissue in its walls (including the blood and vasculature), and external constraints (17). Passive stretch of myofibers results from application of a distending force, for example, a positive pressure gradient across the mitral valve. At any instant in time, the applied distending force, or stress (force/unit area), is exactly balanced by an opposing force in the wall. The relation between pressure and chamber geometry when a stress is applied to the ventricle can be quantified by the LaPlace relationship (17). In its simplest form (for a sphere) the LaPlace equation states that the pressure is proportional to the radius of the chamber divided by its wall thickness. More complicated formulations have been derived for differently shaped chambers, such as an ellipsoid of revolution, but the same basic principles given by the simplified formula apply. The LaPlace relationship quantifies one intuitive feature of the relation between distending pressure and volume, namely, a thicker walled chamber requires a larger distending pressure to achieve a given volume. For nonspherical chambers, other details of geometry (e.g., short/long-axis ratios) also influence the volume resulting from a given distending pressure.

It is also intuitively obvious that the nature of the tissue in the walls determines the distending force required to fill the chamber. Normally, the most important determinant of the PVR at very low pressures is the elastic properties of titin, the same protein responsible for restoring forces when compressed. At higher distending pressures, the myocardial connective tissue matrix assumes a key role. Thus, changes in the amount or composition of Titin or collagen influence the passive PVR. The resistance of the tissue in the walls of the ventricle to passive stretch is quantified as its stiffness, or the change in stress required to produce a given change in stretch (or strain). Biologic tissues usually have a curvilinear (exponential) passive stress-strain relationship, constituting "elastic" behavior. Thus, "operating" elastic stiffness increases at higher strains. By plotting stiffness as a function of stress, a linear relationship is obtained, in contrast to the curvilinear stress-strain relationship. The slope of this linear relationship is one kind of stiffness constant, which in this case characterizes the stiffness of the tissue independent of strain.

Another determinant of stiffness of the myocardial tissue is the amount of blood contained in the vessels of the ventricular wall. Blood vessels occupy a significant volume fraction of the ventricular myocardium and it is therefore not surprising that a greater distending pressure is required to fill the chamber when blood volume increases. This is known as the erectile property of the myocardium (18).

The PVR of the passive left ventricle is curvilinear, paralleling the passive stress-strain relationship of the tissue (17). At any point on this relationship, the instantaneous ratio of change in pressure to change in volume is the operating *chamber stiffness*; its inverse is the *operating compliance*. (Subsequently, we will use the term compliance to refer to the passive PVR.) Similar to the stress-strain relationship, the PVR can be converted into a linear relation by plotting operating chamber stiffness vs. pressure. The slope of this relationship is a *chamber* stiffness constant. It is important to keep in mind that a change in compliance or operating stiffness requires a change in the *slope* of the PVR. A parallel shift (with an accompanying change in Vo) can occur acutely or chronically but does not constitute a compliance change. The term change in diastolic distensibility has been used to denote shifts in the PVR whose details (slope vs. position change) are unknown. This typically applies in situations in which only a small segment of the PVR can be sampled.

The parietal pericardium and right ventricle constitute external constraints to left ventricular filling (conversely, the left ventricle constrains right ventricular filling). Under certain conditions, the lungs within the rigid thoracic cavity may function in the same way. The parietal pericardium has its own PVR, which is very compliant at low volumes but makes a fairly sharp transition to a very steep relation. The details of the normal pericardial PVR are such that it provides only a small reserve volume in relation to the heart. Starting at normal levels of total heart volume, relatively modest increments in total heart volume move the total volume within the pericardial sac to the steep portion of the pericardial PVR. Under these conditions, the pericardium begins to significantly restrain further augmentation of cardiac volume. This is manifested as an increase in the normally low contact pressure between parietal and visceral pericardium, which is in turn transmitted into the cardiac chambers. The result is a progressively increasing, nonparal-

lel upward shift of the *intracavitary* PVR, i.e., a decrease in chamber compliance compared to absence of the pericardium (note that the *transmural* PVR is unaffected by external constraints). Increases in right ventricular diastolic volume and pressure influence the left ventricular PVR in analogous fashion, albeit more modestly under normal conditions since the right ventricle only acts via the interventricular septum. This phenomenon is termed diastolic ventricular interaction. It is important to understand that ventricular and pericardial effects on the PVR are often linked, since the right ventricular diastolic pressure is transmitted through the septum and the right heart also constitutes a large portion of the intrapericardial volume. A good example of this linkage is acute right ventricular infarction, in which the right heart filling pressure can increase due to marked dilatation, causing both increased ventricular interaction and engagement of the steep portion of the pericardial PVR.

Dynamics of Mitral Inflow and Effects of Physiologic Stress

Mitral inflow requires a pressure gradient favoring forward flow across the valve. The pressure gradient is determined in part by the atrial pressure at mitral valve opening, which is a complex function of the filling properties of the left atrium and pulmonary venous bed, the atrial inflow during ventricular systole, and the conduit function of the left atrium. The other component of the gradient of course is the instantaneous time varying filling properties of the ventricle described above. In considering mitral inflow as a marker of altered left ventricular diastolic function, it is important to keep in mind that the ventricle is only one determinant of the inflow pattern. The dynamics of mitral inflow are discussed below and have been the subject of detailed reviews (19–21).

Following the ventriculoatrial pressure crossover at time of mitral valve opening, both atrial and ventricular pressures initially decrease, but the ventricular pressure decreases faster. As a result, a gradient (typically amounting to several mmHg) favoring inflow develops. After reaching a minimum value, left ventricular pressure begins to rise, and then meets and usually transiently recrosses the left atrial pressure. Because the normal mitral valve offers little resistance to inflow, this seemingly small gradient results in rapid inflow of blood into the ventricle early in diastole. Normally, inflow is greatest in volume and velocity at this time, accounting for the dominant E wave of the normal echocardiographic Doppler pattern. The decline of ventricular pressure that occurs after mitral valve opening, despite the fact that the ventricle is filling, is caused by continued relaxation after mitral valve opening. This is modulated by diastolic ventricular suction, providing ESV is less than Vo and restoring forces are present. As mentioned earlier, suction allows filling to occur at lower levels of diastolic pressure than would otherwise be the case. Ventricular pressure reaches its minimum value at a time dictated by opposing effects of relaxation/suction and filling. Relaxation is effectively complete at the end of the rapid filling phase of diastole, when both volume and pressure usually reach a plateau (diastasis). Diastolic suction, if present, is also completed by this time.

As relaxation proceeds to its completion, its influence on the relation between diastolic pressure and volume diminishes whereas the passive PVR becomes progressively more dominant. From the time of diastasis through end-diastole, then, the major determinant of the left ventricular pressure is the PVR of the fully relaxed, or passive ventricle. It is important to remember, however, that the left ventricle, atrium, and pulmonary venous bed are an open system during diastole. Because the left ventricle is the least compliant component of that system, its PVR is the most important determinant of the pressure, but it is not the only one. With diastasis, left ventricular and atrial pressure become essentially identical and mitral inflow becomes negligibly small. At rapid heart rates the diastatic phase shortens and may completely disappear. Atrial contraction causes a second transmitral gradient and corresponding secondary inflow into the ventricle, corresponding to the echocardiographic A wave. The key determinant of the second gradient is the strength of atrial contraction, which is dependent on atrial stretch (preload), contractile function and afterload (dictated largely by left ventricular diastolic pressure).

During endurance exercise, cardiac output increases mainly due to increased heart rate, with relatively small or negligible increases in stroke volume. However, as indicated above, when heart rate increases it does so mainly at the expense of time spent in diastole, with loss of the diastatic period and abbreviation of the early rapid filling phase. As a result, to allow passage of a normal volume of blood across the mitral valve, filling must be augmented, normally without an increase in mean left atrial pressure. This key adaptation is accomplished by adrenergic modulation of left ventricular relaxation and restoring forces (10,14,21,22). With increased adrenergic stimulation, cyclic-AMP-mediated phosphorylation of phospholamban increases the rate of SERCA-2 reuptake of calcium ions by the SR, directly increasing the rate of ventricular relaxation despite the fact that systolic ventricular pressure (contraction load) is increased. In addition, increased contractility results in a smaller ESV and correspondingly greater diastolic suction, which also lowers the ventricular pressure during diastole. This combination of factors lowers left ventricular diastolic pressure in relation to volume, but not at end-diastole, when the ventricle is passive. The net result is a larger and more rapidly developing early diastolic transmitral gradient, due to the more rapid decline to a lower minimum value of ventricular pressure with an essentially unchanged atrial pressure. The strength of atrial contraction and corresponding secondary transmitral gradient and inflow are also augmented during exercise. In heart failure, the early transmitral gradient and filling may be maintained during exercise, but rather than early diastolic left ventricular pressure being lowered, this is accomplished by elevating the left atrial pressure. The latter can cause dyspnea if the increase is sufficiently large (23–26).

ASSESSMENT OF DIASTOLIC FUNCTION

The diseases and pathophysiologic processes that influence relaxation and diastole are numerous. They all have in common an increase in diastolic ventricular pressure in relation to volume. Several of these clinical entities, especially acute and chronic myocardial ischemia and infarction, are discussed elsewhere in this book (see Table 1). For the purposes of this chapter we will concentrate on the role of imaging in processes that cause predominantly or exclusively diastolic heart failure, most typically associated with concentric left ventricular hypertrophy and "hypertensive cardiomyopathy" (27,28). The latter is most commonly observed in elderly patients, especially women, with marked systolic hypertension. This category also includes restrictive cardiomyopathy and constrictive pericarditis. Patients with *combined* systolic and diastolic dysfunction may have similar abnormalities as those described below in patients with predominant diastolic heart failure.

Although some of the specific processes associated with diastolic dysfunction have historic and physical findings suggestive of its presence, it is generally very difficult to confidently diagnose or assess diastolic dysfunction at the bedside. Thus, physical findings such as diastolic gallops at bedside or even radiologic assessment of heart size do not reliably identify patients with diastolic heart failure. However, any method capable of obtaining quantitative, dynamic information about ventricular volume and/or pressure can provide insights into abnormalities of diastolic function. A detailed description of all such methods is beyond the scope of this chapter. Accordingly, we will summarize methods currently available and focus on those in routine clinical use.

Historically, some of the first insights into the pathophysiology of diastole were obtained through invasive procedures (i.e., cardiac catheterization and angiography). In routine clinical practice, cardiac catheterization and left ventricular cineangiography provide direct information by documenting elevated filling pressures (ventricular diastolic, pulmonary capillary wedge) and a normal contraction pattern in patients with diastolic heart failure. Careful attention to the methodologic details of pressure measurement in the cardiac catheter-

---

TABLE 1. *Etiologies of diastolic dysfunction*

- Diastolic dysfunction associated with systolic dysfunction
- Pericardial disease (see Chapters 55 and 56)
- Restrictive cardiomyopathy: idiopathic, amyloidosis, other infiltrative diseases (Chapter 50)
- Ischemic heart disease: chronic stable angina, acute ischemic syndromes, remodeling post-myocardial infarction (see Chapters 38, 39, and 40)
- Hypertrophic heart disease: hypertrophic cardiomyopathy hypertensive cardiomyopathy, aortic stenosis (see Chapters 43 and 44)

ization laboratory are especially important in evaluating diastolic function. By themselves, frame-by-frame quantitative angiographic ventricular volume measurements can be used to estimate diastolic filling rates. Pressure measurements in conjunction with simultaneous angiographic volume estimates allow delineation of the relation between pressure and volume during a single diastolic cycle, i.e., a segment of the diastolic PVR. Delineation of a segment of the PVR can be employed to estimate chamber and myocardial stiffness by fitting the data to appropriate mathematical models. Additionally, indexes of isovolumic ventricular relaxation such as peak (-)dP/dt , a measure of peak relaxation rate, can be obtained (29). However, peak (-)dP/dt is highly dependent on afterload. Mathematical modeling of ventricular isovolumic pressure has been used to partly overcome this limitation and develop more robust measures of relaxation rate, i.e., various estimates of tau (τ), the time constant of left ventricular isovolumic pressure decay (30). Measurements using high fidelity micromanometers are preferable for determination of intraventricular pressure and derived variables during isovolumic relaxation. In general, although still useful in the research setting, the invasive nature and complexity of these procedures imposes significant limitations to their use in routine clinical practice.

Radionuclide ventriculography has been used to estimate both global and regional filling rates (31) by generating gated equilibrium, high-resolution left ventricular time activity curves (32). Diastolic filling parameters derived from mathematical processing of these curves include peak ventricular filling rate (PFR), time-to-peak filling (time to PFR), filling fraction (FF), and the percent of filling occurring during phases of the diastolic filling period, for example, during rapid filling (33,34) (Fig. 1). Use of radionuclide ventriculography has been of particular interest in demonstrating

the relation between regional and temporal inhomogeneities during contraction and abnormal filling rates during early diastole.

Computed tomography (CT) and magnetic resonance imaging (MRI) can be used to generate high-resolution tomographic cardiac images. Ultrafast CT requires intravenous injection of x-ray contrast medium combined with a short image acquisition time (50 msec). MRI does not require contrast injection, but has relatively long acquisition times due to gating. Both technologies can be used to evaluate cardiac chamber dimensions, ventricular hypertrophy and mass, regional and global left ventricular contraction and filling patterns, and the anatomy and thickness of the parietal pericardium, and thus are well-suited for the noninvasive clinical evaluation of patients with suspected diastolic heart failure. Additionally, MRI can be used for detection and semiquantitation of valvular regurgitation.

Modifications of MRI technology may be useful in the evaluation of additional aspects of diastolic function. Thus, breath-hold cine MRI has been used to determine indices of diastolic filling (36) such as time to peak wall thinning rate (TPWR) , regional wall thickness-time curves, radius-time curves, first derivative curves (37), as well as ventricular volumes (38,39). Single-phase MRI employs sequential images throughout the cardiac cycle to significantly reduce the total scanning time. Thus far, it has been used to image the left ventricle at end-diastole for mass estimation. Results compare favorably with echocardiography (40) (see also Chapters 29 and 30).

MRI methods using tagging techniques have been used to measure ventricular geometry and detailed regional wall motion and thickness using manual or automatic edge detection (41). Additionally, this technique has been used to provide information pertinent to elastic recoil by quantifying systolic twist and diastolic untwisting (42) (Fig. 2).

CT and MRI have broad applications for cardiac diagnosis in general, but their high cost currently preclude them from being used routinely for the evaluation of diastolic ventricular function. MRI in addition frequently is problematic because of problems inherent in patients being studied inside a magnet.

Echocardiography and simultaneous Doppler flow velocity measurements have become the most commonly used modalities to evaluate diastolic dysfunction and will be reviewed in detail. Echocardiography has several major advantages. It provides detailed anatomical information, including chamber size, wall thickness, mass, and contraction and filling patterns, as well as transmitral, transtricuspid, and pulmonary vein flow patterns. Thus, the technique is routinely used to document normal or preserved ventricular contractile function and chamber size in patients with diastolic heart failure, as well as the presence of hypertrophy. Moreover, it is noninvasive, relatively inexpensive, and can be performed in physicians' offices. Its chief disadvantage is the fact that even with current generation machines, the transthoracic approach does not yield excellent quality images in a

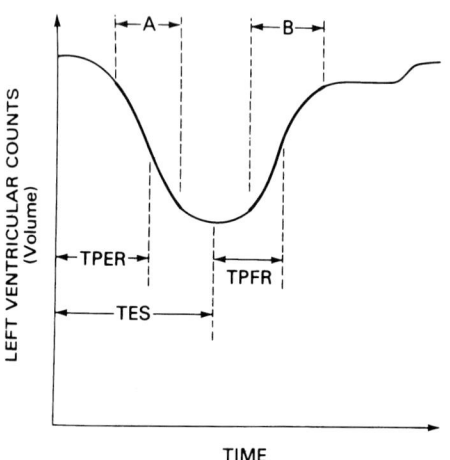

FIG. 1. High temporal resolution time activity curve obtained from radionuclide angiography. Third-order polynomial functions are fitted to the systolic ejection phase (**A**) and the rapid diastolic phase (**B**) of the curve. *TES*, time to the end of systole; *TPER*, time to peak ejection fraction; *TPF*, time to peak filling rate. (From ref. 35, with permission.)

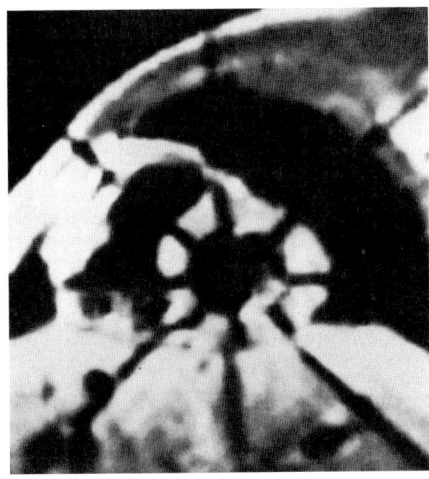 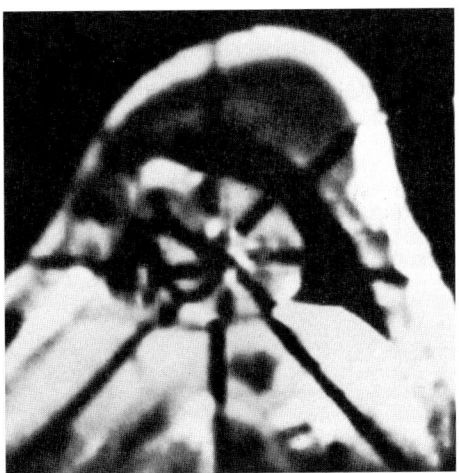

FIG. 2. Magnetic resonance imaging with tagging technique. Short axis of basal slice (**left panel**) and apical slice (**right panel**) of left ventricle at end systole looking from apex to base with tags applied at end diastole. Images were acquired over 512 cardiac cycles. There is counterclockwise rotation of intramyocardial portions of tags of apical slice as compared with basal slice. (From ref. 43, with permission.)

significant minority of patients. In most such patients, however, the transesophageal approach can be used successfully when the transthoracic approach is inadequate. Newer techniques that appear to have a role in clarifying the interpretation of transmitral flow velocity patterns such as Doppler tissue imaging and color M-Doppler have recently become available.

The initial description of transmitral Doppler flow velocity analysis as a tool to assess diastolic filling by Kitabatake et al. (44) was followed by extensive evaluation and development of the technique. The mitral flow velocity pattern is related to the first derivative of diastolic ventricular inflow rates, and closely correlated with inflow rates derived from contrast ventriculography, radionuclide angiography, and digitized M-mode echocardiography.

Transmitral flow velocity may be obtained with the pulsed Doppler method. The rapid velocity of flow in early diastole is known as the early (E) wave. At normal or low heart rates this is followed by a period of slow or negligible velocity (diastasis) and then by a final acceleration, the atrial (A) wave, representing the contribution of left atrial contraction to ventricular filling. These velocities can vary depending on the location of the sample volume. By convention the sample volume is placed at the tips of the mitral valve leaflets as seen in the apical four-chamber view. In some studies (45), the sample volume has been placed at the mitral annulus level, resulting in lower velocities and shorter decay of early diastolic velocity. Several straightforward measurements can be derived from the velocity curves. The maximum E velocity is easily measured and its time velocity integral (TVI) determined from the waveform. The time for velocity to decrease following the maximum E velocity is measured as the deceleration time (DT). The DT is an index of the effective operating chamber compliance of the left ventricle and is also related to the rate of intraventricular pressure increase in early diastole following the pressure nadir (46).

In the normal adult in sinus rhythm, the morphology of the Doppler representation of transmitral flow is character-ized by a rapidly accelerating E wave, which is larger in magnitude than the A wave (Fig. 3A). The downslope of the E wave is more gradual, resulting in a DT of 200 ± 40 msec. At relatively slow heart rates, and depending on the deceleration time, a flat signal indicating a distinct diastatic period may be observed.

With normal aging, ventricular compliance decreases and myocardial relaxation slows. Observational studies have demonstrated a variation in the pattern of transmitral flow velocities that reflect these changes, namely decreased peak E wave, prolonged deceleration time, and increased peak A-wave with an E/A ratio that may be greater than 1 : 1. These normal changes have not been associated with elevated filling pressures or symptoms of heart failure (48).

A primary slowing of relaxation produces specific changes in the mitral flow velocity curve. In conjunction with a slower decrease of isovolumic intraventricular pressure, the duration of relaxation is prolonged. A lower initial atrioventricular pressure gradient driving flow across the mitral valve results from the slower rate of relaxation and causes a lower E-wave velocity. The prolongation of relaxation may continue into mid- or even late diastole, which results in prolongation of the DT of the transmitral flow velocity curve. There is usually a compensatory increase in transmitral flow due to atrial contraction, which is at least in part related to the high atrial preload resulting from slowed ventricular filling earlier in diastole. This results in an increased A wave velocity. Thus, the pattern of slowed relaxation consists of a low E velocity, a high A velocity, E/A ratio less than 1, and prolonged deceleration time (DT ≥ 240 msec) (Fig. 3B).

If left ventricular relaxation slows further and/or passive compliance is progressively reduced such that the left atrial pressure increases even more, the driving force for mitral inflow at the time of mitral valve opening actually begins to increase. As a result, the mitral inflow pattern becomes similar in appearance to normal, and is termed pseudonormalization. Thus, the peak E-wave velocity increases, the deceleration time of the E-wave decreases and the A-wave

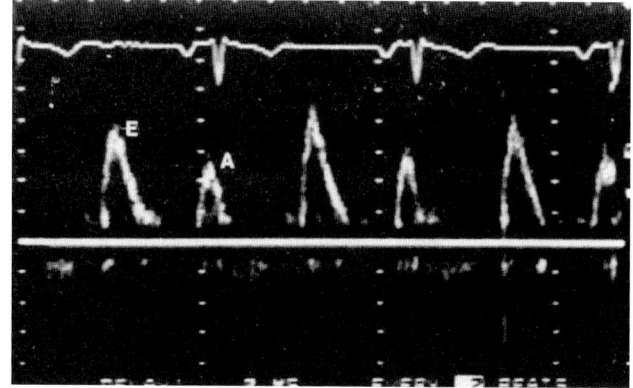

A

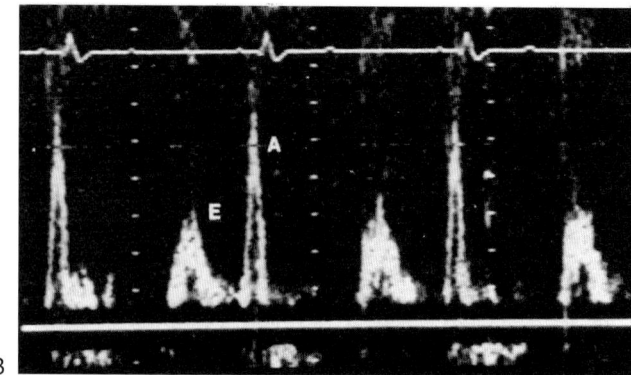

B

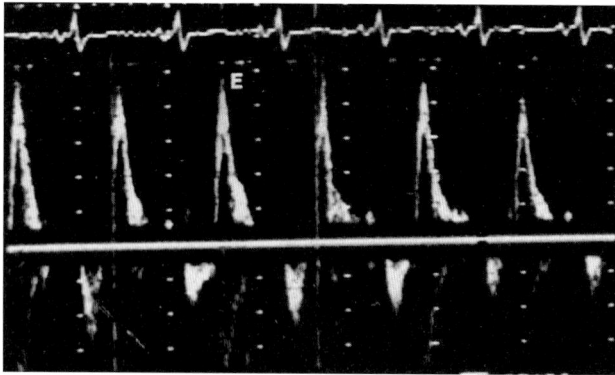

C

FIG. 3. Transmitral Doppler. Typical Doppler mitral inflow patterns. The normal pattern in **A** is characterized by an early E-wave, which is larger than the A-wave in both maximal velocity and in integrated area. Shown in **B** is the filling pattern most commonly associated with diastolic dysfunction: a low amplitude E-wave indicating delayed and reduced early filling, followed by a much larger A-wave. **C** demonstrates an entirely different filling pattern associated most commonly with more advanced diastolic dysfunction and known as a restrictive pattern. The E-wave has an abnormally high peak velocity, but with very rapid deceleration, leading to a brief filling wave. The A-wave is very small (in this case so small it does not rise above the Doppler wall filter). (From ref. 47, with permission.)

decreases such than the E/A ratio reverts to a value greater than 1. Differentiating pseudonormal filling from normal filling is possible with the use of pulmonary vein Doppler flow velocities, triggering maneuvers (e.g., Valsalva) or newer techniques such as Doppler tissue imaging (49). Additionally, patients with the pseudonormalized pattern usually have a clinical history of heart failure.

With further worsening of left ventricular compliance, filling pressures are increased even more, producing more severe symptoms of heart failure. The high left atrial pressure at the time of mitral valve opening contributes to an augmented atrioventricular gradient in early diastole. This results in faster acceleration of blood flow into the ventricle and an even higher E wave velocity. The deceleration time is significantly reduced due to the rapid elevation of ventricular pressure. Because the bulk of ventricular filling now occurs during the rapid filling phase, the atrial contraction is now associated with a lower A velocity or the A wave may even be absent. The E/A ratio is markedly elevated, typically greater than 2:1. This pattern is known as "restriction to filling", and is especially typical of restrictive cardiomyopathy and constrictive pericarditis (Fig. 3C). To the extent that this pattern may reflect an acutely decompensated state, it may improve when treated. Patients with this filling pattern in general have a poor prognosis regardless of the underlying disease.

There are several other echocardiographic-Doppler features that serve to identify constrictive pericarditis and restrictive cardiomyopathy. For example, patients with constrictive pericarditis also may have exaggerated respiratory variation in transmitral and transtricuspid inflow velocity, whereas those with restrictive cardiomyopathy often have marked biatrial enlargement.

With improvement of ultrasound technology transthoracic interrogation of the pulmonary veins and recording of pulmonary venous flow velocity by pulsed-wave Doppler has become possible in a substantial proportion of patients. This technique is achievable in virtually all patients using the transesophageal approach (50). Pulmonary vein velocities can be used in conjunction with transmitral velocities to assess diastolic dysfunction. It is especially useful in distinguishing normal from pseudonormal patterns of left ventricular filling. In normal subjects, pulsed Doppler recording of pulmonary venous flow velocity reveals a triphasic morphology consisting of a systolic wave, S, and a diastolic wave, D, both of which are directed forward, and an atrial reversal wave, A, caused by atrial contraction and retrograde flow. The S wave is caused by atrial filling as left atrial pressure falls during atrial relaxation and the mitral annulus descends during ventricular systole. The D wave represents atrial filling due to the fall in atrial pressure when the mitral valve opens. In normal subjects, the peak systolic and diastolic flow velocities are similar, whereas the peak atrial reversal velocity is low (Fig. 4). In patients with slowed ventricular relaxation and decreased compliance as a result of aging or disease, systolic pulmonary venous flow and reversed atrial

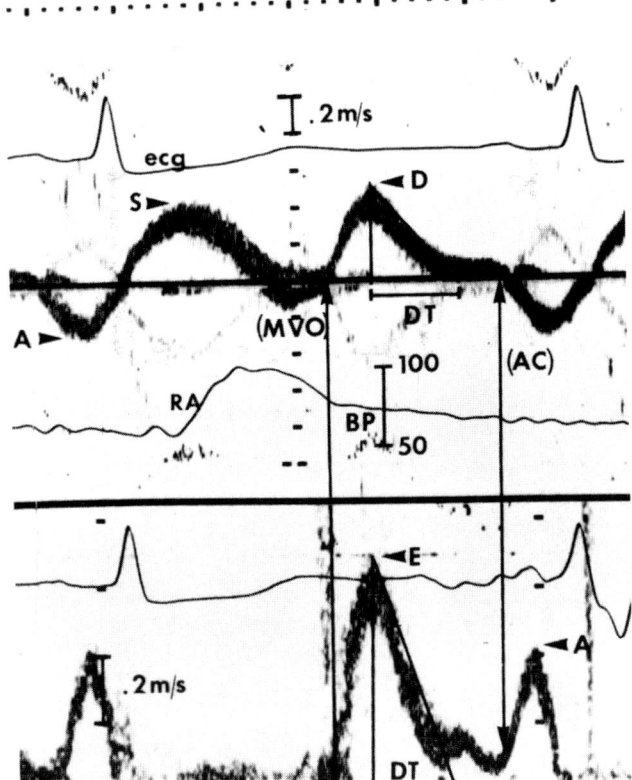

FIG. 4. Recording of a pulmonary vein velocity curve (**top**) aligned with a mitral flow velocity curve (**bottom**) demonstrates Doppler measurements obtained as well as temporal relation between curves. Pulmonary vein velocity consists of retrograde velocity of atrial contraction (*A*) followed by systolic forward flow (*S*) and diastolic forward flow (*D*). Deceleration time (*DT*) is measured from peak of diastolic transmitral forward flow to the extrapolation of slope of velocity deceleration to baseline. In addition, from mitral flow velocity, peak early diastolic velocity (*E*), velocity of atrial contraction (*A*), and deceleration time (*DT*) are measured. Timing of mitral valve opening (*MVO*) and onset of atrial contraction (*AC*) are shown by vertical arrows. Radial artery pressure (*RA*) and electrocardiogram (*ecg*) are shown. Each dot = 0.2 m/s, and blood pressure (*BP*) scale shown is 50–100 mmHg. (From ref. 50, with permission.)

flow increase whereas diastolic flow decreases. A peak atrial reversal flow velocity of greater than 35 cm/s in the setting of a normal appearing transmitral flow profile suggests a pseudonormal state. As the ventricle progresses to a restrictive pattern, diastolic pulmonary venous flow increases markedly, commensurate with increased transmitral flow, systolic flow decreases, and atrial reversal flow increases. Klein et al. (51) have reported that when the duration of the atrial reversal wave exceeds the duration of the transmitral A wave the left ventricular end diastolic pressure is elevated to a value >15 mmHg.

Doppler tissue imaging is a relatively new technology that allows the assessment of velocities of myocardial tissue movement throughout the cardiac cycle. A pulsed Doppler

sample volume is placed in the moving myocardium while filtering out low-amplitude, high-velocity signals from blood cells. Regional systolic and diastolic function can be assessed by placing the sampling volume in different locations. The average of these regions is used to represent global function. In normal subjects the diastolic movement of the myocardium is a mirror image of the transmitral flow pattern. The early diastolic velocity is denoted E_m and the atrial velocity is A_m. Aging is associated with a decreased E_m/A_m ratio. Preliminary studies indicate that E_m velocity changes secondary to abnormalities of relaxation are relatively insensitive to loading conditions (52). Because there is good correlation of these values with τ, regardless of LV filling pressure, differentiating pseudonormal from normal patterns is feasible (53) (Fig. 5**A** and **B**; see also Color Plate 29 following page 758).

Color M-mode Doppler is used to assess the velocity at which the flow propagates in the ventricle throughout diastole. The flow propagation velocity (Vp) has been employed to assess intraventricular gradients using the complete Bernoulli equation. Several studies have found correlations between color-M mode indices and other indices of diastolic function. Brun et al. (55) have demonstrated significant inverse correlations between tau and Vp in ischemic models of diastolic dysfunction and preliminary data suggest that Vp is not strongly load dependent. The time delay between the maximal velocity at the mitral valve and the apex, as measured with color M-mode, has been shown to prolong with slowed relaxation. Despite some promising features of this new technique, there are currently several limitations, including difficulty in obtaining proper alignment and the need for optimal heart rates (Figs. 6 and 7; see also Color Plates 30–31 following page 758).

Continuous Doppler velocity can be measured in a way that includes the transmitral flow profile, the left ventricular outflow, and aortic flow. Isovolumetric relaxation time (IVRT) can then be determined from the time of cessation of aortic flow to the beginning of transmitral flow. The duration of the IVRT often parallels the deceleration time, increasing with delayed relaxation, returning to normal values with pseudonormalization and decreasing with restrictive patterns.

In addition to IVRT, if mitral regurgitation is present and continues beyond aortic valve closure, it is possible to estimate τ noninvasively from transmitral Doppler flow measurements. To accomplish this, the left ventricular-atrial pressure difference is estimated from the modified Bernoulli equation using data from the regurgitant flow velocity profile. The left ventricular pressure is calculated by adding the left atrial pressure, which can be estimated from mitral or pulmonary flow patterns and indices. Alternatively, left atrial pressure has been empirically assigned a value of either 10 mmHg or 20 mmHg. These pressure estimates are combined with the time of pressure fall (from aortic valve closure to the time of mitral valve opening) to calculate τ. The continuous Doppler velocity profile of an aortic regurgitant jet has also been used to calculate τ noninvasively. Other in-

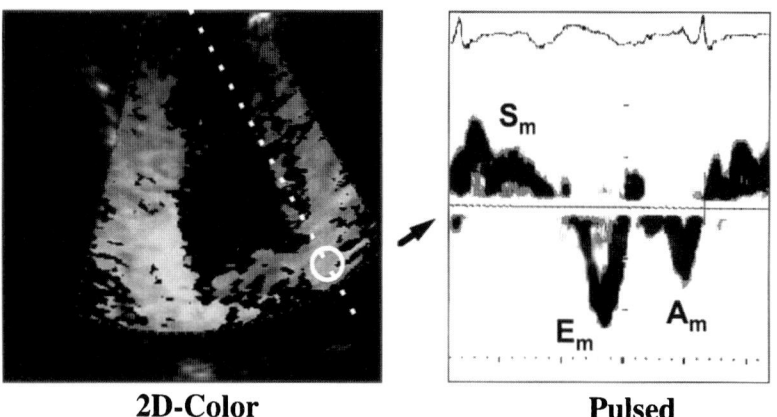

2D-Color   **Pulsed**

FIG. 5. Two-dimensional color and pulsed tissue Doppler axial velocities of the myocardium recorded from the apical four-chamber view. Systolic (*Sm*), early diastolic (*Em*), and atrial contraction (*Am*) velocities are shown in the pulsed Doppler tracing. The two dimensional image was obtained during systole. (See also Color Plate 29 following page 758.) (From ref. 54, with permission.)

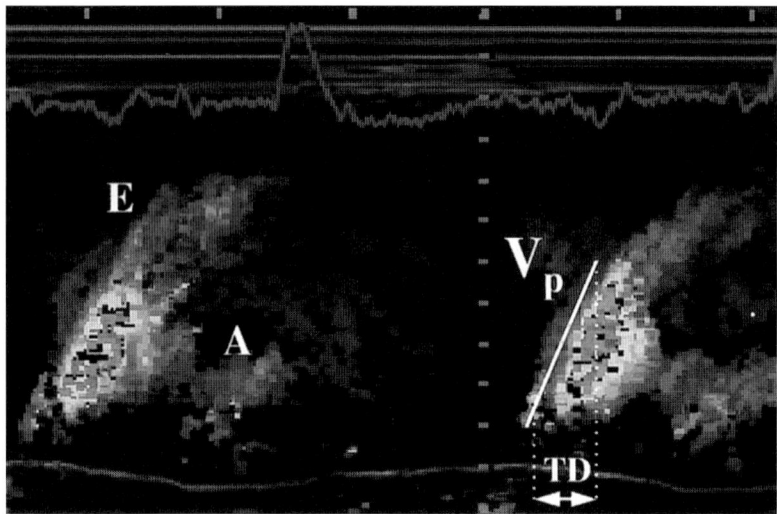

FIG. 6. Color Doppler M-mode recording of transmitral flow velocity. With the cursor line directed through the mitral valve, the spacial-temporal pattern of velocity is shown along a streamline from the mid-atrium to the ventricular apex. *E*, early wave; *A*, atrial contraction wave; *Vp*, flow propagation velocity; *TD*, time delay. (See also Color Plate 30 following page 758.) (From ref. 54, with permission.)

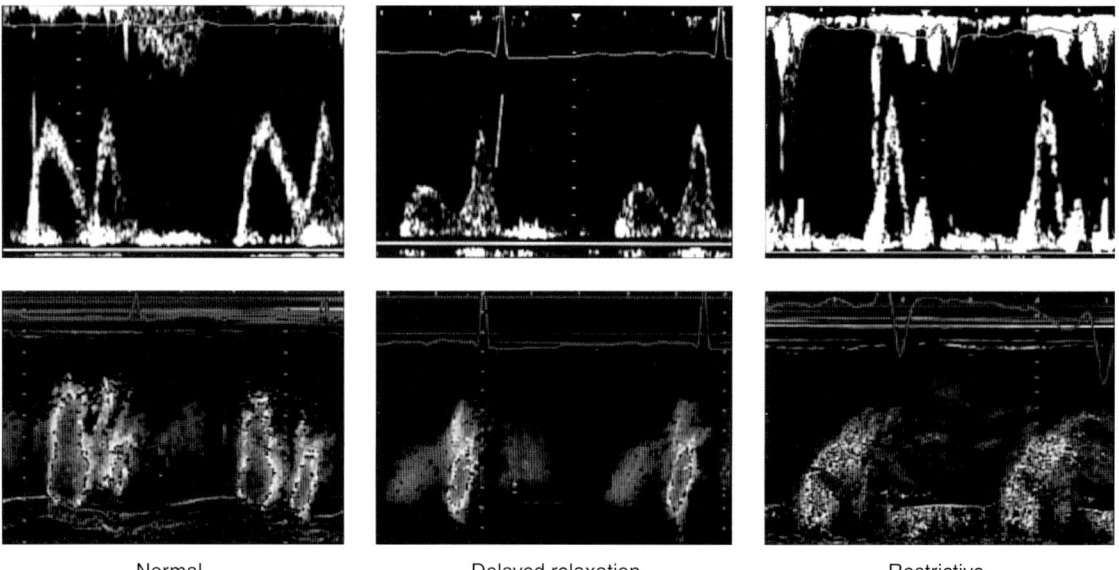

Normal   Delayed relaxation   Restrictive

FIG. 7. Pulsed and color M-mode Doppler recordings of the left ventricular inflow in a subject with normal diastolic function, a patient with delayed relaxation, and a patient with restrictive filling. Notice the delayed apical filling (reduced Vp and prolonged TD in both the delayed relaxation and restrictive cases). (See also Color Plate 31 following page 758.) (From ref. 55, with permission.)

dices of ventricular filling that may be obtained from echo Doppler measurements include peak filling rate (PFR), normalized PFR, and filling fractions at various times in diastole.

REFERENCES

1. Soufer R, Wohlgelernter D, Vita NA, et al. Intact systolic left ventricular function in clinical congestive heart failure. *Am J Cardiol* 1985;55: 1032–1036.

2. Ramachandran S, Vazan MD, Benjamin E, et al. Prevalence, clinical features and prognosis of diastolic heart failure: an epidemiological perspective. *J Am Col Cardiol* 1995;26:1565–1574.

3. Brutsaert DL, Sys SU. Relaxation and diastole of the heart. *Physiol Rev* 1989;69:1228–1315.

4. Little WC, Downes TR. Clinical evaluation of left ventricular diastolic performance. *Prog Cardiovasc Dis* 1990;23:273–290.

5. Wiggers CJ. Studies on the consecutive phases of the cardiac cycle. *Am J Phys* 1921;56:415–459.

6. Brutsaert DL, Rademakers FE, Sys SU. Triple control of relaxation: implications in heart disease. *Circulation* 1984;69:190–196.

7. Leite-Moreira AF, Gillebert TC. Non-uniform course of left ventricular pressure fall and its regulation by load and contractile state. *Circulation* 1994;90:2481–2491.

8. Apstein CS, Grossman W. Opposite initial effects of supply and demand ischemia on left ventricular diastolic compliance. The ischemia-diastolic paradox. *J Mol Cell Cardiol* 1987;19:119–128.

9. Weiss JL, Frederiksen JW, Weisfeldt ML. Hemodynamic determinants of the time course of fall in canine left ventricular pressure. *J Clin Invest* 1976;58:751–760.

10. Gillebert TC, Sys SU, Brutsaert DL. Influence of loading patterns on peak length-tension relation and on relaxation in cardiac muscle. *J Am Coll Cardiol* 1989;13:483–489.

11. Zile MR, Gaasch WH. Load dependent left ventricular relaxation in conscious dogs. *Am J Physiol* 1991;261:H691–H699.

12. Brutsaert DL, Meulemans AL, Sipido KR, et al. Effects of damaging the endocardial surface on the mechanical performance of isolated cardiac muscle. *Circ Res* 1988;62:358–366.

13. Shah AM, Grocott-Mason RM, Pepper CB, et al. The cardiac endothelium: cardioactive mediators. *Prog Cardiovasc Dis* 1996;39:263–284.

14. Yellin EL, Hori M, Yoram C, et al. Left ventricular relaxation in the filling and non-filling intact canine heart. *Am J Physiol* 1986;250: H620–H629.

15. Hori M, Yellin EL, Sonnenblick EH. Left ventricular diastolic suction as a mechanism of ventricular filling. *Jpn Circ J* 1982;46:124–129.

16. Ingels NB Jr, Daughters GT II, Nikolic SD, et al. Left atrial pressure clamp servomechanism demonstrates LV suction in canine hearts with normal mitral valves. *Am J Physiol* 1994;267: H354–H362.

17. Bell SP, Fabian J, LeWinter MM. Effects of dobutamine on left ventricular restoring forces. *Am J Physiol* 1998;275: H190–H194.

18. Solomon SB, Nikolic SD, Glantz SA, et al. Left ventricular diastolic function of remodeled myocardium in dogs with pacing induced heart failure. *Am J Physiol* 1998;274:H945–H954.

19. Ingels NB, Hansen DE, Daughters GT II, et al. Relation between longitudinal, circumferential and oblique shortening and torsional deformation in the left ventricle of the transplanted human heart. *Circ Res* 1989; 64:915–927.

20. Rademakers FE, Buchalter MB, Rogers WJ, et al. Dissociation between left ventricular untwisting and filling. *Circulation* 1992;85:1572–1581.

21. Gaasch WH. Passive elastic properties of the left ventricle. In: Gaasch WH, LeWinter MM, eds. *Left ventricular diastolic dysfunction and heart failure*. Philadelphia: Lea & Febiger, 1994:143–149.

22. LeWinter MM, Myhre ESP, Slinker BK. Influence of the pericardium and ventricular interaction on diastolic function. In: Gaasch WH, Le Winter MM, eds. *Left ventricular diastolic dysfunction and heart failure*. Philadelphia: Lea & Febiger, 1994:103–117.

23. Karliner JS, LeWinter MM, Mahler F, et al. Pharmacologic and hemodynamic influences on the rate of isovolumic left ventricular relaxation in conscious dogs. *J Clin Invest* 1977;60:511–521.

24. Little WC, Rassi A, Freeman GL. Comparison of effects of dobutamine

and ouabain on left ventricular contraction and relaxation in closed chest dogs. *J Clin Invest* 1987;80:613–620.

25. Ross J Jr, Miura T, Kambayashi M, et al. Adrenergic control of the force frequency relation. *Circulation* 1995;92:2327–2332.

26. Miura T, Miyazaky S, Guth BD, et al. Influence of force frequency relation on left ventricular function during exercise in conscious dogs. *Circulation* 1992;86:563–571.

27. Daugherty AH, Naccarelli GV, Gray EL, et al. Congestive heart failure with normal systolic function. *Am J Cardiol* 1984;54:778–782.

28. Iriarte M, Perez Olea J, Sagastagoitia D, et al. Congestive heart failure due to hypertensive ventricular diastolic dysfunction. *Am J Cardiol* 1995;76:43D–47D.

29. Mc Laurin LP, Rolett EL, Grossman W. Impaired left ventricular relaxation during pacing induced ischemia. *Am J Cardiol* 1973;32:751.

30. Mirsky I. Assessment of diastolic function: suggested methods and future considerations. *Circulation* 1984;69:836–841.

31. Udelson JE, Bonow RO. Radionuclide angiographic evaluation of left ventricular diastolic function. In: Gaasch WH, LeWinter MM, eds. *Left ventricular diastolic dysfunction and heart failure*. Philadelphia: Lea & Febiger, 1994:4:167–191.

32. Bacharach SL, Green MV, Borer JS. Instrumentation and data processing in cardiovascular nuclear medicine: evaluation of ventricular function. *Semin Nuc Med* 1979;4:257–274.

33. Bonow RO. Radionuclide evaluation of left ventricular function. *Circulation* 1991;84:1208–1215.

34. Porenta G, Kuhle W, Sinha S. Magnetic resonance imaging vs. ultrafast computed tomography for cardiac diagnosis. *Int J Card Imaging* 1992; 36:217–227.

35. Bonow RO, Bacharach SL, Green MW. Impaired left ventricular diastolic filling. *Circulation* 1981;64:316.

36. Higgins CB, Sakuma H. Heart disease: functional evaluation with MR imaging. *Radiology* 1996;199:307–315.

37. Yamanari H, Morita H, Nakamura K, et al. Assessment of regional early diastolic function using cine magnetic resonance imaging in patients with hypertrophic cardiomyopathy. *Jpn Circ J* 1996;12:917–924.

38. Lawson MA, Blackwell GG, Davis ND, et al. Accuracy of biplane long-axis left ventricular volume determined by cine magnetic resonance imaging in patients with regional and global dysfunction. *Am J Cardiol* 1996;21:1098–1104.

39. Aurigemma GP, Gaasch WH, Villegas B, et al. Noninvasive assessment of left ventricular mass, chamber volume, and contractile function. *Curr Probl Cardiol* 1995;21:361–440.

40. Aurigemma G, Davidoff A, Silver K, et al. Left ventricular mass quantitation using single-phase cardiac magnetic resonance imaging. *Am J Cardiol* 1992;21:259–262.

41. van der Geest RJ, Buller VG, Jansen E, et al. Comparison between manual and semiautomated analysis of left ventricular volume parameters from short-axis MR images. *J Comput Assist Tomogr* 1997;21: 756–765.

42. Buchalter MB, Weiss JL, Rogers, et al. Noninvasive quantification of left ventricular rotational deformation in normal humans using magnetic resonance imaging myocardial tagging. *Circulation* 1990;81: 1236–1244.

43. Bouchalter MB, et al. Noninvasive quantification of left ventricular deformation in normal humans using magnetic resonance imaging myocardial tagging. *Circulation* 1990;81:1238.

44. Kitabatake A, Inoue M, Asao M. Transmitral blood flow reflecting diastolic behavior of the left ventricle in health and disease: a study by pulsed Doppler technique. *Jpn Circ J* 1982;46:92–102.

45. Sagie A, Benjamin E, Galderisi M, et al. Reference values for Doppler indexes of left ventricular diastolic filling in the elderly. *J Am Soc Echocardiogr* 1993;6:570–576.

46. Little WC, Ohno M, Kitzman DW, et al. Determination of left ventricular chamber stiffness from the time for deceleration of early left ventricular filling. *Circulation* 1995;92:1933–1939.

47. Thomas JD, Weyman AE. Echocardiographic Doppler evaluation of left ventricular evaluation of diastolic function: physics and physiology. *Circulation* 1991;84:977.

48. Benjamin E, Levy D, Anderson K, et al. Determinants of Doppler indexes of left ventricular diastolic function in normal subjects (the Framingham study). *Am J Cardiol* 1992;70:508–515.

49. Rodriguez L, Garcia MJ, Ares MA, et al. Assessment of mitral annular dynamics during diastole by Doppler tissue imaging: comparison with mitral Doppler inflow in subjects without heart disease and in patients with left ventricular hypertrophy. *Am Heart J* 1996;131:1982–1987.

50. Nishimura RA, Martin AD, Hatle LK, et al. Relation of pulmonary vein to mitral flow velocities by transesophageal echocardiography. *Circulation* 1990;81:1488–1497.

51. Klein AL, Abdalla I, Murray RD, et al. Age independence of the difference in duration of pulmonary venous atrial reversal flow and transmitral A-wave flow in normal subjects. *J Am Soc Echo* 1998;11: 458–465.

52. Palka P, Lange A, Fleming AD, et al. Differences in myocardial velocity gradient measured throughout the cardiac cycle in patients with hypertrophic cardiomyopathy, athletes and patients with left ventricular hypertrophy due to hypertension. *J Am Coll Cardiol* 1997;30:760–768.

53. Oki T, Tabata T, Yamada H, et al. Clinical application of pulsed Doppler tissue imaging for assessing abnormal left ventricular relaxation. *Am J Cardiol* 1997;79:921–928.

54. Garcia MJ, et al. New Doppler echocardiographic application for the study of diastolic function. *J Am Coll Cardiol* 1998;32:865–875.

55. Brun P, Tribouilloy C, Duval AM, et al. Left ventricular flow propagation during early filling is related to wall relaxation: a color M-mode Doppler analysis. *J Am Coll Cardiol* 1992;20:420–432.

CHAPTER 53

Acute and Chronic Pericardial Disease

Ralph Shabetai

Imaging is playing an increasingly important role in pericardial disease. Appropriate imaging provides information on the anatomy, pathology, function, and pathophysiology of the pericardium itself, and on the effects the pericardium has on the cardiac chambers in health, as well as in the presence of cardiac or pericardial disease. The last half century has witnessed enormous advances in techniques used to visualize the pericardium and the pericardial space, and to elucidate the pathophysiologic changes associated with anomalies and diseases of the pericardium. Some of the more important applications of pericardial imaging are evaluation and treatment of pericardial effusion, cardiac tamponade, and constrictive pericarditis or restrictive cardiomyopathy. Because of the critical importance of diastolic dysfunction in all of these conditions, and because in all of them systolic function is usually preserved, the features of diastolic dysfunction common to all of them, and those abnormalities of diastolic dysfunction that are unique to a specific pericardial disorder will be described in detail (see also Chapter 53).

This chapter is primarily addressed to the clinician. The material is organized along anatomical, physiological, and pathological lines, rather than according to specific imaging entities. For specific clinical entities, only warranted imaging will be discussed. Several imaging modalities have been employed to investigate various abnormal pericardiopathies but, for the most part, one particular modality is most commonly used for a particular pathological entity and will be emphasized in this chapter.

Pericardial imaging finds its principal applications in the diagnosis and evaluation of pericardial effusion and constrictive pericarditis, but also has greatly facilitated the detection and assessment of anatomical abnormalities such as pericar-

R. Shebetai: Department of Medicine, University of California–San Diego; Veterans Administration Health Care System, La Jolla, California 92161.

dial cyst, hematoma, neoplasm of the pericardium, and absence of a part or all of the pericardium.

PERICARDIAL EFFUSION

Echocardiography

Before the advent of numerous imaging modalities, especially echocardiography, the literature described findings that could be elicited by clinical examination, such as dullness to percussion at the lower left scapular border (Ewart sign) (1) and dullness beyond the apex beat, but these and other physical findings are extremely insensitive and nonspecific. The reality is that whenever pericardial effusion is a reasonable explanation for a patient's symptoms, signs, or laboratory abnormalities, echocardiography should be performed as soon as possible. Although pericardial effusion can be suspected from the plain chest radiogram, and can be seen and evaluated on computer-assisted tomography (CT) and magnetic resonance imaging (MRI), in reality, echocardiography is almost always the proper tool with which to establish or exclude the diagnosis and with which to assess the size of an effusion and its hemodynamic effects on the heart and circulation.

At present, echocardiography is virtually 100% specific and sensitive for the diagnosis. Before 2D real-time echocardiography was developed and only M-mode was used to detect pericardial effusion, it was necessary to attenuate the damping and gain in order to visualize the pericardium itself and avoid densities within the pericardium. Lateral orientation of the transducer was employed to avoid false positive diagnosis due to the vertebral column and other mediastinal structures. M-mode studies are still helpful, especially to detect right ventricular diastolic collapse in tamponade and a restrictive filling pattern in restrictive cardiomyopathy or constrictive pericarditis. In the present era, however, the echocardiographic recognition of pericardial effusion relies

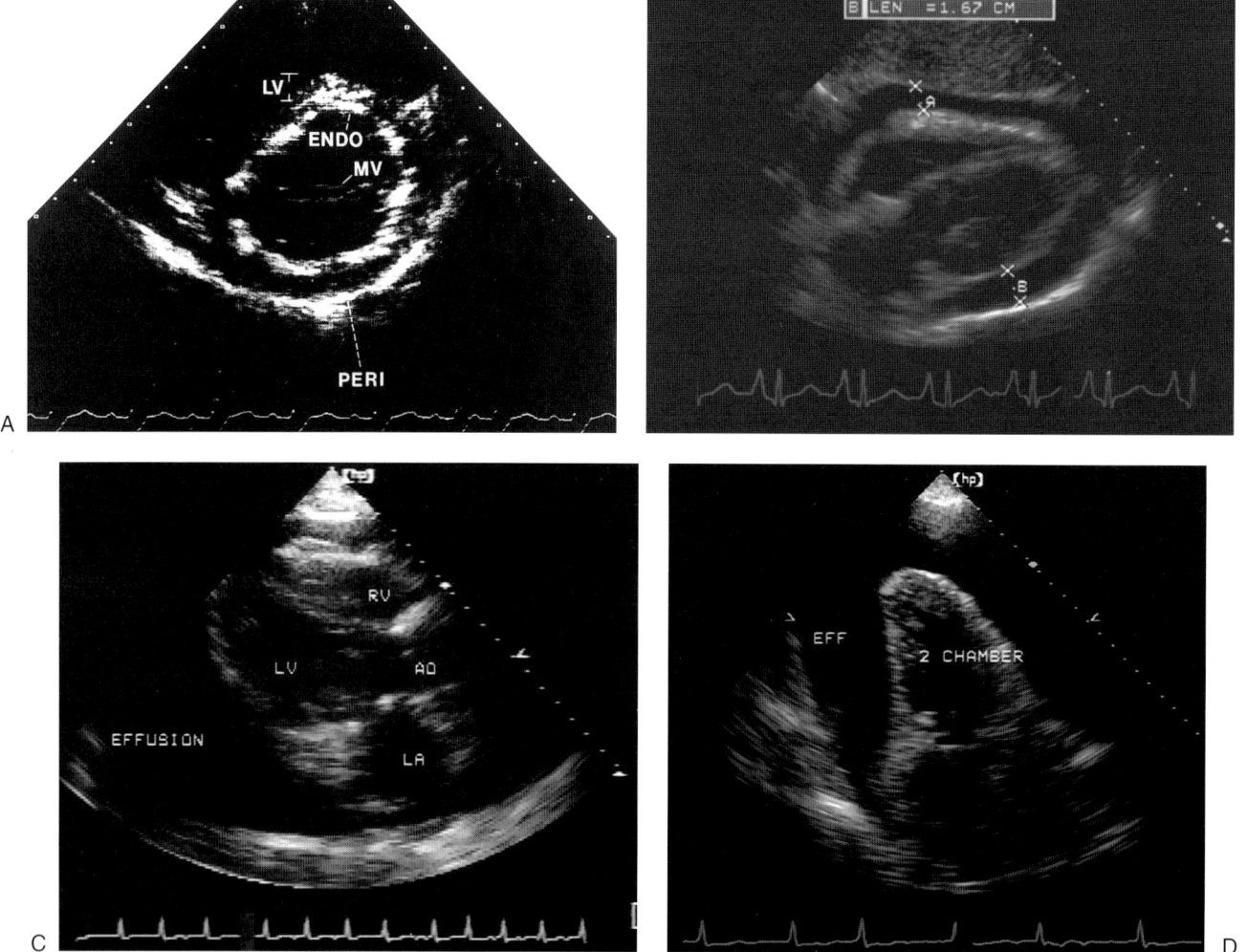

FIG. 1. Two-dimensional echocardiograms of pericardial effusion. **A:** Parasternal short axis. **B:** Subcostal long axis. **C:** Parasternal long axis. **D:** Apical two chamber. *Ao*, aorta; *EFF*, effusion; *ENDO*, endocardium; *LV*, left ventricle; *PERI*, pericardial effusion; *RV*, right ventricle.

more on 2D imaging where it is much simpler to be sure of the diagnosis: the only potential pitfall is mistaking pleural for pericardial effusion. This error is avoided by identifying the descending aorta posterior to a pericardial effusion, but anterior to a pleural effusion. Two-dimensional echocardiograms provide detailed information concerning the size and distribution of pericardial effusion (Fig. 1) and are invaluable in detecting localized loculated effusions, such as commonly occur after cardiac surgery (2). When pericardial effusion begins to organize, fibrin strands and adhesions may be detected in the fluid (Fig. 2) (4) or a massive hematoma may develop and cause localized cardiac compression (Fig. 3). Both real-time two-dimensional and M-mode echo are valuable for assessing pericardial effusion.

A small pericardial effusion is commonly found at autopsy of patients with severe heart failure, but usually is not detected by echocardiography or recognized clinically (5,6). Asymptomatic pericardial effusion may be seen by echocar-

diography in pregnant women, but is only a finding from clinical investigation in which women were screened by echocardiography. A similar situation applies to the small asymptomatic effusion that can be identified after uncomplicated cardiac surgery. Pericardial effusion can also be detected in the second half of gestation of a normal infant (7,8).

Debate persists among echocardiographers regarding the merits of limiting a study to a specific question such as evaluation for left ventricular systolic global and regional function, or determining the presence or absence of pericardial effusion, or exclusion of a cardiac source of an embolus, some holding the view that all studies should be "complete." In patients under 65 years of age with a low pretest probability of having pericardial effusion, a significant incidental diagnosis was found in less than 3% of 40 patients, and sonographer's time was reduced by 93% (9). This question is particularly relevant to the emergency room physician. Here, even more vital is the point that echocardiogra-

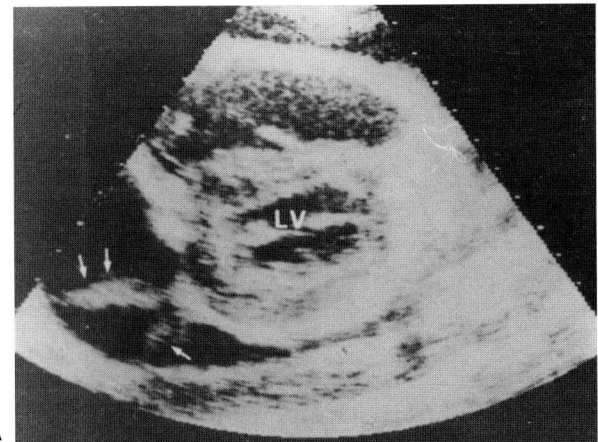

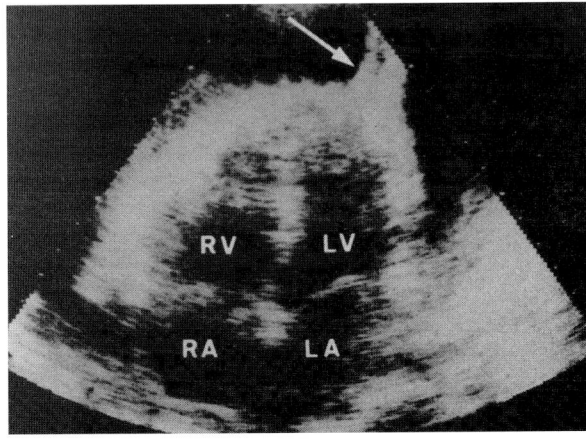

FIG. 2. Organizing pericardial effusion. **A:** Parasternal short axis. **B:** Apical; four chamber. Large pericardial effusion with linear densities (*arrows*) indicating organization of the effusion. *RA*, right atrium; *RV*, right ventricle; *LV*, left ventricle. (From ref. 3, with permission.)

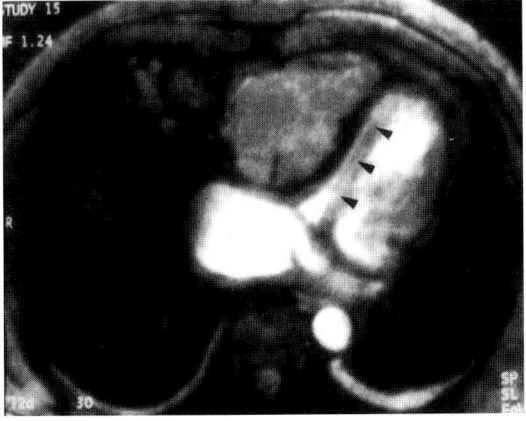

FIG. 3. Axial cine magnetic resonance image demonstrating a massive pericardial hematoma compressing the right ventricle (*arrowheads*). (From ref. 16, with permission.)

phy be performed upon any reasonable suspicion of pericardial effusion and that the study be interpreted and reported by a qualified cardiologist as soon as possible.

Quantification of Pericardial Effusion

By measurement of the anterior posterior dimension of the heart and of the effusion, it is possible to estimate the volume of a pericardial effusion (10). The results correlate fairly well with estimates made at surgery or after pericardiocentesis. For clinical purposes, however, it is sufficient to quantify pericardial effusion as tiny, small, moderate, large, or massive. It should be understood that a small effusion is not necessarily benign. It is important to assess the size of a pericardial effusion before attempting pericardiocentesis. From a practical viewpoint, pericardiocentesis is safe when the effusion at the proposed puncture site is 2-cm wide. A 1-cm width is the lower limit at which most physicians would perform elective pericardiocentesis.

Swinging Heart

With massive pericardial effusion, especially, but not necessarily with tamponade, the heart may swing and twist, such that it occupies a different anatomical position with each alternate systole. When the heart swings within a large effusion, the echocardiogram may be so distorted that interpretation is difficult (Fig. 4). The electrocardiogram shows electrical alternans, commonly regarded as a manifestation of the altered position and orientation of the heart in alternate cardiac cycles. Rarely, alternation is three to one. Other explanations for electrical alternans in cases of pericardial effusion postulate that a change in the depolarization pathway plays a part. Electrical alternans may be accompanied by mechanical alternans in the latest stages of tamponade, indicating a role for increased pericardial pressure in the generation of electrical alternans. Supporting the contribution of raised intrapericardial pressure is the observation that a small reduction of pericardial pressure during pericardiocentesis abolishes alternans. In addition to these mechanical explanations, nonlinear modeling (chaos theory) predicts alternation based on oscillator theory (12). From the practical clinical viewpoint, electrical alternans, when otherwise unexplained, should raise the question of a large pericardial effusion and possible cardiac tamponade. Highly specific, but less sensitive, is total alternans, that is, alternation of all elements of the electrocardiogram (Fig. 5). P-wave alternans, however, is difficult to detect on routine tracings because of low amplitude. Alternans confined to the QRS complex is much more common, but not specific for pericardial effusion. Electrical alternans obscures pulsus paradoxus, but paradox is unmasked after removing a small portion of pericardial fluid to lower pericardial pressure and thus make pulsus alternans disappear.

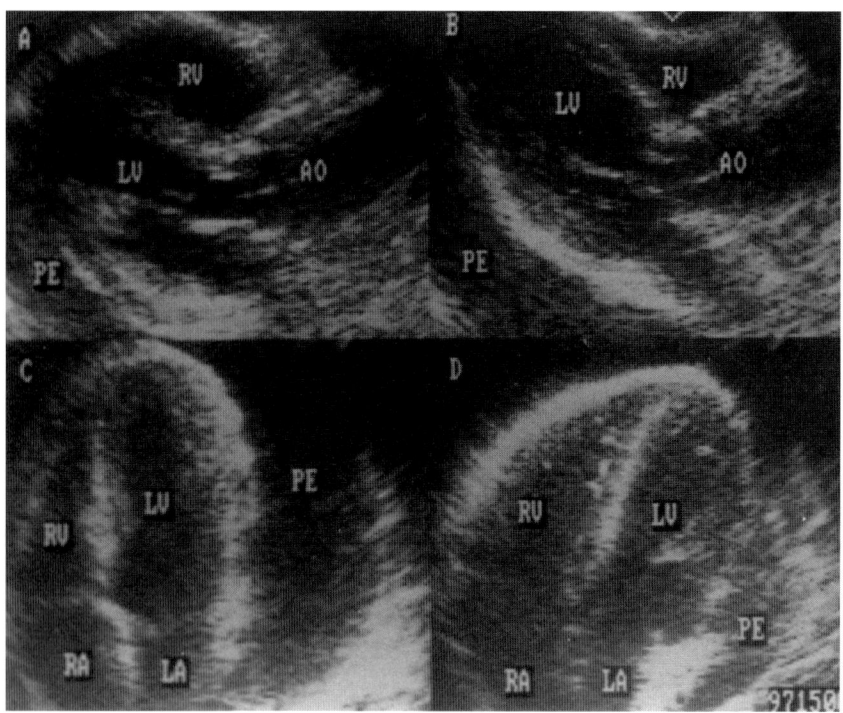

FIG. 4. Swinging heart. **A** and **B**: Parasternal long axis, showing anterioposterior motion. **C** and **D**: Apical four chamber, showing lateral translation. The patient had a large pericardial effusion (*PE*) with tamponade and diastolic collapse of the right ventricle (*arrowhead* at top of **B**). (From ref. 11, with permission.)

Pericardiocentesis

Currently, elective pericardiocentesis is commonly performed in the cardiac catheterization laboratory where physiological monitoring is optimal and the operator can rapidly use fluid samples or contrast injection and pressure measurements to determine whether the pericardium or a cardiac chamber is punctured. Right heart catheterization to confirm and quantify the diagnosis often precedes pericardiocentesis. Fluoroscopy guides the placement of an intrapericardial catheter once the needle puncture has been accomplished. Angiocardiography, obtained by contrast injection at the junction of the superior vena cava and right atrium, shows a pericardial effusion as an area of moderate density surrounding the densely opacified cardiac chambers (Fig. 6). Left ventriculography shows normal systolic function in striking contrast to the immobile pericardial fluid. Echocardiography is often performed when the patient is in the catheterization laboratory; therefore, opacification of the heart with radiopaque material is now very seldom a part of the study of pericardial effusion. Imaging techniques that are now mainly only of historical interest include intravenous injection of CO_2 (14) and induction of pneumopericardium after pericardiocentesis. For the first, the patient was placed left side down on the catheterization table, after which CO_2 was injected into a central vein. Negative contrast was then imaged by fluoroscopy and spot film in the right atrium (the uppermost chamber with the patient in the left lateral decubitus position). The thickness of the pericardium could also be estimated from the image, and occasionally a neoplastic or inflammatory mass was discovered. Another method for estimating the thickness and appearance of the pericardium was to inject CO_2 into the pericardium after completion of pericardiocentesis.

Increasingly, pericardiocentesis is now being carried out in an intensive care unit or emergency room, using echocardiography instead of fluoroscopy to guide the procedure

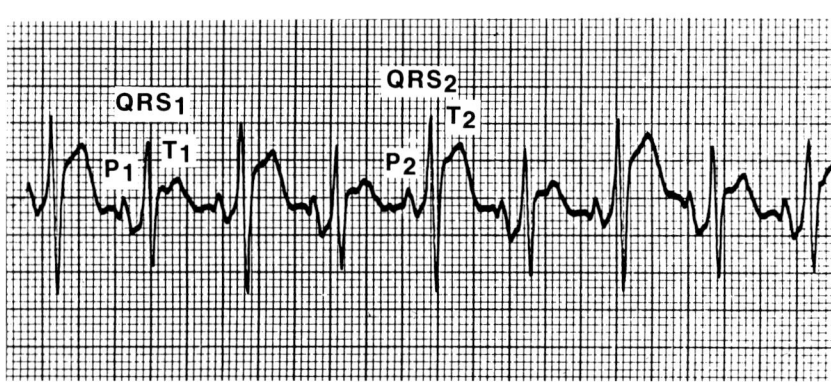

FIG. 5. Total electrical alternans, frequently associated with echocardiographic swinging of the heart. (From ref. 13, with permission.)

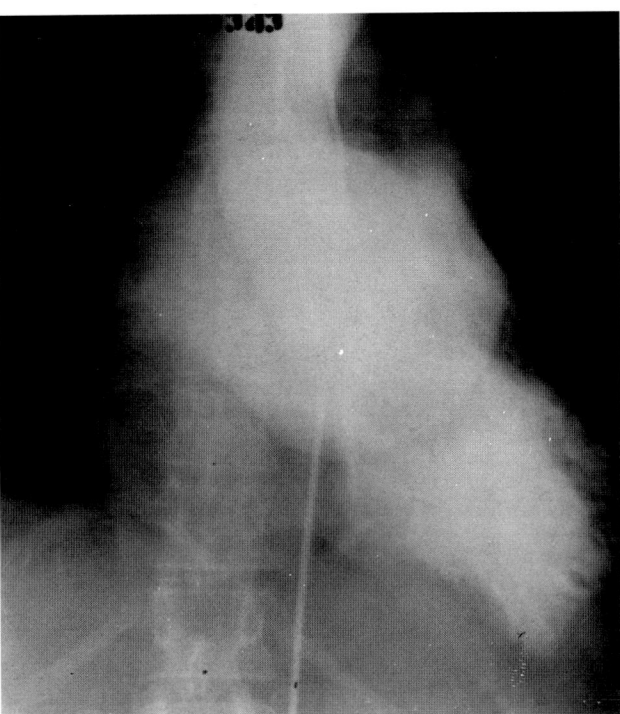

FIG. 6. Angiocardiogram made during hemodynamic study of a patient with a large pericardial effusion. Contrast injected at the junction of the superior vena cava and right atrium densely opacifies the cardiac chambers, which are surrounded by the water density of the effusion. This technique has fallen into disuse.

(15). Bubble contrast is then substituted for radioopaque contrast to ascertain correct placement of a needle or catheter in the pericardial space (Fig. 7). Echo-guided pericardiocentesis has been shown to be as safe and effective as fluoroscopically guided pericardiocentesis (16) and is the preferred

method in many major centers. The choice is largely a matter of local expertise and preference. Echocardiography plays a distinct part even when pericardiocentesis is done in the cardiac catheterization laboratory. By this means the size and distribution of effusion can be estimated, the optimal entry site can be ascertained, the angle and trajectory of the needle can be ascertained before the skin is punctured, and localized effusion, which often is not suitable for tapping, can be avoided. Echocardiography repeatedly has shown that, even in the case of a large effusion, there may be little fluid in the subcostal region, making it preferable to tap from a region near the cardiac apex, not by the classic subxiphoid route.

It is possible to visualize the needle as it punctures the pericardium, but frequently this visualization is inadequate. In this regard, it should be noted that the combined needle and transducer has not found acceptance, because of its complexity and because simple echoguidance has proven satisfactory (17). The real advantage of echoguidance is that the puncture site and the route to the pericardium are preplanned to ensure safe and effective pericardiocentesis while avoiding puncture of other structures that might intervene in the performance of blind pericardiocentesis. Less commonly, pericardiocentesis is guided by CT (Fig. 8) (18). Echocardiography remains the method of choice for the diagnosis and management of all aspects of pericardial effusion, except characterizing the nature of the fluid, for which purpose MRI, or, to a lesser extent, CT is far superior.

Characterizing the Pericardium and Pericardial Fluid

The management of a patient with pericardial effusion may differ, depending upon whether the fluid is a transudate that has a low attenuation value (Fig. 9A), an exudate, or blood with a high attenuation value (Fig. 9B). CT and MRI

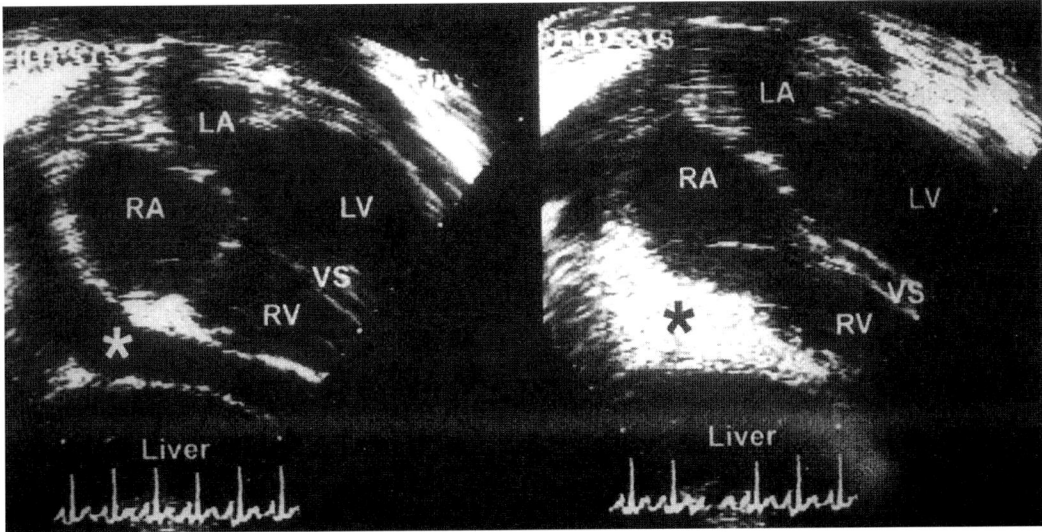

FIG. 7. Bubble contrast confined to the pericardium after injection of agitated saline during echo-guided pericardiocentesis. (From ref. 16, with permission.)

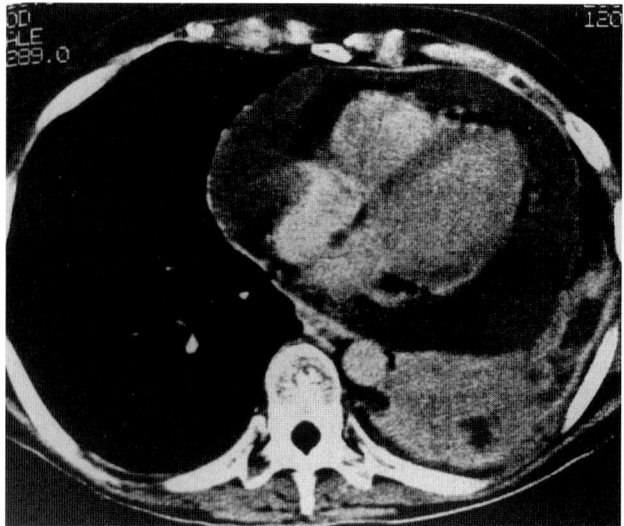

FIG. 8. Computer-assisted tomogram showing a large malignant pericardial effusion. The pericardial thickness is normal. (From ref. 18, with permission.)

both provide noninvasive means of making this important distinction (19).

Spin-echo MRI is accurate for detecting abnormal thickness of the pericardium. On cine magnetic resonance images, the pericardium may appear thicker than on spin-echo images. Using the cine mode, the combination of a pericardial effusion and a thickened pericardium may be found, as in cases with effusive constrictive pericarditis (see below).

Chylopericardium and Cholesterol Pericarditis

Chylopericardium is a pericardial effusion of chyle, high in cholesterol content, some in crystal form, caused by in-

jury, obstruction, or congenital deficiency of the thoracic duct. It is a rare cause of pericardial effusion after thoracic surgery. Contrast-enhanced CT together with lymphangiography (Fig. 10) (20) can help elucidate the responsible etiology and anatomy, and distinguish between the primary and secondary forms. Secondary chylopericardium is more common than primary. The usual cause is injury to the thoracic duct during chest surgery or by trauma. Less commonly, the duct is involved in a neoplastic lesion. The study would then show the obstructing mass and collateral lymph flow. In primary chylopericardium, which tends to occur in younger patients, no mass is present, but the lymphangiogram is abnormal, showing discontinuity of the duct and abnormal collateral flow.

Cholesterol pericarditis, is a different entity and does not implicate abnormality of the thoracic duct. It is a pericardial effusion with high cholesterol content, but no cholesterol crystal formation, that can occur in the course of chronic pericardial inflammation. Lymphangiography, therefore, but not CT, is helpful in the diagnosis.

Instrumenting the Normal Pericardium

Until recently the presence of pericardial effusion was a prerequisite for pericardial puncture. Stimulated by the finding that pharmaceuticals placed in the pericardium exert effects on the myocardium, conduction system, and coronary circulation, investigators have developed techniques to insert catheter delivery systems into the pericardium. One such method, so far reported only for animal studies, but which has proven simple, safe, and effective is via puncture of the right atrial appendage with a fine needle mounted at the end of a number four catheter (22). Another method, with which there is limited clinical and substantial experimental experience, is based on an instrument specially designed for the

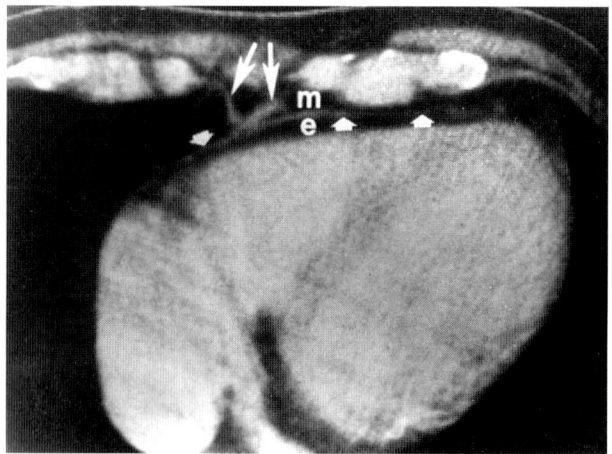
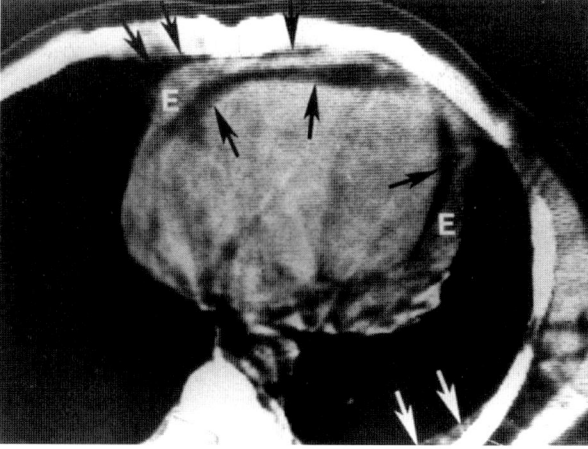

FIG. 9. Computer-assisted tomograms of the pericardium. **A:** Normal. *m,* mediastinal fat; *e,* epicardial fat. *Small arrows* indicate the pericardium and *large arrows* point to the sternopericardial ligaments. **B:** Pericardial effusion (*E*) appears as a water density band between the mediastinal and epicardial fat (*black arrows*). Note also the left pleural effusion (*white arrows*) common in pericardial effusion. (From ref. 19, with permission.)

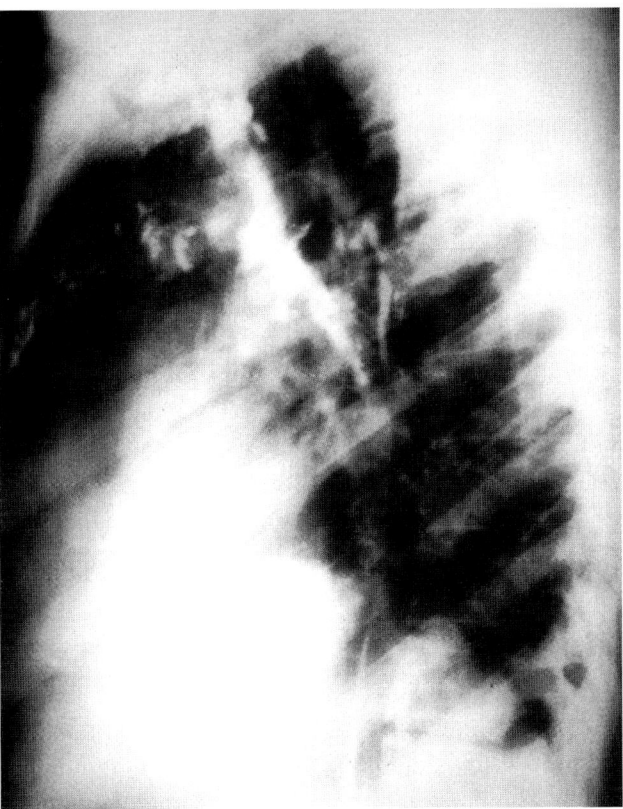

FIG. 10. Lymphangiogram from a patient with chylopericardium secondary to ectasia of the thoracic duct system. The duct was patent up to the level of L5. Radioactivity appears in the anterosuperior region of the thoracic cage in the form of saccules and small vascular channels. (From ref. 21, with permission.)

purpose, the "perducer" (23) passed through a subcostal introducer to the mediastinal trigone, the space bounded by the pleura and pericardium. Suction is applied to raise a bleb that can be seen through the instrument's viewing chamber and the bleb is punctured with a fine needle to permit passage of a catheter into the pericardial space.

The Chest Radiogram

The posterior and lateral chest radiogram ranks a distant second in importance after echocardiography as an imaging modality for detecting pericardial effusion. Chest radiography, nevertheless, has been too much neglected as a simple means to alert the physician to the possibility of pericardial effusion and the need for an echocardiogram. When the clinical circumstances suggest the possibility of pericardial effusion, the chest films should be carefully analyzed for evidence of possible pericardial effusion. Particularly helpful is unexplained increase in the size of the cardio-pericardial silhouette as, for example, after cardiac surgery, myocardial infarction, chest trauma, or in patients undergoing dialysis or experiencing the onset or exacerbation of a collagen-vascular disorder. This sign is of special importance also in

patients with neoplasm or who have had radiation of the mediastinum. The apparent cardiac enlargement makes the silhouette appear globular on a standard film, the contours of the left heart border being blunted (Fig. 11) but pulmonary congestion is absent, or less than expected, a finding that in other circumstances would suggest dilated cardiomyopathy with tricuspid regurgitation. When the radiograph is taken with the patient recumbent, the globular ("water bottle" shape) is not seen, but the base is widened by a shift cephalad in the distribution of fluid. Another, but much less common source of confusion is a giant lipoma that may give a very similar radiological appearance.

Few of the literature citations are current, but the subject has been reviewed recently along with the results of a retrospective analysis of the chest radiogram of 100 patients with pericardial effusion (24). One of the most specific and sensitive findings is posteroinferior bulging of the margin of the cardiac silhouette toward the spine, forming an obtuse angle with the left hemidiaphragm on the lateral projection of the chest radiogram. Left ventricular enlargement may obscure this roentgenographic sign. This sign, described in 1920, has unfortunately been largely forgotten, except by chest radiologists. Better remembered, but often neglected, is the displaced epicardial fat pad sign, a sign sometimes more easily appreciated by fluoroscopy, but cardiac fluoroscopy is little practiced today. In the absence of left atrial enlargement, a widened carinal angle is found in a minority of cases.

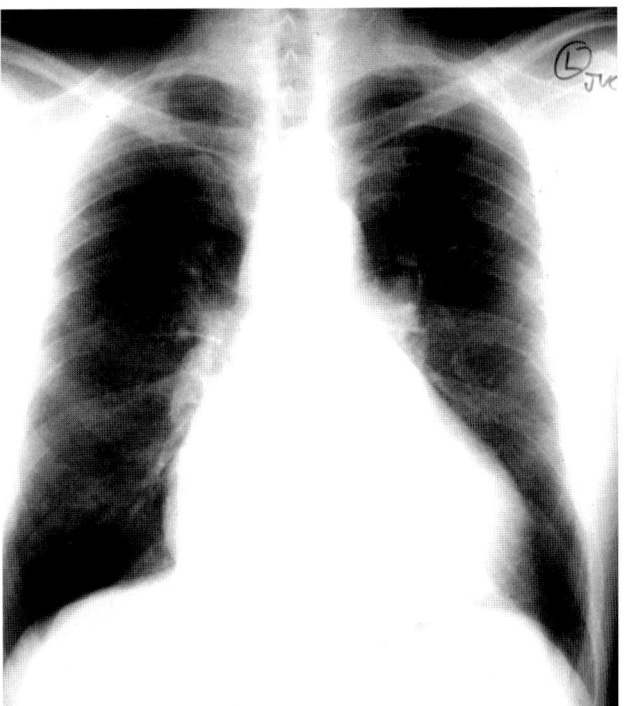

FIG. 11. Chronic pericardial effusion as it may appear on a posterior-anterior projection of a chest radiograph. The cardio-pericardial silhouette is massively enlarged, and the configuration is like a sac of water. Note also that the pericardial effusion is not associated with pulmonary congestion.

Uncommonly, the effusion is visualized as an opacity beyond the cardiac margin, but considerably less dense than the cardiac chambers. This finding is commonly referred to as the double density sign (25).

Fluoroscopy

Pericardial effusion, especially when acute, dampens and finally abolishes cardiac pulsation. This finding, easily observed by fluoroscopy, is particularly important in the cardiac catheterization laboratory where it may indicate or confirm that a cardiovascular perforation has occurred. When cardiac catheterization is being performed using fluoroscopic guidance, it is not possible to make the catheter contact the right heart border. This phenomenon is now less

useful, however, because most right heart catheterization is done using a balloon-tipped catheter that floats through the center of the atrium to the tricuspid valve.

Computerized Tomogram and Magnetic Resonance Imaging

The normal pericardium can be seen on almost every CT scan using appropriate technique (26). The pericardium appears as a thin curvilinear density best seen over the anterior wall of the right ventricle, sandwiched between dark epicardial fat posteriorly and mediastinal fat anteriorly (Fig. 9A). If the pericardium is not seen on any cut, it is safe to assume that the pericardial thickness is not increased and the technique suboptimal.

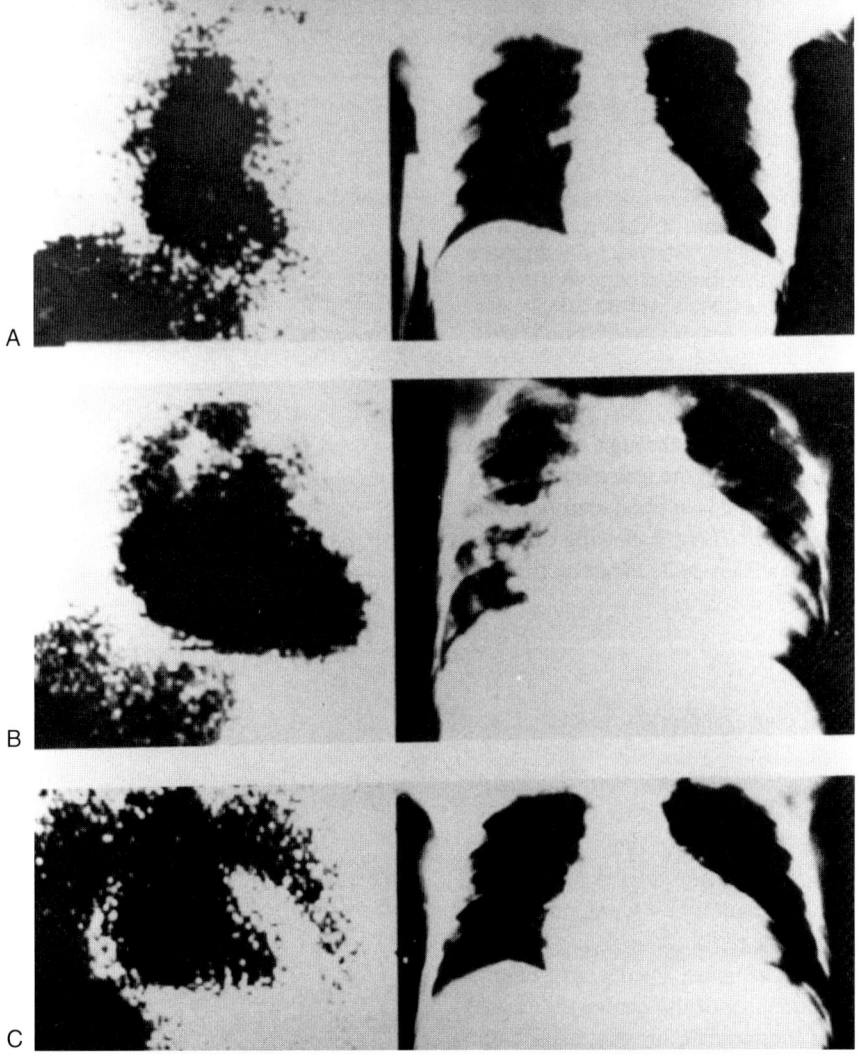

FIG. 12. Pericardial effusion demonstrated during a radionuclide blood pool scan. The scans are shown on the left and the conventional chest radiograms on the right. **A:** Small effusion. **B:** Medium-sized effusion with cardiomegaly. **C:** Large effusion with small heart. (From ref. 27, with permission.)

CT of the heart for evaluating pericardial disease is most often used to detect constrictive pericarditis, but pericardial effusion can be seen as an area of moderate, or water, density between the heart and pericardium (Fig. 9**B**). Effusion is often an incidental finding discovered when the tomography is being performed for some other reason, because echocardiography, not CT or MRI, is the usual primary imaging modality for diagnosing and evaluating pericardial effusion. Nevertheless, CT is an excellent means to image the presence, distribution, and nature of pericardial fluid (Fig. 8). On the CT the pericardium appears as a thin white curvilinear density sandwiched between epicardial and mediastinal fat, which appear dark. On magnetic resonance images, the pericardium appears as a dark line between the two grayish fat densities. In clinical practice, echocardiography is much preferred for this purpose, because it is simpler and can be performed or supervised in a cardiology laboratory by the clinician.

Less Common Modalities: Chance Discovery of Effusion

Pericardial effusion is sometimes discovered accidentally during abdominal ultrasound examination, radionuclide ventriculography (Fig. 12), or scintigraphy for ischemic heart disease (Fig. 13). Gallium-67 citrate, given for investigation of infection of the chest or suspected mediastinitis, may be taken up in the pericardial region, unveiling a pericardial

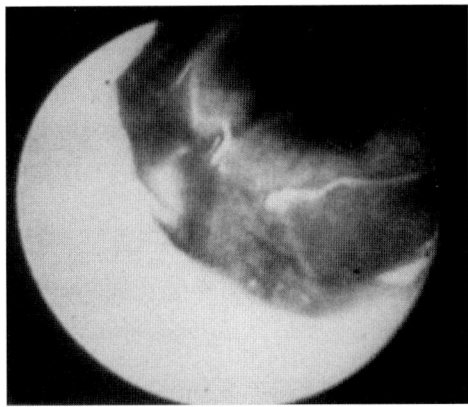
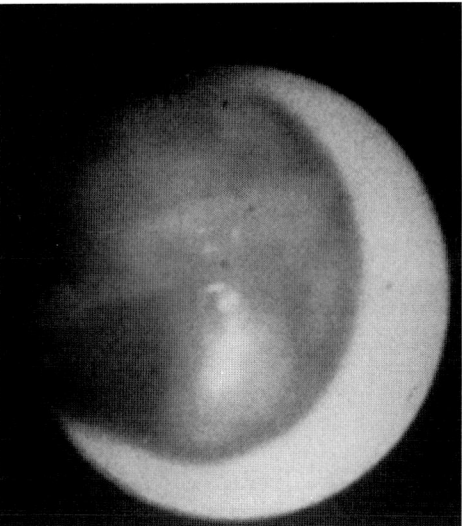

FIG. 14. The pericardium imaged via pericardioscopy. **Top:** fibrin layers in a case of lymphocytic pericarditis; **bottom:** metastatic bronchogenic carcinoma. (See also Color Plate 32 following page 758.) (From ref. 30, with permission.)

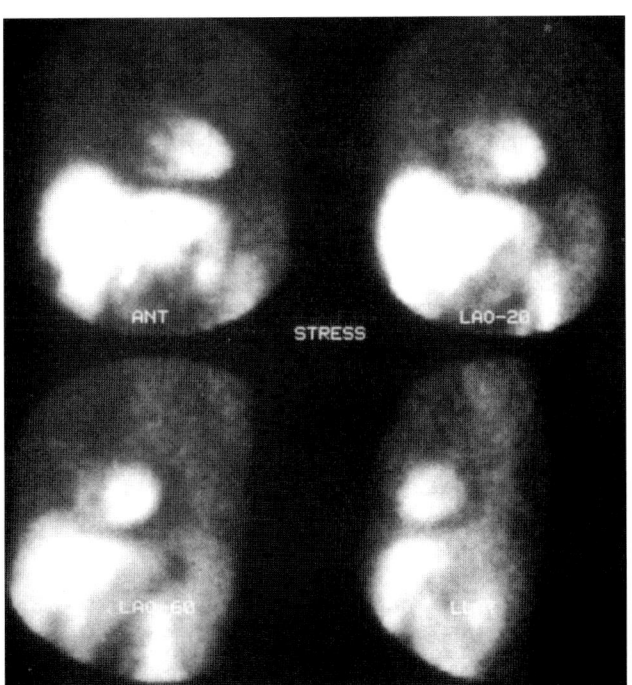

FIG. 13. Stress planar images showing a thick halo of diminished tracer uptake surrounding the heart. The patient had a tuberculous pericardial effusion. (From ref. 28, with permission.)

effusion, or by the myocardium indicating myopericarditis (29). Likewise, pericardial effusion may be revealed incidentally during MRI or CT of the thorax.

Pericardioscopy and Thoracoscopy

The epicardium may be imaged through pericardioscopy and thoracoscopy (Fig. 14; see also Color Plate 32 following page 758) (30). Through this means, sampling errors of biopsy are appreciably reduced.

CARDIAC TAMPONADE

Most of what has been stated above for pericardial effusion applies to cardiac tamponade, because a pericardial effusion or hemorrhage is the cause in virtually every case. In hyperacute tamponade, such as after major trauma, or rup-

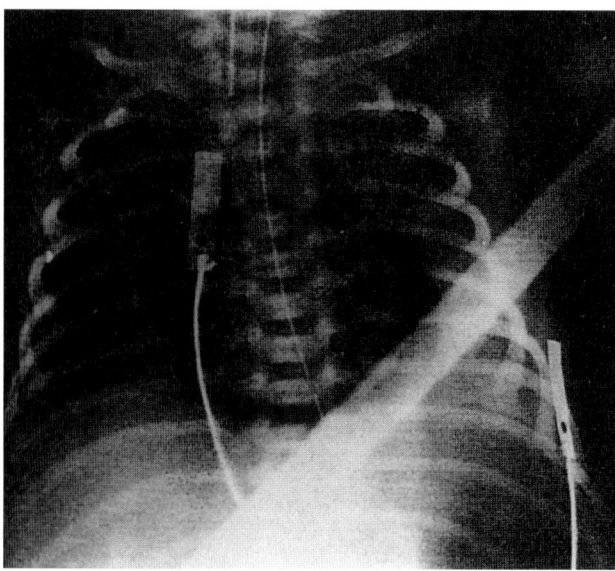

FIG. 15. Tension pneumothorax in a neonate. The resulting cardiac arrest required emergency pericardiocentesis. (From ref. 31, with permission.)

ture of the heart or aorta, cardiac enlargement by chest radiogram may not be apparent. Because the pericardium cannot be stretched acutely, a small volume of blood can cause severe tamponade. With more chronic effusion, varying degrees of enlargement, up to massive, may be present, because a chronic load allows the pericardium to stretch and hypertrophy. As always, careful correlation with the clinical findings is of key importance. An exceedingly rare cause of cardiac tamponade, especially now that diagnostic pneumopericardium is seldom performed, is tension pneumopericardium (Fig. 15). Most patients are premature neonates on mechanical ventilation. The patient illustrated was receiving only CPAP.

A number of echocardiographic abnormalities are highly suggestive of tamponade. A relatively small volume of fluid can cause acute tamponade, as after trauma or rupture of the heart or ascending aorta. In such cases, radiographic enlargement can easily be missed, especially when an earlier film for comparison is not available. More chronic tamponade, as occurs in most patients seen on an internal medical or cardiological service, is caused by considerably larger effusion, because with more gradual fluid accumulation, pericardial compliance increases, the pericardial pressure-volume curve is less steep and shifted rightward on the volume axis. The chest radiograph then shows enlargement of the cardiopericardial silhouette with, in addition, possible prominence of the azygos vein, when central venous pressure is sufficiently elevated.

The two most important echocardiographic signs of tamponade are right ventricular diastolic collapse (32,33) and right atrial compression (34,35). Other abnormalities include inspiratory increase in right ventricular dimension with reduced left ventricular dimension and pseudoprolapse of the

mitral valve. The chief Doppler sign of tamponade is greatly increased respiratory variation of transmitral blood flow velocity with reciprocal changes in transtricuspid blood flow velocity (36). These findings result directly from the altered physiology described in the next section. The final diagnosis of tamponade depends upon thoughtful integration of the clinical with the imaging information.

The Pathophysiologic Basis of Echo Doppler Abnormalities

Echo Doppler evaluation for cardiac tamponade is based on understanding its major pathophysiologic features, which are that the tightly stretched pericardium prohibits change in pericardial volume during the respiratory cycle and that interaction among the cardiac chambers, which in the normal euvolemic subject is weak, becomes powerful. One consequence is that the effects of respiration on the cardiac cycle are greatly intensified. Thus when inspiration increases the volume, atrioventricular valve leaflet excursion, and filling velocity of the right side of the heart, those of the left side must decrease. This enhanced effect of respiration on hemodynamics is manifest on echocardiography by an exaggerated inspiratory bulge of the interventricular septum from the right toward the left ventricle, easily appreciated by M mode and by a dramatic increase in the inspiratory drop in transmitral blood flow velocity, normally less than 10% to as much as 50%. Transtricuspid velocity normally varies more than transmitral with respiration, but in the case of tamponade its inspiratory increase is more pronounced than normal. The enhanced action of respiration on hemodynamics is also manifest clinically as pulsus paradoxus, and by Doppler as increased respiratory variation of semilunar blood flow velocity. Many changes in the cardiac cycle induced by respiration contribute to pulsus paradoxus, but competition for room within a fixed pericardial volume is the dominant one. In cardiac tamponade, as in normal subjects, systemic venous return increases during inspiration secondarily to the drop in intrathoracic pressure. The right heart expansion that therefore occurs with inspiration compresses the left heart, causing its stroke volume and, therefore, systemic arterial pressure to fall. In health, left ventricular compliance is less than right, but in cardiac tamponade, compliance of the two ventricles is identical. This identity of the two ventricular compliances occurs because their diastolic pressures are equal to each other and to pericardial pressure. When cardiac tamponade is superimposed on preexisting heart disease, however, left and right ventricular diastolic compliance may not be equal. When either ventricular diastolic pressure exceeds the pericardial pressure that is causing tamponade, pulsus paradoxus is absent and the expected echo-Doppler findings are attenuated or lost. This interplay between heart and pericardial disease reemphasizes the importance of careful correlation between the echo Doppler and clinical findings.

With cardiac tamponade, pericardial pressure is elevated, and therefore central venous pressure is elevated to the same degree. Consequently, another important echocardiographic sign of tamponade is dilation and a fixed dimension of the inferior vena cava throughout the respiratory cycle (37). A further consequence of equalized pericardial, right atrial, and right ventricular diastolic pressures is the aforementioned compression of the right atrium and ventricle. The atria and right ventricle are thin-walled and in cardiac tamponade their transmural diastolic pressure is essentially zero. Minimal pressure disturbances could then result in a slightly negative transmural pressure in diastole, sufficient to compress these chambers. For moderate and even severe tamponade, the reversal of the pressure difference between the right ventricle and pericardium is too small to measure reliably using conventional technique, but becomes quite evident in extreme or end-stage tamponade (38).

Both right atrial (Fig. 16) and right ventricular diastolic collapse (Fig. 17) are highly specific and highly sensitive markers of tamponade although they can occur with a large pleural effusion (39). Right atrial collapse appears earlier in the course of tamponade and persists longer than ventricular collapse during pericardiocentesis (40). In a study of cardiac tamponade in a canine model, right ventricular diastolic collapse correlated better than pulsus paradoxus with hemodynamic derangement (41), and is a relatively early sign of tamponade, appearing when there is significant but not profound hemodynamic deterioration and before the advent of pulsus paradoxus (42). The collapse occurs at lower pericardial pressure in hypovolemic experimental tamponade. Similarly, diastolic collapse of the right ventricle occurs early in tamponade associated with hemorrhage and in patients with

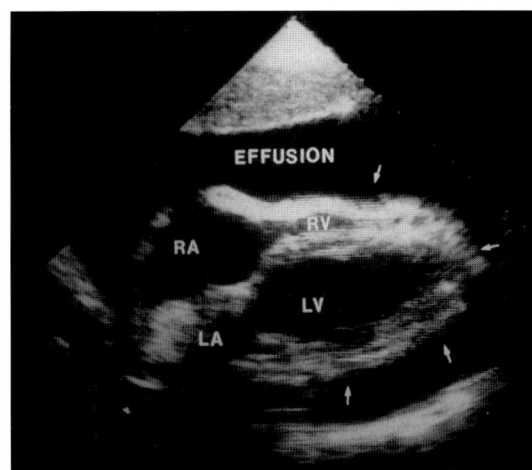

FIG. 17. Subcostal long-axis echocardiogram showing extreme right ventricular compression in a patient with near end-stage tamponade. The chamber appeared normal after pericardiocentesis. *RA*, right atrium; *RV*, right ventricle; *LV*, left ventricle; *LA*, left atrium.

renal disease when hemodialysis is performed too aggressively.

In the present era, right ventricular diastolic collapse is frequently evaluated in real time, but the analysis requires experience. Stop-frame technique is essential to be certain that the collapse is occurring in diastole. M-mode interpretation has much to commend it, as the posterior motion of the anterior wall of the right ventricle is easily recognized and can be seen to correspond with electrical diastole, and can readily be confirmed by simultaneously imaging the open mitral or closed aortic valve (Fig. 17). Right atrial collapse (Fig. 18) is easier to recognize, but still requires experience and should not be attempted by physicians who lack the appropriate training. Most emergency medicine physicians are not trained in echocardiography; therefore, in general, I consider it wise for them to obtain appropriate consultation when the question of tamponade arises in their practice.

In cases of cardiac tamponade in which right ventricular hypertrophy is also present, the increase in pericardial pressure may be insufficient to compress the chamber. Likewise, elevated right heart pressures due to right heart failure can prevent right atrial and ventricular collapse in tamponade. Left atrial or, less commonly, left ventricular collapse may be seen in severe tamponade. Compression may be confined to the left heart chambers when severe right heart disease is present, or involve both sides in severe tamponade.

A less well-appreciated echocardiographic abnormality caused by cardiac tamponade is pseudohypertrophy of the left ventricle. The external pressure exerted on the left ventricle reduces its diastolic volume; consequently, myocardial thickness is increased. Myocardial thickness returns to normal after pericardiocentesis. Calculated myocardial mass is the same before and after tap. This finding, while of physiological interest, is seldom if ever clinically useful.

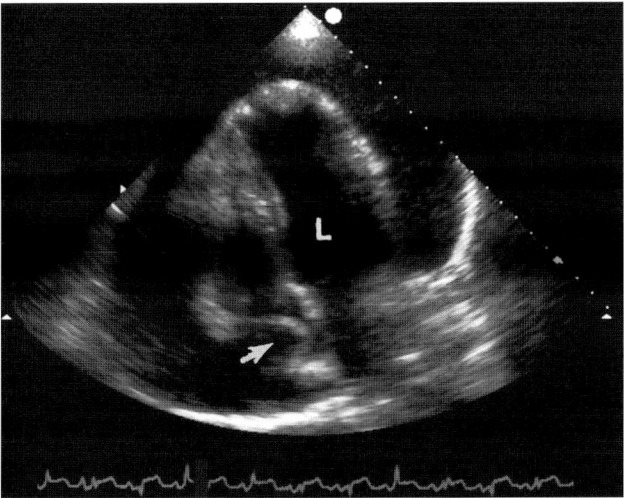

FIG. 16. Echocardiogram showing right atrial compression in a patient with postpericardiotomy cardiac tamponade.

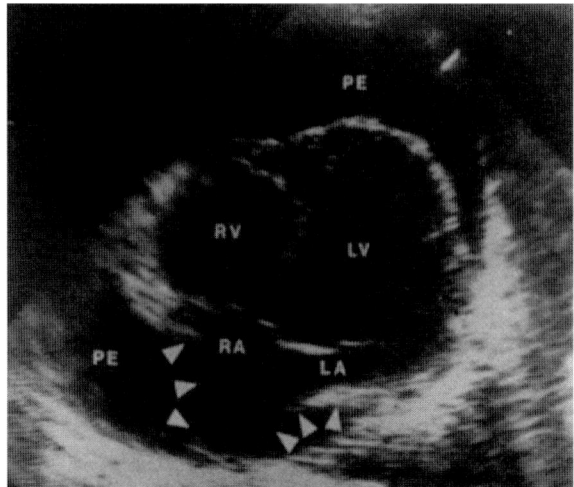

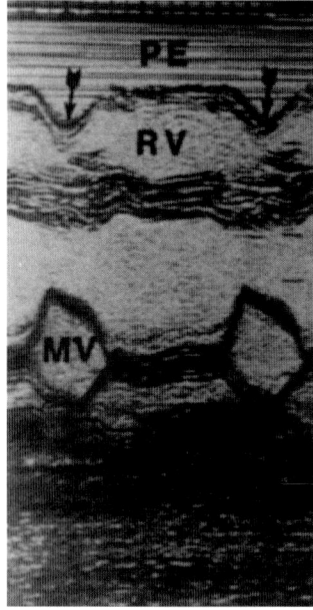
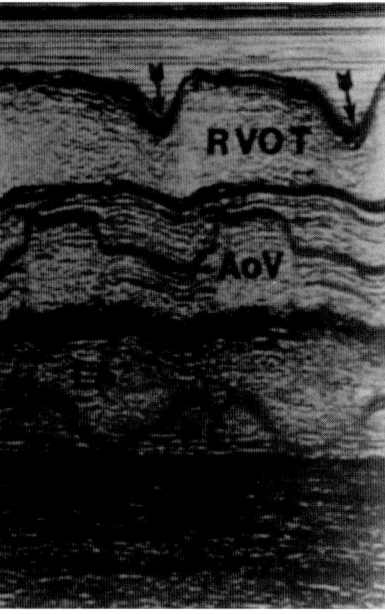

FIG. 18. Apical four chamber (**top**) and M-mode echocardiogram (**bottom**) demonstrating chamber collapse in cardiac tamponade. Diastolic collapse of both atria is shown by the *white arrowheads*. The M-mode (**bottom**) shows that collapse (*black arrows*) coincides with diastole, because the mitral valve is open and the aortic valve is closed. *PE*, pericardial effusion; *RV*, right ventricle; *LV*, left ventricle; *RA*, right atrium; *LA*, left atrium; *MV*, mitral valve; *RVOT*, right ventricular outflow tract; *AoV*, aortic valve. (From ref. 43, with permission.)

CONSTRICTIVE PERICARDITIS

Pathophysiology

Like tamponade, constrictive pericarditis is a disorder of diastole in which total pericardial volume is invariate and therefore ventricular interaction is greatly enhanced. It differs from tamponade in two critical respects. The first is that the heart is not compressed in early diastole, but its volume becomes fixed from the end of the first third of diastole until the ensuing systole. The second difference is that whereas in tamponade, transmural diastolic pressure (cardiac minus pericardial) is a key determinant of the pathophysiology, in constrictive pericarditis, the pericardial space is obliterated, therefore pericardial pressure does not exist. Furthermore, whereas in tamponade changes of intrathoracic pressure induced by respiration are almost completely transmitted to the cardiac chambers, replacement of the pericardial space

with a noncompliant fused pericardium prevents transmission of intrathoracic pressure variations to the cardiac chambers. This transmission failure has profound effects on ventricular filling.

In tamponade, inspiration causes systemic venous return to increase. The decrease of left ventricular filling is a necessary consequence of that increase, because total pericardial volume is fixed. In constriction, on the other hand, the primary, or initiating event is a decrease in left ventricular filling that engenders a secondary increase in right heart volume in the fixed pericardial space. The reason for decreased left ventricular filling and therefore volume is that, because inspiration lowers intrathoracic pressure and, with it, pulmonary venous pressure, while left ventricular diastolic pressure remains constant, the pressure gradient responsible for ventricular filling diminishes with inspiration.

Just as echocardiography is the imaging modality of

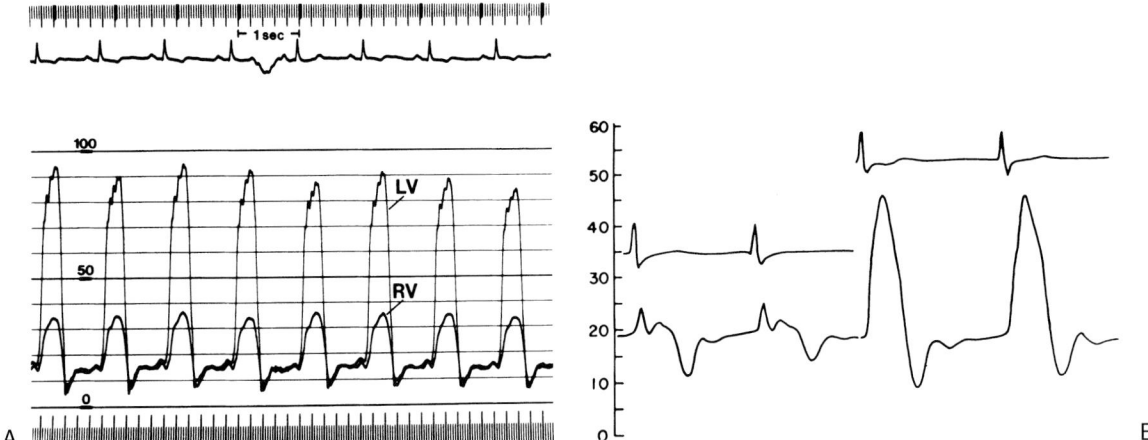

FIG. 19. A: Left and right ventricular pressure recordings from a case of constrictive pericarditis showing an early diastolic dip that corresponds to early rapid ventricular filling, followed by a plateau indicating diastasis from the end of early rapid filling to end-diastole. This pattern of ventricular diastolic pressure predicts the restrictive filling pattern seen on imaging. *LV*, left ventricle; *RV*, right ventricle. **B:** Pressure from right atrium and ventricle in restrictive cardiomyopathy.

choice for pericardial effusion, CT is the preferred method for constrictive pericarditis. Although increased echogenicity of the pericardium by echocardiography may be apparent in gross cases, its absence by no means excludes the diagnosis of constrictive pericarditis. MRI can also be used to excellent effect, but is more disturbing to most patients.

The imaging abnormalities in constrictive pericarditis reflect its pathology and pathophysiology. With varying degrees of sensitivity, imaging modalities demonstrate the abnormal anatomy as a thick, dense, and sometimes calcified structure. In the absence of co-existing heart disease, left ventricular volume is not enlarged, and, in severe cases, may be considerably diminished, with resulting low stroke volume. Ventricular volume increases rapidly in early diastole, only to remain constant for the remainder of diastole, a phenomenon referred to as the restrictive filling pattern, characteristic of constrictive pericarditis, but also seen in restrictive cardiomyopathy. The restrictive filling pattern seen by imaging is reflected by the waveform of atrial and ventricular pressure. During early rapid filling, a sharp dip in left and right ventricular diastolic pressure is inscribed, after the completion of which, ventricular diastolic pressure remains constant (Fig. 19A). The atrial pressure waveform shows a prominent *y* descent, corresponding with the early diastolic dip of ventricular pressure (Fig. 19B). These findings are fundamentally different from those of cardiac tamponade in which compression is present throughout the cardiac cycle and progresses through diastole to become maximal at end diastole. Early rapid filling and with it the early diastolic dip are therefore abolished (Fig. 20). Systemic venous return is limited to ventricular systole. Ventricular diastolic pressure is elevated at early diastole and rises progressively until end diastole. It follows that in cardiac tamponade, a restrictive pattern of ventricular pressure is not observed.

Finally, imaging demonstrates the reciprocity between the respiratory changes in the volume and filling velocities of the two ventricles predicted by tight parallel interaction between the cardiac chambers. Whereas, in cardiac tamponade, the inspiratory increase in right heart volume impedes left ventricular filling, in constrictive pericarditis, the decrease in left ventricular filling allows the right heart volume to increase.

Structure of the Pericardium

The pericardium itself, except when it is calcified, is not visible on the chest radiograph. Calcific constrictive pericarditis is less common now, because tuberculosis is a far less common cause than it used to be, and, partly for this reason, the illness has become less chronic. Extensive curvilinear pericardial calcification is nonetheless highly suggestive of the diagnosis. This calcification is more easily detected in

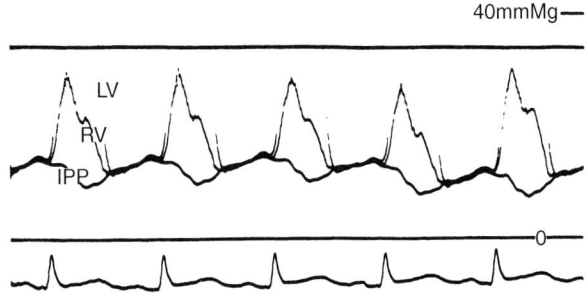

FIG. 20. Right ventricular and pericardial pressure recordings from a patient with cardiac tamponade. Note the absence of an early diastolic dip and a mid-to-late plateau of diastolic pressure that explains the absence of a restrictive filling pattern by imaging. Pericardial pressure is equal to ventricular diastolic pressure. *IPP*, intrapericardial pressure; *LV*, left ventricle; *RV*, right ventricle. (From ref. 44, with permission.)

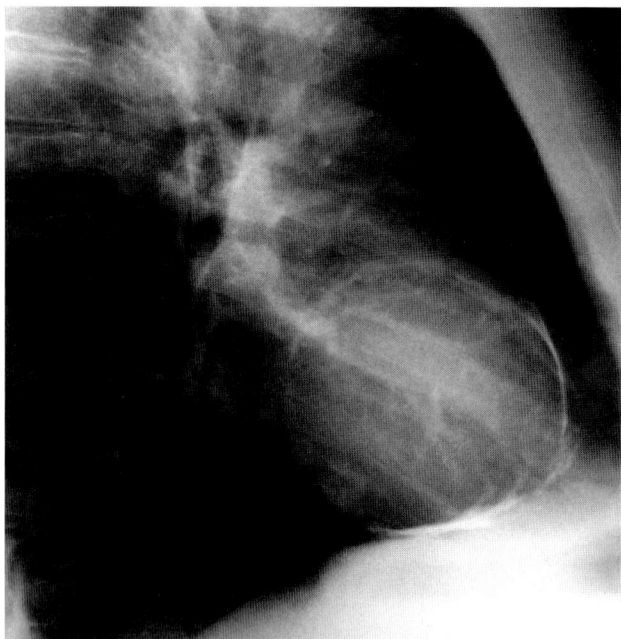

FIG. 21. Calcification by chest radiography: constrictive pericarditis.

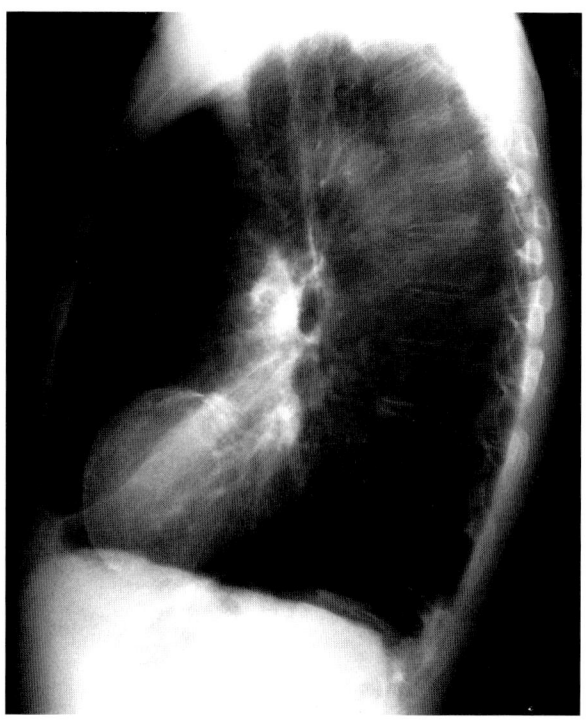

FIG. 22. Calcification by chest radiography: left ventricular aneurysm.

the lateral than in the posteroanterior projection (Fig. 21), and is very evident by fluoroscopy. Absence of pericardial calcification neither supports nor refutes the diagnosis. In an occasional instance, the calcification appears as a large plaque. Specks of calcification can be seen in patients without significant pericardial disease.

It is important not to confuse calcific constrictive pericarditis with calcification of a left ventricular aneurysm (Fig. 22). Other sources of calcification in and around the heart, such as valvular, coronary, or in a mural thrombus or the left atrium are considerably less likely sources of error.

A thick or calcified pericardium is easily imaged on the computerized tomogram (Fig. 23), which therefore is extremely important in distinguishing constrictive pericarditis from restrictive cardiomyopathy, conditions that mimic each other in so many other ways. Fortunately, using this technique, a normal appearance of the pericardium provides strong evidence favoring myocardial over pericardial disease, but false negatives do occur, typically when constriction is caused by a tight visceral pericardium with little or no disease of the parietal pericardium. Constrictive pericarditis without evidence of increased pericardial thickness is found in some cases developing after cardiac surgery.

In contrast to pericardial effusion in which echocardiography is the imaging method of choice, an abnormally thick or a calcified pericardium is effectively imaged on the echocardiogram in only a relatively small proportion of the cases. This lack of sensitivity is to some extent related to the changing etiology that has reduced the chronicity of the disease. It is also explained in part by the high echogenicity of the pericardium, which is a particularly troublesome problem

when the gain and contrast are set high, making the normal pericardium appear abnormal. In some cases, however, characteristic abnormalities of the pericardium are present. The posterior pericardium appears thicker and brighter than normal and is represented as a series of parallel lines, which move with the myocardium instead of remaining flat, as the normal pericardium does. In the subcostal long-axis view, the cardiac image slides along the diaphragm during the cardiac cycle. In constrictive pericarditis, this sliding motion is

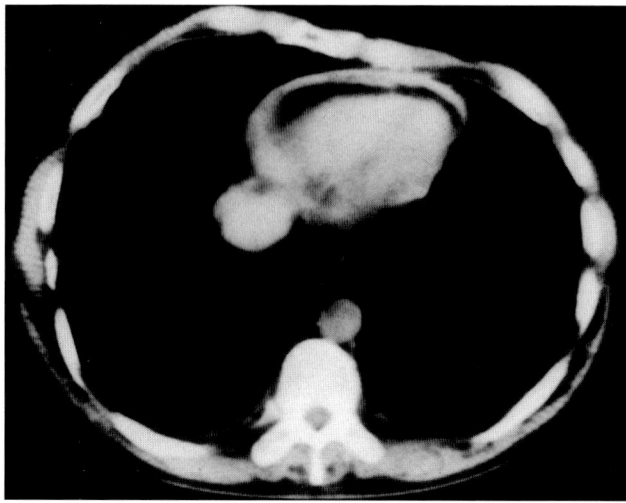

FIG. 23. Computer assisted tomogram showing heavy calcification of the pericardium anterior to the right ventricle.

lost, another sign useful in the differential diagnosis from restrictive cardiomyopathy.

The width of the pericardium, normally less than three mm at its thickest portion, is readily measured by CT, MRI, or transesophageal echocardiography. Likewise, abnormally increased thickness, calcification, irregularities, and masses are well-defined. Of the techniques available for evaluating the anatomy and pathology of the pericardium, CT is the one most often used.

The Restrictive Filling Pattern

The M-mode echocardiogram shows rapid increase in the diameter of the left ventricle in early diastole. Thereafter, the ventricular dimension remains unchanged throughout the remainder of diastole. Numerous real-time imaging techniques can demonstrate the restrictive filling pattern. The rapid filling in early diastole followed by prolonged diastasis can be recognized by experienced observers looking at a two-dimensional echocardiogram or an opaque left ventriculogram. The more painstaking technique of frame-by-frame analysis can be applied to any real-time image of the left ventricle to quantify this abnormality of ventricular filling. Long before the advent of modern cardiac imaging, this filling pattern was hypothesized by investigators studying the diastolic pressure waveform in constrictive pericarditis, showing a rapid narrow dip in early diastole followed by a plateau in mid- and late diastole.

Reciprocity of Left and Right Ventricular Filling Velocities

For reasons comparable to those that apply to cardiac tamponade, namely, a fixed pericardial volume and enhanced ventricular interaction, but with a different underlying mechanism, respiration alters ventricular filling velocities. The inspiratory increase in transmitral velocity and increase in transtricuspid velocity are far greater than normal. In restrictive cardiomyopathy, that frequent mimic of constrictive pericarditis, not only can the pericardium stretch, allowing pericardial volume to change, but also its volume is larger than the volume of its contents (reserve volume). Ventricular interaction therefore is not enhanced and respiratory variation of transatrioventricular velocities remains normal (45). In instances in which atrial pressure is severely elevated, it may be necessary to perform the Doppler evaluation with the patient in the head-up tilt position to demonstrate increased respiratory variation of ventricular filling velocities (46). The inspiratory increase in the constricted right ventricle causes its systolic pressure to increase. Any tricuspid regurgitation that may be present increases in peak velocity and duration (47).

Global and Regional Wall Motion

Overall, systolic function is normal or hyperdynamic, providing co-existing myocardial disease is absent. Severe re-

gional wall motion abnormalities usually are not seen if the patient does not also have coronary arterial disease. In some cases, however, with localized variation in the severity of constriction, the most constricted regions are hypokinetic. The decrease in left ventricular volume that occurs when the patient inspires generates a rapid leftward motion of the interventricular septum, commonly referred to as septal bounce. This abrupt motion contrasts with the more gentle rightward shift of the septum with inspiration in cardiac tamponade.

A number of other abnormalities of the motion of the interventricular septum visible by M-mode have been described (48). Because of their low sensitivity, they are of greater interest to the talmudic echocardiographer than to the pragmatic physician. These abnormalities include an early diastolic notch; an atrial systolic notch, directed either anteriorly or posteriorly; an atrial systolic notch; and premature opening of the pulmonary valve. These abnormalities are thought to result from small transient reversals of the pressure gradient across the atrial and ventricular septa that result from enhanced chamber interaction.

Effusive Constrictive Pericarditis

Effusive constrictive pericarditis, as its name suggests, is a condition in which pericardial effusion and constriction by the visceral pericardium co-exist (49). Commonly, the diagnosis is made during pericardiocentesis because of an abnormal hemodynamic response to the procedure. With uncomplicated cardiac tamponade, pulmonary wedge, right atrial, and pericardial pressures return to normal after pericardiocentesis. In the case of effusive constrictive pericarditis, pericardial pressure falls to normal, but the two cardiac pressures remain elevated and equal (Fig. 24). Furthermore, the right atrial pressure waveform appears characteristic of

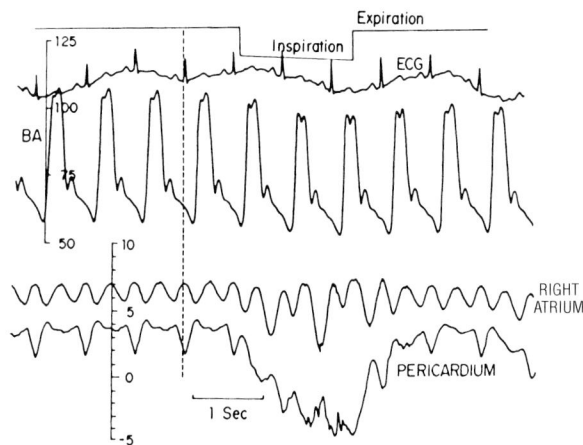

FIG. 24. Pressure recordings from a patient with effusive-constrictive pericarditis made at the completion of pericardiocentesis. Note that the right atrial pressure remains somewhat elevated and shows the waveform of constrictive pericarditis. Pericardial pressure has returned to normal. *BA*, brachial artery.

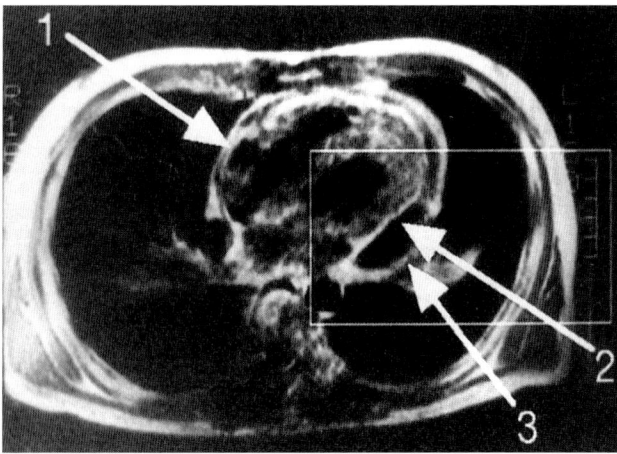

FIG. 25. Gd-DTPA enhanced magnetic resonance image from a patient with effusive-constrictive pericarditis enhances the visceral pericardium (*arrow 2*) and the parietal pericardium (*arrow 3*) and shows local fusion of the two layers (*arrow 1*). (From ref. 50, with permission.)

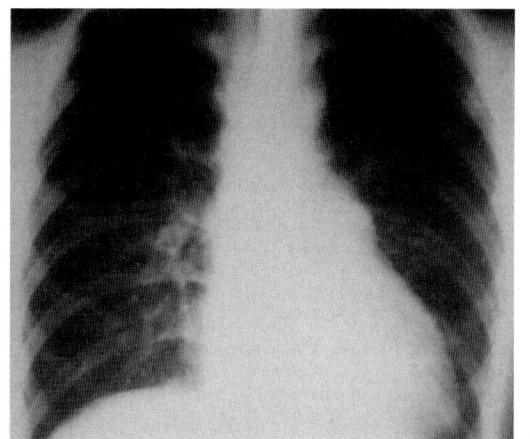

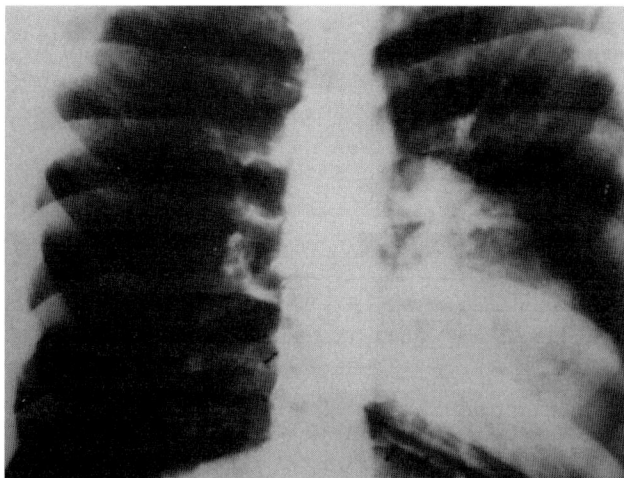

FIG. 26. Congenital absence of the left pericardium, partial (**A**) and complete (**B**). *Arrows* point to the lucency between the heart and diaphragm. (From ref. 27, with permission.)

constriction showing deep x and *y* descents and respiratory variation confined to the *y* descent.

The diagnosis can be suspected before invading the pericardium. It should be sought in subacute pericarditis occurring after radiation therapy and in tuberculous pericarditis. Pulsus paradoxus is much more common, the *y* descent of central venous pressure less prominent, and the heart is usually larger than in classic constrictive pericarditis. The x descent is prominent. Evidence by echocardiography of an organization pericardial effusion suggests the presence or imminence of effusive constrictive pericarditis. The condition may also be recognized by CT or MRI, especially with Gd-DTPA enhancement (Fig. 25) (50).

CONGENITAL ABSENCE OF THE PERICARDIUM

Congenital absence of the pericardium is a rare condition. The deficiency is usually in the left side of the pericardium and may be partial or complete. The first clue is usually obtained from a plain chest radiogram, less often from a systolic murmur or click. A very small defect is of no consequence and total absence, whereas it produces bizarre images, is innocuous. A critically sized defect, however, may permit the left atrium or the left ventricular apex to herniate through it, with the potential for strangulation. These defects must be closed or enlarged so as to eliminate the risk of this surgical emergency.

The radiological abnormalities are most pronounced when absence of the left pericardium (or, rarely, all the pericardium) is complete. In these cases, the heart is markedly displaced to the left (Fig. 26A) and echocardiography shows dramatic shifts of the heart's position when the patient is moved from the supine to the left decubitus position. With partial absence of the left pericardium, the heart's position is normal, but the left atrial appendage and the pulmonary

artery segment are unduly prominent. Lung interposed between the base of the heart and the diaphragm, and between the left atrial appendage and pulmonary artery segments create abnormal lucencies in these locations on the frontal chest radiogram (Fig. 26**B**).

PERICARDIAL CYST

Pericardial cysts are comparatively rare, constituting approximately 5% of mediastinal tumors. The cyst is most often detected in asymptomatic patients on a plain chest radiogram, on which it appears as a small, smooth circular opacity at the right anterior cardiophrenic angle (Fig. 27), or less commonly, at the left. Its opacity is the same as that of the heart, because it contains clear fluid, hence the term "spring water cyst." Much less frequently, pericardial cysts may be found in atypical locations, such as the parasternal area or near the region of the azygos vein, in which case echocardiography, CT (51), or MRI is needed to establish the diagnosis. With the latter two techniques, the cyst shows water density in contradistinction to the blood density of the

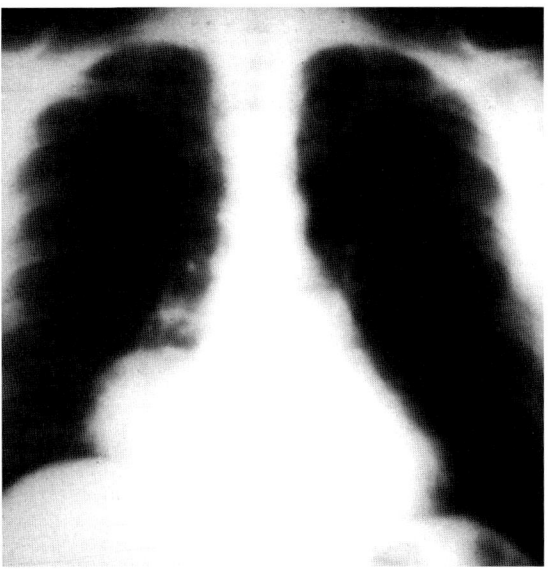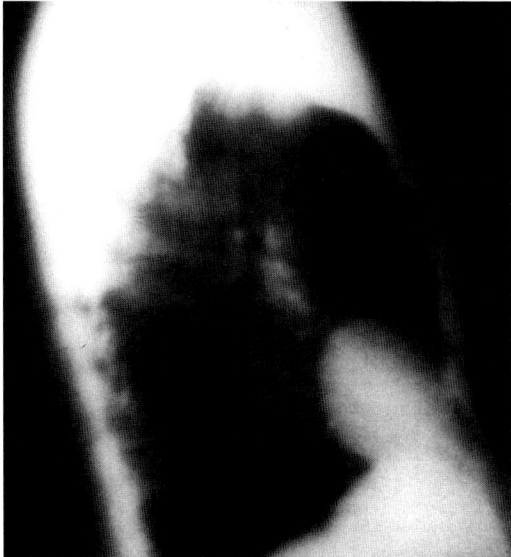

FIG. 27. Pericardial cyst occupying the anterior right cardiophrenic angle. (From ref. 27, with permission.)

contiguous cardiac chamber. Using echocardiography, a cyst can be mistaken for a mass (52). Now, surgical exploration should seldom be necessary, but the lesion should be excised if the diagnosis is not secure. Rarely, a cyst may grow to gigantic proportions and, by compressing the right heart, be responsible for a clinical picture simulating right heart failure, or constrictive pericarditis. Similarly, a large cyst may be the cause of localized extrinsic compression with the murmur of tricuspid or pulmonary valve stenosis (53). Occasionally, a cyst may rupture (54), leaving no trace on a cardiac image, although the tag may be found at operation.

HEMATOMA AND OTHER MASS LESIONS

Bleeding into the pericardium may result in an organized, sometimes calcified hematoma that may simulate constrictive pericarditis. The commonest causes are postoperative complication and trauma (55). Less commonly, the original hemorrhage occurred during a cardiac interventional procedure (56). The lesion can be imaged satisfactorily by any of the modalities, including transesophageal echocardiography (57). Another less common reason for a pericardial mass is neoplasia, but the pericardial manifestation of malignancy usually takes the form of effusion or constriction.

REFERENCES

1. Ewart W. Practical aids in the diagnosis of pericardial effusion, in connection with the question as to surgical treatment. *Brit Med J* 1896; 1:717–772.
2. D'Cruz IA, Overton DH, Ganesh MP. Pericardial complications of cardiac surgery: emphasis on the diagnostic role of echocardiography. *J Cardiac Surg* 1992;7:257–268.
3. Alio-Bosch, et al. *Am Heart J* 1991;21:207–208.
4. Sinha PR, Singh BP, Jaipuria N, et al. Intrapericardial echogenic images and development of constrictive pericarditis in patients with pericardial effusion. *Am Heart J* 1996;132:1268–1272.
5. Enein M, Abou Zina AA, Kassem M, et al. Echocardiography of the pericardium in pregnancy. *Obstet Gynecol* 1987;69:851–853.
6. Abduljabbar HSO, Marzouki KMH, Zawawi TH, et al. Pericardial effusion in normal pregnant women. *Acta Obstet Gynecol Scand* 1991;70: 291–294.
7. Jeanty P, Romero R, Hobbins JC. Fetal pericardial fluid: a normal finding of the second half of gestation. *Am J Obstet Gynecol* 1984; 149:529–532.
8. Dizon-Townson DS, Dildy GA, Clark SL. A prospective evaluation of fetal pericardial fluid in 506 second-trimester low-risk pregnancies. *Obstet Gynecol* 1997;90:958–961.
9. Kimura BJ, Pezeshki B, Frack SA, et al. Feasibility of ''limited'' echo imaging: characterization of incidental findings. *J Am Soc Echocardiogr* 1998;11:746–750.
10. Horowitz MS, Schultz CS, Stinson EB, et al. Sensitivity and specificity of echocardiographic diagnosis of pericardial effusion. *Circulation* 1974;50:239–247.
11. Feigenbaum H. *Echocardiography.* 5th ed. Philadelphia: Lea & Febiger, 1994.
12. Rigney DR, Goldberger AL. Nonlinear dynamics of the heart's swinging during pericardial effusion. *Am J Physiol* 1989;257(Heart Circ Physiol 26): H1292–H1305.
13. Spodick DH. Truly total electrical alternans of the heart. *Clin Cardiol* 1998;21:427–428.
14. Durant TM. Negative (gas) contrast angiocardiography. *Am Heart J* 1961;61:1–4.
15. Taavitsainen M, Bondestam S, Mankinen P, et al. Ultrasound guidance for pericardiocentesis. *Acta Radiol* 1991;32:9–11.
16. Tsang TSM, Freeman WK, Sinak LJ, et al. Echocardiographically guided pericardiocentesis: evolution and state–of-the-art technique. *Mayo Clin Proc* 1998;73:647–652.
17. Drummond JB, Seward JB, Tsang TSM, et al. Outpatient two-dimensional echocardiography-guided pericardiocentesis. *J Am Soc Echocardiogr* 1998;11:433–435.
18. Bellon RJ, Wright WH, Unger EC. CT-guided pericardial drainage catheter placement with subsequent pericardial sclerosis. *J Comput Assist Tomogr* 1995;19:672–673.
19. Silverman PM, Harell GS, Korobkin M. Computed tomography of the abnormal pericardium. *Am J Roentgenol* 1983;140:1125–1129.
20. Hamanaca D, Suzuki T, Kawanishi K., et al. Two cases of primary isolated chylopericardium diagnosed by oral administration of 131 I-triolein. *Radiat Med* 1983;1:65–69.
21. Baratella, et al. *Heart* 1998;80:376.

22. Verrier RL, Waxman S, Lovett EG, et al: Transatrial access to the normal pericardial space: a novel approach for diagnostic sampling, pericardiocentesis, and therapeutic interventions. *Circulation* 1998;98: 2331–2333.

23. Seferovic PM, Ristic AD, Maksimovic R, et al. Initial clinical experience with perducer device promising new tool in the diagnosis and treatment of pericardial disease. *Clin Cardiol* 1999;22(suppl I):I-30–I-35.

24. Woodring JH. The lateral chest radiograph in the detection of pericardial effusion: a reevaluation. *Kentucky Medical Association Journal* 1998;96:218–224.

25. Tehranzadeh J, Kelley MJ. The differential density sign of pericardial effusion. *Radiology* 1979;133:23–30.

26. Silverman PM, Harell GS. Computed tomography of the normal pericardium. *Invest Radiol* 1983;18:141–144.

27. Shabetai R. *The pericardium*. New York: Grune & Stratton, 1980: 109–153.

28. Herzog E, Krasnow N, DePuey G. Diagnosis of pericardial effusion and its effects on ventricular function using gated Tc-99m sestamibi perfusion SPECT. *Clin Nucl Med* 1998;23:361–364.

29. Lin DS, Tipton RE. Ga-67 cardiac uptake. *Clin Nucl Med* 1983;8: 603–604.

30. Maisch B, Pankuweit S, Brilla C, et al. Intrapericardial treatment of inflammatory and neoplastic pericarditis guided by pericardioscopy and epicardial biopsy—Results from a pilot study. *Clin Cardiol* 1999; 22(suppl I):I-17–I-22.

31. Heckmann M, Lindner W, Pohlandt F. Tension pneumopericardium in a preterm infant without mechanical ventilation: a rare cause of cardiac arrest. *Acta Paediatr* 1998;87:346–348.

32. Schiller NB, Botvinick EH. Right ventricular compression as a sign of cardiac tamponade: an analysis of echocardiographic ventricular dimensions and their clinical implications. *Circulation* 1977;56: 774–779.

33. Armstrong WF, Schilt BF, Helper DJ, et al. Diastolic collapse of the right ventricle with cardiac tamponade: an echocardiographic study. *Circulation* 1982;65:1491–1496.

34. Kronzon I, Cohen ML, Winer HE. Diastolic atrial compression: a sensitive echocardiographic sign of cardiac tamponade. *J Am Coll Cardiol* 1983;2:770–775.

35. Gillam LD, Guyer DE, Gibson TC, et al. Hydrodynamic compression of the right atrium: a new echocardiographic sign of cardiac tamponade. *Circulation* 1983;68:294–301.

36. Appleton CP, Hatle LK, Popp RL. Cardiac tamponade and pericardial effusion: respiratory variation in transvalvular flow velocities studied by Doppler echocardiography. *J Am Coll Cardiol* 1988;11:1020–1030.

37. Himelman RB, Kircher B, Rockey DC, et al. Inferior vena cava plethora with blunted respiratory response: a sensitive echocardiographic sign of cardiac tamponade. *J Am Coll Cardiol* 1988;12:1470–1477.

38. Fowler NO, Shabetai R, Braunstein JR. Transmural ventricular pressures in experimental cardiac tamponade. *Circ Res* 1959;7:733–739.

39. Kaplan LM, Epstein SK, Schwartz SL, et al. Clinical, echocardiographic, and hemodynamic evidence of cardiac tamponade caused by large pleural effusions. *Am J Respir Crit Care Med* 1995;151:904–908.

40. Singh S, Wann LS, Schuchard GH, et al. Right ventricular and right atrial collapse in patients with cardiac tamponade—a combined hemodynamic and echocardiographic study. *Circulation* 1984;70:966–971.

41. Klopfenstein HS, Schuchard GH, Wann LS, et al. The relative merits of pulsus paradoxus and right ventricular diastolic collapse in the early detection of cardiac tamponade: an experimental echocardiographic study. *Circulation* 1985;71:829–833.

42. Leimgruber PP, Klopfenstein HS, Wann LS, et al. The hemodynamic derangement associated with right ventricular diastolic collapse in cardiac tamponade: An experimental echocardiographic study. *Circulation* 1983;68:612–620.

43. Lorell B. Pericardial diseases. In: Braunwald E, ed. *Heart disease: a text book of cardiovascular medicine*. 5th ed. Philadelphia: WB Saunders, 1997:1478–1534.

44. Reddy PS, Curtiss EI, O'Toole JD, et al. Cardiac tamponade: hemodynamic observations in man. *Circulation* 1978;58:265–272.

45. Hatle LK, Appleton CP, Popp RL. Differentiation of constrictive pericarditis and restrictive cardiomyopathy by Doppler echocardiography. *Circulation* 1989;79:357–370.

46. Oh JK, Tajik AJ, Appleton CP, et al. Preload reduction to unmask the characteristic Doppler features of constrictive pericarditis. A new observation. *Circulation* 1997;95:796–799.

47. Klodas E, Nishimura RA, Appleton CP, et al. Doppler evaluation of patients with constrictive pericarditis: Use of tricuspid regurgitation velocity curves to determine enhanced ventricular interaction. *J Am Coll Cardiol* 1996;28:652–657.

48. Tei C, Child JS, Tanaka H, et al. Atrial systolic notch on the interventricular septal echogram: An echocardiographic sign of constrictive pericarditis. *J Am Coll Cardiol* 1983;1:907–912.

49. Hancock EW. Subacute effusive-constrictive pericarditis. *Circulation* 1971;43:183–192.

50. Watanabe A, Hara Y, Hamada M, et al. A case of effusive-constrictive pericarditis: an efficacy of GD-DTPA enhanced magnetic resonance imaging to detect a pericardial thickening. *Magn Reson Imaging* 1998; 16:347–350.

51. Rogers CI, Seymour EQ, Brock JG. Atypical pericardial cyst location: the value of computed tomography. *J Comput Assist Tomogr* 1980;4: 683–684.

52. Engle DE, Tresch DD, Boncheck LI, et al. Misdiagnosis of pericardial cyst by echocardiography and computed tomography scanning. *Arch Intern Med* 1983;143:351–352.

53. Ng AF, Olak J. Pericardial cyst causing right ventricular outflow tract obstruction. *Ann Thorac Surg* 1997;63:1147–1148.

54. Kruger SR, Michaud J, Cannom DS. Spontaneous resolution of a pericardial cyst. *Am Heart J* 1985;109:1390–1391.

55. Brown DL, Ivey TD. Giant organized pericardial hematoma producing constrictive pericarditis: a case report and review of the literature. *J Trauma* 1996;41:558–560.

56. Zellner C, Chou TM, Higgins C, et al. Pericardial hematoma after primary angioplasty complicated by coronary rupture. *Circulation* 1998;98:183.

57. Kimura BJ, Paw PT, Shabetai R, et al. Characterization and surgical resection of an organized pericardial hematoma assisted by transesophageal echocardiography. *J Am Soc Echocardiogr* 1996;9:712–715.

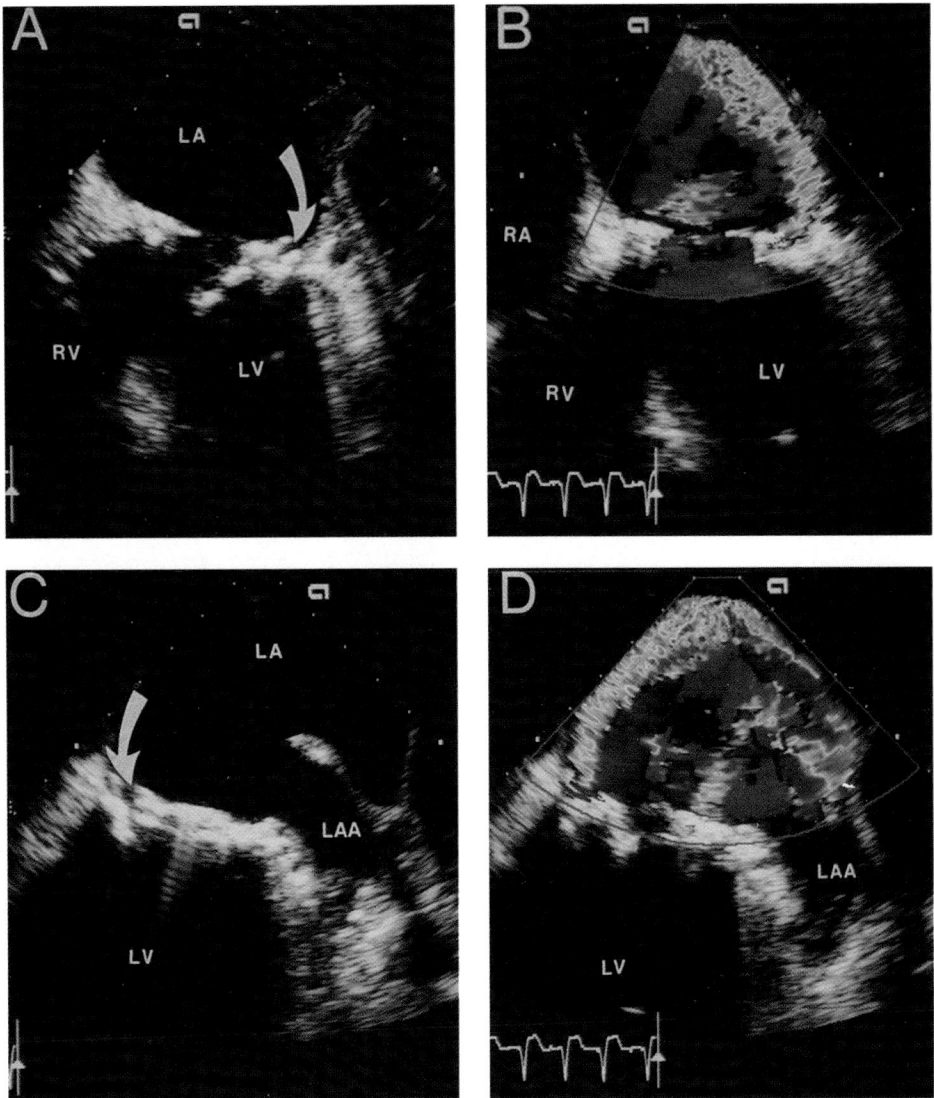

COLOR PLATE 24. Transesophageal imaging in a patient with a dehiscent mitral bioprosthesis. **A** and **C:** Both panels depict a drop-out of echoes (*arrows*) between the sewing ring and the mitral annulus from the transverse and longitudinal views. **B** and **D:** The panels show a large eccentric jet of severe regurgitation that "hugs" the atrial wall. *LA*, left atrium; *LAA*, left atrial appendage; *LV*, left ventricle; *RA*, right atrium; *RV*, right ventricle.

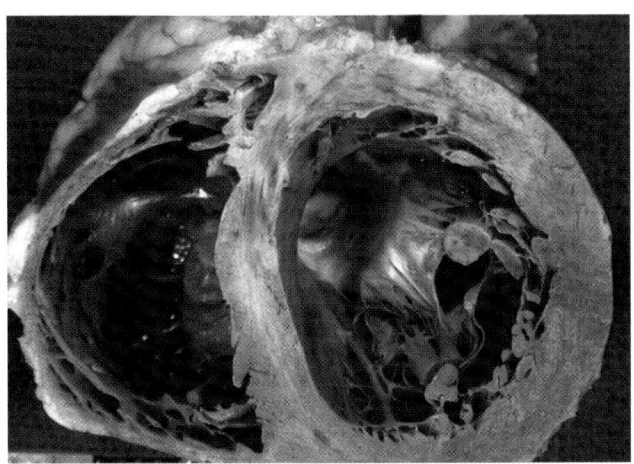

COLOR PLATE 25. MRI of a right ventricular outflow tachycardia located in the conus/ right ventricular outflow tract (RVOT) showing focal thinning 1.5 cm below the pulmonic valve. Interrogation of this area by EPS confirmed the diagnosis of a rapid inducible narrow complex tachycardia, which was subsequently radiofrequency ablated. (From ref. 6, with permission.)

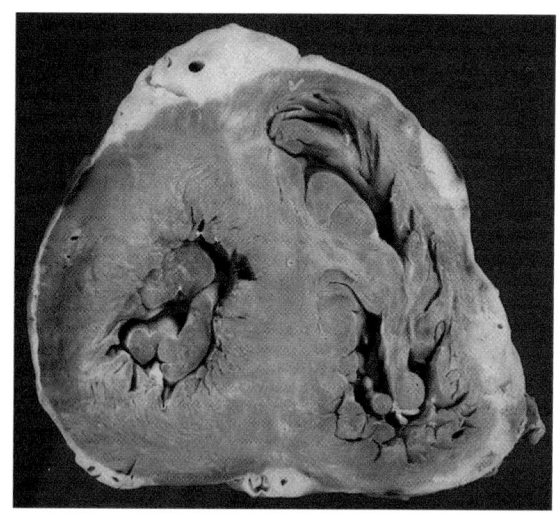

A

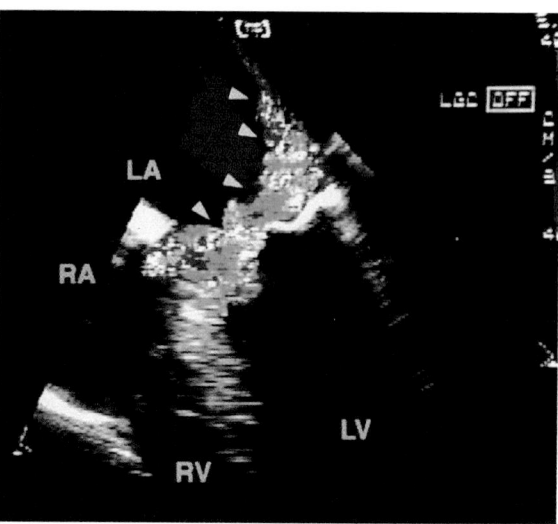

B

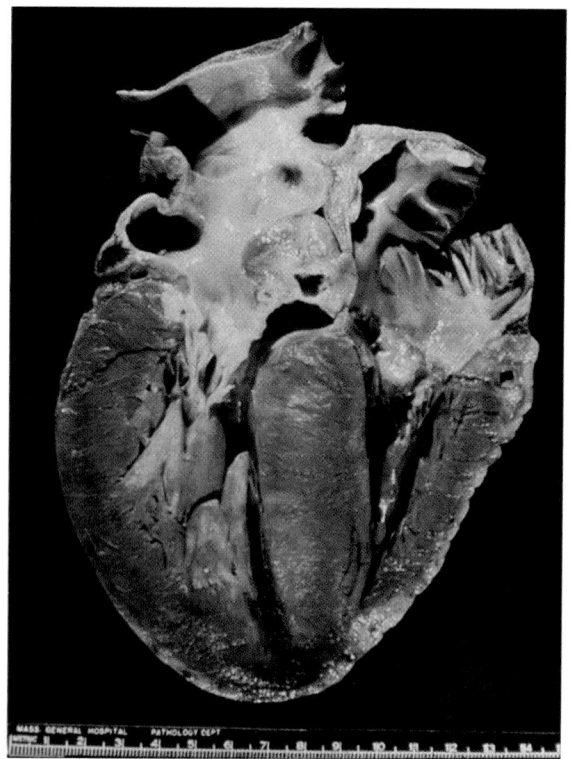

C

COLOR PLATE 26. A: Pathologic specimen of a patient with hypertrophic cardiomyopathy. The LV body weight ratio (g/kg) was in excess of 8:1 (normal 2.5:1). B: Systolic anterior motion (SAM) of the mitral valve is depicted in this patient with a variant of hypertrophic cardiomyopathy, hypertrophic obstructive cardiomyopathy. This was formerly known as idiopathic hypertrophic subaortic stenosis (IHSS). Note, SAM is present in both anterior and posterior mitral leaflets with non-coaptation. The resulting eccentric mitral jet (arrowheads) is demonstrated. M-mode (not shown) echocardiography demonstrated midsystolic preclosure of the aortic valve and course systolic fluttering. C: Pathologic specimen of a hypertrophic cardiomyopathic ventricle (without obstruction) revealing marked concentric hypertrophy. (From ref. 6, with permission.)

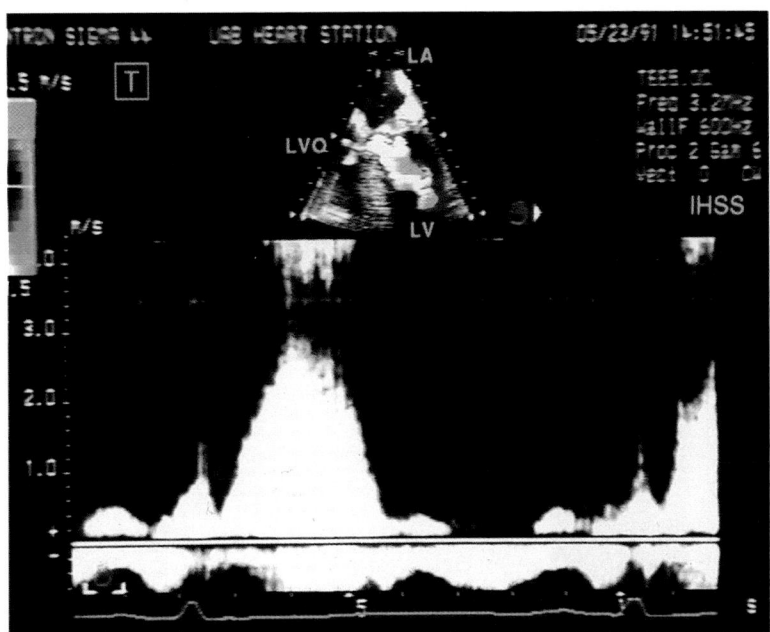

COLOR PLATE 27. Doppler echocardiography demonstrating turbulent systolic flow in the narrowed left ventricular outflow tract (LVOT) and eccentric MR jet. Colorflow-directed continuous-wave Doppler demonstrates high velocities of 3m/sec in the LVOT. Note: the slope of the Doppler velocity upstroke waveform is less than the downstroke, typical of hypertrophic obstructive cardiomyopathy. On transesophageal echocardiography, the classic correlate would be the ``Spanish dagger'' wave form. (From ref. 95, with permission.)

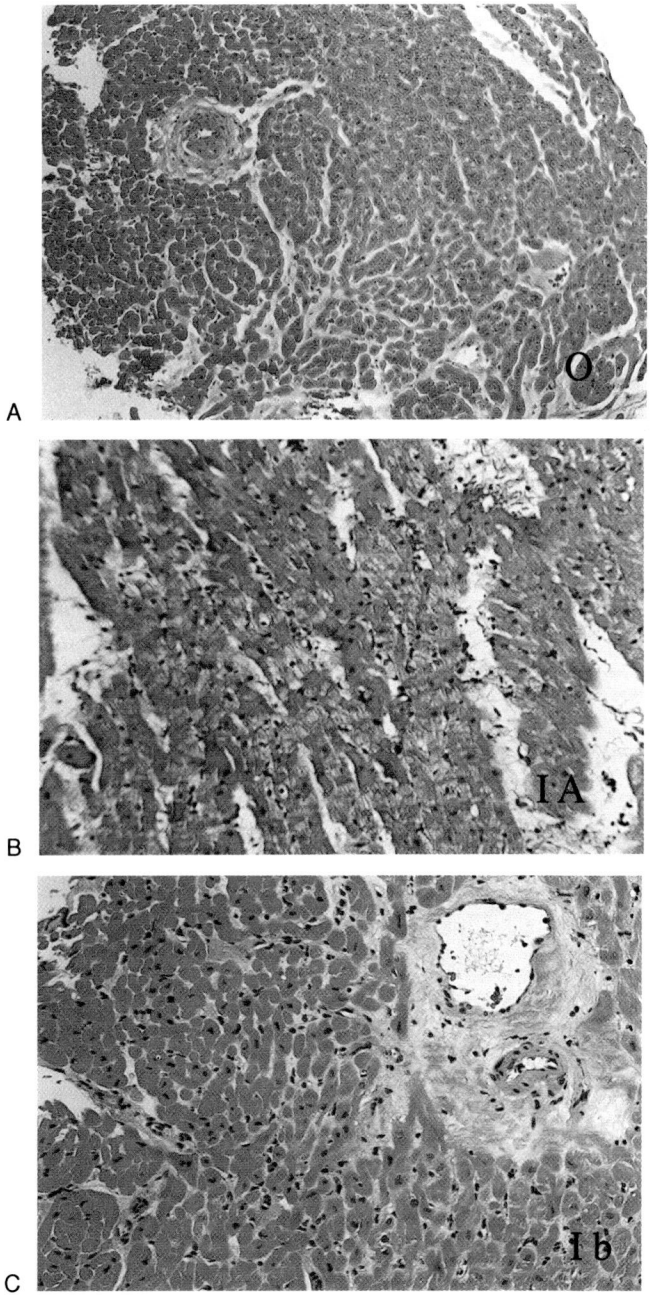

COLOR PLATE 28. Pathology of endomyocardial biopsy. **A:** Grade 0 is normal myocardium. **B:** Grade Ia is mild focal rejection. **C:** Grade Ib is mild diffuse rejection.

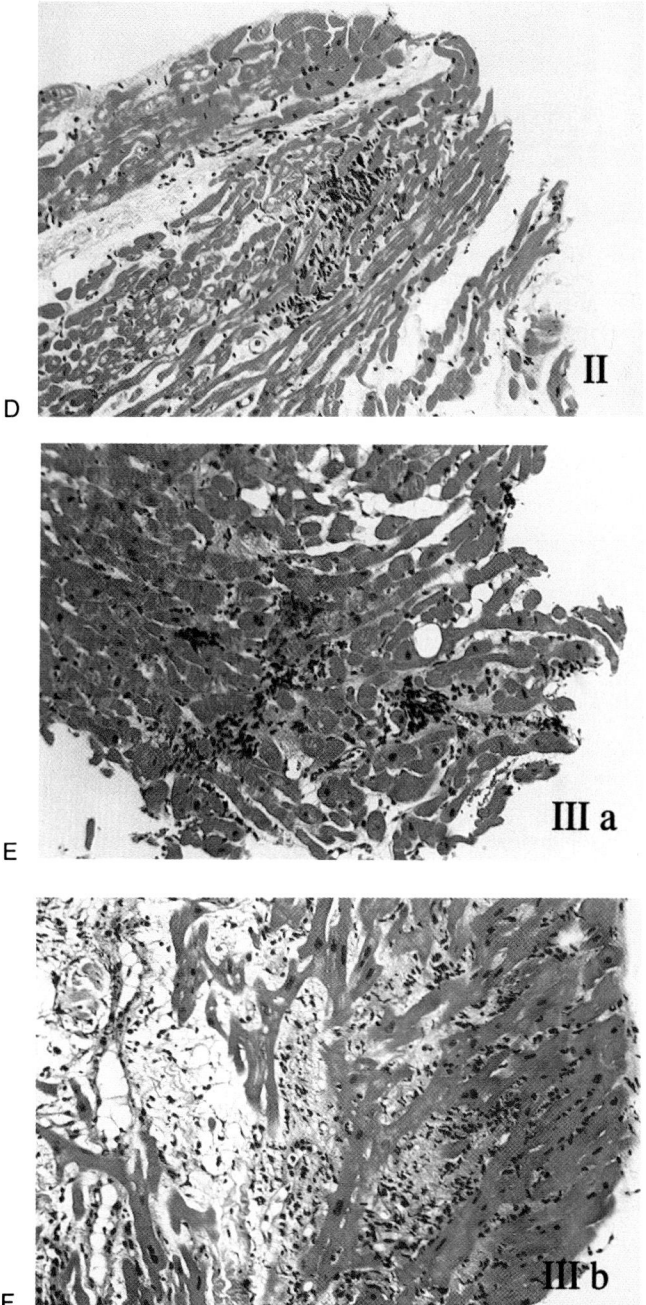

COLOR PLATE 28. *Continued.* **D:** Grade II is a single focus of high-grade rejection in an otherwise grade 0 or 1 biopsy. **E:** Grade IIIa is moderately severe focal rejection. **F:** Grade IIIb is severe diffuse rejection, note the myocyte necrosis. Grade IV is not shown due to its rarity, but has further infiltration than IIIb with more extensive myocyte necrosis diffusely.

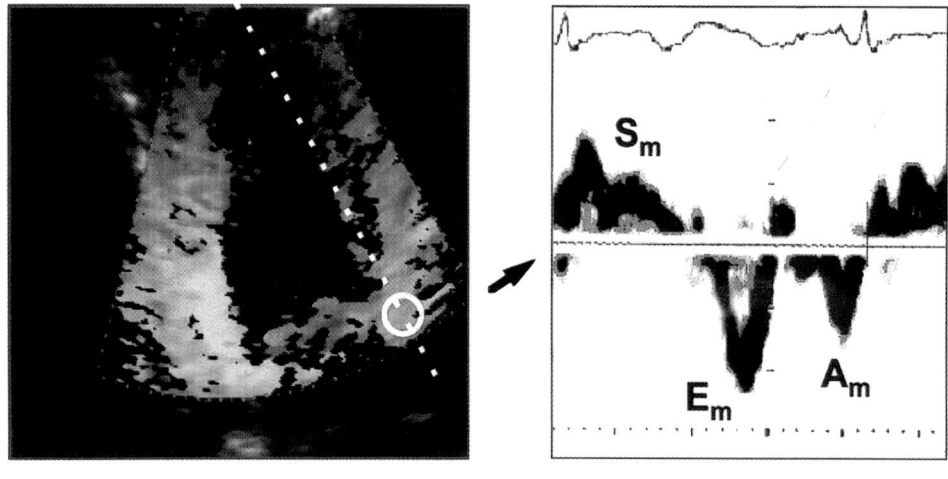

2D-Color   **Pulsed**

COLOR PLATE 29. Two-dimensional color and pulsed tissue Doppler axial velocities of the myocardium recorded from the apical four-chamber view. Systolic (*Sm*), early diastolic (*Em*), and atrial contraction (*Am*) velocities are shown in the pulsed Doppler tracing. The two dimensional image was obtained during systole. (From ref. 54, with permission.)

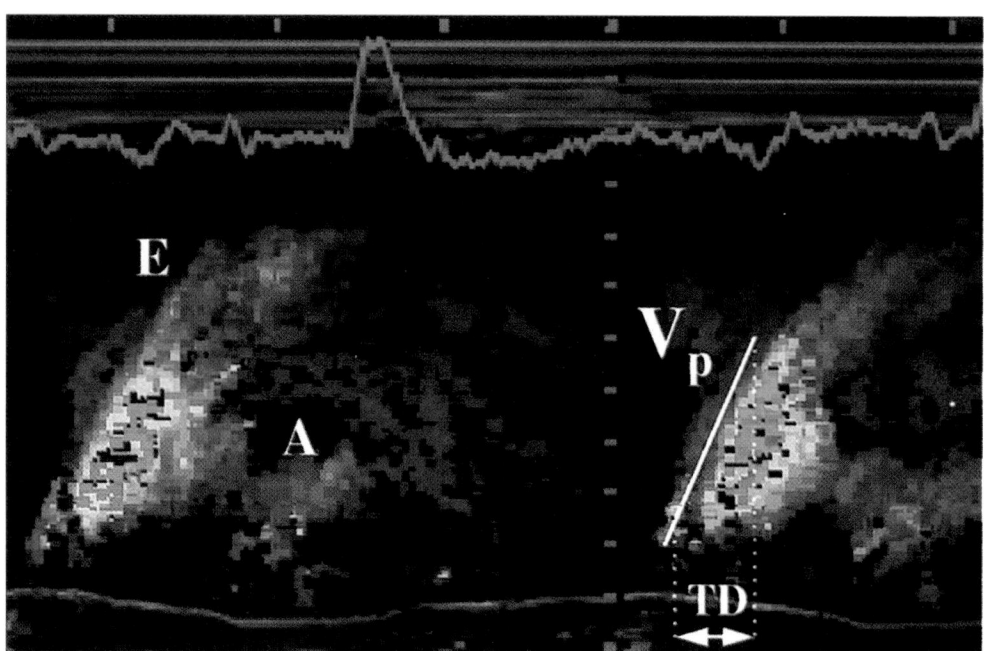

COLOR PLATE 30. Color Doppler M-mode recording of transmitral flow velocity. With the cursor line directed through the mitral valve, the spacial-temporal pattern of velocity is shown along a streamline from the mid-atrium to the ventricular apex. *E*, early wave; *A*, atrial contraction wave; *Vp*, flow propagation velocity; *TD*, time delay. (From ref. 54, with permission.)

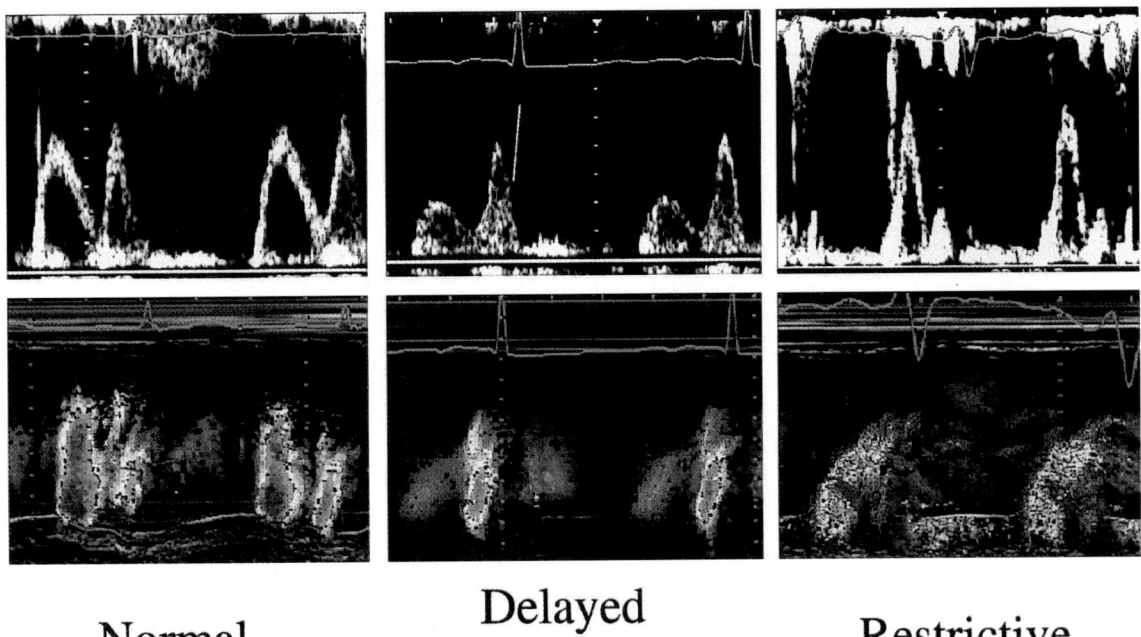

Normal

Delayed
Relaxation

Restrictive

COLOR PLATE 31.   Pulsed and color M-mode Doppler recordings of the left ventricular inflow in a subject with normal diastolic function, a patient with delayed relaxation, and a patient with restrictive filling. Notice the delayed apical filling (reduced Vp and prolonged TD in both the delayed relaxation and restrictive cases). (From ref. 55, with permission.)

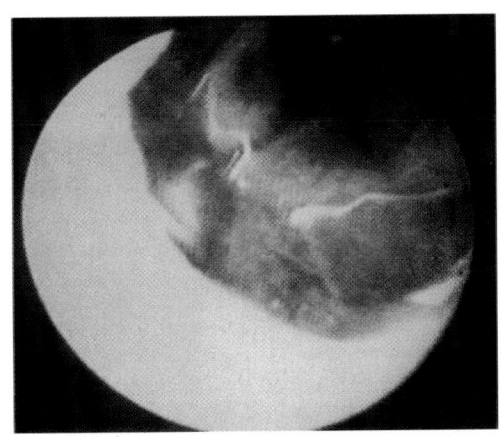

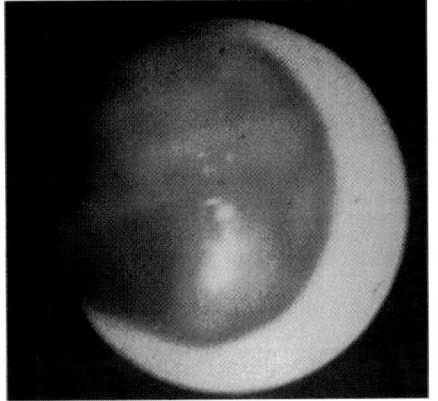

COLOR PLATE 32.   The pericardium imaged via pericardioscopy. **Top:** fibrin layers in a case of lymphocytic pericarditis; **bottom:** metastatic bronchogenic carcinoma. (From ref. 30, with permission.)

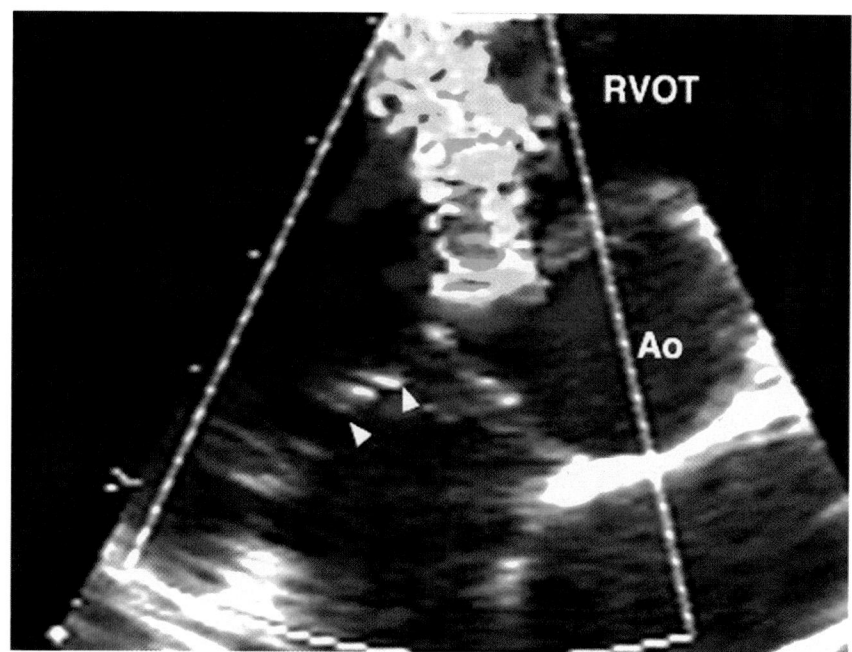

COLOR PLATE 33. Membranous ventricular septal defect (VSD): parasternal short-axis view shows high-velocity left-to-right color flow across a membranous VSD, located anterior to the septal leaflet of the tricuspid valve (*arrowheads*), and between 9 o'clock and 12 o'clock relative to the aortic outflow tract. *RVOT*, right ventricular outflow tract; *Ao*, aortic outflow tract.

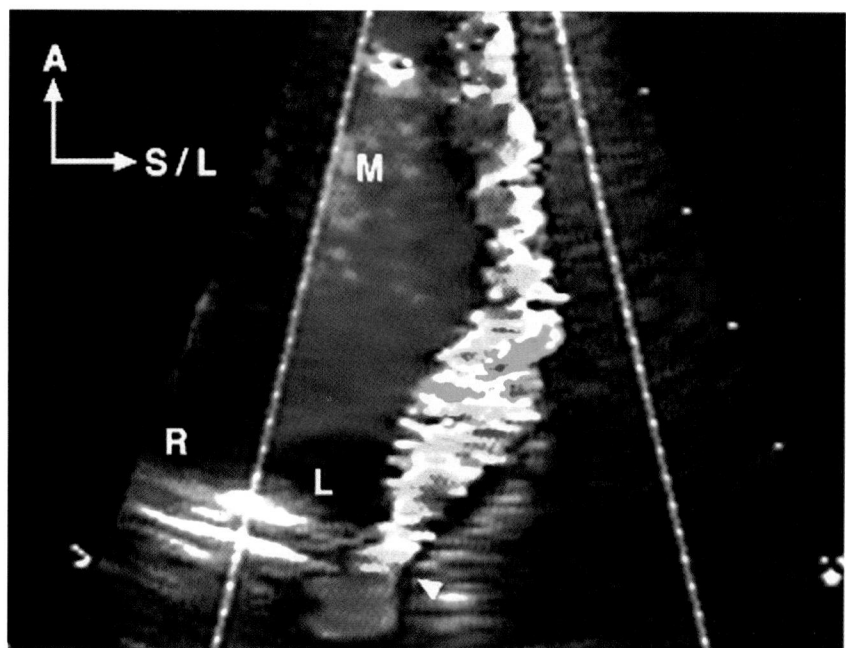

COLOR PLATE 34. Patent ductus arteriosus (PDA): high parasternal short-axis view rotated into a parasagittal plane, showing left-to-right flow across a PDA. *M*, main pulmonary artery; *L*, left pulmonary artery; *R*, right pulmonary artery.

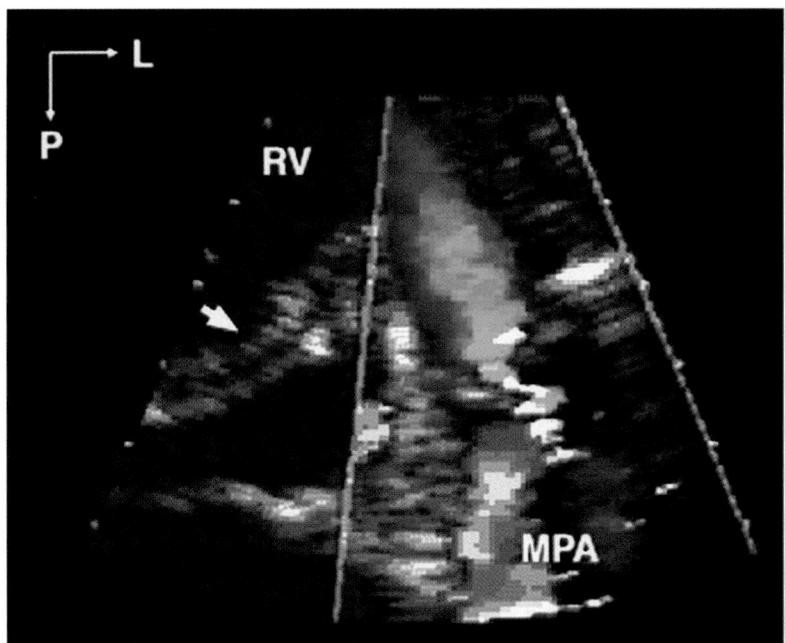

COLOR PLATE 35. Pulmonary stenosis: parasternal short-axis view shows a high-velocity, narrow color flow jet across the stenotic pulmonary valve. The *arrow* points to the paradoxical bulge of the ventricular septum due to suprasystemic RV pressure. *MPA*, main pulmonary artery; *RV*, right ventricle.

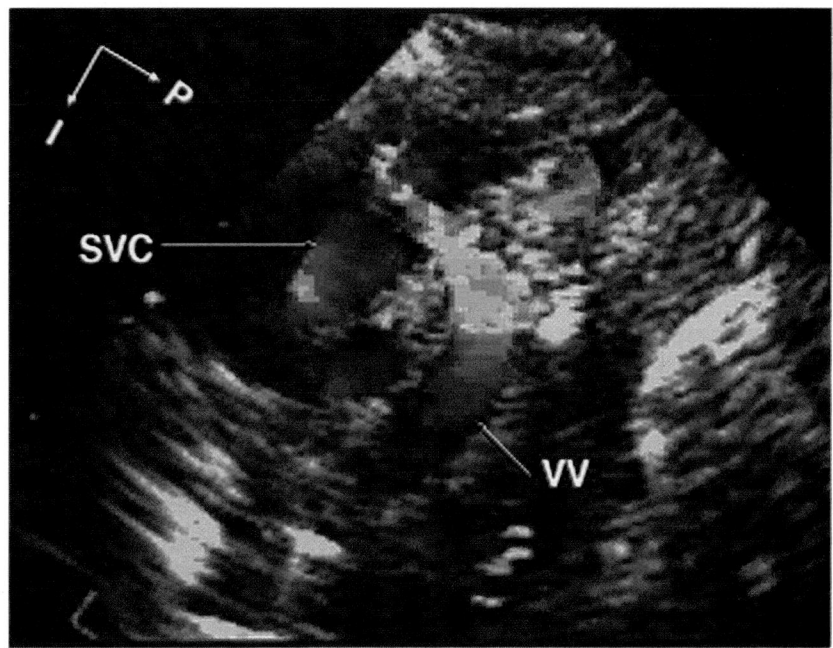

COLOR PLATE 36. Total anomalous pulmonary venous connection: high right parasternal long-axis (parasagittal) view shows a vertical vein (*VV*) that extends superiorly from the pulmonary venous confluence (not shown) to the superior vena cava. Aliasing of color flow at the narrow point of entrance of the vertical vein into the superior vena cava (*SVC*) indicates the location of pulmonary venous obstruction.

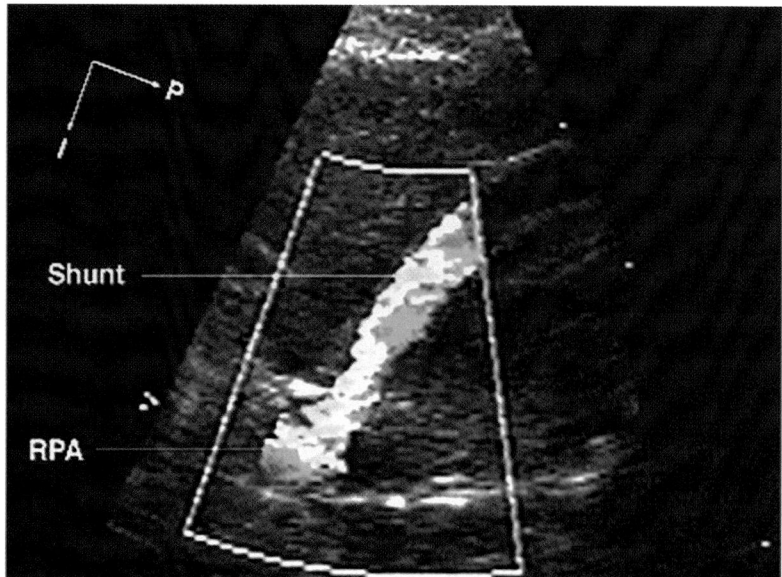

COLOR PLATE 37. Modified Blalock-Taussig shunt: suprasternal long-axis view shows a tubular structure of uniform diameter (a shunt made of prosthetic material) extending from the side of the subclavian artery to the side of the ipsilateral branch PA. There is mild discrete narrowing of the pulmonary end of the shunt.

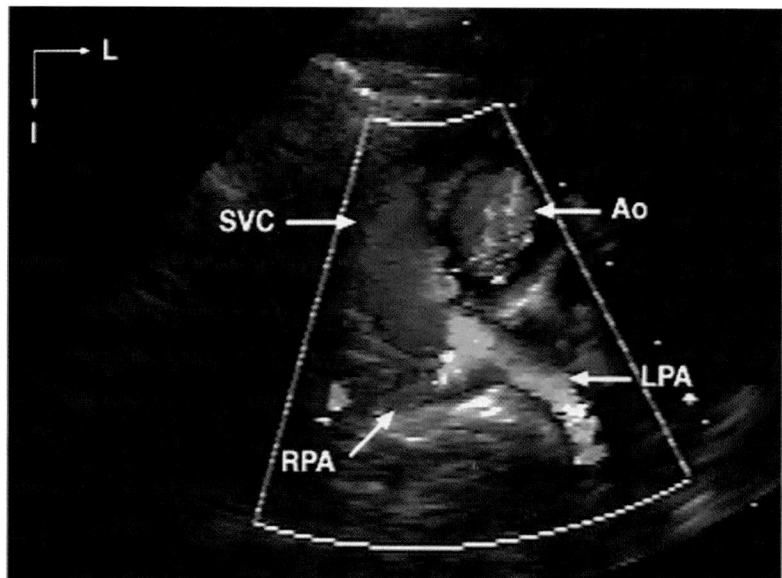

COLOR PLATE 38. Bidirectional Glenn shunt: suprasternal short axis with rightward angulation shows the anastomosis of the superior vena cava (*SVC*) to the right pulmonary artery (*RPA*). The anastomosis and the branch pulmonary arteries are widely patent. *Ao*, aorta; *LPA*, left pulmonary artery; *RPA*, right pulmonary artery; *SVC*, superior vena cava.

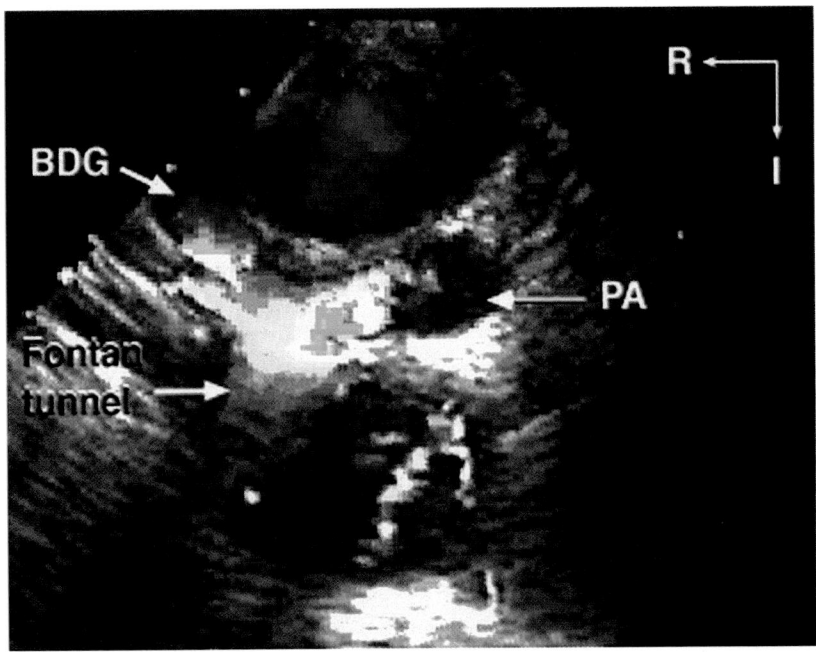

COLOR PLATE 39. Fontan operation: suprasternal short axis with rightward angulation shows the pulmonary connections of the Fontan tunnel and the bidirectional Glenn shunt (*BDG*). The anastomoses and branch pulmonary arteries (*PA*) are widely patent.

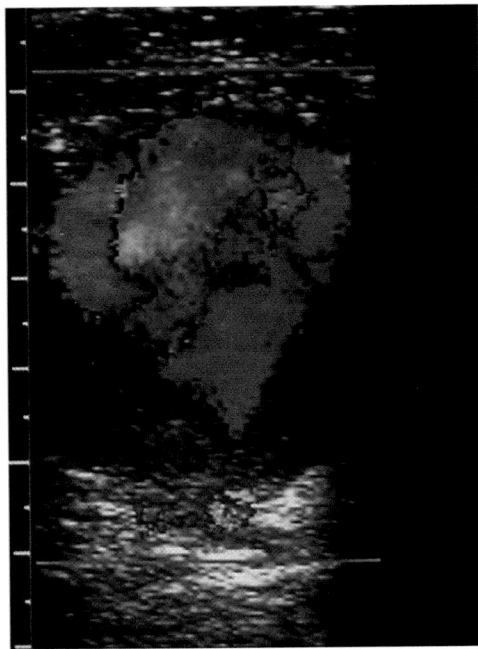

COLOR PLATE 40. Color flow imaging revealing the characteristic nonlaminar, to-and-fro flow within the pseudoaneurysm.

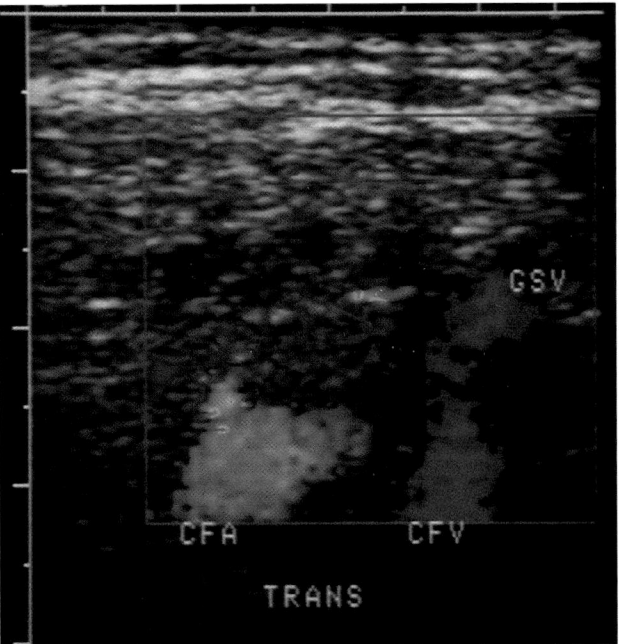

COLOR PLATE 41. Duplex ultrasound and color flow imaging in a patient with a continuous femoral bruit after transfemoral coronary angiography demonstrates an arteriovenous fistula between the right common femoral artery and vein. Note the fistulous tract is well delineated with color flow imaging. *CFA*, common femoral artery; *CFV*, common femoral vein.

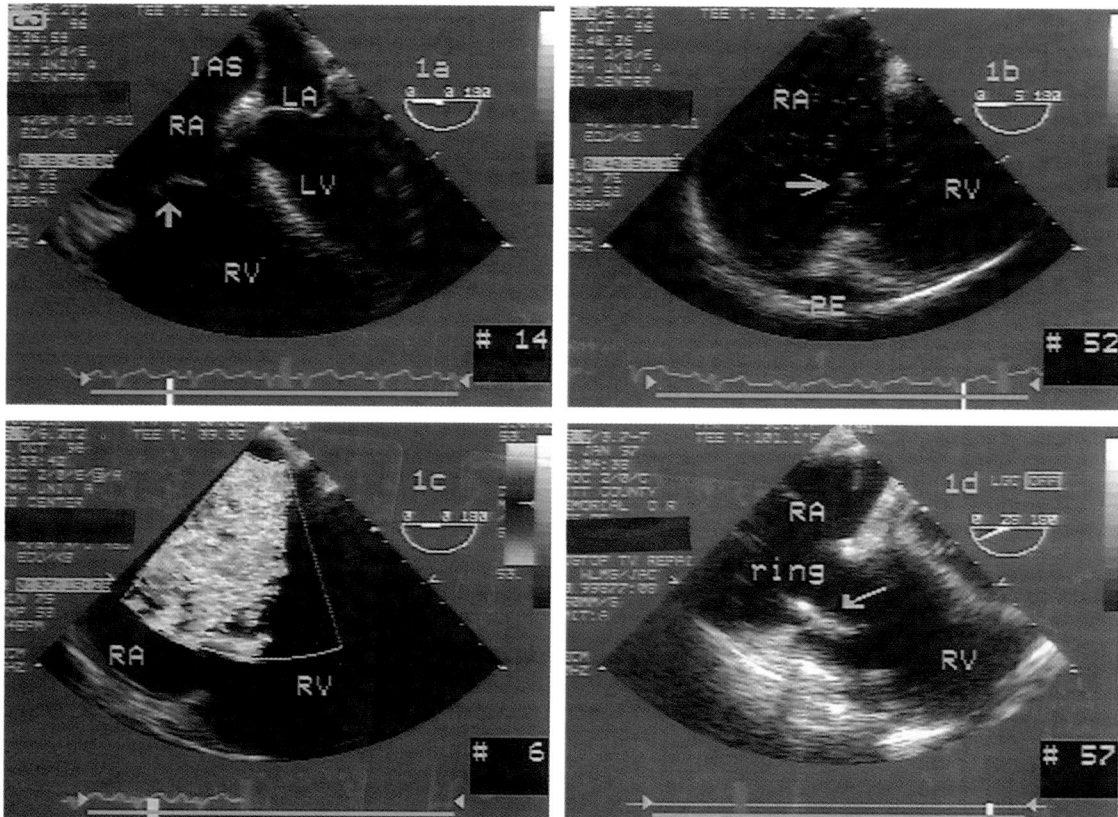

COLOR PLATE 42. **A:** Transesophageal echocardiographic (TEE) examination at the midesophageal plane representing a four-chamber, surface-equivalent view. Note the dramatically enlarged right ventricle (*RV*) and right atrium (*RA*), the deviated interatrial septum (*IAS*) representing markedly elevated RA pressures (exceeding the left-sided pressures), and the flail anterior tricuspid valve leaflet (*arrow*). *LV*, left ventricle; *LA*, left atrium. **B:** Counterclockwise rotation from 1**A**. Note: The right-sided structures are more optimally imaged, and an anterior, loculated pericardial effusion (*PE*) is seen. *Arrow*, flail anterior tricuspid valve leaflet. **C:** Color flow Doppler interrogation of Figure 1**B**. Note: Severe tricuspid regurgitation is seen completely filling the right atrial cavity. **D:** TEE study 3 months later, same orientation as 1**B**. Note: The right atrium (*RA*) and right ventricle (*RV*) are significantly smaller and the pericardial effusion has resolved. *Ring*, tricuspid valve annular ring; *arrow*, repaired chordae tendinea.

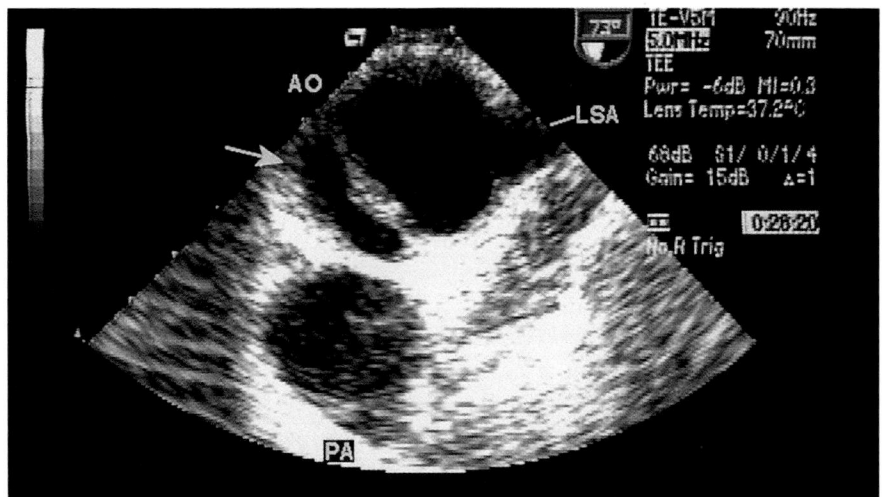

COLOR PLATE 43. Multiplane transesophageal echocardiographic examination demonstrating a traumatic aortic disruption at the aortic isthmus (*arrow*). *Ao*, aorta; *LSA*, left subclavian artery; *PA*, pulmonary artery. (From ref. 98, with permission.)

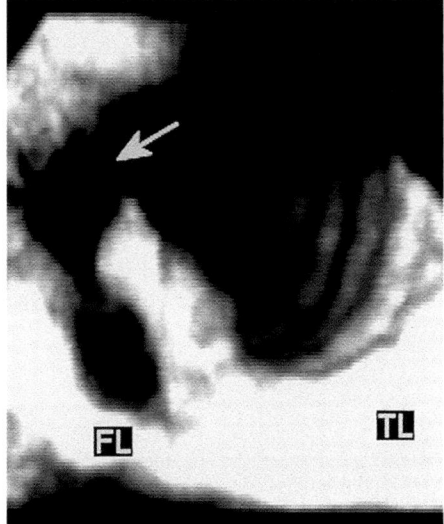

COLOR PLATE 44. Three-dimensionally reconstructed transesophageal echocardiographic examination, performed at the same site as Color Plate 43 demonstrating the circumferential extent of the traumatic aortic disruption (*arrow*). *FL*, false lumen; *TL*, true lumen. (From ref. 98, with permission.)

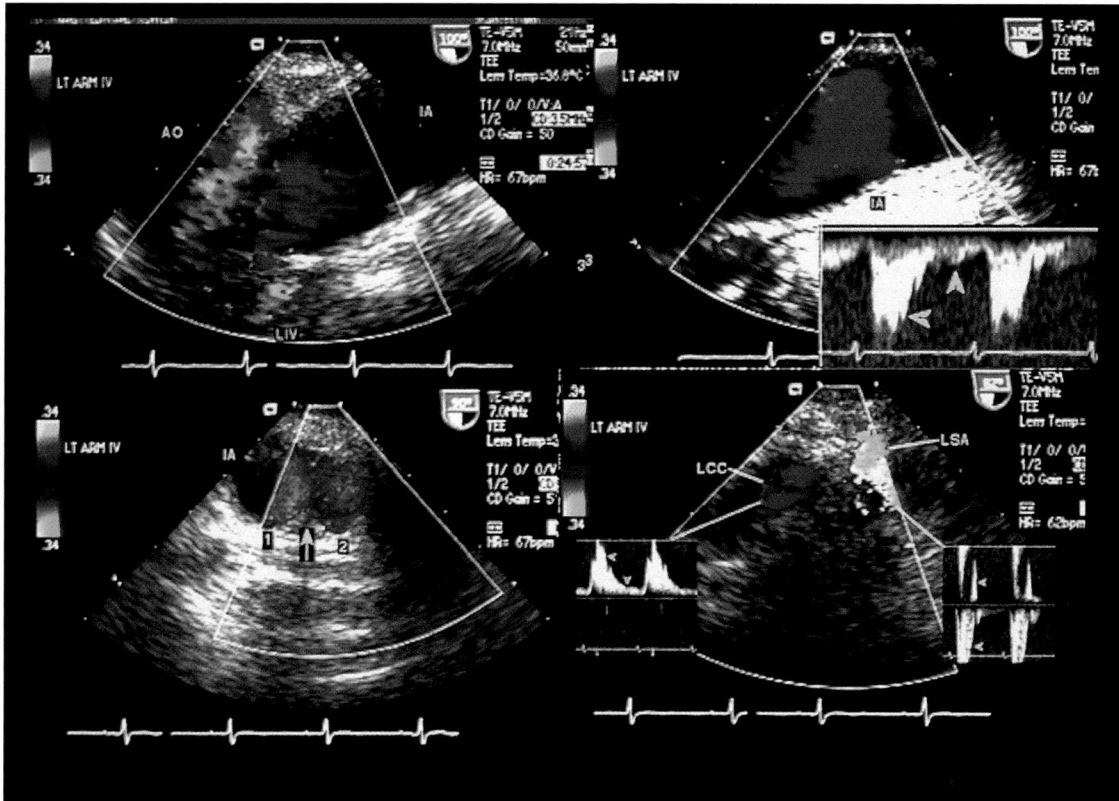

COLOR PLATE 45. Multiplane transesophageal echocardiographic examination of the aortic arch branches (**left upper panel**). The innominate artery (*IA*) is readily visualized (**left lower panel**). *Ao*, aorta; *LIV*, left innominate vein. The innominate artery can be seen to bifurcate into the right common carotid artery (*1*) and the right subclavian artery (*2*) (**right upper panel**). Doppler flow interrogation from the innominate artery shows the antegrade systolic flow signal (*horizontal arrowhead*) and the antegrade diastolic flow signal (*vertical arrowhead*) (**right lower panel**). The left common carotid (*LCC*) and the left subclavian artery (*LSA*) are obtained with counterclockwise rotation of the probe after initially identifying the innominate artery. The relatively low-resistance Doppler flow signals from the left common carotid artery (**left insert**) and the higher resistance profile obtained in the left subclavian artery (**right insert**) are seen. (From ref. 98, with permission.)

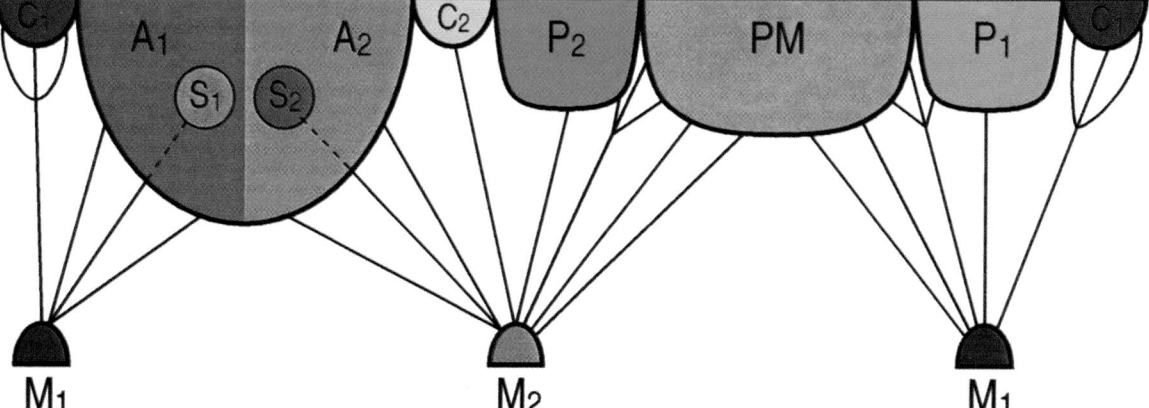

COLOR PLATE 46. The classification of the leaflet components is shown with the valve laid open in order to demonstrate papillary muscle-chordal relationships to the leaflets. The chordae arising from the anterolateral papillary muscle designated as M_1, are inserted to half of anterior leaflet designated A_1 and lateral scallop of posterior leaflet (P_1) and half of middle scallop (*PM*) as well as to small commissural leaflet C_1. Similarly, the chordae arising from the posteromedial papillary muscle M_2 are inserted to A_2, P_2 (medial scallop of posterior leaflet and part of *PM* as well as to C_2). The primary chords are attached to the free edge and secondary chords (S_1 and D_2) to the midportion (i.e., belly) of the leaflets.

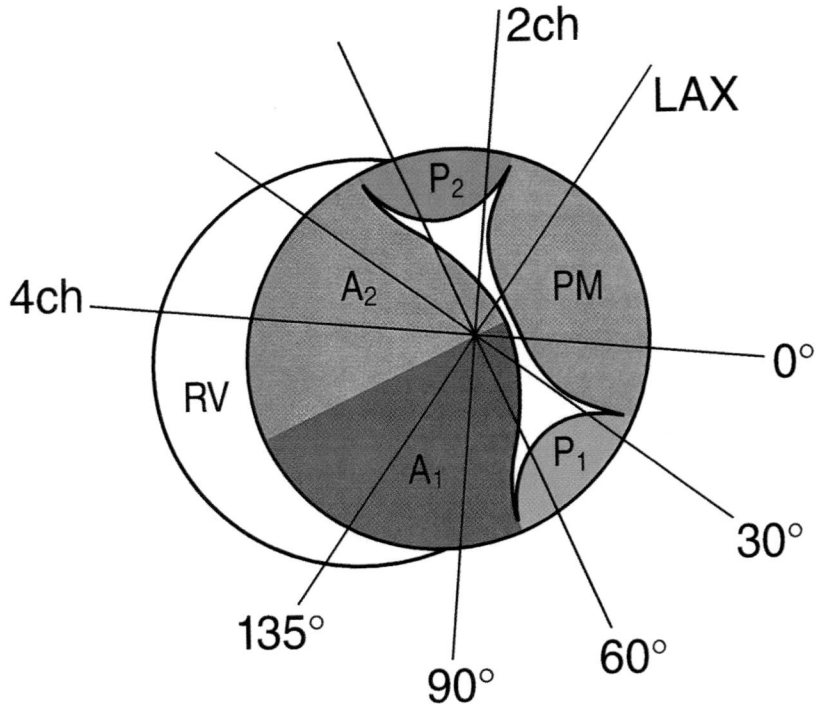

COLOR PLATE 47. A schematic of the mitral leaflet components as obtained from transgastric short axis. The radially placed "clock" diagram represents the corresponding cross sections obtained from midesophageal transducer position using multiplane imaging. Note the portions of valve leaflets visualized in 0 degree or 4-chamber (*4ch*) view, 30 degree to 60 degree or intermediate plane, 90 degree or 2-chamber (*2ch*) view, and approximately 135 degrees in the long-axis plane. The cross sections should image through center of the mitral orifice, and this may be assured by maximizing the left ventricular cavity and the mitral orifice in each of the cross sections imaged. *A*, anterior leaflet; *LAX*, long axis plane; *P*, posterior leaflet; *PM*, middle scallop of posterior leaflet; *RV*, right ventricle.

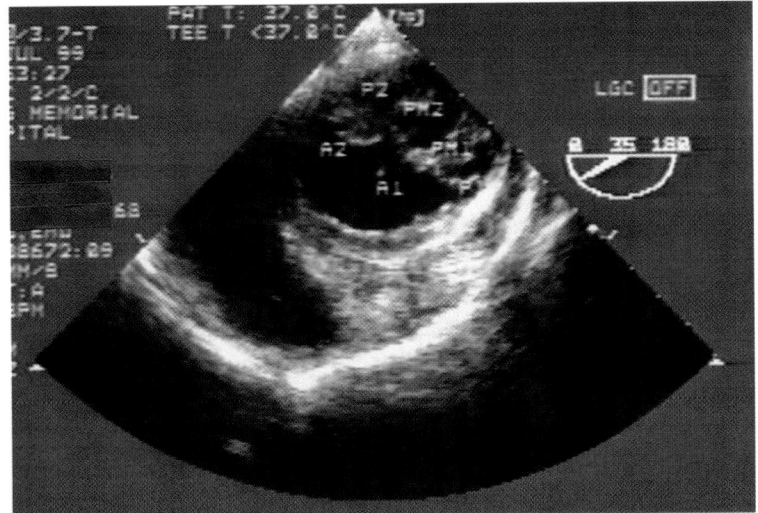

COLOR PLATE 48. The short-axis cross section at the mitral valve level with various components of the valve leaflet labeled. For an explanation of *A1*, *A2*, *P1*, and *P2*, see Color Plate 46. The *PM* is divided into *PM1* and *PM2* based on chordal insertions from *M1* and *M2*, respectively.

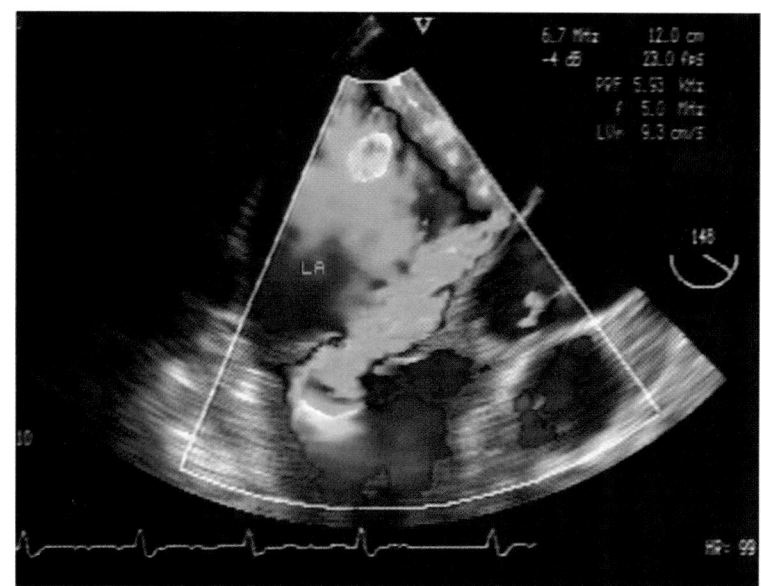

A

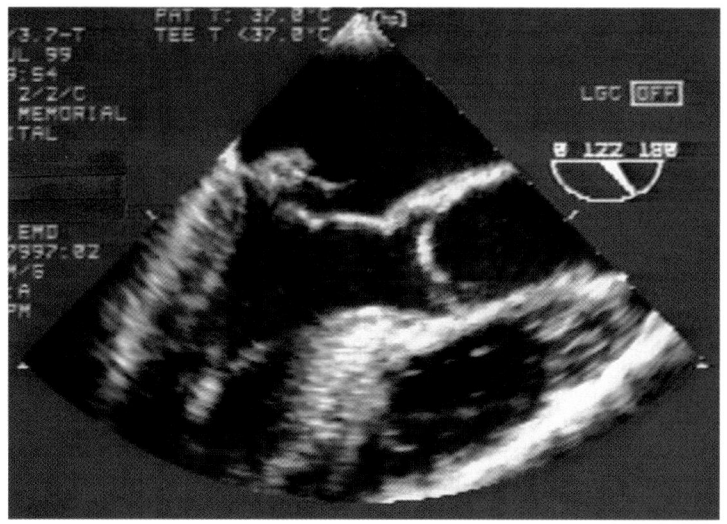

B

COLOR PLATE 49. A: Eccentric mitral regurgitation jet directed anteriorly behind the aorta as seen in transesophageal echocardiography long-axis view. The middle scallop, or *PM*, is flail and severe regurgitation as confirmed by proximal isovelocity surface area (flow convergence) radius of 1.2 cm at a set color scale of 50 cm/sec. *LA*, left atrium. **B:** A flail PM with ruptured chord is demonstrated in the long-axis plane in another patient.

CHAPTER 54

Diagnostic Evaluation in Constrictive Pericarditis and Differentiation from Restrictive Cardiomyopathy

Lieng H. Ling, Jae K. Oh, and A. Jamil Tajik

Although recognized for over a century, constrictive pericarditis continues to evoke a level of clinical interest disproportionate to its frequency, primarily because of the potential for cure once correctly diagnosed (1). Despite the plethora of tests currently available to supplement clinical evaluation, the diagnosis of constriction remains challenging and elusive and may only be resolved after surgical exploration. At operation, the clinical diagnosis is confirmed by herniation of the heart through the pericardial incision accompanied by a fall in right atrial pressure. In the absence of a reliable "gold-standard," various diagnostic modalities have been evaluated by way of surgical validation. "Diagnostic" operative criteria are, however, somewhat subjective, and they may be confounded by hemodynamic fluctuations during cardiac surgery. Reliable preoperative diagnosis is, therefore, essential, especially when thoracotomy in patients with restrictive cardiomyopathy mimicking constriction may have disastrous consequences.

There have been several recent excellent monographs and book chapters (2,3) on the subject of constrictive pericardial disease. This overview discusses the methods currently used to diagnose constriction, emphasising recent advances in understanding of this fascinating syndrome.

CHEST ROENTGENOGRAPHY

The cardiac silhouette in patients with constrictive pericarditis is often described as normal or slightly enlarged (4), but the increasing frequency of associated cardiovascular disease may render this less usual. Pericardial calcification on plain chest films (Fig. 1) strongly implicates constrictive pericarditis in patients presenting with heart failure (5,6). This tends to occur over the right atrium, right ventricle, and diaphragmatic surface, and it may be overlooked without lateral projections. Previous studies (6) have documented calcification in up to 90% of patients, usually due to tuberculous infection. With the decline in tuberculosis, calcific constrictive pericarditis is believed to be uncommon in the United States. However, calcification *per se* is a nonspecific degenerative process (7), and, in our experience, is still encountered relatively frequently, being present in 25% of patients—notwithstanding the rarity of infective causes (8). A recent European series, in which idiopathic constriction comprised 50% of cases, recorded a 53% incidence of calcific disease (9). Therefore, although nonpathognomonic, this simple and low-cost investigation can alert physicians to the diagnosis in a substantial number of patients.

L. H. Ling: Department of Medicine, National University of Singapore, Singapore 119260; Cardiac Department, National University Hospital, Singapore 119074.

J. K. Oh: Department of Internal Medicine, Mayo Medical School; Department of Cardiovascular Diseases, Mayo Clinic, Rochester, Minnesota 55905.

A. J. Tajik: Division of Cardiovascular Diseases, Mayo Clinic; Division of Cardiovascular Diseases, Rochester Methodist and Saint Mary's Hospitals, Rochester, Minnesota 55905.

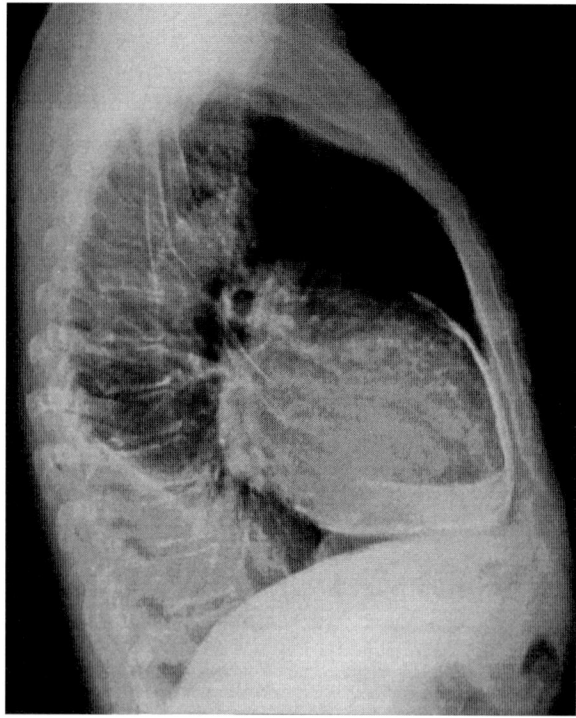

FIG. 1. Lateral chest x-ray from a patient with constrictive pericarditis, demonstrating calcified pericardium.

ECHOCARDIOGRAPHY

Because echocardiography is frequently the initial examination for patients with suspected cardiac disease, it has a central role in the detection of pericardial constriction. Up to 29% of cases of constrictive pericarditis referred on account of congestive heart failure may be picked up incidentally in the echocardiography laboratory (10).

Detection of Constrictive Physiology

Doppler echocardiography is eminently suited to detect respirophasic changes in ventricular filling that uniquely establish the diagnosis of pericardial constriction, and distinguish this condition from restrictive cardiomyopathy. The use of Doppler echocardiography in this role was first described by Hatle et al. (11), and confirmed by other workers (10,12). These consist of an expiratory increase in mitral E velocity of greater than or equal to 25% compared to inspiration and a reciprocal decrease in tricuspid velocity by greater than or equal to 40% (Fig. 2). In addition, there is an expiratory decrease in left ventricular isovolumic relaxation time secondary to an increase in left atrial driving pressure and prolongation of mitral deceleration time, mediated probably by changes in ventricular compliance with septal excursion. Reciprocal changes in these parameters are expected on the right heart. The changes in mitral velocities with respiration in constrictive pericarditis occur abruptly at the onset of inspiration and expiration and should be distinguished from the more gentle respirophasic variation in mitral E velocity

secondary to the prominent intrathoracic pressure shifts in patients with chronic obstructive lung disease (11).

Hepatic venous Doppler shows a reduction in diastolic forward flow velocity with increased diastolic or atrial reversals of greater than or equal to 25% of forward flow during expiration (Fig. 2). Diastolic flow reversal reportedly has a 100% specificity and 68% sensitivity for the diagnosis of constriction (13).

Respirophasic changes affecting diastolic forward flow velocity are also evident in the pulmonary venous Doppler flow velocity curves (Fig. 2) (14–16). Klein et al. (17) performed Doppler transesophageal echocardiography (TEE) in 31 patients with diastolic dysfunction, 14 of whom had constrictive pericarditis and 17, restrictive cardiomyopathy. These authors found a relatively larger pulmonary venous systolic/diastolic flow ratio in both inspiration and expiration and greater respiratory variation in pulmonary venous systolic, and especially diastolic, flow velocities in patients with constrictive pericarditis. The combination of pulmonary venous systolic/diastolic flow ratio greater than or equal to 0.65 in inspiration and percentage increase in peak diastolic flow during expiration of greater than or equal to 40% correctly distinguished 86% of patients with pericardial constriction from restrictive cardiomyopathy.

The clinical utility of Doppler echocardiography was substantiated by Oh et al. (10) who found a diagnostic sensitivity of 88% in a series of 28 patients undergoing exploratory thoracotomy. A small proportion of patients, 12% in a study by Oh et al. (10), will not exhibit classic Doppler-echocardiographic changes. Possible explanations for the lack of respiratory variation are (i) co-existent restrictive myocardial disease, or (ii) extreme elevation of left atrial pressure with mitral valve opening occurring on the steeper slope of the exponential left ventricular pressure decay (18). Reducing preload, either by repeating the Doppler study in the head-up tilt position or after diuresis, will unmask the typical changes in most of these patients (18).

Analysis of superior vena caval flow is helpful in the evaluation of constriction. Using catheter-tip Doppler flowmeters, Fukuda et al. (19) found reduced superior vena caval forward flow velocities in constrictive pericarditis compared to normal controls. Typically, there is little respiratory variation in superior vena caval velocities (19,20). This contrasts with the situation in chronic obstructive lung disease where the large shifts in intrathoracic pressure with respiration result not only in mitral inflow velocity changes with respiration resembling that found in constriction (see above) but also significant augmentation in systolic and diastolic forward flow velocities of the superior vena cava with inspiration or any conditions producing a similar respiratory variation in mitral E velocity due to increased respiratory efforts (21). Thus, evaluation of superior caval Doppler flow should permit distinction between constrictive pericarditis and chronic pulmonary disease.

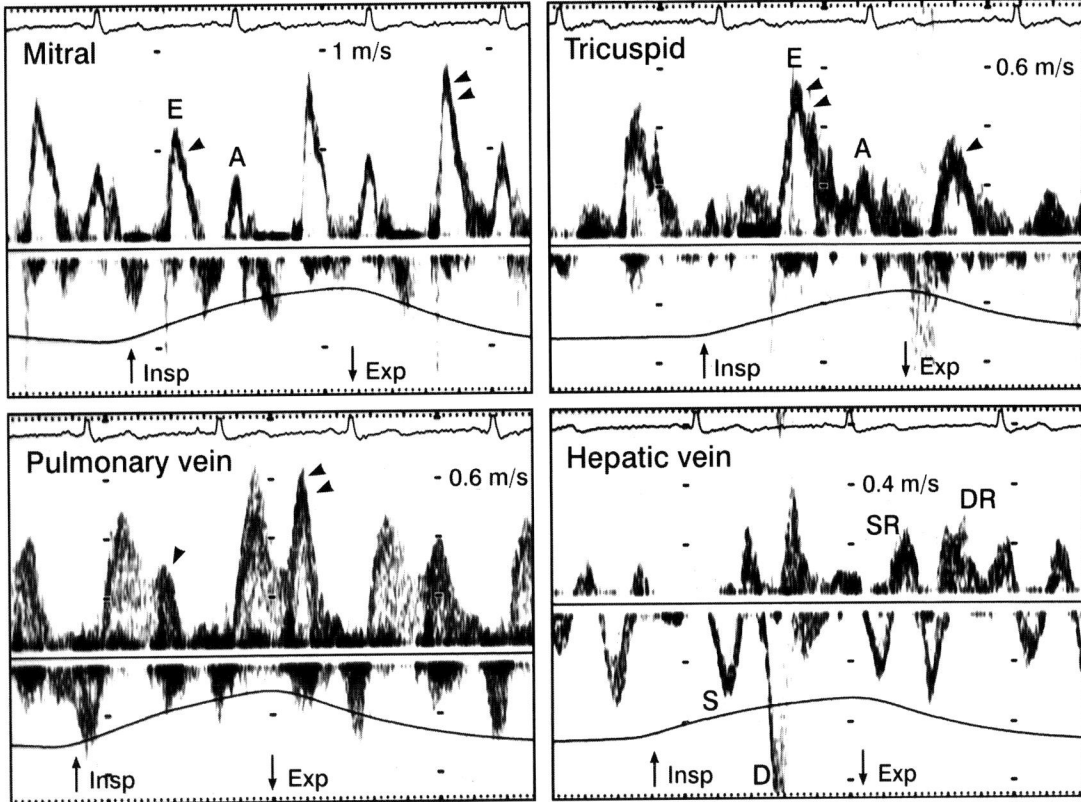

FIG. 2. A composite of characteristic mitral inflow, pulmonary vein flow, tricuspid flow, and hepatic vein flow for constrictive pericarditis. Mitral inspiratory *E* velocity (*single arrowhead*) is 0.6 m/sec and expiratory *E* velocity (*two arrowheads*) is 0.9 m/sec, a 50% increase with expiration. Pulmonary vein inspiratory diastolic forward flow velocity (*single arrowhead*) is 0.3 m/sec, and expiratory diastolic forward flow velocity (*two arrowheads*) is 0.6 m/sec, a 100% respiratory change. Tricuspid flow has an opposite change to mitral inflow velocity change, inspiratory *E* (*two arrowheads*) is 0.6 m/sec and expiratory *E* (*single arrowhead*) is 0.4 m/sec, a 50% change. In hepatic vein velocities, there is a marked decrease in diastolic forward flow and increase in diastolic reversal (*DR*) with expiration.

Detection of Thickened Pericardium

Although surface echocardiography may provide a useful qualitative assessment of the presence or absence of pericardial thickening, direct measurement of pericardial thickness has met with little success. On M-mode echocardiography, the pericardial signal is critically dependent on technical factors such as transducer position, gain and gray scale settings, and ultrasonic reverberation (21). On two-dimensional echocardiography, the pericardium in constrictive pericarditis is visualized as a single or double dense ''immobile'' rind surrounding both ventricles. In a study that correlated surgical or autopsy findings with a prior transthoracic echocardiogram (TTE), Hinds et al. (22) found two-dimensional echocardiography to have a sensitivity of 63% for detection of pericardial thickening greater than 2mm.

TEE, by virtue of superior image resolution, may allow more reliable definition of the pericardium (Fig. 3). Hutchison et al. (23) found thickened pericardium on TEE in 9 patients with suspected constrictive pericarditis, 8 of whom had the diagnosis confirmed by surgery or pathology; TTE identified thickened pericardium in only 4 of these 9 patients.

Recently, we found an excellent correlation between pericardial thickness determined by TEE compared to a gold-standard of electron beam computed tomography (EBCT) (24). The mean normal pericardial thickness was 1.2 mm in this study, identical to pathologic measurements (25). In accord with previous radiologic studies (26), the pericardium in both normal subjects and patients with constrictive pericarditis was best visualized anteriorly over the right ventricular free wall. Various factors conspire to enhance TEE imaging of the anterior pericardium: (i) the abundance of epicardial fat in this location compared to the posterior pericardium (26), (ii) optimal transducer orientation, and (iii) the natural preponderance of pericardial thickening anteriorly in this disease (27). The feasibility of pericardial imaging and performing comprehensive Doppler hemodynamic assessment makes TEE a unique means of demonstrating both the anatomy and physiology of constrictive pericarditis.

Supportive Findings

M-mode echocardiographic features of constrictive pericarditis include normal left ventricular size and systolic func-

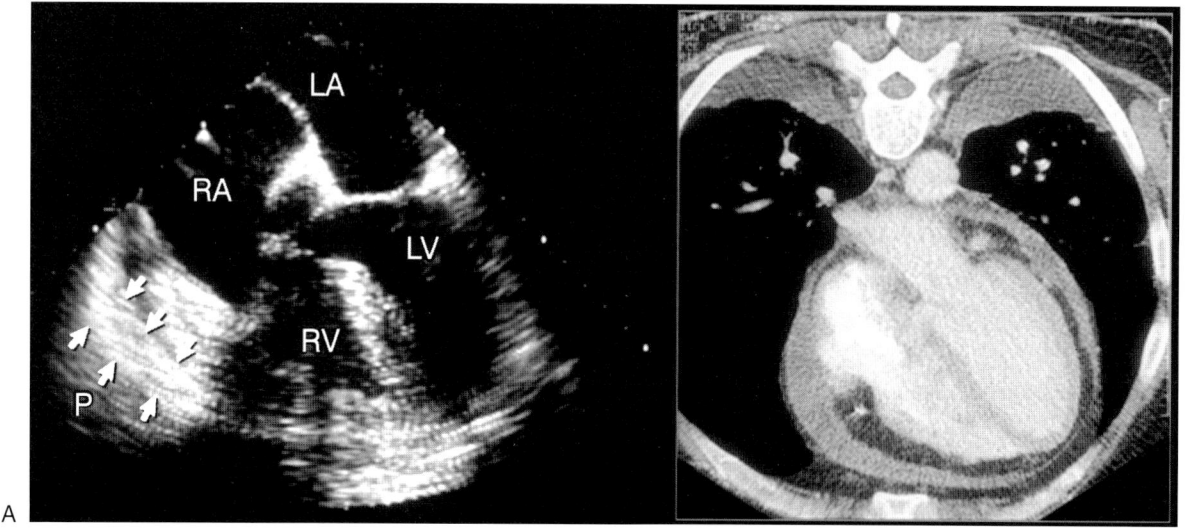

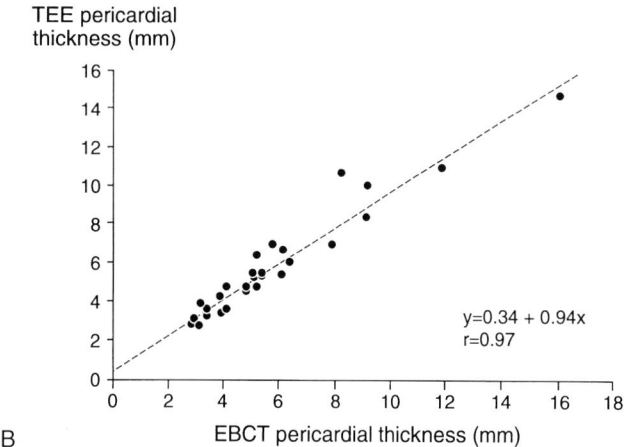

FIG. 3. **A: Left panel:** Transesophageal echocardiographic (TEE) detection of thickened pericardium (*left arrows*), along with electron beam computed tomography (EBCT) of the heart in the same patient, demonstrating thickened pericardium (**right panel**). **B:** Correlation between TEE pericardial thickness and EBCT thickness. *LA*, left atrium; *LV*, left ventricle; *P*, pericardium; *RA*, right atrium; *RV*, right ventricle. (From ref. 24, with permission.)

tion, mild left atrial dilation, and abrupt posterior motion of the left ventricular posterior wall in early diastole followed by a flat segment (28). Abnormalities of interventricular septal motion, occurring during early diastole and following atrial systole, are common. The former consists of a sudden anterior displacement of the interventricular septum followed by a brisk posterior rebound coinciding with the pericardial knock in the phonocardiogram and its peak coinciding with the "Y" trough in the jugular pressure waveform; the latter is probably related to pressure differentials arising from asynchrony of atrial contraction.

Other than pericardial thickening, features of constrictive pericarditis on two-dimensional echocardiography are small ventricles with good ventricular function, enlarged atria and plethora of the inferior vena cava and hepatic veins (29). The septal bounce, an interventricular septal bulge into the left heart on inspiration and vice versa during expiration, is to be differentiated from the septal shudder, a jerky motion of the septum in early diastole. While the latter reflects a nonspecific abnormality of diastolic filling (30), the former reflects the fundamental physiology of constriction and is the two-dimensional equivalent of Doppler variation in intracardiac flow velocities.

COMPUTED TOMOGRAPHY

Computed tomography is a standard technique for detection of pericardial thickening (Fig. 3). However, conventional CT images exhibit motion "blurring," which may lead to failure in recognizing lesser degrees of pericardial thickening. EBCT provides the high spatial resolution (down to 0.7 mm in high resolution mode) required for pericardial detail because of fast scan times (31). Grover-McKay et al. (32) found that the thickness of *ex vivo* pericardium measured by cine EBCT correlated well with pathologic assessment. This modality also remains unsurpassed for detection of pericardial calcification. Where pericardial constriction is the result of compression by a large, partially organized hematoma or tumor infiltration (33,34), computed tomography (CT) or magnetic resonance imaging (MRI) would be the imaging modality of choice. This technique can also define the typical "constricted" cardiac morphology. Other signs, which include inferior vena cava dilatation and deviation of the interventricular septum may also be apparent and corroborate the diagnosis of constriction (35). One limitation of CT is that while it clearly distinguishes mediastinal or epicardial fat from pericardium, small, high-attenuation serous or purulent effusions may be indistinguishable from thickened pericardium (36).

Certain findings on the CT scan may have prognostic and therapeutic implications. Rienmüller et al. (37) found that among 16 patients who had pericardiectomy, all 5 patients with nondetectable posterolateral walls of the left ventricle died at or soon after surgery from myocardial failure. They conclude that nonvisualization of the posterolateral wall suggests myocardial fibrosis or atrophy and defines patients at high operative risk. Asymmetric pericardial thickening or calcification is also readily apparent using CT (or MRI), which provides a circumferential view of the pericardium and may influence the surgical approach for pericardial resection.

MAGNETIC RESONANCE IMAGING

Magnetic resonance imaging (MRI) is another excellent technique for imaging the pericardium, which shows up as a dark low-intensity signal band, consistent with its fibrocalcific nature (Fig. 4). The normal pericardial thickness on MRI is visualized as a curvilinear structure of low signal intensity, not exceeding 3 mm in width (38,39); thickness of up to 8 mm may be normal at the insertion of the central diaphragmatic tendon. The advantages of MRI include excellent contrast resolution with good definition of the pericardium (40), with the ability to demonstrate nonhomogenous thickening or asymmetric compression that may aid the pericardial surgeon in planning surgery (41). This is achieved without the use of contrast medium and radiation.

Because MRI is electrocardiogram-gated, a ''blurring phenomenon'' as with conventional CT may occur. Imaging may be impossible in patients with atrial fibrillation and low voltage ECGs—pertinent points in a population with

constrictive pericarditis. Furthermore, image resolution is inferior to EBCT, scan times are longer, and, unlike CT, MRI cannot reliably detect pericardial calcification (42).

RADIONUCLIDE STUDIES

Physiologic abnormalities have also been reported in constrictive pericarditis using radionuclide angiography, consisting of a short one-third filling rate, a higher peak filling rate, increased one-third filling fractions, and a reduced atrial filling fraction (43,44). These changes indicate rapid early diastolic filling, and, in themselves, are not diagnostic of constrictive physiology. Similar changes are to be expected in restrictive cardiomyopathy, depending on the degree of elevation of left atrial pressure. Accordingly, the role for radionuclide studies in the evaluation of constrictive pericarditis is limited.

CARDIAC CATHETERIZATION

For many years, the hemodynamic features of pericardial constriction were considered to be (i) a rapid Y descent in the right atrial or vena caval waveform and (ii) diastolic equilibration of pressures in all the four chambers of heart. However, it became apparent that these hemodynamic criteria were nonspecific for constriction (45). For instance, equal diastolic pressures on both sides of the heart are compatible with either restrictive cardiomyopathy or constrictive pericarditis, and elevated systemic venous pressure, a Y descent greater than the X descent, and an inspiratory increase in venous pressure may also occur following right ventricular infarction (46).

To more specifically detect the physiology of constriction, Hurrell et al. (47) applied the principles exploited by Doppler

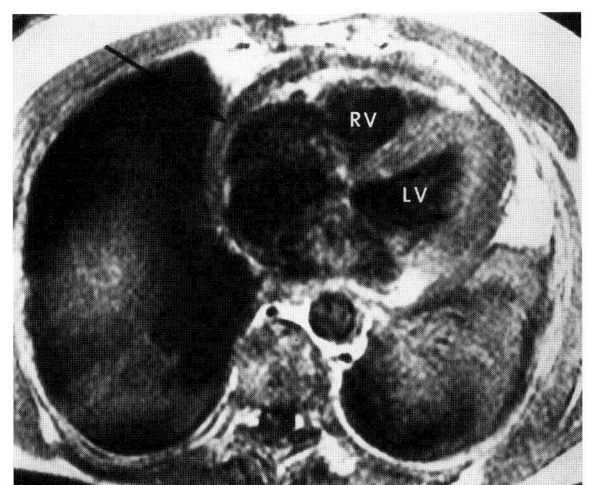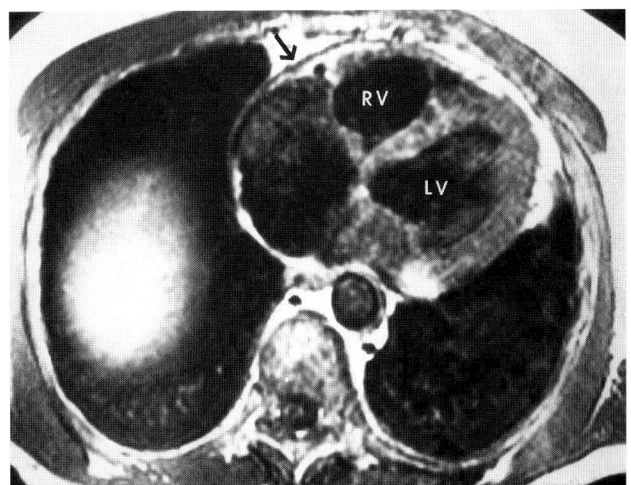

FIG. 4. Magnetic resonance imaging (MRI) of the pericardium. **A:** Thick pericardium (*arrow*) during constrictive phase in a patient with acute pericarditis. **B:** Normal pericardium (*arrow*), after treatment with indomethacine, obtained 2 months after Figure 4**A**. *RV*, right ventricle; *LV*, left ventricle. (From ref. 54, with permission.)

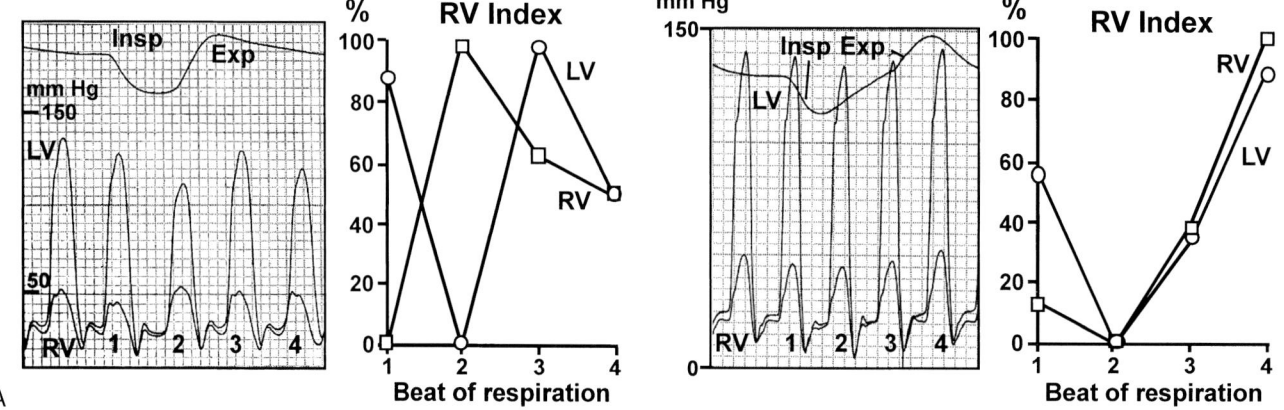

FIG. 5. Differentiation of constrictive pericarditis from restrictive cardiomyopathy by simultaneous left ventricle (*LV*) and right ventricle (*RV*) pressure recording. **A:** In constrictive pericarditis, there is a discordant pressure change in LV and RV. **Left panel:** At end-inspiration (pressure tracing labeled *2*), LV systolic pressure decreases while RV systolic peak pressure increases. **Right panel:** Lowest ventricular systolic pressure was designated as 0% and highest ventricular systolic pressure was designated as 100%. Direction of RV and LV pressure changes are opposite. **B:** In restrictive cardiomyopathy, there is concordant change in LV and RV peak systolic pressure. At end inspiration (pressure tracing *2*), the lowest peak systolic pressure was present in the LV and the RV.

echocardiography to the cardiac catheterization laboratory. Using high-fidelity manometric catheters and respirometry during cardiac catheterization in 15 patients with surgically confirmed constrictive pericarditis and 21 patients with other causes of heart failure, these investigators found that a discordance of right ventricular (RV) and left ventricular (LV) systolic pressures during respiration accurately distinguished between the two groups with no overlap between the groups (Fig. 5). Conventional cardiac catheterization variables were found to be poorly sensitive and nonspecific for the diagnosis of constriction.

DIFFERENTIATION OF CONSTRICTIVE PERICARDITIS FROM RESTRICTIVE CARDIOMYOPATHY

A frequent concern in the evaluation of patients with heart failure and normal ventricular ejection fraction is whether limitation of diastolic filling is the result of constrictive pericarditis or restrictive cardiomyopathy. With the maturation of diagnostic technologies, in particular of echocardiography, differentiating these entities has become less of a clinical challenge since the commonest cause of restrictive cardiomyopathy in the United States, amyloid heart disease, will exhibit increased wall thickness on two-dimensional echocardiography in addition to other classic features (48,49). Some restrictive cardiomyopathies, such as eosinophilic myopathy and other conditions mimicking constrictive pericarditis (such as right ventricular infarction), will also show characteristic echocardiographic features. More challenging, however, is differentiating between constrictive pericarditis and restrictive filling physiology, both of which may co-exist in various disease states, including radiation heart disease.

Although nonspecific in isolation, pericardial thickening in the setting of heart failure strongly suggests the diagnosis of constrictive pericarditis rather than restrictive cardiomyopathy (50).

Distinguishing constrictive pericarditis from restrictive cardiomyopathy on the basis of classic hemodynamic criteria (see above) is not always reliable (Table 1). Vaitkus and Kussmaul reviewed published reports in which hemodynamic criteria were used to distinguish constriction (82 patients) and restriction (37 cases). The predictive accuracies of the difference between right ventricular end-diastolic pressure (RVEDP) and left ventricular end-diastolic pressure (LVEDP) (<5 mm Hg), RV systolic pressure (<50 mm Hg), and the ratio of RVEDP to RV systolic pressure (>0.3) were 85%, 70%, and 76%, respectively. The probability of correct classification exceeded 90%, if all three criteria were concordant, but, disappointingly, 25% of patients could not be so classified. Since constrictive pericarditis has distinct pathophysiologic hallmarks, physiologic differentiation from restrictive cardiomyopathy can be accomplished only by conclusively demonstrating the respiration-mediated changes in intracardiac pressures or ventricular filling, whether by Doppler-echocardiography (10,11) or invasive pressure manometry (47), as described in the preceding sections.

Differences in atrial size have been cited in these conditions, with markedly enlarged atria favoring a diagnosis of restrictive cardiomyopathy. However, in a study comparing echocardiographic left atrial size in 33 cases of constrictive pericarditis, 8 patients with restrictive cardiomyopathy and 33 age- and sex-matched controls, increased left atrial size in both pathologic states was found with no significant differences between the two groups (51). Some investigators

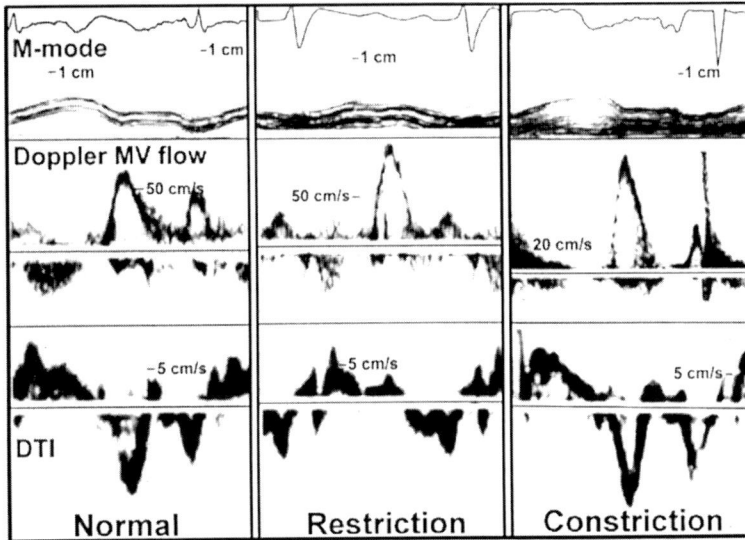

FIG. 6. Doppler tissue imaging (*DTI*) velocity of mitral annulus in normal, restriction, and constrictive pericarditis (see text). *MV*, mitral valve. (From ref. 53, with permission.)

have found significant regurgitation of the atrioventricular valves in patients with restrictive cardiomyopathy (12).

Recently, Garcia et al. (52) described the potential role of Doppler tissue imaging (DTI) in differentiating constrictive pericarditis from restrictive cardiomyopathy (Fig. 6). Using pulsed DTI at the mitral annular region, these investigators found the peak early velocity of longitudinal axis expansion in patients with restrictive disease to be significantly lower than those with constriction. However, overlap was recorded between the constriction and restriction groups, and this may represent the difficulty in distinguishing between these disease entities, particularly in cases where constriction is associated with myocardial disease. A significant correlation was also noted between long-axis expansion as measured by DTI and annular displacement; the usefulness of DTI could possibly be less apparent in advanced cases of constrictive pericarditis where annular motion is severely restricted from myopericardial adhesions and tethering.

Where there is doubt about the diagnosis, endomyocardial biopsy may be necessary. Endomyocardial biopsy has proven useful in establishing the diagnosis of infiltrative cardiomyopathies and may eliminate the need for exploratory thoracotomy. Schoenfeld et al. (5) found that endomyocardial biopsy eliminated the need for exploratory thoracotomy in 39% of 38 patients in whom operation was considered because of severe symptoms. However, a negative biopsy result does not exclude restrictive cardiomyopathy (because of sampling error). Also, the nonspecific finding of myocarditis should not contraindicate thoracotomy if clinical suspicion of constriction remains (5,53).

To conclude, the differentiation between these two disease entities is based on careful clinical evaluation, the demonstration of thickened pericardium, dissociated intrathoracic and intracardiac pressures, and exaggerated ventricular coupling reflecting constriction physiology, and, if necessary, endomyocardial biopsy.

REFERENCES

1. Vaitkus PT, Kussmaul WG. Constrictive pericarditis versus restrictive cardiomyopathy: a reappraisal and update of diagnostic criteria. *Am Heart J* 1991;122:1431–1441.
2. Fowler NO. Constrictive pericarditis: its history and current status. *Clin Cardiol* 1995;18:341–350.
3. Spodick DH. *The pericardium: a comprehensive textbook.* New York: Marcel Dekker, 1996.
4. Wise DE, Conti CR. Constrictive pericarditis. *Cardiovasc Clin* 1976; 7:197–209.
5. Schoenfeld MH, Supple EW, Dec GWJ, et al. Restrictive cardiomyopathy versus constrictive pericarditis: role of endomyocardial biopsy in avoiding unnecessary thoracotomy. *Circulation* 1987;75:1012–1017.
6. Gimlette TMD. Constrictive pericarditis. *Br Heart J* 1959;21:9–16.
7. Brockington GM, Zebede J, Pandian NG. Constrictive pericarditis. *Cardiol Clin* 1990;8:645–661.
8. Ling LH, Oh JK, Seward JB, et al. Clinical profile of constrictive pericarditis in the modern era: a survey of 135 cases. *J Am Coll Cardiol* 1996;27:32A(abst).
9. Rienmüller R, Gürgan M, Erdmann E, et al. CT and MR evaluation of pericardial constriction: a new diagnostic and therapeutic concept. *J Thorac Imaging* 1993;8:108–121.
10. Oh JK, Hatle LK, Seward JB, et al. Diagnostic role of Doppler echocardiography in constrictive pericarditis. *J Am Coll Cardiol* 1994;23: 154–162.
11. Hatle LK, Appleton CP, Popp RL. Differentiation of constrictive pericarditis and restrictive cardiomyopathy by Doppler echocardiography. *Circulation* 1989;79:357–370.
12. Mancuso L, D'Agostino A, Pitrolo F, et al. Constrictive pericarditis versus restrictive cardiomyopathy: the role of Doppler echocardiography in differential diagnosis. *Int J Cardiol* 1991;31:319–327.
13. von Bibra H, Schober K, Jenni R, et al. Diagnosis of constrictive pericarditis by pulsed Doppler echocardiography of the hepatic vein. *Am J Cardiol* 1989;63:483–488.
14. Schiavone WA, Calafiore PA, Salcedo EE. Transesophageal Doppler echocardiographic demonstration of pulmonary venous flow velocity in restrictive cardiomyopathy and constrictive pericarditis. *Am J Cardiol* 1989:1286–1288.
15. Schiavone WA, Calafiore PA, Currie PJ, et al. Doppler echocardiographic demonstration of pulmonary venous flow velocity in three patients with constrictive pericarditis before and after pericardiectomy. *Am J Cardiol* 1989;63:145–147.
16. Meijburg HW, Visser CA, Bredée JJ, et al. Clinical relevance of Doppler pulmonary venous flow characteristics in constrictive pericarditis. *Eur Heart J* 1995;16:506–513.
17. Klein AL, Cohen GI, Pietrolungo JF, et al. Differentiation of constric-

tive pericarditis from restrictive cardiomyopathy by Doppler trans-esophageal echocardiographic measurements of respiratory variations in pulmonary venous flow. *J Am Coll Cardiol* 1993;22:1935–1943.

18. Oh JK, Tajik AJ, Appleton CP, et al. Preload reduction to unmask the characteristic Doppler features of constrictive pericarditis: a new observation. *Circulation* 1997;95:796–799.

19. Fukuda K, Handa S, Abe S, et al. Vena caval flow patterns in patients with constrictive pericarditis: analysis by catheter-tip Doppler flowmetry. *J Cardiol* 1991;21:415–422.

20. Byrd BFI, Linden RW. Superior vena cava Doppler flow velocity patterns in pericardial disease. *Am J Cardiol* 1990;65:1464–1470.

21. Boonyaratavej S, Oh JK, Tajik AJ, et al. Comparison of mitral inflow and superior vena cava Doppler velocities in chronic obstructive pulmonary disease and constrictive pericarditis. *J Am Coll Cardiol* 1998;32:2043–2048.

22. Hinds SW, Reisner SA, Amico AF, et al. Diagnosis of pericardial abnormalities by 2D-echo: a pathology-echocardiography correlation in 85 patients. *Am Heart J* 1992;123:143–149.

23. Hutchison SJ, Smalling RG, Albornoz M, et al. Comparison of transthoracic and transesophageal echocardiography in clinically overt or suspected pericardial heart disease. *Am J Cardiol* 1994;74:962–965.

24. Ling LH, Oh JK, Tei C, et al. Pericardial thickness measured with transesophageal echocardiography: feasibility and potential clinical usefulness. *J Am Coll Cardiol* 1997;29:1317–1323.

25. Elias H, Boyd LJI. Notes on the anatomy, embryology, and histology of the pericardium. *J New York Med Coll* 1960;2:50–75.

26. Silverman PM, Harell GS. Computed tomography of the normal pericardium. *Invest Radiol* 1983;18:141–144.

27. Sutton FJ, Whitley NO, Applefield MM. The role of echocardiography and computed tomography in the evaluation of constrictive pericarditis. *Am Heart J* 1985;109:350–355.

28. Gibson TC, Grossman W, McLaurin LP, et al. An echocardiographic study of the interventricular septum in constrictive pericarditis. *Br Heart J* 1976;38:738–743.

29. Lewis BS. Real time two dimensional echocardiography in constrictive pericarditis. *Am J Cardiol* 1982;49:1789–1793.

30. Chandraratna PA. Echocardiography and Doppler ultrasound in the evaluation of pericardial disease. *Circulation* 1991;84(Suppl 3):I303–I310.

31. Marcus ML, Weiss RM. Evaluation of cardiac structure and function with ultrafast computed tomography. In: *Cardiac imaging: a companion to Braunwald's heart disease.* Philadelphia: WB Saunders Co., 1991:669–681.

32. Grover-McKay M, Burke S, Thompson SA, et al. Measurement of pericardial thickness by cine-computed tomography. *Am J Card Imaging* 1991;5(2):98–103.

33. Dunlap TE, Sorkin RP, Mori KW, et al. Massive organized intrapericardial hematoma mimicking constrictive pericarditis. *Am Heart J* 1982;104:1373–1375.

34. Hartl WH, Kreuzer E, Reuschel-Janetschek E, et al. Pericardial mass mimicking constrictive pericarditis. *Ann Thorac Surg* 1991;52:557–559.

35. Suchet IB, Horwitz TA. CT in tuberculous constrictive pericarditis. *J Comput Assist Tomogr* 1992;16:391–400.

36. Silverman PM, Harell GS, Korobkin M. Computed tomography of the abnormal pericardium. *Am J Roentgenol* 1983;140:1125–1129.

37. Rienmüller R, Doppman JL, Lissner J, et al. Constrictive pericardial disease: prognostic significance of a nonvisualized left ventricular wall. *Radiology* 1985;156:753–755.

38. Furber A, Pézard P, Jeune J, et al. Radionuclide angiography and magnetic resonance imaging: complementary non-invasive methods in the diagnosis of constrictive pericarditis. *Eur J Nucl Med* 1995;22:1292–1298.

39. Stark DD, Higgins CB, Lanzer P, et al. Magnetic resonance imaging of the pericardium: normal and pathologic findings. *Radiology* 1984;150:469–474.

40. White CS. MR evaluation of the pericardium and cardiac malignancies. *Magn Reson Imaging Clin N Am* 1996;4:237–251.

41. D'Silva SA, Nalladaru ZM, Dalvi BV, et al. MRI as guide to surgical approach in tuberculous pericardial abscess. Case report. *Scand J Thorac Cardiovasc Surg* 1992;26:229–231.

42. Sechtem U, Tscholakoff D, Higgins CB. MRI of the abnormal pericardium. *Am J Roentgenol* 1986;147:245–252.

43. Aroney CN, Ruddy TD, Dighero H, et al. Differentiation of restrictive cardiomyopathy from pericardial constriction: assessment of diastolic function by radionuclide angiography. *J Am Coll Cardiol* 1989;13:1007–1014.

44. Gerson MC, Colthar MS, Fowler NO. Differentiation of constrictive pericarditis and restrictive cardiomyopathy by radionuclide ventriculography. *Am Heart J* 1989;118:114–120.

45. Shabetai R. Controversial issues in restrictive cardiomyopathy. *Postgrad Med J* 1992;68:S47–51.

46. Jensen DP, Goolsby JPJ, Oliva PB. Hemodynamic pattern resembling pericardial constriction after acute inferior myocardial infarction with right ventricular infarction. *Am J Cardiol* 1978;42:858–861.

47. Hurrell DG, Nishimura RA, Higano ST, et al. Value of dynamic respiratory changes in left and right ventricular pressures for the diagnosis of constrictive pericarditis. *Circulation* 1996;93:2007–2013.

48. Child JS, Levisman JA, Abbasi AS, et al. Echocardiographic manifestations of infiltrative cardiomyopathy. A report of seven cases due to amyloid. *Chest* 1976;70:726–731.

49. Child JS, Krivokapich J, Abbasi AS. Increased right ventricular wall thickness on echocardiography in amyloid infiltrative cardiomyopathy. *Am J Cardiol* 1979;44:1391–1395.

50. Isner JM, Carter BL, Bankoff MS, et al. Differentiation of constrictive pericarditis from restrictive cardiomyopathy by computed tomographic imaging. *Am Heart J* 1983;105:1019–1025.

51. Mantri RR, Singh M, Radhakrishnan S, et al. Left atrial dilatation in constrictive pericarditis: a pre and post-operative echocardiographic study. *Int J Cardiol* 1994;45:69–75.

52. Garcia MJ, Rodriguez L, Ares M, et al. Differentiation of constrictive pericarditis from restrictive cardiomyopathy: assessment of left ventricular diastolic velocities in longitudinal axis by Doppler tissue imaging. *J Am Coll Cardiol* 1996;27:108–114.

53. Talwar KK, Narula JP, Chopra P. Myocarditis and myocardial interstitial fibrosis in constrictive pericarditis-an extended pathological spectrum? *Int J Cardiol* 1990;29:241–243.

54. Oh JK, Hatle LK, Mulvagh SL, et al. Transient constrictive pericarditis: diagnosis by two-dimensional Doppler echocardiography. *Mayo Clin Proc* 1993;68:1158–1164.

CHAPTER 55

Cyanotic and Acyanotic Defects

Girish S. Shirali and Constance E. Cephus

Every year, between 40,000 and 50,000 newborn babies are diagnosed with congenital heart defects in the United States (1). As diagnostic and treatment modalities continue to advance, increasing numbers of patients with congenital heart defects are diagnosed, treated, and survive into adulthood following corrective or palliative surgery. The historic details of their condition may be unknown to these patients (2), requiring an echocardiogram that starts ''from scratch'' and eventually establishes a complete diagnosis. In addition to patients requiring follow-up care of previously diagnosed conditions, a patient with a previously undiagnosed congenital heart defect may occasionally be encountered. Many of these conditions require vigilant follow-up and serial studies to detect early decompensation. Thus, the task of identification and assessment of patients with operated or native, cyanotic, congenital heart disease takes on added importance. This two-part review discusses imaging techniques that enable assessment of patients with these defects, both in the native state (see Chapter 55) and following surgical/transcatheter defect closure (see Chapter 56). Echocardiography is the imaging modality in widest use, and it will be the only imaging modality discussed here. Other imaging techniques, such as magnetic resonance imaging, are gaining increasing importance in congenital heart disease; however, in the interests of theme consistency and continuity, these techniques are not discussed.

Echocardiography for congenital heart defects is quite different from that performed for other purposes such as assessment of ventricular function and atrioventricular (AV) valve regurgitation. ''Congenital'' echocardiography has three unique characteristics. The fundamental philosophical feature is that the echocardiographer cannot take any structural aspect of the heart for granted. Each cardiac segment and structure must be individually examined and identified. Thus, the echocardiogram is a puzzle consisting of many pieces, each of which must be individually identified, and then placed into perspective. Once all of the structural pieces have been identified in this template, the valves, septa, and great vessels must be evaluated as they relate to the individual heart. Defect associations are useful, but do not always work; therefore, the echocardiographer must interpret a study with no bias toward finding any particular defect or constellation of defects. The second fundamental element that distinguishes echocardiography in congenital heart defects is that, in most cases, the information obtained from a comprehensive echocardiogram is adequate for deciding whether the patient needs surgery and the type of surgery that would be involved. Diagnostic cardiac catheterization has become an infrequent diagnostic modality in the realm of congenital heart defects. In part, this is due to technical advances in the field of echocardiography, including the wide availability of high-resolution echocardiographic equipment. The acceptability of echocardiography for diagnostic purposes is also due, in no small part, to the compulsiveness of the contemporary congenital echocardiographer toward the pursuit of a complete diagnosis. The final feature that distinguishes pediatric echocardiography is the patient: usually, children between 2 months and 3 years of age are uncooperative for echocardiography, and they require conscious sedation for the purposes of a comprehensive test. Children who are older than 3 years are also unlikely to accept a test that may last up to an hour. Performing echocardiograms on children requires patience and understanding on the part of the sonographer and also requires that the echocardiography laboratory be well-equipped with modalities to distract the patient. Videotapes of cartoons work beautifully for this purpose.

G. S. Shirali: Department of Pediatrics, Medical University of South Carolina; Medical University of South Carolina Children's Hospital, Charleston, South Carolina 29425.

C. E. Cephus: Pediatric Cardiology, Loma Linda University Medical Center and Children's Hospital, Loma Linda, California 92354.

The need to establish a complete diagnosis, coupled with the eminent feasibility of achieving this goal, requires that the echocardiographer have a complete understanding of segmental anatomy as a diagnostic approach to assimilate the pieces of this puzzle. In this chapter, which describes echocardiographic findings in most major forms of congenital heart defects, we have presented a concise version of an approach combining pathologic anatomy with corresponding echocardiographic views and images, emphasizing pattern recognition and a discussion of the utility of echocardiography for the comprehensive diagnosis of individual defects.

SEGMENTAL APPROACH

The segmental approach to cardiac diagnosis has been advocated by Van Praagh (3). This approach advocates diagnosing each segment of cardiac anatomy separately based on its own characteristics rather than relying on associations. A brief summary of segmental diagnosis will be presented here; the reader is referred to review articles for further details (3,4). There are three cardiac segments: the atria, the ventricles, and the great arteries. These segments are aligned with each other by "connector" segments; thus, the atria align with the ventricles via the AV canal, and the ventricles align with the great arteries via the conus arteriosus or infundibulum. Complete diagnosis includes determination of cardiac position, visceroatrial situs, the AV canal, the ventricles, conal anatomy, and AV and ventriculoarterial alignments.

Cardiac Position

The position of the heart in the chest is described below.

Levocardia: The heart is predominantly in the left chest, and the cardiac apex points leftward.
Dextrocardia: The heart is predominantly in the right chest, and the cardiac apex points rightward.
Mesocardia: The heart is positioned in the midline, and the cardiac apex points directly inferiorly.
Dextroposition (or dextroversion): The cardiac apex points leftward, but the heart is located predominantly in the right chest (typically due to extrinsic forces such as compression—e.g., by a left-sided pleural effusion or right-sided atelectasis).

Visceroatrial Situs

"Situs" refers to the pattern of anatomic arrangement. Atrial situs is concordant with visceral situs; hence, these two are described together.

Situs solitus: The morphologic right atrium is to the right of the morphologic left atrium. The gastric air bubble is on the left side, and the liver is on the right.
Situs inversus: The morphologic right atrium is to the left

of the morphologic left atrium. The gastric air bubble is on the right side, and the liver is on the left.
Situs ambiguus: This term is used when identification of visceroatrial situs is not possible due to paucity of anatomic markers.

Determination of atrial situs is based on the premise that the morphologic right atrium is that atrium into which the major horn of the sinus venosus (which is the right-sided horn in situs solitus, and the left-sided horn in situs inversus) is incorporated. Thus, the atrium that receives (in order of reliability) the ostium of the coronary sinus, the inferior vena cava and the superior vena cava is the morphologic right atrium. Additional criteria used to identify the right atrium concern the size and anteroposterior location of the atrial appendages; the morphologic right atrial appendage is usually larger and more anterior than the morphologic left atrial appendage. The morphologic right atrium is further defined as the atrium that receives all of the systemic veins, while a separate atrium receives all of the pulmonary veins, or as the atrium that receives all of the systemic veins and some or all of the pulmonary veins without being a common atrium because a second atrium is present. The morphologic left atrium is defined as the atrium that receives all or half of the pulmonary veins and none of the systemic veins (except for a persistent superior vena cava associated with an unroofed coronary sinus in cases with bilateral superior venae cavae), or as the atrium that receives none of the pulmonary veins and none of the systemic veins.

Ventricles

The definition of ventricular anatomy starts with the concept of cardiac looping.

d-loop: In normal embryonic development, the straight heart tube loops to the right at the level of the ventricles. The ventricles loop with the primordium for their corresponding AV valves. This brings the morphologic right ventricle (RV) and tricuspid valve to lie to the right of the morphologic left ventricle (LV), and mitral valve, respectively. This is termed "d-looping."
l-loop: If the straight heart tube were to loop to the left instead of to the right, the morphologic RV and tricuspid valve would lie to the left of the morphologic LV and mitral valve, respectively. This is termed "l-looping."
x-loop: The direction of ventricular looping cannot be surmised from ventricular morphology; this situation typically exists in the setting of a single ventricle.

Evaluation of the direction of cardiac looping is dependent on the ability to recognize the morphologic RV and LV. Briefly, the RV is characterized by a triangular external shape. The interior of the RV consists of an inflow tract, a sinus (or pumping portion), and an outflow tract. The interior of the RV has thick muscle bundles and numerous papillary muscles. The papillary muscles attach to the septal surface;

the tricuspid valve is septophilic, opening toward the ventricular septum. The tricuspid valve forms part of the RV inflow tract and is unrelated to the RV outflow tract. The RV outflow tract has an intricate architecture; it is bounded inferiorly by a circumferential ring consisting of the septal band, moderator band, and parietal band. The septal band runs along the septum and bifurcates superiorly. The gap between the two divisions of the septal band is filled in by the conal septum. The parietal band is continuous with the septal band, and it runs anteriorly onto the RV free wall toward the apex where it is continuous with the moderator band at the base of the anterior papillary muscle. The inferior rim of the infundibular outflow tract is completed by the moderator band, which extends from the parietal band to the inferior aspect of the septal band. Echocardiographic features that help identify the morphologic RV include a trabeculated septal surface and a septophilic tricuspid valve that attaches onto the ventricular septum caudal to the contralateral AV (mitral) valve.

The exterior of the morphologic LV is conical. The septal surface of the LV has numerous fine apical trabeculations and is typically smooth superiorly. The mitral valve has two leaflets: a large, sail-like anterior leaflet and a smaller posterior leaflet; it also has two papillary muscles. These attach to the free wall; the mitral valve is, therefore, septophobic. The anterior mitral leaflet forms a curtain-like boundary between the LV inflow and outflow tracts. Normally, the subaortic conus is resorbed, leading to mitral-aortic fibrous continuity. Echocardiographic features that help identify the morphologic LV include a smooth septal surface and a septophobic mitral valve that attaches onto the ventricular septum cephalad to the contralateral AV (tricuspid) valve.

The direction of ventricular looping can be surmised using the ''chirality'' or ''handedness'' principle, which holds that if the right hand can be positioned in the RV with the palm on the septal surface and the thumb in the inflow and the remaining fingers in the outflow, then the ventricles are d-looped. If this maneuver can be performed with the left hand, then the ventricles are l-looped.

Great Arteries

The position of the aortic valve is described relative to the pulmonary valve.

Solitus: Normally, the aortic valve is posterior and rightward relative to the pulmonary valve.

Inversus: In situs inversus, the aortic valve is posterior and leftward relative to the pulmonary valve.

D-malposition: The aortic valve is anterior and rightward relative to the pulmonary valve.

L-malposition: The aortic valve is anterior and leftward relative to the pulmonary valve.

A-malposition: The aortic valve is directly anterior to the pulmonary valve.

The terminology ''transposed'' aortic valve is not used to describe an anterior aortic valve; instead, the position of the aortic valve relative to the pulmonary valve is described using the terminology listed above. The term ''transposition'' is reserved for ventriculoarterial alignment discordance (see below). Echocardiographic determination of the great artery relationship starts with identification of the individual great arteries by visualization of the branching patterns of the proximal great arteries. Parasternal short-axis and subcostal sweeps are most useful for the echocardiographic determination of the great artery relationship.

Conal Anatomy

This term refers to the structure of the ventricular outflow tracts and, therefore, the orientation of the great arteries.

Normal: The subaortic conus is absent; the subpulmonary conus persists. There is fibrous continuity between the mitral, tricuspid, and aortic valves; the pulmonary valve is anterior, superior, and leftward relative to the aortic valve.

Subaortic conus: The subpulmonary conus is absent; the subaortic conus persists. There is fibrous continuity between the mitral, tricuspid, and pulmonary valves; the aortic valve is anterior and either to the right or the left of the pulmonary valve. This type of conal anatomy is typically seen in association with transposition of the great arteries (TGA).

Bilateral conus: Conal tissue is present beneath the aortic as well as the pulmonary valves. There is no fibrous continuity between the AV valves and the semilunar valves. The aortic valve may be directly anterior or anterior and either leftward or rightward relative to the pulmonary valve. This type of conal anatomy is typically seen in association with double outlet RV.

Bilaterally absent conus: There is no conal tissue beneath either semilunar valve. Both AV valves are in continuity with both semilunar valves. This type of conal anatomy is typically seen in association with double outlet LV.

Echocardiographic determination of conal anatomy requires identification of the individual great arteries by visualization of the branching patterns of the proximal great arteries.

Atrioventricular Alignments

This terminology specifies how the atria are aligned with the ventricles, that is, which atrium opens into which ventricle.

AV concordance: The right atrium opens into the RV and the left atrium opens into the LV.

AV discordance: The right atrium opens into the LV and the left atrium opens into the RV.

Echocardiographic determination of AV alignments requires the identification of atrial situs and identification of each of the ventricles based on morphologic criteria, as detailed previously.

Ventriculoarterial Alignments

This aspect of segmental diagnosis specifies how the ventricles are aligned with the great arteries, that is, which ventricle is aligned with which great artery.

Ventriculoarterial concordance: The RV is aligned with the pulmonary artery and the LV is aligned with the aorta.
Ventriculoarterial discordance (transposition): The RV is aligned with the aorta and the LV is aligned with the pulmonary artery.
Double outlet RV: Both great arteries originate from the RV.
Double outlet LV: Both great arteries originate from the LV.
Truncus arteriosus: A single great artery leaves the heart, and supplies the systemic, pulmonary, and coronary circulations.

In the final three patterns of ventriculoarterial alignment listed above, no decisions can be made regarding concordance or discordance of ventriculoarterial alignments. For example, in a patient with double outlet RV, the origin of the pulmonary artery from the RV would be a concordant alignment; in the same patient, the origin of the aorta from the RV would be a discordant alignment. Thus, the term ''transposition,'' which refers to ventriculoarterial segment discordance, should not be applied to a patient with double outlet right (or left) ventricle.

Echocardiographic determination of ventriculoarterial alignments requires the identification of individual ventricles and great arteries based on morphologic criteria, as detailed previously. Subcostal and parasternal short-axis sweeps are most useful for determining ventriculoarterial alignments.

CLASSIFICATION OF CONGENITAL HEART DEFECTS

A working classification of congenital heart defects is presented below. This is not intended as a comprehensive scheme; it includes the most common forms of congenital heart defects that are encountered, all of which are discussed in this chapter. This classification scheme starts with the clinical presentation (cyanotic versus acyanotic defects); defects are then subclassified based on a combination of physiologic and anatomic criteria. The utility of classifying patients with congenital heart defects based on the presence or absence of cyanosis has a caveat; namely, the range of defects is vast, and this scheme can only address isolated defects. Thus, patients with more than one defect (for example, pulmonary stenosis and a ventricular septal defect [VSD]) may be cyanotic, although each individual defect does not lead to cyanosis.

Congenital Heart Defects

Acyanotic Defects

Left-to-right Shunts

Defects of the interatrial and interventricular septa and PDA represent left-to-right shunts that constitute the three most common forms of congenital heart disease. Outcomes for individual defects range from spontaneous closure to medical management or surgical (or, increasingly, transcatheter) defect closure. Echocardiography is utilized to establish a complete diagnosis, assess the hemodynamic significance of the defect, evaluate associated malformations, and thus help delineate a treatment plan for the individual patient.

Ventricular Septal Defects. These VSDs comprise the most common form of structural congenital heart disease. Echocardiography provides for comprehensive evaluation of these defects (5).

Ventricular septal defect classification. Defects are classified based on their location and embryologic basis (6). Each of the VSD locations (membranous, muscular, canal-type or inlet, supracristal or conal septal, and malalignment type) has specific echocardiographic characteristics.

Membranous defects—pathologic anatomy: Membranous defects are located between the conal septum anteriorly and superiorly, and the trabecular septum and the septal band posteriorly and inferiorly. They are posterior to the septal attachment of the papillary muscle of the conus. The tricuspid valve is intimately involved with the defect; fibrous tissue tags from the tricuspid valve, known as ''aneurysmal tissue formation,'' may result in partial or complete spontaneous closure of the defect.

Echocardiography: Membranous VSDs are best shown in parasternal short axis at the base of the heart (Fig. 1; see

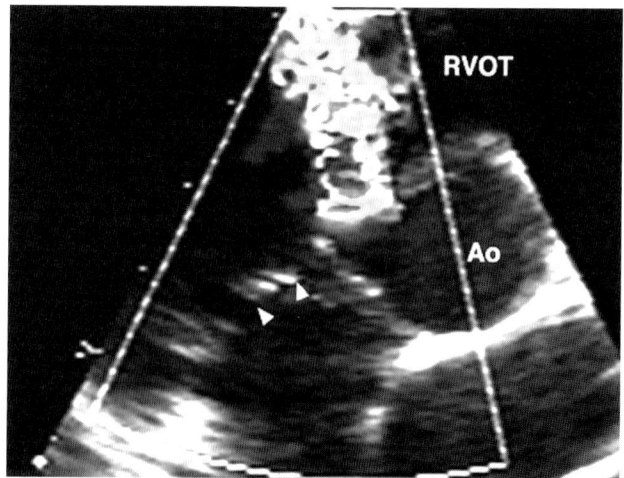

FIG. 1. Membranous ventricular septal defect (VSD): parasternal short-axis view shows high velocity left-to-right color flow across a membranous VSD, located anterior to the septal leaflet of the tricuspid valve (*arrowheads*), and between 9 o'clock and 12 o'clock relative to the aortic outflow tract. *RVOT,* right ventricular outflow tract; *Ao,* aortic outflow tract. (See also Color Plate 33 following page 758.)

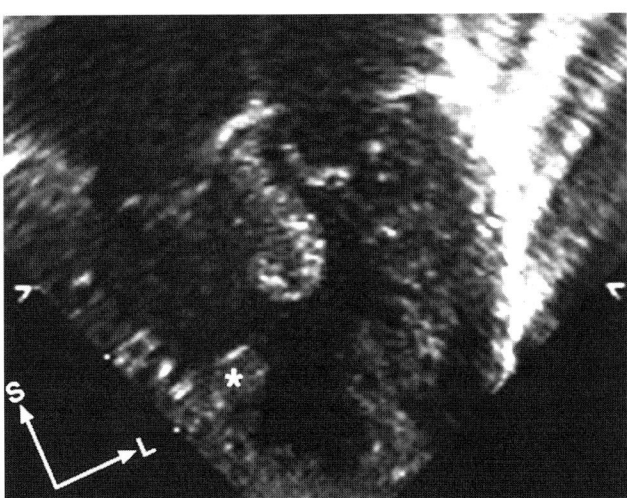

FIG. 2. Muscular ventricular septal defect (VSD): apical four-chamber view shows a large midmuscular VSD, partly obscured by a prominent right ventricular muscle bundle (*asterisk*).

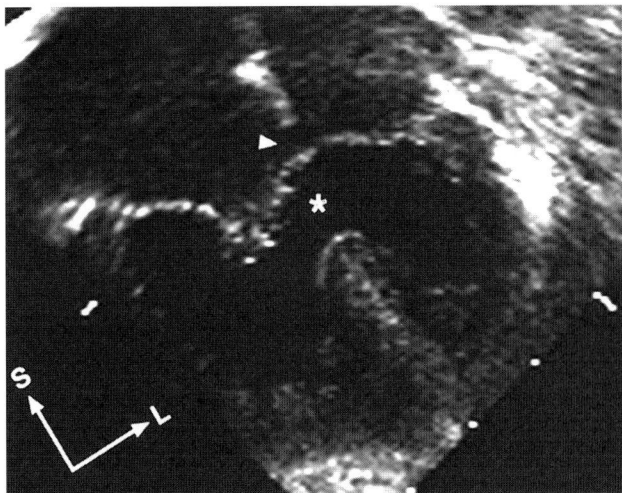

FIG. 3. Complete atrioventricular (AV) canal defect: apical four-chamber view shows complete AV canal defect, consisting of a primum atrial septal defect (ASD) (*arrowhead*), canal-type ventricular septal defect (VSD) (*asterisk*) and a common AV valve.

Color Plate 33 following page 758), immediately anterior and inferior to the septal leaflet of the tricuspid valve (between 9 and 11 o'clock). Other views include subcostal long- and short-axes and apical views with anterior angulation.

Muscular defects—pathologic anatomy: Muscular defects frequently occur in proximity to the septal band. Typically, these VSDs are difficult to identify among the RV trabeculations; they are identified more easily on the LV aspect of the ventricular septum. Multiple muscular VSDs may occur, giving the septum a "Swiss cheese" appearance.

Echocardiography: Muscular VSDs are best shown in parasternal short-axis sweeps from the base to the apex, and in apical views (Fig. 2). Defects may be multiple and are frequently serpiginous, with more than one opening on the RV aspect; overlying RV trabeculations may divide the VSD flow jet on the RV aspect.

Canal-type (inlet) ventricular septal defects—pathologic anatomy: Canal-type VSDs are due to absence of the ventricular component of the septum of the AV canal. They are located posterior and inferior to membranous VSDs, typically beneath the septal leaflet of the tricuspid valve. Chordal attachments of the tricuspid valve may extend to the crest of the ventricular septum, or may straddle the septum.

Echocardiography: Canal-type VSDs are best shown in apical views, in a posterior plane profiling the AV valves (Fig. 3). These defects extend superiorly up to the hinge point of the septal leaflet of the tricuspid valve.

Conal septal (supracristal) ventricular septal defects—pathologic anatomy: Conal septal defects are due to a defect of or within the conal septum. These defects are located in the RV outflow tract, immediately inferior to and in continuity with, the two semilunar valves. Deficiency of the subaortic fibrous supporting structure is frequently associated with prolapse of the right coronary cusp of the aortic

valve into the defect, leading to partial closure of the defect and aortic regurgitation.

Echocardiography: Conal septal defects are best shown in parasternal short-axis views at the base of the heart, between 12 and 2 o'clock (Fig. 4). A parasternal long-axis view helps assess for prolapse of the right coronary cusp of the aortic valve into the VSD. Subcostal sweeps at the base of the heart help to profile these defects and their relationships to the semilunar valves.

Malalignment type (conoventricular) ventricular septal defects—pathologic anatomy: These defects are due to ma-

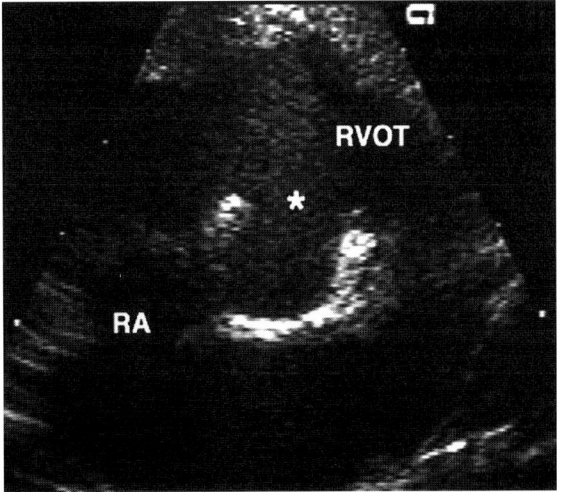

FIG. 4. Supracristal ventricular septal defect (VSD): parasternal short-axis view shows a supracristal (conal septal hypoplasia-type) VSD (*asterisk*), located immediately inferior to the pulmonary valve and between 12 and 2 o'clock relative to the aortic outflow tract. *RVOT*, right ventricular outflow tract; *RA*, right atrium.

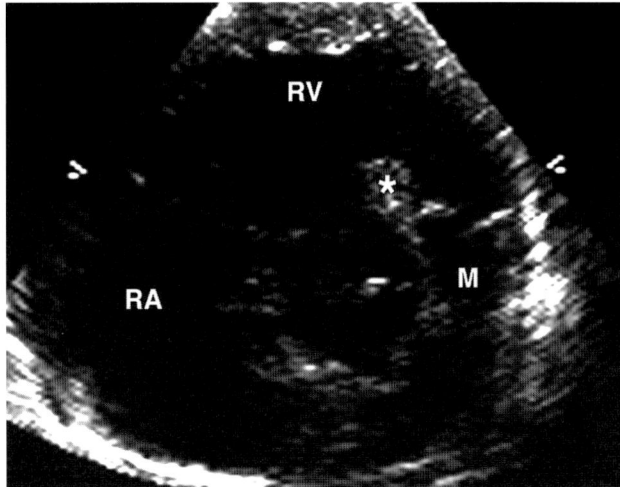

FIG. 5. Malalignment type ventricular septal defect (VSD): parasternal short-axis view shows conal septal malalignment-type VSD from 10 o'clock and 12 o'clock relative to the aortic outflow tract. The malaligned conal septum is marked with an *asterisk*. Right ventricular hypertrophy is present. *RA*, right atrium; *RV*, right ventricle; *M*, main pulmonary artery.

lalignment of the conal septum (which normally occupies the space between the two divisions of the septal band) relative to the trabecular septum. The direction of malalignment is variable; the conal septum may be malaligned anteriorly, superiorly, and leftward, thus raising the "floor" of the RV outflow tract and leading to subpulmonic stenosis (tetralogy of Fallot). Conversely, the conal septum may be malaligned posteriorly, inferiorly, and rightward, thus lowering the "roof" of the LV outflow tract and leading to subaortic stenosis (typically seen in association with interrupted aortic arch).

Echocardiography: The VSD seen in tetralogy of Fallot (anterior malalignment) is best shown in subcostal short axis with anterior angulation and clockwise rotation of the transducer. It is also well profiled from parasternal short axis at the base of the heart (Fig. 5).

The VSD seen with interrupted aortic arch (posterior malalignment) is best shown from parasternal long-axis view. Other views include an apical three-chamber view, which best demonstrates the hypoplastic conal septum.

VSD size and margins. Defect size is critically important in determining prognosis (7). VSDs are typically elliptical and should be measured in two orthogonal planes (8). Defect diameter is measured at end diastole in the widest dimension, using two-dimensional imaging as well as color flow. VSD cross-sectional area, indexed to patient body surface area, has been shown to be an independent predictor of outcome (spontaneous closure versus surgery) (7). VSD margins are evaluated for any chordae or papillary muscles straddling the defect. Structures that may impede surgical visualization of the defect, such as prominent RV muscle bundles, must be recognized. Associated malformations such as subaortic membranes or double-chambered RV, are sought carefully.

Evaluation of the hemodynamic significance of a VSD includes assessment for pulmonary hypertension. If the patient's systolic blood pressure at the time of the study is known, then, in the absence of LV outflow obstruction or coarctation, the simplified Bernoulli equation enables estimation of RV systolic pressure by measuring VSD peak velocity (9). If there is no RV outflow obstruction, then pulmonary arterial and RV systolic pressures should be identical. Similarly, the peak velocity of tricuspid valve regurgitation also enables estimation of RV systolic pressure (10,11).

Left atrial and LV end-diastolic diameter are important, particularly when measured serially and plotted against weight-specific nomograms. The ratio of pulmonary to systemic flow (Qp:Qs) may be estimated by measuring the time-velocity integral of flow across the pulmonary and aortic valves (12). However, this measurement provides data of doubtful utility and unclear reproducibility, and it is not used in most echocardiography laboratories.

Atrial Septal Defects. Patients with these defects (ASD) may be diagnosed late, since they may be asymptomatic and may demonstrate subtle physical findings. ASDs may occur in varying locations; differentiating between these is important because of their specific associations with other defects involving the AV valves and the pulmonary veins.

Atrial septal defect classification. Nomenclature is based on defect location within the atrial septum and the embryological basis or origin of the defect.

Secundum atrial septal defects—pathologic anatomy: Secundum ASDs are due to deficiency of septum primum (the flap valve of the fossa ovalis), deficiency of septum secundum, or both. A fenestrated septum may result from persistent strands of septum primum, with shunting across multiple orifices.

Echocardiography: Secundum ASDs are best shown from subcostal long- and short-axis views (13) (Fig. 6), typically

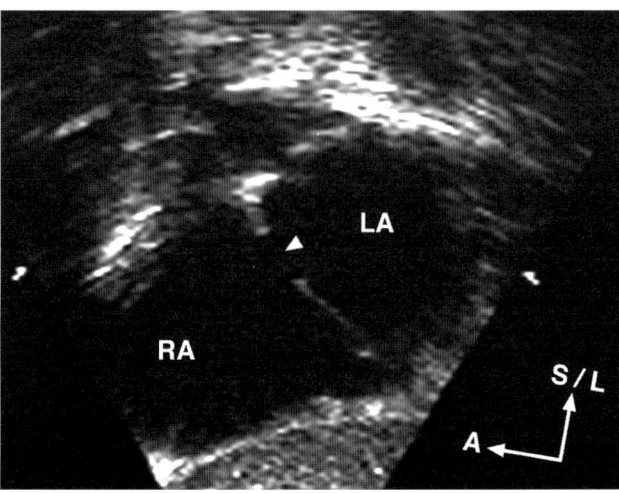

FIG. 6. Secundum atrial septal defect: subcostal short-axis view shows a moderate-sized ("secundum") defect in the midportion of the atrial septum (*arrowhead*). *RA*, right atrium; *LA*, left atrium.

in the midportion of the atrial septum (in the anterior-posterior plane as well as in the superior-inferior plane). If subcostal windows are poor, then a rotated parasternal short-axis view may profile the atrial septum in a plane that is almost perpendicular to the ultrasound beam, thus enabling visualization of the defect. In apical views, the atrial septum is parallel to the ultrasound beam; false dropout of the atrial septum may occur leading to overdiagnosis. Secundum ASDs are typically isolated defects. Defect size is important in determining prognosis and treatment options. ASDs may be elliptical, circular, or crescent-shaped and should be measured in two orthogonal planes. Defect diameter is measured in the widest dimensions at end-diastole, using two-dimensional imaging as well as color flow. If the atrial septum is fenestrated, then the diameter of each of the flow jets is measured. The presence and width of the rims of atrial septum along each of the margins of the defect is important in determining whether the individual defect is amenable to transcatheter device closure.

Primum atrial septal defects—pathologic anatomy: Primum ASDs are the consequence of deficient development of the endocardial cushions and the AV septum. They are located anterior and inferior to the fossa ovalis, and are bordered by a crescent of atrial tissue superiorly (concavity facing inferiorly) and by the AV valves inferiorly. These defects are crescent-shaped, usually larger in the anterior-posterior dimension than they are in the superior-inferior dimension. The septal attachment of the anterior mitral leaflet is apically displaced, leading to loss of the normal mitral-tricuspid valve offset.

Echocardiography: Primum ASDs are best shown from apical (Fig. 3) and subcostal views. Dense AV valve chordal attachments to the septal crest may lead to subaortic stenosis, which should be quantified serially, since it may progress. Associated malformations include a cleft in the anterior mitral leaflet, which must be sought with a slow base-to-apex sweep in parasternal short axis. Since primum ASDs are in proximity to the coronary sinus ostium, they may be mistaken for an enlarged coronary sinus, or, conversely, an enlarged coronary sinus may be mistakenly identified as a primum ASD.

Sinus venosus atrial septal defects—pathologic anatomy: These defects are located posterior to the fossa ovalis. Normally, the right pulmonary veins enter the left atrium immediately to the left of the posterior aspect of the atrial septum; in this location, the anterior wall of the right pulmonary veins is in continuity with the adjacent atrial septum, posterior wall of the venae cavae and the right atrial wall. In this anomaly, the anterior wall of the individual right pulmonary vein is deficient, leading to anomalous drainage of the right pulmonary vein into the right atrium. If the defect is large, the right pulmonary vein may drain into the lateral wall of the right atrium lateral to the entrance of the superior or inferior vena cava, respectively; the defect may similarly involve the right middle pulmonary vein, which may also drain into the right atrium as a result.

Echocardiography: In children, these defects are best shown from subcostal short-axis view with extreme rightward angulation, in a sweep that follows the course of the right upper pulmonary vein. A sagittal view from the right parasternal window is also useful in demonstrating the relationship of the defect to the superior vena cava and the right upper pulmonary vein (14). Anomalous drainage of one or more of the right-sided pulmonary veins is the rule in this defect; thus, comprehensive identification of pulmonary venous anatomy is essential. This has important surgical implications in terms of the orientation of the patch. In adults, transesophageal echocardiography is frequently needed for definition of pulmonary venous anatomy.

Since the right heart chambers cannot be measured reliably, a qualitative assessment for right atrial and/or RV enlargement is performed. Pulmonary hypertension is sought in all patients with ASD, using the echocardiographic techniques described in the preceding section on VSD (10,11). As with VSDs, the Qp:Qs ratio may be estimated echocardiographically (12).

Patent Ductus Arteriosus. The ductus arteriosus develops from the superior portion of the sixth left aortic arch; it connects the main pulmonary artery to the aorta. The ductus is normally patent in utero and undergoes spontaneous closure shortly after birth.

Pathologic Anatomy. The ductus arteriosus arises from the superior and leftward aspect of the bifurcation of the main pulmonary artery and courses inferiorly and leftward, joining the anterior aspect of the descending aorta distal to the origin of the left subclavian artery. The ductus arteriosus is patent in utero, and normally involutes in the early postnatal period, leaving behind a cord-like ligamentum arteriosum. The anatomy and orientation of the ductus arteriosus is variable, particularly in the setting of aortic arch abnormalities (such as a right aortic arch).

Echocardiography. The ductus arteriosus is best seen from high left parasternal short axis with counterclockwise rotation of the transducer (''ductal'' view) (Fig. 7; see also Color Plate 34 following page 758), and from a suprasternal long-axis view profiling the aortic arch (''candy-cane'' view), angling leftward into the long axis of the left pulmonary artery (15). Color flow Doppler is essential for evaluation, particularly when the shunt is small. Patent ductus arteriosus (PDA) flow is typically seen as a flow jet extending between the aorta and the main pulmonary artery. The size of the flow jet and the direction of flow are useful indicators of the hemodynamic significance of the defect. Echocardiographic measurements include the diameter of the ductus at each end and its narrowest diameter, as well as the approximate length of the ductus. Doppler evaluation of flow velocity in the PDA allows for assessment of pulmonary hypertension. Aortic arch situs (right or left arch) and branching pattern are established by echocardiography prior to consideration of surgical intervention. RV pressure and left-sided chamber sizes are measured as detailed in the section on VSD earlier in this lesson (10–12).

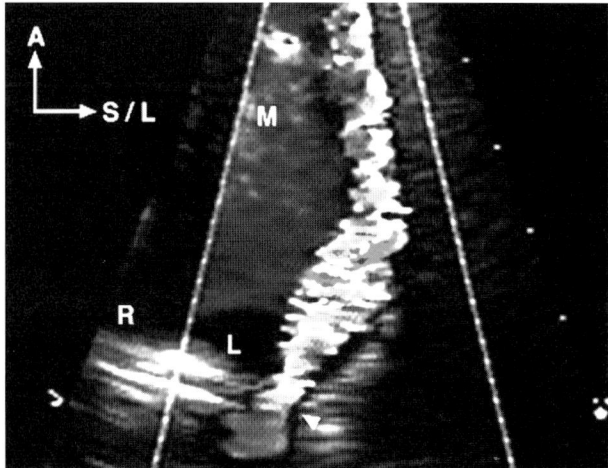

FIG. 7. Patent ductus arteriosus (PDA): high parasternal short-axis view rotated into a parasagittal plane, showing left-to-right flow across a PDA. *M*, main pulmonary artery; *L*, left pulmonary artery; *R*, right pulmonary artery. (See also Color Plate 34 following page 758.)

Atrioventricular Canal Defects. Atrioventricular (AV) canal defects involve the tricuspid and mitral valves, as well as the atrial and ventricular septa. A common AV canal defect exists when the embryonic common AV valve has not divided completely into two AV valves; varying degrees of this abnormality exist. In addition, partial or complete failure of fusion of the superior and inferior components of the anterior mitral leaflet leads to a (partial or complete) cleft in the anterior mitral leaflet. Wakai and Edwards (16) categorized AV canal defects as either partial or complete defects. Partial AV canal is characterized by a primum ASD, cleft anterior mitral leaflet and fibrous continuity between the anterior/superior and the posterior/inferior bridging leaflets; there is no contiguous canal-type VSD. In contrast, complete AV canal defect is characterized by absence of fibrous continuity between the anterior/superior and the posterior/inferior bridging leaflets, presence of an AV canal type VSD (the crest of the ventricular septum is concave superiorly) and a contiguous primum ASD (the free edge of the atrial septum is concave inferiorly). Complete AV canal defect is also evaluated based on the alignments and connections of the common AV valve orifice. Thus, the defect is classified as balanced (where the common AV valve opens approximately equally into both ventricles) or unbalanced, right-dominant versus left-dominant (where the common AV valve opens predominantly into the RV and LV, respectively) (17).

Rastelli et al. (18) classified complete AV canal defect into three types based on differences in the configuration, relationships, and attachments of the anterior leaflet of the common AV valve. Type A is characterized by a divided anterior leaflet, both sides of which attach to (or immediately to the right of) the crest of the ventricular septum by chordae tendineae. In type B, the anterior leaflet is divided, but does

not attach to the ventricular septum; this type is very rare. An anterior leaflet that is undivided and unattached to the ventricular septum characterizes the type C defect. The common AV valve usually has two bridging leaflets and three lateral leaflets.

Associated defects that are related to the basic anomaly include subaortic stenosis, which is more commonly associated with partial AV canal defects and Rastelli type A defects than with Rastelli type C defects (19,20). The presence of dense chordal attachments to the septal crest and the increased separation between the aorta and the left AV valve due to the narrow, elongated LV outflow tract are perceived as the morphologic bases for development of subaortic stenosis (21). David et al. (22) found that 14% of autopsy specimens with complete AV canal had a single focus of LV chordal insertion, not necessarily a single papillary muscle group. This creates the anatomic substrate for a parachute mitral valve when the common AV valve is divided.

Echocardiography. A comprehensive echocardiogram is the definitive preoperative diagnostic test. Each component of the AV canal defect (primum ASD, common AV valve, canal-type VSD) is evaluated (Fig. 3). Sizing of ASD and VSD is performed at end diastole. Since the VSD may be obscured by AV valve chordal attachments, color flow Doppler interrogation is used for VSD sizing. The presence, severity, and morphologic basis for AV valve regurgitation (i.e., annular dilation with a volume-loaded ventricle versus localized clefts) are established. The "*en face*" view of the common AV valve enables assessment of AV valve morphology, number of AV valve orifices, and extent of bridging leaflet tissue. This view is obtained by 45-degree, clockwise rotation of the transducer from the standard subcostal coronal view and then by sweeping from above downward (23). The adequacy and spacing of LV papillary muscles is established. The LV outflow tract is interrogated for evidence of obstruction. Echocardiography should assess for RV pressure overload and for biventricular volume overload.

Recent echocardiographic morphometric studies indicate the importance of quantitative assessment of AV valve morphology. Cohen et al. (24) measured the area of the AV valve overlying each ventricle and calculated an AV valve index as the ratio of the area of the AV valve overlying the LV to the area of the AV valve overlying the RV. They found that an AV valve index greater than 0.67 was consistent with balanced ventricles and predicted successful two-ventricle repair. An AV valve index less than 0.67 in the presence of a large VSD indicated the need for single-ventricle repair. A double-orifice left AV valve was identified as a risk factor that was associated with LV inlet hypoplasia, outflow tract obstruction, aortic arch hypoplasia, and discrete coarctation.

Obstructive Lesions

Pulmonary Valve Stenosis. Pulmonary valvar stenosis is characterized by thickened, doming pulmonary valve leaflets. The valve cusps may be fused, and the commissures may be underdeveloped or hypoplastic, leading to unicuspid or bicuspid valve morphology. The pulmonary valve annulus itself may be hypoplastic and/or dysplastic, with irregular, thick, rolled edges and redundant leaflets that are inherently obstructive to blood flow due to their bulk. Poststenotic dilation of the main pulmonary artery is seen with typical (not dysplastic) pulmonary stenosis, due to the high-velocity jet of prograde flow past the pulmonary valve. Secondary RV hypertrophy is evident, particularly involving the infundibulum. The tricuspid valve may be thickened and regurgitant.

In contrast to the gradual changes in severity at other ages, pulmonary stenosis in infancy may progress rapidly due to inadequate growth of the pulmonary annulus coupled with rapid linear growth that is seen in the first few months of life (25).

Echocardiography. The echocardiographic features of pulmonary stenosis include thickened leaflets and systolic doming of the valve leaflets, as well as variable hypoplasia of the pulmonary annulus (26). Secondary changes include poststenotic dilation and RV hypertrophy. Parasternal short-axis (Fig. 8; see also Color Plate 35 following page 758) and subcostal views are of great utility for demonstrating the features of pulmonary stenosis. Valve leaflet morphology and mobility should be assessed. The severity of stenosis is estimated based on measurement of RV systolic pressure, peak pressure gradient, annular size, RV hypertrophy and function, the presence and severity of tricuspid regurgitation, and the direction of interatrial shunting.

Continuous-wave Doppler estimation of transvalvular gradient by echocardiography has been shown to accurately predict the gradients found at catheterization (27). Suprasys-

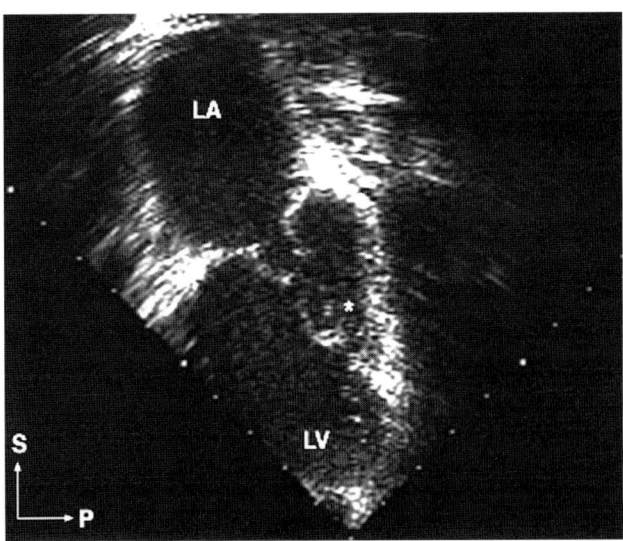

FIG. 9. Parachute mitral valve: apical two-chamber view shows both leaflets of the mitral valve inserting onto a single papillary muscle (*asterisk*). *LA,* left atrium; *LV,* left ventricle.

temic RV pressure or peak systolic gradients greater than 80 mm are findings consistent with severe stenosis.

Mitral Stenosis. Mitral valve morphology in congenital mitral stenosis may be classified as: (i) "typical" mitral stenosis with short chordae tendineae, obliteration of interchordal spaces, closely spaced and underdeveloped papillary muscles; (ii) hypoplastic mitral valve, typically in association with hypoplastic left heart syndrome; (iii) supramitral ring, characterized by a circumferential ridge of tissue originating at the atrial surfaces of the mitral valve, causing varying degrees of mitral inflow obstruction; and (iv) parachute mitral valve, characterized by insertion of all of the chordae tendineae of the mitral valve, predominantly onto a single papillary muscle (28). Isolated mitral stenosis is exceedingly rare; most commonly, the defect is associated with multilevel left heart obstruction.

Echocardiography. The echocardiographic features of congenital mitral stenosis include thickened valve leaflets with restricted excursion (29). The mitral valve leaflets may dome in atrial systole; arcade deformity of the mitral valve may be seen, with short chordae attached to multiple diminutive papillary muscle heads (30). Determination of mitral valve morphology is important because certain types of mitral stenosis, such as supramitral ring and parachute mitral valve (Fig. 9), are not amenable to balloon valvuloplasty (31). Doppler findings include accelerated transmitral flow velocities; however, the utility of quantitative evaluation of the mitral valve is limited by the lack of availability of normal values for the pediatric age group.

Parasternal and apical windows provide excellent visualization of the mitral apparatus. Echocardiographic evaluation of the mitral valve begins with measurement of mitral annulus in two dimensions. The mitral valve leaflets are assessed for mobility, thickening, and redundancy. The sub-

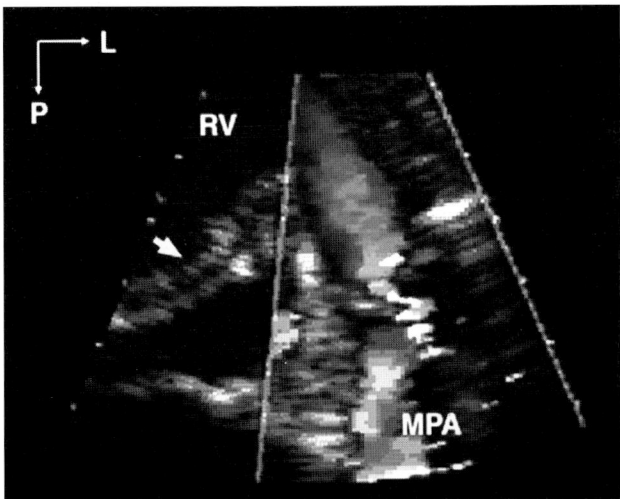

FIG. 8. Pulmonary stenosis: parasternal short-axis view shows a high-velocity, narrow color flow jet across the stenotic pulmonary valve. The *arrow* points to the paradoxical bulge of the ventricular septum due to suprasystemic RV pressure. *MPA,* main pulmonary artery; *RV,* right ventricle. (See also Color Plate 35 following page 758.)

valvar apparatus, consisting of the chordae tendineae and papillary muscles, is evaluated. Chordae tendineae are assessed for foreshortening, fusion, and adequacy of interchordal spaces. The number, spacing, and location of the papillary muscles and the pattern of chordal attachments to the papillary muscles (whether symmetric or predominantly to one papillary muscle) are established. Additional mitral valve pathology (such as a supramitral ring) is sought.

Subvalvar Aortic Stenosis. The morphologic substrate for subaortic stenosis is variable. A discrete membrane in proximity to the valve may progress, tethering the valve cusps, interfering with leaflet coaptation, and causing aortic insufficiency. Long tunnel-like stenosis can occur due to hypertrophy of the basal interventricular septum, exaggeration of the aortoseptal angle, and narrowing of the LV outflow tract. Anomalous attachments of the anterior mitral leaflet to the basal ventricular septum may create the substrate for subaortic stenosis, particularly in patients with AV canal defects (typically, complete Rastelli type A or partial AV canal defects). Posterior deviation of the conal septum can also lead to subaortic stenosis. The progressive nature of membranous, fibromuscular or tunnel-type subaortic stenosis is well known, regardless of whether it occurs in isolation or in association with a VSD (32).

Echocardiography. Weyman et al. (33) first described the echocardiographic findings in subaortic stenosis, classifying this lesion as either a thin, discrete membrane, or a thick or diffuse area of outflow tract narrowing. Other mechanisms of subaortic stenosis, such as mitral valve attachments to the ventricular septum, or conal septal deviation into the aortic outflow tract, are also identifiable by echocardiography.

Parasternal long-axis and apical windows provide excellent views of the subaortic region. The complete extent of the area of stenosis is defined, whether the length of a tunnel or the circumferential extension of a membrane onto the anterior mitral leaflet. Aortic regurgitation may be due to tethering of the aortic valve by a subaortic membrane or due to the impact of the eccentric flow jet across the stenotic subaortic region. The mechanisms, location, and severity of aortic regurgitation are evaluated. Tunnel-type subaortic stenosis may result in a long and tortuous aortic outflow tract, leading to underestimation of pressure gradients by Doppler echocardiography (34). The known progressive nature of subaortic stenosis implies the need for serial study (32).

Recent studies have identified echocardiographic morphometric measurements that allow prediction of development and progression of subaortic stenosis. The future development of subaortic stenosis in children with VSD and/or coarctation of the aorta has been predicted by the echocardiographic appearance of wider mitral-aortic separation, exaggerated aortic override, and a steeper aortoseptal angle (35). Progression of discrete subaortic stenosis is predicted by involvement of the anterior mitral leaflet, proximity of the obstruction to the aortic valve, and initial Doppler gra-

dient (36). Echocardiography is usually adequate for preoperative evaluation of patients with subaortic stenosis.

Valvar Aortic Stenosis. This lesion is characterized by thickened and/or fused aortic valve cusps and underdeveloped commissures, leading to stenosis due to inadequate systolic opening of the valve. The valve annulus itself may be hypoplastic; multiple levels of left heart obstruction may occur in series. Stenotic aortic valves are described by the number of cusps (e.g., bicuspid or unicuspid) or by the number of commissures (e.g., bicommissural or unicommissural). Underdevelopment of a commissure leads to the appearance of fusion of individual cusps. The valve may also be dysplastic, with redundant, irregularly thickened, and nodular appearance of the valve leaflets. In this scenario, the bulk of the valve leaflets causes narrowing of the aortic outflow. In moderate or severe cases, LV hypertrophy is present. Neonates with critical valvar aortic stenosis may exhibit LV systolic dysfunction, dilation, mitral regurgitation, and endocardial fibroelastosis. In a neonate with critical aortic stenosis, the amount of prograde flow through the aortic valve is inadequate for systemic perfusion, thus necessitating patency of the ductus arteriosus for temporarily providing systemic perfusion.

Echocardiography. The echocardiographic features of aortic stenosis include thickened leaflets and systolic doming of the valve leaflets (Fig. 10), as well as variable hypoplasia of the aortic annulus. Secondary changes include poststenotic dilation of the ascending aorta and LV hypertrophy. Echocardiographic evaluation includes assessment of valve leaflet morphology and mobility. The severity of stenosis is estimated based on measurement of peak pressure gradient, annular size, LV hypertrophy and function, and the presence, severity, and peak velocity of mitral regurgitation.

Echocardiography enables measurement of peak and

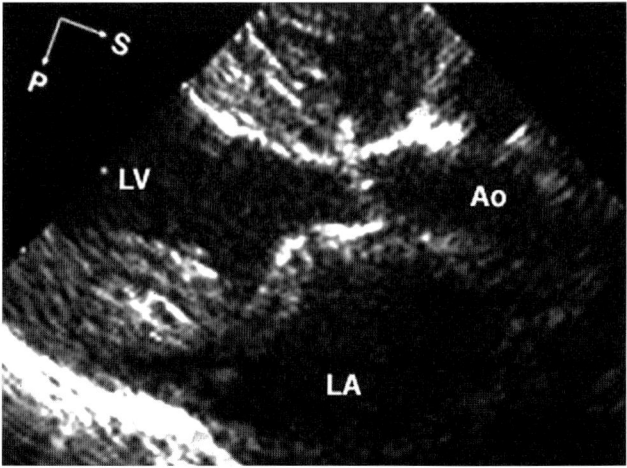

FIG. 10. Aortic stenosis: parasternal long-axis view shows a thickened, hypoplastic aortic valve. Left atrial and LV dilation as well as LV hypertrophy are evident in this neonate with critical aortic valvar stenosis. *Ao,* aorta; *LA,* left atrium; *LV,* left ventricle.

mean transvalvar gradients; careful attention must be paid to the peak velocity proximal to the aortic valve leaflets (37,38). Quantification of aortic stenosis follows the same principles as in adults, with the caveat that the potential for error is larger in smaller patients; in general, the mean transvalvar gradient obtained by echocardiography corresponds closely to the mean transcatheter gradient. Valve annulus is best measured from parasternal long axis, and the commissural arrangement is best shown from parasternal short axis (39).

Transvalvar gradients are best obtained from suprasternal, high right parasternal, and apical views, using the location of post-stenotic dilation of the ascending aorta as a marker that is diametrically opposite the origin of the flow jet through the stenotic aortic valve. Since multiple levels of left heart obstruction may exist in series, these are sought in each case. The presence and severity of aortic regurgitation is noted. Specific morphometric measurements of the LV and outflow tract have been identified as predictors of outcome in neonatal aortic stenosis. Thus, Leung et al. identified LV inflow dimension less than 25 mm, aortic annulus less than 5 mm, and mitral orifice less than 9 mm as predictors of poor results from open valvotomy (40); a single ventricle repair was felt to be more practical in such cases. Rhodes et al. studied 43 infants with critical aortic stenosis and identified four risk factors (41): LV long-axis to heart long-axis length ratio less than or equal to 0.8, indexed aortic root diameter less than or equal to 3.5 cm/m^2, indexed mitral valve area less than or equal to 4.75 cm^2/m^2, and LV mass index less than or equal to 35 g/m^2. The presence of two or more of these risk factors predicted poor outcome from balloon angioplasty.

Supravalvar Aortic Stenosis. Supravalvar aortic stenosis is typically found in patients with Williams' syndrome, although it may be an isolated defect. It is characterized by a diffusely narrow and thick-walled ascending aorta; discrete membranous supravalvar aortic stenosis is far less common. Stenosis is usually most marked at the junction of the sinuses of Valsalva with the ascending aorta (the sinotubular junction), and decreases along the course of the ascending aorta (i.e., the ascending aorta progressively widens as it proceeds cephalad). Secondary hemodynamic effects of supra-aortic stenosis include LV hypertrophy. Associated lesions include coronary artery stenosis or atresia (42).

Echocardiography. The ascending aorta is visualized using a combination of high parasternal long-axis and suprasternal short- and long-axis views to enable identification and quantification of supravalvar aortic stenosis. However, visualization of the ascending aorta may be technically difficult. Color flow and continuous wave Doppler interrogation of the ascending aorta are important tools in the evaluation of supravalvar aortic stenosis. If adequate echocardiographic windows are present, the coronary arteries should also be visualized. Serial study for evaluating the severity of supra-aortic stenosis is important because the stenotic area may not keep pace with the patients' linear growth.

Coarctation of the Aorta. Infantile coarctation is postulated to be due to abnormal embryonic development of the left fourth and sixth aortic arches. In utero, the lower body is perfused via right-to-left shunting at the level of the ductus arteriosus, and the upper body is perfused via prograde flow from the LV into the brachiocephalic vessels. As a result, the aortic isthmus receives only a small portion of cardiac output in fetal life. Any lesion that contributes to a further decrease in prograde flow across the isthmus may adversely affect isthmic growth. Thus, infantile coarctation is frequently seen in the setting of a large VSD with associated hypoplasia of the aortic outflow tract and isthmus. Coarctation is characterized by aortic arch hypoplasia that may include the transverse, proximal, and distal arch. The aortic isthmus is frequently long and narrow. Localized coarctation is seen as a posterior shelf in proximity to the insertion of the ductus arteriosus; contractile tissue from the ductus arteriosus may extend into the adjoining portions of the descending thoracic aorta, thus forming the substrate for coarctation. Coarctation may occur in isolation, or it may be associated with other left-heart obstructive lesions, including supramitral ring, mitral valve stenosis including parachute mitral valve, subaortic stenosis, bicuspid aortic valve, and valvar aortic stenosis (43,44). The complete form of Shone's complex refers to the co-existence of four left-sided obstructive conditions: parachute mitral valve, supramitral ring, subaortic stenosis, and coarctation of the aorta; the presence of two or three of these four lesions is described as a "*forme fruste*" of Shone's complex (44). VSDs are frequent associated findings.

Echocardiography. Coarctation is best shown from suprasternal short- and long-axis (Fig. 11) views (45,46). A high parasternal short-axis view with counterclockwise rotation of the transducer also profiles the isthmus and adjoining

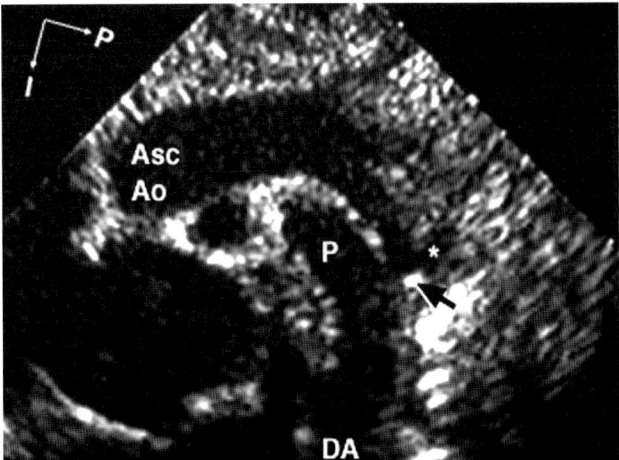

FIG. 11. Coarctation of the aorta: suprasternal long-axis view shows a hypoplastic aortic arch. The *arrow* points to the posterior ledge at the site of coarctation; an *asterisk* marks the origin of the left subclavian artery. A large patent ductus arteriosus (*P*) is continuous with the descending thoracic aorta (*DA*). *Asc Ao*, ascending aorta.

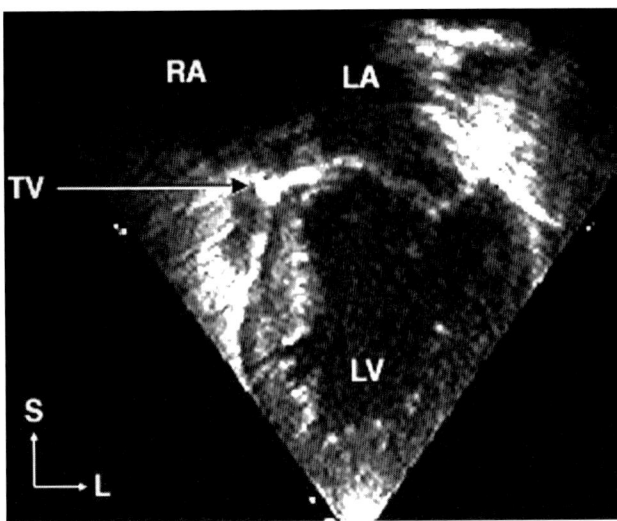

FIG. 14. Tricuspid atresia: apical four-chamber view shows an echodense plate in the normal location of the tricuspid valve (*TV*). An irregularity in the ventricular septal endocardium indicates the site of a muscular ventricular septal defect, which has spontaneously closed. The right ventricle is diminutive. The left-sided heart chambers are dilated. *LA*, left atrium; *LV*, left ventricle; *RA*, right atrium.

degree of pulmonary outflow obstruction. Rao (63) found that in tricuspid atresia, physiologically advantageous VSDs (typically located in the muscular septum) have a 38% incidence of spontaneous closure. This suggests the need for serial evaluation of VSD size in situations where flow across the VSD is an integral part of the blood flow circuit. Associated defects are the rule; septal defects, patency of the ductus arteriosus, TGA, and outflow tract obstruction may be present.

Echocardiography. Seward et al. (64) noted that the tricuspid valve is not visualized echocardiographically (Fig. 14); there is no tricuspid valve orifice, and no communication between the right atrium and the hypoplastic RV. The RV is usually hypoplastic; the degree of hypoplasia depends on the size of interventricular communication(s). The ASD represents the only egress from the right atrium and demonstrates obligate right-to-left flow. The left atrium and ventricle are typically dilated due to volume overload, and the mitral valve may exhibit redundant chordae. A VSD is frequently present. Ventriculoarterial alignments may be concordant or discordant. Tricuspid atresia with D-TGA is frequently associated with left juxtaposition of the right atrial appendage (65). The echocardiographic features of a left juxtaposed right atrial appendage include visualization of the malpositioned right appendage extending leftward from the right atrium, behind both great arteries, interposed between the posterior great artery and the left atrium. When the right atrial appendage is juxtaposed to the left, the atrial septum has a horizontal right-to-left orientation, which is best shown from parasternal short-axis and apical views (66).

Parasternal short-axis and apical windows provide excel-

lent views of the tricuspid valve. Characterization of segmental anatomy is important, since d- or l-looping of the ventricles and D-TGA or L-TGA may be present. All septal defects are measured, and the direction of flow across these defects is determined. Serial evaluation of VSDs is important since these defects are prone to spontaneous diminution in size and even spontaneous closure. Aortic outflow tract (multilevel) obstruction is frequently seen in association with tricuspid atresia, D-TGA, and a small VSD. Pulmonary outflow tract (multilevel) obstruction is typically seen with tricuspid atresia with ventriculoarterial concordance and a small VSD.

Pulmonary Atresia with Intact Ventricular Septum

This lesion represents the extreme end of the spectrum of pulmonary valve stenosis with an intact ventricular septum. Absence of prograde flow across the pulmonary valve is associated with varying degrees of hypoplasia of the tricuspid valve and RV. The RV continues to attempt to eject against the imperforate pulmonary valve, resulting in high (even suprasystemic) RV pressure; this results in RV hypertrophy and tricuspid regurgitation.

Pulmonary atresia with intact ventricular septum typically occurs in the setting of normal cardiac segmental arrangement (67,68). The right atrium is usually dilated; the tricuspid valve (annulus, leaflets and chordae) is hypoplastic, and tricuspid annular size correlates with RV size (69). The RV is hypertrophied and hypoplastic; rarely, it may be dilated. RV hypoplasia is global, involving the inlet, trabecular, and infundibular components of the normally tripartite RV. Endocardium-lined outpouchings of the RV into adjoining myocardium—so-called sinusoids—may be present. Fistulous communications may connect the RV cavity to the right and/or left coronary artery. The involved coronary arteries may be stenotic, and they may lack connection with the aorta. This condition, termed RV-dependent coronary circulation, is associated with the propensity for myocardial ischemia and infarction (68).

Echocardiography. Leung et al. (70) showed an excellent correlation between echocardiographic and angiocardiographic measurements of the tricuspid valve annulus diameter. Small RV size, quantified by tricuspid valve diameter and RV volume (indexed to body surface area), is associated with coronary artery fistulae with stenoses to multiple coronary arteries (RV-dependent coronary circulation) (71). Echocardiography alone is of doubtful value in comprehensive assessment for RV-dependent coronary circulation; angiographic evaluation of the coronary arteries is essential for this purpose (72).

Parasternal short-axis and apical views (Fig. 15) provide excellent visualization of the echocardiographic features of this lesion. The tricuspid annulus z value must be measured since RV size correlates with this measurement (73). Comprehensive echocardiography includes evaluation of the (obligate right-to-left) interatrial shunt and the ductus arteriosus.

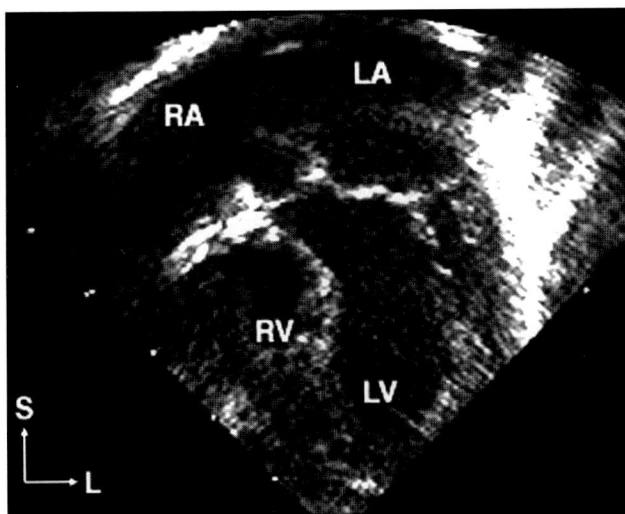

FIG. 15. Pulmonary atresia with intact ventricular septum: apical four-chamber view shows a hypertrophic, hypoplastic right ventricle (*RV*). The ventricular septum bulges paradoxically into the left ventricle (*LV*) outflow tract due to suprasystemic RV pressure. *LA*, left atrium; *RA*, right atrium.

The length of the atretic segment (that is, the distance between the blind-ending pulmonary outflow tract and the main pulmonary artery) must be measured. This has important implications with regard to the type of initial palliation, since a localized atretic plate is amenable to transcatheter perforation and dilation, while long-segment atresia that includes absence of the proximal main pulmonary artery would necessitate surgical repair. The presence of ventriculocoronary connections may be suspected based on low-velocity flow within the RV myocardium, shown by adjusting color flow Doppler to a low Nyquist limit (74). RV systolic pressure is quantified by using the peak velocity of tricuspid regurgitation. The severity of tricuspid regurgitation and the degree of right atrial dilation are also assessed. LV dysfunction and mitral regurgitation must be sought, since these may be markers for coronary insufficiency.

Ventricular Malformations

Single Ventricle. Van Praagh et al. (75) define a single ventricle by the absence of the contralateral ventricle; thus, single ventricles are classified by their morphology as either single RV or as single LV. An opposing school of thought defines a single ventricle based on the arrangement of the AV valves, thus designating as "single ventricle" an arrangement wherein both AV valves or a common AV valve open into one ventricular chamber (76). The type of AV connection may be one of three types: double-inlet (via two AV valves), single inlet (via one AV valve, with atresia of the second AV valve), or common inlet (via a common AV valve) (77). Single LV is more common than is single RV, and it may occur with either d-loop or, more commonly, with l-loop ventricles. The septal surface of this single LV

separates it from the infundibulum, which is also termed the "rudimentary outlet chamber." There is frequently a defect in the septum that separates the LV from the infundibulum; this defect is termed the bulboventricular foramen. The origin of the great arteries is variable. Thus, either or both of the great arteries may originate from either the LV or the infundibulum. If a great artery originates from the infundibulum, then the bulboventricular foramen is an important site for potential outflow tract obstruction ("restrictive bulboventricular foramen"). In patients with double-inlet single LV, the AV valve that is concordant with the ventricular loop is frequently abnormal; thus, the right AV valve in d-loop is typically regurgitant, and the left AV valve in l-loop is typically stenotic (78). VSD is most commonly either subaortic (with infundibular septal malalignment and/or hypoplasia) or muscular. Muscular defects are more frequently obstructive than are subaortic defects. Patients with origin of the aorta from the infundibulum exhibit a strong correlation between VSD size and aortic annulus diameter, coarctation, or arch interruption (78).

Echocardiography. Echocardiography enables evaluation of ventricular morphology, detection of bulboventricular foramen obstruction, great artery position, pulmonary outflow obstruction, and AV valve abnormalities, including abnormal chordae, hypoplasia, or dysplasia (77,79). Apical (Fig. 16) and subcostal views are most useful for evaluating ventricular morphology. Outflow tract obstruction is variable; the presence, severity, location, and morphologic basis for outflow tract obstruction must be defined. Serial levels of obstruction are sought specifically. Ventricular function and AV valve regurgitation are also sought. Matitiau et al. (80) demonstrated an excellent correlation between *antemortem* echocardiographic measurements of bulboventricu-

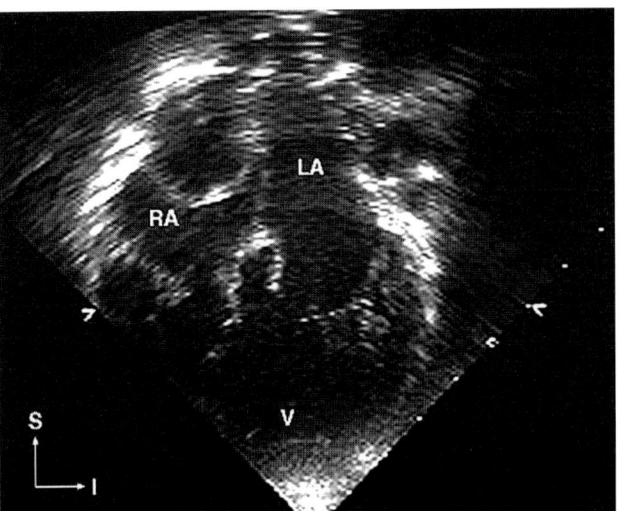

FIG. 16. Single left ventricle: apical four-chamber view shows a single smooth-walled ventricular chamber. The offset of the atrioventricular valves is normal, consistent with d-loop ventricles. These characteristics indicate that this is a morphologic left ventricle. *LA*, left atrium; *RA*, right atrium; *V*, ventricle.

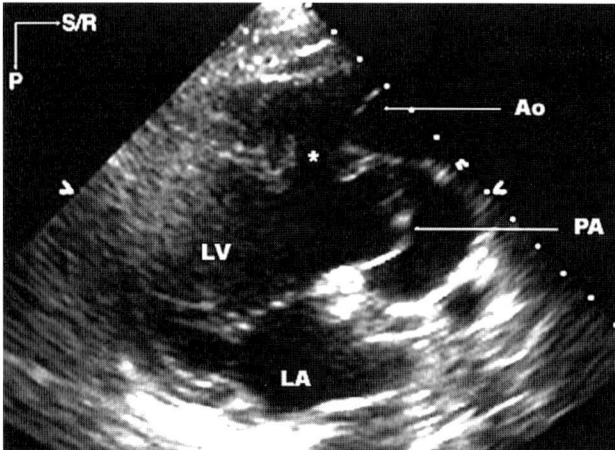

FIG. 17. Bulboventricular foramen: parasternal long-axis view shows the connection of the pulmonary valve to the morphologic LV. The aorta (*Ao*) connects to the infundibulum, which is located anterosuperiorly. LV output must pass through the bulboventricular foramen (*asterisk*) in order to reach the aortic valve. *LA*, left atrium; *LV*, left ventricle; *PA*, pulmonary artery.

lar foramen area and the dimensions measured at autopsy. If one or both great arteries originate from the infundibulum, the cross-sectional area of the bulboventricular foramen should be measured and plotted against available nomograms to predict future restriction. Shiraishi (81) showed that restriction at the level of the bulboventricular foramen is associated with a significantly smaller bulboventricular foramen area (normalized by body surface area); foramen area less than 2 cm^2/m^2 indicated a restrictive communication. The bulboventricular foramen (Fig. 17) may also fail to grow commensurate with linear growth. Serial echocardiograms are important in this situation since progressive diminution of the bulboventricular foramen may occur—both absolutely and relative to the patient's linear growth.

Hypoplastic Left Heart Syndrome. This term refers to a spectrum of malformations that share underdevelopment of the left heart, including the left atrium, mitral valve, LV, aortic valve, and aortic arch. Circulation depends on the patency of the ductus arteriosus, utilizing the RV as the combined systemic and pulmonary ventricle.

The left atrium may be hypoplastic and thick-walled, or, less commonly, dilated and thin-walled. The mitral valve may be stenotic, hypoplastic, or atretic. The entire mitral valve apparatus may be abnormally formed, with annular hypoplasia, short chordae leading to direct attachment of the mitral valve leaflets onto the papillary muscles, obliteration of interchordal spaces, and closely spaced papillary muscles, or a single papillary muscle (parachute mitral valve).

The LV is almost always hypoplastic; it may be completely absent. A well developed LV is usually seen in association with VSD. LV endocardial fibroelastosis may be seen, particularly if there is prograde flow through the mitral valve in the setting of aortic atresia. Atresia of the aortic

valve may be due to complete absence of recognizable valve tissue, which is represented by a membrane or a shelf or due to diminutive and imperforate valve structure. When the aortic valve is patent, the leaflets are usually thick and most frequently obstructive. The ascending aorta and aortic arch are hypoplastic, frequently with an associated coarctation of the aorta. Typically, the ascending aorta is miniscule and serves only as a main coronary artery with retrograde filling via the ductus arteriosus.

The morphology of the atrial septum is an important determinant of clinical manifestations and management outcomes in patients with hypoplastic left heart syndrome. Variations of atrial septal morphology include (i) a large secundum ASD, (ii) an intact atrial septum, (iii) an aneurysm of septum primum, and (iv) leftward malalignment of the septum primum with direct attachment of the left atrial wall to the left of septum secundum (82). In the presence of an intact atrial septum, pulmonary venous return to the right atrium may occur via anomalous pulmonary venous drainage (e.g., scimitar syndrome), or through persistence of primitive venous channels between the left atrium and the systemic veins (e.g., the levoatriocardinal vein), or an unroofed coronary sinus that allows decompression of the left atrium.

The right heart chambers are enlarged, more noticeably so due to left heart hypoplasia. The RV is hypertrophic and may be dysfunctional. Tricuspid regurgitation may be present. The pulmonary valve may be regurgitant, or, rarely, stenotic. Abnormalities of systemic venous drainage may also be present.

Echocardiography. The apical view of hypoplastic left heart syndrome is diagnostic (Fig. 18). The LV may be diminutive and difficult to identify. An echocardiographic search for the LV should focus on the AV groove, since the hypoplastic LV is not apex forming. The presence of

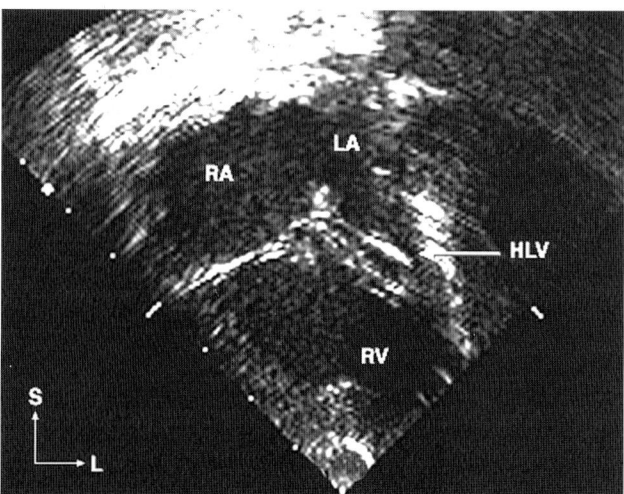

FIG. 18. Hypoplastic left heart syndrome: apical four-chamber view shows a hypoplastic left ventricle (HLV). The right atrium (*RA*) and right ventricle (*RV*) are dilated, and the RV is apex forming. The left atrium (*LA*) and mitral valve are hypoplastic.

endocardial fibroelastosis is noted. LV size and function are assessed. If the mitral valve is atretic and the LV is not correspondingly hypoplastic, additional sources of LV filling, such as VSDs, are sought.

Aortic arch diameter is measured at multiple levels. The presence, location, and severity of coarctation are defined. In the setting of a large PDA, two-dimensional imaging, and color flow Doppler are more helpful in identifying coarctation than are Doppler flow patterns.

Leftward malalignment and anomalous attachment of septum primum to the left atrial wall is sought. The location and size of all atrial-level shunts are noted, for purposes of serial comparison as well as for interventions such as balloon atrial septostomy. Small perforations of the atrial septum may be located posterior and superior to the usual location of the foramen ovale; these are evaluated using color flow Doppler. Dilation of the pulmonary veins, which may occur secondary to a restrictive atrial septum, is sought specifically.

If the atrial septum appears intact, sources of pulmonary venous drainage into the right heart are sought. Each of the pulmonary veins is tracked. Thus, a subcostal sweep beginning in the transverse abdominal plane, sweeping up to the heart, will identify scimitar syndrome, with anomalous entry of the right-sided pulmonary veins into the right atrium. Interrogation of the coronary sinus septum helps evaluate for a coronary sinus septal defect. Lowering the Nyquist limit for color sweeps from suprasternal imaging helps identify levoatriocardinal veins or anomalies of pulmonary venous return.

RV systolic function and the severity of tricuspid regurgitation are difficult to quantify and are evaluated qualitatively. Pulmonary valve stenosis or regurgitation is also evaluated. Systemic venous drainage is completely defined; and the surgical implications of systemic venous abnormalities that are identified must be understood, e.g., persistent left superior vena cava with absence of the left innominate (''bridging'') vein may necessitate bilateral bidirectional Glenn shunts.

Conotruncal Malformations

Tetralogy of Fallot. Fallot described the four components of a cardiac malformation that, he noted, was the most common cause of cyanotic congenital heart disease (83). These components are pulmonary stenosis, VSD, overriding aorta, and concentric RV hypertrophy. It is currently believed that Fallot's tetralogy has a single basis; it is thus a monology, based on hypoplasia of the subpulmonary infundibulum (84). The constellation of features that comprise tetralogy of Fallot is attributed to anterior, superior, and leftward malalignment of the conal septum, which results in a large malalignment type VSD that is committed to the RV outflow tract. The deviated conal septum raises the floor of the RV outflow tract leading to pulmonary outflow tract obstruction and a smaller subpulmonary infundibulum (85). Malalignment of

the conal septum carries the aorta with it; as a result, the aorta overrides the ventricular septum. Varying degrees of conal septal malalignment and hypertrophy lead to varying severity of pulmonary outflow obstruction; subpulmonary stenosis may be progressive (85). The classic form of tetralogy consists of subpulmonary stenosis, with prograde pulmonary blood flow, a large malalignment type VSD, and an overriding aorta. The pulmonary annulus may be hypoplastic; valve leaflets may be thickened, and commissural underdevelopment may result in a bicuspid pulmonary valve. The branch pulmonary arteries are usually of normal size. RV hypertrophy is maintained by the pressure load placed upon the ventricle by the subpulmonary stenosis, as well as that transmitted from the LV through the VSD. Associated defects include coronary artery anomalies (origin of the left anterior descending coronary artery from the right coronary artery, single coronary artery—either right or left, or dual anterior descending coronary arteries), which are seen in approximately 5% of patients with tetralogy of Fallot (86).

Echocardiography. Tetralogy of Fallot can be adequately evaluated by echocardiography, including the various levels of potential RV outflow tract obstruction. This includes subvalvar pulmonary stenosis due to conal septum deviation and muscular hypertrophy (Fig. 5), valvar pulmonary stenosis due to annular hypoplasia and/or fused, dysplastic leaflets, supravalvar pulmonary stenosis, and branch pulmonary artery stenosis or hypoplasia. Additional VSDs are sought using color flow Doppler with low Nyquist limits. Potential sources of additional pulmonary blood flow, such as a PDA or aortopulmonary window, can be identified by echocardiography. Determination of coronary artery origin and course is an important aspect of echocardiographic evaluation (87). One of the limitations of echocardiography in tetralogy of Fallot is the inability of the technique to evaluate the distal branch pulmonary arteries and aortopulmonary collaterals.

Dextro-transposition of the Great Arteries. Dextro-transposition of the great arteries (D-TGA) is defined as ventriculoarterial discordance (that is, the aorta arises from the morphologic RV, and the pulmonary artery arises from the morphologic LV) in the setting of d-loop ventricles (88,89). Therefore, the pulmonary and systemic circulatory systems function in parallel, i.e., systemic venous blood flows to the aorta, while pulmonary venous blood flows to the pulmonary artery. In order to evaluate for the feasibility and nature of surgical repair, echocardiography for patients with D-TGA must include comprehensive segmental analysis of the great arteries, conal anatomy, evaluation for outflow tract obstruction, and assessment of the ventricular septum and other potential sources of mixing of the circulations (such as ASD, PDA, or aortopulmonary window).

Conal Anatomy, Great Arterial Relationship. Pathologic anatomy: Conal anatomy is variable in patients with D-TGA. Presence of subaortic conus and absence of subpulmonary conus is the most common conal pattern (88.2%), followed by presence of bilateral conus (6.7%), and presence of subpulmonary conus with absent subaortic conus (3.4%) (90).

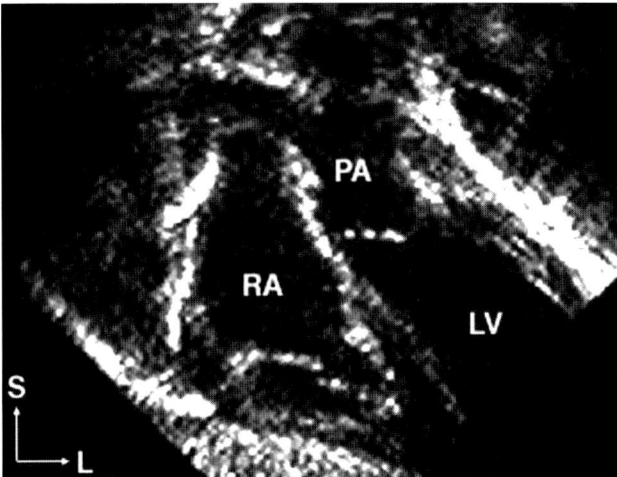

FIG. 19. Dextro-transposition of great arteries (D-TGA): subcostal long-axis view, angled posteriorly, shows the origin of the main pulmonary artery (*PA*) from the left ventricle (*LV*). The *LV* is identified as such based on the smooth septal surface; the main pulmonary artery is identified by its branching pattern (dividing into the branch pulmonary arteries). *RA*, right atrium.

With the most common conal anatomy, persistence of the subaortic conus lifts the aortic valve anteriorly, superiorly, and rightward, relative to the pulmonary valve, and it leads to alignment of the aorta with the RV. Absence of the subpulmonary conus leads to mitral-pulmonary valve fibrous continuity and alignment of the pulmonary valve with the LV. The great arteries are parallel in their course.

Echocardiography: Accurate identification of the great artery relationships requires localization of the semilunar valves, the ventricular attachments of these valves, and visualization of the branching patterns of the proximal great arteries (Fig. 19). The utility of the subxiphoid windows in establishing the diagnosis of transposition has been long recognized (91). King et al. (92) first described the echocardiographic features of TGA, including parallel alignment of the outflow tracts and great arteries and directly anterior or rightward position of the anterior great artery—the aorta (contrasted with the normal leftward position of the anterior great artery—the pulmonary artery).

Ventricular Septal Defects. Pathologic anatomy: VSDs occur in about one third of patients with D-TGA. Defect location is variable; malalignment-type defects are common. Posterior, inferior, and rightward deviation of the conal septum can lead to pulmonary outflow tract obstruction associated with valvar pulmonary stenosis, potentially making these patients ineligible for a simple arterial switch operation wherein the LV outflow tract would become the neoaortic outflow tract. Anterior, superior, and leftward deviation of the conal septum may lead to RV outflow tract obstruction. This may be associated with aortic valvar hypoplasia and stenosis as well as coarctation of the aorta, which must be identified preoperatively. Canal-type or inlet VSD may also

occur in patients with TGA. These defects are large, and may be associated with straddling of the tricuspid valve across the ventricular septum. Finally, muscular VSD (single or multiple) may also occur in patients with TGA, complicating the nature of any planned repair.

Echocardiography: VSDs are best seen from subcostal and apical views. To identify structures that may impede future VSD closure to the (neo)aorta, the VSD must be profiled from views that simultaneously show the (neo)aortic valve. The echocardiographer has to draw a mental picture of the orientation of the VSD patch. Sweeps from multiple planes of interrogation at the level of the VSD are used to evaluate for structures (such as AV valve attachments and chordae tendineae) that cross the VSD and may complicate defect closure.

Outflow Tract Obstruction. Pathologic anatomy: Dynamic pulmonary outflow tract obstruction is seen in patients with an intact ventricular septum due to elevated (systemic) RV pressure, causing the ventricular septum to bulge into the LV (pulmonary) outflow tract. Fixed outflow tract obstruction may be due to subvalvar membranes, fibromuscular ridges, AV valve attachments, or semilunar valve stenosis. In patients with a VSD, outflow tract obstruction may be due to conal septal malalignment.

Echocardiography. Visualization and assessment of the nature and severity of outflow tract obstruction are all performed using standard echocardiographic windows. In the presence of a VSD, anatomic definition of the substrate for outflow tract obstruction is more meaningful than are Doppler gradients. Preoperative echocardiograms should evaluate for actual obstruction as well as the potential for future (postoperative) obstruction. The presence of a malalignment type VSD should lead to evaluation for multilevel outflow tract obstruction in series. Preoperative echocardiograms should evaluate for all sites of potential mixing of the two parallel circuits: ASD, VSD, and the ductus arteriosus.

Coronary artery anatomy can be evaluated reliably by echocardiography (93). Unusual coronary artery patterns are found more commonly in patients with side-by-side great arteries or a posterior aorta, or a VSD, or both. A detailed description of the variations of coronary artery anatomy encountered in patients with D-TGA is outside the scope of this text; the reader is referred to excellent studies on the subject (93,94).

Truncus Arteriosus. Truncus is defined as a single arterial trunk leaving the base of the heart, with no remnant of atretic pulmonary artery or aorta; this single arterial trunk must supply the coronary, pulmonary, and systemic circulations (95). Collett and Edwards (95) classified truncus based on the embryologic stages in the development of the pulmonary arteries from the sixth aortic arches. Truncus type 1 is characterized by a single pulmonary trunk (main pulmonary artery, which bifurcates) and ascending aorta arising from the truncus arteriosus. In type 2, the right and left pulmonary arteries arise close together from the dorsal wall of the truncus arteriosus. Type 3 is characterized by origin of the branch pulmonary arteries independently from either side of the truncus arteriosus. In type 4 truncus, there are no pulmonary arteries; the sixth aortic arches are apparently congenitally absent, and pulmonary blood flow is provided by bronchial arteries. The existence of this type as a specific diagnostic entity is open to doubt, and it is probably identical to tetralogy of Fallot with pulmonary atresia. Becker et al. (96) evaluated the semilunar valve in truncus arteriosus and found it to have 1 to 6 cusps, occasionally with unequal cusp length, and frequently associated with cusp prolapse. Cusps were found to be nodular, with imperfect formation of commissures. Truncus arteriosus may occur in association with interrupted aortic arch type B (97).

Echocardiography. Riggs and Paul (98) described the echocardiographic features of truncus. These include a single great artery that overrides the ventricular septum (Fig. 20), with origin of the pulmonary arteries from this artery and the almost-invariable presence of a VSD. The VSD and great artery override are best shown from parasternal long axis. Truncal valve cusps are best shown from parasternal long axis (prolapse, thickening, coaptation, doming, regurgitation) and short axis (number of cusps and commissures, eccentric orifice, morphologic basis for regurgitation or stenosis). The pattern of pulmonary artery branching is best shown from a combination of parasternal short-axis and subcostal views. Associated anomalies of the aortic arch, including a right aortic arch or interrupted aortic arch, are also easily visualized by echocardiography.

Double-outlet Right Ventricle. In this type of ventriculoarterial alignment, both great arteries arise primarily from the RV. Double-outlet RV is a "basket term," including a spectrum of great artery relationships, conal anatomy, outflow tract obstructions, AV valve abnormalities and associated septal defects. Evaluation of a patient with double-outlet RV includes complete segmental diagnosis, with particular attention to the great artery relationship and the outflow

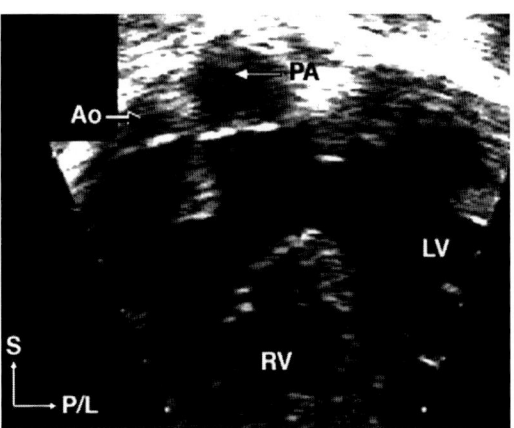

FIG. 21. Double-outlet right ventricle (*RV*): subcostal short-axis view shows both semilunar valves aligned with the anterior RV. Muscular conus is seen below each of the semilunar valves; this conal tissue separates the semilunar valves from the atrioventricular valves. *Ao,* aorta; *LV,* left ventricle; *PA,* pulmonary artery.

tracts. The echocardiographic features of double-outlet RV include origin of both great arteries from the anterior RV, absence of LV outflow other than through a VSD, and mitral-semilunar valve discontinuity due to interposition of a muscular conus (Fig. 21) (99).

Any of the five patterns of great artery relationship (solitus, inversus, d-(right and anterior), l-(left and anterior), or a-(directly anterior) malposition of the aortic valve) may occur in patients with double outlet RV. Echocardiographic windows that best demonstrate the great artery relationship include subcostal (Fig. 15) and parasternal sweeps.

VSD is almost invariably present in association with this defect. One critical issue in patients with double-outlet RV is the feasibility of biventricular repair, wherein VSD closure is achieved by means of a patch that directs LV outflow into the aorta. Therefore, VSD location, size, and relationship to the great arteries are critical issues. Evaluation of VSD location must include a description of the relationship of the VSD to the great arteries. In this context, the VSD may be subaortic, subpulmonary (Taussig–Bing defect), doubly committed (related to both semilunar valves), or noncommitted (distant from both semilunar valves, e.g., muscular or AV canal-type). VSD size is important; patients with a small interventricular communication or with far rightward malposition of the aortic valve may require VSD enlargement to avoid postoperative subaortic stenosis. The relationship of the VSD to the individual semilunar valves determines the type of surgical procedure, e.g., patch closure of a subaortic VSD versus patch closure with arterial switch operation for a subpulmonary VSD. Patients with double-outlet RV may also exhibit straddling of the AV valves across the ventricular septum. Echocardiographic evaluation includes profiling the VSD from multiple planes that also simultaneously show the aortic valve (or the pulmonary valve, if an arterial switch operation is considered). Structures that cross the VSD in

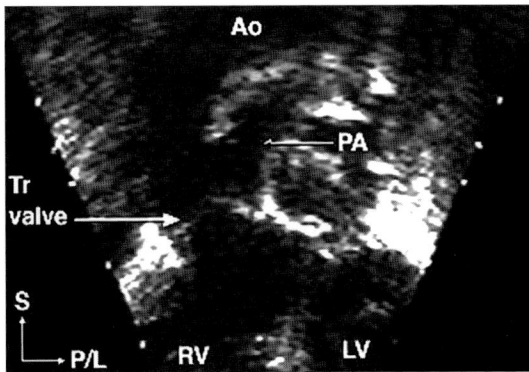

FIG. 20. Truncus arteriosus: subcostal short-axis view shows origin of a single great artery from the heart. This semilunar (truncal, *Tr*) valve overrides the ventricular septum. The valve domes in systole. The truncus continues cephalad as the ascending aorta (*Ao*) after giving origin to the main pulmonary artery (*PA*), which courses posteriorly. *LV,* left ventricle; *RV,* right ventricle.

these planes may complicate or contraindicate VSD closure. In order to identify potential sources of postoperative outflow tract obstruction, the preoperative echocardiograms must include a mental picture of the orientation of the VSD patch. In order to ensure that there are no AV valve attachments straddling the ventricular septum, echocardiography utilizes sweeps from multiple planes of interrogation at the level of the VSD.

Up to 50% of patients with double-outlet RV have pulmonary outflow tract obstruction, usually due to deviation of the conal septum causing subpulmonary stenosis; subaortic stenosis may also occur (100). Outflow tract obstruction may also be due to AV valve attachments, usually beneath the posterior great artery; multilevel obstruction may occur. Thus, a patient with a subaortic VSD and subpulmonary outflow obstruction may have pulmonary valvar, supravalvar, and/or branch pulmonary artery stenosis. Similarly, a patient with a subpulmonary VSD (Taussig–Bing defect) may have mitral stenosis, parachute mitral valve, straddling mitral valve, subaortic stenosis, valvar aortic stenosis, and/or coarctation of the aorta. Echocardiographic evaluation of the outflow tracts is best performed from subcostal and parasternal views and includes assessment for actual obstruction as well as the potential for future obstruction (e.g., following VSD closure).

Total Anomalous Pulmonary Venous Connection. In this malformation, the pulmonary veins do not communicate with the left atrium; instead, drainage is to the right atrium, either directly or via venous tributaries. This defect is due to failure of development of the common pulmonary vein (101). As a consequence, the primitive anastomosis between the pulmonary venous plexus in the lungs and the systemic veins persists and enlarges. Such anastomoses may be at the supracardiac (anterior cardinal), cardiac (sinus venosus), or subdiaphragmatic (omphalomesenteric) level, or at several of these levels—so-called mixed type of total anomalous pulmonary venous connection (102). Supracardiac connections may drain to the left innominate vein, right or left superior vena cava, or the azygous vein. Common sites of obstruction for this type of total anomalous pulmonary venous connection include the junction of the right-sided vertical vein with the right superior vena cava, or where the left-sided vertical vein crosses the left pulmonary artery (103,104). Intracardiac total anomalous pulmonary venous return may drain to the coronary sinus or the right atrium. Obstruction of this type of connection is rare. Infradiaphragmatic connections may drain into the ductus venosus and thence into the portal vein or inferior vena cava. Obstruction of this type of connection is the rule, and it may occur at the level of the diaphragm or at the junction between the descending vein and the left portal vein. Functional obstruction of infradiaphragmatic total anomalous pulmonary venous return is due to the length of the connection and the hepatic capillary bed, both of which impose increased resistance to flow.

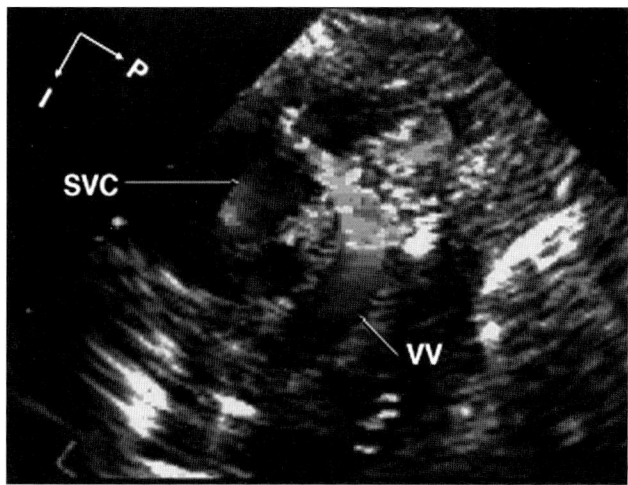

FIG. 22. Total anomalous pulmonary venous connection: high right parasternal long-axis (parasagittal) view shows a vertical vein (*VV*) that extends superiorly from the pulmonary venous confluence (not shown) to the superior vena cava. Aliasing of color flow at the narrow point of entrance of the vertical vein into the superior vena cava (*SVC*) indicates the location of pulmonary venous obstruction. (See also Color Plate 36 following page 758.)

In all cases of total anomalous pulmonary venous connection (except intracardiac and occasionally mixed), the pulmonary veins form a horizontal confluence behind the left atrium.

Echocardiography: The echocardiographic evaluation of pulmonary venous drainage is based on identification of anatomic connection and flow patterns within individual pulmonary venous drainage from each of the lung lobes. Supportive features include dilation of the right atrium and ventricle, the pulmonary annulus and proximal branch pulmonary arteries, and a restrictive ASD coupled with a relatively small left atrium and LV (105). The presence of complex congenital heart disease (heterotaxy) with decreased pulmonary blood flow, mixed type of total anomalous pulmonary venous connection, and pulmonary vein atresia may be associated with diagnostic errors in echocardiography. The application of color flow (Fig. 22; see also Color Plate 36 following page 758) and pulsed Doppler echocardiography has improved the ease and efficacy of diagnosis of pulmonary venous drainage and obstruction; these modalities provide information on the normal phasicity of pulmonary venous flow and its alterations under conditions of decreased prograde flow or pulmonary venous obstruction (106). Echocardiographic features that should lead to a suspicion of pulmonary venous obstruction include the following: (i) a continuous, nonphasic, high-velocity Doppler flow signal and nonlaminar flow are noted anywhere along the path of pulmonary venous drainage; and (ii) systolic flattening of the ventricular septum or high-velocity tricuspid regurgitation suggesting pulmonary hypertension (107).

SUMMARY

The segmental approach to echocardiographic diagnosis provides a systematic understanding of congenital heart defects. Pathologic anatomy must be integrated with echocardiographic appearance in order to achieve a complete three-dimensional picture of individual defects. Comprehensive echocardiographic evaluation is the only cardiac imaging study needed prior to palliative and corrective surgery for a wide range of congenital heart defects.

REFERENCES

1. Guyer B, Martin JA, MacDorman MF, et al. Annual summary of vital statistics—1996. *Pediatrics* 1997;100:905–918.
2. Kantoch MJ, Collins-Nakai RL, Medwid S, et al. Adult patients' knowledge about their congenital heart disease. *Can J Cardiol* 1997;13:641–645.
3. Van Praagh R. Segmental approach to diagnosis. In: DC Fyler, ed. *Nadas' pediatric cardiology.* Philadelphia: Hanley & Belfus, 1992:27–35.
4. Van Praagh R, Van Praagh S. Atrial isomerism in the heterotaxy syndromes with asplenia, or polysplenia, or normally formed spleen: an erroneous concept. *Am J Cardiol* 1990;60:1504–1506.
5. Bierman FZ, Fellows K, Williams RG. Prospective identification of ventricular septal defects in infancy using subxiphoid two-dimensional echocardiography. *Circulation* 1980;62:807–817.
6. Van Praagh R, Geva T, Kreutzer J. VSD: how shall we describe, name and classify them? *J Am Coll Cardiol* 1989;14:1298–1299.
7. Shirali GS, O'Brian Smith E, Geva T. Quantitation of echocardiographic predictors of outcome in infants with isolated ventricular septal defect. *Am Heart J* 1995;130:1228–1235.
8. Sharif DS, Huhta JC, Marantz P, et al. Two-dimensional echocardiographic determination of ventricular septal defect size: correlation with autopsy. *Am Heart J* 1989;117:1333–1336.
9. Marx GR, Allen HD, Goldberg SJ. Doppler echocardiographic estimation of pulmonary artery pressure in pediatric patients with ventricular communications. *J Am Coll Cardiol* 1985;6:1132–1137.
10. Yock PG, Popp RL. Noninvasive estimation of right ventricular systolic pressure by Doppler ultrasound in patients with tricuspid regurgitation. *Circulation* 1984;70:657–662.
11. Currie PJ, Seward JB, Chan K-L, et al. Continuous wave Doppler determination of right ventricular pressure: a simultaneous Doppler-catheterization study in 127 patients. *J Am Coll Cardiol* 1985;6:750–756.
12. Vargas Barron J, Sahn DJ, Valdes-Cruz LM, et al. Clinical utility of two-dimensional Doppler echocardiographic techniques for estimating pulmonary to systemic blood flow ratios in children with left to right shunting atrial septal defect, ventricular septal defect or patent ductus arteriosus. *J Am Coll Cardiol* 1984;3:169–178.
13. Shub C, Dimopoulos IN, Seward JB, et al. Sensitivity of two-dimensional echocardiography in the direct visualization of atrial septal defect utilizing the subcostal approach: experience with 154 patients. *J Am Coll Cardiol* 1983;2:127–135.
14. McDonald RW, Rice MJ, Reller MD, et al. Echocardiographic imaging techniques with subcostal and right parasternal longitudinal views in detecting sinus venosus atrial septal defects. *J Am Soc Echocardiogr* 1996;9:195–198.
15. Huhta JC, Cohen M, Gutgesell HP. Patency of the ductus arteriosus in normal neonates: two-dimensional echocardiography versus Doppler assessment. *J Am Coll Cardiol* 1984;4:561–564.
16. Wakai CS, Edwards JE. Pathologic study of persistent common atrioventricular canal. *Am Heart J* 1958;56:779–794.
17. Bharati S, Lev M. The spectrum of common atrioventricular orifice (canal). *Am Heart J* 1973;86:553–561.
18. Rastelli GC, Kirklin JW, Titus JL. Anatomic observations on complete form of persistent common atrioventricular canal with special reference to atrioventricular valves. *Mayo Clin Proc* 1966;41:296–308.
19. DeLeon SY, Ilbawi MN, Wilson WR Jr, et al. Surgical options in subaortic stenosis associated with endocardial cushion defects. *Ann Thorac Surg* 1991;52:1076–1083.
20. Reeder GS, Danielson GK, Seward JB, et al. Fixed subaortic stenosis in atrioventricular canal defect: a Doppler echocardiographic study. *J Am Coll Cardiol* 1992;20:386–394.
21. Ebels T, Ho SY, Anderson RH, et al. The surgical anatomy of the left ventricular outflow tract in atrioventricular septal defect. *Ann Thorac Surg* 1986;41:483–488.
22. David I, Castaneda AR, Van Praagh R. Potentially parachute mitral valve in common atrioventricular canal. Pathologic anatomy and surgical importance. *J Thorac Cardiovasc Surg* 1982;84:178–186.
23. Minich LA, Snider AR, Bove EL, et al. Echocardiographic evaluation of atrioventricular orifice anatomy in children with atrioventricular septal defect. *J Am Coll Cardiol* 1992;19:149–153.
24. Cohen MS, Jacobs ML, Weinberg PM, et al. Morphometric analysis of unbalanced common atrioventricular canal using two-dimensional echocardiography. *J Am Coll Cardiol* 1996;28:1017–1023.
25. Rowland DG, Hammill WW, Allen HD, et al. Natural course of isolated pulmonary valve stenosis in infants and children utilizing Doppler echocardiography. *Am J Cardiol* 1997;79:344–349.
26. Weyman AE, Hurwitz RA, Girod DA, et al. Cross-sectional echocardiographic visualization of the stenotic pulmonary valve. *Circulation* 1977;56:769–774.
27. Lima CO, Sahn DJ, Valdes-Cruz LM, et al. Noninvasive prediction of transvalvular pressure gradient in patients with pulmonary stenosis by quantitative two-dimensional echocardiographic Doppler studies. *Circulation* 1983;67:866–871.
28. Ruckman RN, Van Praagh RV. Anatomic types of congenital mitral stenosis: report of 49 autopsy cases with consideration of diagnosis and surgical implications. *Am J Cardiol* 1978;42:592–601.
29. Snider RA, Roge CL, Schiller NB, et al. Congenital left ventricular inflow obstruction evaluated by two dimensional echocardiography. *Circulation* 1972;61:848–852.
30. Grenadier E, Sahn DJ, Valdes-Cruz LM, et al. Two-dimensional echo Doppler study of congenital disorders of the mitral valve. *Am Heart J* 1984;107:319–325.
31. Spevak PJ, Bass JL, Ben-Shachar G, et al. Balloon angioplasty for congenital mitral stenosis. *Am J Cardiol* 1990;66:472–476.
32. Freedom RM, Pelech A, Brand A, et al. The progressive nature of subaortic stenosis in congenital heart disease. *Int J Cardiol* 1985;8:137–143.
33. Weyman AE, Feigenbaum H, Hurwitz RA, et al. Cross-sectional echocardiography in evaluating patients with discrete subaortic stenosis. *Am J Cardiol* 1976;37:358–365.
34. Yoganathan AP, Valdes-Cruz LM, Schmidt-Dhona J, et al. Continuous-wave Doppler velocities and gradients across fixed tunnel obstructions: *in vitro* and *in vivo*. *Circulation* 1987;76:657–666.
35. Kleinert S, Geva T. Echocardiographic morphometry and geometry of the left ventricular outflow tract in fixed subaortic stenosis. *J Am Coll Cardiol* 1993;22:1501–1508.
36. Bezold LI, O'Brian Smith E, Kelly K, et al. Development and validation of an echocardiographic model for predicting progression of discrete subaortic stenosis in children. *Am J Cardiol* 1998;81:314–320.
37. Hagler DJ, Tajik AJ, Seward JB, et al. Noninvasive assessment of pulmonary valve stenosis, aortic valve stenosis, and coarctation of the aorta in critically ill neonates. *Am J Cardiol* 1986;57:369–372.
38. Vered Z, Schneeweiss A, Meltzer RS, et al. Echocardiographic assessment of left ventricular outflow tract obstruction. *Am Heart J* 1983;106:177–181.
39. Huhta JC, Gutgesell HP, Latson LA, et al. Two-dimensional echocardiographic assessment of the aorta in infants and children with congenital heart disease. *Circulation* 1984;70:417–424.
40. Leung MP, McKay R, Smith A, et al. Critical aortic stenosis in early infancy. Anatomic and echocardiographic substrates of successful open valvotomy. *J Thorac Cardiovasc Surg* 1991;101:526–535.
41. Rhodes LA, Colan SD, Perry SB, et al. Predictors of survival in neonates with critical aortic stenosis. *Circulation* 1991;84:2325–2335.
42. Allen HD, Moller JH, Formanek A, et al. Atresia of the proximal left coronary artery associated with supravalvular aortic stenosis: surgical treatment. *J Thorac Cardiovasc Surg* 1974;67:266–271.
43. Becker A, Becker J, Edwards JE. Anomalies associated with coarctation of the aorta: particular reference to infancy. *Circulation* 1970;41:1067–1075.

44. Shone JD, Sellers RD, Anderson RC, et al. The developmental complex of "parachute mitral valve," supravalvular ring of left atrium, subaortic stenosis and coarctation of the aorta. *Am J Cardiol* 1963; 11:714–725.
45. Sahn DJ, Allen HD, McDonald G, et al. Real-time cross-sectional echocardiographic diagnosis of coarctation of the aorta. A prospective study of echocardiographic-angiographic correlations. *Circulation* 1977;56:762–769.
46. Nihoyannopoulos P, Karas S, Sapsford RN, et al. Accuracy of two-dimensional echocardiography in the diagnosis of aortic arch obstruction. *J Am Coll Cardiol* 1987;10:1072–1077.
47. George B, DiSessa TG, Williams RG, et al. Coarctation repair without cardiac catheterization in infants. *Am Heart J* 1987;114:1421–1425.
48. Morrow RW, Huhta JC, Murphy DJ Jr, et al. Quantitative morphology of the aortic arch in neonatal coarctation. *J Am Coll Cardiol* 1986;8: 816–820.
49. Hagler DJ. Echocardiographic assessment of Ebstein's anomaly. *Prog Pediatr Cardiol* 1993;2:28–37.
50. Matsumoto M, Matsuo H, Nagata S, et al. Visualization of Ebstein's anomaly of the tricuspid valve by two-dimensional and standard echocardiography. *Circulation* 1976;53:69–79.
51. Shiina A, Seward JB, Edwards WD, et al. Two-dimensional echocardiographic spectrum of Ebstein's anomaly: detailed anatomic assessment. *J Am Coll Cardiol* 1984;3:356–370.
52. Hurwitz RA. Left ventricular function in infants and children with symptomatic Ebstein's anomaly. *Am J Cardiol* 1994;73:716–718.
53. Celermajer DS, Dodd SM, Greenwald SE, et al. Morbid anatomy in neonates with Ebstein's anomaly of the tricuspid valve: pathophysiologic and clinical implications. *J Am Coll Cardiol* 1992;19: 1049–1053.
54. Roberson DA, Silverman NH. Ebstein's anomaly: echocardiographic and clinical features in the fetus and neonate. *J Am Coll Cardiol* 1989; 14:1300–1307.
55. Van Praagh R. What is congenitally corrected transposition? *N Engl J Med* 1970;282:1097–1098.
56. Allwork SP, Bentall HH, Becker AE, et al. Congenitally corrected transposition of the great arteries: morphologic study of 32 cases. *Am J Cardiol* 1976;38:910–922.
57. Van Praagh R, Papagiannis J, Grunenfelder J, et al. Pathologic anatomy of corrected transposition of the great arteries: medical and surgical implications. *Am Heart J* 1998;135:772–785.
58. Hagler DJ, Tajik AJ, Seward JB, et al. Atrioventricular and ventriculo-arterial discordance (corrected transposition of the great arteries). Wide-angle two-dimensional echocardiographic assessment of ventricular morphology. *Mayo Clin Proc* 1981;56:591–600.
59. Silverman NH, Gerlis LM, Horowitz ES, et al. Pathologic elucidation of the echocardiographic features of Ebstein's malformation of the morphologically tricuspid valve in discordant atrioventricular connections. *Am Heart J* 1995;76:1277–1283.
60. Orie JD, Anderson C, Ettedgui JA, et al. Echocardiographic-morphologic correlations in tricuspid atresia. *J Am Coll Cardiol* 1995;26: 750–758.
61. Van Praagh R, Ando M, Dungan WT. Anatomic types of tricuspid atresia: clinical and developmental implication. *Circulation* 1971;44: II-115.
62. Edwards JE, Burchell HB. Congenital tricuspid atresia: a classification. *Med Clin North Am* 1949;33:1177–1196.
63. Rao PS. Natural history of the ventricular septal defect in tricuspid atresia and its surgical implications. *Br Heart J* 1977;39:276–288.
64. Seward JB, Tajik AJ, Hagler DJ, et al. Echocardiographic spectrum of tricuspid atresia. *Mayo Clin Proc* 1978;53:100–112.
65. Melhuish BPP, Van Praagh R. Juxtaposition of the atrial appendages: a sign of severe cyanotic congenital heart disease. *Br Heart J* 1968; 30:269–284.
66. Rice M, Seward JB, Hagler DJ, et al. Left juxtaposed atrial appendages: diagnostic two-dimensional echocardiographic features. *J Am Coll Cardiol* 1983;1:1330–1336.
67. Freedom RM, Wilson G, Trusler GA, et al. Pulmonary atresia and intact ventricular septum. A review of the anatomy, myocardium, and factors influencing right ventricular growth. *Scand J Thorac Cardiovasc Surg* 1983;17:1–28.
68. Freedom RM, Culham JAG, Moes CAF. *Angiocardiography of congenital heart disease.* New York: Macmillan, 1984.
69. Zuberbuhler JR, Anderson RH. Morphological variations in pulmo-nary atresia with intact ventricular septum. *Br Heart J* 1979;41: 281–288.
70. Leung MP, Mok CK, Hui PW. Echocardiographic assessment of neonates with pulmonary atresia and intact ventricular septum. *J Am Coll Cardiol* 1988;12:719–725.
71. Giglia TM, Jenkins KJ, Matitiau A, et al. Influence of right heart size on outcome in pulmonary atresia with intact ventricular septum. *Circulation* 1993;88(Pt I):2248–2256.
72. Giglia TM, Mandell VS, Connor AR, et al. Diagnosis and management of right ventricle-dependent coronary circulation in pulmonary atresia with intact ventricular septum. *Circulation* 1992;86:1516–1528.
73. Hanley FL, Sade RM, Blackstone EH, et al. Outcomes in neonatal pulmonary atresia with intact ventricular septum. A multiinstitutional study. *J Thorac Cardiovasc Surg* 1993;105:406–423.
74. Sanders SP, Parness IA, Colan SD. Recognition of abnormal connections of coronary arteries with the use of Doppler color flow mapping. *J Am Coll Cardiol* 1989;13:922–926.
75. Van Praagh R, David I, Van Praagh S. What is a ventricle? The single-ventricle trap. *Pediatr Cardiol* 1982;2:79–84.
76. Wilkinson JL, Becker AE, Tynan M, et al. Nomenclature of the univentricular heart. *Herz* 1979;4:107–112.
77. Huhta JC, Seward JB, Tajik AJ, et al. Two-dimensional echocardiographic spectrum of univentricular atrioventricular connection. *J Am Coll Cardiol* 1985;5:149–157.
78. Bevilacqua M, Sanders SP, Van Praagh S, et al. Double-inlet single left ventricle: echocardiographic anatomy with emphasis on the morphology of the atrioventricular valves and ventricular septal defect. *J Am Coll Cardiol* 1991;18:559–568.
79. Sahn DJ, Harder JR, Freedom RM, et al. Cross-sectional echocardiographic diagnosis and subclassification of univentricular hearts: imaging studies of atrioventricular valves, septal structures and rudimentary outflow chambers. *Circulation* 1982;66:1070–1077.
80. Matitiau A, Geva T, Colan SD, et al. Bulboventricular foramen size in infants with double-inlet left ventricle or tricuspid atresia with transposed great arteries: influence on initial palliative operation and rate of growth. *J Am Coll Cardiol* 1992;19:142–148.
81. Shiraishi H, Silverman NH. Echocardiographic spectrum of double inlet ventricle: evaluation of the interventricular communication. *J Am Coll Cardiol* 1990;15:1401–1408.
82. Chin AJ, Weinberg PM, Barber G. Subcostal two-dimensional echocardiographic identification of anomalous attachment of septum primum in patients with left atrioventricular valve underdevelopment. *J Am Coll Cardiol* 1990;15:678–681.
83. Fallot A. Contribution a l'anatomie pathologique de la maladie bleue. *Marseille-Medical* 1888;25:77–93, 136–158, 207–223, 270–286, 341–354, 403–420.
84. Van Praagh R. Etienne-Louis Arthur Fallot and his tetralogy: a new translation of Fallot's summary and a modern reassessment of this anomaly. *Eur J Cardiothorac Surg* 1989;3:381–386.
85. Geva T, Ayres NA, Pac FA, et al. Quantitative morphometric analysis of progressive infundibular obstruction in tetralogy of Fallot. A prospective longitudinal echocardiographic study. *Circulation* 1995;92: 886–892.
86. Fellows KE, Freed MD, Keane JF, et al. Results of routine preoperative coronary angiography in tetralogy of Fallot. *Circulation* 1975; 51:561–566.
87. Jureidini SB, Appleton RS, Nouri S, et al. Detection of coronary artery abnormalities in tetralogy of Fallot by two-dimensional echocardiography. *J Am Coll Cardiol* 1989;14:960–967.
88. Van Praagh R, Perez-Trevino C, Lopez-Cuellar M, et al. Transposition of the great arteries with posterior aorta, anterior pulmonary artery, subpulmonary conus and fibrous continuity between aortic and atrioventricular valves. *Am J Cardiol* 1971;28:621–631.
89. Van Praagh R. Transposition of the great arteries: history, pathologic anatomy, embryology, etiology, and surgical considerations. *Cardiac Surg: State of the Art Rev* 1991;5:7–82.
90. Pasquini L, Sanders SP, Parness IA, et al. Conal anatomy in 119 patients with d-loop transposition of the great arteries and ventricular septal defect: an echocardiographic and pathologic study. *J Am Coll Cardiol* 1993;21:1712–1721.
91. Bierman FZ, Williams RG. Prospective diagnosis of d-transposition of the great arteries in neonates by subxiphoid, two-dimensional echocardiography. *Circulation* 1979;60:1496–1502.

92. King DL, Steeg CN, Ellis K. Demonstration of transposition of the great arteries by cardiac sonography. *Radiology* 1973;107:181–186.
93. Pasquini L, Sanders SP, Parness IA, et al. Coronary echocardiography in 406 patients with d-loop transposition of the great arteries. *J Am Coll Cardiol* 1994;24:763–768.
94. Pasquini L, Parness IA, Colan SD, et al. Diagnosis of intramural coronary artery in transposition of the great arteries using two-dimensional echocardiography. *Circulation* 1993;88:1136–1141.
95. Collett RW, Edwards JE. Persistent truncus arteriosus: A classification according to anatomic types. *Surg Clin North Am* 1949;29:1245–1270.
96. Becker AE, Becker MJ, Edwards JE. Pathology of the semilunar valve in persistent truncus arteriosus. *J Thorac Cardiovasc Surg* 1971;62:16–26.
97. Moes CAF, Freedom RM. Aortic arch interruption with truncus arteriosus or aorticopulmonary septal defect. *Am J Roentgenol* 1980;135:1011–1016.
98. Riggs TW, Paul MH. Two-dimensional echocardiographic prospective diagnosis of common truncus arteriosus in infants. *Am J Cardiol* 1982;50:1380–1384.
99. Hagler DJ, Tajik AJ, Seward JB, et al. Double-outlet right ventricle: wide-angle two-dimensional echocardiographic observations. *Circulation* 1981;63:419–428.
100. Van Praagh S, Davidoff A, Chin A, et al. Double-outlet right ventricle: anatomic types and developmental implications based on a study of 101 cases. *Coeur* (Paris) 1982;12:389–439.
101. Lucas RV, Woolfrey BF, Anderson RC, et al. Atresia of the common pulmonary vein. *Pediatrics* 1962;29:729–739.
102. Darling RC, Rothney WB, Craig JM. Total pulmonary venous drainage into the right side of the heart. *Lab Invest* 1957;6:44–64.
103. Delisle G, Ando M, Calder AL, et al. Total anomalous pulmonary venous connection: report of 93 autopsied cases with emphasis on diagnostic and surgical considerations. *Am Heart J* 1976;91:99–122.
104. Brown VE, De Lange M, Dyar DA, et al. Echocardiographic spectrum of supracardiac total anomalous pulmonary venous connection. *J Am Soc Echocardiogr* 1998;11:289–293.
105. Huhta JC, Gutgesell HP, Nihill MR. Cross sectional echocardiographic diagnosis of total anomalous pulmonary venous connection. *Br Heart J* 1985;53:525–534.
106. Smallhorn JF, Freedom RM. Pulsed Doppler echocardiography in the preoperative evaluation of total anomalous pulmonary venous connection. *J Am Coll Cardiol* 1986;8:1413–1420.
107. Van der Velde ME, Parness IA, Colan SD, et al. Two-dimensional echocardiography in the pre- and postoperative management of totally anomalous pulmonary venous connection. *J Am Coll Cardiol* 1991;18:1746–1751.

CHAPTER 56

Palliated and Corrected Congenital Heart Disease

Girish S. Shirali and Anne P. Osher

As cardiac diagnostic, interventional, and surgical modalities continue to improve, the growing population of patients with palliated or corrected congenital heart defects requires increasing numbers of care providers who are experienced in the care of these patients. Expertise is required in multiple modalities, including clinical follow-up, cardiac imaging, patient management, and interventional or surgical procedures. Echocardiography in patients who have undergone treatment for structural cardiac defects is challenging. The surgical or transcatheter treatment, palliation, or correction of congenital heart defects represents an ongoing effort toward excellence. Unusual surgical approaches may be devised for individual defects, resulting in unique postoperative echocardiographic appearances. The echocardiographer must be able to use his knowledge of normal and abnormal cardiac anatomy to mentally construct an image of the native defect, the repair, and the residua. To this end, the echocardiographer must master the evaluation of native congenital heart defects in terms of imaging of cardiac structure. A thorough knowledge of hemodynamics and pathophysiology is essential. Armed with this knowledge, the echocardiographer must understand the objectives and structural results of surgical repair or palliation. He must be cognizant of the untoward effects of certain surgical repairs, and be able to master the echocardiographic views used to demonstrate postoperative anatomy. The limitations of echocardiographic evaluation, particularly with large adult patients, must be understood as well.

This chapter is an overview of surgical procedures and postsurgical echocardiographic imaging for the forms of congenital heart disease that were discussed in Chapter 55. For each defect, description of surgical treatment is coupled with echocardiographic findings, with emphasis on visual pattern recognition. The components of postoperative echocardiography that are of particular relevance to an individual palliative or corrective operation are emphasized with a view toward developing a methodical process of comprehensive imaging for individual patients.

VENTRICULAR SEPTAL DEFECT

Surgery

The objective of surgery is to achieve closure of the ventricular septal defect (VSD). This is indicated for patients with symptoms of congestive heart failure, pulmonary hypertension, aortic regurgitation [typically with supracristal (conal septal) defects], and subaortic membranes or double-chambered right ventricle (RV) (typically with membranous defects).

Surgery consists of closure of the VSD using a prosthetic patch, which is sutured onto the right side of the ventricular septum. An important part of the conduction system, namely the bundle of His, typically courses along the posterior, inferior rim of a membranous defect to reach the septal surface of the left ventricle (LV). Patch sutures are placed at a safe distance from this rim; as a result, residual shunts following patch closure of membranous defects are more likely to occur along the posterior, inferior rim of the patch. Small residual defects are frequently seen following surgical closure of large VSDs; these defects may exhibit spontaneous closure at follow-up evaluation (1). Echocardiographic studies performed following VSD closure have revealed residual VSD and predominantly left-sided sequelae, including mitral or aortic regurgitation, subaortic stenosis, LV dilation, hypertrophy, or dysfunction (2).

Echocardiography

A VSD patch appears as a linear echo-density in the ventricular septum (Fig. 1). Postoperative echocardiograms

G. S. Shirali: Department of Pediatrics, Medical University of South Carolina; Medical University of South Carolina Children's Hospital, Charleston, South Carolina 29425.

A. P. Osher: Pediatric Echograph Laboratory, Loma Linda Children's Hospital, Loma Linda, California 92354.

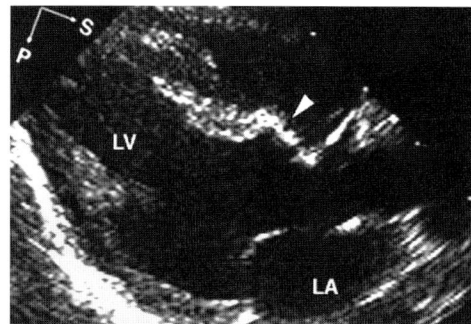

FIG. 1. Ventricular septal defect (VSD) patch: parasternal long-axis view shows a linear echodensity (*arrowhead*) in the ventricular septum, where a VSD patch has been placed. *LA*, left atrium; *LV*, left ventricle.

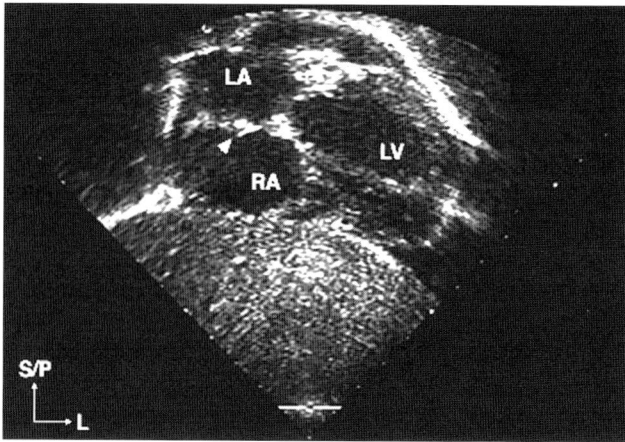

FIG. 2. Atrial septal defect (ASD) patch: subcostal long-axis view shows a linear echodensity (*arrowhead*) in the atrial septum, where an ASD patch has been placed. *LA*, left atrium; *LV*, left ventricle; *RA*, right atrium.

should evaluate the VSD patch, and include two-dimensional imaging and color flow Doppler interrogation of all the margins of the patch, looking for residual defects. Free mobility of the patch margin(s), coupled with a large left-to-right shunt, is consistent with patch dehiscence, which usually requires reoperation. The outflow tracts are assessed for obstruction (which may be unmasked following VSD closure), and the atrioventricular (AV) and semilunar valves are evaluated for regurgitation and stenosis. The tricuspid valve is assessed closely for stenosis or regurgitation, particularly if valve leaflets were detached in order to visualize VSD margins. Assessment for pulmonary hypertension is performed as detailed in the previous chapter. Chamber sizes and ventricular function should be assessed serially.

ATRIAL SEPTAL DEFECT

Surgery

Closure of atrial septal defect (ASD) is undertaken to prevent the long-term consequences of atrial dysrhythmias secondary to right atrial dilatation and pulmonary hypertension.

Conventional treatment consists of surgical closure, utilizing either direct suture apposition or a prosthetic/pericardial patch. The treatment of secundum ASD is being revolutionized by the availability of transcatheter device closure of these defects. Sinus venosus defects are closed with a patch that directs pulmonary venous flow to the left atrium.

Echocardiography

An ASD patch is seen as a linear echodensity in the atrial septum (Fig. 2). Long-term echocardiographic studies following ASD closure have revealed RV dilatation and, less frequently, residual ASD (3,4); echocardiographic evaluation following ASD closure includes assessment for residual defects, right-sided chamber enlargement, and elevated RV pressure. Following closure of sinus venosus defects, the pulmonary veins are evaluated for obstruction or abnormal drainage; transesophageal echocardiography may be re-

quired for this purpose. Echocardiograms obtained following transcatheter device closure of an ASD include evaluation for residual leak, device position (ideally straddling the atrial septum with device arms on the appropriate sides of the septum), and device impingement on the atrial inflow and outflow tracts.

PATENT DUCTUS ARTERIOSUS

Treatment

The indications for treatment of a patent ductus arteriosus (PDA) include congestive heart failure due to pulmonary over-circulation and pulmonary hypertension. Because the procedure of PDA closure is associated with minimal risk, the list of indications for PDA closure has grown to include elimination of the lifelong risk of infectious endocarditis (in this case, infectious endarteritis), even when the PDA is detected as an incidental finding.

Elimination of ductal patency is achieved via surgical ligation/division or transcatheter (coil) occlusion.

Echocardiography

Echocardiograms obtained following occlusion of a PDA should evaluate for residual shunt, left-sided chamber sizes, ventricular function, and RV pressure. The left pulmonary artery (PA) may undergo inadvertent distortion during the procedure, and should be evaluated for stenosis. When a coil is employed for ductal occlusion, it is visualized as an echodense shadow in a plane between the left PA and the descending thoracic aorta. Echocardiograms following coil occlusion should (in addition to evaluation for residual shunt) assess specifically for protrusion of the coil causing obstruction to flow in the left PA or the aorta.

AV CANAL DEFECTS

Surgery

Surgery is undertaken in order to prevent or treat pulmonary overcirculation, pulmonary hypertension, and AV valve regurgitation. The goals of surgical repair are closure of the ASD and VSD, division of the common AV valve into two competent and nonstenotic AV valves, and repair of associated defects. Surgical repair of complete AV canal defects consists of single- or double-patch closure of the ASD and VSD, with reconstruction or division and resuspension of the common AV valve (5). Postoperative findings of hemodynamic significance may include mitral regurgitation, VSD, and subaortic stenosis. Rarely, AV valvar stenosis may occur following repair of complete AV canal defect, due to unequal partitioning of the common AV valve.

Echocardiography

Echocardiography following repair of complete AV canal defect reveals the echodense, linear prosthetic patch(es) used to close the contiguous ASD, and VSD; the two AV valves are seen in the same horizontal plane (absence of AV valve offset) (Fig. 3). Postoperative echocardiography includes evaluation of each component of the repair (ASD and VSD closure, AV valve resuspension or repair), and assessment for new lesions. The morphologic basis for mitral regurgitation (residual cleft in the anterior leaflet versus annular dilation) is established. Serial echocardiographic evaluation following repair of AV canal defects is important because certain associated lesions (such as subaortic stenosis) may progress even after repair of these defects. In addition, the operated heart is subjected to the stresses of linear growth of the patient; thus, AV valves, in particular, may be competent initially following repair, but may subsequently become re-

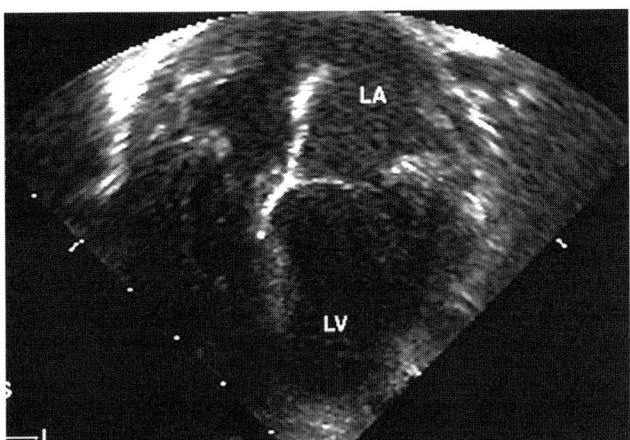

FIG. 3. Arterioventricular (AV) canal repair: apical four-chamber view shows a linear echodensity in the atrial and (contiguous) ventricular septa, representing patch closure of complete AV canal defect. The AV valves insert onto the cardiac crux at the same horizontal level. *LA*, left atrium; *LV*, left ventricle.

gurgitant. In the setting of Down syndrome, it is especially important to serially evaluate PA pressures to detect pulmonary hypertension.

PULMONARY STENOSIS

Treatment

Treatment of pulmonary valve stenosis is undertaken to pressure unload the RV. Relief of stenosis is achieved via transcatheter balloon valvuloplasty or surgical repair consisting of pulmonary valvotomy or valvectomy and a transannular patch. Surgical treatment is usually needed in the setting of a dysplastic and/or hypoplastic pulmonary valve (6). Hemodynamic sequelae encountered following balloon pulmonary valvuloplasty include residual valvar and infundibular stenosis, and pulmonary regurgitation. Right heart structures (tricuspid and pulmonary valve annulus) and the main and branch PAs have been shown to grow at rates similar to or exceeding those of normal control subjects (7).

Echocardiography

Echocardiography following transcatheter or surgical relief of valvar pulmonary stenosis includes evaluation for residual stenosis, and assessment of the presence and severity of pulmonary insufficiency. Relief of valvar pulmonary stenosis may unmask proximal (subvalvar) or distal (supravalvar or branch PA) stenosis. Clinically useful parameters that must be evaluated by serial echocardiography include estimation of RV pressure, assessment of the presence and severity of tricuspid regurgitation, and evaluation of right-sided chamber sizes and the branch PA.

MITRAL STENOSIS

Treatment

Mitral stenosis usually occurs in association with other defects, which frequently include hemodynamically significant hypoplasia of the left heart structures; the nature and severity of associated defects is likely to determine the nature and timing of intervention. Thus, a neonate with mitral stenosis as part of hypoplastic left heart syndrome would be placed in the treatment algorithm for the entire complex of defects. The goals for treatment of isolated mitral stenosis are to establish unobstructed prograde flow across the mitral valve, while maintaining valvar competence. Transcatheter balloon or surgical valvuloplasty is the procedure of choice; mitral valve replacement may be needed in some cases. Residual stenosis, or new or increased mitral regurgitation may develop following any intervention to relieve mitral stenosis.

Echocardiography

Echocardiograms obtained following treatment of mitral stenosis should evaluate for residual or recurrent stenosis, and for new or increased regurgitation. Serial studies are needed due to the potentially impaired ability of the repaired mitral valve to keep pace with linear growth of the patient.

SUBAORTIC STENOSIS

Surgery

The objectives of surgery in patients with subaortic stenosis include relief of LV pressure overload, and removal of the substrate for aortic insufficiency (which is attributed either to the impact of the eccentric LV outflow jet on the aortic valve, or to extension of a subaortic membrane tethering the aortic valve leaflets). Membranous subaortic stenosis is treated by resecting the membrane. Tunnel-type subaortic stenosis necessitates enlargement of the entire LV outflow tract including the frequently hypoplastic aortic valve and annulus. The preferred technique for relief of tunnel-type subaortic stenosis consists of resection of the obstruction and enlargement of the LV outflow tract with a prosthetic patch (8), retaining the integrity of the aortic annulus and thus maintaining the native aortic valve. If the native aortic annulus is hypoplastic, enlargement of the aortic root via septal myomectomy (and patch closure of the resulting VSD) is coupled with replacement of the aortic valve with either a mechanical prosthesis, the Konno-Rastan procedure (9) or a pulmonary autograft, the Konno-Ross procedure (10).

Echocardiography

Serial postoperative echocardiograms should assess for residual or recurrent stenosis (which is frequently encountered in this condition) and for new or increased aortic and/or mitral regurgitation. The location and width of regurgitant jets is best evaluated from parasternal short-axis views. Obstruction at levels proximal or distal to the LV outflow tract may be unmasked following relief of subaortic stenosis. Thus, mitral inflow patterns should be evaluated for mitral stenosis, and flow profiles in the ascending and descending aorta should be evaluated for supravalvar aortic stenosis and coarctation of the aorta, respectively.

VALVAR AORTIC STENOSIS

Treatment

The goals of treatment for valvar aortic stenosis are to pressure-unload the LV by providing unobstructed LV outflow with a competent (nonregurgitant) aortic valve. Preintervention echocardiographic quantification of the degree of left heart hypoplasia (represented by LV cavity size, inflow and outflow) helps decide between biventricular repair and the option of a single-ventricle (Norwood-type) approach (11). Treatment choices that follow the biventricular route are either transcatheter (balloon) or surgical aortic valvuloplasty; the choice between these two modalities is unrelated to echocardiographic parameters and is outside the scope of this chapter. Regardless of whether balloon or surgical valvuloplasty is utilized, recurrence of stenosis and pro-

gressive increase in the severity of aortic regurgitation should be sought on follow-up (12,13).

Echocardiography

Postintervention echocardiograms should assess for aortic valve cusp mobility, coaptation, and residual stenosis. New or increased aortic insufficiency is sought; the location and width of the regurgitant jet and the morphologic substrate for aortic regurgitation are evaluated. As for other obstructive lesions, obstruction at levels proximal or distal to the aortic valve may be unmasked following relief of valvar aortic stenosis; these are sought specifically. The value of serial study cannot be overemphasized; aortic valvar stenosis or regurgitation may recur and progress, and other levels of LV inflow or outflow tract obstruction may manifest themselves with linear growth.

SUPRAVALVAR AORTIC STENOSIS

The goals of surgery are to achieve an unobstructed path for LV ejection into the aorta. Since supravalvar aortic stenosis is a diffuse process typically affecting the length of the ascending aorta, surgery typically consists of patch augmentation extending from the sinuses of Valsalva into the ascending aorta beyond the distal extent of the stenotic segment. This lesion may recur; surgery in proximity to the aortic valve may adversely affect valvar competence.

Postoperative echocardiograms should evaluate for residual stenosis and for new or increased aortic insufficiency. Proximal and distal levels of obstruction such as mitral stenosis, valvar aortic stenosis, and coarctation of the aorta may be unmasked after repair of supravalvar aortic stenosis, and should be sought specifically.

COARCTATION OF THE AORTA

Treatment

The goals for treatment of coarctation of the aorta consist of establishing an unobstructed communication from the ascending aorta to the descending thoracic aorta. This is usually performed surgically, with resection of the coarctation and either an end-to-end anastomosis or a subclavian artery flap. Transcatheter balloon angioplasty is being utilized for treatment of coarctation of the aorta in some centers. The choice between these two modalities is unrelated to echocardiographic parameters and is outside the scope of this chapter. The outcome following balloon angioplasty of native coarctation of the aorta can be predicted by preangioplasty echocardiographic measurement of aortic isthmus diameter and aortic valve annulus diameter (14). Regardless of the modality used, the treatment of coarctation may be inadequate (residual coarctation); alternatively, growth of the coarctation site may fail to keep pace with linear growth (recurrent coarctation). Intimal tears or either dissecting or true aneurysms may develop at the site of repair. Obstruction at proximal or distal sites may be unmasked by relieving coarctation.

Echocardiography

Postintervention or postoperative echocardiograms should assess for residual or recurrent coarctation; serial studies are essential in this context. Luminal irregularities may be difficult to detect even with the use of high-frequency transducers; magnetic resonance imaging may be more useful for this purpose. Residual or new proximal and distal obstructions are sought as well.

EBSTEIN ANOMALY

Surgery

The goals of surgery for Ebstein anomaly of the tricuspid valve are to achieve a competent, nonstenotic tricuspid valve, and to treat associated defects such as ASD (a frequent finding in this condition). Surgery consists of tricuspid valve repair (annuloplasty and/or valvuloplasty, fashioning a "monocusp" from the anterior leaflet of the tricuspid valve), or replacement with a prosthetic valve if repair is not an option. Neonates with severe forms of Ebstein anomaly may be staged toward a single-ventricle (Fontan) repair.

Echocardiography

Echocardiographic evaluation of tricuspid valve function following surgery for Ebstein anomaly includes assessment of prograde and regurgitant tricuspid valve flow. Enlargement of the right atrium may persist following surgical repair of Ebstein anomaly. The repair of associated defects (such as ASD) should be evaluated as well. RV function is evaluated qualitatively. Because the natural history of Ebstein anomaly includes the possibility of progressive LV dysfunction, this should be sought with serial studies.

L-LOOP VENTRICLES ("VENTRICULAR INVERSION") WITH L-TRANSPOSITION OF THE GREAT ARTERIES

Because the pattern of blood flow is "physiologically corrected," surgery is not performed for this lesion per se; it may be required for associated defects, which are frequently encountered. The RV and tricuspid valve are subjected to systemic workloads, with the long-term eventuality of ventricular dysfunction and tricuspid valve regurgitation. One aggressive surgical approach has been to perform a "double-switch" operation, consisting of an arterial switch coupled with an atrial switch (Senning or Mustard) operation. The potential advantages of this surgical approach are that it reverts to physiologically normal ventricular loading patterns, that is, the LV is converted into the systemic ventricle; however, the double switch operation is not widely accepted. Echocardiographic features following the atrial and arterial

switch procedures are discussed individually in the section "d-transposition of the Great Arteries" later in this chapter.

TETRALOGY OF FALLOT

Surgery

Corrective surgery for tetralogy of Fallot may be preceded by a palliative aortopulmonary shunt procedure to augment pulmonary blood flow. Direct end-to-side anastomosis of the subclavian artery to the ipsilateral branch PA was devised by Blalock and Taussig (the classic Blalock-Taussig shunt) (15). A modification of this procedure, utilizing a Gore-Tex tube graft that extends from the side of the subclavian artery to the side of the ipsilateral branch PA (the modified Blalock-Taussig shunt) is used today to augment pulmonary blood flow.

The goals of corrective surgery in tetralogy of Fallot are to provide an unobstructed pulmonary outflow tract and to eliminate intracardiac shunting. As originally described, repair of tetralogy of Fallot consisted of VSD closure through a RV anterior free-wall incision, extensive resection of hypertrophied obstructive infundibular muscle, and patch augmentation of the RV outflow tract. The pulmonary valve was excised, and the patch was carried across the level of the pulmonary valve into the main PA (transannular patch) (16). Currently, VSD closure is performed via the right atrium. Obstructive RV muscle is excised via a limited incision in the RV outflow tract or via the RA. This technique has been associated with less RV dilation and dysfunction (17); however, it may result in inadequate relief of RV outflow tract obstruction. Associated cardiac defects are addressed at the time of corrective surgery, and previously placed aortopulmonary shunts are taken down. Patients with tetralogy of Fallot with pulmonary atresia require the placement of a conduit, typically a homograft, from the RV to the branch PAs.

The components of surgical repair of tetralogy of Fallot are associated with inherent sequelae that may adversely affect the RV. Removal of the pulmonary valve allows free pulmonary regurgitation, resulting in a volume-overloaded, dilated RV. The combination of subpulmonary muscle resection and impaired concentric muscle contraction due to the right ventriculotomy and transannular patch may contribute to depressed RV systolic function (18). RV dilation results in dilation of the tricuspid annulus; over time, this may result in a progressive increase in the severity of tricuspid regurgitation and right atrial enlargement. RV hypertrophy typically regresses after surgical correction of tetralogy of Fallot (19). Recurrence or an increase in RV hypertrophy at any time following surgery should raise the suspicion of recurrent RV outflow tract obstruction, due to failure of the outflow tract structures to keep pace with linear growth or due to scarring. Pulmonary homografts may exhibit calcification or scarring affecting the entire homograft including the valve, resulting in progressive obstruction to flow. Decreased coaptation of the homograft valve leaflets may lead to pulmonary insufficiency. Between 10 and 15% of patients may require reoperation for residual pulmonary stenosis or insufficiency, residual VSD and true or false aneurysms of the RV outflow tract (20,21). RV systolic and diastolic function is impaired in most patients following repair (22). LV function may be impaired, particularly after corrective surgery at an older age (23).

Echocardiography

Palliative aortopulmonary shunts are seen as tubular echodense structures extending from the undersurface of the subclavian artery to the side of the ipsilateral branch PA (Fig. 4; see also Color Plate 37 following page 758). The entire length of the shunt is examined for kinks or areas of stenosis. The PA should be carefully evaluated for distortion or stenosis in the immediate vicinity of the shunt.

Certain typical echocardiographic features are evident following complete repair of tetralogy of Fallot. The VSD patch is seen as a linear echodensity in the ventricular septum (Fig. 5). The specific findings on evaluation of the RV outflow tract are widely variable, depending on what specific levels of obstruction existed preoperatively, the extent of surgical relief and the degree of recurrence of obstruction. Each component of the repair, including assessment for residual VSD, is evaluated. Residual or recurrent RV outflow tract obstruction is assessed by interrogating the subvalvar region, the pulmonary annulus and valve leaflets (if present), and the main and branch PAs. Any of these areas may be narrowed, reflecting obstruction to flow; enlargement of these areas, reflecting aneurysm formation or dilatation, may be indicators of distal obstruction. Stenosis and obstruction to flow may be progressive, necessitating serial studies. Serial echocardiographic evaluation includes assessment for RV size,

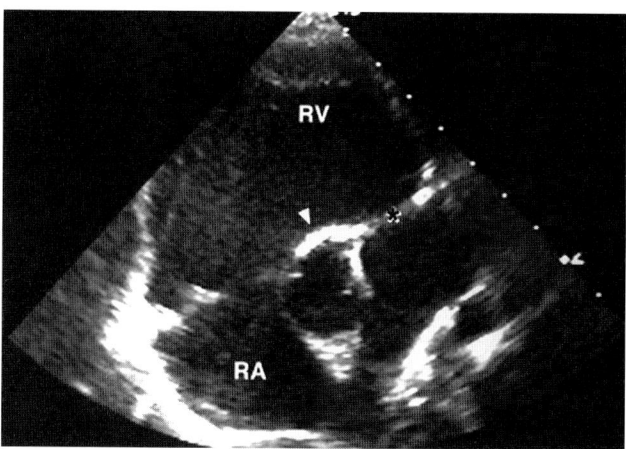

FIG. 5. Tetralogy of Fallot repair: parasternal short-axis view shows a linear echodense ventricular septal defect patch (*arrowhead*). The pulmonary valve (*asterisk*) is rudimentary. The right ventricle is dilated and hypertrophic. The main and proximal right pulmonary arteries are of good size. *RA*, right atrium; *RV*, right ventricle.

pressure, and systolic function. Echocardiography has been found to be a reliable method for distinguishing between true or pseudo-aneurysms of the RV, either of which may occur following repair of tetralogy of Fallot, particularly if a homograft is placed (24).

PULMONARY ATRESIA WITH INTACT VENTRICULAR SEPTUM

Treatment

The widely variable severity of right heart (tricuspid valve and RV) hypoplasia results in a wide range of treatment options, all of which start in infancy. Thus, a mild case with an adequate-sized tricuspid valve and RV is treated by establishing prograde flow from the RV across the pulmonary valve to the main PA to encourage right heart growth (25,26). Transcatheter perforation of the atretic pulmonary valve plate, or surgical placement of a transannular patch may be undertaken for this purpose. An aortopulmonary shunt may be placed simultaneously to ensure adequate flow into the branch PAs (27). An ASD may be created via balloon atrial septostomy or open surgical atrial septectomy.

The rate of subsequent right heart growth is variable, resulting in a range of future treatment choices. If right heart growth is adequate, a complete biventricular repair may be achieved by closing the previously created ASD and elimination of the aortopulmonary shunt. In intermediate cases, where the right heart can handle part (but not all) of the systemic venous return, a "one and a half ventricle" type repair may be undertaken. In this procedure, superior vena cava (SVC) flow is directed into the PA (the SVC is divided, and its cranial end is connected to the side of the right PA: the bidirectional Glenn shunt), coupled with closure of the ASD and closure of the aortopulmonary shunt. This operation leaves only inferior vena caval and coronary sinus flow

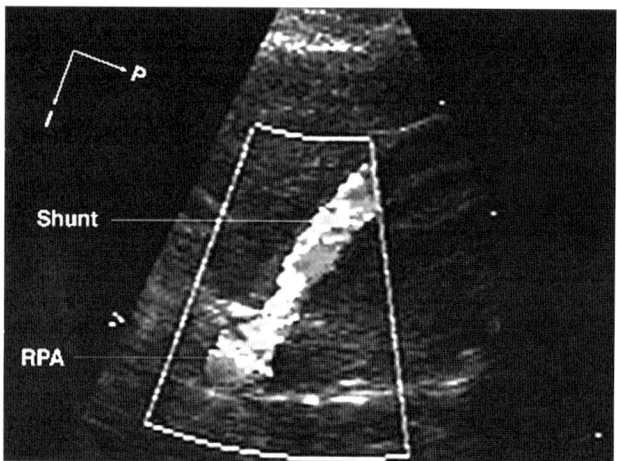

FIG. 4. Modified Blalock-Taussig shunt: suprasternal long-axis view shows a tubular structure of uniform diameter (a shunt made of prosthetic material) extending from the side of the subclavian artery to the side of the ipsilateral branch PA. There is mild discrete narrowing of the pulmonary end of the shunt. (See also Color Plate 37 following page 758.)

returning to the RV-an arrangement, which is viable in the setting of a moderately hypoplastic RV.

Institutional practices vary for patients with severe degrees of right heart hypoplasia. In some centers, staged reconstruction aimed at Fontan-type single-ventricle repair is undertaken in all cases. Other centers perform RV decompression (as noted above) regardless of right heart size, except in the presence of a right-ventricle dependent coronary circulation (28,29). When the latter exists, coronary perfusion may be compromised if the RV is decompressed; therefore, treatment consists of a staged single-ventricle (Fontan) type of repair. The first stage, in this situation, would consist of an atrial septostomy and an aortopulmonary (modified Blalock-Taussig type) shunt. The subsequent stages of the Fontan series of operations are described in the "Functionally Single Ventricle" section later in this chapter. Finally, in severe cases with myocardial ischemia and infarction, cardiac transplantation may be the only viable option.

Echocardiography

Regardless of the treatment path for the individual patient, serial echocardiography plays a critical role in the evaluation and management of patients with pulmonary atresia with intact ventricular septum. Comprehensive echocardiograms are an important part of the process that determines when further intervention is required and what is the most appropriate form of intervention. Echocardiography allows for accurate measurement of tricuspid valve annulus size, which has been shown to be the only patient-specific predictor of success of biventricular repair in this condition (27). Evaluation of the adequacy of surgically created communications (such as interatrial or aortopulmonary shunts, or a transannular patch to enable prograde flow from the RV to the main PA) is of great importance. Qualitative assessment of RV size and quantitation of RV pressure and LV function are important parameters. Serial echocardiography must also evaluate for branch PA growth, stenosis, or distortion. Finally, the velocity of flow across surgically created aortopulmonary shunts allows estimation of PA pressure. The echocardiographic evaluation of patients being staged toward a single-ventricle type of repair is discussed in the "Functionally Single Ventricle" section later in this chapter.

D-TRANSPOSITION OF THE GREAT ARTERIES

The objectives of surgery in patients with d-transposition of the great arteries (TGA) have evolved greatly in the last three decades. From the 1960s to the 1980s, surgery consisted of physiologic correction by switching the ventricular inflows (the "atrial switch"), thus placing the pulmonary and systemic circulations in series. The hemodynamic drawback to this approach is that the tricuspid valve and RV are subjected to systemic loading conditions, with resulting long-term sequelae including tricuspid regurgitation and RV dysfunction.

Surgery today achieves anatomic as well as physiologic correction via an arterial switch operation, wherein the great arteries are switched to "correct" transposition. In patients with d-TGA and a VSD that is committed to an unobstructed semilunar valve and outflow tract, surgical repair may consist of closing the VSD to that (unobstructed) outflow tract (the Rastelli repair, which is discussed in the "Double-outlet RV" section later in this chapter). This procedure may be combined with an arterial switch operation if needed.

THE ATRIAL SWITCH (MUSTARD OR SENNING PROCEDURE)

Surgery

The two types of atrial switch procedures differ in the anatomy of the baffles that redirect venous flows. Following an atrial septectomy, pericardium or prosthetic material (Mustard procedure) or excised atrial septum (Senning procedure) is used to fashion an intraatrial baffle along the posterior wall of the atria. This baffle directs superior and inferior vena caval blood to the mitral valve, and also directs pulmonary venous blood to the tricuspid valve. In the Mustard procedure, the SVC baffle makes a sharp turn immediately inferior to the entrance of the right upper pulmonary vein; the inferior vena caval baffle makes a gentler curve between the orifice of the coronary sinus and the right inferior pulmonary vein. These two locations are likely areas of future baffle obstruction. The technical details of the baffle used in the Senning procedure are quite complex, and are not discussed in this text. Systemic and pulmonary venous obstruction are both more likely following the Mustard procedure than following the Senning procedure. The RV performs systemic work following the atrial switch operation; RV hypertrophy is inevitable. Conversely, the LV performs low-pressure work, pumping into the pulmonary circulation; as a result, disproportion between the right and LV walls is evident. RV pressure-loading causes the ventricular septum to bulge into the pressure-deconditioned LV, which assumes a "pancaked" shape. This paradoxic bulge of the ventricular septum leads to dynamic LV outflow tract obstruction, which tends to progress with time. Progressive RV systolic dysfunction and tricuspid regurgitation occur frequently.

Echocardiography

The echocardiographic evaluation of a patient who has undergone an atrial switch operation requires a complete understanding of pathologic anatomy and the unique postoperative hemodynamics seen in this condition. The difference between the Mustard and Senning baffles cannot be ascertained by echocardiography. Echocardiography is used for serial evaluation of baffle patency and leaks, systemic (right) ventricular function and tricuspid valvar regurgitation, and acquired outflow tract obstruction. The systemic venous (su-

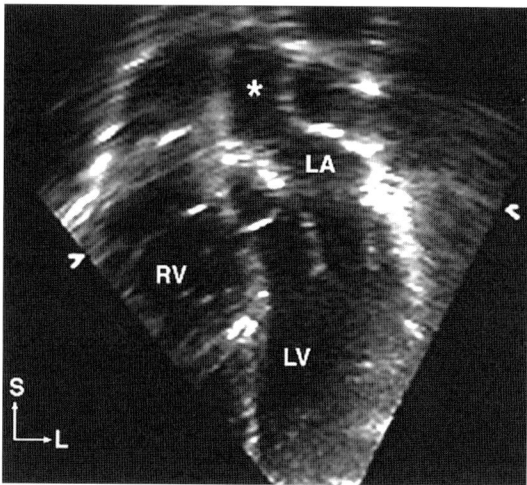

FIG. 6. Mustard operation, superior vena cava (SVC) baffle: apical four-chamber view shows the SVC baffle (*asterisk*) draining into the left ventricle (*LV*) via the mitral valve. The right ventricle (*RV*) is hypertrophied. The ventricular septum bulges into the LV due to elevated RV pressure. *LA*, left atrium.

perior and inferior vena caval) baffles (Fig. 6) and pulmonary venous drainage (Fig. 7) are all well seen using transthoracic echocardiography. Injection of echocardiographic contrast material into a systemic vein is used to evaluate for baffle leaks. Both the systemic venous baffles and the pulmonary venous drainage channel should allow low velocity, unobstructed flow without baffle leaks. Superior and, less commonly, inferior vena caval baffle obstruction may occur at the locations described above. Rarely, pulmonary venous drainage obstruction usually occurs anterior to the entrance of the right lower pulmonary vein. A caveat in

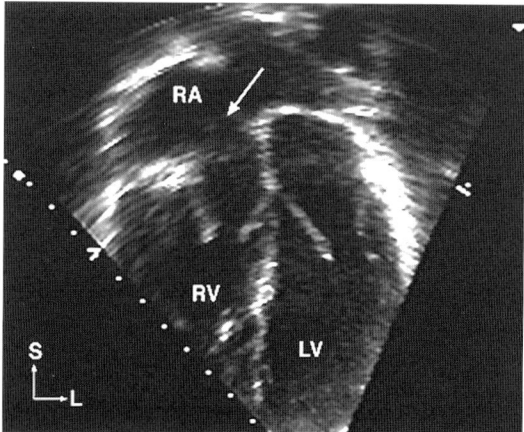

FIG. 7. Mustard operation, pulmonary venous baffle: Apical four-chamber view with posterior angulation shows the pulmonary venous drainage (*arrow*) into the leftward superior aspect of the right atrium. Pulmonary venous flow is directed into the right ventricle (*RV*) via the tricuspid valve. *LV*, left ventricle; *RA*, right atrium.

evaluation for baffle obstruction is the low velocity of venous flows; thus, localized alteration in phasicity of flow or localized turbulence of flow at a site of anatomic narrowing is much more important than arbitrary Doppler threshold values for determining venous baffle obstruction.

No criteria exist for the quantitative evaluation of RV function under systemic loading pressures; besides, the shape of the RV does not easily lend itself to geometric modeling. Therefore, serial qualitative evaluations of RV function and of the severity of tricuspid regurgitation are performed to enable early detection of RV decompensation. The echocardiographer must note that following the atrial switch operation, the velocity of mitral regurgitation reflects systolic PA pressure; conversely, the velocity of tricuspid regurgitation reflects systemic pressures.

THE ARTERIAL SWITCH PROCEDURE

Surgery

This procedure allows for anatomic correction of d-TGA. The aorta and main PA are transected just distal to the respective valves; the coronary arteries are mobilized from the native aorta, and are sutured into place into the "neo-aorta" (the native main PA, which arises from the LV). In order to provide adequate length of the main PA to connect it to the anteriorly placed RV outflow tract, the PA confluence and the right PA are moved anterior to the aortic root (Lecompte maneuver). The great arteries are then sutured into their anatomically "correct" locations; thus, the aorta and coronary arteries are aligned with the LV outflow tract, and the PA is aligned with the RV outflow tract. This "anatomic correction" has resulted in excellent survival (30) and good late hemodynamic results. Thus, over a 10-year follow-up period, Colan et al. (31) demonstrated that these patients have normal LV size, mass, and contractility, with no evidence of time-dependent deterioration of function. Longitudinal studies have revealed growth of the aortic anastomosis commensurate with linear growth (32). However, progressive dilation of the neoaortic annulus and root has been encountered, particularly in patients with neoaortic regurgitation or a history of PA banding. The cause-effect relationship between neoaortic root/annulus dilation and aortic regurgitation has not been clarified.

Echocardiography

Echocardiography provides for comprehensive evaluation following the arterial switch operation. The main and branch PAs have an unusual course following the Lecompte maneuver. The PA confluence is anterior to the ascending aorta, and the proximal branch PAs wrap around the ascending aorta as they dive posteriorly (Fig. 8). The left PA is stretched anteroposteriorly by this procedure, and may become stenotic or fail to develop adequately. Anastomotic suture lines are seen in both great arterial roots, and may be the sites of supravalvar (aortic or pulmonary) stenosis. Serial evaluation for neoaortic root dilation and valvar insuffi-

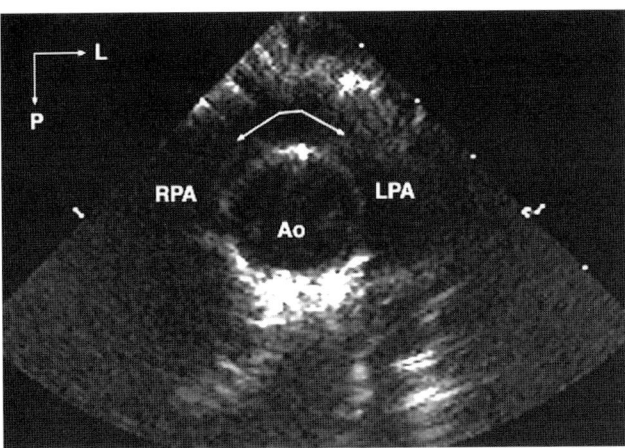

FIG. 8. Arterial switch operation, Lecompte maneuver: parasternal short-axis view shows the PA confluence anterior to the ascending aorta (*Ao*). The proximal branch pulmonary arteries (*arrows*) straddle the aorta to reach the pulmonary hilum. *LPA*, left pulmonary artery; *RPA*, right pulmonary artery.

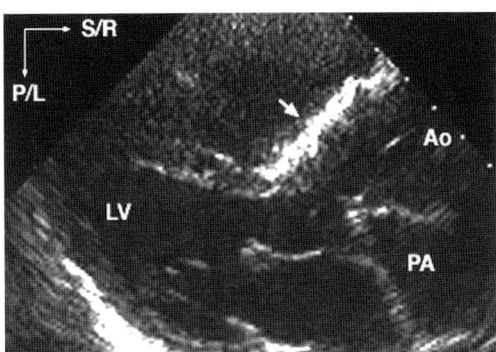

FIG. 9. Rastelli operation, VSD patch: parasternal long-axis shows a linear echodense patch (*arrow*) that has been directed to close the ventral septal defect (VSD) to the aorta (*Ao*). The (atretic) pulmonary outflow tract connects to the main pulmonary artery. See companion view (Fig. 10). *LV*, left ventricle; *PA*, pulmonary artery.

confluence. Stretching, kinking, and focal stenosis or diffuse hypoplasia of the branch PAs may also develop.

TRUNCUS ARTERIOSUS

Surgery

The objectives of surgery for truncus arteriosus are to separate the systemic and pulmonary circulations and to provide unobstructed ventricular outflows. Surgery for truncus arteriosus consists of patch closure of the VSD, disconnection of the PA from the truncal root, and reconstruction of the RV outflow tract with a pulmonary or aortic homograft, which is connected distally to the PA confluence (33). Repairs of associated defects, including a stenotic or regurgitant truncal valve, are also performed as needed. Repair of truncus arteriosus is typically undertaken within the first few months of life, with good prospects for survival (34,35). The presence of severe truncal insufficiency or associated defects such as an interrupted aortic arch or PA anomalies are preoperative predictors of poor surgical outcome.

Reoperation is frequently needed for patients who undergo repair of truncus arteriosus. Indications for reoperation include conduit/homograft obstruction (requiring conduit replacement), worsening truncal valve insufficiency (requiring valve replacement) and residual VSD (36). The homograft that is placed as part of the repair has no growth potential; this leads to inevitable "relative" stenosis with the patient's continued linear growth. Progressive homograft stenosis may also be due to scarring, fibrosis, and calcification. Stenosis may develop at various sites along the homograft: proximally at its RV attachment, or diffusely along its course, or distally at its attachment to the branch PA

Echocardiography

The typical echocardiographic appearance following repair of truncus arteriosus consists of the VSD patch, which channels LV outflow to the aorta, and the homograft conduit from the RV outflow tract to the PA confluence. This appearance is similar to that seen following the Rastelli operation for double-outlet RV with pulmonary outflow tract obstruction (discussed in the next section) (Figs. 9 and 10). Postoperative echocardiography can comprehensively assess repair of truncus arteriosus. The conduit/homograft requires careful evaluation for diffuse narrowing as well as focal stenosis at the anastomotic sites. Evaluation for homograft stenosis or regurgitation, residual VSD and for branch PA stenosis or distortion are also part of the postoperative echocardio-

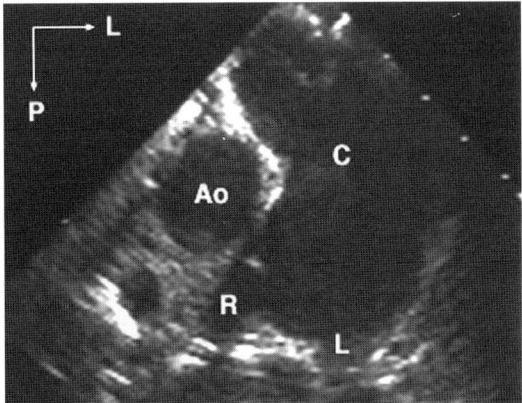

FIG. 10. Rastelli operation, RV-to-PA conduit: parasternal short-axis view shows the widely patent conduit (*C*) connecting the RV outflow tract to the branch pulmonary arteries (right [*R*] and left [*L*], respectively). See companion view (Fig. 9). *Ao*, aorta.

ciency (32), growth of the coronary anastomoses and evaluation of LV systolic function are other long-term issues that emphasize the need for serial study.

graphic evaluation. Truncal valvar stenosis or regurgitation may be progressive, and is assessed serially. Secondary effects of semilunar valvar stenosis or regurgitation, including progressive (right and/or left) ventricular hypertrophy, dilation, and dysfunction, are also sought.

DOUBLE-OUTLET RV

Surgery

Whereas the goal in all patients is successful completion of biventricular repair, the wide range of associated defects, especially outflow tract obstruction, VSD, and ventricular hypoplasia necessitates a range of options for surgical repair. Thus, a patient with a subaortic VSD and no outflow tract obstruction needs VSD closure to the aorta, allowing the LV to eject into the aorta. With a subpulmonary defect, the VSD is closed to the pulmonary valve; in addition, an arterial switch operation is performed. If pulmonary outflow obstruction is present with a malalignment-type VSD, the Rastelli procedure is performed. In this procedure, the VSD is closed to the aorta, and a conduit or homograft is placed from the RV to the main PA. Some patients may not be candidates for biventricular repair; this includes patients with a noncommitted (muscular or AV canal-type) VSD, or with hypoplasia of one (either the right or the left) ventricle. In such cases, the only surgical option is the staged reconstructive (Fontan) approach to single ventricle repair.

Residual VSD may occur following repair of double-outlet RV. These may be "intramural," around the edges of the patch anchored to the RV free wall near the aortic root. These defects are probably due to suturing of the VSD patch to trabeculations within the ventriculoinfundibular fold, rather than to the ventriculoinfundibular fold itself. As a result, blood flows from the neo-LV outflow tract, between the trabeculae, into the RV. The sites of entry of these flow channels into the RV sinus tends to be more lateral and posterior than the edge of the VSD patch, making for an unusual location of residual VSD flow (37). Other concepts of importance in patients following repair of double-outlet RV include the need for growth of cardiac structures commensurate with linear growth. In addition, structures distal to a site of obstruction may themselves be hypoplastic.

Echocardiography

The typical echocardiographic appearance following the Rastelli operation for double-outlet RV with pulmonary outflow tract obstruction is described in the previous section ("Truncus Arteriosus," Figs. 9 and 10). Comprehensive postoperative echocardiography requires a thorough understanding of native anatomy and surgical techniques. Echocardiographic evaluation is tailored to the specific operation(s) undertaken in an individual case. The principles of postoperative echocardiograms include evaluation for residual VSD, and evaluation of the outflow tracts for evidence of

progressive obstruction. The plane of the native ventricular septum is a common site of LV outflow tract obstruction, particularly when the aorta arises far rightward from the RV. As is true for other repairs, relief of outflow tract obstruction at one level may unmask obstruction at other levels proximally or distally, necessitating serial evaluation for multiple levels of obstruction.

FUNCTIONALLY SINGLE VENTRICLE

This category includes patients with tricuspid atresia, hypoplastic left heart syndrome, pulmonary atresia with intact ventricular septum with RV-dependent coronary circulation, and patients with true "single ventricle" (absent RV or LV). The goal of staged reconstruction is completion of the Fontan operation, separating the systemic and pulmonary venous circulations (38). This operation is based on the principle that within certain anatomic and physiologic constraints, systemic venous blood can pass through the PAs and pulmonary vascular bed and into the pulmonary venous atrium without being propelled by a ventricle or "pump." Only pulmonary venous (oxygenated) blood returns to the heart; therefore, the Fontan series of operations requires one atrium, one AV valve, one ventricle, and one semilunar valve. Oxygenated blood flows through these structures and is delivered to the body. The separation of circulations is performed in a staged fashion, typically involving two or three operations. The specifics of these stages are tailored to the individual patient. Completion of staged reconstruction in early life is associated with improved ventricular contractile mechanics (39). Thus, the first stage is usually undertaken in the neonate; the second stage is performed at age 6 to 9 months, and the final stage is performed at 18 to 24 months of age.

Hypoplasia of the PAs may be hemodynamically disadvantageous following the Fontan operation (40,41). In the presence of these and other conditions that hinder pulmonary blood flow, the Fontan operation may be completed with a fenestration in the systemic venous baffle to allow right-to-left shunting. This enables maintenance of cardiac output at the expense of oxygenation, and also limits elevation of right atrial pressure (42). The surgically created fenestration can be closed subsequently via transcatheter or other techniques.

STAGE 1: AORTOPULMONARY SHUNT

Surgery

Patients with pulmonary outflow tract obstruction and decreased pulmonary blood flow (such as patients with tricuspid atresia with ventriculoarterial concordance and a restrictive VSD or those with pulmonary atresia and an intact ventricular septum) may need an aortopulmonary shunt to provide controlled augmentation of pulmonary blood flow. The modified Blalock-Taussig shunt (using a Gore-Tex tube from the side of the subclavian artery to the side of the ipsilateral branch PA) is commonly used for this purpose.

Echocardiography

The echocardiographic appearance of the shunt is discussed in the "Tetralogy of Fallot" section earlier in this chapter. The entire length of the shunt (Fig. 4) must be visualized, because narrowing or kinking of the shunt may be localized and severe. PA distortion or stenosis may develop, particularly in the vicinity of the shunt; serial evaluation for this purpose is important. Measurement of the peak flow velocity in the shunt with concomitant recording of systemic blood pressure allows estimation of PA pressure; however, due to the long tubular nature of the shunt, the simplified Bernoulli equation may underestimate the gradient and therefore overestimate PA pressure.

STAGE 1: NORWOOD OPERATION

Surgery

Patients with hypoplastic left heart syndrome, or other similar conditions with hypoplasia of the LV and the aortic outflow tract and arch, require the Norwood operation as the first stage toward completing single-ventricle palliation. The goals of the Norwood operation are to allow unobstructed RV ejection into the systemic circulation, to establish unrestricted mixing at the atrial level, and to provide pressure- and volume-controlled PA blood flow. The components of this operation include aortic arch augmentation and use of the pulmonary valve as the "neo-aortic" valve. The main PA is transected, thus eliminating prograde flow into the branch PAs. Controlled PA blood flow is provided by means of an aortopulmonary shunt. An atrial septectomy is performed to ensure free mixing at the atrial level.

Echocardiography

All of the components of the Norwood operation may be imaged by echocardiography. The atrial septectomy leads to a wide-open interatrial communication. The aortopulmonary shunt is seen connecting to the isolated branch PAs. The contour of the reconstructed aortic arch is unusual (Fig. 11), with disproportion between the augmented ascending aorta and the normal-sized native descending thoracic aorta. Each of these components of the Norwood operation is individually assessed. PA size, distortion, and stenosis are sought. PA systolic pressures are estimated using the peak systolic gradient across the shunt, which probably underestimates the gradient due to the length of the shunt. The adequacy of the interatrial communication is assessed. Systemic ventricular function and systemic AV valve regurgitation are evaluated. The patency of the entire length of the aortopulmonary shunt is serially evaluated. The neoaortic arch is interrogated throughout its length for coarctation, which can occur at any location along the anastomosis. The echocardiographic diagnosis of neoaortic arch obstruction by echocardiography is highly specific but relatively insensitive; supportive criteria such as new AV valve regurgitation, new systemic ven-

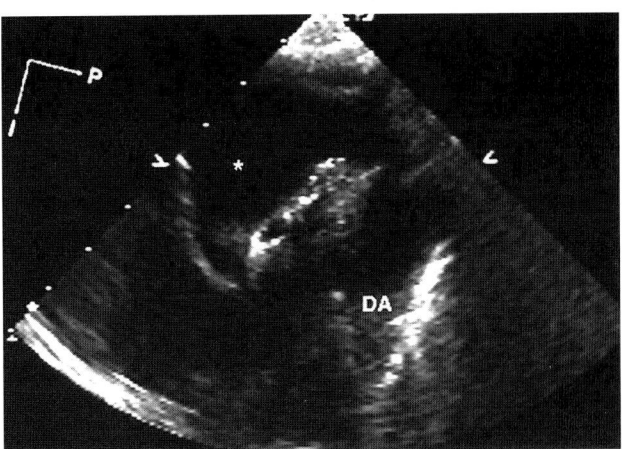

FIG. 11. Aortic arch reconstruction with the Norwood operation: suprasternal long-axis view shows the generously reconstructed ascending aorta and aortic arch. The right pulmonary artery (*PA*) is seen in cross-section immediately posterior to the proximal ascending aorta. The descending aorta is widely patent, without any evidence of recoarctation.

tricular dysfunction and altered flow profiles in the descending aorta have been suggested as additional indicators of arch obstruction (43).

STAGE 1: PULMONARY ARTERY BAND

Surgery

This is performed in patients who have a functionally single ventricle with excessive pulmonary blood flow. The purpose of this operation is to control the volume and pressure of PA blood flow; this is accomplished by placing a band around the proximal main PA. An alternative approach consists of PA isolation to eliminate prograde flow into the branch PAs, and placement of an aortopulmonary shunt to provide controlled pulmonary blood flow.

Echocardiography

Serial study is important because the band may migrate either proximally or distally with linear growth. Postoperative echocardiograms should evaluate for band location, including its proximity to the pulmonary valve leaflets and to the branch PAs, encroachment onto the origin or the lumen of either branch PA, and any erosion of the band into the main or branch PA. In the absence of aortic outflow obstruction, the peak velocity of flow across the band, together with measurement of systemic systolic blood pressure, provides an estimate of PA systolic pressure distal to the band. Serial study of the aortic outflow tract must evaluate for progressive subaortic outflow obstruction, which may be exacerbated following placement of a PA band (44).

STAGE 1: DAMUS-KAYE-STANSEL PROCEDURE

Surgery

This is indicated for patients who have subaortic obstruction and yet have a well-developed aortic arch. This situation typically occurs in the setting of a single LV where the aorta arises from an infundibular chamber that communicates with the underlying ventricle via a restrictive bulboventricular foramen, causing progressive (sub)aortic outflow obstruction. This surgical procedure uses the pulmonary outflow tract, pulmonary valve, and main PA to bypass this level of aortic outflow obstruction. The operation consists of transection of the main PA, thus isolating the branch PAs. The cardiac end of the main PA is anastomosed to the side of the ascending aorta. Prosthetic material may be needed to augment this anastomosis. An aortopulmonary shunt is placed to provide controlled pulmonary blood flow. Following this operation, both the pulmonary and aortic valves function as "aortic" valves.

Echocardiography

Visualizing the Damus-Kaye-Stansel anastomosis in its entirety can be a challenge (particularly in older children and adults) due to the three-dimensional nature of the connection. Echocardiography includes evaluation for obstruction to flow. Since both semilunar valves function as "aortic" valves, regurgitation of either valve represents aortic regurgitation; the neoaortic (native pulmonary) valve is particularly prone to distortion and regurgitation.

STAGE 2: SUPERIOR CAVOPULMONARY SHUNT: HEMI-FONTAN OR BIDIRECTIONAL GLENN SHUNT

Surgery

This is an intermediate stage in the completion of the Fontan series of operations, originally proposed as interim palliation for high-risk patients but now widely used for most patients in most centers (45,46). Although the specifics of the operation may differ among centers and among individual patients, it is designed to direct SVC blood directly into the branch PAs. This allows partial separation of the circulations, and achieves partial volume-unloading of the systemic ventricle. For each patient, this operation serves as a test of future success along the Fontan pathway; thus, failure to adapt to this (hemi-Fontan or bidirectional Glenn) physiology is an indication of the inadvisability of proceeding to completion of the Fontan operation. The PAs are usually isolated in this operation. The SVC is divided, and its cranial end is connected to the side of the ipsilateral branch PA. The cardiac end of the divided SVC is either oversewn (bidirectional Glenn shunt) or maintained in external continuity with the side of the ipsilateral branch PA (hemi-Fontan), while allowing inferior vena caval and hepatic venous return

into the heart. Wide augmentation of the branch PAs may be part of the operation (hemi-Fontan) or may be performed in addition (bidirectional Glenn shunt). Additional surgery is performed as needed to correct ASD restriction, AV valve regurgitation or aortic arch obstruction. The specifics of the operation vary based on systemic venous anatomy in the individual patient. Thus, if bilateral SVCs exist, bilateral cavopulmonary (bidirectional Glenn) anastomoses would be needed. In situations with a small but usable "pulmonary" ventricle, prograde flow from this ventricle into the branch PAs may be maintained.

Echocardiography

Comprehensive echocardiography is performed prior to the superior cavopulmonary anastomosis. This includes evaluation for PA growth, distortion, and stenosis. Patients who have previously undergone aortic arch reconstruction should have a complete assessment of the neoaortic arch for coarctation. The adequacy of interatrial communication, systemic ventricular size and function, and the presence and severity of AV valve regurgitation are also evaluated. PA pressures are assessed using the peak systolic gradient across any previously placed aortopulmonary shunt (keeping in mind that the gradient probably is an underestimate due to the length of the shunt).

PA pressures and resistance cannot be adequately measured by echocardiography. Therefore, cardiac catheterization is routinely performed for hemodynamic assessment prior to the superior cavopulmonary anastomosis (and also prior to the Fontan operation).

Echocardiograms obtained following the superior cavopulmonary shunt should assess the patency of this latter shunt in addition to the above components (as individually applicable). With careful imaging, the bidirectional Glenn shunt (Fig. 12; see also Color Plate 38 following page 758)

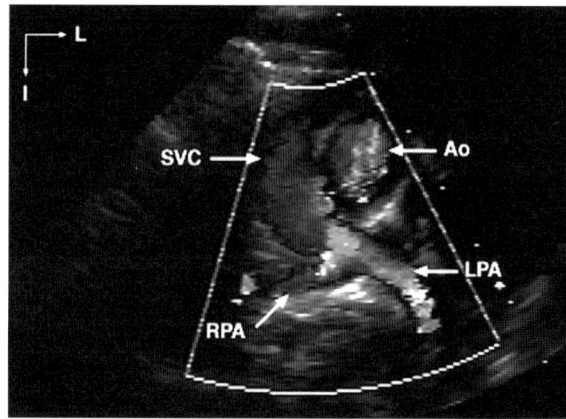

FIG. 12. Bidirectional Glenn shunt: suprasternal short axis with rightward angulation shows the anastomosis of the superior vena cava (*SVC*) to the right pulmonary artery (*RPA*). The anastomosis and the branch pulmonary arteries are widely patent. *Ao*, aorta; *LPA*, left pulmonary artery; *RPA*, right pulmonary artery; *SVC*, superior vena cava. (See also Color Plate 38 following page 758.)

and the hemi-Fontan shunt are seen echocardiographically from the suprasternal and high right parasternal windows. Patency of this shunt is determined echocardiographically based on direct visualization of the anastomosis. Because the systemic veins have high compliance, SVC obstruction may be more evident on the basis of dilation of the cranial portions of the SVC and the azygous vein rather than by Doppler gradients. Although PA pressures cannot be measured by echocardiography following cavopulmonary anastomoses, elevated PA pressures are suggested by a dilated SVC without evidence of anatomic obstruction.

STAGE 3: FONTAN OPERATION

Surgery

This is the final stage in surgical palliation for patients with a functionally single ventricle. The goals of surgery are to achieve complete separation of the pulmonary and systemic circulations. This operation consists of placement of a baffle or tunnel to direct hepatic venous and inferior vena caval blood into the ipsilateral branch PA. The combination of this operation with the superior cavopulmonary anastomosis (Stage 2 detailed above) would channel all systemic venous flow directly into the PAs. Only oxygenated pulmonary venous blood would return to the heart. Additional surgery is simultaneously performed as needed to correct atrial septal restriction, PA distortion, or distortion or stenosis of the superior cavopulmonary anastomosis. Residual aortic arch obstruction and regurgitant AV valves are also repaired as indicated. Successful completion of Fontan pathway staging surgery unfortunately does not represent a cure. Thus, systemic ventricular function and AV valve regurgitation may worsen progressively even after completion of the Fontan operation.

Echocardiography

Echocardiograms performed prior to the Fontan operation should include comprehensive evaluation of prior repairs as noted in the previous section ("Superior Cavopulmonary Anastomoses"). Patency of the previously completed superior cavopulmonary anastomosis is confirmed.

Post-Fontan echocardiograms should, in addition to the above, assess for patency and size of the Fontan tunnel or baffle, which may become very dilated and occasionally may contain thrombi. The Fontan baffle may be difficult to visualize, and is best shown by a combination of suprasternal (Fig. 13; see also Color Plate 39 following page 758) and subcostal imaging. Transesophageal echocardiography is frequently needed for comprehensive evaluation of the Fontan tunnel. If a fenestration has been placed in the Fontan baffle, right-to-left flow across this orifice may be visualized by echocardiography. Measurement of the velocity of this flow jet is part of the post-Fontan evaluation, because it provides an estimate of transpulmonary gradient. Inadvert-

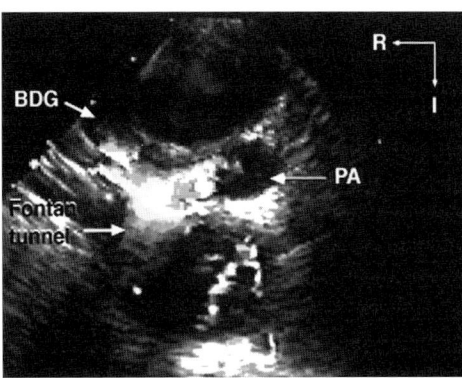

FIG. 13. Fontan operation: suprasternal short axis with rightward angulation shows the pulmonary connections of the Fontan tunnel and the bidirectional Glenn shunt (*BDG*). The anastomoses and branch pulmonary arteries (*PA*) are widely patent. (See also Color Plate 39 following page 758.)

leaks in the Fontan baffle should also be sought by echocardiography; contrast echocardiography may be useful in this context.

Evaluation of systemic ventricular function and AV valve regurgitation is an important aspect of serial postoperative echocardiography. Branch PA stenosis or obstruction may develop or worsen. Thus, patients who have achieved successful completion of the Fontan pathway must undergo lifelong serial study.

In summary, the hemodynamics of the functionally single ventricle are based on a delicate balance between the factors that propel pulmonary blood flow forward (ultimately, the function of the single ventricle) and factors that retard prograde pulmonary blood flow (including PA hypoplasia or stenosis and elevated pulmonary resistance). The size and anatomy of the PA, the size and function of the ventricle, the competence of the AV and semilunar valve(s), and patency of the outflow tract(s) are among the factors critical to the successful maintenance of hemodynamics, either prior to or following palliation. These issues are most effectively evaluated by serial echocardiographic studies.

TOTAL ANOMALOUS PULMONARY VENOUS CONNECTION

Surgery

Treatment of this condition consists of establishing an unobstructed communication via direct anastomosis between the pulmonary venous confluence and the posterior wall of the left atrium. The anatomic adequacy of the anastomosis depends on the native anatomy. Thus, a wide and horizontal pulmonary venous confluence constitutes a more desirable surgical substrate than a narrow and vertical confluence.

Pulmonary venous obstruction may develop after surgical repair. The most common site of obstruction is the venoatrial anastomosis. Obstruction of the orifices of single or multiple

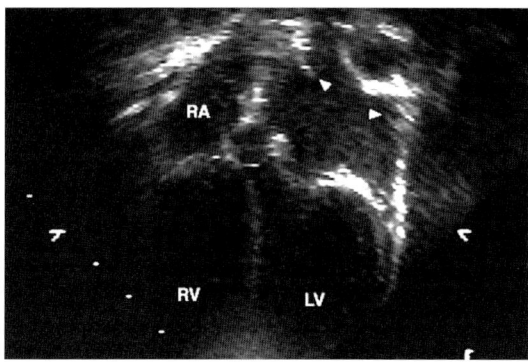

FIG. 14. Repair of total anomalous pulmonary venous connection: apical four-chamber view shows the anastomosis of the pulmonary venous confluence (*arrowheads*) to the posterior wall of the left atrium. *LV*, left ventricle; *RA*, right atrium; *RV*, right ventricle.

individual pulmonary veins, or long-segment stenosis of the individual pulmonary veins may also occur.

Echocardiography

Echocardiography following repair of total anomalous pulmonary venous connection reveals the anastomosis of the confluence to the posterior wall of the left atrium, leading to an unusual left atrial contour (Fig. 14). Serial postoperative echocardiographic evaluation includes assessment of flow in individual pulmonary veins and through the venoatrial anastomosis into the left atrium. Following successful repair, phasic and low-velocity flow is seen in the individual pulmonary veins and the venoatrial anastomosis, with no aliasing noted on color flow Doppler mapping. Serial evaluation of RV size, function, and pressure is performed, because residual or recurrent pulmonary venous obstruction may lead to progressive pulmonary hypertension and (secondary) RV dysfunction (47). Following successful repair, the pattern of pulmonary venous flow is altered compared to normals (48). Thus, although normal children have greater prograde pulmonary venous flow during ventricular systole than during ventricular diastole, patients who have undergone repair of total anomalous pulmonary venous connection exhibit reversal of this pattern; this alteration in pattern is felt to be due to a possible decrease in left atrial compliance. Serial evaluation is important because obstruction at any level (most commonly at the level of the anastomosis between the left atrium and the pulmonary venous confluence) may be progressive and unpredictable.

CONCLUSIONS

Evaluation of patients who have undergone corrective repair or palliation of structural congenital heart defects requires that the echocardiographer possess a thorough knowledge of native anatomy and surgical procedures. The echocardiographer must also be aware of the potential unto-

ward effects of individual interventions, and be conversant with the role (and limitations) of echocardiographic techniques in the detection and quantification of postoperative residua. Echocardiograms are required to monitor lesions that are progressive or tend to recur, and for detection of pulmonary hypertension and ventricular dysfunction. The value of serial echocardiograms in evaluation of palliated or corrected structural heart defects cannot be overemphasized.

REFERENCES

1. Rychik J, Norwood WI, Chin AJ. Doppler color flow mapping assessment of residual shunt after closure of large ventricular septal defects. *Circulation* 1991;84(Suppl III):153–161.
2. Meijboom F, Szatmari A, Utens E, et al. Long-term follow-up after surgical closure of ventricular septal defect in infancy and childhood. *J Am Coll Cardiol* 1994;24:1358–1364.
3. Meijboom F, Hess J, Szatmari A, et al. Long-term follow-up (9 to 20 years) after surgical closure of atrial septal defect at a young age. *Am J Cardiol* 1993;72:1431–1434.
4. Pastorek JS, Allen HD, Davis JT. Current outcomes of surgical closure of secundum atrial septal defect. *Am J Cardiol* 1994;74:75–77.
5. Rastelli GC, Ongley PA, Kirklin JW, et al. Surgical repair of complete form of persistent common atrioventricular canal. *J Thorac Cardiovasc Surg* 1968;55:299–308.
6. McCrindle BW, Valvuloplasty and Angioplasty of Congenital Anomalies (VACA) Registry Investigators. Independent predictors of long-term results after balloon pulmonary valvuloplasty. *Circulation* 1994; 89:1751–1759.
7. Kovalchin JP, Forbes TJ, Nihill MR, et al. Echocardiographic determinants of clinical course in infants with critical and severe pulmonary valve stenosis. *J Am Coll Cardiol* 1997;29:1095–1101.
8. Vouhe PR, Ouakniue R, Pulaui H, et al. Diffuse subaortic stenosis: modified Konno procedures with aortic valve preservation. *Eur J Cardiothorac Surg* 1993;7:132–136.
9. Konno S, Imai Y, Iida Y, et al. A new method for prosthetic valve replacement in congenital aortic stenosis associated with hypoplasia of the aortic valve ring. *J Thorac Cardiovasc Surg* 1975;70:909–917.
10. Calhoon JH, Bolton JW. Ross/Konno procedure for critical aortic stenosis in infancy. *Ann Thorac Surg* 1995;60(Suppl 6):S597–599.
11. Rhodes LA, Colan SD, Perry SB, et al. Predictors of survival in neonates with critical aortic stenosis. *Circulation* 1991;84:2325–2335.
12. Justo RN, McCrindle BW, Benson LN, et al. Aortic valve regurgitation after surgical versus percutaneous balloon valvotomy for congenital aortic valve stenosis. *Am J Cardiol* 1996;77:1332–1338.
13. Rocchini AP, Beekman RH, Ben Shachar G, et al. Balloon aortic valvuloplasty: results of the valvuloplasty and angioplasty of congenital anomalies registry. *Am J Cardiol* 1990;65:784–789.
14. Kaine SF, O'Brian Smith E, Mott AR, et al. Quantitative echocardiographic analysis of the aortic arch predicts outcome of balloon angioplasty of native coarctation of the aorta. *Circulation* 1996;94: 1056–1062.
15. Blalock A, Taussig HB. The surgical treatment of malformations of the heart in which there is pulmonary stenosis or pulmonary atresia. *JAMA* 1945;128:89.
16. Castaneda A, Atai M, Varco RL. Technical consideration in the correction of Fallot's tetralogy. *Chest* 1965;47:223–230.
17. Atallah-Yunes NH. Postoperative assessment of a modified surgical approach to repair of tetralogy of Fallot. Long-term follow-up. *Circulation* 1996;94(Suppl):I122–126.
18. Jonsson H, Ivert T, Brodin L-A. Echocardiographic findings in 83 patients 13–26 years after intracardiac repair of tetralogy of Fallot. *Eur Heart J* 1995;16:1255–1263.
19. Mitsuno M, Nakano S, Shimazaki Y, et al. Fate of right ventricular hypertrophy in tetralogy of Fallot after corrective surgery. *Am J Cardiol* 1993;72:694–698.
20. Zhao HX, Miller DC, Reitz BA, et al. Surgical repair of tetralogy of Fallot: long-term follow-up with particular emphasis on late death and reoperation. *J Thorac Cardiovasc Surg* 1985;89:204–220.
21. Murphy JG, Gersh BJ, Mair DD, et al. Long-term outcome in patients

undergoing surgical repair of tetralogy of Fallot. *N Engl J Med* 1993; 329:593–599.

22. Redington AN. Determinants of short- and long-term outcome in the surgical correction of tetralogy of Fallot. *Curr Opin Pediatr* 1993;5: 619–622

23. Borow KM, Green LH, Castaneda AR, et al. Left ventricular function after repair of tetralogy of Fallot and its relationship to age at surgery. *Circulation* 1980;61:1150–1158

24. Levine JC, Mayer JE Jr, Keane JF, et al. Anastomotic pseudoaneurysm of the ventricle after homograft placement in children. *Ann Thorac Surg* 1995;59:60–66.

25. Hanseus K, Bjorkhem G, Lundstrom N-R, et al. Cross-sectional echocardiographic measurements of right ventricular size and growth in patients with pulmonary atresia and intact ventricular septum. *Pediatr Cardiol* 1991;12:135–142.

26. Ovaert C, Qureshi SA, Rosenthal E, et al. Growth of the right ventricle after successful transcatheter pulmonary valvotomy in neonates and infants with pulmonary atresia and intact ventricular septum. *J Thorac Cardiovasc Surg* 1998;115:1055–1062.

27. Hanley FL, Sade RM, Blackstone EH, et al. Outcomes in neonatal pulmonary atresia with intact ventricular septum. A multiinstitutional study. *J Thorac Cardiovasc Surg* 1993;105:406–427.

28. Giglia TM, Mandell VS, Connor AR, et al. Diagnosis and management of right ventricle-dependent coronary circulation in pulmonary atresia with intact ventricular septum. *Circulation* 1992;86:1516–1528.

29. Giglia TM, Jenkins KJ, Matitiau A, et al. Influence of right heart size on outcome in pulmonary atresia with intact ventricular septum. *Circulation* 1993;88(Pt I):2248–2256.

30. Kirklin JW, Blackstone EH, Tchervenkov CI, et al. Clinical outcomes after the arterial switch operation for transposition: patient, support, procedural and institutional risk factors. *Circulation* 1992;86: 1501–1515.

31. Colan SD, Boutin C, Castaneda AR, et al. Status of the left ventricle after arterial switch operation for transposition of the great arteries. Hemodynamic and echocardiographic evaluation. *J Thorac Cardiovasc Surg* 1995;109:311–321.

32. Hourihan M, Colan SD, Wernovsky G, et al. Growth of the aortic anastomosis, annulus, and root after the arterial switch procedure performed in infancy. *Circulation* 1993;88:615–620.

33. McGoon DC, Rastelli GC, Ongley PA. An operation for the correction of truncus arteriosus. *JAMA* 1968;205:69–73.

34. Hanley FL, Heinemann MK, Jonas RA, et al. Repair of truncus arteriosus in the neonate. *J Thorac Cardiovasc Surg* 1993;105:1047–1056.

35. Heinemann MK, Hanley FL, Fenton KN, et al. Fate of small homograft conduits after early repair of truncus arteriosus. *Ann Thorac Surg* 1993; 55:1409–1412.

36. Di Donato RM, Fyfe DA, Puga FJ, et al. Fifteen-year experience with surgical repair of truncus arteriosus. *J Thorac Cardiovasc Surg* 1985; 89:414–422.

37. Preminger TJ, Sanders SP, van der Velde ME, et al. "Intramural" residual interventricular defects after repair of conotruncal malformations. *Circulation* 1994;89:236–242.

38. Fontan F, Baudet E. Surgical repair of tricuspid atresia. *Thorax* 1971; 26:240–248.

39. Sluysmans T, Sanders SP, van der Velde M, et al. Natural history and patterns of recovery of contractile function in single left ventricle after Fontan operation. *Circulation* 1992;86:1753–1761.

40. Senzaki H, Isoda T, Ishizawa A, et al. Reconsideration of criteria for the Fontan operation. Influence of pulmonary artery size on postoperative hemodynamics of the Fontan operation. *Circulation* 1994;89:266–271.

41. Fontan F, Fernandez G, Costa F, et al. The size of the pulmonary arteries and the results of the Fontan operation. *J Thorac Cardiovasc Surg* 1989;98:711–724.

42. Bridges ND, Lock JE, Castaneda AR. Baffle fenestration with subsequent transcatheter closure. Modification of the Fontan operation for patients at increased risk. *Circulation* 1990;82:1681–1689.

43. Fraisse A, Colan SD, Jonas RA, et al. Accuracy of echocardiography for detection of aortic arch obstruction after stage I Norwood procedure. *Am Heart J* 1998;135:230–236.

44. Freedom RM, Benson LN, Smallhorn JF, et al. Subaortic stenosis, the univentricular heart, and banding of the pulmonary artery: an analysis of the courses of 43 patients with univentricular heart palliated by pulmonary artery banding. *Circulation* 1986;73:758–764.

45. Bridges ND, Jonas RA, Mayer JE Jr, et al. Bidirectional cavopulmonary anastomosis as interim palliation for high-risk Fontan candidates: early results. *Circulation* 1990;82(Suppl IV):170–176.

46. Pridjian AK, Mendelsohn AM, Lupinetti FM, et al. Usefulness of the bidirectional Glenn procedure as a staged reconstruction for the functional single ventricle. *Am J Cardiol* 1993;71:959–962.

47. van der Velde ME, Parness IA, Colan SD, et al. Two-dimensional echocardiography in the pre- and postoperative management of totally anomalous pulmonary venous connection. *J Am Coll Cardiol* 1991;18: 1746–1751.

48. Minich LL, Tani LY, Hawkins JA, et al. Abnormal Doppler pulmonary venous flow patterns in children after repaired totalanomalous pulmonary venous connection. *Am J Cardiol* 1995;75:606–610.

CHAPTER 57

Pulmonary Embolism

Daniel F. Worsley and Abass Alavi

Pulmonary embolism (PE) is a relatively common and potentially fatal disorder for which treatment is highly effective and improves patient survival. The accurate and prompt diagnosis of acute PE requires an interdisciplinary team approach and may be difficult because of nonspecific clinical, laboratory, and radiographic findings (1,2). The incidence of venous thromboembolism is approximately 1 in 1,000 per year (3). Approximately 10% of patients with PE die within 1 hour of the event (4). For those patients who survive beyond the first hour, following PE, treatment with heparin or thrombolytic agents are both effective therapies (4–6). The mortality in patients with PE who are untreated has been reported to be as high as 30% (4). In contrast, the correct diagnosis and appropriate therapy significantly lowers mortality to between 2.5 and 8% (5,7). Although anticoagulant therapy is effective in treating PE and reducing mortality, it is not without some risk. The prevalence of major hemorrhagic complications has been reported to be as high as 10 to 15% among patients receiving anticoagulant therapy (8,9). In one study investigating drug-related deaths among hospital patients, heparin was responsible for the majority of drug-related deaths in noncritically ill patients (10). Therefore, the accurate and prompt diagnosis of PE is not only essential to prevent excessive mortality but also to avoid complications related to unnecessary anticoagulant therapy.

CLINICAL DIAGNOSIS OF PULMONARY EMBOLISM

In the clinical evaluation of patients with established PE risk factors, clinical signs and symptoms were similar in males and females (11). The risk of pulmonary embolism does increase with age (12,13). Sedentary lifestyle, pro-

longed recovery phase following illness, congestive heart failure, malignancy, and increased hip fracture rates in the elderly are factors that increase the likelihood of pulmonary embolism. The clinical findings of patients with suspected PE and no preexisting cardiac or pulmonary disease were evaluated in a subset of the Prospective Investigation of Pulmonary Embolism Diagnosis (PIOPED) study population (14). The most common symptoms of patients with PE and no preexisting cardiac or pulmonary disease were dyspnea, pleuritic chest pain, and cough (14). However, the prevalence of these symptoms were not significantly different when compared with patients in whom PE was excluded. Dyspnea, tachypnea, or pleuritic chest pain alone or in combination were present in 97% of patients with PE (15). Like the symptoms, the clinical signs associated with acute PE are also nonspecific. The prevalence of tachypnea, tachycardia, and fever were similar among patients with PE when compared with those in whom the disease was excluded. Increased intensity of the pulmonic component of the second heart sound was more commonly heard in patients with PE. However, this finding was only present in 23% of patients (14). The prevalence of immobilization (strict bed rest for more than 3 continuous days) and surgery (an incision under regional or general anesthesia) within 3 months were more common in patients with PE compared to those without (14). The frequency of other risk factors recorded during the PIOPED study were approximately the same between the two groups.

More recently, neural networks have been developed to aid in the clinical diagnosis of PE. In simplistic terms, neural networks are computer programs that are capable of processing information similar to the way the human brain processes information. A more detailed description of the application of neural networks in radiologic diagnoses can be found elsewhere (16). A neural network for the clinical diagnosis of PE has been developed utilizing 50 variables that were available from patients enrolled in the PIOPED study (17). These variables included information obtained from history, physical examination, chest radiograph, electrocardiograph,

D. F. Worsley: University of British Columbia; Division of Nuclear Medicine, Vancouver General Hospital, Vancouver, British Columbia V5Z 1M9, Canada.
A. Alavi: Department of Radiology, University of Pennsylvania School of Medicine; Department of Radiology, Hospital of the University of Pennsylvania, Philadelphia, Pennsylvania 19104.

and room air arterial blood gas measurements. The likelihood of PE based on clinical findings as predicted by the neural network was similar to that predicted by experienced clinicians. Therefore, neural networks can provide a reproducible assessment of the clinical likelihood of PE and may aid in the diagnostic evaluation of patients suspected of having acute pulmonary embolism. However, the clinical manifestations of PE were quite variable and lack the specificity to reliably diagnose or exclude clinically significant PE.

D-DIMER

D-dimer is a plasmin-mediated degradation product of circulating cross-linked fibrin. Elevated D-dimer levels are not specific for venous thromboembolism and may occur in any condition in which fibrin has been formed and degraded by plasmin. Arterial thrombosis, disseminated intravascular coagulation, infections, sepsis, recent trauma, and postoperative states may all cause elevated D-dimer levels. D-dimer levels are commonly measured using either latex agglutination or ELISA-based methods. The ELISA-based methods are more sensitive and can detect D-dimer concentration levels as low as 30 ng/mL. However, the test is labor-intensive and may take over 36 hours to perform; therefore, these methods are not appropriate for emergency use. The latex agglutination method is a more rapid, semiquantiative test that can detect D-dimer concentration levels in the 200 to 500 ng/mL range. In a consensus statement from the American College of Chest Physicians, there was general agreement that an ELISA-based assay that measures D-dimer excluded PE in 90 to 95% of patients and that a normal latex agglutination D-dimer was unreliable for excluding PE and should not be performed (18). There is currently no method to standardize D-dimer results from different manufacturers, and high variations in assay results have been reported (19,20). In an attempt to overcome the problems of low specificity, it has been recommended that the test be performed only on outpatients and used to exclude the diagnosis of PE. In spite of this, a recent metaanalysis of 29 D-dimer studies concluded that the clinical utility of the D-dimer assay remains unproven (21).

ELECTROCARDIOGRAM

The main value of the electrocardiogram in the evaluation of patients with suspected PE is the diagnosis of other conditions that may mimic PE. Both pericarditis and acute myocardial infarction can mimic the symptoms of PE and are readily diagnosed with an electrocardiogram. Electrocardiographic evidence of acute cor pulmonale (P pulmonale, right-axis deviation, right bundle-branch block, or S1Q3T3 pattern are infrequent and nonspecific findings in patients with PE). The most common electrocardiographic pattern in patients with PE was nonspecific ST segment or T-wave changes. A normal electrocardiogram was present in 6% of

patients with massive PE and 23% of patients with submassive PE (14,22). Therefore, while an electrocardiogram can help substantiate an alternative diagnosis, it can not reliably diagnose or exclude pulmonary embolism.

CHEST RADIOGRAPHIC FINDINGS IN PULMONARY EMBOLISM

Similar to electrocardiography, chest radiographs are helpful in excluding diseases that clinically mimic PE. In the PIOPED study, chest radiographs were obtained within 24 hours of angiography and, among patients with angiographically documented PE, only 12% (45 of 383) of patients had chest radiographs interpreted as normal (23). The positive and negative predictive values of a normal chest radiograph were 18% and 74%, respectively. In patients with PE and no preexisting cardiac or pulmonary disease only 16% had chest radiographs interpreted as normal (14). The most common chest radiographic findings in patients with PE were atelectasis and/or parenchymal opacities in the affected lung zone (14,23). However, atelectasis and/or parenchymal opacities were also the most common finding in patients in whom PE was excluded. Pleural effusions within the affected hemithorax occurred in approximately 35% of patients with PE. The majority of pleural effusions were small, causing only blunting of the costophrenic angles (23). Therefore, chest radiographic findings alone were nonspecific for PE. However, chest radiographs are essential in the evaluation of patients with suspected PE to diagnose conditions that can clinically mimic PE and aid in the interpretation of the V/Q lung scans.

VENTILATION-PERFUSION LUNG SCANNING IN PULMONARY EMBOLISM

The ventilation-perfusion (V/Q) lung scan has been shown to be a safe noninvasive technique to evaluate regional pulmonary perfusion and ventilation. The technique has been widely used in the evaluation of patients with suspected PE. Despite these attributes and studies suggesting the under diagnosis of PE, critics have suggested that V/Q scanning has been overutilized and has minimal impact on patient management (24–26).

RADIOPHARMACEUTICALS AND TECHNIQUES IN V/Q LUNG SCANNING

Perfusion lung scanning was first described in 1964 when Wagner et al. (28) and Taplan et al. (27) reported on the use of iodine-131-labeled macroaggregates of albumin in the evaluation of pulmonary perfusion. Currently, the agents of choice for perfusion imaging are either Tc-99m-labeled human albumin microspheres (Tc-99m HAM) or macroaggregated albumin (Tc-99m MAA). Technetium-99m MAA particles range in size from 10 to 150μ; however, over

90% of injected particles measure between 10 and 90μ. Technetium-99m HAM particles are more uniform in size and range from 35 to 60μ. The injection of labeled particles should be performed with the patient in the supine position, which limits the effect of gravity on regional pulmonary arterial blood flow. Following the intravenous administration of Tc-99m MAA, particles are mixed within the heart, then lodge within precapillary arterioles in the lungs. The usual administered activity is between 74 to 148 MBq (2 to 4 mCi). The distribution of particles within the lungs is proportional to regional pulmonary blood flow at the time of injection. Approximately 200,000 to 500,000 particles are injected during a routine clinical perfusion lung scan. The normal adult human lung contains approximately 300 million precapillary arterioles and 300 billion capillaries; therefore, in routine clinical use only about 0.1% of precapillary arterioles are blocked. In addition, the blockage of pulmonary precapillary arterioles by Tc-99 MAA is transient, and the biological half-life within the lung ranges between 2 and 6 hours. In pediatric patients, patients with right-to-left shunts, patients with pulmonary hypertension, or patients who have undergone pneumonectomy or single lung transplantation, the number of particles injected should be reduced. A minimum of 60,000 particles is required to obtain an even distribution of activity within the pulmonary arterial circulation and avoid potential false-positive interpretations (29).

When performing for perfusion scintigraphy, at least six views of the lungs should be obtained. These include anterior, posterior, right and left lateral, and right and left posterior oblique views. Additionally, right and left anterior oblique views may be helpful in selected cases. Animal studies have demonstrated that perfusion imaging will detect greater than 95% of emboli that completely occlude pulmonary arterial vessels greater than 2 mm in diameter (30). In spite of imaging in multiple projections the perfusion scan may underestimate perfusion abnormalities. A solitary segmental perfusion defect within the medial basal segment of the right lower lobe is completely surrounded by normal lung, consequently a perfusion defect in this segment will not be detected on planar perfusion imaging (31).

Perfusion scintigraphy is sensitive but not specific for diagnosing pulmonary diseases. Virtually all parenchymal lung diseases (including tumors, infections, chronic obstructive pulmonary disease (COPD), or asthma) can cause decreased pulmonary arterial blood flow within the affected lung zone. Consequently, shortly after the introduction of perfusion scintigraphy, Wagner et al. (33) and DeNardo et al. (32) combined ventilation and perfusion scintigraphy to improve the diagnostic specificity for diagnosing pulmonary embolism (PE). The pathologic basis for combining ventilation and perfusion scintigraphy was that PE characteristically causes abnormal perfusion with preserved ventilation (mismatched defects; Fig. 1), whereas parenchymal lung disease would most often cause both ventilation and perfu-

sion abnormalities in the same lung region (matched defects). Conditions in which the ventilation abnormality appears larger than the perfusion abnormality (reverse mismatch) include airway obstruction, mucous plug, airspace disease, atelectasis, or pneumonia and following treatment with bronchodilators, such as albuterol.

Xenon-133 is most frequently utilized for demonstration of regional ventilation to the lungs. Alternative ventilation imaging agents include xenon-127, krypton-81m, technetium-99m aerosols, technegas, or pertechnegas, which have not been as extensively tested as Xe-133. Studies that have compared various ventilation agents are limited in number, but based on the data, no major diagnostic differences appear to exist among the various agents with regard to their diagnostic efficacy (34,35).

With Xe-133 or Xe-127 first breath or washin images demonstrate regional lung ventilation. Equilibrium images are obtained while the patient rebreathes the gas for at least 4 minutes. Regions of the lung that appear as defects on the breath-hold image may normalize on the equilibrium image because of collateral air drift. During washout imaging, the patient breathes in room air and regional air-trapping can be detected as focal areas of retained activity. The diagnostic performance of the V/Q lung scan was significantly better in patients who had ventilation studies performed in the erect position compared with the supine position (36). Generally, ventilation images with Xe-133 are obtained prior to perfusion imaging.

As indicated above, the imaging technique with Xe-133 and Xe-127 is identical, but because of the higher energy of the latter with this gas, ventilation imaging can be performed following perfusion scan utilizing Tc-99m MAA. The advantages of performing a ventilation scan following a perfusion study include positioning the patient such that the lung demonstrating the greatest perfusion abnormality can be optimally examined, and, also, ventilation imaging may be avoided altogether in cases when the perfusion scan appears normal. However, Xe-127 does have several disadvantages; namely, it is more costly than Xe-133 and requires medium energy collimation. When performing ventilation imaging with either Xe-133 or Xe-127 initial breath-hold or washin images are generally obtained only in a single projection, which limits the comparison with perfusion images that are obtained in multiple projections.

Krypton-81m is another noble gas used to evaluate regional ventilation. This agent has a very short physical half-life (13 sec), and, therefore, only washin or breath-hold images can be obtained. However, the short physical half-life of Kr-81m enables one to obtain images in multiple projections. Krypton-81m is produced from a rubidium-81 generator. The parent radionuclide has a physical half-life of 4.7 minutes; therefore, the useful lifetime of the generator is only 1 day. Similar to Xe-127, ventilation imaging with Kr-81m is generally performed following perfusion imaging.

Ventilation imaging with Tc-99m radiolabeled aerosols

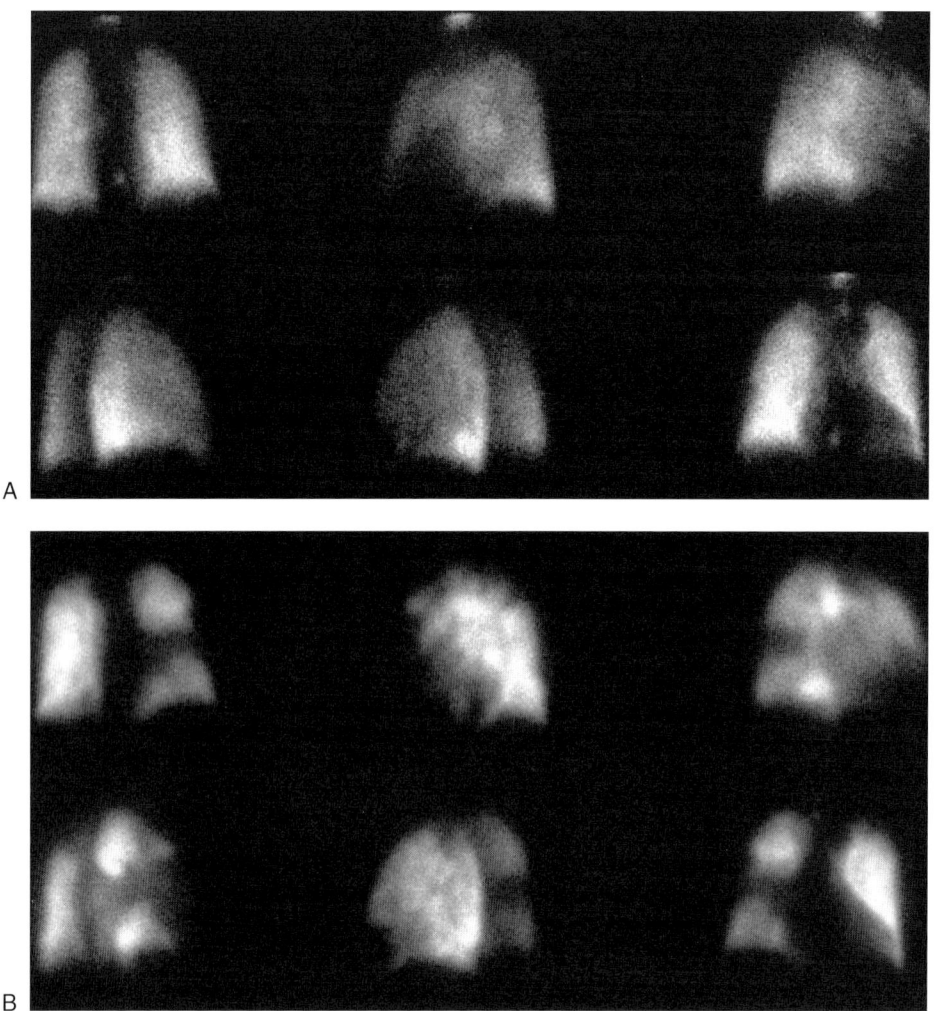

FIG. 1. Tc-99m DTPA aerosol (**A**) and Tc-99m MAA perfusion (**B**) images demonstrate multiple segmental and subsegmental perfusion defects in regions that are ventilated normally (V/Q mismatch). The findings indicate a high probability of acute pulmonary embolism.

can be performed with several radiopharmaceuticals including Tc-99m DTPA, Tc-99m sulfur colloid, Tc-99m pyrophosphate, Tc-99m MDP, or Tc-99m glucoheptanate. The most popular agent is Tc-99m DTPA, which has a relatively short residence time within the lung, especially in smokers where Tc-99m-labeled sulfur colloid or pyrophosphate may be the preferred agents. Technetium-99m-labeled radioaerosols are between 0.5 to 3 microns in size and are produced by a commercially available nebulizer. For a routine ventilation study, 1.11 GBq (30 mCi) of Tc-99m DTPA in 3 mL of saline is placed in the nebulizer. Oxygen is then forced through the nebulizer at high pressure to produce aerosolized droplets that are inhaled by the patient through a mask or mouthpiece. The patient generally breathes from the nebulizer for 3 to 5 minutes or until 37 MBq (1 mCi) of activity is deposited within the lungs. The distribution of activity within the lungs is proportional to regional ventilation. Multiple image projections can be obtained that correspond to those obtained during subsequent perfusion imaging. In contrast to Xe imaging, ventilation studies with Tc-99m-labeled radioaerosols require minimal patient cooperation and portable studies or studies in patients on respirators can be successfully performed. Disadvantages of Tc-99m labeled radioaerosols include central deposition of activity in patients with COPD or airway obstruction and the amount of radioactive material that remains and is wasted in the nebulizer. In general, aerosol ventilation studies are performed prior to perfusion imaging; however, the order can be reversed, and, in patients with a normal or near normal perfusion study, a ventilation scan can be avoided (36,37).

Central deposition of Tc-99m-labeled radioaerosol in patients with COPD results in suboptimal studies, and, to overcome this problem, newer agents have been developed. These include Tc-99m technegas and Tc-99m pertechnegas.

Both of these agents are performed by burning Tc-99m pertechnetate in a carbon crucible at very high temperatures to produce an ultrafine radiolabeled aerosol (particle size 0.02 to 0.2 microns). Pertechnegas is purged with 5% oxygen and 95% argon, compared with technegas, which is purged with 100% argon. This relatively minor difference causes profound changes in the biological behavior of the preparation. When inhaled, both agents distribute homogeneously within the lung proportional to regional lung ventilation, and very little central deposition of activity is seen even in patients with COPD. Pertechnegas readily penetrates the alveolar membrane, and, therefore, its biological half-life in the lungs is quite short, measuring approximately 6 to 10 minutes. On the other hand, there is very little transalveolar or mucociliary clearance of technegas, and the effective half-life approximates the physical half-life of Tc-99m. Both agents require minimal patient cooperation, and only 2 to 3 breaths are required to obtain sufficient counts in the lungs to perform ventilation imaging. In general, ventilation imaging with both technegas and pertechnegas is performed prior to perfusion imaging, and multiple views of the lungs corresponding to those of the perfusion study are obtained.

CLINICAL TRIALS USING LUNG SCANNING AND PULMONARY EMBOLISM

The first large-scale study that utilized perfusion lung scanning as a screening test for the diagnosis of PE was the Urokinase Pulmonary Embolism Trial (UPET). In more than 90% of the patients enrolled in the trial perfusion, lung scanning was performed following the intravenous administration of I-131-labeled MAA. Perfusion scanning was accomplished with rectilinear scanners and, as such, no ventilation imaging was performed. Despite utilizing suboptimal techniques as judged by today's standards, the UPET study established perfusion lung scanning as an effective technique for both screening for PE and for assessing the restoration of pulmonary blood flow following an embolic event (38). The majority of patients with acute PE either completely or partially lyse their thrombi. Approximately 75 to 80% of perfusion defects resolved by 3 months, and perfusion defects that did not resolve by 3 months remained mostly persistent when followed for 1 year. The amount of clot resolution observed in the UPET is likely to be underestimated, since ventilation scanning was not performed, and many of the unresolved perfusion defects might have been due to preexisting chronic obstructive lung disease. Based on the data from the UPET, the American College of Chest Physicians consensus statement would still recommend performing a follow-up V/Q lung scan at 3 months following the initial diagnosis to evaluate clot resolution and to serve as a baseline for future comparisons when recurrent emboli are suspected (18). If the patient is unable to return in 3 months, a V/Q scan at discharge may also be useful.

Data from other large studies using modern imaging techniques have reported on the efficacy of V/Q scanning in patients suspected of having acute PE (39–41). In a prospective study by Hull et al., 874 patients with ventilation-perfusion scan interpretations were grouped into three diagnostic categories; normal, nonhigh probability, and high probability (mismatch defect involving at least 75% of a segment). The purpose of the study was to determine if anticoagulation therapy could be withheld in patients with a nonhigh probability V/Q scan, adequate cardiorespiratory reserve, and absent proximal lower extremity venous thrombosis as determined by negative serial impedance plethysmography (IPG). This diagnostic approach emphasized the importance of the basic pathophysiologic concept that venous thromboembolism is a systemic disease process and that pulmonary embolism is merely a manifestation of the disorder that results in initiating the diagnostic work-up. High probability and normal V/Q scans were interpreted in 8% and 36% of patients, respectively. Nine percent of patients had nonhigh probability V/Q scans and inadequate cardiorespiratory reserve as defined by the presence of pulmonary edema, right ventricular failure, systolic BP less than 90 mm Hg, syncope, acute tachyarrhythmia, and very abnormal arterial blood gases. Most patients (47%) had nonhigh probability V/Q scans and adequate cardiorespiratory reserve. The outcome in each group was assessed during a 3-month follow-up period. In patients with nonhigh probability lung scan interpretation, adequate cardiorespiratory reserve, and negative serial IPG studies, anticoagulants were withheld. Only 2.7% of these patients had evidence of thromboembolism on follow-up. The conclusion from this study was that patients with a nonhigh probability V/Q scan, adequate cardiorespiratory reserve, and negative serial IPG studies could be managed safely without anticoagulation. In addition, these results also confirm findings from previous studies that suggested that the incidence of recurrent PE is very low in the absence of proximal lower extremity venous thrombus. Unfortunately, the interpretation criteria used to categorize the probability of PE were, to some extent, unconventional (normal, nondiagnostic, or high). Consequently, comparison of these results with the PIOPED study is not directly possible.

More recently, Hull et al. (40) have prospectively examined 1,564 consecutive patients with suspected pulmonary embolism who underwent both V/Q scanning and IPG of the lower extremities. In 40% (627 of 1,564), V/Q scans were interpreted as nondiagnostic and serial IPG studies were negative. All of these patients had an adequate cardiorespiratory reserve and were managed without anticoagulation. Only 1.9% (12 of 627) of this population developed evidence of either DVT or PE on follow-up. As Hull and his colleagues have demonstrated, the combination of V/Q scan findings and IPG can be very useful in selecting patients who have not had substantial PE and in whom there is no evidence of proximal lower extremity venous thrombi. In these patients, the risk of recurrent embolic events is low and anticoagulation may not be required (39,40,42,43).

PISA-PED

In the prospective investigative study of acute pulmonary embolism diagnosis (PISA-PED), which utilized perfusion scanning alone in conjunction with the chest radiograph, the sensitivity and specificity of scintigraphy was 92% and 87%, respectively (44). The prevalence in their population was relatively high at 39%. By combining the clinical assessment of the likelihood of PE (very likely, possible, or unlikely), the positive predictive value of a positive perfusion scan was 99%. A near-normal or abnormal perfusion scan without segmental defects combined with a low clinical likelihood of PE had a negative predictive value of 97%.

PIOPED STUDY

To date, the most comprehensive prospective study addressing the role of V/Q scanning in the diagnosis of PE has been the PIOPED study (41). The prospective investigation of pulmonary embolism diagnosis (PIOPED) study was a multiinstitutional study designed to evaluate the efficacy of various conventional methods for diagnosing acute PE. In particular, the study was designed to determine the sensitivity and specificity of V/Q lung scanning for diagnosing acute PE. In addition, the relative contributions of the clinical assessment, chest radiograph, and other routine studies were assessed. The PIOPED study also provided an opportunity to assess the validity of pulmonary angiography for diagnosing acute PE and determine the incidence of complications related to this procedure.

The sensitivity, specificity, and positive predictive value of a high probability V/Q scan interpretation for detecting acute PE are 40%, 98%, and 87%, respectively. The diagnostic accuracy of V/Q scanning was not significantly different in women compared with men (11). Similarly, the overall diagnostic performance of the V/Q scan was similar among patients with varying ages (45,46). The diagnostic utility of V/Q scanning for detecting PE was similar among patient with preexisting cardiac or pulmonary disease compared with patients with no underlying cardiac or pulmonary disease (46,47). In a subset of patients with chronic obstructive pulmonary disease, the sensitivity of V/Q scan interpretation for PE was significantly lower than in patients with no preexisting cardiopulmonary disease (48). However, the positive predictive value of a high probability V/Q scan interpretation in this subset was 100%, and the negative predictive value of a low or very low probability V/Q scan interpretation was 94%.

Although the clinical diagnosis of PE is not diagnostic in most instances, the results from the PIOPED study emphasized the importance of incorporating the clinical assessment data into the utilization scheme of V/Q results when evaluating patients suspected of having acute PE. As expected, combining clinical assessment with the V/Q scan interpretation improved the diagnostic accuracy. In patients with low or

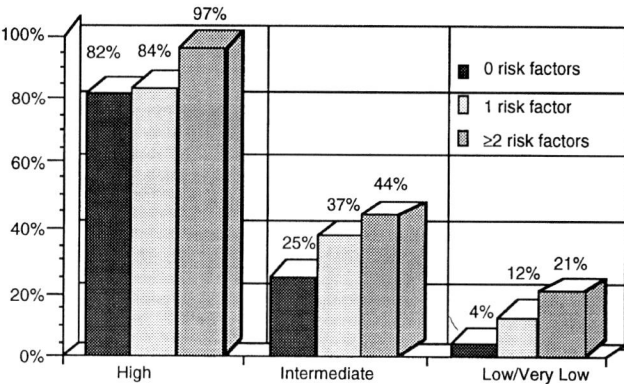

FIG. 2. Prevalence of pulmonary embolism. Value of combining selected risk factors and the V/Q lung scan interpretation. Selected risk factors include immobilization, trauma to the lower extremities, recent surgery, or central venous instrumentation.

very low probability V/Q scan interpretations and no history of immobilization, recent surgery, trauma to the lower extremities, or central venous instrumentation, the prevalence of PE was only 4.5% (49,50). Whereas in patients with low or very low probability V/Q lung scan interpretations and one or more than one of the above mentioned risk factors, the prevalences of PE were 12% and 21%, respectively (Fig. 2). However, in PIOPED, the majority of patients had intermediate probability V/Q scans and an intermediate clinical likelihood of PE. For these patients, the combination of clinical assessment and V/Q scan interpretation is not adequate for optimal management, and further investigations with peripheral venous studies and CT and/or pulmonary angiography are usually required.

The most common cause of V/Q mismatch in patients who do not have acute PE are due to chronic or unresolved PE. Other causes include: compression of the pulmonary vasculature (mass lesions, adenopathy, mediastinal fibrosis), vessel wall abnormalities (pulmonary artery tumors, vasculitis), intraluminal obstruction (tumor emboli, foreign body emboli), congenital vascular abnormalities (pulmonary artery agenesis or hypoplasia). In patients with unilateral V/Q mismatch (hypoperfusion or absent perfusion) within an entire lung or multiple contiguous segments and normal perfusion in the contralateral lung, extrinsic compression of the pulmonary vasculature, congenital abnormalities or proximal PE all need to be considered in the differential diagnosis. These patients will often require further imaging with computed tomography (CT) or angiography.

INTERPRETATION CRITERIA AND AMENDMENTS OF ORIGINAL PIOPED CRITERIA

Several diagnostic criteria have been suggested for the interpretation of V/Q lung scans. In a study comparing the various interpretation algorithms, the original PIOPED crite-

TABLE 1. *Revised PIOPED criteria*

High probability (>80%)
  ≥2 Large (>75% of a segment) segmental perfusion defects without matching ventilation or chest x-ray abnormalities
  1 Large segmental perfusion defect and ≥2 moderate (25%–75% of a segment) segmental perfusion defects without matching ventilation or chest x-ray abnormalities
  ≥4 Moderate segmental perfusion defects without matching ventilation or chest x-ray abnormalities

Intermediate probability (20%–79%)
  1 moderate to <2 large segmental perfusion defects without matching ventilation or chest x-ray abnormalities
  Matching V/Q defects and chest x-ray parenchymal opacity in lower lung zone
  Matching V/Q defects and small pleural effusion
  Single moderate matched V/Q defects with normal chest x-ray findings in the lower lobes
  Difficult to categorize as normal, low, or high probability

Low probability (10%–19%)
  Multiple matched V/Q defects, regardless of size, with normal chest x-ray findings
  Matching V/Q defects and with or without chest x-ray parenchymal opacity in upper or middle lung zone
  Matching V/Q defects and large pleural effusion
  Defects surrounded by normally perfused lung (stripe sign)

Very low (<10%)
  Nonsegmental perfusion defects (cardiomegally, aortic impression, enlarged hilia)
  Any perfusion defects with substantially larger chest x-ray abnormality
  Single or multiple small (<25% of a segment) segmental perfusion defects with a normal chest x-ray

Normal
  No perfusion defects and perfusion outlines the shape of the lung seen on chest x-ray

---

ria had the highest likelihood ratio for predicting the presence of PE on pulmonary angiography (51). However, the PIOPED criteria also had the highest proportion of V/Q scans interpreted as representing an intermediate probability of acute PE (51). Several revisions of the original PIOPED criteria have been made based on the observations from the PIOPED study, as illustrated in Table 1. By and large, with these revisions, it is possible to decrease the number of intermediate V/Q scan interpretations and increase the number considered as low probability of acute PE. The use of revised PIOPED criteria has already been shown to provide a more accurate assessment of angiographically proven PE compared with the original criteria (52,53).

Currently accepted modifications of the original PIOPED criteria include the following:

1. Single, moderate, mismatched perfusion abnormality, initially considered to be low probability, is now considered intermediate probability (Fig. 3);
2. Intermediate probability is now a well-defined category with clear criteria;
3. Single matched defects are better defined. Those present

in the upper and middle lobes can be classified as low probability, and those in the lower lobes as intermediate probability.

In patients with single segmental V/Q mismatch and multiple risk factors, the prevalence of PE is higher; these patients should be considered to have PE until proven otherwise (Fig. 3).

In patients with matching V/Q defects and chest radiographic opacities (triple matches) the overall prevalence of PE was 26% (54). However, triple matches within the upper and middle lung zone has a lower prevalence of PE compared with triple matches in the lower lung. When triple matches were present within the upper and middle lung zones, the prevalences of PE were 11% and 12%, respectively, whereas PE was present in 33% of lower lung zones with such findings (54). Therefore, patients with matching V/Q defects and chest radiographic opacities isolated to the upper or middle lung zones can be interpreted as representing a low probability for acute PE.

A single moderate-sized V/Q mismatch was classified as representing a low probability of PE using the original PIOPED criteria. However, 36% of patients with a moderate-sized V/Q mismatch had PE; therefore, this finding represents an intermediate probability for acute PE (55).

Among patients with no previous cardiopulmonary disease, no patient with PE had radiographic evidence of a pleural effusions that occupied more than one third of the hemithorax (14). Therefore, V/Q defects with large pleural effusion represent a low probability of acute PE. In contrast, the majority of patients with PE and pleural effusions had small effusions that caused blunting of the costophrenic angles. The prevalence of PE within the lower lung zones in patients with small pleural effusions was 32% in the right hemithorax and 25% in the left hemithorax (23). Therefore, matching V/Q defects with a small effusion represents an intermediate probability of acute PE.

The stripe sign is defined as a rim of perfused lung tissue between the perfusion defect and the adjacent pleural surface. The presence of the sign excluded the diagnosis of PE within the effected zone in 93% of cases (56). Therefore, perfusion defects that demonstrate a stripe sign are unlikely to be due to PE, and, in the absence of perfusion defects elsewhere, they should be interpreted as representing a low probability for PE. Patients with partially resolving perfusion defects may have a similar appearance to the stripe sign; therefore, this sign should be interpreted with caution in patients with chronic symptoms of PE.

The nuclear medicine physician's subjective estimate of the likelihood of PE (without using specific interpretation criteria) correlated well with the fraction of patients with angiographic evidence of PE (57). Thus, experienced readers (such as the PIOPED investigators) can provide an accurate estimate of the probability of PE based on radiographic and scintigraphic findings.

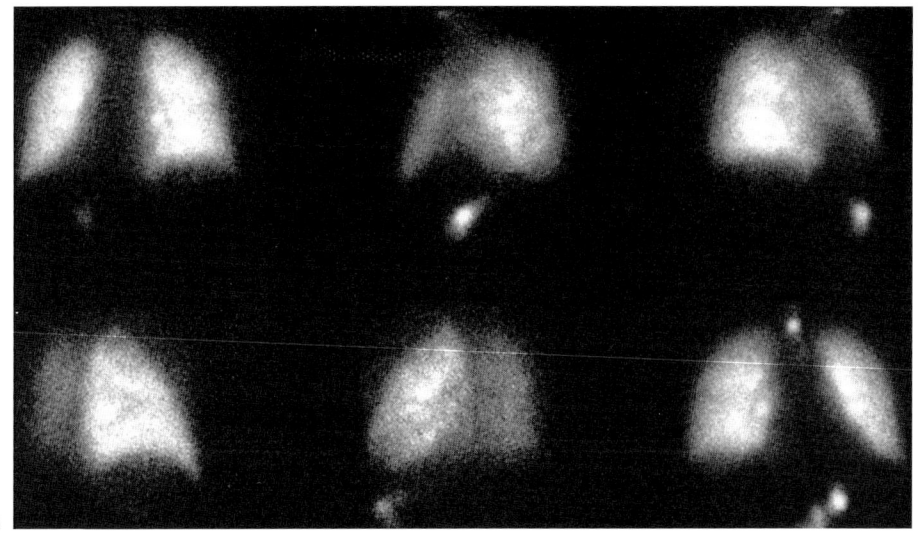

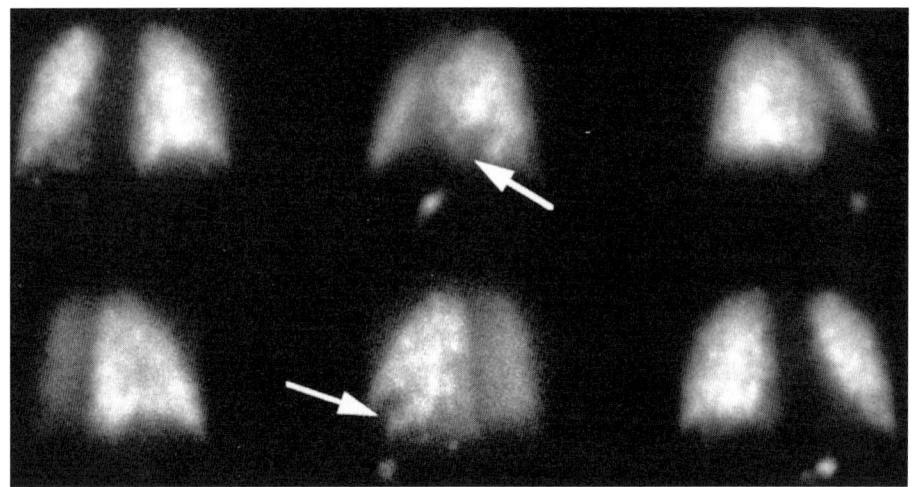

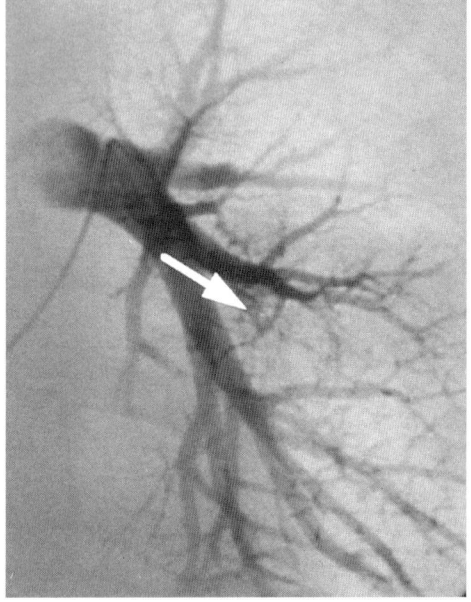

FIG. 3. Tc-99m DTPA ventilation (**A**) and Tc-99m MAA perfusion (**B**) images demonstrate a single segmental V/Q mismatch (*arrows*) within the superior lingular segment in this patient who is 3 days postoperative following surgery for a fractured hip. Matching decreased ventilation and perfusion was also present within multiple segments of the left lower lobe. A spiral CT performed within 1 hour of the ventilation/perfusion scan was normal. A subsequent pulmonary angiogram (**C**) demonstrated an intraluminal filling defect and abrupt vascular cutoff within a lingular artery (*arrow*) confirming pulmonary embolism.

COMPUTED TOMOGRAPHIC ANGIOGRAPHY IN PULMONARY EMBOLISM

Both spiral CT angiography and electron beam CT have been used to diagnose PE and visualize associated parenchymal and pleural changes (58–64). With spiral CT angiography, data is continuously and rapidly collected as the patient moves through the gantry. Volumetric data sets of the entire lungs can generally be acquired during a single breath, which eliminates respiratory misregistration (Fig. 4**D**). Electron beam CT is less widely available and has superior temporal resolution but inferior spatial resolution compared with spiral CT. Electron beam CT does not acquire a true volumetric data set but rather acquires overlapping transaxial images that can be reformatted to be viewed as multiplanar or three-dimensional images. In animal models, CT has been shown to detect thrombi in central to fourth division (segmental) pulmonary arteries (65,66).

The sensitivity and specificity of CT angiography for detecting central PE is 86 to 95% and 75 to 97%, respectively (58,60,63,64,67–69). The diagnostic performance of CT for detecting subsegmental thrombi is lower. In a prospective comparison of spiral CT and pulmonary angiography in 20 patients, Goodman et al. (67) reported that the sensitivity for detecting PE decreased from 86 to 63% when all vessels (segmental and subsegmental) were included. Similarly, Teigen et al. (63), utilizing electron beam CT, reported that

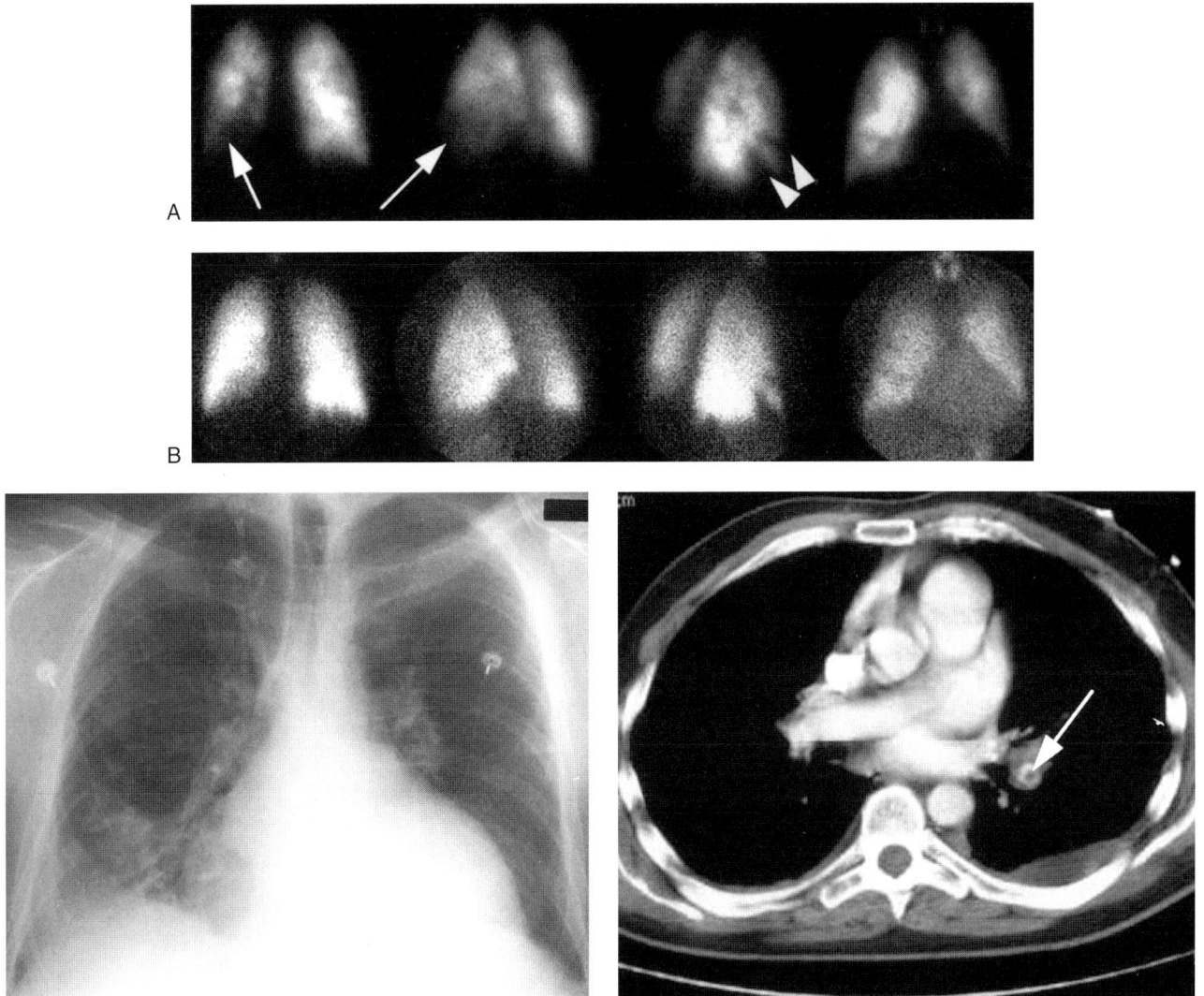

FIG. 4. Tc-99m MAA perfusion (**A**) and Tc-99m Pertechnegas (**B**) images demonstrate a matching ventilation, perfusion, and chest x-ray opacity within the right middle and lower lobes (*arrowheads*) (Q defect equals V defect equals chest x-ray opacity). Within the left lower lobe and lingula, the perfusion abnormalities (*arrow*) appear more extensive than the corresponding ventilation and chest radiograph (**C**) opacity (Q defect > V defect > chest x-ray opacity). The corresponding spiral CT (computed tomographic) image (**D**) on vascular windows demonstrates partially occlusive thrombus within the left lower lobe pulmonary artery (*arrow*).

the sensitivity for the detection of PE decreased from 88 to 65% when subsegmental vessels were evaluated. In a prospective study comparing spiral CT angiography and V/Q scintigraphy, Mayo et al. (70) reported that spiral CT angiography had a higher sensitivity compared with a high probability V/Q scan interpretation. The specificity, positive predictive value, and negative predictive value were similar between the two modalities. An advantage of spiral CT angiography compared with V/Q scanning is higher interobserver agreement and the ability to provide an alternative diagnosis for patients with suspected PE (68,70).

The performance of optimum CT angiography for detection of PE is technically demanding and several examination parameters need to be considered. Scans are generally performed from the level of the aortic arch to below the inferior pulmonary veins. Imaging can be performed during a single breath hold or during shallow respiration. Nonionic iodinated contrast is injected with a power injector through a well-established 18-gauge intravenous line. A total of 120 to 160 mL of contrast is injected at 4 to 5 mL/sec through a central line or at 3 mL/sec into a peripheral line. A "test dose" of contrast may be given to determine the optimum scan delay time, or scanning is performed 15 to 20 seconds after the initiation of the contrast injection. Images are acquired with a 3-mm collimation, with a pitch of 1.8 to 2 for nonbreath-holding sequences. Images are reconstructed at 1.5–3 mm intervals. Scan volumes are generally 12 to 15 cm in the caudal-cranial direction. For optimum reporting, images should be viewed on both pulmonary vascular and lung parenchymal settings on a workstation.

Acute PE appears as an intraluminal filling defect, which partially or completely occludes the pulmonary artery, as shown in Figure 4**D**. Commonly, mild vascular distention is present within the effected vessel at the site of the thrombus. Segmental pulmonary arteries are located in close proximity to their accompanying bronchus on the corresponding lung window. Upper and lower lobe arteries run perpendicular to the scan plane, whereas lingular and right middle lobe arteries tend to run parallel to the scan plane, and, in these vessels, the sensitivity for detecting PE is lower (64,67) (Fig. 3). Other limitations of CT angiography include technical failures and incomplete examinations. Patient-related factors, which can result in incomplete or suboptimal examinations, include: orthopnea, poor intravenous access, or severe shortness of breath. In patients who are unable to breath hold, respiratory misregistration may occur and degrade image quality. Poor signal-to-noise ratio or vascular enhancement may occur in patients with right heart failure, large right-to-left shunts or extravasated intravenous lines. An imaging artifact called flow phenomenon, which produces a central low density within the vessels oriented perpendicular to the scan, has been described. This is most often seen in vessels scanned either too early or too late following intravenous contrast. The mechanisms causing this artifact have not been fully elucidated. However, it is likely in part due to laminar flow and uneven mixing of contrast within the vessel. In spite of the technical demands, CT angiography can provide a prompt and accurate diagnosis of PE in most patients. Some authors have suggested that CT angiography be the first line test in patients with suspected PE (71). However, its routine use for this purpose is not widely accepted at this time.

PULMONARY ANGIOGRAPHY IN PULMONARY EMBOLISM

Pulmonary angiography has remained the definitive gold standard test for the diagnosis or exclusion of PE, as illustrated in Figure 4**C**. The angiographic diagnosis of acute PE in PIOPED was based on the identification of an intraluminal filling defect or the trailing edge of a thrombus obstructing a vessel. In patients who had angiographic evidence of PE, reader agreement among angiographers was noted to be 86% (331 of 383) of cases. In patients with angiograms interpreted as negative or uncertain for PE, reader agreement was noted to be 80% (544 of 681) and 40% (14 of 35) of cases, respectively. In PIOPED, pulmonary angiography was completed in 99% (1,099 of 1,111) of patients who consented to undergo the procedure (72). In the majority of patients in whom angiography was not completed, a complication was encountered during the procedure. Nondiagnostic pulmonary angiograms were obtained in only 3% (35 of 1,111) of patients.

The validity of pulmonary angiography was assessed by the outcome classification committee. In 681 patients whose angiograms were interpreted as being negative for PE, only 4 patients had their diagnosis reversed by the outcome classification committee. Thus, a negative pulmonary angiogram excluded the diagnosis of acute PE in 99% (667 of 681) of cases. Since angiography was considered the gold standard in the PIOPED study, the validity of a positive angiogram representing PE could not be assessed.

An analysis of the regional distribution of PE on angiography demonstrated that PE occurred more frequently on the right compared with the left and more frequently in the lower lung zones compared with the middle or upper lung zones (73).

The complications related to pulmonary angiography have been well documented by Stein et al. (72). Death attributed to pulmonary angiography occurred in 0.5% (5 of 1,111) of patients. Nonfatal major complications including respiratory distress, severe renal failure, or hematoma requiring transfusion occurred in 1% (14 of 1,111) of patients. The frequency of major complications was higher in patients from the medical intensive care unit compared with patients from other hospital locations. Minor complications, which were not life threatening and responded promptly to pharmaceutical therapy, occurred in 5% (60 of 1,111) of patients. The most common minor complications were urticaria or pruritus and mild renal dysfunction. The frequency of complications was not related to patient age, the presence of PE, or pulmonary artery pressure.

OUTCOME IN PULMONARY EMBOLISM

Of the 399 patients in the PIOPED study who had confirmed PE, treatment was initiated for 94% (375 of 399). Among the 24 patients who were not treated, 19 patients had negative angiogram interpretations at the local hospital that were in disagreement with the final angiogram interpretation. Death attributed to pulmonary embolism occurred in only 2.5% (10 of 399) of patients with PE (7). Patients were far more likely to die from comorbid conditions rather than PE. Among the patients who died of PE only, 1 was untreated and 9 of the deaths were due to clinically suspected recurrent PE. Therefore, when properly diagnosed and treated, death attributed to PE was relatively uncommon.

From the prospective and outcome-based studies that have been carried out in the past few years, the following conclusions regarding the diagnostic evaluation of patients with suspected PE can be made:

1. A normal V/Q scan interpretation excludes the diagnosis of clinically significant PE.
2. Patients with very low or low probability V/Q scan interpretation and low clinical likelihood of PE do not require angiography or anticoagulation.
3. Patients with very low or low probability V/Q scan interpretation, intermediate or high clinical likelihood of PE, and negative serial noninvasive venous studies of the lower extremities generally do not require anticoagulation or angiography. If serial noninvasive venous studies of the lower extremities are positive, patients should be treated.
4. Clinically stable patients with an intermediate probability V/Q scan interpretation require noninvasive venous studies of the legs and, if negative, require CT angiography or pulmonary angiography for a definite diagnosis.
5. Clinically stable patients with a high probability V/Q scan interpretation and a high clinical likelihood of PE require treatment and generally need no further diagnostic tests to confirm the diagnosis.
6. Clinically stable patients with a high probability V/Q scan interpretation and a low or intermediate clinical likelihood of PE require noninvasive venous studies of the legs and, if negative, often require CT angiography or pulmonary CT for a definitive diagnosis.

V/Q LUNG SCANNING IN THE EVALUATION OF PULMONARY HYPERTENSION

Chronic pulmonary thromboembolism is a serious and potentially curable cause of pulmonary hypertension (PHT). It has been estimated that between 0.5 and 4% of patients with acute pulmonary emboli will eventually develop chronic thromboembolic PHT (74). Unfortunately, the clinical features, laboratory investigations, and other noninvasive investigations are often unreliable in distinguishing chronic thromboembolic PHT from primary and nonthromboembolic secondary PHT. Evaluation with pulmonary angiogra-

phy is usually required to confirm the diagnosis and to determine whether surgical intervention is indicated. Although some authors have reported that pulmonary angiography can be performed safely in patients with severe PHT, others have documented a higher frequency of complications, including death (72,75). Ventilation/perfusion lung scanning provides a safe, noninvasive technique that effectively selects which patients with PHT require pulmonary angiography to confirm the diagnosis of chronic PE and determine surgical intervention for cure. However, both V/Q lung scanning and pulmonary angiography may underestimate the severity of chronic thromboembolic material within the pulmonary vasculature as determined during thromboendarterectomy (76).

When performing the V/Q lung scan in patients with PHT, it is important that the number of Tc-99m MAA particles injected is reduced to avoid possible hemodynamic effects. It is recommended that patients with PHT be injected with between 60,000 particles of Tc-99m MMA. Several studies have documented the safety of perfusion lung scanning in patients with PHT when the number of particles are reduced (77,78). In patients with chronic thromboembolic PHT, 96% had V/Q lung scans that were interpreted as representing a high probability of pulmonary embolism (77). In the remaining 1 patient from this group, the V/Q lung scan was interpreted as representing an intermediate probability of pulmonary embolism. Therefore, based on this retrospective study, pulmonary angiography was justified in patients with intermediate or high probability V/Q lung scan interpretations to confirm the diagnosis of chronic PE. Most patients with primary PHT and nonthromboembolic secondary PHT had low probability V/Q lung scan interpretations. Patients with PHT rarely, if ever, have normal or very low probability V/Q lung scan interpretations; however, a low probability V/Q lung scan interpretation effectively excludes chronic thromboembolism as the cause of PHT.

REFERENCES

1. Palevsky HI. The problems of the clinical and laboratory diagnosis of pulmonary embolism. *Semin Nucl Med* 1991;21:276–280.
2. Wigton RS, Hoellerich VL, Patil KD. How physicians use clinical information in diagnosing pulmonary embolism: an application of conjoint analysis. *Med Decis Making* 1986;6:2–11.
3. Silverstein MD, Heit JA, Mohr DN, et al. Trends in the incidence and of deep vein thrombosis and pulmonary embolism: a 25-year population-based study. *Arch Intern Med* 1998;158:585–593.
4. Dalen JE, Alpert JS. Natural history of pulmonary embolism. *Prog Cardiovasc Dis* 1975;17:257–270.
5. Alpert JS, Smith R, Carlson J, et al. Mortality in patients treated for pulmonary embolism. *JAMA* 1976;236:1477–1480.
6. Hirsh J, Hoak J. Management of deep vein thrombosis and pulmonary embolism. A statement for healthcare professionals. *Circulation* 1996; 93(12):2212–2245.
7. Carson JL, Kelley MA, Duff A, et al. The clinical course of pulmonary embolism. *N Engl J Med* 1992;326:1240–1245.
8. Mant MJ, O'Brien BD, Thong KL, et al. Haemorrhagic complications of heparin therapy. *Lancet* 1977;1:1133–1135.
9. Nelson PH, Moser KM, Stoner C, et al. Risk of complications during intravenous heparin therapy. *West J Med* 1982;136:189–197.
10. Porter J, Jick H. Drug-related deaths among medical inpatients. *JAMA* 1977;237:879–881.

11. Quinn DA, Thompson BT, Terrin ML, et al. A prospective investigation of pulmonary embolism in women and men. *JAMA* 1992;268: 1689–1696.

12. Goldhaber SZ. Pulmonary embolism. *N Engl J Med* 1998;339(2): 93–104.

13. Anderson FA Jr., Wheeler HB, Goldberg RJ, et al. A population-based perspective of the hospital incidence and case-fatality rates of deep vein thrombosis and pulmonary embolism. The Worcester DVT Study. *Arch Intern Med* 1991;151(5):933–938.

14. Stein PD, Terrin ML, Hales CA, et al. Clinical, laboratory, roentgenographic, and electrocardiographic findings in patients with acute pulmonary embolism and no pre-existing cardiac or pulmonary disease. *Chest* 1991;100:598–603.

15. Stein PD, Saltzman HA, Weg JG. Clinical characteristics of patients with acute pulmonary embolism. *Am J Cardiol* 1991;68:1723–1724.

16. Boone JM, Gross GW, Greco-Hunt V. Neural networks in radiologic diagnosis: I. Introduction and illustration. *Invest Radiol* 1990;25: 1012–1016.

17. Patil S, Henry JW, Rubenfire M, et al. Neural network in the clinical diagnosis of acute pulmonary embolism. *Chest* 1993;104:1685–1689.

18. Anonymous. Opinions regarding the diagnosis and management of venous thromboembolic disease. ACCP Consensus Committee on Pulmonary Embolism. *Chest* 1996;109:233–237.

19. van Beek EJ, van den Ende B, Berckmans RJ, et al. A comparative analysis of D-dimer assays in patients with suspected pulmonary embolism. *Thromb Haemost* 1993;70(3):408–413.

20. Heaton DC, Billings JD, Hickton CM. Assessment of D dimer assays for the diagnosis of deep vein thrombosis. *J Lab Clin Med* 1987;110(5): 588–591.

21. Becker DM, Philbrick JT, Bachhuber TL, et al. D-dimer testing and acute venous thromboembolism. A shortcut to. *Arch Intern Med* 1996; 156:939–946.

22. Stein PD, Dalen JE, McIntyre KM, et al. The electrocardiogram in acute pulmonary embolism. *Prog Cardiovasc Dis* 1975;17:247–257.

23. Worsley DF, Alavi A, Aronchick JM, et al. Chest radiographic findings in patients with acute pulmonary embolism: observations from the PIOPED study. *Radiology* 1993;189:133–136.

24. Hull RD, Raskob GE. Low-probability lung scan findings: a need for a change. *Ann Intern Med* 1991;114:142–143.

25. Robin ED. Overdiagnosis and overtreatment of pulmonary embolism: the emperor may have no clothes. *Ann Intern Med* 1977;87:775–781.

26. Robinson PJ. Lung scintigraphy-doubt and certainty in the diagnosis of pulmonary embolism. *Clin Radiol* 1989;40:557–560.

27. Taplin GV, Johnson DE, Dore EK, et al. Suspensions of radioalbumin aggregates for photoscanning the liver, spleen, lung and other organs. *J Nucl Med* 1964;5:259–275.

28. Wagner HN, Sabiston AC, McAfee JG, et al. Diagnosis of massive pulmonary embolism in man by radioisotope scanning. *N Engl J Med* 1964;271:377–384.

29. Heck LL, Duley JW. Statisical considerations in lung scanning with Tc-99m albumin particles. *Radiology* 1975;113:675–679.

30. Alderson PO, Doppman JL, Diamond SS, et al. Ventilation-perfusion lung imaging and selective pulmonary angiography in dogs with experimental pulmonary emboli. *J Nucl Med* 1978;19:164–171.

31. Morrell NW, Roberts CM, Jones BE, et al. The anatomy of radioisotope lung scanning. *J Nucl Med* 1992;33:676–683.

32. DeNardo GL, Goodwin DA, Ravasini R, et al. The ventilatory lung scan in the diagnosis of pulmonary embolism. *N Engl J Med* 1970; 282(24):1334–1336.

33. Wagner HN Jr, Lopez-Majano V, Langan JK, et al. Radioactive xenon in the differential diagnosis of pulmonary embolism. *Radiology* 1968; 91:1168–1174.

34. James JM, Herman KJ, Lloyd JJ, et al. Evaluation of 99Tcm Technegas ventilation scintigraphy in the diagnosis of pulmonary embolism. *Br J Radiol* 1991;64:711–719.

35. Alderson PO, Biello DR, Gottschalk A, et al. Tc-99m-DTPA aerosol and radioactive gases compared as adjuncts to perfusion scintigraphy in patients with suspected pulmonary embolism. *Radiology* 1984;153(2): 515–521.

36. Worsley DF, Alavi A. Does patient position affect the diagnostic performance of the V/Q lung scan for detecting acute pulmonary embolism. *J Nucl Med* 1994;35:24P(abst).

37. Anonymous. Opinions regarding the diagnosis and management of venous thromboembolic disease. ACCP Consensus Committee on Pulmonary Embolism. *Chest* 1998;113(2):499–504.

38. UPET Investigators. The urokinase pulmonary embolism trial. A national cooperative study. *Circulation* 1973;47[Suppl 2]:46–50.

39. Hull RD, Raskob GE, Coates G, et al. A new noninvasive management strategy for patients with suspected pulmonary embolism. *Arch Intern Med* 1989;149:2549–2555.

40. Hull RD, Raskob GE, Ginsberg JS, et al. A noninvasive strategy for the treatment of patients with suspected pulmonary embolism. *Arch Intern Med* 1994;154:289–297.

41. PIOPED Investigators. Value of the ventilation/perfusion scan in acute pulmonary embolism. *JAMA* 1990;263:2753–2759.

42. Hull RD, Feldstein W, Stein PD, et al. Cost-effectiveness of pulmonary embolism diagnosis. *Arch Intern Med* 1996;156:68–72.

43. Kelley MA, Carson JL, Palevsky HI, et al. Diagnosing pulmonary embolism: new facts and strategies. *Ann Intern Med* 1991;114:300–306.

44. Miniati M, Pistolesi M, Marini C, et al. Value of perfusion lung scan in the diagnosis of pulmonary embolism: results of the prospective investigative study of acute pulmonary embolism diagnosis (PISA-PED). *American Journal of Respiratory and Critical Care Medicine* 1996;154:1387–1393.

45. Stein PD, Gottschalk A, Saltzman HA, et al. Diagnosis of acute pulmonary embolism in the elderly. *J Am Coll Cardiol* 1991;18:1452–1457.

46. Worsley DF, Alavi A, Palevsky HI, et al. Comparison of the the diagnostic performance of ventilation/perfusion lung scanning in different patient populations. *Radiology* 1996;199(2):481–483.

47. Stein PD, Coleman RE, Gottschalk A, et al. Diagnostic utility of ventilation/perfusion lung scans in acute pulmonary embolism is not diminished by pre-existing cardiac or pulmonary disease. *Chest* 1991; 100:604–606.

48. Lesser BA, Leeper KV Jr, Stein PD, et al. The diagnosis of acute pulmonary embolism in patients with chronic obstructive pulmonary disease. *Chest* 1992;102:17–22.

49. Worsley DF, Palevsky HI, Alavi A. Clinical characteristic of patients with pulmonary embolism and low or very low probability lung scan interpretations. *Arch Intern Med* 1994;154:2737–2741.

50. Worsley DF, Alavi A, Palevsky HI. Clinical characteristic of patients with pulmonary embolism and low or very low probability lung scan interpretations. *J Nucl Med* 1994;35:25P(abst).

51. Webber MM, Gomes AS, Roe D, et al. Comparison of Biello, McNeil, and PIOPED criteria for the diagnosis of pulmonary emboli on lung scans. *Am J Roentgenol* 1990;154:975–981.

52. Freitas FE, Sarosi MG, Nagle CC, et al. The use of modified PIOPED criteria in clinical practice. *J Nucl Med* 1995;36:1573–1578.

53. Sostman HD, Coleman RE, Delong DM, et al. Prospective trial of revised PIOPED criteria for lung scan interpretation in clinically selected patients. *J Nucl Med* 1994;35:25P(abst).

54. Worsley DF, Kim CK, Alavi A, et al. Detailed analysis of patients with matched ventilation-perfusion defects and chest radiographic opacities. *J Nucl Med* 1993;34:1851–1853.

55. Gottschalk A, Sostman HD, Coleman RE, et al. Ventilation-perfusion scintigraphy in the PIOPED study. Part II. Evaluation of the scinitigraphic criteria and interpretations. *J Nucl Med* 1993;34:1119–1126.

56. Sostman HD, Gottschalk A. Prospective validation of the stripe sign in ventilation-perfusion scintigraphy. *Radiology* 1992;184:455–459.

57. Sostman HD, Coleman RE, Delong DM, et al. Evaluation of revised criteria for ventilation-perfusion scintigraphy in patients with suspected pulmonary embolism. *Radiology* 1994;193:103–107.

58. van Rossum AB, Pattynama PM, Ton ER, et al. Pulmonary embolism: validation of spiral CT angiography in 149 patients. *Radiology* 1996; 201:467–470.

59. van Erkel AR, van Rossum AB, Bloem JL, et al. Spiral CT angiography for suspected pulmonary embolism: a cost-effectiveness analysis. *Radiology* 1996;201:29–36.

60. Remy-Jardin M, Remy J, Deschildre F, et al. Diagnosis of pulmonary embolism with spiral CT: comparison with pulmonary angiography and scintigraphy. *Radiology* 1996;200:699–706.

61. Remy-Jardin M, Remy J, Artaud D, et al. Peripheral pulmonary arteries: optimization of the spiral CT. *Radiology* 1997;204:157–163.

62. Remy-Jardin M, Duyck P, Remy J, et al. Hilar lymph nodes: identification with spiral CT and histologic. *Radiology* 1995;196:387–394.

63. Teigen CL, Maus TP, Sheedy PF, et al. Pulmonary embolism: diagnosis with contrast-enhanced electron-beam CT and comparison with pulmonary angiography. *Radiology* 1995;194:313–319.

64. Teigen CL, Maus TP, Sheedy PF, et al. Pulmonary embolism: diagnosis with electron-beam CT. *Radiology* 1993;188:839–845.

65. Stanford W, Reiners TJ, Thompson BH, et al. Contrast-enhanced thin slice ultrafast computed tomography for the detection of small pulmonary emboli. Studies using autologous emboli in the pig. *Invest Radiol* 1994;29:184–187.

66. Geraghty JJ, Stanford W, Landas SK, et al. Ultrafast computed tomography in experimental pulmonary embolism. *Invest Radiol* 1992;27:60–63.

67. Goodman LR, Curtin JJ, Mewissen MW, et al. Detection of pulmonary embolism in patients with unresolved clinical and scintigraphic diagnosis: helical CT versus angiography. *Am J Roentgenol* 1995;164:1369–1374.

68. van Rossum AB, Treurniet FE, Kieft GJ, et al. Role of spiral volumetric computed tomographic scanning in the assessment of patients with clinical suspicion of pulmonary embolism and an abnormal ventilation/perfusion lung scan. *Thorax* 1996;51:23–28.

69. Remy-Jardin M, Remy J, Cauvain O, et al. Diagnosis of central pulmonary embolism with helical CT: role of two-dimensional multiplanar reformations. *Am J Roentgenol* 1995;165:1131–1138.

70. Mayo JR, Remy-Jardin M, Muller NL, et al. Pulmonary embolism: prospective comparison of spiral CT with ventilation-perfusion scintigraphy. *Radiology* 1997;205(2):447–452.

71. Goodman LR, Lipchik RJ. Diagnosis of acute pulmonary embolism: time for a new approach. *Radiology* 1996;199:25–27.

72. Stein PD, Athanasoulis C, Alavi A, et al. Complications and validity of pulmonary angiography in acute pulmonary embolism. *Circulation* 1992;85:462–468.

73. Barrett T, Tangoren A, Worsley DF, et al. Regional distribution of pulmonary emboli: an observation from the PIOPED study. *J Nucl Med* 1993;34:16P-17P(abst).

74. Moser KM, Auger WR, Fedullo PF, et al. Chronic thromboembolic pulmonary hypertension: clinical picture and surgical treatment. *Eur Respir J* 1992;5:334–342.

75. Nicod P, Peterson K, Levine M, et al. Pulmonary angiography in severe chronic pulmonary hypertension. *Ann Intern Med* 1987;107:565–568.

76. Ryan KL, Fedullo PF, Davis GB, et al. Perfusion scan findings understate the severity of angiographic and hemodynamic compromise in chronic thromboembolic pulmonary hypertension. *Chest* 1988;93:1180–1185.

77. Worsley DF, Palevsky HI, Alavi A. Ventilation/perfusion lung scanning in the evaluation of pulmonary hypertension. *J Nucl Med* 1994;35:793–796.

78. Rich S, Dantzker DR, Ayres SM, et al. Primary pulmonary hypertension: a national prospective study. *Ann Intern Med* 1987;107:216–223.

CHAPTER 58

Aortic Diseases

Radd H. Mohiaddin, Philip J. Kilner, and Dudley J. Pennell

IMAGING THE AORTA

A number of imaging modalities may be used in the assessment of aortic disease. The chest x-ray is sometimes useful. However, the proximal portion of the ascending aorta adjacent to the aortic annulus may not be seen, and it is less sensitive to change than other modalities. Dissection is not easily detected by conventional transthoracic echocardiography, and limited acoustic windows may restrict its use in patients with Marfan chest deformity or emphysematous lungs, making accurate measurement of aortic root diameter difficult. Although, transesophageal echocardiography is better (1), the technique is invasive, the risk of aortic rupture is greater due to the risk of a hypertensive response to probe insertion (2), and visualization of aortic arch vessels is frequently problematic. Catheter lab angiography and, more recently, fast computed x-ray tomographic methods (electron-beam and spiral) have been used, but catheterization requires the administration of iodinated contrast medium, which may have a deleterious effect on renal function or aggravate heart failure. With these caveats in mind, magnetic resonance imaging (MRI) has become an important modality for aortic disease because it offers accurate images that can be quantified without the need for catheterization, contrast medium administration, or x-ray irradiation. The high spatial resolution, the good signal-to-noise ratio, the large field of view, and the ability to obtain images in any orientation or plane are also relevant advantages of MRI. However, the need to place the patient within the enclosed magnet resulting in difficult access in emergency situations, the altered ECG configuration, and the resultant time delay for resusci-

tation are disadvantages of MRI. Thus, none of these modalities are ideal, and knowledge of advantages and limitations of each method is required when deciding which imaging approach to use for a particular patient. This chapter reviews diseases of the aorta and discusses the useful imaging modalities.

THE AGING AORTA

A popular saying is that a man is as old as his arteries. Aortic size is dependent on age, and age-related dimensional changes in the thoracic aorta have been determined by echocardiography, CT, and MRI (3). These changes should be considered when evaluating aortic size. Aortic cross-sectional area increases with age (Table 1), and the area of descending thoracic aorta increases disproportionately to the ascending aorta and aortic arch. There is also elongation and unfolding of the thoracic aorta with age. The significance of these changes on the hemodynamics in the thoracic aorta is not known and needs further investigation. Structural, physiologic, and biochemical alterations of the vascular wall associated with aging of the large arteries (4–6) are principally responsible for these morphological changes. Such fac-

R. H. Mohiaddin: Cardiovascular Magnetic Resonance Unit, Royal Brompton Hospital, London, England SW3 6NP.

P. J. Kilner: Cardiovascular Magnetic Resonance Unit, Royal Brompton Hospital, London, England SW3 6NP.

D. J. Pennell: National Heart and Lung Institute, Imperial College, London, England SW7 2AZ; Cardiovascular Magnetic Resonance Unit, Royal Brompton Hospital, London, England SW3 6NP.

TABLE 1. *Age-related changes in aortic cross-sectional area*[a]

Age	AA(cm^2/m^2)	AR(cm^2/m^2)	DA(cm^2/m^2)
10–19	2.13 ± 0.35	1.65 ± 0.24	1.09 ± 0.21
20–29	2.33 ± 0.53	1.62 ± 0.19	1.23 ± 0.21
30–39	2.64 ± 0.48	2.17 ± 0.33	1.57 ± 0.20
40–49	3.27 ± 0.60	1.96 ± 0.37	1.89 ± 0.22
50–59	3.64 ± 0.40	2.26 ± 0.35	1.88 ± 0.19
>60	4.82 ± 1.56	2.91 ± 0.90	2.82 ± 0.90

[a] Age-related changes in the cross-sectional areas (Mean ± SD) of ascending aorta (AA), aortic arch (AR), and descending thoracic aorta (DA). The measurements were normalized for body surface area.

tors are also responsible for the progressive increase in aortic stiffness associated with aging, and this can be measured by echocardiography and MRI.

STUDIES OF AORTIC WALL MECHANICS

The wall of the aorta contains a variety of tissues, each with its own characteristic properties. Smooth muscle is the physiologically active element, and, by contracting, it can alter the diameter of the vessel or the tension in the wall. The other components include endothelial cells, connective tissue, bands of elastin, and fibers of collagen, which are essentially passive in their mechanical behavior. Aortic compliance depends on the proportions and interconnections of these tissue components and on the contractile state of the vascular smooth muscle. Effectively, the aorta is an elastic tube whose diameter varies with pulsatile pressure. The aorta also propagates pressure and flow waves at certain velocities with the ejection of blood from the heart, which are largely determined by the elastic properties of the wall. Flow waves are propagated in much the same way as pressure waves. The propagation of flow waves has not been studied as extensively as that of pressure (pulse) waves, partly because, unlike flow, accurate methods of pulsatile pressure measurements have been available for a long time and partly because the distinction between flow wave velocity and blood velocity has not always been clearly recognized. Blood velocity means the speed of an average drop of blood, while flow wave velocity means the speed with which motion is transmitted. Methods for measurement of arterial compliance can be divided into two main groups: those relating the radial expansion of the artery to the change in the distending pressure (pressure-volume curve) and those measuring pressure wave and flow wave velocities.

Previous workers have measured human arterial compliance from pressure-volume curves of postmortem arteries

(7). *In vivo* estimation has also been performed using indirect and invasive techniques, including pulse wave velocity measurements in animals and in man (8), the pressure-radius relationship using the Peterson transformer coil in animals, x-ray contrast angiography in humans (9), and pulsed ultrasound aortography.

Regional Aortic Compliance

MRI and echocardiography provide a direct noninvasive means for studying regional aortic compliance (10). Echocardiography, generally uses measurements of aortic *diameter,* whereas MRI uses measurement of cross-sectional area. The technique will be described for MRI. Briefly, high resolution cine or spin-echo images in a plane perpendicular to the aorta allows measurement of aortic cross-sectional area during systole and diastole. The lumen of the aorta can be outlined manually on the computer screen to measure the change in aortic area (ΔA) between diastole and systole. Regional aortic compliance (C) (microl/mm Hg) can be calculated from the change in volume ($\Delta V = \Delta A \times$ slice thickness) of the aortic segment (Fig. 1) divided by the aortic pulse pressure (ΔP) measured by a sphygmomanometer. Automated measurement of aortic cross-sectional area is also possible (11). Other indices of aortic stiffness that can be derived from these measurements include: distensibility (cross-sectional area strain / pulse pressure), elastic modulus (pulse pressure / area strain), and stiffness index β ([systolic blood pressure/diastolic blood pressure] / area strain).

Limitation of Studies of Aortic Distensibility

Measurement of regional aortic compliance by MRI or by echocardiography is calculated from the observed changes in the volume or diameter of an aortic segment and from aortic pulse pressure measured by a sphygmomanometer.

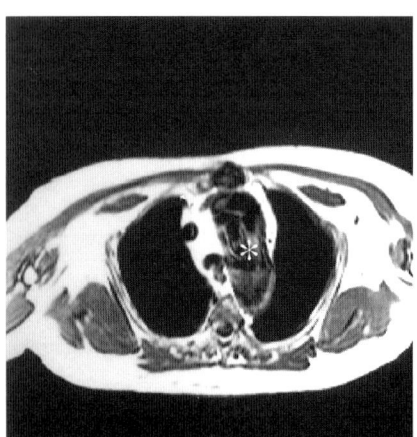
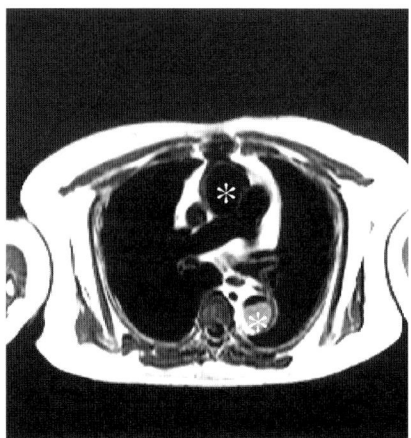
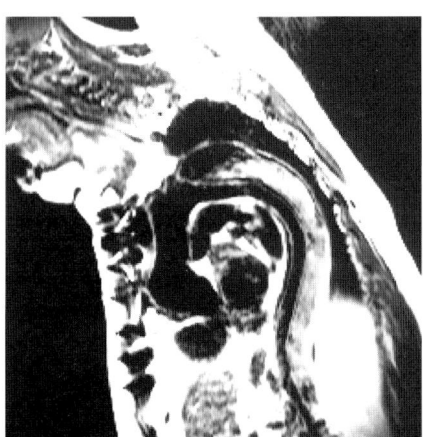

A,B   C

FIG. 1. A stack of transverse images can be used to define an oblique plane through the aortic arch. Three points (*asterisk*) are placed on the arch (**A**), the ascending and descending thoracic aorta (**B**) of patient with type B aortic dissection. **C:** Oblique plane through the aortic arch shows the origin and extension of a dissection with the smaller true lumen anterior to the larger partially thrombosed false lumen.

However, the accuracy of the indirect measurement of the pressure change needed to compute compliance is limited since the pressure wave changes as it propagates through the arterial tree. Despite the limitations of the pressure measurement, there is a good correlation between measurement of regional aortic compliance and measurement of global compliance from the speed of the propagation of the flow wave within the vessel (12). Furthermore, Bohning et al. (13) derived aortic compliance from the aortic flow wave velocity and showed a good agreement between their measurement and those previously reported by Mohiaddin et al. (10).

Aortic Flow Wave Velocity

Doppler echocardiography and MR velocity mapping can be used to acquire high temporal resolution velocities in the aorta, and the time taken for the flow wave to travel between the two points can be determined. For MRI, the instantaneous flow (L/sec) in the ascending and descending aorta can be calculated from aortic cross-sectional area and the mean velocity within that area. Aortic flow wave velocity (FWV) is calculated in m/sec from the transit time (T) of the foot of the flow wave (Fig. 2) and from the distance (D) between the two points obtained from an oblique sagittal spin-echo image. The distance is determined manually on the computer screen by drawing a line in the center of the aorta joining the two points. The foot of the flow wave is defined by extrapolation of the rapid upstroke of the flow wave to the baseline.

$$FWV = D/T$$

Mohiaddin et al. showed the feasibility of using MR velocity mapping for measurement of aortic flow wave velocity. Aortic flow wave velocity increased linearly with age, and there was a significant difference between the youngest decade and the oldest decade studied. Flow wave velocity was negatively correlated with regional ascending aortic compliance measured in the same subjects. Kupari et al. (14) demonstrated that aortic flow wave velocity was more reproducible (with lower inter- and intra-oberver variability) than measurement of the pulsatile aortic area change or the elastic modulus.

Clinical Importance of Aortic Mechanical Properties and Its Application

The combination of elastic arteries and resistant arterioles constitutes a hydraulic filter enabling the intermittent cardiac output to be converted to a steady capillary flow. Part of the energy of left ventricular contraction produces forward flow during systole, but the remainder is stored as potential energy in the distended arteries. During diastole, elastic recoil converts this potential energy again into forward flow (the Windkessel effect). A fall in aortic compliance, therefore, increases the impedance to ventricular ejection and decreases capillary blood flow (15). In addition, reduced compliance may also decrease myocardial oxygen supply through its effect on the normal aortic diastolic back flow that aids coronary perfusion (16,17). The association between atheromatous vascular disease and arterial wall stiffness, or sclerosis, has been recognized for many decades (18,19). Arterial wall stiffness can be demonstrated with experimental disease in both animals (20) and man (21), and regression leads to reduced stiffness (22).

Mohiaddin et al. (10) were the first to use MRI for measurement of aortic compliance. They demonstrated that aortic compliance in asymptomatic subjects decreases with age and that patients with coronary artery disease have abnormally low compliance. The results suggest a possible role for the determination of compliance in the assessment of cardiovascular fitness and as a risk factor for coronary artery disease. Since there is overlap between normal compliance

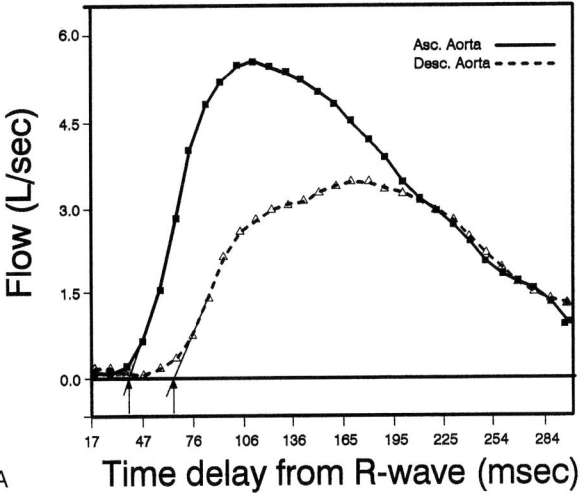

A

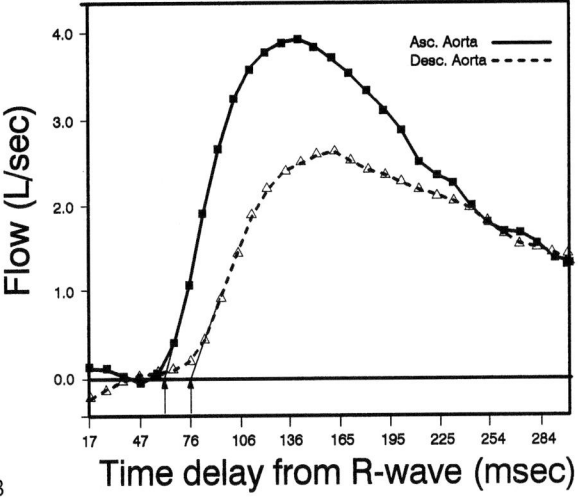

B

FIG. 2. A: Data obtained from a young normal subject with good aortic compliance. **B:** Data obtained from an elderly normal subject with poor compliance and a reduced flow wave velocity. (From ref. 12, with permission.)

and compliance in patients with coronary artery disease above the age of 50, the test is not highly sensitive or specific. Below the age of 50, however, there is much less overlap, and the test is more specific. Abnormally low aortic compliance has also been demonstrated in patients with aortic coarctation (23) and in patients with Marfan syndrome (24).

Kupari et al. (25) measured aortic elastic modulus by MRI in asymptomatic subjects and correlated these measurements with physical activity, ethanol consumption, systolic blood pressure, fasting blood lipids, and serum insulin. They showed that the average value of the ascending and descending aortic elastic modulus was associated positively and statistically significantly with blood pressure, physical activity, serum insulin, and high density lipoprotein (HDL). The elastic modulus was associated negatively with LDL/HDL cholesterol ratio. No association between aortic elastic modulus and either smoking or ethanol consumption was demonstrated. A higher aortic elastic modulus is present in patients with Marfan syndrome than normal healthy subjects, indicating a relative decrease in the distensibility of the thoracic aorta (14).

FLOW IN THE AORTA

MRI is better suited than other techniques to assess aortic flow because it can measure the cross-sectional area and velocity simultaneously. Quantitative analysis of aortic flow using MRI has been a subject of considerable interest in health and disease. Blood flow in the ascending and descending thoracic aorta is phasic. Although the average resting flow measured by MR velocity mapping in the ascending portion and descending portion of the thoracic aorta of normal subjects is 6.0 L/min and 3.9 L/min, respectively, instantaneous peak systolic flow in these aortic segments can reach over 40 L/min and 30 L/min, respectively (26). Qualitative studies of flow in the aorta show normal systolic flow in the ascending aorta as plug flow with a skewed velocity profile that has higher velocities around the inside of the arch. Throughout diastole the blood continues to move with simultaneous forward and reverse channels (27,28). In normal subjects, the reverse flow channel is closely associated with the left coronary sinus, and it is tempting to speculate that it augments flow in the left coronary artery by imparting momentum to the blood that is destined to enter it. In patients with coronary artery disease, the reverse flow channel is smaller and may enter any of the coronary sinuses (29). Ascending and descending aortic flow shows helical flow patterns during systole. The helical flow is clockwise in the ascending aorta and counterclockwise in the descending aorta (Fig. 3). In aortic valve regurgitation, the magnitude of the reverse flow is understandably increased, and aortic valve regurgitation may be quantified from the back flow of blood in the proximal great vessels assessed by velocity mapping (30).

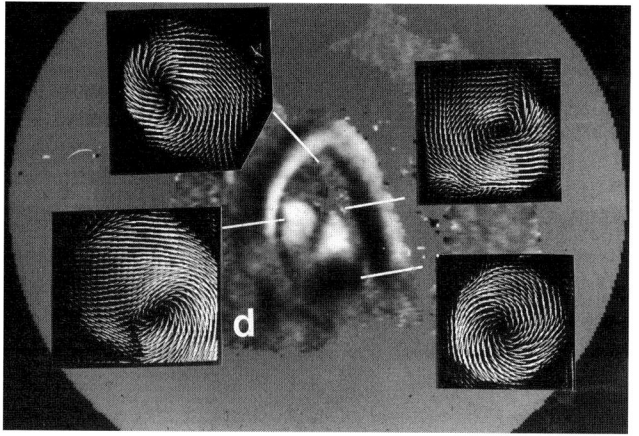

A

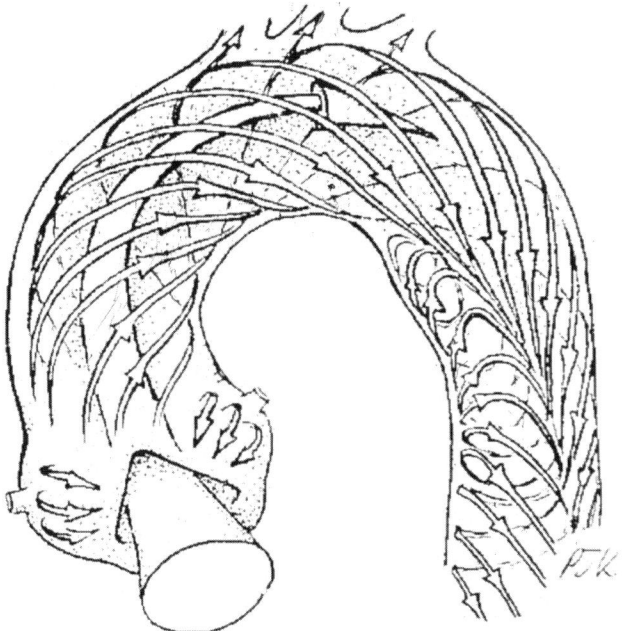

B

FIG. 3. A: Helical flows in the aorta. The late systolic magnetic resonance velocity map in a plane aligned with the aortic arch of a healthy adult is viewed from the left side, *d* is located anterior to the aortic valve. Velocity is encoded through-plane to record nonaxial blood movements: movement toward the viewer appears dark, away, light. Vector maps in four planes transecting the lumen are shown in the black squares. All are viewed in the direction of forward flow, showing evidence of right-handed helical flow in the ascending but left-handed helical flow in the descending aorta at this phase in this subject. B: Drawing representing streamlines in an aortic arch in late systole, based on velocity and vector maps of Figure 4, together with similar studies in additional volunteers.

AORTIC FLOW VECTOR MAPPING

Visualization of Aortic Flow in Health and Disease

Visualization of aortic flow has been a subject of considerable interest for centuries and has attracted enormous experimental and theoretical research. Leonardo da Vinci

(1452–1519) was the first to sketch the profiles of free jets and the formation of eddies near the aortic valve. The classical methods for flow visualization rely largely on optical techniques, often involving introduction of particles or other materials in the flow field. While useful for studying steady flow in phantoms, these techniques are not suited for *in vivo* visualization of pulsatile flow in the human vessels. Magnetic resonance phase shift velocity mapping has unique capability for the acquisition of multidirectional and multidimensional velocity data. Velocities can be then represented by multiple computer-generated streaks whose orientation, length, and movement corresponded to velocity vectors in the chosen plane (31). Magnetic resonance velocity vector mapping is well-suited for studying spatial and temporal patterns of flow in the cardiovascular system (32).

The Healthy Aorta

Vector analysis of multidirectional cine MR velocity mapping of blood flow passing through the aortic valve of a normal subject shows the primary and secondary flow structure clearly, with two vortices near the aortic valve (33). These rotating vortices could be identified flowing back into each sinus in late systole. These trapped vortices carry a momentum that contributes to efficient valve closure at end systole. Flow in the ascending aorta and aortic arch shows arrows orientated predominantly parallel to the wall curvature, with longer arrows toward the outer wall of the descending arch, relatively lower velocities following the inner curvature. There is a small channel of retrograde flow in the ascending and descending aorta during diastole. This retrograde flow is predominately posterior in the ascending aorta and predominately anterior in the descending thoracic aorta (33,34). Ascending and descending aortic flow, acquired in a plane transecting these vessels, shows circular distributions of velocity vectors representing helical flow patterns in the ascending limb, a pair of counter-rotating helices formed in early systole, with the more anterior, clockwise movement dominating in late systole (as viewed from below). In the descending limb, helical movement, as viewed from above in the direction of flow, is counterclockwise.

Aortic Aneurysms

Visualization of aortic flow pattern in patients with aortic aneurysms and grafts by MR velocity vector mapping has been described (35). In patients with atherosclerotic aortic aneurysm who had severely dilated thoracic aorta, the flow pattern in the ascending aorta was shown to be different from that of normals. During left ventricular systole, blood is ejected as a narrow jet into the ascending aorta. The jet is directed toward the anterior aortic wall creating vortices of secondary flow in a clockwise direction (Fig. 4). These

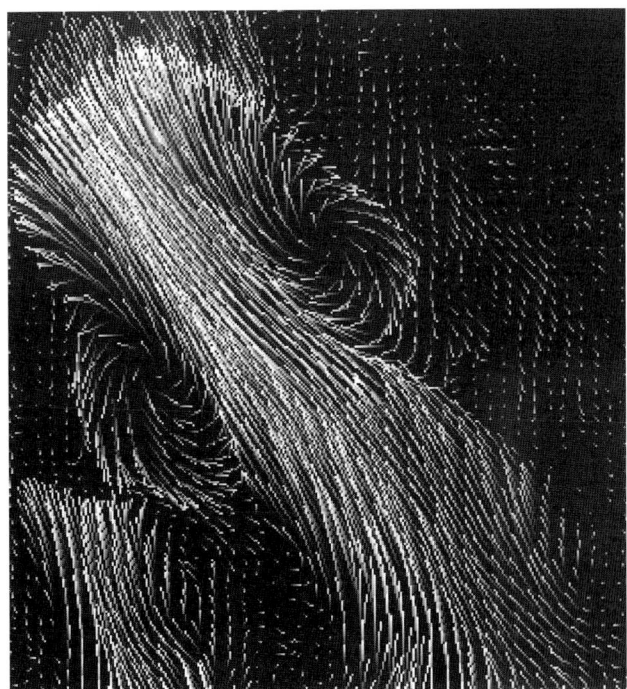

FIG. 4. A blood flow vector map reconstructed from late systolic magnetic resonance velocity data in a plane aligned with flow through the aortic valve in a healthy volunteer. Vectors pass upward and left through the valve, but curl back in sinuses above the two of the cusps that lie in the image plane, confirming Leonardo's deduction.

vortices migrate distally during the course of ventricular systole. On the other hand, patients with Marfan syndrome had a central jet and two large vortices in the dilated segment of the ascending aorta.

Clinical Importance Flow Patterns in the Pathophysiology of Aortic Aneurysms

The role of the hydraulic forces in the formation and propagation of aortic aneurysms has long been discussed but is still poorly understood (36). The initial change in the formation of an aneurysm is structural and results from a degenerative process in the vascular wall. Once the morphologic change has occurred, the blood flow pattern is likely to alter, which may cause altered shear stresses and consequent strains and accelerate the propagation of the aneurysm, so that a vicious cycle is created. The geometry of the aorta is altered in aneurysmal degeneration and the geometric relationship between the left ventricle valve and the ascending aorta becomes more and more distorted during the propagation of an ascending aortic aneurysm. Similar changes occur in aneurysm of the aortic arch and descending thoracic aorta that are likely to influence blood flow patterns and change the hydraulic forces. The interplay and counterplay between morphologic changes and hydrodynamic forces in the development of aortic dissection are unknown and increased knowledge about blood flow patterns in dissections might increase our understanding of the pathophysiologic features of this disease process. The final scenario in the natural history of aneurysm is aortic rupture causing death or that they are surgically replaced with graft. In the latter case, what are the blood flow patterns in surgical grafts? Do they restore normal flow patterns or do they create their own hydrodynamic problems? Magnetic resonance imaging with velocity vector mapping may help to answer these questions.

AORTIC FLOW DURING STRESS

The steady-state hemodynamics created by dobutamine infusion allow the measurement of aortic flow during stress by MRI velocity mapping. By measuring the heart rate and blood pressure during stress, the stroke volume, cardiac output, aortic acceleration, cardiac power output, and flow wave velocity may be calculated. Pennell et al. (37) have reported studies in normal subjects and patients with coronary artery disease. The data so obtained were examined to determine which parameters were predictive of the extent of reversible myocardial ischemia determined from dobutamine thallium tomography. A fall in peak flow and peak flow acceleration at peak stress was found to occur significantly more frequently in patients with moderate and severe ischemia than in patients with mild or no ischemia (Fig. 5). Using a multivariate analysis, the peak flow acceleration was found to be the most predictive variable ($P < 0.00001$), and it alone explained 58.4% of the variation in the observed myocardial ischemia. Only the cardiac power output retained predictive significance after allowing for the peak flow acceleration, but its contribution to the predictive accuracy of the model was small (4.2%).

This study showed that an assessment of aortic flow during dobutamine stress could be used to evaluate global ventricular function, and similar studies of peak acceleration with echocardiography have also been performed (38). Aortic flow has also been measured during exercise stress using devices fitted to the rear of the magnet made from nonferromagnetic materials, and faster imaging techniques have been used to reduce movement artefact (39). Mohiaddin et al. (12) imaged flow in the aorta throughout systole from a single heartbeat in normals. Significant increases were documented in mean and peak aortic flow, while the time to peak flow fell (Fig. 6). Oshinski et al. (40) used restraints across the hips and shoulder to restrict motion, and achieved a heart rate of 65% of maximum predicted for age. Fast gradient echo acquisitions were used to obtain six short-axis slices at rest and three during stress to estimate the ejection fraction. The ejection fraction rose from 55 to 62% in normals, but remained at 44% in patients with coronary artery disease. Scan quality was not sufficient to allow regional wall motion analysis, however. These ejection fraction response differences are compatible with the findings long established using

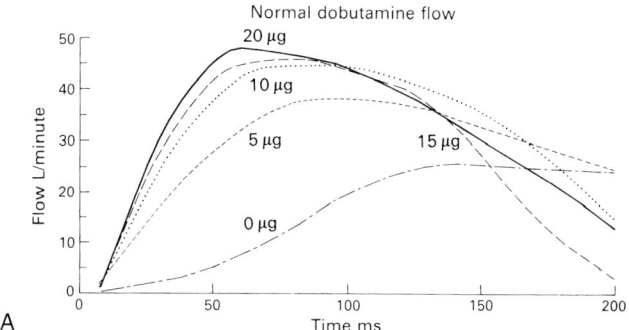

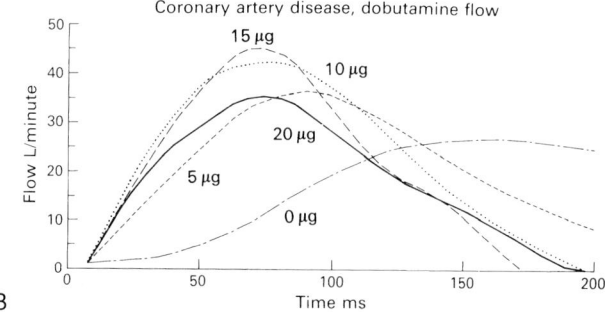

FIG. 5. A: Normal pattern of aortic flow during dobutamine stress. The flow curves are shown for the first 200 msec of the cardiac cycle during baseline and four stages of dobutamine stress. There is progressive increase in peak flow and peak flow acceleration (rate of change of flow). **B:** Abnormal pattern of aortic flow during dobutamine stress in a patient with two-vessel coronary artery disease and moderate reversible ischemia on thallium single-photon emission computed tomography. The peak flow increases until 15 μg/kg/min, and then decreases. There is an associated fall in peak flow acceleration. (From ref. 94, with permission.)

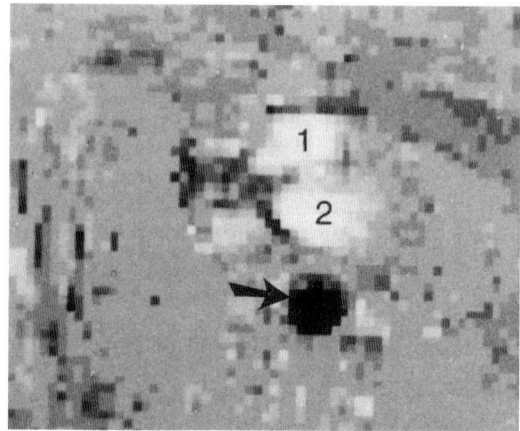

FIG. 6. Peak systolic frames from a cine spiral echo planar velocity study in a transverse plane transecting the descending thoracic aorta at midventricular level acquired at rest (**A**). *(continued)*

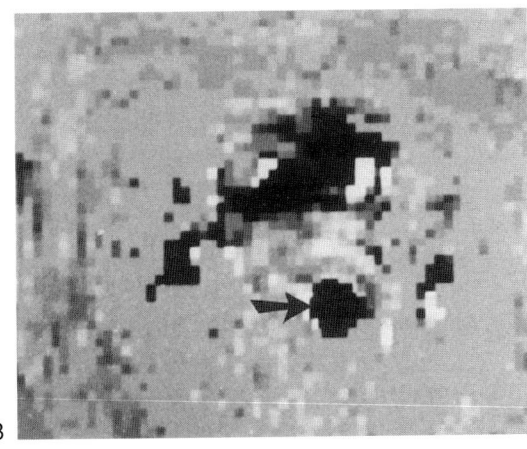
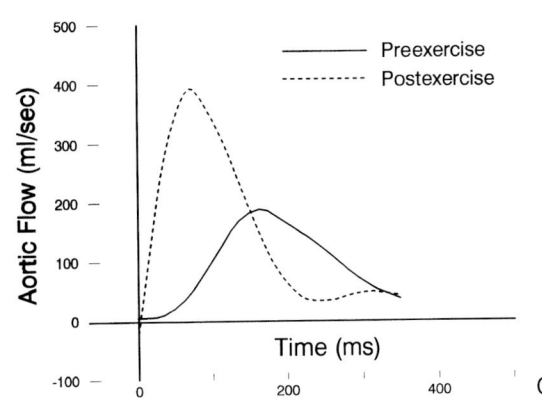

FIG. 6. *Continued.* **B:** Following exercise. **C:** Resting and postexercise time-related flow in the descending thoracic aorta. Instantaneous flow at each frame was calculated from the cine acquisition partly shown in Figure 1**A** and **B**. The velocity maps indicate zero velocity as midgray, cranial velocities in lighter shades of gray, and caudal velocities in darker shades of gray. Following exercise, the cranial velocities in the right (*1*) and left (*2*) ventricular outflow tracts appear with a dark signal because of aliasing. Descending thoracic aorta (*arrow*). (From ref. 95, with permission.)

nuclear cardiology and are encouraging; but improvements in image resolution are necessary, and direct comparisons need to be made with the pharmacologic techniques in the induction of ischemia.

AORTIC ANGIOGRAPHY

It is possible to perform aortic angiography with spiral CT, and, of course, with invasive catheter techniques. The disadvantages of spiral CT include the limited images planes, the x-ray irradiation and the relatively toxic contrast agent, while catheter angiography suffers from a small incidence of serious complications and is a projection technique. More recently, high-performance and fast gradient MR systems have become available allowing the use of fast gradient echo MR techniques during a breath hold (approximately 20 seconds) to acquire images of preselected volumes during bolus administration of the safe gadolinium chelates, such as Gd-DTPA (41). This technique is commonly known as three-dimensional contrast-enhanced magnetic resonance angiography (CE-MRA), and it is fast replacing other techniques of aortic angiography. Following the appropriate intravenous injection of Gd, local blood signal is substantially enhanced due to the shortening of the T1 relaxation time of blood. The result is optimal when data collection (in particular the center of the k space) occurs when the contrast agent arrives at the targeted vessel. Therefore, timing of the scan with respect to the intravenous injection of contrast agent is important. CE-MRA has become an increasingly popular angiographic technique—in particular for assessment of vessels in areas of major physiologic motion, such as the thorax and abdomen (42).

The Gd is injected through a plastic cannula in an antecubital vein. A flow rate of 2.0 mL/sec is usually maintained

through an automatic power injector, which provides both the contrast injection and a saline flush. Various dosages of Gd have been used from 0.05 to 0.2 mmol/kg body weight, followed by 15 to 20 mL of normal saline. To calculate the arrival time of the Gd to the targeted area, a 2 mL test bolus of Gd followed by 10 to 15 mL of normal saline is injected at the start of 30 to 40 fast gradient echo images in the area of interest at a rate of one image per second. This test enables the observation of the arrival of the Gd to the area of interest. The interval between the peripheral injection and the initial signal increase at the volume under the investigation defines the bolus transit time for a given patient. In order to achieve the maximum vascular signal at the central 20% of the k-space it is necessary to time the bolus to arrive at the middle of center of the k-space minus 10%.

Clinical Application of Aortic CE-MRA

Although aortic aneurysms or dissection can be assessed by CE-MRA, including the definition of type A and type B dissection (43), these can be readily assessed using a combination of spin-echo and gradient-echo images. CE-MRA is particularly useful for assessing the origin of the arch vessels, the renal arteries, and the tortuous aorta where conventional tomographic imaging is less helpful (Figs. 7 and 8). Because the anatomy of the aorta and its branches can be displayed in three dimension, this technique is also useful for planning surgery or stenting of aortic aneurysm.

CE-MRA of the renal artery has been shown to be accurate for detection of renal artery stenosis when compared with conventional methods (44). There are several indications for noninvasive renal MRA. Patients with hypertension may require renal MRA because renal artery stenosis is the cause in 2 to 5% of patients, and these patients are difficult to

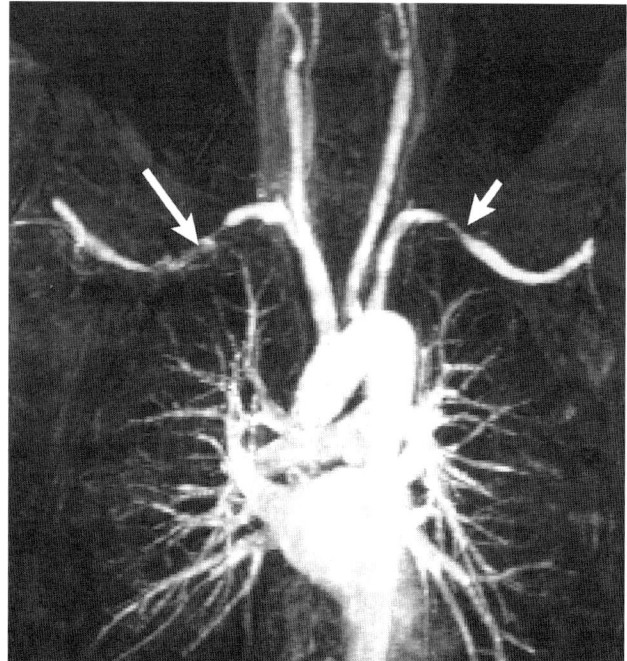

FIG. 7. Three-dimensional contrast-enhanced magnetic resonance angiography of the thoracic aorta and arch vessels showing right and left subclavian artery stenosis (*arrows*) in a patient with scleroderma.

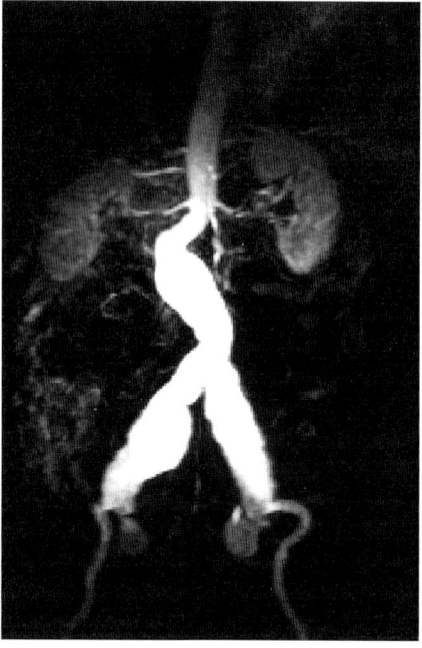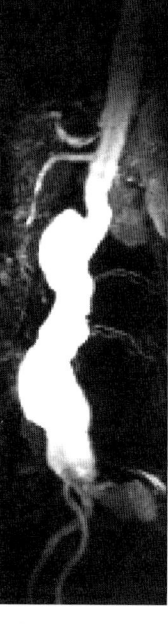

A,B

FIG. 8. Three-dimensional contrast-enhanced magnetic resonance angiography of the abdominal aorta in a patient with aneurysm of the abdominal aorta and iliac arteries. Anteroposterior view (**A**) and (**B**) lateral view. The morphology of the aneurysm is well-defined and the origin of renal arteries is clearly seen.

control with medical therapy (45). MRA is also helpful in patients with worsening renal function where it can be used to exclude bilateral renal artery stenosis (46). This is a reversible cause of renal failure and, when corrected, could avoid the need for, or could delay, dialysis. In patients with abdominal aortic aneurysm, MRA is important in identifying the number of renal arteries, their location relative to the aneurysm, and whether significant atherosclerotic disease is present. In patients who have undergone renal revascularization, MRA may be useful in assessing the revascularization.

AORTIC ANEURYSM

An aneurysm is a sac filled with blood in direct communication with the arterial lumen. A true aneurysm is due to local dilatation of the artery, whereas a false aneurysm is a sac with its walls formed by condensed connective tissue that communicates with the lumen of the artery through an aperture in its wall. Atherosclerosis is the leading cause of aortic aneurysm and usually involves the complete circumference of long segments of the aorta (fusiform shape). When an ascending aortic aneurysm results from atherosclerosis, it usually involves the arch and the descending aorta as well. Aneurysms localized in the ascending aorta are generally saccular in configuration and, in these cases, other less common causes of aneurysms should be considered. These include Marfan syndrome and other degenerative processes of the media, syphilis, cystic medial necrosis, and dilatation caused by valvular stenosis. Poststenotic aortic aneurysm distal to aortic coarctation or recoarctation, following intervention, are common, and these patients need regular follow-up.

In evaluating aortic aneurysms by imaging methods, it is important to localize the lesion, to describe its shape and its relation to branch vessels, and to measure luminal dimensions and blood flow. Assessment of the aortic wall for possible dissection, aortitis, mural thrombosis, paraaortic hematomas, and pericardial effusion is also required. In addition, involvement of coronary arteries and evaluation of the aortic valve are important. This information is useful to delineate etiology, to assess a patient's prognosis, and to define the roles of surgical intervention. This information can be gained from echocardiography, x-ray CT, and MRI (see below), but for long-term follow-up, MR is usually the technique of choice.

Marfan Syndrome

The cardiovascular manifestations of Marfan syndrome are very important, and they result in 95% of deaths in this condition (Fig. 9) (47). The common complications are prolapse of the mitral or tricuspid valves with or without regurgitation, dilatation or dissection of the aortic root, and aneurysm or dissection of the ascending, descending, and

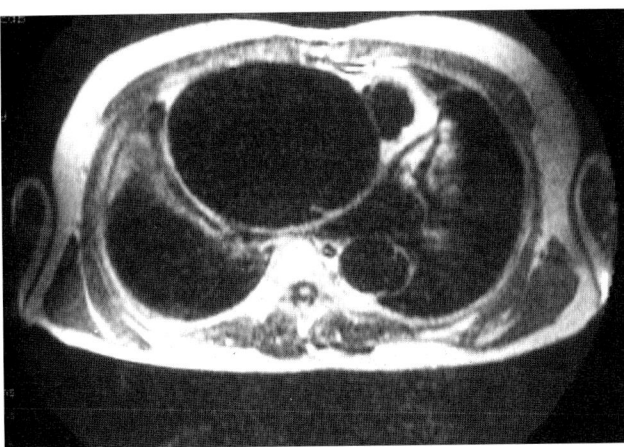

FIG. 9. Transaxial spin-echo image of a patient with Marfan syndrome and a large ascending aortic aneurysm. Note the small dissection flap just anterior and to the left of the spine. The left anterior coronary artery and great cardiac vein are also clearly seen.

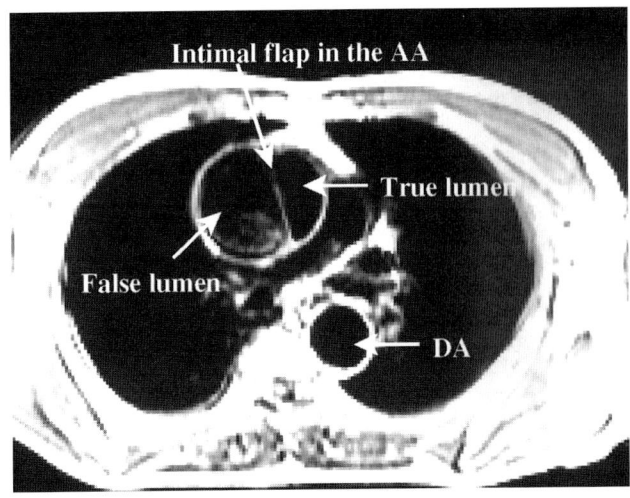

FIG. 10. Spin-echo image in a transverse plane at the level of pulmonary bifurcation in a patient with "type A" aortic dissection. The true and false lumen and the intimal flap are clearly seen. *AA*, ascending aorta; *DA*, descending aorta.

abdominal aorta. The most important of these is dilatation of the thoracic aorta, which can lead to dissection or rupture. The importance of early diagnosis and follow-up of these complications is clear. Therefore, elective repair of aortic aneurysm before dissection occurs is clinically important. The aortic root dimension and its rate of increase are the best predictors so far available. The current recommendation is that patients with Marfan syndrome should have their aortic size monitored so that prophylactic surgery can be considered when the aortic diameter exceeds 55 mm (this is equivalent to cross-sectional area of 23.8 cm^2) (48,49). MRI is a valuable screening method in these patients, although it is not well known at what age aortic involvement develops in symptomatic patients; therefore, the age for starting use of screening MRI is still debatable. Furthermore, the noninvasive nature of MRI allows frequent follow-up studies of Marfan patients following surgical or medical interventions.

AORTIC DISSECTION

MRI has been shown to be the most accurate imaging technique for dissection (50,51). Both MRI and transesophageal echocardiography are highly sensitive methods for identifying and classifying acute dissections of the thoracic aorta, but MRI has a better specificity. False-positive diagnoses may result in unnecessary surgery. In a well-organized general hospital, it has been shown that MRI can be safely and very effectively offered as the first line investigation (52). Often in practice, however, because of ease of access, transoesophageal echocardiography is performed first, with MRI used in cases of doubt. However, MRI is certainly the technique of choice in long-term follow-up after surgery to exclude new aneurysm formation or dissection (53). There is

no doubt that invasive investigation can be avoided with a combination of echocardiography and MRI (54). X-ray computed tomography is also a useful first-line investigation with an accuracy not far behind MRI, but it has the disadvantages of potentially renotoxic contrast injection in a compromised patient and imaging planes limited to transaxial or near transaxial.

MRI can display the entire thoracic and abdominal aorta in the true long axis of the vessel, which is very helpful. Sometimes, a thin intimal flap may not be shown by spin-echo images unless static blood in the false lumen provides natural contrast with the true lumen, but if there is any doubt, then the flap will be more easily seen using a gradient echo sequence, and velocity mapping will confirm the diagnosis by demonstrating the different flow velocities in each lumen (Figs. 10–12) (55,56). The entry and exit points are often successfully found using gradient echo images with velocity measurements. Aortic dissection may be classified according to the site and extent of aortic involvement (DeBakey classification) into: Type I involves the ascending aorta with extension beyond the arch, type II involves the ascending aorta only, and type III involves the descending aorta only (57). An alternative classification is that of Stanford, which categorizes aortic dissection into two types according to prognosis: type A, which involves the ascending aorta, or type B, which does not involve the ascending aorta (58).

Intramural Hematoma

It is also now recognized that aortic hematoma behaves clinically like dissection with a similar prognosis, and this is well assessed by echocardiography, x-ray CT, and MRI (Fig. 13) (59–61).

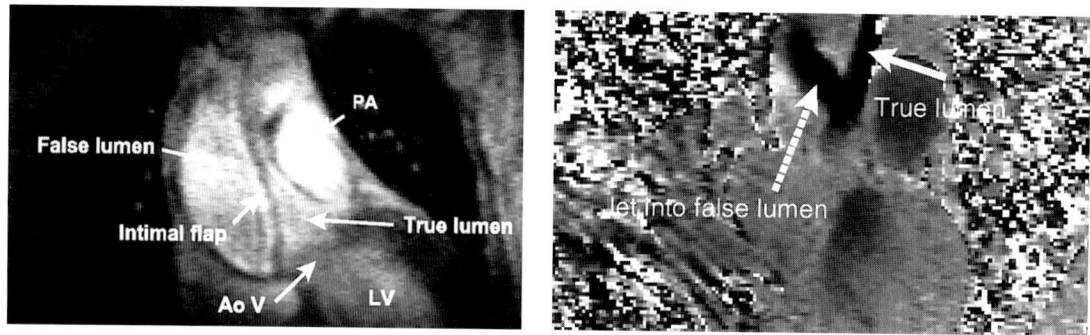

FIG. 11. A: Coronal gradient echo image (echo time 14 msec) of the ascending aorta acquired in diastole showing the intimal flap (*arrow*) and true and false lumina. **B:** Velocity map (echo time 3.6msec) in the same plane as (**A**) with vertical velocity encoding. The image has been rotated clockwise to align the true lumen of the aorta with the velocity encoding gradient. In systole, there are two clear jets of blood flow, in the true lumen (*solid arrow*) and through an intimal tear into the false lumen (*dashed arrow*). *LV*, left ventricle; *PA*, pulmonary artery; *AoV*, aortic valve. (From ref. 96, with permission.)

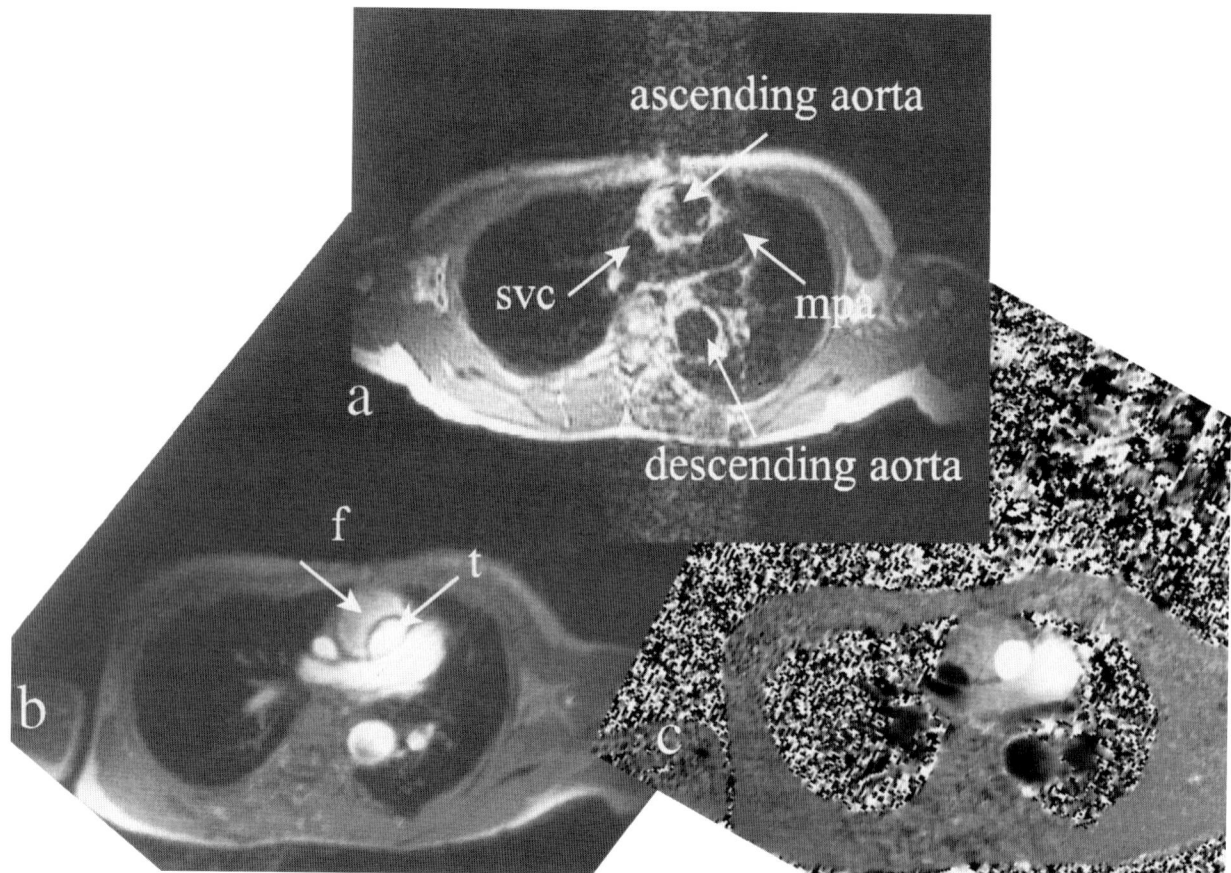

FIG. 12. A spin-echo image (*a*) in a transverse plane through the ascending aorta and descending thoracic aorta in a patient with aortic dissection (type A). The intimal flap is not clearly seen. The corresponding systolic gradient echo (*b*) and velocity images (*c*) identify the dissection clearly by showing high velocity in the true lumen (*t*) and low velocity in the false lumen (*f*). The velocity maps in this study indicate zero velocity as midgray, cranial velocities in lighter shades of gray, and caudal velocities in darker shades of gray. *svc*, superior vena cava. (From ref. 97, with permission.)

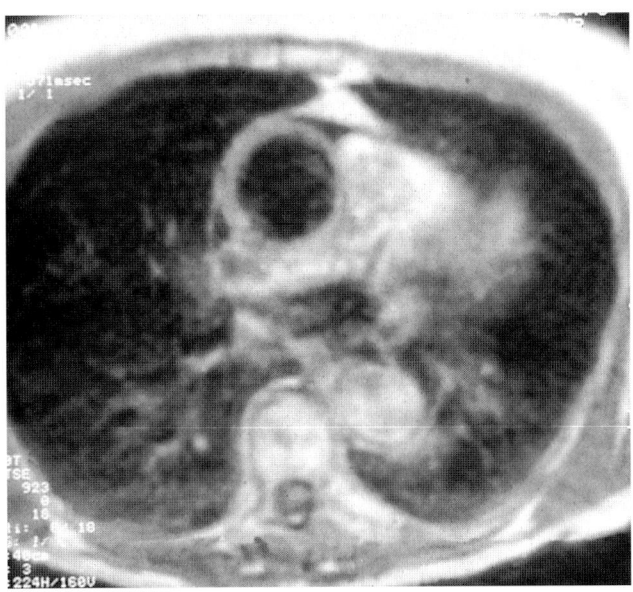

FIG. 13. Intramural hematoma of the ascending aorta. Note that there is no dissection flap, but clear thickening of the aortic wall in a patient with symptoms suggestive of dissection.

POSTTRAUMATIC AORTIC ANEURYSM

Aortic rupture is a major cause of death following serious road traffic accidents. The common sites for involvement are the ascending aorta just proximal to the innominate artery (about 30%) and the descending aorta just distal to the left subclavian artery (about 70%). Of patients with aortic rupture, 90% die before hospital admission. Of those surviving the initial injury, 30% die within 24 hours and 90% within 12 months due to secondary hemorrhage from walled-off tears. Transthoracic echocardiography is usually the best first-line approach for assessing patients with a question of posttraumatic aortic aneurysm, and catheter angiography is performed in patients that are unstable. X-ray CT would also be of value in the more stable patient. Although patients with serious traffic accidents usually have other life-threatening injuries making MRI impractical, MRI is appropriate in patients with chronic or missed aortic tears.

AORTITIS

A variety of inflammatory disorders may affect blood vessels. Takayasu's syndrome (pulseless disease; aortic arch syndrome) is a rare disorder characterized by thickening of the wall of the aorta and the origin of its main branches, particularly in the neck, leading to stenosis, thrombosis, and occlusion of the vessels (62). The disease may also affect the pulmonary arteries and other vessels. While catheter angiography has been the standard approach to assess such patients, MRI can be a useful first-line method. MRI shows diffuse thickening of the thoracic (Fig. 14) and abdominal aorta as well as stenosis and occlusion of the branch vessels.

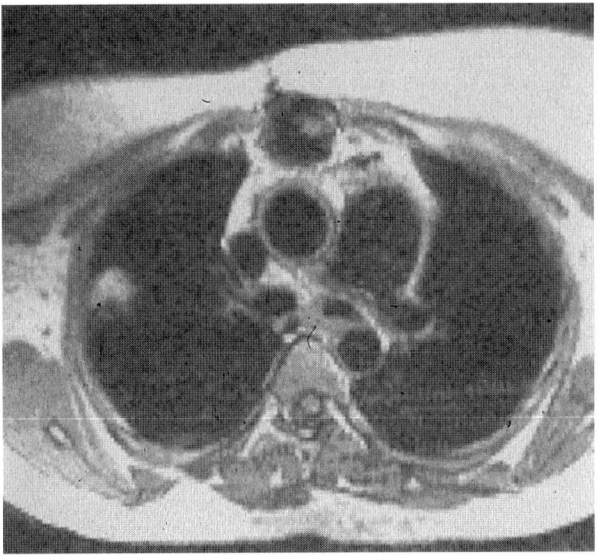

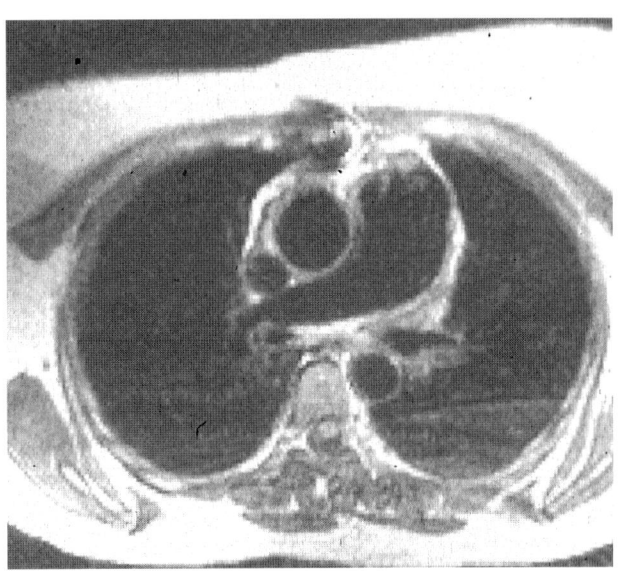

FIG. 14. Two transaxial images of a patient with Takayasu's aortitis. Marked thickening of the wall of the aorta and pulmonary artery are clearly seen, and a small midzone pulmonary infarct is present.

There is often a symmetric thickening of the aortic wall caused by fibrosis.

AORTIC ATHEROMATA

Echocardiography, x-ray CT, and MRI are all useful methods to detect aortic atheromata. MRI is also capable of determining the composition of atheromatous plaques of the aorta. Although this can be performed invasively with intravascular echocardiography and MRI (63), there is considerable interest in the noninvasive approach. Several groups have shown the potential of MRI for investigating atherosclerotic vascular disease and, in particular, imaging of the arterial wall. Early investigations were done on cadaveric atherosclerotic plaques. Most of the early studies relied on imaging of distortion of the arterial wall and did not exploit the ability of the technique to study the key components of atheroma (64,65).

Maynor (66) studied cadaveric fibrous atherosclerotic plaques, periaortic fat, and cholesterol standards using a 7.0 Tesla imaging spectrometer. Fibrous plaques and fat were shown to have unique spectra, differing in the ratios of water and various components of fat. These two tissues had different T2 relaxation times of their components, with fibrous plaques having a short T2 compared with fat—15.9 versus 46.2 milliseconds. Signal intensity of the fat resonance of fibrous plaque increased with increasing temperature from 24°C to 37°C.

Carpenter et al. (67) used an animal model of atherosclerosis by placing a collar around the carotid artery of a New Zealand white rabbit. Transverse cardiac gated images were obtained from the neck of the rabbit, both in normal animals and those with irritating carotid constrictions. Animals were fed normal and high cholesterol diets. The spatial resolution and sensitivity were investigated at a field strength of 2T using a large radiofrequency transmitter system and a surface coil receiver. A resolution of $200\mu m$ was readily obtained, but even this was insufficient for delineating pathology within the arterial wall, such as intimal thickening. Comparison with histopathology confirmed that morphologic changes were smaller than the pixel resolution of the image and that to detect atherosclerotic changes a resolution of $50\mu m$ would be necessary.

Characterization of atherosclerotic plaques has been performed in animal and human models with magnetic resonance chemical shift imaging (CSI) and spectroscopy (68). Atherosclerosis was induced in the abdominal aorta of four rabbits by a combination of balloon denudation and cholesterol supplemented diet. In vivo spin-echo and fat/water suppressed images of rabbit aortas were obtained at 1.5T. Chemical shift imaging was achieved using a hybridization of selective excitation and modified Dixon techniques. These techniques were then used to image atherosclerotic lesions in the carotid arteries of 4 patients before endarterectomy. The MRI results were confirmed by histology and by high resolution proton MR spectroscopy (8.5T) of rabbit aortas, human carotid endarterectomy, and six additional human superficial femoral and iliac atherectomy specimens. All animal and human lesions were classified as either fatty streaks or fibrous plaques. When compared with spin-echo images, fat suppression by CSI substantially improved the measured contrast-to-noise ratio between plaque and vessel lumen, and enhanced discrimination of perivascular fat. In contrast, water suppression eliminated signal from plaque because of the negligible amount of isotropic (liquid-like) signal from the immobilized lipid in the lesion. Magnetic resonance spectroscopy confirmed the CSI results by demonstrating broad fat resonances characteristic of nonmobile lipids in both human and rabbit atherosclerotic lesions. These findings indicated that in vivo MRI of plaque is technically feasible and could be improved using CSI.

To determine the lipid content of atheroma, Mohiaddin (69) evaluated the use of proton magnetic resonance chemical shift imaging for assessment of lipid content in atheromatous plaques in cadaver human arteries. After imaging, the postmortem specimens were examined histologically and the lipid content of the plaque was assessed using a semiquantitative scale. The distribution of lipid within the plaque and between intima and media was also noted. The findings of chemical shift imaging agreed well with histologic examination both for total lipid content and for distribution within each plaque. They also applied this method for evaluation of the aortoiliac region of patients with peripheral vascular disease and compared the finding with healthy volunteers (70). The majority of aortic plaques studied were classified by MRI as fibrous plaque, but there was no histologic validation (Fig. 15).

Gold et al. (71) characterized ex vivo atherosclerotic lesions at 1.5T. Fresh human aortic tissue with atheroma was suspended in solutions of agarose and manganese chloride and heated to body temperature. The specimens were imaged with modified Dixon and projection-reconstruction imaging sequences and then examined histologically to obtain direct correlation between images, spectra, and histologic characteristics. The vessel wall and plaque components could be identified by means of their MR characteristics and correlated with histologic appearance. Calcification and fibrous tissue appear with signal loss or attenuated signal on the Dixon water image and perivascular and intimal lipid appear with a high signal on the lipid image.

To address whether magnetic resonance imaging is capable of imaging progression of atherosclerosis noninvasively, Skinner et al. (72) used high resolution MRI to serially image advanced lesion of atherosclerosis in the rabbit abdominal aorta. They demonstrated that progression of disease resulted in increased lesion mass and intralesion complications with decreased in arterial lumen. Images acquired in vivo correlated with the fine structure of the lesions of atherosclerosis, including the fibrous cap, necrotic core, and lesion fissures, as verified by gross examination, dissection microscopy, and histology. In vivo imaging using T1 and T2 weighting has also been performed by Toussaint et al. (73), with good discrimination of lipid cores, fibrous caps, calcification, media, and adventitia in humans.

Bulte et al. (74) used human peripheral blood mononuclear cells labeled with dextran-magnetite particles and concluded that the labeling of these cells may be used in future studies of selective MRI of in vivo cell migration in a variety of immunologically compromised tissue states, e.g., tumors, transplants, and abscesses. Atherosclerotic lesions may be an important area of future investigation.

Magnetic Resonance Microscopy

In parallel with the developments in MRI, magnetic resonance microscopy (MRM) has emerged as an interesting

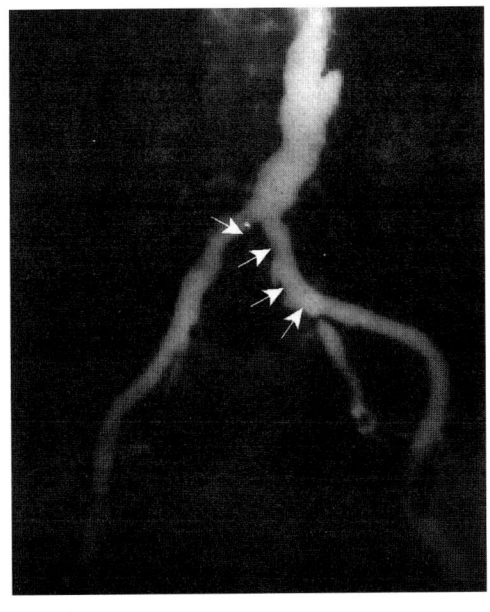

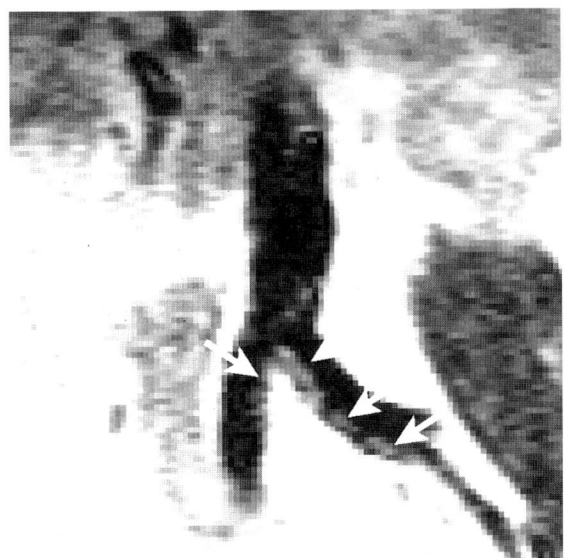

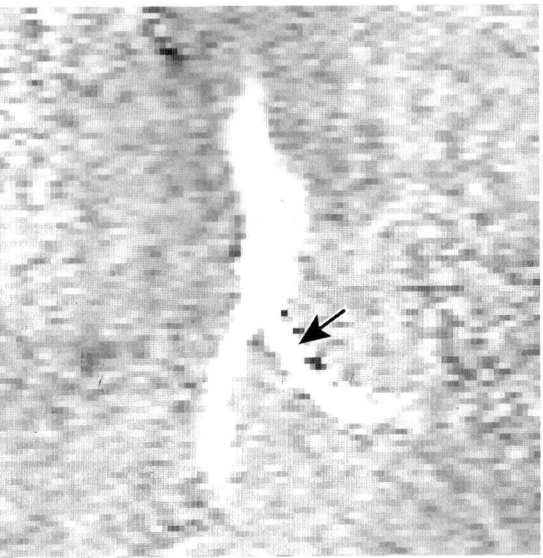

FIG. 15. Multiple atheromatous plaques (*arrows*) causing stenoses of both common iliac arteries in a patient with peripheral vascular disease. **A:** X-ray angiogram. Spin-echo image (**B**) and corresponding velocity map (**C**). The peak velocity in both iliac arteries is higher than in the aorta. (From ref. 70, with permission.)

research tool for basic science. Initially applied in experimental studies of models of various diseases in small animals, MRM has grown to include applications ranging from histology and plant anatomy to fluid dynamics. Resolution limits imposed by motion *in vivo* have been overcome by improved physiologic monitoring. Resolution *in vivo* is now down to 50μm, and *in vitro* 10μm can be detected. The many forms of contrast provided by MRM (T1, T2, and diffusion weighting), permit direct examination of the state of water in tissues, which is not possible by other microscopic techniques. With this in mind, one may consider a range of applications covering the spectrum of resolution available with current MR microscopes, including athero-

sclerosis. The unique features that distinguish MRM from conventional light microscopy are that MRM is nondestructive, it differentiates tissue structure on the basis of "proton stain," and it is inherently three dimensional.

Pearlman et al. (75) investigated the use of MRM to quantify and image atheroma lipids in human coronary arteries and to validate the results by comparison with histology. MRM was performed on an experimental MR imaging system operating at 2.0T with a probe designed for short echo time, strong B1 field strength, and small samples. Data acquisition used multiple-offset chemical encoding with offsets based on the thermotropic spectral signature of atheroma lipids within the human arterial wall. Perimeters, areas, and a shape index of lumen, atheroma, and outer wall were determined and compared for MRI versus histology. There was no significant difference in the measurements with the exception of luminal shape indices, which were uniformly larger by histology, attributable to flattening of the vessel during histologic preparation. MR measurement of atheroma content of coronary artery wall agreed with histology. More recently, Fayad et al. (76) used MRM to investigate atherosclerotic lesions in genetically engineered apolipoprotein-E knockout mice and used the technique to follow changes in plaque morphology in the intact animal.

Practical Considerations for Chemical Shift Imaging of Atheroma

Several factors need careful attention if this technique is to be used routinely. Motion artifact can be a problem in long scans, and subtraction of two images makes this more severe unless interleaved acquisition of the images is used. If signal is obtained from slow-moving blood it may mimic or obscure areas of atheroma. This can be avoided by using a presaturation band to reduce the blood signal, or by acquiring images during diastole where blood is almost still and gives an unmistakably high signal. Another factor influencing the ease of chemical shift imaging is magnetic field strength and homogeneity. The absolute chemical shift (in Hertz) depends on field strength and greater separation is obtained between the water and fat peaks at higher fields. High field would therefore make the technique more reliable for static specimens. At all field strengths, however, careful adjustment of shimming for good homogeneity is vital. Knowledge of the quality of the main field is necessary before embarking on these studies (77,78). Another factor to be considered is that eddy currents created by the gradient pulses can affect the field homogeneity during the sequence.

CONGENITAL MALFORMATIONS OF THE AORTA

All imaging modalities have their place in investigating congenital heart disease, but invasive angiography in the 1990s is now mainly reserved for invasive pressure measurements because most anatomical and flow information can be gained from noninvasive techniques. The noninvasive techniques have varying strengths and limitations, and these also vary according to the age of the subject. In children, transthoracic echocardiography is the technique of choice, but MRI can be very helpful in selected cases. However, in adolescents and adults, particularly after operative repairs, a combination of techniques is often necessary. Transesophageal echocardiography is particularly helpful for intracardiac structures including valves and septa, while MRI is preferable for extracardiac connections, conduits, and flow. MRI is also very helpful in complex congenital disease, where the contiguous slices and wide field of view help in the appreciation of the anatomy. Although x-ray CT scans can provide anatomic information in these conditions, it is not widely used because of the limited imaging planes and the need for contract and x-rays. However, it is helpful in determining calcification of extracardiac conduits. It should be remembered that plain film chest x-rays may provide inexpensive diagnostic clues to the presence of most of these abnormalities (79,80) and that MRI can provide detailed and clinically useful information in most cases (81,82).

Aortic Coarctation

Aortic coarctation is one of the most frequently encountered congenital malformations. It consists of narrowing or interruption of the aortic lumen, usually just distal to the origin of the left subclavian artery, although occasionally there is narrowing proximal to the left subclavian artery. Narrowing is typically adjacent to what was the origin of the arterial duct, which normally closes spontaneously at birth. The narrowing of aortic coarctation may appear as a narrowed segment or as a partial or complete membrane obstructing the lumen. Where coarctation is severe or complete, collateral arteries develop, connecting arteries arising proximal to the lesion with ones that then reenter the descending aorta distally. A well-developed collateral system is usually associated with enlarged aortic arch branches, particularly the left subclavian artery, and with enlargement and tortuosity of intercostal and other thoracic arteries that carry collateral flow, this being the cause of rib-notching that can be identified on a chest x-ray.

Though often symptom-free, patients with aortic coarctation are prone to hypertension in arteries arising proximal to the lesion, and hence to cerebro-vascular accidents. Aortic coarctation therefore needs investigation, leading to surgical repair or catheter intervention if aortic obstruction is considered to contribute significantly to hypertension. A bicuspid aortic valve, prone to stenosis, is also present in approximately half of all patients with aortic coarctation.

MRI is often used for investigation of adolescents or adults with coarctation, but because infants and young children need sedation or anaesthesia and because echocardiography is relatively straightforward, MRI tends to be requested less in the pediatric age group. With appropriately small receiver coils (an adult head receiver set may accommodate an infant), useful images can be acquired (Fig. 16), but adequate sedation is needed in patients who are too young to lie still.

When investigating aortic coarctation in adults (unoperated, balloon dilated, or operated) there are a number of questions to be considered:

- Is blood pressure elevated in one or both arms?
- To what extent is it caused by obstruction due to coarctation?
- If operated, what type of surgery?
- Is there diastolic prolongation of forward flow?
- Do blood pressure and ''gradient'' rise markedly with exercise?

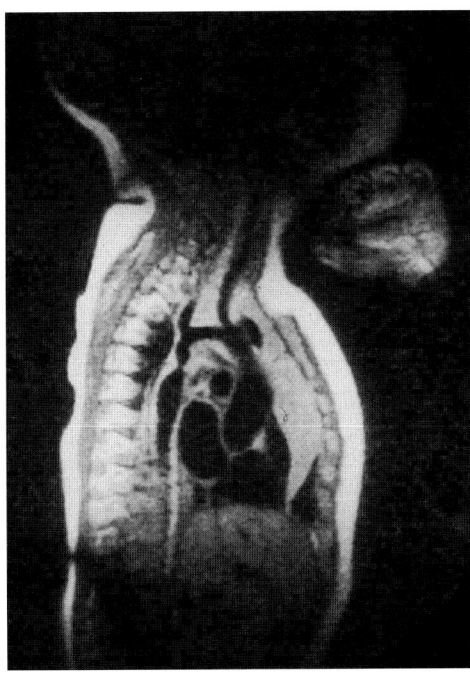

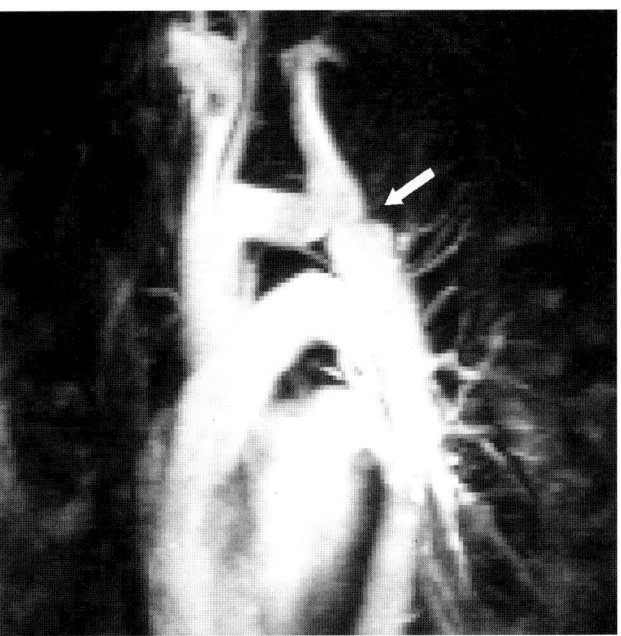

A

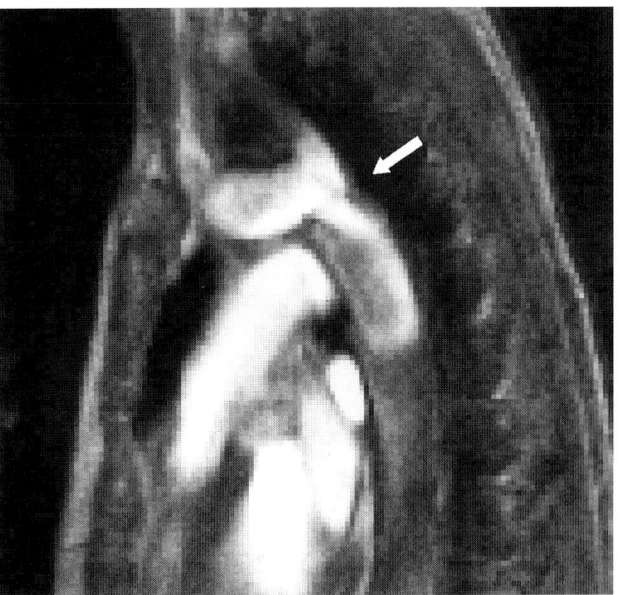

B

FIG. 16. Aortic coarctation in an infant. The spin-echo image is aligned with the plane of the aortic arch in a sedated 1-year-old baby unoperated coarctation. Image acquisition at 0.5 Tesla with a small chest surface receiver coil.

- Is there associated aortic valve disease?
- Is the left ventricle hypertrophied?
- How extensive is collateral flow?
- What is the location and severity of coarctation?
- Of what type is it? (e.g., membrane or narrow segment)
- What is the geometry of aorta and branches in the vicinity of coarctation?
- Is there a dissection, aneurysm, or false aneurysm of the aorta?

No single modality answers all these questions (83), but MRI with velocity mapping, in addition to blood pressure measurements and perhaps Doppler echocardiography (with stress, if appropriate), should give enough information to proceed to surgery. Invasive angiography should not be needed unless coronary artery disease is suspected. CE-MRA or computed x-ray tomography, with three-dimensional reconstruction, can provide impressive images of aortic arch geometry (Fig. 17), but these approaches may not adequately demonstrate dissecting or false aneurysms or determine the severity of coarctation. There is, however, a case for combining CE-MRA, which clearly displays lumen geometry and collateral arteries, with spin echo, cine gradient echo imaging, and velocity mapping in appropriately selected planes, for assessment of extra-luminal tissue, and the obstructive significance of coarctation (Figs. 18 and 19).

MRI of coarctation generally begins with acquisition of multislice spin-echo images in standard planes, with oblique acquisition in the plane of the arch. Spin-echo images are useful for visualizing the location, but not necessarily the

FIG. 17. A: Magnetic resonance three-dimensional contrast angiography, a maximum intensity projection, in a patient with unoperated aortic coarctation (*arrow*). Aortic arch geometry and site of coarctation are well shown, but the severity of coarctation is not easily assessed from the angiogram alone. **B:** Gradient-echo cine imaging—a systolic frame—in a plane aligned with the orifice and the jet passing through it. The width of the jet (*arrow*) indicates relatively mild coarctation, confirmed by velocity mapping that recorded a peak velocity no higher than 2.2 m/sec.

severity of coarctation. Gradient-echo cine imaging, preferably with jet velocity mapping, can contribute to assessment of severity. To achieve this, a useful approach is to identify a plane aligned with the lumen at its narrowest point and with the jet beyond, passing into the descending aorta. This allows visualization of the location, width, and duration of

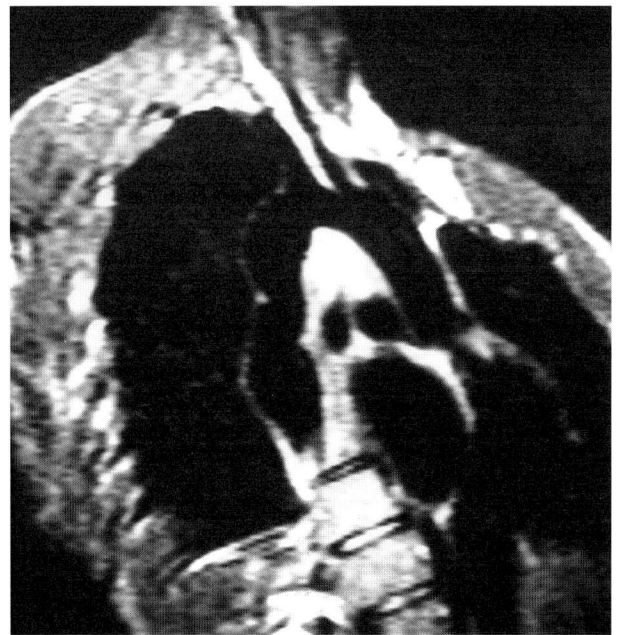
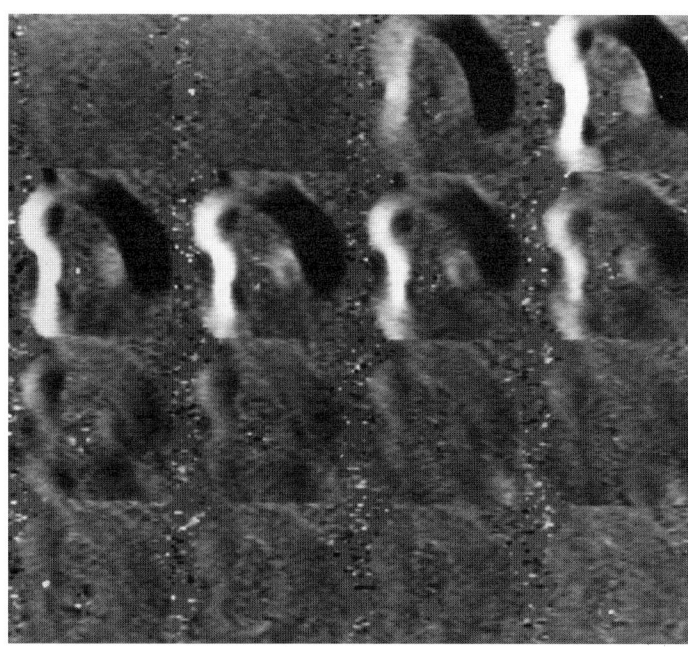

A

B

FIG. 18. Mild recoarctation studied by magnetic resonance imaging with velocity mapping. **A:** Spin-echo image aligned with the aortic arch and repaired descending aorta, viewed from the right, 12 years after internal mammary artery patch repair of coarctation. **B:** Detail from all 16 frames of the velocity map acquisition, velocity encoded in the vertical read gradient direction. Downward velocities appear white and upward velocities, dark. The 16 frames run from left to right in lines ordered from above downward. Systolic forward flow is seen in frames 3 to 8, after which slight swirling of blood persists for a few frames. The lumen is tortuous, but not severely narrowed. The peak recorded velocity was 2 m/sec, without significant diastolic prolongation of forward flow.

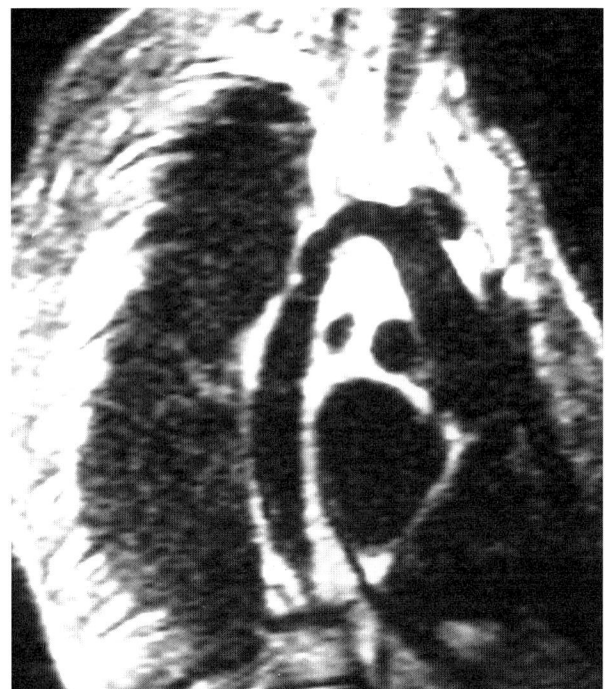
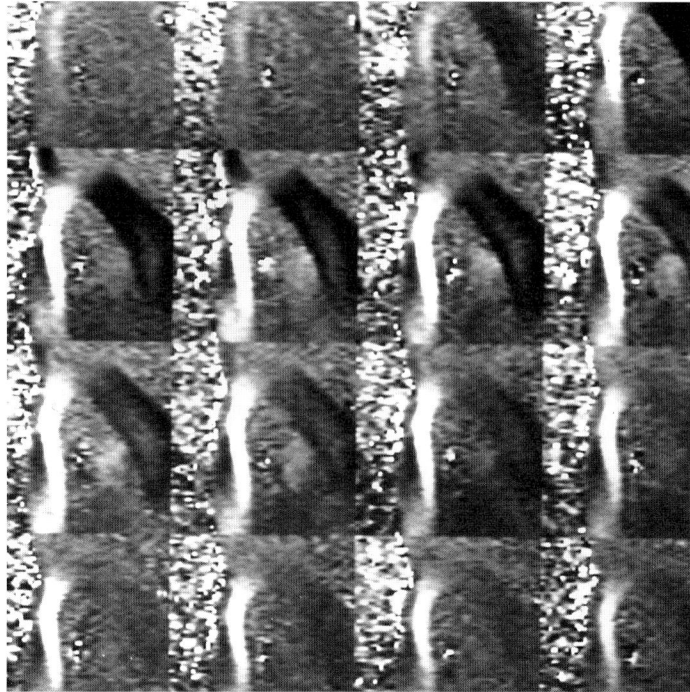

A

B

FIG. 19. Significant recoarctation shown by magnetic resonance imaging with velocity mapping. **A:** Spin-echo image aligned with the arch and descending aorta 12 years after Dacron tube repair of recoarctation at 4 years of age. The narrowed lumen suggests significant stenosis, which was confirmed by velocity mapping. **B:** Detail from all 16 velocity map frames in the same patient, encoded and ordered as in Figure 1**B**. A peak jet velocity of 3.4 m/sec is recorded in frame 6. Forward flow does not cease at the end of systole (frame 10), but continues throughout diastole, showing significant diastolic prolongation of forward flow.

the jet. The way to align the plane is to use two or more orthogonal cine acquisitions (TE equals 5 to 8 msec) to home in on the line of the jet, starting from suitable transaxial or oblique spin-echo images. Once the line of the jet core has been identified, in-plane velocity maps may be acquired (TE equals 3 to 5 msec) for measurement of jet velocity. In this setting, a resting peak velocity of 3 m/sec or more generally represents significant obstruction, particularly if associated with diastolic prolongation of forward flow (a diastolic "tail"), which is a useful indicator of the obstructive significance (compare Figs. 18 and 19) (84). Peak velocity measured by MR, if acquired appropriately, agrees well with peak velocity measured by continuous-wave Doppler ultrasound (85), although peak pressure differences ("gradients") calculated from these velocity measurements by application of the modified Bernoulli equation tend to give higher results than measurements made at catheterization. There are several potential reasons for this discrepancy:

- Catheterization may have been performed under sedation or anesthesia.
- Peak-to-peak rather than peak instantaneous gradients may have been measured at catheterization.
- There may be a degree of "pressure recovery" distal to the jet, particularly if the narrowing is gradual rather than abrupt (86).
- Localized indentation of the lumen in the absence of severe coarctation may be associated with a localized but unrepresentative peak of velocity due to localized, asymmetric convergence of streamlines (85,87).

These potential discrepancies mean that caution is needed when comparing "gradients" arrived at by different means. Magnetic resonance has the advantage of providing good anatomic images for consideration in relation to velocity measurements.

It should also be kept in mind that peak velocity and peak pressure difference depend not only on the degree of narrowing, but also on the rate of flow through the orifice, which tends to be diminished if narrowing is severe. A well-developed collateral system bypasses the coarctation, so reducing flow through it. MR measurements of volume flow in the ascending and descending thoracic aorta have shown that normal proportions of about 3:2 change toward 3:1 in the presence of significant coarctation, reflecting reduced volume flow through the narrowed region (88,89).

Aneurysms Associated with Coarctation

Dissecting aneurysm is a relatively frequent complication of attempted balloon dilatation (Fig. 20). True or false aneurysms may also complicate surgical repairs (Fig. 21), particularly those incorporating patches of incompliant fabric such as Dacron (90). The cause of this is probably related stress between the incompliant patch and compliant aortic wall,

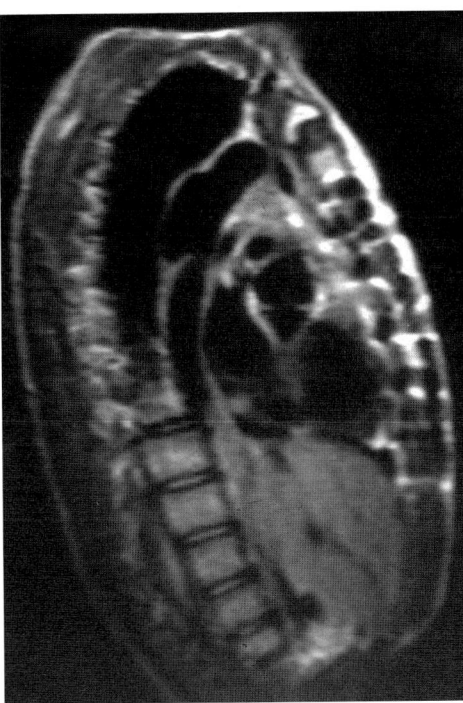

FIG. 20. Dissecting aneurysm of descending aorta following attempted balloon dilatation of aortic coarctation.

the aneurysm typically developing adjacent to the patch. Patients with such patches should be reinvestigated regularly by MRI. Infected false aneurysms can complicate native or repaired coarctation. Poststenotic dilatation also occurs, appearing as smooth, fusiform dilatation beyond the coarctation, usually distinguishable by location and shape from a more clearly demarcated and asymmetric bulge that may be presumed to pose greater risk of rupture, although adequate research on this subject is lacking.

Surgery for coarctation or recoarctation in adults may not be straightforward. Imaging has important roles in foreseeing or identifying complications. Hemoptysis, early or late after coarctation repair, is an ominous sign. It may result from blood leaking from aorta to bronchi by way of a false aneurysm, which is most readily demonstrated by MRI (91,92).

Bicuspid Aortic Valve

Because of the high incidence of bicuspid aortic valve, it is good practice to perform Doppler echocardiography or cine MRI (TE equals 14 msec) in a plane to visualize flow through the aortic valve in all patents studied for aortic coarctation. The presence of turbulent systolic or diastolic jets can then be followed up with measurements of peak velocity or, more rarely, regurgitant fraction using phase velocity mapping (82). For cine imaging, an oblique sagittal plane aligned from coronal pilots to show flow from left ventricular outflow tract to aortic root is advantageous as it also

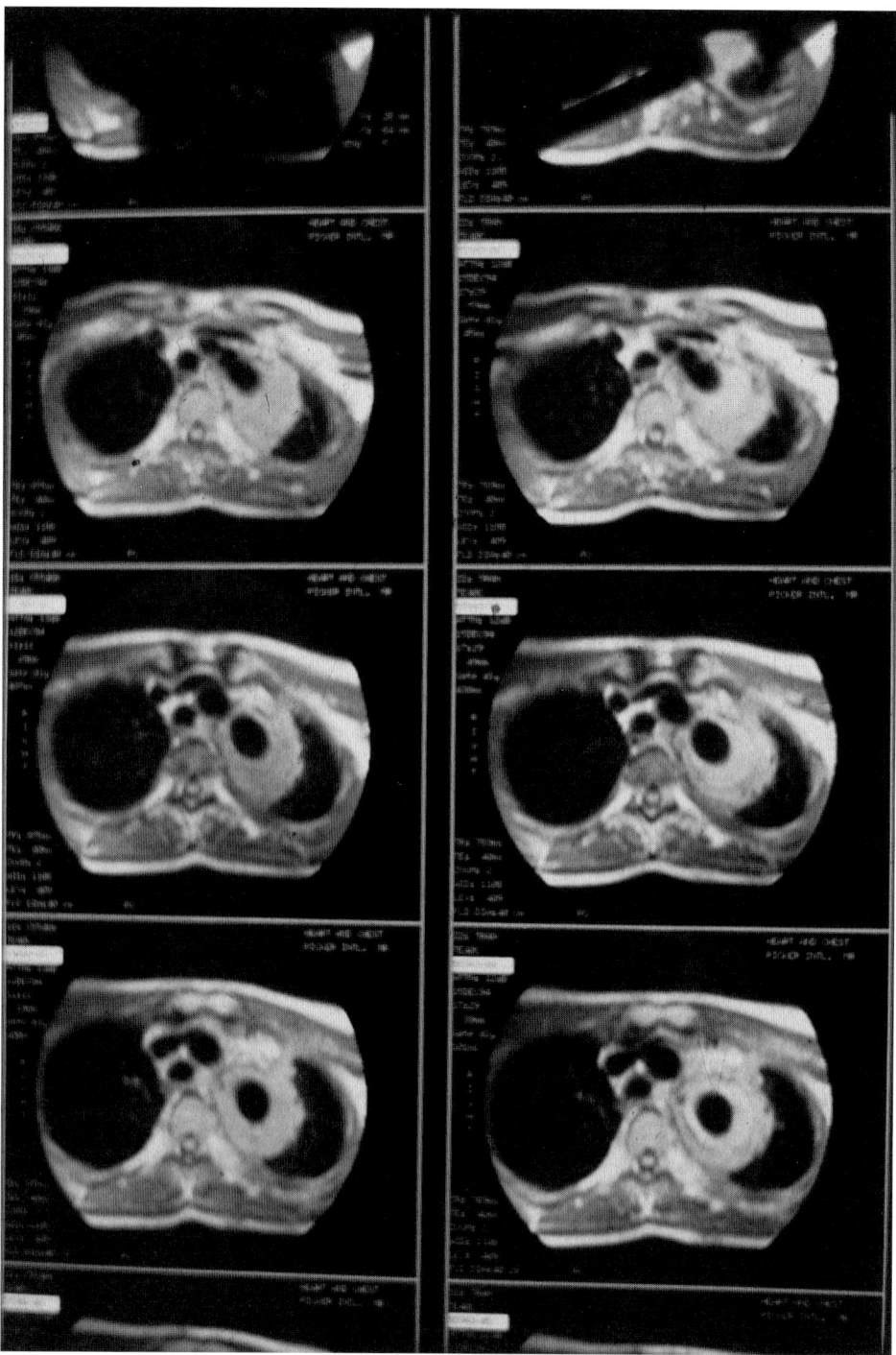

FIG. 21. A false aneurysm due to leakage from a suture line after surgery for recoarctation using an interposition graft. The three transaxial spin-echo images on the left show appearances 3 weeks after surgery, the patient having developed hemoptysis. Equivalent images on the right were acquired 3 days later after further hemoptysis. They show increase in the volume of signal surrounding the graft, with a slightly brighter inner layer suggestive of fresh hematoma. The graft and hematoma were removed at emergency reoperation, and a jump graft inserted from the ascending to descending aorta.

provides a view of mitral inflow, left ventricular movement, and left ventricular hypertrophy, if present.

Patent Arterial Duct

The arterial duct, patent before birth, can persist after birth to give rise to a murmur. If the duct is of sufficient size, the aortopulmonary shunt can lead to pulmonary hypertension. A patent duct is easily missed with echocardiography or MRI unless specifically looked for. Its location is between the region of the pulmonary artery bifurcation, usually slightly to the left, and the descending aortic arch. Apparent communication or deformation between pulmonary artery bifurcation and the aorta on spin-echo images should raise the suspicion, which can be followed up by cine imaging (TE equals 14 msec) in a plane aligned with suspected duct flow (Fig. 22). Interpretation may still be difficult if pulmonary pressure is near systemic, with little flow through the patent duct. Flow through a narrow duct may give rise to a turbulent jet directed anteriorly from the pulmonary artery bifurcation region. Shunt flow can potentially be measured by phase velocity mapping of flow through planes transecting the ascending aorta and pulmonary trunk (93). It should be remembered, however, that aortopulmonary shunting at duct level leads to increased volume flow in the ascending aorta relative to that in the pulmonary trunk and that turbulence in the pulmonary trunk could compromise the accuracy of flow measurement.

Right-sided Aortic Arch

Location of the aortic arch to the right of the trachea is, in itself, a benign anatomic variant that may be associated with other more serious cardiovascular abnormalities.

Double Aortic Arch

Persistence of a right as well as left-sided aortic arch results in an aortic "ring" surrounding the lower trachea and esophagus (Fig. 23). Presenting symptoms may be dyspnea or dysphagia. Left and right sides of a double arch generally each give rise to a carotid and a subclavian artery branch. The arch on one side may persist less completely than on the other, for example, with occlusion of the lumen between one of the subclavian arteries and the descending aorta.

Anomalous Aortic Arch Branches

Minor variants of aortic branch anatomy are relatively frequent and insignificant, but a peculiarity to be aware of is anomalous origin of the *right* subclavian artery from the proximal descending aorta on the *left* side. This anomalous vessel passes across obliquely toward the right axilla, behind the airways, and it may contribute to airway compression.

Systemic-pulmonary Collaterals

Lung tissue deprived of its pulmonary blood supply, for example, through congenital atresia of the pulmonary valve or through severe pulmonary valve or pulmonary arterial stenosis, can acquire systemic-pulmonary collateral vessels. These most commonly arise from the sides or front of the descending aorta. Catheterization with X-ray angiography, in skilled hands, remains the most informative way to assess the presence and size of collaterals and of stenoses that may develop in them. CE-MRA, particularly when the raw data are studied tomographically, may also provide useful information of the distribution of collaterals, expediting subsequent catheter intervention.

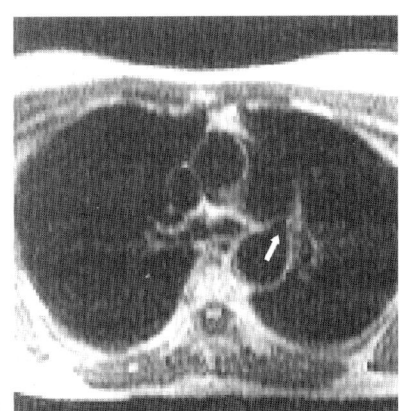
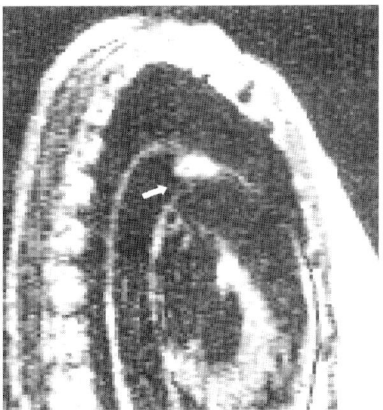
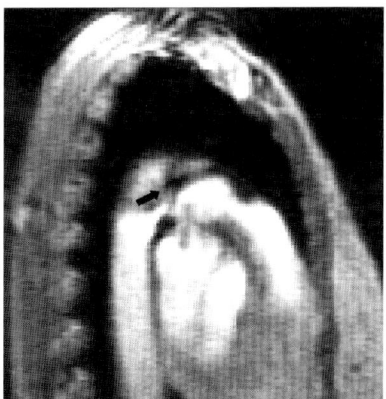

A   B,C

FIG. 22. A narrow, patent arterial duct in an adult. On transaxial (**A**) and sagittal (**B** and **C**) spin-echo images, an apparent diverticulum from the front of the descending aortic arch to the top of the pulmonary artery bifurcation indicates the location of the duct (*arrow*). Gradient-echo cine imaging (TE equals 14 msec) shows a narrow, continuous jet, maximum in systole, directed forward into the pulmonary trunk (*arrow*).

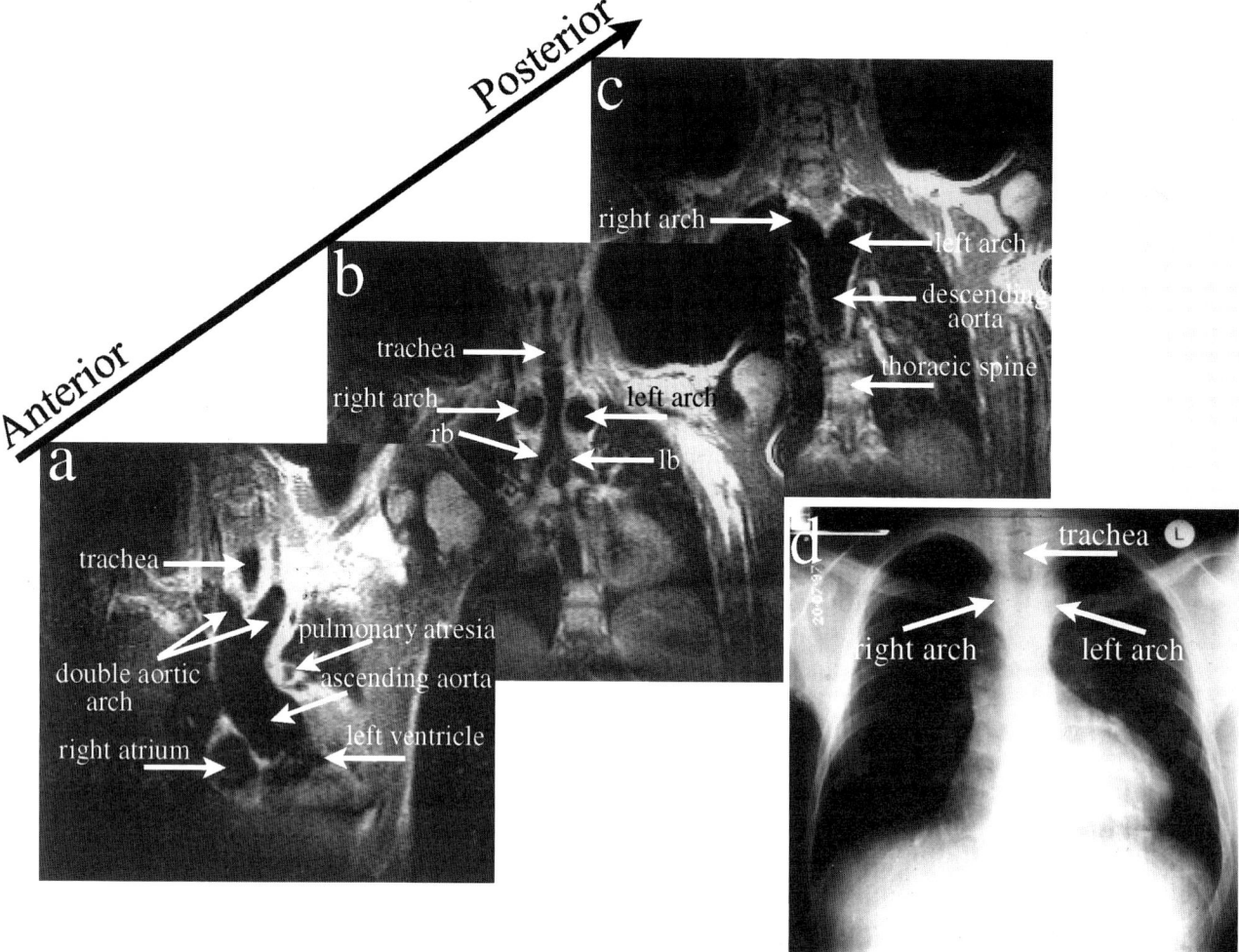

FIG. 23. Double aortic arch. Coronal spin-echo images (**a–c**) show appearances of a double aortic arch in a patient who also has pulmonary atresia with large aortopulmonary collaterals. One of these can be seen passing through the plane immediately below the carina. *rb*, right main bronchus; *lb*, left main bronchus.

REFERENCES

1. Simpson IA, de Belder MA, Treasure T, et al. Cardiovascular manifestations of Marfan's syndrome: improved evaluation by transesophageal echocardiography. *Br Heart J* 1993;69:104–108.
2. Silvey SV, Stoughton TL, Pearl W, et al. Rupture of the outer partition of aortic dissection during transesophageal echocardiography. *Am J Cardiol* 1991;68:286–287.
3. Mohiaddin RH, Shoser K, Amanuma M, et al. Magnetic resonance imaging of age-related dimensional changes of thoracic aorta. *J Comput Assist Tomogr* 1990;14(5):748–752.
4. Schlatmann TJ, Becker AE. Histologic changes in the normal aging aorta: implications for dissecting aortic aneurysm. *Am J Cardiol* 1977; 39:1320.
5. Homebeck W, Adnet J, Robert L. Age-dependent variation of elastin and elastase in aorta and human breast cancers. *Exp Gerontol* 1978; 13:293–298.
6. Robert L, Moczar M. Age related changes of proteoglycans and glycosaminoglycans. In: Varma RS, Varma R, eds. *Glycosaminoglycans and proteoglycans in physiological and pathological processes of body system.* Basel: Karger, 1982:440–460.
7. Hallock P, Benson IC. Studies on the elastic properties of human isolated aorta. *J Clin Invest* 1937;15:595–602.
8. Hallock P. Arterial elasticity in man in relation to age as evaluated by the pulse wave velocity method. *Arch Int Med* 1934;54:770–798.
9. Luchsinger PC, Sachs M, Patel D. Pressure-radius relationship in large blood vessels of man. *Circ Res* 1962;11:885–887.
10. Mohiaddin RH, Underwood SR, Bogren HG, et al. Regional aortic compliance studied by magnetic resonance imaging: the effects of age, training, and coronary artery disease. *Br Heart J* 1989;62:90–96.
11. Rueckert D, Burger P, Yang GZ, et al. Automatic tracking of the aorta in cardiovascular MR images using deformable models. *IEEE Transact Med Imag* 1997;16:581–590.
12. Mohiaddin RH, Firmin DN, Longmore DB. Age-related changes of human aortic flow velocity measured non-invasively by magnetic resonance imaging. *J Applied Physiol* 1993;74:492–497.
13. Bohning DE, Wood ML, Poon PY, et al. Aortic compliance by pulse wave speed. *Magn Res Med* 1992;720(abst).
14. Kupari K, Keto P, Hekali P, et al. Cine magnetic resonance imaging in the assessment of aortic diensibility. In: Boudoulas P, Toutouzas PK, Wooley C, eds. *Functional abnormality of the aorta.* Armonk, NY: Futura Publishing, 1996:247–268.
15. Wilcken DE, Charlier AA, Hoffman JI, et al. Effect of alterations in aortic impedance on the performance of the ventricles. *Circ Res* 1964; 14:283–293.
16. Bogren HG, Mohiaddin RH, Klipstein RH, et al. The function of the aorta in ischemic heart disease: a magnetic resonance and angiographic study of aortic compliance and blood flow patterns. *Am Heart J* 1989; 118:234–247.
17. Klipstein RH, Firmin DN, Underwood SR, et al. Blood flow patterns

in the human aorta studied by magnetic resonance. *Br Heart J* 1987; 58:316–323.

18. Aschoff L. In: Cowdry EV, ed. *Arteriosclerosis: a survey of the problem.* New York: Macmillan, 1933:1–8.

19. Blankenhorn DH, Kramsch DM. Reversal of atherosis and sclerosis. *Circulation* 1989;79:1–7.

20. Band W, Goedhard WJ, Knoop AA. Comparison of effects of high cholesterol intake on viscoelastic properties of the thoracic aorta in rats and rabbits. *Atherosclerosis* 1973;18:163–172.

21. Banga I, Balo J. Elasticity of the vascular wall. 1. The elastic tensibility of the human carotid as a function of age and arteriosclerosis. *Acta Physiol Acad Sci Hung* 1961;20–21:237–247.

22. Farrar DJ, Bond GM, Riley WA, et al. Anatomic correlates of aortic pulse wave velocity and carotid artery elasticity during atherosclerosis progression and regression in monkeys. *Circulation* 1991;83:1754–1763.

23. Rees RSO, Somerville J, Ward C, et al. Magnetic resonance imaging in late post-operative assessment of coarctation of the aorta. *Radiology* 1989;173:499–502.

24. Manzara CC, Mohiaddin RH, Pennell DJ, et al. Magnetic resonance assessment of thoracic aorta in Marfan's syndrome. American Heart Association, Dallas. *Circulation* 1990;82[Suppl III]:497(abst).

25. Kupari K, Hekali P, Keto P, et al. Relation of aortic stiffness to factors modifying the risk of atherosclerosis in healthy persons. *Arterioscler Thromb* 1994;14:386–394.

26. Mohiaddin RH, Kilner PJ, Rees RSO, et al. Magnetic resonance volume flow and jet velocity mapping in aortic coarctation. *J Am Coll Cardiol* 1993;22:1515–1521.

27. Klipstein RH, Firmin DN, Underwood SR, et al. Blood flow patterns in the human aorta studied by magnetic resonance. *Br Heart J* 1987; 58:316–323.

28. Kilner PJ, Yang GZ, Mohiaddin RH, et al. Helical and retrograde secondary flow patterns in the aortic arch studied by three-directional magnetic resonance velocity mapping. *Circulation* 1993;88:2235–2247.

29. Bogren HG, Mohiaddin RH, Klipstein RH, et al. The function of the aorta in ischemic heart disease: a magnetic resonance and angiographic study of aortic compliance and blood flow patterns. *Am Heart J* 1989;118:234–247.

30. Dulce MC, Mostbeck GH, O'Sullivan RN, et al. Severity of aortic regurgitation: Interstudy reproducibility of measurements with velocity-encoded cine MR imaging. *Radiology* 1992;185:235–240.

31. Yang GZ, Burger P, Mohiaddin RH. *In vivo* blood flow analysis and animation for magnetic resonance imaging. *Proc Int Soc Optic Eng (SPIE)* 1990;1233:176–182.

32. Mohiaddin RH, Yang GZ, Kilner PJ. Visualization of flow by vector analysis of multidirectional cine magnetic resonance velocity mapping. *J Comput Assist Tomogr* 1994;18:383–392.

33. Kilner PJ, Yang GZ, Mohiaddin RH, et al. Helical and retrograde secondary flow patterns in the aortic arch studied by three-directional magnetic resonance velocity mapping. *Circulation* 1993;88:2235–2247.

34. Bogren HG, Mohiaddin RH, Kilner PJ, et al. Blood flow patterns in the thoracic aorta studied with three-directional magnetic resonance velocity mapping: the effect of age and coronary artery disease. *J Magn Reson Imag* 1997;7:784–793.

35. Bogren HG, Mohiaddin RH, Yang GZ, et al. Magnetic resonance velocity vector mapping of blood flow in thoracic aortic aneurysms and grafts. *J Thorac Cardiovasc Surg* 1995;110:704–714.

36. Holman E. The development of arterial aneurysms. *J Surg Gyn Obstr* 1955;100:599–611.

37. Pennell DJ, Firmin DN, Burger P, et al. Assessment of magnetic resonance velocity mapping of global ventricular function during dobutamine infusion in coronary artery disease. *Br Heart J* 1995;74:163–170.

38. Fisman EZ, Ben-Ari E, Pines A, et al. Pronounced reduction of aortic flow velocity and acceleration during heavy isometric exercise in coronary artery disease. *Am J Cardiol* 1991;68:485–491.

39. Gatehouse PD, Firmin DN, Collins S, et al. Real time blood flow imaging by spiral scan phase velocity mapping. *Magn Reson Med* 1994;31:504–512.

40. Oshinski JN, Ferichs F, Doyle JA, et al. Exercise stress measurements of cardiac performance using an MR compatible cycle ergometer. *Proc Int Soc Magn Reson Med* 1997;900(abst).

41. Prince MR, Grist TM, Debatin JF. *3D contrast MR angiography.* Berlin: Springer Verlag, 1997.

42. Prince MR, Yucel EK, Kaufman JA, et al. Dynamic gadolinium-enhanced three-dimensional abdominal MR arteriography. *J Magn Reson Imaging* 1993;3:877–881.

43. Bongartz GM, Boos M, Winter K, et al. Clinical utility of contrast-enhanced MR angiography. *Eur Radiol* 1997;7[Suppl 5]:S178–S186.

44. Bakker J, Beek FJ, Beutler JJ, et al. Renal artery stenosis and accessory renal arteries: accuracy of detection and visualization with gadolinium-enhanced breath-hold MR angiography. *Radiology* 1998;207(2):497–504.

45. Badr KF, Brenner BM. Vascular injury to the kidney. In: Isselbacher KJ, Braunwald E, Wilson JD, eds. *Harrison's principles of internal medicine,* vol. 2. New York: McGraw-Hill, 1994:1320.

46. Ghantous VE, Eisen TD, Sherman AH, et al. Evaluating patients with renal failure for renal artery stenosis with gadolinium-enhanced magnetic resonance angiography. *Am J Kidney Dis* 1999;33(1):36–42.

47. Murdoch JL, Walker BA, Halpern BL, et al. Life expectancy and causes of death in the Marfan's syndrome. *N Engl J Med* 1972;286:804–808.

48. Murgatroyd F, Child A, Poloiecki J, et al. Does routine echo cardiographic assessment of the aortic root diameter help predict the risk of dissection in Marfan's syndrome? *Eur Heart J* 1991;12[Suppl]:410(abst).

49. Treasure T. Elective replacement of the aortic root in Marfan's syndrome. *Br Heart J* 1993;69:101–103.

50. Nienaber CA, von Kodolitsch Y, Nicolas V, et al. The diagnosis of thoracic aortic dissection by noninvasive imaging procedures. *N Engl J Med* 1993;328:1–9.

51. Nienaber CA, Spielmann RP, von Kodolitsch Y, et al. Diagnosis of thoracic aortic dissection: magnetic resonance imaging versus transesophageal echocardiography. *Circulation* 1992;85:434–447.

52. Panting JR, Norell MS, Baker C, et al. Feasibility, accuracy and safety of magnetic resonance imaging in acute aortic dissection. *Clin Radiol* 1995;50:455–458.

53. Moore NR, Parry AJ, Trottman-Dickenson B, et al. Fate of the native aorta after repair of acute type A dissection: a magnetic resonance imaging study. *Heart* 1996;75:62–66.

54. Goldman AP, Kotler MN, Scanlon MH, et al. Magnetic resonance imaging and two dimensional echocardiography. Alternative approach to aortography in diagnosis of aortic dissecting aneurysm. *Am J Med* 1986;80:1225–1229.

55. Bogren HG, Underwood SR, Firmin DN, et al. Magnetic resonance velocity mapping in aortic dissection. *Br J Radiol* 1988;61:456–462.

56. Chang JM, Friese K, Caputo GR, et al. MR measurement of blood flow in the true and false channel in chronic aortic dissection. *J Comput Assist Tomogr* 1991;15:418–423.

57. DeBakey ME, Henley WS, Cooley DA, et al. Surgical management of dissecting aneurysms of the aorta. *J Thorac Cardiovasc Surg* 1965;49:130.

58. Dailey PO, Trueblood HW, Stinson EB, et al. Management of acute dissection. *Am J Thorac Surg* 1970;10:237.

59. Nienaber CA, von Kodolitsch Y, Petersen B, et al. Intramural hemorrhage of the thoracic aorta: diagnostic and therapeutic implications. *Circulation* 1995;92:1465–1472.

60. Robbins RC, McManus RP, Mitchell RS, et al. Management of patients with intramural hematoma of the thoracic aorta. *Circulation* 1993;88:1–10.

61. von Kodolitsch Y, Spielmann RP, Petersen B, et al. Intramural hemorrhage as a precursor of aortic dissection. *Z Kardiol* 1995;84:939–946.

62. Ito I. Aortitis syndrome (Takayasu's arteritis). A historical perspective. *Jpn Heart J* 1995;36:273–281.

63. Zimmermann GG, Erhart P, Schneider J, et al. Intravascular MR imaging of atherosclerotic plaque: ex-vivo analysis of human femoral arteries with histologic correlation. *Radiology* 1997;204:769–774.

64. Kaufman L, Crooks L, Sheldon P, et al. Evaluation of NMR imaging for the detection and quantification of obstruction in vessels. *Invest Radiol* 1982;17:554–560.

65. Herfkens R, Higgins C, Hricak H, et al. Nuclear magnetic resonance imaging of atherosclerotic disease. *Radiology* 1983;148:161–166.

66. Maynor CH, Charles HC, Herfkens RJ, et al. Chemical shift imaging of atherosclerosis at 7.0 Tesla. *Invest Radiol* 1989;24:52–60.

67. Carpenter TA, Hodgson RJ, Herrod NJ, et al. Magnetic resonance imaging in a model of atherosclerosis: use of collar around the rabbit carotid artery. *Magn Reson Imag* 1991;9:365–371.

68. Vinitski S, Consigny M, Shapiro MJ, et al. Magnetic resonance chemi-

cal shift imaging and spectroscopy of atherosclerotic plaque. *Invest Radiol* 1991;26:703–714.

69. Mohiaddin RH, Firmin DN, Underwood SR, et al. Magnetic resonance chemical shift imaging of human atheroma. *Br Heart J* 1989;62:81–90.

70. Mohiaddin RH, Sampson C, Firmin DN, et al. Magnetic resonance morphological, chemical shift and flow imaging in peripheral vascular disease. *Eur J Vasc Surg* 1991;5:383–396.

71. Gold GE, Pauly JM, Glover GH, et al. Characterization of atherosclerosis with a 1.5T imaging system. *J Magn Reson Imag* 1993;3:399–407.

72. Skinner MP, Yuan C, Mitsunori L, et al. Serial magnetic resonance imaging of experimental atherosclerosis detect lesion fine structure, progression and complications *in vivo*. *Nature Med* 1995;1:69–73.

73. Toussaint JF, LaMuraglia GM, Southern JF, et al. Magnetic resonance imaging lipid, fibrous, calcified, hemorrhagic and thrombotic components of human atherosclerosis *in vivo*. *Circulation* 1996;94:932–938.

74. Bulte JW, Ma LD, Magin RL, et al. Selective MR imaging of labelled human peripheral blood mononuclear cells by liposome mediated incorporation of dextran-magnetite particles. *Magn Reson Med* 1993;29:32–37.

75. Pearlman JD, Southern JF, Ackerman JL. Nuclear magnetic resonance microscopy of atheroma in human coronary arteries. *Angiology* 1991;42:726–733.

76. Fayad ZA, Fallon JT, Shinnar M, et al. Non-invasive *in vivo* high resolution magnetic resonance imaging of atherosclerotic lesions in genetically engineered mice. *Circulation* 1998;98:1541–1547.

77. Yeung HN, Kormos DW. Separation of true fat and water images by correcting magnetic field inhomogeneity in situ. *Radiology* 1986;159:783–786.

78. Yang GZ, Firmin DN, Mohaiddin RH, et al. BO Inhomogeneity correction for two point Dixon chemical shift imaging. *Magn Res Med* 1992;11:3819(abst).

79. Elliott LP. *Cardiac imaging in infants, children and adults*. Philadelphia: Lippincott, 1991.

80. Steiner RM, Gross GW, Flicker S, et al. Congenital heart disease in the adult patient: the value of plain film chest radiology. *J Thorac Imaging* 1995;10:1–25.

81. Wexler L, Higgins CB. The use of magnetic resonance imaging in adult congenital heart disease. *Am J Card Imag* 1995;9:15–28.

82. Kilner PJ. Imaging of adults with congenital heart disease. In: Lima J, ed. *Diagnostic imaging in clinical cardiology*. London: Martin Dunitz, 1998:211–233.

83. Sechtem U. Imaging of aortic coarctation—difficult choices. *Eur Heart J* 1995;16:1315–1316.

84. Carvalho JS, Redington AN, Shinebourne EA, et al. Continuous wave Doppler echocardiography and coarctation of the aorta: gradients and flow patterns in the assessment of severity. *Br Heart J* 1990;64:133–137.

85. Kilner PJ, Shinohara T, Sampson C, et al. Repaired aortic coarctation in adults—MRI with velocity mapping shows distortions of anatomy and flow. *Cardiol Young* 1996;6:20–27.

86. Baumgartner H, Schima H, Tulzer G, et al. Effect of stenosis geometry on the Doppler-catheter relation *in vitro*: a manifestation of pressure recovery. *J Am Coll Cardiol* 1993;21:1018–1025.

87. Migliavacca F, Kilner PJ, Dubini GG, et al. Localised peaks of computed flow velocity through asymmetric stenoses in large vessel models could have implications for "pressure gradient" estimation. *J Vasc Invest* 1997;3:17–25.

88. Mohiaddin RH, Kilner PJ, Rees S, et al. Magnetic resonance volume flow and jet velocity mapping in aortic coarctation. *J Am Coll Cardiol* 1993;22:1515–1521.

89. Steffens JC, Bourne MW, Sakuma H, et al. Quantification of collateral blood flow in coarctation of the aorta by velocity encoded cine magnetic resonance imaging. *Circulation* 1994;90:937–943.

90. Rees S, Somerville J, Ward C, et al. Coarctation of the aorta: MR imaging in late postoperative assessment. *Radiology* 1989;173:499–502.

91. Holdright DR, Kilner PJ, Somerville J. Haemoptysis from false aneurysm: near fatal complication of repair of coarctation of the aorta using a Dacron patch. *Int J Cardiol* 1991;32:406–408.

92. Lo SSS, Kilner PJ, Somerville J. Leaking aortic aneurysm after repair of aortic coarctation—the significance of MRI. *Cardiol Young* 1997;7:340–343.

93. Hundley WG, Li HF, Lange RA, et al. Assessment of left to right arterial shunting by velocity encoded, phase-difference magnetic resonance imaging: a comparison with oximetric and indicator dilution techniques. *Circulation* 1995;91:2955–2960.

94. Pennell DJ, Underwood SR. Magnetic resonance imaging of the heart. *Postgrad Med J* 1991;67:S1–9.

95. Mohiaddin RH, Gatehouse PD, Firmin DN. Exercise-related changes in aortic flow. *J Magn Reson Imag* 1995;5:159–163.

96. Forbat SM, Thorne S, Underwood SR, et al. Magnetic resonance phase velocity mapping in dissecting aortic aneurysm: demonstration of a proximal intimal tear. *Circulation* 1995;91:236–237.

97. Mohiaddin RH, Pennell DJ. MR blood flow measurement: clinical application in the heart and circulation. *Cardiol Clin North America* 1998;16:161–187.

CHAPTER 59

Peripheral Vascular Disease

Peter C. Spittell

Peripheral vascular disease is frequently encountered in current cardiovascular practice. Characteristic clinical findings identify patients with peripheral arterial disease, and, usually, further noninvasive testing to quantify disease severity is pursued. Several noninvasive tests currently available allow for accurate diagnosis of peripheral arterial diseases with angiography being reserved for patients requiring revascularization and for patients suspected of having an uncommon type of arterial disease.

LOWER EXTREMITY ARTERIAL DISEASE

Intermittent claudication, the symptomatic hallmark of lower extremity arterial occlusive disease, has a classic clinical presentation: lower extremity discomfort that occurs with walking and is relieved by rest, standing still. Physical examination often reveals arterial pulse deficits and the presence of arterial bruits. The most common cause of intermittent claudication is atherosclerosis that tends to affect the proximal arterial segments (aortic bifurcation to popliteal artery level), but, in patients with diabetes mellitus, a different pattern of arterial involvement occurs with predominant infrapopliteal disease. Disease localized to the distal abdominal aorta and iliac arteries is a pattern often seen in younger patients (<55 years old) who smoke tobacco.

Although the clinical diagnosis of intermittent claudication is accurate, noninvasive testing is often indicated to confirm the diagnosis and to quantify disease severity. Several noninvasive methods are accurate in the diagnosis of lower extremity arterial occlusive disease, providing functional and/or anatomic information. Angiography is indicated in patients with critical limb ischemia (ischemic rest pain, ulceration and/or gangrene) prior to revascularization,

and in patients suspected of having an uncommon type of arterial disease.

Noninvasive Methods

Continuous-Wave Doppler and Blood Pressure Methods

A complete lower extremity arterial evaluation frequently includes a continuous-wave Doppler assessment in addition to measurement of the ankle:brachial systolic pressure index (ABI), segmental pressures, and pulse-volume recordings. Continuous-wave Doppler evaluation of the arterial velocity patterns of the external iliac-common femoral artery; superficial femoral artery; popliteal artery; and pedal arteries (dorsalis pedis and posterior tibial arteries) are readily obtainable with a hand-held continuous-wave Doppler device. The normal pattern of flow in the lower extremity arteries is triphasic (forward flow during systole, a late systolic and early diastolic reverse-flow component, and mid-to-late diastolic forward flow). When there is a proximal arterial stenosis greater than 50% or if there is proximal arterial occlusion, blunting of the early systolic peak occurs, and there is loss of the reverse-flow component resulting in a monophasic waveform. The monophasic waveform distal to a hemodynamically significant stenosis has a characteristic tardus and parvus appearance (lower amplitude and late or absent systolic peak) (Fig. 1).

Following the continuous-wave Doppler assessment, ABI testing is performed. Measurement of lower extremity blood pressure is the most commonly used test to detect lower extremity arterial occlusive disease. When an area of arterial narrowing exceeds 50%, a reduction in systolic blood pressure distal to the narrowing occurs, the magnitude of the reduction providing an estimate of disease severity and the presence or absence of an adequate collateral circulation. Most commonly, systolic blood pressure at the level of the ankle is compared to the brachial artery systolic blood pres-

P. C. Spittell: Mayo Medical School; Department of Internal Medicine, Division of Cardiovascular Diseases, Mayo Medical Center, Rochester, Minnesota 55905.

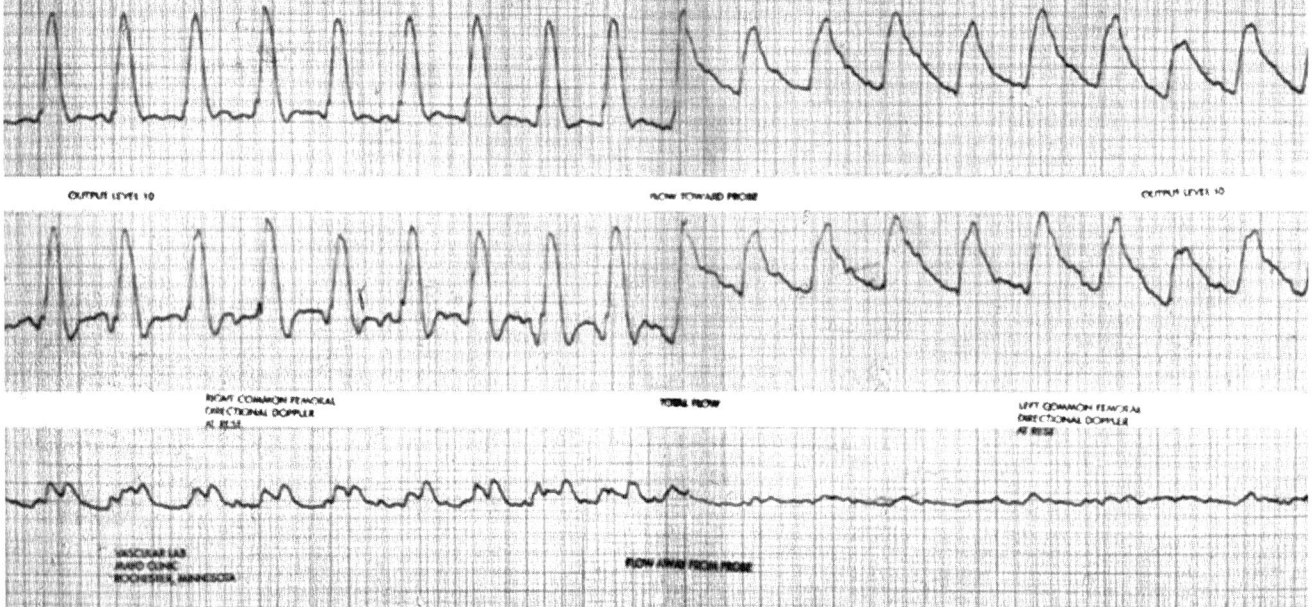

FIG. 1. Continuous-wave Doppler tracings of the common femoral arteries in a patient with intermittent claudication. The tracings on the **left** demonstrates the normal pattern of triphasic flow of a peripheral artery. On the **right**, the waveform is monophasic (lower amplitude and has a delayed systolic peak characteristic of a hemodynamically significant stenosis proximal to this signal).

sure, the ankle:brachial systolic blood pressure index (ABI). The ABI is defined as the ratio of ankle systolic pressure (dorsalis pedis artery or posterior tibial artery) to the brachial artery systolic blood pressure. The ankle systolic pressure is measured with a hand-held continuous-wave Doppler flowmeter and a standard arm blood pressure cuff. The systolic blood pressure is measured in both arms (brachial arteries) and both tibial arteries at the ankle and is taken at the point at which flow is first detected during cuff deflation, not at the point the Doppler signal disappears during cuff inflation. The ankle and brachial systolic pressures are obtained in the supine position, the higher of the brachial systolic pressures is used to calculate the ABI. A normal ABI is 1.0; an ABI of 0.8 to 0.9, 0.5 to 0.8, and less than 0.5 correlates with mild, moderate, and severe lower extremity arterial occlusive disease, respectively. In general, a resting ABI less than 0.9 suggests the presence of significant lower extremity arterial occlusive disease.

Because the resting ABI may be normal or only minimally reduced in patients with isolated proximal aortoiliac disease and in patients with femoral and popliteal disease and an adequate collateral circulation, exercise testing (usually treadmill walking) is often performed to provide a more accurate assessment of disease severity. A standard exercise test includes walking on a treadmill (1 to 2 mph, 10% incline) for up to 5 minutes (symptom-limited). Supine ABIs are measured before and immediately after the treadmill exercise, and the time of appearance of any lower extremity symptoms is recorded. ABIs before and after treadmill exercise provide an estimate of both disease severity and the functional significance of disease, as well as aiding in the

differential diagnosis of leg pain (e.g., pseudoclaudication due to lumbar spinal stenosis). In patients unable to walk on a treadmill (such as patients with orthopedic or neurologic limitations) active pedal plantarflexion, i.e., having the patient stand with fingertip support against a wall and perform up to 50 repetitions of ankle dorsiflexion, can be performed. ABI testing before and immediately following active pedal plantarflexion provides results similar to treadmill testing.

Limitations of the ABI include its inability to accurately localize the arterial segments involved by occlusive disease. In addition, when medial calcification of the tibial arteries is present (Monkeberg's medial calcification or calcification secondary to diabetes mellitus or advanced age), the pedal arteries become noncompressible (i.e., the ankle systolic pressure usually exceeds 300 mm Hg or is >50 mm Hg higher than the brachial artery systolic pressure) making calculation of an ABI inaccurate. When medial calcification is suspected, the systolic pressure should be measured from the toe, which is then compared to the arm (the toe:brachial systolic pressure index), a value that is normally greater than 0.6. The absolute levels of pressure at the ankles (and the digits) may also be useful in providing an estimate of the extent of the perfusion deficit in patients with ischemic ulceration. For example, a toe systolic pressure less than 30 mm Hg predicts nonhealing of an ischemic ulcer unless peripheral arterial revascularization is performed.

Segmental blood pressure measurements are usually performed in conjunction with ABI testing to further localize the arterial segment(s) involved by the occlusive disease. Pneumatic cuffs are applied to various points on the lower extremity (thigh, calf, ankle, transmetatarsal, toe) to determine systolic pressure at several levels. This is performed by placing the pneumatic cuffs at these levels and inflating them to suprasystolic pressures to interrupt flow. When there are multiple levels of stenosis, the systolic pressure level measured distal to the last area of involvement will reflect the additive resistances offered by the collateral circuits. Segmental blood pressure measurements are typically obtained in both lower extremities and are interpreted by comparing the pressure gradient between two adjacent sites in an extremity, by comparing the values in opposite limbs, or by calculating the pressure ratio with reference to brachial systolic readings. Segmental pressures recorded by this method will be artifactually high because the cuffs used may not effectively transmit the pressure to the vessels deep in the leg, a factor that must be taken into account when this technique is used.

The pulse-volume recorder (PVR) is another noninvasive method used to assess lower extremity arterial occlusive disease. The PVR device records the pulsatile volume changes that occur in the lower extremity arteries with each cardiac cycle. The pneumatic cuffs used to measure a PVR are placed in the same locations as when performing segmental pressures. A measured quantity of air is injected into each cuff until a preset pressure is reached. As the lower extremity volume increases during systole, the pressure in the cuff changes, and this change is recorded on a strip chart. A 1-mm Hg pressure change in the cuff produces a 20-mm chart deflection. The amplitude of the pulse-volume recording reflects local arterial pressure, vascular wall compliance, the number of arterial vessels beneath the cuff, and the severity of atherosclerotic disease. The phasic characteristics of the arterial waveform provide further information on the presence of lower extremity arterial occlusive disease.

Ultrasound Imaging in Lower Extremity Arterial Occlusive Disease

The development of peripheral arterial ultrasonography (Duplex ultrasound) represented a major advance in the noninvasive diagnosis of lower extremity arterial occlusive disease. By combining two-dimensional (B-mode) ultrasound imaging with pulsed-wave Doppler and color flow Doppler imaging, the ability to accurately localize the arterial segment(s) involved by disease and provide an estimate of hemodynamic significance of the arterial stenosis became possible. With two-dimensional imaging as an anatomic guide, a pulsed-wave Doppler sample volume can be used to sample flow along the visualized artery. Color flow Doppler is utilized in positioning the pulsed-wave Doppler sample volume within the axis of the vessel lumen and to aid in detecting arterial stenosis (color flow aliasing). The angle between the pulsed-wave Doppler sample volume and the vessel axis is measured and used to derive velocity information, which is recorded graphically as a function of time. Normal laminar flow in an artery produces a narrow range of modal veloci-

ties, whereas flow through a stenosis is accelerated and turbulent flow immediately distal to a stenosis results in spectral broadening of the velocity display.

A standard ultrasound examination of the lower extremity arteries is performed with the patient in the supine position. The abdominal aorta is imaged in the midline beginning just below the level of the xiphoid process and followed distally to the level of the iliac artery bifurcation. Longitudinal and transverse views of the abdominal aorta (supraceliac aorta to aortic bifurcation) are recorded, and assessment of any aneurysmal disease and /or atherosclerotic disease is made. The common iliac and external iliac artery are then examined to the level of the groin. The common femoral, deep (profunda) femoral, and superficial femoral arteries are imaged to the level of the adductor hiatus. The patient is then positioned prone with the feet elevated approximately 30 degrees for examination of the popliteal artery and origins of the tibial arteries. Pulsed-wave Doppler spectral velocity data is recorded from each accessible arterial segment, and a more detailed analysis is performed for each area in which disturbed flow is detected.

The absolute peak systolic velocity in any single arterial segment shows such wide variability between patients that it is necessary to compare velocity information from one arterial segment to the next in each individual. When a stenosis is present, the peak systolic velocity increases, allowing an estimate of the degree of stenosis at the site at which the velocity increase occurred. As previously mentioned, normal velocity patterns in the lower extremity arteries are triphasic and have a clear spectral velocity envelope. When minimal arterial disease (1 to 19% stenosis) is present, there is spectral broadening without a significant increase in peak systolic velocity, and the reverse-flow component is preserved. With mild occlusive arterial disease (20 to 49% stenosis), the peak systolic velocity increases greater than 30% but less than 100% from the proximal arterial segment, with preservation of the reverse-flow component. When an arterial stenosis greater than 50% is present, the increase in peak systolic velocity is greater than 100% in the stenosis, and there is marked spectral broadening and loss of the reverse-flow component. With arterial occlusion, there is no detectable flow within the visualized arterial segment. The accuracy of ultrasound in detecting greater than 50% stenosis can be further improved when the increase in peak systolic velocity is greater than 150% from one arterial segment to another, resulting in a sensitivity of greater than 90% and specificity greater than 98% in the aortoiliac and femoropopliteal segments (1,2). Diagnostic velocity criteria such as these for grading the severity of lower extremity arterial stenosis with ultrasonography and validation of the criteria with angiography have previously been published (3).

The overall sensitivity of ultrasonography in patients with lower extremity arterial occlusive disease is 82%, specificity 92%, positive predictive value 80%, and negative predictive value 93% in predicting stenosis severity. Ultrasound is the most sensitive in the iliac and femoral artery territories as compared to the popliteal and infrapopliteal segments. Ultra-sonography is also often able to accurately predict which patients with iliac arterial occlusive disease are candidates for percutaneous transluminal angioplasty and is able to follow the results of percutaneous and surgical interventions over time, thereby reducing the long-term complications of these procedures (4–7).

Although the resolution of current ultrasound instruments continues to improve the ability to visualize arterial plaque, spectral waveform analysis and a sequential velocity assessment are currently required to quantify lower extremity arterial occlusive disease. Ultrasound tissue-characterization techniques and utilization of harmonic imaging will hopefully allow for a more precise definition of the atherosclerotic lesions themselves as fibrotic, ulcerated, lipoid, thrombotic, hyperplastic, or calcific, leading to improved and more timely interventional techniques and improved patient outcomes.

Magnetic Resonance Angiography

Magnetic resonance angiography (MRA) is increasingly being used to diagnose and treat patients with lower extremity arterial occlusive disease. Detailed anatomic and functional information can be noninvasively obtained from the abdominal aorta to the smaller arteries of the foot with an accuracy equal to contrast angiography (Fig. 2). Recent advances in MRA technology resulting from fast gradients and use of intravenous contrast agents have allowed MRA to make substantial advances in providing the preoperative "road map" required before intervention. The inherent advantages of MRA (noninvasive technique; ability to provide three-dimensional, high resolution images; exquisite flow sensitivity (<10 cm/sec) and no absolute need for contrast material) make MRA useful in the evaluation of patients with contraindications to standard angiography. The contrast media in MRA, flowing blood, causes a projected three-dimensional "flow map" of the vasculature. The flow-map incorporates information about both anatomic and physiologic effects of arterial stenoses. Initially, time-of-flight flow effects and phase effects were the two general approaches utilized to provide projection images of the infrainguinal arteries. Time-of-flight flow effects are associated with the increase in amplitude of the signal returning from flowing blood entering the imaged area. Phase effects are associated with the increase in phase angle of this returning signal that is proportional to the velocity of flowing blood. Several studies comparing two-dimensional time-of-flight peripheral MRA with conventional x-ray angiography have demonstrated good agreement in the majority of patients. Furthermore, two-dimensional time-of-flight MRA is able to identify "angiographically occult" runoff vessels more often than standard contrast angiography (8–10). Although time-of-flight and phase effects can produce magnetic resonance angiograms, undesirable flow phenomena, such as turbulence, cause signal loss, and visual overestimation of the severity

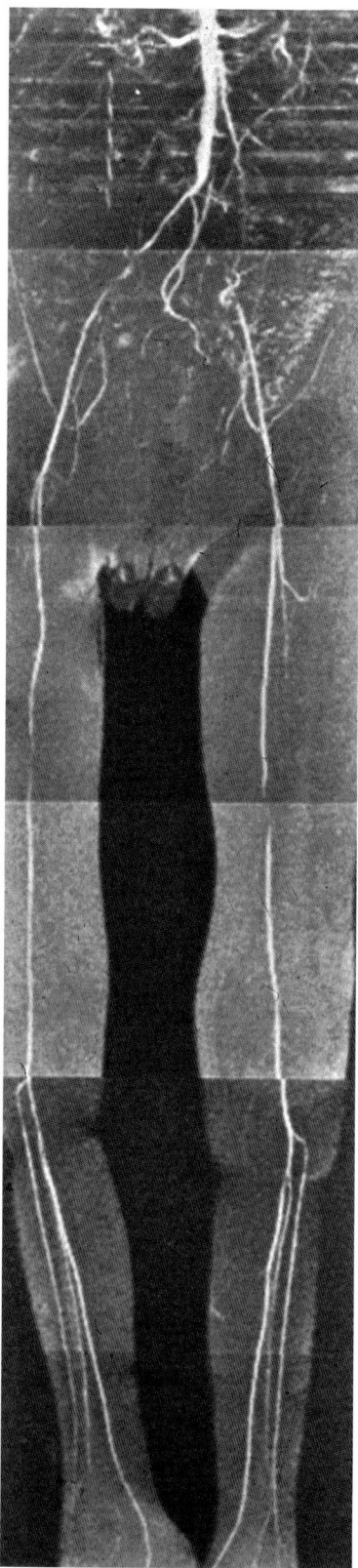

FIG. 2. Reconstructed photograph of a contrast-enhanced magnetic resonance angiogram of the lower extremity arteries demonstrating occlusion of the left common iliac artery, high-grade stenosis of the right common iliac artery, bilateral superficial femoral artery stenoses, and occlusion of the peroneal artery on the right.

of a stenosis can occur. For this reason, the findings on magnetic resonance angiography alone can sometimes be misleading in terms of the hemodynamic importance of a stenosis. To overcome the flow-related artifacts and prolonged imaging times that have plagued two-dimensional time-of-flight MRA, several variations in imaging techniques have been examined. Developments such as velocity-encoded cine MR imaging, combined with magnetic resonance angiography, allow detection of the monophasic waveforms associated with significant arterial stenosis and have improved the assessment of the hemodynamic importance of a peripheral arterial stenosis (11). Contrast-enhanced (gadolinium-DTPA) MRA improved image quality but limitations remained, such as venous overlap, imaging artifacts, and suboptimal visualization of subtle lesions (12). There has been rapid progress in peripheral MRA since its introduction and, at select centers with significant expertise, peripheral MRA has been able to replace standard contrast angiography for patients with symptomatic peripheral arterial occlusive disease.

MRA has also been shown to be accurate and effective when used to follow the results of peripheral arterial interventions. For example, in patients with iliofemoral disease, contrast-enhanced MRA is comparable to digital subtraction angiography for the detection of stenosis greater than 50% and occlusion in the iliofemoral arteries (13). Although MRA can accurately determine stent patency and provide information about the vascular anatomic areas proximal and distal to the stent, some stents made of stainless steel and some nitinol stents cause signal intensity dropout, making determination of stent patency difficult. Tantalum stents are not associated with a significant metallic artifact, and stent patency can be determined accurately with MRA.

MRA is indicated in patients being considered for peripheral revascularization in whom contraindications to standard contrast angiography exist. Typical indications for MRA in patients with lower extremity arterial occlusive disease are preexisting renal disease, especially in the setting of diabetes mellitus; and severe contrast allergy. Magnetic resonance angiography is contraindicated in patients with pacemakers, internal cardiac defibrillators, or ferromagnetic cerebral aneurysm clips. The presence of surgical clips, vascular coils, and metallic orthopedic implants are not a contraindication to MRA; however, all may produce artifacts on the images potentially causing false-positive findings for the presence of an arterial stenosis. With the exception of patients with an older Starr-Edwards (pre-6000) valve and suspected dehiscence of that valve, magnetic resonance angiography is generally regarded as safe in patients with prosthetic heart valves. MRA is not currently cost-effective as a screening method for patients with lower extremity arterial occlusive disease, as compared to ABI measurement or duplex ultrasonography.

Indications for x-ray contrast angiography in patients with lower extremity arterial occlusive disease include: critical limb ischemia (ischemic rest pain, ulceration, and/or gan-grene); disabling symptoms of intermittent claudication; definition of vascular grafts and their associated native vessels; following acute trauma if distal pulses are diminished or absent; and when an uncommon type of arterial occlusive disease is suspected.

Aneurysmal Disease

Peripheral artery aneurysms involving the iliac, superficial femoral, and popliteal arteries can occur in isolation, but they are more common in patients who have aneurysms in other locations, with disorders of connective tissue, and following trauma. An iliac artery aneurysm usually occurs in association with an abdominal aortic aneurysm, but it may occur as an isolated finding. Iliac artery aneurysms are usually asymptomatic but they may cause atheroembolism, obstructive urologic symptoms, unexplained groin or perineal pain, iliac vein obstruction, or rupture. Iliac artery aneurysms are often occult, but a pulsatile mass in the lower abdominal quadrants may be evident on clinical examination. Computed tomography with intravenous contrast or MRI/MRA is the preferred diagnostic procedure. The diagnosis can also be confirmed with ultrasonography. The criteria used to diagnose a peripheral artery aneurysm relate the dimension of the artery proximal to the dilated segment. An artery that is $1\frac{1}{2}$ to 2 times the diameter of the artery immediately proximal to it should be considered aneurysmal.

Popliteal artery aneurysms can be complicated by thrombosis, venous obstruction, embolization, popliteal neuropathy, popliteal thromobophlebitis, rupture, and infection. They are bilateral in 50% of patients, and 40% of patients have one or more aneurysms at other sites, usually of the abdominal aorta. The diagnosis is readily made with ultrasonography, but angiography is necessary before surgical treatment to evaluate the proximal and distal arterial circulation. Spiral computed tomography and MRA are also accurate noninvasive methods used in the diagnosis of popliteal artery aneurysms.

Peripheral Arterial Complications of Interventional Procedures

Peripheral vascular complications as a result of an interventional procedure deserve special mention. The most clinically significant complications are not uncommon with an incidence ranging from 1.5 to 9% (14). Following any interventional procedure, the clinical finding of a groin mass or a bruit should raise the possibility of a hematoma, pseudoaneurysm, or arteriovenous (AV) fistula. Ultrasonography is diagnostic in most cases.

Groin hematomas are the most common complication of the transfemoral angiographic approach. Large hematomas (>6 cm) occur in 6 to 12% of patients, with blood transfusion or surgical repair required in less than 1.4% of patients. A groin hematoma is clinically manifest as a localized swelling at the femoral puncture site, and is confirmed by ultrasonography demonstrating absence of blood flow from the artery to a perivascular hematoma, thereby differentiating the hematoma from a pseudoaneurysm or AV fistula.

Femoral pseudoaneurysm occurs with an incidence of 0.5 to 6.3% following interventional coronary angiographic procedures, and it is usually manifest as a tender, pulsatile groin mass with an overlying bruit. Ultrasound is diagnostic, demonstrating a hypoechoic cavity communicating with an artery by a narrow neck and demonstrating to-and-fro flow with pulsed-wave Doppler and color flow imaging (Fig. 3; see also Color Plate 40 following page 758). Small, asymptomatic femoral pseudoaneurysms commonly undergo spontaneous closure upon cessation of anticoagulant therapy. Nonsurgical closure by ultrasound-guided compression of the neck of the pseudoaneurysm is a noninvasive alternative treatment to surgery and is effective in over 90% of patients (15). Contraindications for ultrasound-guided compression of an iatrogenic femoral artery pseudoaneurysm include infection, cutaneous ischemia, large hematomas with compartment syndrome, aneurysms originating proximal to the inguinal ligament, and excessive discomfort precluding adequate compression. Surgical repair is indicated in patients who are not candidates for ultrasound-guided compression therapy.

Arteriovenous fistula complicating an interventional procedure can result from puncture and subsequent placement of the sheath through the anterior and posterior wall of the femoral artery and then into the femoral vein. It occurs with a reported incidence of 0.2 to 2.1% in patients undergoing coronary interventional procedures (16). Physical examination usually discloses a palpable thrill and continuous bruit overlying the fistula. Distal arterial insufficiency, high-output congestive heart failure, deep venous thrombosis, or lower extremity pain may complicate an untreated arteriovenous fistula. The diagnosis is confirmed by duplex ultrasonography that demonstrates "arterialization" of the venous waveform and often can demonstrate the fistulous tract (Fig. 4; see also Color Plate 41 following page 758). Ultrasound-guided compression of iatrogenic AV fistula in the groin has a reported 75% success rate (17). Elective surgical repair is indicated when contraindications to ultrasound-guided compression therapy are present.

Acute arterial occlusion complicating interventional angiographic procedures usually results from thromboembolism from a cardiac chamber, proximal aneurysm, or aortic atherosclerotic plaque. Thromboemboli can also develop at a sheath site or catheter tip, embolizing during sheath removal. Although ultrasonography can accurately identify lower extremity arterial occlusion, angiography is required to precisely localize the site of occlusion and define the arterial circulation proximal and distal to the occlusion, as well as to guide subsequent thrombolytic therapy, percutaneous aspiration thromboembolectomy, or surgical embolectomy.

Aortic dissection is an uncommon but potentially serious complication of invasive angiographic procedures. Catheter-induced dissection can originate at any location, most com-

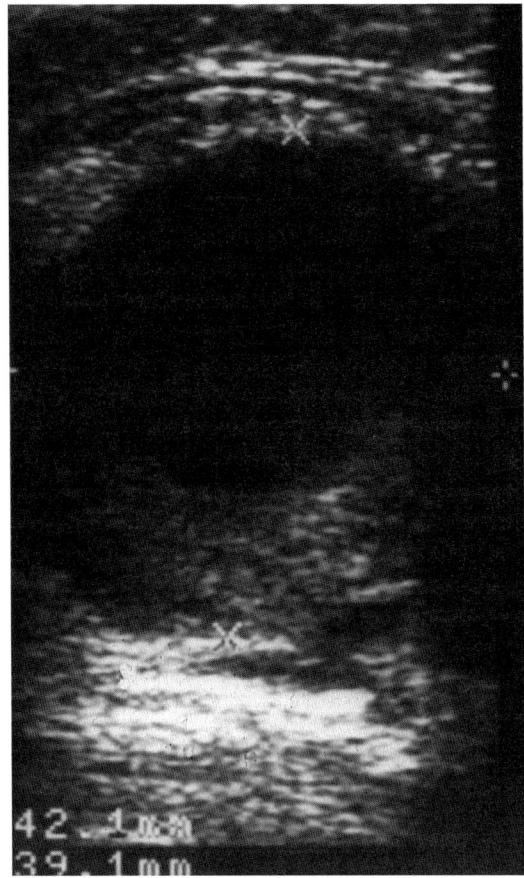

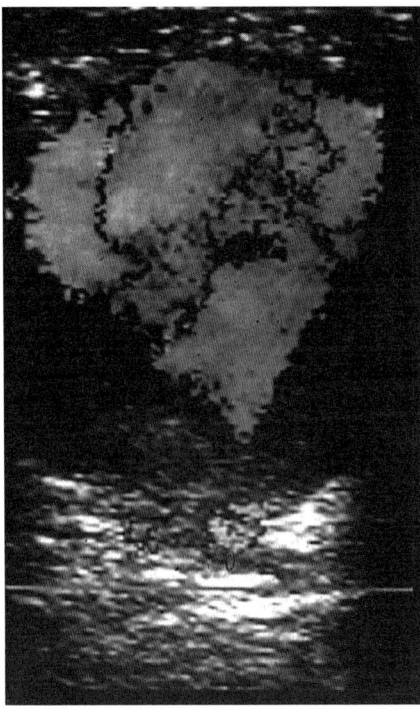

FIG. 3. Duplex ultrasound demonstrating (**A**) a large pseudoaneurysm of the left common femoral artery with a large amount of mural thrombus and (**B**) color flow imaging revealing the characteristic nonlaminar, to-and-fro flow within the pseudoaneurysm. (See also Color Plate 40 following page 758.)

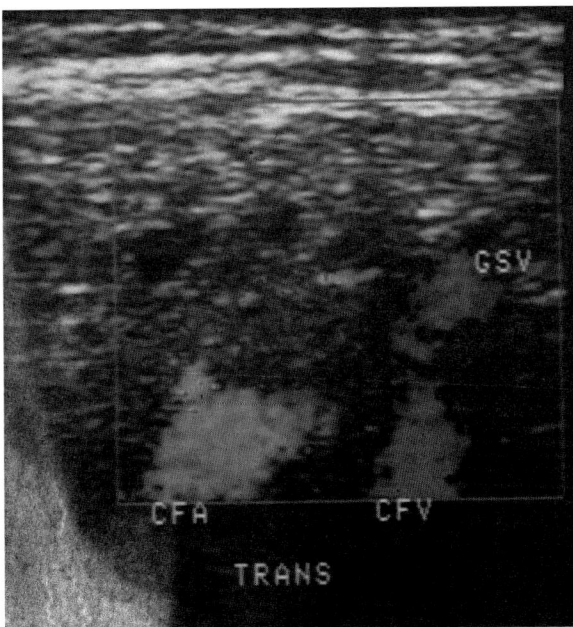

FIG. 4. Duplex ultrasound and color flow imaging in a patient with a continuous femoral bruit after transfemoral coronary angiography demonstrates an arteriovenous fistula between the right common femoral artery and vein. Note the fistulous tract is well delineated with color flow imaging. *CFA,* common femoral artery; *CFV,* common femoral vein, *GSV,* greater saphenous vein. (See also Color Plate 41 following page 758.)

monly in the sinus of Valsalva, brachiocephalic arteries, descending thoracic aorta, abdominal aorta, and iliac or femoral arteries. The majority of catheter-induced dissections are retrograde dissections and tend to decrease in size over time due to thrombosis of the false lumen, whereas anterograde dissections tend to persist on follow-up. Nearly all iatrogenic aortic dissections can be treated medically with serial clinical examinations and noninvasive testing used to identify those in need of surgical therapy.

UPPER EXTREMITY ARTERIAL DISEASE

Noninvasive Methods

Diseases of the upper extremity arteries can be evaluated with the noninvasive tests previously described for the lower extremity arteries. Atherosclerotic disease of the upper extremity arteries most commonly involves the subclavian arteries or the more proximal brachiocephalic artery origins. Normal arterial velocity patterns in the upper extremity arteries are either triphasic or biphasic, and the reverse-flow component is absent in about 50% of healthy individuals, presumably due to lower arterial resistance in the upper extremity arteries. Segmental pressures (brachial, forearm, digital levels) are performed, usually in association with a continuous-wave Doppler assessment of flow in the subclavian, brachial, radial, and ulnar arteries. Digital systolic pres-

sures are obtained and compared to brachial systolic pressure as an index of the severity of digital occlusive arterial disease. An assessment of the superficial palmar arch and digital arteries is also possible with these techniques, using radial or ulnar artery compression while measuring digital pressure or pulse volume recordings. In patients with a suspected vasospastic disorder, digital temperatures and/or laser Doppler blood flow are measured before and following a thermal challenge, most commonly immersion of the hands in ice water. In patients without vasospasm, digital temperature recovers to within 1 degree centigrade of the baseline (preimmersion) temperatures within 10 minutes following removal from the cold water stimulus. In patients with a vasospastic disorder, digital temperature recovery is significantly prolonged beyond 10 minutes. In patients with digital ischemia, angiography is indicated to diagnose the underlying disease and plan appropriate therapy.

Upper extremity arterial aneurysms are rare. They may arise as pseudoaneurysms secondary to trauma or iatrogenic complications, or as degenerative lesions often secondary to chronic external trauma, such as in the thoracic outlet syndrome or secondary to the chronic use of crutches. Upper extremity arterial aneurysms can be complicated by distal embolization, cause external compression of a surrounding structure, or undergo rupture or thrombosis. Diagnosis of upper extremity aneurysmal disease can be made with ultrasonography, computed tomography, and MRA. Angiography is indicated preoperatively to define the circulation proximal and distal to the aneurysm.

Uncommon Types of Arterial Occlusive Disease

The clinical features that suggest an uncommon type of peripheral arterial disease include young age at the onset of symptoms, acute ischemia without a history of occlusive arterial disease, and involvement of only the upper extremity or digits. Further objective testing is indicated when an uncommon type of peripheral arterial disease is suspected to establish the diagnosis and direct treatment. These disorders may result in occlusive arterial disease and/or aneurysmal disease, the arterial segment involved being relatively specific for each disease. It is important to remember that all connective tissue disorders and giant cell arteritides can involve peripheral arteries, and symptoms of peripheral arterial involvement may dominate the clinical picture. Peripheral arterial occlusive disease that occurs secondary to connective tissue disorders requires angiography for definitive diagnosis. Because the upper extremity digits are frequently involved, upper extremity angiography with magnified hand views is often performed.

Thromboangiitis obliterans (Buerger's disease) is an uncommon type of arterial occlusive disease that most often affects young men (<40 years of age) who smoke tobacco. Episodes of migratory superficial thrombophlebitis, intermittent claudication involving the arch or calf, and/or Raynaud's phenomenon in the appropriate patient population suggest the diagnosis. More definitive diagnosis of Buerger's disease requires angiography, which usually reveals multiple focal segments of stenosis or occlusion involving the smaller arteries of the upper and lower extremities, with normal proximal vessels.

Popliteal artery entrapment characteristically affects young men and results in intermittent claudication in the arch of the foot or calf. If the popliteal artery is not already occluded, the finding of diminished pedal pulses with sustained active pedal plantarflexion may be noted. The diagnosis of popliteal artery entrapment may be confirmed with ABI measurement, pulse volume recordings, duplex ultrasonography, computerized axial scanning, magnetic resonance imaging, and magnetic resonance angiography (18–22). All of these methods rely on demonstrating popliteal artery compression, with reduced or abolished popliteal artery blood flow occurring with forced active plantar flexion or dorsiflexion of the foot against resistance. Despite the availability of noninvasive testing, the most widely used diagnostic method is contrast angiography, particularly when surgical therapy is anticipated (23). As with noninvasive testing, angiographic results may show an apparently normal popliteal artery at rest and usually necessitate forced active plantar flexion or dorsiflexion of the foot against resistance to show the arterial compression, provided the artery has not already undergone degenerative changes. In contrast, cases of popliteal adventitial cystic disease will usually show the characteristic angiographic abnormality, both at rest and on stress views.

Compression of the subclavian artery in the thoracic outlet (thoracic outlet compression syndrome) can occur at several points, but the most common site of compression is in the costoclavicular space between the uppermost rib (cervical rib or first rib) and the clavicle. Thoracic outlet compression syndrome can have diverse presentations, including Raynaud's phenomenon in one or more fingers of the ipsilateral hand, digital cyanosis or ulceration, upper extremity emboli, and ''claudication'' of the arm or forearm. Compression of the subclavian artery in the thoracic outlet can be demonstrated by noting a decreased or absent pulse in the ipsilateral radial artery during performance of thoracic outlet maneuvers. The diagnosis can be confirmed by pulse volume recordings, duplex ultrasonography, helical computed tomography, MRI and MRA, and standard contrast angiography (24,25) (Fig. 5). All of these methods rely on demonstrating subclavian artery compression with reduced or abolished subclavian artery blood flow occurring with the arm in the hyperabducted position. Contrast angiography is required before surgical therapy to define the arterial circulation proximal and distal to the compressed arterial segment.

Extracranial Arterial Disease

Carotid artery disease has a wide spectrum of clinical presentations ranging from the asymptomatic cervical bruit to cerebrovascular accident. The prevalence of significant in-

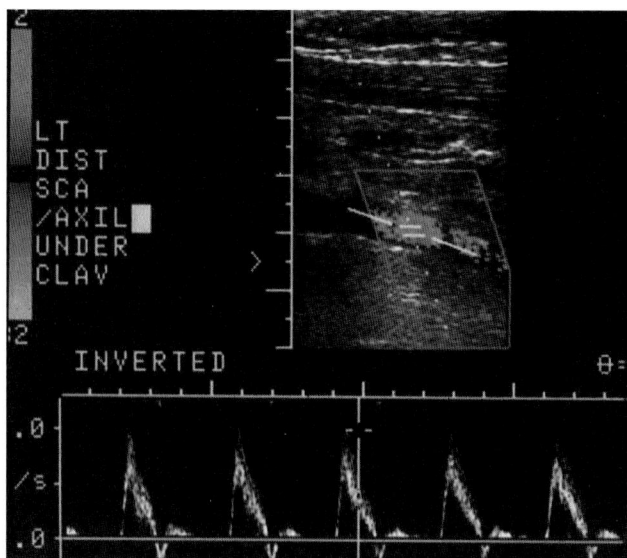

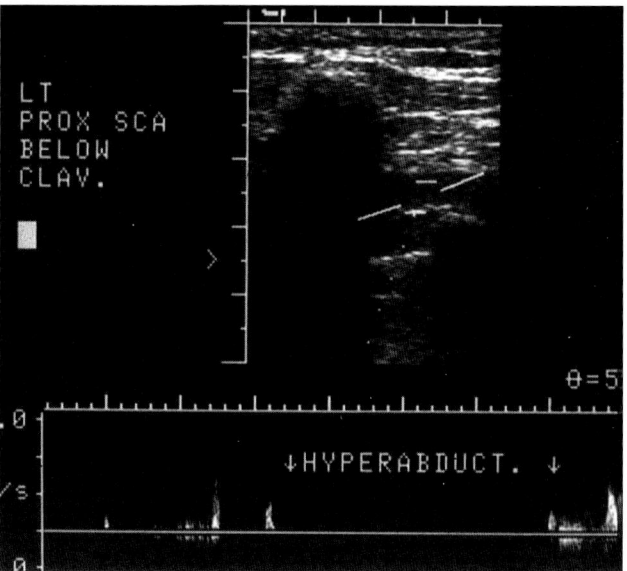

FIG. 5. Duplex ultrasound examination in a patient with suspected thoracic outlet syndrome demonstrates normal triphasic flow in the left subclavian artery with the arm in the neutral position (**A**) and cessation of subclavian artery flow with hyperabduction of the left arm (**B**), consistent with dynamic occlusion of the subclavian artery.

ternal carotid artery stenosis is related to patient age, gender, and traditional cardiovascular risk factors such as hypertension, hyperlipidemia, and tobacco use. An asymptomatic carotid bruit is present in 10% of elderly persons. Transient ischemic attack (TIA) refers to focal neurologic symptoms that last less than 24 hours. The episodes are rapid in onset and occur spontaneously. Patients remain conscious during the attack and are normal between attacks. Clinical features of a TIA in a carotid artery territory that may occur singly or in combination include mono- or hemiparesis, unilateral numbness, unilateral impairment of vision, aphasia (when the dominant hemisphere is involved), a carotid bruit, and retinal findings (cholesterol emboli). Features of a TIA in the vertebrobasilar system include paresis of 1, 2, or 4 limbs, "drop attacks," numbness of the limbs and face, diplopia or bilateral visual field defects, vertigo, nausea, dysarthria, and/or ataxia.

The presence of significant carotid artery stenosis has been causally related to the subsequent development of cerebrovascular events. Data from two large randomized trials in North America, the North American Symptomatic Carotid Endarterectomy Trial (NASCET) and the Asymptomatic Carotid Artery Stenosis (ACAS) trial have demonstrated the efficacy of carotid endarterectomy in preventing future stroke and death in both symptomatic and asymptomatic patients with a high degree of stenosis in the common carotid artery and have emphasized the importance of screening tests to be accurate in the diagnosis of significant carotid occlusive disease (26,27). Guidelines for carotid endarterectomy have been clarified by these and other randomized studies published during the past 5 years (28).

Noninvasive Tests

Noninvasive screening of patients for the presence of a hemodynamically significant carotid stenosis was developed in response to the availability of an effective treatment for symptomatic high-grade stenosis (carotid endarterectomy) and the small yet nonnegligible risk of stroke with carotid angiography.

Oculoplethysmography

Oculoplethysmography (OPG) is an indirect test of occlusive disease of the extracranial arteries. OPG detects the hemodynamic effect of a significant carotid artery stenosis as a decrease in the arterial pulse pressure wave that reaches the ipsilateral ocular globe. In the OPG method most commonly employed (OPG-Gee), a negative pressure of 300 mm Hg is applied to suction cups placed on both ocular globes. The negative pressure occludes blood flow through the retina from the ophthalmic artery. Increasing the negative pressure within the suction cup leads to a loss in the pulse transmitted to the ocular globe. The negative pressure is then slowly released, and the time at which arterial pulsations reappear in the eye is measured. A significant (>75% stenosis) of the common, internal, or ophthalmic artery will result in a pressure difference in the reappearance of these pulsations. Contraindications to OPG include glaucoma and recent ophthalmologic surgery. A second OPG method (OPG-Zira) also utilizes pressure cups placed on the eyes, but only a small amount of negative pressure is applied to them (40 to 60 mm Hg). Tracings are made of the arterial waveform at both ocular globes and utilize an ear lobe as a reference point. A delay in the waveform of 5 msec is considered to be indicative of an ipsilateral pressure significant carotid stenosis. OPG is accurate in detecting those lesions that are both pressure and flow reducing. Both OPG methods are accurate in

detecting significant lumen diameter narrowing of the internal carotid artery when the stenosis exceeds 75%. Potential problems arise with both techniques in the presence of significant bilateral internal carotid artery stenoses, when disease severity is often underestimated. Furthermore, localization of the involved arterial segment(s) cannot be determined, and, therefore, the technique cannot differentiate between significant obstructive lesions within the internal carotid artery, the ophthalmic artery, the common carotid artery, or even the innominate artery.

Ultrasonography

Duplex ultrasonography has been extensively studied and validated in the evaluation of extracranial carotid artery disease and is currently the best single method of screening for carotid bifurcation disease. It can provide information about the location of disease and extent of disease, using categories that are of clinical value.

A standard imaging protocol for examining the extracranial carotid artery system is able to visualize the common carotid artery, carotid bulb, the origin of the internal and external carotid arteries, and the origin and midportion of the vertebral arteries. Initially, transverse views are obtained from the lowest portion of the neck, just superior to the clavicle, to a point 4 to 6 cm above the carotid bifurcation, near the angle of the jaw. This initial scan helps to determine the course of the carotid artery and to determine the location and extent of atherosclerotic plaque within the common and internal carotid arteries. Atherosclerotic lesions are more likely to occur near the origin of the internal carotid artery or within the carotid bulb. The transducer is then rotated longitudinally and the same arterial segments are imaged to allow measurements of the Doppler spectral velocity waveforms using pulsed-wave Doppler. Color flow Doppler is often utilized during these longitudinal images to identify regions of turbulent flow.

The normal flow patterns within the common, internal, and external carotid arteries have a typical appearance on the pulsed-wave Doppler spectral waveform. Unlike flow in peripheral arteries, the common carotid, internal carotid, and vertebral arteries have forward flow throughout the cardiac cycle. Flow reversal (flow away from the head) is uncommon and, when present, suggests the presence of significant aortic regurgitation. In the internal carotid artery, the low vascular resistance of the intracerebral branches results in a monophasic flow pattern with a smooth contour. The peak systolic velocities normally range from 60 to 100 cm/sec. The external carotid artery has a different pattern of flow due to the increased resistance of the smaller arteries supplying the neck and face. Flow is predominantly antegrade, with a smaller diastolic component. The flow pattern within the common carotid artery represents a hybrid between the internal carotid and external carotid arteries. A zone of flow separation typically occurs at the origin of the normal internal carotid artery. This is caused by the loss of normal laminar flow as the common carotid artery branches into the internal and external carotid arteries.

Occlusive atherosclerotic lesions are most commonly located at the origin of the internal carotid artery. Although atherosclerotic plaque deposition is thought to first occur within the carotid bulb, the larger diameter of this portion of the common carotid artery makes it less likely for a hemodynamically significant stenosis to develop at this site. As a stenosis in the proximal internal carotid artery increases to occupy approximately 20 to 30% of the lumen diameter, the velocity spectrum develops a broader distribution in the velocity of blood cells due to loss of the normal laminar pattern of blood flow. This is measured on the Doppler waveform as spectral broadening. As the stenosis becomes hemodynamically significant (50% lumen diameter narrowing), an elevation in the systolic velocity occurs. A peak systolic velocity greater than 125 cm/sec is recognized as a reliable indicator of significant internal carotid artery stenosis. Using spectral waveform analysis of velocity data recorded from the proximal internal carotid artery, categories of disease severity can be determined. Clinically significant stenosis of the internal carotid artery can be categorized as severe (50 to 79% narrowing) when the peak systolic velocity exceeds 125 cm/sec or extreme (80 to 99% narrowing) when the end-diastolic velocity exceeds 140 cm/second. Internal carotid artery occlusion is diagnosed when no blood flow is detected and there is often an occlusive "thump" present proximal to the occlusion. To estimate the degree of narrowing in reference to recently published prospective trials, the ratio of the peak systolic velocity at the site of the narrowing to that measured from the common carotid artery proximal to the lesion is used. For example, the ACAS study noted that in asymptomatic patients, a 60% lesion of the internal carotid artery was clinically significant. If one uses a ratio of 3.2 for the peak systolic velocity at the site of the stenosis divided by that from the common carotid artery, a sensitivity of 92% and a specificity of 86% can be achieved. This results in a positive predictive value of 93%, with an overall accuracy of 89% (29).

An important application of duplex ultrasound of the extracranial circulation is for the evaluation of patients who have undergone carotid endarterectomy. In the immediate perioperative period, if an ischemic event occurs, duplex ultrasound can readily determine patency of the surgical site. In later postoperative follow-up (i.e., 3 months or longer) duplex examinations can detect the development of myointimal hyperplasia and the development of new atherosclerotic plaques.

Limitations of duplex ultrasonography in carotid occlusive disease are particularly evident with two types of lesions, ulcerated plaques and subtotal occlusions of the internal carotid artery. The sensitivity of carotid ultrasound in detecting ulcerated plaque is approximately 40%, compared to angiography with a sensitivity estimated at between 60 and 70%. Detection of ulcerated plaque is important as these lesions serve as a source of embolic stroke and may not be associated with significant internal carotid artery stenosis. Extremely high-grade lesions of the internal carotid artery may also be difficult to detect with ultrasonography. These lesions are associated with such a profound reduction in blood flow that the Doppler sample volume may not detect the zone of slow flow in a small residual lumen. Although the ability to detect subtotal occlusions with ultrasound is improved somewhat with low-velocity color flow Doppler imaging, a significant number of these lesions may be inappropriately classified as total occlusions. In patients with a suspected total occlusion by ultrasound, MRA or x-ray contrast angiography is usually indicated. Future developments in the use of intravenous contrast agents may improve the accuracy of duplex ultrasound in detecting ulcerated plaque and subtotal occlusion. Furthermore, overestimation of a stenosis in the internal carotid artery by duplex sonography can occur when a contralateral high-grade carotid artery stenosis or occlusion is present.

Another application of carotid ultrasonography gaining increased attention is in the detection of early atherosclerotic lesions and in following progression or regression of atherosclerotic disease. Ultrasound measurement of the thickness of the intima-media complex has been shown to be associated with early atherosclerotic change. This measurement is more accurate when performed on the far wall of the carotid artery where artifacts secondary to gain settings are less likely to obscure the interfaces. Thickening of the wall to greater than 0.6 mm in younger patients is thought to represent evidence of early atherosclerosis. An association between increased carotid intimal-medial thickness and coronary artery calcification (a marker of early atherosclerosis) and between cardiovascular risk factors and increased intimal-medial thickness in young adults has been reported (30). This finding may be of importance in determining the response of patients to aggressive risk factor modification, such as pharmacologic and lifestyle interventions (31).

Additional applications of carotid ultrasonography include evaluation of inflammatory diseases of the brachiocephalic arteries, such as Takayasu's disease and giant cell arteritis. These disorders affect the adventitia and media of the extracranial arteries manifest ultrasonographically as a diffuse thickening of the arterial wall readily perceived on high resolution real-time ultrasonography. Evaluation of a pulsatile neck mass is also a common referral diagnosis for carotid ultrasonography. True aneurysms of the carotid arteries are very rare and usually occur secondary to trauma. They are readily detected with duplex ultrasonography. In older patients, a pulsatile neck mass is most often due to increased vessel tortuosity or ectasia secondary to atherosclerosis. Other neck masses readily diagnosed with carotid ultrasonography include carotid body tumors and thyroid masses.

Evaluation of the vertebral arteries by ultrasonography is more challenging. Ultrasound assessment of these arteries is limited to visualization of short segments that are visible between the cervical vertebral lamina. The ability to evaluate vertebral flow and vessel patency is approximately 71%. The presence of antegrade flow within the vertebral artery normally guarantees against occlusion. The inability to detect flow may signify occlusion or represent a technical limitation. Furthermore, there are no diagnostic ultrasound criteria for determining severity of vertebral artery disease. A reversed pattern of vertebral artery flow suggests a pathologic process such as an ipsilateral subclavian artery stenosis. An association between this phenomenon and neurologic symptoms has been termed the subclavian steal syndrome, suggesting that blood is stolen by the ipsilateral vertebral artery from the contralateral vertebral artery by way of the basilar artery (32–34). The mechanism is as follows. The subclavian artery stenosis results in a lower pressure in the distal subclavian artery; as a result, blood flows in a retrograde direction down the ipsilateral vertebral artery away from the brain stem. Reversed vertebral artery flow, although it may have deleterious effects, serves as an important collateral artery for the arm in the setting of a significant stenosis or occlusion of the subclavian artery. The incidence of a subclavian steal appears to be much higher than the clinical syndrome. In the majority, the finding of an ''angiographic steal'' appears to be clinically insignificant and is not associated with an increased risk of vertebrobasilar ischemia (35). Symptoms of vertebrobasilar insufficiency are rare and tend to develop only when there are concurrent cerebrovascular lesions. As an example, anomalies of the circle of Willis, the most important collateral route in the cerebrovascular circulation, occur with increased frequency in patients with symptomatic subclavian steal (36).

The most common cause for a subclavian steal syndrome is atherosclerosis. Subclavian steal is more common on the left side, possibly due to a more acute origin of the subclavian artery, resulting in accelerated atherosclerosis from increased turbulence (37). Conditions other than atherosclerosis that may cause hemodynamically significant subclavian artery stenosis include Takayasu's disease, congenital isolation of the subclavian artery, chronic aortic dissection, and compression of the subclavian artery in the thoracic outlet, and certain forms of congenital heart disease. In addition, a coronary-subclavian steal phenomenon has been described in patients who have undergone prior coronary artery bypass surgery (CABG) utilizing the internal mammary artery (IMA) (38,39). When a hemodynamically significant subclavian artery stenosis is present ipsilateral to the IMA graft, flow through the internal mammary artery may reverse or ''steal'' during upper extremity exercise. Coronary and graft angiography demonstrate retrograde flow in the involved IMA during injection of the grafted coronary artery (38). Simultaneous coronary and cerebrovascular insufficiency has also been reported (39). Vertebral steal, as determined by continuous-wave Doppler, is apparent in approximately 6% of patients with asymptomatic neck bruits, but in one series, none of the patients developed symptoms during a 2-year follow-up period (40). Continuous-wave Doppler examination has shown that, even when reversed flow occurs

in the vertebral artery, antegrade basilar arterial flow persists and may even be increased (41). Duplex ultrasonography can readily diagnose and semiquantify proximal subclavian artery stenosis and demonstrate reversal of flow, if present, in the ipsilateral vertebral artery. Duplex ultrasound can also evaluate the origin of the vertebral artery for evidence of occlusive disease, as well as diagnose significant coincident extracranial carotid artery occlusive disease. When severe stenosis (>80% narrowing) of the proximal subclavian artery is present, 65% of patients have permanent flow reversal in the ipsilateral vertebral artery, and 30% have intermittent flow reversal (42). In patients with moderate subclavian artery stenosis (approximately 50% narrowing), flow reversal in the vertebral artery is permanent in 56% and intermittent in 36%.

MRA is an accurate noninvasive test in patients with suspected subclavian steal syndrome and can demonstrate proximal subclavian artery stenosis or occlusion and flow reversal in the ipsilateral vertebral artery (43). An advantage of MRA is its ability to provide detailed anatomic information regarding both the extracranial and intracranial cerebrovascular circulation. Subclavian artery stenosis and reversal of flow in the ipsilateral vertebral artery, if present, can readily be demonstrated by angiography. Concurrent intracranial atherosclerotic disease and anomalies of the circle of Willis are also identified.

Magnetic Resonance Angiography

MRA from the aortic arch to the circle of Willis may be accomplished by several different MRI techniques, including two-dimensional time-of-flight, three-dimensional time-of-flight, and contrast-enhanced MRA (44–46) (Fig. 6). Carotid MRA correlates well with duplex ultrasound and expands the anatomic information obtained, and it identifies tandem lesions from the aortic arch to the circle of Willis that can affect surgical management. As a result of time constraints, only the cervical carotid artery is usually studied. A full study of the brain, intracranial vessels, bifurcation, and aortic arch requires that the patient spend more than 1 hour in the magnet. Technical factors that may affect MRA are excessive patient motion and the presence of ferromagnetic metal in the neck. Furthermore, special care should be taken to avoid overestimation of stenosis severity in an area of turbulent flow (47).

Prospective studies comparing MRA and contrast angiography for the evaluation of carotid bifurcation disease have demonstrated a median sensitivity for a high-grade lesion of 93% and a median specificity of 88% (48). When surgical specimens, rather than contrast angiography, are used as the gold standard, duplex sonography and MRA correlate better with the endarterectomy specimen than does contrast angiography (49).

A combined noninvasive evaluation of the patient with suspected carotid artery stenosis should begin with duplex sonography. MRA is indicated in patients with technically

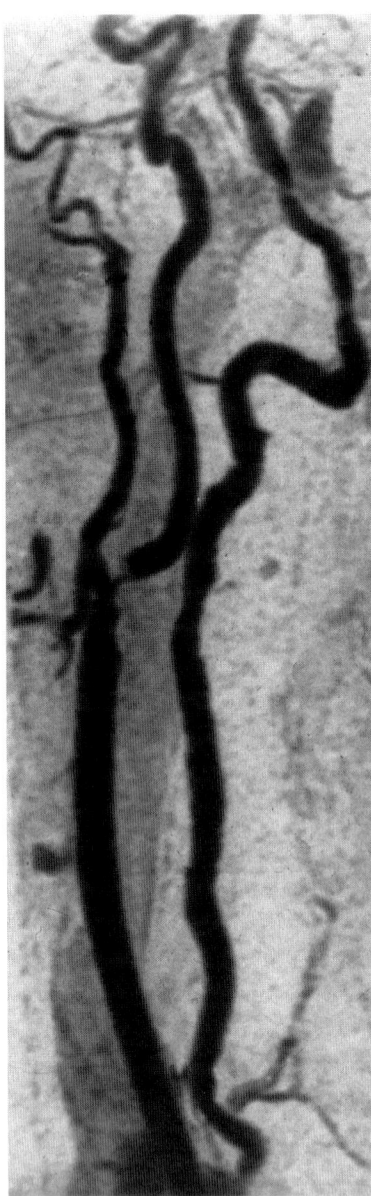

FIG. 6. Gadolinium bolus magnetic resonance angiography of the extracranial arteries shows circumferential plaque at the origin of the right internal carotid artery resulting in a high-grade stenosis (>75%). There was high velocity signal loss on the time-of-flight images.

limited ultrasound examinations, such as acoustic shadowing by a calcified plaque, a deep course of the internal carotid artery, discordant gray-scale and Doppler measurements, as well as in those patients with evidence of tandem lesions. Patients with atypical symptoms of cerebral ischemia in whom ultrasonography shows insignificant disease should also probably be considered for MRA. Carotid angiography should be considered when the results of duplex ultrasonography and MRA are discordant and in cases of possible extreme stenosis (angiographic string sign). Helical computed tomography is also a safe, noninvasive technique that precisely measures carotid artery area reduction and highly correlates to conventional arteriography (50). The precise role for helical computed tomography in the evaluation of patients with carotid artery disease requires further study.

X-ray contrast cerebral angiography is generally reserved for patients with equivocal noninvasive findings, as in preoperative evaluation, and for patients with questionable intracerebral vascular disease. The aim of angiography is to define the severity of carotid artery disease. Noninvasive studies may not be able to distinguish between very tight stenosis and occlusion, the treatment of the two being markedly different. Angiography may also be important for studying the intracerebral vasculature to ensure that repair of extracranial disease is likely to be beneficial. Angiography is also important in the assessment of aneurysms in defining their location and relationship to major arteries. Although cerebral angiography as a diagnostic modality is less useful than it was prior to the availability of computed tomography and MRA, angiographic treatment is increasing in importance, in the form of angioplasty of the carotid, vertebral, and subclavian arteries, as well as transcatheter ablation of aneurysms and vascular malformations.

REFERENCES

1. Legemate DA, Teeuwen C, Hoeneveld H, et al. The potential of duplex scanning to replace aortoiliac and femoropopliteal angiography. *Eur J Vasc Surg* 1989;3:49–54.
2. Moneta GL, Yeager RA, Antonovic R, et al. Accuracy of lower extremity arterial duplex mapping. *J Vasc Surg* 1992;15:275–284.
3. Jager KA, Ricketts HJ, Strandness DE Jr. Duplex scanning for the evaluation of lower limb arterial disease. In: Bernstein EF, ed. *Noninvasive diagnostic techniques in vascular disease,* 3rd ed. St. Louis: Mosby, 1985.
4. Edwards JM, Coldwell DM, Goldman ML, et al. The role of duplex scanning in the selection of patients for transluminal angioplasty. *J Vasc Surg* 1991;13:69–74.
5. Mattos MA, van Bemmelen PS, Hodgson KJ, et al. Does correction of stenoses identified by color duplex scanning improve infrainguinal graft patency? *J Vasc Surg* 1993;17:54–66.
6. Bandyk DF, Schmitt DD, Seabrook GR, et al. Monitoring functional patency of in-situ saphenous vein bypasses: the impact of a surveillance protocol and elective revision. *J Vasc Surg* 1989;9:286–296.
7. Idu MM, Blankenstein JD, de Gier P, et al. Impact of color-flow duplex surveillance program on infrainguinal vein graft patency. *J Vasc Surg* 1993;17:42–53.
8. Owen RS, Carpenter JP, Baum RA, et al. Magnetic resonance imaging of angiographically occult runoff vessels in peripheral arterial occlusive disease. *N Engl J Med* 1992;326:1577–1581.
9. Baum RA, Rutter CM, Sunshine JH, et al. Multicenter trial to evaluate vascular magnetic resonance angiography of the lower extremity. *JAMA* 1995;274:875–880.
10. Hoch JR, Kennell TW, Hollister MS, et al. Comparison of treatment plans for lower extremity arterial occlusive disease made with electrocardiographically-triggered two-dimensional time-of-flight magnetic resonance angiography and digital subtraction angiography. *Am J Surg* 1999;178:166–172.
11. Caputo GR, Masui T, Gooding GAW, et al. Popliteal and tibioperoneal arteries: feasibility of two-dimensional time-of-flight MR angiography and phase velocity mapping. *Radiology* 1992;182:387–392.
12. Lossef SV, Rajan SS, Patt RJ, et al. Gadolinium-enhanced magnitude contrast MR angiography of popliteal and tibial arteries. *Radiology* 1992;184:349–355.
13. Link J, Steffens JC, Brossmann J, et al. Iliofemoral arterial occlusive disease: contrast-enhanced MR angiography for pre-interventional evaluation and follow-up after stent placement. *Radiology* 1999;212:371–377.

14. Nasser TK, Mohler ER, Wilensky RL, et al. Peripheral vascular complications following coronary interventional procedures. *Clin Cardiol* 1995;18:609–614.
15. Agrawal SK, Pinheiro L, Roubin GS, et al. Nonsurgical closure of femoral pseudoaneurysms complicating cardiac catheterization and percutaneous transluminal coronary angioplasty. *J Am Coll Cardiol* 1992;20:610–615.
16. Pompa JJ, Satler LF, Pichard AD, et al. Vascular complications after balloon and new device angioplasty. *Circulation* 1993;88:1569–1576.
17. Feld R, Patton G, Carabasi RA, et al. Treatment of iatrogenic femoral artery injuries with ultrasound-guided compression. *J Vasc Surg* 1992; 16:832–840.
18. di Mrazo L, Cavallaro A, Sciacca V, et al. Surgical treatment of popliteal artery entrapment syndrome: a ten year experience. *Eur J Vasc Surg* 1991;5:59–64.
19. Akkersdijk WL, de Ruyter JW, Lapham R, et al. Colour duplex ultrasonographic and provocation of popliteal artery compression. *Eur J Vasc Endovasc Surg* 1995;10:342–345.
20. Rizzo RJ, Flinn WR, Yao JST, et al. Computed tomography for evaluation of arterial disease in the popliteal fossa. *J Vasc Surg* 1990;11:112–119.
21. Fujiwara H, Sugano T, Fujii N. Popliteal artery entrapment syndrome: accurate morphological diagnosis utilizing MRI. *J Cardiovasc Surg* 1992;33:160–162.
22. Turnipseed WD, Pozniak M. Popliteal entrapment as a result of neurovascular compression by the soleus and plantaris muscles. *J Vasc Surg* 1992;15:285–294.
23. Levien LJ, Veller MG. Popliteal artery entrapment syndrome: more common than previously recognized. *J Vasc Surg* 1999;30:587–598.
24. Matsumura JS, Rilling WS, Pearce WH, et al. Helical computed tomography of the normal thoracic outlet. *J Vasc Surg* 1999;26:776–783.
25. Dymarkowski S, Bosmans H, Marchal G, et al. Three-dimensional MR angiography in the evaluation of thoracic outlet syndrome. *Am J Roentgenol* 1999;173:1005–1008.
26. North American Symptomatic Carotid Endarterectomy Trial Collaborators. Beneficial effect of carotid endaraterectomy in symptomatic patients with high-grade carotid stenosis. *N Engl J Med* 1991;325:445–453.
27. Executive Committee for the Asymptomatic Carotid Atherosclerosis Study. Endarterectomy for asymptomatic carotid artery stenosis. *JAMA* 1995;273:1421–1428.
28. AHA Scientific Statement: Guidelines for Carotid Endarterectomy. A statement for healthcare professionals from a special writing group of the stroke council, American Heart Association. *Circulation* 1998;97:501–509.
29. Strandness DE Jr. Noninvasive vascular laboratory and vascular imaging. In: Young JR, Olin JW, Bartholomew JE, eds. *Peripheral vascular disease*, 2nd ed. St. Louis: Mosby, 1996.
30. Davis PH, Dawson JD, Mahoney LT, et al. Increased carotid intimal-medial thickness and coronary calcification are related in young and middle-aged adults. The Muscatine Study. *Circulation* 1999;100:838–842.
31. Hodis HN, Mack WJ, LaBreel, et al. Reduction in carotid arterial wall thickness using lovastatin and dietary therapy: a randomized, controlled clinical trial. *Ann Intern Med* 1996;124:548–556.
32. Contorni L. Il circolo collaterale vertebro-vertebrale nelle obliterazione dell'arteria succlavia alla sua origine. *Minerva Chir* 1960;15:268–273.
33. Reivich M, Holling HE, Roberts B, et al. Reversal of blood flow through the vertebral artery and its effect on cerebral circulation. *N Engl J Med* 1961;265:878–886.
34. Fisher CM. A new vascular syndrome: "the subclavian steal." *N Engl J Med* 1961;265:912–917.
35. Bornstein NM, Krajewski A, Norris JW. Basilar artery blood flow in subclavian steal. *Can J Neurol Sci* 1988;15:417–422.
36. Lord RSA, Adar R, Stein RL. Contribution of the circle of Willis to the subclavian steal syndrome. *Circulation* 1969;40:871–879.
37. Kesteloot H, Houte OV. Reversed circulation through the vertebral artery. *Acta Cardiol* 1963;18:285–292.
38. Ochi M, Yamauchi S, Yajima T, et al. Simultaneous subclavian artery reconstruction in coronary artery bypass grafting. *Ann Thorac Surg* 1997;5:1284–1287.
39. Takach TJ, Beggs ML, Nykamp VJ, et al. Concomitant cerebral and coronary subclavian steal. *Ann Thorac Surg* 1997;3:853–854.
40. Nguyen NH, Reeves F, Therasse E, et al. Percutaneous transluminal angioplasty in coronary-internal thoracic-subclavian steal syndrome. *Can J Cardiol* 1997;13:285–289.
41. Borstein NM, Norris JW. Subclavian steal: a harmless hemodynamic phenomenon. *Lancet* 1986;2:303–308.
42. Hennerici M, Klemm C, Rautenberg W. The subclavian steal phenomenon: a common vascular disorder with rare neurologic deficits. *Neurology* 1988;38:669–673.
43. Carriero A, Salute L, Tartaro A, et al. The role of magnetic resonance angiography in the diagnosis of subclavian steal. *Cardiovasc Intervent Radiol* 1995;18:87–91.
44. Keller PJ, Drayer BP, Fram EK, et al. MR angiography with two-dimensional acquisition and three-dimensional display: work in progress. *Radiology* 1989;173:527–532.
45. Masaryk TJ, Modic MT, Ruggieri PM, et al. Three-dimensional (volume) gradient echo imaging of the carotid bifurcation: preliminary clinical experience. *Radiology* 1989;171:801–806.
46. Cloft HJ, Murphy KJ, Prince MR, et al. 3D gadolinium-enhanced MR angiography of the carotid arteries. *Magn Reson Imaging* 1996;14:593–600.
47. Yucel EK, Anderson CM, Edelman RR, et al. Magnetic resonance angiography: update of applications for extracranial arteries. *Circulation* 1999;100:2284–2301.
48. Pan XM, Saloner D, Reilly LM, et al. Assessment of carotid artery stenosis by ultrasonography, conventional angiography, and magnetic resonance angiography: correlation with ex vivo measurement of plaque stenosis. *J Vasc Surg* 1995;21:82–88.
49. Urchuk SN, Plewes DB. Mechanisms of flow-induced signal loss in MR angiography. *J Magn Reson Imaging* 1992;2:453–462.
50. Cinat ME, Pham H, Vo D, et al. Improved imaging of carotid artery bifurcation using helical computed tomographic angiography. *Ann Vasc Surg* 1999;13:178–183.

CHAPTER 60

Imaging Techniques in Cerebrovascular Disorders

Camilo R. Gomez and Marco A. Zenteno

Cerebrovascular disorders (i.e., stroke) continue to be the third cause of death in the United States and the most important cause of disability of adults. The last decade has brought with it significant progress in the diagnosis and treatment of cerebrovascular disorders. Advances in imaging technology have played a key role in some of the progress made, facilitating the identification, classification, and documentation of the different clinical entities that represent the subject of study by physicians involved in this field. In fact, as we approach the turn of the century, the subspecialty of vascular neurology is becoming recognized, and specialized training in this growing field of clinical medicine is being offered at many centers of excellence. Imaging, more specifically neuroimaging, is an integral part of both the training and practice of this specialty, with many of the specialists in vascular neurology also spending a considerable portion of their time in the application of imaging techniques for the diagnosis and treatment of their patients.

The importance of neuroimaging parallels both historically and practically that of imaging in cardiovascular medicine. The utilization by cardiac specialists of echocardiography, nuclear cardiac imaging, magnetic resonance imaging (MRI), and angiography has been trailed by similar use of comparable imaging techniques by neurologists. The present chapter will address the most important concepts about imaging in cerebrovascular disorders. We will explore the rules that guide the selection of appropriate imaging modalities for specific clinical scenarios. We will also discuss the most important characteristics of the techniques with greatest practical value, pointing out their advantages and disadvantages.

C. R. Gomez: Department of Neurology, Comprehensive Stroke Center, University of Alabama at Birmingham, Birmingham, Alabama 35294.

M. A. Zenteno: Department of Radiology, Neuroimaging Service, Instituto Nacional de Neurologia y Neurocirugia, DF CP 10700 Mexico City, Mexico.

PURPOSE OF IMAGING: TASK-ORIENTED CHOICES

The most practical approach to a discussion of the application of imaging techniques in cerebrovascular disorders is to first address the tasks, diagnostic or therapeutic, that require the utilization of imaging. It is only this type of approach that will allow the issuing of guidelines for choosing the appropriate technique for each clinical situation. From this perspective, the clinical scenarios in which imaging techniques are likely to be needed must be assessed along the following lines: (1) what information is being sought, and how quickly is it needed? (2) which of the available imaging techniques is most likely to answer the question being asked? and (3) how will the information obtained by imaging impact further diagnostic algorithms, the treatment, and the prognosis of the patient? Based on these considerations, the following tasks require the utilization of imaging during clinical care of cerebrovascular patients.

Imaging of the Brain

Direct imaging of the brain is necessary in order to assess the status of the tissue, often documenting the damage caused by the stroke, and also to differentiate between ischemic and hemorrhagic strokes. The techniques available to complete this task include x-ray computed tomography (CT) and MRI. As discussed below, choosing between one and another involves considerations of speed, sensitivity, type of stroke, and temporal profile of the event.

Imaging of the Brain Vessels

Imaging of the brain blood vessels is part of the standard risk stratification algorithm that every stroke patient must undergo. As such, documentation of vascular abnormalities causally associated to the stroke allows not only determination of the level of risk for subsequent stroke, but helps plan preventive therapy. In general, the tests that are available for the completion of this task are divided into two groups: (1) those that are noninvasive (currently encompassing ultrasonic and magnetic-based techniques), and (2) one that is invasive: catheterization and angiography. In addition to its diagnostic capabilities, the latter also allows the application of endovascular therapeutic techniques.

Documentation of the Ischemic Process

Although, as we noted earlier, documentation of the ischemic injury to tissue can be accomplished using CT and MRI, the possibility of visually demonstrating ischemic-yet-not-damaged tissue is gaining increasing popularity. At first, radionuclide-based imaging techniques such as single-photon emission computed tomography (SPECT) and positron emission tomography (PET) were the most studied methods for functional imaging of the brain. Then, a combination of radionuclide and radiographic techniques (i.e., xenon CT) was introduced as a more practical tool for the assessment of emergency stroke situations. More recently, the use of more sophisticated magnetic-based techniques (diffusion- and perfusion-weighted MRI) promises to assist in the identification of ischemic tissue that may be salvageable, possibly having a role in the selection of patients for specific types of therapy.

Documentation of Cardiac Sources of Embolism

Although this section is not on imaging of the brain, it is an important aspect of the application of imaging to the care of the neurologic patient. The last decade has shown how cardiogenic embolism is more frequent than was once suspected (1). The introduction and development of transesophageal echocardiography (TEE) represented a major advance in the identification of cardiac sources of cerebral embolism, and changed how stroke patients are typically evaluated (2–4). However, the reader is referred to the chapters on echocardiography and MRI as the methods of choice for defining the source of cardioembolic strokes.

SCENARIOS OF IMAGING: DIMENSIONS OF PRACTICE

The tasks noted above must also be placed in the practical context of two distinct clinical scenarios: (1) the emergency care of a stroke victim, and (2) the nonemergent risk stratification of patients with cerebrovascular disorders. Depending upon the scenario, the choice of imaging technique is then guided by the question being asked, the diagnostic characteristics inherent to each imaging modality, and the expectations of results based upon the natural history of the process being investigated.

Emergency Imaging of Stroke Victims

The majority of patients with acute stroke are initially evaluated in emergency departments by physicians whose priorities include answering specific questions with direct relevance to the management of the patient, both immediate and within the days that follow. The first set of clinical questions confronted by stroke specialists is:

• Does the patient have a stroke?
• Is it an ischemic or a hemorrhagic stroke?
• What vascular territory has been compromised?
• What is the risk of death or significant neurologic disability?
• What is the likelihood of neurologic deterioration?

Once the first question is answered, and the presumptive diagnosis of stroke is made, imaging of the brain becomes essential. It is important to know if: (1) the event is ischemic or hemorrhagic; (2) the brain has already undergone damage; and (3) there is any alternative diagnostic possibility. In the past, it was thought that astute clinicians could easily differentiate between hemorrhagic and ischemic stroke at the bedside. The introduction of x-ray CT in the 1970s, however, clearly showed the inaccuracies of clinical differentiation, while it provided an easy method for making this diagnostic distinction. In fact, at present, emergency CT imaging is of paramount importance in the early evaluation of patients with acute stroke, as well as a pivoting point in any emergency stroke treatment algorithm (5). New technologic advances, including helical CT scanning and 3D reconstruction add to the ability of this test to be used in emergency situations.

Imaging and Risk Stratification Algorithms

The diagnostic perspective of patients with cerebrovascular disorders revolves around defining the ''stroke subtype'' (i.e., identifying the cause and mechanism of the stroke) (1). This leads to a somewhat educated prediction of the risk of subsequent strokes, while it allows the implementation of secondary prevention strategies tailored to the individual patient. In this context, the importance of imaging techniques cannot be overemphasized. Three categories of disorders are capable of leading to the production of stroke: cardiac abnormalities, cerebrovascular abnormalities per se, and hematologic disorders. Cardiac imaging will be addressed elsewhere in the book. Vascular imaging includes all techniques designed to display the cerebral vessels and their abnormalities.

COMPUTED TOMOGRAPHY: THE BEGINNING OF CONTEMPORARY NEUROIMAGING

Every discussion about imaging techniques in cerebrovascular disorders must begin with CT. The introduction of CT in the 1970s changed the way all neurologic diseases are diagnosed and treated. Suddenly, it was possible to directly look at the brain tissue and document the damage caused both by cerebral infarction and cerebral hemorrhage. Furthermore, CT allowed a rapid differentiation between these two main types of stroke and has ultimately provided the avenue for the application of aggressive treatment strategies, such as thrombolysis.

The usefulness of CT for the evaluation of cerebrovascular disorders is primarily related to the emergency assessment of acute patients. It is in this context that the technique allows the determination of hemorrhagic changes and the identification of early signs of ischemic tissue damage. Most recently, it has become a determining factor for the selection of patients for specific types of treatment (e.g., thrombolysis). The CT findings in patients with acute stroke can be divided into six categories:

1. *Normal brain tissue.* A large number of patients presenting early with acute or hyperacute ischemic brain processes have normal CT scans. This results from the low sensitivity of the test for the detection of ischemic tissue within the first few hours of evolution. A normal CT scan in the context of a patient with an acute focal neuro-

logic deficit by no means excludes the diagnosis of ischemic stroke and, in fact, should be considered a good sign. Indeed, the fact that the tissue is not shown as irreparably damaged should open numerous possibilities for therapeutic intervention. Clearly, for patients suspected of having hemorrhagic stroke, a normal CT scan almost completely excludes the diagnosis.

2. *Abnormal, demonstrating the acute stroke.* The appearance of infarction on CT during the first few hours largely depends upon the size and location of the effected tissue (Fig. 1) (6). Large territories supplied by the carotid artery system (e.g., middle cerebral artery) have a tendency to be displayed earlier than smaller territories supplied by the vertebrobasilar system (e.g., penetrating pontine arteries). The early signs of infarction include changes of gray matter density with loss of gray-white matter differentiation, evolving into frank hypodensity and early signs of edema over the next 12–24 hours (Fig. 1). Hemorrhagic strokes are displayed as hyperdense areas corresponding to the extravasated blood, for which CT is highly sensitive.

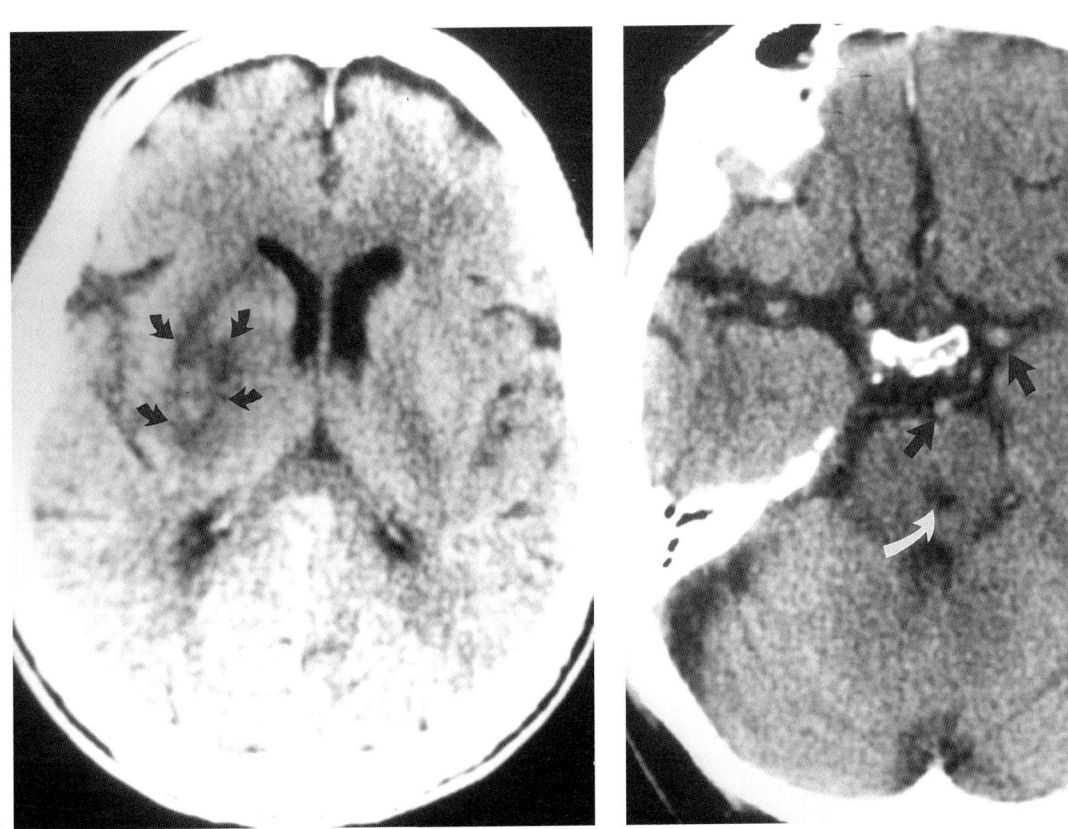

A   B

FIG. 1. A: Computed tomography (CT) of a patient with a left hemiparesis of a few hours of evolution. It is possible to see infarction of the right lenticulostriate territory (*black arrows*) with questionable hemorrhagic transformation in its center. This type of stroke is most commonly due to embolic occlusion of the middle cerebral artery, with subsequent recanalization and distal migration of the embolic material. **B:** Sometimes the CT does not show the lesion responsible for the patient's presentation, but shows associated relevant findings. For example, it may disclose old infarctions (*white arrow*), which often have been undetected. Also, relative hyperdensity of the basal arteries (*black arrows*) has been associated with atherosclerotic lesions or occlusion. *(continued)*

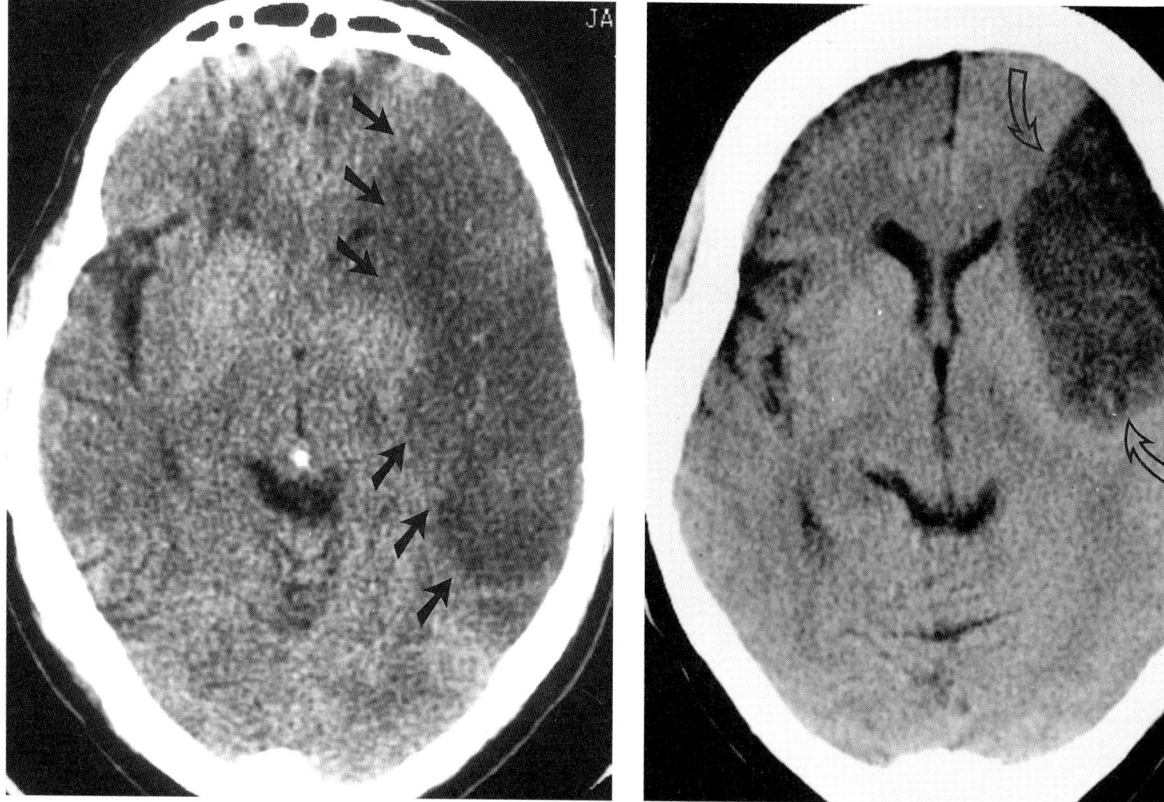

FIG. 1. *Continued.* **C:** One of the advantages of CT is that it facilitates the follow-up of patients destined to deteriorate and to require intensive therapy. The typical finding of a large hemispheric infarction (*black arrows*) during the first 24 to 36 hours is a sign of evolving edema with significant potential for secondary injury due to intracranial hypertension. **D:** Once the tissue is damaged, it acquires a well-demarcated and very hypodense appearance on CT (*black arrows*).

3. *Abnormal, with findings related to the acute stroke.* Frequently, CT scans show abnormalities that bear a relationship with the ischemic stroke. For example, in patients with occlusion of the middle cerebral artery, the "hyperdense MCA" sign has been described. This exemplifies the appearance of a vessel acutely occluded by a thrombus as a hyperdense structure within the Sylvian fissure. Also, a more common finding is that of calcification of the brain arteries (e.g., carotid or vertebral), implying the presence of atherosclerotic plaques that are capable of causing narrowing of these vessels (Fig. 1). For patients with hemorrhagic strokes, it is possible sometimes to identify an aneurysm by its calcification and location.

4. *Abnormal, displaying previous strokes.* Often, patients who present with acute stroke are found to have abnormal CT scans that demonstrate preexisting strokes (Fig. 1). These represent the evidence of cerebrovascular abnormalities, either intrinsic or secondary to other processes, and they can help in the diagnosis. For example, evidence of infarctions in multiple bilateral territories may represent evidence of a cardiogenic or aortogenic source of embolism. On the other hand, previous infarctions clustered within one hemisphere may represent the effect of unilateral severe carotid stenosis.

5. *Abnormal, displaying an alternative diagnostic process.* Some patients who present with a clinical syndrome suggestive of stroke might have an alternative diagnostic process. CT is helpful in uncovering such conditions that mimic stroke and require alternative treatment (e.g., subdural hematoma).

6. *Abnormal, a combination of the above.*

The routine utilization of radiopaque contrast medium during CT examination of the emergency stroke patient is unwarranted in our opinion. The potential enhancement of any of the tissue in patients with acute ischemia serves no clinical purpose because it does not help guide treatment. Furthermore, there is at least some suggestion in the literature that contrast media are somewhat neurotoxic to ischemic tissue. For the patient with hemorrhagic stroke, it adds even less. Furthermore, in certain clinical scenarios, it is dangerous. The intense nausea that can be produced by intravenous contrast administration, in fact, can jeopardize the outcome of patients with ruptured aneurysms.

As time elapses, the appearance of the two major forms of stroke on CT scanning changes. Infarcted tissue develops swelling and its margins become progressively demarcated. Its density decreases as the damaged tissue shrinks, producing *ex vacuo* enlargement of adjacent structures (i.e., ventricles).

Another practical aspect of CT in the management of patients with cerebrovascular disorders is the ease with which it allows follow-up imaging in patients who evolve, either positively or negatively. An example of the former is the resolution of hydrocephalus in a patient who requires a ventriculostomy following an intraventricular hemorrhage. On the other hand, the latter is best exemplified by the follow-up of a patient with malignant brain edema secondary to a large hemispheric infarction.

CT Angiography

CT angiography is a relatively new noninvasive technique that couples helical CT scanning with contrast enhancement to obtain vascular images. It is performed by first obtaining a series of axial images. These are then reconstructed into three-dimensional angiographic images. The development of this technique required the introduction of a scanner that allowed the patients to be translated through a continuously rotating gantry, with very rapid data acquisition. The operator controls several variables that determine the protocol to be utilized for each region of interest to be imaged, including duration of the scan, speed of movement of the table, and collimation. Several recount studies have compared CT angiography with conventional angiography, finding agreement of 80–95% between the two techniques, when studying extracranial carotid atherosclerotic stenotic plaques. As with any other technique, CT angiography has advantages and disadvantages (7,8). It is not susceptible to flow perturbations and complex flow patterns like MRI. On the other hand, it utilizes ionizing radiation and iodinated radiopaque contrast medium administration, which limit is use in patients with azotemia and contrast allergy.

MAGNETIC RESONANCE IMAGING: VERSATILITY IN ACTION

The utilization of MRI in clinical medicine became widespread during the 1980s. The increased sensitivity of this technique, as compared with CT, for the detection of abnormalities in brain structure made it an immediate candidate for the imaging modality of choice to demonstrate infarction of the brain parenchyma. With time, MRI has allowed the demonstration of ischemic brain lesions earlier and more precisely, particularly in regions that had remained relatively unavailable to previous imaging modalities, such as the brain stem. More recently, new MRI pulse sequences have resulted in the ability to image the cerebral vasculature, the degree of ischemia, and the viability of the tissue.

The detection of abnormalities in patients with acute stroke, using MRI, depends upon both alteration of flow within the vessels, and on the changes induced by the disease process upon the parenchyma. Alterations of flow, when present, can be detected immediately. Normally, high velocity flow generally associated with turbulence is displayed as a "flow-void" on conventional MRI sequences. This is easily seen both in T2- and T1-weighted images. On the other hand, increased MR signal implies slowed or stagnant flow within the vessel. In fact, arterial "enhancement" has been described among the MRI findings of patients with acute ischemic stroke as a sign of vascular occlusion or flow stagnation.

Parenchymal abnormalities in patients with ischemic stroke responds to the accumulation of water or edema within the ischemic cells as a result of all membrane incompetence, later due to breakdown of the blood–brain barrier (BBB). Increased tissue signal on T2-weighted, proton density, and fast low-angled inversion recovery (FLAIR) images, as well as a less pronounced drop in signal, accompany this pathophysiologic process on T1-weighted imaging (Fig. 2). As opposed to the flow-related findings noted earlier, the parenchymal changes evolve over a period of hours to days. As time goes by, the changes observed on MRI give way to a picture most representative of encephalomalacia, necrosis, and gliosis (Fig. 2). Thus, in the chronic stages, infarcted tissue appears as an area of high intensity on T2-weighted images, low intensity on T1-weighted images, and moderate intensity on proton density imaging.

The MRI appearance of hemorrhagic stroke is even more complex because it largely depends upon the natural evolution of hemoglobin degradation within the tissue and the strength of the magnetic field. Typically, the sequence of conversion from oxyhemoglobin to deoxyhemoglobin (first intracellular and then extracellular, as the erythrocytes disappear), and then from deoxyhemoglobin to methemoglobin and, finally, to hemosiderin, occurs as part of a continuum over weeks to months. Acute hemorrhage varies from isointense to slightly hypointense on T1-weighted images and from isointense (low field strength) to markedly hypointense on T2-weighted images. These findings represent the presence of intracellular deoxyhemoglobin. As the erythrocytes undergo lysis, extracellular deoxyhemoglobin is converted to aqueous methemoglobin, and a peripheral ring of hyperintensity develops first on T1-weighted images and later on T2-weighted images. Then, the center of the lesion progressively becomes hyperintense due to subsequent oxidation. Finally, the rim becomes extremely hypointense on T2-weighted images due to the deposit of hemosiderin.

Diffusion-weighted MRI

Ischemia of brain tissue results in inhibition of oxidative phosphorylation due to impaired oxygen delivery to tissue. For energy production, brain cells must resort to anaerobic glycolysis, less efficient for energy production. These changes lead to impaired function of the Na-K ATPase system in the cell membrane with resultant accumulation of intracellular sodium. The more labile high-energy phos-

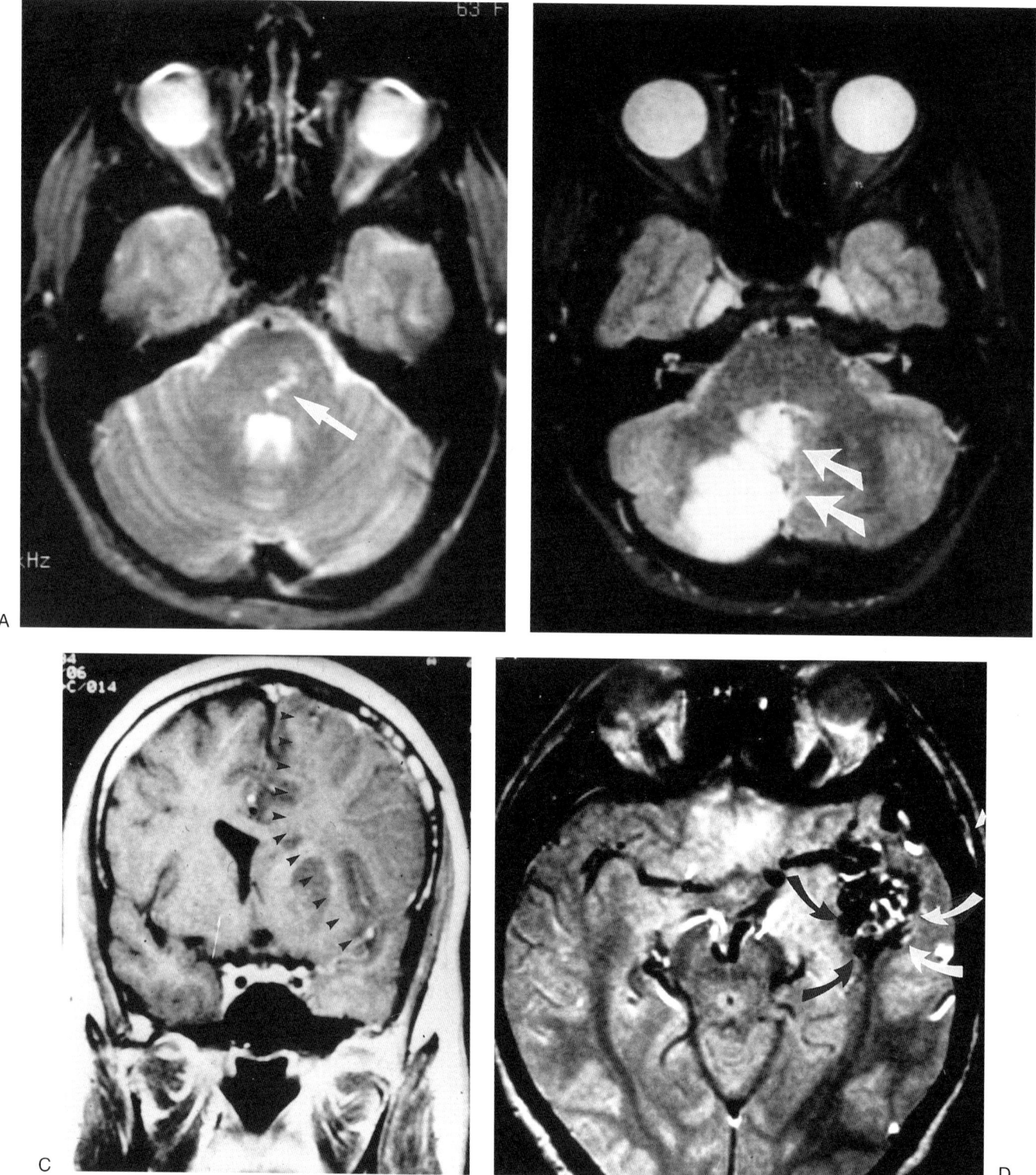

FIG. 2. A: Magnetic resonance imaging (MRI) is more sensitive than computed tomography, particularly for the detection of small infarcts in the brain stem (*white arrow*). The example is a T2-weighted axial image of a patient with a small lacunar infarct in the pons (*white arrow*). **B:** Larger infarcts can also be detected easily using T2-weighted imaging (*white arrows*). The advantage of MRI is that it helps to precisely define the vessel affected by the process, a critical step in the planning of therapy. **C:** Although T2-weighted imaging is very sensitive for detection of vascular lesions, T1-weighted imaging can also display the extent of the damage, particularly in large infarcts (*arrowheads*). **D:** In addition, MRI can detect other specific vascular lesions, such as arteriovenous malformations (*arrows*), which are displayed as a convolution of vessels with a "flow-void" due to the rapid blood flow through them.

phates are resultant with accumulation of inorganic phosphate and lactic acid within the tissue. The reduced osmotic gradient created by the accumulation of intracellular sodium results in the influx of water into the cells with the production of cytotoxic edema.

Signal intensity on diffusion-weighted MRI (DW-MRI) is related to the random microscopic motion of water protons (brownian motion), whereas conventional MRI sequences depend upon the accumulation of water within the tissue. It is thus possible to detect slower proton motion within the ischemic tissue, with lower diffusion coefficients, as early as minutes following the onset of ischemia (9). Regardless of the exact cause of these findings, it is apparent that DW-MRI findings represent the earliest sign of ischemic injury, perhaps at a stage in which the tissue can still recover. Regions of ischemia have a decreased apparent diffusion coefficient (ADC) and high signal intensity on DW-MRI, reflecting restricted proton diffusion (10–13). Further research is currently being conducted in this area and the future utilization of this technique in the algorithms for imaging cerebrovascular disorders is yet to be defined.

Perfusion-weighted MRI

The ability to induce enhancement of MRI with magnetic susceptibility agents (paramagnetic contrast agents) that facilitate T2* relaxation provides a method for assessing cerebral blood volume and tissue perfusion. These agents, dysprosium (Dy) or gadolinium (Gd) DTPA-BMA are confined to the intravascular space by the intact blood-brain barrier. A field gradient is created at the capillary level, resulting in significant signal loss in regions with normal blood flow. In contrast, nonperfused areas appear relatively hyperintense. This technique has been shown to significantly advance the time of detection of focal brain ischemia and reveal small infarctions not shown by conventional MRI sequences. In addition, ultrafast MRI techniques (i.e., echo planar or turbo FLASH) allow tracking of the passage of contrast agents through the vascular bed, using kinetic modeling of regional blood flow and volume.

MR Spectroscopy

Clinical spectroscopy has been the best studied of all the magnetic resonance techniques. Cerebral ischemia leads to a decrease in phosphocreatine (PC) to a fall in PCr/ATP and to an increase in inorganic phosphate (P) using ^{31}P spectroscopy. A shift in the position of the inorganic phosphate peak indicates a change in intracellular pH. The acidosis associated with ischemia induces a shift in P, detectable by spectroscopy. With the development of better techniques for spectral editing and localization, it will be possible to generate spectra from ischemic infarcted or normal tissue. This technique may be most useful in the assessment of the reversibility of ischemic brain damage. Although ^{31}P spectroscopy

appears to have great clinical potential, the methodology, is not yet widely available on commercial systems.

Magnetic Resonance Angiography

The discussion of MRI only applies to spin-echo pulse sequences. These produce images in which there is "negative" visualization of the cerebral blood vessels owing to their characteristic signal-void. Although recognized early in the development of MRI, such "negative" visualization did not seem to provide a reliable means for evaluating the cerebral vasculature. The advent of fast scanning MRI pulse sequencing, particularly the gradient-echo and the bipolar flow-encoding gradient methods, has allowed direct vascular imaging, resulting in the development of magnetic resonance angiography (MRA).

Cerebrovascular MRA uses two different techniques: time-of-flight (TOF) or phase contrast (PC) angiography. The technique is based upon the phenomenon of flow-related enhancement, and can be performed with either two- or three-dimensional volume acquisitions (14). It utilizes flip angles of less than 60 degrees and no refocusing 180-degree pulse (the echo is refocused by reversing the readout gradient). This technique, also known as the gradient refocused echo (GRE) approach can use one of several methods, including "fast low-angle shot (FLASH)," free-induction steady-state precession (FISP) and "gradient-recalled acquisition study state (GRASS)." On the other hand, phase contrast angiography is based upon the detection of velocity-induced phase shifts to distinguish flowing blood from the surrounding stationary tissue. By using bipolar flow-sensitized gradients it is possible to subtract the two acquisitions of opposite polarity and no net phase (stationary tissue) from one another. The data that remain reflect the phase shift induced by flowing blood. The use of cardiac gating helps overcome the sensitivity of PC angiography to pulsatile and nonuniform flow. From this point of view, however, PC is somewhat impractical for three-dimensional imaging.

Using MRA, it is possible to study the extracranial carotid artery system and obtain reasonable information about morphologic changes and stenosis (Fig. 3) (15,16). On the other hand, with the improvement in sensitivity of ultrasonic techniques and the recent report of angiographic criteria suitable for intervention, together with the detailed visualization provided by digital subtraction angiography, MRA has become somewhat less useful for the evaluation of extracranial carotid disease (17), although it is better in vertebrobasilar insufficiency (Fig. 3) (18,19). It is in the noninvasive assessment of intracranial vascular disorders that MRA appears to have its most useful potential application because it allows the detection of stenotic lesions of first-order vessels, as well as the identification of the patterns of resultant collateral flow (7,20,21). In our center, the preliminary MRA experience in stroke patients has been encouraging particularly when complemented by other noninvasive tests (16,22,23).

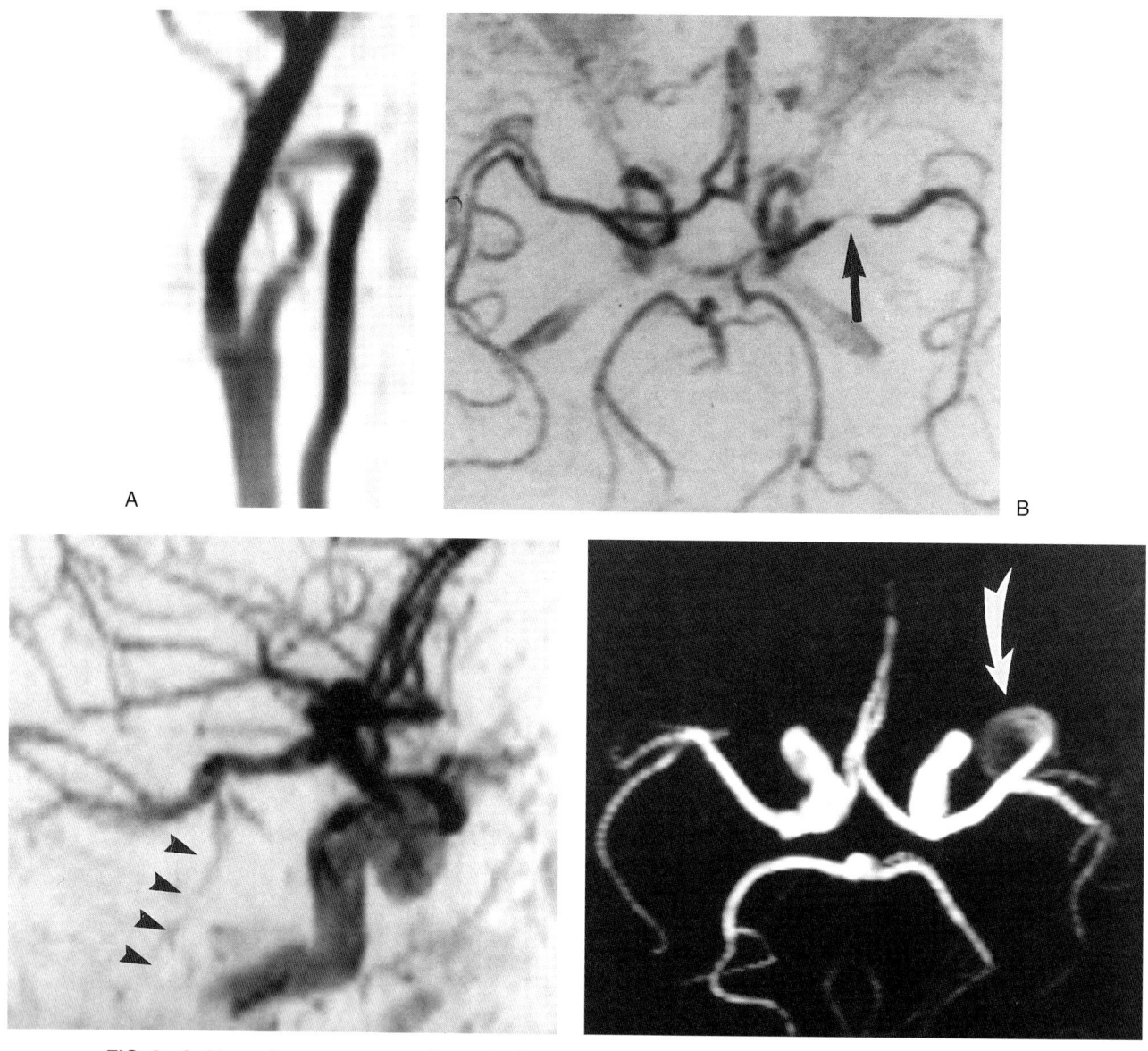

FIG. 3. A: Magnetic resonance angiography (MRA) allows visualization of the extracranial vessels with exquisite detail. It allows screening of patients with cerebral ischemia and selection of those requiring invasive diagnosis and treatment. **B:** Intracranial phase-contrast MRA assists in detecting focal stenosis of the major cerebral arteries, such as the middle cerebral artery (*arrow*). **C:** Because MRA provides more physiologic than strictly anatomic information, extracranial lesions that decrease intracranial arterial perfusion can be also identified. In this case, the conspicuous loss of signal in the vertebrobasilar system (*arrowheads*) helps diagnose slow flow in that territory, caused by proximal flow-reducing vertebral lesions. **D:** MRA can also detect other vascular anomalies, such as giant aneurysms (*white arrow*).

NEUROVASCULAR ULTRASONOGRAPHY: NONINVASIVE FLEXIBILITY

Ultrasound provides a noninvasive means to obtain diagnostic anatomic and physiologic information. Vascular ultrasonography is used to study blood vessel morphology and blood flow (24). The principles of vascular ultrasonography can be applied to the evaluation of patients with disorders of the cerebral circulation.

In the assessment of carotid atherosclerosis, at first, Dopp-

ler techniques were utilized to document reversal of periorbital flow direction. This, at least theoretically, indicates high-grade internal carotid artery stenosis. Later, continuous-wave (CW) Doppler transducers allowed the direct study of the extracranial carotid arteries and the detection of stenoses greater than 50% by the flow acceleration they caused. Small plaques that had no hemodynamic effect, however, were commonly missed. Conversely, ultrasonic real-time B-mode imaging of the extracranial vessels was able to identify smaller carotid artery plaques but failed to provide dynamic information about flow disturbances. The sensitivity and specificity of either of the Doppler or B-mode technique were so low that they prevented their unconditional acceptance by many clinicians. In the late 1970s, the technique of real-time imaging was combined with pulsed-wave Doppler and a new, more reliable, system was introduced: duplex ultrasound. This combined the sensitivity of high resolution real-time B-mode imaging for small plaques, with the ability of pulsed-wave Doppler for assessing flow velocity characteristics at specific points within the blood vessels. The introduction of duplex ultrasound resulted in an immediate increase in the confidence with which noninvasive evaluation was considered, particularly in the outpatient setting. The technologic step that followed conventional duplex ultrasound was an imaginative, yet improbable one: color Doppler imaging (CDI). Until 1982, the use of ultrasound to study the cerebral blood vessels was limited to their extracranial segments. The sonic barrier represented by the skull was first crossed by Aaslid and his collaborators (25) when, using a low frequency (2 MHz) pulsed Doppler ultrasonic transducer, they were able to noninvasively study the hemodynamic characteristics of the basal cerebral blood vessels. This marked the introduction of transcranial Doppler (TCD) as a research and, later, a clinical tool (24).

Extracranial Ultrasound

The association between ischemic cerebrovascular events and atherosclerosis of the extracranial portion of the carotid arteries has been the main factor behind the development of neurovascular ultrasonography. In theory, carotid atheromatous plaques can be assessed using: (a) the degree of stenosis they cause, (b) their surface characteristics, and (c) their histomorphology. Using duplex ultrasound, plaques can be fully studied by direct visualization, both sagittally and transversely. It is also possible to assess the hemodynamic compromise caused by atheromatous plaques, and help in the risk stratification of the patient.

The degree of stenosis caused by atheromatous plaques can be readily evaluated by duplex ultrasound, as follows: the B-mode image displays the spatial relationship between the plaque and the vessels (Fig. 4), whereas the PW Doppler shows the turbulence and flow acceleration caused by it. This acceleration, accompanied by disruption of normal laminar flow, increases progressively as the lumen narrows and allows estimation of the degree of stenosis and hemodynamic impact of the plaque (26). The evaluation of plaque surface characteristics is geared toward the determination of whether the plaque is "ulcerated," a factor that has been believed to contribute to the increased risk for arterial occlusion and stroke (Fig. 4). Unfortunately, ulceration implies a disruption in the endothelium continuity, a characteristic not easily discernible by any of the available diagnostic techniques. From this perspective, ulcers would have to be differentiated from plaque surface irregularities ("craters"), which are

probably more frequent and which are associated with an intact endothelium. The ability of B-mode ultrasound to identify "ulcers" is not considered optimal, although it is similar to that of angiography. With regard to the assessment of plaque morphology, the literature suggests that soft plaques, as well as unstable plaques, represent a greater risk for the development of stroke (27–29). Currently, plaque morphology can only be assessed ultrasonically, as follows: the B-mode images show whether the plaque is soft (fibrofatty), fibrous, or calcific depending upon its echogenic characteristics (i.e., fibrofatty plaques are echolucent, while calcific plaques are echodense). Other characteristics, such as intraplaque hemorrhage, another finding believed to be a risk factor for stroke (30,31), can also be identified by B-mode ultrasound.

The main role of duplex ultrasound is the early assessment (screening) of patients at risk of ischemic stroke, and their follow-up. The recent results of multicenter studies designed to assess the effectiveness of carotid endarterectomy have placed significant pressure upon clinicians due to the need for quick identification of patients with ischemic brain events resulting from atheromatous plaques that meet criteria for surgical treatment. In spite of suggestions that these results (which are based on strict and often peculiar angiographic criteria) demand the absolute need for angiographic evaluation, clinical practice has demonstrated that duplex ultrasound is a reliable enough tool that allows clinicians to plan for further evaluation and care. Finally, the discussion so far has been centered on the ultrasonic evaluation of the carotid artery system. It must be noted, however, that the flow direction and velocity of the vertebral arteries within the vertebral canal of the cervical spine can also be assessed with duplex ultrasound.

Color Doppler Imaging

Color Doppler imaging (CDI) presents two-dimensional cross-sectional Doppler shift information superimposed upon gray-scale anatomic images. It utilizes the pulse-echo imaging principle, in which a pulse of ultrasound is emitted into the tissues and its echoes are then received and analyzed. Echoes returning from stationary tissues are detected and presented in gray scale in appropriate locations within the scan line. When a returning echo has a frequency different from when it was transmitted, it implies the occurrence of a Doppler shift. Such Doppler shift can be detected along the scan line and its sign (positive or negative), magnitude, and variance are recorded. These variables are utilized by the instrument to determine the hue, saturation, and luminance of the color pixel at its location on the display. Each pixel is then updated multiple times per second, creating dynamic images of the flowing blood. Recently, instrumentation capable of performing direct color velocity imaging (rather than frequency shift imaging) has also been intro-

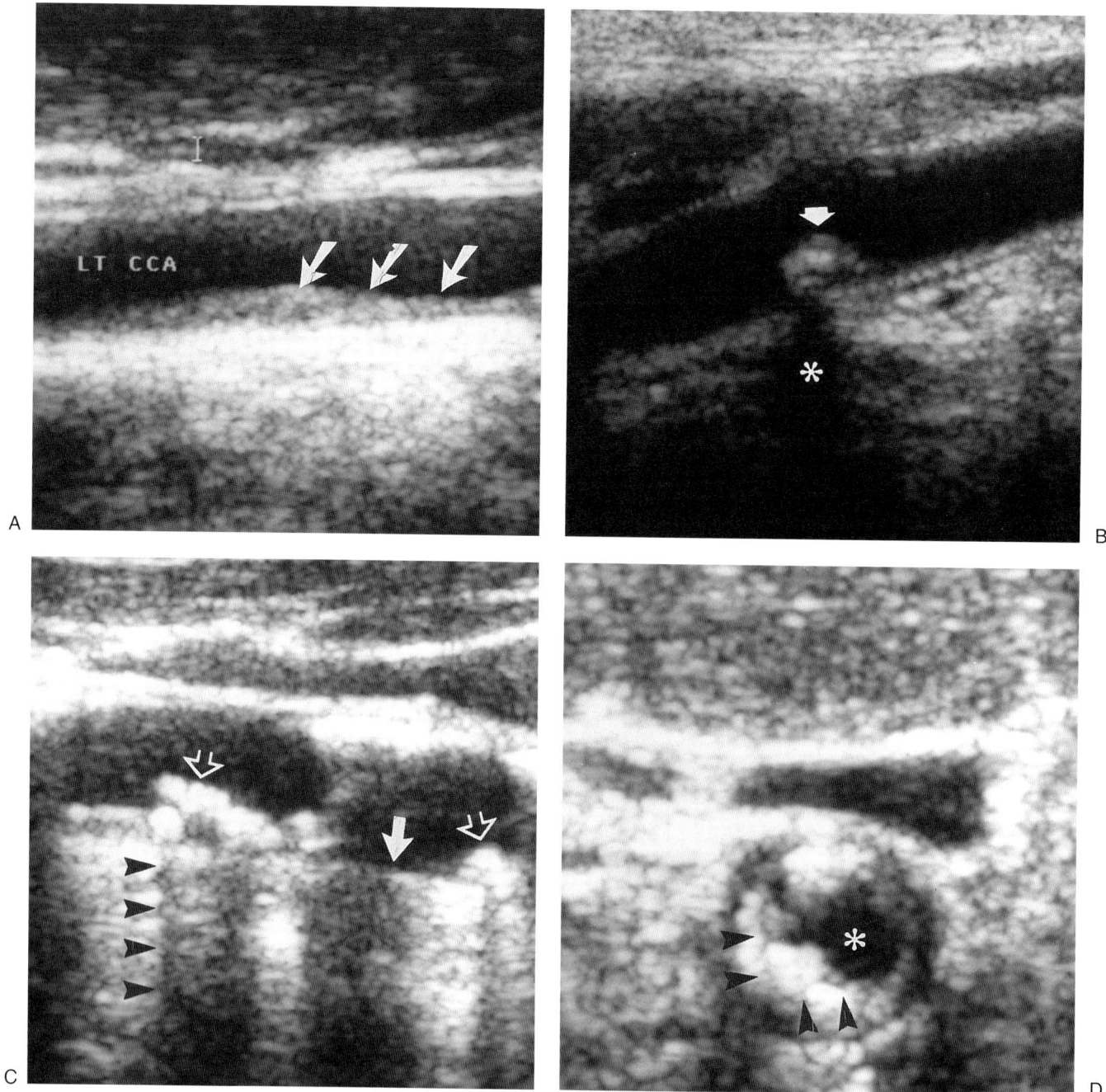

FIG. 4. **A:** B-mode ultrasound displays soft (i.e., fibrofatty) plaque with smooth surface (*white arrows*) that causes moderate diffuse narrowing of a common carotid artery. **B:** A focal calcific plaque (*white arrow*) in the carotid bulb presents with smooth surface and casts acoustic shadows into the tissue (*asterisk*). **C:** A more complex plaque, with elements of calcification (*white open arrows*) and acoustic shadows (*black arrowheads*), also presents an irregular surface, with the possibility of a crater (*solid white arrow*). **D:** An advantage of ultrasound is that it also allows transverse imaging of vessels. In this case, a carotid artery is affected by an irregular, eccentric, and complex plaque (*black arrowheads*), which narrows the lumen moderately. The true lumen is marked by the *asterisk*.

duced. Recent reviews suggest that the main advantages of CDI over duplex are that:

1. It allows easier identification of vascular structures, leading to faster scan times
2. It is helpful in differentiating plaque stenoses from other problems, such as kinks
3. It allows appreciation of flow disturbances, even in the absence of stenosis
4. It helps identify very small amounts of flow (e.g., critical stenosis or ''string sign'')
5. It rapidly identifies echolucent plaques based upon the absence of flow
6. It allows better delineation of surface features

In general, the application of CDI is quite similar to that of conventional duplex ultrasound. However, the sophisticated nature of the images produced has resulted in its application in the evaluation of conditions other than carotid atherosclerosis, including carotid body tumors, intimal fibroplasia, and dissection. Finally, CDI has expanded the ability to evaluate the vertebral arteries as they course through the vertebral canal of the cervical spine extracranially.

Transcranial Doppler

Transcranial Doppler (TCD) ultrasound is based upon the use of a range-gated pulse-Doppler ultrasonic beam of 2 MHz frequency to assess the hemodynamic characteristics of the major cerebral arteries (25). The ultrasonic beam crosses the intact adult skull at points known as *windows,* bounces off the erythrocytes flowing within the arteries at the base of the brain, and allows the determination of blood flow velocity, direction of flow, collateral patterns, and state of cerebral vasoreactivity. By sampling multiple cerebral blood vessels using TCD, it is possible to identify patterns suggesting intra- or extracranial lessons, follow-up their natural history over time, and even monitor the effects of therapeutic strategies. Although certainly having its own inherent limitations, TCD provides physiologic information about the brain circulation that cannot be obtained by any other means. In addition to the uniqueness of the information gathered by TCD, other attractive characteristics are that it is noninvasive, reproducible, versatile, and dynamic.

The role of TCD in clinical practice has changed over the past decade. The technique, somewhat of an ancillary procedure, is best conceived as a specialized ''stethoscope'' that allows clinicians to ''listen'' to the hemodynamic changes of the brain blood vessels, and to follow changes over time. Indeed, the best approach to TCD is to consider it an extension of the clinical examination, analogous to the way in which electromyography has been regarded for many years. From the clinical point of view, TCD is an ideal tool not only for diagnosis, but also for follow-up. Just as cardiologists have previously performed sequential auscultatory examinations of patients looking for new murmurs that would

suggest the development is advancement of valvular dysfunction, it is also possible to use TCD to alert us about the presence of hemodynamic disturbances representative of cerebrovascular pathology.

The clinical context in which TCD was introduced was the detection of vasospasm in victims of aneurysmal subarachnoid hemorrhage (25,32–34). Since then, however, there has been an explosion in its utilization in a variety of clinical and research scenarios. Time and time again the versatility of TCD has prevailed, and the technique has been able to show aspects of various clinical disorders, which previously were not fully understood. The most important established (Class II and III evidence) clinical applications of TCD are the evolution of schemic cerebrovascular disorders, the evaluation of cerebral vasospasm, and the assessment of arteriovenous malformations.

Evaluation of Ischemic Cerebrovascular Disorders

Atherosclerosis of the cerebral vasculature is by no means restricted to the common carotid bifurcation. In fact, the second most common location of atherosclerotic plaques in the carotid circulation is the cavernous portion of the internal carotid artery. Intracranial atherosclerotic stenosis is relatively common in blacks and Orientals, and can certainly alter prognosis and management (35). TCD provides a noninvasive way of screening and following these patients. Characteristically, TCD shows that the intracranial stenotic vessel displays increased blood flow velocities to levels greater than two standard deviations of normal (Fig. 5). In addition to local stenosis causing increased velocities in the vessel affected, other patterns of collateralization may be identified. In addition to intracranial lesions, those causing significant hemodynamic narrowing of the extracranial portions of the cerebral blood vessels lead to decreased TCD velocities (36,37). The degree of the decrement depends upon the existence of collateral flow through the communicating arteries. Such a pattern, in turn, will be characterized by increased blood flow velocities in the vessel acting as the collateral supplier. In these patients, it is also possible to show reduced vasoreactivity in the hemisphere ipsilateral to the stenosis (36,37).

The capability of TCD to detect embolic particles as they traverse the cerebral blood vessels has become a subject of intense investigation, and one with a potentially significant impact on the care of patients with ischemic brain events (Fig. 5) (38). Due to the differences in impedance between the embolic material and the red blood cells, the ultrasound beam is reflected with greater intensity from embody, leading to characteristic signature signals within the Doppler waveform. These signals are known as high intensity transients (HITs) and they vary in intensity, duration, and appearance within the cardiac cycle. Not only has it been possible to detect HITs during surgical procedures that place patients at risk for cerebral embolism (e.g., carotid endarter-

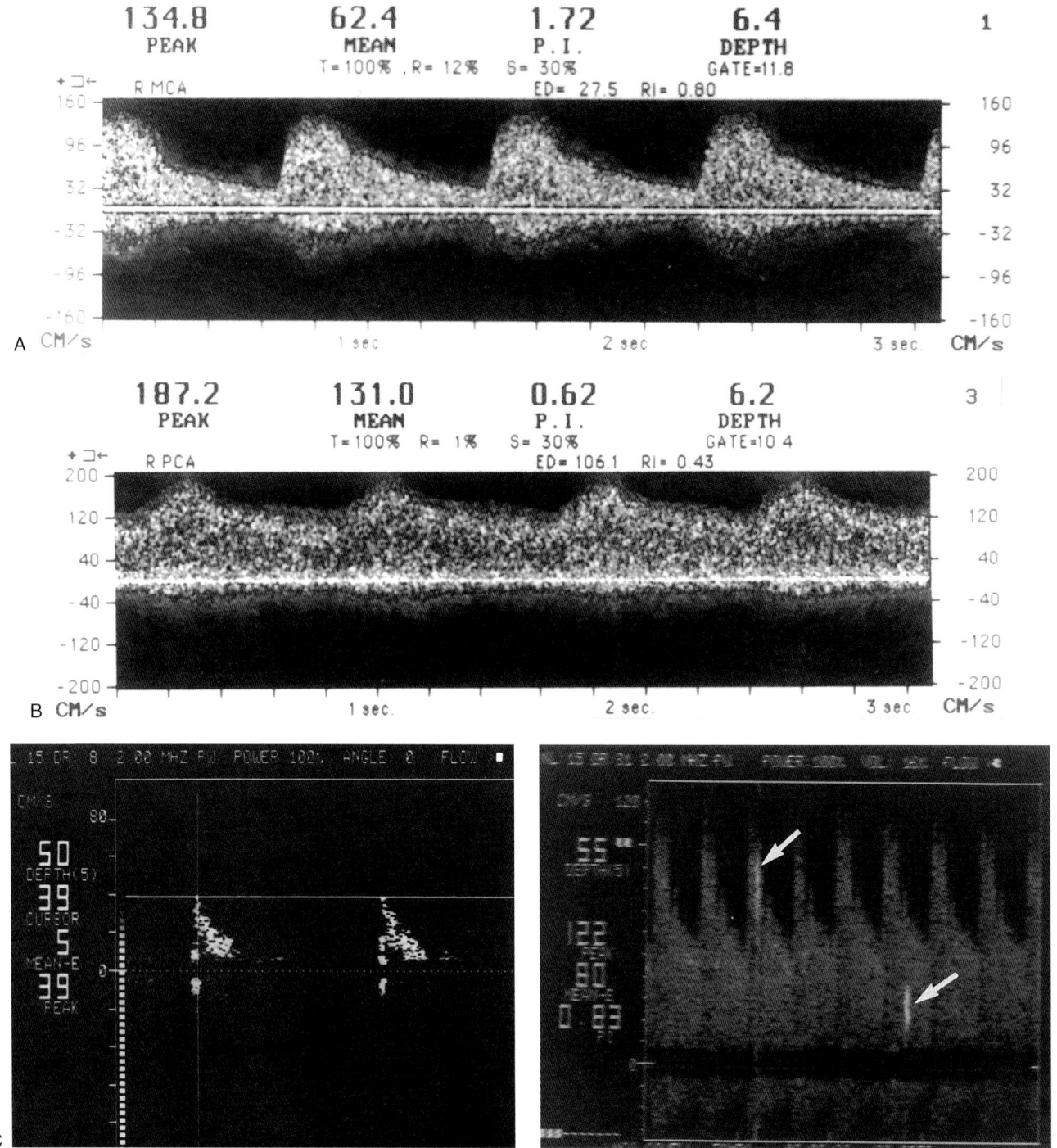

FIG. 5. A: Normal TCD waveform and velocities from a primary cerebral artery (Vm = 62 cm/s). **B:** Focal stenosis is detected by the elevation in blood flow velocities it causes. In this case, Vm = 131 cm/s is highly suggestive of a focal stenosis. **C:** TCD sampling of a acutely occluded cerebral vessel often discloses a "drumbeat" signal, with a characteristic appearance and sound. **D:** One of the most interesting applications of TCD is the detection of emboli based upon the finding of high intensity transients (HITs) (*white arrows*) in the TCD waveform.

ectomy or cardiopulmonary bypass), but also at the bedside (38–42). It has been possible to visualize spontaneous asymptomatic emboli in patients with atrial fibrillation and/or mechanical heart valves. Such a finding has carried with it the implication that cerebral embolic may occur continuously under certain circumstances, and that the factors that lead to the development of symptoms could be determined. Further work is being done in order to define the role of TCD for the identification of sources of embolism from more than one site. Additionally, the technique can be combined with the intravenous injection of agitated saline solution, allowing diagnosis of patent foramen ovale (PFOs) and other etiologic right-to-left shunts of that could lead to paradoxical embolic.

Evaluation of Cerebral Vasospasm

The diagnosis of vasospasm by TCD is made by the observation of velocities greater than two standard deviations over normal, in a given arterial segment (25,32–34). Vasospasm, under any circumstance, is a dynamic process that requires serial evaluation for adequate documentation and follow-up. It is because of these characteristics that TCD is so useful in the assessment of patients with vasospasm. The test should be performed immediately after a condition known to be associated with vasospasm is diagnosed (e.g., subarachnoid hemorrhage). A follow-up TCD study must be repeated as often as necessary. For example, in patients with aneurysmal subarachnoid hemorrhage or closed head injury, daily TCD studies should be performed in order to identify trends that will alert the clinician to the presence of vasospasm and that therapeutic measures should be instituted (43). Also, TCD can be used to follow-up the response to treatment, particularly in the case of interventional procedures (44–47).

Assessment of Arteriovenous Malformations

Although the diagnosis of arteriovenous malformations is most commonly performed by imaging procedures, TCD can be used to assess the flow characteristics of anomalies greater than 2 cm in diameter. Such hemodynamic evaluation can be used to assess the effects of certain therapeutic procedures such as embolization, for AVM. Finally, TCD can also help determine the degree of dysregulation existing in the brain region where the malformation is located, an important variable in planning surgery and preventing the hyperemic syndrome that sometimes follows (48–50).

CATHETERIZATION AND ANGIOGRAPHY: BACK TO THE FUTURE!

Cerebral angiography was introduced in 1927 by Egas Moniz, a Portuguese neurologist, as a method for neurologic diagnosis. Originally angiography was performed by direct carotid puncture and injection of relatively toxic contrast agents. The introduction of guidewires and catheters allowed access to the cerebral blood vessels from the femoral arteries, facilitating the performance of angiography, and contributing to its widespread utilization. The development of CT in the early 1970s and of MRI approximately a decade later, has resulted in decreased utilization of diagnostic angiography. Nevertheless, there are situations in which angiography must be performed and the information it provides, unique. The materials for cerebrovascular angiography have become increasingly sophisticated leading to the progressive reduction of risk during the last few years.

Cerebral angiography carries with it a certain amount of risk and potential complications (51,52). In the first place, just as any other type of angiography, allergic reactions to iodinated contrast can occur. Anaphylactic reactions are less frequent (in the range of 1 out of every 50,000 patients). Another negative aspect of contrast agents is their potential nephrotoxic effect. Finally, the most dreaded complication of cerebral angiography is stroke. This is related to either clot formation in the catheterization instruments or dislodging of plaque material during catheter and wire manipulation. Emboli are probably quite common during angiography and yet, only occasionally become symptomatic (53). One factor that seems to make the patient prone to develop neurologic symptoms during angiography is the state of hydration. The current incidence of permanent neurologic complications following diagnostic angiography is less than 1% (51,52, 54,55).

Cerebral angiography allows clear visualization of the lumen of the cerebral blood vessels, arteries, arterioles, capillaries, veins, and venous sinuses. From this point of view, the technique can be considered "lumenography." It is the technique that provides the most precise detail of a wide range of neurovascular structures. This makes it sometimes essential in the planning of therapy. However, angiography per se does not provide information about the vascular wall. For this, ultrasound and ultimately magnetic resonance angiography are much better tools (Fig. 4).

It is said that another limitation of angiography is the lack of physiologic information. We feel that this is not the case, and that there is dynamic information available with the angiographic procedure. The technique allows the assessment of pressure gradients, collateral patterns, competitive flow patterns, hemodynamic compromise patterns, and even tissue perfusion. The latter stems from the concept of digital parenchymography, championed by Theron and his collaborators. By digitally manipulating the angiographic data, it is possible to obtain information about the perfusion of tissue distal to stenotic lesions. This can sometimes be used to assess the potential value of revascularization of arteries with moderate degrees of stenosis (Fig. 6). Despite the relatively low risk, cerebral catheterization and angiography should only be utilized if it is the only or best method to obtain information key to treating the patient (56), or if it is used to treat the patient (57,58) (Fig. 6).

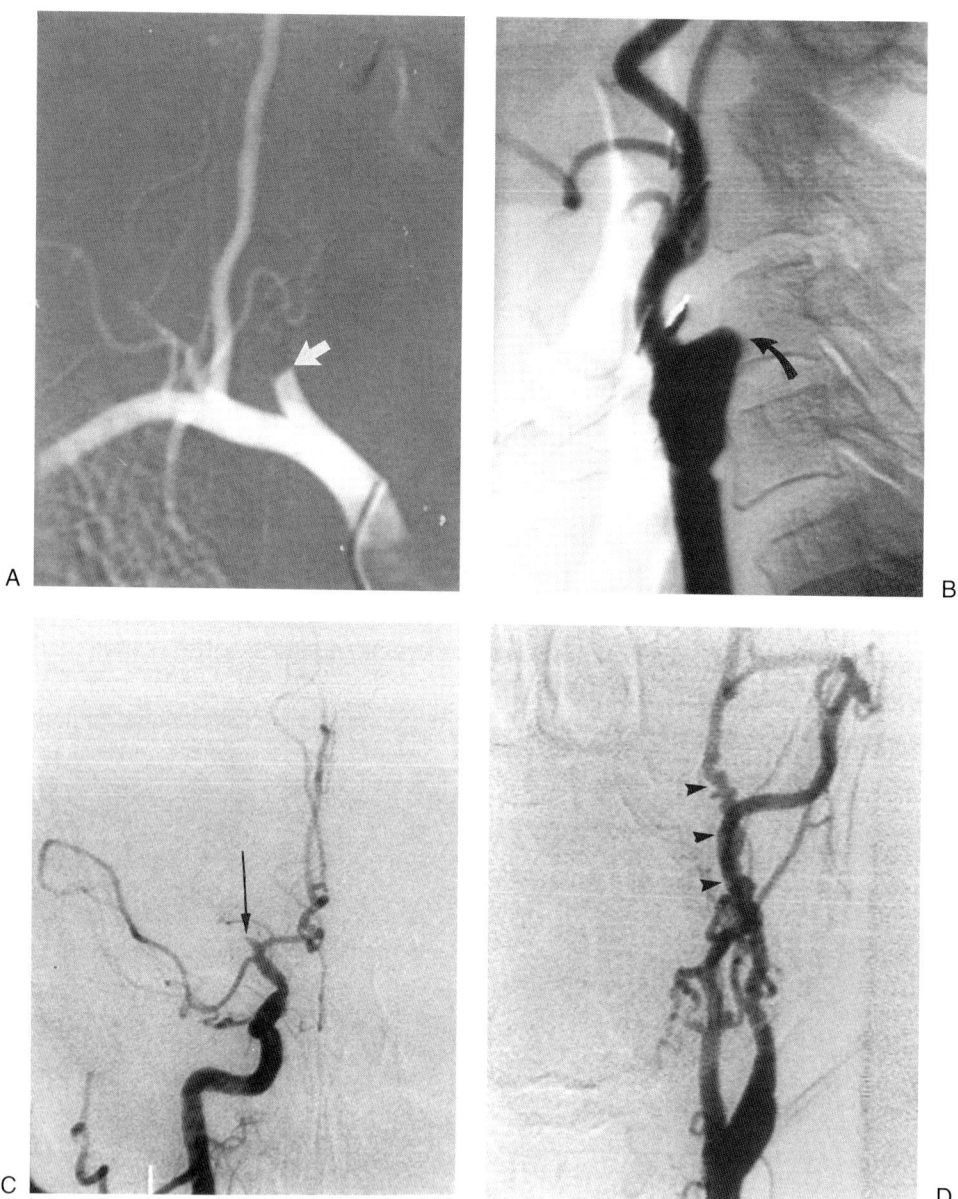

FIG. 6. Angiography is the definitive test for diagnosis of both acute (**A**, *white arrow*) and chronic (**B**, *black curved arrow*) occlusion of extracranial arteries. It is also diagnostic of occlusion of intracranial arteries (**C**, *black thin arrow*). Angiography helps diagnose nonatherosclerotic lesions of the cerebral vasculature, such as fibromuscular dysplasia (**D**, *black arrowheads*). *(continued)*

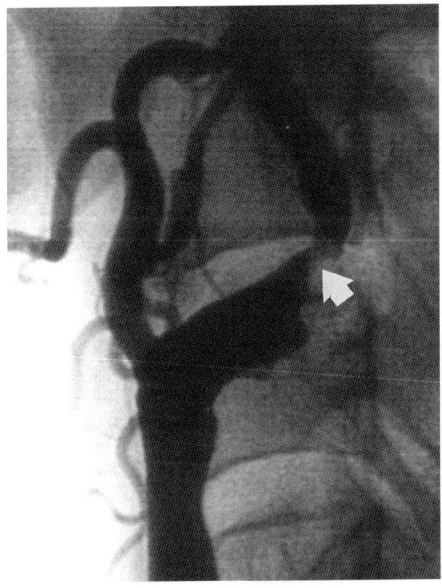
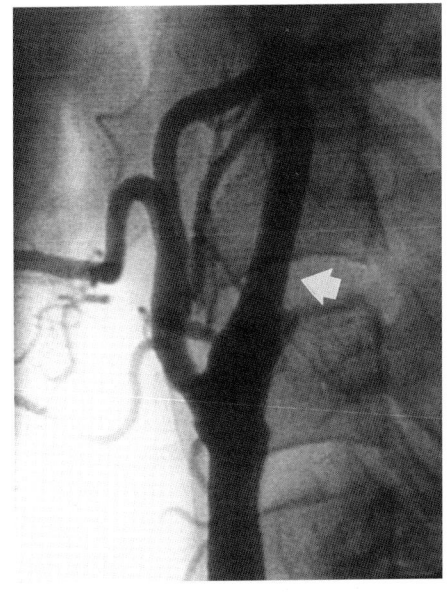

E   F

FIG. 6. *Continued.* Finally, the technique also allows detection of lesions suitable for endovascular treatment. A stenotic internal carotid artery (**E**) is also shown following elective stenting (**F**). The point of stenosis is shown by the *white arrow* in both images.

CONCLUSIONS AND RECOMMENDATIONS

The utilization of imaging techniques for the evaluation of patients with cerebrovascular disorders must be guided by the specific needs of the clinical situation. Newer tests being introduced will not necessarily replace the old ones but rather will provide additional dimensions to our ability to diagnose and treat different conditions capable of causing stroke. It is important to keep in mind that every one of these diagnostic techniques is operator-dependent. As such, another aspect of choosing the appropriate diagnostic technique requires the recognition of the quality of the resources available.

REFERENCES

1. Gomez C, Tulyapronchote R, Malkoff M, et al. Changing trends in the etiologic diagnosis of ischemic stroke. *J Stroke Cerebrovasc Dis* 1994; 4:169–173.
2. Amarenco P, Cohen A, Baudrimont M, et al. Transesophageal echocardiographic detection of aortic arch disease in patients with cerebral infarction. *Stroke* 1992;23:1005–1009.
3. Labovitz AJ, Camp A, Castello R, et al. Usefulness of transesophageal echocardiography in unexplained cerebral ischemia. *Am J Cardiol* 1993;72:1448–1452.
4. Acarturk E, Ozeren A, Sarica Y. Detection of aortic plaques by transesophageal echocardiography in patients with ischemic stroke. *Acta Neurol Scand* 1995;92:170–172.
5. Gomez CR, Malkoff MD, Sauer CM, et al. Code stroke. An attempt to shorten inhospital therapeutic delays. *Stroke* 1994;25:1920–1923.
6. Wardlaw JM, Lewis SC, Dennis MS, et al. Is visible infarction on computed tomography associated with an adverse prognosis in acute ischemic stroke. *Stroke* 1998;29:1315–1319.
7. Wong KS, Lam WW, Liang E, et al. Variability of magnetic resonance angiography and computed tomography angiography in grading middle cerebral artery stenosis (see comments). *Stroke* 1996;27:1084–1087.
8. Leclerc X, Godefroy O, Salhi A, et al. Helical CT for the diagnosis of extracranial internal carotid artery dissection. *Stroke* 1996;27:461–466.

9. Vaneverdingen KJ, Vanderground J, Kappelle LJ, et al. Diffusion-weighted magnetic resonance imaging in acute stroke. *Stroke* 1998;29: 1783–1790.
10. Chong J, Lu D, Aragao F, et al. Diffusion-weighted MR of acute cerebral infarction: comparison of data processing methods. *Am J Neuroradiol* 1998;19:1733–1739.
11. Warach S, Chien D, Li W, et al. Fast magnetic resonance diffusion weighted imaging of acute human stroke. *Neurology* 1992;42: 1717–1723.
12. Warach S, Gaa D, Siewert B, et al. Acute human stroke studied by whole brain echoplanar diffusion weighted magnetic resonance imaging. *Neurology* 1995;37:231–241.
13. Warach S, Boska M, Welch K. Pitfalls and potential of clinical diffusion weighted MR imaging in acute stroke. *Stroke* 1998;28:481–482.
14. Chiesa R, Melissano G, Castellano R, et al. Three dimensional time-of-flight magnetic resonance angiography in carotid artery surgery: a comparison with digital subtraction angiography. *Eur J Vasc Surg* 1993;7:171–176.
15. Anson JA, Heiserman JE, Drayer BP, et al. Surgical decisions on the basis of magnetic resonance angiography of the carotid arteries (see comments). *Neurosurgery* 1993;32:335–343; discussion 343.
16. Erdoes LS, Marek JM, Mills JL, et al. The relative contributions of carotid duplex scanning, magnetic resonance angiography, and cerebral arteriography to clinical decision making: a prospective study in patients with carotid occlusive disease. *J Vasc Surg* 1996;23:950–956.
17. Vanninen RL, Manninen HI, Partanen PK, et al. How should we estimate carotid stenosis using magnetic resonance angiography? *Neuroradiology* 1996;38:299–305.
18. Yamasoba T, Kikuchi S, O'Uchi T, et al. Magnetic resonance angiographic findings in vertiginous patients with slow vertebrobasilar blood flow. *Acta Oto-Laryngologica* 1995;520(suppl Pt 1):153–156.
19. Gomez C, Cruz-Flores S, Malkoff M, et al. Isolated vertigo as a manifestation of vertebrobasilar ischemia. *Neurology* 1996;47:94–97.
20. Rother J, Wentz KU, Rautenberg W, et al. Magnetic resonance angiography in vertebrobasilar ischemia. *Stroke* 1993;24:1310–1315.
21. Barona R, Martinez Sanjuan V, Campos A, et al. (Assessment of vertebrobasilar insufficiency using magnetic resonance angiography). (Spanish). *Acta Otorhinolaringol Española* 1994;45:329–334.
22. Freeman J, Free T, Payne H, et al. Assessing extracranial carotid stenosis: magnetic resonance angiography, duplex scanning, and digital angiography. *S D J Med* 1993;46:53–56.
23. Kenton AR, Martin PJ, Abbott RJ, et al. Comparison of transcranial color-coded sonography and magnetic resonance angiography in acute stroke. *Stroke* 1997;28:1601–1606.

24. Grolimund P, Seiler RW, Aaslid R, et al. Evaluation of cerebrovascular disease by combined extracranial and transcranial Doppler sonography. Experience in 1,039 patients. *Stroke* 1986;18:1018–1024.
25. Aaslid R, Huber P, Nornes H. A transcranial Doppler method in the evaluation of cerebrovascular spasm. *Neuroradiology* 1986;28:11–16.
26. Carpenter JP, Lexa FJ, Davis JT. Determination of duplex Doppler ultrasound criteria appropriate to the North American Symptomatic Carotid Endarterectomy Trial. *Stroke* 1996;27:695.
27. Gray-Weale AC, Graham JC, Burnett JR, et al. Carotid artery atheroma: comparison of preoperative B-mode ultrasound appearance with carotid endarterectomy specimen pathology. *J Cardiovasc Surg* 1988;29: 676–681.
28. O'Farrell CM, FitzGerald DE. Prognostic value of carotid ultrasound lesion morphology in retinal ischaemia: result of a long term follow up. *Br J Ophthalmol* 1993;77:781–784.
29. Anonymous. Carotid artery plaque composition—relationship to clinical presentation and ultrasound B-mode imaging. European Carotid Plaque Study Group. *Eur J Vasc Endovasc Surg* 1995;10:23–30.
30. Aburahma AF, Robinson P, Decanio R. Prospective clinicopathologic study of carotid intraplague hemorrhage. *Am Surg* 1989;55:169–173.
31. Geroulakos G, Domjan J, Nicolaides A, et al. Ultrasonic carotid artery plaque structure and the risk of cerebral infarction on computed tomography. *J Vasc Surg* 1994;20:263–266.
32. Bartels RH, Verhagen WI, Van der Spek JA, et al. Transcranial Doppler ultrasonography: influence on scheduling of angiography and delayed surgery for ruptured intracranial aneurysms. *J Neurosurg Sci* 1994;38: 21–27.
33. Compton JS, Teddy PJ. Cerebral arterial vasospasm following severe head injury: a transcranial Doppler study. *Br J Neurosurg* 1987;1: 435–439.
34. Compton JS, Redmond S, Symon L. Cerebral blood velocity in subarachnoid haemorrhage: a transcranial Doppler study. *J Neurol Neurosurg Psychiatry* 1987;50:1499–1503.
35. de Bray JM, Missoum A, Dubas F, et al. Detection of vertebrobasilar intracranial stenoses: transcranial Doppler sonography versus angiography. *J Ultrasound Med* 1997;16:213–218.
36. Giller CA. A bedside test for cerebral autoregulation using transcranial Doppler ultrasound. *Acta Neurochir Wien* 1991;108:7–14.
37. Chimowitz MI, Furlan AJ, Jones SC, et al. Transcranial Doppler assessment of cerebral perfusion reserve in patients with carotid occlusive disease and no evidence of cerebral infarction. *Neurology* 1993;43: 353–357.
38. Ackerstaff RG, Jansen C, Moll FL, et al. The significance of microemboli detection by means of transcranial Doppler ultrasonography monitoring in carotid endarterectomy (see comments). *J Vasc Surg* 1995; 21:963–969.
39. van Zuilen EV, Moll FL, Vermeulen FE, et al. Detection of cerebral microemboli by means of transcranial Doppler monitoring before and after carotid endarterectomy. *Stroke* 1995;26:210–213.
40. Spencer MP, Thomas GI, Nicholls SC, et al. Detection of middle cerebral artery emboli during carotid endarterectomy using transcranial Doppler ultrasonography (see comments). *Stroke* 1990;21:415–423.
41. Achtereekte HA, van der Kruijk RA, Hekster RE, et al. Diagnosis of traumatic carotid artery dissection by transcranial Doppler ultrasound:

case report and review of the literature. (Review) (11 refs). *Surg Neurol* 1994;42:240–244.
42. Gaunt ME, Brown L, Hartshome T, et al. Unstable carotid plaques: preoperative identification and association with intraoperative embolisation detected by transcranial Doppler. *Eur J Vasc Endovasc Surg* 1996;11:78–82.
43. Kilic T, Pamir MN, Ozek MM, et al. A new, more dependable methodology for the use of transcranial Doppler ultrasonography in the management of subarachnoid haemorrhage. *Acta Neurochirurgica* 1996; 138:1070–1077; discussion 1077–1078.
44. Hurst RW, Schnee C, Raps EC, et al. Role of transcranial Doppler in neuroradiological treatment of intracranial vasospasm. *Stroke* 1993;24: 299–303.
45. Bracard S, Ducrocq X, Picard L, et al. (Transluminal angioplasty in the treatment of vasospasm. Value of transcranial Doppler in the diagnosis and follow-up). (French). *Neuro-Chirurgie* 1992;38:165–169.
46. Rowe JG, Byrne JV, Molyneux A, et al. Haemodynamic consequences of embolizing aneurysms: a transcranial Doppler study. *Br J Neurosurg* 1995;9:749–757.
47. Seiler RW, Grolimund P, Zurbruegg HR. Evaluation of the calcium-antagonist nimodipine for the prevention of vasospasm after aneurysmal subarachnoid haemorrhage. A prospective transcranial Doppler ultrasound study. *Acta Neurochirurgica* 1987;85:7–16.
48. Fleischer LH, Young WL, Pile-Spellman J, et al. Relationship of transcranial Doppler flow velocities and arteriovenous malformation feeding artery pressures (see comments). *Stroke* 1993;24:1897–1902.
49. Diehl RR, Henkes H, Nahser HC, et al. Blood flow velocity and vasomotor reactivity in patients with arteriovenous malformations: a transcranial Doppler study. *Stroke* 1994;25(8):1574–1580.
50. De Salles AA, Manchola I. CO2 reactivity in arteriovenous malformations of the brain: a transcranial Doppler ultrasound study [see comments]. *J Neurosurg* 1994;80(4):624–630.
51. Dion J, Gates P, Fox AJ, et al. Clinical events following neuroangiography: a prospective study. *Acta Radiologica* 1986;369(Suppl):29–33.
52. Warnock NG, Gandhi MR, Bergvall U, et al. Complications of intraarterial digital subtraction angiography in patients investigated for cerebral vascular disease. *Br J Radiol* 1993;66(790):855–858.
53. Markus H, Loh A, Israel D, et al. Microscopic air embolism during cerebral angiography and strategies for its avoidance [see comments]. *Lancet* 1993;341(8848):784–787.
54. Kachel R, Ritter H, Schiffmann R, et al. [Complications following cerebral angiography. Report on 4181 cerebral angiographies] [German]. *Zentralblatt fur Chirurgie* 1980;105(8):504–512.
55. Kachel R, Jahn U, Schiffmann R, et al. [Complications in cerebral angiography. A study of 6698 cerebral angiographies] [German]. *Revista Medico-Chirurgicala a Societatii de Medici Si Naturalisti Din Iasi* 1991;95(1–2):97–105.
56. Donaldson MC, Ivarsson BL, Mannick JA, et al. Impact of completion angiography on operative conduct and results of carotid endarterectomy. *Ann Surg* 1993;217(6):682–687.
57. Vinuela F, Dion J, Lylyk P, et al. Update on interventional neuroradiology [review]. *AJR* 1989;153(1):23–33.
58. Khayata M, Aymard A, Guichard JP, et al. Interventional neuroradiology. *Current Opinion in Radiology* 1992;4(1):71–78.

CHAPTER 61

Cardiac Tumors

Ernesto E. Salcedo

OVERVIEW AND CLASSIFICATION

Cardiac tumors, although relatively rare, represent an important group of cardiac abnormalities. Untreated they usually have an indolent or even fatal outcome, whereas the possibility of cure with timely excision makes their diagnosis challenging and consequential (1–5). Early diagnosis and accurate characterization of cardiac tumors is essential for effective patient management. Cardiac tumors are important in the differential diagnosis of valvular heart disease, congestive heart failure, systemic and pulmonary emboli, syncope, ventricular and supraventricular arrhythmias, and conduction defects. In addition, cardiac tumors may mimic a systemic, infective or immunologic disease.

A detailed medical history and a thorough physical examination are the first required steps for the diagnosis of cardiac tumors. The emergence of sophisticated imaging techniques has significantly enhanced the detection and management of patients with cardiac neoplasms (4).

In this chapter we describe the role of cardiac imaging techniques in the diagnosis and characterization of cardiac tumors. Emphasis is placed on assisting the clinician in selecting the most appropriate imaging tool for this purpose.

For this discussion we will consider as ''cardiac tumors'' not only primary or secondary neoplasms of the heart, but also some cardiac and paracardiac ''masses'' that can be visualized with imaging techniques. Therefore we will include lesions such as pericardial cyst, lipomatous hypertrophy of the interatrial septum, and fibroelastomas. Vegetations and thrombosis, although ''cardiac masses,'' are described in Chapters 46 and 64. The classification of primary and secondary cardiac tumors is indicated in Tables 1

and 2. The incidence of primary tumors of the heart is quite low. McAllister (6) reported an incidence between 0.0017 and 0.28% in reported or collected autopsy series (17 to 2,800 tumors in 1 million autopsies). Reymen (7), based upon the data of 22 large autopsy series, reported a frequency of primary cardiac tumors at approximately 0.02% (200 tumors in 1 million autopsies). In adults, almost 50% of the primary benign tumors are myxomas.

Approximately 25% of all primary tumors are malignant; most of these are sarcomas (Fig. 1).

Secondary tumors of the heart are comparatively more frequent (8) occurring 20 to 40 times more often than primary cardiac tumors. Carcinoma of the lung and breast, because of their prevalence, are the most common to metastasize to the heart. Melanomas, leukemias, and lymphoma have the greatest propensity to metastasize to the heart (Fig. 2).

Cardiac tumors may affect the pericardium, the myocardium, or they can be intracavitary. Benign tumors are usually circumscribed to one area, whereas malignant tumors frequently are more invasive and affect multiple planes and structures. Table 3 summarizes the most frequent locations for cardiac tumors.

TABLE 1. *Primary tumors of the heart*

Benign	Malignant
Myxoma	Sarcomas
Pericardial Cyst	Angiosarcoma
Lipoma	Rhabdomyosarcoma
Fibroelastoma	Fibrosarcoma
Rhabdomyoma	Osteosarcoma
Fibroma	Unclassified
Hemangioma	Mesothelioma
Other	Lymphoma
	Other

E. E. Salcedo: Echocardiography Laboratory, Department of Cardiology, St. Vincent's Medical Center, Jacksonville, Florida 32204.

TABLE 2. *Secondary tumors of the heart*

Direct extension	Venous extension	Metastatic spread
Lung carcinoma	Renal cell	Melanoma
Breast carcinoma	carcinoma	Leukemia
Esophageal	Adrenal carcinoma	Lymphoma
carcinoma	Hepatoma	Gastrointestinal
Mediastinal	Lung carcinoma	tract
tumors	Thyroid carcinoma	Genitourinary
	Uterine carcinoma	tract

TABLE 3. *Cardiac tumors by location*

Pericardium	Right Ventricle	Left Ventricle
Mesothelioma	Rhabdomyoma	Rhabdomyoma
Angiosarcoma	Fibroma	Papilloma
Mediastinal tumors	Lipoma	Fibroma
Right Atrium	Sarcomas	Sarcoma
Myxoma	Hepatoma	Lipoma
Sarcomas	Hypernephroma	Melanoma
Hypernephroma	**Left Atrium**	Myxoma
Hepatoma	Myxoma	**Valves**
Mediastinal	Mediastinal	Fibroelastoma
malignancies	malignancies	Fibrolipoma
		Myxoma

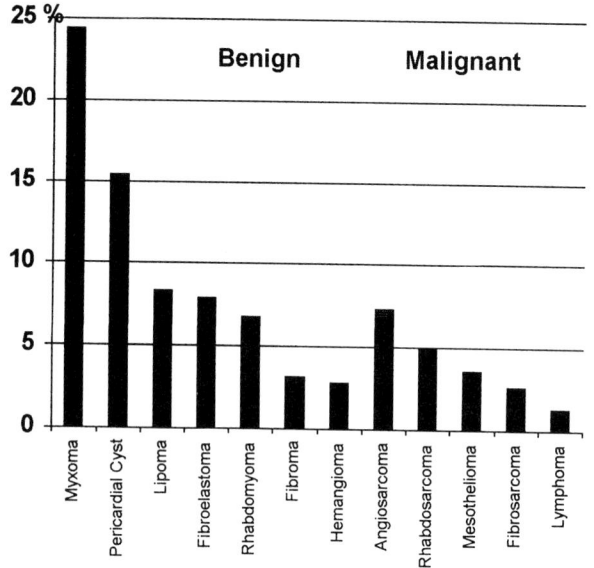

FIG. 1. Incidence of primary cardiac tumors. The *solid bars* depict the frequency of benign primary cardiac tumors. As can be seen, myxomas comprise about a quarter of all tumors. The *striped bars* depict the malignant tumors, the majority of which are sarcomas.

IMAGING TECHNIQUES FOR DIAGNOSING CARDIAC TUMORS

Cardiac tumors remained clinically esoteric entities until the development of modern cardiac imaging techniques in the 1960s and 1970s. Current interest lies in new technologies including transesophageal and three-dimensional echocardiography (9,10), magnetic resonance imaging, and ultrafast computed tomography.

The first report of the diagnosis of cardiac tumors by echocardiography was made in 1959 by Effert and Domanig (12). However, until two-dimensional echocardiography became well established in the 1970s, conventional chest radiographs (11), fluoroscopy, and angiography were the mainstays of the diagnosis.

The *chest radiograph* has low diagnostic yield for tumor detection; nevertheless, it may direct the clinician toward a more precise diagnostic imaging test. Calcification of cardiac tumors is not common but has been described in teratomas, sarcomas, and myxomas. If present it may be detectable by conventional x-ray and fluoroscopy.

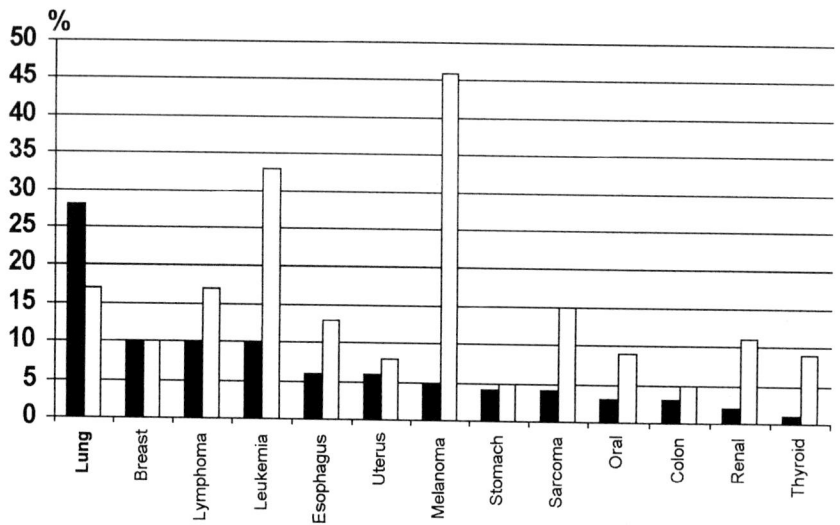

FIG. 2. Frequency of secondary cardiac tumors. The *solid bars* represent the order of frequency of cancers encountered at autopsy with metastatic heart disease. The *white bars* represent the order of frequency of metastasis of each primary tumor. As can be seen, carcinomas of the lung and breast, because of their prevalence, are the most frequent to metastasize to the heart (*solid bars*). Whereas, the tumors with the greatest propensity to metastasize to the heart are melanoma, leukemia, and lymphoma (*white bars*).

Angiography, once the standard for cardiac tumor diagnosis has waned in importance due to the emergence of reliable noninvasive diagnostic methods. Angiography is now mainly used to define coronary anatomy prior to cardiac surgery and to delineate sites of peripheral tumor emboli occlusion. *Digital subtraction angiography,* which provides high-resolution images of all four cardiac chambers, and has been used effectively for the diagnosis of cardiac tumors (13). However, transesophageal echocardiography (TEE) and MRI have largely replaced intravenous digital subtraction angiography as alternatives to suboptimal transthoracic echocardiography.

In 1962, Isley and Reinhardt (14) reported the first description of a myxoma diagnosed through *radionuclear intravascular scanning.* However, because of its relative low resolution, nuclear techniques are of only limited value for the management of patients with cardiac tumors. Computed tomography (CT) has found its greatest role in assessing paracardiac masses, often found in the pericardium (15). Conventional CT permits some degree of tissue characterization. The low density of fatty material can be distinguished from higher densities as seen in myxomas and other tumors. CT is clearly superior to echocardiography in determining the degree of myocardial, pericardial, and mediastinal tumor extension, but provides little or no information regarding intracavitary tumors.

Ultrafast CT (cine CT), facilitates the evaluation of intracardiac tumors that appear as filling defects within the cardiac chambers. Similar to conventional CT, cine CT can be used to identify the tissue type of intracardiac masses and distinguish them from extracardiac masses. The real-time nature of cine CT allows a time-density curve analysis for assessing the vascular nature of a cardiac mass.

The high resolution offered by magnetic resonance imaging makes it the most accurate diagnostic technique to evaluate the presence of cardiac and paracardiac tumors (16,17). The ability to identify a variety of benign and malignant cardiac tumors has been well documented (18). Their differentiation from abnormal intracavitary signal, caused by either thrombus or slow flow of blood may be achieved by both spin-echo and cine MRI (19). Cine MRI also permits visualization of the movement of an intracardiac mass such as a pedunculated atrial myxoma prolapsing into the left ventricle.

Two-dimensional echocardiography (20) is the procedure of choice for detection of cardiac neoplasias because it demonstrates precise anatomical details in real time. Its diagnostic value is greatest for endocardial lesions, where the contrast between the mass and the echolucent chamber is most apparent. Intramyocardial lesions, such as rhabdomyomas or fibromas, can also be well demarcated, especially with transesophageal echocardiography (TEE). Pericardial lesions are the most difficult to characterize by echocardiography, and CT or MRI provide a better diagnostic yield.

TEE is ideally suited for the detection, or confirmation, of cardiac tumors. It is superior to transthoracic echocardiog-

TABLE 4. *Imaging techniques for diagnosing cardiac tumors*

	X-ray	CT	Angio	MRI	ECHO
Primary benign					
Myxoma	E	D	C	B	A
Pericardial cyst	C	B	O	A	D
Lipoma	E	B	E	A	B
Fibroelastoma	O	O	O	C	A
Rhabdomyoma	O	E	E	B	A
Fibroma	O	E	E	B	A
Primary malignant					
Sarcoma	E	D	D	A	B
Mesothelioma	E	C	E	A	C
Lymphomas	D	C	E	A	C
Secondary tumors					
Direct extension	E	C	D	A	B
Venous extension	O	E	C	B	A
Metastatic spread	E	C	E	A	B

A, preferred diagnostic tool; *B,* very useful; *C,* useful; *D,* may be of use; *E,* of limited use; *O,* of no use.

raphy (TTE) in the detection of tumors in the superior vena cava, pulmonary artery, descending aorta, and right atrium. TEE is useful for detecting right-sided cardiac tumors and differentiating the benign from the malignant ones. Most tumors arising within the right atrium are benign, whereas those extending into the right atrium from outside are malignant. Right ventricular tumors are rarely encountered, and when present, they are likely to be malignant.

TEE has also been invaluable for the evaluation and clarification of "pseudomasses." With the advent of three dimensional echocardiography the size of cardiac neoplasms can be measured in three dimensions (9,10), and conceptualization of tumor involvement of adjacent structures is improved.

However, the differential diagnosis between primary and secondary cardiac tumors, malignant and benign forms, and nonneoplastic masses can be achieved with certainty only though surgical pathology. The specific diagnosis of cardiac tumors by current imaging techniques should only be consider presumptive.

Echocardiography remains the most useful imaging diagnostic tool for the diagnosis and management of cardiac tumors, and MRI may be reserved for better definition of paracardiac or infiltrative tumors.

Table 4 summarizes the current imaging techniques and their relative value for diagnosing cardiac tumors.

SPECIFIC CARDIAC TUMORS

Pseudomases

The high resolution of the new diagnostic imaging techniques has introduced a new problem, that is the visualization of many structures within the heart that may be confused with cardiac masses. It is imperative that physicians dealing with cardiac imaging techniques for the diagnosis of cardiac

TABLE 5. *Pseudo cardiac masses*

Foreign Bodies	AV groove	Interatrial septum
Catheters	Lipomatosis	Membrane of fossa ovalis
Pacing wires	Mitral annular calcification	Septal aneurysm
Right Atrium	Descending aorta	**Valves**
Crista terminalis	Dilated circumflex	Lambl excrescences
Thebezian valve	Dilated coronary sinus	Annular calcification
Eustachian valve	Persistent left superior cava	Flail leaflets
Chiari network	Anomalous pulm. veins	Accessory leaflets
Inferior vena cava orifice	Mitral valve abscess	**Extracardiac**
Right ventricle	**Left Ventricle**	Descending aorta
Moderator band	Papillary muscles	Hiatal hernia
Left atrium	False tendons	Epicardial fat
Left upper pulmonary vein	Accessory chordae	Thymus
Coronary sinus		Collapsed lung

masses be well acquainted with these "pseudomasses." Table 5 summarizes the most common cardiac structures and abnormalities that can be confused with cardiac neoplasms.

Primary Benign Tumors

Myxomas

Myxomas account for approximately 25% of all cardiac neoplasms and for 50% of benign tumors of the heart. They occur more often in women and most patients are middle aged. Cardiac myxomas occur predominately in the left atrium (75%); some occur in the right atrium and very few in the left or right ventricle and mitral valve (21).

Myxomas can be sporadic (most common), familial (earlier in life—mean 25 years—multiple and recurrent) and be complex (22) or in Carney syndrome (lentiginosis, fibroadenomas of the breast, skin myxomas, tumor of the pituitary, and primary pigmented modular adrenocortical disease and multiple and recurrent cardiac myxomas) (23).

The diagnosis of a cardiac myxoma requires the appropriate use of imaging techniques. TTE and especially TEE offer the best diagnostic yield for the evaluation of a patient with suspected myxoma. Often the first diagnostic clue of the presence of a myxoma is provided by echocardiography. Echocardiography is used to define the tumor's location, size, number, consistency, and presence or absence of stalk; it also demonstrates valvular obstruction and regurgitation. In the familial and complex form, TTE is a convenient method during follow-up to search for recurrences and for the screening of first-degree relatives. Spectral and color Doppler provide information regarding associated mitral regurgitation and presence and severity of transmitral flow obstruction. Three-dimensional echocardiography permits fairly accurate volumetric determination of myxomas.

Echo-gated MRI has several attributes that make it useful for the evaluation of atrial myxomas. The excellent anatomic detail provided by spin-echo (dark blood) MRI allows full assessment of atrial myxomas. Cinegradient-echo ("bright blood") MRI provides additional information concerning the movement of myxomas relative to the cardiac chambers

(see Chapters 29–31). Although the resolution of MRI is superior to that of echocardiography, in practice its use for the diagnosis and management of patients with myxoma is appropriate only when examination by echocardiography is equivocal or inadequate, which is a rare occurrence.

Conventional CT permits some degree of soft tissue characterization with internal references being provided by subcutaneous fat and normal myocardium. The low radiodensity of fatty material can be distinguished from higher radiodensities of myxomas. Delineation of cardiac mass by CT may be facilitated by using contrast enhancement. With ultrafast CT the mobility of a pedunculated myxoma and the site of its attachment to the walls of the heart can be assessed. The tissue radiodensities are readily measured and the real-time nature of CT allows a time-density curve analysis for assessing the possible vascular nature of a cardiac mass. Cine CT compares well to echocardiography for the diagnosis of myxomas but at present this method is not widely available. There have been several reports of the diagnosis of atrial myxoma by nuclear techniques including the intravenous injection of radioactive ionated albumin and technetium-gated equilibrium blood pool scanning. However, the relative low resolution of these techniques permits visualization of only a relatively large tumor.

Conventional cineangiography and digital subtraction angiography have been used in the diagnosis of myxoma but, with the advances in noninvasive imaging techniques, are rarely needed for the diagnosis of myxomas. Sessile myxomas are more vascularized than pedunculated ones and usually get their vascular supply from the right coronary artery or circumflex. This information may be of use in detecting a left atrial mass during coronary arteriography.

Pericardial Cyst

Although pericardial cysts are usually outside the pericardial cavity and, therefore should not be considered true cardiac tumors, their frequency is important in the imaging evaluation of cardiac and paracardiac masses.

Pericardial cysts are relatively common, usually asymptomatic, and often discovered during a routine chest x-ray as a round sharply demarcated mass along the right cardiac silhouette. They are most commonly located in the right costophrenic angle, followed by the left costophrenic angle, and rarely in the anterior or posterior mediastinum. The diagnosis is made by the typical x-ray appearance and location. Echocardiography is of limited value in the diagnosis of pericardial cysts. When pericardial cysts are visualized by echocardiography, they appear as echolucent masses usually in close proximity to the right atrium. Pericardial cysts can be easily recognized and characterized by MRI and CT. MRI and CT also allows for differentiating benign pericardial cysts from intrapericardial lesions.

Lipomas and Lipomatous Hypertrophy of the Interatrial Septum

Cardiac lipomas occur as circumscribed, encapsulated, usually solitary, intramuscular, subendocardial, or subepicardial tumors. They are similar to lipomas elsewhere in the body; histologically they consist of mature fat cells within a matrix of myxoid fibrous tissue and blood vessels. Clinical manifestations are usually absent or minimal although there have been a few case reports of pericardial effusion, tricuspid valve compression, cardiac enlargement, murmurs, and conduction abnormalities. A fibrolipoma appearing as a nodular mass on the tricuspid valve, mimicking a vegetation has been described (23).

Cardiac lipomas may be associated with rhabdomyoma and/or tuberous sclerosis. These lipomas are usually an incidental finding during an echocardiographic study, appearing as nodular echodensities without other distinct qualities. The ability of MRI to characterize fat makes it the preferred technique to diagnose cardiac lipomas. If the patient is asymptomatic and the lipomas are not causing any hemodynamic or anatomic derangement, treatment is not indicated but serial follow-up is indicated.

Lipomatous hypertrophy of the interatrial septum is a more common and more clinically relevant diagnosis because of the patient's predisposition to cardiac arrhythmias. The lesion appears as a nonencapsulated fatty mass within the atrial septum in continuity with the epicardial fat of the transverse pericardial sinus anteriorly and the atrioventricular groove posteriorly. The fossa ovalis itself is usually spared (24–26). Microscopically, the presence of fetal fat is a hallmark of lipomatous hypertrophy of the interatrial septum. Myocardial cells are usually seen entrapped in the mass.

Lesions other than lipomatous hypertrophy of the interatrial septum (including thrombi, amyloidosis, metastatic tumors, myxomas, and septal aneurysms) can present as septal masses. Although echocardiography may help distinguish these abnormalities, CT and MRI improve specificity by their ability to identify adipose tissue. The diagnosis of lipomatous hypertrophy of the interatrial septum by TTE has been well described by Fyke et al. (26). A high incidence of atrial arrhythmias has been described in these patients,

including multifocal atrial tachycardia and sinus arrest. Treatment is limited to controlling arrhythmias; surgical removal of fatty tissue is not indicated.

Papillary Fibroblastoma

Papillary fibroblastomas are the third most common histologic type of the benign cardiac tumors. Fibroelastomas were previously discovered as incidental finding at autopsy or during cardiac surgery, but now these masses are increasingly identified during TTE and TEE (27).

Echocardiography is the imaging technique of choice for the diagnosis and management of patients with fibroelastoma (Fig. 3A). By echo these tumors appear as small pedunculated mobile echo dense mass with a cystic appearance. Differential diagnosis include myxomas (rarely affecting

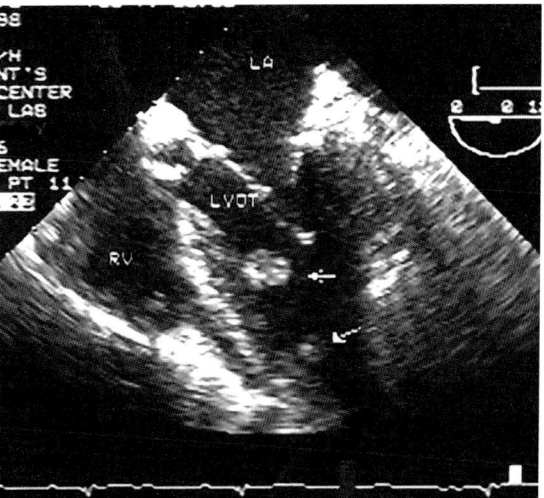

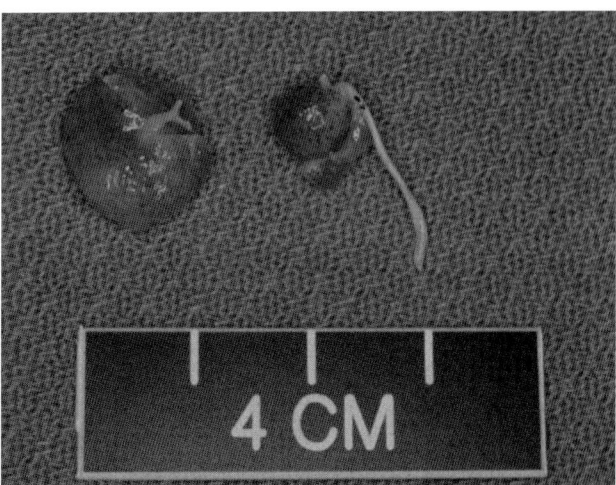

FIG. 3. A: Transesophageal echocardiogram demonstrating two small round masses (*arrowheads*) attached to the mid and lower portion of the interventricular septum. **B:** These masses were removed at the time of aortic valve replacement for aortic stenosis and by histology they were confirmed to be papillary fibroblastomas. *LA*, left atrium; *RV*, right ventricle; *LVOT*, left ventricular outflow tract.

valves), fibromas (nonencapsulated highly reflective), and Lambl excrescences (usually multiple and attached to either side of the leaflets).

Because of the propensity of fibroelastomas to embolize, prompt identification and localization of this tumor is essential so that surgical resection may be contemplated. TTE and TEE play a very important role in the management of patients with fibroelastomas.

Rhabdomyoma

Primary cardiac tumors of the heart are quite rare in infants and children, with rhabdomyomas comprising the most common group (more than 60% of pediatric tumors are rhabdomyomas). Rhabdomyomas can present at birth, in early infancy, or in childhood. Most cases present before 1 year of age. Usually, rhabdomyomas are multiple and occur with equal frequency in the right and left ventricle. They can also involve the atria but not the valves. Macroscopically these tumors are white to yellow and vary in size from a few millimeters to a few centimeters in diameter. They are circumscribed but not encapsulated. Microscopically they are characterized by large cells (spider cells) with vacuoles and a high glycogen content. Clinical presentation is quite varied ranging from absence of symptoms to acute severe heart failure and sudden death. Tuberous sclerosis and cardiac rhabdomyoma are frequently associated. Bass et al. (28) described the echocardiographic incidence of cardiac rhabdomyoma in tuberous sclerosis at 50%. An autopsy series by Fenoglio et al. (29) revealed a 30% incidence. Single or multiple echo-dense masses are detected in the ventricular septum or ventricular walls; they appear well circumscribed and are slightly brighter than the surrounding myocardium.

In the past, rhabdomyomas have been associated with a poor prognosis if untreated. However, recent studies advocate an expectant approach for the asymptomatic patient. Smythe et al. (30) followed 9 patients using echocardiography over a 2- to 15-year period. Diagnosis of rhabdomyoma was based on echocardiographic and angiographic criteria, not histology, but 78% had resolution whereas only 1 patient required surgery.

Fibromas

Cardiac fibromas are rare, benign neoplasms found primarily in children in a ratio of approximately 3:1 compared with adults. They are almost always solitary and located in the ventricular myocardium. Most grow to a diameter of 4 to 7 cm but they range in size from a few millimeters to over 10 cm in their greatest dimension. These tumors most often involve the anterior wall of the left ventricle and interventricular septum, the right ventricle, and rarely the atria.

Fibromas are the second most common benign cardiac tumor of childhood and are also associated with lethal ventricular arrhythmias and heart failure. Rarely, the tumor is also found in adults. Timely excision is indicated as the risk

of sudden death is significant. The tumor displaces rather than destroys adjacent tissue. Thus, the fibroma may be dissected from surrounding muscle by an epicardial approach with subsequent reapposition of the myocardium. A report of a right ventricular fibroma presenting as tricuspid stenosis and diagnosed by echocardiography was reported by Bapat et al. (31).

Fibromas have a characteristic echocardiographic appearance, typically hyperrefractile, solitary well demarcated, homogeneous intramural left ventricular masses. TTE has been used in planning surgical removal of an interventricular fibroma (32).

Over 50% of cardiac fibromas occur in the left ventricle. When localized in the apex of the left ventricle, fibromas need to be differentiated from other apical masses such as thrombus, eosinophilic cardiomyopathy, endomyocardial fibrosis, and malignant tumors.

Hemangiomas

Hemangiomas are comprised of benign proliferation of endothelial cells forming blood-containing channels. They occur in any site of the heart and pericardium, they are usually single, but can be multiple and are usually an incidental finding during autopsy. The echocardiographic finding of a solitary, nonpedunculated, nonhomogeneous right-sided mass, particularly when associated to a pericardial effusion, is more suggestive of a hemangioma than any other primary cardiac tumor. On coronary arteriography these tumors yield a characteristic ''tumor blush.''

Primary Malignant Tumors

Approximately 25% of primary cardiac tumors are malignant and most of these are sarcomas. Any of the cardiac chambers can be affected and because of their rapid proliferation primarily malignant tumors commonly extend through different anatomic planes, into the cardiac chambers and pericardium. There is some predilection for right heart structures.

MRI provides the best diagnostic tool for the evaluation of patients with known or suspected primary malignant tumors. Siripornpitak and Higgins (33) have described the MRI features of 7 patients with primary malignant cardiac tumors. By analyzing the length of attachment to cardiac structures, size of tumors, involvement of more than one chamber, extension to the pericardium or beyond the heart, and necrosis of the mass, they felt there were distinctive MR features to differentiate them from primary benign tumors. Lepore et al. (34) have described their surgical experience with primary malignant cardiac tumors and reported that a preoperative diagnosis of cardiac ''tumor'' was established by echocardiography in each of the 6 patients they treated surgically. Intramural tumor infiltration of the myocardium appears on echocardiography as localized wall thickening, a segment of hypocontractility, or areas of increased reflectivity.

Sarcomas

All primary malignant tumors are rare. Of these, the sarcomas comprise the largest proportion. Angiosarcomas are the most common, followed by rhabdomyosarcomas, fibrosarcomas, and osteosarcomas. The rest of the sarcomas are exceedingly rare and include leiomyosarcoma, liposarcoma, and synovial sarcoma. Regardless of the histological type cardiac sarcomas have a rapidly deteriorating clinical course and are uniformly fatal. The role of cardiac imaging in the management of these patients is directed to the initial diagnosis, evaluation of complications such as pericardial effusion and tamponade, palliative measurements, and assessment of prognosis.

Angiosarcomas (35) occur two to three times more often in adult men than in women and usually originate in the right atrium or pericardium. Clinically most patients present with right-sided heart failure or signs and symptoms of pericardial disease, or vena cava obstruction. A small proportion of patients present with systemic symptoms. Metastasis occurs most commonly to the lungs, lymph nodes, liver, and rarely, the brain. The high malignancy of this tumor is illustrated by a median survival of 3 months.

Histologically angiosarcomas are composed of anastomosing vascular channels formed by malignant cells, including spindle cells and anaplastic cells.

Rhabdomyosarcomas (36) originate with equal frequency in the left or right side of the heart, though involvement at multiple sites is common. Although rare in children, rhabdomyosarcomas have been reported in all decades of life and have a slight male predominance with a male-to-female ratio of 1.4:1. Clinically most patients present with systemic symptoms associated with findings of pericardial disease, pleuritic chest pain, dyspnea, and embolic phenomena.

The microscopic diagnosis of rhabdomyosarcomas is based on the demonstration of rhabdomyoblasts. Associated foci of necrosis and hemorrhage are common as well as pleomorphic tumor cells with cross-striations.

Various conditions have been reported in association with rhabdomyosarcomas, including hypertrophic osteoarthropathy, polyarthritis, amyloidosis, neurofibromatosis, eosinophilia, and mammopathy.

Fibrosarcomas also arise with equal frequency on the left and right side of the heart. Involvement of multiple sites is common. The tumor frequently protrudes into a cardiac chamber and affects a valve in approximately 50% of cases. Histologically, fibrosarcomas consists of spindle-shaped cells with elongated nuclei. In contrast to the rhabdomyosarcomas, pleomorphism is only minimal and necrosis is rare.

Osteosarcomas usually originate in the posterior wall of the atrium near the entrance of the pulmonary veins. They can be intramural or intracavitary. The clinical features of intramural sarcomas include conduction defects, arrhythmias, and asystole. The manifestations of an intracavitary osteosarcoma are similar to those of other sarcomas, including left ventricular inflow tract obstruction. Histologically, these tumors have areas of osteoid and malignant osteoblasts mixed with fibrosarcomatous zones.

Lymphomas

Of all lymphoma (37) patients, approximately 25% have cardiac involvement on autopsy, whereas primary lymphoma of the heart is exceedingly rare. There were only 7 patients described in the Armed Forces Institute of Pathology Series report by McAllister. All areas of the heart are involved including the pericardium. The lymphoma may become intracavitary and produce obstruction. Chou et al. (38) described a patient with primary cardiac lymphoma who presented with acute myocardial infarction and heart failure. Gallium and blood-pool scintigraphy suggested the diagnosis of primary cardiac lymphoma.

A variety of histologic types of cardiac lymphoma, including Hodgkin disease, lymphosarcoma, and reticulum cell sarcoma have been described. The lesions appear as nodules and rarely as polypoid growths in the endocardial surface.

Secondary Tumors of the Heart

Whereas primary tumors of the heart are rare, secondary tumors are common (39–41). Among unselected autopsied, the incidence is about 4% and this rises to about 20% in patients dying from malignancies. Tumors spread to the heart the same ways they spread elsewhere: direct extension, venous extension, and metastatic spread.

Direct Extension

The most common secondary tumors of the heart originate from continuous spread of tumors in the chest cavity. Carcinoma of the breast and carcinoma of the lung extend to the heart in this fashion. Because the atria are in direct contact with the pericardium, are less muscular, and have less vigorous contractions, they are more likely than the ventricles to be initially affected by the neoplasms. The initial clinical manifestation of these tumors is due to pericardial involvement with pericardial effusion and tamponade.

Venous Extension

Another form of direct extension of the tumors into the heart is through tumor growth along and within blood vessels. Renal cell carcinoma (42), Wilm tumor (43), adrenal carcinoma, hepatocellular carcinoma, and uterine leiomyosarcoma represent abdominal tumors that reach the heart through the inferior vena cava. Thyroid carcinoma has been described growing through the superior vena cava into the right atrium (44).

Echocardiographically these tumors appear as large masses extending from the vena cava into the right atrium. They may prolapse through the tricuspid valve partially occluding its orifice. Carcinoma of the lung may extend into the

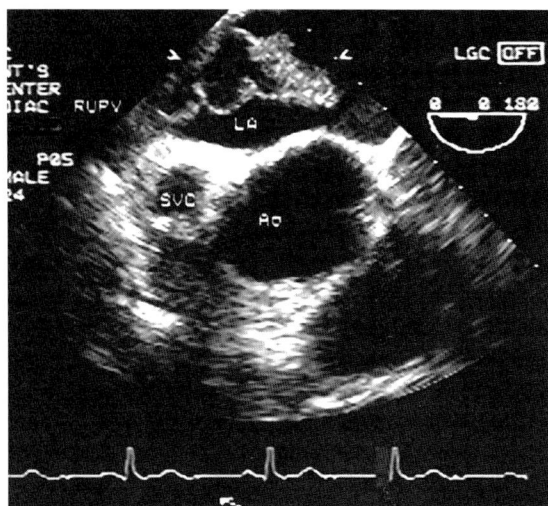

FIG. 4. Transesophageal echocardiogram demonstrating a left atrial mas invading the left atrium (*LA*) trough the right upper pulmonary vein (*RUPV*) in this patient with carcinoma of the lung. *Ao*, aorta; *SVC*, superior vena cava.

left atrium through the pulmonary veins (45) as illustrated in Figure 4. A report of a bronchogenic carcinoma reaching the left atrium through the pulmonary veins and embolizing to the aorta was described by Isada et al. (46).

Metastatic Spread

The hematogenous route is probably the most common form of metastatic spread. Tumor cells origination in the lung or breast pass through the lungs into the systemic circulation and reach the myocardium through the coronary arteries. In most series an equal number of right- and left-sided metastases are reported.

Most patients with cardiac metastasis have concomitant involvement of their mediastinal lymph nodes. These fill with tumor and eventually obstruct the lymphatics. Stagnated lymph flow allows for retrograde extension of the tumor. The leukemias and lymphomas have the greatest potential to involve the heart. By this route Mousseaux et al. (47) have recently described the use of MRI for the diagnosis of cardiac metastasis from malignant melanoma, and its superiority to echocardiography. By precisely detecting the extent of the tumors, MRI can be of great help in management, especially when an isolated metastasis may be suitable for surgical ablation.

REFERENCES

1. Bloor CM, O'Rourke RA. Cardiac tumors: clinical presentation and pathologic correlations. *Curr Probl Cardiol* 1984;9:7–48.
2. Endo A, Shigemasa C, Mashiba H, et al. Characteristics of 161 patients with cardiac tumors diagnosed during 1993 and 1994 in Japan. *Am J Cardiol* 1997;79:1708–1711.
3. Perchinsky MJ, Tyers GF, Lichtenstein SV. Primary cardiac tumors: forty years' experience with 71 patients. *Cancer* 1997;79:1809–1815.
4. Salcedo EE, Cohen GI, White RD, et al. Cardiac tumors: diagnosis and management. *Curr Probl Cardiol* 1992;17:2.
5. Roberts WC. Primary and secondary neoplasms of the heart. *Am J Cardiol* 1997;80:671–682.
6. McAllister HG Jr. Primary tumors and cysts of the heart and pericardium. *Curr Problems Cardiol* 1979; May.
7. Reymen K. Frequency of primary tumors of the heart. *Am J Cardiol* 1966;77:107.
8. Abraham DP, Reddy V, Gattusa P. Neoplasms metastatic to the heart: review of 3314 consecutive autopsies. *Am J Cardiovasc Path* 1990;3: 195–198.
9. Borges AC, Witt C, Bartel T, et al. Preoperative two- and three-dimensional transesophageal echocardiographic assessment of heart tumors. *Ann Thorac Surg* 1996;61:1163–1167.
10. Kupferwaser I, Mohr-Kahaly S, Erbel R, et al Three-dimensional imaging of cardiac mass lesions by transesophageal echocardiographic computed tomography. *Am Soc Echocardiogr* 1994;7:561–570.
11. Abrams HL, Adams DF, Grant HA. The radiology of tumors of the heart. *Radiol Clin North Am* 1971;9:299–326.
12. Effert S, Domanig E. The diagnosis of intra-atrial tumors and thrombi by the ultrasound echo method. *Ger Med Mon* 1959;4:1–3.
13. Detrano R, Salcedo BE, Simpfendorfer C, et al. Digital subtraction angiography in the evaluation of right heart tumors. *Am Heart J* 1985; 109:366–368.
14. Isley, Reinhardt. Intracardiac myxoma diagnosed by nuclear scanning. *Am J Roentgen* 1962;88:70–72.
15. Moncada R, Baker M, Salinas M, et al. Diagnostic role of computed tomography in pericardial heart disease: Congenital defects, thickening, neoplasms and effusions. *Am Heart J* 1982;103:263.
16. White RD, Zisch RJ. Magnetic resonance imaging of pericardial disease and paracardiac and intracradiae masses. In: Elliot LP, ed. *The fundamentals of cardiac imaging in infants, children, and adults*. Philadelphia: JB Lippincott Company, 1991:420–433.
17. Go RT, O'Connell JK, Underwood DA, et al. Comparison of gated cardiac MRI and 2D echocardiography of intracardiac neoplasms. *Am J Roentgenol* 1985;145:21–25.
18. Barakos JA, Brown JJ, Higgins CB. MR imaging of secondary cardiac and pericardiac lesions. *Am J Roentgenol* 1989;153:47–50.
19. Brown JJ, Barakos JA, Higgins CB. Magnetic resonance imaging of cardiac and pericardiac masses. *J Thorac Imag* 1989;4:58–64.
20. Pyke FE, Seward JB, Edwards WD, et al. Primary cardiac tumors: experience with 30 consecutive patients since the introduction of two-dimensional echocardiography. *J Am Coll Cardiol* 1985;5:1465–1473.
21. Gosse P, Herpin D, Roudault R, et al. Myxoma of the mitral valve diagnosed by echocardiography. *Am Heart J* 1986;111:803–805.
22. McCarthy PM, Piehler JM, Schaff HV, et al. The significance of multiple, recurrent, and complex cardiac myxomas. *J Thorac Cardiovas Surg* 1986;91:389–396.
23. Carney JA, Gordon H, Carpenter PC, et al: The complex of myxomas, spotty pigmentation and endocrine overactivity. *Medicine (Baltimore)* 1985;64:270–283.
24. Benvenuti LA, Campos RV, Lopes DO, et al. Primary lipomatous tumors of the cardiac valves. *South Med J* 1996;89:1018–1020.
25. Levine RA, Weyman AE, Dinsmore RE, et al. Noninvasive tissue characterization: Diagnosis of lipomatous hypertrophy of the atrial septum by nuclear magnetic resonance imaging. *J Am Coll Cardiol* 1986;7: 688–692.
26. Fyke FE III, Tajik AJ, Edward WD, et al. Diagnosis of lipomatous hypertrophy of the atrial septum by two-dimensional echocardiography. *J Am Coll Cardiol* 1983;1:1352–1357.
27. Shub C, Tajik AJ, Seward JB, et al. Cardiac papillary fibroelastomas. Two-dimensional echocardiographic recognition. *Mayo Clin Proc* 1981;56:629.
28. Bass JL, Breningstall GN, Swairman KF. Echocardiographic incidence of cardiac rhabdomyoma in tuberous sclerosis. *Am J Cardiol* 1985;53: 978–979.
29. Fenoglio JJ, McAllister HA, Ferrans VJ. Cardiac rhabdomyoma: a clinicopathologic and electron microscopic study. *Am J Cardiol* 1976;38: 241–251.
30. Smythe JF, Dick JD, Smallhorn JF, et al. Natural history of cardiac

rhabdomyoma in infancy and childhood. *Am J Cardiol* 1990;66: 1247–1249.

31. Bapat VN, Varma GG, Hordikar AA, et al. Right ventricular fibroma presenting as tricuspid stenosis: a case report. *Thorac Cardiovasc Surg* 1996;44:152–154.

32. Reece IJ, Houston AB, Pollack JCS. Interventricular fibroma: echocardiographic diagnosis and successful surgical removal in infancy. *Br Heart J* 1983;50:590.

33. Siripornpitak S, Higgins CB. MRI of primary malignant cardiovascular tumors. *J Comput Assist Tomogr* 1997;21:462–466.

34. Lepore V, Wallentin I, Bugge M, et al. Primary malignant cardiac tumors. *Minerva Cardioangiol* 1996;44:353–359.

35. Glancy EL, Morales JB, Roberts WC. Angiosarcoma of the heart. *Am J Cardiol* 1968;21:413–419.

36. Hui KS, Green LK, Schmidt WA. Primary cardiac rhabdomyosarcoma: definition of a rare entity. *Am J Cardiovascular Pathol* 1988; 2:19–29.

37. Roberts WC, Glancy DL, DeVita VT. Heart in malignant lymphoma (Hodgkin's disease, lymphosarcoma, reticulum cell sarcoma and mycosis fungoides): a study of 196 autopsy cases. *Am J Cardiol* 1968;22: 85–107.

38. Chou ST, Arkles LB, Gill GD, et al. Primary lymphoma of the heart: a case report. *Cancer* 1983;52:744–747.

39. Cohen GU, Perry TM, Evans JM. Neoplastic invasion of the heart and pericardium. *Ann Int Med* 1955;42:1238–1245.

40. Brian S, Hocbman A, Levij IS, et al. Clinical-diagnosis of secondary tumors of the heart and pericardium. *Dis Chest* 1959;55:202.

41. Smith LH. Secondary tumors of the heart. *Rev Surg* 1976;33:223–231.

42. Choh JH, Gurney R, Shenoy SS, et al. Renal-cell carcinoma. *N Y State J Med* 1981;929–932.

43. Murphy DA, Rabinovitch H, Chevalier L, et al. Wilm's tumor in right atrium. *Am J Dis Child* 1973;126:210–211.

44. Kim RH, Mautner L, Henning J. An unusual case of thyroid carcinoma with direct extension in to great veins right heart and pulmonary arteries. *Can Med Assoc J* 1966;94:238.

45. Gandhi AK, Pearson AC, Orsinelli DA. Tumor invasion of the pulmonary veins: a unique source of systemic embolism detected by transesophageal echocardiography. *J Am Soc Echocardiog* 1995;8:97–99.

46. Isada LR, Salcedo EE, Homa DA, et al. Intraoperative transesophageal echocardiographic localization of tumor embolus during pneumonectomy. *J Am Soc Echocardigr* 1992;5:551–554.

47. Mousseaux E, Meunier P, Azancott S, et al. Cardiac metastatic melanoma investigated by magnetic resonance imaging. *Magn Reson Imaging* 1998;16:91–95.

CHAPTER 62

Cardiac Thrombi

Michael J. Longo and Michael D. Ezekowitz

Intracardiac thrombi are most frequently located in the left ventricle after acute transmural myocardial infarction or in patients with dilated cardiomyopathy and in the left atrium in association with atrial fibrillation or rheumatic mitral valve disease. Less frequently, thrombi are found in the right atrium and ventricle. The detection of cardiac thrombi is of importance given the risk of embolization. Several imaging techniques are available to identify intracardiac thrombi. This chapter evaluates the merits of these imaging techniques, with special focus on echocardiography, which is the technique of choice in most instances.

LEFT VENTRICULAR THROMBUS

Left ventricular thrombi occur most commonly in association with acute myocardial infarction (1,2), chronic left ventricular aneurysm (3), and dilated cardiomyopathy (4,5). Less commonly, thrombi have been reported with trauma and in the antiphopholipid antibody syndrome (6). Left ventricular thrombus develops in approximately 30% of patients after acute myocardial infarction and occurs almost exclusively with anterior myocardial infarction (7). Factors associated with thrombus formation after transmural myocardial infarction are those related to local stasis; reduced global ventricular function, larger infarction, atrial fibrillation, and focal areas of apical akinesis or dyskinesis (8). Left ventricular thrombus must be differentiated from tumors, normal cardiac structures—in particular, muscle trabeculations, papillary muscles, and the mitral valve supporting structures—and artifacts produced from the imaging techniques used in their diagnosis. Several imaging techniques are available for the detection of left ventricular thrombus, including two-dimensional echocardiography, platelet scintigraphy, computed tomography, magnetic resonance imaging, contrast angiography, and radionuclide angiography.

M. J. Longo: Virginia Mason Medical Center, Seattle, Washington 98111.
M. D. Ezekowitz: Department of Cardiology, Clinical Trials Office, Yale University, New Haven, Connecticut 06510.

Echocardiography

Transthoracic echocardiography (TTE) is the most widely used technique for the diagnosis of the left ventricular clot. Its popularity is based on favorable cost, general availability, and its noninvasive nature that is free of known dangers. Most instruments are compact and portable; thus, studies can be performed at the patient's bedside in the intensive care unit. This is particularly important when considering patients who are unstable. Although echocardiography is often superfluous for the diagnosis of acute infarction (9), it frequently provides important diagnostic information, however. There is an important relationship between the extent of acute left ventricular dysfunction and serious complications, such as death, heart failure, and arrhythmia (10,11). Patients with a detectable anatomic impairment have a 4-to-5-fold higher risk for major in-hospital complications (12). This information is obtainable by a skilled echocardiographer in a few minutes. A baseline study also serves as a frame of reference for specific complications that may occur later.

For the evaluation of the left ventricle, a 2- or 2.25-mHz transducer is used. This represents an acceptable compromise between adequate penetration of the ultrasonic beam and the resolution of the image. For the evaluation of the left ventricle for thrombus, it is critical to evaluate the anterior-apical segment, the most important site of thrombus formation (Fig. 1). The apical two- and four-chamber views are most commonly used. Careful adjustment of gain and the use of multiple views are necessary for an accurate diagnosis. In addition, the use of a high-frequency transducer (5 mHz) with a short focus and a high near-field resolution is useful to obtain optimal and detailed apical imaging.

Accuracy of Echocardiography Detection of Thrombi

Over the past decade, numerous studies have been performed that have defined the accuracy of this technique in identifying thrombi in the left ventricle. Early studies using

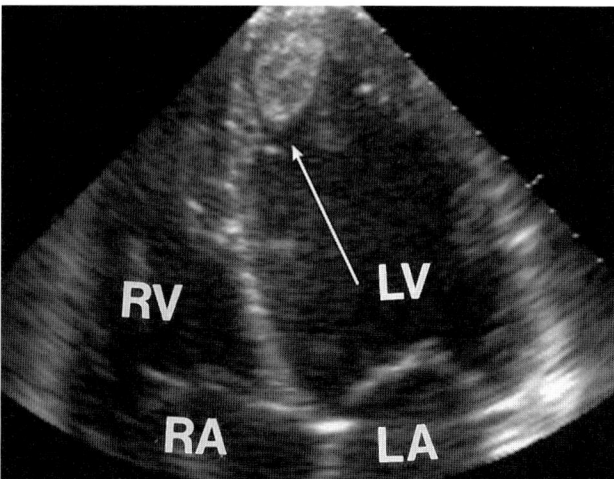

FIG. 1. Transthoracic apical four-chamber view. *Arrow* points to a thrombus at the apex of the left ventricle in a patient after anterior wall myocardial infarction. *LV*, left ventricle; *LA*, left atrium; *RV*, right ventricle; *RA*, right atrium.

M-Mode echocardiography were neither sensitive nor specific for identifying left ventricular thrombus because it is seldom possible to examine the cardiac apex, where more than 90% of thrombi occur (13–15). Therefore, the modality of choice is TTE. It offers spatial resolution enabling examination of the apex of the heart in most patients from either the apical or subxyphoid transducer positions. To distinguish a thrombus from an artifact, it is important to use strict criteria for thrombus diagnosis (16). The thrombus should be adjacent to (but distinct from) abnormal contracting myocardium, be seen in at least two transducer positions, and be distinguished by a clear thrombus blood interface. The interior of the thrombus may be highly echogenic. If the thrombus is homogenous, the interior may be relatively echo free. The thrombus may be classified as mural, protuberant, or mobile (17–19). The accuracy of two-dimensional echocardiography in diagnosing thrombus has been assessed in several surgical and autopsy studies with a reported sensitivity of 77 to 95% and specificity of 86 to 100% (20–23). In addition, the presence of abnormal spatial patterns of mitral inflow accessed by color Doppler provides additive information for the prediction of left ventricular thrombus formation after myocardial infarction (24). Thus, for the vast majority of patients, echocardiography is a very accurate technique for the identification of left ventricular thrombus.

Optimal Timing for Echocardiographical Imaging of Thrombi following Myocardial Infarction

The optimal timing for echocardiography in acute myocardial infarction depends not only on when thrombi can be visualized, but also on when emboli occur and on the expected effect of therapy. Several prospective studies in patients with acute myocardial infarction have shown that ap-

proximately half of all left ventricular thrombi develop between 48 and 72 hours, and approximately 80% develop within the first week (2,25–29). It is important to recognize that very early studies, i.e., within the first 48 to 72 hours after the infarction, may fail to identify thrombi that may form later. Therefore, in patients with large myocardial infarction who are at high risk for developing a thrombus, echocardiographic examinations should be performed within 48 to 72 hours of the acute episode; if no thrombus is detected, the echocardiogram should be repeated, if there is a clinical need, at 1 week to 2 weeks after infarction. Later studies should be reserved for patients with predischarge left ventricular aneurysm, severe congestive heart failure, and deteriorating systolic function, because, in these patients, the risk of late development of ventricular thrombosis remains high (30). In many patients, the decision to anticoagulate is independent of the presence of clot. Thus, clinical judgment should be used regarding the necessity for future examinations.

In patients with acute myocardial infarction, the risk of embolization is highest in the first few days and decreases over time with approximately two thirds of systemic emboli occurring within the first week after the index infarction (18,19,31–34). Patients with left ventricular thrombi continue to be at increased risk of embolization as long as 5 years after myocardial infarction, although the risk is less than in the acute period (35). Thus, the risk of embolization is highest immediately after infarction; emboli may occur as early as the first day, and the presence of thrombus indicates a persistently increased risk.

Echocardiographic Stratification of Risk for Thromboembolism

Because the overall risk of embolization following myocardial infarction is low, it is important to identify subgroups of patients at higher risk of embolization. A number of investigators have identified anterior transmural myocardial infarction as the major source of intracardiac thrombi, and, therefore of systemic embolization (36,37). The risk of systemic embolization in patients with inferior myocardial infarction and subendocardial myocardial infarction is small (36,37). Large inferior myocardial infarction that involves the anteroapical segment has the same risk of developing intraventricular thrombi and systemic embolization as anterior myocardial infarction and should be treated accordingly.

The presence of thrombus indicates a significant risk for subsequent embolization in both the chronic setting, as well as in the acute setting (33,36). In addition, the morphology and mobility of the thrombus both predict risk for embolization. Several studies have shown a positive correlation between the mobility of the clot, its protuberance into the ventricular cavity, and the risk of subsequent embolization (31–33,38,39). These studies show that the more mobile and protuberant the thrombus, the more likely it is to embolize. An extensive and prospective evaluation of the morphologic characteristics of left ventricular clot showed considerable spontaneous variation in the characteristics of a thrombus (29). Mobile thrombi may become immobile, and mural thrombi may become protuberant and vice versa. These changes may occur over widely disparate times. Therefore, caution must be exercised in the analysis of the morphologic features of thrombi.

Transesophageal Echocardiography

In some patients, TTE is technically inadequate or cannot confirm the presence of a thrombus. Transesophageal echocardiography (TEE) has better resolution and signal-to-noise ratio than transthoracic echocardiography and thus can be helpful in differentiating left ventricular thrombus from other structures. In a study of 36 patients with equivocal results for the diagnosis of left ventricular thrombus by TTE, Chen et al. (40), using TEE identified thrombus in 19 of the 36 patients (53%), with 6 patients (31%) experiencing arterial embolization. To date, the sensitivity and specificity of TEE for the detection of left ventricular thrombi has not been determined, but it remains a reasonable alternative to transthoracic echocardiography in patients with technically inadequate or nondiagnostic studies. It will frequently miss left ventricular (LV) thrombus localized to the apex.

Indium 111 Platelet Scintigraphy

Thakur et al. (41) first chelated 111 indium, a gamma-emitting radioisotope with 8-hydroxy quinoline, a molecule that permitted passage of the isotope into the cell and the labeling of platelets with an imageable isotope. The labeling procedure did not alter the physiologic function of the cells. Thus, it was possible to inject labeled platelets into patients and image clot in (theoretically) any location in the body. This technique depends on the active exchange of platelets between the blood and the thrombus surface and, thus, not only allows identification of the thrombus, but also reflects its activity (42,43). In patients with left ventricular aneurysm, this technique has been found to be highly specific, with a figure that approached 100% (20). The sensitivity for clot detection was lower, 72%, reflecting the relative inactivity of clot that is long-standing (20). Although comparative studies have not been performed in patients with acute infarction, one would anticipate that sensitivity would be higher because of the active formation of clot.

Interpretation of Platelet Scintigraphic Images

Thrombi are most often represented as a single "hot spot." Multiple hot spots may be seen, but this is less common. A thrombus may be imaged tangentially, in which case a linear area of increased activity is depicted. Occasionally, in a clot that is laminated against an aneurysm, a doughnut-shaped image is seen. Increased activity caused by a thrombus tends to be maximal 3 to 4 days after injection of the

platelet suspension. Occasionally, cardiac myxomas may accumulate platelets on their surface and be mistaken for thrombi. With attention to these details, errors with interpretation are unusual. It must also be noted that antiplatelet and anticoagulant drugs may suppress the activity of labeled platelets and cause false-negative results (43,44).

Platelets interact in a dynamic manner at the blood thrombus interface and therefore, platelet scintigraphy might be used as a direct index of thrombus activity and provide information that is complementary to that offered by echocardiography. In patients with left ventricular thrombus diagnosed by echocardiography, it has been shown that platelet scintigraphy can be used as an excellent predictor of embolic risk and enhances the risk stratification of patients, thus permitting the selection of high-risk patients for therapy (45).

Although it is true that platelet scintigraphy offers functional information on thrombus activity that is not provided by echocardiography, its relatively low sensitivity, high cost, and the extended period of time required for the acquisition and interpretation of images limits it clinical utility.

Magnetic Resonance Imaging and Computed Tomography

Magnetic resonance imaging (MRI) and computed tomography (CT) generate high-resolution images of the cardiovascular system and are very effective techniques for the detection of left ventricular thrombi (46–48) (see Chapters 28 and 29). CT has been shown to be as sensitive and more specific for the identification of left ventricular thrombus than echocardiography (49). However, systematic studies during the acute stage of myocardial infarction have not been performed. This is likely because of the fact that these techniques are costly and cumbersome, and it is not feasible to transport sick patients to the imaging facilities. MRI and CT are expensive imaging alternatives to echocardiography that are not routinely used for identifying left ventricular thrombus, but may be a useful test if the echocardiographic examination is suboptimal (see Chapter 46).

Contrast Ventriculography

Contrast ventriculography was the first technique used for the diagnosis of left ventricular clot. The reported sensitivity is 31 to 75%, and specificity of 67 to 100% (3,22,50). The insensitivity of this technique is because clots are often laminated against the wall of the ventricle and cannot be seen. It is not specific because thrombi form in large-volume ventricles that are incompletely opacified with contrast material and therefore, apparent filling defects caused by incomplete mixing often lead to overdiagnosis. Furthermore, there is an added risk of precipitating systemic embolization with this technique.

Radionuclide Angiography

Stranton and Ritchie (51) evaluated the use of radionuclide angiography as a means of identifying left ventricular thrombi. The diagnosis of a left ventricular thrombus should be considered if a discreet filling defect or a square ventricular apex is identified on routine images. However, the technique has proved insensitive to small thrombi and was only able to detect those that protrude significantly into the ventricular cavity. From a practical standpoint, the low sensitivity (31 to 62%) (56) of this technique precludes its use as a routine clinical test, although the reported sensitivity is high at 92 to 100% (51).

LEFT ATRIAL THROMBI

Thrombus in the left atrium (LA) is most commonly associated with atrial fibrillation, mitral valve disease (in particular, rheumatic mitral stenosis), and dilated cardiomyopathy (52). Less frequently, left atrial thrombi have been reported with atrial septal aneurysm, heart transplantation (53), and the antiphospholipid antibody syndrome (6). The incidence of thrombus in the left atrium in patients with mitral valve disease and/or atrial fibrillation reported by autopsy and surgical studies ranges from 16 to 64% (56–59). There is an inverse relation between the severity of mitral regurgitation and the prevalence of left atrial thrombi. This protective effect has been hypothesized as being related to the mixing of atrial contents as blood from the left ventricle is injected into the atrium at high velocity during ventricular systole (58).

Thrombus in the left atrium may be located in the body of the left atrium, the left atrial appendage (LAA), or on the interatrial septum. Thrombus in the LAA is frequently attached to the tip or the lateral wall, but it may also completely fill the lumen of the appendage. Left atrium thrombus must be differentiated from tumors, especially myxomas, normal anatomic structures, and artifacts produced by the various imaging techniques used for their detection. The classic appearance of a left atrial myxoma is an irregularly shaped mobile mass attached to the interatrial septum in the region of the fossa ovalis that lies in the atrial cavity during systole and prolapses through the mitral valve during diastole. These features usually allow atrial myxomas to be accurately differentiated from thrombus. Echocardiograpy, CT, MRI, platelet scintigraphy, radionuclide angiography, coronary angiography, and pulmonary arteriography can be used to diagnose left atrial thrombi. Of these techniques, TEE and CT are the most useful with TEE the most widely employed.

Echocardiography

Detection of left atrial thrombi with transthoracic echocardiography is limited due to the posterior location of the left atrium and the difficulty in imaging of the LAA. Herzog et al. (60) reported a modified short-axial parasternal view to improve detection of thrombi in the LAA. Even with this approach, however, the LAA may be visualized in less than

20% of cases. The reported sensitivity and specificity for transthoracic echocardiography and the detection of left atrial thrombi are 28% to 59% and 99%, respectively (54,61–63), with the majority of false-negative cases due to thrombi located in the LAA.

Transesophageal Echocardiography

TEE can overcome the limitation of the transthoracic approach and has emerged as the technique of choice for the detection of clot in the left atrium and LAA (Fig. 2). With the left atrium being adjacent to the esophagus, it is easily accessible to the transducer, and various tomographic sections can be readily obtained with a biplane or multiplane probe. The left atrium and LAA are visualized in the basal short-axis, four-chamber, and longitudinal two-chamber view (see Chapter 4). For the evaluation of thrombus, the left atrium and LAA are initially viewed in the horizontal (0 degree) plane, and the probe is slowly withdrawn until the bifurcation of the pulmonary artery is visualized. The left atrium and LAA are then viewed in the vertical plane (90%) followed by posterior and anterior rotation of the probe until the coronary sinus and aorta are visualized respectively. Using a multiplane probe the above steps are followed with 5- to 10-degree stepwise rotation of the imaging sector from 0 to 180 degrees.

It must be emphasized that the LAA is a complex structure with a wide variability in size and configuration. The greatest difficulty arises in distinguishing thrombus from the pectinate muscles of the LAA. By visualizing the LAA in multiple planes, however, the pectinate muscles can usually be

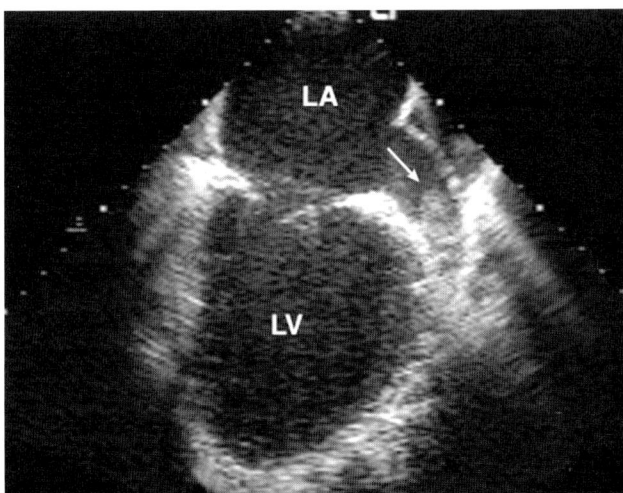

FIG. 2. Transesophageal two-chamber view. *Arrow* points to a thrombus in the left atrial appendage in a 40-year-old patient with nonischemic cardiomyopathy admitted with new onset atrial fibrillation and abdominal pain. *LA*, left atrium; *LV*, left ventricle.

clearly visualized and accurately distinguished from thrombus. Additionally, the presence of an infolding ridge of tissue separating the left upper pulmonary vein from the LAA is now well recognized and should not be misinterpreted as thrombus. The presence of spontaneous echo contrast may conceal the presence of thrombi. The reported sensitivity and specificity for TEE in the detection of left atrial thrombi is 83 to 100%, and 97 to 100% (56,57,64,65). The presence on TEE of a mobile thrombus or a maximal thrombus dimension greater than 1 centimeter has been shown to be an independent predictor of embolization (66). TEE is commonly performed in a search for atrial thrombi among patients presenting with thromboembolism and also to exclude atrial thrombi before procedures that are associated with increased risk of embolization if atrial thrombi are present, such as cardioversion from atrial fibrillation and percutaneous balloon mitral valvuloplasty.

Computed Tomography

CT is a very effective technique for the detection of left atrial thrombi (67), even if thrombi are located in the LAA or lateral wall of the left atrium (Fig. 3). Recent studies have shown CT to be more sensitive than transthoracic echocardiography for the detection of left atrial thrombi (68); however, the diagnostic accuracy of CT compared with TEE has yet to be determined. Theoretically, it may be possible to differentiate a new thrombus from an old thrombus by virtue of the increased density of the latter due to a higher percentage of fibrous tissue and the presence of calcification or capillary blood supply, but this remains to be determined. CT has the advantage of offering uniform slices of the heart in an attempt to detect thrombi in unknown areas of the heart. Its

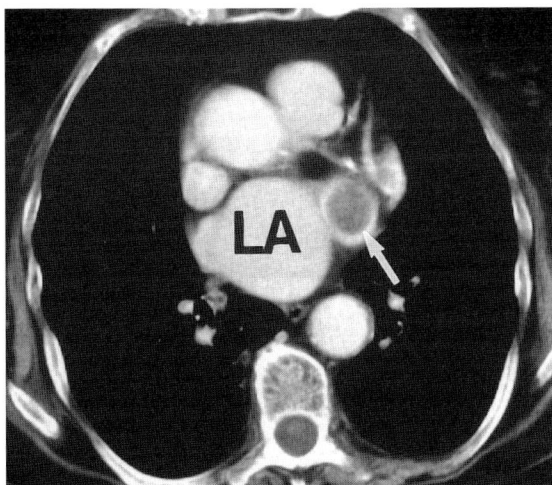

FIG. 3. Computed tomography with *arrow* pointing to a thrombus in a dilated left atrial appendage in a patient with atrial fibrillation. *LA*, left atrium.

use is limited by the need for the injection of approximately 70 mL of contrast material, its cost, and its failure to provide information about thrombus mobility and embolization, although cine CT using short scan times may be able to overcome this limitation. Despite these concerns, CT remains a reasonable alternative when the results of TEE are equivocal or left atrial thrombus is strongly suspected, but not detected by TEE.

Radionuclide Studies

When the left atrium and LAA are enlarged, they may be visualized with radionuclide angiography. Using the criteria of nonvisualization of the left atrium or of LAA, Uehara et al. (69), in a group of patients undergoing surgery for mitral valve disease, reported a sensitivity of 83% and a specificity of 79% for first-pass radionuclide angiography for the detection of left atrial thrombus. A higher diagnostic accuracy with 100% sensitivity and 80% specificity was reported when only thrombi in the LAA were considered.

Experience with I-111 platelet scintigraphy is limited. Yamada et al. (70) reported a sensitivity of 80% and specificity of 100% for platelet scintigraphy in diagnosis of left atrial thrombi. Despite the favorable results of these studies, given the limited experience with these techniques and the superiority of TEE and CT, it is difficult to advocate their use in the diagnosis of left atrial thrombi.

Coronary Angiography

Left atrial thrombus may be detected on coronary angiography by the presence of neovascularization and fistula formation between the coronary arteries and the left atrium (71,72). This may be the result of partial necrosis of the thrombus that allows the contrast medium to pass into the left atrial cavity (71). Cardiac tumors, particularly myxomas, and congenital anomalies, may also have this angiographic appearance and must be differentiated from thrombus. Angiography has a reported sensitivity of 33 to 70% and specificity of 55 to 95% (71,72). The invasive nature of coronary angiography is a drawback to its potential as a screening test for left atrial thrombi. However, since coronary angiography is often performed prior to surgery in patients with mitral valve disease, these signs should be looked for and may raise suspicion for the presence of left atrial thrombi.

RIGHT ATRIAL THROMBI

Right atrial (RA) thrombi are most frequently associated with indwelling central venous catheters (73), dilated cardiomyopathy, and constrictive pericarditis (74). They have also been reported in association with atrial fibrillation, atrial septal aneurysm, and the antiphospholipid antibody syndrome (6). Of great clinical importance, thrombi may be transiently located in the right atrium, having already embolized from a distant source. Right atrial thrombi are rare, but recent studies suggest that the incidence of right atrial thrombus may be higher than previously appreciated. Korones et al. (75) demonstrated a 9% incidence of right atrial thrombi in children with acute leukemia and indwelling venous catheters using transthoracic echocardiography. Gilon et al. (73) showed a 12.5% incidence of right atrial thrombus in bone marrow transplantation patients with central venous catheters using TEE. Furthermore, transthoracic echocardiogram studies of patients with acute pulmonary embolism have shown the presence of right heart thrombi in 7 to 11% of patients (76).

Echocardiography, CT, and MRI have detected right atrial thrombi. Although no comparative studies exist, TEE appears to be the imaging modality of choice for detecting right atrial thrombi. Right atrial thrombi must be differentiated from other right atrial masses—such as myxoma and other primary and secondary tumors, particularly hypernephroma, tricuspid valve endocarditis as well as normal anatomic structures such as the eustachian valve, chiari network and tricuspid valve and supporting structures that may mimic their appearance. It is likely that small thrombi are underdiagnosed due to the difficulties in differentiating sessile thrombi from the atrial wall and because small thrombi may exceed the resolution capabilities of these techniques.

RIGHT VENTRICULAR THROMBI

Right ventricular thrombi are rarely diagnosed antemortem. They are most commonly seen in association with right ventricular infarction (77), cardiomyopathy (78), and indwelling venous catheters or pacemakers (5). Right ventricular thrombi have also been reported with blunt chest trauma (79), endomyocardial fibroelastosis (80), and in the antiphospholipid antibody syndrome (6). Echocardiography is used most commonly to make the diagnosis, although CT and MRI are reasonable alternative approaches. Right ventricular thrombus must be differentiated from tumors, tricuspid valve vegetations, and the tricuspid valve supporting structures.

REFERENCES

1. Keeley EC, Hillis LD. Left ventricular mural thrombus after acute myocardial infarction. *Clin Card* 1996;19:83–89.
2. Asinger RW, Mikell FL, Elsperger J, et al. Incidence of left ventricular thrombus after acute transmural myocardial infarction: serial evaluation by two dimensional echocardiography. *N Engl J Med* 1981;305:297–304.
3. Reeder GS, Lengyl M, Tajic AJ, et al. Mural thrombus in left ventricular aneurysm: incidence, role of angiography and relation between anticoagulation and embolization. *Mayo Clin Proc* 1981;56:77–84.
4. Gottdeiner JS, Gay JA, VanVorhees L, et al. Frequency and embolic potential of left ventricular thrombus in dilated cardiomyopathy as-

sessed by two dimensional echocardiography. *Am J Cardiol* 1983;52:1281–1289.
5. Waller BF, Grider L, Rohr JM, et al. Intracardiac thrombi: frequency, location, etiology, and complications: a morphologic review. *Clin Cardiol* 1995;18:477–486.
6. Kaplan SD, Chartash E, Pizzarello RA, et al. Cardiac manifestations of the antiphospholipid syndrome. *Am Heart J* 1992;124:1331–1338.
7. Dantzig JM, Delewarre BJ, Bot H, et al. Left ventricular thrombus in acute myocardial infarction. *Eur Heart J* 1996;17:1640–1649.
8. Weinrich DJ, Bricke JF, Pauletto FJ. Left ventricular mural thrombi complicating myocardial infarction. Long term follow up with serial echocardiography. *Ann Intern Med* 1984;100:789–794.
9. Kloner RA, Parisi AS. Acute myocardial infarction: diagnostic and prognostic applications of two-dimensional echocardiography. *Circulation* 1987;75:521–524.
10. Horowitz RS, Morganroth J, Parrotto C, et al. Immediate diagnosis of acute myocardial infarction by two-dimensional echocardiography. *Circulation* 1982;65:323–329.
11. Gibson RS, Bishop HL, Stamm RB, et al. Value of early two-dimensional echocardiography in patients with acute MI. *Am J Cardiol* 1982;49:1110–1116.
12. Nishimura RA, Tajik AJ, Shub C, et al. Role of two-dimensional echocardiography in the prediction of in hospital complications after myocardial infarction. *J Am Coll Cardiol* 1984;4:1080–1089.
13. Horowitz RS, Morganroth J. Immediate detection of high risk patients with acute myocardial infarction using two-dimensional echocardiographic evaluation of left ventricular regional wall motion abnormalities. *Am Heart J* 1982;103:814–823.
14. Horgan JH, O'Mshiel F, Goodman AC. Demonstration of left ventricular thrombus by conventional echocardiography. *J Clin Ultrasound* 1976;4:287–288.
15. Kramer NE, Rathod R, Chawla KK, et al. Echocardiographic diagnosis of left ventricular mural thrombi occurring in cardiomyopathy. *Am Heart J* 1978;96:381–383.
16. Dejoseph RL, Shiroff FA, Levenson LW, et al. Echocardiographic diagnosis of intraventricular clot. *Chest* 1977;71:417–419.
17. van den Bos AA, Vletter WB, Hagemeijer F. Progressive development of left ventricular thrombus. Detection and evolution studied with echocardiographic techniques. *Chest* 1978;74:307–309.
18. Meltzer RS, Visser CA, Kan G, et al. Two-dimensional echocardiographic appearance of left ventricular thrombi with systemic emboli after myocardial infarction. *Am J Cardiol* 1984;53:1511–1513.
19. Haugland JM, Asinger RW, Mikell FL, et al. Embolic potential of left ventricular thrombi detected by two-dimensional echocardiography. *Circulation* 1984;70:588–598.
20. Ezekowitz MD, Wilson DA, Smith EO, et al. Comparison of indium-111 platelet scintigraphy and two-dimensional echocardiography in the diagnosis of left ventricular thrombi. *N Engl J Med* 1982;306:1509–1513.
21. Visser CA, Kan G, David GK, et al. Two-dimensional echocardiography in the diagnosis of left ventricular thrombus. A prospective study of 67 patients with anatomic validation. *Chest* 1983;83:228–232.
22. Stratton JR, Lighty GW, Pearlman AS, et al. Detection of left ventricular thrombus by two-dimensional echocardiography: sensitivity, specificity and causes of uncertainty. *Circulation* 1982;66:156–166.
23. Sheiban I, Casarotto D, Trevi G, et al. Two-dimensional echocardiography in the diagnosis of intracardiac masses: a prospective study with anatomic validation. *Cardiovasc Intervent Radiol* 1987;10:157–161.
24. Maze SS, Kotler MA, Pavy WR. The contribution of color flow Doppler imaging to the assessment of left ventricular thrombus. *Am Heart J* 1988;115:479–482.
25. Jordan RA, Miller RD, Edwards JE, et al. Thromboembolism in acute and healed myocardial infarction. Intracardiac mural thrombosis. *Circulation* 1952;6:1–6.
26. Gueret P, Duborg O, Ferrier A, et al. Effects of full dose heparin anticoagulation on the development of left ventricular thrombosis in acute transmural myocardial infarction. *J Am Coll Cardiol* 1986;8:419–426.
27. Davis MJE, Ireland MA. Effect of early anticoagulation on the frequency of left ventricular thrombi after anterior wall acute myocardial infarction. *Am J Cardiol* 1986;57:1244–1247.

28. Spirito P, Bellotti P, Chiarella F, et al. Prognostic significance and natural history of left ventricular thrombi in patients with acute anterior myocardial infarction. A 2D echocardiographic study. *Circulation* 1985;72:774–780.

29. Domenicucci S, Bellotti P, Chiarella F, et al. Spontaneous morphologic changes in left ventricular thrombi: a prospective two-dimensional echocardiographic study. *Circulation* 1987;75:737–743.

30. Keren A, Goldberg S, Gottlieb S, et al. Natural history of left ventricular thrombi: their appearance and resolution in the posthospitalization period of acute myocardial infarction. *J Am Coll Cardiol* 1990;15:790–800.

31. Stratton JR, Resnick AD. Increased embolic risk in patients with left ventricular thrombi. *Circulation* 1987;75:1004–1011.

32. Lary BG, deTakats G. Peripheral arterial embolism after myocardial infarction: occurrence in unsuspected cases and ambulatory patients. *JAMA* 1954;155:10.

33. Thompson PL, Robinson JS. Stroke after myocardial infarction: relation to infarct size. *BMJ* 1978;2:457–459.

34. Darling RC, Austen G, Linton RR. Arterial embolism. *Surg Gynecol Obstet* 1967;124:106–114.

35. Visser CA, Kan G, Meltzer RS, et al. Embolic potential of left ventricular thrombus after myocardial infarction: a two-dimensional echocardiographic study of 119 patients. *J Am Coll Cardiol* 1985;5:1276–1280.

36. Johannessen KA, Nordrehaug JE, Lippe G. Left ventricular thrombosis and cerebrovascular accident in acute myocardial infarction. *Br Heart J* 1984;51:553–556.

37. Keating EC, Gross SA, Schlamowitz RA, et al. Mural thrombi in myocardial infarctions: prospective evaluation by two-dimensional echocardiography. *Am J Med* 1983;74:989–995.

38. Weinreich DJ, Burke JF, Pauletto FJ. Left ventricular mural thrombi complicating acute myocardial infarction: long term follow up with serial echocardiography. *Ann Intern Med* 1984;100:789–794.

39. Johannessen K. Peripheral emboli from left ventricular thrombi of different echocardiographic appearance in acute myocardial infarction. *Arch Intern Med* 1987;147:641–644.

40. Chen C, Koschyk D, Hamm C, et al. Usefulness of transesophageal echocardiography in identifying small left ventricular apical thrombus. *J Am Coll Cardiol* 1993;21:208–215.

41. Thakur ML, Welch MJ, Joist JM, et al. Indium-111 labeled platelets: studies on the preparation and evaluation of *in vitro* and *in vivo* functions. *Thromb Res* 1976;9:345–357.

42. Stratton JR. Indium-111 platelet imaging of left ventricular thrombi: predictive value for systemic emboli. Presented at the International Meeting on Left Ventricular Thrombosis after Myocardial Infarction. Genoa, Italy, October 21, 1988.

43. Stratton JR, Ritchie JL. The effects of antithrombotic drugs in patients with LV thrombi: assessment with indium-111 platelet imaging and two-dimensional echocardiography. *Circulation* 1984;69:561–568.

44. Bellotti P, Claudiani F, Chiarella F, et al. Left ventricular thrombi: changes in size and platelet deposition during treatment with indobufen and ticlopidine. *Cardiology* 1990;77:272–279.

45. Stratton JR, Ritchie JL. 111 In platelet imaging of left ventricular thrombi: predictive value for systemic emboli. *Circulation* 1990;81:1182–1189.

46. Gomes AS, Lois JF, Child JS, et al. Cardiac tumors and thrombus: evaluation with MR imaging. *Am J Roentgenol* 1987;149:895–899.

47. Tomada H, Hoshai M, Furuya M, et al. Evaluation of left ventricular thrombus with computed tomography. *Am J Cardiol* 1981;48:573–577.

48. Goldstein JA, Schiller NB, Lipton MJ, et al. Evaluation of left ventricular thrombi by contrast enhanced computed tomography and two-dimensional echocardiography. *Am J Cardiol* 1986;57:757–760.

49. Tomora H, Hoshia M, Furuya H, et al. Evaluation of intracardiac thrombus with computed tomography. *Am J Cardiol* 1983;51:843–851.

50. Raphael MJ, Steiner RC, Goodwin JF, et al. Cineangiography of left ventricular aneurysm. *Clin Radiol* 1972;23:129–139.

51. Stratton JR, Ritchie JL, Hammermeister KE, et al. Detection of left ventricular thrombi with radionuclide angiography. *Am J Cardiol* 1981;48:565–572.

52. Chiarella F, Bellone P. The diagnosis of left atrial thrombus. *G Ital Cardiol* 1994;24:303–314.

53. Derumeaux G, Mouton-Schleifer D, Soyer R, et al. High incidence of left atrial thrombus detected by transesophageal echocardiography in heart transplant recipients. *Eur Heart J* 1995;16:120–125.

54. Shrestha NK, Moreno FL, Narciso FV, et al. Two-dimensional echocardiographic diagnosis of left atrial thrombosis in rheumatic heart disease: a clinicopathologic study. *Circulation* 1983;67:341–347.

55. Jordan RA, Scheifley C, Edwards JE. Mural thrombosis and arterial embolism in mitral stenosis. A clinicopathologic study of fifty-one cases. *Circulation* 1951;3:363–367.

56. Manning WJ, Weintraub RM, Waksmouski CA, et al. Accuracy of transesophageal echocardiography in identifying left atrial thrombi. *Ann Intern Med* 1995;123:817–822.

57. Hwang JJ, Chen JJ, Lin SC, et al. Diagnostic accuracy of transesophageal echocardiography for detecting left atrial thrombi in patients with rheumatic heart disease having undergone mitral valve operations. *Am J Cardiol* 1993;72:677–681.

58. Movsowitz C, Meyerowitz CB, Jacobs LE, et al. Significant mitral regurgitation is protective against left atrial spontaneous echo contrast and thrombus as assessed by transesophageal echocardiography. *J Am Soc Echocardiogr* 1993;6:107–114.

59. Wrisley D, Giambartolomei A, Lee I, et al. Left atrial ball thrombus: review of clinical and echocardiographic manifestations with suggestion for management. *Am Heart J* 1991;121:1784–1790.

60. Herzog CA, Bass D, Kane M, et al. Two-dimensional echocardiographic imaging of left atrial appendage thrombi. *J Am Coll Cardiol* 1994;5:1340–1344.

61. DePace NL, Soulen RL, Kolter MN, et al. Two-dimensional detection of intraatrial masses. *Am J Cardiol* 1981;48:954–960.

62. Schweizer P, Bardos F, Erbel R, et al. Detection of left atrial thrombi by echocardiography. *Br Heart J* 1981;45:148–156.

63. Baker KM, Martin RP. Two-dimensional echocardiographic detection of left atrial thrombi in rheumatic mitral valve disease. *J Am Coll Cardiol* 1983;1:703(abst).

64. Aschenberg W, Schluter M, Kremer P, et al. Transesophageal two-dimensional echocardiography for the detection of left atrial appendage thrombus. *J Am Coll Cardiol* 1986;7:163–166.

65. Archer SL, James KE, Kvernen LR, et al. Role of transesophageal echocardiography in the detection of left atrial thrombus in patients with chronic nonrheumatic atrial fibrillation. *Am Heart J* 1995;130:287–295.

66. Leung DY, Davidson PM, Cranney GB, et al. Thromboembolic risks of left atrial thrombus detected by transesophageal echocardiogram. *Am J Cardiol* 1997;79:626–629.

67. Tomoda H, Hoshiai M, Tagawa R, et al. Evaluation of left atrial thrombus with computed tomography. *Am Heart J* 1980;100:306–309.

68. Foster CJ, Sekiya T, Love MG, et al. Identification of intracardiac thrombus: comparison of computed tomography and cross sectional echocardiography. *Br J Radiol* 1987;60:327–331.

69. Uehara T, Nashimura T, Hayashida K, et al. Diagnostic value of technetium-99m radionuclide angiography for detecting thrombosis in left atrial appendage. *J Nucl Med* 1992;33:365–372.

70. Yamada M, Hori N, Ishikawa K, et al. Detection of left atrial thrombi in man using Indium-111 labelled autologous platelets. *Br Heart J* 1984;51:298–305.

71. Parker BM, Friedenberg MJ, Templeton AW, et al. Preoperative angiocardiographic diagnosis of left atrial thrombi in mitral stenosis. *N Engl J Med* 1956;273:136–138.

72. Fu M, Hung J, Lee C, et al. Coronary neovascularization as a specific sign of left atrial appendage thrombus in mitral stenosis. *Am J Cardiol* 1991;67:1158–1160.

73. Gilon D, Schechter D, Rein AJ, et al. Right atrial thrombi are related to indwelling central venous catheter position: insights into time course and possible mechanism of formation. *Am Heart J* 1998;135:457–462.

74. Crowley JJ, Kenny A, Dardas P, et al. Identification of right atrial thrombi using transesophageal echocardiography. *Eur Heart J* 1995;16:708–710.

75. Korones DN, Buzzard CJ, Asselin BL, et al. Right atrial thrombi in children with cancer and indwelling catheters. *J Pediatr* 1996;128:841–846.

76. Chapoutot L, Nazeyrollas P, Metz D, et al. Floating right heart thrombi and pulmonary embolism: diagnosis, outcome and therapeutic management. *Cardiology* 1996;87:169–174.

77. Stowers SA, Leiboff RH, Wasserman AG, et al. Right ventricular thrombus formation in association with acute myocardial infarction: diagnosis by two-dimensional echocardiography. *Am J Cardiol* 1983; 52:912–913.

78. Kawamura Y, Nakamura Y, Handa S. Right ventricular thrombosis. *Chest* 1978;73:435–437.

79. Kessler KM, Mallon SM, Bolooki H, et al. Pedunculated right ventricular thrombosis due to repeated blunt chest trauma. *Am Heart J* 1981; 102:1064–1066.

80. Guimaraes AC, Esteves JP, Filho AS, et al. Clinical aspects of endomyocardial fibrosis in Bahia, Brazil. *Am Heart J* 1971;81:7–19.

CHAPTER 63

Cardiac Arrhythmias

Hasan Garan and Szilard Voros

The evaluation of cardiac arrhythmias is a complex clinical task. It includes the identification and characterization of the rhythm disturbance by electrocardiography and the identification of an anatomic substrate using various cardiac imaging modalities. In the first section of this chapter, we describe specific cardiac conditions associated with arrhythmias, with an emphasis on the imaging modalities useful for diagnostic evaluation. In the second section, we describe the role of imaging modalities in the evaluation of syncope, focusing on arrhythmogenic etiologies.

SPECIFIC DISEASES ASSOCIATED WITH ARRHYTHMIAS

Table 1 provides a classification of specific cardiac diseases that are commonly associated with disturbances in cardiac rhythm, including selected anatomic substrates that can be evaluated by noninvasive cardiac imaging modalities. Although coronary artery disease is responsible for ischemic arrhythmias, its description is beyond the scope of this chapter and is described in detail elsewhere in this book (see Chapters 37–40).

Patients might present with any number of cardiac signs or symptoms, including arrhythmias. In general, patients may be evaluated by conventional radiography, radionuclide imaging, echocardiography, computed tomography (CT), or magnetic resonance imaging (MRI), as dictated by the clinical scenario. In some cases, the underlying heart disease is already known and different imaging modalities can be used to identify complications or to determine further management decisions. In other patients, an arrhythmia is the initial presentation of a cardiac disorder, and imaging modalities are necessary to define the underlying heart disease. In the

TABLE 1. *Classification of arrhythmias with selected anatomic substrates*

1. Tachyarrhythmias
   a. Supraventricular arrhythmias:
      Atrial fibrillation (ischemic, cardiomyopathy, "lone")
      Atrial flutter
      Atrial tachycardia
      Atrioventricular nodal tachycardias (AVNRT)
      Preexcitation syndromes (WPW, AVRT)
   b. Ventricular arrhythmias:
      Ischemic heart disease
      Cardiomyopathies
      Idiopathic
2. Bradyarrhythmias (sinoatrial and conduction disease):
   Ischemic heart disease
   Cardiomyopathies (infiltrative)
   Subaortic abscess
   Idiopathic

AVNRT, atrioventricular nodal reentrant tachycardia; *AVRT*, atrioventricular reentrant tachycardia; *WPW*, Wolff-Parkinson-White syndrome.

first section, we describe strategies of diagnostic imaging in specific cardiac disorders.

TACHYARRHYTHMIAS

Supraventricular Tachycardias

Atrial Fibrillation

Except for extrasystoles, atrial fibrillation (AF) is the most common cardiac arrhythmia encountered in clinical practice (1). Nuclear modalities are generally problematic because of difficulties with gating. Echocardiography is the most commonly applied imaging technique. Experience with MRI is limited, and unless difficulties with gating are overcome, it is unlikely to be widely used in AF in the near future. Several structural parameters associated with AF have been

H. Garan: Department of Medicine, University of Texas at Houston; Department of Cardiac Electrophysiology, University of Texas at Houston, Houston, Texas 77030.

S. Voros: Department of Medicine, University of Alabama at Birmingham, Birmingham, Alabama 35233.

TABLE 2. *Morphologic and functional predictors in atrial fibrillation*

1. Predictors of atrial fibrillation:
   Left atrial size
   Left ventricular function
   Left ventricular hypertrophy
2. Predictors of restoration and maintenance of normal sinus rhythm:
   Left atrial size
   Left atrial function
   Left atrial appendage function
3. Predictors of thromboembolism:
   Recent congestive heart failure
   History of hypertension
   History of thromboembolism
   Left atrial size
   Left and right atrial thrombus
   Spontaneous echo contrast
   Left atrial function
   Left atrial appendage function
   Left ventricular function

described (Table 2) (2–5). Some of these findings are predictors of AF, some are predictive of recurrence after cardioversion, and some indicate high risk for thromboembolic complications. Because most of these findings have been described by echocardiography, the following sections focus on echocardiographic predictors in AF.

Predictors of Atrial Fibrillation

Several studies have shown that mitral stenosis had by far the highest odds ratio of all parameters in predicting AF (2). In nonvalvular forms, left atrial enlargement, decreased left ventricular contractility, and left ventricular hypertrophy appeared to be the strongest indicators, at least in elderly populations. Although these parameters are independent predictors, they are also additive. Mitral annular calcification, mitral regurgitation, aortic stenosis, and aortic regurgitation have been implicated in some, but not all, studies (2–5).

Left Atrial Enlargement. It has been long proposed that left atrial enlargement is associated with chronic AF, based on radiologic, autopsy, and angiographic data. Several investigators have shown in a prospective manner that there is an incremental relationship between left atrial size and the occurrence of AF (5). It is difficult to determine a specific value for the upper limit above which AF will occur, but most reports agree on 40–45 millimeters as a reference. Importantly, it has also been shown that patients with AF and left atrial enlargement have a higher risk for cerebral embolism (5). In contrast to chronic AF, paroxysmal cases are not always associated with left atrial enlargement (6).

Decreased Left Ventricular Contractility and Left Ventricular Hypertrophy. Similar to atrial enlargement, decreased left ventricular contractility and left ventricular hypertrophy have been shown to predict a higher risk of AF and thromboembolic complications in the Stroke Prevention in Atrial Fibrillation (SPAF) trial (7).

Predictors of Restoration and Maintenance of Normal Sinus Rhythm

To assess the need for long-term antiarrhythmic treatment and anticoagulation, it is desirable to identify patients at high risk for recurrence of AF. The echocardiographic parameter most strongly associated with recurrence, which can be evaluated prior to cardioversion, is left atrial size. Transmitral flow characteristics that reflect atrial function after cardioversion are also useful in predicting recurrence.

Left Atrial Size. Left atrial size before or after cardioversion has been proposed as a predictor of recurrence. Henry et al. noted that in patients with valvular disease and hypertrophic obstructive cardiomyopathy, left atrial size greater than 45 millimeters predicted a high rate of recurrence. This original suggestion has been confirmed by most, but not all, investigators (3). A study by Mattioli et al. (8) confirmed the predictive value of left atrial size after cardioversion in a univariate analysis. They found that left atrial size of 50 millimeters or greater was associated with recurrence. Another study, using internal atrial defibrillation with a 6-month follow-up, showed that there was an overlap between left atrial size in patients who remained in sinus rhythm and those in whom AF recurred. However, they noted that none of the patients whose left atrial dimension was greater than 5 centimeters remained in sinus rhythm (9). In summary, although left atrial size might be difficult to interpret in some patients, in those with considerable left atrial enlargement (>45–50 mm), it might be a useful predictor.

Left Atrial Function. Left atrial function immediately after cardioversion assessed by pulsed-wave Doppler evaluation of the left ventricular filling pattern is a reliable predictor of recurrence. The time required for normal function to return following cardioversion is a function of the duration and the underlying cause of AF. Mattioli et al. (8) examined the predictive value of this pattern in patients with chronic, nonvalvular AF. Using univariate analysis, they demonstrated that characteristics of the A-wave were the strongest predictors. Peak A-wave velocity and A-wave time integral were significantly lower in patients who subsequently reverted to AF (8).

Left Atrial Appendage Function. Left atrial appendage function prior to cardioversion has been shown to be a reliable predictor of the maintenance of normal sinus rhythm, at least in patients with internal atrial defibrillation (9). Omran et al. (9) studied the predictive value of left atrial diameter, left ventricular ejection fraction, maximum left atrial appendage area, and left atrial appendage function using TEE by measuring the inflow and outflow velocities of the left atrial appendage at its ostium. They found that peak emptying velocities were significantly lower in patients with recurrence, compared with patients who maintained normal sinus rhythm. They determined a peak emptying velocity less than 36 cm/s to be the best cut-off value for the prediction of recurrence. Using this value, the sensitivity and specificity of this method was 82% and 83%, respectively.

Return of Normal Atrial Function after Cardioversion

Normal sinus rhythm returns in 90% of patients following electrical cardioversion, as evidenced by the appearance of P-waves on the electrocardiogram (3). However, atrial and appendage contractile function might not be restored immediately; rather, it might return gradually within a few hours to several weeks (8,10). This has been known for a long time, based on the evaluation of intracardiac pressure recordings. When sinus rhythm is restored without complete restoration of atrial and atrial appendage function, the patient is still at risk for thromboembolic complications. Atrial function can be assessed during transthoracic echocardiography by analyzing transmitral flow patterns, whereas atrial appendage function can be evaluated by TEE.

Electrical Cardioversion. Bellotti et al. (11) studied left atrial appendage function immediately before and the day after electrical cardioversion. Electrical normal sinus rhythm was restored in all patients, as shown by the appearance of P-waves on the electrocardiogram. Moreover, left atrial function was also restored in all patients, which was evidenced by the appearance of an A-wave following the E-wave on the transmitral flow pattern. Following cardioversion, organized appendage contraction was found in 68% of patients, confirmed by appendage filling and emptying synchronous with the P-wave on the electrocardiogram, whereas disorganized appendage activity was found in 32%. Of the precardioversion parameters, smaller maximal left atrial appendage area was a significant predictor of the restoration of normal appendage function. On the postcardioversion echocardiogram, peak filling velocity, peak emptying velocity, and the ejection fractional area were significantly higher in patients with organized appendage activity than in patients with disorganized activity. Moreover, spontaneous echo contrast was present more frequently in patients with unsynchronized appendage function.

These data demonstrated that atrial or appendage standstill is present in some patients following electrical cardioversion, and that echocardiography can identify patients in whom the restoration of normal atrial function is delayed. These patients might need longer periods of anticoagulation, but definite recommendations cannot be made until data from controlled studies are available (10).

Pharmacological Cardioversion. Jovic et al. (10) studied the time course of atrial functional recovery following pharmacological cardioversion by serial evaluation of the contribution of atrial contraction to left ventricular filling on the transmitral flow pattern on day 1, 8, 15, and 30. Atrial contraction returned in all patients following pharmacological cardioversion. This finding was different from electrical cardioversion, where atrial standstill was observed in some patients (see above). Jovic et al. found that there was a serial increase in peak A-wave velocity from day 1 through day 30, with the largest incremental increase between day 1 and 8. At the same time, there was a serial decrease in the peak E-wave velocity, with the largest incremental decrease between day 1 and 8 as well. These data confirm that even though electrical sinus rhythm is restored immediately, mechanical atrial function recovers gradually. This period is characterized by a low-flow state, which increases the risk for thromboembolic complications. Such data confirm the need for anticoagulation for at least 4 weeks following cardioversion (10).

Predictors of Thromboembolism

Beyond the hemodynamic compromise associated with the loss of atrial contraction, cerebral thromboembolism is the most devastating consequence of AF. It has long been known that valvular AF carries a very high incidence of stroke (1,3). Nonvalvular AF is also associated with a high incidence of stroke, approximately 7% per year, which is about 5 to 6 times higher than in patients with normal sinus rhythm. Because the hazards associated with chronic anticoagulation are substantial, identification of patients in the high risk category is of great clinical importance. For this purpose, clinical and echocardiographic predictors have been identified in clinical trials. The largest series was the SPAF Investigators study (7,12).

As mentioned above, one of the most important predictors is the cause of AF. Valvular AF is associated with a much higher risk for thromboembolic complications. Echocardiographic predictors in nonvalvular AF are discussed below.

Echocardiographic Predictors. Prior to the SPAF investigation, at least eight relatively large series attempted to identify echocardiographic predictors of thromboembolism in nonvalvular chronic AF. Four studies found no such parameters, three reported the predictive value of left atrial enlargement, and one noted the role of mitral annular calcification. Using multivariate analysis, the SPAF investigators found that if only echocardiographic parameters were considered, left atrial enlargement on M-mode and left ventricular dysfunction assessed by two-dimensional real-time imaging were independent predictors of thromboembolism. When clinical parameters were also taken into consideration, only left ventricular dysfunction was an independent predictor. A scheme for risk stratification using these clinical and echocardiographic variables was published by the SPAF investigators (7). More recently, with the widespread use of TEE, newer echocardiographic features have been proposed, including left atrial thrombi, left atrial and appendage function, and left atrial spontaneous echo contrast (Fig. 1).

Left Atrial Size. Increased left atrial size is a strong predictor of thromboembolism in patients with AF. From the data available, it seems that the risk is proportional to the degree of enlargement. In the SPAF trial, the relative risk was 1.6 and 2.7 for left atrial sizes of 2.4 cm/m^2 (4.7 cm) and 2.9 cm/m^2 (5.7 cm), respectively. Values corrected for body surface area were stronger predictors than noncorrected ones.

Left Atrial Thrombus. The most common site for thrombus formation in atrial fibrillation is the left atrial appendage

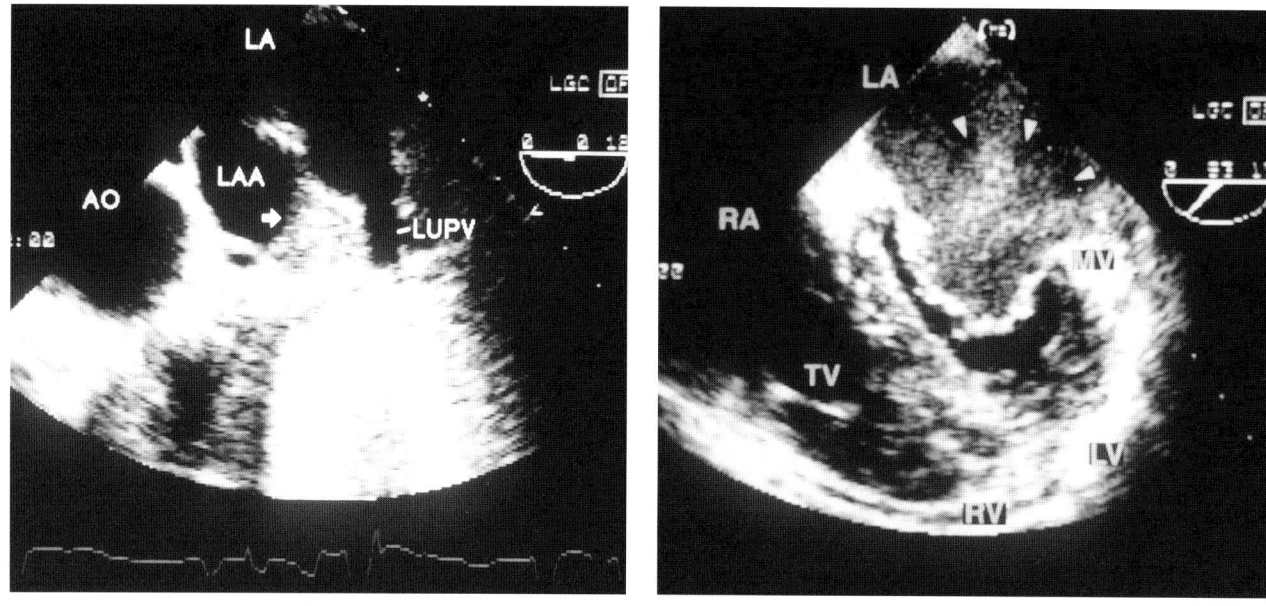

FIG. 1. Transesophageal echocardiographic findings in atrial fibrillation. **A:** Thrombus in the left atrium (*LA*), predicting a high risk of systemic thromboembolism (*arrow*). **B:** Spontaneous echo contrast in the *LA* of a patient with atrial fibrillation, representing a low-flow state. *AO*, aorta; *LAA*, left atrial appendage; *LUPV*, left upper pulmonary vein; *MV*, mitral valve; *RA*, right atrium; *RV*, right ventricle; *TV*, tricuspid valve. (From ref. 13, with permission.)

(Fig. 1**A**). TEE is superior to the transthoracic approach in visualizing both the appendage and intracardiac thrombi (3). The reported prevalence of echocardiographically detected atrial thrombi in AF ranges from 4 to 27% (14). Tsai et al. (14) studied the prevalence and clinical significance of atrial thrombi in chronic nonvalvular AF in a large, consecutive, unselected patient population. In their series, atrial thrombi were found in 6.8% of patients, and 80% of these thrombi were present in the left atrial appendage. They also pointed out that the use of multiplane transesophageal probes dramatically increased the detection rate. In predicting thromboembolic complications, the sensitivity, specificity, positive predictive value and negative predictive value of the presence of a left atrial thrombus was 14%, 97%, 73%, and 68%, respectively. Compared to spontaneous echo contrast, the presence of thrombus was more specific, but less sensitive in predicting thromboembolism.

It is important to distinguish between atrial thrombi and other similar structures in the left atrium, including prominent trabeculations, adipose tissue, and duplication artifacts (3). The appendage should be interrogated from multiple views, using a multiplane probe (Fig. 1**A**). In addition, the right atrial appendage should be examined. The prevalence of right atrial appendage thrombi is not well known.

Spontaneous Echo Contrast. Spontaneous echo contrast is a smoke-like, swirling effect in the cardiac chambers (Fig. 1**B**). *In vitro* observations suggest that it is a result of increased ultrasound backscatter from aggregated red blood cells, and it is usually an indicator of a low-flow state (3).

Initially, it was described in the left ventricle associated with severe dysfunction, and in the left atria of patients with severe mitral stenosis, using transthoracic echocardiography. With the advent of TEE, it has been seen frequently in patients with AF. The reported prevalence of spontaneous echo contrast ranges from 25 to 68% in patients with valvular, and from 24 to 59% in nonvalvular AF. Tsai et al. (14) detected spontaneous echo contrast in 39% of patients, with an interobserver variability of 0.9%. All patients with atrial thrombi had spontaneous echo contrast. Moderate or moderate-to-severe mitral regurgitation was an independent predictor of the absence of echo contrast, presumably due to the regurgitant flow through the valve. In predicting thromboembolism, the sensitivity, specificity, positive predictive value, and negative predictive value of spontaneous echo contrast was 73%, 80%, 66%, and 84%, respectively. Compared to the presence of left atrial thrombi, spontaneous echo contrast is more sensitive and less specific, with a lower positive and a higher negative predictive value (Fig. 1**B**).

Left Atrial and Atrial Appendage Function. Because atrial echo contrast or thrombus cannot be demonstrated in all patients who are at increased risk for thromboembolic complications, the evaluation of atrial and atrial appendage function has been proposed to identify patients at high risk. Two parameters might be used to evaluate the function of the atrial appendage: appendage ejection fraction and ostial flow velocities. Appendage ejection fraction might be measured by using the area of the appendage before and after contraction. During sinus rhythm, the normal range is 45 to

55%. Patients with lower atrial appendage ejection fraction are at increased risk for thromboembolism (3).

In normal sinus rhythm, the flow at the ostium of the appendage shows a biphasic pulsed-wave Doppler pattern, with flow velocities exceeding 40 cm/s. In AF, ostial flow varies from normal to absent, and the velocity seems to correspond with the duration of the arrhythmia (3). More studies are needed to determine the role of measuring ostial flow in these patients.

As was described earlier, the time for atrial and atrial appendage functional recovery after cardioversion is prolonged, and this transitional period is associated with a higher rate of embolic events. Clinical recommendations, however, cannot be made at this time.

Role of Echocardiography in Cardioversion

The role of echocardiography in elective cardioversion has been investigated by Silverman and Manning (15). Spontaneous, pharmacological, or electrical cardioversion is associated with thromboembolism in a substantial number of patients. Based on several studies, the incidence of thromboembolism in sustained AF (duration 2 days or more) was 5 to 7% (1,14). To avoid embolic events, patients are fully anticoagulated with warfarin for 4 weeks prior to cardioversion. Although this approach has reduced the risk of embolism to approximately 1.2%, it delays the restoration of normal atrial activity by 4 weeks. Also, it is associated with some minor and major bleeding complications (6 to 18% and 1 to 2%, respectively). It has been shown that chronic maintenance of normal sinus rhythm after cardioversion is inversely related to the duration of AF (15). Similarly, the rate and degree of atrial mechanical recovery is also inversely related to the duration of the arrhythmia with an elevated risk of systemic embolization during the period of abnormal atrial function. Considering these problems, Silverman and Manning proposed the strategy of early cardioversion using TEE (15). Based on their recommendations, in patients with AF for 2 days or more, if they are candidates for long-term anticoagulation, heparin and warfarin should be started immediately. TEE should then be performed, and in the absence of thrombi, cardioversion can be done. If the TEE reveals the presence of a thrombus, cardioversion should be delayed, and the patient should be anticoagulated for 4 weeks. At the end of the 4 weeks, the echocardiogram should be repeated; if the thrombus has resolved, cardioversion might be performed. In patients who are not candidates for long-term anticoagulation, TEE should be performed; if no thrombus is detected, cardioversion can be attempted. The authors concluded that this approach of TEE-guided early cardioversion should be considered to have a safety profile similar to, but not better than, conventional therapy. Currently, the Assessment of Cardioversion Using Transesophageal Echocardiography (ACUTE) is an ongoing trial to answer remaining questions regarding this strategy.

Atrial Flutter, Atrial Tachycardia, Atrioventricular Nodal Reentrant Tachycardia (AVNRT)

The role of noninvasive imaging modalities in atrial tachycardias is somewhat limited but emerging, especially with the use of intracardiac echocardiography (ICE) in the electrophysiology laboratory. Similar to AF, perfusion scintigraphy may be used to diagnose concomitant coronary artery disease. Unlike in AF, gating is not an issue in atrial tachycardias.

Conventional surface echocardiography has been used in atrial flutter to aid noninvasive diagnosis in cases in which the surface electrocardiogram was limited. In such instances, atrial septal wall motion could be easily visualized from a subcostal view, and atrial flutter could be clearly diagnosed based on the septal contraction pattern. Similarly, dissimilar atrial rhythms have been demonstrated using the same technique. Because atrial thrombosis is much less common in these supraventricular arrhythmias than in atrial fibrillation, a search for intracardiac thrombi is usually not indicated.

Over the past few years, ICE has gained a role in the electrophysiology laboratory (16). Conventional surface echocardiography and TEE have been used to guide catheter ablation procedures. However, it was the introduction of intracardiac ultrasound probes that made invasive echocardiography possible. ICE has two major roles in the hands of the electrophysiologist. First, similar to other imaging modalities, it is able to identify an anatomic substrate for given arrhythmias. Surgical scars left behind from cardiac surgery have been demonstrated by ICE as the anatomic substrate for atrial tachycardias. Catheter ablation of these foci using ICE guidance was curative. The second role of ICE is direct visualization of anatomic landmarks, helping the electrophysiologist in correct catheter placement, in transseptal crossing, and in ensuring adequate endocardial contact (16). The addition of ICE to conventional fluoroscopy can reduce fluoroscopy time, decreasing radiation exposure to both patient and physician.

Atrial Flutter

Typical atrial flutter is caused by a counterclockwise reentrant circuit around the tricuspid annulus. This circuit contains a protected zone of conduction in an anatomic area defined by the coronary sinus ostium, the tricuspid valve annulus and the inferior vena cava (isthmus). ICE allows for excellent visualization of this area in most patients, with the exception of patients with significant right atrial enlargement, in whom the depth of penetration of the ultrasound might be inadequate. Traditionally, detailed endocardial mapping is necessary prior to ablation procedures. However, ICE-guided ablation has been used instead of endocardial mapping procedures (16).

Atrial Tachycardias

As mentioned earlier, ICE has been used to identify the anatomic substrate for reentrant atrial tachycardias. Abnormal atrial wall scarring related to prior septal defect repair has been identified in 2 patients, with subsequent successful catheter ablation guided by the intracardiac probe (16).

Other Supraventricular Arrhythmias

Similarly, ICE has been successfully used in other catheter ablation procedures, including atrioventricular nodal reentrant tachycardia (AVNRT), sinus nodal reentrant tachycardia, and the Wolff-Parkinson-White syndrome (16).

Wolff-Parkinson-White Syndrome

In manifest ventricular preexcitation (Wolff-Parkinson-White syndrome; WPW), the electrical impulse reaches the basal segments of the ventricles through an accessory pathway (AP), whereas other parts of the ventricles are activated through the normal conduction system, resulting in a ventricular fusion beat. The gold standard for localizing these pathways used to be epicardial mapping during surgery, which has been replaced by transcatheter endocardial mapping and recording of AP potentials. Less invasive methods, such as functional nuclear angiography and echocardiography, have also been used to localize APs (16,18). These methods are described in the following sections.

Phase Image Analysis of the Radionuclide Cineangiogram in the Localization of Accessory Pathways

Kent Bundles. Several investigators have studied the accuracy of phase image analysis of blood pool images in localizing APs in WPW syndrome (17–23). In general, left or right free wall pathways could be localized with a high degree of accuracy. By contrast, patients with septal/paraseptal pathways could not be separated from patients with normal conduction based on the nuclear scans alone, if the investigators were blinded to the ECG.

Botvinick et al. (24) found that in left-sided free wall pathways, the site of earliest activation was always in the region of the left ventricle, away from the septum, and the localization of the pathways using triangulation was in good agreement with the electrophysiologic findings. In fact, the phase image was more accurate than the surface ECG in localizing the pathways. Similarly, in patients with right ventricular free wall pathways, the site of earliest phase angle appeared in the right ventricle, away from the septum. The onset and upstroke of the right ventricular phase histogram preceded that of the left ventricle. In patients with septal/paraseptal pathways, the earliest phase angle was localized to the septum, but neither the phase image, nor the phase histogram values, were able to differentiate patients with septal/paraseptal tracts from those with normal conduction.

Similar results were reported by Johnson et al. (22), who found that all free wall pathways were correctly identified, whereas the localization of septal/paraseptal pathways was less reliable.

Mahaim Fibers. Mahaim fibers can also be identified using phase analysis (25). In patients with ventricular preexcitation via atriofascicular connections, the site of earliest activation is the septal/paraseptal region. The activation spreads asymmetrically, first to the ipsilateral and then to the contralateral ventricle. Correct localization of AP in patients with more than one abnormal connection has not been reliable (26).

Although phase patterns associated with the WPW syndrome are well-described, the method is not widely used in clinical practice. One potential clinical application might be serial evaluation of patients following catheter ablation.

Myocardial Perfusion Imaging Using Radionuclides

Myocardial perfusion images with thallium- or technetium-labeled agents must be interpreted with caution in patients with WPW (27). It has been known for a long time that preexcitation causes false-positive results on exercise stress testing, and ST segment depression observed in these patients during exercise is not a result of myocardial ischemia. Similarly, myocardial perfusion scans are also influenced by the presence of accessory atrioventricular connections. The first reported series of thallium perfusion imaging in patients with WPW noted that of patients with preexcitation and ST segment depression during exercise, 20% had perfusion defects. On the other hand, of patients in whom preexcitation disappeared during exercise, but who had ST segment depression, 63% had perfusion defects on thallium scanning. However, these results were not compared to x-ray cineangiography with radioopaque contrast medium. Archer et al. (27) studied 8 patients with WPW syndrome by exercise thallium testing. Seven of the 8 patients demonstrated at least 1-mm ST segment depression during exercise, and 2 patients had stress perfusion defects, while 5 demonstrated delayed thallium clearance. Delayed thallium clearance has also been associated with different intraventricular conduction disturbances, including right and left bundle branch block, left anterior fascicular block, and APs. Because the diagnosis of coronary disease by perfusion imaging may be problematic in preexcitation syndromes, other modalities should be used to detect ischemic myocardium in these patients.

Echocardiography

As the myocardial contraction sequence follows the electrical activation sequence, direct visualization of the myocardium during echocardiography can trace the electrical activation pattern, identifying the earliest site of contraction in the basal segments of the left ventricle in patients with APs. Several echocardiographic modalities have been used, including M-mode, two-dimensional echocardiography, Doppler, and phase analysis. Newer techniques, such as TEE and myocardial Doppler imaging, have recently been described.

M-mode Echocardiography. DeMaria et al. (28) noted that in WPW with left-sided pathways, the most striking feature was the presence of a 2–3 millimeter, early anterior systolic movement of the left ventricular posterior wall (LVPW) during the first 100 ms of the QRS complex (i.e., during the delta wave). Also, the onset and the peak of contraction of the LVPW occurred earlier than in normal subjects. This early movement of the LVPW was accompanied by a simultaneous paradoxical anterior motion of the interventricular septum (IVS), which was not observed in normal patients. On the other hand, the initial posterior movement of the IVS and the contraction of the right ventricular (RV) wall were delayed, compared to normal subjects. These findings were consistent with the theory that in manifest WPW with left AP, the left ventricle is prematurely activated, resulting in early contraction, whereas the activation of the IVS and RV anterior wall is delayed. In this study by DeMaria et al., (28) the echocardiographic features of manifest WPW with right-sided pathways were less well characterized due to the low number of patients with this pattern. Similar findings were reported by Hishida et al. (29) both for left and right APs, with almost identical numeric values. They also studied the effects of ajmaline (which blocks conduction through the AP) on the echocardiographic patterns of ventricular preexcitation, and found that it reversed the early LVPW and IVS motion in patients with left and right APs, respectively. Also, a report by Ng et al. showed similar findings with right-sided APs, demonstrating an early posterior movement of the IVS (30).

All these early reports pointed out that the role of echocardiography in WPW is mainly to exclude co-existing cardiac abnormalities and perhaps to aid in the localization of the APs (31). MRI also should be useful for this application.

Two-dimensional Echocardiography. The first two-dimensional echocardiographic study of WPW syndrome was reported by Windle et al. (32) using cine-loops of digitized images, primarily in the short-axis view of the ventricles. They identified three regions of the right ventricle and five regions of the left ventricle around the mitral valve annulus, and the site of earliest contraction was determined by a frame-by-frame analysis of these digitized images. The echocardiographic analysis localized 82% of pathways to the correct segment as determined by electrophysiologic testing, while in the remaining 18% the pathway was localized to an adjacent segment. When compared to M-mode, two-dimensional echocardiography was superior in accurately localizing these pathways.

Doppler Echocardiography. Jue et al. (33) reported that following catheter ablation, there was a significant increase in peak A-wave velocity and its time integral, atrial filling fraction, and total mitral inflow velocity integral, while the E-to-A wave ratio decreased significantly. In another Doppler study, there was a significant decrease in left ventricular output during sinus rhythm with preexcitation, mostly with right ventricular free wall pathways. Antidromic tachycardia resulted in a significant decrease in left ventricular output, while the decrease in ventricular output was less marked during ortodromic tachycardia (34).

Echocardiographic Phase Imaging. Similar to blood pool scintigraphy, phase image analysis using the Fourier transform has been applied to echocardiographic images (35,36). In patients with WPW and normal sinus rhythm, the phase image did not differ significantly from normal patients. However, during maximal preexcitation as a result of atrial pacing, the delay of mean phase angle between earliest and latest contracting regions and the delay of minimal phase angle between the earliest and latest contracting regions increased significantly. In the focal segments that were identified as the earliest contracting segments on the static phase image, the delay of mean phase angle also increased significantly.

In these series, the accuracy of echocardiographic phase analysis in localizing APs was quite high, especially when preexcitation was enhanced by atrial pacing. Using electrophysiologic mapping as a reference standard, surface electrocardiography identified 53% of the pathways correctly. Conventional two-dimensional echocardiography was correct in 58% and phase imaging in 82%. When all three methods were combined, 94% of pathways could be accurately localized.

Phase analysis has also been applied to transesophageal images. Kuecher et al. (36) investigated the accuracy of transesophageal echocardiographic phase imaging for localizing APs. During maximal preexcitation following an intravenous bolus of adenosine, visual identification of the earliest site of contraction was easy, and 75% of pathways could be accurately localized. Moreover, all midseptal and anteroseptal pathways were correctly localized, whereas none of these could be classified based on the surface electrocardiogram.

Color Doppler Imaging of the Myocardium. Color Doppler imaging of the myocardium has been used to localize APs in WPW syndrome. To date, the largest series was reported by Nakayama et al. (37), which included 42 patients with WPW syndrome. In patients with WPW syndrome, unlike in controls, there was an early ventricular contraction that followed the ventricular expansion caused by atrial emptying, usually just below the mitral annulus. In case of left-sided pathways, the site of early contraction was coded in red in the left posterior or lateral wall and was coded in blue in the septum or in the anterior wall. The site of earliest contraction was observed in the endocardium, from where it spread toward the epicardial surface. Overall, 25 of the 29 left sided pathways were identified correctly. In right-sided pathways, the site of earliest contraction was recognized as an abnormal inward motion of either the right ventricular free wall (which appeared in blue) or of the septum (which appeared in blue or red, depending on septal orientation). In contrast to left-sided pathways, only 5 of 13 right-sided pathways could be accurately localized. Although other investigators reported similar results, the clinical role of myocardial Doppler imaging is yet to be determined.

Echocardiography in the Electrophysiology Laboratory. Echocardiography may be used as an adjunct in the electrophysiology laboratory to facilitate catheter placement in difficult cases (38). It is most useful during ablation of left-sided pathways, and it has been used both in adult and pediatric populations. Because the patient is usually already sedated, a transesophageal probe can be passed without difficulty. TEE provides additional imaging planes that cannot be well-visualized on traditional fluoroscopic images. Echocardiography is synergistic with fluoroscopy, and it can decrease fluoroscopic time in complicated situations. Visualization of the valvular apparatus and the fibrous annulus can guide catheter placement, and inadequate contact with the myocardium can be avoided (38). Longitudinal views of the atria are helpful during transseptal procedures, while modified short-axis views can be useful when ablating right anterior paraseptal pathways. In addition, postablation echocardiographic studies can immediately rule out possible complications of ablation procedures, such as valvular perforation or thrombus formation. In addition to TEE, ICE has been used to facilitate identification of landmarks and catheter placement (see Atrial tachycardias). However, the future role of echocardiography in the electrophysiology laboratory is yet to be determined.

Ventricular Arrhythmias

Ventricular Tachycardia Associated with Postinfarction Left Ventricular Aneurysm

Cardiac imaging modalities for the evaluation of ischemic heart disease are discussed in detail elsewhere (see Chapters 37–40). However, the evaluation of patients with ventricular tachycardia (VT) associated with a left ventricular aneurysm is described briefly, since noninvasive imaging is crucial for their management (Fig. 2).

Sustained, monomorphic VT is commonly seen with ventricular aneurysm. It is generally accepted that the aneurysm provides the anatomic substrate for the arrhythmia on the basis of a reentrant circuit. Endocardial mapping can localize the arrhythmogenic focus to an area close to the aneurysm in most patients (39).

After myocardial infarction, patients suspected of having developed a left ventricular aneurysm based on persistent ST-elevations on the electrocardiogram, or based on the known site of coronary obstruction, should undergo noninvasive diagnostic imaging, especially in the presence of ventricular arrhythmias. Radionuclide blood-pool imaging, echocardiography, or MRI can be used to identify a ventricular aneurysm (Fig. 2). If a patient presents with VT and a left ventricular aneurysm, invasive electrophysiologic testing is

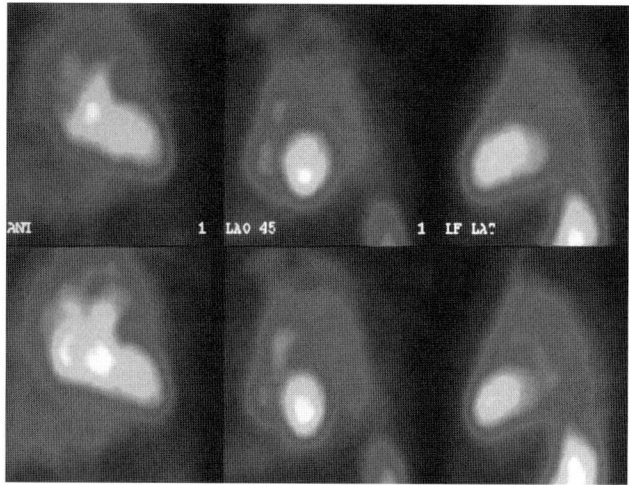

A

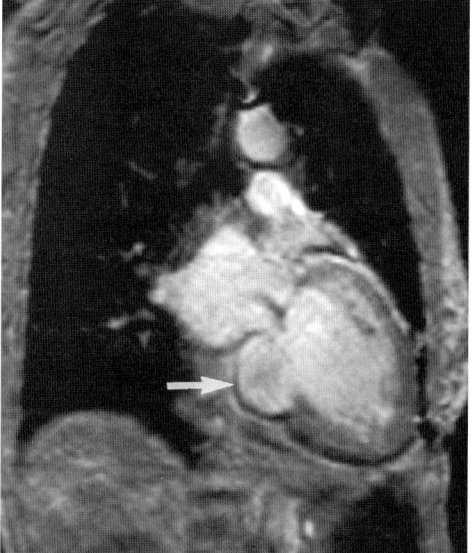

B

FIG. 2. Postinfarction left ventricular aneurysm. **A:** Radionuclide blood pool image of an apical left ventricular aneurysm in the anterior, 45-degree left anterior oblique, and left lateral projections in systole and diastole. (Courtesy of Ami E. Iskandrian, M.D., University of Alabama at Birmingham.) **B:** Magnetic resonance imaging of a large left ventricular aneurysm in the inferior wall in the two-chamber view (*arrow*).

warranted. Map-guided resection of the aneurysm may cure the VT (39,40).

Over the past years, left ventricular volume reduction surgery has been used in patients with ischemic cardiomyopathy to improve left ventricular function by resecting aneurysmal components (40). MRI has been used to evaluate the detailed left ventricular geometry prior to such surgery. It is now recommended that patients who are referred for volume reduction surgery on the basis of appropriate anatomy, as defined by MRI, should undergo invasive electrophysiologic testing prior to surgery, even in the absence of spontaneous VT. Thus, the site of the arrhythmogenic focus can be taken into consideration during surgery. Using this approach, VT could not be induced in 92% of patients after surgery (40).

Such results underlie the importance of noninvasive imaging modalities in the management of patients with a left ventricular aneurysm and VT.

Hypertrophic Cardiomyopathy

Hypertrophic cardiomyopathy (HCM) is characterized by thickening of the myocardial wall, with increased propensity for the interventricular septum. HCM is described in detail in Chapter 48. Cardiac arrhythmias are common in HCM, and they have been implicated as the cause of sudden cardiac death. Several clinical features have been reported to predict sudden cardiac death. In addition, arrhythmias discovered during ambulatory electrocardiographic monitoring or electrophysiologic testing might help in risk-stratification. Cardiac imaging modalities such as echocardiography, radionuclide imaging, and MRI are crucial in the diagnosis and in further risk stratification.

Echocardiography

Echocardiographic Features Predicting Arrhythmias and Sudden Death. General echocardiographic features of HCM are described in Chapter 48. There have been several attempts to identify echocardiographic features that predict ventricular arrhythmias and sudden death. In general, myocardial thickness does not correlate with the occurrence of such events (41,42). In contrast, Lazzeroni et al. (43) reported that the extent of hypertrophy correlates with the occurrence of serious arrhythmias. They classified 77 patients in three groups: septal hypertrophy (43%), extensive hypertrophy (septal and free wall) (49%), and apical hypertrophy (8%). They found that higher grade PVCs were more frequent in patients with extensive hypertrophy than with septal hypertrophy (73 vs. 33%; $p < 0.001$). Also, AF was more frequent in extensive hypertrophy compared to septal hypertrophy (24 vs. 3%; $p < 0.01$). In this series, 3 patients died in the follow-up period. All 3 patients had extensive hypertrophy (43).

Almost identical results were reported by Cheng et al. (44). High-grade PVCs were more common in patients with extensive hypertrophy, compared to septal hypertrophy (87 vs. 40%; $p < 0.05$). There was a trend toward a higher incidence of AF in extensive hypertrophy, but this was not statistically significant. In addition, they found that high-grade PVCs were more common in patients with the obstructive form than with the nonobstructive form (92 vs. 43%; $p < 0.01$) (44). In contrast, it appears that apical hypertrophy is associated with a more benign course (43,44). Although echocardiography has been useful as a means to assess the extent and distribution of myocardial hypertrophy, MRI is probably a better choice.

Magnetic Resonance Imaging

Until recently, echocardiography had been the "gold-standard" in the diagnosis of HCM. However, over the past few years, MRI has emerged as an important tool in the diagnosis. The general features of HCM, including myocardial hypertrophy, small ventricular cavity, and narrow outflow tract, are readily recognized on MRI studies. Pons Llado et al. (45) compared the accuracy of echocardiography and MRI. They found that of 330 myocardial segments, thickness could be measured in 67% by echocardiography and in 97% by MRI. MRI was superior in visualizing the anterolateral and apical aspects of the left ventricle. In cases in which echocardiography cannot provide the necessary anatomical information, MRI should be performed. To the present time, no studies have evaluated MRI predictors of arrhythmias or sudden death in HCM.

Radionuclide Imaging

Fixed and reversible defects on thallium- or technetium-labeled sestamibi imaging are common in HCM, even in the absence of epicardial coronary disease, suggesting the presence of intramural coronary artery disease and myocardial ischemia. It is controversial whether perfusion defects are predictive of arrhythmias or of sudden death. Fixed defects have been associated with a history of syncope and decreased systolic function. Reversible ischemia has been reported to be associated with syncope and sudden death by some authors (42), but the opposite has been shown by others.

Using gated radionuclide cardiac blood pool imaging in 22 patients with HCM, Pohost et al. (46) found disproportionate upper septal thickening in 11, septal flattening in 16, cavity obliteration in 17, and LVOT filling defects in 16 patients, demonstrating the complimentary role of radionuclide imaging and echocardiography.

Dilated Cardiomyopathy

Dilated cardiomyopathy (DCM) is characterized by the enlargement of all cardiac chambers, decreased systolic function, multivalvular regurgitation, and arrhythmias. The incidence of DCM is about 5 to 8 per 100,000. DCM appears to be the final common pathway for various specific cardiac diseases, leading to clinical congestive heart failure (see Chapter 47).

Imaging Modalities

DCM is readily diagnosed by chest x-ray, which is characterized by a grossly enlarged cardiac silhouette, quantified by a cardiothoracic ratio greater than 0.5.

Echocardiography is the most widely used modality. General echocardiographic features of DCM are described in Chapter 47. A large, ongoing study (MACAS) was designed to determine echocardiographic predictors of arrhythmias in DCM (48). Preliminary results suggest that left ventricular ejection fraction less than 30% was associated with a higher incidence of left bundle branch block (43 vs. 25%; $p < 0.05$)

and nonsustained VT (44 vs. 22%; $p < 0.05$). The prognostic significance of these findings will be evaluated at the completion of the study (48).

Radionuclide ventriculography can be carried out in patients in whom echocardiography yields suboptimal images. It provides parameters similar to echocardiography, including increased left ventricular end-systolic and diastolic dimensions, decreased ejection fraction, and regional wall motion abnormalities. Perfusion scintigraphy should be performed in most patients to exclude ischemic origin of the cardiomyopathy.

MRI has emerged as an important tool in the evaluation of DCM. Four-chamber enlargement, decreased left ventricular function and panvalvular regurgitation are easily recognized and quantified by MRI. In contrast to echocardiography, optimal thoracic "window" is not a concern. Furthermore, MRI recognition of intracardiac thrombi can be diagnostic in cases when echocardiography is equivocal. Atrial fibrillation, which is common in DCM, might make gated MRI more problematic.

Arrhythmogenic Right Ventricular Dysplasia

Arrhythmogenic right ventricular dysplasia (ARVD) is characterized by progressive replacement of the right ventricular myocardium by fibroadipose tissue, which can lead to right ventricular enlargement and recurrent ventricular tachycardias (VT) (49). Because it can be associated with sudden cardiac death in healthy, young individuals, identification and treatment of this disorder is extremely important. The prevalence of ARVD was recently reviewed by Dalal et al. (49). In a series of 9,000 consecutive echocardiograms at the Duke University Medical Center, 2 patients met criteria for ARVD (50). Buja et al. studied the prevalence in patients in whom the disease was suspected on clinical grounds (49). Of 268 preselected patients, 126 were diagnosed with right ventricular dysplasia (not necessarily associated with arrhythmias). In the well-known Venetian Regional Program on Juvenile Sudden Death registry, ARVD was diagnosed in 12 cases out of 60 subjects between ages 14 and 38 who suffered sudden death. Overall, ARVD is common in young, otherwise healthy individuals who present with ventricular arrhythmias and no other apparent heart disease. Moreover, it is one of the leading causes of VT with left bundle branch morphology (49). Different modalities of cardiac imaging play important roles in the diagnosis and management of ARVD. These are discussed below.

Radionuclide Angiography

The diagnosis of ARVD requires the demonstration of right ventricular morphologic and functional abnormalities in the appropriate clinical setting. Conventional first-pass or equilibrium radionuclide angiography at rest and during exercise have been used to evaluate right ventricular structure and function in these patients (49,51). It has been pro-

posed that radionuclide angiography might have an advantage over other techniques, including contrast angiography, CT, or MRI, because the heart can be evaluated not only at rest, but also during exercise (49). Four radionuclide angiographic criteria have been proposed for the diagnosis of ARVD: (i) right ventricular ejection fraction less than 50% during exercise, (ii) failure to increase right ventricular ejection fraction by more than 6% during exercise, (iii) right ventricular wall motion abnormality during exercise, and (iv) ratio of right ventricular to left ventricular volume more than 1.8. Decreased right ventricular function with normal left ventricular function and without another explanation for right ventricular dysfunction, in the right clinical setting, is diagnostic of ARVD. Based on radionuclide imaging, the most frequently involved regions of the right ventricle are the basal part of the inferior wall, the apex and the infundibulum, corresponding to the previously described "triangle of dysplasia" based on histologic examinations.

More recently, LeGuludec et al. (51) evaluated the value of radionuclide angiography using multiharmonic Fourier analysis against contrast angiography as a reference standard. Right ventricular regional wall motion abnormalities could be identified on the phase images of patients with abnormal right ventricles, and the difference of mean right and left ventricular end-systolic time angles differed significantly between patients and controls. Using contrast angiography as a reference standard, the sensitivity and specificity of radionuclide angiography was 94.3% and 90%, respectively. Positive predictive value was 96% and negative predictive value was 85.7%. The best agreement in the location of regional wall motion abnormalities between the methods was in the inferior wall (82%) and the poorest was in the apex (60%).

123-I Meta-Iodobenzylguanidine (MIBG) Radionuclide Imaging

In patients with ARVD, VT frequently starts during exercise. Also, such tachycardias are commonly inducible by catecholamines, whereas they may be improved by beta adrenergic antagonists. These observations have suggested the role of the sympathetic nervous system in the development of these arrhythmias. Imaging of the sympathetic nervous system of the heart has been possible since the introduction of tracers that are selectively taken up and stored by the sympathetic nerve endings.

Wichter et al. (52) extensively studied patients with ARVD by MIBG scintigraphy. In normal controls, 123-I MIBG uptake was homogeneous, except for some decline in activity toward the apex. Of the patients with ARVD, 83% demonstrated regional reduction in MIBG uptake. Tracer uptake was significantly lower than in normal controls in the basal septal, posteroseptal, and posterior segments of the right ventricle. Because there were no perfusion defects in the given segments as assessed by thallium scintigraphy, these segments were considered to have scan evidence of regional sympathetic denervation, as shown by the ''thallium-MIBG mismatch.'' All these patients were studied by electrophysiologic testing. In 95% of patients, endocardial mapping localized the arrhythmogenic focus to the right ventricular outflow tract, correlating with the site of decreased MIBG uptake. On the other hand, when the tachycardia originated at sites other than the right ventricular outflow tract, MIBG scintigraphy identified only 40% of the sites correctly. MIBG scintigraphy might be able to identify patients with ARVD in whom no morphologic abnormalities can be demonstrated by other imaging modalities. Furthermore, it has been proposed that decreased MIBG uptake might be able to identify patients who might benefit from antiadrenergic therapy for the prevention of arrhythmias (52).

Echocardiography

Two-dimensional Echocardiography. Several two-dimensional echocardiographic features have been associated with ARVD (50,53,54). These findings can be classified as global or localized abnormalities (Table 3). In general, echocardiographic findings are sensitive, but not specific, for ARVD. However, in the appropriate clinical setting, two-dimensional echocardiographic findings may suggest the diagnosis.

Doppler Echocardiography. Iliceto et al. (53) found no significant difference between transmitral flow patterns in patients with ARVD and controls. On the other hand, right ventricular filling was altered in patients with ARVD, as evidenced by a significantly decreased E-to-A ratio on the transtricuspid flow pattern.

Diagnostic Accuracy of Echocardiography in ARVD. The diagnostic accuracy of echocardiography in ARVD is difficult to establish, due to lack of a reliable reference standard. So far, contrast angiography has been considered the gold standard, but interobserver reproducibility is low. Endomyocardial biopsy is specific, but not sensitive enough, due to

a large number of sampling errors. Nevertheless, several studies have evaluated the value of echocardiography in predicting ARVD (50,54).

Kisslo (50) found that global abnormalities detected by two-dimensional echocardiography correlated well with angiographic findings, and in the appropriate clinical setting, they were diagnostic of ARVD. While the presence of localized abnormalities (sacculations, bulges) also predicted similar findings on the angiogram, the two methods generally did not agree on the precise location.

Scognamiglio et al. (54) investigated the value of echocardiography in asymptomatic patients with high likelihood of ARVD, using endomyocardial biopsy as a reference standard. In their series, 29% of patients had echocardiographic evidence of right ventricular dysplasia. Moreover, 90% of these patients with echocardiographic evidence of ARVD had serious arrhythmias on 24-hour Holter monitoring. Another study also looked at the accuracy of echocardiography in identifying right ventricular disease in patients with right ventricular tachycardia, using endomyocardial biopsy as a reference standard. Echocardiography was 80% sensitive and 94% specific in predicting abnormal biopsy findings, with a positive predictive value of 88%. Right ventricular abnormalities were present in all patients in whom VT manifested left bundle mimicry with a superior frontal plane axis, suggesting a site of origin in the right ventricular inferior wall or apex. On the other hand, in patients with an inferior frontal axis, echocardiographic abnormalities were uncommon, and when present, they were confined to the outflow tract. The authors concluded that right ventricular tachycardia with a superior axis was associated with a more generalized, global right ventricular involvement, whereas an inferior axis was indicative of a localized process, usually in the region of the outflow tract. The same group found similar results in a more comprehensive study of ARVD, in which they found that an abnormal echocardiogram, along with the sustained nature of tachycardia, superior axis, and abnormal signal-averaged EKG, was associated with positive biopsy findings (54).

Computed Tomography

Computed tomography, just like MRI, is an excellent tool in the evaluation of ARVD because it is tissue specific (Table 3). Using densitometric analysis, it is possible to differentiate between fat and myocardium, and the exact location and extent of myocardial involvement can be assessed (49). One of the earliest reports on the CT features of ARVD comes from Klersy et al. (56). Using densitometric tissue analysis, CT is able to demonstrate the presence of subepicardial fibroadipous tissue, which is the sine qua non of ARVD. Although right ventricular morphologic and functional abnormalities are suggestive in the appropriate clinical setting, the demonstration of intracardiac fibroadipous tissue is more specific for the diagnosis of ARVD. However, the presence of subepicardial fat is a late manifestation, and in

TABLE 3. *Ability of different noninvasive imaging modalities in recognizing characteristic abnormalities in ARVD*

	ECHO	CT	MRI
1. Global abnormalities:			
RV enlargement	Yes	Yes	Yes
RV dysfunction	Yes	Yes	Yes
2. Localized abnormalities:			
Regional RV wall thinning	Yes	Yes	Yes
Regional WMA	Yes	Yes	Yes
Sacculations, bulges	Yes	Yes	Yes
Trabecular disarray	Yes	Yes	Yes
Abnormal moderator band	Yes	Yes	Yes
Intramyocardial fat	No	Yes	Yes

ARVD, arrhythmogenic right ventricular dysplasia; *ECHO,* echocardiography; *CT,* computed tomography; *MRI,* magnetic resonance imaging; *RV,* right ventricle; *WMA,* wall motion abnormality.

the earlier stages one must rely on more general morphologic and functional criteria. Of note, the authors also found occasional left ventricular involvement, which seemed to be present in more advanced cases, in agreement with earlier histologic reports on ARVD.

More recently, electron beam CT (EBCT) has been used in patients with ARVD. Tada et al. (57) proposed that EBCT has better temporal and spatial resolution than conventional CT and attempted to identify characteristic EBCT criteria. The following criteria were identified: abundant epicardial adipose tissue, conspicuous trabeculations with low attenuation, scalloped appearance of the right ventricular free wall, and intramyocardial fat deposits. In addition, from cine-mode images, they detected decreased right ventricular ejection fraction in all patients. None of these features were observed in normal subjects or in patients with RV abnormalities due to reasons other than RV dysplasia. In addition, they observed similar left ventricular involvement in 21% of their patients. Cine-mode imaging confirmed left ventricular dysfunction in these cases.

During electrophysiologic testing there was good correlation between the site of myocardial involvement as determined by EBCT and sites identified by endocardial mapping. EBCT was less reliable in identifying myocardial abnormalities in the diaphragmatic portion of the right ventricle. Based on this one study, the sensitivity and specificity of EBCT appears to be comparable to MRI, but its true clinical role for the diagnosis of ARVD must be determined by further studies.

Magnetic Resonance Imaging

Magnetic resonance imaging is emerging as a gold standard for the evaluation of ARVD, since its sine qua non, intramyocardial adipous tissue, is readily recognizable (Fig. 3). In contrast to fibrous tissue it appears as an area of high signal intensity. In general, sites of right ventricular abnormalities detected by MRI correlate well with arrhythmogenic foci found on electrophysiologic mapping (49). In addition to the ability to characterize tissue, MRI appears to be superior in imaging the right ventricle when compared to echocardiography and x-ray contrast angiography. Several MRI features have been proposed to be characteristic of ARVD (Table 3). General features, similar to those observed by echocardiography and CT, include global or localized abnormalities of right ventricular structure and function. However, the most specific finding is the presence of adipous infiltration of the myocardium, which is readily recognizable on MRI images (49,58,59). Adipous tissue appears as an increase in signal intensity on T1- and T2-weighted images, with a slight increase with T2 weighting. In contrast, fibrous tissue has low signal intensity compared to the myocardium, which makes its differentiation from fat very easy. It is important to note that the high resolution of MRI allows one to differentiate between epicardial fat pads and intracardiac adipous replacement (Fig. 3).

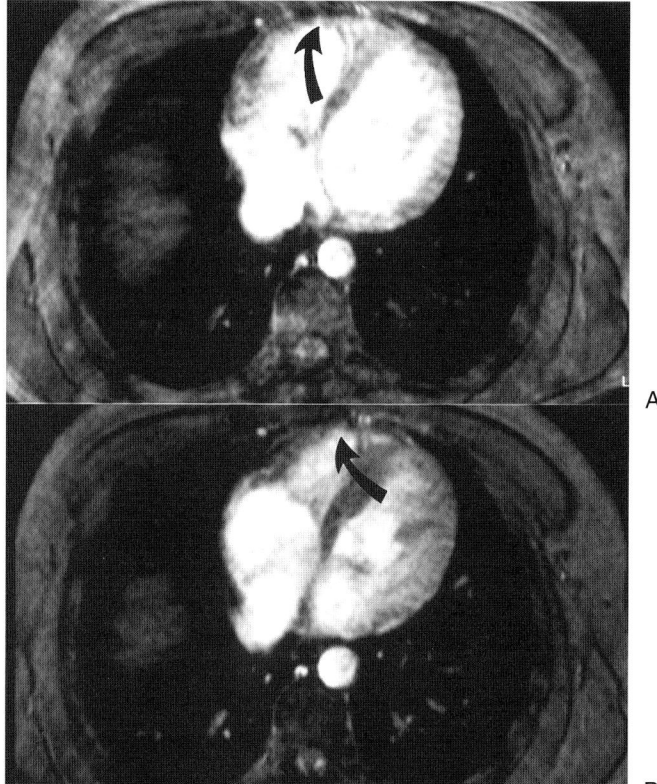

FIG. 3. Arrhythmogenic right ventricular dysplasia (ARVD) in an asymptomatic 14-year-old boy who was referred for magnetic resonance imaging screening after his brother was diagnosed with ARVD. **A, B:** Focal thinning of the right ventricular wall and intramyocardial fat is clearly demonstrated on these multislice axial images (*arrows*).

Auffermann et al. (58) evaluated the accuracy of MRI in diagnosing ARVD, using a combination of contrast angiography and endomyocardial biopsy as reference standard. MRI features associated with right ventricular disease were the following: global right ventricular dilatation, focal wall motion abnormalities, dilatation of the right ventricular outflow tract (RVOT), systolic bulging, regional wall thinning, and increased signal intensity, consistent with fatty infiltration. Patients with electrically inducible tachycardia had significantly more right ventricular dilatation, focal wall motion abnormalities, right ventricular outflow tract enlargement, regional wall thinning, and fatty infiltration, compared to patients with no inducible VT. Fatty infiltration was present in 33% of patients with inducible VT, compared to 11% of noninducible patients. When compared to contrast angiography, MRI detected 86% of regional wall motion abnormalities.

Using MRI in a cohort of patients with documented episodes of VT with left bundle branch morphology, precordial repolarization abnormalities during sinus rhythm and RV abnormalities detected by echocardiography and contrast angiography, Midiri et al. (59) found fatty infiltration of the myocardium in 47%, right ventricular outflow tract enlargement in 27%, dyskinetic bulges in 13%, and right atrial enlargement in 27%. They concluded that although fatty infiltration of the myocardium is the most specific feature of ARVD, it was only present in more advanced cases, and they proposed that the diagnosis should be based on the presence of multiple abnormalities, not solely on the presence of adipous tissue.

In the differential diagnosis of ARVD, idiopathic right ventricular outflow tract (RVOT) tachycardia is a common rhythm disturbance, and its anatomic substrate is not well known. The usual form of this arrhythmia originates in the right ventricular outflow tract, as evidenced by left bundle branch morphology and an inferior axis in the frontal plane. Cardiac MRI has been used to investigate its anatomic substrate and to clarify its relationship to ARVD (60).

Carlson et al. (60) found right ventricular abnormalities on MRI in 95% of patients with RVOT tachycardia, such as focal wall thinning, regionally decreased systolic wall thickening and systolic wall motion abnormalities. Because they did not exclude patients with precordial repolarization abnormalities, even though they did not observe fatty infiltration, it is not clear that cases with early forms of ARVD were not part of their study population. Another group evaluated MRI features in patients with RVOT tachycardia, excluding patients with precordial repolarization abnormalities. MRI was normal in 96% of the cases. In the only patient who had fatty replacement of the myocardium, it was located in the interventricular septum. They concluded that in patients with normal precordial repolarization during sinus rhythm, localized form of RVD was not the etiology of the arrhythmia.

In a similar study, patients with frequent PVCs (average 544 per hour) originating in the RVOT were evaluated. Patients with precordial repolarization abnormalities were excluded. Criteria for right ventricular dysplasia were similar to the ones described above. They found right ventricular enlargement in patients when compared to normal subjects. Also, wall motion abnormalities and regional morphological abnormalities were found in 84% of patients. None of the patients had fatty infiltration. Based on these findings, they concluded that morphologic abnormalities might be responsible for the development of these arrhythmias.

From the above papers MRI appears to be useful both in the clinical and research setting for the evaluation of ARVD, and could become the reference standard for the diagnosis. Because ARVD is a progressive disease usually affecting young individuals, serial evaluation and follow-up is necessary, and invasive studies such as angiography and endomyocardial biopsy are less suitable for such interval evaluations. Instead, noninvasive tests should be considered in this setting. For this purpose, MRI has several advantages over other studies, including CT. It has better soft tissue definition, there is no need for contrast medium, and image planes can be selected freely. The only disadvantage of MRI compared to CT is its relatively long acquisition time. Whereas CT images are obtained during one single beat, MRI images

are a composite of 128 to 256 cardiac cycles, influenced by respiratory and patient motion artifacts, translational movements, and arrhythmias. However, with the recent introduction of systems capable of high-speed acquisition, many of these issues may be overcome.

In conclusion, ARVD is a complex clinical entity, and in the absence of a gold standard, its diagnosis requires the presence of anatomic, imaging and electrophysiologic criteria. The most specific finding is the presence of intramyocardial adipose tissue, but this might not be present until more advanced stages. For this reason, integration of data from different modalities is essential in the clinical diagnosis.

Idiopathic Left Ventricular Tachycardia (ILVT)

Two studies specifically evaluated whether false tendons provide an anatomic substrate for this arrhythmia by comparing their incidence in patients with ILVT to normal subjects. Both studies used two-dimensional echocardiography, either by a transthoracic or transesophageal approach (61). Thakur et al. (61) found fibromuscular bands in 100% of patients with ILVT, compared to 5% in normal subjects. Lin et al. also found a similarly high incidence of false tendons in ILVT patients (94%), however, the incidence in their control population was comparably high (87%). The role of fibromuscular bands in ILVT will need further clarification by electrophysiologic and imaging studies.

BRADYARRHYTHMIAS

Bradyarrhythmias may be caused by ischemic heart disease. However, ischemic heart disease is discussed elsewhere in this book. Clinically significant bradyarrhythmias, in which noninvasive imaging modalities play an important role, are observed in patients with restrictive or infiltrative cardiomyopathy and subaortic abscess. These are described below.

Restrictive Cardiomyopathy

Restrictive cardiomyopathy can be caused by fibrosis or by the deposition of various materials in the myocardium and in the specialized conduction tissue. We describe cardiac amyloidosis as an example of restrictive cardiomyopathy, but other conditions can lead to the same pathophysiologic and clinical picture, including sarcoidosis, hemochromatosis, Fabry's disease, glycogen storage diseases, endocardial fibroelastosis, and others.

Echocardiography

Echocardiography is useful in the diagnosis of restrictive cardiomyopathy (62–64). In general, it usually reveals restrictive physiology based on the analysis of the transmitral flow pattern. In some cases, mostly in cardiac amyloidosis, a specific diagnosis can be made based on further morphologic criteria.

Echocardiographic features of restrictive cardiomyopathies are described in Chapter 49. In general, amyloid cardiomyopathy is characterized by normal end-systolic and end-diastolic dimensions, decreased left ventricular ejection fraction, increased atrial septal thickness and increased echogenicity of the myocardium. This latter is thought to be highly specific for cardiac amyloidosis and is generally referred to as a "granular sparkling" or "speckled appearance," caused by amyloid deposition within the myocardium. With the advent of tissue harmonic imaging, caution must be used when interpreting images using this feature, since it gives the myocardium a speckled appearance, similar to amyloid deposition.

Echocardiography is invaluable in assessing diastolic physiology based on the transmitral flow pattern (63). In the early stages of the disease, a pattern of abnormal relaxation can be observed, while in the later stages, restrictive physiology ensues. It is important to differentiate between restrictive and constrictive disease. The lack of significant respiratory variation on the transmitral and transtricuspid flows suggests restrictive disease. However, in some instances this difference might not be apparent by echocardiography. In those situations, MRI is frequently useful. It is important to bear in mind that Doppler echocardiography can help establish the presence of restrictive cardiomyopathy, but a specific etiology must be made by other means (e.g., amyloidosis in the presence of increased myocardial echogenicity).

Falk et al. (64) evaluated the sensitivity and specificity of the echocardiographic features using endomyocardial biopsy as the reference standard. They found that the presence of increased myocardial echogenicity was 87% sensitive and 81% specific. Furthermore, increased atrial septal thickness (>6 mm) in the presence of increased myocardial echogenicity was 60% sensitive and 100% specific in the diagnosis. Using these criteria, they were able to distinguish between increased ventricular wall thickness caused by amyloid versus other causes (hypertension, etc).

Echocardiographic Features Predicting Arrhythmias

Falk et al. (62) evaluated echocardiographic features that predicted clinically significant arrhythmias in patients with primary and familial amyloidosis. They found that an abnormal echocardiogram (defined as increased myocardial thickness in the absence of obvious causes, thickened atrial septum and increased myocardial echogenicity) predicted arrhythmias and cardiac events with the following frequency: high-grade (grade 3 to 4b) PVCs in 71%, cardiac death in 41%, and sudden cardiac death in 24% of patients. They concluded that echocardiographic evidence of cardiac amyloidosis identifies patients at high risk for cardiac events caused by tachyarrhythmias. However, due to the low number of bradyarrhythmias in their series, they could not comment on the predictive value of echocardiography in bradyarrhythmias.

Magnetic Resonance Imaging

Magnetic resonance imaging has emerged as an invaluable tool in the diagnosis of restrictive cardiomyopathy, including cardiac amyloidosis (63). Although diastolic physiology cannot be assessed as precisely as with echocardiography, its excellent tissue resolution makes it superior in imaging the pericardium. MRI is usually able to differentiate between restrictive cardiomyopathy and constrictive pericarditis, based in part on pericardial thickness and appearance. Furthermore, myocardial tissue characterization can help to identify the nature of the infiltrative process.

In a recent study, Celetti et al. (63) evaluated the role of MRI in the differential diagnosis of restrictive cardiomyopathy, as an adjunct to echocardiography. They studied patients who were found to have restrictive cardiomyopathy based on echocardiographic criteria. They found that MRI was very important in excluding constrictive pericarditis, which was ruled out when pericardial thickness was less than 4 millimeters. They used conventional morphologic criteria and myocardial tissue characterization to differentiate between cardiac amyloidosis and idiopathic restrictive cardiomyopathy. Patients with cardiac amyloid had increased atrial septal thickness and increased right atrial free wall thickness when compared to normal controls or to patients with idiopathic restrictive cardiomyopathy. Furthermore, in cardiac amyloidosis, they observed a significant decrease in the signal intensity ratio of myocardium to skeletal muscle when compared to controls or to patients with idiopathic restrictive cardiomyopathy.

Overall, MRI provides clinically relevant morphologic information in patients who are suspected of having cardiac amyloid or other restrictive cardiomyopathy on the basis of clinical suspicion or echocardiography.

In addition to cardiac amyloidosis, MRI is diagnostic in patients with myocardial dysfunction due to hemochromatosis. The iron present in the myocardium and liver markedly reduces signal, leading to disappearance of tissues on usual clinical magnetic resonance images. In this condition, MRI is the diagnostic study of choice.

Radionuclide Imaging

Several radionuclide approaches have been used in amyloidosis. In general, they provide little additional information compared to echocardiographic and MRI findings. However, it has been proposed that since some tracers are specific for cardiac amyloidosis, they could replace the invasive endomyocardial biopsy, at least in some selected cases. An example of "amyloid specific" tracers is iodine-123 or iodine-131 labeled serum amyloid component. Although it might be useful in identifying extracardiac amyloidosis, it is limited

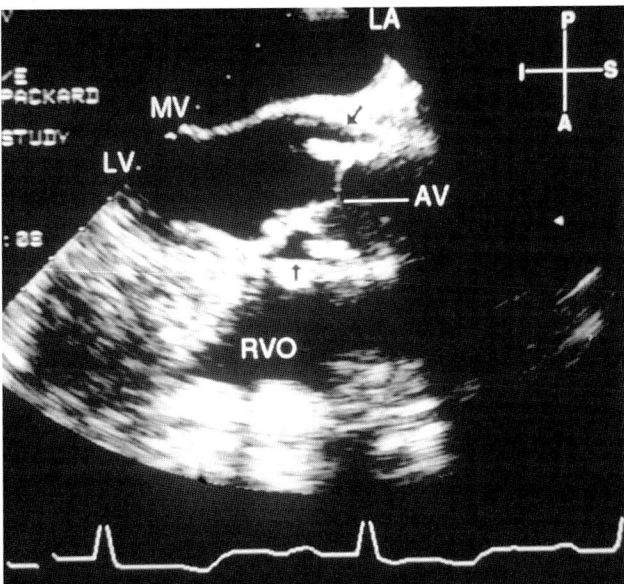

FIG. 4. Transesophageal echocardiographic image of a subaortic abscess in a patient with a prosthetic aortic valve (*AV*) (*arrows*). *LA*, left atrium; *LV*, left ventricle; *MV*, mitral valve; *RVO*, right ventricular outflow tract. (From ref. 13, with permission.)

in detecting myocardial involvement. On the other hand, scanning with labeled antimyosin antibodies was positive in all patients in one series. Several investigators showed abnormal MIBG-uptake in most patients with cardiac amyloid, suggesting derangements in sympathetic innervation. Similarly, technetium-99 pyrophosphate imaging is positive in most patients.

Perivalvular Abscess

Patients with mechanical aortic prosthetic valves are at high risk for developing an abscess in the subaortic region in close proximity to the septal conduction system. Conduction abnormalities are common in these patients, manifesting in various degrees of atrioventricular block. Patients with a history of aortic valve replacement, unexplained fever, and conduction abnormalities should undergo emergent TEE to rule out perivalvular extension of endocarditis (Fig. 4). Patients with a documented perivalvular abscess should be referred for surgical excision immediately.

SYNCOPE

Syncope is a common and frequently complex medical problem. In a cohort of individuals followed for 26 years in the Framingham study, at least one episode of syncope was observed in 3% of the study population during this time period (65). It is responsible for approximately 3% of emergency room visits, and for approximately 1 to 6% of hospital admissions. It is important to realize that syncope is not a

disease, but a symptom that can be seen in a wide variety of disorders, ranging from benign conditions such as situational syncope to life-threatening illnesses such as VT.

Syncope is defined as a sudden, temporary loss of consciousness, accompanied by the loss of postural tone (66). Consciousness is usually rapidly regained upon recumbency. This is an important feature, because cerebral hypoperfusion is usually transient even in sustained, ongoing tachy- or bradyarrhythmias (65). This information from the history might help to differentiate cardiogenic syncope from true seizure disorders, which are usually followed by a prolonged period of decreased consciousness. The definition of syncope also includes the fact that it does not require chemical or electrical cardioversion, unlike sudden cardiac death.

The differential diagnosis of syncope is extensive; it is beyond the scope of this chapter. The four main categories include reflex-mediated syncope (neurocardiogenic syncope), orthostatic hypotension, central nervous system abnormalities, and cardiogenic syncope. In a recent metaanalysis (66), the most frequent causes of syncope were as follows (mean; range in parentheses): vasovagal in 18% (8–37%), cardiac arrhythmias in 14% (4–38%), central nervous system abnormalities in 10% (3–32%), and orthostatic hypotension in 8% (4–10%). No specific etiology could be found in approximately 34% (13–41%) (66). In the following discussion, we focus on cardiogenic syncope (Table 4). Cardiogenic syncope is generally divided into two major categories. A sudden fall in cardiac output may be caused

TABLE 4. *Classification of cardiogenic syncope and noninvasive imaging modalities*

1. Decreased cardiac output resulting from obstruction to flow: ECHO, MRI
   a. Left ventricular outflow obstruction
      Valvular disease (acute regurgitation, stenosis)
      Functional obstruction (hypertrophic obstructive cardiomyopathy)
      Myxoma
      Aortic dissection
   b. Right ventricular outflow tract obstruction: ECHO, MRI
      Valvular disease
      Myxoma
      Paricardial tamponade
      Acute pulmonary thromboembolism
   c. Systolic dysfunction: ECHO, MRI, RNI
      Coronary artery disease (acute ischemia)
      Cardiomyopathy
2. Decreased cardiac output resulting from rhythm disturbances
   a. Bradyarrhythmias
      Sinoatrial disease (sick sinus syndrome, etc)
      Atrioventricular nodal disease (2nd-, 3rd-degree atrioventricular block)
      Pacemaker malfunction
   b. Tachyarrhythmias
      Supraventricular tachycardia
      Ventricular tachycardia

ECHO, echocardiography; *MRI*, magnetic resonance imaging; *RNI*, radionuclide imaging.

by obstruction to flow, or by disturbances in cardiac rhythm. This distinction, however, is artificial, because many conditions causing obstruction to flow (like hypertrophic cardiomyopathy or mitral stenosis) are associated with a variety of arrhythmias.

The diagnostic evaluation of syncope is complex, and its extent is dictated by the individual circumstances (66). The cornerstone of the decision pathway is to determine whether or not the patient has organic heart disease (65,66). For the purposes of this discussion, an expert panel defined organic heart disease, including coronary artery disease, congestive heart failure, valvular heart disease, cardiomyopathy, and congenital heart disease in the definition. Importantly, conduction system disease was not included (66). The role of cardiac imaging modalities in most of these conditions has been described in detail previously. In the following section we focus on the diagnostic assessment of syncope, with a special emphasis on the crucial role of echocardiography in the decision algorithm.

Initial evaluation includes a thorough history, physical exam, and a resting EKG. The combined diagnostic yield of these three modalities is about 50%. Interestingly, the history and physical exam alone had a diagnostic yield of 45%, and the electrocardiogram only provided an additional 5%. Nevertheless, a resting electrocardiogram should be obtained in all patients with syncope, given the virtual lack of potential complications, its low cost, and its ability to reveal potentially life-threatening, reversible conditions (66). In the expert position paper referred to earlier, organic heart disease was excluded if the history and physical exam were negative for cardiovascular symptoms and signs. However, there is some debate as to whether an echocardiogram is necessary to exclude organic heart disease. Regardless, an echocardiogram is obtained further down in the decision pathway.

In patients in whom the initial evaluation is diagnostic, specific treatment should be implemented. Patients with features suggestive of a specific condition should undergo specific testing such as perfusion scintigraphy or cardiac catheterization, if the history is suspicious for coronary artery disease. Patients in whom the initial evaluation is neither diagnostic nor suggestive are considered to have unexplained syncope.

In the group of patients with unexplained syncope, diagnostic imaging of the heart is in the center of the decision pathway. Although no studies have been specifically designed to evaluate the usefulness of echocardiography in syncope, it is very helpful in further risk stratification and management. Unsuspected abnormalities are usually found in 5 to 10% of unselected patients undergoing echocardiography (67). This diagnostic yield is similar to electrocardiography, but it is unclear that echocardiography is cost-effective when used in all patients with unexplained syncope.

Despite these concerns, echocardiography or MRI has a twofold role in the evaluation of unexplained syncope. First, they can identify organic heart disease, revealing conditions that are associated with obstruction to flow, including aortic stenosis, hypertrophic cardiomyopathy, pericardial tamponade, and others. Second, imaging modalities identify patients with organic heart disease, in whom an anatomic substrate might exist for clinically significant arrhythmias. Patients suspected of having significant arrhythmias on the basis of organic heart disease should undergo further evaluation to identify their rhythm disturbance. Exercise testing is recommended if the patient has exertional syncope or if the history is suspicious for coronary artery disease. However, patients should undergo echocardiography prior to exercise stress testing to exclude significant left ventricular outflow tract obstruction caused by hemodynamically significant aortic stenosis or hypertrophic cardiomyopathy, because exercise testing is contraindicated in these patients.

Patients in whom echocardiography or MRI reveals organic heart disease should undergo 24-hour ambulatory electrocardiographic monitoring to identify significant arrhythmias. The lack of symptomatic arrhythmias on Holter monitoring does not exclude the possibility of potentially significant arrhythmias. If the Holter examination is nondiagnostic, the patient should be considered for invasive electrophysiologic testing. Because intracardiac electrophysiologic testing is not free of complications, is quite expensive, and time-consuming, it should be used judiciously based on the initial evaluation and echocardiography. Intracardiac electrophysiologic testing is unlikely to yield positive results in the absence of organic heart disease (67). For this reason, it is recommended that patients with clinically normal hearts and a normal echocardiogram should not undergo invasive electrophysiologic testing. Such patients should be considered for loop electrocardiographic monitoring to rule out idiopathic ventricular tachycardia or other arrhythmias, tilt-table testing to investigate orthostatic hypotension, or psychiatric testing to evaluate possible contributing psychiatric features.

In conclusion, syncope is a common and complicated clinical entity. However, a structured diagnostic evaluation based on the history, physical exam, electrocardiogram, echocardiogram, MRI, and noninvasive or invasive electrophysiologic testing yields a diagnosis in most cases.

REFERENCES

1. Prystowsky EN, Benson DW, Fuster V, et al. Management of patients with atrial fibrillation. *Circulation* 1996;93:1262–1277.
2. Aronow WS, Ahn C, Kronzon I. Echocardiographic findings associated with atrial fibrillation in 1,699 patients aged >60 years. *Am J Cardiol* 1995;76:1191–1192.
3. Dent JM. Role of echocardiography in the evaluation and management of atrial fibrillation. *Cardiol Clin* 1996;14:543–553.
4. Slany J, Stollberger C, Kronik G. Value of echocardiography in atrial fibrillation. *Wien Klin Wochenschr* 1992;10410–10415.
5. Vaziri SM, Larson MG, Benjamin EJ, et al. Echocardiographic predictors of nonrheumatic atrial fibrillation. *Circulation* 1994;89:724–730.
6. Villecco AS, Pilati G, Bianchi G, et al. Left atrial size in paroxysmal atrial fibrillation: echocardiographic evaluation and follow-up. *Cardiology* 1992;80:89–93.
7. The Stroke Prevention in Atrial Fibrillation Investigators. Predictors

of thromboembolism in atrial fibrillation, II: echocardiographic features of patients at risk. *Ann Intern Med* 1992;116:6–12.

8. Mattioli AV, Vivoli D, Bastia E. Doppler echocardiographic parameters predictive of recurrence of atrial fibrillation of different etiologic origins. *J Ultrasound Med* 1997;16:695–698.

9. Omran H, Jung W, Schimpf R, et al. Echocardiographic parameters for predicting maintenance of sinus rhythm after internal atrial defibrillation. *Am J Cardiol* 1998;81:1446–1449.

10. Jovic A, Troskot R. Recovery of atrial systolic function after pharmacological conversion of chronic atrial fibrillation to sinus rhythm: a Doppler echocardiographic study. *Heart* 1997;77:46–49.

11. Bellotti P, Spirito P, Lupi G, et al. Left atrial appendage function assessed by transesophageal echocardiography before and on the day after elective cardioversion for nonvalvular atrial fibrillation. *Am J Cardiol* 1998;81:1199–1202.

12. The Stroke Prevention in Atrial Fibrillation Investigators. Predictors of thromboembolism in atrial fibrillation, I: clinical features of patients at risk. *Ann Intern Med* 1992;116:1–5.

13. Nanda NC, Domanski M. *Atlas of transesophageal echocardiography.* Baltimore: Williams & Wilkins, 1998.

14. Tsai LM, Lin LJ, Teng JK, et al. Prevalence and clinical significance of left atrial thrombus in nonrheumatic atrial fibrillation. *Int J Cardiol* 1997;58:163–169.

15. Silverman DI, Manning WJ. Role of echocardiography in patients undergoing elective cardioversion of atrial fibrillation. *Circulation* 1998;98:479–486.

16. Chu E, Kalman JM, Kwasman MA. Intracardiac echocardiography during radiofrequency catheter ablation of cardiac arrhythmias in humans. *J Am Coll Cardiol.* 1994;24:1351–1357.

17. Swiryn S. Nuclear electrophysiology. *PACE* 1993; 6:1171–1180.

18. Botvinick E, Dunn R, Frais M, et al. The phase image: its relationship to patterns of contraction and conduction. *Circulation* 1982;65:551–560.

19. Yiannikas J, Eastway RJ, MacIntyre WJ, et al. Phase imaging: a new, noninvasive method for diagnosis, localization of accessory pathways, and serial assessment of therapy in patients with Wolff-Parkinson-White syndrome. *Cleveland Clin Q* 1982;49:61–72.

20. Botvinivck EH, Frais MA, Shosa D, et al. An accurate means of detecting and characterizing abnormal patterns of ventricular activation by phase image analysis. *Am J Cardiol* 1982;50:289–298.

21. Dormehl IC, Bitter F, Henze E, et al. An evaluation of the diagnostic efficacy of phase analysis of data from radionuclide ventriculograms in patients with Wolff-Parkinson-White syndrome. *Eur J Nucl Med* 1985;11:150–155.

22. Johnson LL, Seldin DW, Yeh HL, et al. Phase analysis of gated pool scintigraphic images to localize bypass tracts in Wolff-Parkinson-White syndrome. *J Am Coll Cardiol* 1986;8:67–75.

23. Rakovec P, Kranjec I, Fettich J, et al. Localization of accessory pathways in Wolff-Parkinson-White syndrome by phase imaging. *Cardiology* 1983;70:138–144.

24. Botvinick EH, Frais M, O'Connell W, et al. Phase image evaluation of patients with ventricular preexcitation syndromes. *J Am Coll Cardiol* 1984;3:799–814.

25. Schechtmann N, Botvinick EH, Dae M, et al. The scintigraphic characteristics of ventricular preexcitation through Mahaim fibers with use of phase analysis. *J Am Coll Cardiol* 1989;13:882–891.

26. Rakovec P, Kranjec I, Fettich JJ, et al. Multiple accessory pathways: a combined electrophysiological and radionuclide study. *PACE* 1985; 8:60–65.

27. Archer S, Gornick C, Grund F, et al. Exercise thallium testing in ventricular preexcitation. *Am J Cardiol* 1987;59:1103–1106.

28. DeMaria AN, Vera Z, Neumann A, et al. Alterations in ventricular contraction pattern in the Wolff-Parkinson-White syndrome. *Circulation* 1976;53:249–257.

29. Hishida H, Sotobata I, Koike Y, et al. Echocardiographic patterns of ventricular contraction in the Wolff-Parkinson-White syndrome. *Circulation* 1976;54:567–571.

30. Ng WH, Kew ST. Cardiac arrhythmias and echocardiographic features in Wolff-Parkinson-White syndrome. *Med J Malaysia* 1980;35:41–45.

31. Chandra M, Kerber RE, Brown DD, et al. Echocardiography in Wolff-Parkinson-White syndrome. *Circulation* 1976;53:943–946.

32. Windle JR, Armstrong WF, Feigenbaum H, et al. Determination of the earliest site of ventricular activation in Wolff-Parkinson-White syndrome: Application of digital continuous loop two-dimensional echocardiography. *J Am Coll Cardiol* 1986;7:1286–1294.

33. Jue J, Winslow T, Ossipov M, et al. Effect of preexcitation on Doppler indexes of left ventricular filling. *Am J Cardiol* 1993;71:1462–1464.

34. Vaskelyte J, Bredikis J. Correlations between the localization of accessory atrioventricular pathway and Doppler indexes of left ventricular output and function in patients with Wolff-Parkinson-White syndrome. *Pacing Clin Electrophysiol* 1992;15:268–273.

35. Kuercher HF, Abbott JA, Botvinick EH, et al. Two dimensional echocardiographic phase analysis. *Circulation* 1992;85:130–142.

36. Kuercher HF, Kleber GS, Melichercik J, et al. Transesophageal echo phase imaging for localizing accessory pathways during adenosine induced preexcitation in patients with the Wolff-Parkinson-White syndrome. *Am J Cardiol* 1996;77:64–71.

37. Nakayama K, Miyatake K, Uematsu M, et al. Application of tissue Doppler imaging technique in evaluating early ventricular activation associated with accessory atrioventricular pathways in Wolff-Parkinson-White syndrome. *Am Heart J* 1998;135:99–106.

38. Lai WW, Al-Khatib Y, Klitzner TS, et al. Biplanar transesophageal echocardiographic direction of radiofrequency catheter ablation in children and adolescents with the Wolff-Parkinson-White syndrome. *Am J Cardiol* 1993;71:872–874.

39. Sosa E, Scanavacca M, d'Avila A, et al. Long-term results of visually guided left ventricular reconstruction as single therapy to treat ventricular tachycardia associated with postinfarction anteroseptal aneurysm. *J Cardiovasc Electrophysiol* 1998;9:1133–1143.

40. Dor V. The treatment of refractory ischemic ventricular tachycardia by endoventricular patch plasty reconstruction of the left ventricle. *Sem Thorac Cardiovasc Surg* 1997;9:146–155.

41. Kuck KH. Arrhythmias in hypertrophic cardiomyopathy. *PACE* 1997; 20(pt. II):2706–2713.

42. Leier CV. The cardiomyopathies: mortality, sudden death, and ventricular arrhythmias.

43. Lazzeroni E, Domenicucci S, Finardi A, et al. Severity of arrhythmias and extent of hypertrophy in hypertrophic cardiomyopathy. *Am Heart J* 1989;118:734–738.

44. Cheng XS, Kusachi S, Urabe N, et al. Association between high grade ventricular arrhythmias and extent of ventricular hypertrophy in hypertrophic cardiomyopathy. *Acta Med Okayama* 1991;45:155–159.

45. Pons-Llado G, Carreras F, Borras X, Palmer J, Llauger J, Bayes de Luna A. Comparison of morphologic assessment of hypertrophic cardiomyopathy by magnetic resonance versus echocardiographic imaging. *Am J Cardiol* 1997;79:1651–1656.

46. Pohost GM, Vignola PA, McKusick KE, et al. Hypertrophic cardiomyopathy. Evaluation by gated cardiac blood pool scanning. *Circulation* 1977;55:92–99.

47. Brachmann J, Hilbel T, Grunig E, et al. Ventricular arrhythmias in dilated cardiomyopathy. *PACE* 1997;20(pt.II):2714–2718.

48. Grimm W, Glaveris C, Hoffmann J, et al. Noninvasive arrhythmia risk stratification in idiopathic dilated cardiomyopathy: design and first results of the Marburg Cardiomyopathy Study. *Pacing Clin Electrophysiol* 1998;21(11 pt 2):2551–2556.

49. Dalal P, Fujisic K, Hupart P, et al. Arrhythmogenic right ventricular dysplasia: a review. *Cardiology* 1994;85:361–369.

50. Kisslo J. Two-dimensional echocardiography in arrhythmogenic right ventricular dysplasia. *Eur Heart J* 1989;10:22–26.

51. LeGuludec D, Slama MS, Frank R, et al. Evaluation of radionuclide angiography in diagnosis of arrhythmogenic right ventricular cardiomyopathy. *J Am Coll Cardiol* 1995;26:1476–1483.

52. Wichter T, Hindricks G, Lerch H, et al. Regional myocardial sympathetic dysinnervation in arrhythmogenic right ventricular cardiomyopathy. *Circulation* 1994;89:667–683.

53. Iliceto S, Izzi M, Martine D, et al. Echo Doppler evaluation of right ventricular dysplasia. *Eur Heart J* 1989;10(suppl D):29–32.

54. Scognamiglio R, Fasoli G, Nava A, et al. Contribution of cross-sectional echocardiography to the diagnosis of right ventricular dysplasia at the asymptomatic stage. *Eur Heart J* 1989;10:538–542.

55. Mehta D, Davies MJ, Ward DE, et al. Ventricular tachycardias of right ventricular origin: Markers of subclinical right ventricular disease. *Am Heart J* 1994;127:360–366.

56. Klersy C, Raisaro A, Salerno JA, et al. Arrhythmogenic right and left ventricular disease: evaluation by computed tomography and nuclear magnetic resonance imaging. *Eur Heart J* 1989;10:33–36.

57. Tada H, Shimizu W, Ohe T, et al. Usefulness of electron-beam computed tomography in arrhythmogenic right ventricular dysplasia. Rela-

tionship to electrophysiological abnormalities and left ventricular involvement. *Circulation* 1996;94:437–444.

58. Auffermann W, Wichter T, Breithardt G, et al. Arrhythmogenic right ventricular disease: MR imaging vs angiography. *Am J Roentgenol* 1993;161:549–555.
59. Midiri M, Finazzo M, Brancato M, et al. Arrhythmogenic right ventricular dysplasia: MR features. *Eur J Radiol* 1997;7:307–312.
60. Carlson MD, White RD, Trohman RG, et al. Right ventricular outflow tract ventricular tachycardia: detection of previously unrecognized anatomic abnormalities using cine magnetic resonance imaging. *J Am Coll Cardiol* 1994;24:720–727.
61. Thakur RK, Klein GJ, Sivaram CA, et al. Anatomic substrate for idiopathic left ventricular tachycardia. *Circulation* 1996;93:497–501.
62. Falk RH, Rubinow A, Cohen AS. Cardiac arrhythmias in systemic amyloidosis: correlation with echocardiographic abnormalities. *J Am Coll Cardiol* 1984;3:107–113.
63. Celetti F, Fattori R, Napoli G, et al. Assessment of restrictive cardiomyopathy of amyloid or idiopathic etiology by magnetic resonance imaging. *Am J Cardiol* 1999;83:798–801.
64. Falk RH, Plehn JF, Deering T, et al. Sensitivity and specificity of the echocardiographic features of cardiac amyloidosis. *Am J Cardiol* 1987;59:418–422.
65. Benditt DG, Lurie KG, Fabian WH. Clinical approach to diagnosis of syncope. *Cardiol Clin* 1997;15:165–176.
66. Linzer M, Yang EH, Estes M, et al. Diagnosing syncope. Part 1: value of history, physical examination, and electrocardiography. *Ann Intern Med* 1997;126:989–996.
67. Linzer M, Yang EH, Estes M, et al. Diagnosing syncope. Part 2: unexplained syncope. *Ann Intern Med* 1997;127:76–86.

CHAPTER 64

Cardiovascular Trauma

Role of Imaging

Vincent L. Sorrell and Navin C. Nanda

BACKGROUND

This century has witnessed a faster and more violent world than ever before and cardiac trauma is increasing. Proportionate mortality trends have shown a war-like involvement of urban streets with a much higher likelihood than ever before of encountering a gunshot or knife wound in the emergency department (1). Automobiles continue to impact with each other and with pedestrians at an alarming rate.

Cardiovascular trauma remains a leading cause of death in patients arriving in the emergency department, but with decreasing prehospital scene times, patients are now arriving in the emergency department in a premorbid state (2). Furthermore, the advancement of knowledge and technology in the field of emergency medicine has allowed more of these patients to be stabilized and survive long enough to be surgically corrected.

In the last century, a noted surgeon, Billroth (3), stated that ''the surgeon who should attempt to suture a wound of the heart would lose the respect of his colleagues.'' This is certainly not the case anymore. Each day someone else survives a motor vehicle accident or gunshot wound because of the advances in cardiac trauma surgery. Indeed, the cardiothoracic surgeon maintains the greatest burden of care, but the medical physician can be an integral member of the trauma team. The role of this physician is to assist in the diagnosis of cardiac trauma, recognize unsuspected participating injuries, clarify the cardiac pathophysiology in stabilized patients, and provide important insight in the intra-

V. L. Sorrell: Section of Cardiology, East Carolina University Brody School of Medicine; Graphics and Exercise Physiology Laboratories, Greenville, North Carolina 27858.

N. C. Nanda: Department of Medicine, Heart Station, Echocardiography Laboratories, University of Alabama at Birmingham, Birmingham, Alabama 35249.

operative, early and late postoperative care of the trauma patient.

INTRODUCTION

The cardiologist or cardiovascular internist must have an understanding of the types of injuries likely to invoke specific cardiac complications. In addition, they must have a working familiarity of the various diagnostic tools available to assist in this critical triage. Numerous algorithms have been proposed involving electrocardiography, cardiac enzyme analysis, echocardiography, aortography, computed tomography (CT) scan, and even cardiorrhaphy, but all lack sufficient accuracy to be routinely performed on each patient (4–9). This is in part due to individual patient circumstances, but also the various institutional capabilities and local expertise.

Only through a combined understanding of the numerous cardiac injuries in addition to the multiple diagnostic tools is the managing physician capable of determining when best to utilize which tool.

This chapter provides the reader with an understanding of the various types of cardiac injuries that may occur. The diagnostic tools available for cardiac imaging are discussed with specific insight into the advantages and disadvantages of each as they relate to cardiac trauma. Finally, the various clinical settings that often require the use of these diagnostic imaging devices are separately discussed to help the reader consider the types of cardiac pathology most likely encountered.

DIFFERENTIAL DIAGNOSES

Nonpenetrating (Blunt) versus Penetrating Trauma

Blunt cardiac trauma constitutes less than 10% of cardiac injuries, and the majority of cardiac trauma result from penetrating etiologies (2). Closed thoracic injuries result in cardiac trauma 10 to 16% of the time (10).

The common separation by many authors into blunt and penetrating wounds was not used in this chapter to avoid limiting the reader in their diagnostic considerations. Although cardiac tamponade and coronary laceration occur with greater frequency after penetrating wounds, essentially all cardiac injuries can occur with both penetrating and blunt wounds, and an extensive differential diagnosis must be considered despite this classification.

Myocardial Contusion

Myocardial contusion is a histologic diagnosis (11). An absolute clinical diagnosis of myocardial contusion is lacking. Without a definite diagnosis in living patients, the actual incidence, clinical significance, and prognosis remain poorly defined. A commonly used clinical diagnosis is the identification of a new wall motion abnormality first seen after cardiac trauma and associated with significantly elevated cardiac isoenzymes that suggest a cardiac injury.

Despite the clinical diagnosis of a contusion, the prognosis is routinely good with usually no cardiac deaths or complications (12). It is still important to diagnose, not because of its poor outcome, but to prevent aggravating the situation through the inadvertent use of anticoagulation or thrombolytic therapy, and to council the patient to limit excessive activities. A dilemma is when the wall motion abnormality results in the formation of an intracardiac thrombus. In this situation, the clot must be recognized and treated with anticoagulation, since the incidence for embolic events is probably high (13).

Both echocardiography and radionuclide angiography are more diagnostic than electrocardiography (ECG) (14). It is important to maintain a broad differential diagnosis for the finding of a wall motion abnormality. Although a myocardial contusion with normal coronary arteries is one such possibility, a number of ischemic etiologies must be considered. An acute myocardial infarction should be considered. Whether primarily occurring and possibly contributing to the trauma, or secondary to the trauma resulting in a coronary injury, is sometimes difficult to confirm. The location of hypokinesis resulting from trauma may be helpful in differentiating myocardial ischemia or infarction (15). Typically, traumatic injury affects the apical septal region in addition to the distal, or less often, the entire, right ventricular (RV) anterior free wall. Myocardial ischemic injury usually involves the RV basal wall.

''And always with a heart contusion, arise both doubt and much confusion.'' Although true for nearly half a century, this is much less valid now given the currently available tools. In the only metaanalysis to date, ECG and enzymatic testing were highly useful in detecting clinically significant myocardial contusions (16). It seems reasonable to anticipate an even greater benefit with the increased usage of more sophisticated evaluations such as troponin isoenzymes combined with some method of wall motion assessment.

Myocardial Concussion

Similar to a contusion, a wall motion abnormality must be present for this diagnosis. However, unlike a contusion, histologic findings of cellular injury are absent (17). The clinical value of this clarification is not known.

Pericardial Injury

The pericardium is subjected to direct injury from penetrating chest trauma and indirect damage from blunt chest trauma. Myocardial injuries may slowly bleed into the pericardial sac causing large effusions, or rapid bleeding may result in clinical tamponade with minimally sized effusions. Depending on the degree of the myocardial injury, local hemorrhage may be controlled by the development of an intrapericardial thrombus. It is important to properly diagnose cardiac tamponade prior to the induction of anesthesia in preparation for surgery. The removal of the sympathetic support may result in immediate cardiovascular collapse.

Early pericardial bleeding without tamponade, may result in an inflammatory response with subsequent late tamponade days to weeks later (18). Systematic follow-up is required for several weeks after any evidence of pericardial trauma.

A pericardial laceration may occur and usually involves the left pleuropericardium (55%); the next most common injury is the diaphragmatic pericardium (27%), and least common is the right pleuropericardium (19%) (19). If small, it may cause no problems. Interestingly, very large lacerations also cause minimal problems and may heal uneventfully. However, intermediate lacerations measuring 8 to 12 cm in diameter may result in cardiac herniation or strangulation of the left ventricle. This may impair chamber filling or may compress the coronary arteries leading to ischemia or infarction.

The chest x-ray, CT scan, and echocardiogram have each provided important diagnostic information in these patients.

Traumatic Aortic Dissection

The paucity of specific physical examination and chest x-ray findings in acute aortic rupture, coupled with the markedly increased mortality in delaying the diagnosis may warrant the routine evaluation of severe truncal deceleration injuries with advanced techniques.

The physical examination may reveal elevated arm pressures compared with leg pressures. If significant aortic regurgitation exists, then a widened pulse pressure and sometimes a new holodiastolic murmur is found.

Patients who survive acute aortic rupture long enough to be evaluated, have a 95% likelihood of the aortic tear occurring at the aortic isthmus, just distal to the left subclavian artery origin (20). Aortic aneurysms classically develop near the ligamentum arteriosum and are frequently associated with hematomas. If encapsulated by adjacent tissues, a great vessel wound may partially heal and form a pseudoaneurysm. The instability of this defect warrants appropriate diagnosis and surgical repair.

Transesophageal echocardiography (TEE) and CT scanning are the most commonly used noninvasive tools for investigations of aortic injuries. The most cited gold standard is still invasive—aortography.

Great Vessel Injury

Rupture or avulsion of the innominate, carotid, or left subclavian arteries, and the inferior or superior vena cava may occur. The proximal portions of these vessels are seen equally well with TEE and CT scanning, but aortography is required for greater resolution or for suspected distal vessel trauma.

Foreign Body Emboli

Bullets and other projectiles may be found anywhere after penetration and entry into the human body. It is important to confirm their presence outside of the cardiovascular system. If found within an artery or heart chamber, they may embolize and cause further damage (21). If juxtapositioned near an artery, these may penetrate over time and lead to distal embolization. In these situations, the foreign body requires identification and removal. Also, if an operation is required for other purposes and the projectile is readily located, or if an infection is suspected, the foreign body should be removed.

Indeed, this was the concern by the physicians caring for President Ronald Reagan after the assassination attempt on his life (22). On entering the operating room, the surgeons were aware of the bullet location in the left chest by chest x-ray. After initially being unable to locate it where anticipated, they considered distal embolization a possibility. Further searching confirmed its position in the left lower lobe, and they did not need to perform any additional evaluations with either direct intraoperative sterile echo, transesophageal echocardiography, or fluoroscopy, which may at times be necessary for this purpose (23).

Cardiac Rupture

Rupture of the heart may occur and involve the right ventricle; ventricular septum; mitral, tricuspid, or aortic valves; or the aorta and the other great vessels. It is important to remember that cardiac rupture may occur up to 2 weeks after the initial trauma (24). The same diagnostic tools helpful in the evaluation for a myocardial contusion are useful in this assessment.

Valvular Injury

The atrioventricular valves are more commonly involved than the semilunar valves (25). Acute mitral regurgitation is usually a result from disruption of the chordae tendinae or papillary muscles and, much less commonly, the leaflets themselves (26). The etiology is thought to be related to the sudden decompression of a distended heart chamber at late diastole or early systole at a time when the mitral valve is closed. This degree of injury is often not compatible with survival, and, therefore, mitral regurgitation is actually more frequently encountered in surviving patients.

Acute tricuspid regurgitation is less frequently reported (27). This may be related to the less severe and more tolerable symptoms, or it may actually occur less commonly since the right ventricle is a lower pressure chamber with less stress generated during sudden cardiac compression. A patient with continued right heart failure symptoms, despite medical treatment, was found to have a flail anterior tricuspid valve leaflet and severe tricuspid regurgitation 3 months after a motor vehicle accident. This patient underwent successful valve repair (Fig. 1A–D; see also Color Plate 42 following page 758). With acute aortic regurgitation, congestive heart failure (CHF) symptoms are common. Echocardiography is the noninvasive diagnostic modality of choice to determine the etiology of valvulopathy and the degree of regurgitation. Ventriculography is also useful.

Coronary Artery Injury

The various types of coronary lesions that can occur include coronary laceration or tear, fistula formation, or the development of an intracoronary thrombus. Artery lacerations from direct penetration or indirect alterations from abrupt deceleration of cardiac structures remain uncommon.

There is limited data on the natural history of coronary artery fistulas or ventricular septal defects, especially when left surgically unrepaired (28). One report documented persistence of the left-to-right shunt using echocardiography at 15 months follow-up (29). This suggests that spontaneous closure is unlikely, and, since the development of endocarditis or heart failure is significantly increased, finding these on diagnostic imaging should probably lead to surgical repair.

The most common coronary artery injured through noniatrogenic trauma is the left anterior descending (LAD) coronary artery. Subsequently, the anterior myocardial wall becomes hypokinetic or akinetic. A fistula may develop between the right coronary artery and the right ventricle or the coronary sinus and may result in a new continuous murmur (30). Although a dilated coronary sinus may be seen with echocardiography or identified with contrast-enhanced CT scanning, the absolute diagnosis is still made with cardiac catheterization and coronary angiography.

Acute myocardial infarctions have been reported to occur from partial coronary tears, activated thrombotic alterations in the presence of preexisting atherosclerotic disease, or im-

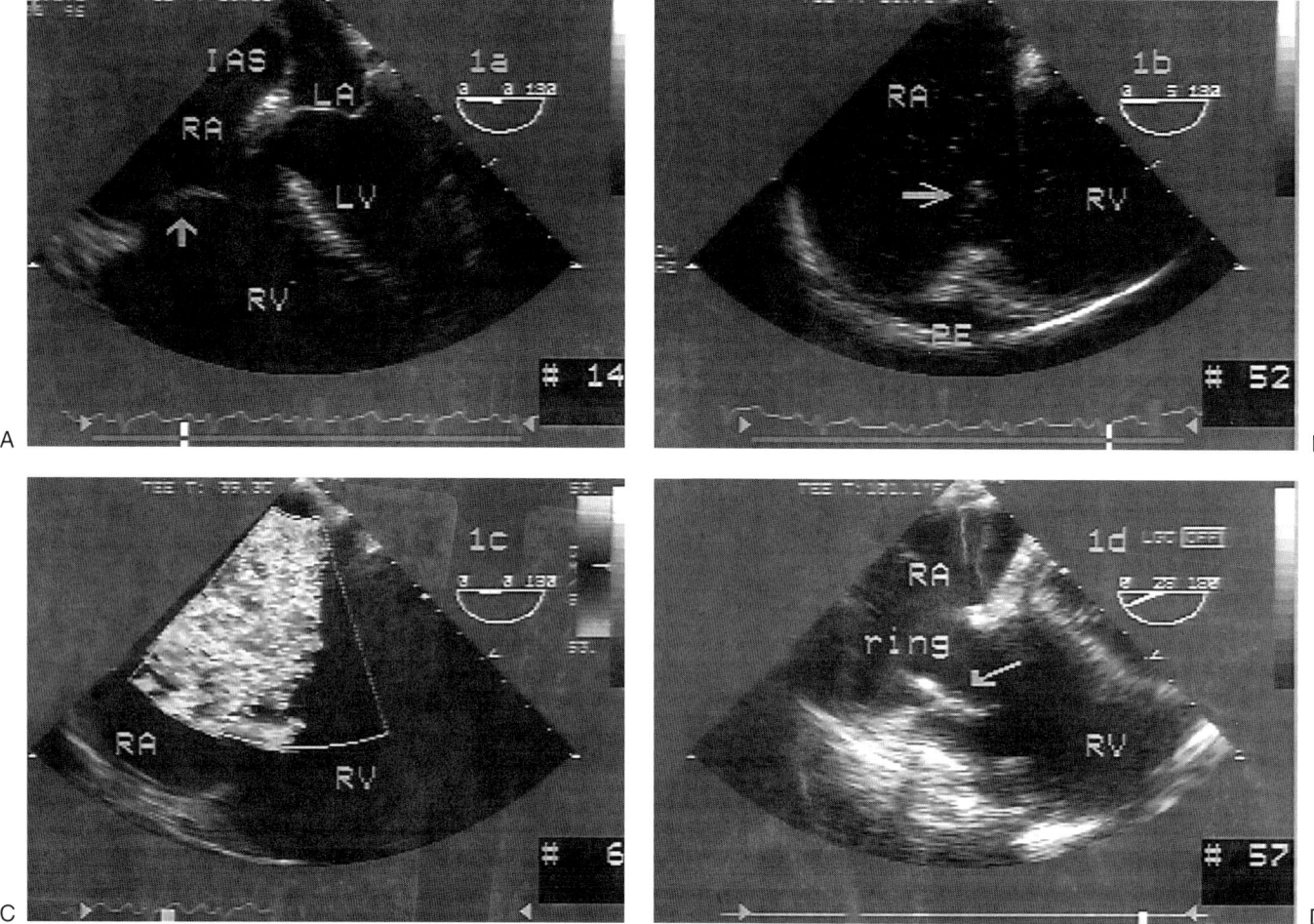

FIG. 1. A: Transesophageal echocardiographic (TEE) examination at the midesophageal plane representing a four-chamber, surface-equivalent view. Note the dramatically enlarged right ventricle (*RV*) and right atrium (*RA*), the deviated interatrial septum (*IAS*) representing markedly elevated RA pressures (exceeding the left-sided pressures), and the flail anterior tricuspid valve leaflet (*arrow*). *LV*, left ventricle; *LA*, left atrium. **B:** Counterclockwise rotation from 1**A**. Note: The right-sided structures are more optimally imaged, and an anterior, loculated pericardial effusion (*PE*) is seen. *Arrow*, flail anterior tricuspid valve leaflet. **C:** Color flow Doppler interrogation of Figure 1**B**. Note: Severe tricuspid regurgitation is seen completely filling the right atrial cavity. **D:** TEE study 3 months later—same orientation as 1**B**. Note: The right atrium (*RA*) and right ventricle (*RV*) are significantly smaller and the pericardial effusion has resolved. *Ring*, tricuspid valve annular ring; *arrow*, repaired chordae tendinea. (See also Color Plate 42 following page 758.)

mediate thrombus formation. The end result of each is myocardial dysfunction of varying degrees. Cardiac isoenzymes, ECG testing, echo, radionuclide perfusion imaging, and coronary angiography are each helpful in this setting.

CARDIAC IMAGING

The diagnostic process begins with the history and physical examination, usually followed by blood work , the electrocardiogram, and the chest x-ray. The following sections describe the various advantages and disadvantages of the diagnostic tools available to assist in the evaluation of suspected cardiac trauma (Table 1).

Physical Examination

One should suspect a cardiac injury when a penetrating wound occurs within "the box," defined by the Cook County Hospital as follows: superiorly, as the clavicles; laterally, the nipples; and, inferiorly, the lower rib margins (31). Sometimes, external evidence of injury is undetectable, despite heart or great vessel injury. The often sought after but rarely found finding of aortic dissection, termed "pseudocoarctation" (isolated reduced blood pressure in the left arm), is only present in approximately 5% of these patients (32).

Classically described findings for chronic aortic regurgitation are not present when this lesion is acute. Often the mur-

TABLE 1. *Useful diagnostic tools for the various types of cardiac injuries*

Cardiac injury	Commonly used imaging tools								
	CXR	ECG	Echo	TEE	Nuc	CT	MRI	Angio	Fluoro
Contusion	−	+/−	+ +	+ +	+	−	ID	+/−	−
Pericardial									
Effusion	+	−	+ +	+ +	−	+ +	+ +	−	−
Tamponade	−	−	+ + +	+ + +	−	−	−	−	−
Rupture	+ +	−	+ +	+ +	−	+ +	+ +	−	−
TAD	+	−	+	+ + +	−	+	+ +	+ + +	−
Valvular injury	−	−	+ + +	+ + +	+/−	−	ID	+ +	−
Cardiac rupture	+	−	+ +	+ +	−	+ +	+ +	+	−
Coronary injury	−	+ +	+/−	+	+/−	+/−	−	+ + +	−
Foreign body	+/−	−	+ +	+ +	−	+ +	+ +	−	+ +

CXR, roentgenography; *ECG,* electrocardiography; *Echo,* surface echocardiography; *TEE,* Transesophageal echocardiography; *Nuc,* radionuclide angiography or perfusion imaging; *CT,* computed tomography; *MRI,* magnetic resonance imaging; Angio, coronary or ventricular angiography; *Fluoro,* fluoroscopy; *TAD,* traumatic aortic dissection; + + +, recommended; + +, clinically useful; +, some benefit; +/−, possible benefit; −, no benefit; ID, insufficient data.

mur of acute, severe aortic or mitral regurgitation is absent. Other findings of acute mitral regurgitation are the signs and symptoms of congestive heart failure. If the tricuspid valve is damaged, then the findings are predominantly right-sided heart failure.

With acute tricuspid regurgitation, patients may have a soft holosystolic murmur that increases with respirations, elevated neck veins, fatigue, dyspnea, and peripheral edema. Cyanosis may occur if a significant patent foramen ovale is present, due to the sudden increase in right atrial pressures with resultant shunting across the atrial septum to the left atrium.

Despite hemodynamically significant cardiac tamponade, significant hemorrhage, and volume, depletion may prevent the elevation of the neck veins. Hypotension and distant heart sounds are often present for other reasons unrelated to tamponade.

The patient with a pericardial rupture often complains of coughing and dyspnea. A consistent finding in a literature review of 40 patients with this abnormality revealed that rib fractures were universal (33). Cyanosis with hypotension is common. The apex may be deviated significantly if the myocardium has protruded beyond the pericardial border. A pericardial friction rub may also be detected. An unusual, but helpful, finding, related to the intermittent myocardial evulsion, is the development of hemodynamic instability only during certain patient positions (34).

The differential appearance of upper torso cyanosis has been described as a frequent occurrence after blunt cardiac rupture, and should be recognized (35).

A number of trauma indices that combine the age of the victim, the mechanism of injury, other associated injuries, and specific pathophysiologic findings are frequently used by trauma teams (36). These have been shown to provide a reasonably accurate prediction of clinical outcomes.

Overall, there generally remains a poor correlation between the mechanism of injury, the symptoms, the physical examination findings, the chest x-ray appearance, and the likelihood of myocardial damage or cardiac morbidity and mortality (37). The lack of evidence of chest wall injuries or symptoms may impede the diagnosis of a cardiac injury, and, therefore, a high index of suspicion must remain throughout the evaluation process.

Usually, the finding of significant congestive heart failure warrants the investigation for mechanical disruption (left-sided valve regurgitation; free wall or septal rupture; etc.), since this is an exceedingly rare finding from myocardial contusion alone.

Cardiac Blood Work

The MB fraction of creatine phosphokinase (MB-CPK) is the most commonly measured cardiac isoenzyme. It is commonly elevated from associated muscle injury and does not accurately reflect the degree of myocardial contusion. This is in part due to the proportionately limited quantity of MB isoenzyme that is released compared to the MM isoenzyme from the surrounding muscle injury. The ratio of MB-CPK to total CPK improves the specificity at the expense of sensitivity.

Although MB-CPK is imperfect, it has correlated with morbidity and mortality, even when more sophisticated nuclear or echocardiographic imaging was unable to do so (38,39).

Troponin I (TnI) and T isoenzymes are probably more specific and should be considered the standard of care in most trauma situations (40). These should be measured in addition to, or in place of, the MB-CPK. In a study using echo-defined wall motion abnormalities (WMA) as evidence of myocardial contusion, both MB-CPK and Tn I were increased (41). In 26 of the 37 patients without a WMA, the MB-CPK isoenzyme was inappropriately increased. The TnI isoenzyme was normal in all 37 patients. Using a TnI level of 1.1 mg/L and a MB-CPK level of 18 mg/L, a specificity of 100% and 80%, respectively, was obtained (42).

Newer cardiac markers, such as the immunohistochemical detection of C5b-9(m), are in development and may further improve the diagnosis of cardiac injuries (43).

Electrocardiography

Despite the presence of a myocardial contusion, the electrocardiogram (ECG) is usually nonspecific and of minimal diagnostic contribution. This may be related to the commonly involved right ventricle, which is thinner and has minimal electrical contribution to the ECG. Sinus tachycardia is usual, but the ECG may remain entirely normal, despite cardiac damage. Right ventricular leads have been attempted but have not significantly helped (44,45). Serial abnormalities are probably more important than a single ECG finding, since this suggests an acute, on-going process.

Almost any abnormality can occur, and old ECG findings must be compared to be certain that any pathologic findings are new. The ECG may also be altered by hypoxia, pulmonary contusion, acid-base disturbances, anemia, or elevated catecholamines, which commonly co-exist. Global or focal ST-segment elevations provide evidence of pericarditis or myocardial injury, respectively.

Holter monitoring devices have also been used to provide a longer ECG evaluation, but thus far have been similarly nonspecific and are not routinely recommended.

An important, but ominous finding, is electromechanical dissociation, which most often results from cardiac tamponade.

Roentgenography

This remains an important diagnostic tool in the evaluation of the trauma patient (see Chapter 24). It is universally available and rapidly performed. Although not always diagnostic, it remains a vital complimentary tool to the other techniques discussed.

An enlarged heart with a rounded cardiac silhouette ("water flask" appearance), associated with a prominent superior vena cava and azygous vein, suggests a hemodynamically significant pericardial effusion—cardiac tamponade (46).

The chest x-ray should be specifically interrogated for any of the following findings associated with aortic injuries: widened mediastinum (most common and least accurate finding); apical "cap" of extrapleural hematoma; depression of the left mainstem bronchus greater than 140 degrees; opacification of the aortic-pulmonary window; abnormal aortic knob (loss of normal contour or double density); pulmonary congestion; massive pleural effusion (particularly left); pneumo- or hemopericardium; esophageal deviation to the right (displaced nasogastric tube: most accurate and least common) (47,48).

The greatest disadvantage of this technique is the low specificity. Nearly one third of patients with a diagnosed aortic rupture will have a normal chest x-ray (49,50).

If abdominal contents are identified in the pericardial silhouette, this signifies an inferior pericardial rupture with a diaphragmatic rent. Leftward deviation of the left ventricle (LV) apex or spontaneous pneumopericardium are also supportive of this diagnosis (51).

Echocardiography

This is currently the most widely utilized tool due to its nearly universal accessibility, excellent safety profile, portability, and the immediate availability of real-time images (see Chapter 2). Other technical advantages allow the interrogation of the global and regional, left and right ventricular function, pericardium and pericardial space, and valve structure and competence (52–56) (see Chapter 3). Color flow Doppler provides accurate quantitation of the severity of traumatic valvular regurgitation or acute cardiac shunting (57). Conventional Doppler echo provides an accurate assessment of the hemodynamic significance of constrictive pericarditis or cardiac tamponade.

Echo is optimally suited for serial evaluations when required. The disadvantage is related to the lack of prospective investigations proving its role in this clinical arena and also to the incidence of nearly 25% technically suboptimal studies in the trauma patient.

With the recent Food and Drug Administration (FDA) approval of the first of a new line of late generation contrast agents, the ventricular endocardial borders are better visualized, and the number of suboptimal studies may be reduced (58). These agents may also provide additional information when myocardial rupture or other mechanical complications are suspected. Additionally, most of newer ultrasound systems are providing novel, improved techniques that use Doppler devices and harmonic imaging to better visualize the cardiac chamber and determine the systolic function (see Chapter 10). An unexpected finding, now being realized with these newer techniques originally developed to enhance the contrast image, is an improved cardiac image even without contrast injection. Better anatomic resolution with these newer devices will only further enhance our evaluation of the cardiac trauma patient.

Although concern has been raised that the identification of a wall motion abnormality is nonspecific—possibly related to a cardiac contusion, an old myocardial infarction, or a metabolic abnormality—the absence of such a finding is usually helpful to the managing physician.

A single echocardiogram after a penetrating chest injury is only 40% accurate for diagnosing cardiac tamponade (59). With serial echo studies, the accuracy was increased to 96% when the second examination was performed 8 to 10 hours after the first (60). With a pneumopericardium, echocardiography may detect air between the pericardium and myocardium.

Recent data suggests increased blood flow to the damaged zone of myocardial contusion with preferential shunting to the epicardium and an actual decline in flow to the subendocardium (61). This heterogeneous blood flow pattern raises the possibility of eventually using myocardial contrast perfusion echocardiography (or radionuclide perfusion imaging) to evaluate these individuals. Although not ready for routine clinical use, myocardial perfusion agents are close to release and are undergoing extensive research investigations.

When a left pleural effusion is present, retrocardiac imaging from a parascapular approach may reveal important images of the ascending, transverse, and descending thoracic aorta (62). The posterior pericardium is often difficult to see with standard echo and is better visualized through this approach allowing localized, posterior pericardial effusions an improved chance of detection.

Unfortunately, major intrapericardial injuries have been found at surgery after an entirely normal echo (31). Reports such as these require the maintenance of a high index of suspicion and a low threshold for exploratory surgery.

Intracardiac Ultrasound

Although not widely available, this device uses a small piezoelectric ultrasound transducer placed on the end of a cardiac catheter (see Chapter 7). By manipulating the catheter within the cardiac chambers, specific cardiac anatomy is randomly interrogated. This was used to identify a localized pericardial effusion adjacent to the right atrium resulting from perforation of this chamber after an iatrogenic injury (63). It has also been used to investigate the aorta during an acute aortic dissection (64).

As this technique improves and devices become more portable, this may provide a rapid, accurate cardiac diagnosis for the trauma patient.

Transesophageal Echocardiography

There are several distinct advantages of transesophageal echocardiography (TEE) compared to the other commonly utilized diagnostic techniques available (see Chapter 4). TEE images are real-time, allowing immediate interpretations. The procedure is quick, portable, and semiinvasive, with emergency studies usually completed within 10 to 20 minutes. Importantly, simultaneous procedures can be performed. For instance, if an emergency laparotomy is required, the TEE can be performed without delaying both potentially life-saving studies.

A recent investigation was completed in 80 patients with blunt chest trauma and suspected myocardial contusion each of whom received a TEE within 48 hours (65). A wall motion abnormality was detected in 19%, and each had right ventricular (RV) involvement—one third had an LV abnormality extending from the adjacent septal WMA. An interesting and clinically important finding was that in 40% of patients, the only RV abnormality was the finding of ''tardokinesis'' (RV contraction begins after the QRS and peaks after the T wave). Each of these patients, particularly the group with tardokinesis, had clinically significant hypotension requiring treatment and a trend to more frequent arrhythmias. Again,

there was no increase in mortality—a repeated finding in myocardial contusion studies.

TEE has the greatest advantage in its ability to interrogate the entire aorta for the suspicion of a dissection, subintimal hematoma, or intraluminal thrombi. The transesophageal approach is necessary in the 25% of patients that have suboptimal standard echo images. The sensitivity and specificity for aortic injury is 100% and 98%, respectively (66).

Earlier reports of blind areas related to interference from the left mainstem bronchus have essentially been eliminated with the use of a multiplane imaging probe (67,68). The sensitivity and specificity remains similar to magnetic resonance imaging (MRI) and is probably better than CT scanning with experienced operators (6,69,70).

In a direct comparison of TEE and aortography, TEE was actually superior, with a greater statistical accuracy. There were fewer false negatives with TEE, but a slightly greater chance for a false positive (71).

This technique requires advanced skills and is highly operator dependent (as are all standard ultrasound modalities). The ability to intubate the esophagus usually reflects the experience of the performer—the inability to routinely intubate the esophagus is more likely to occur with less experienced operators. This was evident in another comparison of TEE with aortography, where the authors were unable to intubate 5 of the 34 patients attempted (15% failure rate) (72). They obtained a sensitivity and specificity of only 57% and 91%, respectively. Additionally, the importance of the learning curve was illustrated by Vignon et al. (73), when a single center retrospective review was performed. The accuracy improved, and the number of inconclusive studies decreased over the 4-year study period.

Three-dimensional TEE remains an investigational tool that may provide additional value in the detection of small traumatic ruptures of the aorta (Figs. 2 and 3; see also Color Plates 43 and 44 following page 758). This technique was

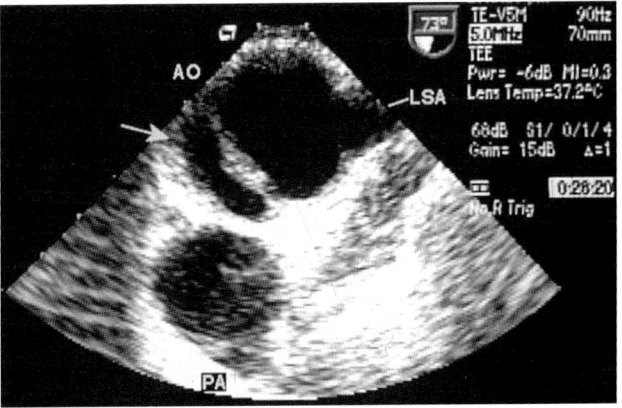

FIG. 2. Multiplane transesophageal echocardiographic examination demonstrating a traumatic aortic disruption at the aortic isthmus (*arrow*). *Ao*, aorta; *LSA*, left subclavian artery; *PA*, pulmonary artery. (From ref. 98, with permission.) (See also Color Plate 43 following page 758.)

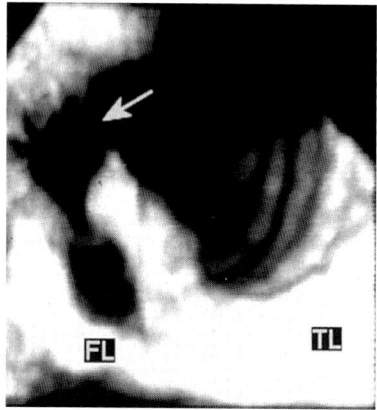

FIG. 3. Three-dimensionally reconstructed transesophageal echocardiographic examination, performed at the same site as Figure 2 demonstrating the circumferential extent of the traumatic aortic disruption (*arrow*). *FL*, false lumen; *TL*, true lumen. (From ref. 98, with permission.) (See also Color Plate 44 following page 758.)

able to accurately identify the location and extent of this traumatic rupture, measuring less than 1 cm, despite a normal CT scan.

In addition to the operator dependence, other disadvantages are related to its semiinvasive placement within the esophagus. This technique usually requires sedation. With esophageal injury, further trauma may occur from probe manipulation. Anteflexion of the cervical spine is required, and severe cervical neck trauma should be considered a contraindication. With severe maxillofacial injuries, it may be contraindicated or simply impossible to pass the probe. With continued development and clinical experience of a prototype, minature, transnasal TEE probe, this device may allow esophageal intubation when not possible by standard imaging probes (74).

Another disadvantage is the absence of optimal visualization of the great vessels. With experience, the origins and proximal few centimeters of the great vessels are routinely imaged (Fig. 4; see also Color Plate 45 following page 758) (75). If clinical suspicion warrants investigation of the great vessels, an angiogram or MRI is often more diagnostic.

Despite these potential problems with TEE, it has repeatedly been shown to be more accurate than transthoracic echocardiography (TTE) for contusion and aortography for aortic trauma, and it had no complications when evaluated in 68 consecutive trauma patients (76).

Radionuclide Angiography

Either the first-pass or equilibrium-gated radionuclide angiographic (RNA) techniques provides direct evaluation of LV and RV regional and global wall motion, size, and function (see Chapters 18 and 19). This technique was accurately used to evaluate for LV aneurysm formation and was able to determine the cause of hemodynamic instability in the

majority of study patients (38). Unfortunately, the identification of a wall motion abnormality with this technique does not correlate well with clinical outcome (77). In 77 consecutive patients with possible cardiac contusions, a wall motion abnormality was identified in 55%. Only 3 of these patients experienced sudden cardiac death, but a contusion was confirmed at pathology in each.

Using first-pass imaging techniques, Harley (78) found 74% with a reduced right ventricular function. At a three-week follow up study, all patients had returned to normal function. This method can also quantitate the severity of traumatic ventricular septal shunts or regurgitant lesions (79). It is rarely suboptimal and could be considered a substitute for echo.

The advantages of this type of imaging is its ability to reproducibly calculate the right and left ventricular global and regional function and guide surgery. Disadvantages are related to the required time delay from technical reconstruction for image display and subsequent delay in image availability, lack of high quality portable imaging systems requiring transportation of the trauma patient, and difficulty in gating when the cardiac rhythm is irregular.

Radionuclide Perfusion Imaging

Myocardial contusion in patients with blunt chest trauma has been evaluated by thallium-201 chloride and technetium-99m myocardial scintigraphy (80,81) (see Chapter 13). Animal studies have suggested that this technique is only accurate with transmural, or "full-thickness," myocardial contusions, which are probably not common clinically (82).

Technetium 99m pyrophosphate imaging should also reveal myocardial injury, but is significantly limited by the thinner RV wall and extensive overlying boney injuries that make it difficult to distinguish from cardiac involvement (see Chapter 16). Despite its accuracy in animals, only 6% of patients with probable myocardial injury detected by other means were predicted with this technique (83).

Monoclonal antimyosin imaging with indium-111 was previously considered a sensitive method for the detection of myocardial injuries (see Chapter 21) (84). However, this technique has not been extensively evaluated and is not universally available; therefore, many nuclear physicians have very little if any experience in this technique, which further limits its clinical application.

A significant disadvantage of this technique, as well as all techniques that are not portable, is the need to transport the trauma patient to areas less fit to supervise the critically injured patient. Additionally, nuclear images, by design, require the patient to remain motionless while specialized gamma cameras acquire radioactive count profiles. These patients with multiple traumas are likely to have difficulty remaining still long enough not to produce motion artifacts.

Computerized Tomography

Computed tomographic (CT) systems have become ultrafast with concomitantly improved image quality, but rapid

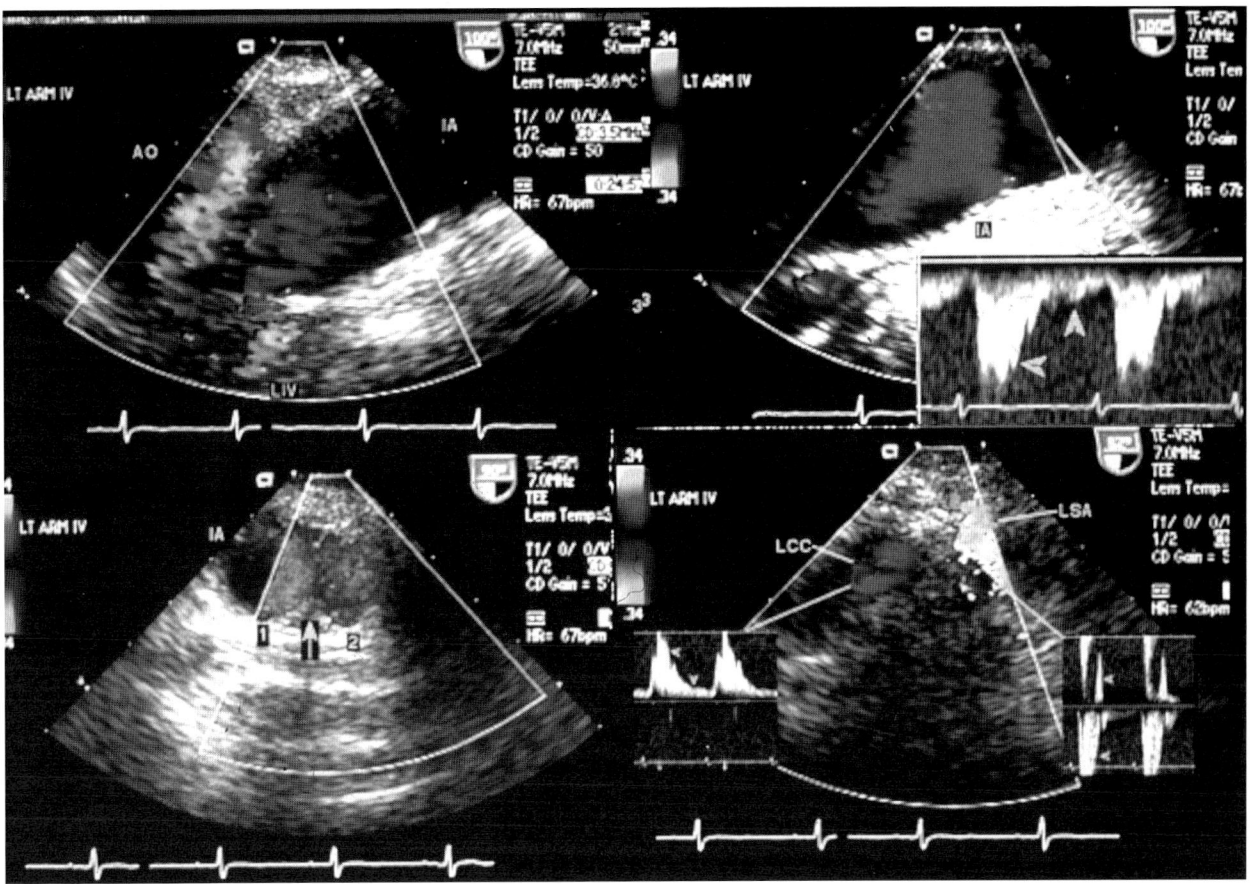

FIG. 4. Multiplane transesophageal echocardiographic examination of the aortic arch branches (**left upper panel**). The innominate artery (*IA*) is readily visualized (**left lower panel**). *Ao*, aorta; *LIV*, left innominate vein. The innominate artery can be seen to bifurcate into the right common carotid artery (*1*) and the right subclavian artery (*2*) (**right upper panel**). Doppler flow interrogation from the innominate artery shows the antegrade systolic flow signal (*horizontal arrowhead*) and the antegrade diastolic flow signal (*vertical arrowhead*) (**right lower panel**). The left common carotid (*LCC*) and the left subclavian artery (*LSA*) are obtained with counterclockwise rotation of the probe after initially identifying the innominate artery. The relatively low resistance Doppler flow signals from the left common carotid artery (**left insert**) and the higher resistance profile obtained in the left subclavian artery (**right insert**) are seen. (From ref. 98, with permission.) (See also Color Plate 45 following page 758.)

cardiac movements still provide some motion artifacts (see Chapter 26). The CT image is well designed to also evaluate for the presence of associated injuries, extent of hematoma, and the presence of pericardial effusions.

Contrast enhanced image protocols are necessary for vascular definition and determine if an aortic leak is present. Extravasation of contrast material beyond the confines of the aortic wall is a definite sign of rupture. Other indirect signs include obliteration of periaortic tissue planes.

A traumatic aortic dissection (TAD) and intimal flap is readily detected with both enhanced and unenhanced protocols. An unenhanced image is first obtained to assist in the identification of calcification within the vessel lumen.

The interpreter must keep a high index of suspicion when evaluating for TAD and realize that indirect signs from aortic rupture may be all that is seen. A periaortic hematoma is one such finding. Loss of periaortic tissue planes from local inflammation, pleural effusions or atelectasis, cardiomegaly suggesting aortic regurgitation, compression of the esophagus or left atrium, and lack of organ perfusion are other indirect findings suggesting TAD (85).

Very thin slices are mandatory, especially near the region of clinical suspicion. This technology remains limited by this defined thickness at each level that is imaged. Even with very thin cuts, an arterial tear may be missed (86).

This technique provides excellent anatomic relationships and has been shown to assist in the diagnosis of a pericardial rupture (87). The ability to provide axial images is unique and may provide a clearer anatomic relationship to the managing physician or surgeon. The great vessels are difficult to optimally visualize and injuries may be missed. Helical CT scanning, however, should improve the detection rate of these arterial lesions (88).

Contrast enhanced CT was directly compared to aortography in 104 stable patients suspected of blunt aortic injuries (85). The sensitivity and specificity of detecting major thoracic injury was 55% and 65%, respectively. Had CT alone been used, two transected aortas and three major aortic branch injuries would have been missed in their investigation.

Despite these limitations, CT imaging provides high-resolution images with minimal motion artifact, excellent vessel opacification, and it allows a high degree of interpretive accuracy. At many institutions, this is probably the only tool available, and it may provide insightful information prior to transport to trauma centers.

The major disadvantages are less resolution than angiography, the requirement for contrast material with renal compromise and allergy risks, and the required transport to the imaging suite.

Magnetic Resonance Imaging

This is an excellent imaging modality that provides superb quality images with outstanding, well-delineated anatomic relationships (see Chapters 28 and 29). In the trauma patient, it remains of limited practicality due to its reliance on a magnetic field, its inability to be used near metal (mechanical ventilators, certain chest tubes and lines, etc.), requirement for patient cooperation, and time delay for image reconstruction. It also requires a high level of interpreter experience.

Serial magnetic resonance imaging (MRI) studies were utilized to delay emergency surgery for traumatic aortic ruptures in over 20 patients allowing recovery from other injuries (89). Elective surgery proceeded an average of 7 months later with no mortality. Patients were medically treated, and the serial MRI was performed to detect any unstable, rapidly changing traumatic lesions. Their data suggests that emergency surgery may not always be necessary if careful, serial follow-up images are obtained with MRI and aggressive, adequate medical management occurs (90).

This technique was also utilized to diagnose an intrapericardial hematoma and was combined with Doppler echocardiography to confirm the hemodynamic presence of delayed constrictive pericarditis (91). It has also been educational in describing the finding of a pariaortic fat pad misinterpreted by TEE as an intramural hematoma (92). Through the excellent anatomic images provided by MRI, surgery was avoided. Through this example, the investigators were able to recommend careful inspection of the line separating the aortic wall near the adjacent periaortic fat pad. If separate movement is noticed, this suggests that this is not an intramural hematoma.

With the recent development of cardiac gating capabilities, magnetic resonance evaluation of the cardiac and pericardiac structures is now possible (see Chapter 30). Current research is concentrating on the development of a portable, hand-held MRI magnet that would greatly expand the use of this device and may allow this tool to eventually become

the gold standard for evaluating the trauma patient. With technological improvements in cardiac imaging, shortening of the examination times, and the development of cost-effective strategies, this tool will merge further into the clinical mainstream.

Contrast Angiography

Coronary angiography remains an important, albeit invasive, diagnostic tool in the evaluation of the trauma patient (see Chapter 32). It provides important, otherwise unobtainable, data on the coronary artery anatomy. This is necessary to help determine the etiology of an identified wall motion abnormality.

Aortography remains the gold standard for the detection of aortic disease at most trauma centers in the United States. With injection of contrast at the aortic root, the presence and degree of aortic regurgitation is determined.

Thoracoscopy

Recent developments in fiberoscopic imaging devices have allowed cardiothoracic surgeons to place intrathoracic video-assisted probes in the mediastinum to visually explore the surface of cardiac structures. This technique was recently used to diagnose a traumatic pericardial rupture and assist with the selection of the most appropriate location of the surgical incision (93). More clinical trials are needed before this technique can be recommended for this purpose.

Flouroscopy

Standard fixed and portable flouroscopic systems are widely available and may be complementary in the investigation to the trauma patient. They provide the physician with the opportunity to evaluate many body regions rapidly and with one imaging device. When foreign bodies are not readily found by other means, this may provide the location, if they are radioopaque and dense enough to be spotted.

The major disadvantage is that it is limited by markedly inferior resolution by most imaging standards, which does not allow it to be used except for the most crude investigations.

CLINICAL SETTINGS

Acutely Unstable, "In Extremis" Patients

Acutely ill patients remain in the direct care of the cardiothoracic surgeon and require immediate surgical intervention for any opportunity to survive. The mortality of these patients remains 50%, despite the numerous improvements in diagnostic and therapeutic capabilities previously described. When patients with blunt trauma present acutely ill (''*in extremis*''), the mortality is nearly 100% and reflects the significant diffuse body trauma (94).

Many of these trauma patients will be subjected to postoperative evaluations, and specific postoperative complications must be considered. At immediate entry into the hospital setting, a brief physical examination should be performed with concentration on the location of the injuries. An ECG and chest x-ray should only be obtained if there is a delay into the operating room. Upon arrival in the operating room, an intraoperative TEE should be utilized. It provides an opportunity to identify unanticipated cardiac injuries as well as diverse interrogation of multiple other potentially involved cardiac structures. It also provides the surgeon and anesthesiologist immediate knowledge of the right and left ventricular systolic function.

Critical, but Stabilized (Detectable, but Reduced Blood Pressure)

The mortality is approximately 25% in these patients, and pericardial tamponade is not uncommon. These patients require quick evaluation to rule out tamponade prior to transport into the operating room. When identified, the anesthesia should be appropriately modified to prevent rapid induction with removal of sympathetic support that may result in sudden hemodynamic collapse and cardiac arrest. Pericardial fluid should first be removed prior to the induction of anesthesia.

Echocardiography plays an increasingly valuable role in this triage. The surface study, even when suboptimal, will often reveal a large pericardial effusion. The subsequent TEE study in the operating room will confirm other cardiac pathology and the integrity of the aorta.

Hemodynamically Stable (Normal Blood Pressure)

These patients have a low mortality, and, therefore, diagnostic investigations should be used as clinically warranted. Prior to the development and use of these diagnostic tools, the stable patient presented a considerable dilemma. With only the option of careful observation or exploratory surgery, the outcomes were less predictable. With echocardiography, patients are triaged to either surgery or observation with significantly less risk of predictable deterioration (95).

Optimal physical examinations are recommended for these patients. The finding of an elevated central venous pressure, tachycardia, and S3 gallop should stimulate an investigation to confirm the presence or absence of a myocardial contusion, LV dysfunction and CHF, or cardiac tamponade. Echocardiography is well designed to specifically look for each cause of the physical findings. One must remember the potential for an iatrogenic cause for these findings from ''over-resuscitation'' by aggressive intravenous fluid administration.

These patients may develop sudden deterioration despite only mild evidence of trauma. It still remains difficult to determine which patients require admission with intensive monitoring and who can be safely discharged.

Delayed Symptoms (Weeks to Years)

Patients who present with potential cardiovascular symptoms late after their trauma, usually as outpatients, should be evaluated carefully. Previously utilized diagnostic tools should be reviewed and compared for significant changes. Delayed pericardial tamponade, ventricular and atrial septal defects, aortic and mitral regurgitation, pericarditis, myocarditis, intracardiac thrombi, and heart blocks have all been reported as potential late complications (13,18,96).

Routine follow-up should be arranged for patients with complicated or uncomplicated myocardial contusions or pericardial effusions. Physical examinations, ECG, chest x-ray, and echo at 4 to 6 weeks are usually sufficient to identify late complications.

Posttraumatic pericarditis has been identified as late as 6 months after trauma and may precede the development of constrictive pericarditis months to years later. Patients with traumatic wall motion abnormalities are also subjected to LV thrombus formation and embolic events from either the RV or LV months to years later. Patients with abnormal wall motion and the development of aneurysmal formation are subject to LV rupture at the time of maximal necrosis, which usually occurs 1 to 2 weeks after trauma.

CONCLUSIONS

Cardiac trauma has a large spectrum of morbidity and mortality, with partial thickness myocardial contusions resulting in no symptoms and nearly impossible to diagnose to cardiac rupture with a high incidence of sudden death.

All patients with the potential of a cardiac contusion should receive serial ECGs, cardiac troponins, a chest x-ray, and an echocardiogram. An adequate echo is available in 75% of trauma patients, and the finding of normal LV function, normal valvular function, and no pericardial effusion is helpful to the managing physician.

A stable patient with a normal chest x-ray should probably just be observed. If an aortic injury is suspected and the chest x-ray is entirely normal, then additional evaluation should proceed with either TEE or CT scan, depending on local preferences. A stable patient with an abnormal x-ray should undergo a TEE or a CT scan, depending on local expertise and other issues discussed above. An unstable patient with an abnormal CXR should probably receive an aortogram without delay.

With early, rapid evaluation by TEE, the trauma team will have either a greatly enhanced or reduced suspicion for aortic trauma, myocardial contusion, and pericardial damage, allowing time to either stabilize the patient or to arrange for emergency surgery. A normal finding requires no further investigation and allows obvious trauma elsewhere to proceed to surgery unimpeded. Any ill-defined, nonspecific aortic abnormalities should be followed with aortography.

In addition to the specific differences related to the techniques, local personnel and other institutional considerations are important modifiers in any algorithm. Issues related to the transportation of critical patients to radiology and other less emergency-oriented settings, which study that can be obtained most rapidly at each institution, and the local expertise must all be considered. All imaging tools that are not portable are at a significant disadvantage for this reason. Improving the mobility of these tools should be an area of continued research and may eventually provide enhanced outcomes in the trauma patient.

Physicians using TEE for these important evaluations must initially compare their findings to aortography and determine their individual accuracy rates. Continuous quality improvement techniques should be employed to maintain a high level of accuracy and reproducibility. Despite the excellent high quality images and reproducible accuracy provided by TEE, eliminating the need for aortography to less than 10% in experienced operators, there remain certain circumstances that require additional testing (97). Significant atheromatous debris and technical factors may prevent an optimal study from being obtained, and an aortogram should be performed to evaluate this potentially fatal injury.

If significant hemorrhage is present and immediate repair of abdominal or extremity lesions are required, then an abnormal chest x-ray should prompt evaluation by TEE, since this can proceed simultaneously with ongoing surgery.

Since cardiac trauma is likely to remain a relatively common cause of mortality in the emergency room and our diagnostic armamentarium is continuing to improve, clinical investigations of the cardiac trauma patient are strongly encouraged to determine if clinical outcomes can be improved.

Cardiac imaging provides a multitude of reliable techniques, each with its own specific advantages and limitations, but no single tool providing all the necessary diagnostic capabilities is needed. As newer cardiac imaging tools are developed and found to have additional diagnostic capabilities, our accurate diagnosis and effective treatment of cardiac injuries should also improve.

REFERENCES

1. James S. *Injury mortality: national summary of injury mortality data, 1987–1993.* Washington DC: U.S. Department of Health and Human Services, Public Health Service Center for Disease Control and Prevention, June 1996.
2. Mattox KL, Feliciano DV, Burch J, et al. Five thousand seven hundred sixty cardiovascular injuries in 4459 patients. Epidemiologic evolution 1958 to 1987. *Ann Surg* 1989;209(6):698–705.
3. Jeger E. *Die Chirurgie der Blutgefasse und des Herzens.* Berlin: A. Hirschwald, 1913:295.
4. Freshman SP, Wisner DH, Weber CJ. 2D-Echocardiography: emergent use in the evaluation of penetrating precordial trauma. *J Trauma* 1991;31(7):902–906.
5. Rosenthal MA, Ellis JI. Cardiac and mediastinal trauma. *Adv Update Cardiovasc Emerg* 1995;13(4):887–902.
6. Buckmaster MJ, Kearney PA, Johnson SB, et al. Further experience with transesophageal echocardiography in the evaluation of thoracic aortic injury. *J Trauma* 1994;37(6):989–995.
7. Mattox KL, Limacher MC, Feliciano DV, et al. Cardiac evaluation following heart injury. *J Trauma* 1985;25(8):758–765.
8. Cheitlin MD. The internist's role in the management of the patient with traumatic heart disease. *Acute Cardiol Care* 1991;9(4):675–688.
9. Miller FB, Shumate CR, Richardson D. Myocardial contusion. *Arch Surg* 1989;124:805–808.
10. Glinz W. Injuries to the heart by blunt trauma. In: Glinz W, ed. *Chest trauma.* Berlin: Springer-Verlag, 1981:180–209.
11. Roxburgh JC. Myocardial contusion. *Injury* 1996;27(9):603–605.
12. Cachecho R, Gindlinger GA, Lee VW. The clinical significance of myocardial contusion. *J Trauma* 1992;33:1.
13. Timberlake GA, McSwain NE Jr. Thromboembolism as a complication of myocardial contusion: a new capricious syndrome. *J Trauma* 1988;28:535–540.
14. Coleman J, Gonzalez A, Harlafter N, et al. Myocardial contusion: diagnostic value of cardiac scanning and echocardiography. *Surg Forum* 1976;27:293–294.
15. Karalis DG, Victor MF, Davis GA, et al. The role of echocardiography in blunt chest trauma: a transthoracic and transesophageal echocardiographic study. *J Trauma* 1994;36(1):53–58.
16. Maenza RL, Seaberg D, D'Amico F. A meta-analysis of blunt cardiac trauma: ending myocardial confusion. *Am J Emerg Med* 1996;4(3):237–241.
17. Rudesky BM. More on myocardial contusion—with additional insight on myocardial concussion [letter; comment]. *Chest* 1997;112(2):570–572.
18. Raney JL, Kennedy ES. Delayed cardiac tamponade following a stab wound: a case report. *J Ark Med Soc* 1997;93(12):589–591.
19. Feczko JD, Lynch L, Pless JE, et al. An autopsy review of 142 nonpenetrating (blunt) injuries of the aorta. *J Trauma* 1992;33(6):846–849.
20. Symbas MD, Tyras DH, Ware RE, et al. Traumatic rupture of the aorta. *Ann Surg* 1973;178:6–12.
21. Wascher RA, Gwinn BC. Air rifle pellet injury to the heart with retrograde caval migration. *J Trauma* 1995;38(3):379–381.
22. Aaron BL, Rockoff SD. The attempted assassination of President Reagan. *JAMA* 1994;272:1689–1693.
23. Hassett A, Moran J, Sabiston DC, et al. Utility of echocardiography in the management of patients with penetrating missile wounds of the heart. *J Am Coll Cardiol* 1986;7:1151–1156.
24. Olsovsky MR, Wechsler AS, Topaz O. Cardiac trauma: diagnosis, management, and current therapy. *Angiology* 997;48(5):423–432.
25. Parmley LF, Manion WC, Mattingly TW. Nonpenetrating traumatic injury to the heart. *Circulation* 1958;18:371–396.
26. McDonald ML, Orszulak TA, Bannon MP, et al. Mitral valve injury after blunt chest trauma. *Ann Thorac Surg* 1996;61(3):1024–1029.
27. Prenger KB, Ophius TO, van Dantzig JM. Traumatic tricuspid valve rupture with luxation of the heart. *Ann Thorac Surg* 1995;59(6):1524–1527.
28. Cooper MJ, Berstein D, Silverman NH. Recognition of left coronary artery fistula to the left and right ventricles by contrast echocardiography. *J Am Coll Cardiol* 1985;6:923–926.
29. Kwan T, Salciccioli L, Elsakr A, et al. Coronary artery fistula coexisting with a ventricular septal defect due to a penetrating gunshot wound. *Cath Cardiovasc Diag* 1995;34(3):235–239.
30. MacMillan RM, Shahriari A, Sumithisena, et al. Contrast-enhanced cine computed tomography for diagnosis of right coronary artery to coronary sinus arteriovenous fistula. *Am J Cardiol* 1985;56:997–998.
31. Farkas LM, Martin M. Is two-dimensional echocardiography reliable in detecting cardiac injury? *J Thorac Cardiovasc Surg* 1993;106:2.
32. Cowley RA, Turney SZ, Hankins JR, et al. Rupture of the thoracic aorta caused by blunt cardiac trauma: a fifteen year experience. *J Thorac Cardiovasc Surg* 1990;100:652–660.
33. Galindo Gallego M, Lopez-Cambra MJ, Fernandez-Acenero MJ, et al. Traumatic rupture of the pericardium. Case report and literature review. *J Thorac Cardiovasc Surg* 1996;37(2):187–191.
34. Bogers AJ, Zweers DJ, Vroom EM, et al. Cardiac subluxation in traumatic rupture of diaphragm and pericardium. *J Thorac Cardiovasc Surg* 1986;34(2):132–134.
35. Rogers FB, Leavitt BJ. Upper torso cyanosis: a marker for blunt cardiac rupture. *Am J Emerg Med* 1997;15(3):275–276.
36. Coimbra R, Pinto MC, Razuk A, et al. Penetrating cardiac wounds: predictive value of trauma indices and the necessity of terminology standardization. *Amer Surg* 1995;61(5):448–452.
37. Soliman MH, Waxman K. Value of a conventional approach to the diagnosis of traumatic cardiac contusion after chest injury. *Crit Care Med* 1987;15(3):218–220.

38. Fenner JE, Knopp R, Lee B, et al. The use of radionuclide angiography in the diagnosis of cardiac contusion. *Ann Emerg Med* 1984;13(9)[Pt 1]:688–694.

39. Kettunen P, Nieminen M. Creatine kinase Mb and M-modeechocardiographic changes in cardiac contusion. *Ann Clin Res* 1985;17:292–298.

40. Adams JE, Davila-Roman VG, Bessey PQ, et al. Improved detection of cardiac contusion with cardiac troponin I. *Am Heart J* 1996;131(2):308–312.

41. Adams JE, Bodor GS, Davila-Roman VG, et al. Cardiac troponin I: a marker with high specificity for cardiac injury. *Circulation* 1993;88:101–107.

42. Ognibene A, Mori F, Santoni R, et al. Cardiac troponin I in myocardial contusion [letter]. *Clin Chem* 1998;44(4):889–890.

43. Thomsen H, Held H. Immunohistochemical detection of C5b-9(m) in myocardium: an aid in distinguishing infarction-induced ischemic heart muscle necrosis from other forms of lethal myocardial injury. *Forensic Sci Int* 1995;71(2):87–95.

44. Mooney RJ, Nieman JT, Bessen HA, et al. Conventional and right precordial ECG's, creatine kinase and radionuclide angiography in post-traumatic ventricular dysfunction. *Ann Emerg Med* 1988;17:890.

45. Potkin RT, Werner JA, Trobaugh GB, et al. Evaluation of noninvasive tests of cardiac damage in suspected cardiac contusion. *Circulation* 1982;66(3):627–631.

46. Mirvis SE. Traumatic disruption of the thoracic aorta: imaging diagnosis. *Trauma Quarterly* 1988;4:2.

47. Hipona FA, Paredes S. The radiologic evaluation of patient with chest trauma. *Med Clin North Am* 1975;59:65–93.

48. Dee PM. The radiology of chest trauma. *Radiology Clin North Am* 1992;30(2):297–300.

49. Goarin J, Le Bret F, Riou B, et al. Early diagnosis of traumatic thoracic aortic rupture by transesophageal echocardiography. *Chest* 1993;103:618–620.

50. Rose CC, Delbridge TR, Mosesso VN. The portable chest film. *Emerg Med Clin North Am* 1991;9(4):776–778.

51. Van GW. Stab wounds of the heart: two new signs of pneumopericardium. *Br J Radiol* 1993;66:789.

52. Pandian NG, Skorton DJ, Doty DB, et al. Immediate diagnosis of acute myocardial contusion by two-dimensional echocardiography: studies in a canine model of blunt chest trauma. *J Am Coll Cardiol* 1983;2:488–496.

53. King RM, Mucha P Jr, Seward JB, et al. Cardiac contusion: a new diagnostic approach utilizing two-dimensional echocardiography. *J Trauma* 1983;23:610–614.

54. Markiewicz W, Best LA, Burstein S, et al. Echocardiographic evaluation after blunt trauma of the chest. *Int J Cardiol* 1985;8:269–274.

55. Hiatt JR, Yeatman LA, Child JS. The value of echocardiography in blunt chest trauma. *J Trauma* 1988;28(7):914–922.

56. Reid CL, Rahimtoola SH, Chandraratna AN. Chest trauma: evaluation by two-dimensional echocardiography. *Am Heart J* 1987;113(4):971–976.

57. Goldman AP, Kotler MN, Goldberg SE, et al. The uses of two-dimensional Doppler echocardiographic techniques preoperatively and postoperatively in a ventricular septal defect caused by penetrating trauma. *Ann Thorac Surg* 1985;40:625–627.

58. Wei K, Kaul S. Recent advances in myocardial contrast echocardiography. *Curr Opinion Cardiol* 1997;12(6):539–546.

59. Bolton JWR, Bynoe RP, Lazar HL, et al. Two-dimensional echocardiography in the evaluation of penetrating intrapericardial injuries. *Ann Thorac Surg* 1993;53:506–509.

60. Jimenez E, Martin M, Krukenkamp T. Subxiphoid pericardiotomy versus two-dimensional echocardiography: a prospective evaluation. *Surgery* 1990;108:676–680.

61. Liedtke AJ, Allen RP, Nellis SH. Effects of blunt cardiac trauma on coronary vasomotion, perfusion, myocardial mechanics and metabolism. *J Trauma* 1980;20:277.

62. Waggoner AD, Baumann CM, Stark PA. Views from the back by subscapular, retrocardiac imaging: technique in clinical application. *J Am Soc Echocardiogr* 1995;8(3):257–262.

63. Weintraub AR, Schwartz SL, Smith J, et al. Intracardiac two-dimensional echocardiography in patients with pericardial effusion and cardiac tamponade. *J Am Soc Echocardiogr* 1991;4(6):571–576.

64. Weintraub AR, Erbel R, Gorge G, et al. Intravascular ultrasound imaging in acute aortic dissection. *J Am Coll Cardiol* 1994;24:495–503.

65. Lau S, Moloney J, Palac R, et al. Prevalence and prognostic significance of segmental ventricular wall motion abnormalities in blunt chest trauma. *J Am Soc Echocardiogr* 1998;11(3).

66. Smith MD, Cassidy JM, Souther S, et al. Transesophageal echocardiography in the diagnosis of traumatic rupture of the aorta. *N Engl J Med* 1995;332:356–362.

67. Blanchard D, Kimura B, Dittrich H. Transesophageal echocardiography of the aorta. *JAMA* 1994;272:7.

68. Miller FA Jr, Seward JB, Gersh BJ, et al. Two-dimensional echocardiographic findings in cardiac trauma. *Am J Cardiol* 1982;50:1022–1027.

69. Karalis DG, Victor MF, Davis GA, et al. The role of echocardiography in blunt chest trauma: a transthoracic and transesophageal echocardiographic study. *J Trauma* 1994;36(1):53–58.

70. Vignon P, Lagrange P, Boncoeur MP, et al. Routine transesophageal echocardiography for the diagnosis of aortic disruption in trauma patients without enlarged mediastinum [comments]. *J Trauma* 1997;42(5):969–972.

71. Skoularigis J, Essop MR, Sareli P. Usefulness of transesophageal echocardiography in the early diagnosis of penetrating stab wounds to the heart. *Am J Cardiol* 1994;73:407–409.

72. Minard G, Schurr MJ, Croce MA, et al. A prospective analysis of transesophageal echocardiography in the diagnosis of traumatic disruption of the aorta. *J Trauma* 1996;40(2):225–230.

73. Vignon P, Francois B, Gastinne H. Diagnosis of traumatic aortic disruption using transesophageal echocardiography: importance of the learning curve. *J Am Soc Echocardiogr* 1998;11(3):558.

74. Spencer KT, Krauss D, Thurn J, et al. Transnasal transesophageal echocardiography. *J Am Soc Echocardiogr* 1997;10(7):728–737.

75. Agarwal G, LaMotte LC, Nanda NC, et al. Identification of the aortic branches using transesophageal echocardiography. *Echocardiography* 1997;14:461–466.

76. Brooks SW, Young JC, Cmolik B, et al. The use of transesophageal echocardiography in the evaluation of chest trauma. *J Trauma* 1992;32(6):761–765.

77. Schamp DJ, Plotnik GD, Croteau D, et al. Clinical significance of radionuclide angiographically-determined abnormalities following acute blunt chest trauma. *Am Heart J* 1988;116:500–504.

78. Harley DP, Mena I, Narahara KA, et al. Traumatic myocardial dysfunction. *J Thorac Cardiovasc Surg* 1994;87(3):386–393.

79. Szabo JR, Chen JT, Putman CE, et al. New murmur following blunt chest trauma. *Invest Radiol* 1984;19:163–167.

80. Go RT, Doty DB, Chiu CL, et al. A new method of diagnosing myocardial contusion in man by radionuclide imaging. *Radiology* 1975;116:107–110.

81. Brantigan CO, Burdick D, Hopeman AR, et al. Evaluation of technetium scanning for myocardial contusion. *J Trauma* 1978;18:460–463.

82. Gonzalez AC, Waldo W, Harlaftis N, et al. Imaging of experimental myocardial contusion: observations and pathologic correlations. *Am J Roentgenol* 1977;128:1039–1040.

83. Rodriguez A, Shatney C. The value of technetium 99m pyrophosphate scanning in the diagnosis of myocardial contusion. *Am Surg* 1982;48:472–474.

84. Hendel RC, Cohn S, Aurigemma G, et al. Focal myocardial injury following blunt chest trauma: a comparison of indium-111 antimyosin scintigraphy with other noninvasive methods. *Am Heart J* 1992;123(5):1208–1215.

85. Miller FB, Richardson JD, Thomas HA, et al. Role of CT in diagnosis of major arterial injury after blunt thoracic trauma. *Surgery* 1989;106(4):596–603.

86. McClean TR, Olinger G, Thorsen K. Computed tomography in the evaluation of the aorta in patients sustaining blunt chest trauma. *J Trauma* 1991;31:2.

87. Kirsch JD, Escarous A. CT diagnosis of traumatic pericardium rupture. *J Comput Assist Tomogr* 1989;13:523–524.

88. Gavant ML, Menke PG, Fabian T, et al. Blunt traumatic aortic rupture: detection with helical CT of the chest. *Radiology* 1995;197:125–133.

89. Fattori R, Celleti F, Bertaccini P, et al. Early and late follow-up of untreated aortic lesion: a support to delayed surgery. *J Am Coll Cardiol* 1998;31[Suppl A]:325A.

90. Walker WA, Pate JW. Medical management of acute rupture of the aorta. *Ann Thorac Surg* 1990;50:965–967.

91. Maleca MJ, Hoit BD. Previously unrecognized intrapericardial hema-

toma leading to refractory abdominal ascites. *Chest* 1995;108(6):
1747–1748.

92. Ionescu AA, Virereanu D, Wood A, et al. Periaortic fat pad mimicking
an intramural hematoma of the thoracic aorta: lessons for transesophageal echocardiography. *J Am Soc Echocardiogr* 1998;11(3):487–490.

93. Thomas P, Saux P, Lonjon T, et al. Diagnosis by video-assisted thoracoscopy of traumatic pericardial rupture with delayed luxation of the
heart: case report. *J Trauma* 1995;38(6):967–970.

94. Leavitt BJ, Meyer JA, Morton JR, et al. Survival following nonpenetrating traumatic rupture of cardiac chambers. *Ann Thorac Surg* 1987;
44:532–535.

95. Aaland MO, Bryan FC, Sherman R. Two-dimensional echocardiogram in hemodynamically stable victims of penetrating precordial
trauma. *Am Surg* 1994;60:412–415.

96. Larrea JL, Silvestre J, Oliver J, et al. Delayed papillary muscle rupture
following mild chest trauma. *J Heart Valve Dis* 1995;4(3):291–
292.

97. Smith MD, Xie GY, Charash WE, et al. Transesophageal characteristics of traumatic aortic injury: can we eliminate the need for aortography? *J Am Soc Echocardiogr* 1998;11(5):503(abst 5B).

98. Samal AK, et al. Traumatic rupture of atherosclerotic plaque producing aortic isthmus dissection. *Echocardiography* 1998;15:695–701.

CHAPTER 65

Intraoperative Echocardiography

Pravin M. Shah

Early work using transesophageal echocardiography (TEE) was carried out in the operating room more than 15 years ago (1). The initial observations consisted of monitoring left ventricular function by M-mode echo transducer placed in the esophagus. Subsequently, a transesophageal probe was developed to provide a single-plane, two-dimensional echocardiographic image. Omoto and colleagues from Japan were instrumental in early development of biplane TEE probes and a pediatric probe. The technology was further advanced to multiplane imaging, which currently is state of the art in routine intraoperative imaging. The applications in the field have been fostered by cardiac anesthesiologists needing to monitor ventricular size and function and by cardiac surgeons in concert with echocardiographers exploring functional anatomy of pathologic valves being considered for innovative surgical approaches such as valve repair. Although the intraoperative TEE is firmly established in most major medical centers, its use in community hospitals has become more widespread in the last 3 to 5 years. The major uses of intraoperative TEE may be grouped under four categories: (i) monitoring of cardiac function, (ii) planning appropriate surgical approaches, (iii) assessment of the immediate results of cardiac operation, and (iv) additional applications, such as detection of air bubbles. Each category will be examined in some detail after discussing issues of personnel, equipment, and techniques.

PERSONNEL

Intraoperative echocardiography is not fully claimed by the cardiologist-echocardiographer, the cardiac anesthesiol-

ogist, or by the cardiothoracic surgeon. A cardiologist experienced in echocardiography would be a logical person to assume responsibility; however, time constraints and lack of availability when called into the operating room are two of the factors that make it an impractical proposition. Ability to transmit live echo images for immediate interpretation should make it possible for an echocardiographer to play an active role in the future. It must, however, be recognized that a cardiologist–echocardiographer will have to develop skills in imaging and interpretation beyond mere detection and quantification of valvular stenosis and regurgitation. The assessment of surgical anatomy, understanding relevant information sought by surgeons, and developing a common language of communication and team approach toward surgical management of patients are all requirements for using intraoperative TEE for improved patient outcome. This relationship must develop not only in the academic centers, where it is already set in motion, but also in all centers where open-heart surgery is carried out. The cardiac anesthesiologist is an obvious practical choice to interpret intraoperative echo, and, indeed, this is provided in a small number of institutions. The monitoring of cardiac function is clearly within the purview of cardiac anesthesiologists. Besides the issue of training, the anesthesiologist is also busy providing and monitoring anesthetics and cannot be diverted for too long in a careful performance of TEE, especially in valvular and congenital cases. The cardiac surgeon with knowledge of cardiac anatomy would be well suited to assess echocardiographic anatomy. Since this requires time and the commitment to learn nuances of imaging techniques and evidence of artifacts, few surgeons have ventured into this field. Nevertheless, it is important for a surgeon to develop sufficient interpretive skills, so as to be able to communicate with the echocardiographer about the significance of preoperative or postoperative findings, which may impact management decisions.

P. M. Shah: Loma Linda University School of Medicine, Loma Linda, California 92350; Noninvasive Cardiac Imaging and Academic Programs, Hoag Memorial Hospital Presbyterian, Newport Beach, California 92663.

EQUIPMENT

Dedicated cardiac ultrasound equipment with multiplane TEE capabilities is required. If epicardial or epiaortic echocardiography is to be employed, a higher frequency transducer (7.5 to 10.0 MHz) should be available. Cable appropriate for obtaining electrocardiographic (ECG) signal from the monitor should be used, since accurate diagnosis generally requires accurate timing of events. Data should be recorded on videotape and stored for diagnostic interpretations and for future reference. Single-plane and biplane TEE probes have limited place in modern intraoperative application, since accurate information is often required in as short a time as possible.

TECHNIQUES

The patient's chart should be carefully scanned to exclude pathologies that may contraindicate TEE examination. The introduction of a TEE probe in the intubated, anesthetized patient is generally easy. It should not be advanced against resistance, as esophageal trauma can result, especially in an anesthetized setting. A comprehensive evaluation of the cardioaortic pathologies should be carried out, especially if the patient has not undergone a recent TEE examination. Unsuspected pathologies, such as left atrial thrombus or mobile aortic atheroma may be important in intraoperative and postoperative management. Subsequently, the probe should be positioned for a detailed assessment based on the clinical circumstance.

Epicardial Echocardiography

Need for direct epicardial placement of a transducer (wrapped in a long sterile sheath) in the current era of multiplane TEE rarely arises. One important application is epiaortic imaging of the mid- and distal ascending aorta prior to aortic cross clamping in order to prevent iatrogenic embolism or dissection of the proximal aorta. A special transducer designed for this application is commercially developed. Alternately, a 7.5- to 10.0-MHz transducer may be placed on the aorta with a small balloon filled with sterile water (a sterile glove may be improvised) acting as an offset between the transducer and the wall of the aorta. This approach is especially indicated in elderly subjects, in whom the incidence of postoperative stroke is relatively high.

INDICATIONS

Monitoring Left Ventricular Function

TEE is ideally suited for continuous monitoring of the left ventricle in high-risk patients undergoing major noncardiac surgery (2). These are patients with advanced ischemic heart disease and/or severely depressed left ventricular function undergoing major operations such as abdominal aortic aneurysm resection, aortic-iliac disease, major lung operation, etc. It has been clearly demonstrated that detection of abnormality by conventional monitoring of pulmonary artery

TABLE 1. *Indications of intraoperative monitoring of left ventricular function by transesophageal echocardiography*

High-risk cardiac patients
    Unstable coronary syndromes with resting electrocardiogram changes and/or enzyme elevation
    Recent myocardial infarction (<3 months)
    Left main coronary occlusion
    Multivessel disease with subtotal occlusions
    Ejection fraction <30%
High-risk noncardiac surgery
    Aortic aneurysm resection
    Peripheral vascular surgery
    Major abdominal/pelvic surgery in patients with known cardiac history

wedge pressure using a balloon floatation catheter is associated with considerable time lag following deterioration of segmental or global ventricular function. Since the outcome in the operating room setting depends on an immediate correction of abnormal function, TEE is clearly superior for real-time assessment of left ventricular volume and function. The indications for intraoperative monitoring of left ventricular (LV) function by TEE is summarized in Table 1.

Transducer placement in a transgastric location to obtain short-axis cross section at papillary muscle level is often favored. The left ventricular size may be monitored by a cursor-derived M-mode dimension or by planimetered end-diastolic area computation. The loading conditions as well as systolic ejection performance may be rapidly evaluated. This approach is excellent for global assessment of ventricular volume and function; it is somewhat limited for segmental analysis. Since left ventricular apical segments are often poorly visualized from the transgastric approach. The longitudinal plane may be combined to visualize the anterior and inferior walls, but not the interventricular septum and the lateral walls. For a detailed evaluation of segmental function, the probe may be withdrawn to the midesophageal level, and multiple cross sections examined. The transverse four-chamber view permits assessment of the interventricular septum and lateral walls along the proximal, mid- and apical segments. An intermediate plane at approximately 45 to 60 degrees visualizes the posterior interventricular septum and anterolateral wall. The vertical plane (at aproximately 90 degrees) providing a two-chamber cross section demonstrates posteroinferior and anterior walls. The long-axis plane cross section (at aproximately 120 to 150 degrees) displays inferolateral wall and anterior interventricular septum. These cross sections are better suited to demonstrate development of segmental asynergy using multiplane imaging from the midesophageal position. The basal septum in the four-chamber plane (0 degrees), being the posterior basal septum, is perfused by the right coronary artery (RCA); while the mid- and apical septum are served by left anterior descending (LAD) coronary artery. The lateral wall, similarly at the basal level, represents the posterolateral segment and is perfused by the left circumflex (LCX) coronary artery,

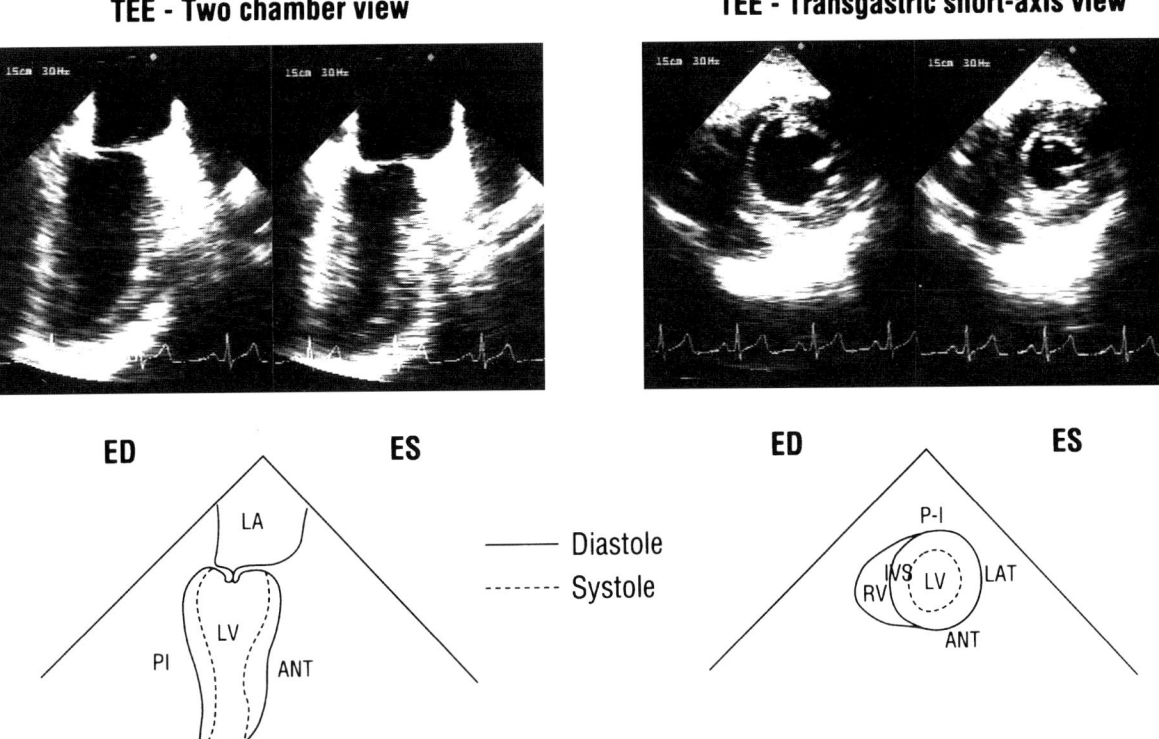

TEE - Two chamber view

TEE - Transgastric short-axis view

FIG. 1. An example of asynergy induced by a distal left anterior descending coronary artery occlusion observed in distal anterior, apical, and inferoapical segments as visualized in the longitudinal or two-chamber view. Note that the transgastric short-axis view failed to show any evidence of asynergy because of distal occlusion. This occlusion was induced during off-pump coronary bypass (MIDCAB) surgery, and the asynergy fully recovered within seconds after reperfusion. *ANT,* anterior; *ED,* end diastole; *ES,* end systole; *IVS,* interventricular septum; *LA,* left atrium; *LV,* left ventricle; *LAT,* lateral; *P1,* lateral scallop ; *P-I,* posteroinferior; *RV,* right ventricle; *TEE,* transesophageal echocardiography.

whereas the midlateral wall segment is perfused by either LCX or LAD; and the apical lateral segment by LAD. In the cross section at 45 degrees, the posterior septum is generally RCA territory, while the anterolateral wall segments are served by LAD. In the two-chamber view (90 degrees), the basal and midsegments of the posteroinferior wall are RCA territory, while the anterior wall segments and, frequently, the apical inferior segments are LAD-served territories. In the long-axis equivalent view, the posteroinfero lateral wall segments are LCX territories, and the anterior interventricular septum are LAD territories. There are, of course, individual variations in perfusion territories based on anatomic dominance of left versus right circulations and on the number and size of diagonal or obtuse marginal branches. Similarly, in the presence of chronic total occlusion, an entire territory may be served by collaterals arising from another artery. An overall road map of expected coronary distribution is useful, especially in patients undergoing coronary bypass surgery (Fig. 1). Frequently, coronary artery bypass is undertaken on a beating heart without use of cardiopulmonary bypass. Myocardial segmental function returns within minutes of bypass grafting. Persistent asynergy would lead to examination of the graft for possible technical reasons for poor flow

rate, preventing permanent dysfunction. Similarly, segmental asynergy may be noted following traditional coronary artery surgery with the patient coming off bypass as a result of a technical fault. This may be appropriately remedied in the operating room, resulting in an improved outcome.

Quantitation of Left Ventricular Function

Determination of Volumes and Ejection Fraction

Quantitation of left ventricular function is summarized in Table 2. The visual "eye ball" assessment of left ventricular volumes and ejection fraction are usually carried out using transgastric short- and long-axis views or midesophageal plane views (3). Should a need for quantitation arise, Sha-

TABLE 2. *Quantitation of left ventricular function by transesophageal echocardiography*

1. Left ventricular end-diastolic, end-systolic volumes and ejection fraction
2. Cardiac output
3. Filling pressures—pulmonary artery "wedge" pressure
4. Left ventricular end-diastolic pressures

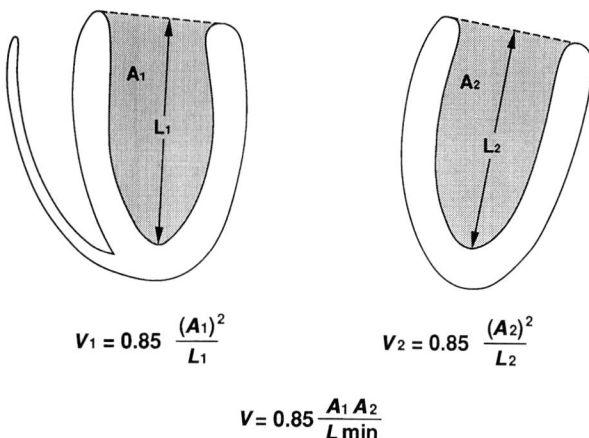

$$V_1 = 0.85 \frac{(A_1)^2}{L_1} \qquad V_2 = 0.85 \frac{(A_2)^2}{L_2}$$

$$V = 0.85 \frac{A_1 A_2}{L \, min}$$

FIG. 2. A schematic to show use of transverse plane (**left,** four-chamber view) and longitudinal plane (**right,** two-chamber view) from the midesophageal TEE to calculate volume (*V*) using the area (*A*) / length (*L*) method.

kudo and co-workers (4) from our laboratory have demonstrated the feasibility of calculating end-diastolic and end-systolic volumes of the left ventricle using four- and two-chamber images (0-degree and 90-degree cross sections, respectively). After tracing end-diastolic and end-systolic images in the two planes, one may employ a modified Simpson approach or ellipsoid assumption with the area/length method to calculate the volumes (Fig. 2). When these volumes were compared to those obtained from apical four- and two-chamber transthoracic echocardiography (TTE) in the same subjects, a good correlation was obtained, but with consistent underestimation of TEE volumes. This results from foreshortened cross sections using TEE. However, ejection fraction by TEE correlated well with that obtained by TTE. Thus, TEE may be employed for measuring volumes while recognizing a systematic underestimation, and it may be relied on for accurate quantitation of ejection fraction.

Quantitation of Cardiac Output

Cardiac output is often measured invasively during surgery using a thermodilution technique with a right-heart catheter for functional monitoring. Cardiac output can be easily measured using a pulsed-Doppler approach across the mitral annulus. The method consists of placing a sample volume at the level of the mitral annulus in the four-chamber view (midesophageal 0-degree plane). The mitral annulus area is obtained by measuring diameter of the annulus in the four-chamber and the two-chamber planes (0 degrees and 90 degrees, respectively). Since the mitral annulus is often more ovoid than circular, these two diameters are used to calculate the mitral annulus area.

$$Cardiac \; Output = CSA_{MA} \times TVI_{MA} \times HR$$

where CSA_{MA} equals the *cross sectional area of the mitral*

annulus; TVI_{MA} equals the *velocity time integral at annulus level* and *HR* equals *heart rate.*

Hozumi et al. (5) compared this Doppler approach with thermodilution cardiac output measured in the operating room on 14 consecutive patients. The two correlated well: $r = 0.81$ for single-plane imaging (SEE = 0.72 L/min) and $r = 0.93$ for biplane imaging (SEE = 0.47 L/min). Thus, the biplane approach outlined provided accurate quantitation of cardiac output in the operating room setting.

Filling Pressures

The pulmonary artery wedge pressure is often measured using right-heart catheterization in the operating room in order to monitor fluid volume status (preload) and as an index of left ventricular failure or reduced compliance. An estimation of filling pressure and altered compliance of the left ventricle can be provided by Doppler parameters using intraoperative TEE.

Mitral inflow pulsed-wave Doppler tracings can be obtained by placing the sample volume at the tip of the open-valve leaflets. A tall E wave (early diastolic filling wave) and shortened E-deceleration time (<130 msec) generally reflect elevated left atrial (i.e., pulmonary wedge) pressure in absence of significant mitral regurgitation. On the other hand, a tall A wave with prolonged E-wave deceleration time (>250 msec) reflects impaired ventricular compliance, which often is secondary of ventricular hypertrophy or ischemia. A second important parameter providing an estimation of filling pressures consists of pulmonary venous Doppler profile. A reduced systolic component of pulmonary venous flow reflects elevated "wedge" pressure, while a dominant systolic flow with reduced diastolic flow is indicative of reduced "wedge" pressures. These parameters can be obtained within a few minutes and provide useful hemodynamic information (6,7).

A feasibility of measuring cardiac output and assessing filling pressures using Doppler parameters from TEE makes it redundant to utilize swan-ganz or balloon flotation catheter, with its potential for complications.

Left Ventricular End-Diastolic Pressure

A useful indicator of elevated left ventricular end-diastolic pressure (LVEDP) consists of analyzing mitral inflow A-wave duration and comparing it to pulmonary venous A_r (A reversal) duration. Normally, the A-wave duration of the mitral inflow filling wave form is longer than A_r duration. As the left ventricular end-diastolic pressure is increased, the A-wave duration is abbreviated, and the A_r longer in duration than A wave generally indicates LVEDP to be in excess of 15 mm Hg.

Intraoperative monitoring of functions is often done in setting of rapidly changing clinical parameters and a rapid convenient assessment of global and segmental function is required for prompt intervention.

Surgical Planning and Intraoperative Evaluation of Results

Multiplane TEE is extremely useful in providing a map to the surgeon in planning specific surgical procedures and subsequently confirming surgical outcome in the operating room. Some of the surgical operations for which TEE is clearly indicated include those discussed below.

Mitral Valve Repair

Mitral valve repair, whenever feasible, has been increasingly recognized as a surgical procedure of choice for mitral valve disease. Transesophageal echocardiography plays a crucial role in preoperative identification of patients likely to be suitable candidates for valve repair. Intraoperatively, TEE provides valuable information on the nature and extent of surgical pathology and the type of surgical procedure needed. This information is generally gathered prior to thoracotomy and communicated to the surgeon.

The communication between the echocardiographer describing echo anatomy and the cardiac surgeon visualizing surgical anatomy is facilitated by using nomenclature and classification proposed by Duran and colleagues, N. Kumar and M. Kumar (8). The following description is based on their recommendation.

Normal Mitral Valve Anatomy

The nomenclature and classification proposed by Duran and his colleagues will be used as a reference (Fig. 3; see also Color Plate 46 following page 758). A surgeon inspecting the mitral valve from the left atrium views lateral commissure (C_1) to his left and medial commissure (C_2) to his right. The posterior leaflet commonly has three identifiable scallops, lateral scallop (P_1), medial scallop (P_2) and middle scallop (PM). PM may be divided into PM_1 with chordal attachments to anterolateral papillary muscle and PM_2 with chordal attachments to posteromedial papillary muscle. The anterior leaflet has a smoother nonscalloped surface and is divided into lateral half (A_1) and medial half (A_2). The anterolateral papillary muscle is designated as M_1, and medial as M_2. The chordae from M_1 are inserted in A_1, P_1, and PM_1, whereas those from M_2 attach to A_2, P_2, and PM_2. The primary chords are attached near free margins of the leaflets; and the secondary chords are inserted to the base of the leaflets from corresponding papillary muscle. The tertiary chords arise from the left ventricular free wall and are inserted to the ventricular surface of the leaflets. The precise function of the tertiary chords is not known. The primary and secondary chords are important in maintaining valve competence.

Echocardiographic Anatomy by TEE

Since TEE provides two-dimensional imaging, it is essential to obtain several different cross sections to accurately define the three-dimensional aspects of valvular anatomy. The mitral valve complex comprises not only the leaflets, the chords, and the papillary muscles, but, in addition, includes the annulus, the left ventricular size and function, as well as the left atrial size and function. TEE should be used to provide systematic evaluation of all components of the valve complex.

The leaflet anatomy can be evaluated using a systematic imaging using midesophageal and transgastric views. Figure 4 (see also Color Plate 47 following page 758) shows the valve leaflet anatomy from a transgastric short-axis view

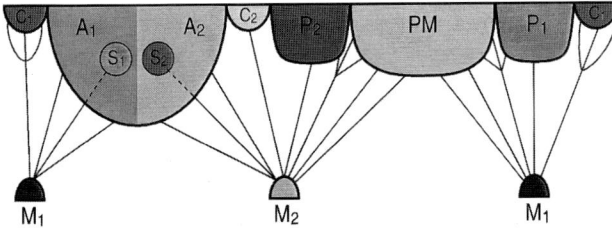

FIG. 3. The classification of the leaflet components is shown with the valve laid open in order to demonstrate papillary muscle-chordal relationships to the leaflets. The chordae arising from the anterolateral papillary muscle designated as M_1, are inserted to half of anterior leaflet designated A_1 and lateral scallop of posterior leaflet (P_1) and half of middle scallop (*PM*) as well as to small commissural leaflet C_1. Similarly, the chordae arising from the posteromedial papillary muscle M_2 are inserted to A_2, P_2 (medial scallop of posterior leaflet) and part of *PM* as well as to C_2. The primary chords are attached to the free edge and secondary chords (S_1 and D_2) to midportion (i.e., belly) of the leaflets. (See also Color Plate 46 following page 758.)

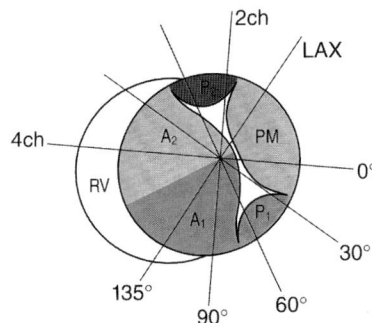

FIG. 4. A schematic of the mitral leaflet components as obtained from transgastric short axis. The radially placed "clock" diagram represents the corresponding cross sections obtained from midesophageal transducer position using multiplane imaging. Note the portions of valve leaflets visualized in 0 degree or 4-chamber (*4ch*) view, 30 degree to 60 degree or intermediate plane, 90 degree or 2-chamber (*2ch*) view, and approximately 135 degrees in the long-axis plane. The cross sections should image through center of the mitral orifice, and this may be assured by maximizing the left ventricular cavity and the mitral orifice in each of the cross sections imaged. *A*, anterior leaflet; *LAX*, long axis plane; *P*, posterior leaflet; *PM*, middle scallop of posterior leaflet; *RV*, right ventricle. (See also Color Plate 47 following page 758.)

and clockwise orientations of leaflet anatomy encountered in different cross sections using the midesophageal views.

In each of the *midesophageal views*, it is important to maximize the chamber dimension in order to avoid off-axis imaging.

View 1—The horizontal plane (0 degrees) displays A2 at base and A1 at free margin, and PM1. This is the four-chamber view, without imaging the aorta, and both atrio-ventricular valves are seen.

View 2—A 40-degree to 60-degree cross-section cuts through P2 and P1 and the free margins of A2 and A1. This is an intermediate cross section between the four- (0 degrees) and the two- (90 degrees) chamber views. P2 is seen on left side of the cross section, P1 on the right, and an anterior leaflet goes in and out of the image during cardiac cycle.

View 3—A 90-degree cross section (longitudinal plane) displays P2 or PM2, and predominantly A1. This is the two-chamber view imaging the left atrium and the left ventricle only.

View 4—A 120-degree to 140-degree cross section (long-axis equivalent) displays PM2 and A2 at its free margin and A1 at base. This long-axis view visualizes left ventricular inflow and outflow with the left ventricular cavity maximized by rotation of the probe.

Transgastric views should be obtained at proximal and midgastric levels to demonstrate valvular and subvalve pathology.

View 1—Short axis at mitral valve level (Fig. 5; see also Color Plate 48 following page 758) displays surface anat-omy of both leaflets, but since the valve moves toward the apex in systole, it is difficult to visualize throughout the cardiac cycle. The posterior leaflet is to the right with P2 in near field, P1 far field, and PM in the middle. The anterior leaflet is seen on the left, A2 in the near field, and A1 in far field.

View 2—Sixty-degree to 90-degree cross sections permit visualization of M2 and M1, including chordal attachments to both leaflets. This view is especially used to measure chordal lengths and attachments.

Color Doppler Flow Imaging

The valve anatomy is mentally reconstructed using the two-dimensional echo approach as outlined above. However, color flow imaging can be used not only to quantify the severity of regurgitation, but also to provide insight into the anatomic site from where regurgitation originates.

The cross section with a fully developed flow convergence map (proximal isovelocity surface area or PISA) best displays the regurgitation orifice, besides providing an important clue as to severity of the regurgitation. This approach is especially useful in the presence of perforation or a small cleft that may be difficult to image and may be mistaken as image dropouts.

The jet direction provides a clue of anatomic site of origin of the regurgitation jet, e.g., anteromedial and medial jet from PM pathology, posterolateral from A2 and posterome-dial or posterior jet from A1 pathology. Multiple jets generally indicate multiple pathologic sites responsible for valve regurgitation.

Common Reconstructive Procedures

Mitral valve repair or reconstruction (Table 3) is carried out to address the specific pathology responsible for valve regurgitation. Each patient presents with unique problems, and an experienced surgeon adapts his techniques for repair to the underlying anatomy (9–11). However, there are several broad approaches that are commonly undertaken. These most common procedures include those discussed below.

Quadrangular resection of the flail posterior mitral leaflet followed by plication of the edges and supporting the repair

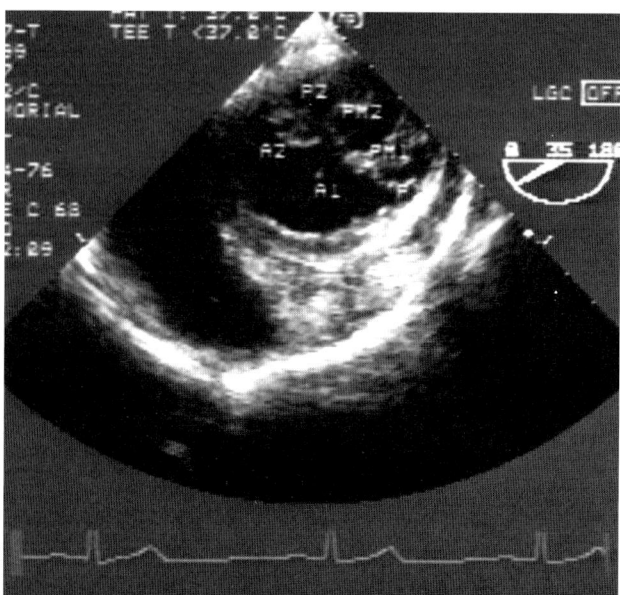

FIG. 5. The short-axis cross section at the mitral valve level with various components of the valve leaflet labeled. For an explanation of *A1, A2, P1,* and *P2,* see Figure 3. The *PM* is divided into *PM1* and *PM2* based on chordal insertions from *M1* and *M2,* respectively. (See also Color Plate 48 following page 758.)

TABLE 3. *Mitral valve repair—common procedures*

1. Quadrangular resection of posterior mitral leaflet (PML) with plication and ring annuloplasty
2. Quadrangular resection of anterior mitral leaflet with leaflet-chordae transfer from a corresponding segment of posterior leaflet, plication of PML, and ring annuloplasty
3. Same as 1, plus sliding annuloplasty
4. Chordal shortening
5. Artificial chords (e.g., Gore-Tex chords)
6. Ring annuloplasty—annular reduction
7. Pericardial patch over perforation or cleft
8. Chordal splitting, commissurotomy
9. Mitral homograft surgery

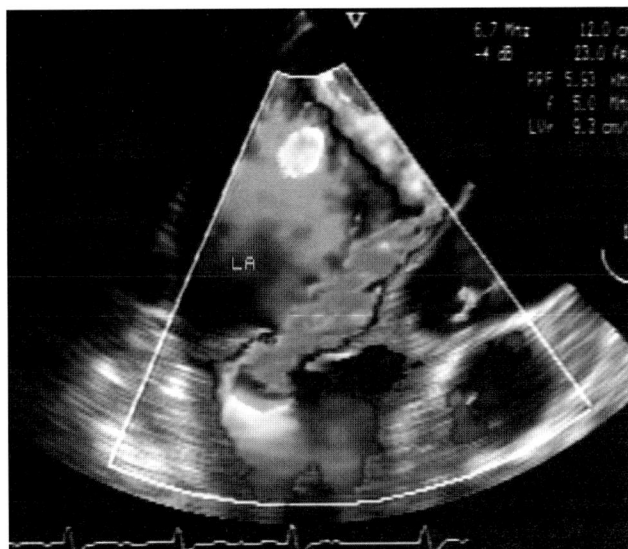

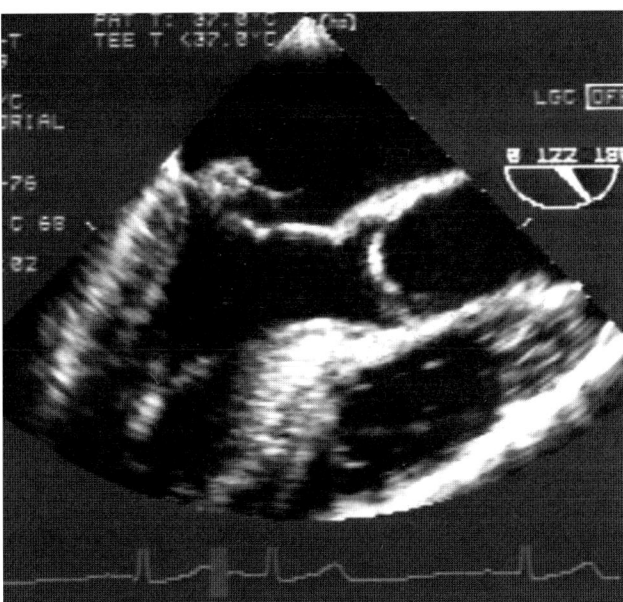

FIG. 6. A: Eccentric mitral regurgitation jet directed anteriorly behind the aorta as seen in transesophageal echocardiography long-axis view. The middle scallop, or *PM*, is flail and severe regurgitation as confirmed by proximal isovelocity surface area (flow convergence) radius of 1.2 cm at a set color scale of 50 cm/sec. *LA,* left atrium. **B:** A flail PM with ruptured chord is demonstrated in the long-axis plane in another patient. (See also Color Plate 49 following page 758.)

with annuloplasty ring. This is the most frequently performed repair procedure, since the posterior leaflet middle scallop is the most common site of prolapse or flail (Fig 6; see also Color Plate 49 following page 758). The feasibility of this procedure partly depends on the extent of posterior leaflet involvement. If P2 and PM or P1 and PM are extensively involved, it may be difficult to find the widely resected edges for plication. This, however, is only rarely the case. The application and success of this operation is based on

the fact that the posterior leaflet does not contribute significantly to the normal functioning of the mitral valve, i.e., it does not permit unobstructed inflow in diastole and prevent valve regurgitation in systole.

Quadrangular resection of the anterior mitral leaflet is followed by the transfer of a corresponding segment of the posterior leaflet with intact chords (chordal transfer or "flip over" technique). The resected posterior leaflet is plicated and subsequently a ring annuloplasty is performed. This approach utilizing the "flip over" technique is predicated on the fact that anterior mitral leaflet in the open position is a curtain that permits unobstructed diastolic inflow. A compromise in the surface area of this leaflet would result in obstruction to inflow. The size of the anterior leaflet that can be safely resected to perform this procedure is somewhat limited by the size and integrity of the posterior leaflet segment available for transfer.

Sliding annuloplasty of the posterior leaflet. This is carried out as an added procedure in response to a special circumstance of elongated height of the posterior mitral leaflet. A tall posterior leaflet in excess of 1.0 cm after completion of resection and plication is often associated with systolic anterior motion (SAM) of the anterior mitral leaflet. This may result in outflow obstruction and mitral regurgitation. The precise mechanism of this dynamic obstruction complicating the repair is not known, but the combined lengths or heights of posterior and anterior leaflet in relation to the annular ring appear to be contributory. TEE permits measurements of the heights of the posterior leaflet middle scallop and the anterior leaflet, thus suggesting a need for such a procedure.

Chordal shortening is carried out when prominent leaflet billowing is associated with regurgitation. The base of the chords to be shortened is looped around a papillary muscle and anchored in place. The extent of shortening to be undertaken depends on how elongated the chords are. This may be best judged by measuring the extent of leaflet billowing above the annular plane by intraoperative TEE. This is a difficult parameter to assess at surgery with the heart emptied while on cardiopulmonary bypass. Thus, TEE is ideally suited to provide this practical information intraoperatively.

Placement of artificial chords or Gore-Tex chords is carried out when the underlying redundant chords are attenuated and thin. These chords, if left unstrengthened, have potential for rupture. There are no real criteria to predict a need for placement of artificial chords, short of direct inspection at time of surgery.

Ring annuloplasty is nearly always carried out following mitral valve repair, especially in myxomatous valves with dilated annulus. The size of the ring is selected by the surgeon on basis of intertrigonal distance, which is measured at surgery. In general, most surgeons favor placement of a flexible ring, such as Duran ring, so that normal mitral annular "contraction" and "dilatation" during cardiac cycle would be maintained. In some cases where annular dilatation is a primary pathology (e.g., dilated cardiomyopathy), annular reduction is undertaken by selecting a smaller annular ring (approximately 25 mm) in order to provide improved coaptation surface.

Pericardial patch is placed over a localized perforation or a small cleft in the mitral valve leaflet. The exact location and size of the perforation or cleft can be assessed by TEE utilizing multiple cross sections and flow convergence by color flow imaging.

Chordal splitting and thinning are carried in rheumatic mitral valve disease with combined stenosis and regurgitation. This procedure makes the leaflet more pliable and mobile, providing a more competent valve. This procedure can only be carried out if the chords are not so shortened as to bring the tip of the papillary muscle in close proximity to the valve leaflet. This distance from the papillary muscle apex to the valve leaflet can be assessed by TEE using appropriate cross sections.

Mitral homograft surgery is currently undertaken at few centers in highly selected patients with suitable pathology. Partial homograft involves the use of one papillary muscle and the corresponding portions of the leaflet tissues of both leaflets. Complete homograft replacement involves both papillary muscles and both leaflets.

Suitability for Valve Repair

Transesophageal echocardiography provides important clues to predict suitability for mitral valve repair. This is especially relevant since the timing of surgery in an asymptomatic patient is in part influenced by demonstrating a feasibility of valve repair. The following echocardiographic appearances portend a high likelihood of repair, although the final decision is made by the surgeon.

- Myxomatous mitral valve disease with localized flail segment of posterior leaflet with chordae rupture
- Myxomatous mitral valve disease with localized flail segment of the anterior leaflet with preserved opposing segment of the posterior leaflet
- Myxomatous mitral valve disease with billowing of portions of the valve leaflets localized to segments having chordal attachments from one papillary muscle
- Rheumatic valve disease with thickened but not markedly foreshortened chordal structures and with restricted leaflet mobility
- Dilated or "ischemic" cardiomyopathy with ventricular enlargement and annular dilatation with severe mitral regurgitation
- Localized perforation of the mitral valve, commonly involving the anterior mitral leaflet and generally secondary to endocarditis
- Congenital cleft of the mitral valve, when localized with well developed adjacent leaflet tissue

Postrepair Evaluation

TEE is essential to determining the status of attempted valve repair. A competent valve repair shows normal inflow without valve regurgitation. The modern echocardiographic equipment is able to demonstrate trivial "stitch" regurgitation along the orifice margins where sutures are placed. This may be ignored since they eventually disappear spontaneously. Residual valve regurgitation, when significant, is associated with turbulent jets.

Central valve regurgitation. This occurs through the orifice either as a result of residual billowing or excessive correction and restriction of the valve. It is important to assess the severity under appropriate loading conditions, especially the systolic blood pressure brought up to between 120 to 140 mm Hg. The severity index will depend on the size of the turbulent jet, as well as the proximal flow convergence assessment.

Paravalvular mitral regurgitation. This type of regurgitation can be imaged and carefully localized as to the exact site. If severe, it needs to be dealt with on a second pump run.

Systolic anterior motion of the mitral valve. This may be observed and, if pronounced, it is associated with left ventricular outflow obstruction and mitral regurgitation. It is exaggerated in the presence of an unloaded hyperdynamic ventricle. It is, therefore, important to assess the effect of increasing preload as well as afterload and withdrawing the use of inotropes. If the SAM persists with outflow gradient and mitral regurgitation, additional repair in the form of sliding annuloplasty may be undertaken.

Mitral Valve Replacement

When the mitral valve pathology is considered unsuitable for repair, replacement with a prosthetic device is undertaken. Key information with potential impact on surgical technique relates to morphology of the mitral annulus. A heavily calcified mitral annulus may modify the approach to the seating of the valve. The valve function following replacement should be assessed for appropriate disc motion and the absence of pathologic regurgitation. A low velocity jet with uniform color is considered physiologic and represents washing jets designed in bileaflet mechanical prostheses.

Aortic Valve Repair

The aortic valve, despite a deceptively simpler design—or perhaps because of it—is difficult to repair. Attempted repair has been successful for rheumatic commissural fusion, for bicuspid valve with a raphe, and mild-to-moderate calcification of the valve. A major concern is postrepair valve regurgitation, which may persist or become more severe. Aortic cusp prolapse valve repair is currently undertaken for moderate degrees of regurgitation and a suitable pathology, especially in combination with mitral valve repair or coronary bypass surgery.

Aortic Valve Replacement

The information from TEE that is most likely to influence surgical technique consists of the following major considerations:

Aortic annulus diameter;
Dilatation and pathology of the sinuses of Valsalva;
Sinotubular junction;
Origin of coronary arteries; and
LV outflow tract dimension and septal hypertrophy in the subaortic region.

The aortic annulus diameter is best measured by multiplane TEE in long-axis cross sections (approximately 130 to 140 degrees) and in anteflexed four-chamber view (0 degrees) with visualization of aortic root. Several measurements are made by manipulating the probe to maximize the diameter. The measurement is made between the point of cusp attachments at the annulus, and the largest diameter recorded should be taken as accurate (Fig. 7). Calcification of the aortic annulus may make it difficult to obtain accurate measurements. The annulus measurement reflects within 1 mm the size of the aortic annulus as measured with a surgical sizer and, hence, the size of the prosthesis to be implanted. Since a cryopreserved homograft needs to be thawed for several minutes, a surgeon could use the aortic annulus diameter obtained by TEE to select the appropriate prosthesis.

The origin of coronary arteries may play an important role in aortic homograft or autograft (Ross operation) surgery. Anomalous origin, unusually high or low origin, multiple orifices, proximity to the commissures, and significant aortic calcification at the ostia will influence surgical technique in root replacements, which are commonly undertaken with the aortic homograft and autograft replacement operations.

The left ventricular outflow tract (LVOT) in the subvalvular region may be markedly narrowed due to severe septal hypertrophy, especially in the elderly. Similarly, hypertro-

phic cardiomyopathy may co-exist with aortic valve disease. When associated with aortic stenosis, LVOT obstruction with SAM may become evident after aortic valve replacement. These patients require myectomy to be undertaken at the time of the aortic valve replacement for optimal results.

Hypertrophic Cardiomyopathy with Subaortic Obstruction

Surgical myectomy is an established procedure designed to relieve LVOT obstruction in symptomatic patients who are not relieved by medical management. The technique consists of resecting a wedge of hypertrophied septum under direct vision through an aortotomy. TEE is capable of providing invaluable information that can guide the surgeon as to how long and deep a myectomy needs to be undertaken to relieve obstruction, while avoiding iatrogenic ventricular septal defect. The information from TEE of use to a surgeon consists of the following considerations:

Interventricular septal thickness 0.5 cm, 1.0 cm, and 2.0 cm below the aortic annulus. This provides a guide to location, and extent of myectomy that would be safe to undertake and needed for effective relief of obstruction.

Mitral valve morphology to assess independent co-existent pathology, although in most cases the severity of mitral regurgitation is secondary to SAM. A successful myectomy provides relief of SAM and mitral regurgitation.

Mitral regurgitation and its association with outflow obstruction. This may be readily assessed in the operating room by using a vasoactive agent such as neosynephrine, which by increasing arterial blood pressure tends to reduce or eliminate SAM and mitral regurgitation associated with it. On the other hand, mitral regurgitation of independent etiology will increase or remain unchanged.

Aortic Dissection, Aneurysm, and Traumatic Disruption

The role of TEE in assisting the surgical treatment of these conditions, which often present as cardiovascular emergencies, is well established. TEE can identify the extent and location of pathology prior to surgical correction. It is also useful for confirming the adequacy of surgical procedure, and it provides intraoperative detection of complications. In patients with aortic dissection, TEE can be used to assess the entry and exit sites and the nature of the intimal flap and the false lumen.

Congenital Heart Disease

A variety of congenital disorders benefit from intraoperative TEE in order to assess the exact anatomic site of the anomaly, associated anomalies, and postsurgical outcome (12). Some of the more common uses of intraoperative TEE are discussed briefly below.

Atrial septal defect (ASD). The location of ASD has an important bearing on the surgical approach. The common

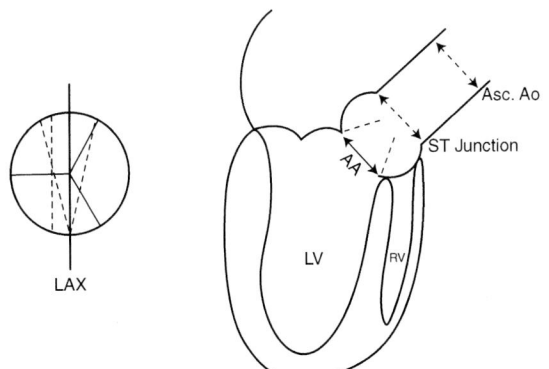

FIG. 7. A schematic diagram to show the measurement technique of the aortic annulus (*AA*) in the long-axis plane (*LAX*) with the largest diameter being more accurate for determining the annulus. The additional measurements relevant to surgery include sinotubular (*ST*) junction and ascending aorta (*Asc. Ao*). *LV*, left ventricle; *RV*, right ventricle.

types are ostium secundum, ostium primum, and sinus venosus. A fourth type, which is the least common, is an inferiorly placed defect near the inferior vena caval entrance into the right atrium.

Besides ascertaining the absence of residual shunting, TEE is useful in the delineation of anomalous pulmonary venous drainage, which is commonly associated with sinus venosus atrial septal defect. A rare complication of surgical closure of inferiorly placed ASD is diversion of inferior vena cava into the left atrium. This can be immediately identified and corrected during surgery. The ostium primum is often associated with cleft mitral and/or tricuspid valves. These need to be identified and corrected.

Ventricular septal defect (VSD). The types of VSD, as based on location, consist of perimembranous, infracristal or subpulmonic, inflow type near the tricuspid orifice and the muscular VSD.

Following a successful patch closure of VSD, TEE may be helpful in the detection of unsuspected smaller muscular VSDs.

Transposition of great arteries. Evaluation of the baffle operation, as in the Mustard operation for complete transposition of the great vessels, can be carried out for possible obstruction or leaks.

Single ventricle or hypoplastic right ventricle. Conduit function, as in the hypoplastic right heart, can be assessed intraoperatively.

Patent ductus arteriosus. TEE provides an accurate assessment of the location, size, and length of the ductus. A successful closure can be confirmed following surgery by intraoperative TEE.

Aortic coarctation. Its location, length, and the proximity of the left subclavian artery can be evaluated by imaging the aortic arch and the upper thoracic aorta. A successful repair can be confirmed intraoperatively.

CONCLUSION

Intraoperative transesophageal echocardiography is indicated under a variety of cardiac surgery procedures. Its use in valvular heart disease, congenital heart disease, hypertrophic obstructive cardiomyopathy, diseases of the aorta, and selected cases with high-risk or unstable coronary artery disease patients is likely to be associated with improved outcome and should be strongly encouraged. It is often necessary for the cardiologists and sonographers to be associated with the cardiac surgery program in order to facilitate communication and provide for optimal outcome. The intraoperative TEE is often considered a gold standard, since evaluation of pathology and success of operation cannot otherwise be determined in an arrested heart.

REFERENCES

1. Matsumoto M, Oka Y, Strom J, et al. Application of transesophageal echocardiography to continuous intraoperative monitoring of left ventricular performance. *Am J Cardiol* 1980;46:95–105.
2. Savage RM, Lytle BW, Aronson S. Intraoperative echocardiography is indicated in high risk coronary artery bypass grafting. *Ann Thorac Surg* 1997;64:367–374.
3. Shah PM, Kyo S, Matsumura M, et al. Utility of biplane transesophageal echocardiography in left ventricular wall motion analysis. *J Cardiothorac Vasc Anesth* 1991;5:316–319.
4. Shakudo M, Shah P, Bansal RC, et al. Biplane transesophageal echocardiography for estimation of left ventricular volumes and ejection fraction. *Circulation* 1990;82(4):III-669.
5. Hozumi T, Shakudo M, Applegate R, et al. Accuracy of cardiac output estimation with biplane transesophageal echocardiography. *J Am Soc Echocardiogr* 1993;6:62–68.
6. Kuecherer HF, Muhiudeen IA, Kusumoto FM, et al. Estimation of mean left atrial pressure from transesophageal pulsed Doppler echocardiography of pulmonary venous flow. *Circulation* 1990;82:1127–1139.
7. Nishimura RA, Abel MD, Hatle LF, et al. Relation of pulmonary vein to mitral flow velocities by transesophageal Doppler echocardiography. *Circulation* 1990;81:1488–1497.
8. Kumar N, Kumar M, Duran CMG. A revised terminology for recording surgical findings of the mitral valve. *J Heart Valve Dis* 1995;4:70–75.
9. Carpentier A. Cardiac valve surgery—the ''French Correction.'' *J Thorac Cardiovasc Surg* 1983;86:323–333.
10. Chitwood WR, Wixon CL, Elbeery JR, et al. Video assisted minimally invasive mitral valve surgery. *Thorac Cardiovasc Surg* 1997;114:773–783.
11. Foster GP, Isselbacher EM, Rose GA, et al. Accurate localization of mitral regurgitation defects using multiplane transesophageal echocardiography. *Ann Thorac Surg* 1998;65:1025–1031.
12. Muhiudeen IA, Roberson DA, Silverman NH, et al. Intraoperative echocardiography for evaluation of congenital heart defects in infants and children. *Anesthesiology* 1992;76:165–172.

SECTION III

The Implication of Health Care Delivery System on Imaging Applications

CHAPTER 66

Principles of Imaging Applications under Managed Care[1]

Joseph R. Carver

"It was the best of times, it was the worst of times" (1). For the cardiologist approaching the end of the 20th century, a more accurate description of the practice of medicine in the United States is not possible. New technology, genetically engineered drugs, gene therapy, and advanced diagnostic capabilities all contribute positively to the excitement of medical practice. A focus on cost containment, loss of autonomy, fears of income reduction and economic credentialing have produced a fear of imposed change and questionable future survival. In the midst of this complex dichotomy, how can cardiac imaging continue to thrive? What are the trends and the strategic decisions that are mandated? What tools must be developed not only to remain viable, but also to deliver high quality care at an affordable cost. This chapter will examine the major trends affecting cardiac imaging and physician imagers and attempt to offer some suggestions for success in this ever-changing environment.

MAJOR TRENDS, 2000

In 2000, health care is responsible for almost 14% of the gross national product of the United States (2). Considering a broad definition that includes a plan type with a network or with precertification requirements, approximately 85% of the population is under the umbrella of some form of managed care. The progressive growth of managed care has developed largely at the expense of traditional indemnity coverage and now includes the Medicare and Medicaid populations (3,4).

Although there is regional variation in the definition, ac-

tivity, maturity, and impact of managed care (5), several trends that dominate each marketplace relate to finances, the structure of medical practice, care delivery, quality, and physician accountability. To understand how to prepare for the future, it is necessary to understand the influence of these forces in relation to physician behavior and decision-making. In broad terms, the trends are listed in Table 1 and are discussed below. Although discussed separately, the dissection is artificial and the whole picture can only be understood in the context of the whole being more than the sum of the individual parts.

Application of Classic Economic Rules to the Practice of Medicine and the Delivery of Health Care

At the present time, the practice of medicine does not follow the same economic rules as the rest of the business world. Although the gaps have narrowed in the last 5 years, significant differences remain. Teisberg et al. (6) recently identified the following:

- Consumers (patients and physicians) do not have a financial stake in what they purchase, i.e., the cost is generally the responsibility of a third party (employer). Consumers are not responsible for paying for the product. Given the choice between a luxury limousine and an economy sedan, who would take the latter if someone else is paying?
- Consumers do not always purchase care on the basis of objective measures of outcomes or quality. When they comparison shop, it is more often for price. Most shoppers have no idea of the relationship between price and quality for a given treatment or procedure. This observation becomes universal when applied to emergency situations when "need clearly equals want" with a resultant inelasticity that cripples the controls that the laws of economics

J. R. Carver: AETNA U.S. Health Care, Blue Bell, Pennsylvania 19422.

[1] The observations and opinions expressed in this chapter are those of Joseph R. Carver only and do not represent the policy or views of AETNA U.S. Health Care® or its affiliates.

TABLE 1. *Current trends in health care*

- Application of classic economic rules to the practice of medicine and the delivery of health care
- Increased penetration of managed care
- Consolidation and integration at every level
- Accountability at every level
- Focus on cost-effectiveness
- Focus on quality
- Focus on data and management
- Shift of service from in-patient to other sites
- Changing role of primary care and specialty physicians
- Influence of fourth parties on the practice of medicine
- Capitation and risk assumption
- Electronic commerce

traditionally supply—sick people do not want to shop around especially when the ability to gather the information to make the "right" choice may not be easily obtained. Because of this, some suppliers (doctors and hospitals) have remained economically successful, independently setting fees at random, charging more than a competitor for equal or even lesser quality.

- Prices have continually risen faster than the general cost of living increases, remaining high even in the presence of excess capacity. The laws of supply and demand have not applied, and this results in an ineffective market.
- Physicians and hospitals have previously lacked the incentive or need to refer or purchase services (i.e., laboratory studies, x-rays, or specialist consultation) from a more cost-competitive, less expensive, or more cost-efficient vendor of equal quality.
- Irrational duplication is unchecked and not governed by market forces.
- Other forces—pharmaceutical industry, imaging equipment, and device companies—exert a significant force on the expectation and the subsequent delivery of care.

Managed care has attempted to "heal" economic illnesses in medical care delivery. This has moved through several distinct stages. The first stage was *purchasing the services at a wholesale rate*. This was accompanied and followed by a *focus on utilization* (stage two). We are in the midst of the simultaneous transition to the third *proactive* stage that begins to use data for identification and risk stratification of the population and a fourth *best practice* stage. The former is attempting to try to answer the question "Who will be sick tomorrow?" to create a milieu of service coordination between patients and their physicians at an early phase of illness to prevent or slow complications and improve the quality of life. The latter stage superimposes evidence-based algorithms and pathways on clinical decision-making and creates new consumer expectations and provider accountability. As this stage matures, best practice medicine will smooth the impact of economic issues and transcend all of the various forms of payment to align incentives properly as a correction to the laws of economics. It is not likely that the third and fourth stages of this evolution will be achieved

by individual practitioners or small groups, but will depend on the systems, infrastructure, and data capabilities of insurers.

A fundamental truth in today's world is that medicine is a business, and the recognition of this reality is the first step for correction. It is also crucial to manage the business while continuing to manage the delivery of high quality care where decision-making rests on evidence-based principles. These deviations from the "laws" that govern other businesses are slowly being restored to match the rest of the business world. Understanding that the future business of medicine will more closely resemble the real world of business that follows classic economic theory is crucial for any practice reorganization or posturing decisions that are made today. Supply and demand rules will apply; purchasers will look to a "Medicine Consumers Report" to pick a doctor or imaging modality that will be accountable for cost and quality. A major step in preparing for the future is acknowledging that the current chaotic application of the laws of economics is ending rapidly.

Increased Penetration of Managed Care

Since 1973, the ratio of people enrolled in managed care plans compared to traditional indemnity plans has reversed. In 2000, almost 85% of the insured population is enrolled in some form of managed care. The important point of emphasis is the increased penetration of managed care and the expanded new definition of managed care. The latter has matured from "managed care equals HMO" to "managed care equals anything that is not traditional indemnity insurance." Even with this distinction, the lines of difference are further blurred whenever anyone with any insurance is hospitalized—concurrent or retrospective utilization review is an equal opportunity activity that crosses all product lines in remarkably similar ways. The expectations for the physician treatment of patients hospitalized as in-patients is remarkably consistent across all plan types.

As the price differential continues to increase dramatically between some form of managed versus unmanaged (indemnity) care, there will be further growth of managed care and erosion into the remaining 15% market share that indemnity plans have today.

Consolidation and Integration at Every Level

There is a slowly evolving trend for individual practitioners, smaller groups, single hospitals, and independent insurers to merge to deliver their product (8). In the United States today, "bigger is better." For physicians, efficiencies of service delivery, coverage, and access to technology can be more logically achieved through group compared to solo practice. The phenomenon takes health-care delivery beyond the balance sheet to integration, coordination, and defragmentation. This sets the stage for integration for the delivery of care. One could argue or at least question whether this is better than the perceived friendliness or personalized vision of the solo practice of the "old days." The advantage of moving through an integrated group of physicians for the efficient approach to diagnosis and treatment is obvious. This has also expanded to another larger level as medical practices integrate with hospitals and hospitals consolidate into grouped systems. A similar trend has also occurred among insurers with the expansion of some regional insurers to the national level and the expansion of national insurers to new locations and populations through merger and acquisition. The latter phenomenon has led to more portability for the insured population with the conceptual ability to reduce regional variation of care delivery through the distribution of evidence-based clinical practice guidelines for uniform implementation across the country. There has been static from nationally organized representatives of medicine regarding nonexistent gag clauses, misunderstood all product contracts, and the fear that physicians will be limited in their ability to make medical decisions. In reality, this has had little impact in reversing or modifying this trend of integration/consolidation.

Accountability at Every Level

An increased responsibility has accompanied this increased membership. At every level, there is third-party oversight demanding accountability for activity. It has been said that the practice of medicine used to be "doctors in ivory towers." Today, we all live in "glass houses." Doctors are accountable for their medical activity not only to patients, but also to the government, hospitals, and insurers. Someone scrutinizes everything done by physicians, hospitals, and insurers in health care. Hospitals compete for Joint Commission accreditation and are under a similar watchful eye from their financiers. Insurers compete for National Committee for Quality Assurance (NCQA) and American Accreditation Health Care Commission Utilization/URAC accreditation, and they compile data for the Health Plan Employer Data Information Set (HEDIS) and Health Compass reporting. Although this has added some level of bureaucracy to the practice of medicine, the overall value is a constant challenge to raise the bar of care delivery to higher levels.

Focus on Cost-Effectiveness

The medical literature has been invaded by discussions about cost-effectiveness (9,10). The marked regional variation in care delivery and the enlarging menu of diagnostic and therapeutic options have fueled this interest. Current levels of understanding and measurement are basic relative to other process measures and questions that seem intuitively simple have difficult-to-unravel answers. It does, however, indicate a broad awareness of the cost of health-care delivery at every level that has been embraced by all communities including the purchasers of health care.

What is cost-effectiveness? Providing evidence-based care to achieve the best statistical outcome in comparison to other treatments at the lowest cost. For example, ask a simple question like "What is the cost-effectiveness of treating coronary artery disease with or without a stent?" Providing the answer is not so simple because of the low event rate of subsequent events and the heterogeneity of interventionalists and coronary artery disease. The current state is now more theoretical than operational. It is clear that without near-universal agreement on practice guidelines, the world will continue to be bridled with marked variation in care delivery.

What is driving the concern and emphasis on cost-effectiveness? Many would blame managed care. In reality, there has been concern about the rising proportion of the gross national product (GNP) attributed to medical care. People will cite under- and overutilization in every sector to push cost-effectiveness. The reality is, the right medical care is affordable and dictates cost-effectiveness. Using resources to get the most payback with regard to outcomes and the chance for a successful outcome should drive the system.

Focus on Quality

Quality assessment has become a major focus of clinical practice (11–14). When all other things are equal, the differentiation of a health system, health plan, individual provider, or imaging facility is reduced to quality. Like the discussion about cost-effectiveness, quality is easy to talk about, slightly more difficult to agree on a definition, and markedly more difficult to measure. A working definition should include access to care, appropriateness of care, outcomes of care, measurement of satisfaction at every level, and value (i.e., cost). Currently, most measurements of quality either come from survey data or administrative data. We can answer questions about access to care, satisfaction, and value with more ease than evaluating appropriateness and most outcomes.

Focus on Data and Measurement

How can the delivery of care be cost-effective and improve quality? This critical question cannot be answered without data. The infrastructure to record, warehouse, and analyze these data does not universally exist today. Most practices, whether solo or group, are not "in this business." Integrated systems have the ability to gather these data. To date, the major focus has been productivity rather than quality assessment and improvement. Insurers have the requisite infrastructure populated by administrative data, but sometimes lack access to the clinical data necessary to refine and severity adjust data to reliably answer questions. In spite of this limitation, report cards of various sophistication and content are generated today (15,16). They may or may not have practical implications for network participation and/or reimbursement. National societies, such as the American

College of Cardiology, have taken an interest in this activity and have begun to invest resources in national databases to enable their membership to begin their data collection and analysis. Thus far, there has been only modest buy-in and participation from their membership. In spite of these barriers, there is more focus on data and its use today than ever before. In rudimentary small steps, medical practitioners are entering this world and beginning to let data modify the way that they deliver care. Iezzoni (17) has recently reviewed issues around administrative data collection, validation, and pitfalls in interpretation.

The average group of doctors with access to clinical data can begin to ask the right questions about their practice. Today, there is only minimal incentive to gather, warehouse, and analyze these data. It is an incremental expense (systems, dedicated personnel) that in today's world may not contribute directly to revenue. The implications:

- Entry level data collection can be done simply and without adding cost to doing business. Ask simple straightforward questions and analyze the answers to reinforce practices or improve the delivery of care.
- In reality, data-derived and data-driven analysis of the practice can be profitable in today's market by improving productivity and the quality of the care that is delivered.
- In the future, patient selection of doctors, volume, and, ultimately, reimbursement will flow from the profile of the practice that these data reflect.

In the end, one thing is clear—it is not possible to move to a quality, cost-effective system of care delivery without data to establish benchmarks, best practices, and produce report cards.

Shift of Site of Service from Inpatient to Other Sites

As managed care markets mature, there is a concomitant shift in service site from the hospital to the outpatient setting (18). This has led to shorter lengths of stay. The latter has produced an excess bed capacity and the explosion of outpatient cardiac imaging laboratories. The latter perform diagnostic and therapeutic cardiovascular procedures that previously were the domain of hospitals and associated with an inpatient stay. They now compete with the hospital laboratories for market share and bring a fundamental advantage to the bargaining table. As freestanding and specialized units, they are able to operate more economically than the hospital laboratory and can offer to provide their services at a lower cost. Often, they offer "one stop shopping" and can deliver a full range of cardiology services in the office, a short procedure unit, freestanding diagnostic center, or heart hospital. All of these are associated with new economic relationships that range from nonphysician-owned ventures to risk-sharing arrangements with hospitals. An additional outgrowth of this trend has been the emergence and reliance on an expanded corps of health-care attorneys and new volumes of health-care law.

Changing Role of Primary Care and Specialist Physicians

The role of the primary care physician (PCP) as gatekeeper and coordinator of care continues to be an essential and fixed element of managed care (19). There are currently several variations of this concept:

- The traditional HMO model in which access to cardiology care and cardiac imaging services are managed by the primary care physician through the referral process. In the tightly managed HMO model, the PCP may have to call the HMO to generate the referral. The HMO may judge the appropriateness of the referral against an objective set of criteria, e.g., Milliman and Robertson (M&R). In a less restrictive model, the PCP may have the autonomy to make a referral to any cardiologist in the network or order any imaging test based solely on clinical judgment.
- The interposition of a management group between the patient and the physician, i.e., an Independent Practice Association (IPA) or a Management Services Group (MSO). This model adds another layer between the physician and the patient. Access to specialty care and cardiac imaging services has to be approved by this group prior to referral: the PCP has to call the intermediary who judges the appropriateness of the referral and then directs the patient to an appropriate participating cardiologist or imaging center in the network.
- A cardiologist gatekeeper for additional diagnostic or therapeutic services. This currently in-vogue model places a noninvasive cardiologist gatekeeper to allow access to invasive cardiology procedures. The concept can be extended to a nonimaging cardiologist gatekeeper to allow access to diagnostic imaging services.
- Direct access to specialty care is another emerging alternative. In this construct, patients who meet certain eligibility criteria (e.g., chronicity, severity, comorbidity, utilization triggers) may be able to access cardiology care (visits, diagnostic and therapeutic services) after an initial referral. The patient, the PCP, the specialist, or the health plan may be able to initiate this direct access enrollment. The identification and referral can be proactive or reactive. Regardless of the health plan's specific detail and variation, the cardiologist, often without an intermediary, drives access to cardiac imaging. For these patients, the cardiologist acts like the traditional PCP (gatekeeper) for cardiology care. As of mid-1999, a version of this direct access alternative had been mandated in more than a dozen states and by the federal government for Medicare members and federal employees enrolled in managed care plans.

Influence of Fourth Parties on the Practice of Medicine

With the realization of managed care in 1973, the practice of medicine was given an added dimension. Oversight and quality initiatives led to reductions in length of stay, the achievement of new targets for preventive care (e.g., mammography, immunizations), and the introduction of accountability. In the past 3 years, there has been a dramatic shift regarding the influence of fourth parties on the practice of medicine. These include:

- Employers—the largest private purchasers of health care. In 1997, they purchased 90.5% of all nonelderly private health insurance. Coalitions of large employers have been instrumental in bringing quality to the forefront (HEDIS measures) and many choose their health plan on the basis of quality measures and satisfaction rather than on cost alone (20–22). At present, this direction/involvement represents only a small fraction of the health care that is purchased.
- Government—as the largest purchaser of health services in the United States (22,23), local, state and the federal governments have had a significant influence on the practice of medicine. CPT (Current Procedural Terminology) codes, the relative value system (RBRVS), and the Health Care Financing Agency (HCFA) have changed and continue to change the "rules" of practice with no likelihood that this will diminish in the foreseeable future. On another level, legislative interference with the practice of medicine continues to exponentially expand. Many states and the federal government have passed health-care delivery legislation and promulgated regulations in the past 5 years altering coverage policy, clinical relationships, and clinical decision-making. Of interest, legislated benefit enhancements have contributed to the recent increase in health-care insurance premiums.
- Public interest groups—there has been a parallel increase in consumer influence on health care. Lay groups have lobbied legislators, brought their causes to the mainstream through the media, and worked with established groups to bring the patient's point of view to discussions about molding and modeling health care. In Seattle, Washington, members of the Pudget Sound Health Plan sit on the board of directors and are equal and active participants in the health plan's policy formation. The Foundation for Accountability (FACCT), founded by Paul Ellwood in 1995, has become a nationally known and influential forum for patient advocacy. Their purpose is to develop measures of performance that are relevant to consumers and to educate consumers about how to use this information. Other groups include the National Patient Safety Foundation, the National Roundtable on Health Care Quality, and the Institute of Medicine. With the ever increasing and near universal access to the Internet for medical information, this empowerment trend will only continue to produce a new type of medical consumer (and help in the economic correction previously discussed) and medical practitioner.

Capitation and Risk Assumption

Many payment models have been suggested to replace the fee for service system. They include:

- "Fee for time," in which payment is based on a relative time value for each type of encounter. There is recognition of cognitive interventions and a devaluation of testing (25,26).
- "Fee for benefit," in which payment is based on the outcome and long-term benefit of a procedure. For example, the reimbursement for coronary artery bypass surgery would be more for a 40-year-old male with unstable angina and left main disease than for a 80-year-old male with lung cancer and single right coronary artery disease (27).
- Case rates or episode of care payment, in which a single all-inclusive payment is made for a defined time period. This is based on a diagnosis, an all-inclusive Diagnosis-Related Group (DRG) for all sites of care; for example, $100 for the x-ray evaluation of a headache or $400 for the 4-month treatment and evaluation of chest pain. Another variation of this is "contact capitation" in which the fee for a period of time is set regardless of the amount of activity that is generated;
- Capitation, which in its simplest form prepays a fixed amount of money on a regular basis for the care of a defined population. The dollar figure is independent of the type or quantity of the services rendered. The amount can be a fixed amount for each patient "assigned" per month, or a percentage of the premium dollar.

In 2000, there is still a great but waning interest in "taking risk," i.e., taking some form of member-based payment (capitation) with the risk taker believing that they can manage the care better than the current manager and either share or keep all of the projected savings. What are the implications? For the doctor and patient, this almost always adds another management layer to influence care delivery, the quantity of services delivered, and diverts a portion of the health-care dollar from the delivery to the management of care. Successful endeavors are few. Recent experiences in Pennsylvania with the Allegheny Health system and elsewhere in the country have added reticence and caution to those thinking about similar risk relationships in the future. The trend may be reversing with a correction back to the traditional role of doctors delivering care to patients and insurers taking the financial risk for that care.

Electronic Commerce

Beyond the new consumerism described above, as we enter the millennium, the use of computers and the Internet to enhance the practice of medicine has exploded. A partial list of applications in medicine include, but are not limited to:

- Billing and scheduling
- Electronic medical records
- Digital transmission of images for primary and secondary opinions

- Creation of a virtual office, giving patients access to scheduling, lab results, medical information, answers to questions, prescription refills
- Data bases and quality improvement
- On-line provider and payer report cards
- Disease/case management

TRENDS AND CARDIAC IMAGING

The performance and reimbursement of cardiac imaging has been influenced by the aforementioned trends.

Michnich and colleagues (28) asked several crucial questions about nuclear cardiology in 1996, and I would like to extend their discussion to the whole universe of cardiac imaging from the perspective of the current trends and the environment that exists as we enter the 21st century.

Who Will Deliver the Service?

Excluding cardiac echocardiography, there is an ongoing turf battle between radiologists and cardiologists. Whose domain is the nonechocardiography cardiac imaging laboratory? Each proponent has cogent arguments to exclude the other. The solution is simply stated. From the standpoint of training and experience, who can meet credentialing guidelines? The simplicity is lost after the statement of concept. Beyond training and experience, a whole series of apropo questions emerge: Who will develop the credentialing standards? Should image quality, interpretation, and appropriateness of testing be part of the process? What is the relative role of quality improvement? Who will operationalize the credentialing process? Will credentialing provide adequate access to services from the perspective of technicians, physicians, and facilities? Should this be a cardiology or radiology process? Some believe cardiologists should drive nuclear cardiology. This is based on the theory that they bring an understanding of cardiac physiology, an ability to better interpret the nonimaging portion of the study (the stress electrocardiogram), more specific and intensive training to evaluate the patient with a cardiology complaint or diagnosis, and that they have the ability to participate in the continuum of care from pretest, test interpretation, and posttest therapy. Nevertheless, there is acceptance that radiologists as well as cardiologists can be qualified to perform and interpret these studies.

It is incumbent on the professional community, rather than nonprofessional forces, to establish the standards for credentialing. Nuclear cardiology has taken the lead in the imaging area. The Certification Board of Nuclear Cardiology was established to credential physicians in the practice of nuclear cardiology. They offer an annual examination. Today, this process is in its infancy and the number of credentialed physicians and accredited laboratories cannot justify a mandate that only allows those credentialed individuals to perform,

read, and interpret studies. Therefore, the impact of this process is a future consideration and not an operative credentialing mechanism for insurers to utilize. As the numbers of physicians and laboratories achieve a critical number to allow adequate access for patients to have cardiac imaging studies in these qualified laboratories, the marketplace will demand that insurers adopt this third party imprimatur for network participation.

What is needed is an agreed upon set of standards, a form of data collection, and a credentialing body—what is not needed is a separate radiology initiative and a separate cardiology initiative to achieve this end.

With the assumption that some cardiologists will indeed be actively involved in cardiac imaging, which cardiologist is going to deliver it? Will it be the generalist or a specially trained cardiologist, i.e., a nuclear cardiologist, a magnetic resonance imaging cardiologist? A trend for the future is that only those people who have been specifically trained and certified through a certifying or credentialing examination will perform imaging studies. At present, the only modality that has an active program is nuclear cardiology. The Certification Board of Nuclear Cardiology offers the current examination. As of June 1999, 1,262 physicians have been credentialed in nuclear cardiology.

This shift to subspecialty certification is in contrast to today's acceptance of cardiology board certification as a license to do everything in cardiovascular diagnosis and treatment. Just because a cardiology fellowship was completed in the past does not mean the automatic capability to open a nuclear lab, perform cardiac magnetic resonance imaging (MRI) studies, or interpret any or all of the imaging studies available today. Like the credentialing discussion, this concept, although logical, has not been adopted by the national cardiology or radiology societies. It, therefore, remains a theoretical construct for the future. This is a dramatic shift in expectations, and it's going to move cardiology to a new level, enhancing the value of all modes of cardiac imaging. Ultimately, there will be group recognition of the value of subspecialty credentialing, and the official position will become: "you can't do it unless you are board certified (or at least board qualified) and not only in cardiology, but in a recognized subspecialty of cardiology." Just because training was completed doesn't mean the trainee is ready to perform and interpret all modalities of cardiac imaging.

Credentialing generally refers to the professional component of imaging (the imager/interpreter). The credentialed person has met or exceeded established standards for the imaging modality. The parallel process for the technical component, i.e., the laboratory, is defined as accreditation. Issues and controversies are similar to those described for credentialing. The current process can range from a self-assessment questionnaire (American Society of Nuclear Cardiology Report Card) to the review of clinical studies with or without a nuclear phantom image. The review may be a paper process or include a site visit. Since 1997, the Intersocietal Commission for the Accreditation of Nuclear Laboratories (ICANL) has provided a mechanism to independently confirm the technical, professional, and administrative expertise of nuclear laboratories. The ICANL consists of a broad base of sponsoring organizations that includes the American Society of Nuclear Cardiology, the American College of Cardiology, the Society of Nuclear Medicine, the Technologist Section of the Society of Nuclear Medicine, the American College of Nuclear Physicians, and the Institute for Clinical Positron Emission Tomography. The purpose of the ICANL is to provide a program by which facilities can be accredited in Nuclear Medicine, Positron Emission Tomography, and Nuclear Cardiology. Similar collaborative efforts are under way for Echocardiography and Cardiac MRI laboratories, and, for the most part, these efforts suffer from the same lack of penetration/volume of accredited laboratories as the nuclear cardiology initiative.

The accreditation process has recently been outlined by Wackers (29). The process includes an examination of physical facilities, personnel and their supervision, imaging services, nonimaging medical services, safety and confidentiality, procedures, image interpretation and reporting, quality assessment measures, and satisfaction. As of July 1999, 12 Nuclear Cardiology laboratories have been accredited by ICANL and more than 250 orders for accreditation materials have been fulfilled. The cost for "Essentials and Standards" and the Application Book is $200, and the application fee for accreditation is $2,000. A similar joint accreditation process exists for echocardiography laboratories, and preliminary discussions are under way for cardiac MRI imaging accreditation.

Another issue around "Who is going to do it?" originates from the payer practice of global radiology contracting and risk assumption. When a managed care organization contracts with a radiology group for all of the radiology CPT codes, cardiac MRI, nuclear cardiology, and echocardiography may be "carved-in" or "carved-out." If it is "in," then the opportunity to do these studies belongs to radiologists rather than cardiologists. The latter may actually be excluded or "locked-out," depending on the contract, the makeup of the radiology group, and the payer. In rare cases, the contractor may not even understand the difference between a chest x-ray and a stress perfusion study, although I believe that this is the exceptional health plan rather than a universal scenario. However, it remains a theoretical pitfall for cardiac imaging, which can easily be overcome through dialogue and education between those performing cardiac imaging and the health plans that contract for these services. Who is doing the study may depend on managed care contracting and not credentialing/accreditation or proven expertise. In spite of this possible roadblock to cardiologists, a recent survey suggests that cardiologists are conducting 78% of nuclear studies (30).

After "you build it"—achieve provider credentialing, laboratory accreditation, and a contract with an insurer to be part of a network—"will they come?" Will the service be accessed in your laboratory? This relates to the role of the managed care gatekeeper. For cardiac imaging testing, the gatekeeper may be:

- A primary care physician generating a request;
- A primary care physician only able to make the request following input from a cardiologist;
- A primary care physician only able to make the request following the approval of a third party, i.e., an MSO, IPA, or MCO;
- A cardiologist (31).

To be successful in cardiac imaging, it is critical to understand credentialing and accreditation requirements as well as how each MCO's system operates. It is critical to know and develop relationships with the gatekeeper. It is critically important as part of that relationship to promote and "sell" your expertise and value by providing data about your laboratory's sensitivity, specificity, false and true negative/positive rates, and predictive accuracy, i.e., your lab's report card. Mastering each component is critical to having access to patients to provide these services.

Where Will the Service Be Delivered?

The current trends that shape the delivery of cardiac imaging services are the shift of service site and the process of consolidation. To some extent, the delivery site may be defined by the answer to the previous question. Assuming all credentialing and accreditation issues are moot, it is clear that almost all cardiac imaging services with the possible exception of cardiac MRI will be delivered in the outpatient setting and more often in a freestanding (nonhospital) facility. The latter may be a cardiology or radiology office or a dedicated cardiology imaging center. Consistent with current merger and consolidation activity, it is most likely that the delivery site will be part of a larger system—single or multispecialty group or hospital. These larger systems take advantage of pooled resources to have the most current and modern equipment, and an economy of scale for staffing and purchasing with flexibility of scheduling not available in small practices or hospital-based laboratories. Larger groups can also dedicate appropriately trained and credentialed physicians to maximize quality and have the system resources to collect and analyze data for quality assessment and approval.

The future site of delivery of imaging services will continue to be outpatient. Bateman et al. (32) recently reviewed design and implementation models for nuclear cardiology testing facilities. The concepts and recommendations can be universally applied to other diagnostic imaging modalities.

An interesting issue, which is beyond the scope of this chapter, relates to ownership and referral. It is sufficient to recognize that cardiac imaging today is a business that has the potential for return on investment independent of the owner.

How Will the Service Be Paid For?

Traditionally, the piecework concept has dominated reimbursement for cardiac imaging procedures. The Health Care Financing Administration (HCFA) model of payment based on the combination of a series of CPT-4 codes is the "gold standard" and dominant model today. To participate and obtain reimbursement for a cardiac imaging study, a laboratory generally has to contract with each individual insurer in the marketplace. Many of these contracts are obtained based on the existence of the laboratory, a perceived need by the health plan for the available services, the laboratory's ability to meet the then-current credentialing criteria and the ability of both parties to agree on a reimbursement package. A more sophisticated second-level approach would include the achievement of laboratory accreditation and physician credentialing as a threshold for contracting and participation. As previously discussed, this could be the domain and the direct activity of an individual health plan or a more far reaching national body with delegated responsibility for the development and implementation of the approval process. At this level, access to begin the contracting process is variable and may depend on:

- Market penetration
- Need for choice
- Cost of the procedures
- Who holds any capitated radiology or cardiology contract and what is included and carved out

The addition of quality-based contracting accelerates this process to the third level. This is based on performance data that may include:

- Access—Can the laboratory provide all the testing that is desired?
- Appropriateness of testing—Are there processes and procedures in place to do the right test and not the test that may provide less information or that may be inappropriate for the patient's condition?
- Outcomes—What is the laboratory's track record for predictive accuracy, false-positive and negative testing rates? Is there consistency and accuracy of interpretation (over reading, outside review of studies and interpretation)
- Patient satisfaction—What do the consumers (patients and referring physicians) think of the services that are provided?
- Referring physician satisfaction—What does the referring physician think of the service provided, the quality of testing, and the resultant communication?

The ability to provide these data may ultimately be the key to contracting and network participation.

At each of these levels for participation, the payment system may be fee for service or a member-based payment. It is critical to recognize that as financial risk increases in member-based payment relationships, utilization predictably decreases. The decreases are modest and most pronounced in the first year of the transition and then level off to a new baseline in subsequent years. This has obvious implications for staffing and operating costs as these relationships are established. Safeguards for underutilization and quality oversight need to be built into all of these arrangements.

The recognition of the value of these quality data may be the key to more sophisticated quality-based compensation. At this level, quality-based compensation can actually transcend and overlay the payment system (fee for service, a fixed payment for all nuclear cardiology studies done for a defined population [carve-out], a radiology contract, a cardiology services contract, a total health-care delivery contract).

Movement to this third level of compensation is dependent on the provider's willingness and ability to gather and report data, the insurer's ability to understand the value of the data, and the initial ability for both to have the conversation. This requires the development of a relationship with the health plan. It should begin with a nonadversarial dialogue, which focuses on quality and evolves to reimbursement rather than to a discussion that begins with the attitude that the provider thinks that reimbursement is too low and the insurer thinks that the reimbursement is already too high. Communication and the ability to objectively demonstrate the quality of the laboratory with data and reports are the keys to future success.

Is Cardiac Imaging Cost-Effective?

There is an abundance of literature that documents the worth of cardiac imaging in answer to clinical questions about cost-effectiveness (33–36). These issues have been discussed in previous chapters with affirmative answers for the mature imaging techniques (echocardiography, positron emission tomography, and nuclear cardiology) with an abundance of questions for emerging imaging techniques (ultrafast CT and cardiac MRI). For all, evidence-based guidelines for test appropriateness will ultimately dictate cost-effective use of these and new imaging technologies.

Each imaging modality will have to compete regarding sensitivity and specificity as well as its effects on clinical decision-making, and outcomes and cost (37). For any given clinical presentation, the cardiology community will continue to measure and assess any emerging imaging modality against existing diagnostic tests for cost-effectiveness (38). Ultimately, for comparable sensitivity, specificity, and predictive accuracy, a new imaging technology must be less expensive than currently available technology to be deemed "cost-effective," and it must be able to reach the marketplace.

Will the Technologies Survive?

The answer to this question is intimately linked to the preceding question about cost-effectiveness and discussions about data and guidelines. Each cardiac imaging technique needs to satisfy a simple generic construct for continued survival. Either the imaging technique has to provide a unique answer not obtainable through the use of another technique or it must provide a cost-effective answer relative to other technology in the solution of a clinical problem. How do we get to that point? The solution hinges on the collection of data and the application of those data to achieve the appropriate balance between cost and quality. The beauty of this construct is that it allows decision-making today as well as in the future as new cardiac imaging techniques emerge.

Who Will Develop Future Guidelines?

If evidence-based medicine is the final stage in the evolution of managed care, the development of guidelines and clinical pathways assumes a crucial role.

Guidelines will be developed from the focus on data and measurement. Guidelines will be developed from evidence-based data. Cardiac imaging is suited for this—there is a clear-cut starting point and the ability to follow patients longitudinally from an event or a test to determine standard measures of test accuracy and value: false-positive, false-negative rates, and predictive accuracy. Collecting data in real time and prospectively is what cardiac imaging is all about. Does the test lead to or drive a clinical decision tree and can a clinician rely on the results for treatment that offers the patient the optimal chance of a good outcome? The answers only come from data that are clinically and statistically accurate.

It is also crucial that this effort must be driven and completed by physicians in concert with all of the stakeholders. This cannot be done without physicians.

CONCLUSIONS

Providers and payers have preconceived and often divergent opinions about noninvasive cardiology imaging. Many cardiologists and radiologists look at one or more of these tests as another revenue center and another way to maintain a practice. These modalities are more than a revenue center. They are an important delivery component of health care that are selectively cost-effective when used according to evidence-based guidelines. Everyone is currently fixated on and complaining about reimbursement. "We are losing money doing the study with what we are paid." Clearly, doctors are saying managed care doesn't understand the value of noninvasive cardiac imaging. Managed care views these noninvasive testing modalities as a cost center that can be controlled by cutting the unit price. "Too many tests are done, there are too many labs all over the place, and we can't deal with quality." The perception of and approaches to cardiac imaging are currently stuck in the first stage of

managed care—discount contracting. We need to move to a different level that attempts to balance cost and quality in accordance with the laws of economics that govern other nonmedical services.

Depending on the maturity of the market place, there is marked variation in the impact of the trends described in this chapter. The impact of these trends on cardiac imaging in California is different from the impact in rural Montana, rural Mississippi, or central Pennsylvania. Even small geographical differences produce potentially disparate effects on the practice of cardiology. The ultimate way in which clinical decisions are made and care is delivered may depend in part on the product, the geography, the compensation mechanism, and the managed care company. Regardless of the reimbursement method, the managed care organization will monitor cardiac imaging trends for under- and overutilization and to educate imaging providers about evidence-based best practice and appropriate utilization of imaging modalities. Is it quality? Is it saving money? Is it making money? Is it increasing membership? All of these drive the payment strategies, the number of tests performed, and the usefulness of any of the discussed imaging modalities in any local area.

Payers and providers have shared goals. In regard to cardiology testing, all of the stakeholders want the opportunity to have access to high quality studies. Everyone also desires to do it at a cost that's affordable to keep everyone financially viable. As a provider, you might believe that your product is the best or even that your laboratory produces the best study around. If you can not prove it with outcomes data and if other labs that you perceive are not as good as yours can produce these data, the flow of testing may be away from you and toward your competitor. Your perception of, and even measurement of, the quality of the tests that come from your laboratory may also lead to little consideration and market share if a competitor with comparable results can do it less expensively. This will have more impact as the world moves toward correction to market-based economics: if it's too expensive, nobody will use it. Each test has to be understood based on real value or its cost-effectiveness. The real costs of a stress myocardial perfusion study or a cardiac MRI are not the $600 to $2,000, but that direct cost plus the costs that follow downstream. A high quality study for $1,000, for example, might save money in the future by preventing an unnecessary procedure or operation or a subsequent study because the information for a clinical decision was not provided the first time. Doing it right the first time is a lot cheaper then paying a discounted $400 (based on cost alone) for a poor study that provides the wrong information (poor quality).

In a rapidly evolving world of technology where everything seems to be improving (cameras, isotopes, hardware, and software) we must be able to support the basic research to continue moving testing to a higher level. At every juncture, we must not be content with the status quo. We must continue to ask the right questions to improve imaging quality, imaging value at an affordable cost.

Rx FOR SUCCESS

For cardiac imaging to be successful in an environment dominated by the current, expanded definition of managed care, there is a need to understand this environment both globally and locally. How is the world defined in general and at the individual practice site? To be successful, imagers and imaging centers need to define the strengths and weaknesses of practice partners, colleagues, competitors, other facilities, etc., and place more emphasis on strengths and shore up the weaknesses. The latter may mean abandoning those weak or second-level activities. It may mean concentrating efforts on a single imaging modality rather than trying to provide everything that exists. The latter, without specific expertise in each modality is a formula for future failure. With this in mind, everyone needs to have a long-term plan that is built with "San Francisco construction": strong enough to meet today's needs with the flexibility to survive any "earthquake" in the health-care system. Long-term planing is difficult to define—it might be 8 months, or 16 months, or 5 years. The mandate is to constantly change with the times and be open-minded enough to recognize the opportunities that emerge. Building and strengthening relationships at all levels, beginning with referring physicians and the payers, is at the foundation. The building comes together with the addition of the ability to collect data and to develop a data base on top of that foundation. The data will demonstrate the value brought to the marketplace and the clinical practice of cardiology by each imaging modality. The laws of economics are catching up with cardiac imaging—rather than this being a threat or "the worst of times," a few basic, midcourse corrections to the foundation and structure suggested in this chapter can create a path to the "best of times."

In the future, the surviving testing modalities will recognize the niche that they occupy in the continuum of cardiology care by demonstrating value. In this new world, accreditation will be mandatory; there will be a gatekeeper; testing protocols will be evidence-based; data will reign; and reimbursement will be enhanced based on quality and outcomes.

In the future, the promise of market reform will hopefully not be legislated but be successfully achieved through the cooperative efforts of physicians working with insurers pushing evidence-based change.

REFERENCES

1. Dickens CA. *A tale of two cities*. New York: Puffin Books, 1996:1.
2. Levit KR, Lazenby HC, Braden BR, et al. National health expenditures. 1996. *Health Aff* 1998;17(1):35–51.
3. Schreiber G, Poullier JP, Greenwald L. US health expenditure performance: an international comparison and data update. *Health Care Financ Rev* 1992;13:1–15.
4. Inglehart JK. The American health care system—managed care. *N Engl J Med* 1992;327:742–747.
5. Murray D. The four market stages, and where you fit it. *Med Econ* 1995;72(5):44–57.
6. Teisberg EO, Porter ME, Brown GB. Making competition in health care work. *Harvard Bus Rev* 1994;4:131–141.
7. Becker ER, Morris DC, Culler SD, et al. The changing healthcare market and how it has influenced the treatment of cardiovascular disease—part 1. *Am J Man Care* 1999;5:1119–1124.
8. Bodenheimer T. The American health care system. Physicians and the changing medical marketplace. *N Engl J Med* 1999;340:584–588.
9. Woodall ML. Cost-effectiveness studies in interventional cardiology. *J Inv Cardiol* 1998;10(6):366–369.
10. Hachamovitch R, Shaw LJ, Berman DS. The ongoing evolution of risk stratification using myocardial perfusion imaging in patients with known or suspected coronary artery disease. *ACC Cur J Rev* 1999;8(1):66–74.
11. Blumenthal D. Total quality management and physician's clinical decisions. *JAMA* 1993;269:2775–2778.
12. Kassirer JP. The quality of care and the quality of measuring it [editorial]. *N Engl J Med* 1993;329:1263–1265.
13. Blummenthal D, Epstein A. Quality of health care. Part 6: the role of physicians in the future of quality management. *N Engl J Med* 1996;335:1328–1331.
14. Bodenheimer T. The American health care system. The movement for improved quality in health care. *N Engl J Med* 1999;340:488–492.
15. Hannan EL, Kilburn H Jr, O'Donnell JF, et al. Adult open heart surgery in New York State: an analysis of risk factors and hospital mortality rates. *JAMA* 1990;264:2768–2774.
16. Report Card Pilot Project. *Key findings and lessons learned: 21 plans' performance profiles.* Washington, DC: National Committee for Quality Assurance, 1995.
17. Iezzoni LI. Assessing quality using administrative data. *Ann Int Med* 1997;127:8(2):666–673.
18. Levit K, Cowan C, Braden B, et al. National health expenditures in 1997: more slow growth. *Health Aff* 1998;17(6):99–110.
19. Franks P, Clancy CM, Nutting PA. Gatekeeping revisited—protecting patients from over treatment. *N Engl J Med* 1992;327:424–427.
20. Schaufler HH, Rodriquez T. Exercising purchasing power for preventive care. *Health Aff* 1996;15(1):73–85.
21. Carrasquillo O, Himmelstein DU, Woolhandler S, et al. A reappraisal of private employers' role in providing health insurance. *N Engl J Med* 1999;340:109–114.
22. Kuttner R. The American health care system. Employer-sponsored health coverage. *N Engl J Med* 1999;340:248–352.
23. Iglehart JK. The American health care system. Medicaid. *N Engl J Med* 1999;340:403–408.
24. Iglehart JK. The American health care system. Medicare. *N Engl J Med* 1999;340:327–332.
25. Wachtel TJ, Stein MD. Fee for time system: a conceptual framework for an incentive neutral method of physician payment. *JAMA* 1993;270:1226–1229.
26. Lasker RD, Marquis MS. The intensity of physicians' work in patient visits. Implications for the coding of patient evaluation and management services. *N Engl J Med* 1999;341:337–341.
27. Diamond GA, Denton TA, Matloff JM. Fee for benefit: a strategy to improve the quality of healthcare and control costs through reimbursement incentives. *Am J Cardiol* 1993;22:343–352.
28. Michnich ME, Mills PS, Seidman JJ. The effect of managed care on nuclear cardiology. *J Nucl Cardiol* 1996;3:65–71.
29. Wackers FJ Th. Blueprint of the accreditation program of the Intersocietal Commission for the Accreditation of Nuclear Medicine Laboratories. *J Nucl Cardiol* 1999;6:372–374.
30. Sorrell VL, Reeves WC. Who is interpreting nuclear cardiology studies in the United States, and what are the requirements for privileges? A national survey of institutional policies from 80 major medical centers. *J Nucl Cardiol* 1997;4:309–315.
31. Stein JH, Uretz EF, Parrillo JE, et al. Cost and appropriateness of radionucleotide exercise stress testing by cardiologists and non-cardiologists. *Am J Cardiol* 1996;77:139–142.
32. Bateman TM, O'Keede JH Jr, Williams ME. Design and implementation of a nuclear cardiology testing facility in a private-practice cardiology office setting. *J Nucl Cardiol* 1997;4:156–163.
33. Berman DS, Kiat H, Friedman JD, et al. Clinical applications of exercise nuclear cardiology studies in the era of healthcare reform. *Am J Cardiol* 1995;75:3D–13D.

34. Maddahi J, Gambhir SS. Cost-effective selection of patients for coronary arteriography. *J Nucl Cardiol* 1997;4(2):S141–151.
35. Mattera JA, Arain SA, Sinusas AJ, et al. Exercise testing with myocardial perfusion imaging in patients with normal baseline electrocardiograms: cost savings with a stepwise diagnostic strategy. *J Nucl Cardiol* 1998;5:498–506.
36. Patterson RE, Eisner RL, Horowitz SF. Comparison of cost-effectiveness and utility of exercise ECG, single photon emission computed tomography, positron emission tomography as a diagnostic modality for diagnosis of coronary artery disease. *Circulation* 1995;91:54–65.
37. Steinberg EP. Magnetic resonance coronary angiography—assessing an emerging technology [editorial]. *N Engl J Med* 1993;328:879–880.
38. Phelps CE, Mushlin AI. Focusing technology assessment using medical decision theory. *Med Decis Making* 1988;8:279–289.

Subject Index

Autografts, 621
A-wave, 33

B

Backprojection, tomographic transaxial
images, 143
Backscatter
cyclic variation of integrated, 116
extracellular matrix and, 116
integrated, 115
cardiac function and, 117
dilated cardiomyopathy and, 119
experimental cardiomyopathy and,
119
hypertrophic cardiomyopathy and,
119
technology, endocardial border
detection and, 30
Backscattering, 115
Bacteremia, persistent, infective
endocarditis and, 631
Bacterial infection, heart muscle disease
and, 646
Balatine coli, heart muscle disease and,
646
Ball-in-cage valve, 620
Balloon valvuloplasty, transesophageal
echocardiography and, 45
Barium swallow, left atrial enlargement
and, 339
Basal septum, five-chamber view, 24
BATO compounds, 166
B bump, 14
Beriberi, heart muscle disease and, 646
Bernoulli equation, 6
modified, 617
Beta blockers, 556
mitral valve prolapse and, 587
BGO crystals, 196
Bibasilar pulmonary disease, 344
Bicycle exercise testing, 152
first-pass radionuclide angiography and,
262
stress echocardiography and, 67
Bidirectional Glenn shunt
echocardiography, 802
surgery, 802
Biopsy
endomyocardial, 696
myocardial, 695
BiSphere, 86
Biventricular failure, 335
Blastomycosis, heart muscle disease and,
646
Blood cells' velocity, 5
Blood flow
coronary
cardiac output and, 152
MR phase velocity evaluation, 459
coronary angiography assessment, 362
Doppler, 20
measurements of, 3
hemodynamics, echocardiography role
in, 3
myocardial, 117

exercise and, 151
flow tracers and, 196
PET assessment of, 195–212
PET measurements of, 205
radiopharmaceuticals and, 196
myocardial retention and, 195
physiology of, 3
pulmonary, 342
pregnancy and, 343
reversal of, 343
regional, 160
structural abnormality visualization
and, 3
threshold value for, 225
washout kinetics and, 195
Blood motion, at endocardial borders, 243
Blood pool imaging, 137
gated, 243
regional function measurement, 251
regional ventricular function
analysis, 254
planar gated
counts-based method, 249
gamma camera and, 244
gating the data, 245
image acquisition, 244
LV function parameters, 248
LV volume curve in, 247
ventricular function assessment, 244
tomographic gated, 251
Blood pressure
exercise testing and, 153
lower extremity arterial disease, 843
Blood pressure gradient, Doppler
evaluation of, 20
Blood volume, myocardial vascular, CT
measurement of, 384
BMIPP (15-(p-iodophenyl)-3R, S-methyl
pentadecanoic acid)
basic analysis of, 299
clinical applications of, 299
B-mode echocardiography, 4–5
artificial heart valves and, 5
cardiac events and, 4
hemodynamics and, 5
reverberations, 5
spatial resolution and, 4
stenotic valves and, 5
transducer and, 4
BOLD imaging, 441
BR14, 86
Bradyarrhythmias, 903
restrictive cardiomyopathy, 903
Bradycardia, dipyridamole and, 70
Brain
imaging of, 857
ischemic process, documentation of,
858
Brain–heart interactions, 307
Brain vessels, imaging of, 857
Breast carcinoma, 874
Bronchospasm, dipyridamole and, 70
Bronchus, left atrial enlargement and, 339
Brucellosis, heart muscle disease and, 646
Bundle branch block
left, 32
stress echocardiography and, 65

right, coronary artery disease and, 504
BY963, 86

C

CABG: *see* Coronary artery bypass grafts
C-11 acetate, 197
CAD: *see* Coronary artery disease
Calcification, 339–342
annulus, 340
aortic valve, 340
calcium levels and, 340
coronary artery, 340
dystrophic, 340
image interpretation and, 99
metastatic, 340
mitral valve, 340
myocardial, 340
pericardial, 341
phosphate levels and, 340
radiographic evaluation of, 335
Calcium
cardiac calcification and, 340
coronary, 380
Calcium antagonists, 556
Calcium deposits, image interpretation
and, 99
Calcium-phosphate abnormality, mitral
valve calcification and, 340
Camera
dual-detector, 140
gamma: *see* Gamma camera
multidetector, SPECT and, 141
ring PET, 196
single-detector vs. multidetector, 278
SPECT, future perspectives in, 317
Candidiasis, heart muscle disease and,
646
Capillary wedge pressure, pulmonary, 342
Capitation, 939
[11]Carbon acetate, myocardial viability
assessment, 224
Carbon monoxide
blood pool imaging, 256
heart muscle disease and, 646
[11]Carbon palmitate, myocardial viability
assessment, 225
Carbon tetrachloride, heart muscle disease
and, 646
Carcinoid syndrome, 692
Cardiac allograft rejection
electrical characteristics and, 709
hemodynamic changes and, 707
MRI and, 706
MRS and, 707
tissue characterization in, 705
echocardiography, 705
Cardiac apex, inspiration and, 337
Cardiac arrhythmias, 891–908
atrial fibrillation, 891
classification of, 891
diseases associated with, 891
supraventricular tachycardias, 891
tachyarrhythmias, 891
Cardiac axis, left ventricular enlargement
and, 339

ultrasound interaction with, 115
vascular blood volume and perfusion, measurement of, 384
viability assessment, 177
Myocyte relaxation, cellular determinants of, 730
Myopathy, familial centronuclear, heart muscle disease and, 646
Myopericarditis, myocardial edema and, 701
Myxoma, 873, 874, 876

N

N-13 ammonia, 197
Nausea
    arbutamine and, 70
    dobutamine and, 69
Necrosis
    myocardial: see Myocardial necrosis
    myocyte, antimyosin antibody cardiac imaging, 697
Necrotic myocytes, 240
Neoplasm
    heart muscle disease and, 646
    pericardial, 741
Neuroimaging, 858
Neuromuscular disease, cardiomyopathy and, 653
    imaging of, 666
Niemann-Pick disease, heart muscle disease and, 646
Nitrate therapy, 556
Nitrogen-13, 147
Nitroglycerin, 556
NMR: see Nuclear magnetic resonance
Node of Arantius, 591
Norepinephrine, MIBG and, 307
Norwood operation
    echocardiography, 801
    surgery, 801
Nuclear cardiology
    ALARA principle, 149
    after CABG, 552
    camera/computer systems for, 137, 147
    cardiac disease evaluation and, 335
    clinical applications, future directions in, 319–320
    collimator and, 137
    cost findings related to, 491
    description of, 137
    dimensionality of protocols, 147
    ECG-gating: see ECG-gating
    exposure of workers, 148
    future perspectives in, 315–321
    gamma camera and, 137
    image acquisition, 137
    image matrix size in, 137
    integration of information, 181
    myocardial perfusion imaging and, 137
    planar vs. single-photon emission computed tomography, 138
    principles of, 137
    processing workstations for, 147
    protocols in, 148

future perspectives, 317–318
after PTCA, 545
    prognostic impact and, 548
radioisotopes used in, 147
radiopharmaceuticals and, 137
risk stratification in, myocardial perfusion SPECT and, 189
safety of, 137, 147–148
single-photon emission computed tomography: see Computed tomography, single-photon emission
software, future developments in, 318–319
techniques of, 137
Nuclear magnetic resonance, 389
    cardiovascular magnetic resonance and, 471
    safety of, 401–402
Nuclear magnetic resonance signal detection of, 390
MRI and, 393
Nuclear magnetic resonance spectroscopy cardiac ^{31}P, 463
^{31}P
    dilated cardiomyopathy and, 466
    exercise testing and, 465
    heart failure and, 466
    hypertrophic cardiomyopathy, 466
    microvascular disease and, 467
    myocardial energy metabolism and, 467
    transplanted hearts and, 467
Nuclear stress, stress echocardiography and, 80
Nyquist transition, 8

O

Obesity
    cardiac size/configuration, 337
    cardiomyopathy, 648
    heart muscle disease and, 646
Ochronosis, heart muscle disease and, 646
Oculoplethysmography, 851
Oligemia
    peripheral, pulmonary arterial hypertension and, 345
    pulmonary, pericardial calcification and, 342
    radiographic diagnosis of, 343
Optison, 86
Oropharyngeal distortion, transesophageal echocardiography and, 44
Oscilloscopic image, 13
Osmolar agents, 357
Osteosarcoma, 873
OUC 82755, 86
Outflow tract
    left ventricular, obstruction of, 16
    obstruction, echocardiography, 784
Oxalosis, heart muscle disease and, 646
Oxygen consumption
    exercise testing and, 153
    myocardial, exercise and, 151

P

C-11 Palmitate, 296
Palpitation
    arbutamine and, 70
    dobutamine and, 69
Papaverin, myocardial perfusion assessment and, 195
Papillary muscles, 2-D echocardiography assessment, 18
Papilloma, 874
Paracardiac masses, MRI evaluation of, 410
Paragonimiasis, heart muscle disease and, 646
Paravalvular abscess, transesophageal echocardiography and, 45
Paresthesia, arbutamine and, 70
Patent arterial duct, 839
Patent ductus arteriosus, 773
    echocardiography, 773, 792
    transesophageal echocardiography and, 59
    treatment, 792
Patent foramen ovale, transesophageal echocardiography and, 49
Patient motion, myocardial perfusion SPECT and, 168
PCr/ATP ratio, handgrip exercise and, 465
Pectus excavatum, right ventricle and, 338
Pellagra, 646
Penn convention, left ventricular mass and, 15
Pericardium, hematoma of, 741
Percutaneous transluminal coronary angioplasty
    clinical follow-up after, 544
    complications of, intravascular ultrasound role in detection, 108
    coronary angiography and, 348
    echocardiography follow-up after, 548
    exercise testing after, 545
    follow-up after, 544
        recommendations for, 549
    frequency of, 544
    intracoronary stenting and, 544
    intravascular ultrasound and, 106
    myocardial infarction in angina and, 187
    nuclear cardiology after, 545
    prognostic impact by nuclear cardiology, 548
    restenosis rates, 544
    stress echocardiography after, 548
Perfusable tissue index, 201
    myocardial viability and, 226
Perfusion agents, myocardial
    technetium-99m, 162
    technetium-99m furifosmin, 168
    technetium-99m-NOET, 168
    technetium-99m sestamibi, 163
    technetium-99m teboroxime, 166
    technetium-99m tetrofosmin, 166
    thallium-201, 159